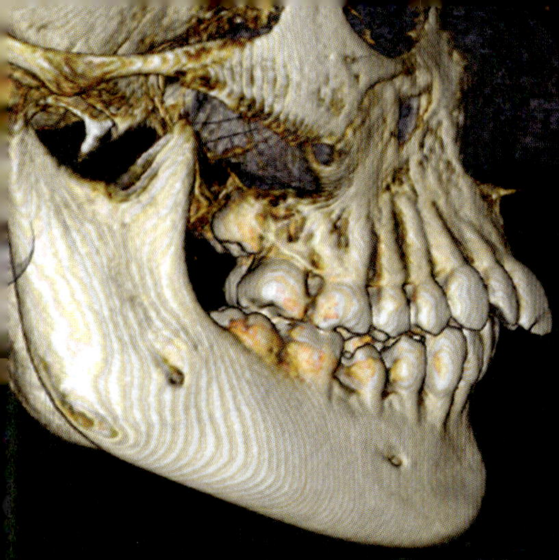

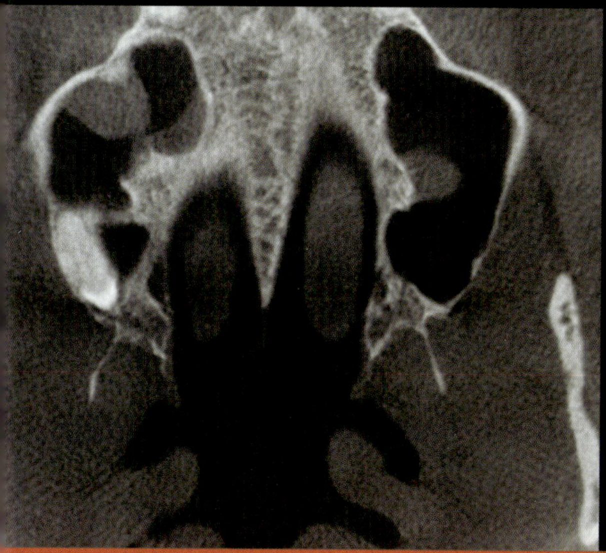

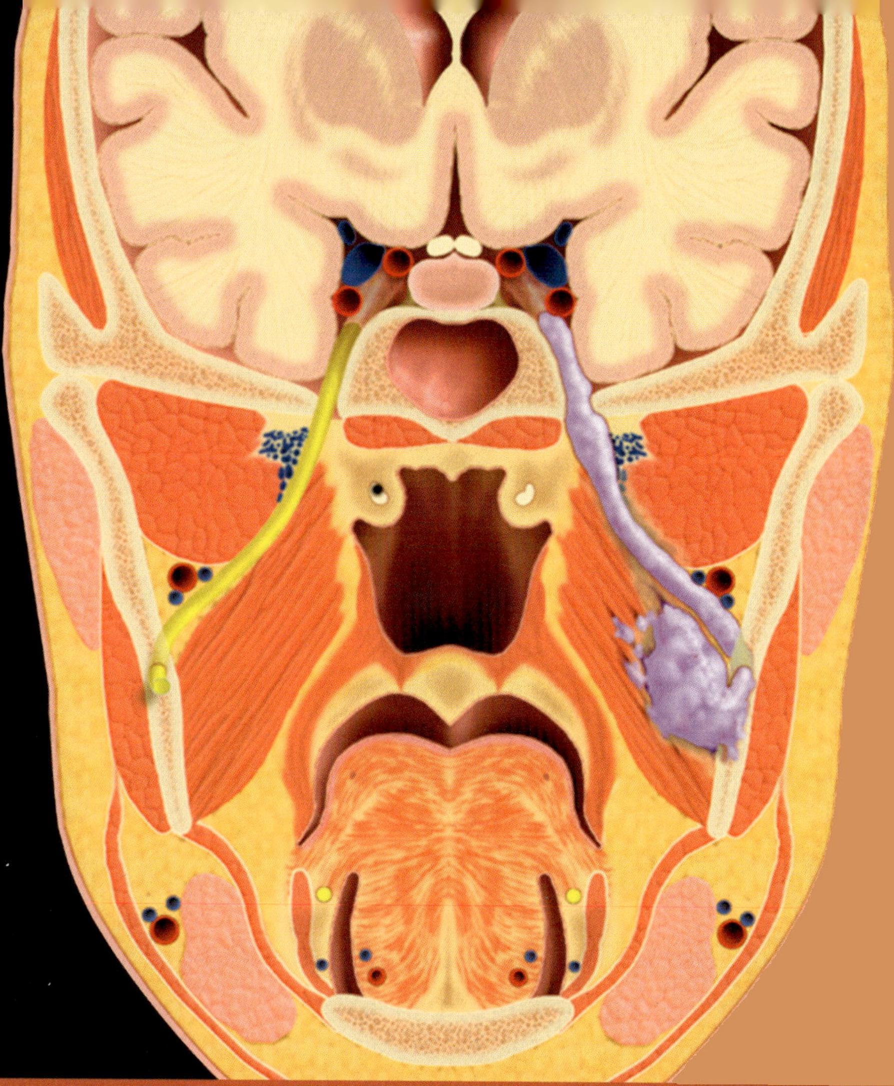

Diagnostic Imaging

Oral and Maxillofacial

SECOND EDITION

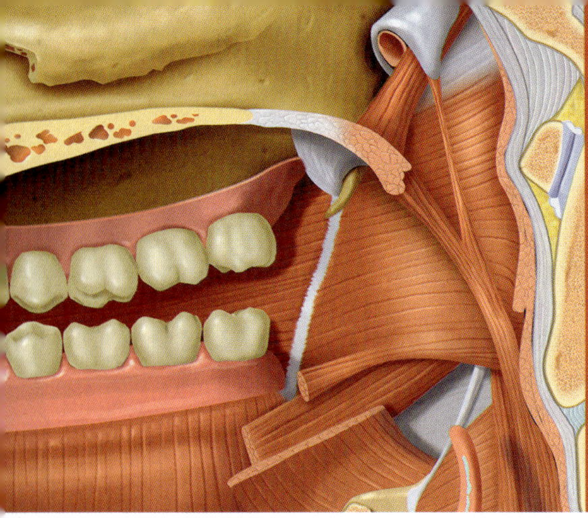

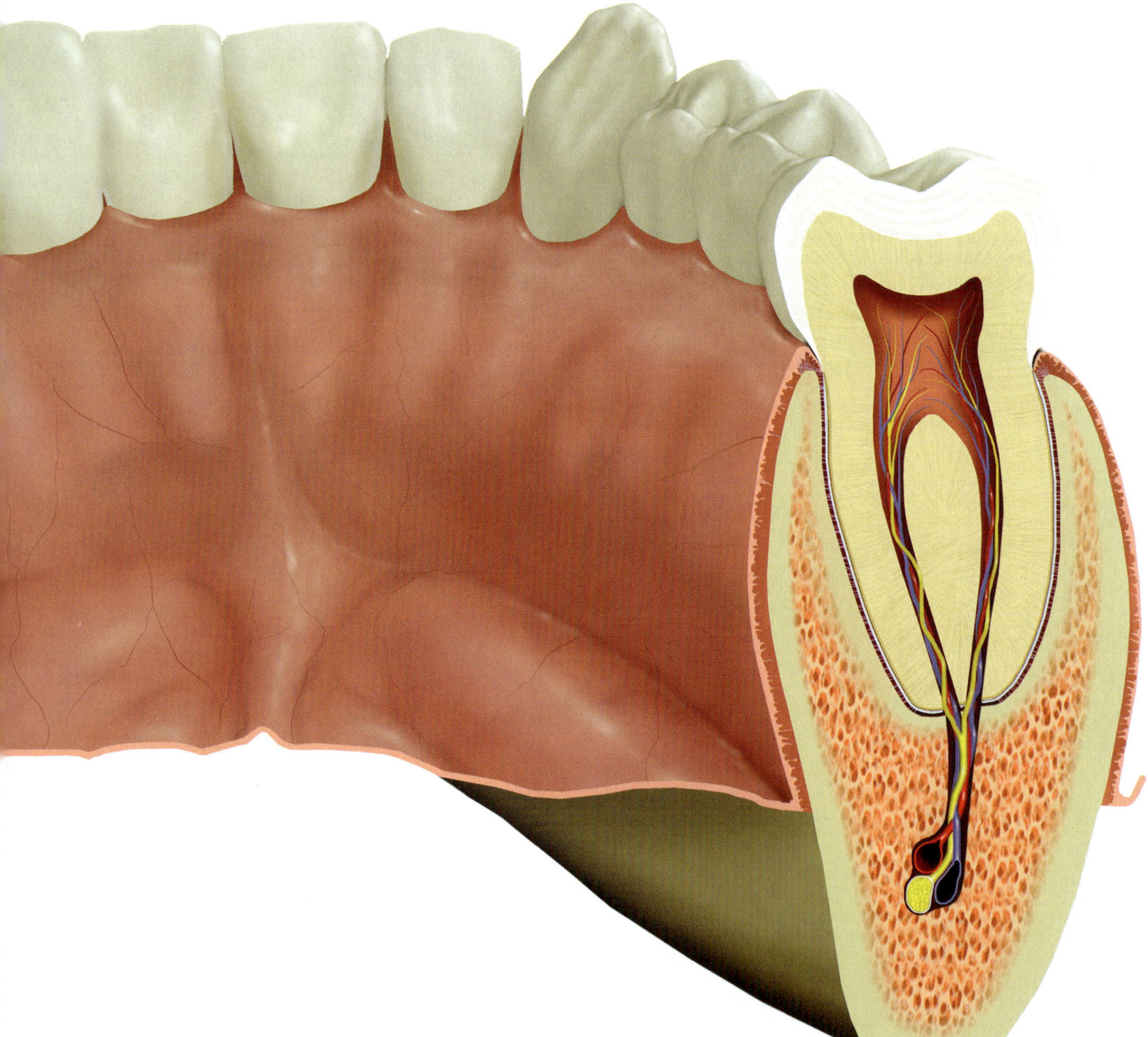

Diagnostic Imaging

Oral and Maxillofacial

SECOND EDITION

Lisa J. Koenig, BChD, DDS, MS

Associate Dean for Academic Affairs
Professor, Oral Medicine and Oral Radiology
Marquette University School of Dentistry
Milwaukee, Wisconsin

Dania Tamimi, BDS, DMSc

Oral and Maxillofacial Radiology Consultant
Private Practice
Orlando, Florida
Adjunct Assistant Professor
Department of Comprehensive Dentistry
University of Texas Health Science Center
San Antonio, Texas

C. Grace Petrikowski, DDS, MSc, FRCD(C)

Oral and Maxillofacial Radiologist
Huronia Maxillofacial Radiology
Toronto, Ontario, Canada

Susanne E. Perschbacher, DDS, MSc, FRCD(C)

Assistant Professor
Oral & Maxillofacial Radiology
University of Toronto, Faculty of Dentistry
Toronto, Ontario, Canada

Axel Ruprecht, DDS, MScD, FRCD(C)

Professor Emeritus of Oral
and Maxillofacial Radiology
Professor Emeritus of Radiology
Professor Emeritus of Anatomy
and Cell Biology
The University of Iowa
Adjunct Clinical Professor of Oral
and Maxillofacial Radiology
University of Florida
Gainesville, Florida

Byron W. Benson, DDS, MS

Regents Professor and Vice Chair
Department of Diagnostic Sciences
Texas A&M University
College of Dentistry
Dallas, Texas

David Hatcher, DDS, MSc

Clinical Professor, Orofacial Sciences
School of Dentistry
University of California, San Francisco
San Francisco, California
Clinical Professor, School of Dentistry
University of California, Los Angeles
Los Angeles, California
Adjunct Professor, School of Dentistry
Department of Orthodontics
University of the Pacific
San Francisco, California
Clinical Professor Volunteer, Department of
Surgical & Radiological Sciences
School of Veterinary Medicine
University of California, Davis
Davis, California
Clinical Professor, School of Dentistry
Roseman University of Health Sciences
Henderson, Nevada
Private Practice, Diagnostic Digital Imaging
Sacramento, California

Brad J. Potter, DDS, MS

Professor and Director of Oral
and Maxillofacial Radiology
Department of Diagnostic
and Biological Sciences
University of Colorado
School of Dental Medicine
Aurora, Colorado

H. Ric Harnsberger, MD

R.C. Willey Chair in Neuroradiology
Professor of Radiology and Otolaryngology
University of Utah School of Medicine
Salt Lake City, Utah

ELSEVIER

1600 John F. Kennedy Blvd.
Ste 1800
Philadelphia, PA 19103-2899

DIAGNOSTIC IMAGING: ORAL AND MAXILLOFACIAL, SECOND EDITION ISBN: 978-0-323-47782-6

Notices

Knowledge and best practice in this field are constantly changing. As new research and experience broaden our understanding, changes in research methods, professional practices, or medical treatment may become necessary.

Practitioners and researchers must always rely on their own experience and knowledge in evaluating and using any information, methods, compounds, or experiments described herein. In using such information or methods they should be mindful of their own safety and the safety of others, including parties for whom they have a professional responsibility.

With respect to any drug or pharmaceutical products identified, readers are advised to check the most current information provided (i) on procedures featured or (ii) by the manufacturer of each product to be administered, to verify the recommended dose or formula, the method and duration of administration, and contraindications. It is the responsibility of practitioners, relying on their own experience and knowledge of their patients, to make diagnoses, to determine dosages and the best treatment for each individual patient, and to take all appropriate safety precautions.

To the fullest extent of the law, neither the Publisher nor the authors, contributors, or editors, assume any liability for any injury and/or damage to persons or property as a matter of products liability, negligence or otherwise, or from any use or operation of any methods, products, instructions, or ideas contained in the material herein.

Publisher Cataloging-in-Publication Data

Names: Koenig, Lisa J. | Tamimi, Dania Faisal | Petrikowski, C. Grace | Perschbacher, Susanne E.
Title: Diagnostic imaging. Oral and maxillofacial / [edited by] Lisa J. Koenig, Dania Tamimi, C. Grace Petrikowski, and Susanne E. Perschbacher.
Other titles: Oral and maxillofacial.
Description: Second edition. | Salt Lake City, UT : Elsevier, Inc., [2017] | Includes bibliographical references and index.
Identifiers: ISBN 978-0-323-47782-6
Subjects: LCSH: Mouth--Surgery--Handbooks, manuals, etc. | Maxilla--Surgery--Handbooks, manuals, etc. | Face--Surgery--Handbooks, manuals, etc. | MESH: Radiograophy--Atlases. | Stomatognathic Diseases--diagnostic images--Atlases. | Imaging, Three-Dimensional--Atlases. | Radiography, Panoramic--Atlases.
Classification: LCC RK529.D52 2017 | NLM WU 140 | DDC 617.5'22059--dc23

International Standard Book Number: 978-0-323-47782-6

Cover Designer: Tom M. Olson, BA
Cover Art: Richard Coombs, MS

Printed in Canada by Friesens, Altona, Manitoba, Canada

Last digit is the print number: 9 8 7 6 5 4 3 2 1

Dedications

To my children, Sophie, Ben, Alex, Jack, and especially Natalie and baby Raphi, who have kept me grounded; my friend Esme, who made me food; and my students and patients who inspire me.

LJK

Dedicated to all the incredible teachers I've had in my life, most notably my parents and children. Time management and compassion are the most precious of skills.

DT

Thank you to my parents for encouraging me to pursue a career in dentistry during a time when women comprised only a small minority in dental school classes. Thanks also to my teachers and mentors during my oral radiology training, as well as my coauthors, colleagues, and editors, who so generously shared their knowledge and experience as this book was being written. My biggest thanks go to my husband and best friend, Eggert Boehlau, who has so generously supported me, both in my work as a radiologist, which puts food on the table, and my passion as a musician, which feeds the soul.

CGP

To my teachers: For showing me the path.
To my students: For keeping me on it
To Mom, Dad, and Kristina: For your enthusiasm.
To Anya and Daphne: For always sleeping while I wrote.
To Mark: For always staying up…I love you.

SEP

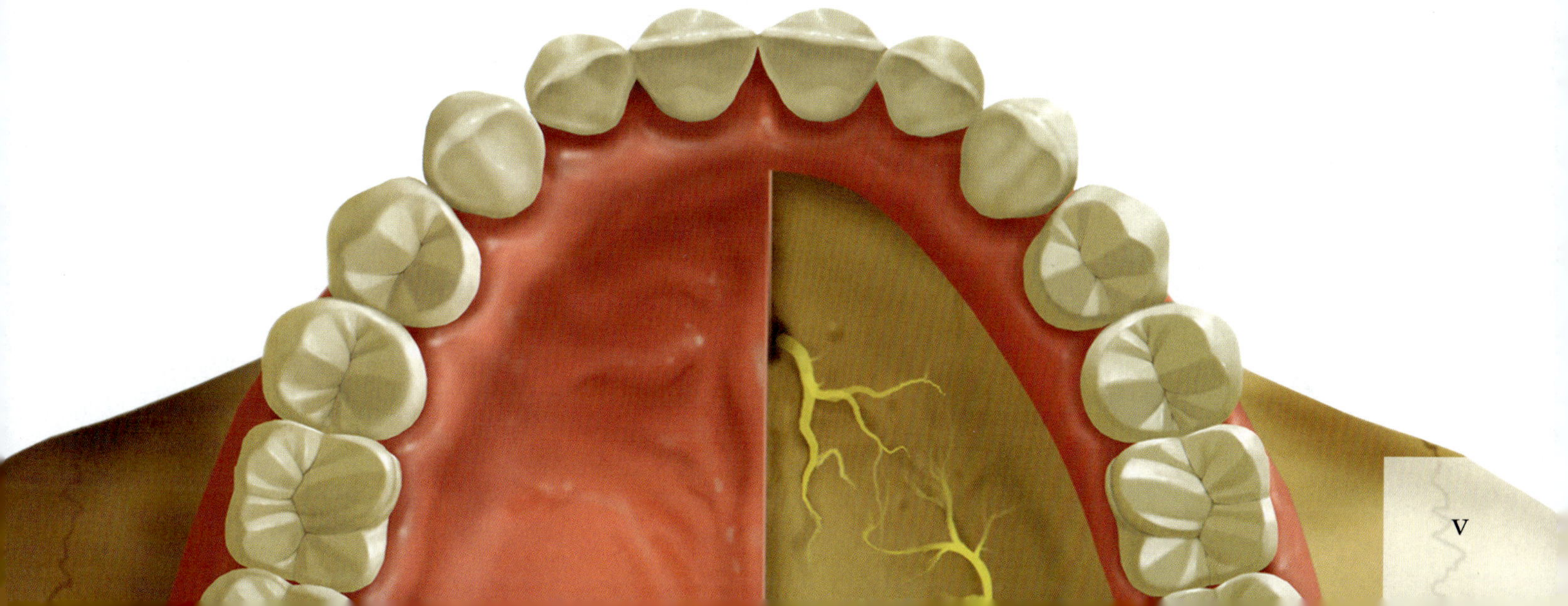

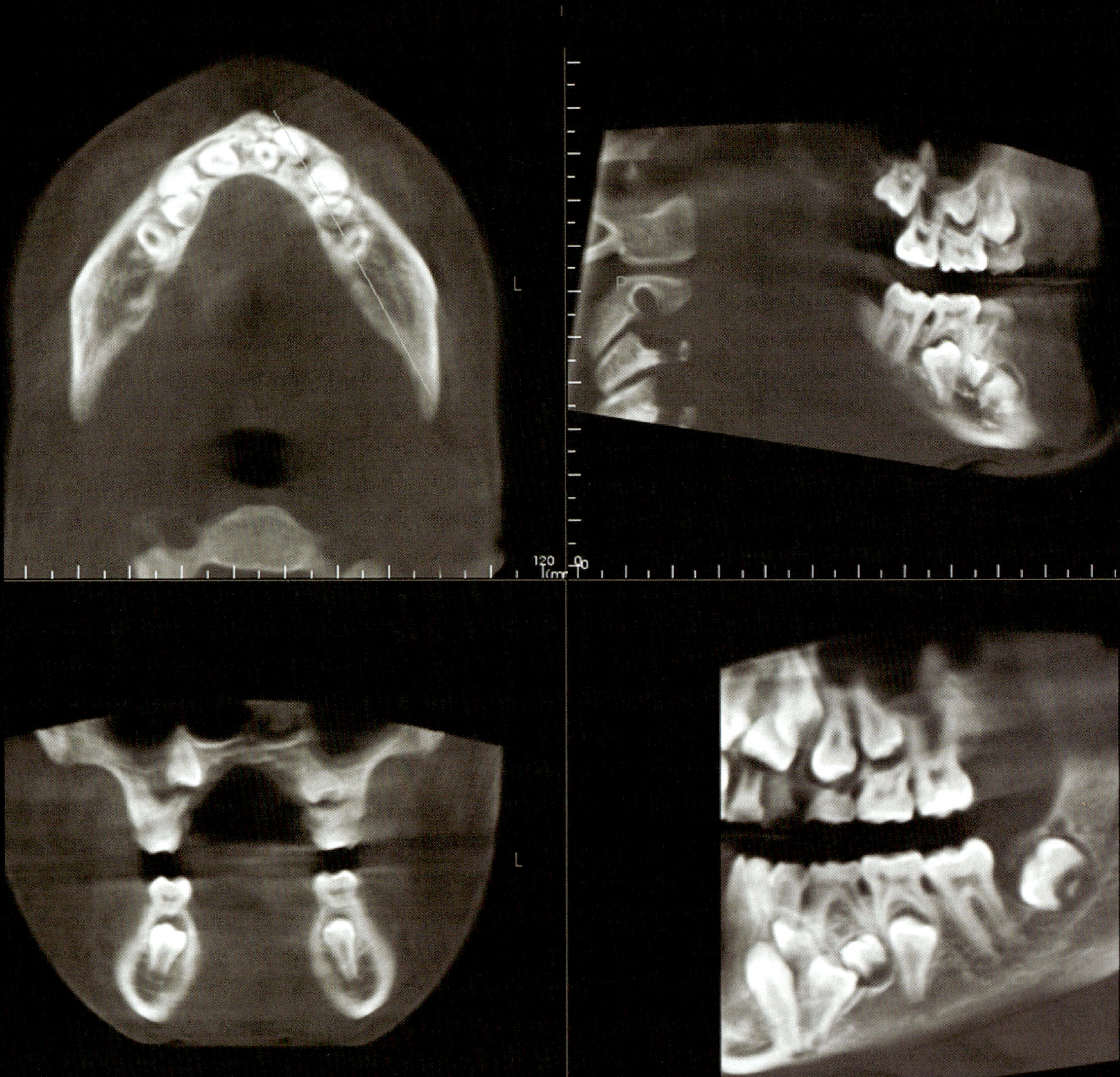
L
120
L

Additional Contributors

Barton F. Branstetter, IV, MD, FACR
Rebecca S. Cornelius, MD, FACR
Julia Crim, MD
H. Christian Davidson, MD
Joanne Ethier, DMD, MBA, MS
Bronwyn E. Hamilton, MD
Patricia A. Hudgins, MD, FACR
Richard W. Katzberg, MD
Bernadette L. Koch, MD
Nicholas A. Koontz, MD
Luke N. Ledbetter, MD
Daniel E. Meltzer, MD
Michelle A. Michel, MD
Kevin R. Moore, MD
Kristine M. Mosier, DMD, PhD
Cheryl A. Petersilge, MD, MBA
Caroline D. Robson, MBChB
Jeffrey S. Ross, MD
Lubdha M. Shah, MD
Deborah R. Shatzkes, MD
Hilda E. Stambuk, MD
Margot L. Van Dis, DDS, MS
Richard H. Wiggins, III, MD, CIIP, FSIIM

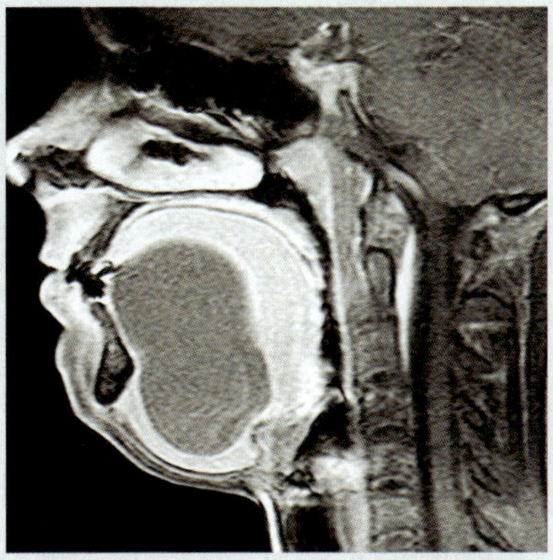

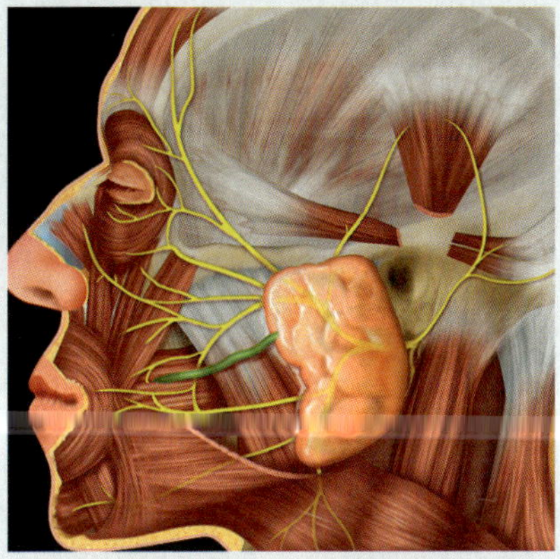

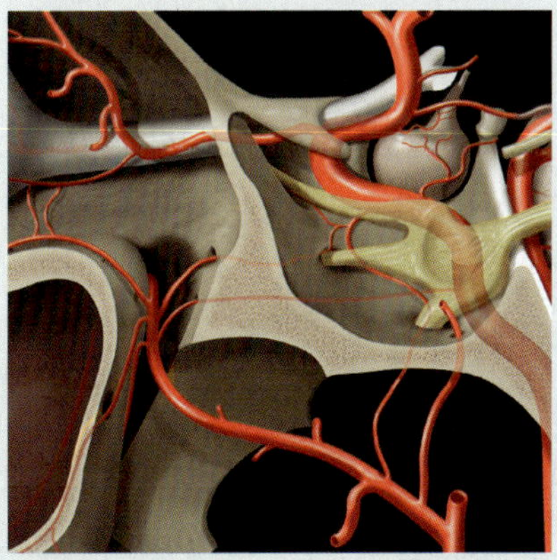

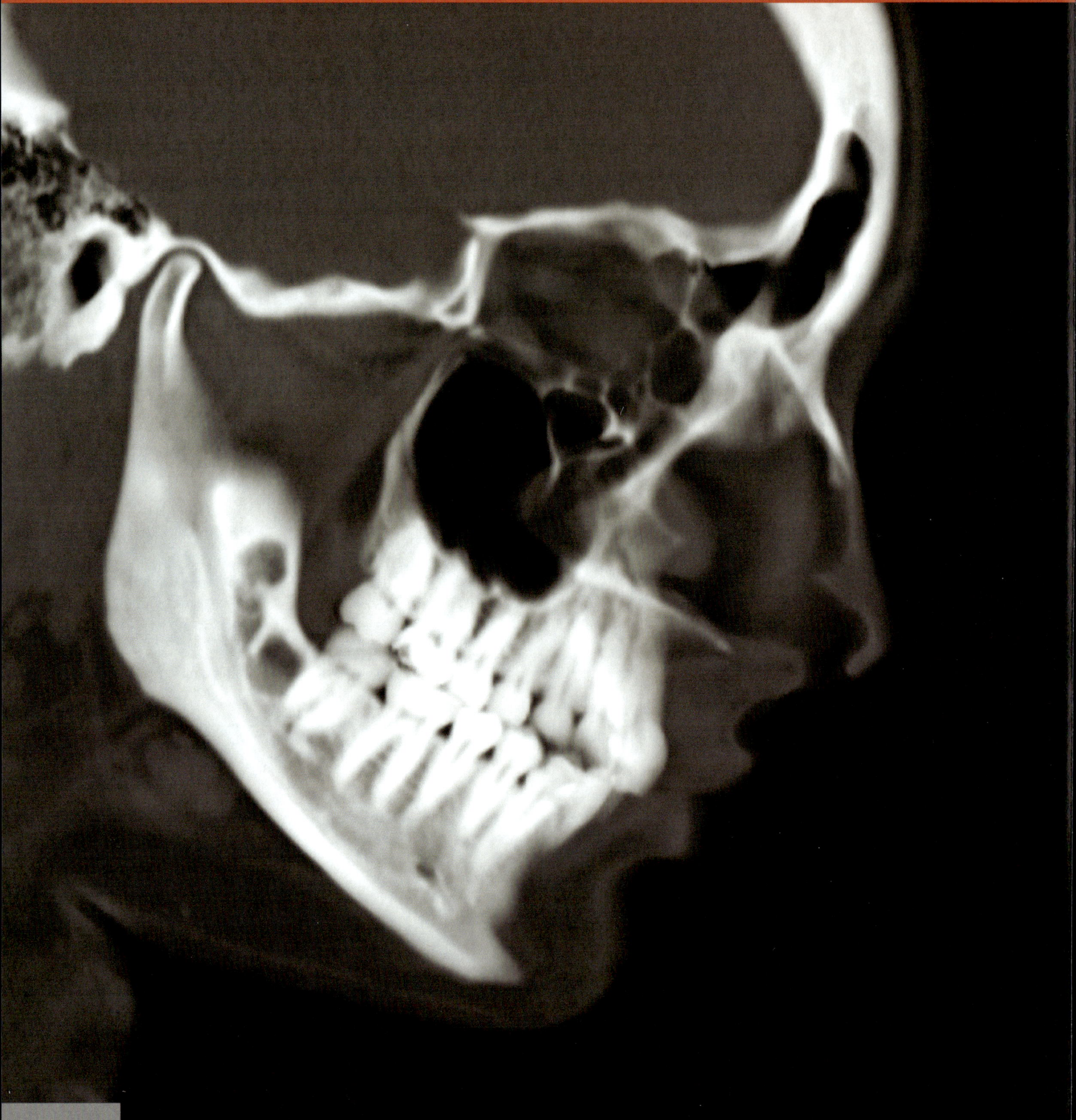

Preface

We are very proud to present the second edition of our Diagnostic Imaging text dedicated to oral and maxillofacial radiology. As in the first edition, the book is divided into three parts: Anatomy, Diagnoses, and Differential Diagnoses. The Anatomy part has seen the addition of a chapter on the posterior skull base that reflects the increasing need for oral and maxillofacial radiologists to interpret larger fields of view. In this regard, the Diagnoses part includes 18 new chapters dedicated to the more common findings in the cervical spine. There are also extended chapters on TMJ and airway evaluation. The Diagnoses part now contains over 200 chapters.

You will also find in this second edition new graphics from our expert illustrators, exquisitely detailing the Anatomy and Diagnoses parts and serving to enhance the learning experience. Each chapter has been meticulously updated with the addition of new references and images wherever possible.

Purchase of the book comes with an electronic version, Expert Consult, that allows for easy navigation between chapters and access to many more images, as well as text that was excluded from the print version due to page constraints.

We trust that this second edition, like the first, will appeal to both the beginning and the experienced radiologist, as well as the increasing number of general dental practitioners and specialists who are using CBCT technology in their offices. For medical radiologists, the book will also serve as a valuable companion text to *Diagnostic Imaging: Head and Neck*, third edition.

Lisa J. Koenig, BChD, DDS, MS
Associate Dean for Academic Affairs
Professor, Oral Medicine and Oral Radiology
Marquette University School of Dentistry
Milwaukee, Wisconsin

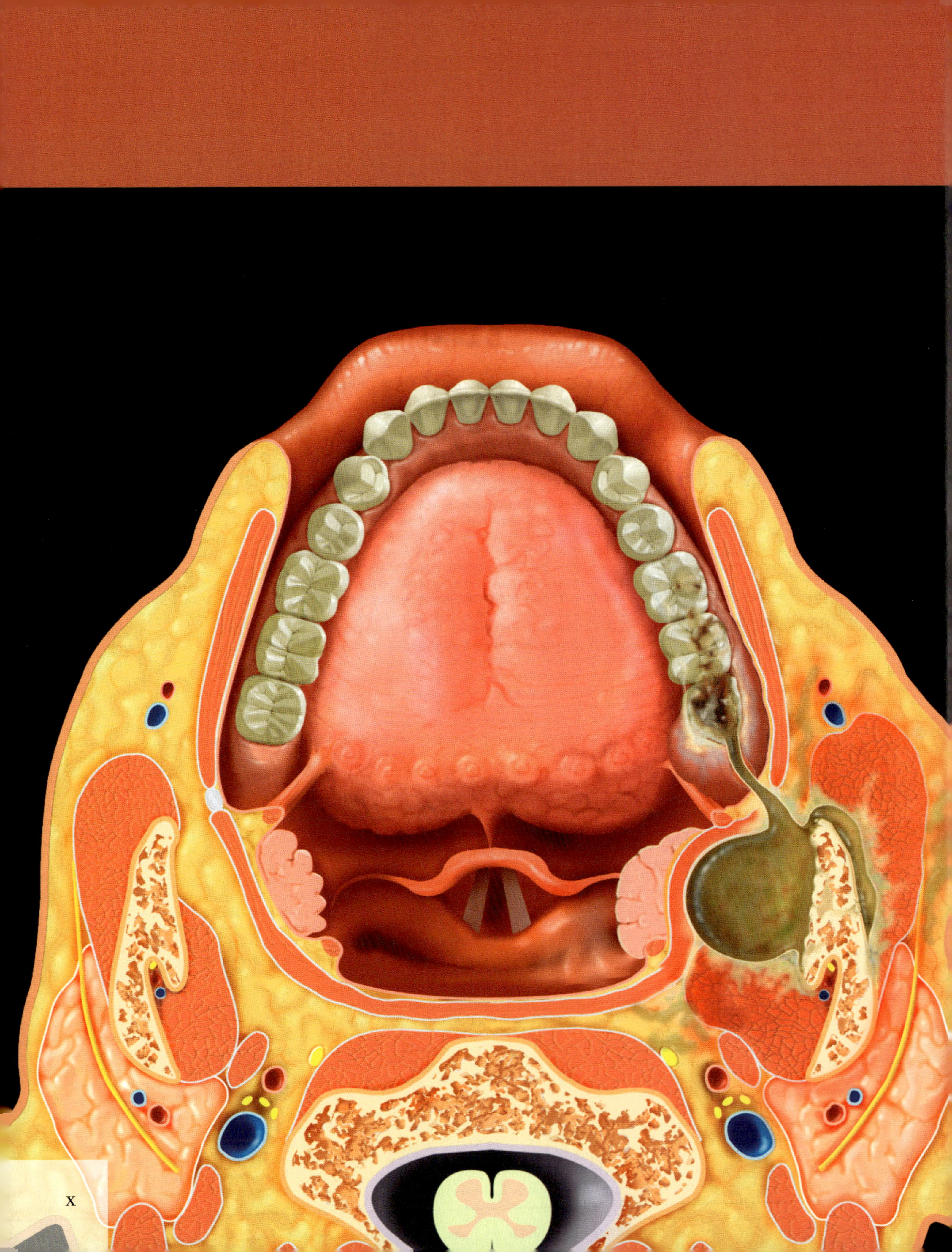

Acknowledgments

Text Editors

Arthur G. Gelsinger, MA
Nina I. Bennett, BA
Terry W. Ferrell, MS
Karen E. Concannon, MA, PhD
Matt W. Hoecherl, BS
Megg Morin, BA

Image Editors

Jeffrey J. Marmorstone, BS
Lisa A. M. Steadman, BS

Illustrations

Lane R. Bennion, MS
Richard Coombs, MS
Laura C. Wissler, MA

Art Direction and Design

Tom M. Olson, BA
Laura C. Wissler, MA

Lead Editor

Lisa A. Gervais, BS

Production Coordinators

Rebecca L. Bluth, BA
Angela M. G. Terry, BA
Emily C. Fassett, BA

ELSEVIER

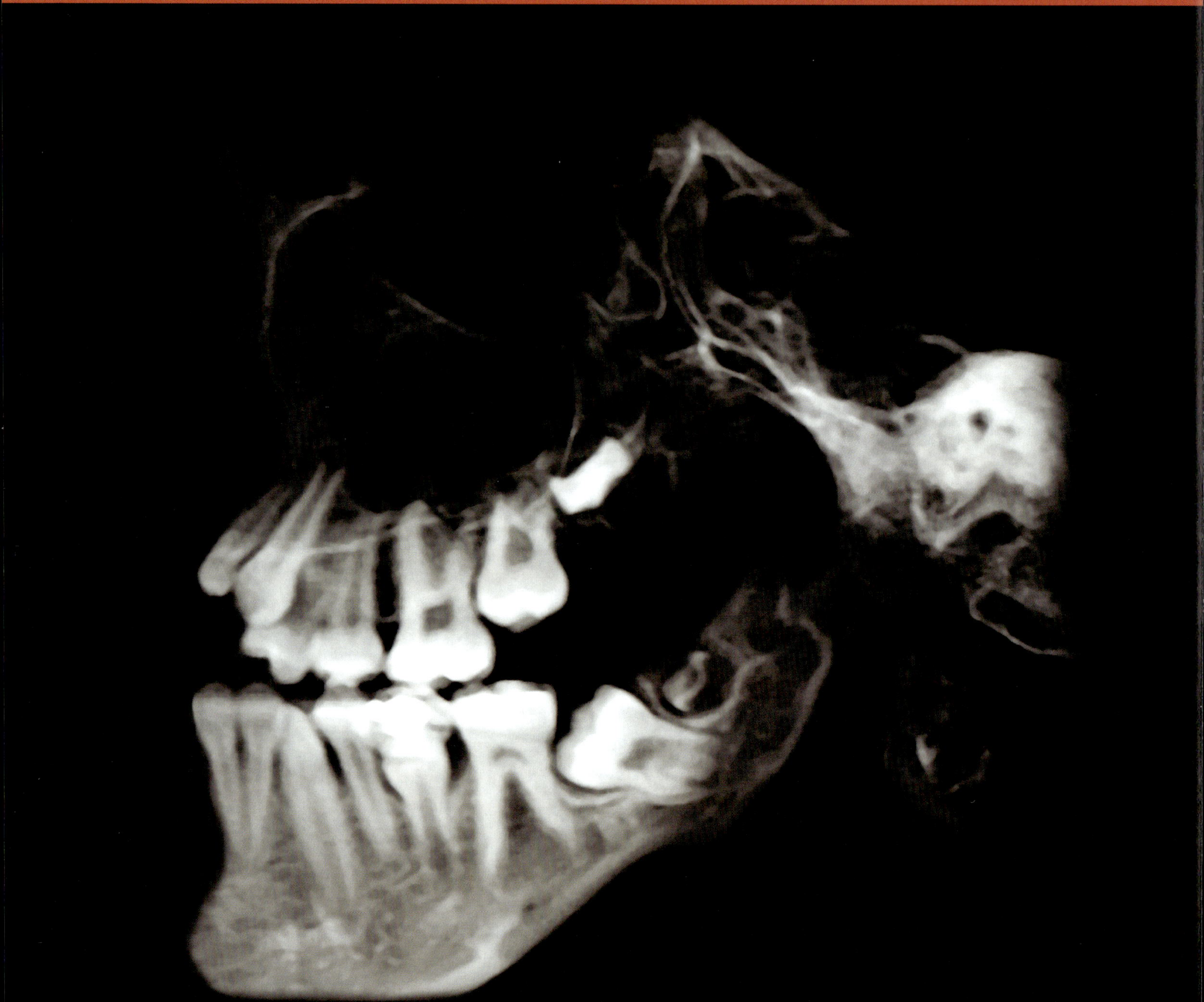

Sections

Part I: Anatomy

SECTION 1: Oral Cavity
SECTION 2: Nose and Sinuses
SECTION 3: Temporal Bone
SECTION 4: Base of Skull
SECTION 5: Cranial Nerves
SECTION 6: Cervical Spine
SECTION 7: Suprahyoid Neck

Part II: Diagnoses

SECTION 1: Teeth
SECTION 2: Oral Cavity
SECTION 3: Mandible and Maxilla
SECTION 4: Temporomandibular Joint
SECTION 5: Maxillary Sinus and Nasal Cavity
SECTION 6: Masticator Space
SECTION 7: Parotid Space
SECTION 8: Cervical Spine

Part III: Differential Diagnoses

SECTION 1: Teeth
SECTION 2: Mandible and Maxilla
SECTION 3: Oral Cavity
SECTION 4: Temporomandibular Joint
SECTION 5: Maxillary Sinus and Nasal Cavity

TABLE OF CONTENTS

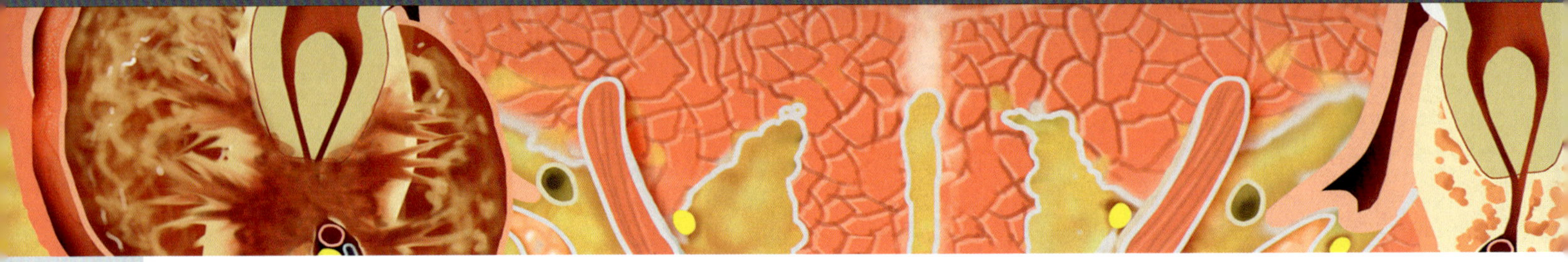

Part I: Anatomy

SECTION 1: ORAL CAVITY

4 **Teeth**
Dania Tamimi, BDS, DMSc

14 **Dental Restorations**
Dania Tamimi, BDS, DMSc

22 **Maxilla**
Dania Tamimi, BDS, DMSc

30 **Mandible**
Dania Tamimi, BDS, DMSc

36 **Tongue**
H. Ric Harnsberger, MD

40 **Retromolar Trigone**
H. Ric Harnsberger, MD

44 **Sublingual Space**
H. Ric Harnsberger, MD

48 **Submandibular Space**
H. Ric Harnsberger, MD

52 **Oral Mucosal Space/Surface**
H. Ric Harnsberger, MD

SECTION 2: NOSE AND SINUSES

56 **Sinonasal Overview**
Susanne E. Perschbacher, DDS, MSc, FRCD(C)

72 **Ostiomeatal Complex**
H. Ric Harnsberger, MD

76 **Pterygopalatine Fossa**
H. Ric Harnsberger, MD

SECTION 3: TEMPORAL BONE

82 **Temporomandibular Joint**
Susanne E. Perschbacher, DDS, MSc, FRCD(C)

90 **External, Middle, and Inner Ear**
H. Ric Harnsberger, MD

SECTION 4: BASE OF SKULL

98 **Anterior Skull Base**
H. Ric Harnsberger, MD

104 **Central Skull Base**
H. Ric Harnsberger, MD

110 **Posterior Skull Base**
H. Ric Harnsberger, MD

118 **Styloid Process and Stylohyoid Ligament**
Susanne E. Perschbacher, DDS, MSc, FRCD(C)

SECTION 5: CRANIAL NERVES

124 **Cranial Nerve V**
H. Ric Harnsberger, MD and Susanne E. Perschbacher, DDS, MSc, FRCD(C)

138 **Cranial Nerve VII**
H. Ric Harnsberger, MD and Susanne E. Perschbacher, DDS, MSc, FRCD(C)

SECTION 6: CERVICAL SPINE

150 **Craniocervical Junction**
H. Ric Harnsberger, MD

SECTION 7: SUPRAHYOID NECK

162 **Suprahyoid Neck Overview**
H. Ric Harnsberger, MD

168 **Parapharyngeal Space**
H. Ric Harnsberger, MD

172 **Nasopharynx and Oropharynx**
H. Ric Harnsberger, MD and Susanne E. Perschbacher, DDS, MSc, FRCD(C)

180 **Masticator Space**
H. Ric Harnsberger, MD

184 **Parotid Space**
H. Ric Harnsberger, MD

188 **Carotid Space**
H. Ric Harnsberger, MD

192 **Retropharyngeal Space**
H. Ric Harnsberger, MD

196 **Perivertebral Space**
H. Ric Harnsberger, MD

200 **Lymph Nodes**
H. Ric Harnsberger, MD

204 **External and Internal Carotid Arteries**
Lisa J. Koenig, BChD, DDS, MS

Part II: Diagnoses

SECTION 1: TEETH

DEVELOPMENTAL ALTERATIONS IN SIZE AND SHAPE OF TEETH

212 **Hypodontia**
Brad J. Potter, DDS, MS and Margot L. Van Dis, DDS, MS

214 **Hyperdontia**
Brad J. Potter, DDS, MS and Margot L. Van Dis, DDS, MS

216 **Macrodontia, Gemination, and Fusion**
Brad J. Potter, DDS, MS and Margot L. Van Dis, DDS, MS

TABLE OF CONTENTS

218 **Microdontia**
Brad J. Potter, DDS, MS and Margot L. Van Dis, DDS, MS

219 **Concrescence**
Brad J. Potter, DDS, MS and Margot L. Van Dis, DDS, MS

220 **Talon Cusp**
Brad J. Potter, DDS, MS and Margot L. Van Dis, DDS, MS

221 **Dens Invaginatus**
Brad J. Potter, DDS, MS and Margot L. Van Dis, DDS, MS

222 **Enamel Pearls**
Brad J. Potter, DDS, MS and Margot L. Van Dis, DDS, MS

223 **Taurodontism**
Brad J. Potter, DDS, MS and Margot L. Van Dis, DDS, MS

224 **Dilaceration**
Brad J. Potter, DDS, MS and Margot L. Van Dis, DDS, MS

225 **Supernumerary Roots**
Brad J. Potter, DDS, MS and Margot L. Van Dis, DDS, MS

DEVELOPMENTAL ALTERATIONS IN STRUCTURE OF TEETH

226 **Amelogenesis Imperfecta**
Brad J. Potter, DDS, MS and Margot L. Van Dis, DDS, MS

230 **Dentinogenesis Imperfecta**
Brad J. Potter, DDS, MS and Margot L. Van Dis, DDS, MS

232 **Dentin Dysplasia**
Brad J. Potter, DDS, MS and Margot L. Van Dis, DDS, MS

233 **Regional Odontodysplasia**
Brad J. Potter, DDS, MS and Margot L. Van Dis, DDS, MS

234 **Segmental Odontomaxillary Dysplasia**
Lisa J. Koenig, BChD, DDS, MS

ACQUIRED ALTERATIONS OF TEETH AND SUPPORTING STRUCTURES

236 **Attrition**
Dania Tamimi, BDS, DMSc

238 **Abrasion**
Dania Tamimi, BDS, DMSc

239 **Erosion**
Dania Tamimi, BDS, DMSc

240 **Abfraction**
Dania Tamimi, BDS, DMSc

241 **Turner Dysplasia**
Dania Tamimi, BDS, DMSc

242 **Internal and External Resorption**
Dania Tamimi, BDS, DMSc

248 **Hypercementosis**
Dania Tamimi, BDS, DMSc

TRAUMA

249 **Concussion**
Dania Tamimi, BDS, DMSc

250 **Luxation**
Dania Tamimi, BDS, DMSc

254 **Dentoalveolar Fractures**
Dania Tamimi, BDS, DMSc

INFECTION/INFLAMMATION

260 **Dental Caries**
Dania Tamimi, BDS, DMSc

264 **Periapical Rarefying Osteitis**
Dania Tamimi, BDS, DMSc

268 **Periapical Sclerosing Osteitis**
Dania Tamimi, BDS, DMSc

270 **Periodontal Disease**
Dania Tamimi, BDS, DMSc

MISCELLANEOUS

276 **Gubernaculum Dentis**
Lisa J. Koenig, BChD, DDS, MS

SECTION 2: ORAL CAVITY

CONGENITAL/GENETIC

280 **Submandibular Space Accessory Salivary Tissue**
Daniel E. Meltzer, MD

282 **Lingual Thyroid**
Deborah R. Shatzkes, MD

284 **Dermoid and Epidermoid**
Bernadette L. Koch, MD

288 **Submandibular Gland Aplasia-Hypoplasia**
Byron W. Benson, DDS, MS

290 **Foregut Duplication Cyst in Tongue**
Byron W. Benson, DDS, MS

INFECTION

292 **Oral Cavity Soft Tissue Infections**
Byron W. Benson, DDS, MS and Richard H. Wiggins, III, MD, CIIP, FSIIM

INFLAMMATION

296 **Ranula**
Richard H. Wiggins, III, MD, CIIP, FSIIM

300 **Submandibular Gland Sialadenitis**
Richard H. Wiggins, III, MD, CIIP, FSIIM

302 **Oral Cavity Sialocele**
Richard H. Wiggins, III, MD, CIIP, FSIIM

304 **Submandibular Gland Mucocele**
Byron W. Benson, DDS, MS

NEOPLASM, BENIGN

306 **Sublingual Gland Benign Mixed Tumor**
Byron W. Benson, DDS, MS

308 **Submandibular Gland Benign Mixed Tumor**
Richard H. Wiggins, III, MD, CIIP, FSIIM

310 **Palate Benign Mixed Tumor**
Byron W. Benson, DDS, MS and Richard H. Wiggins, III, MD, CIIP, FSIIM

NEOPLASM, MALIGNANT

312 **Oral Cavity Minor Salivary Gland Malignancy**
Bronwyn E. Hamilton, MD

314 **Sublingual Gland Carcinoma**
Hilda E. Stambuk, MD

316 **Submandibular Gland Carcinoma**
Hilda E. Stambuk, MD

TABLE OF CONTENTS

318 **Submandibular Space Nodal Non-Hodgkin Lymphoma**
Bronwyn E. Hamilton, MD
320 **Oral Tongue Squamous Cell Carcinoma**
Nicholas A. Koontz, MD
324 **Floor of Mouth Squamous Cell Carcinoma**
Nicholas A. Koontz, MD
326 **Gingival Squamous Cell Carcinoma**
C. Grace Petrikowski, DDS, MSc, FRCD(C)
328 **Retromolar Trigone Squamous Cell Carcinoma**
Nicholas A. Koontz, MD
330 **Submandibular Space Nodal Squamous Cell Carcinoma**
Bronwyn E. Hamilton, MD
332 **Buccal Mucosa Squamous Cell Carcinoma**
Nicholas A. Koontz, MD
334 **Hard Palate Squamous Cell Carcinoma**
Nicholas A. Koontz, MD

MISCELLANEOUS/IDIOPATHIC

336 **Motor Denervation CNXII**
Richard H. Wiggins, III, MD, CIIP, FSIIM
338 **Submandibular Sialoliths**
Byron W. Benson, DDS, MS

SECTION 3: MANDIBLE AND MAXILLA

NORMAL VARIANTS

342 **Buccal and Palatal Exostoses**
Lisa J. Koenig, BChD, DDS, MS
344 **Mandibular Torus**
Lisa J. Koenig, BChD, DDS, MS
346 **Palatal Torus**
Lisa J. Koenig, BChD, DDS, MS
348 **Accessory Mandibular Canal**
Lisa J. Koenig, BChD, DDS, MS
350 **Mandibular Salivary Gland Defect (Stafne)**
Lisa J. Koenig, BChD, DDS, MS
354 **Mandible-Maxilla Idiopathic Osteosclerosis**
Lisa J. Koenig, BChD, DDS, MS

CONGENITAL/GENETIC

356 **Clefts**
Brad J. Potter, DDS, MS and Margot L. Van Dis, DDS, MS
358 **Cherubism**
C. Grace Petrikowski, DDS, MSc, FRCD(C)
362 **Basal Cell Nevus Syndrome**
Susanne E. Perschbacher, DDS, MSc, FRCD(C)
364 **Cleidocranial Dysplasia**
Brad J. Potter, DDS, MS and Margot L. Van Dis, DDS, MS
366 **Pierre Robin Sequence**
Caroline D. Robson, MBChB and Dania Tamimi, BDS, DMSc
368 **Treacher Collins Syndrome**
Brad J. Potter, DDS, MS, Margot L. Van Dis, DDS, MS, and Caroline D. Robson, MBChB

TRAUMA

370 **Mandible Fracture**
Byron W. Benson, DDS, MS and Michelle A. Michel, MD
374 **Nasoethmoid Complex Fracture**
Byron W. Benson, DDS, MS and Michelle A. Michel, MD
376 **Complex Midfacial Fracture**
Byron W. Benson, DDS, MS and Michelle A. Michel, MD
378 **Zygomaticomaxillary Complex Fracture**
Byron W. Benson, DDS, MS and Michelle A. Michel, MD
380 **Transfacial Fracture (Le Fort)**
Byron W. Benson, DDS, MS and Kristine M. Mosier, DMD, PhD

INFECTION/INFLAMMATION

384 **Mandible-Maxilla Osteomyelitis**
Susanne E. Perschbacher, DDS, MSc, FRCD(C)
388 **Mandible-Maxilla Osteoradionecrosis**
Susanne E. Perschbacher, DDS, MSc, FRCD(C)
392 **Mandible-Maxilla Osteonecrosis**
Susanne E. Perschbacher, DDS, MSc, FRCD(C)

CYSTS, ODONTOGENIC

396 **Dentigerous Cyst**
Lisa J. Koenig, BChD, DDS, MS
400 **Odontogenic Keratocyst**
Susanne E. Perschbacher, DDS, MSc, FRCD(C)
404 **Lateral Periodontal Cyst**
Lisa J. Koenig, BChD, DDS, MS
406 **Residual Cyst**
Lisa J. Koenig, BChD, DDS, MS
408 **Buccal Bifurcation Cyst**
Lisa J. Koenig, BChD, DDS, MS
412 **Calcifying Odontogenic Cyst**
Lisa J. Koenig, BChD, DDS, MS

CYSTS, NONODONTOGENIC

414 **Mandible-Maxilla Aneurysmal Bone Cyst**
Lisa J. Koenig, BChD, DDS, MS
418 **Nasopalatine Duct Cyst**
Lisa J. Koenig, BChD, DDS, MS
422 **Nasolabial Cyst**
Lisa J. Koenig, BChD, DDS, MS and Kristine M. Mosier, DMD, PhD
424 **Mandible-Maxilla Simple (Traumatic) Bone Cyst**
Lisa J. Koenig, BChD, DDS, MS

FIBROOSSEOUS LESIONS

428 **Periapical Osseous Dysplasia**
C. Grace Petrikowski, DDS, MSc, FRCD(C)
432 **Florid Osseous Dysplasia**
C. Grace Petrikowski, DDS, MSc, FRCD(C)
436 **Ossifying Fibroma**
C. Grace Petrikowski, DDS, MSc, FRCD(C)
440 **Mandible-Maxilla Fibrous Dysplasia**
C. Grace Petrikowski, DDS, MSc, FRCD(C) and Dania Tamimi, BDS, DMSc

TABLE OF CONTENTS

METABOLIC/SYSTEMIC

446 **Paget Disease**
C. Grace Petrikowski, DDS, MSc, FRCD(C)

NEOPLASM, BENIGN, ODONTOGENIC

450 **Odontoma**
Dania Tamimi, BDS, DMSc

454 **Adenomatoid Odontogenic Tumor**
Dania Tamimi, BDS, DMSc

456 **Ameloblastoma**
Susanne E. Perschbacher, DDS, MSc, FRCD(C)

460 **Ameloblastic Fibroma**
Lisa J. Koenig, BChD, DDS, MS

464 **Ameloblastic Fibroodontoma**
Dania Tamimi, BDS, DMSc

466 **Calcifying Epithelial Odontogenic Tumor**
Dania Tamimi, BDS, DMSc

468 **Cementoblastoma**
Brad J. Potter, DDS, MS and Margot L. Van Dis, DDS, MS

470 **Odontogenic Myxoma**
Brad J. Potter, DDS, MS and Margot L. Van Dis, DDS, MS

472 **Central Odontogenic Fibroma**
Dania Tamimi, BDS, DMSc

NEOPLASM, BENIGN, NONODONTOGENIC

474 **Central Hemangioma**
Byron W. Benson, DDS, MS

476 **Osteoid Osteoma**
Lisa J. Koenig, BChD, DDS, MS

478 **Osteoblastoma**
Lisa J. Koenig, BChD, DDS, MS

480 **Mandible-Maxilla Osteoma**
Lisa J. Koenig, BChD, DDS, MS

482 **Nerve Sheath Tumor**
Lisa J. Koenig, BChD, DDS, MS

486 **Neurofibromatosis Type 1**
Lisa J. Koenig, BChD, DDS, MS

490 **Desmoplastic Fibroma**
Lisa J. Koenig, BChD, DDS, MS

NEOPLASM, MALIGNANT, ODONTOGENIC

492 **Malignant Ameloblastoma and Ameloblastic Carcinoma**
Byron W. Benson, DDS, MS

NEOPLASM, MALIGNANT, NONODONTOGENIC

494 **Mandible-Maxilla Metastasis**
C. Grace Petrikowski, DDS, MSc, FRCD(C)

500 **Mandible-Maxilla Osteosarcoma**
C. Grace Petrikowski, DDS, MSc, FRCD(C)

504 **Mandible-Maxilla Chondrosarcoma**
C. Grace Petrikowski, DDS, MSc, FRCD(C)

508 **Primary Intraosseous Squamous Cell Carcinoma**
C. Grace Petrikowski, DDS, MSc, FRCD(C)

510 **Central Mucoepidermoid Carcinoma**
C. Grace Petrikowski, DDS, MSc, FRCD(C)

512 **Burkitt Lymphoma**
C. Grace Petrikowski, DDS, MSc, FRCD(C)

516 **Non-Hodgkin Lymphoma of Pharyngeal Mucosal Space**
Patricia A. Hudgins, MD, FACR

520 **Multiple Myeloma**
Lisa J. Koenig, BChD, DDS, MS

524 **Ewing Sarcoma**
Axel Ruprecht, DDS, MScD, FRCD(C)

528 **Leukemia**
Byron W. Benson, DDS, MS

TUMOR-LIKE LESIONS

530 **Mandible-Maxilla Central Giant Cell Granuloma**
Susanne E. Perschbacher, DDS, MSc, FRCD(C)

534 **Langerhans Histiocytosis**
Lisa J. Koenig, BChD, DDS, MS

SECTION 4: TEMPOROMANDIBULAR JOINT

CONGENITAL DISORDERS

540 **Condylar Aplasia**
David Hatcher, DDS, MSc

542 **Hemifacial Microsomia**
David Hatcher, DDS, MSc

DEVELOPMENTAL ACQUIRED DISORDERS

546 **Condylar Hyperplasia**
David Hatcher, DDS, MSc and Lisa J. Koenig, BChD, DDS, MS

552 **Coronoid Hyperplasia**
Lisa J. Koenig, BChD, DDS, MS, David Hatcher, DDS, MSc, and Dania Tamimi, BDS, DMSc

556 **Condylar Hypoplasia**
David Hatcher, DDS, MSc, Lisa J. Koenig, BChD, DDS, MS, and C. Grace Petrikowski, DDS, MSc, FRCD(C)

560 **Fibrous Ankylosis**
David Hatcher, DDS, MSc and Lisa J. Koenig, BChD, DDS, MS

562 **Bony Ankylosis**
C. Grace Petrikowski, DDS, MSc, FRCD(C)

TRAUMA

564 **TMJ Fractures**
David Hatcher, DDS, MSc and C. Grace Petrikowski, DDS, MSc, FRCD(C)

570 **TMJ Dislocation**
C. Grace Petrikowski, DDS, MSc, FRCD(C)

572 **Bifid Condyle**
C. Grace Petrikowski, DDS, MSc, FRCD(C)

576 **TMJ Osteochondritis Dissecans**
David Hatcher, DDS, MSc

INFLAMMATION

578 **TMJ Rheumatoid Arthritis**
David Hatcher, DDS, MSc

TABLE OF CONTENTS

584 **TMJ Juvenile Idiopathic Arthritis**
Lubdha M. Shah, MD and David Hatcher, DDS, MSc

590 **TMJ Pigmented Villonodular Synovitis**
David Hatcher, DDS, MSc and Kristine M. Mosier, DMD, PhD

DEGENERATIVE DISORDERS

592 **Degenerative Joint Disease**
David Hatcher, DDS, MSc

596 **TMJ Synovial Cyst**
David Hatcher, DDS, MSc

598 **Progressive Condylar Resorption**
David Hatcher, DDS, MSc

DISC DERANGEMENT DISORDERS

604 **Disc Displacement With Reduction**
Richard W. Katzberg, MD, David Hatcher, DDS, MSc, and Joanne Ethier, DMD, MBA, MS

610 **Disc Displacement Without Reduction**
Richard W. Katzberg, MD, David Hatcher, DDS, MSc, and Joanne Ethier, DMD, MBA, MS

616 **Adhesions**
David Hatcher, DDS, MSc

NEOPLASM, BENIGN

618 **TMJ Osteoma**
Lisa J. Koenig, BChD, DDS, MS and H. Ric Harnsberger, MD

620 **TMJ Osteochondroma**
David Hatcher, DDS, MSc and C. Grace Petrikowski, DDS, MSc, FRCD(C)

TUMOR-LIKE LESIONS

626 **TMJ Calcium Pyrophosphate Dihydrate Deposition Disease**
C. Grace Petrikowski, DDS, MSc, FRCD(C)

630 **TMJ Primary Synovial Chondromatosis**
C. Grace Petrikowski, DDS, MSc, FRCD(C) and David Hatcher, DDS, MSc

NEOPLASM, MALIGNANT

634 **TMJ Osteosarcoma**
C. Grace Petrikowski, DDS, MSc, FRCD(C)

636 **TMJ Chondrosarcoma**
C. Grace Petrikowski, DDS, MSc, FRCD(C)

640 **TMJ Metastasis**
C. Grace Petrikowski, DDS, MSc, FRCD(C) and Lisa J. Koenig, BChD, DDS, MS

MISCELLANEOUS

642 **TMJ Simple (Traumatic) Bone Cyst**
C. Grace Petrikowski, DDS, MSc, FRCD(C) and Lisa J. Koenig, BChD, DDS, MS

644 **Aneurysmal Bone Cyst**
David Hatcher, DDS, MSc

SECTION 5: MAXILLARY SINUS AND NASAL CAVITY

NORMAL VARIANTS

650 **Deviated Nasal Septum**
Axel Ruprecht, DDS, MScD, FRCD(C)

652 **Concha Bullosa**
Axel Ruprecht, DDS, MScD, FRCD(C)

656 **Accessory Ostia**
Axel Ruprecht, DDS, MScD, FRCD(C)

DEVELOPMENTAL

658 **Hypoplasia/Aplasia**
Axel Ruprecht, DDS, MScD, FRCD(C)

INFLAMMATION

662 **Mucus Retention Pseudocyst**
Axel Ruprecht, DDS, MScD, FRCD(C)

664 **Sinonasal Mucocele**
Axel Ruprecht, DDS, MScD, FRCD(C) and Michelle A. Michel, MD

668 **Sinonasal Granulomatosis With Polyangiitis (Wegener Granulomatosis)**
Axel Ruprecht, DDS, MScD, FRCD(C) and Michelle A. Michel, MD

672 **Sinonasal Polyposis**
Michelle A. Michel, MD

676 **Acute Rhinosinusitis**
Axel Ruprecht, DDS, MScD, FRCD(C) and Michelle A. Michel, MD

680 **Chronic Rhinosinusitis**
Axel Ruprecht, DDS, MScD, FRCD(C) and Michelle A. Michel, MD

684 **Odontogenic Sinusitis**
Axel Ruprecht, DDS, MScD, FRCD(C)

686 **Allergic Fungal Sinusitis**
H. Christian Davidson, MD

688 **Invasive Fungal Sinusitis**
Michelle A. Michel, MD

692 **Mycetoma**
Michelle A. Michel, MD

694 **Invasive Pseudotumor**
Axel Ruprecht, DDS, MScD, FRCD(C)

NEOPLASM, BENIGN

696 **Sinonasal Inverted Papilloma**
Axel Ruprecht, DDS, MScD, FRCD(C) and Michelle A. Michel, MD

700 **Sinonasal Osteoma**
Axel Ruprecht, DDS, MScD, FRCD(C)

NEOPLASM, MALIGNANT

704 **Sinonasal Squamous Cell Carcinoma**
Axel Ruprecht, DDS, MScD, FRCD(C)

706 **Sinonasal Adenoid Cystic Carcinoma**
Axel Ruprecht, DDS, MScD, FRCD(C) and Michelle A. Michel, MD

TABLE OF CONTENTS

708 Nasopharyngeal Carcinoma
Luke N. Ledbetter, MD
712 Sinonasal Malignant Melanoma
Axel Ruprecht, DDS, MScD, FRCD(C)

FIBROOSSEOUS LESIONS

714 Sinonasal Fibrous Dysplasia
Axel Ruprecht, DDS, MScD, FRCD(C)
718 Sinonasal Ossifying Fibroma
Axel Ruprecht, DDS, MScD, FRCD(C) and Michelle A. Michel, MD

SECTION 6: MASTICATOR SPACE

INFECTION

724 Masticator Space Abscess
Rebecca S. Cornelius, MD, FACR

DEGENERATIVE

728 Masticator Muscle Atrophy
Rebecca S. Cornelius, MD, FACR

NEOPLASM, BENIGN

732 Masticator Space CNV3 Schwannoma
Rebecca S. Cornelius, MD, FACR

NEOPLASM, MALIGNANT

734 Masticator Space Chondrosarcoma
Rebecca S. Cornelius, MD, FACR
738 Masticator Space Sarcoma
Rebecca S. Cornelius, MD, FACR
742 Masticator Space CNV3 Perineural Tumor
Rebecca S. Cornelius, MD, FACR

MISCELLANEOUS/IDIOPATHIC

746 Benign Masticator Muscle Hypertrophy
Rebecca S. Cornelius, MD, FACR

SECTION 7: PAROTID SPACE

INFLAMMATION

750 Benign Lymphoepithelial Lesions: HIV
Barton F. Branstetter, IV, MD, FACR
754 Parotid Sialadenitis
Byron W. Benson, DDS, MS

NEOPLASM, BENIGN

756 Parotid Benign Mixed Tumor
Barton F. Branstetter, IV, MD, FACR
760 Warthin Tumor
Barton F. Branstetter, IV, MD, FACR
764 Parotid Schwannoma
Barton F. Branstetter, IV, MD, FACR

NEOPLASM, MALIGNANT

766 Parotid Malignant Mixed Tumor
Barton F. Branstetter, IV, MD, FACR
768 Parotid Mucoepidermoid Carcinoma
Barton F. Branstetter, IV, MD, FACR
772 Parotid Adenoid Cystic Carcinoma
Barton F. Branstetter, IV, MD, FACR
774 Parotid Non-Hodgkin Lymphoma
Barton F. Branstetter, IV, MD, FACR
778 Metastatic Disease of Parotid Nodes
Barton F. Branstetter, IV, MD, FACR

AUTOIMMUNE

782 Sjögren Syndrome
Byron W. Benson, DDS, MS

MISCELLANEOUS/IDIOPATHIC

784 Parotid Sialoliths
Byron W. Benson, DDS, MS

SECTION 8: CERVICAL SPINE

DEVELOPMENTAL ALTERATIONS

788 C2-C3 Fusion
Kevin R. Moore, MD
790 C1 Assimilation
Kevin R. Moore, MD
792 Ponticulus Posticus
Kevin R. Moore, MD
794 Ossiculum Terminale
Kevin R. Moore, MD
796 Split Atlas
Kevin R. Moore, MD
798 Os Odontoideum
Kevin R. Moore, MD
802 Os Avis (Fused to Clivus)
Kevin R. Moore, MD
804 Odontoid Hypoplasia/Aplasia
Kevin R. Moore, MD
806 Failure of Formation
Kevin R. Moore, MD
810 Failure of Segmentation
Kevin R. Moore, MD

DEGENERATIVE DISORDERS

814 Degenerative Joint Disorders of Craniovertebral Junction
Cheryl A. Petersilge, MD, MBA
818 Ossification of Posterior Longitudinal Ligament
Cheryl A. Petersilge, MD, MBA
822 Diffuse Idiopathic Skeletal Hyperostosis
Cheryl A. Petersilge, MD, MBA
826 Cervical Facet Arthropathy
Jeffrey S. Ross, MD

TUMOR AND TUMOR-LIKE LESIONS

830 Hemangioma, Cervical Spine
Cheryl A. Petersilge, MD, MBA
834 Lytic and Blastic Metastases
Cheryl A. Petersilge, MD, MBA

TABLE OF CONTENTS

FIBROOSSEOUS

838 **Fibrous Dysplasia, Cervical Spine**
Cheryl A. Petersilge, MD, MBA and Julia Crim, MD

MISCELLANEOUS

840 **Tumoral Calcinosis**
Jeffrey S. Ross, MD and Lubdha M. Shah, MD

Part III: Differential Diagnoses

SECTION 1: TEETH

ALTERATIONS IN TOOTH NUMBER

844 **Extra Teeth**
Brad J. Potter, DDS, MS and Margot L. Van Dis, DDS, MS

846 **Missing Teeth**
Brad J. Potter, DDS, MS and Margot L. Van Dis, DDS, MS

ALTERATIONS IN TOOTH MORPHOLOGY/SHAPE

848 **Crown Changes**
Brad J. Potter, DDS, MS and Margot L. Van Dis, DDS, MS

850 **Root Changes**
Brad J. Potter, DDS, MS and Margot L. Van Dis, DDS, MS

SECTION 2: MANDIBLE AND MAXILLA

ALTERATIONS IN SUPPORTING STRUCTURES OF TEETH

856 **Periapical Radiolucencies**
Dania Tamimi, BDS, DMSc

860 **Periapical Radiopacities and Mixed Lesions**
Dania Tamimi, BDS, DMSc

862 **Floating Teeth**
Lisa J. Koenig, BChD, DDS, MS

864 **Widened Periodontal Ligament Space**
Lisa J. Koenig, BChD, DDS, MS

866 **Lamina Dura Changes**
Lisa J. Koenig, BChD, DDS, MS

RADIOLUCENCIES

870 **Well-Defined Unilocular Radiolucencies**
Lisa J. Koenig, BChD, DDS, MS

874 **Pericoronal Radiolucencies Without Radiopacities**
Lisa J. Koenig, BChD, DDS, MS

876 **Pericoronal Radiolucencies With Radiopacities**
Lisa J. Koenig, BChD, DDS, MS

878 **Multilocular Radiolucencies**
Brad J. Potter, DDS, MS and Margot L. Van Dis, DDS, MS

882 **Ill-Defined Radiolucencies**
Byron W. Benson, DDS, MS

888 **Generalized Rarefaction**
Dania Tamimi, BDS, DMSc

RADIOPACITIES

892 **Well-Defined Radiopacities**
Brad J. Potter, DDS, MS and Margot L. Van Dis, DDS, MS

896 **Ground-Glass and Granular Radiopacities**
Dania Tamimi, BDS, DMSc

902 **Generalized Radiopacities**
Dania Tamimi, BDS, DMSc

PERIOSTEAL REACTIONS

906 **Periosteal Reactions**
Dania Tamimi, BDS, DMSc

SECTION 3: ORAL CAVITY

ANATOMICALLY BASED LESIONS

914 **Submandibular Space Lesions**
Byron W. Benson, DDS, MS

918 **Parotid Space Lesions**
Byron W. Benson, DDS, MS

922 **Sublingual Space Lesions**
Byron W. Benson, DDS, MS

926 **Oral Mucosal Space/Surface Lesions**
Byron W. Benson, DDS, MS

930 **Root of Tongue Lesions**
Byron W. Benson, DDS, MS

MISCELLANEOUS

934 **Soft Tissue Calcifications**
Brad J. Potter, DDS, MS and Margot L. Van Dis, DDS, MS

SECTION 4: TEMPOROMANDIBULAR JOINT

CHANGES IN CONDYLAR SIZE AND FUNCTION

940 **Small Condyle**
C. Grace Petrikowski, DDS, MSc, FRCD(C) and Dania Tamimi, BDS, DMSc

946 **Large Condyle**
C. Grace Petrikowski, DDS, MSc, FRCD(C) and Dania Tamimi, BDS, DMSc

950 **Limited Condylar Translation**
C. Grace Petrikowski, DDS, MSc, FRCD(C)

MASS LESIONS

954 **TMJ Radiolucencies**
C. Grace Petrikowski, DDS, MSc, FRCD(C)

956 **TMJ Radiopacities**
C. Grace Petrikowski, DDS, MSc, FRCD(C) and Dania Tamimi, BDS, DMSc

MISCELLANEOUS

960 **TMJ Articular Loose Bodies**
C. Grace Petrikowski, DDS, MSc, FRCD(C) and Dania Tamimi, BDS, DMSc

TABLE OF CONTENTS

SECTION 5: MAXILLARY SINUS AND NASAL CAVITY

NASAL LESIONS

964 **Perforated Nasal Septum**
Axel Ruprecht, DDS, MScD, FRCD(C)

966 **Nasal Lesion Without Bony Destruction**
Axel Ruprecht, DDS, MScD, FRCD(C)

970 **Nasal Lesion With Bony Destruction**
Axel Ruprecht, DDS, MScD, FRCD(C)

974 **Sinonasal Fibroosseous and Cartilaginous Lesions**
Axel Ruprecht, DDS, MScD, FRCD(C)

SINUS LESIONS

976 **Paranasal Sinus Lesions Without Bony Destruction**
Axel Ruprecht, DDS, MScD, FRCD(C)

980 **Paranasal Sinus Lesions With Bony Destruction**
Axel Ruprecht, DDS, MScD, FRCD(C)

MISCELLANEOUS

984 **Displaced Dental Structures Into Antrum**
Axel Ruprecht, DDS, MScD, FRCD(C)

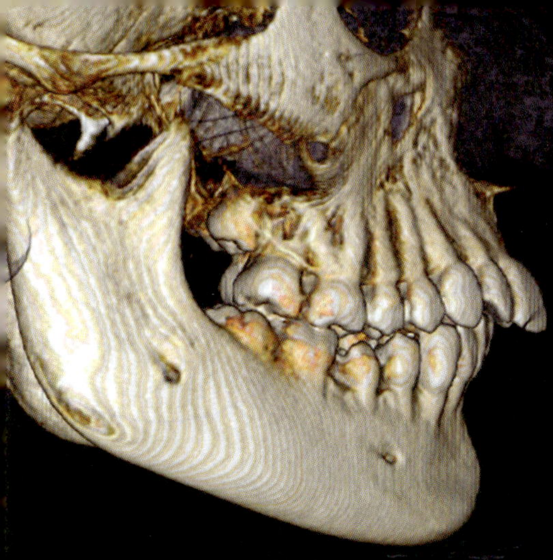

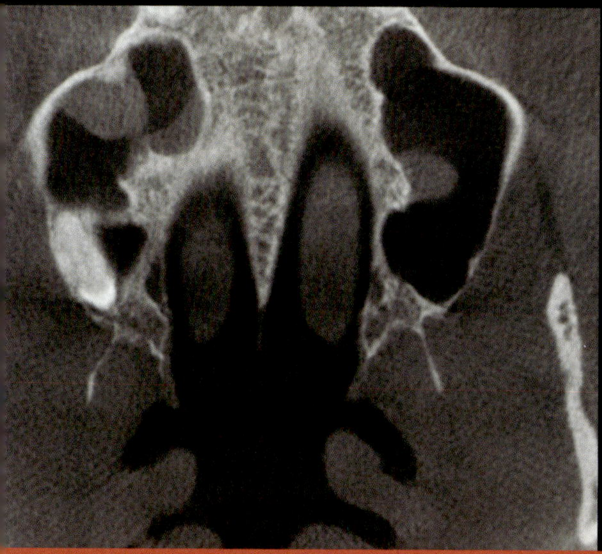

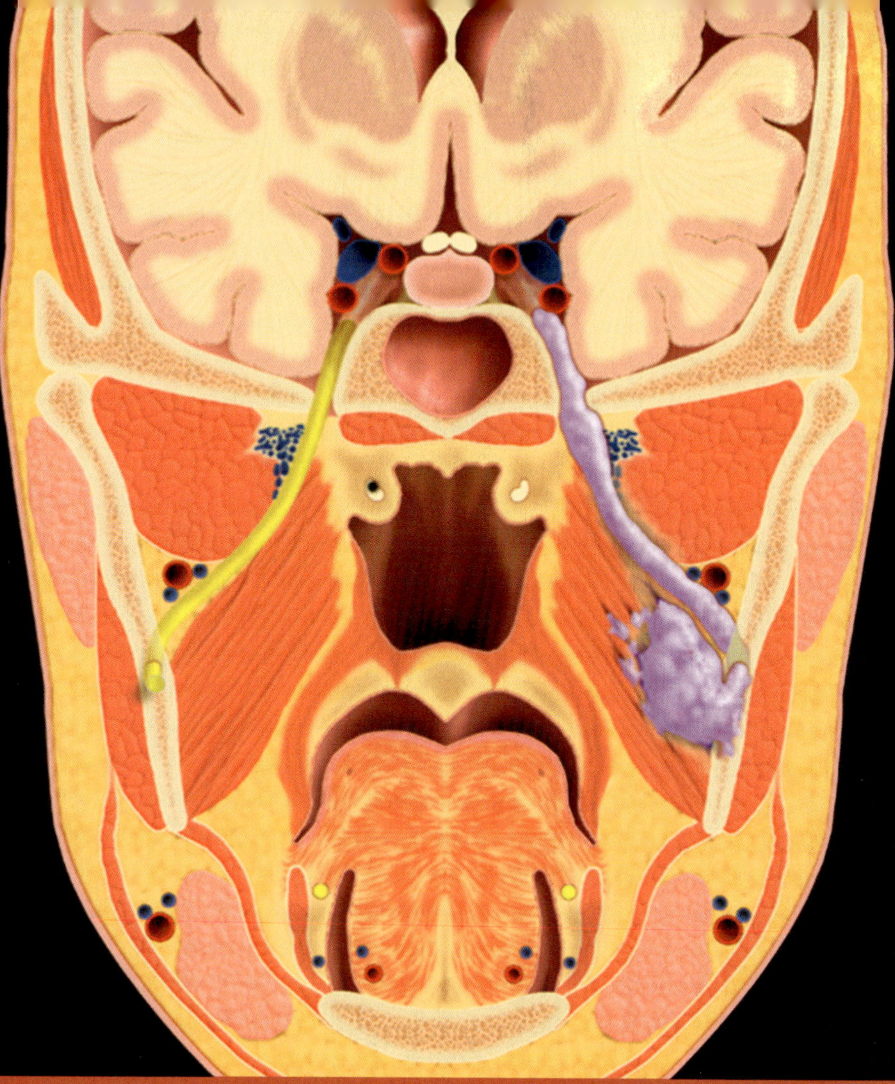

Diagnostic Imaging

Oral and Maxillofacial

SECOND EDITION

PART I

SECTION 1

Oral Cavity

Teeth	**4**
Dental Restorations	**14**
Maxilla	**22**
Mandible	**30**
Tongue	**36**
Retromolar Trigone	**40**
Sublingual Space	**44**
Submandibular Space	**48**
Oral Mucosal Space/Surface	**52**

Teeth

TERMINOLOGY

Abbreviations

- Incisor (Inc), canine (C), premolar (PM), molar (M)

Synonyms

- Cuspid = canine
- Bicuspid = premolar

IMAGING ANATOMY

Overview

- Humans have 2 dentitions: **Primary** and **permanent**
- Teeth are divided into **maxillary** (upper) and **mandibular** (lower)
- Each jaw is divided into 2 quadrants: **Right** and **left** separated by midline
- Each quadrant has **5 primary** and **8 permanent teeth**
  - **Primary**: 2 Incs (central and lateral), 1 C, 2 Ms (1st and 2nd)
  - **Permanent**: 2 Incs (central and lateral), 1 C, 2 PMs (1st and 2nd), 3 Ms (1st, 2nd, and 3rd)
- Teeth can be **named** or **numbered**
- Naming teeth should follow this sequence: Dentition → jaw → side → tooth name
  - Example: **Primary maxillary right 1st M**; permanent mandibular left C
  - Exceptions are PMs and 3rd Ms: Only present in permanent dentition, so no need to use "permanent"
  - If only permanent teeth are present (all primary teeth have been exfoliated), no need to use "permanent"
- **Numbering teeth depends on country**
  - Most countries use **FDI (Federation Dentaire International) system for numbering**
    - **Quadrants are numbered**
    - Permanent: Upper right (UR) = 1, upper left (UL) = 2, lower left (LL) = 3, lower right (LR) = 4
    - Primary: UR = 5, UL = 6, LL = 7, LR = 8
    - **Teeth are numbered**
    - Permanent: Central Inc = 1, lateral Inc = 2, C = 3, 1st PM = 4, 2nd PM = 5, 1st M = 6, 2nd M = 7, 3rd M = 8
    - Primary: Central Inc = 1, lateral Inc = 2, C = 3, 1st M = 4, 2nd M = 5
    - Example: Permanent mandibular right 1st M = tooth #46 **(pronounced four six)**
  - United States uses **universal system**
    - **Only teeth are numbered**
    - Permanent teeth start with #1 (maxillary right 3rd M) and go to #16 (maxillary left 3rd M) pronounced **sixteen**
    - Mandibular left 3rd M is #17 **(seventeen)** and goes to mandibular right 3rd M #32 **(thirty two)**
    - Primary teeth are labeled with letters A → T starting with last M on UR: UR → UL→ LL → LR
  - Other tooth numbering systems exist; check with local dental organization
  - When in doubt, **describe teeth by name**

Anatomy Relationships

- When describing teeth or objects in relation to teeth, **conventional anatomic positions** (inferior, posterior, medial, lateral, anterior, posterior) **are not used**
- Position is described in relation to
  - **Midline of arch** (i.e., line between central Incs), **not anatomical midline**
    - All **surfaces** of teeth that are **in direction** of midline of arch are **"mesial"**
    - All **surfaces** of teeth **away** from midline of arch are **"distal"**
  - **Inside or outside of arch**
    - Surfaces toward face are **facial** (can use buccal if posterior, labial if anterior)
    - Surfaces toward tongue are **lingual** (can use palatal if maxillary)
  - **Anatomic tooth**
    - If **above crown** of tooth, use **"coronal to"**
    - If **below apices** of tooth, use **"apical to"**

Eruption Patterns

- 3 phases of eruption: Primary, mixed, and permanent dentitions
- **Primary dentition**
  - **Starts to erupt between 6-12 months**
  - 1st teeth are usually lower central Incs; last teeth are 2nd Ms
- **Mixed dentition**
  - **Combination of primary and permanent teeth** have erupted
  - 1st permanent teeth are permanent 1st Ms at 6 years
  - Exfoliation of primary Incs followed by eruption of permanent Incs (6-9 years)
  - Exfoliation of primary mandibular Cs followed by eruption of permanent mandibular Cs (9-10 years)
  - Exfoliation of primary Ms followed by eruption of PMs (10-12 years)
  - Exfoliation of primary maxillary Cs followed by eruption of permanent Cs (11-12 years)
    - **May get crowded out of arch**, either impacted or malerupted
    - **High incidence of dentigerous cyst formation** with impaction of these teeth
- **Permanent dentition**
  - **No more primary teeth in jaws**
  - Eruption of permanent 2nd Ms (11-13 years)
  - Eruption of 3rd Ms (17-21 years)
    - **Impactions are common**; **dentigerous cysts** may occur around crown of impacted tooth

Tooth Anatomy

- Teeth are made up of 4 basic anatomic structures: Enamel, dentin, cementum, and pulp
  - **Enamel**
    - Hardest substance in body = most mineralized (95% calcified) = highest radiographic density
    - Covers crown of tooth; contacts dentin at **dentinoenamel junction**
    - Contacts cementum at **cementoenamel junction (CEJ)**
    - Develops from ameloblasts
  - **Dentin**
    - Makes up majority of tooth; provides resiliency to hard overlying enamel; 75% calcified

    - Contains dentinoblastic processes: Tooth becomes sensitive when dentin is exposed
  - **Cementum**
    - Thin layer of calcified material covering root of tooth and providing attachment for periodontal ligament (PDL)
    - Not visible radiographically unless hypercementosis occurs
  - **Pulp** (a.k.a. "nerve")
    - Vital portion of tooth (tooth "dies" when pulp dies)
    - Contains nerves and vessels that enter and emerge through **apical foramen** of tooth
    - Most radiolucent portion of tooth
    - Crown portion called **pulp chamber** with pointy **pulp horns**; root portion called **pulp canal**
- Teeth are made up of **crown** and **root**
  - **Crown**: Everything above CEJ
    - Further subdivided into **occlusal/incisal, middle, and cervical 1/3rds**
    - Incs have incisal edges as functional component; all other teeth have cusps
  - **Root**: Everything below CEJ
    - Further subdivided into **cervical, middle, and apical 1/3rds**
    - Teeth can have single root or be multirooted; area between roots of tooth is called **furcation area**
    - Roots are named according to location in alveolar process: **Buccal, lingual, mesial, distal, mesiobuccal, distobuccal**

Periodontium

- Primary function is to support teeth; **when teeth are lost, periodontal bone recedes**
- Made up of **periodontal bone**, **PDLs**, and **gingiva**
  - **Periodontal bone**
    - Portion of alveolar processes of maxilla and mandible that come in direct contact with teeth
    - Most cervical aspect called **crest**; **corticated when healthy**
    - If **tooth is lost**, most cervical aspect of bone is called **residual ridge**
    - Bone at apex of tooth called **periapical bone**
    - Bone in furcation area called **furcal bone**
    - Thin radiopaque line seen radiographically lining tooth socket is called **lamina dura**
  - **PDL**
    - Multidirectional fibers that attach tooth to socket; offer resilience to tooth during function
    - Radiographically seen as uniform **radiolucent line on inside of lamina dura**
    - **If loses uniformity, suspect pathology**
    - Houses **epithelial rests of Malassez**, which may contribute to formation of cyst lining for odontogenic cysts
    - Position in relation to tooth can determine if lesion is attached to tooth structure (inside PDL) or not (outside PDL)
  - **Gingiva** (a.k.a. gums)
    - Soft tissue component covering periodontal bone
    - Attaches to root to form small gingival sulcus with crown; **cannot be visualized radiographically**

Tooth Development and Tumorigenesis

- Potential sources for development of tumors
  - **Prefunctional dental lamina** (odontogenic epithelium with ability to produce tooth); more abundant distal to lower 3rd Ms
  - **Postfunctional dental lamina**: Epithelial remnants, such as rests of Serres, in fibrous gingival tissue; epithelial cell rests of Malassez in PDL and reduced enamel organ epithelium (covers enamel surface until tooth eruption)
  - **Basal cell layer of gingival epithelium** (source of dental lamina)
  - **Dental papilla** (origin of dental pulp); can be induced to produce odontoblasts and synthesize dentin &/or dentinoid material
  - **Dental follicle**
  - **PDL**: Can induce production of fibrous and cemento-osseous mineralized material

ANATOMY IMAGING ISSUES

Imaging Recommendations

- For imaging of teeth for **caries, periapical or periodontal disease, intraoral radiography** is recommended
  - **Horizontal bitewings for caries** and early periodontal disease detection
  - **Vertical bitewings** for moderate to severe **periodontal disease**
  - **Periapical radiographs** if **periapical pathology** is suspected
  - **Pros**: High-resolution images showing fine changes in demineralization; low radiation dose, especially if F-speed film or digital radiography is used
  - **Cons**: Limited to dimensions of intraoral film, cannot see lesions or impacted teeth if they extend beyond
- **For general overview of teeth in jaws**: **Panoramic radiography**
  - Shows eruption pattern and impactions of teeth; presence of intraosseous pathology
  - **Pros**: Cost effective; lower radiation dose when compared to CBCT
  - **Cons**: Distortion, magnification, and blurring can impede evaluation
- **For relationship of impacted teeth with vital anatomic structures: CBCT**
  - Can show inferior alveolar nerve canals in relation to 3rd Ms if extraction is planned
  - Can show relationship of impacted Cs to anterior superior alveolar canal, nasopalatine canal, and floor of nasal cavity
  - **Pros**: 3D representation of 3D structures; 3D reformations can be obtained to give exact visualization of anatomy
  - **Cons**: Expensive imaging modality, generally not covered by insurance; higher radiation dose
  - If unable to obtain CBCT or CT, use intraoral radiography and **SLOB** (**s**ame **l**ingual, **o**pposite **b**uccal) **rule** and **2 images at right angles** to one another

TOOTH DEVELOPMENT

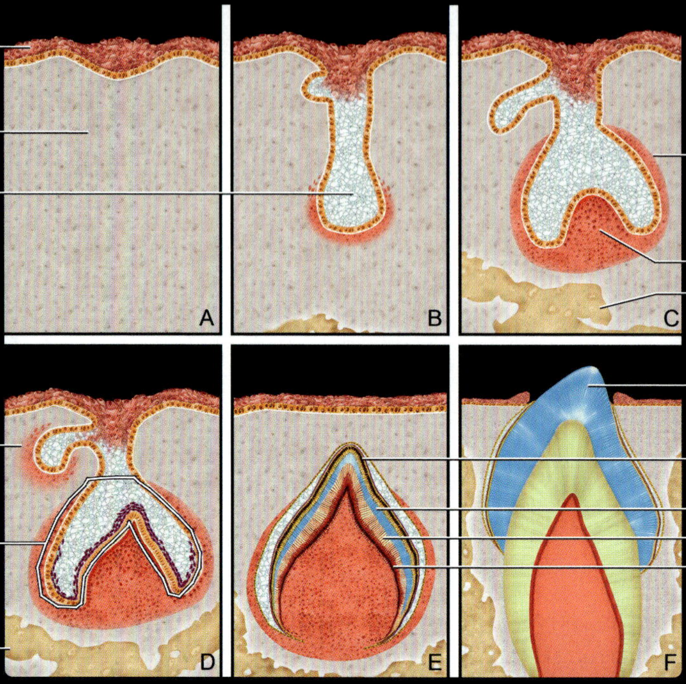

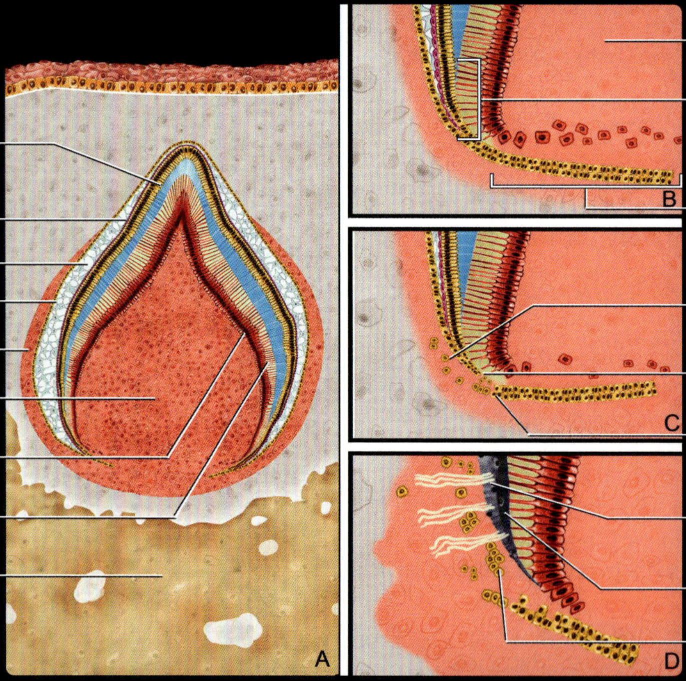

(Top) *Graphic shows stages of tooth development: (A) Initiation: Ectoderm develops oral epithelium and dental lamina, (B) bud stage: Dental lamina grows into bud penetrating the ectomesenchyme, (C) cap stage: Enamel organ forms cap surrounding dental papilla and surrounded by dental sac, (D) bell stage: Differentiation of enamel organ and dental papilla into different cells types, (E) apposition stage: Secretion of dental tissue matrix, and (F) maturation: Full mineralization of dental tissues.* **(Bottom)** *Graphic shows stages of root development: (A) Apposition stage, (B) enamel deposition completion at the cervical loop and formation of Hertwig epithelial root sheath from inner and outer enamel epithelium cells, (C) root sheath disintegration and fragmentation of some of its cells into epithelial rests of Malassez, and (D) formation of cementum and periodontal ligaments with persistence of these epithelial remnants, which may be the source of the epithelial component of some odontogenic cysts and tumors.*

TOOTH ERUPTION

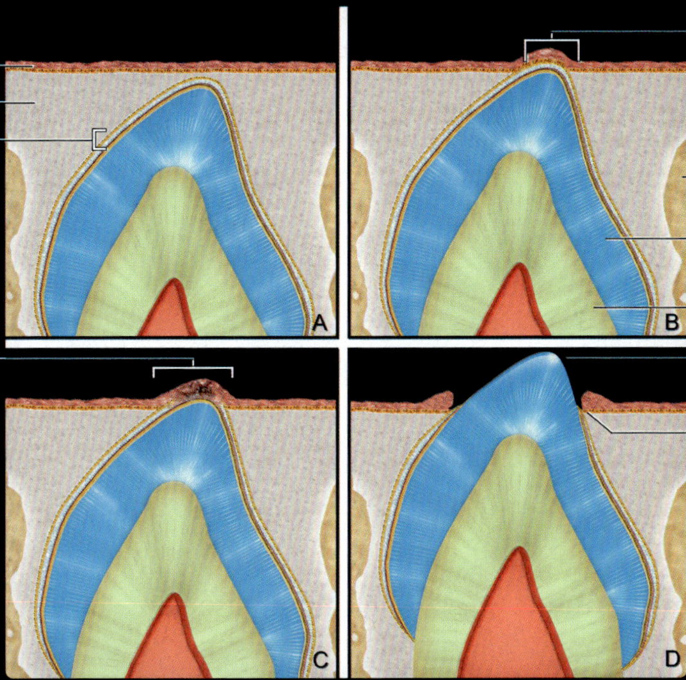

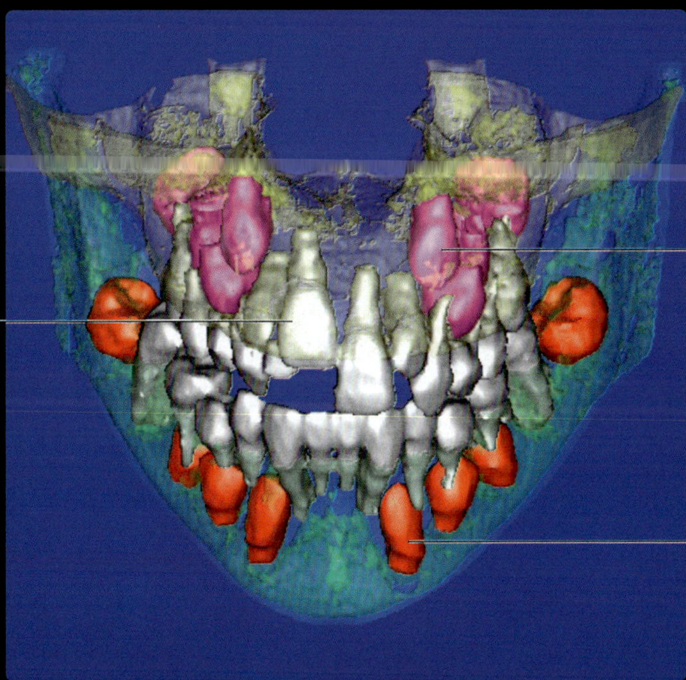

(Top) *Graphic shows process of tooth eruption: (A) Enamel organ reduces to thin layers covering enamel and secretes enzymes, (B) fusion of the reduced enamel epithelium with the oral epithelium, (C) disintegration of the central fused tissues, leaving a canal for tooth movement, and (D) peripheral-fused tissues peel back from the crown as the tooth erupts and form initial junctional epithelium that migrate cervically to cementoenamel junction.* **(Bottom)** *The age of the patient can be determined by examining the eruption of the teeth. This CBCT 3D reformation shows that the permanent incisors and 1st molars have erupted, but the premolars have not. This puts the patient's age at between 8-10 years. 3D reformations can be helpful in evaluation of erupting teeth if malocclusion and malalignment are present. Note that the maxillary right central incisor has not fully erupted, although the apical foramen is almost closed. This may be due to ankylosis (loss of periodontal ligament) of the tooth. (Courtesy 3D Diagnostix, Inc.)*

TEETH NOMENCLATURE AND ERUPTION AGES

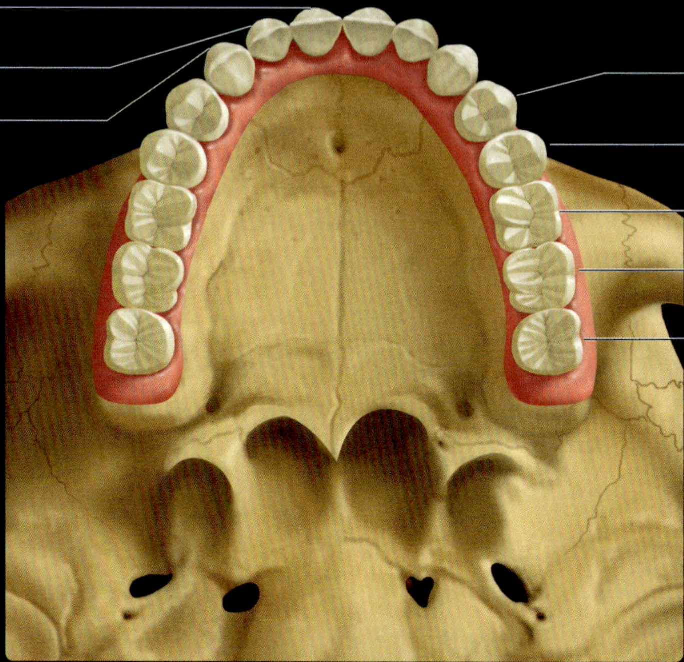

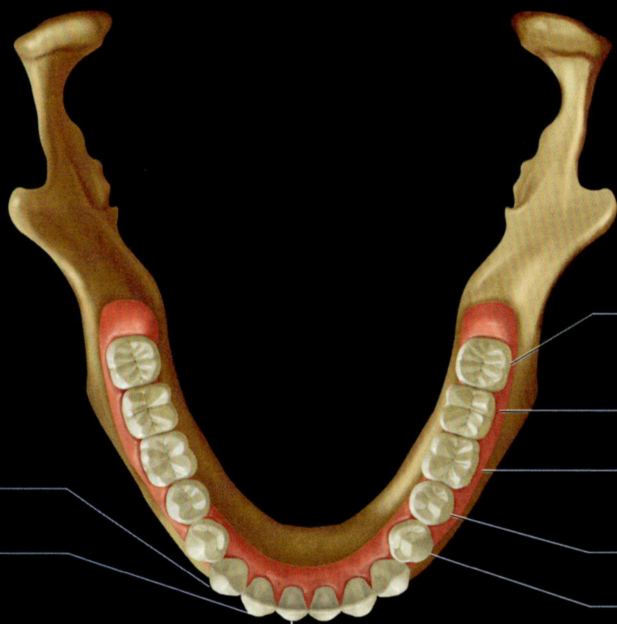

(Top) *The maxilla has 16 permanent teeth arranged in 2 quadrants: The upper right quadrant, also known as quadrant 1, and the upper left quadrant, also known as quadrant 2. Eruption ages are in parenthesis. The functional cusps on the maxillary posterior teeth are lingual (palatal) cusps.* **(Bottom)** *The mandible has 16 permanent teeth arranged in 2 quadrants: The lower left quadrant, also known as quadrant 3, and the lower right quadrant, also known as quadrant 4. Eruption ages are noted in parenthesis. The functional cusps on the mandibular posterior teeth are the buccal (facial) cusps. The permanent maxillary and mandibular incisors and canines have similarly named deciduous predecessors. The predecessors of the 1st and 2nd premolar teeth are the 1st and 2nd deciduous molars, respectively. The deciduous incisors and canines have a single root, the mandibular deciduous molars have 2 roots, and the maxillary deciduous molars have 3 roots.*

HUMAN DENTITIONS

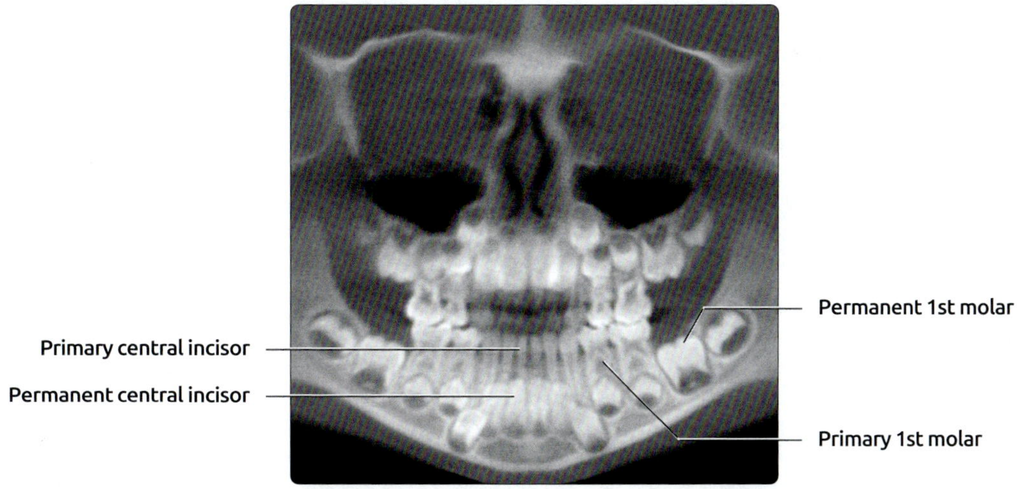

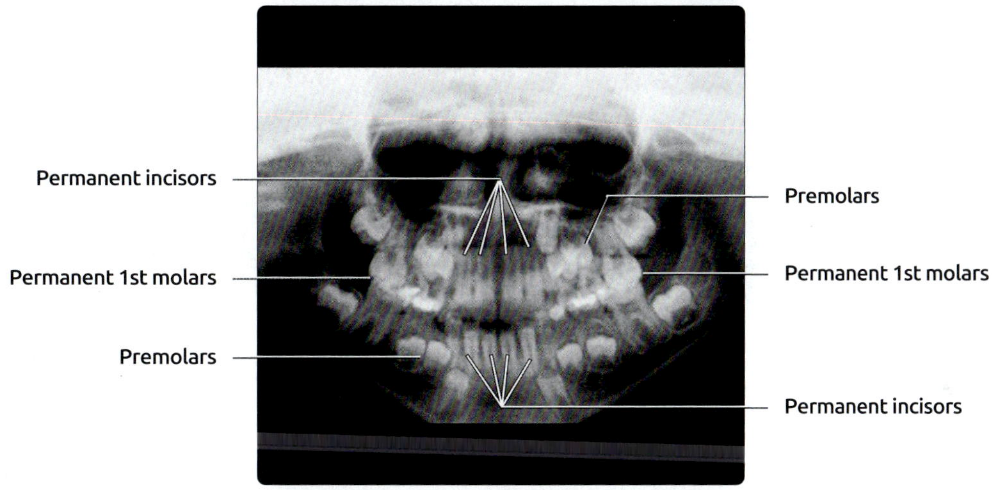

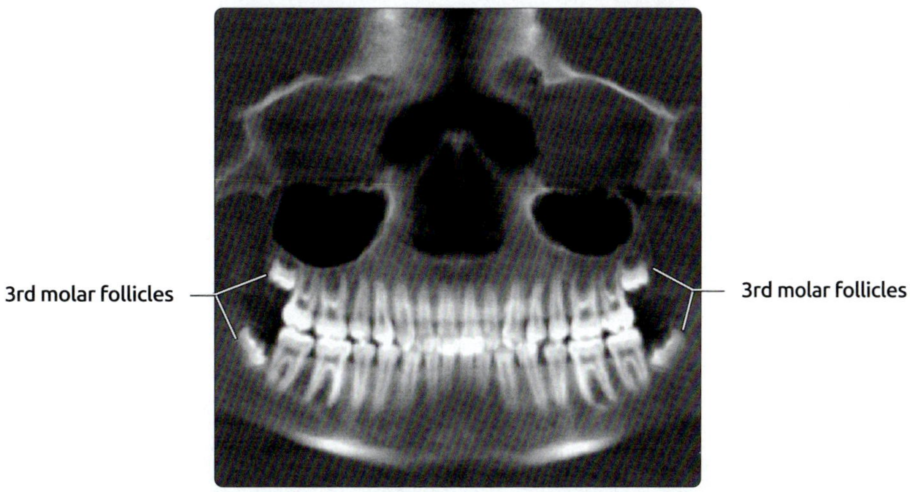

(Top) *Panoramic reformat of CBCT data shows a patient at the primary dentition stage. All 20 primary teeth have erupted into the oral cavity and are in occlusion, but all permanent teeth are still unerupted. Examination of the follicles of the permanent teeth for any displacement or expansion is recommended when evaluating images for the primary dentition phase. It is also important to note any missing permanent teeth to aid in future orthodontic treatment planning.* **(Middle)** *Panoramic radiograph shows a patient at the mixed dentition stage. The upper and lower permanent 1st molars have erupted as well as the upper and lower incisors. As the premolars have not erupted yet, it means the patient's age is between 8-10 years.* **(Bottom)** *CBCT panoramic reformat shows a patient in the permanent dentition/late adolescence stage. All erupted teeth are permanent. The developing 3rd molars are present but unerupted. The stage of 3rd molar development indicates that the patient's age is between 17-20 years.*

DENTAL ANATOMY

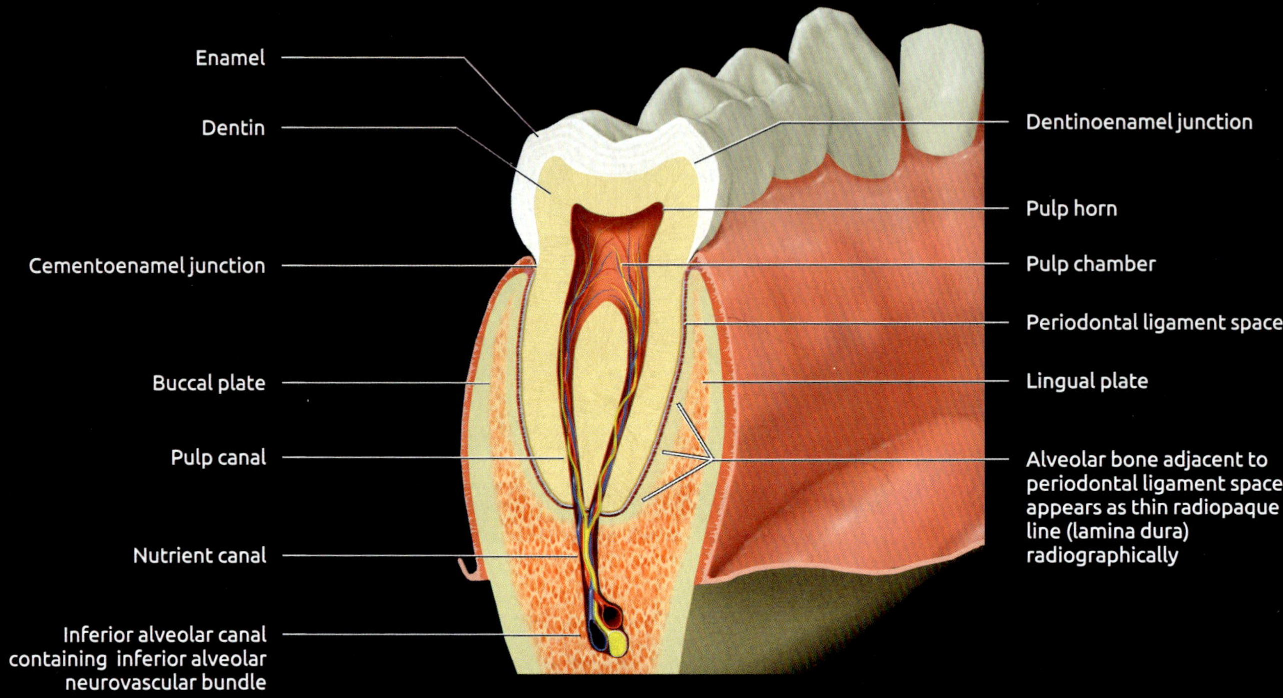

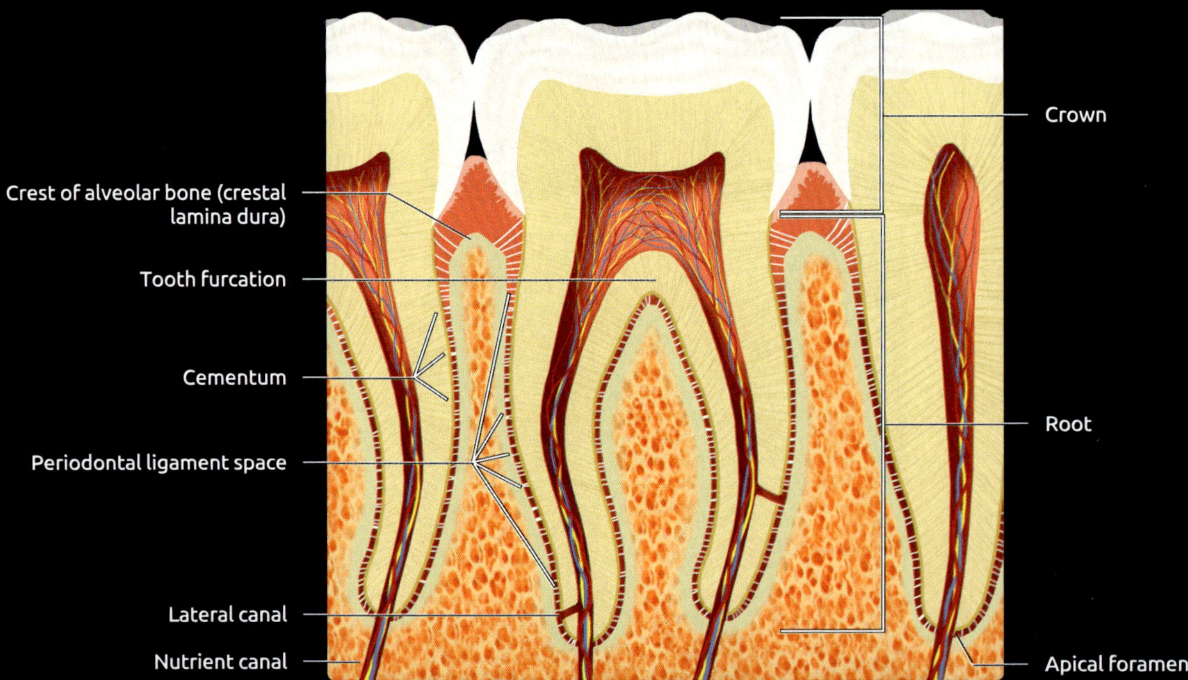

(Top) *Graphic representation shows a mandibular 1st molar in coronal cross section through the mesial root. Identification of the location of pathology in relation to the DEJ and CEJ helps in classifying caries and periodontal disease. Cross sections of the teeth are the most common reformation for dental applications, such as implant and impaction analysis, as they allow for evaluation of alveolar bone width and height and accurate localization of the inferior alveolar nerve canal.* **(Bottom)** *Graphic representation shows sagittal cross section of a mandibular 1st molar. The tooth is attached to the socket through the periodontal ligaments. The crest of the healthy alveolar bone is located about 1-2 mm apical to the CEJ of a tooth. Innervation and vasculature exit through the apical foramen, but on occasion, lateral canals may exit through the lateral aspects of the root. If pulpal death occurs, bacteria can seep through the lateral canals, causing lateral radicular abscesses and cysts, and through the apical foramina, causing periapical inflammation.*

DENTAL RADIOGRAPHIC ANATOMY

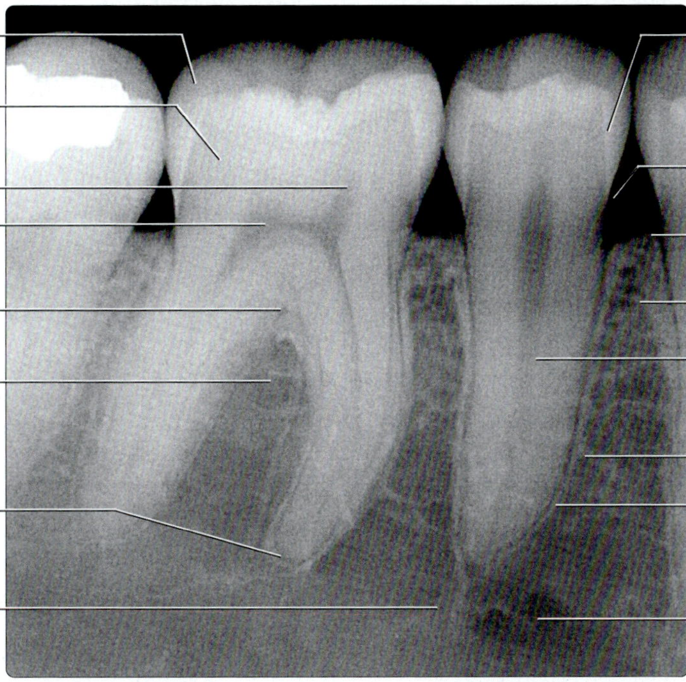

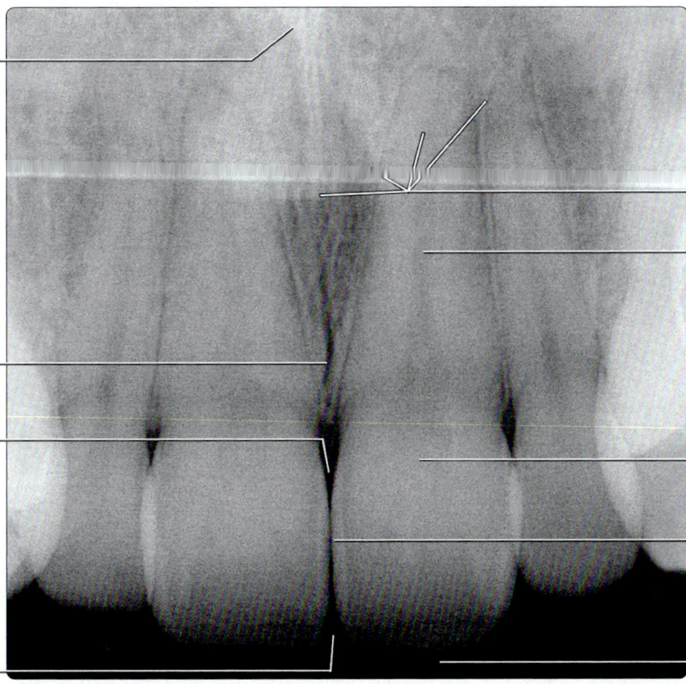

(Top) *Periapical radiograph shows normal dental and periodontal anatomy. The periodontal ligament space is a thin radiolucent line that surrounds the root of the tooth. The lamina dura is a thin radiopaque line that surrounds the tooth socket radiographically. Healthy alveolar bone crests (crestal laminae dura) are corticated. Nutrient canals may appear as small corticated canals within the bone connected to the apical foramen. (Courtesy M. Kroona, DXT.)* **(Bottom)** *Periapical radiograph of the central incisors shows the normal anatomic landmarks in this area. It is important to realize that soft and hard tissue superimpositions may occur when imaging teeth, and their recognition is necessary to determine normal from abnormal. Evaluation of the interproximal contact point and crown contours is important as caries tends to occur cervical to the contact point, and incomplete contact or improper crown contour may lead to plaque accumulation and resulting caries and periodontal disease. (Courtesy M. Kroona, DXT.)*

TOOTH IMPACTIONS

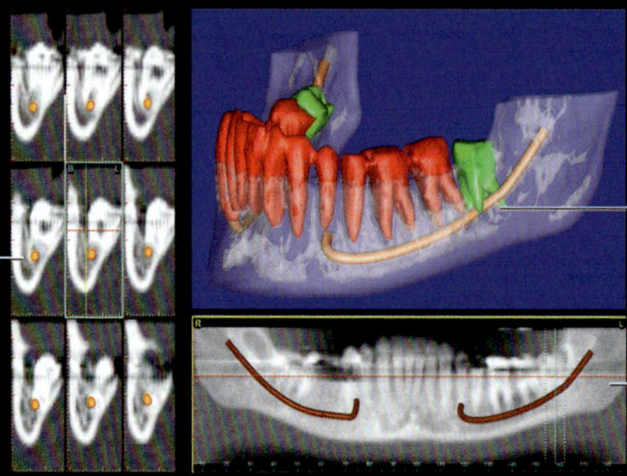

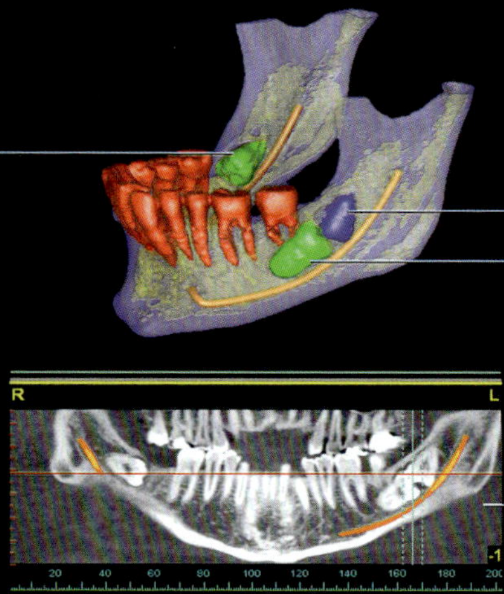

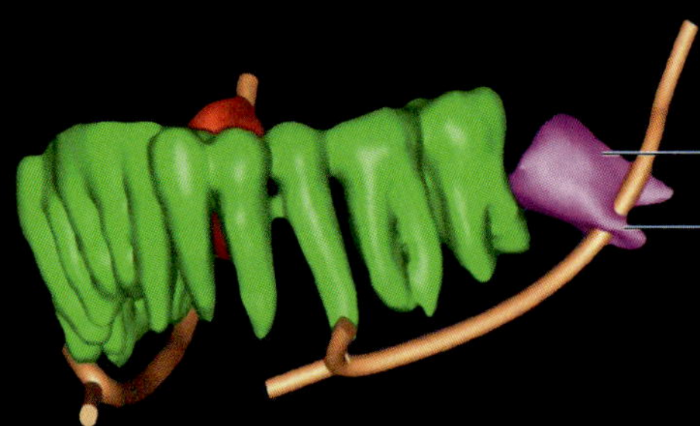

(Top) *Cross sections, panoramic, 3D reformations using Simplant software show the inferior alveolar nerve canal traveling between the roots of the distoangularly impacted mandibular left 3rd molar. (Courtesy 3D Diagnostix, Inc.)* **(Middle)** *Panoramic and 3D reformations show a horizontally impacted left 3rd molar with its crown oriented distally and an impacted supernumerary tooth (4th molar) with its crown oriented mesially, both lying on top of the left inferior alveolar nerve canal. The right 3rd molar is horizontally impacted with its crown oriented mesially. CBCT imaging can aid in predicting and preventing nerve damage when removing 3rd molars surgically. (Courtesy 3D Diagnostix, Inc.)* **(Bottom)** *3D reformation shows the left inferior alveolar nerve going through the mesial root of the mesioangularly impacted mandibular left 3rd molar. This occurs during tooth development due to proximity of the tooth follicle to the inferior alveolar nerve, which is engulfed by the root as it develops and calcifies. (Courtesy 3D Diagnostix, Inc.)*

TOOTH IMPACTIONS

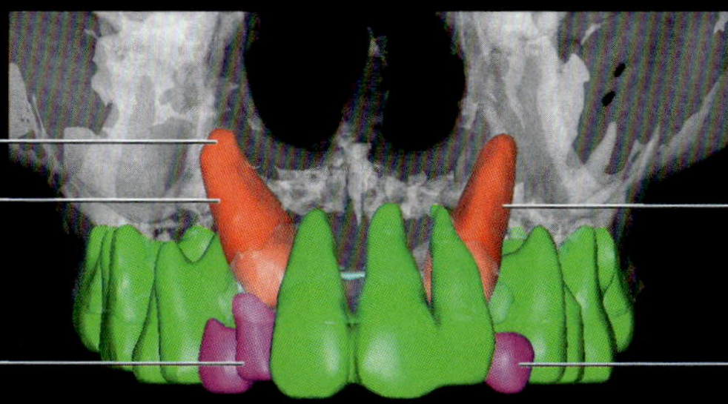

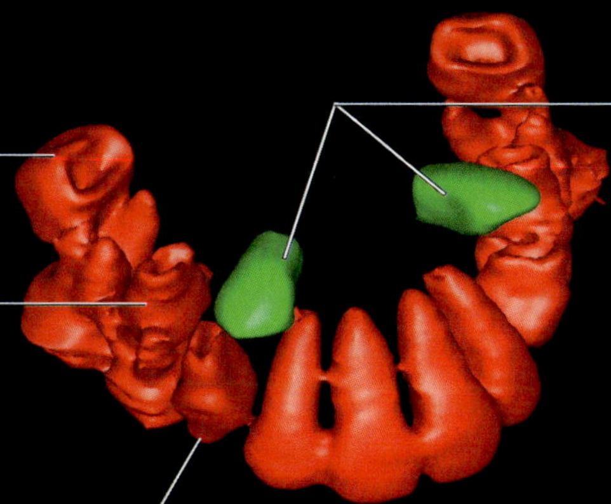

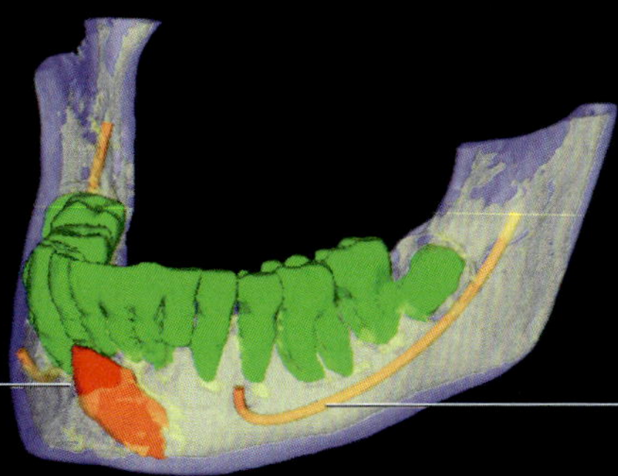

(Top) *CBCT 3D reformation with transparent bone shows the vertical impaction of the permanent canines with lingual placement of the crowns and slight facial tipping of the roots. Knowledge of this orientation aids the surgeon in deciding on the entry point for either extraction or exposure of the crowns for placement of an orthodontic bracket. (Courtesy 3D Diagnostix, Inc.)* **(Middle)** *The bone can also be made transparent on CBCT 3D reformations and segmentations to further visualize the relationship of the teeth with one another. This image shows unerupted maxillary canines with the crowns oriented facially. The roots are not completely formed. (Courtesy 3D Diagnostix, Inc.)* **(Bottom)** *CBCT 3D reformation and segmentation using Simplant software shows an impacted mandibular canine. The position of the impacted tooth in relation to the erupted dentition can easily be determined with 3D reformation. Virtual extractions (digital removal of teeth) can also be performed. (Courtesy 3D Diagnostix, Inc.)*

TERMINOLOGY

Definitions

- Materials used to restore form and function of teeth or to enhance dental aesthetics

IMAGING ANATOMY

Restorative Materials

- **Amalgam**
  - Traditional silver filling material; **metallic** in density
  - Combination of silver, mercury, tin, and copper and sometimes zinc, indium, and palladium
- **Composite**
  - Tooth-colored restoration that binds to enamel through acid-etching bonding
  - **Historically radiolucent, now mixed with radiopaque fillers**
  - More radiodense than enamel, but less than metal
- **Glass ionomer**
  - Tooth-colored restoration that binds to dentin chemically
  - **Used on root lesions** where there is no enamel present for acid etching
  - Also used as **base** under other large restorations

Prosthetic

- **Crowns**
  - Full or partial tooth coverage
  - **Full cast metal**, full **porcelain**, or porcelain fused to metal
  - Tooth must be **prepped**: Ground down to specific dimensions to create space for crown material
- **Bridges**
  - Replace missing teeth by crowning at least 2 adjacent teeth (**abutments**)
  - Portion that replaces missing tooth called **pontic**
  - Bridge can be supported by implants
- **Post and core**
  - **Post**: Metal rod affixed to, or cast with, core to anchor it to root canal
  - **Core**: Cast metal replacement of tooth structure to mimic crown prep; crown placed on top of it
- **Implants**
  - Osseointegrated root form replacement of teeth restored with crown
- **Complete and partial dentures**
  - Removable dentures used when several or all teeth are missing
  - Should be removed from mouth prior to imaging to prevent metal artifact unless scan with denture is requested

Endodontics

- **Gutta percha**
  - Cone-shaped flexible radiopaque material that can be condensed to fill tapering prepared root canal
  - Should be ≤ 1 mm from apex within root
    - 0.5 mm is ideal
  - If it extends beyond apex, called overfill
    - If it is 1 mm from apex (within root canal), called underfilled or short
- **Sealer cement**
  - Viscous radiopaque material that seals gaps between gutta percha cones
  - May extend beyond apex of tooth and cause rarefaction of bone; most are biocompatible

Orthodontics

- **Brackets**
  - Traditionally fixed to facial aspect of teeth with resin; lingual brackets available
- **Bands**
  - Placed on posterior teeth as anchors for appliance
- **Archwire**
  - Stainless steel wires that follow outline of arch fixed to brackets and bands with elastic &/or ligature wire
- **Other fixed appliances**
  - Anchored to posterior teeth through bands
  - May have several metallic spring and loop components as well as acrylic components

Pediatrics

- **Stainless steel crown**
  - Prefabricated crown
  - Used when tooth structure cannot be restored by amalgam alone or when tooth is root canal-treated (pulpotomy or pulpectomy)
- **Space maintainer**
  - Teeth will drift mesially when adjacent mesial tooth is extracted
  - To ensure enough space for permanent successor tooth, space maintainer is placed on tooth adjacent to edentulous space
  - Many different types: Fixed and removable; unilateral and bilateral
  - Band and loop space maintainer: Made of band soldered to thick wire formed to abut with tooth mesial to edentulous space, thus preventing drift

ANATOMY IMAGING ISSUES

Imaging Recommendations

- **MR for orthodontic patients**
  - If MR of head and neck
    - **Temporary removal** of orthodontic appliances to prevent signal void artifact
  - If MR of other body structures
    - **Stainless steel archwire is magnetic** and should be removed
    - All orthodontic brackets and bands **should be secured**

Imaging Pitfalls

- Dental restorations can cause metal streaking and beam-hardening artifact on CT and signal voids on MR, thus marring evaluation of adjacent bone and soft tissue
  - 2D imaging radiographic and clinical examination is recommended for evaluation of bone and dental lesions if artifact is excessive on CBCT or CT
  - To reduce artifact when examining oral cavity soft tissues on CT and MR, obtain scans without teeth crowns in field of view (modified axial)

PERIAPICALS AND AXIAL CBCT

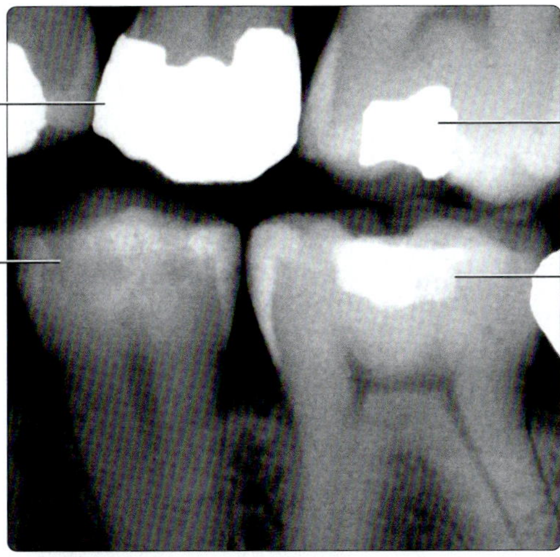

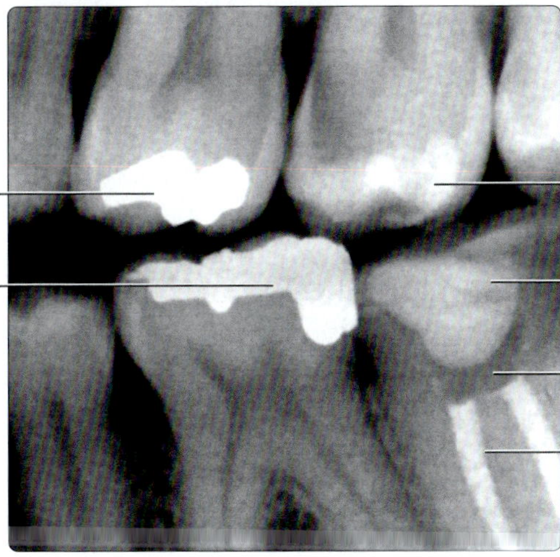

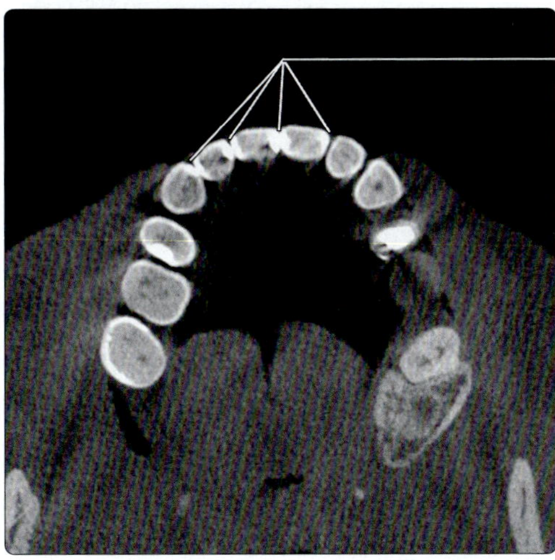

(Top) *Bitewing radiograph shows several posterior restorations. Amalgam is metallic and, therefore, appears completely radiopaque (image void). Posterior composite restorations can be used for more aesthetic results if clinically indicated and appear radiolucent (if of 1st-generation composites), posing a diagnostic challenge if evaluating for recurrent caries. Composites with radiopaque fillers appear moderately radiopaque. (Courtesy B. Friedland, BDS.)* **(Middle)** *Bitewing radiograph shows 2 types of amalgam restorations that are named according to surfaces replaced [occlusal (class I), mesio- or disto-occlusal (class II), amalgam build-up, etc.]. If treatment of a tooth has not been completed or if a period of pulpal healing is required after deep caries excavation, a temporary (interim) filling may be placed. If a root canal-treated tooth is awaiting a crown, a cotton ball is placed to separate the gutta percha from the sticky temporary filling. (Courtesy B. Friedland, BDS.)* **(Bottom)** *Axial CBCT shows several anterior composite restorations.*

AXIAL CBCT AND PERIAPICALS

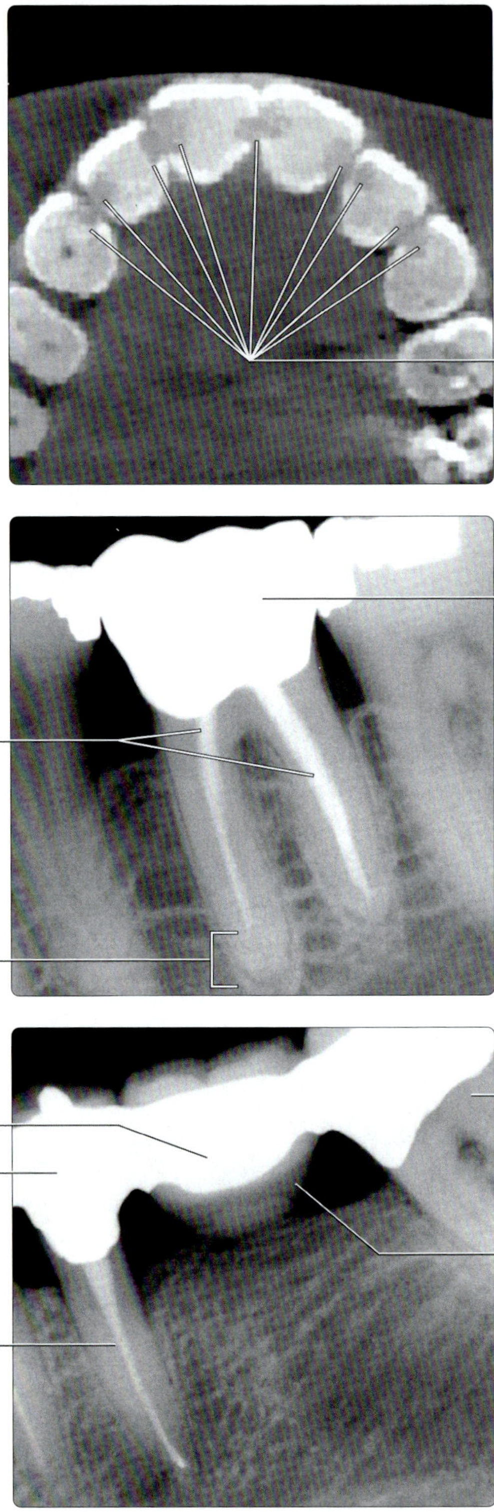

(Top) *Axial CBCT shows multiple rounded well-defined radiolucencies on the proximal surfaces of the teeth, representing radiolucent old-generation composite restorations.* **(Middle)** *A periapical radiograph shows a full metal coverage crown on the mandibular left 1st molar. The contours of the crown should follow the original contours of the tooth with no overhangs or open margins. This tooth is root canal treated, and the filling material in the mesial root is short, which may mean that a portion of the root canal was not instrumented to remove debris, presenting a risk for periapical rarefying osteitis. (Courtesy B. Friedland, BDS.)* **(Bottom)** *A periapical radiograph shows a porcelain fused to metal (PFM) bridge. The teeth onto which the bridge is fixed are called abutments and are covered with crowns. The portion that replaces the missing tooth is called a pontic. According to the number of teeth involved and replaced, the bridge is called a 3-unit, 4-unit, 5-unit, etc. bridge. (Courtesy B. Friedland, BDS.)*

CBCT REFORMATS

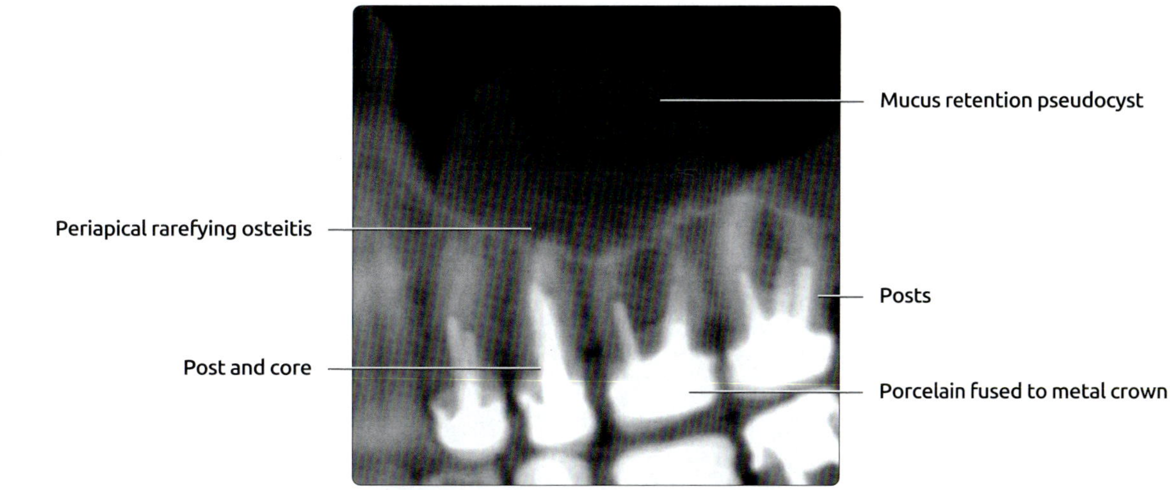

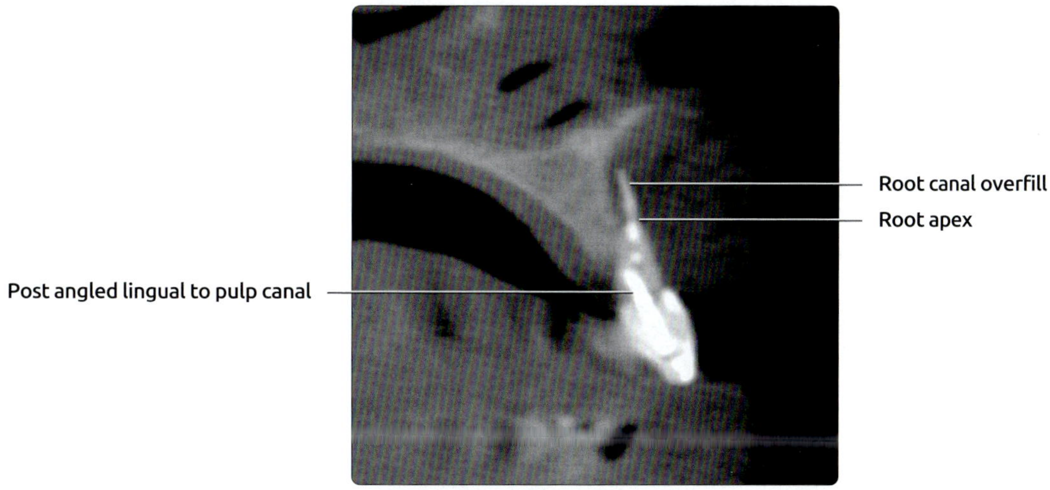

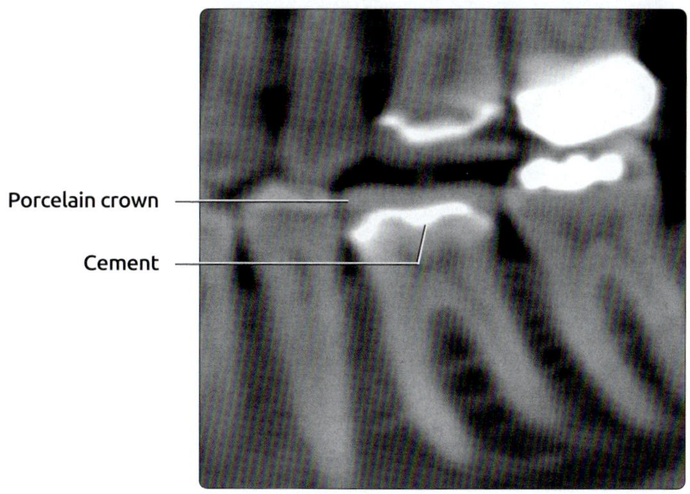

(Top) *CBCT cropped panoramic reformat shows multiple root canal-treated teeth that have been restored with post and core restorations followed by crowns. A core recreates proper crown preparation outline when tooth structure is inadequate to support seating of the crown restoration. A post anchors the core to the root and should not extend more than 2/3 of the root length. Note large mucus retention pseudocyst in left maxillary sinus.* **(Middle)** *CBCT sagittal section shows root canal overfill of the central incisor with post and core not in line with the pulp canal. Perforation of the tooth structure with the post can occur during preparation of the tooth. Root canal filling in the periapical tissues may be attached to the apex or may be dissociated from it. This foreign body may illicit an inflammatory reaction with symptoms of pain, or it may be asymptomatic.* **(Bottom)** *CBCT panoramic reformat shows full porcelain coverage crowns in the maxillary and mandibular 1st molars. These are cemented to the tooth with radiopaque cement.*

CBCT REFORMATS

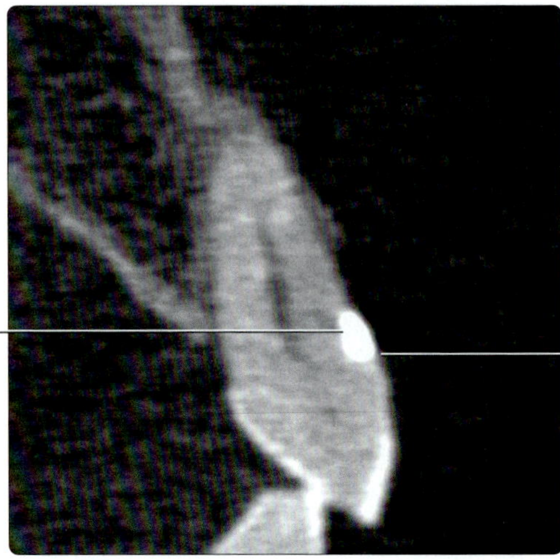

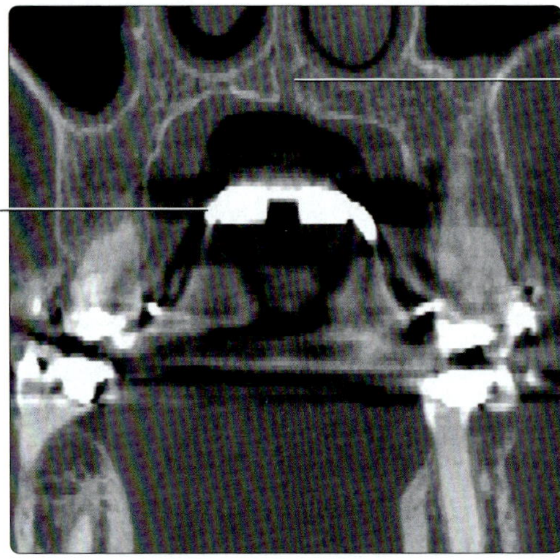

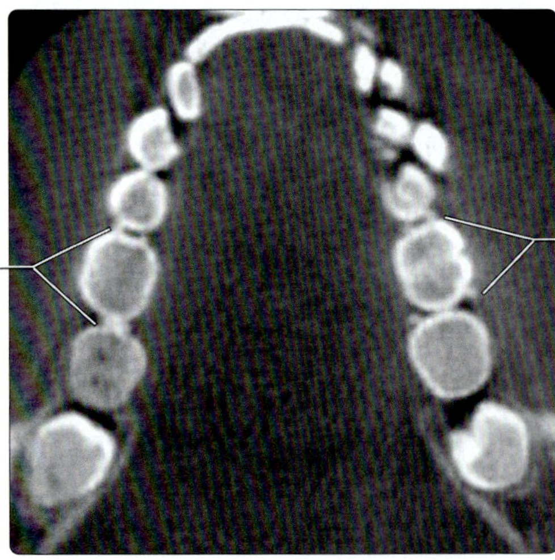

(Top) *CBCT sagittal reformat shows a restoration of glass ionomer cement (GIC) in the buccal cervical region of this anterior tooth. GICs are used to restore carious or tooth wear lesions that occur on the root surface of the tooth, or partially in enamel and partially in dentin.* **(Middle)** *Coronal CBCT shows a rapid palatal expander, which is a type of fixed appliance that is used to quickly increase the width of the maxillary arch by splitting the intermaxillary suture before puberty. It is cemented onto the posterior teeth of the patient.* **(Bottom)** *Axial CBCT shows orthodontic separators (spacers) that are placed between the molars before fixed appliances, such as a palatal expander or orthodontic bands, are applied. Spacers are circular rubber bands about a centimeter in diameter placed between adjacent molars. There may be 1-12 spacers applied. The spacers stay between the teeth for 1-2 weeks and move the teeth apart slowly until they are far apart enough so that the dentist can fit an orthodontic band in between them.*

CBCT REFORMATS

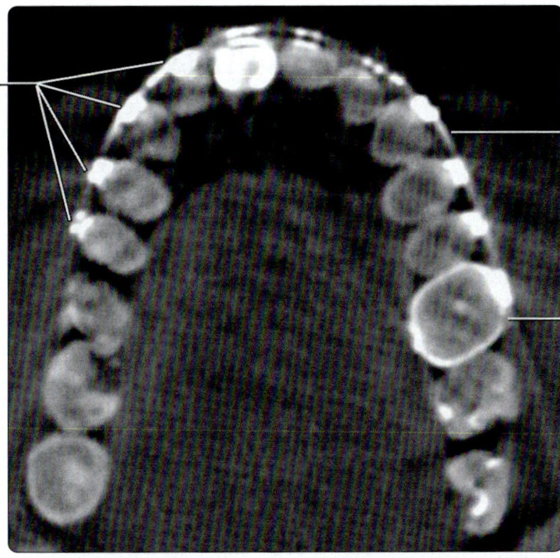

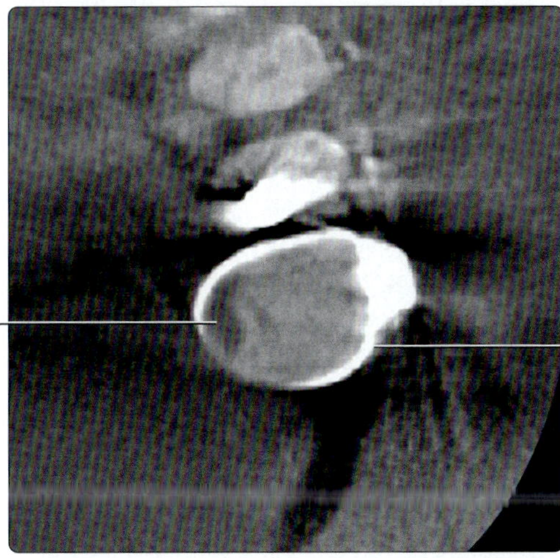

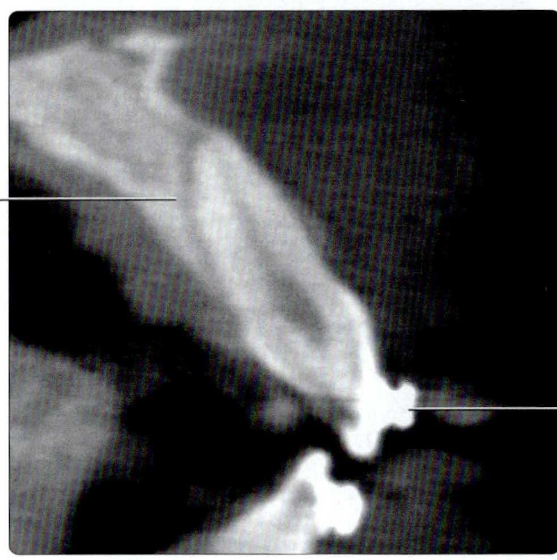

(Top) *Axial CBCT shows a traditional fixed orthodontic appliance, which consists of brackets fixed to the facial surfaces of teeth, bands that are cemented to 1 posterior tooth bilaterally, and archwire that is fixed to the brackets with elastic bands. Stainless steel archwire is ferromagnetic, and metal hardware may cause degradation of image quality on MR.* **(Middle)** *Axial CBCT shows caries in a tooth with an orthodontic band and bracket. Meticulous oral hygiene should be maintained for the duration of the orthodontic treatment to prevent plaque accumulation and the development of caries.* **(Bottom)** *Orthodontic brackets are placed on the crown of the tooth, and force is applied through the tightening of the orthodontic wire attached to them. With the movement of the teeth, widening of the periodontal ligament (PDL) space along the surface of the tooth away from the direction of the movement of the root is commonly seen. In this cross-sectional CBCT, the widening is noted on the lingual surface of the root due to the facial torquing of the root.*

CBCT REFORMATS

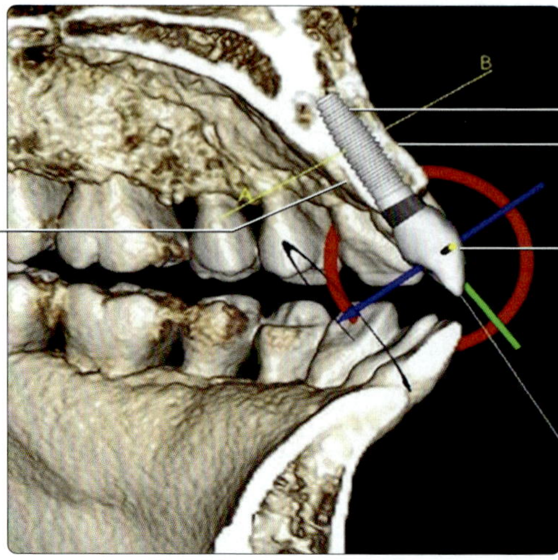

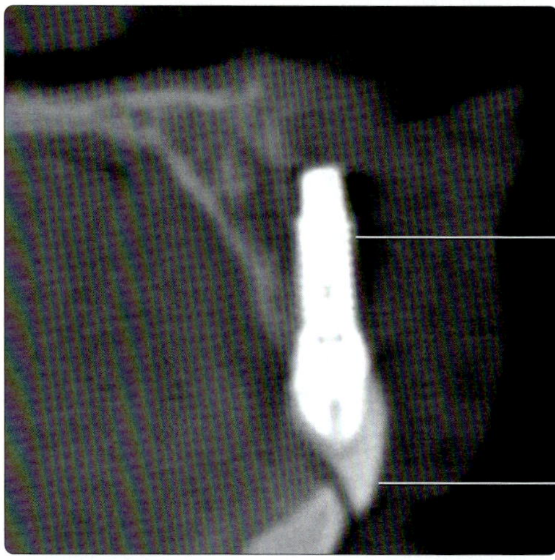

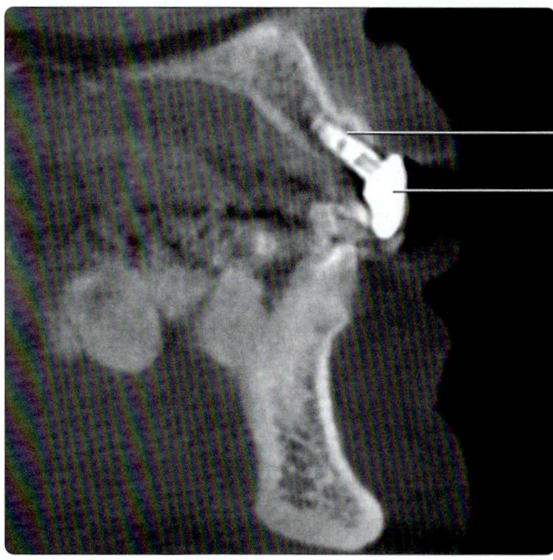

(Top) *CBCT 3D surface rendering shows implant planning for an edentulous maxillary anterior alveolar process. The simulated implant is positioned in the alveolar process following several rules: The crown restoration should function against the opposing dentition, there should be at least 2 mm of facial alveolar bone and 1 mm of lingual alveolar bone, and there should be 1.5- to 2.0-mm between the implant and the adjacent teeth. The anatomy should be evaluated to prevent violation of vital anatomical structures. (Courtesy D. Chenin, DDS.)* **(Middle)** *CBCT cross section of a central incisor implant that was positioned to bring the crown into contact with the opposing teeth, but no ridge augmentation, was performed, resulting in no bone coverage on the facial aspect of the implant.* **(Bottom)** *Sagittal CBCT shows an implant that was centered in the alveolar process but without considering the position of the final restoration. A tilted abutment was used to bring the crown into occlusion (in this case, not biomechanically ideal for load distribution).*

PERIAPICAL RADIOGRAPH AND CBCT REFORMATS

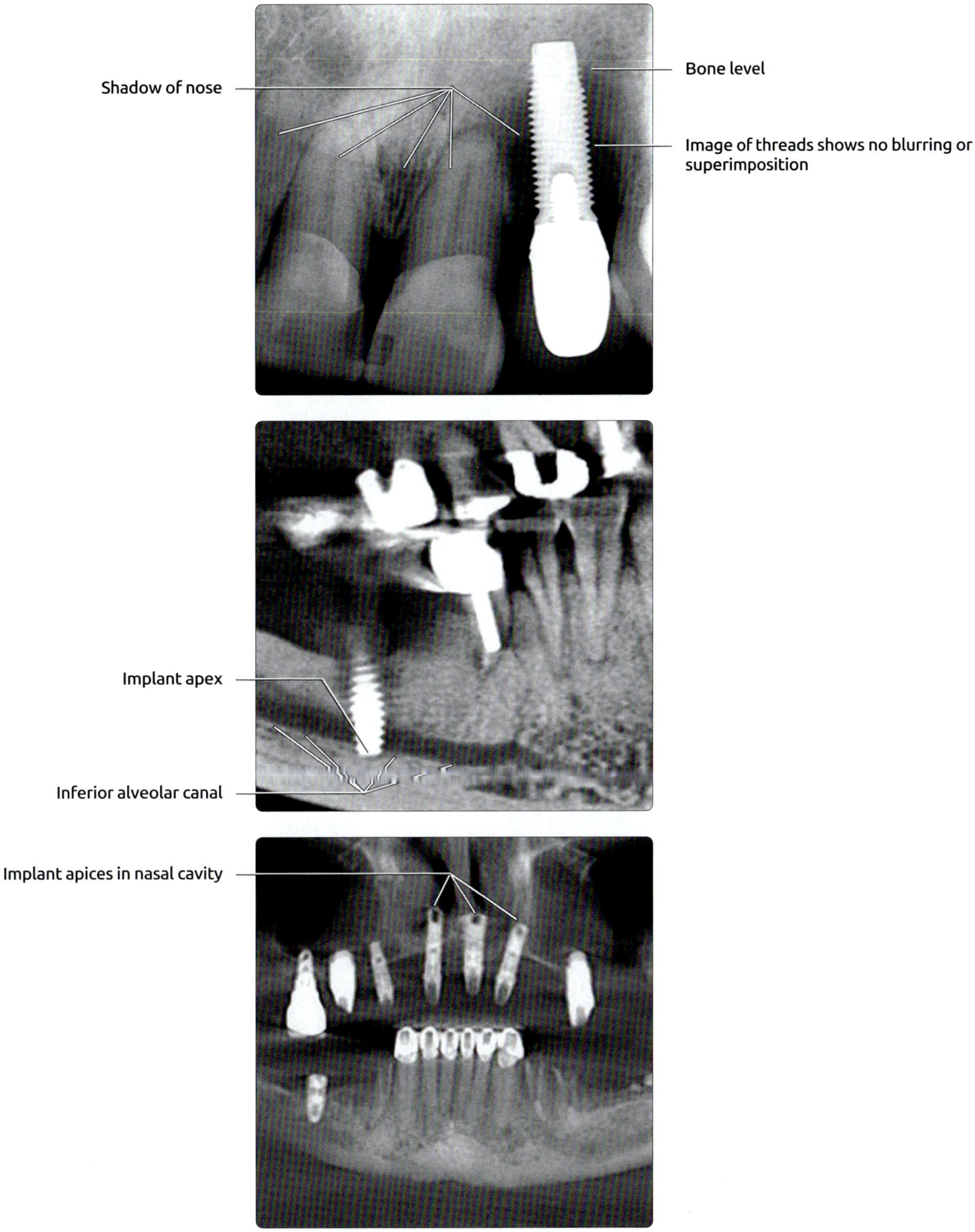

(Top) *Periapical radiograph of an implant replacing the left lateral incisor shows severe peri-implant bone loss, extending to the apical portion of the implant. Vertical bitewings or periapical radiographs in which the central x-ray beams pass through the threads (resulting in a crisp image of the threads) are ideal for evaluation of peri-implant bone loss, as metal artifact does not obscure evaluation on these intraoral 2D imaging.* **(Middle)** *CBCT panoramic reformat shows the apex of an implant passing through the right inferior alveolar canal. Cross-sectional reformations of the alveolar process are the gold standard during implant treatment planning to avoid violating important anatomy.* **(Bottom)** *CBCT panoramic reformation shows maxillary anterior implants placed in the right and left nasal cavities. Evaluation of the amount of bone present and its angulation in relation to the opposing dentition is necessary prior to placement of implants to determine the need for alveolar process augmentation. (Courtesy T. Sawisch, DDS.)*

TERMINOLOGY

Abbreviations

- Maxilla (Mx)

IMAGING ANATOMY

Overview

- Forms majority of midface skeleton and upper jaw
- Contains maxillary sinuses
- There are 2 maxillae that fuse in midline (intermaxillary suture)
- Presence of "premaxilla" in humans widely contested
  - Exists in early embryonic human development
  - Disappears early by fusing to anterior aspect of maxillary bones
  - Has implications for cleft palate development

Anatomy Relationships

- Articulates with
  - Opposite Mx
  - Frontal, sphenoid, nasal, vomer, and ethmoid bones
  - Inferior nasal concha
  - Palatine, lacrimal, and zygomatic bones
  - Septal and nasal cartilages

Internal Contents

- **Maxillary bone**
  - **Body**
    - Major part of bone
    - Pyramid-like shape
    - Gives borders to 4 different regions: Orbit, nasal cavity, infratemporal fossa, middle 1/3 of face
    - Infraorbital canal and foramen pass from orbit region to face region
    - Anterior nasal spine: Pointed prominence in midline
    - Nasal notch: Concave rims lateral to anterior nasal spine that form floor of piriform aperture
  - **Frontal process**
    - Articulates superiorly with nasal, frontal, ethmoid, and lacrimal bones
    - Forms posterior boundary of lacrimal fossa and houses lacrimal canal
  - **Zygomatic process**
    - Articulates laterally with maxillary process of zygomatic bone
  - **Palatine process**
    - Extends medially to form majority of hard palate
    - Articulates with palatine process of opposite Mx in midline
    - Articulates with horizontal plate of palatine bone posteriorly
    - Incisive foramen located anteriorly and **may be in midline or slightly shifted**
    - In axial plane, palate may be U shaped or V shaped (high palatal vault)
  - **Alveolar process**
    - Supports maxillary teeth
    - Extends inferiorly from Mx
    - Each maxillary bone **normally contains 5 primary and 8 permanent teeth**
    - Alveolar bone is resorbed when tooth is lost
    - Bone overlying tooth roots forms wave-like eminences
    - Bulky part surrounding facial aspect of canine called **canine eminence**
    - Concavity noted on facial surface mesial to canine called **incisive fossa** (a.k.a. lateral fossa)
    - Concavity noted on facial surface distal to canine called **canine fossa**
    - Most posterior aspect called **maxillary tuberosity**
    - Site of extracted tooth called **tooth or extraction socket**
    - Early tooth extractions may cause localized developmental hypoplasia
- **Innervation**
  - **Infraorbital nerve**
    - Continuation of V2
    - Passes anteriorly through infraorbital groove and infraorbital canal and exits onto face via infraorbital foramen
    - Gives rise to 2 alveolar branches: Middle superior and anterior superior
  - **Middle superior alveolar nerve**
    - May or may not be present
    - As it descends to form superior dental plexus, innervates part of maxillary sinus, premolars, and mesiobuccal root of 1st molar, and gingiva and mucosa of same teeth
    - Not usually visualized radiographically
  - **Anterior superior alveolar nerve**
    - As it descends to form superior dental plexus, innervates part of maxillary sinus, maxillary anterior teeth, and gingiva and mucosa of these teeth
    - Vertical component may be seen on coronals and cross sections lateral to lateral wall of nasal cavity in canine/premolar region
    - Horizontal component may be seen on axials extending from inferior aspect of vertical component to midline
  - **Posterior superior alveolar nerve**
    - Branch of V2
    - In infratemporal fossa: Passes on posterior surface of Mx along region of maxillary tuberosity
    - Gives rise to gingival branch that innervates buccal gingiva alongside maxillary molars
    - Enters posterior surface of Mx and supplies maxillary sinus and maxillary molars, except mesiobuccal root of 1st molar
  - **Nasopalatine nerve** (V2 sensory branch) travels from superior portion of nasal cavity to nasal septum, then travels anteroinferiorly to go through incisive (nasopalatine) canal and exit through incisive foramen (foramen of Stenson)
    - Supplies sensory fibers to gingiva and mucosa of anterior hard palate from central incisor to canine
    - May be single, fused, paired, or have multiple canals ± single large incisive canal
    - Canals located lateral to incisive foramen are called foramina of Scarpa
  - **Greater palatine nerve** descends palatine canal in palatine bone

- Exits greater palatine foramen at junction of palatine and maxillary bones and passes anteriorly to hard palate and gingival mucosa
- Supplies palatal gingiva and mucosa from premolar region to posterior border of hard palate to midline

- **Minor salivary glands**
  - Numerous minor salivary glands live in mucosa of hard palate
  - Supplied by postganglionic parasympathetic fibers that arise from pterygopalatine ganglion and are distributed by V2
  - Predominantly mucous secretions
  - Usually not visible on imaging unless affected by salivary gland pathology; on CBCT, will not show unless causing remodeling or erosion of underlying bone

ANATOMY IMAGING ISSUES

Imaging Recommendations

- Intraoral 2D imaging for caries, periapical, and periodontal disease
- CBCT
  - Dental cross sections for implant analysis, 3rd molar analysis
- CECT or MR if soft tissue tumor or malignancy suspected

CLINICAL IMPLICATIONS

Clinical Importance

- Pain in maxilla can refer to TMJ
  - Sources of pain that may refer to TMJ
    - Pulpal or periodontal disease
    - Suboptimal root canal filling procedure (overfill, underfill)
    - Sinus inflammation
- Temporalis middle and posterior attachment trigger points can refer pain to maxilla
- Masseter superficial layer musculotendinous junction trigger points can refer pain to maxilla
- **Proximity of apices of maxillary teeth to maxillary sinus and nasal cavity**
  - Spread of odontogenic infection **(odontogenic sinusitis)**
  - Spread of odontogenic tumors
  - Displacement of tooth or tooth root into maxillary sinus
  - Root canal filling may be found in maxillary sinus if tooth is overfilled
- **V2 perineural spread of malignant tumor**
  - If malignancy affects skin of upper lip, **hard palate**, soft palate, or cheek overlying infraorbital foramen, check for V2 perineural tumor (PNT) spread
  - Major locations to identify V2 PNT extend from incisive canal to greater palatine foramen or infraorbital foramen to root entry zone of V nerve in lateral pons
  - If imaging for V2 PNT, check incisive canal, greater and lesser palatine foramen, pterygopalatine canal and fossa, foramen rotundum, Meckel cave, preganglionic segment of CNV, and root entry zone
  - Advanced imaging, such as C+ MR, recommended if suspected
- **Minor salivary gland pathology**
  - Due to proximity to hard palate, large pathology can be visualized on CBCT as remodeling or destruction of bony cortices of hard palate
  - On coronal, evaluate palatine processes of maxillae for asymmetry or erosion of bony cortices
  - Conditions that may occur include pleomorphic adenoma, necrotizing sialometaplasia, adenoid cystic carcinoma, and mucoepidermoid carcinoma
  - Salivary gland malignancy more common in these glands than other salivary glands
  - Aggressive soft tissue pathology should be imaged with imaging techniques that show soft tissue extent &/or perineural spread
- **Maxillary 3rd molar evaluation should include relationship to**
  - Greater palatine nerve
  - Maxillary sinus
  - Pterygopalatine fissure
  - Posterior border of maxillary tuberosity
  - Adjacent tooth
- **Maxillary midline suture** (intermaxillary suture, midpalatine suture, median suture)
  - Can be site of developmental or acquired pathology
    - Cleft palate can run along entire length of maxillary midline suture
    - Nasopalatine duct cyst develops in midline
    - Wegener granulomatosis or midline lethal granuloma develop in midline
- **Fracture of maxilla analysis**
  - In cases of trauma (motor vehicle accident or otherwise), evaluation for fractures should involve maxilla
  - Should put into consideration major nerves that run in areas of fracture
    - **Le Fort 1**: Incisive, posterior superior alveolar and greater palatine nerves
    - **Le Fort 2**: Infraorbital nerve
    - **Le Fort 3**: Can involve V2 distribution at level of V2 as it exits foramen rotundum; may sever lacrimal duct
- **Maxillary hypoplasia (micrognathia)**
  - Underdevelopment of maxillary bone
  - Gives appearance of concave profile ("dish face") clinically and on sagittal view
  - Mandibular protrusion is illusion; cephalometric analysis shows retruded relationship of maxilla to skull base
  - Associated with Crouzon syndrome, Apert syndrome, Binder syndrome, cleft palate, cleidocranial dysplasia
- **Anterior nasal spine hypoplasia**
  - May require augmentation
- **Bimaxillary protrusion**
  - Increased protrusion and proclination of maxillary and mandibular incisors
  - Etiology: Genetic and environmental (mouth breathing, thumb sucking, and other oral habits), size of tongue
  - Associated with short posterior cranial base, longer Mx, and mild class II skeletal pattern

GRAPHICS

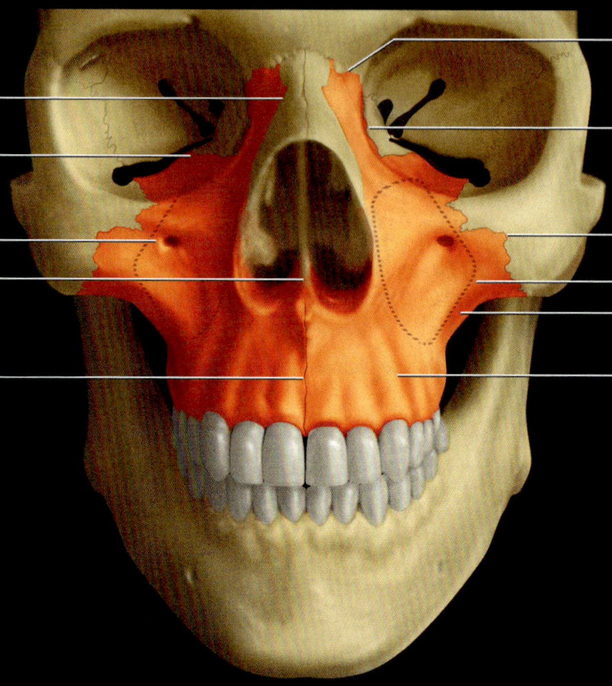

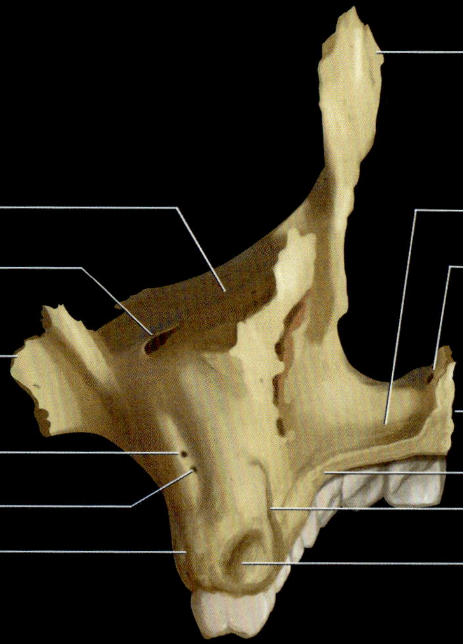

(Top) *Graphic shows an anterior view of the maxilla (highlighted in orange) and its relationship to the other facial bones. There are 2 maxillae that meet in the midline. These house the maxillary sinuses and make up the majority of the midface. The extent of the maxilla and its relationships with the adjacent bones should be considered when planning a palatal expansion to increase its transverse dimension.* **(Bottom)** *Graphic depicts one disarticulated maxilla as viewed from the posterior aspect. The foramina for multiple branches of CNV2 and the maxillary artery are seen. The greater palatine nerve branches off the pterygopalatine ganglion and courses down the greater palatine canal, partially formed by the maxilla. The nasopalatine nerve also branches off the pterygopalatine ganglion, runs along the nasal septum, and enters the nasopalatine canal. The middle superior alveolar neurovascular bundle may or may not be present. The posterior alveolar neurovascular bundle enters the posterior aspect of the maxilla.*

GRAPHICS

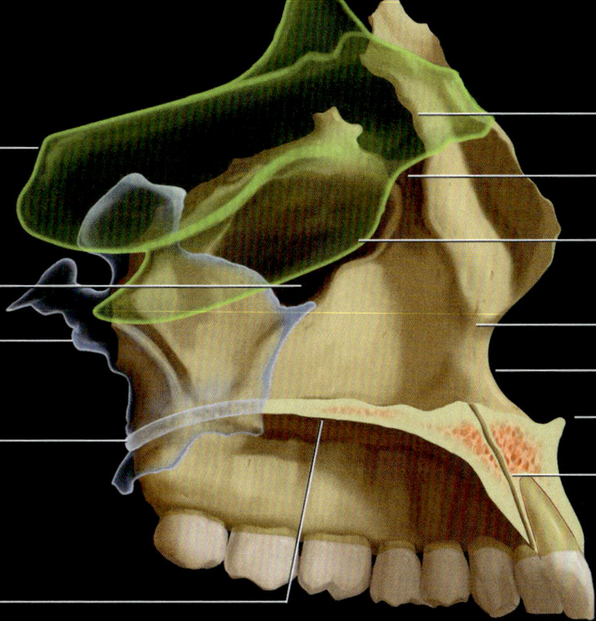

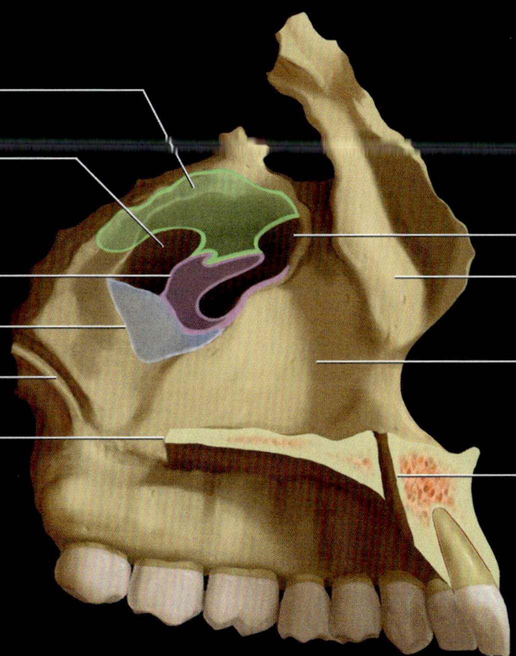

(Top) *Graphic of the medial aspect of the maxilla shows its relationship to the ethmoid (transparent green) and palatine (transparent blue) bones. The inferior nasal concha articulates at the conchal crest. The hard palate line passes through 2 anatomic points: The anterior nasal spine, which is part of the maxilla, and the posterior nasal spine, which is part of the palatine bone.* **(Bottom)** *Graphic of the medial aspect of the maxilla shows the bones that partially cover the maxillary hiatus and form the ostiomeatal complex.*

GRAPHICS

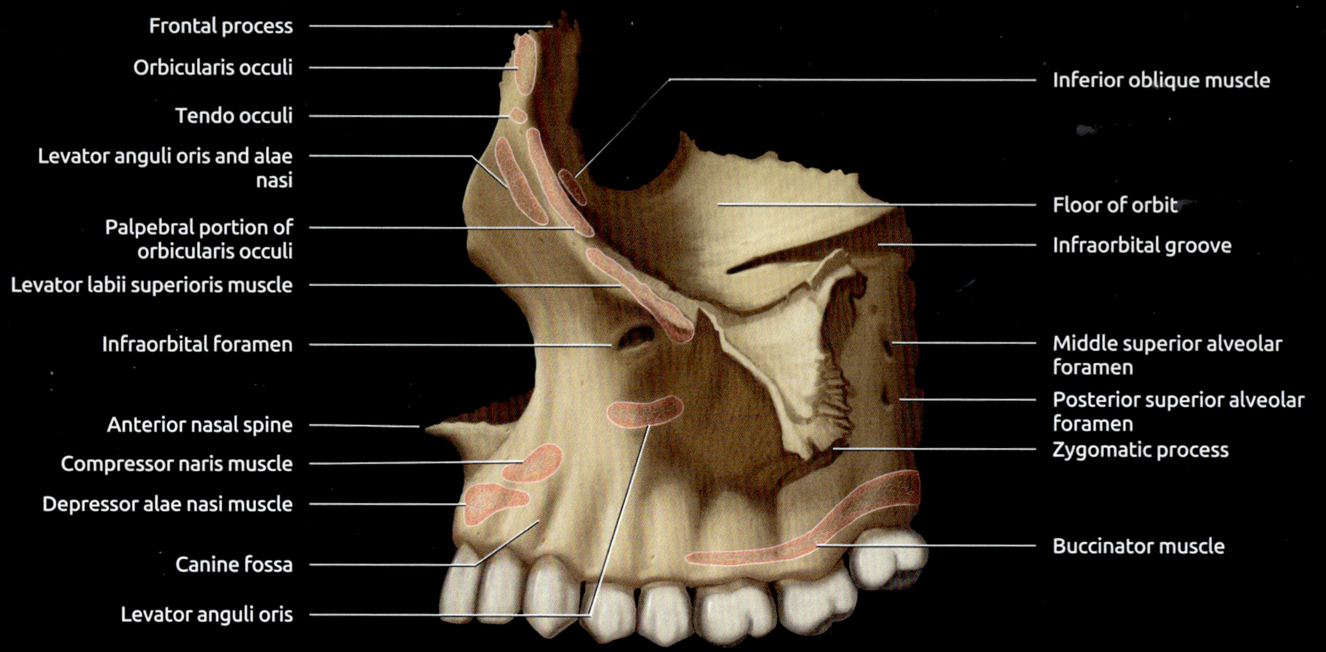

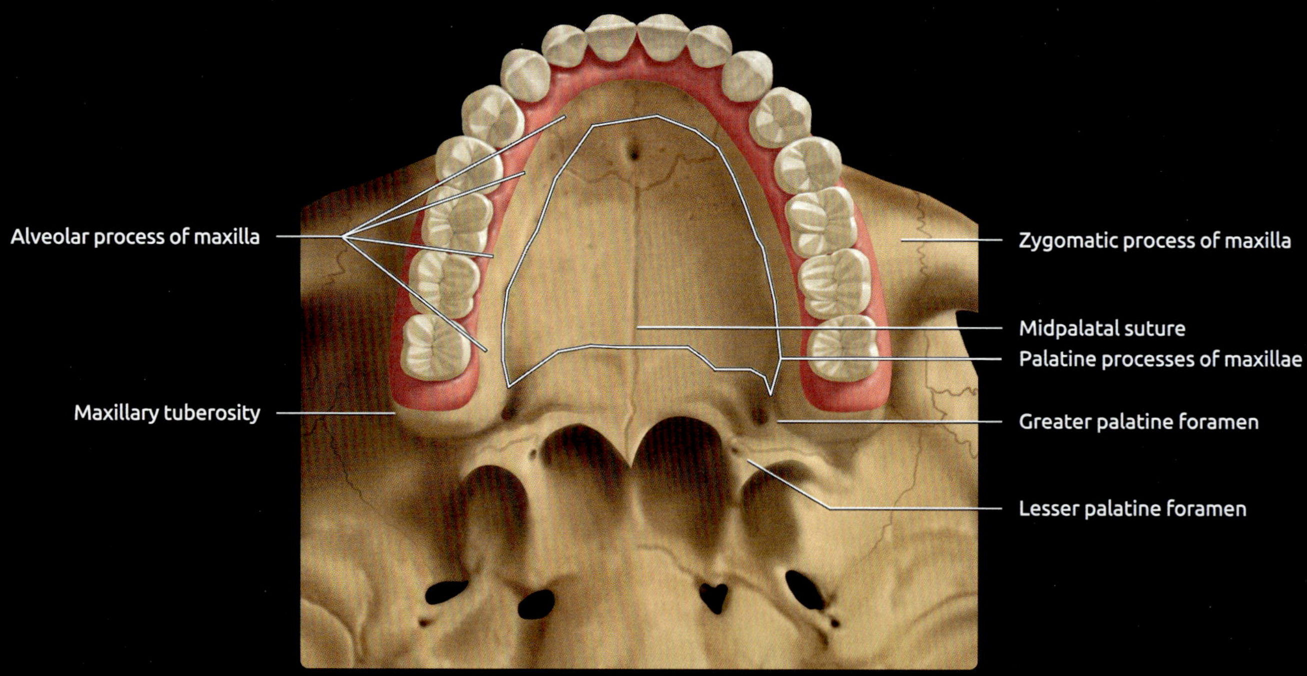

(Top) *Graphic shows the lateral aspect of a disarticulated maxilla with muscle origins and insertions outlined. CNV2 enters through the posterior aspect of the orbital floor, courses anteriorly in a groove or fully formed infraorbital canal, and exits anteriorly through the infraorbital foramen. The zygomatic process of the maxilla is a thick portion of bone that is usually avoided during LeFort 1 osteotomies or Caldwell-Luc procedures.* **(Bottom)** *Graphic of hard palate and maxillary alveolar ridge viewed from below shows the palatine processes of the maxillary bone. The premaxilla is an embryonic process and does not form a separate bone in adult humans. The 2 palatine processes meet in the midline in the maxillary midline suture (midpalatal suture, intermaxillary suture, or median suture). The horizontal plate of the palatine bone completes the hard palate posteriorly. Note the incisive foramen in the anterior midline and the greater and lesser palatine foramina at the junction of the maxilla and the palatine bones and in the palatine bone, respectively.*

GRAPHIC AND BONE CT

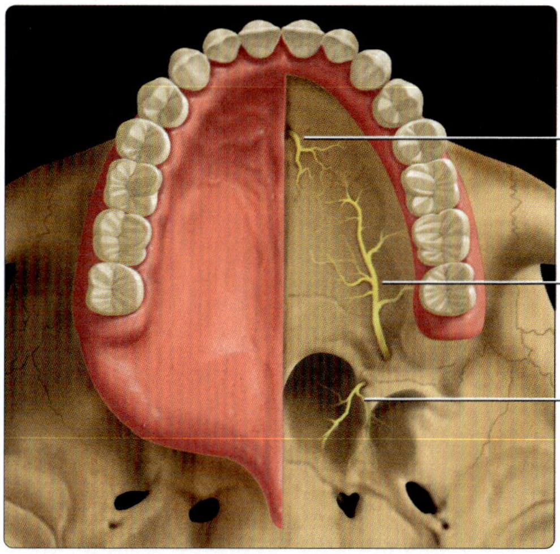

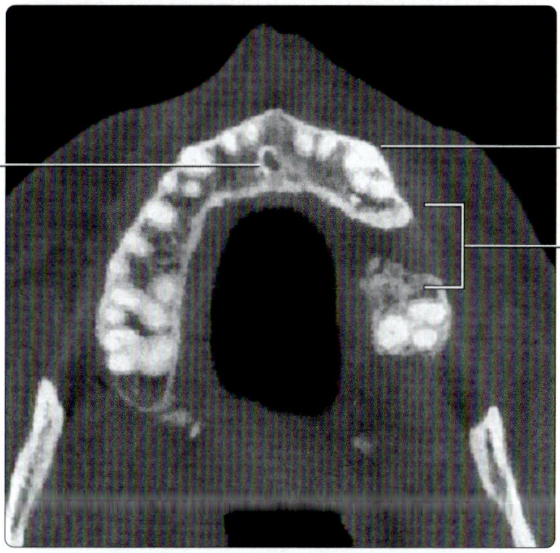

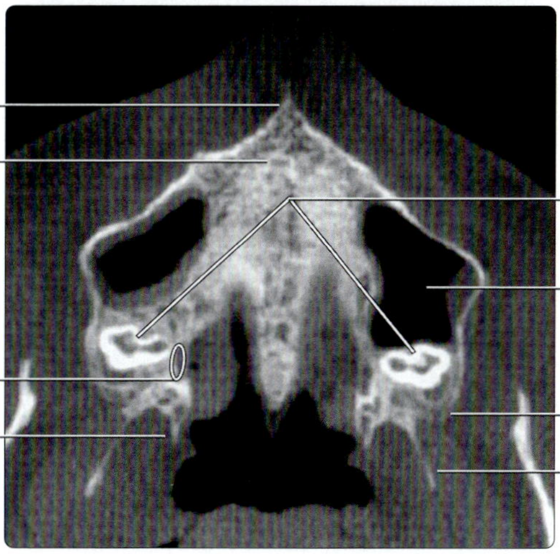

(Top) *Graphic of the hard palate viewed from below, with mucosa removed on right side, shows the hard palate sensory innervation. The anterior 1/3 of the hard palate is supplied by the nasopalatine nerve, and the posterior 2/3 of the hard palate is supplied by the greater palatine nerve. The greater palatine nerve often indents the junction of the palatine and the alveolar processes of the maxilla (greater palatine groove), as can be seen on coronal series.* **(Middle)** *The incisive foramen may be single (as shown) or paired and may be centered or slightly lateral to the midline (as shown). There may be several canals seen lateral to the main canal(s), the foramina of Scarpa.* **(Bottom)** *When examining the maxilla for 3rd molar impactions, it is important to localize the adjacent anatomical structures and note proximity to teeth if removal is planned. These structures are the maxillary sinuses, the greater palatine canals and foramina, the pterygoid plates, and the maxillary tuberosities. Axial CBCT shows the relation of the developing 3rd molars to these structures.*

AXIAL AND CORONAL CBCT

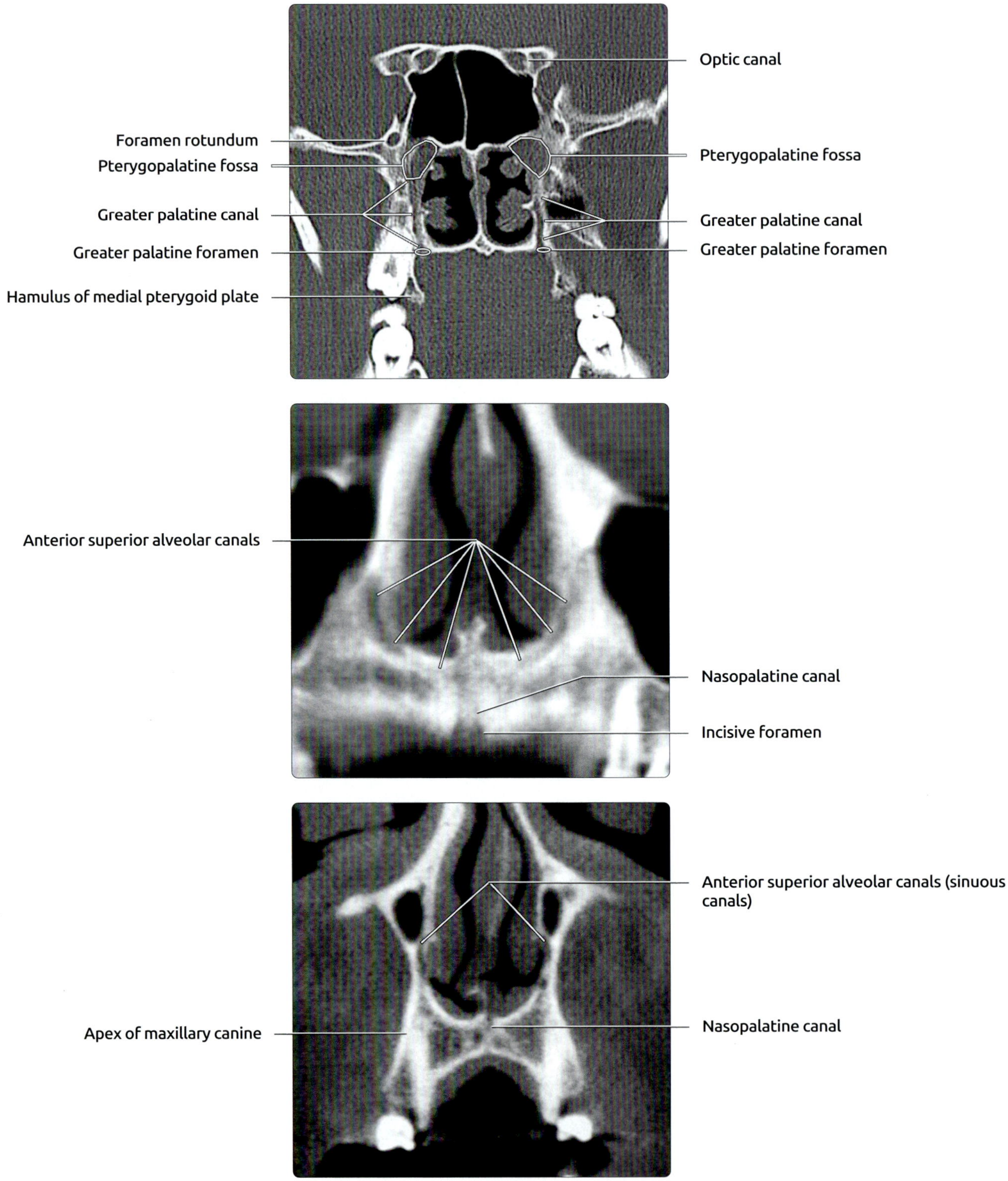

(Top) *Coronal bone CT through the vertical aspect of greater palatine canal shows this canal connecting the pterygopalatine fossa above with the greater palatine foramen below. The greater palatine nerve uses the greater palatine canal to access the palate.* **(Middle)** *Panoramic 1.5-mm reformat shows the right and left anterior superior alveolar canals descending to form the superior dental plexus. These can meet in the midline in the area of the nasopalatine canal as seen in this image. Care should be taken if implant placement is planned in this area.* **(Bottom)** *Coronal CBCT shows the anterior superior alveolar canal after it leaves the infraorbital canal and descends along the anterior aspect of the lateral wall of the nasal cavity. The course of this nerve often comes close to the apices of the maxillary canines.*

PERIAPICAL AND PANORAMIC

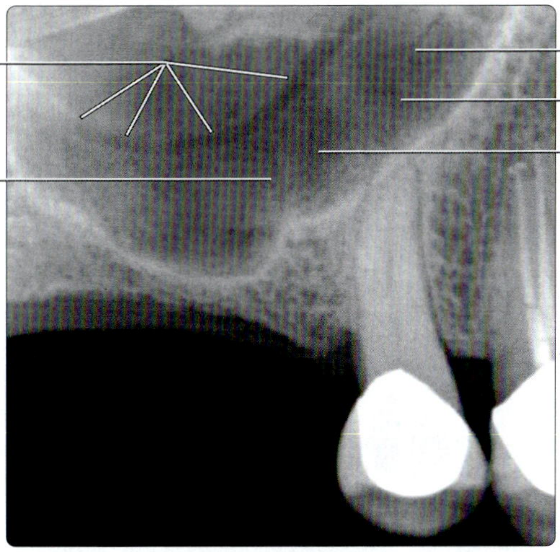

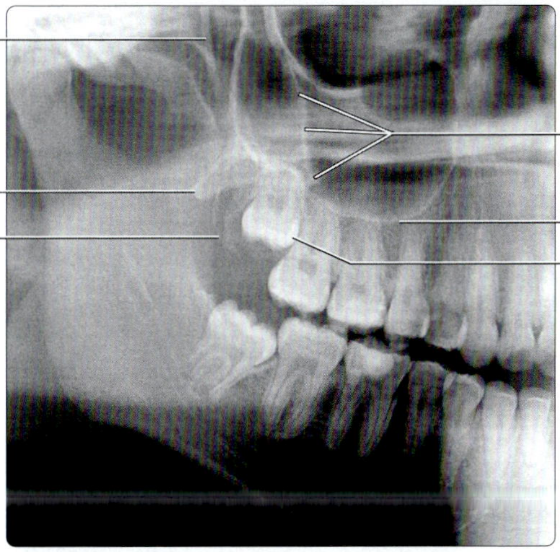

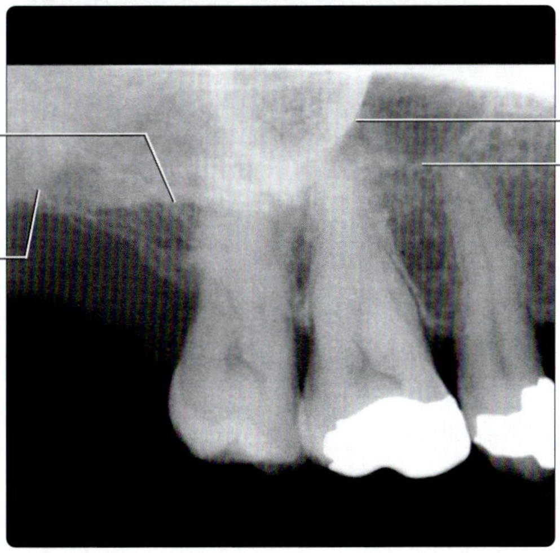

(Top) *The posterior superior alveolar canal may sometimes be visible as a radiolucent curved line that appears to be inside the sinus on periapical radiographs of the posterior maxilla. The canal is usually located along the lateral wall of the sinus. The middle superior alveolar nerve, when present, supplies the maxillary premolars and the mesiobuccal root of the maxillary 1st molar. These nerves are usually difficult to visualize on CBCT. (Courtesy I. Angel, DDS.)* **(Middle)** *Cropped panoramic radiograph shows normal maxillary anatomical landmarks commonly encountered when evaluating this type of image. Superimposition of structures may confound evaluation.* **(Bottom)** *Periapical radiograph shows the zygomatic process of the maxilla and the inferior border of the zygomatic bone superimposing over the inferior aspect of the maxillary sinus, the apices of the maxillary molars, and the maxillary tuberosity.*

TERMINOLOGY

Abbreviations

- Mandible (Md)

IMAGING ANATOMY

Overview

- Unpaired horseshoe-shaped bone

Anatomy Relationships

- All muscles of mastication attach to Md

Internal Contents

- Bone
  - **Mandibular body**
    - U-shaped, horizontal body; fuses in early childhood in anterior midline at **symphysis**
    - **Mental protuberance**: Bony prominence of chin; more prominent in males
    - **Mental foramen**: Transmits mental nerve; located buccally in premolar/1st molar regions
    - **Genial tubercles (mental spines)**: Small projections on lingual aspect of anterior Md; genioglossus and geniohyoid attach here
    - **Lingual foramen**: Small foramen on lingual aspect of anterior Md in midline; conducts terminal branch of incisive nerve and often small branch of lingual artery
    - **Internal oblique/mylohyoid ridge**: Bony ridge on lingual Md body; origin of mylohyoid muscle and divides sublingual from submandibular fossae
    - **Mylohyoid groove**: Impression of nerve to mylohyoid as it leaves V3 before V3 enters mandibular foramen
    - **Submandibular fossa**: Indentation on lingual aspect of Md inferior to mylohyoid ridge; impression of submandibular salivary gland
    - **Antegonial notch**: Indentation in inferior border anterior to angle; masseter insertion
    - **External oblique ridge/line**: Bony ridge on lateral posterior aspect adjacent to molars; buccal shelf is superior to it
  - **Ramus**
    - Meets body of Md at angle of Md on each side
    - Masseter muscle attaches to lateral side
    - Medial pterygoid muscle and sphenomandibular ligament attach to medial side
    - Mandibular ramus divides masticator space into lateral and medial compartments
    - **Mandibular foramen**: Center medial surface of ramus
    - **Lingula**: Small, osseous lip on medial surface of ramus extending from anterior aspect of mandibular foramen
    - **Antilingula**: Anatomic and surgical landmark on lateral surface of ramus at level of lingula
    - **Coronoid notch**: Deepest point on anterior border of ramus
  - **Condylar process**
    - **Condyle**: Articulates with temporal bone in TMJ
    - **Condylar neck**: Attaches condylar head to ramus
    - Superior belly and most of inferior belly of lateral pterygoid muscle insert into **pterygoid fovea** on neck
  - **Coronoid process**
    - Temporalis attaches here
    - **Mandibular (sigmoid) notch** separates coronoid process and condylar neck
  - **Alveolar process**
    - Bone that supports teeth with thick facial and thin lingual cortical plates
    - Alveolar bone is resorbed when teeth are lost
  - **Inferior alveolar (mandibular) canal**
    - Lies within distal ramus and proximal body of Md
    - Extends from mandibular to mental foramen
    - Contains inferior alveolar nerve (IAN) and vessels
    - May have anomalous branches and foramina
- **Nerves**
  - **IAN**
    - Extends from mandibular foramen through mandibular canal to mental foramen
    - Innervates ipsilateral premolars and molars
    - Divides into mental and incisive branches
  - **Mental nerve**
    - Anterior extraosseous branch of IAN
    - Exits mental foramen
    - Provides sensory innervation to skin and mucosa of lower lip and labial gingiva
  - **Incisive nerve**
    - Anterior intraosseous branch of IAN
    - Innervates ipsilateral canine and incisors
    - May reach midline → cross-innervation

ANATOMY IMAGING ISSUES

Questions

- **Deepened mandibular notch**
  - Consider **neurofibromatosis**
- **Deepened antegonial notch**
  - Consider conditions that cause **clockwise growth pattern of Md due to condylar height reduction** (juvenile idiopathic arthritis or progressive condylar resorption), masseteric hyperfunction, scleroderma
  - Check TMJs for dysfunction or degenerative changes
- **Coronoid hyperplasia**
  - Consider if limitation of opening is noted clinically
- **Asymmetrical mandibular ramus and body height**
  - Degenerative disease of TMJ or condylar hypoplasia on smaller side
  - Condylar hyperplasia on larger side
  - Hemifacial microsomia
- **Steep mandibular plane**
  - May be associated with small condyles bilaterally
    - Bilateral small condyles may be due to degenerative changes, juvenile idiopathic arthritis, rheumatoid arthritis
- **V3 malignant perineural tumor (PNT) spread**
  - If malignant tumor of skin of chin, mandibular alveolar ridge, or masticator space, check for V3 PNT
  - If imaging for V3 PNT, check entire length of V3 to root entry zone
    - Pay special attention to mental foramen, mandibular canal, mandibular foramen, and masticator space

GRAPHIC, 3D REFORMATION

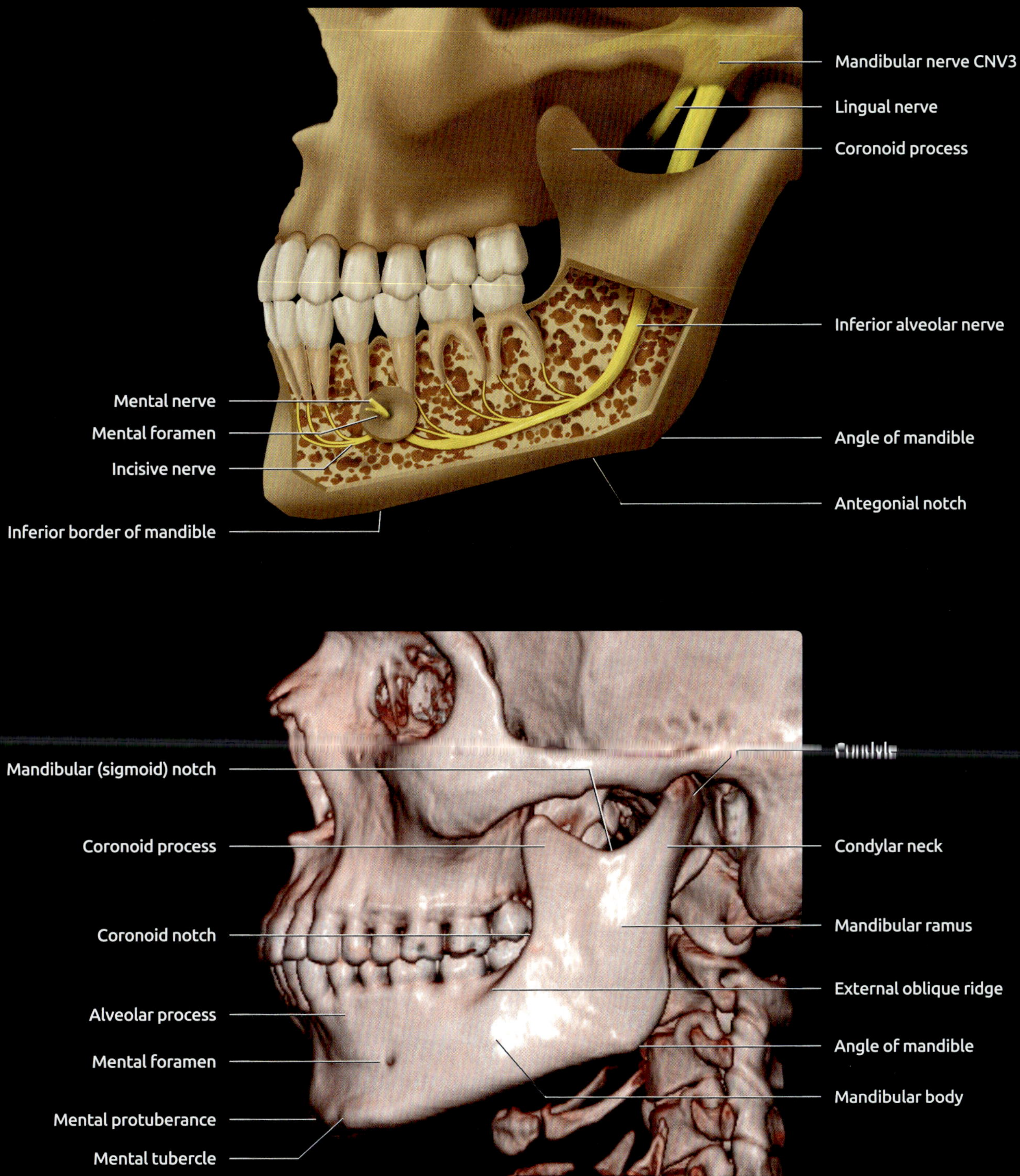

(Top) *Lateral graphic of the mandible with the buccal cortex removed reveals the mandibular nerve entering the mandible as the inferior alveolar nerve. The inferior alveolar nerve divides anteriorly into mental and incisive branches. The mental nerve branch reaches the superficial chin through the mental foramen. The incisive nerve continues to the areas of the incisors, sometimes reaching the midline and providing cross-innervation to the contralateral side. This may or may not be visible radiographically.* **(Bottom)** *Lateral view shows 3D reconstruction of facial bones. The mandible can be divided into condylar process, coronoid process, ramus, body, and alveolar process. The mental foramen is seen in the anterior portion of the body and transmits the mental nerve, which is sensory to the skin and mucosa of the lower lip. The coronoid notch is an important landmark when determining the entry point for an inferior alveolar nerve block anesthesia.*

GRAPHICS

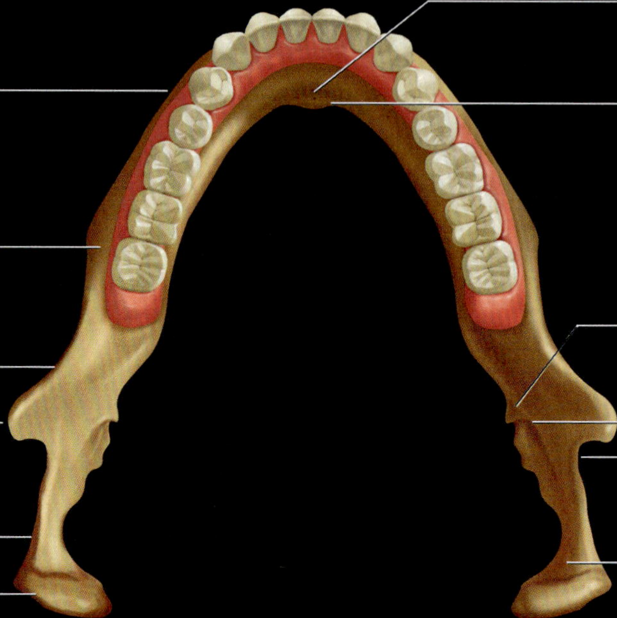

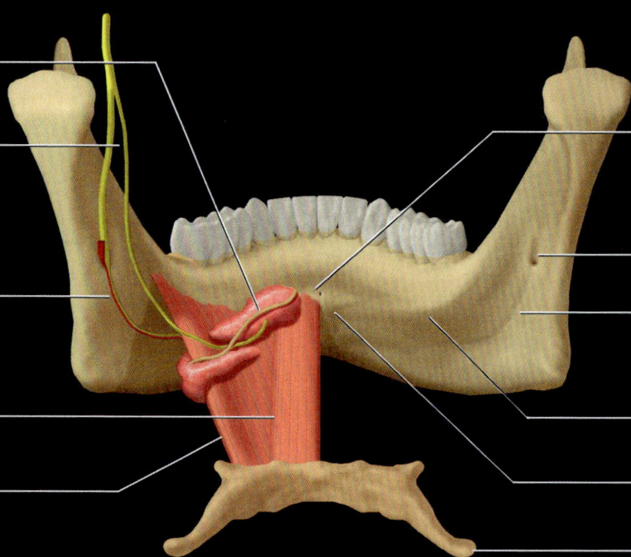

(Top) *Axial graphic of the mandible seen from above demonstrates the condyle and condylar neck leading to the more inferior ramus. The mandibular foramen is seen on the inner surface of the mandibular ramus. The superiorly projecting coronoid processes attach the temporalis muscle tendons. The lateral pterygoid muscle (superior belly and most of the inferior belly) inserts in the pterygoid fovea. The lingula is a lip-like projection at the inferior anterior aspect of the mandibular foramen.* **(Bottom)** *Graphic shows the posterior view of the mandible. The nerve to the mylohyoid muscle branches off V3 before it enters the mandibular canal and creates a slight impression in the bone called the mylohyoid groove. The mylohyoid muscle attaches to the mylohyoid ridge, and the geniohyoid muscle attaches to the genial tubercles. The lingual foramen exits superior to the genial tubercles in the midline.*

3D REFORMATION, PANORAMIC, PANORAMIC REFORMAT

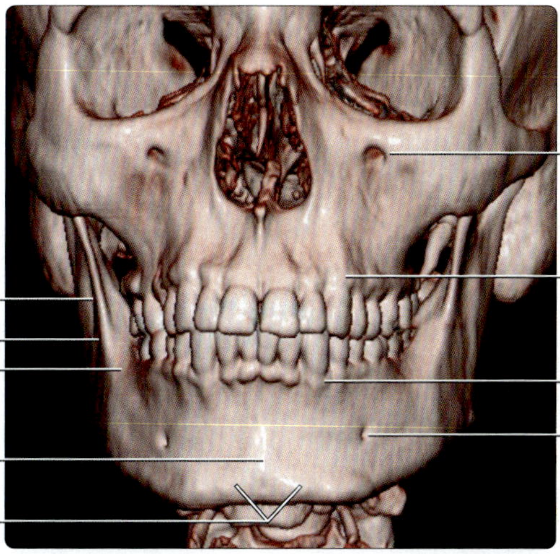

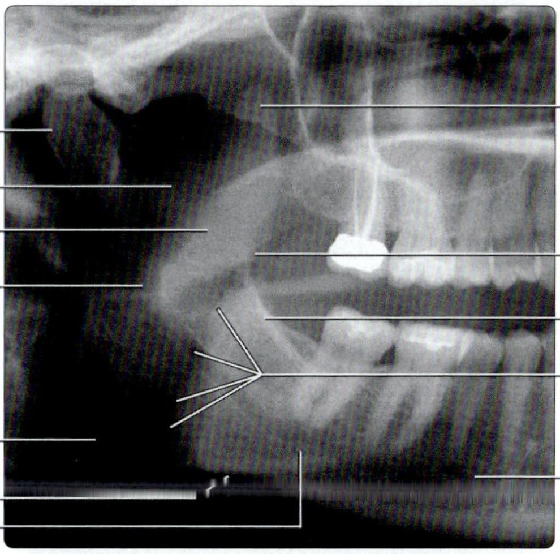

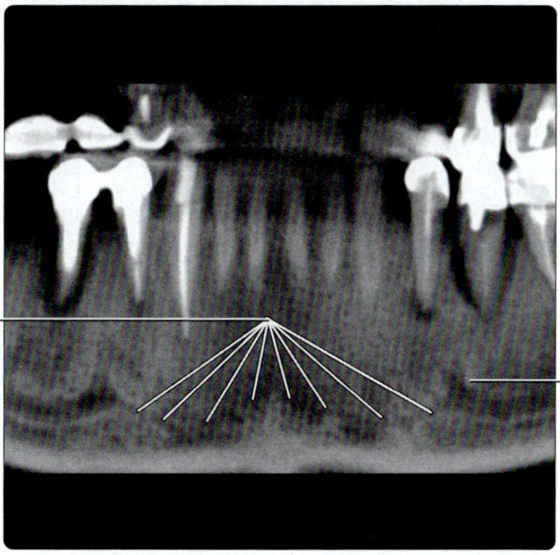

(Top) *Frontal view shows 3D reconstruction of the facial bones. The mandible anterior body is best delineated with the paired mental foramina evident. The infraorbital nerves are transmitted via the paired infraorbital foramina.* **(Middle)** *Panoramic radiograph shows normal mandibular anatomy. One of the limitations of panoramic radiography is the superimposition of structures and ghost images that can obscure evaluation of areas of interest. The superimposition of soft tissues, such as the soft palate and the tongue, gives the appearance of denser bone, whereas bone that has the airway superimposed on it appears less radiopaque.* **(Bottom)** *Panoramic reformation of CBCT data shows the inferior alveolar canals emerging through the mental foramina, then a continuation of the canals is seen reaching the midline (incisive canals). These may terminate within the bone or may join fiber emerging through the lingual canal. This is of importance if implant placement is planned in the anterior region.*

CBCT, PERIAPICAL RADIOGRAPH

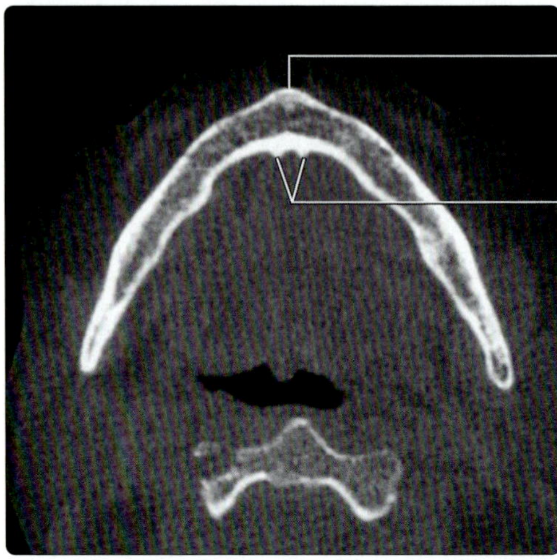

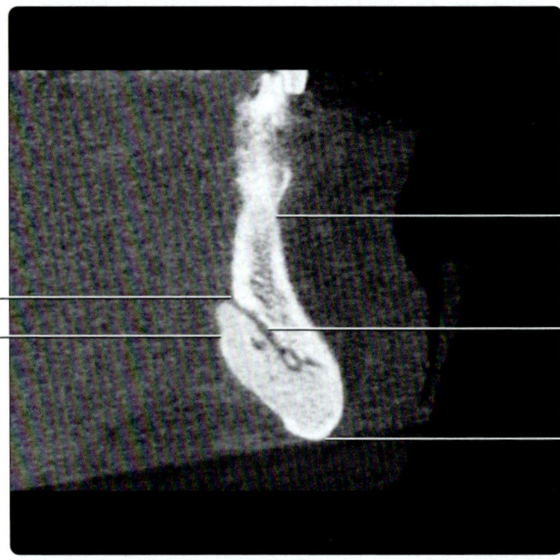

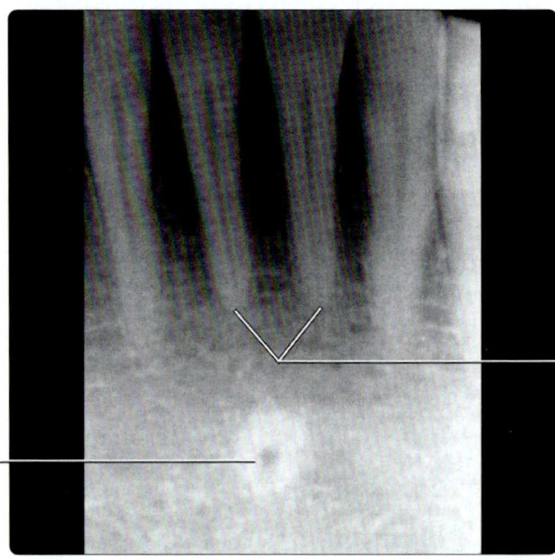

(Top) *Axial CBCT shows the genial tubercles on the lingual surface of the anterior mandible. This is the site of attachment of the genioglossus and geniohyoid muscles. These tubercles vary in appearance. They may be nonexistent, a small bump, a set of paired bony protrusions (as seen here), which can vary in size, or 2 sets (inferior and superior) of bony protrusions.* **(Middle)** *Sagittal CBCT of the anterior mandible shows the lingual canal emerging through the lingual foramen superiorly to the genial tubercles. Variations of this canal may occur, and there may be multiple canals emerging superiorly and inferiorly to the genial tubercles.* **(Bottom)** *Periapical radiograph of the anterior mandibular teeth shows a densely corticated lingual foramen in the symphyseal region of the mandible inferior to the apices of the central incisors. This is a normal anatomic landmark in the anterior mandible and may vary in size or may not be apparent at all on this exposure.*

PERIAPICAL RADIOGRAPH, CBCT

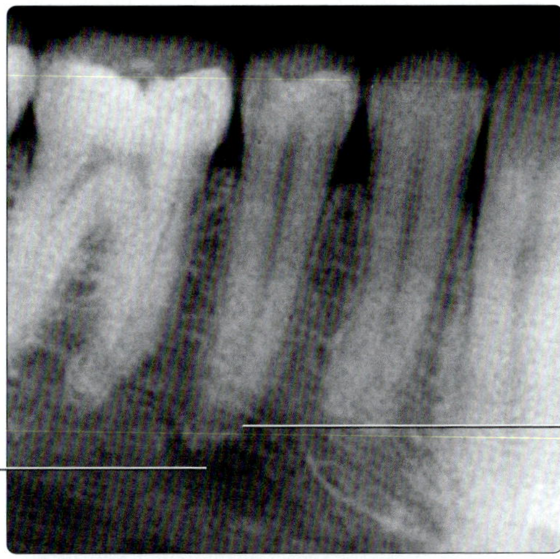

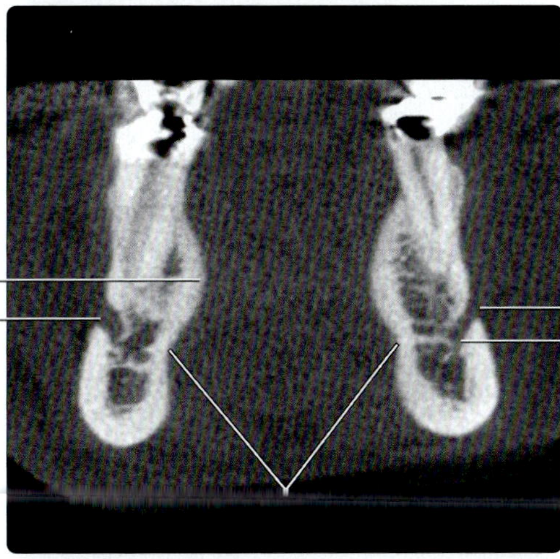

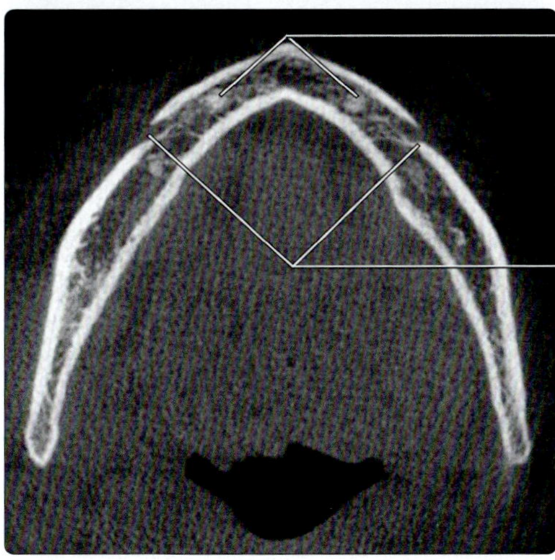

(Top) *Periapical radiograph shows the position of the mental foramen in the mandibular premolar region. This may be present between the 1st molar and the canine regions but is most commonly in the premolar region. The image of the foramen may superimpose on the apices of the mandibular teeth (as shown) and should not be mistaken for pathology. Careful evaluation of the lamina dura of the related tooth should show continuous apical lamina dura.* **(Middle)** *Coronal CBCT shows the normal appearance of the region of the mental foramina. The inferior alveolar nerve canal runs superiorly and laterally to emerge through the buccal cortex of the mandible. The medial aspect of the mandibular body shows a depression in the premolar/molar region caused by the presence of the submandibular gland underneath the mylohyoid ridge. This creates a lingual undercut that should be considered if implant planning is being performed.* **(Bottom)** *Axial CBCT shows the position & shape of normal mental foramina. There can be variations to their location.*

TERMINOLOGY

Abbreviations

- Oral mucosal space/surface (OMS)
- Root of tongue (ROT)
- Floor of mouth (FOM)
- For muscles: Origin (O), insertion (I), function (F), innervation (N)

Definitions

- **Oral tongue**: Anterior 2/3 of tongue not including tongue base
  - Includes freely mobile portion of tongue anterior to lingual tonsil
- **ROT**: Undersurface of oral tongue at its junction with anterior FOM and mandible
  - Includes lingual septum, genioglossus muscles, and geniohyoid muscles
- **FOM**: Crescent-shaped region of tissue, including mylohyoid and hyoglossus muscles
  - Extends from inner aspect of lower alveolar ridge to undersurface of anterior oral tongue
  - Includes mylohyoid muscle as it hangs from side-to-side from medial mandible (mylohyoid ridge) to medial mandible and hyoglossus muscle
- **Base of tongue**: Posterior 1/3 of tongue in oropharynx
  - Includes **lingual tonsil**

IMAGING ANATOMY

Overview

- Oral tongue sits centrally within oral cavity
  - Mucosal covering of oral tongue part of OMS
  - Sublingual space (SLS) is nonfascia-lined space within oral tongue
- Surfaces of oral tongue are covered with mucosa

Anatomy Relationships

- **SLS**
  - Part of oral tongue between mylohyoid muscle inferolaterally and genioglossus medially
  - Communicates with contralateral SLS beneath **frenulum** anteriorly
  - Empties posteriorly into posterosuperior aspect of submandibular space and inferior parapharyngeal space
- **ROT**
  - Inferiorly ROT ends at mylohyoid sling
  - Superiorly ends at intrinsic tongue muscles
  - Anteriorly ends at mandibular symphysis

Internal Contents

- **Oral tongue**: Consists of 4 anatomic regions
  - Tip of oral tongue
  - Lateral borders of oral tongue
  - Dorsum of oral tongue
  - Undersurface (nonvillous surface) of oral tongue
- **SLS**
  - Anterior hyoglossus muscle
  - Lingual nerve; CNIX and XII
  - Lingual artery and vein
  - Sublingual glands and ducts
  - Submandibular gland duct
- **Extrinsic tongue muscles**: Move tongue body and alter its shape
  - **Genioglossus**: Large, fan-shaped muscle lying parallel to median plane in sagittal plane
    - O: Upper genial tubercle and internal surface of symphysis menti of mandible
    - I: Along entire length of under surface of tongue
    - F: Protrudes tongue
    - N: CNXII
  - **Hyoglossus**: Thin and quadrilateral-shaped muscle; "arms reaching up" from posteroinferior FOM into posterior SLS
    - O: Body and greater cornu of hyoid bone
    - I: Passes vertically upward to insert into side of tongue
    - F: Depresses tongue
    - N: CNXII
  - **Styloglossus**
    - O: Arises from styloid process and stylomandibular ligament
    - I: Passes anteroinferiorly between internal and external carotid arteries to insert into side of tongue, merging with hyoglossus muscle
    - F: Retracts tongue upward and backward
    - N: CNXII
  - **Palatoglossus**
    - O: Undersurface of palatine aponeurosis
    - I: Side and dorsum of tongue
    - F: Forms palatoglossal arch (anterior tonsillar pillar)
    - N: CNX; pharyngeal plexus branch
- **Intrinsic tongue muscles**: Alters shape of tongue during deglutition and speech
  - Complicated bundles of interlacing fibers innervated by CNXII
  - Superior and inferior longitudinal
  - Transverse and vertical
- **N of tongue**
  - Sensory supply (touch, pain, temperature, and **taste**)
    - Anterior 2/3: Lingual nerve (taste fibers are from chorda tympani branch of CNVII)
    - Posterior 1/3: CNIX
  - **Motor supply: Hypoglossal nerve** (CNXII)
    - Emerges from nasopharyngeal carotid space
    - Receives fibers from 1st and 2nd cervical nerves
    - Loops inferiorly to level of hyoid bone
    - Rises anteriorly to enter posterior SLS just lateral to hyoglossus muscle
    - Runs in SLS on lateral surface of genioglossus muscle
    - Innervates extrinsic and intrinsic tongue muscles
- **Vasculature of tongue**
  - Lingual artery: 2nd branch of external carotid artery
    - Divides in SLS into sublingual and deep lingual branches
  - Lingual vein: Parallels lingual artery; drains into internal jugular or facial veins
- **Oral tongue lymph vessels**
  - 2 systems: Superficial mucosa and deep collecting
  - Superficial system: Crossing vessels in anterior FOM drain bilaterally into anterior submandibular nodes
  - Deep collecting system: Drain into ipsilateral anterior submandibular nodal chain only

ANATOMY OF TONGUE

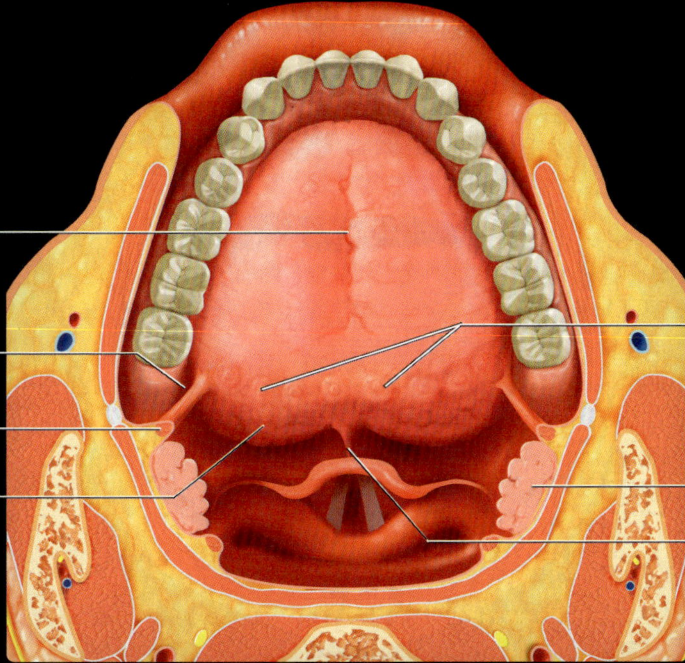

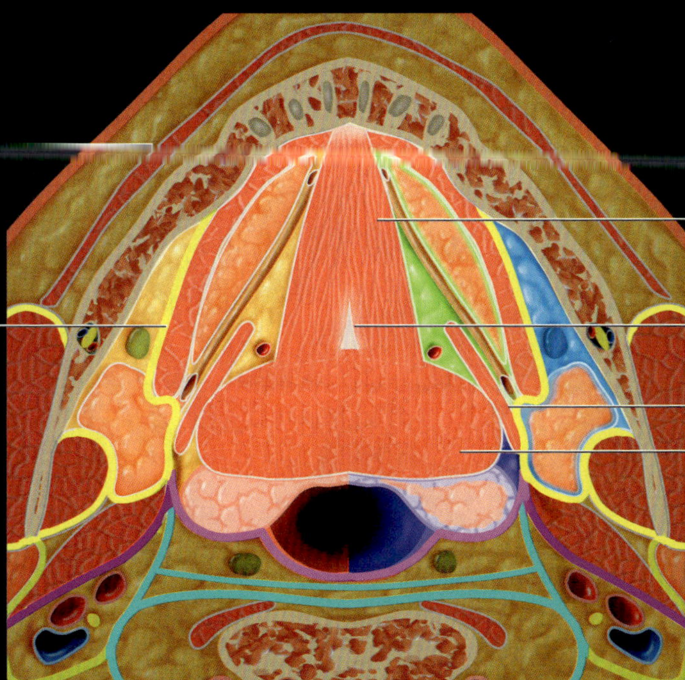

(Top) *Axial graphic shows the surface of the oral tongue. The oral tongue sits anterior to the oropharyngeal lingual tonsil. The line of the circumvallate papillae delineates the mucosal surface transition to the more anterior oral cavity.* **(Bottom)** *In this axial graphic through the deep portion of the oral tongue, it is possible to see the large, bilateral paramedian genioglossus muscles bordering the midline lingual septum. The genioglossus muscles rise to mingle with the complex tangle of intrinsic tongue muscles. The hyoglossus muscles are also seen rising from the hyoid bone below into the posterior sublingual space. The sublingual space is shaded in green on the patient's left.*

ANATOMY OF TONGUE

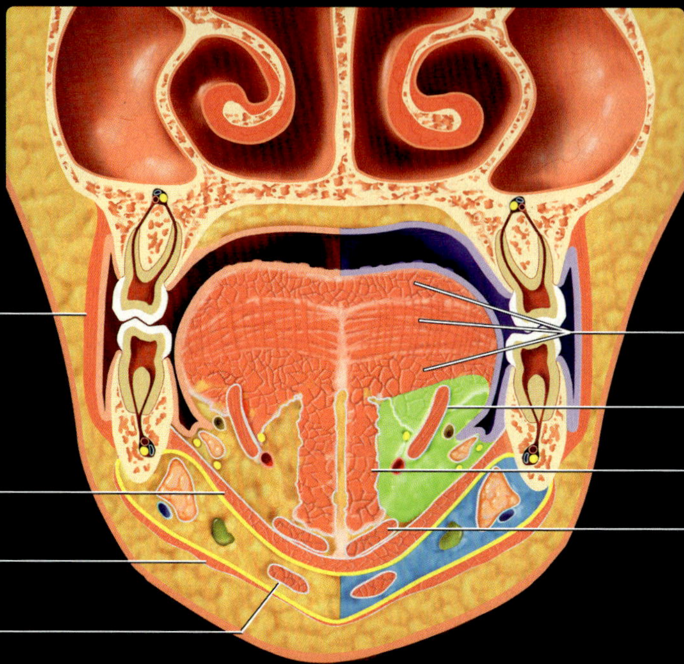

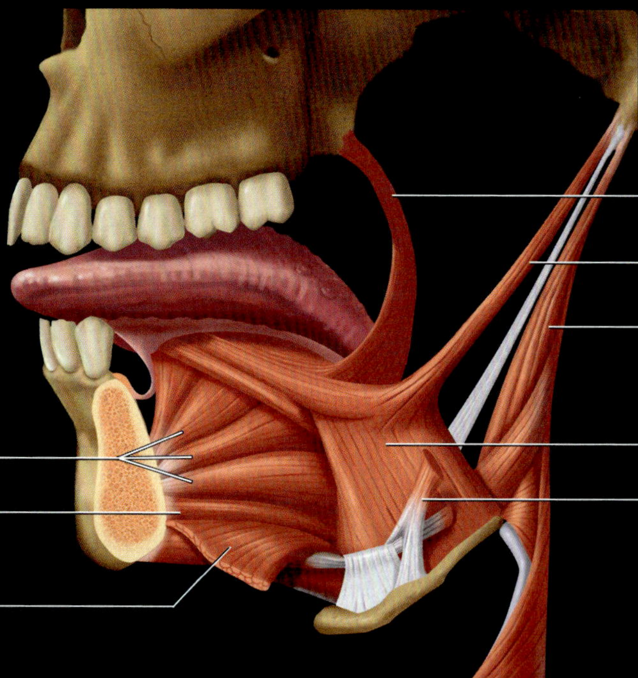

(Top) *Coronal graphic through the oral cavity highlights all major muscles with their innervations indicated in parenthesis. Note all intrinsic and extrinsic (genioglossus, hyoglossus, styloglossus, palatoglossus) tongue muscles are innervated by CNXII except palatoglossus. The buccinator and platysma, both muscles of facial expression, are innervated by CNVII.* **(Bottom)** *Sagittal graphic shows muscles of the tongue area. Each muscle is labeled and its innervating nerve is shown in parenthesis. Pay attention to the fan-shaped genioglossus, which represents much of the oral tongue extrinsic musculature. Note the hyoglossus muscle projecting upward from the hyoid bone like 2 big arms into the oral tongue's posterior sublingual space. The geniohyoid muscle is not considered part of the extrinsic muscles of the tongue but instead is a suprahyoid neck muscle innervated by the CNXII branch with 1st cervical nerve root in it.*

SAGITTAL, CORONAL, & AXIAL T1 MR

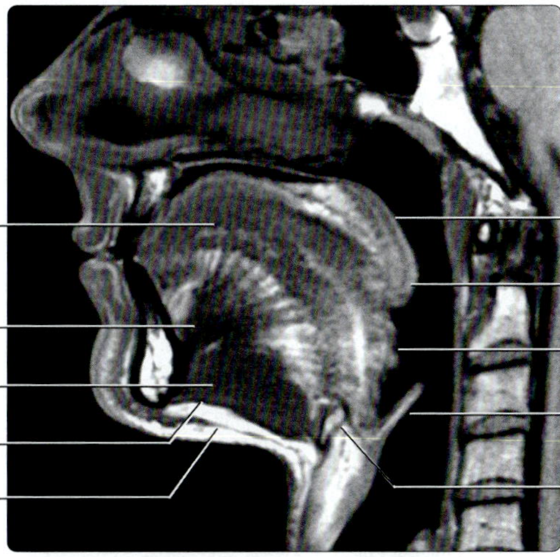

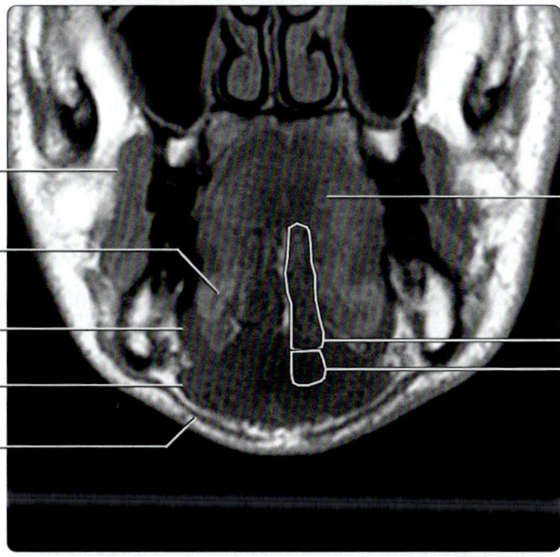

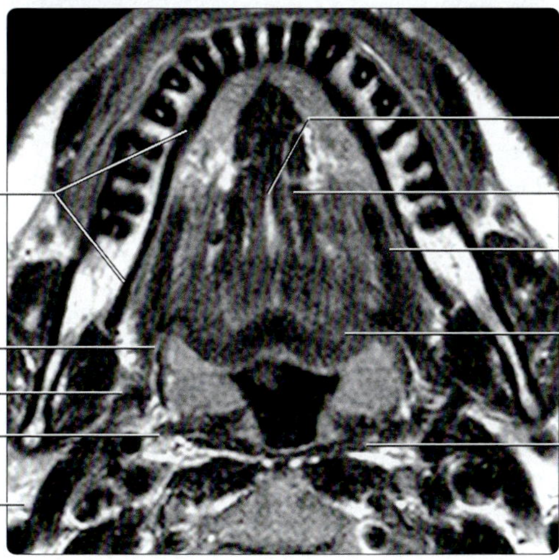

(Top) *In this sagittal T1 MR, the full extent of the genioglossus muscle can be seen extending cephalad in a fan shape from its attachment to the posteroinferior mandible. Notice that it is difficult to distinguish the mylohyoid, geniohyoid, and inferior genioglossus muscles.* **(Middle)** *In this coronal T1 MR, 4 muscles can be identified from inferior to superior, namely the anterior belly of digastric, mylohyoid, geniohyoid, and genioglossus muscles. The anterior belly of the digastric and mylohyoid muscles are innervated by the mandibular division of the trigeminal nerve. The geniohyoid and genioglossus muscles are innervated by the hypoglossal nerve.* **(Bottom)** *In this axial T1 MR, the hyoglossus upper margin is seen rising into the posterior sublingual space. The genioglossus is now readily apparent on either side of the fibrofatty lingual septum.*

TERMINOLOGY

Abbreviations

- Retromolar trigone (RMT)

Definitions

- Triangle-shaped area of mucosa posterior to last mandibular molar that covers anterior surface of lower ascending ramus of mandible

IMAGING ANATOMY

Overview

- Pterygomandibular raphe (PMR) lies beneath mucosa of RMT
    - PMR: Thick fascial band that extends between posterior border of mandibular mylohyoid ridge and hamulus of medial pterygoid plate
        - Fascial band represents thickening of middle layer of deep cervical fascia condensed between posterior margin of buccinator muscle and anterior margin of superior constrictor muscle
- If RMT is affected by squamous cell carcinoma (SCCa), PMR is involved early
- PMR provides both inferior and superior routes of spread for SCCa

Extent

- RMT extent
    - Cephalad tip is at level of base of pterygoid plate
    - Base of mucosal triangle is posterior margin of last mandibular molar tooth
- PMR extent
    - Fascial band extends from **posterior border of mylohyoid ridge of mandible** to hamulus of medial pterygoid plate

Anatomy Relationships

- RMT relationships
    - Deep to RMT mucosa is posterior mandibular body
    - Also covers anterior surface of inferior ascending ramus of mandible
- PMR can be located at line of junction between buccinator (posterior margin) muscle and superior constrictor muscle (anterior margin)

Internal Contents

- **RMT**
    - Paired triangle-shaped mucosal surface in posterolateral oral cavity
- **PMR**
    - PMR forms line of attachment for buccinator and superior constrictor muscles
    - Represents junction of oropharynx posteriorly and oral cavity anteriorly
    - Lies between anterior tonsillar pillar and RMT

Fascia

- PMR: **Thick fascial band formed at junction of buccinator and superior constrictor muscles**
    - Fascia made up of focally thickened middle layer of deep cervical fascia
    - Middle layer of deep cervical fascia runs along superficial margin of buccinator muscle and along deep and lateral margins of superior constrictor muscle

ANATOMY IMAGING ISSUES

Questions

- RMT SCCa can spread in multiple directions
    - Posterior spread of SCCa: May involve mandibular ramus, masticator space, and perineural CNV3
    - Anterior spread of SCCa: Along alveolar ridge
    - Inferior spread of SCCa
        - If directly into mandible, may extend anteriorly via perineural spread along inferior alveolar nerve
        - If caudal spread along PMR, reaches posterior mylohyoid line of mandible and, thereby, posterior margin of mylohyoid muscle
    - Superior spread of SCCa: Cephalad spread along PMR to inferior margin of medial pterygoid plate at hamulus

Imaging Recommendations

- CECT provides both soft tissue and bone information
    - May be severely degraded by dental amalgam artifact
- MR less affected by dental amalgam artifact in most cases
    - Reserve for invasive RMT SCCa
    - Axial T2 and T1 fat-saturated enhanced MR sequences best for evaluation of cephalad PMR

Imaging Pitfalls

- Dental amalgam artifact on CECT may obscure RMT primary SCCa primary site ± spread along PMR in cephalad direction
    - Key CT observation
        - Always check **above CT artifact** in oral cavity in area of cephalad PMR (inferior margin of pterygoid plate) for evidence of tumor spread if primary RMT SCCa is known to be present

CLINICAL IMPLICATIONS

Clinical Importance

- SCCa of RMT may spread along PMR
    - Cephalad spread along PMR takes tumor up to inferolateral pterygoid plate-anteromedial masticator space
        - Tumor is seen at level of inferior pterygoid plate involving posterior buccinator muscle and anterior superior constrictor muscle
        - Enlarging tumor involves maxillary sinus, buccal and masticator spaces
    - Caudal spread along PMR takes tumor inferiorly to posterior margin of mylohyoid muscle
        - Enlarging tumor in this location involves floor of mouth of oral cavity

AXIAL & SAGITTAL GRAPHICS, RETROMOLAR TRIGONE & PTERYGOMANDIBULAR RAPHE

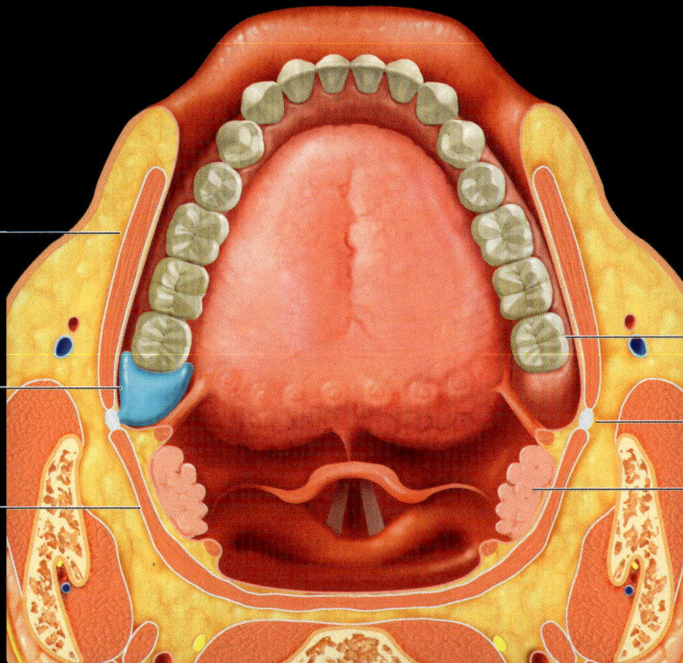

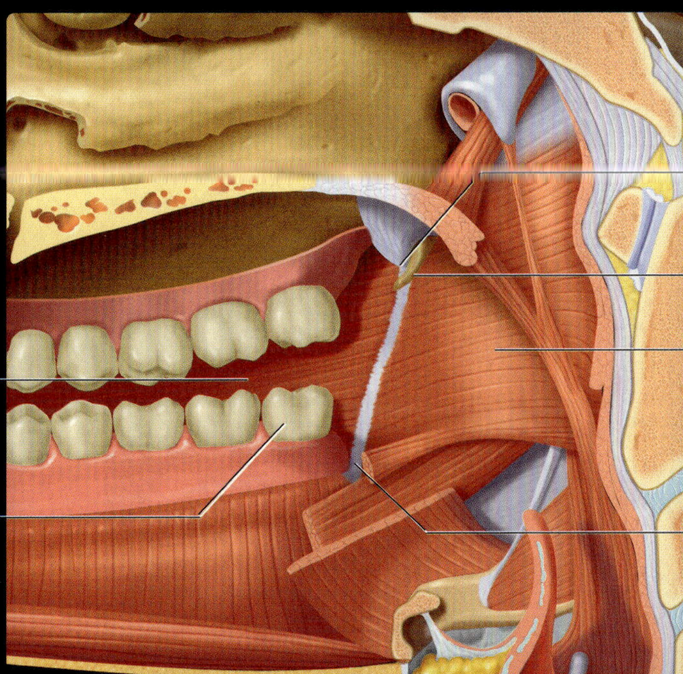

(Top) *Axial graphic highlights the retromolar trigone (shaded in blue on patient's right) and the pterygomandibular raphe. Notice that the mucosal surface of the retromolar trigone is found directly behind the mandibular 3rd molar. Its proximity to the pterygomandibular raphe (fascial band connecting buccinator and superior pharyngeal constrictor muscles) is important when squamous cell carcinoma occurs here because of this tumor's propensity for spreading cephalad on this fascia.* **(Bottom)** *Sagittal graphic viewed from inside the mouth delineates the full extent of the pterygomandibular raphe. Note the cephalad pterygomandibular raphe attachment to the hamulus of the medial pterygoid plate and its inferior attachment to the posterior aspect of the mylohyoid ridge on the mandibular lingual cortex. The pterygomandibular raphe "connects" the buccinator muscle to the superior pharyngeal constrictor muscle.*

NORMAL AXIAL T2 MR PTERYGOMANDIBULAR RAPHE

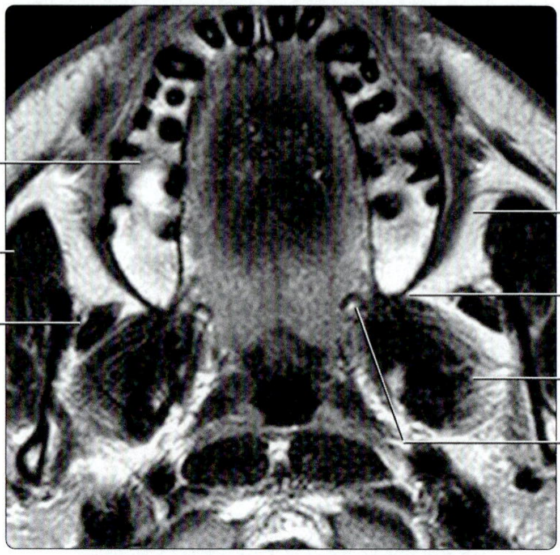

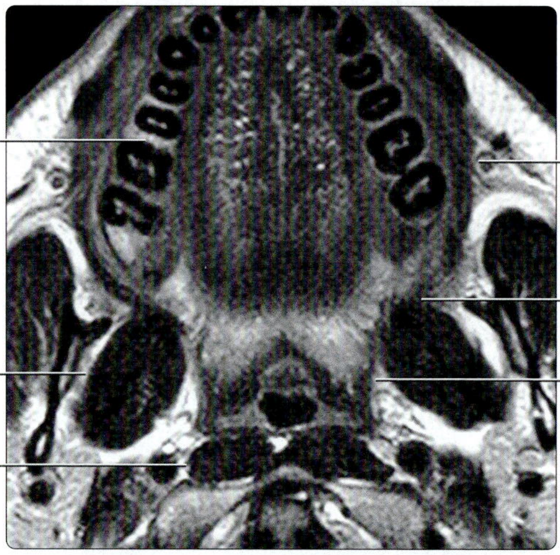

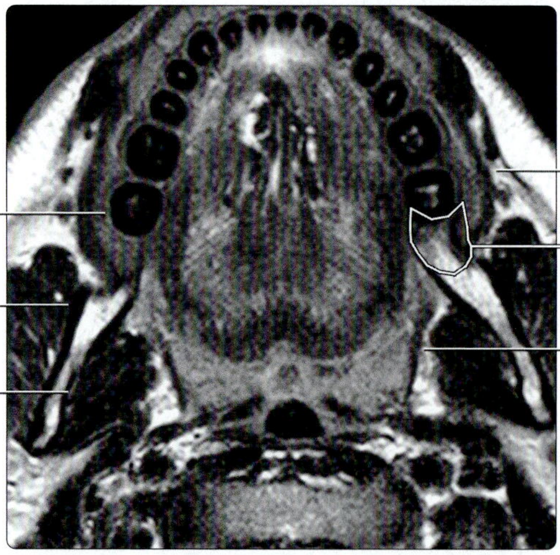

(Top) *First and most superior of 3 axial T2 MR images (presented from superior to inferior) shows the point of attachment of the pterygomandibular raphe to the hamulus of the medial pterygoid plate.* **(Middle)** *On this more inferior image, the buccinator can be seen meeting the superior pharyngeal constrictor muscle at the pterygomandibular raphe. The raphe itself is difficult to visualize.* **(Bottom)** *At the level of the mandibular alveolar ridge, the area of the retromolar trigone can be outlined. Notice it is found directly behind the mandibular 3rd molar tooth. The buccinator is seen along its lateral margin, while the superior pharyngeal constrictor can be seen approaching its medial margin. Just above this slice these 2 muscles meet at the pterygomandibular raphe. Squamous cell carcinoma of the retromolar trigone often spreads cephalad along this raphe.*

AXIAL T1 MR

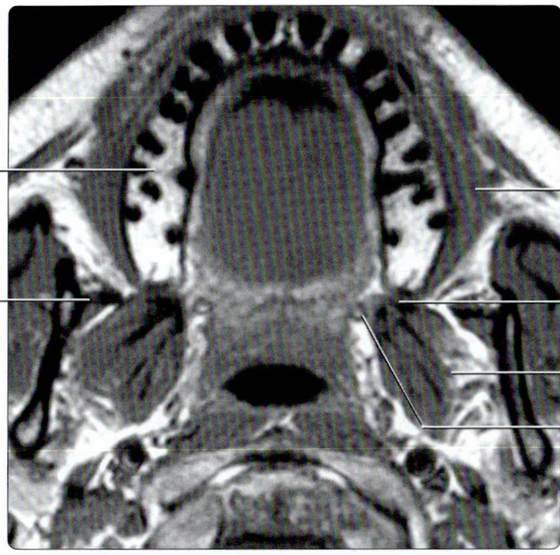

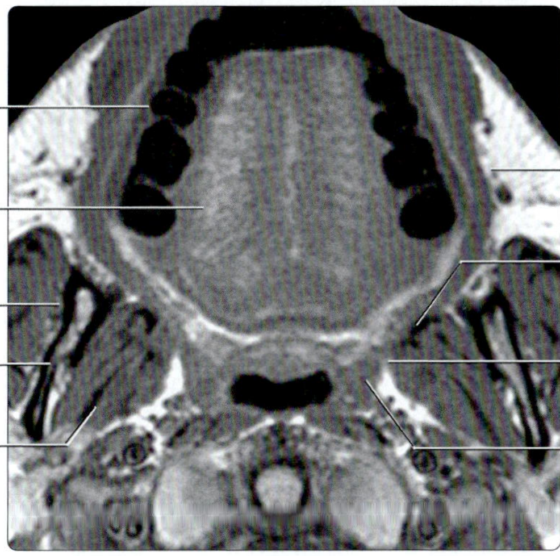

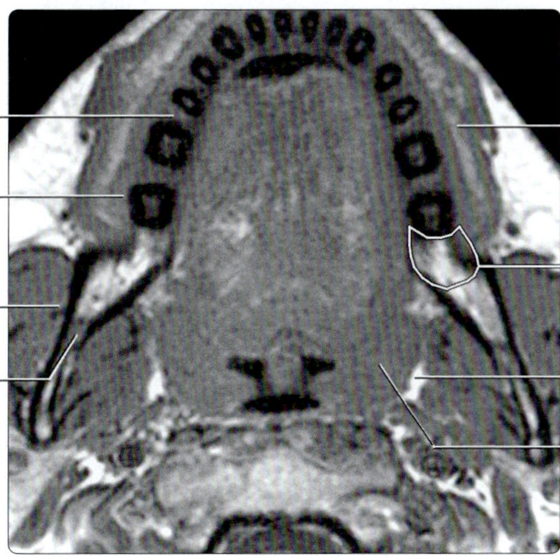

(Top) *First of 3 axial T1 MR images, presented from superior to inferior, shows the oropharynx-oral cavity. On this most superior image the buccinator can be seen inserting at the inferolateral margin of the pterygoid plate with the most superior aspect of the pterygomandibular raphe.* **(Middle)** *Inferiorly, at the level of the mandibular teeth, the buccinator and the superior constrictor muscle meet at the pterygomandibular raphe. The superior constrictor muscle cannot be differentiated from the palatine tonsil on T1 images.* **(Bottom)** *On this most inferior image at the level of the mandibular alveolar ridge, the area of the retromolar trigone is outlined on the patient's left. Note that the retromolar trigone is found directly behind the 3rd mandibular molar tooth. Squamous cell carcinoma can spread up the pterygomandibular raphe from this location.*

TERMINOLOGY

Abbreviations

- Sublingual space (SLS)
- Submandibular space (SMS)

Definitions

- SLS: Paired nonfascial-lined spaces of oral cavity in deep oral tongue above floor of mouth superomedial to mylohyoid muscle

IMAGING ANATOMY

Overview

- SLS contains key neurovascular structures of oral cavity
  - Includes glossopharyngeal nerve (CNIX), hypoglossal nerve (CNXII), lingual nerve (branch of V3), lingual artery and vein
- When lesion involves both SLSs across anterior isthmus, it appears as **horizontal horseshoe** parallel to line of inferior mandibular surface

Anatomy Relationships

- SLS relationships
  - SLS in deep oral tongue **superomedial to mylohyoid muscle** and lateral to genioglossus-geniohyoid muscles
  - Communication between SLSs occurs in midline anteriorly as narrow **isthmus** beneath frenulum
  - SLS communicates with SMS and inferior parapharyngeal space (PPS) at posterior margin of mylohyoid muscle
    - There is **no fascia** dividing posterior SLS from adjacent SMS; therefore, there is direct communication with SMS and PPS in this location

Internal Contents

- Posterior aspect of SLS is divided into medial and lateral compartments by hyoglossal muscle
- Lateral compartment contents
  - **Hypoglossal nerve**: Motor to intrinsic and extrinsic muscles of tongue
    - Intrinsic muscles of tongue include inferior lingual, vertical, and transverse muscles
    - Extrinsic muscles of tongue include genioglossus, hyoglossus, styloglossus, and palatoglossus muscles
  - **Lingual nerve**: Branch of mandibular division of trigeminal nerve (CNV3) combined with chorda tympani branch of facial nerve
    - Lingual nerve branch of CNV3: Sensation to anterior 2/3 of oral tongue
    - Chorda tympani branch of facial nerve: Carries anterior 2/3 of tongue taste centrally and parasympathetic secretomotor fibers peripherally to submandibular ganglion/gland
  - **Sublingual glands and ducts**
    - Lie in anterior SLS bilaterally
    - ~ 5 small ducts open under oral tongue into oral cavity
    - With age, sublingual glands atrophy, becoming difficult to see on imaging
  - **Submandibular gland deep portion and submandibular duct**
    - Submandibular gland deep margin extends into posterior opening of SLS
    - Enlarging lesions of SLS in effect push deep margin of submandibular gland out of way as they emerge from SLS into SMS
    - Submandibular duct runs anteriorly to papillae in anteromedial subfrenular mucosa
- Medial compartment contents
  - **Glossopharyngeal nerve** (CNIX)
    - Provides sensation to posterior 1/3 of tongue
    - Carries taste input from posterior 1/3 of tongue
    - Located more cephalad in medial compartment compared to lingual artery and vein
  - **Lingual artery and vein**
    - Vascular supply to oral tongue
    - Seen running just lateral to genioglossus muscle

Fascia

- SLS is **not fascia-lined** space but instead is **potential space** only

ANATOMY IMAGING ISSUES

Questions

- What defines mass as primary to SLS
  - Center of lesion is superomedial to mylohyoid muscle and lateral to genioglossus muscle
- Besides spilling out back of SLS into posterior SMS, how can lesion of SLS access SMS
  - **Mylohyoid** muscle has variably sized **cleft** between its anterior 1/3 and posterior 2/3 area
  - Lesions may "escape" SLS into SMS through this cleft
  - When this occurs, lesion is found in anterior SMS **in front of** submandibular gland

Imaging Recommendations

- CECT or T1 C+ MR with fat saturation are both excellent imaging tools to evaluate SLS lesions
- MR better in cooperative patient
  - MR less affected by dental amalgam artifact compared to CT
  - MR permits direct coronal imaging to assess relationship of lesion to mylohyoid muscle

Imaging Pitfalls

- Extension of oral cavity squamous cell carcinoma (SCCa) into floor of mouth or root of tongue can be obscured by dental amalgam on CECT

CLINICAL IMPLICATIONS

Clinical Importance

- Since neurovascular bundle to tongue travels in SLS, oral cavity SCCa involving posterior SLS is challenging to treat
- If SCCa crosses lingual septum to contralateral SLS, lesion becomes unresectable for cure
- When dental infection is present, SLS may be affected by abscess
  - This is particularly true when tooth socket drains medially above mylohyoid ridge (mylohyoid muscle attachment area)

AXIAL GRAPHIC, NORMAL AXIAL CECT OF SUBLINGUAL SPACE

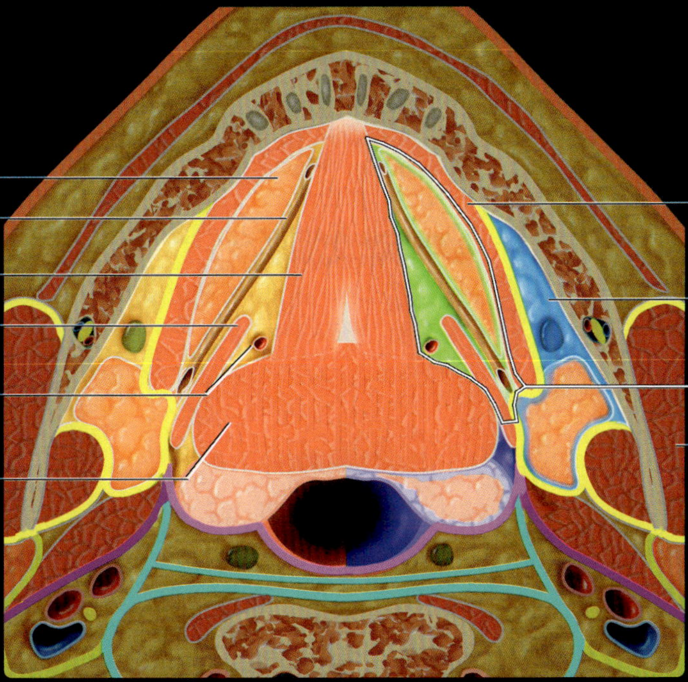

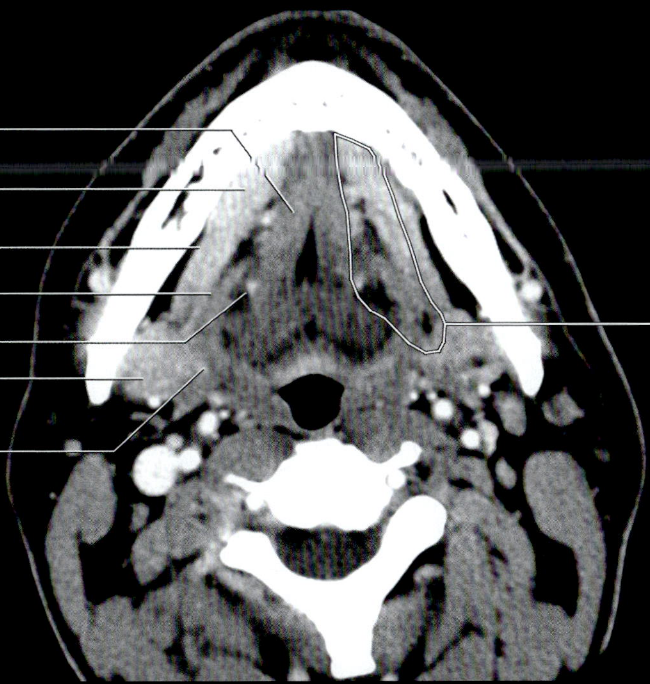

(Top) *Axial graphic through the body of the mandible shows the sublingual space (on patient's left, shaded in green) situated superomedial to the mylohyoid muscle and lateral to the genioglossus muscle. Notice the absence of fascia surrounding the sublingual space. The yellow line represents the superficial layer of deep cervical fascia.* **(Bottom)** *Axial CECT shows the sublingual space outlined on the patient's left. On enhanced CT, it is difficult to separate the mylohyoid muscle from the sublingual gland. The deep portion of the submandibular gland projects into the posterior margin of the sublingual space.*

CORONAL GRAPHIC, NORMAL CORONAL T1 MR OF SUBLINGUAL SPACE

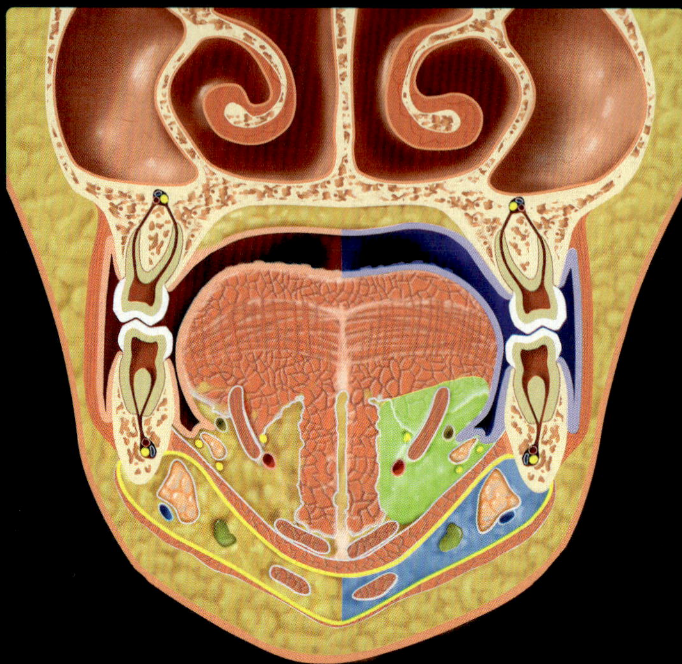

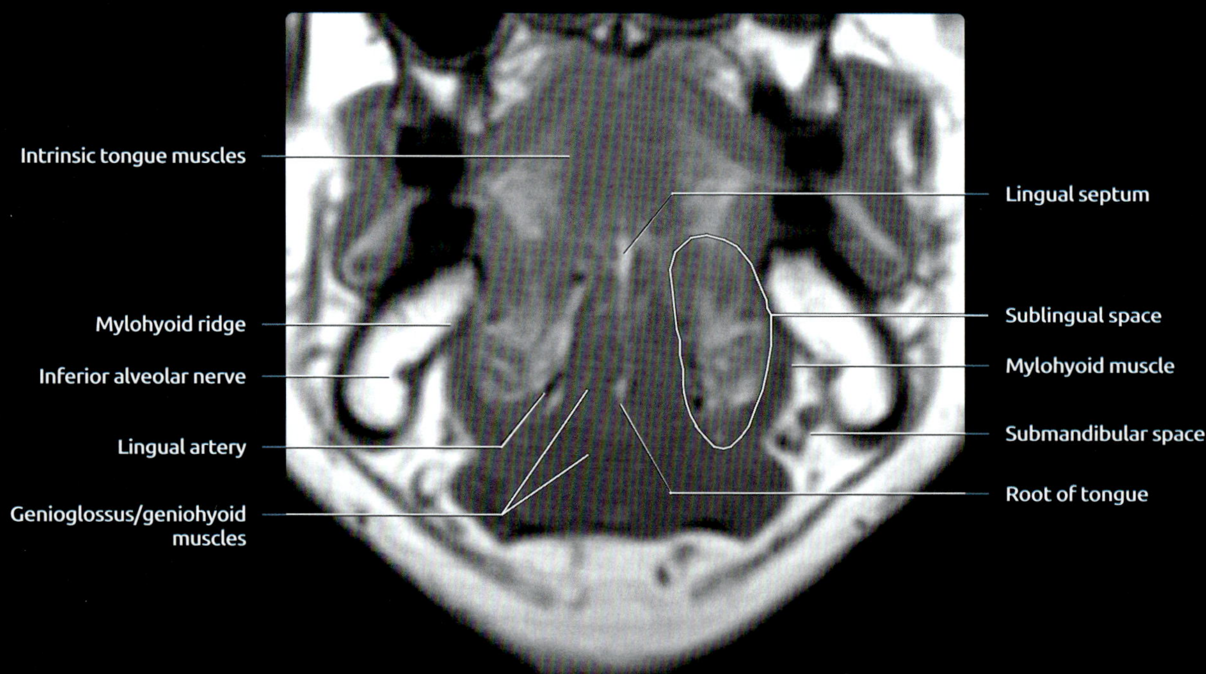

(Top) *In this coronal graphic through the oral cavity, the sublingual space is shaded in green. The sublingual space medial compartment contents include the glossopharyngeal nerve (CNIX) and lingual artery/vein. The lateral sublingual space compartment contents include the submandibular duct, sublingual gland, lingual nerve, and hypoglossal nerve (CNXII). The fascia-lined (yellow line) submandibular space is inferolateral to the mylohyoid muscle.* **(Bottom)** *In this coronal T1 MR image, the "potential" sublingual space is superomedial to the mylohyoid muscle and lateral to the genioglossus muscle. It is difficult to identify the margins of the genioglossus muscles.*

NORMAL AXIAL CECT OF SUBLINGUAL SPACE

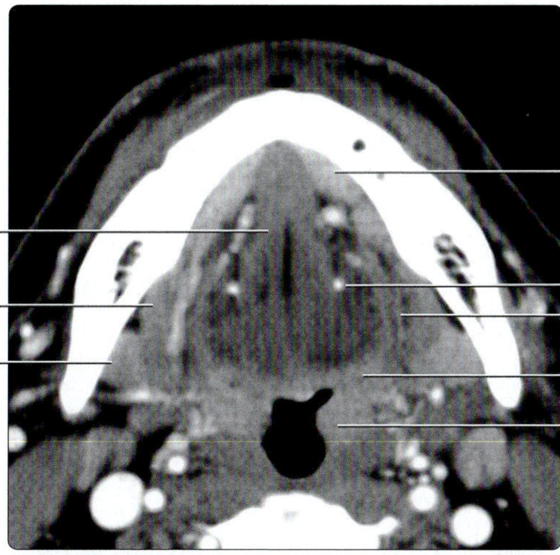

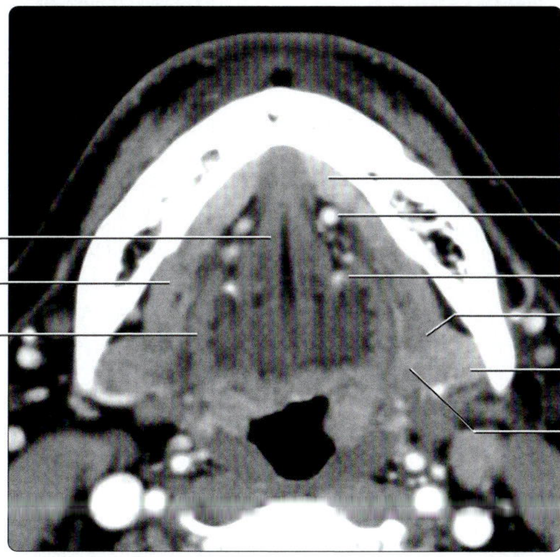

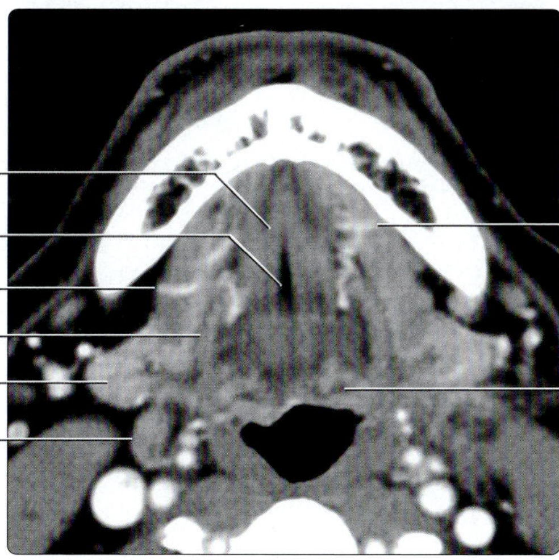

(Top) *First of 3 axial CECT images shows the sublingual space within the oral cavity. This most superior image shows that the medial border of the sublingual spaces is the genioglossus muscle. The mylohyoid muscle forms the lateral boundary of the sublingual spaces. The hyoglossus muscles are seen projecting into the posterior sublingual spaces.* **(Middle)** *More inferiorly, a larger portion of the mylohyoid muscle can be seen forming the inferolateral border of the sublingual space. Notice the submandibular gland wrapping around the posterior margin of this muscle on the patient's left. The deep portion of the submandibular gland is found in the posterior sublingual space.* **(Bottom)** *Inferiorly, the sublingual spaces become smaller with the hyoglossus muscle filling most of these spaces. Both mylohyoid muscles demonstrate small clefts with a vessel present bilaterally.*

TERMINOLOGY

Abbreviations

- Submandibular space (SMS)

Synonyms

- Term submaxillary space used by surgeons

Definitions

- SMS: Fascial-lined space inferolateral to mylohyoid muscle containing submandibular gland, nodes, and anterior belly of digastric muscles

IMAGING ANATOMY

Overview

- SMS is 1 of 4 distinct locations within oral cavity (OC) that may be used to develop location-specific differential diagnoses
  - Other 3 locations include oral mucosal space/surface, sublingual space, and root of tongue

Extent

- SMS is defined as superficial space above hyoid bone deep to platysma and superficial to mylohyoid sling

Anatomy Relationships

- **Inferolateral to mylohyoid muscle** of floor of mouth
- Deep to platysma muscle
- Cephalad to hyoid bone
- **Vertical horseshoe-shaped** space between hyoid bone below and mylohyoid sling above
- Communicates posteriorly with sublingual space and inferior parapharyngeal space at posterior margin of mylohyoid muscle
- Continues inferiorly into infrahyoid neck as anterior cervical space

Internal Contents

- **Submandibular gland**
  - Superficial portion is larger and in SMS itself
    - Superficial layer, deep cervical fascia (SL-DCF) forms submandibular gland capsule
    - Crossed by facial vein and cervical branches of facial nerve (marginal mandibular branch)
  - Smaller deep portion often called deep process
    - Deep process is tongue-like extension of gland
    - Wraps around posterior margin of mylohyoid muscle
    - Projects into posterior aspect of sublingual space
    - Submandibular duct projects off deep process into sublingual space
  - Submandibular gland innervation
    - Parasympathetic secretomotor supply from chorda tympani branch of facial nerve
    - Comes via lingual branch of cranial nerve V3
- **Submental (level IA) and submandibular (level IB) nodal groups**
  - Receive lymph drainage from anterior facial region
    - Including OC, anterior sinonasal, and orbital areas
- Facial vein and artery pass through SMS
- **Caudal loop of CNXII** passes through SMS before looping anteriorly and cephalad into tongue muscles
- **Anterior belly of digastric muscles**
- Tail of parotid may "hang down" into posterior SMS

Fascia

- **SMS is lined by SL-DCF**
  - Superficial surface of mylohyoid muscle is covered by SL-DCF
  - Deep surface of platysma covered by SL-DCF
- There is **no midline fascia** separating 2 sides of SMS
  - Consequently, lesion growth from side to side in SMS is unobstructed

ANATOMY IMAGING ISSUES

Questions

- Major clinical-imaging question when mass present in SMS: Is lesion nodal or submandibular gland in origin
  - Fatty cleavage plane between mass and submandibular gland identifies lesion as nodal in origin
    - If facial vein separates lesion from submandibular gland, then lesion is from node
  - "Beaking" of submandibular gland tissue around lesion margin identifies lesion as submandibular gland in origin
- What are major diagnoses in SMS differential diagnoses list
  - Congenital: Epidermoid, cystic hygroma
  - Inflammatory: Submandibular gland sialoadenitis with ductal calculus; diving ranula; reactive or suppurative adenopathy
  - Benign tumor: Benign mixed tumor of submandibular gland, lipoma
  - Malignant tumor: Salivary gland carcinomas; nodal squamous cell carcinoma and non-Hodgkin lymphoma

Imaging Recommendations

- CECT or T1 C+ fat-saturated MR both effective in SMS
- Ultrasound with needle aspiration of lesion also used

Imaging Pitfalls

- Do not mistake obstructed, enlarged submandibular gland for malignant node in setting of anterior floor of mouth primary squamous cell carcinoma

CLINICAL IMPLICATIONS

Clinical Importance

- Majority of lesions of SMS are either from submandibular gland or nodes
  - Sorting lesions into these 2 categories helps work through imaging differential diagnosis
- Remember, clinicians can see and feel area of SMS
  - Fine-needle cytopathology may have already been done at time of imaging
- Lesions of parotid tail may appear in posterior SMS clinically

AXIAL GRAPHIC, NORMAL AXIAL T2 MR

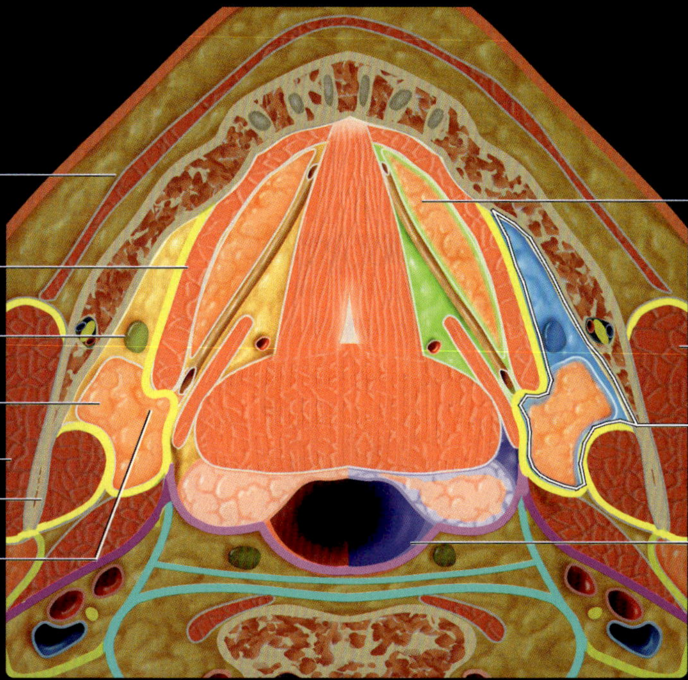

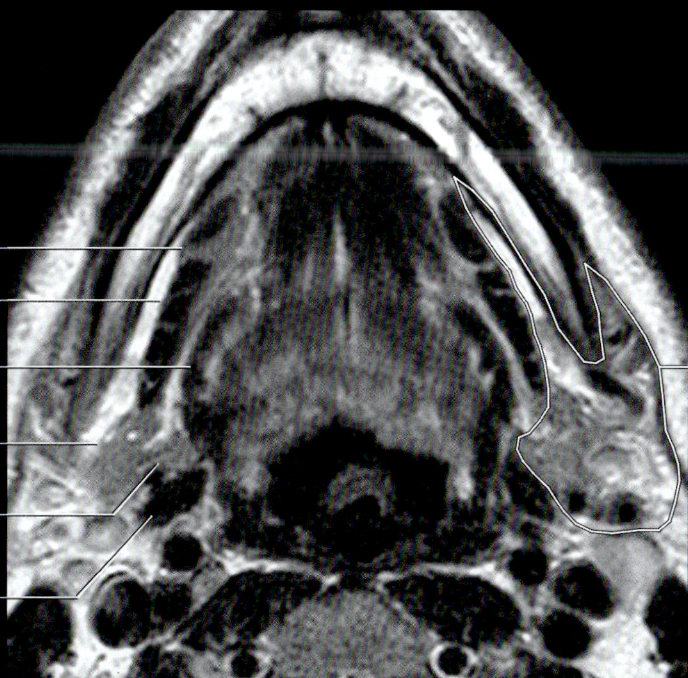

(Top) *Axial graphic of oral cavity with emphasis on the submandibular space is shaded in light blue on patient's left. The submandibular space is inferolateral to the mylohyoid muscle. Note the principal occupants of the submandibular space are the submandibular gland and nodes.* **(Bottom)** *Axial T2 MR demonstrates the axial appearance of the submandibular space outlined on the patient's left. The principal occupants of the submandibular space are the submandibular gland and nodes. Consequently, the differential diagnosis of lesions of this space includes gland tumors and lymph node diseases.*

CORONAL GRAPHIC, NORMAL CORONAL T1 MR

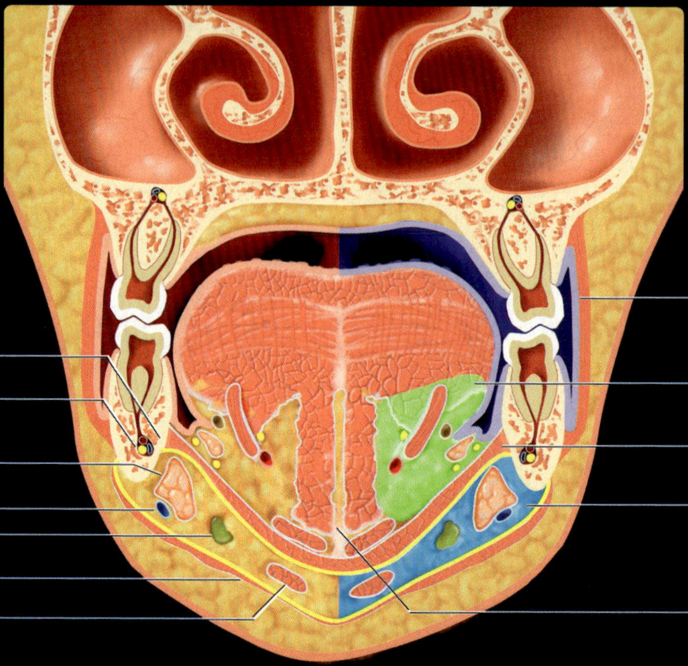

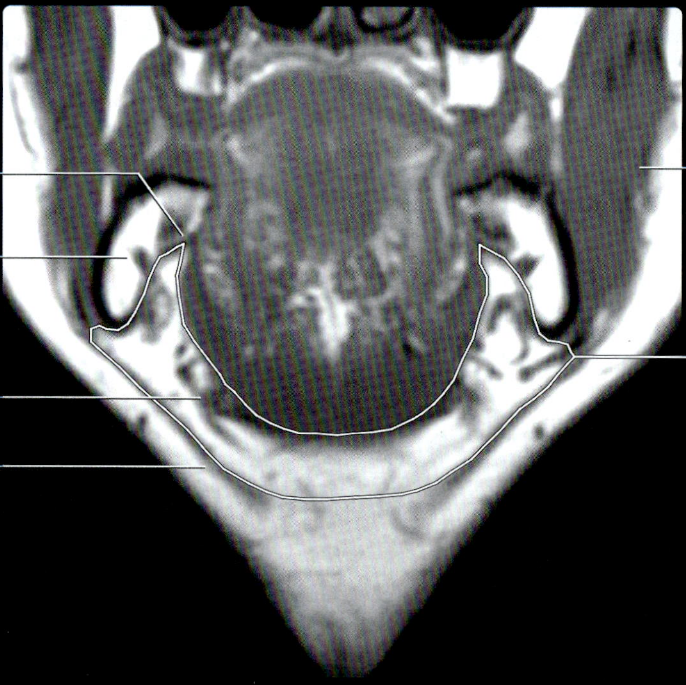

(Top) *In this coronal graphic through the oral cavity, the submandibular space is shaded in light blue. The superficial layer of deep cervical fascia (yellow line) is seen lining the vertical horseshoe-shaped submandibular space inferolateral to the mylohyoid muscle. Contents of submandibular space are the anterior belly of digastric muscle, submandibular nodes, submandibular gland, and facial vein. Notice the platysma forms the superficial margin of the submandibular space.* **(Bottom)** *Coronal T1 MR shows the horseshoe-shaped submandibular space extending from side to side inferior and inferolateral to the mylohyoid muscle and deep to the platysma muscle. Notice the lack of vertical fascia or septation. Consequently, lesions of the submandibular space spread readily across the midline.*

NORMAL AXIAL CECT SUPRAHYOID SMS

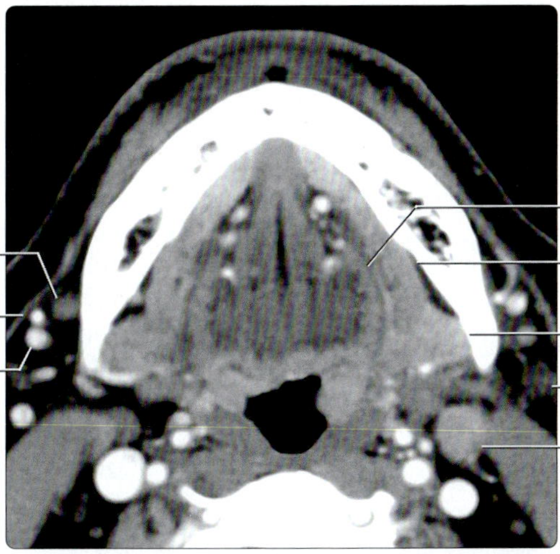

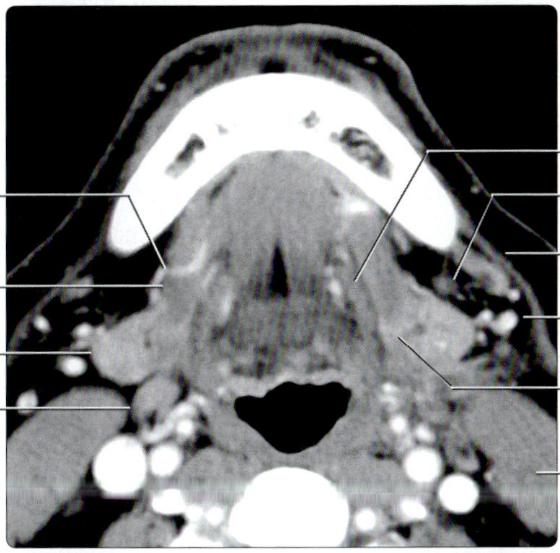

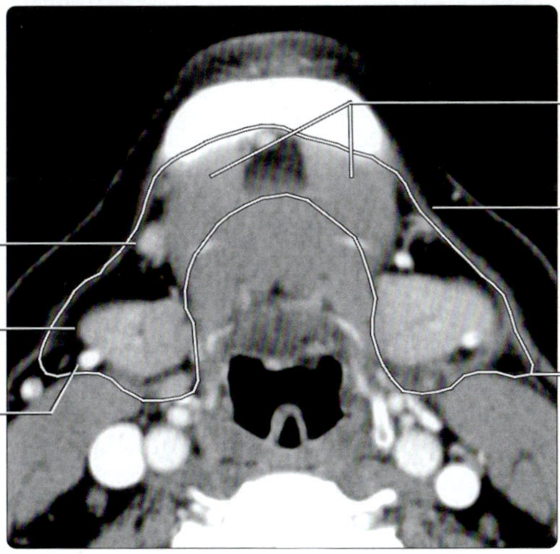

(Top) *First and most superior of 3 axial CECT images (presented from superior to inferior) reveals the uppermost portion of the submandibular space. Notice the parotid gland tail projecting into the posterior submandibular space on the patient's left.* **(Middle)** *More inferiorly, this image shows the enlarging submandibular space filled with the submandibular gland, nodes, and facial vein. The submandibular gland, deep portion, extends to fill the posterior margin of the sublingual space on the patient's left.* **(Bottom)** *Low submandibular space axial CECT highlights the full extent of these spaces. Notice how large the submandibular glands become inferiorly. Also note that the anterior bellies of the digastric muscles fill the anteromedial submandibular space.*

TERMINOLOGY

Abbreviations

- Oral mucosal space/surface (OMS)

Definitions

- OMS: Mucosal surface of oral cavity (OC) extending from skin-vermilion junction of lips to junction of hard and soft palate above and to line of circumvallate papillae below

IMAGING ANATOMY

Overview

- OMS is constructed to complete radiologist's thinking regarding OC locations where specific lesions primarily occur
- Since OMS describes mucosal surface of entire oral cavity, it represents continuous sheet of mucosa where squamous cell carcinoma (SCCa) may originate

Extent

- Anterior extent of OMS: Skin-vermilion junction of upper and lower lips
- Posterior extent of OMS
  - Posterosuperior extent: Junction of hard and soft palate
  - Posteroinferior extent: Junction of anterior 2/3 of tongue and posterior 1/3 of tongue at circumvallate papillae
    - Anterior 2/3 of tongue is **oral tongue**
    - Posterior 1/3 of tongue is **lingual tonsil**; part of **oropharynx**

Anatomy Relationships

- OMS represents continuous mucosal surface of OC, which sits anterior to mucosal surface of oropharynx
- Superior OMS overlies hard palate
  - Floor of nose and maxillary sinuses (palatine process of maxillary palatine bones) lie deep to this mucosa
- Inferior OMS overlies sublingual spaces and mylohyoid muscles

Internal Contents

- Oral mucosal space/surface divided into 8 specific areas
  - **Mucosal lip**
    - Lip begins at vermilion border junction with skin
    - Includes only vermilion surface or portion of lip that makes contact with opposing lip
  - **Upper alveolar ridge mucosal surface**
    - Refers to mucosa (gingiva) overlying alveolar process of maxilla
    - Extends from line of attachment of mucosa in upper gingival buccal vestibule to junction of hard palate
    - Posterior margin is upper end of pterygopalatine arch
  - **Lower alveolar ridge mucosal surface**
    - Refers to mucosa (gingiva) overlying alveolar process of mandible
    - Extends from line of attachment of mucosa in buccal vestibule to line of free mucosa of floor of mouth
    - Posteriorly extends to ascending ramus of mandible
  - **Retromolar trigone** mucosal surface
    - Attached mucosa overlying ascending ramus of mandible
    - Extends from level of posterior surface of last molar tooth to apex superiorly, adjacent to tuberosity of maxilla
  - **Buccal mucosa**
    - Includes all membranes that line inner surface of cheeks and lips
    - Extends from line of contact of opposing lips to line of attachment of mucosa of alveolar ridge (upper and lower) and pterygomandibular raphe
  - **Floor of mouth, mucosal surface**
    - Semilunar mucosal surface overlying mylohyoid and hyoglossus muscles
    - Extends from inner surface of lower alveolar ridge to undersurface of tongue
    - Posterior boundary is base of anterior pillar of tonsil
    - Divided into 2 sides by tongue **frenulum**
    - Contains ostia of submandibular and sublingual salivary glands
  - **Hard palate mucosal surface**
    - Semilunar mucosal area between upper alveolar ridge and mucous membrane covering palatine process of maxillary palatine bones
    - Extends from inner surface of superior alveolar ridge to posterior edge of palatine bone
  - **Anterior 2/3 of tongue (oral tongue) mucosal surface**
    - Mucosal surface overlying oral tongue
    - Extends anteriorly from line of circumvallate papillae (anterior edge of lingual tonsil) to undersurface of tongue at junction of mucosal surface of floor of mouth
    - Composed of 4 areas including tongue tip, lateral borders, dorsum, and undersurface (nonvillous oral tongue ventral surface)
- Contents of OMS
  - Mucosal surface of OC
  - **Minor salivary glands** (MSG)
    - Lie within submucosa of OC, paranasal sinuses, pharynx, larynx, trachea, and bronchi
    - Particularly concentrated in buccal, palatal, and lingual submucosal regions
    - Mucinous or seromucinous in nature

Fascia

- **No** fascia exists to define OMS

CLINICAL IMPLICATIONS

Clinical Importance

- Primary malignancies arising from OMS include SCCa and MSG malignancy
- Vast majority of malignancies of OMS are SCCa, while MSG malignancy is relatively rare

GRAPHICS

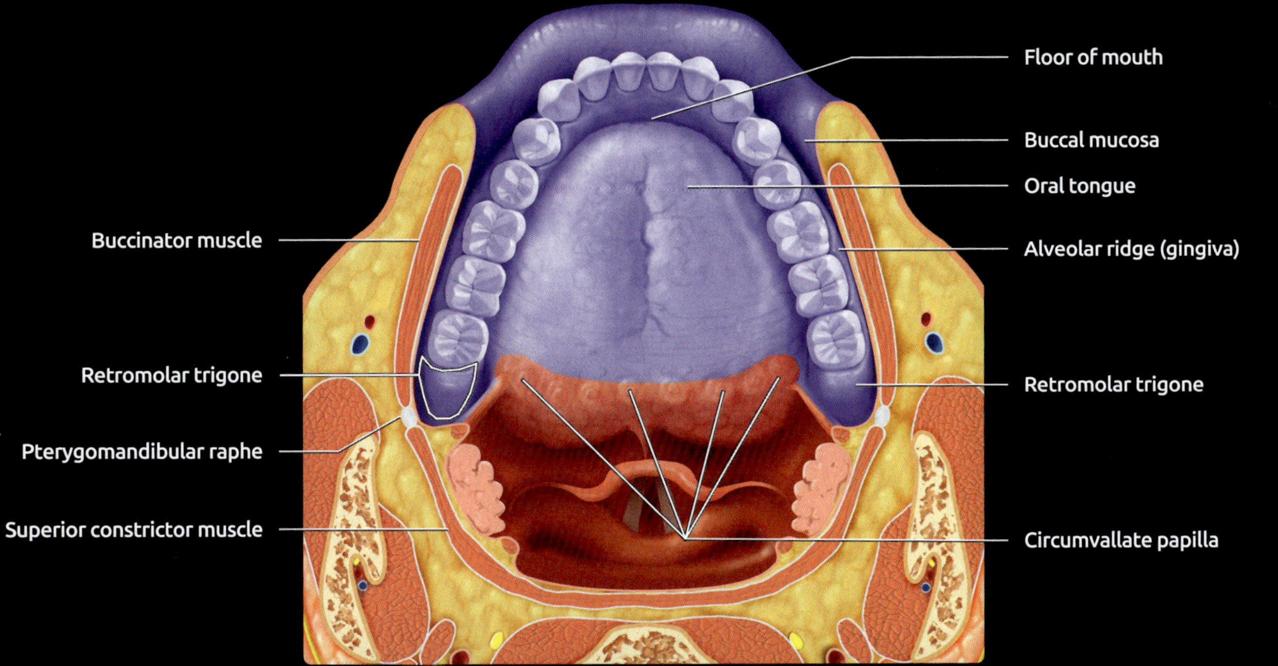

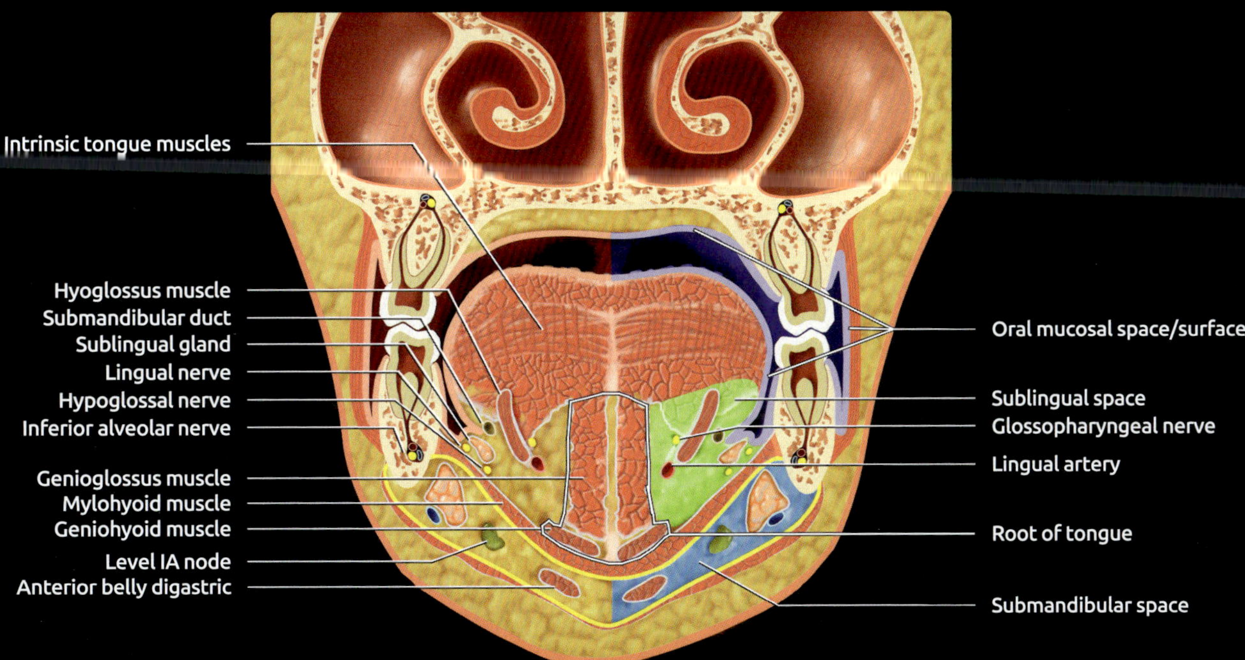

(Top) *View from above shows oral mucosal space/surface shaded in blue. Note that circumvallate papilla, a superficial line of taste buds, divides anterior oral cavity from posterior oropharynx. The lingual tonsil is part of the oropharynx, not the oral cavity. Five squamous cell carcinoma (SCCa) subsites are labeled on the right including the floor of the mouth, buccal mucosa, oral tongue, alveolar ridge (gingiva), and retromolar trigone. Note the pterygomandibular raphe connects the posterior margin of buccinator muscle to anterior margin of the superior pharyngeal constrictor muscle.* **(Bottom)** *In this coronal graphic through the oral cavity, the oral mucosal space/surface is again highlighted in blue. The hard palate, oral tongue, upper and lower alveolar ridge, buccal, and floor of mouth mucosal surfaces are seen. The 4 main areas of the oral cavity [oral mucosal space/surface (blue), sublingual space (green), submandibular space (light blue), and root of tongue] are all present.*

PART I
SECTION 2

Nose and Sinuses

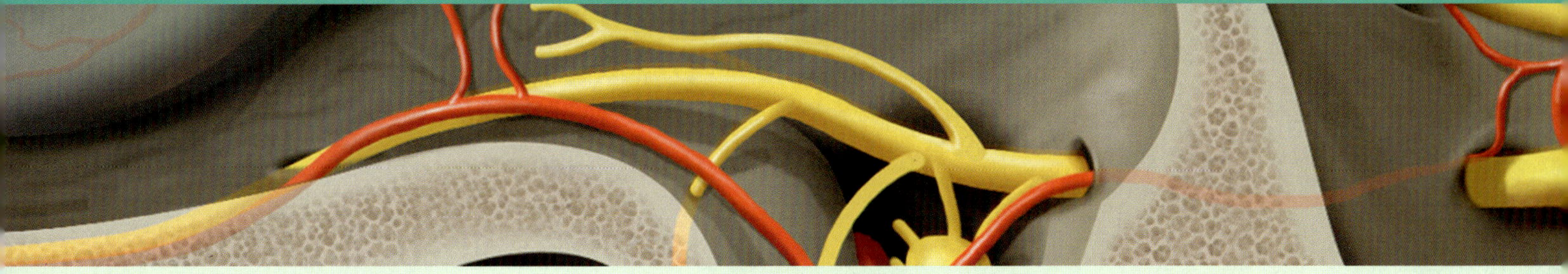

Sinonasal Overview **56**
Ostiomeatal Complex **72**
Pterygopalatine Fossa **76**

TERMINOLOGY

Definitions

- Nasal cavity, paranasal sinuses (maxillary, frontal, ethmoid, and sphenoid), and surrounding structures

IMAGING ANATOMY

Overview

- Nasal cavity: Triangle divided in midline by septum
  - Roof: Cribriform plate
  - Floor: Hard and soft palate
  - Lateral: Lateral nasal wall with attached turbinates
  - Nasal septum
    - Bony septum: Perpendicular plate of ethmoid posterosuperiorly and vomer posteroinferiorly
    - Cartilage: Septal cartilage anteriorly
  - Turbinates
    - Bony superior, middle, and inferior turbinates project inferomedially into nasal cavity
    - Region below each turbinate defined as superior, middle, and inferior meati, respectively
    - Middle turbinate attaches superiorly to cribriform plate via vertical lamella and posteriorly and laterally to lamina papyracea via basal lamella
  - Meati
    - **Superior meatus**: Receives drainage from posterior ethmoid cells at sphenoethmoidal recess
    - **Middle meatus: Ethmoid bulla** is large ethmoid air cell positioned at superior aspect of ostiomeatal complex; receives drainage from anterior ethmoid air cells
    - **Middle meatus: Hiatus semilunaris** is semilunar region between uncinate process and ethmoid bulla; receives drainage from anterior ethmoid air cells and maxillary sinus via infundibulum
    - **Inferior meatus**: Receives drainage from nasolacrimal duct anteriorly

Extent

- Nasal cavity and paranasal sinuses aerate maxillary, frontal, sphenoid, and ethmoid bones

Anatomy Relationships

- **Maxillary sinus**: Paired air cells within maxillary bone
  - Drain via maxillary ostium located along superior aspect of medial wall into infundibulum then into hiatus semilunaris at middle meatus
  - May pneumatize alveolar, zygomatic, frontal, or palatal processes (sinus expansion phenomenon)
  - Septa and grooves of neurovascular canals are commonly seen on intraoral images
- **Ethmoid sinus**: Paired groups of 3-18 air cells within ethmoid labyrinths
  - Separated into anterior and posterior groups divided by basal lamella (lateral attachment of middle turbinate to lamina papyracea)
  - Ethmoid bulla: Dominant anterior ethmoid air cell that protrudes inferomedially into infundibulum or hiatus semilunaris
  - Anterior drainage: Anterior recess of hiatus semilunaris and middle meatus via ethmoid bulla
  - Posterior drainage: Superior meatus and sphenoethmoidal recess
- **Frontal sinus**: Paired air cells within frontal bone
  - Drainage through frontal recess into middle meatus
- **Sphenoid sinus**: Paired air cells within sphenoid bone
  - Drainage into sphenoethmoidal recess
  - Pneumatizes pterygoid process
- Extramural paranasal air cells
  - **Infraorbital ethmoid cells (Haller)**: Ethmoid cells that extend into inferomedial orbital floor
  - **Agger nasi cells**: Most anterior air cells that involve lacrimal bone or maxilla
  - **Sphenoethmoidal cells (Onodi)**: Posterior ethmoid air cells with prominent superolateral pneumatization; close relationship to optic nerve

ANATOMY IMAGING ISSUES

Questions

- Majority of sinonasal imaging depicts complete absence or sporadic (nonobstructive) mild disease

Imaging Recommendations

- Common rhinosinusitis symptoms are best imaged with NECT, bone algorithm, or CBCT
- Sinusitis complications can be imaged with CECT, but CEMR better evaluates surrounding structures

Imaging Approaches

- Coronal sinus CT used in presurgical work-up and follow-up of inflammatory sinonasal disease
- MR: If enhanced scan needed to define complex inflammatory or neoplastic disease, use enhanced MR
  - Fat-saturation should be utilized on at least 1 postcontrast sequence
- Maxillary sinus imaged on intraoral and panoramic radiographs
  - Must be assessed when imaged but insufficient for full evaluation
  - **Identification of all sinus boundaries on panoramic radiographs is imperative**
    - **Absent cortices may be subtle but could be only sign of destructive lesion**
    - Assess zygomatic process of maxilla and pterygomaxillary fissure simultaneously

Imaging Pitfalls

- **Be aware of variations in sinus pneumatization**

CLINICAL IMPLICATIONS

Clinical Importance

- Rhinosinusitis accounts for over 2 million office visits and $2 billion in direct medical costs yearly
- Close proximity between maxillary molar roots and maxillary sinus can lead to referred pain between them
- Risk of displacement of tooth/roots into maxillary sinus or oral-antral communication during extraction
- Dental disease or neoplasm in alveolar process may extend into maxillary sinus
  - Look for periosteal new bone or elevated floor to indicate lesion extrinsic to sinus
  - Sinus loculation may mimic appearance of cyst

GRAPHICS

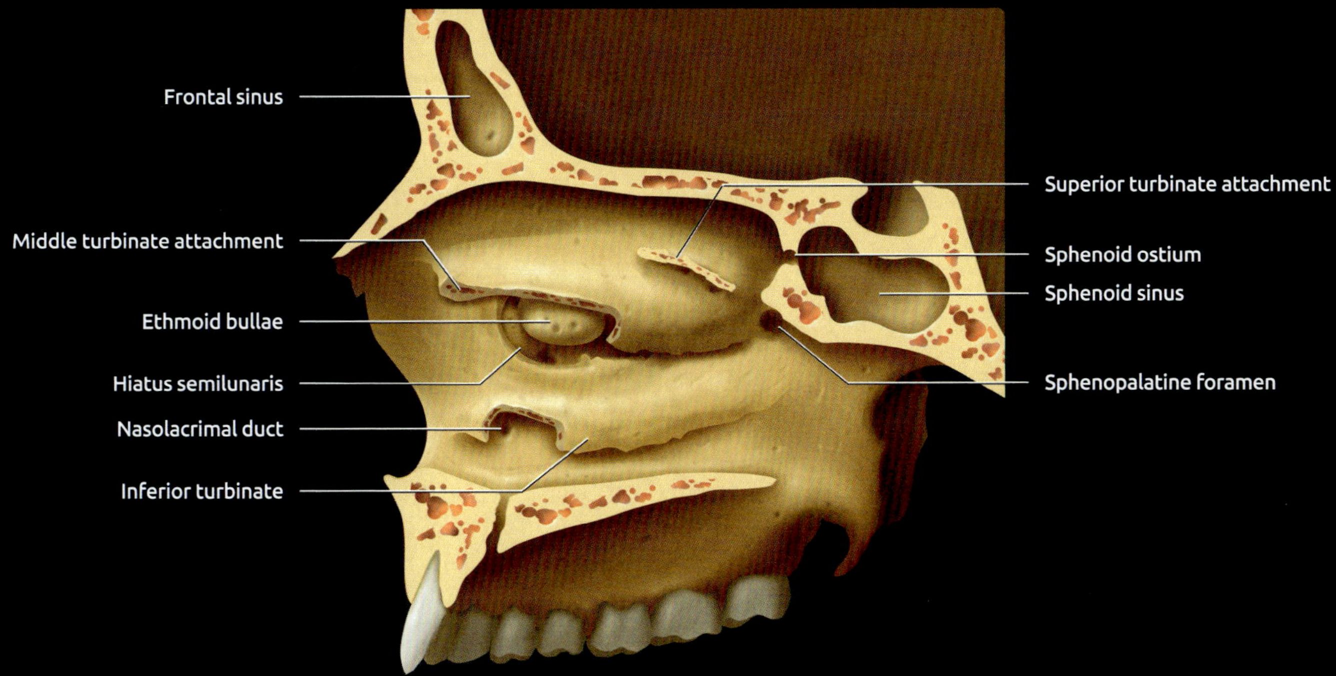

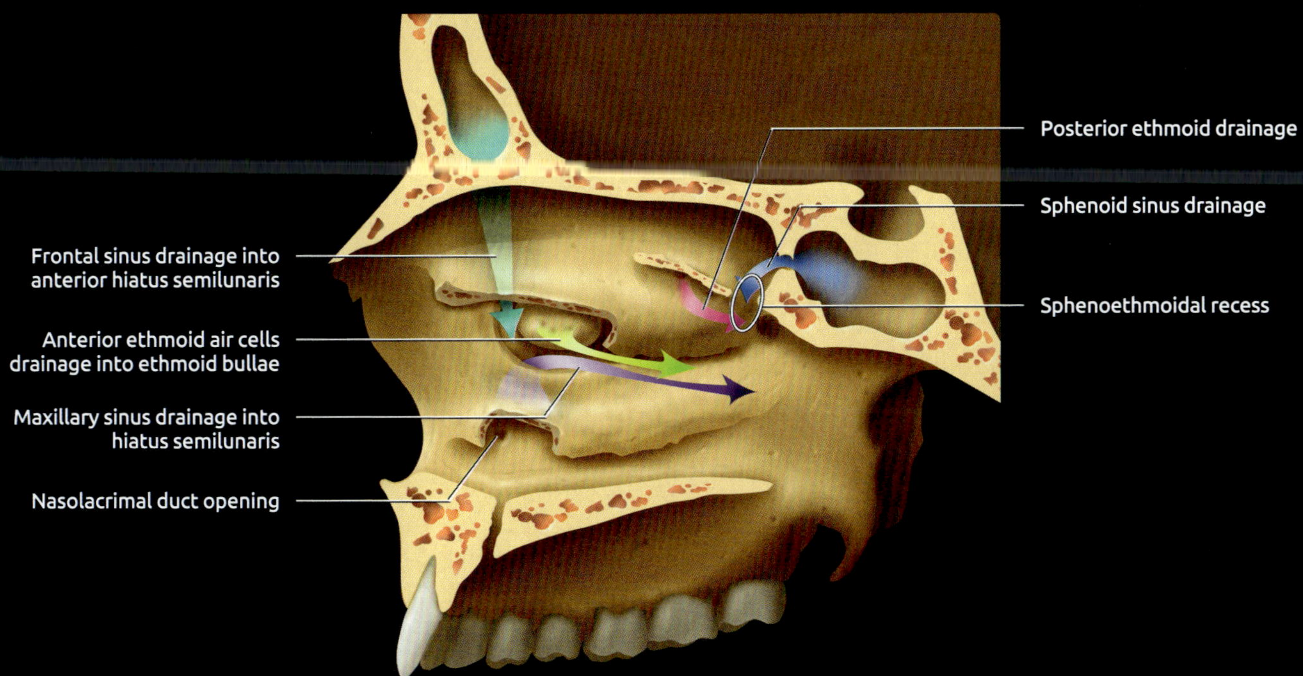

(Top) *Sagittal graphic demonstrates the osseous anatomy of the lateral wall of the nose. The superior and middle turbinates have been resected. The ethmoid bullae and hiatus semilunaris are seen below the middle turbinate attachment. The inferior turbinate has been partially resected to reveal the nasolacrimal duct, which empties into the anterior aspect of the inferior meatus.* **(Bottom)** *Sagittal graphic of the lateral wall of the nose shows the drainage pathways of the sinuses. The sphenoid and posterior ethmoid sinuses drain into the sphenoethmoidal recess in the posterior nasal cavity. The maxillary sinus drains via the maxillary infundibulum while the anterior ethmoids mostly drain through the ethmoid bullae into the ostiomeatal complex/middle meatus. The frontal sinus drains into the anterior middle meatus through the nasofrontal drainage system.*

GRAPHICS

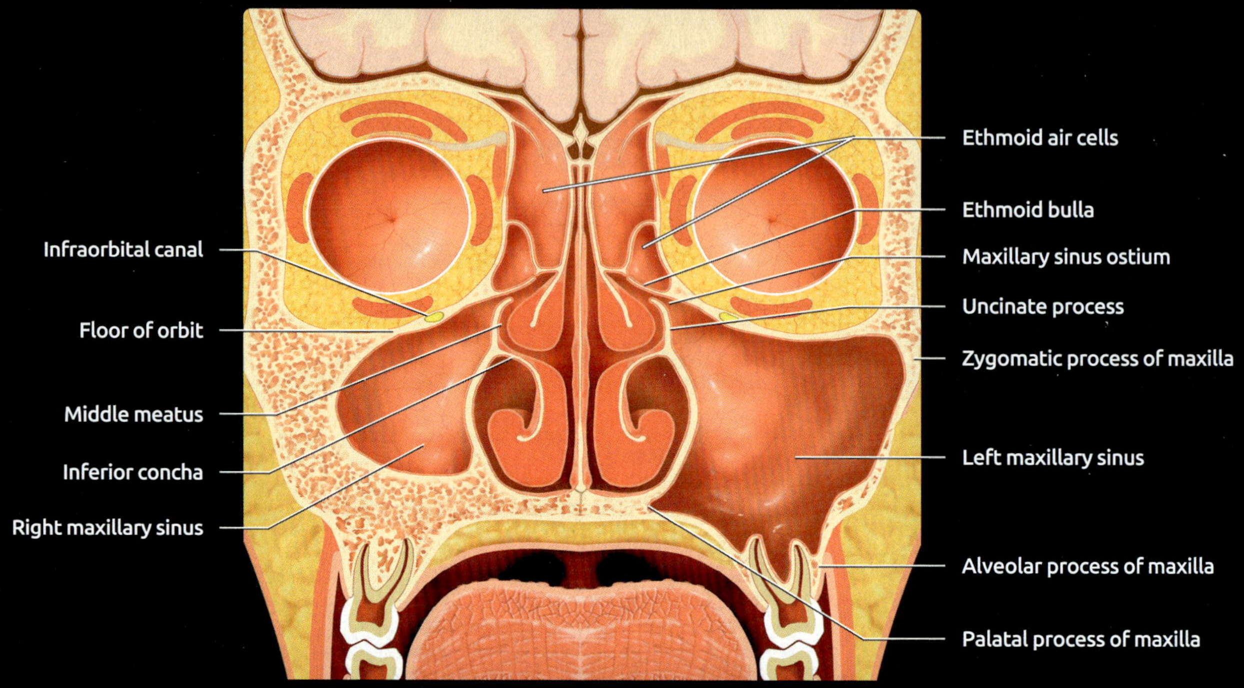

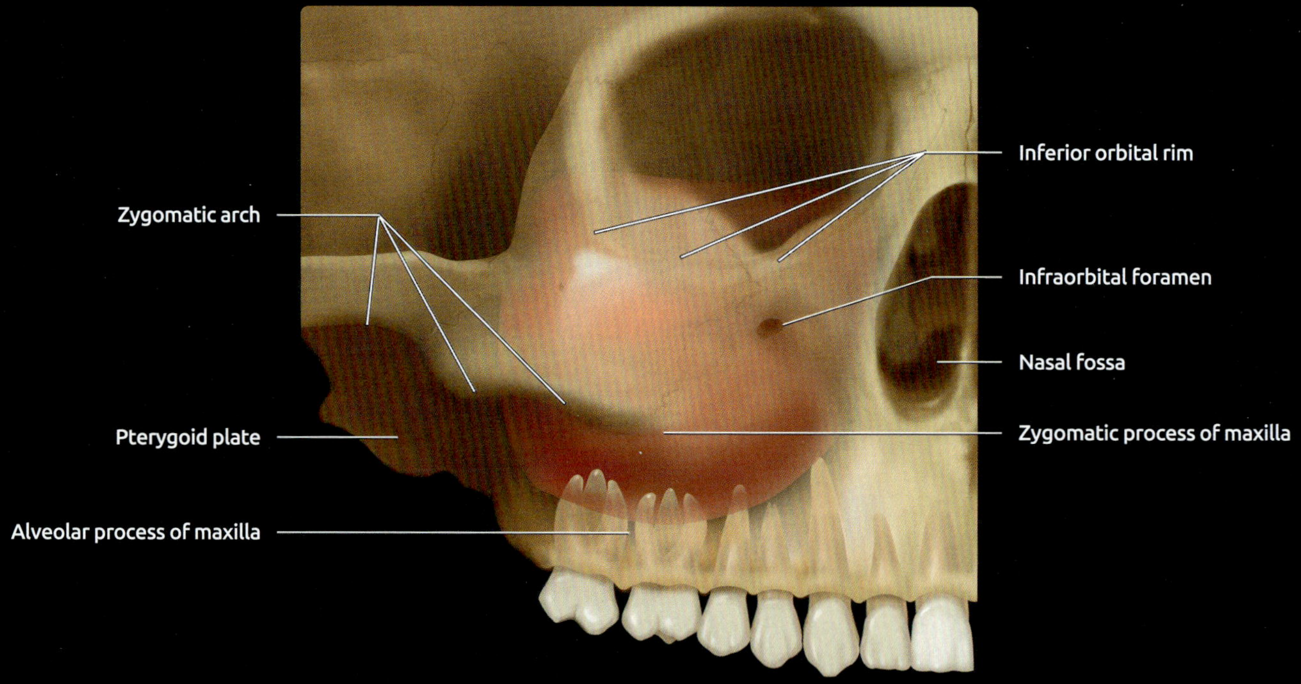

(Top) *Coronal graphic depicts normal size variations of the maxillary sinuses. The right maxillary sinus is hypoplastic while the left sinus has pneumatized the zygomatic, palatal, and alveolar processes. Note the close relationship of the maxillary molar roots to the sinus when the sinus extends into the alveolar process. This may more easily result in the spread of dental disease to involve the sinus. Oral surgical procedures in the region are also more likely to create an oral-antral communication in this situation.* **(Bottom)** *Graphic depicts the relationship of the maxillary sinus to the surrounding osseous structures and teeth from the perspective of a panoramic radiograph. The sinus generally extends anteroposteriorly from the lateral nasal wall to the posterolateral wall of the maxilla and superoinferiorly from the floor of the orbit to the alveolar process. The zygomatic process of the maxilla and zygomatic arch are superimposed over the sinus.*

MAXILLARY SINUS VARIATIONS

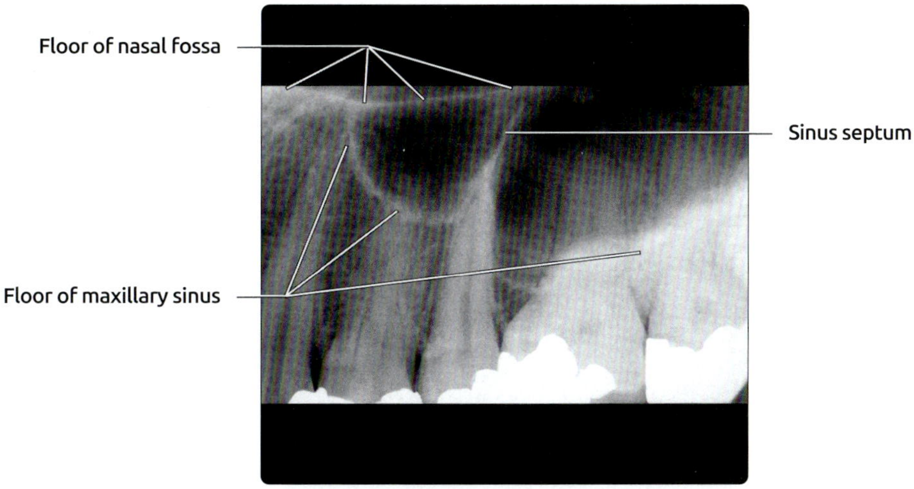

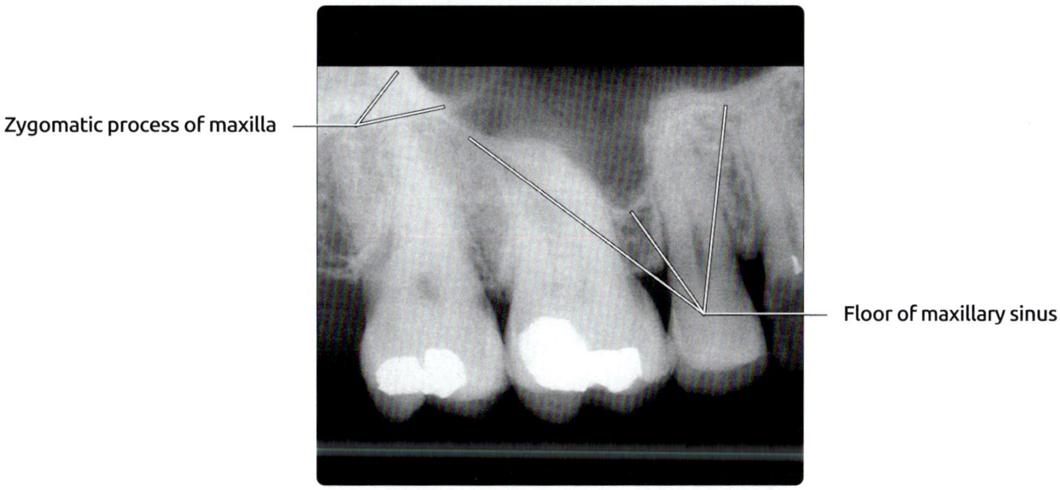

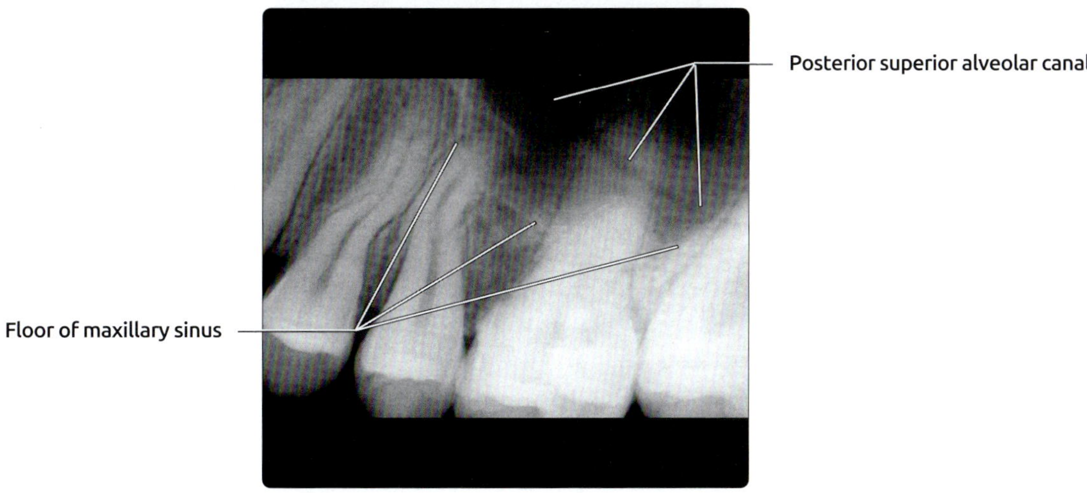

(Top) *This is the 1st of 3 periapical radiographs showing normal variations of the maxillary sinus. This image demonstrates the "inverted Y" created where the floor of the nasal fossa crosses the floor of the maxillary sinus. A sinus septum is also seen apical to the 2nd premolar tooth.* **(Middle)** *This periapical radiograph shows a normal variation in the morphology of the floor of the maxillary sinus, which has pneumatized the alveolar process between the 1st molar and 2nd premolar teeth. The zygomatic process of the maxilla, which is commonly superimposed on the sinus in posterior maxillary periapical radiographs as a thick, curved radiopaque line, is also seen in this image.* **(Bottom)** *This radiograph shows a linear radiolucency crossing the maxillary sinus. This represents the posterior superior alveolar canal, found in the wall of the sinus, which carries the posterior superior alveolar nerves and vessels. This structure may be mistaken for a fracture if not recognized as normal anatomy.*

MAXILLARY SINUS VARIATIONS

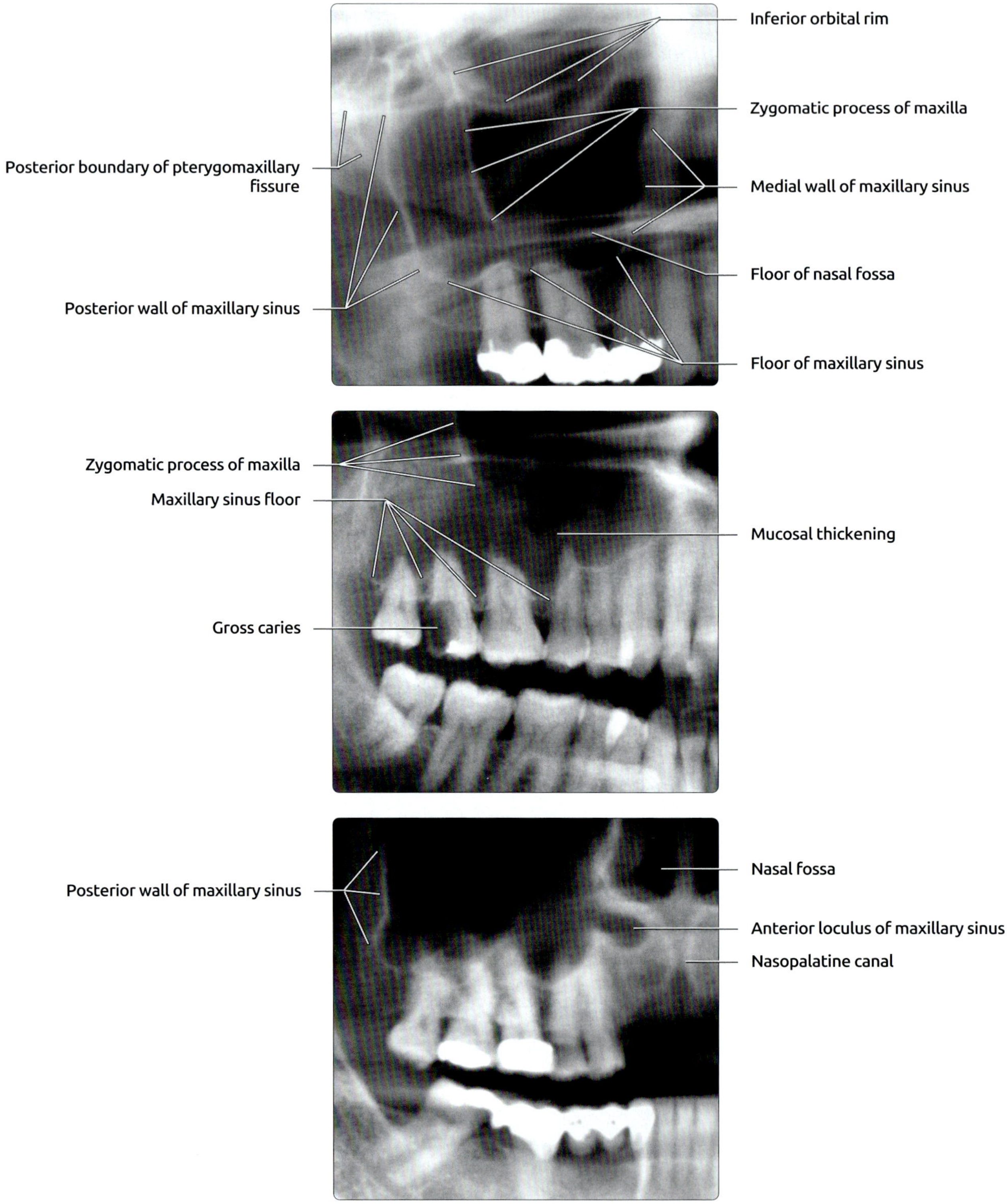

(Top) *Cropped panoramic radiograph shows a normal appearance of the maxillary sinus. Note there are many structures superimposed on the image of the sinus, making its visualization challenging. When examining a panoramic radiograph, it is essential to always assess the cortical boundaries of the maxillary sinus to rule out any pathology that could cause their destruction. The radiopaque lines formed by the images of the zygomatic process of the maxilla and the posterior boundary of the pterygomaxillary fissure run nearly parallel to the posterior wall of the maxillary sinus. These 3 lines should be assessed together to ensure they are all present and normal.* **(Middle)** *Cropped panoramic radiograph shows a maxillary sinus that has pneumatized the alveolar process around the molars. Mucosal thickening is noted and is suggestive of sinus inflammation.* **(Bottom)** *CBCT panoramic reformat shows anterior sinus extension to the anterior maxilla. This is an important variation to note when treatment planning an implant fixture in the incisor region.*

MAXILLARY SINUS VARIATIONS

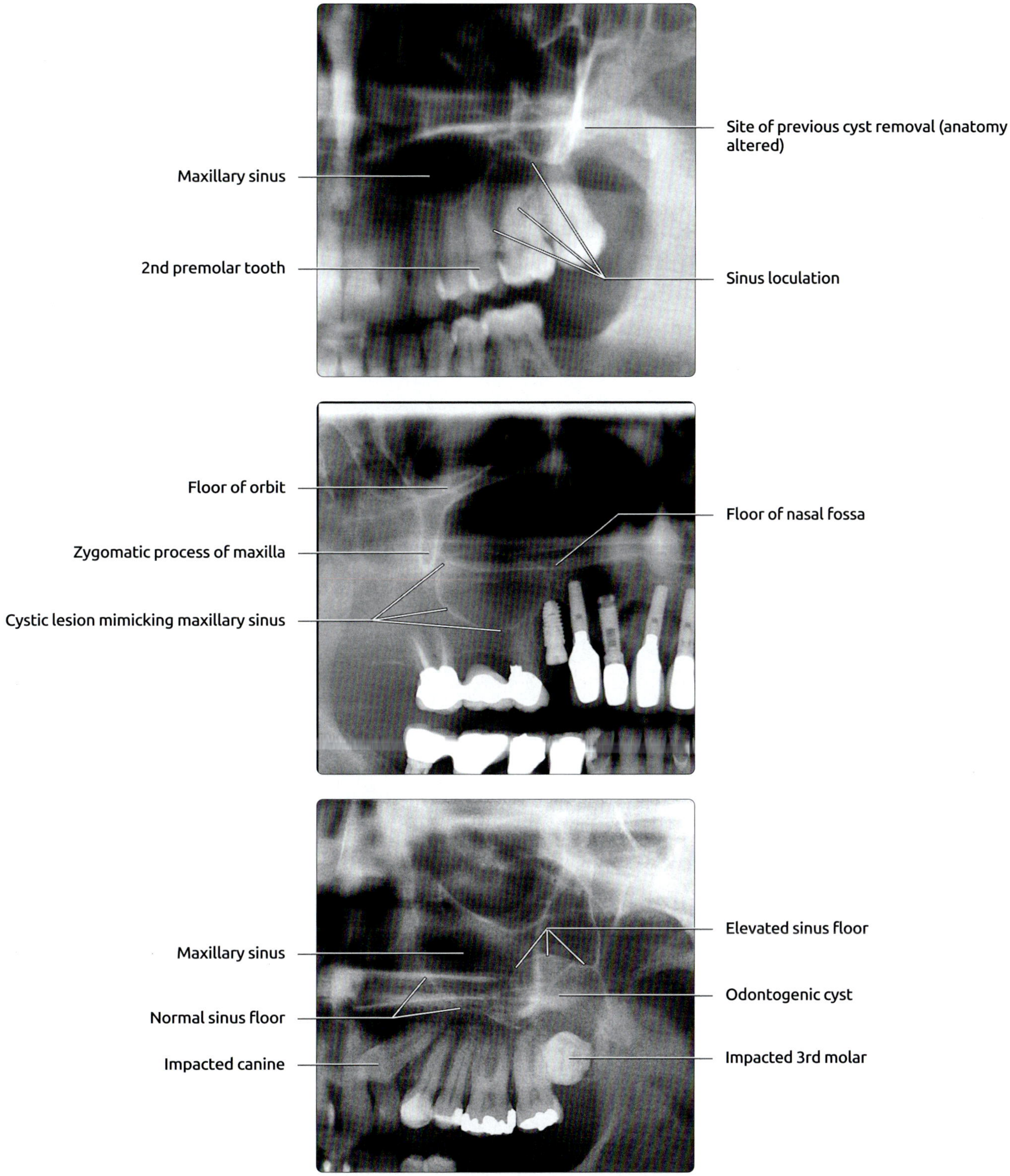

(Top) *Cropped panoramic radiograph in a patient under investigation for recurrent odontogenic cysts is shown. This well-defined, corticated radiolucency between the 2nd premolar and 1st molar proved to be a sinus loculation. Note that there are no effects on the teeth (displacement or resorption), which supports this diagnosis of an anatomic variation.* **(Middle)** *Cropped panoramic radiograph demonstrates a well-defined, corticated radiolucency in the right alveolar process where the normal maxillary sinus would be expected. In this case, this was a cystic lesion mimicking a normal sinus floor. The patient's right maxillary sinus is hypoplastic.* **(Bottom)** *Cropped panoramic radiograph demonstrates elevation of the floor of the maxillary sinus caused by an odontogenic cyst related to the impacted 3rd molar. Lesions in the maxillary sinuses that originate outside the sinus and those coming from the alveolar process will appear corticated when they extend into the sinus due to periosteal reaction appearing as a displacement of the cortical boundary.*

SINONASAL VARIATIONS

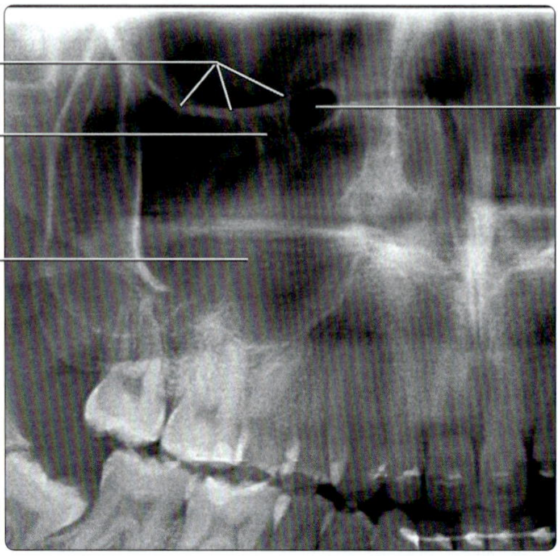

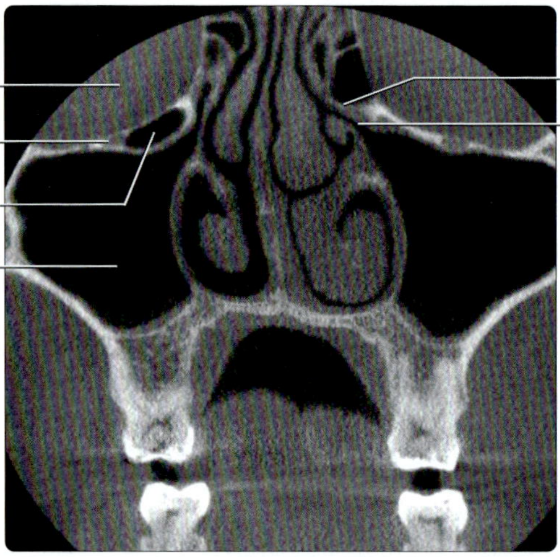

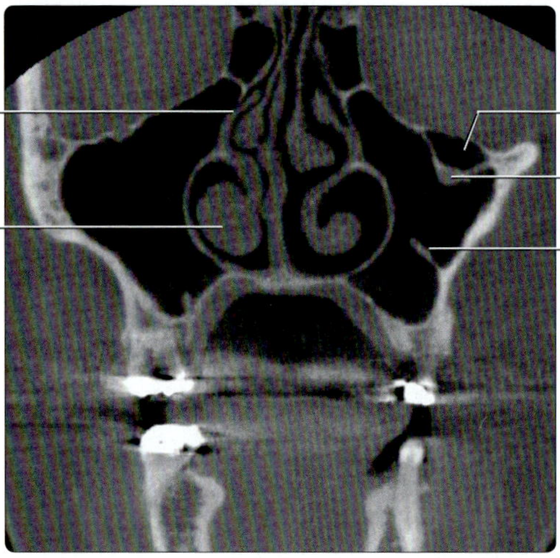

(Top) *Cropped panoramic radiograph shows an infraorbital ethmoid (Haller) cell just medial to the infraorbital canal. This is a variation of normal.* **(Middle)** *Coronal CBCT shows an infraorbital ethmoid (Haller) cell on the right side. This is a variation of normal anatomy that should be considered in the case of large Haller cells blocking the infundibulum and compromising the drainage pathway of the maxillary sinus. This should also be considered if sinus surgery is planned to avoid entering the orbit.* **(Bottom)** *Coronal CBCT shows an infraorbital ethmoid (Haller) cell on the left. Note that the left infraorbital canal is displaced inferiorly due to this air cell. There is also a sinus septum extending from the anterolateral border of the left maxillary sinus. These anatomic variants should be considered if sinus surgery is planned.*

SINONASAL VARIATIONS

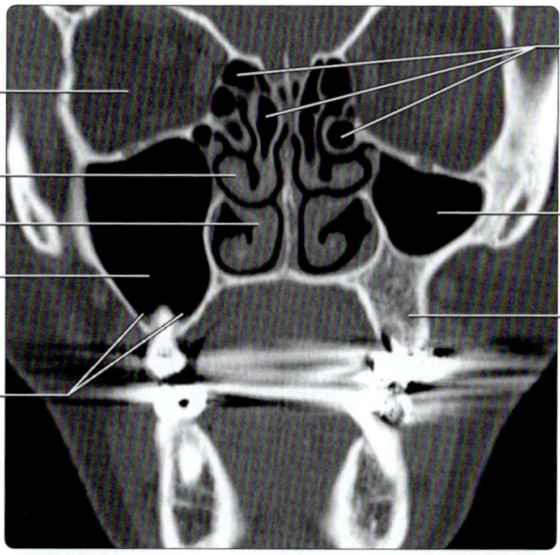

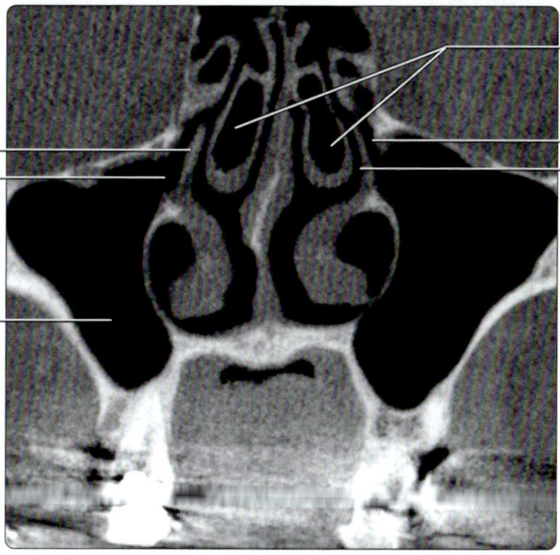

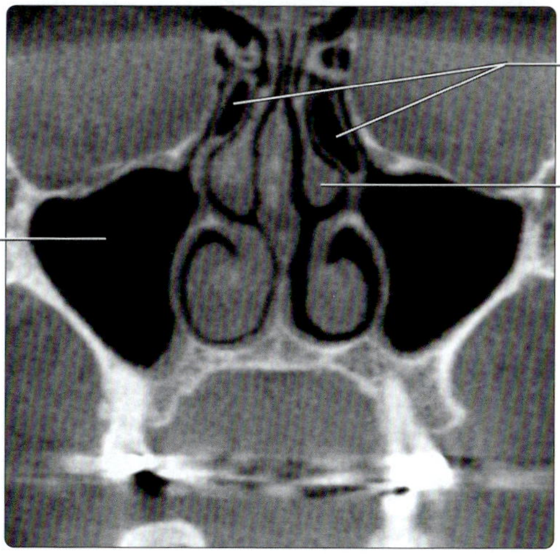

(Top) *Coronal CT shows asymmetry in the size of the right and left maxillary sinuses. The left sinus is hypoplastic. This is a normal anatomic variation. Maxillary sinus hypoplasia can in some cases result in a change of the maxillary boundaries and alveolar process dimensions (maxillary hypoplasia).* **(Middle)** *Coronal CBCT shows pneumatization of the middle turbinates of the ethmoid bone. These are known as concha bullosa. This is a variation of normal anatomy, but in some patients the bulk of these concha may block normal drainage of the maxillary sinus into the middle meatus or narrow the lumen of the nasal cavity reducing the flow of air.* **(Bottom)** *Coronal CBCT shows pneumatization of the uncinate processes of the ethmoid bones. This variation could also potentially obstruct maxillary sinus drainage. There is no sinus disease evident in this patient.*

CORONAL BONE CT

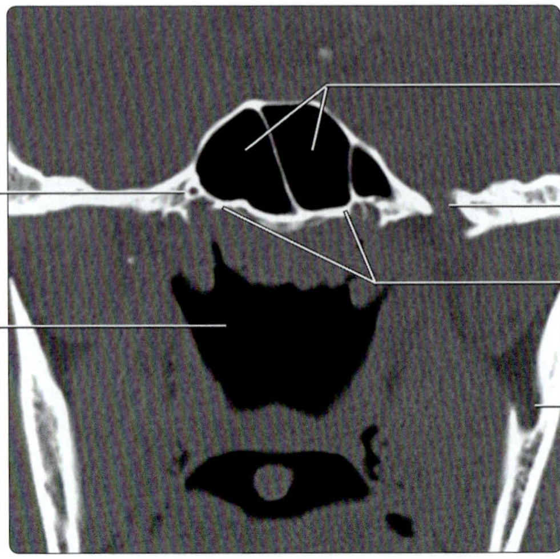

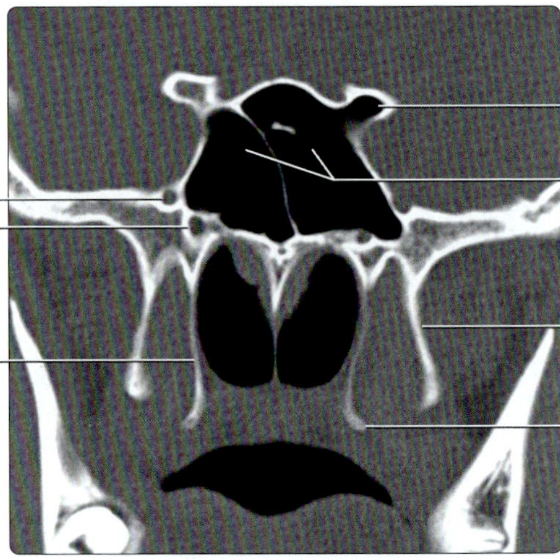

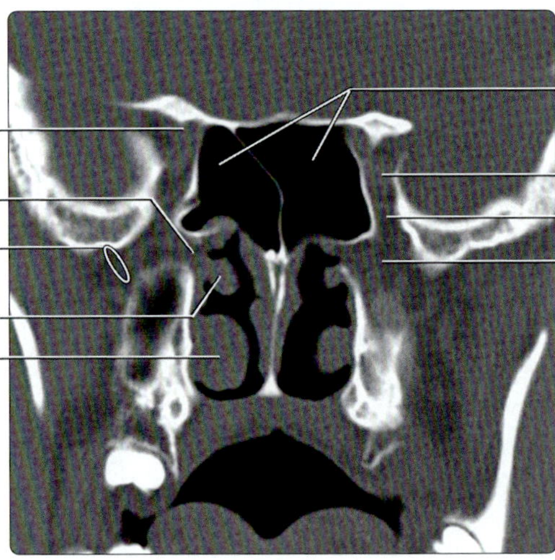

(Top) *This is the 1st of 9 coronal bone CT noncontrast images through the paranasal sinuses, presented from posterior to anterior. This image shows the sphenoid sinuses, superior to the nasopharynx.* **(Middle)** *This image shows the pterygoid plates, posterior to the maxillary sinuses. Note the foramen rotundum and the vidian canal inferolateral to the sphenoid sinus.* **(Bottom)** *This image shows the complex anatomic landscape surrounding the pterygopalatine fossa (PPF). The lateral exit of the PPF is the pterygomaxillary fissure through which it enters into the masticator space. Superiorly, the PPF exits into the inferior orbital fissure. The medial exit from the PPF is through the sphenopalatine foramen into the posterolateral nose.*

CORONAL BONE CT

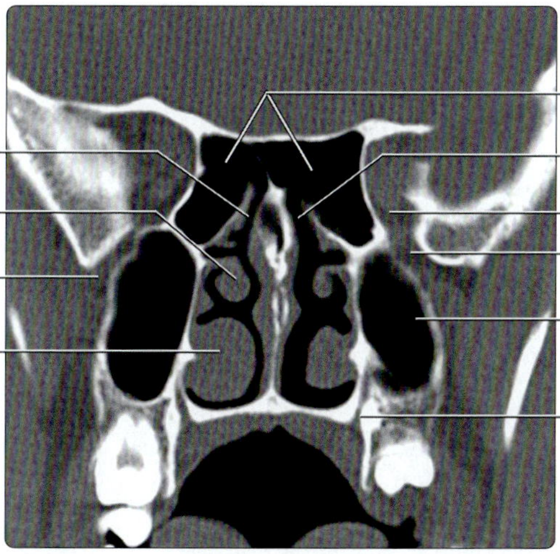

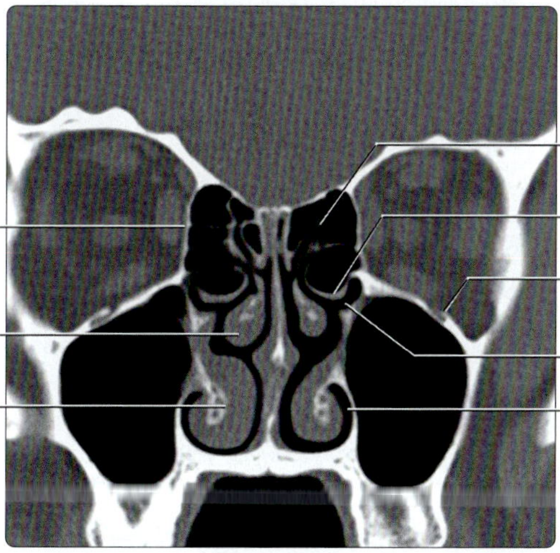

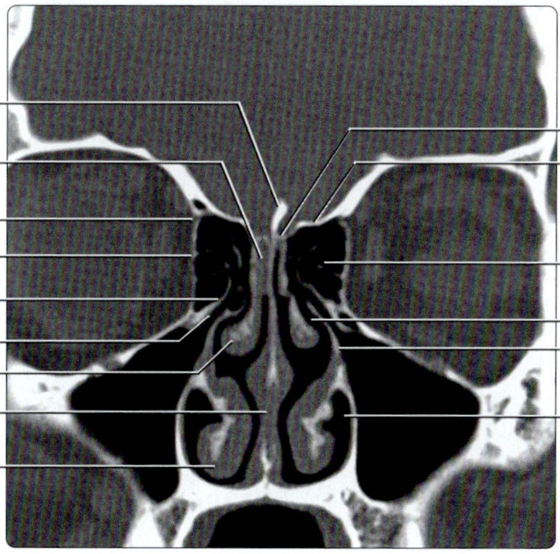

(Top) *In this image, the sphenoethmoidal recesses are visible as vertical, air-filled slits in the posterosuperior nose into which both the posterior ethmoid sinus and the sphenoid sinus empty. Note the greater palatine canal exiting the lateral hard-soft palate junction. Perineural malignancy may travel from the palate to the pterygopalatine fossa via the greater palatine nerve.* **(Middle)** *In this image through the anterior ethmoid air cells, the ethmoid bulla is seen projecting inferiorly into the middle meatus. The shared wall between the anterior ethmoid air cells and the orbit is paper thin, hence the term lamina papyracea.* **(Bottom)** *Image through the ostiomeatal complex (OMC) shows the maxillary infundibulum draining the maxillary sinuses into the middle meatus. The uncinate process, middle meatus, maxillary infundibulum, and ethmoid bulla are the components of the OMC.*

CORONAL BONE CT

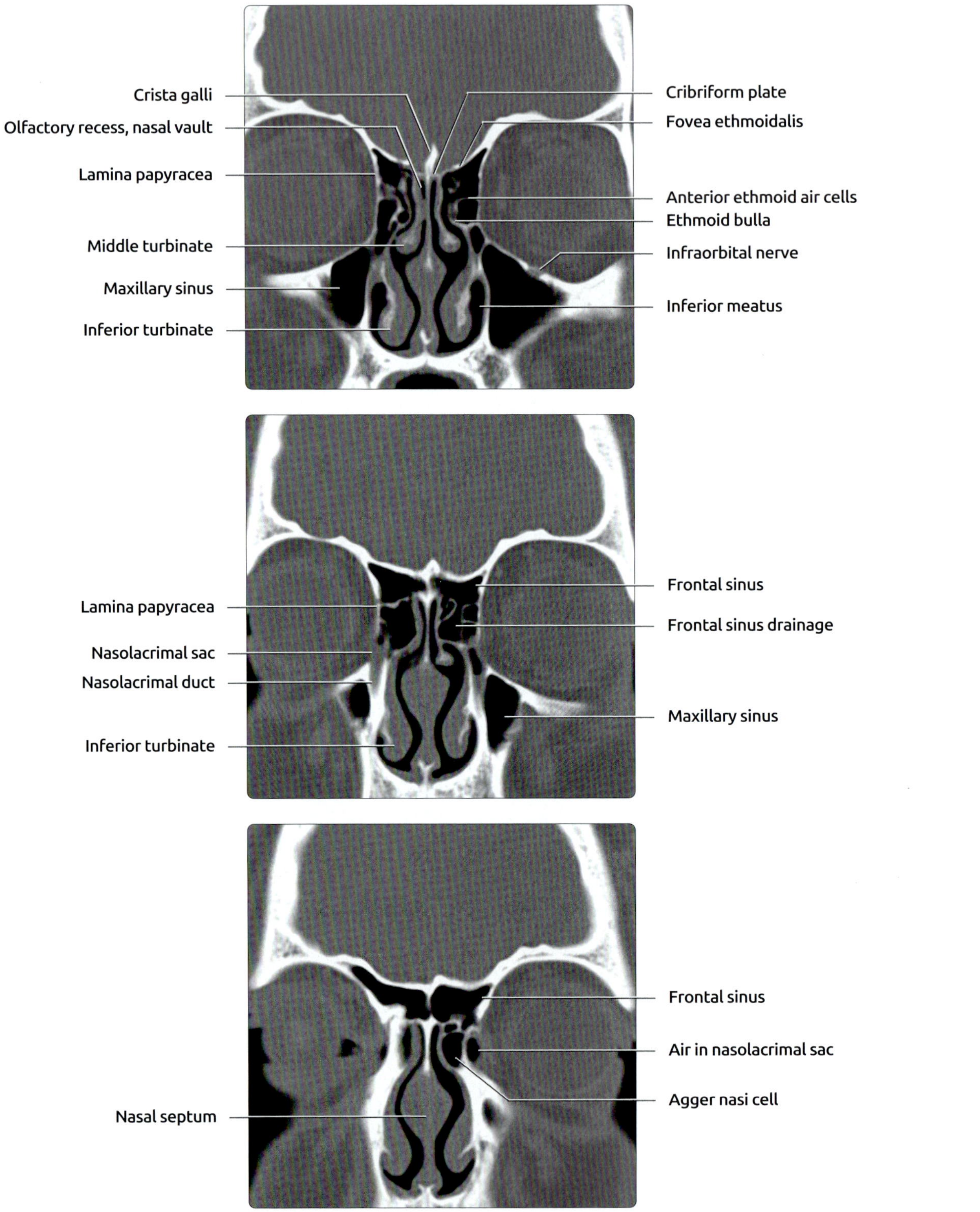

(Top) *In this image through the anterior aspect of the anterior ethmoid complex, the fovea ethmoidalis (roof of ethmoid), cribriform plate, and crista galli can all be seen along the roof of the sinuses and nose from lateral to medial. The olfactory recess of the nasal vault contains the nasal mucosa. From the nasal mucosa arises esthesioneuroblastoma.* **(Middle)** *This image shows the close relationship of the nasolacrimal ducts to the maxillary sinuses. Remember that the nasolacrimal duct drains into the anterior recess of the inferior meatus.* **(Bottom)** *In this image through the frontal sinuses, the anteroinferior extramural ethmoid air cells (a.k.a. agger nasi air cells) can be seen. Notice the normal, air-filled, left nasolacrimal sac just lateral to the agger nasi cells.*

AXIAL T1 MR

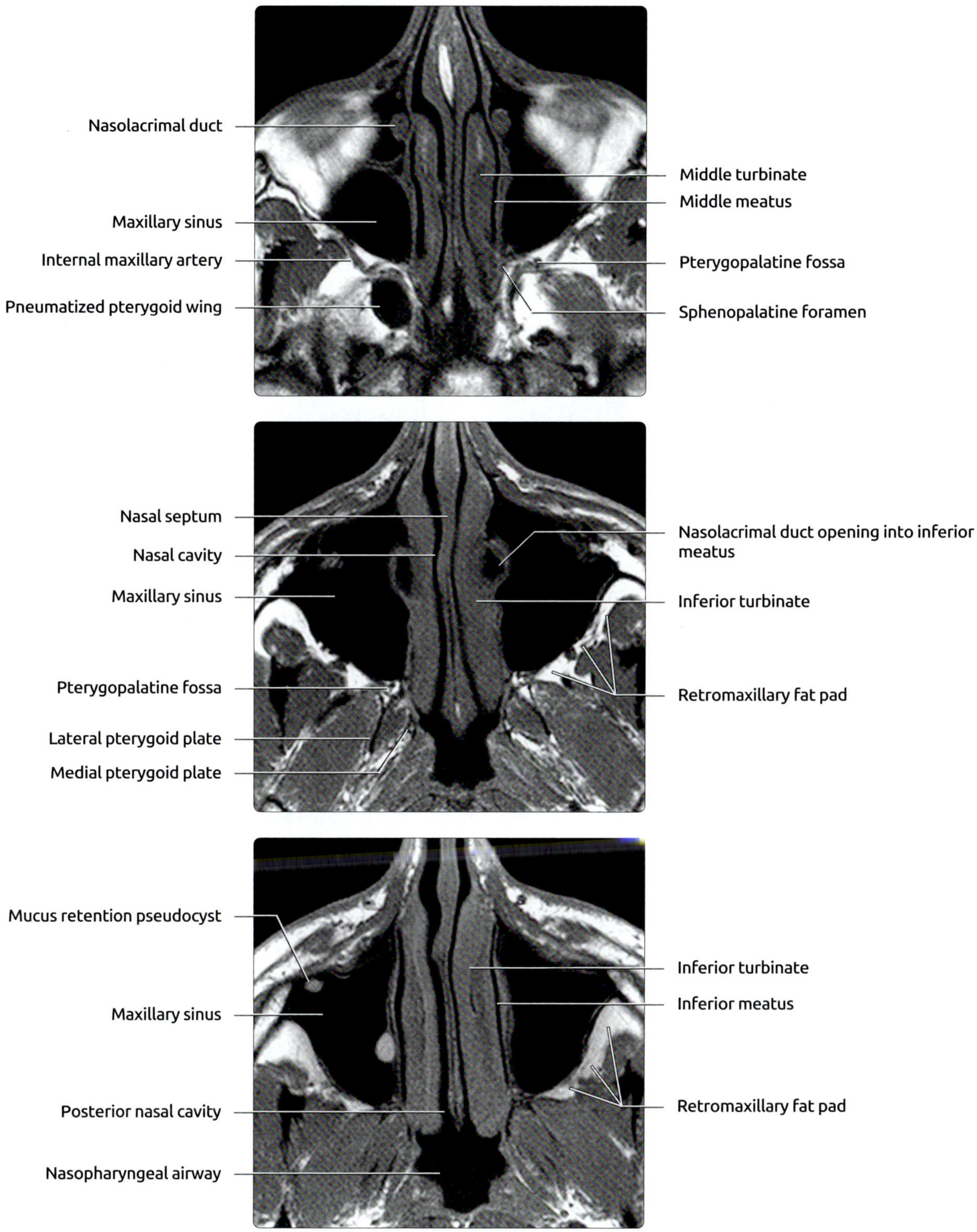

(Top) *At the level of the pterygopalatine fossa, the internal maxillary artery can be seen as its principal occupant. The medial exit from the pterygopalatine fossa is the sphenopalatine foramen. Juvenile angiofibroma originates along the nasal margin of the sphenopalatine foramen. Often, the 1st route of spread for this tumor is through this foramen into the pterygopalatine fossa.* **(Middle)** *In this image, the nasolacrimal duct is visible emptying inferiorly into the anterior recess of the inferior meatus. The inferior turbinate is the largest of the turbinates and can be mistaken for a mass when large and asymmetric.* **(Bottom)** *At the level of the mid maxillary sinus, the posterior nasal cavity can be seen in direct continuity with the nasopharyngeal airway. The retromaxillary fat pad sits behind the maxillary sinus. It is the superior extension of the buccal space.*

TERMINOLOGY

Abbreviations

- Ostiomeatal complex (OMC)

Definitions

- Ostiomeatal unit (OMU): Complex anatomic region where drainage of frontal, anterior ethmoid, and maxillary sinuses occurs

IMAGING ANATOMY

Overview

- OMU includes superomedial maxillary sinus, maxillary infundibulum, uncinate process, ethmoid bulla, hiatus semilunaris, and middle meatus

Extent

- OMU is area superolateral to middle meatus that receives drainage of frontal, anterior ethmoid, and maxillary sinuses

Anatomy Relationships

- **Middle meatus** is most complicated of meati, receiving drainage from multiple sinuses
  - **Anterior ethmoid air cells** drain mostly into **ethmoid bulla**
    - **Ethmoid bulla**: Large ethmoid air cell positioned at superior aspect of OMU, immediately superior to hiatus semilunaris
  - **Frontal sinus** drains into anterior aspect of middle meatus
    - If uncinate process inserts on middle turbinate or skull base, frontal sinus drains through **frontal recess** into ethmoid infundibulum and then middle meatus
    - If uncinate process inserts on lamina papyracea, frontal recess drains into anterior middle meatus directly
    - **Frontal recess**: Drainage funnel for frontal sinus
  - **Maxillary sinus** drains through maxillary infundibulum into middle meatus via maxillary ostium
- **Hiatus semilunaris**: Semilunar trough between tip of uncinate process and ethmoid bulla seen best from endoscopic vantage point
  - Hiatus semilunaris difficult to see on coronal sinus CT

Internal Contents

- **Middle meatus**: Space between middle turbinate and medial wall of maxillary sinus
- **Maxillary infundibulum**: Drainage channel of maxillary sinus
  - Defined laterally by orbit and medially by uncinate process
  - Drains into middle meatus via **maxillary ostium**
- **Uncinate process**: Upper medial maxillary sinus wall
  - Defines medial wall of maxillary infundibulum
- **Ethmoid bulla**: Dominant anterior ethmoid air cell that protrudes inferomedially into infundibulum and upper middle meatus
- Normal aeration variants in vicinity of OMU
  - **Concha bullosa**: Aeration of nasal turbinate, most commonly **middle turbinate**
    - When inflamed, concha bullosa may obstruct OMU at middle meatus
    - Complete obstructive OMU pattern with frontal, maxillary, and anterior ethmoid opacification
  - **Haller cell** (infraorbital ethmoid air cell): Air cell located inferolateral to orbit and lateral to maxillary infundibulum
    - When inflamed, may obstruct maxillary infundibulum creating isolated maxillary infundibular pattern of sinus disease
    - Infundibular pattern: Only maxillary sinus is diseased with sparing of ethmoid sinuses
  - **Agger nasi** air cells: Most anterior ethmoid air cells
    - Found lateral to lamina papyracea, adjacent to frontal recess
    - When inflamed, agger nasi air cells may obstruct frontal recess, causing isolated opacification of frontal sinus without involving anterior ethmoid or maxillary sinuses

ANATOMY IMAGING ISSUES

Questions

- Sinus CT used in presurgical work-up and follow-up of inflammatory sinonasal disease

Imaging Recommendations

- Common rhinosinusitis symptom cases are best imaged with bone algorithm CT or CBCT
  - Coronal plane CT optimally depicts OMU

Imaging Approaches

- Multislice scanners can acquire thin (1 mm) supine sections with reconstruction of coronal and sagittal images
- If only older scanner available, prone hyperextended coronal acquisitions may be preferable to move potential fluid in maxillary sinus away from OMU
- CBCT in upright position moves fluid away from OMU

CLINICAL IMPLICATIONS

Clinical Importance

- Sinus disease is single most common chronic complaint in USA
  - OMU is most important anatomic region for potential surgical treatment
- Clinical presentation of OMU obstruction
  - Facial fullness, pressure, loss of sense of smell, and postnasal drainage
- OMU can also be obstructed secondary to anatomic variations or local noninfectious inflammatory processes, such as allergic rhinitis

Function Dysfunction

- Normal mucociliary pattern within paranasal sinuses is movement of secretions toward natural ostia
- Recirculation disorders may result despite endoscopic creation of surgical ostia

CORONAL AND SAGITTAL OSTIOMEATAL COMPLEX GRAPHICS

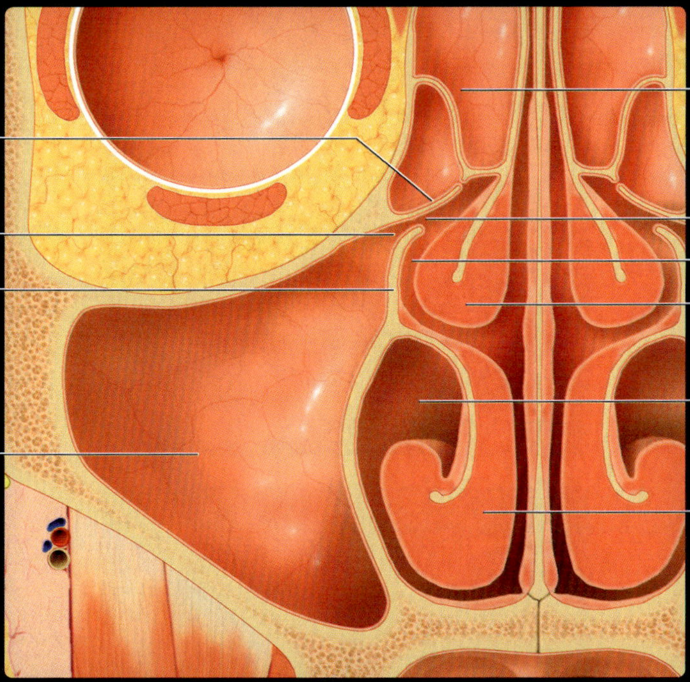

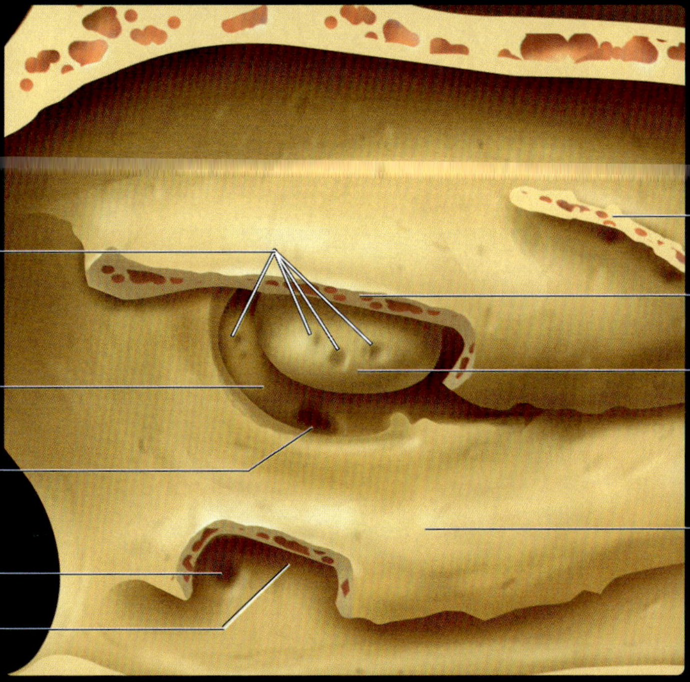

(Top) *Coronal graphic of the magnified right sinonasal area illustrates the important structures of the ostiomeatal unit. Note that the maxillary infundibulum provides drainage for the maxillary sinus, while the ethmoid bulla (dominant ethmoid air cell of anterior ethmoid complex) protrudes inferomedially into the upper middle meatus. The middle meatus is the key area for drainage of normal secretions of the anterior ethmoid sinuses and the maxillary sinus.* **(Bottom)** *Graphic of the lateral wall of the nose is focused on the region of the middle meatus with the superior turbinate removed as well as part of the middle turbinate. Note that the anterior ethmoid ostia drain into the middle meatus as does the maxillary sinus via the maxillary infundibulum. The nasolacrimal duct drains into the inferior meatus.*

NORMAL CORONAL BONE CT OF OSTIOMEATAL COMPLEX

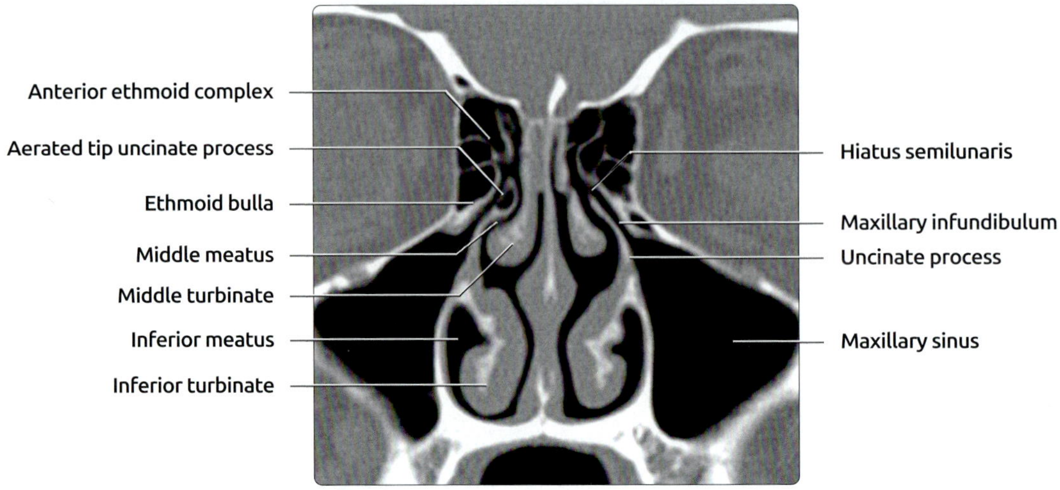

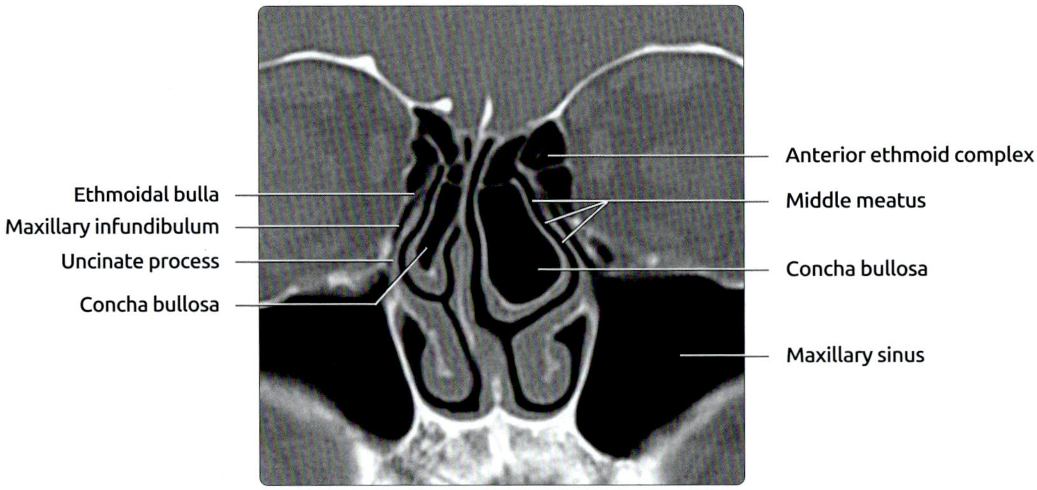

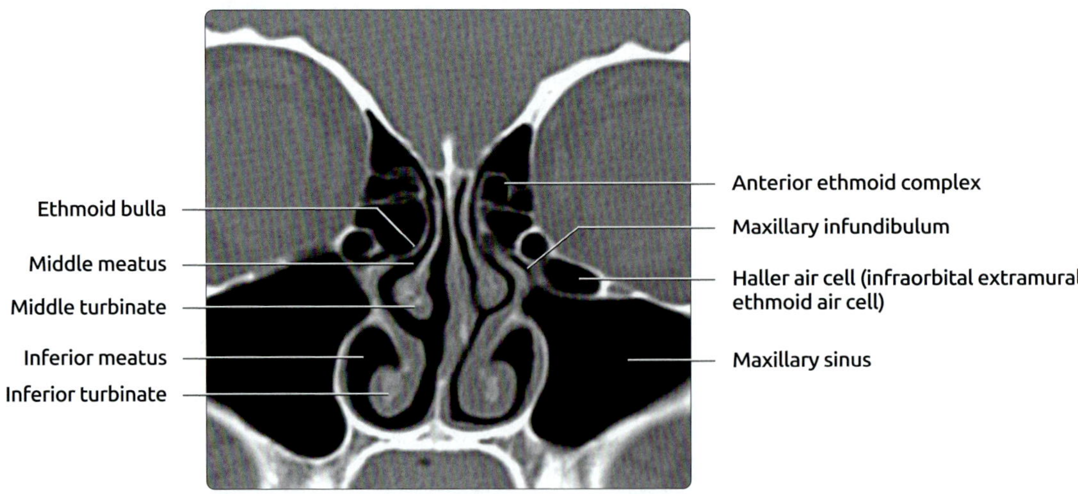

(Top) *First of 3 coronal bone CT images through the normal ostiomeatal complex shows the typical appearance of the maxillary infundibulum and ethmoid bulla. Notice that the right superior tip of the uncinate process is pneumatized.* **(Middle)** *In this image, bilateral aerated uncomplicated concha bullosa are visible. Notice the attenuated maxillary infundibulum. If the concha bullosa becomes infected (complicated), early obstruction of the middle meatus causes opacification of the ipsilateral maxillary, anterior ethmoid, and frontal sinuses.* **(Bottom)** *Image through a normal ostiomeatal unit shows a Haller air cell (infraorbital air cell) protruding into the maxillary infundibulum. If the Haller cell becomes infected, it can cause an infundibular pattern of sinus disease where the maxillary sinus is opacified without ethmoid involvement.*

NORMAL SAGITTAL BONE CT OF OSTIOMEATAL COMPLEX

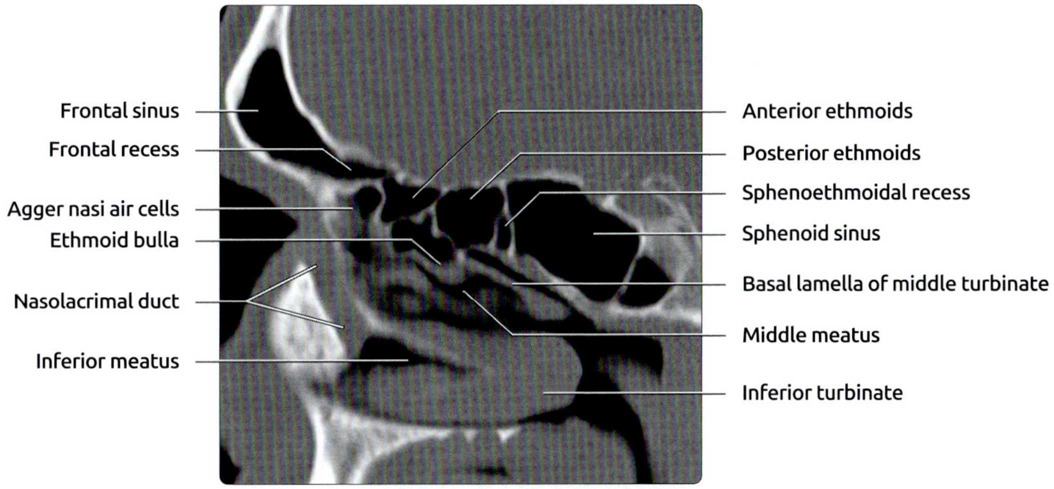

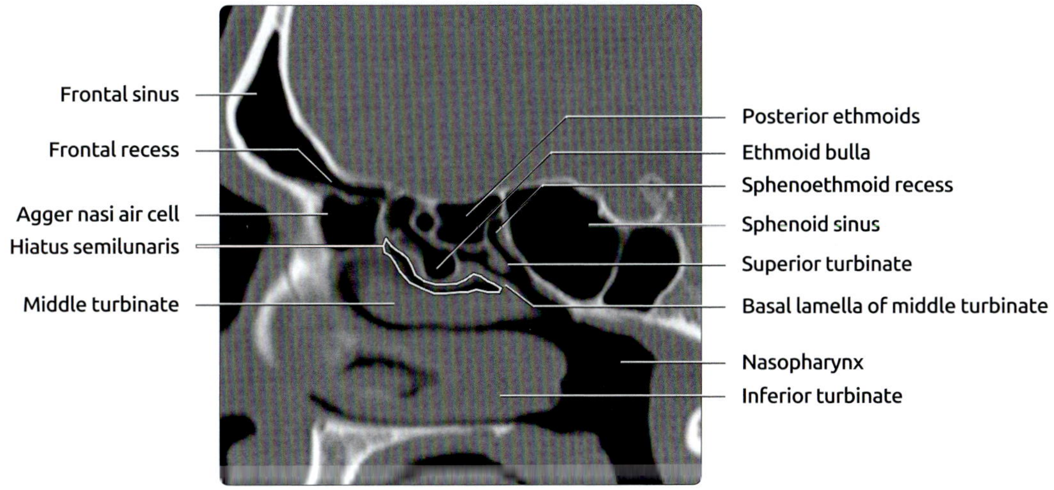

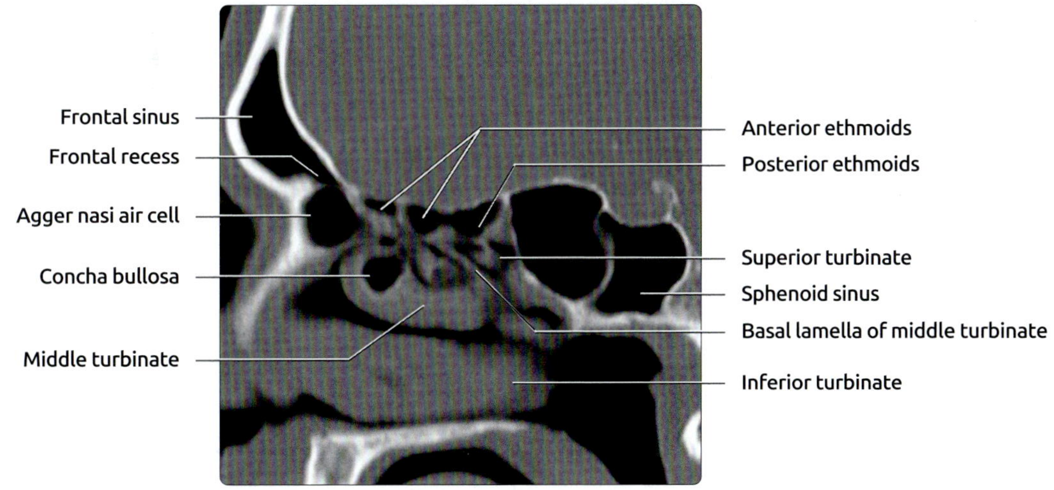

(Top) *First of 3 sagittal bone CT reformations of the sinonasal region presents from lateral to medial, demonstrating the structures of the ostiomeatal unit and its vicinity. In this image, the middle meatus can be seen just inferior to the ethmoid bulla. The nasolacrimal duct is visible emptying inferiorly into the anterior aspect of the inferior meatus.* **(Middle)** *In this image, middle and inferior turbinates, as well as the basal lamella of the middle turbinate, are seen. Also note the curvilinear hiatus semilunaris. The frontal recess is visible extending around the agger nasi air cell. The sphenoethmoid recess receives the secretions of the posterior ethmoid and sphenoid sinuses.* **(Bottom)** *Notice the air cell in the anterior middle turbinate (concha bullosa) in this image. The basal lamella of the middle turbinate is also visible.*

TERMINOLOGY

Abbreviations

- Pterygopalatine fossa (PPF)

Synonyms

- Sphenopalatine fossa

Definitions

- **PPF**: Major crossroads deep within deep face between nasal cavity, oral cavity, masticator space, orbit, and middle cranial fossa

GROSS ANATOMY

Overview

- PPF is 3D box
  - Anterior wall: Posterior wall of maxillary sinus
  - Posterior wall: Pterygoid plates and inferior aspect of lesser wing of sphenoid bone
  - Roof: Inferior orbital fissure
  - Floor: Narrowing to palatine canals
  - Medial wall: Perpendicular plate of palatine bone with sphenopalatine foramen
  - Lateral wall: Narrowing to pterygomaxillary fissure

IMAGING ANATOMY

Overview

- PPF is important anatomic landmark for potential routes of spread of disease throughout deep face

Extent

- Small, but important, deep face cavity with osseous borders

Anatomy Relationships

- Boundaries
  - Anterior: Posterior wall maxillary sinus
  - Posterior: Pterygoid process of sphenoid bone
  - Medial: Perpendicular plate of palatine bone

Internal Contents

- Pterygopalatine ganglion
- Maxillary nerve (CNV2) enters via foramen rotundum
- Distal internal maxillary artery enters via pterygomaxillary fissure

ANATOMY IMAGING ISSUES

Questions

- Communications
  - **Pterygomaxillary fissure**: Lateral opening into nasopharyngeal masticator space, between maxilla and lateral pterygoid plate
  - **Sphenopalatine foramen**: Medial opening into superior meatus; covered with mucosa
  - **Foramen rotundum**: Posterior opening to middle cranial fossa that transmits maxillary nerve (CNV2)
  - **Vidian canal**: Posterior opening below foramen rotundum that extends posteriorly to foramen lacerum (transmits vidian nerve)
  - **Inferior orbital fissure**: Anterior opening into orbit (transmits infraorbital nerve and artery)
  - **Pterygopalatine canal**: Inferior canal leading to greater and lesser palatine foramina to oral cavity (transmits descending palatine nerve and artery)

Imaging Recommendations

- Like many lesions near skull base, both bone CT (for bone evaluation) and enhanced MR (for soft tissue evaluation) may be required for complete evaluation of PPF mass

Imaging Approaches

- Thin (1 mm or less), bone algorithm, noncontrasted axial sections best delimitate osseous structures surrounding PPF
- Contrasted MR of deep face best evaluates soft tissue abnormalities of PPF
  - Similar to many lesions of extracranial head and neck, precontrasted T1 MR series often best show lesions of PPF

Imaging Sweet Spots

- Axial T1-weighted precontrasted images often best demonstrate subtle lesions of PPF
- Similar to most of head and neck imaging, clinical information is critical

Imaging Pitfalls

- Beware of fat saturation artifact
  - Blooming at air-tissue interface may obscure PPF as result of maxillary sinus air directly anterior to PPF
- Dental amalgam artifact may also obscure subtle lesions of PPF

CLINICAL IMPLICATIONS

Clinical Importance

- PPF serves as crossroads of deep face
  - **Perineural tumor** from hard/soft palate may follow **palatine nerves** superiorly into PPF
  - **Perineural tumor** from cheek skin, maxillary sinus, or orbit may follow **infraorbital nerve** to PPF
  - PPF tumor may access intracranial compartment via foramen rotundum or vidian canal

Function Dysfunction

- Pterygopalatine ganglion contains postsynaptic parasympathetic nerve cell bodies and sympathetic fibers
  - Parasympathetic fibers from superior salivatory nucleus in brainstem enter via vidian nerve, greater superficial petrosal nerve, and nervus intermediate root of facial nerve
  - Sympathetic fibers from vidian nerve communicate autonomic impulses to greater and lesser palatine nerves and branches of CNV2
    - Supply lacrimal gland, glands of nasal cavity, paranasal sinus, and roof of oral cavity

PART I
SECTION 3
Temporal Bone

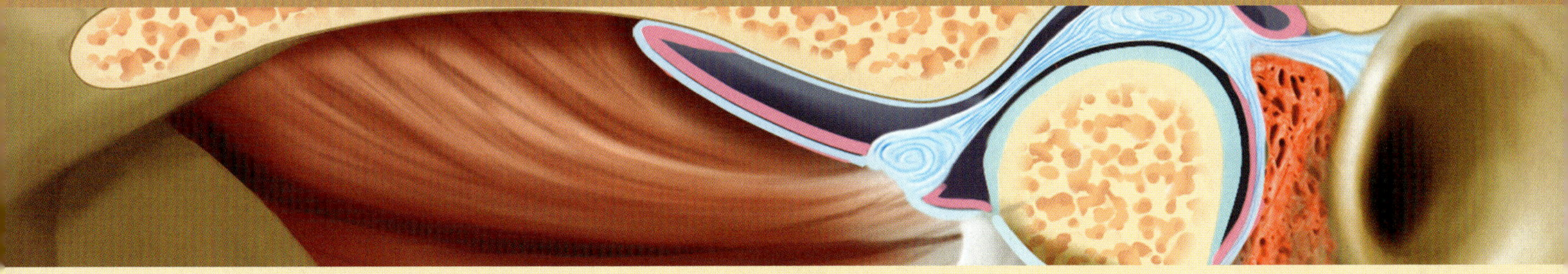

Temporomandibular Joint 82
External, Middle, and Inner Ear 90

TERMINOLOGY

Abbreviations

- Temporomandibular joint (TMJ)

Definitions

- Articulation between mandible and temporal bone
  - Bilateral but work in tandem due to mandible being single bone

GROSS ANATOMY

Overview

- Complex diarthrodial joint with 2 functional movements
  - Rotatory movement in inferior compartment between mandibular condyle and articular disc
  - Sliding (translational) movement in superior compartment between disc and temporal component

Internal Contents

- **Temporal osseous component**
  - Undersurface of squamosal portion of temporal bone contains glenoid fossa and articular eminence
  - **Glenoid fossa** (mandibular fossa, articular fossa) located anterior to external auditory meatus
    - Oval concavity forms "socket"
    - Thin roof of glenoid fossa forms part of floor of middle cranial fossa
    - Tympanic plate forms posterior boundary
    - Squamotympanic fissure extends mediolaterally, posterior to glenoid fossa
  - **Articular eminence** located anterior to glenoid fossa
    - Most inferior aspect termed "summit," "apex," or "crest"
    - Prominence at lateral aspect termed "articular tubercle" or "lateral rim"
    - Posterior surface and summit of eminence are primary sites of articulation for mandibular condyle
    - Lined by articular fibrocartilage
    - Development relies on functional stimulus from condyle
- **Mandibular osseous component**
  - **Mandibular condyle**
    - Bilateral ellipsoid processes of mandible that articulate with cranium
    - Attached to mandibular ramus at narrow condylar neck
    - Condyle generally has convex superior surface between medial and lateral poles
      - May show flat, angular, or round variations in coronal plane
    - Long axis oriented such that medial pole is angled posteriorly, toward foramen magnum
    - Anterior and superior surfaces primarily involved in articulation
    - Capped with articular fibrocartilage
    - Prominent anterior ridge
      - Extends mediolaterally at anteroinferior limit of articulating surface
      - May appear as anterior lip in sagittal oblique view
      - Forms superior limit of pterygoid fovea
  - **Pterygoid fovea**
    - Small depression on anterior surface at junction of condyle and neck
    - Site of attachment of superior head of lateral pterygoid muscle
- **Articular disc**
  - Biconcave oval in shape
  - Avascular dense fibrous connective tissue
  - Thickened anterior and posterior zones of disc termed **"anterior band"** and **"posterior band,"** respectively
    - Conform to contours of articulating surfaces
  - **Intermediate zone**
    - Thin central portion between anterior and posterior bands
    - Fits convex surfaces of opposing articulating components
  - **Attachments**
    - Periphery of articular disc attaches to temporal bone and condyle through blending with fibers of capsule
    - Medial and lateral collateral ligament attach disc to condylar neck, inferior to poles
    - Anterior portion of disc has superior and inferior attachments
    - **Posterior attachment = bilaminar zone = retrodiscal tissue**
      - Superior **temporal posterior attachment** composed of **loose** fibroelastic tissue; attached to squamotympanic fissure
      - Inferior **condylar posterior attachment** portion composed of **taut** fibrous connective tissue; attached to condylar neck
      - Between these attachments are loose, vascular tissues
- **TMJ compartments**
  - Disc divides joint space into superior and inferior compartments
  - **Superior joint compartment**
    - Between disc and temporal component; 2 distinct recesses
  - **Inferior joint compartment**
    - Between disc and condyle; 2 distinct recesses
    - **Anterior and posterior recesses**: Separated by condylar head; size varies with position during translation
  - **Synovial membrane** lines nonarticulating surfaces of superior and inferior compartments

Peripheral Components

- **TMJ capsule and ligaments**
  - **Joint capsule**
    - Funnel-shaped, surrounds joint
    - Attachments
      - Superiorly to temporal articulating components (fossa and eminence)
      - Inferiorly to neck of condyle
      - Posteromedially to squamotympanic fissure
    - Functions to provide stability and limit range of movement
  - **TMJ ligaments**
    - Temporomandibular ligament

- Lateral thickening of capsule with fibers angled inferiorly and posteriorly from articular eminence to posterior condylar neck
  - Other ligaments
    - Sphenomandibular, stylomandibular, discomalleolar
- **Muscles of mastication**
  - Temporalis, masseter, medial and lateral pterygoids

Vascular Supply and Innervation

- Vascular supply from branches of external carotid artery
  - Superficial temporal artery
  - Maxillary artery branches
- Innervation via mandibular division of trigeminal nerve (CNV3)
  - Auriculotemporal nerve
  - Posterior deep temporal nerve
  - Masseteric nerve

IMAGING ANATOMY

Overview

- Osseous anatomy best visualized with CT/CBCT
- Soft tissues/articular disc visualized with MR

CT/CBCT Appearances

- **Normal osseous structures**
  - Both articular eminence and mandibular condyle should have smooth convex contours on sagittal views
    - Flattening of articular surfaces indicates loss of structure due to remodeling or degenerative changes
  - Covered with thin, even, uninterrupted cortices
    - Cortices of articular eminence are thicker than condyle
  - Medullary bone shows even trabeculation around marrow spaces
- Radiographic joint space
  - Radiolucent area between condyle and temporal bone
  - Contains soft tissue components
  - **Normal: Superior > posterior ≥ anterior**
    - Reduced radiographic joint space may indicate disc displacement or perforation
- Condylar position
  - Shape of condyle does not need to match shape of glenoid fossa
  - Some variation of positioning of condyle from center is normal
  - Marked eccentric condylar positioning suggests abnormality
    - Posterior position may correlate with anterior disc displacement
    - Anterior position occurs with severe degeneration of articular eminence

MR Appearances

- **Normal osseous structures**
  - PD or T1
    - Even, uninterrupted low-signal cortices around high-signal cancellous bone
- **Condylar head movement**
  - Initially upon mouth opening, condyle rotates in inferior compartment
  - When mouth fully opens, mandibular condyle translates forward and downward along articular eminence
  - Normal range of motion upon maximal opening brings condyle to level of summit of articular eminence
    - May be posterior at or anterior to summit
  - Condylar translation to anterior and superior to summit indicates hypermobility
- **Disc appearance on sagittal MR**
  - Low signal on PD, T1, and T2
  - Normal disc has **bow tie** shape
  - In closed position, posterior band sits between 11 and 12 o'clock positions relative to condyle
  - More importantly, intermediate thin zone sits at point where maximum force is directed between condyle and eminence
  - Upon opening, intermediate zone of disc translates with condyle against eminence
- **Joint compartments**
  - Intraarticular soft tissues are low to intermediate signal on all sequences
  - Small amount of high-signal fluid on T2 is normal
  - Large area of high signal on T2 indicates pathology (i.e., effusion)

ANATOMY IMAGING ISSUES

Imaging Recommendations

- Panoramic radiographs depict overview of TMJs and can serve to rule out gross disease during initial examination
  - However, distortions and superimpositions render them inadequate for definitive imaging assessment
- MR is best imaging modality to evaluate TMJ soft tissues, especially articular disc position
- **Sagittal MR** is mainstay of TMJ imaging evaluation
  - Coronal closed mouth T1/PD, sagittal T1/PD, and T2 with closed- and open-mouth acquisitions needed
  - Fat-saturated T2 best for evaluation of joint effusion
- Bone CT/CBCT to assess osseous structures
  - CBCT = lower dose
  - Sagittal and coronal reformations required
- All image reconstructions should be made on planes axially corrected for angulation of condyle

Imaging Pitfalls

- In cases with apparent limited motion between open- and closed-mouth series, look closely for articular disc abnormalities
  - Entire sagittal series from lateral to medial should be evaluated for disc displacement, which can occur in any direction
  - Not acquiring axially corrected images may lead to missed or incorrect diagnosis
- Condylar cortical borders may not complete calcification **until age 20**; less cortication in children is normal finding
- Pterygoid fovea superior border (anterior lip) may resemble osteophyte (spur) and should not be mistaken as sign of degenerative joint disease
- Pneumatization of temporal articular component by mastoid air cells is common normal variation

3D-VRT BONE CT

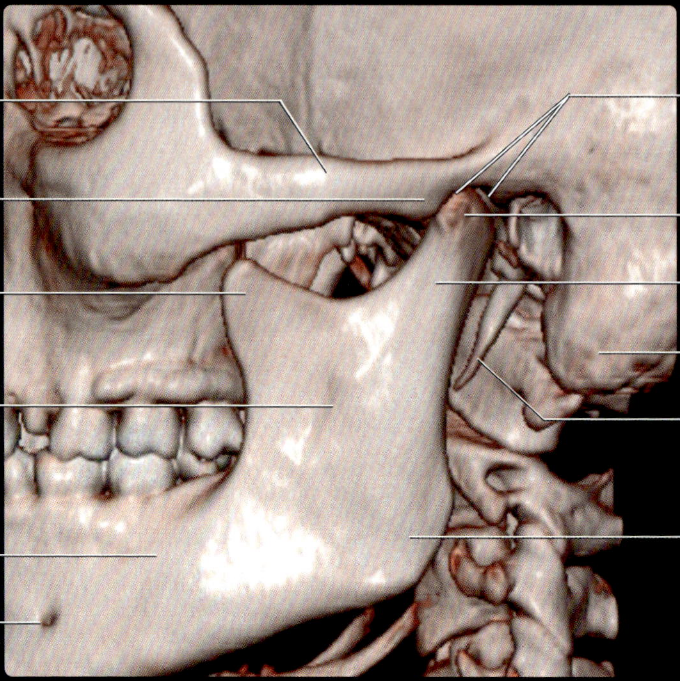

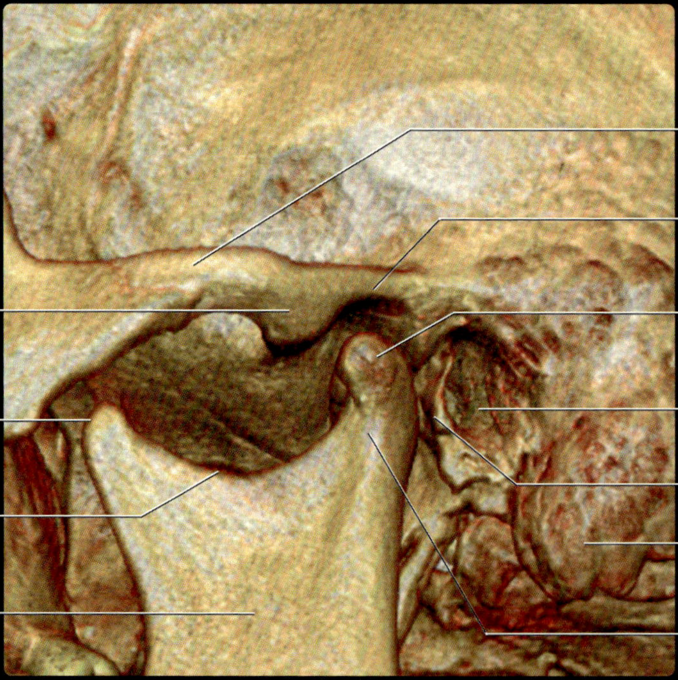

(Top) *Sagittal 3D-VRT image shows the osseous anatomy of the TMJ. The condyle is situated in the glenoid fossa deep to the posterior zygomatic arch. The zygomatic arch provides some protection laterally for the TMJ in the setting of trauma. Because forces to the mandible are transmitted through the joints, the TMJ must be fully evaluated on all mandibular trauma cases to ensure that fractures or central dislocation of the mandibular condyle have not occurred.* **(Bottom)** *Sagittal 3D-VRT magnified image shows the osseous anatomy of the TMJ area. In this closed or occlusal position, the condyle is within the glenoid fossa. In the open-mouth position (not shown), the condyle translates anteroinferiorly onto the articular eminence. Notice the close relationship between the condyle and tympanic bone of the external auditory canal. An upward blow to the mandible can easily fracture the bony external auditory canal.*

TMJ GRAPHICS

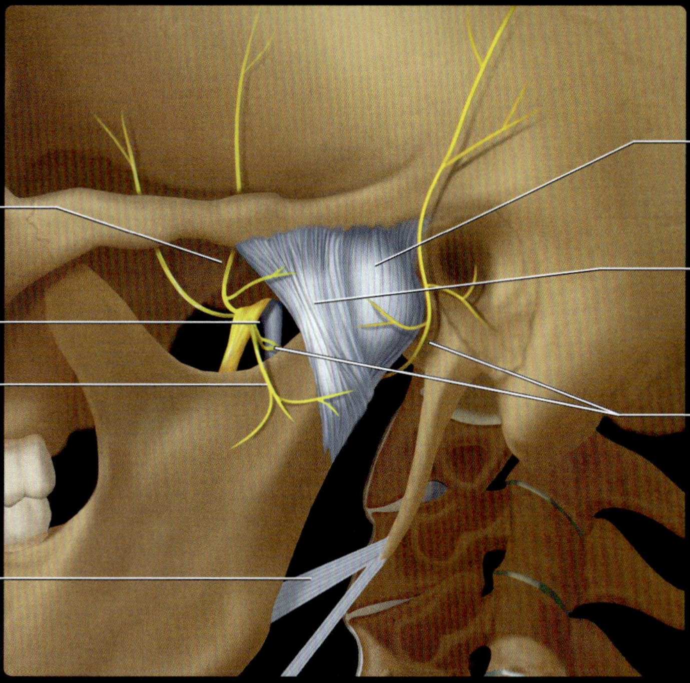

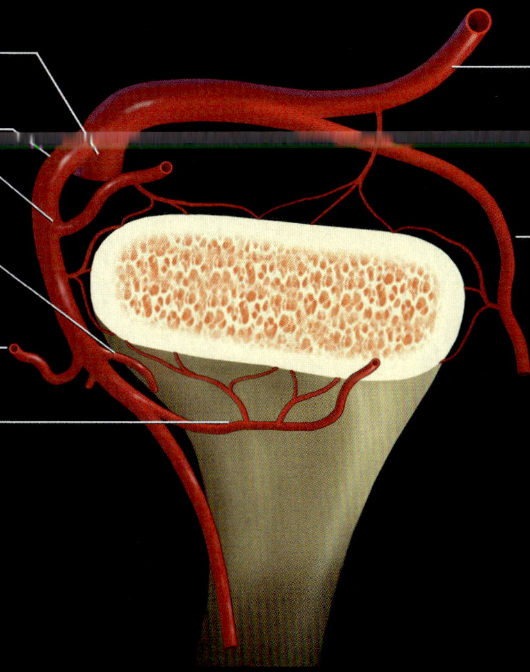

(Top) *Lateral graphic depicts the ligaments and nerves of the temporomandibular joint. The lateral temporomandibular ligament is a thickening of the joint capsule. Sensory innervation to the joint comes from branches of the auriculotemporal, masseter, and posterior temporalis nerves of CNV. (From SI: TMJ.)* **(Bottom)** *Graphic shows the arterial blood supply of the TMJ from the superior view. The condyle is circumferentially supplied with blood coming from the superficial temporal artery and the maxillary artery, both branches of the external carotid artery. In addition to these branches, the inferior alveolar artery anastomoses within the mandible supplies the marrow spaces of the condyle and condylar neck. (From SI: TMJ.)*

TMJ GRAPHICS

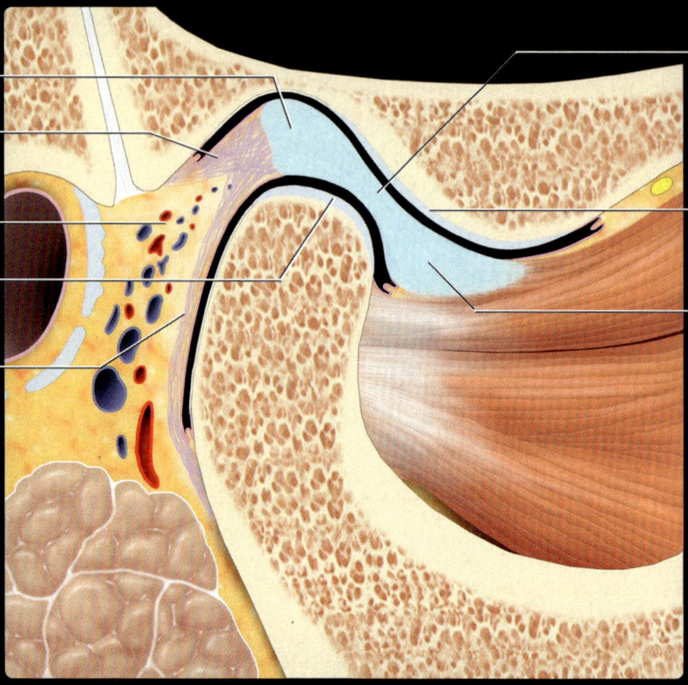

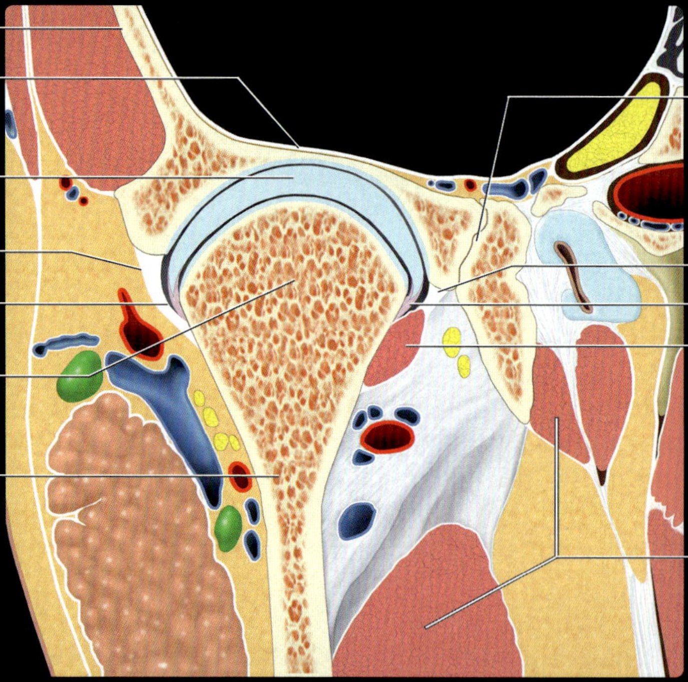

(Top) *Sagittal oblique graphic shows the TMJ with the focus on the structures of the disc and fibrocartilage. These are optimally evaluated by MR. The molecular structure and orientation of these soft tissue elements give the tissues their MR properties and appearance. Any change in the signal intensity may indicate a structural abnormality. The morphology and position of these tissues can also be anatomically evaluated using MR. (From SI: TMJ.)* **(Bottom)** *Coronal oblique graphic of a TMJ shows the condyle centered in the fossa. The posterior band of the disc is sitting on top of the condyle. The disc tapers medially and laterally and is attached to the condyle at the medial and lateral collateral ligaments.*

CBCT OF NORMAL TMJ

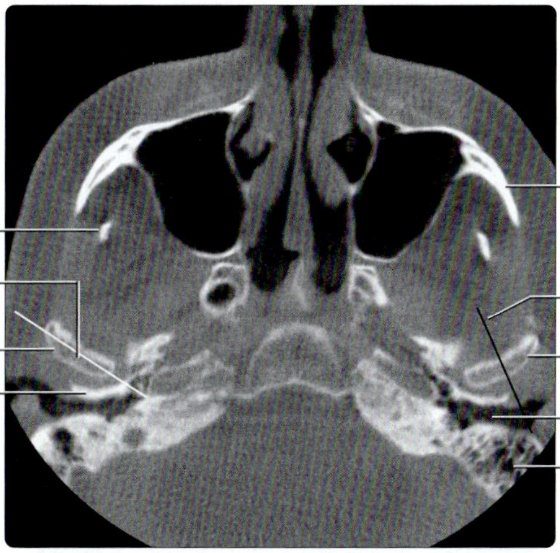

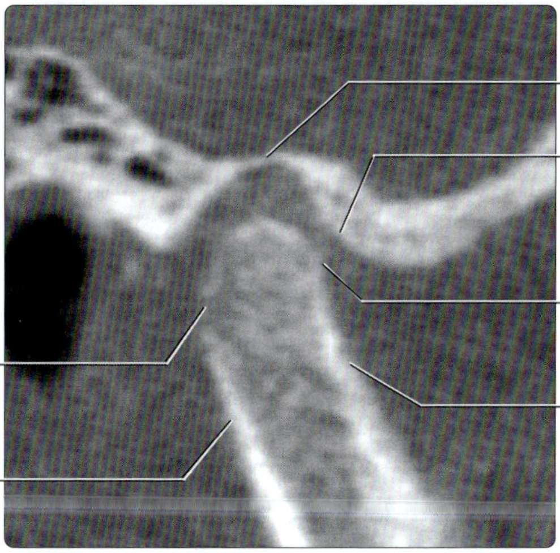

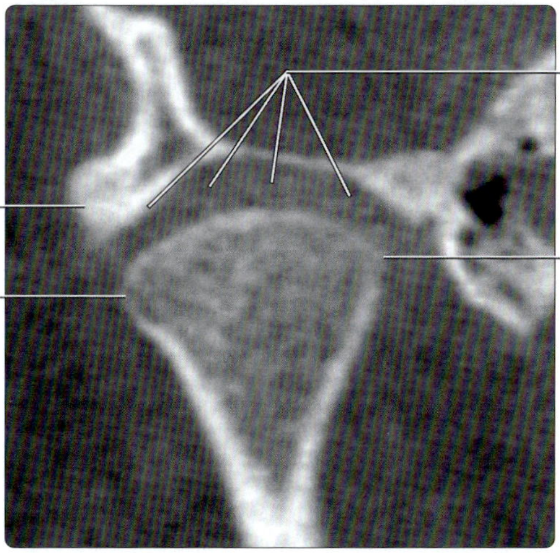

(Top) *Axial CBCT through the TMJ condyles shows their long axis angled with the medial poles positioned more posteriorly. Correcting for this angulation to the sagittal and coronal oblique planes during image reformation is important for accurate representation.* **(Middle)** *Sagittal oblique CBCT of the right TMJ shows the normal morphology and spatial relationships of the condylar process and fossa. The cortices of the condylar neck taper toward the condyle into the posterior and anterior heights of contour and becomes eggshell thin superiorly (subchondral bone). The anterior height of contour of the condyle and the posterior height of contour of the eminence form an incongruent articulation.* **(Bottom)** *Coronal oblique CBCT of a normal condyle shows the normal bone morphology of the condyle and fossa as well as the spatial relationships between the 2 structures. The contours of the condyle relatively follow the contours of the fossa and the condyle is centered in the fossa with uniform joint space seen between the 2 structures.*

CBCT OF NORMAL TMJ

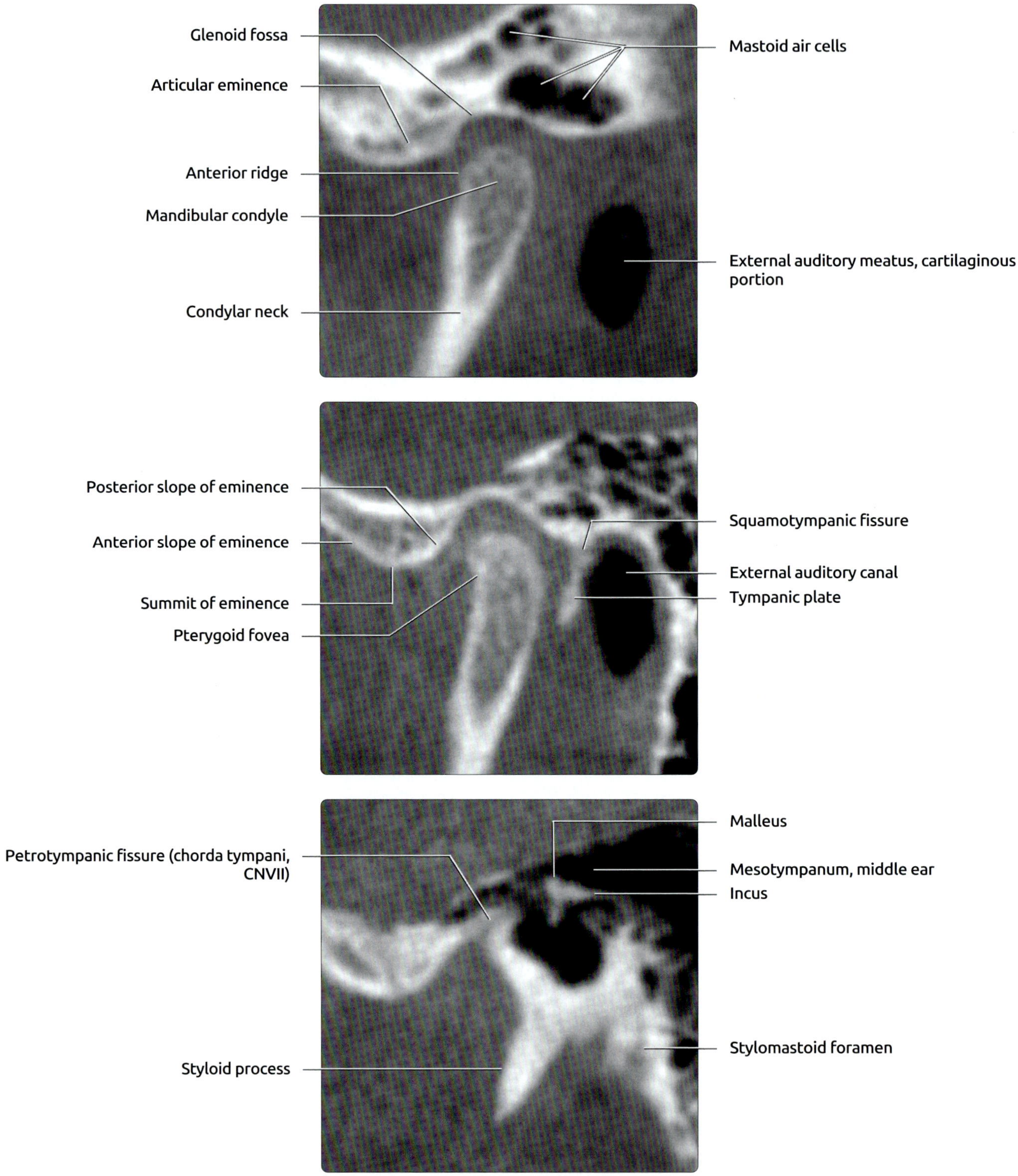

(Top) *First of 3 oblique sagittal images through the TMJ from lateral to medial is shown. The anterior ridge forms the anterior boundary of the articulating surface of the condyle. Pneumatization of the roof of the glenoid fossa and eminence is a normal variation.* **(Middle)** *Section through the midjoint region shows normal morphology of the osseous articular components. The posterior slope of the eminence should assume a rounded morphology with a gently rounded crest. The subchondral bone of the eminence is normally thicker than that of the condyle.* **(Bottom)** *This section medial to the condyle shows the petrotympanic fissure, middle ear, and ossicles in close relationship. The styloid process is found medial and posterior to the glenoid fossa. It is a process of the temporal bone with varying degrees of length and thickness. The stylomastoid foramen is seen posterior to it and is where the facial nerve (CNVII) exits the temporal bone.*

MR OF NORMAL TMJ

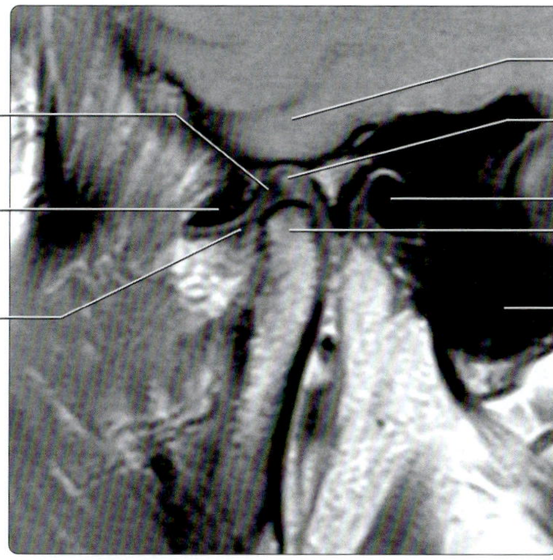

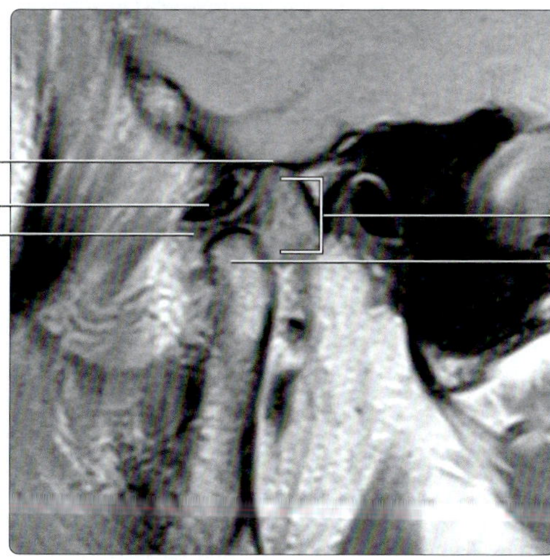

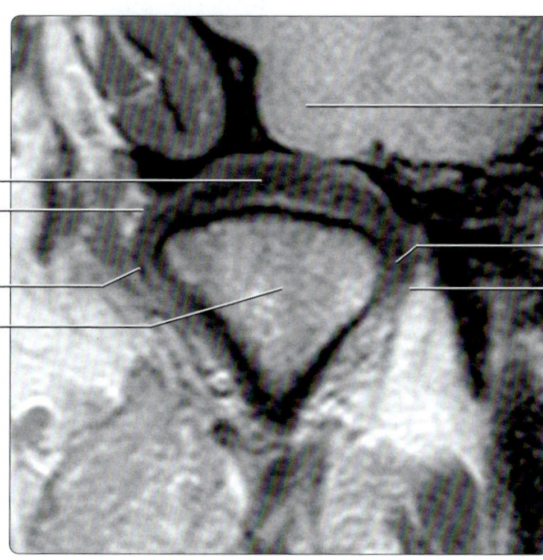

(Top) *Sagittal proton-density MR shows a normal TMJ in the closed position. The articular disc has a low signal and is bow tie-shaped. The posterior band is sitting at ~ the 11 o'clock position and the intermediate thin zone is positioned between the loading points of the condylar head and articular eminence. The osseous structures have thin low-signal cortical outlines. The trabecular bone of the condyle has a high signal due to the fatty marrow.* **(Middle)** *Sagittal proton-density MR shows the same joint in the open position. The condyle has translated to the summit of the articular eminence. Note the condyle has also rotated within the inferior joint space. The articular disc has translated with the condyle and remains with its thin zone positioned between the articular surfaces.* **(Bottom)** *Coronal proton-density MR of a normal right TMJ is shown. The medial and lateral capsule and collateral ligaments are seen in this view. The collateral ligaments present as low to intermediate signal tapering inferior to the poles of the condyles.*

TERMINOLOGY

Abbreviations

- Temporal bone (T-bone)
- Middle ear (ME)

Definitions

- Ossicles: 3 smallest bones in human body (malleus, incus, & stapes) in ME that amplify sound vibrations, conveying them from tympanic membrane (TM) to oval window
- ME: 6-sided cavity between external ear & inner ear, containing 3 ossicles, 2 muscles, & opening to eustachian tube

IMAGING ANATOMY

Anatomy Relationships

- ME sits in T-bone between external & inner ears

Internal Contents

- **ME subdivisions**
  - **Epitympanum** (attic): Tegmen tympani is roof with floor defined by line between scutum & tympanic segment of facial nerve
    - **Prussak space**: Lateral epitympanic recess
    - **Anterior epitympanic recess**: Epitympanic recess anteromedial to epitympanic "cog"; medial wall made up of anterior tympanic segment of CNVII
    - **Tegmen tympani** (Latin for roof of cavity): Thin bony roof between epitympanum & middle cranial fossa dura
    - **Aditus ad antrum** (Latin for entrance to cave): Connects epitympanum of ME to mastoid antrum
  - **Mesotympanum**: ME cavity between line connecting scutum & tympanic segment CNVII above & line connecting tympanic annulus & base of cochlear promontory below
    - Posterior wall (posterior tympanum) has 3 important structures: Facial nerve recess, pyramidal eminence, & sinus tympani
    - Medial wall: Lateral semicircular canal, tympanic segment CNVII, oval & round window found here
  - **Hypotympanum**: Shallow trough in floor of ME cavity
- **ME muscles**
  - **Tensor tympani muscle**
    - Muscle found anteroinferior to anterior tympanic segment CNVII
    - Tendon passes through cochleariform process then attaches to neck of malleus
    - Innervated by CNV3
  - **Stapedius muscle**
    - Muscle found just medial to upper mastoid segment CNVII
    - Tendon emerges from apex of pyramidal eminence, then attaches to head or posterior crura of stapes
    - Innervated by CNVII motor branch of mastoid segment
- **Ossicles of ME**
  - **Malleus** (hammer)
    - Location: Anterior epitympanum & mesotympanum
    - Components: Head, neck, lateral process, anterior process, manubrium, & umbo
    - Ligaments: Superior, anterior, lateral mallear ligaments & tendon of tensor tympani muscle
  - **Incus** (anvil)
    - Location: Posterior epitympanum & mesotympanum
    - Components: Body, short, long, & **lenticular processes**
    - Ligament: Posterior incudal ligament
  - **Stapes** (stirrup)
    - Location: Medial mesotympanum
    - Components: Head, anterior & posterior crura, & footplate
    - Ligament: Ligament of stapedius muscle attaches to stapes
    - **Stapes superstructure**: Stapes portion derived from 2nd branchial arch = head, crura, tympanic portion of footplate
    - Vestibular portion of footplate of stapes & annular ligament derived from otic capsule
- **TM**
  - Separates external from ME
  - Upper 1/3 = **pars flaccida**; lower 2/3 = **pars tensa**
  - Malleus umbo & lateral process embedded in TM
  - 3 layers of TM
    - External layer continuous with skin of external auditory canal (EAC) = ectoderm
    - Inner layer continuous with ME mucosa = endoderm
    - Intermediate fibrous layer = mesoderm
  - Superior attachment: **Scutum** (Latin for shield)
  - Inferior attachment: **Tympanic annulus**

CLINICAL IMPLICATIONS

Clinical Importance

- EAC-TM-ossicles-oval window
  - Conductive chain disruption results in conductive hearing loss

EMBRYOLOGY

Embryologic Events

- EAC forms from 1st branchial groove
- ME forms from 1st branchial pouch
- Ossicles form from 1st & 2nd branchial arches
  - 1st branchial arch: Head & neck of malleus, body & short process of incus
  - 2nd branchial arch: Manubrium of malleus, long & lenticular processes of incus, stapes superstructure

Practical Implications

- EAC atresia is 1st & 2nd branchial apparatus lesions
- Ossicular rotation & deformity part of imaging appearance
- Oval window atresia may or may not be associated with EAC atresia

GRAPHICS

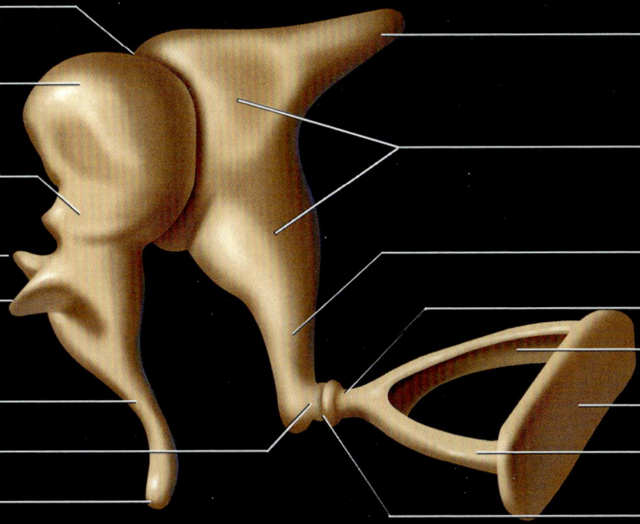

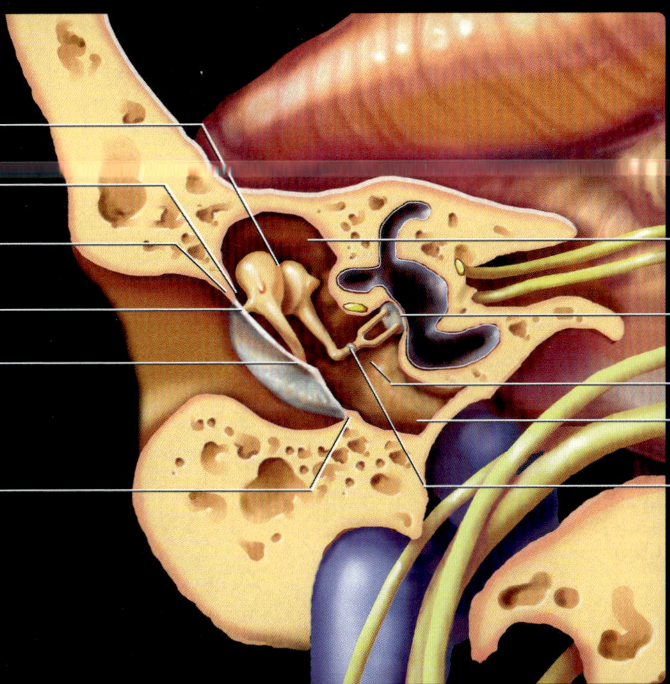

(Top) *Graphic shows right middle ear ossicles viewed from the front. The anterolateral malleus has a head, neck, and manubrium with lateral and anterior processes. The inferior malleus tip is called the umbo. The umbo and lateral process are embedded in the tympanic membrane (TM). The incus is the largest ossicle with a large body, a short and long process, and a lenticular process. The lenticular process and stapes hub meet at a 90° angle. The stapes has a head, crura, and a footplate. The space between stapes crura is called the obturator foramen.* **(Bottom)** *Coronal graphic of right temporal bone shows the conductive chain from the TM to the oval window. Notice the lateral process and umbo of the malleus are embedded in the TM. The TM is attached superiorly to the scutum and inferiorly to the tympanic annulus. The 2 joints between the ossicles are the malleoincudal and incudostapedial articulations.*

AXIAL BONE CT

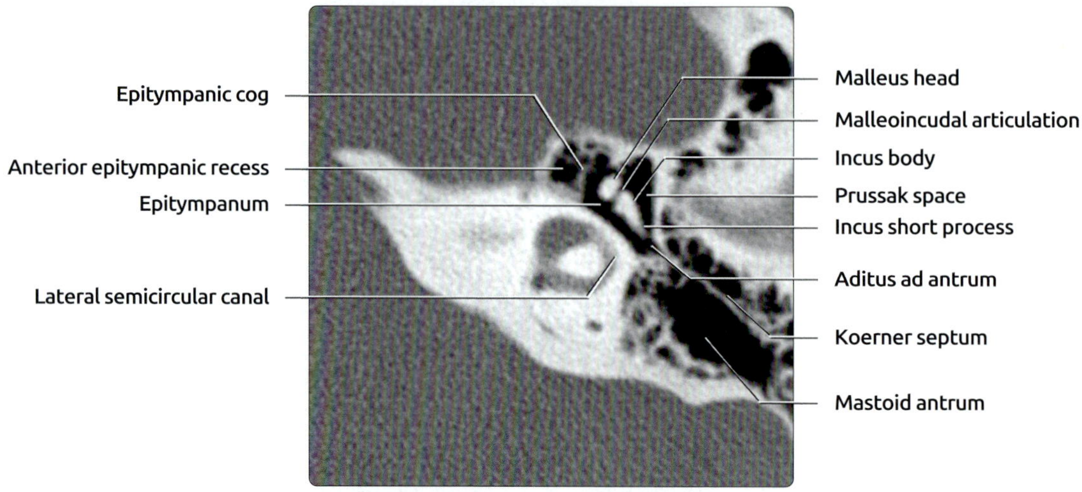

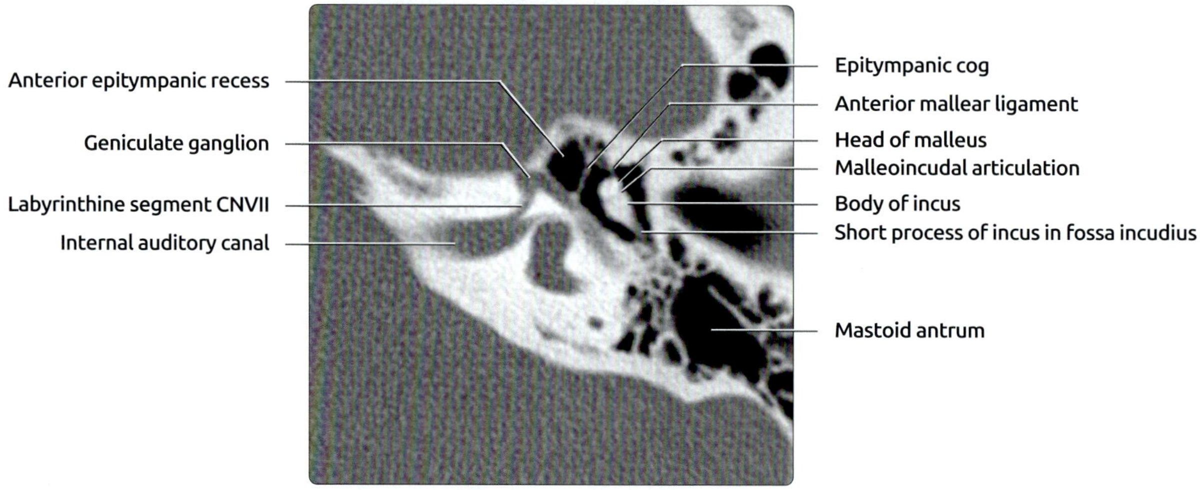

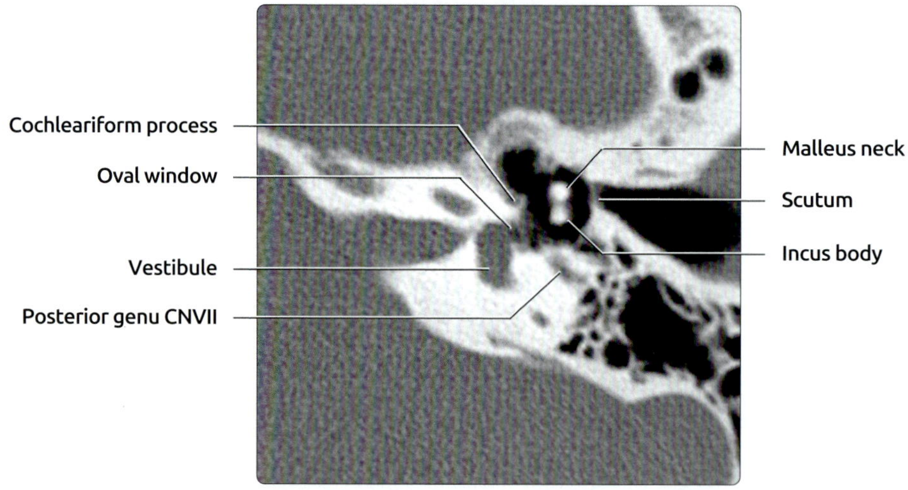

(Top) *First of 6 magnified axial bone CT images of the left ear from superior to inferior shows the malleus head articulating with the body of the incus at the malleoincudal articulation. Prussak space (lateral epitympanic recess) is seen lateral to the ossicles. The short process of the incus is "pointing" into the aditus ad antrum.* **(Middle)** *In this image through the level of the geniculate ganglion, it is possible to see the anterior epitympanic recess defined by the epitympanic cog laterally and the anterior tympanic segment of the facial nerve. Diseases affecting this area may cause facial nerve paralysis.* **(Bottom)** *At the level of the oval window, the malleus neck and incus body are seen in the upper mesotympanum. The facial nerve is transitioning from its tympanic segment to its mastoid segment as the posterior genu.*

AXIAL BONE CT

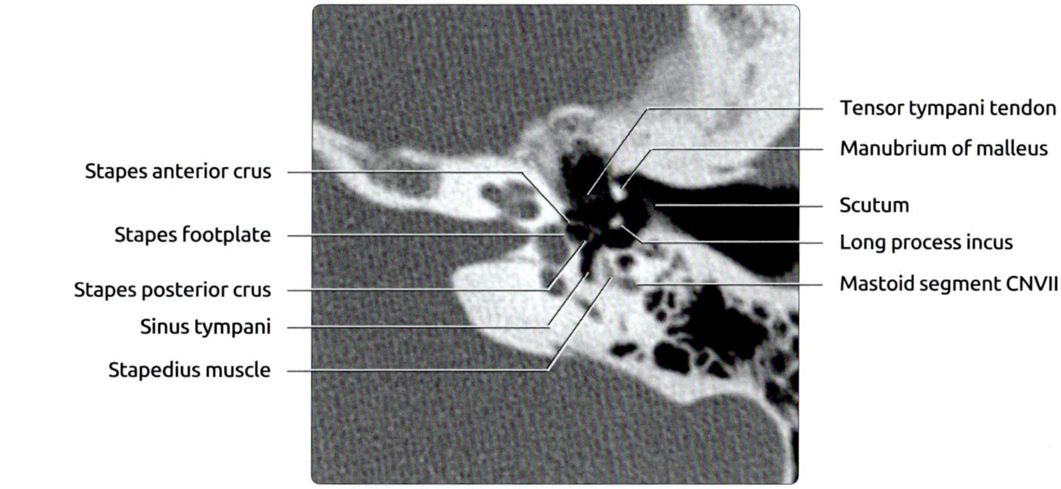

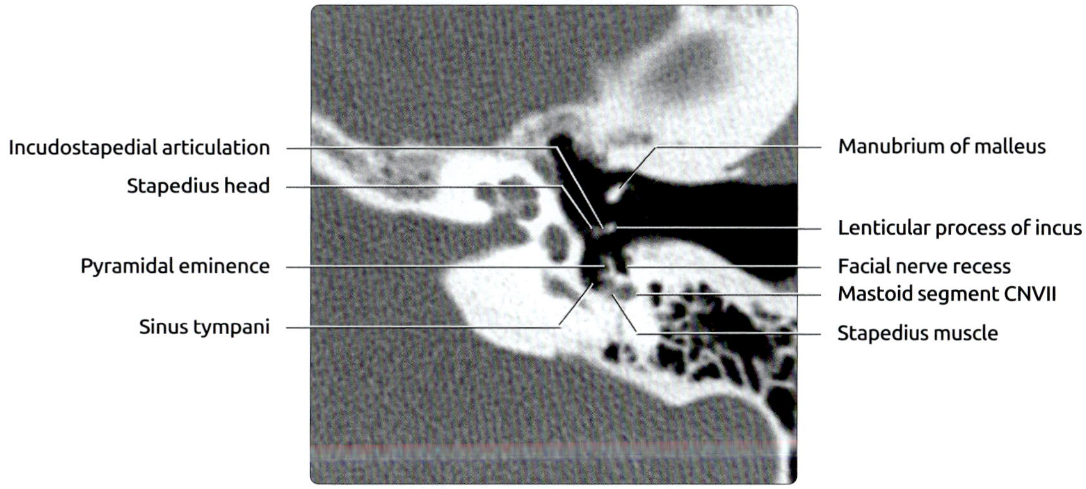

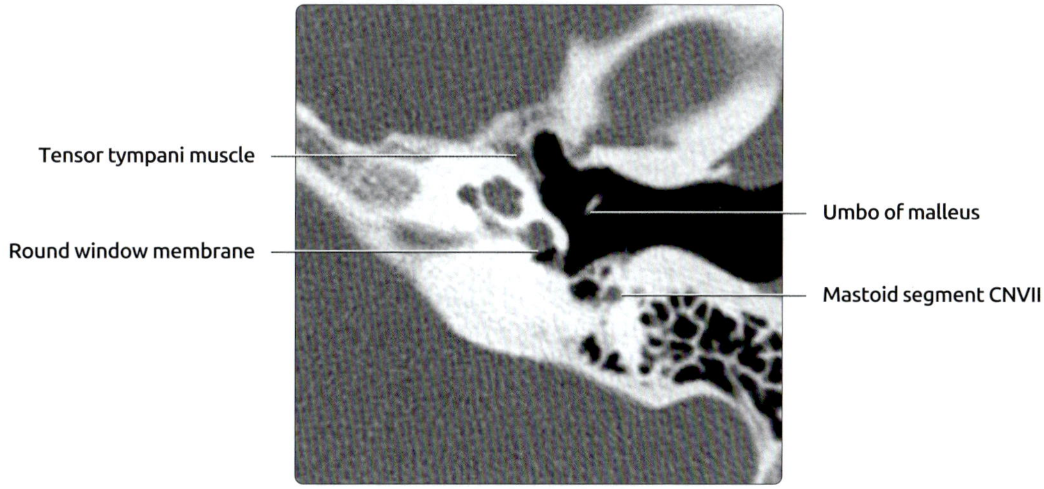

(Top) *In this image, the anterior and posterior crura of the stapes are visible with the stapes footplate/oval window in between. The tensor tympani tendon can be seen reaching from the cochleariform process to the manubrium of the malleus. Both the stapedius muscle and mastoid segment of the facial nerve are seen in the posterior tympanum wall.* **(Middle)** *In this image, the ridges and recesses of the posterior tympanum are well seen. From medial to lateral, they are the sinus tympani, pyramidal eminence, and facial nerve recess. Behind these structures, observe the stapedius muscle and the mastoid segment of CNVII. Note the incudostapedial articulation connecting the lenticular process of the incus to the head of the stapes.* **(Bottom)** *The inferior tip of the manubrium is the umbo. At the round window membrane level, the mastoid segment of CNVII is now seen without the stapedius muscle.*

CORONAL BONE CT

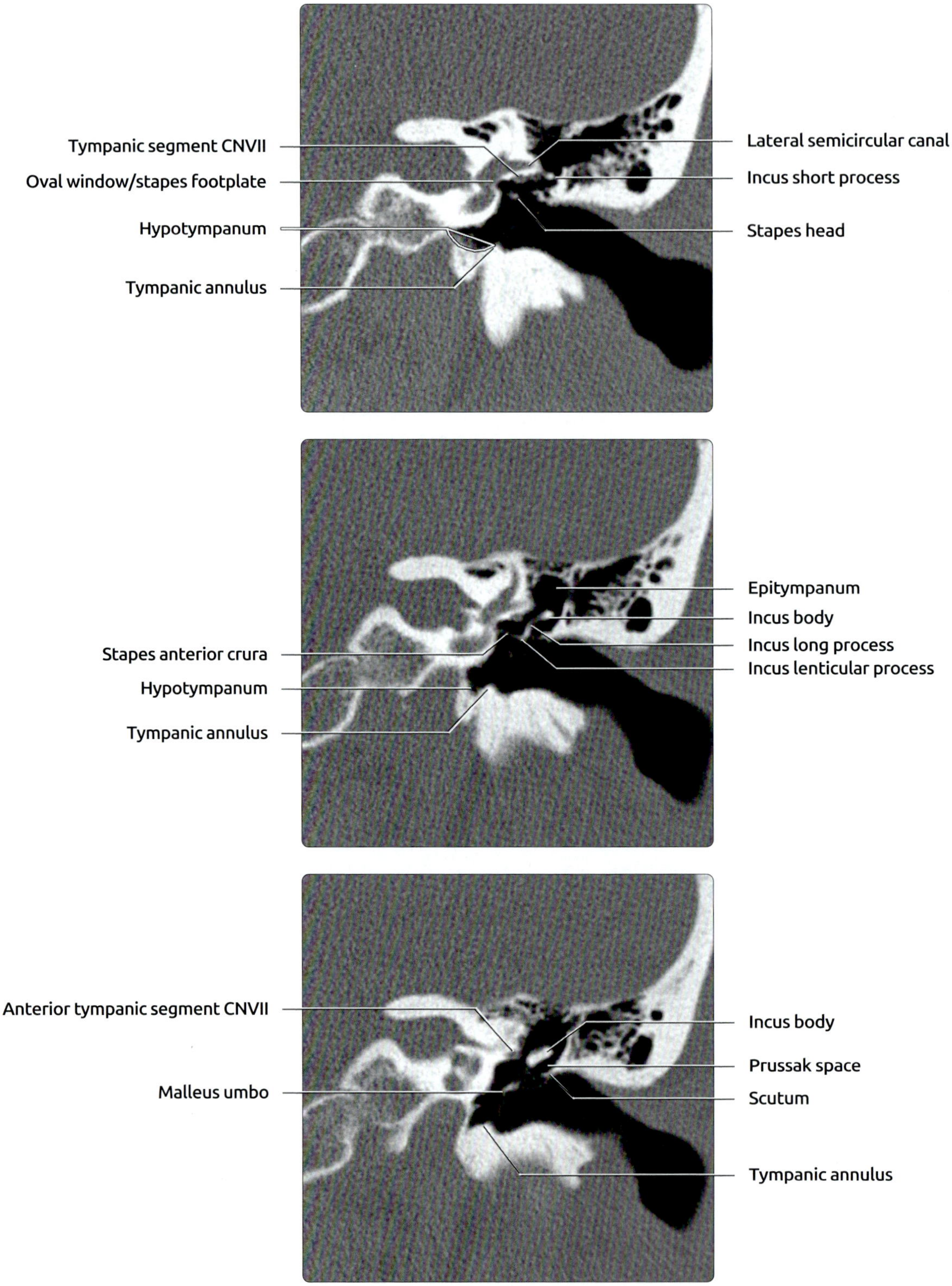

(Top) *This is the 1st of 6 coronal bone CT images of the left ear presented from posterior to anterior. In this image through the oval window, notice how thin the normal stapes footplate appears.* **(Middle)** *At the level of the anterior oval window margin, the body, long process, and lenticular process of the incus can be seen.* **(Bottom)** *In this image, the body of the incus is seen at the same level as the umbo of the malleus. The TM is barely visible, strung between the superior scutum and inferior tympanic annulus. The epitympanum is defined as the area of the middle ear cavity above a line drawn between the tip of the scutum and the tympanic segment of the facial nerve.*

CORONAL BONE CT

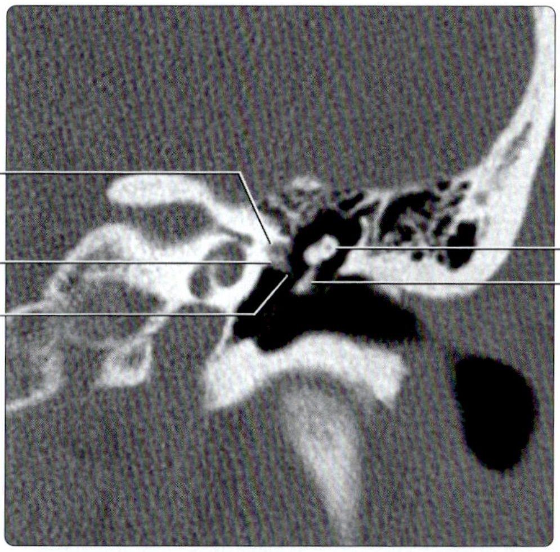

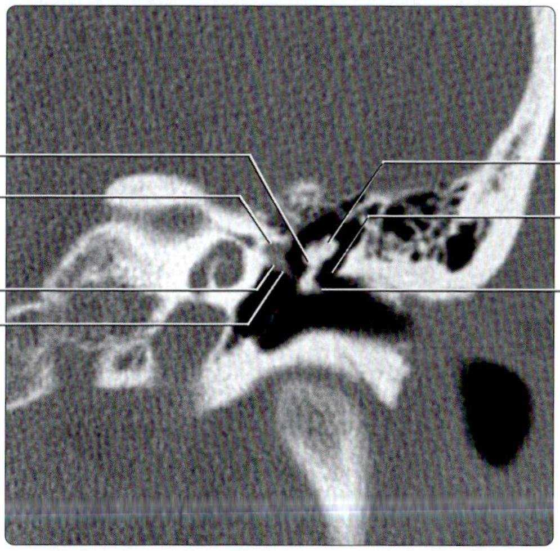

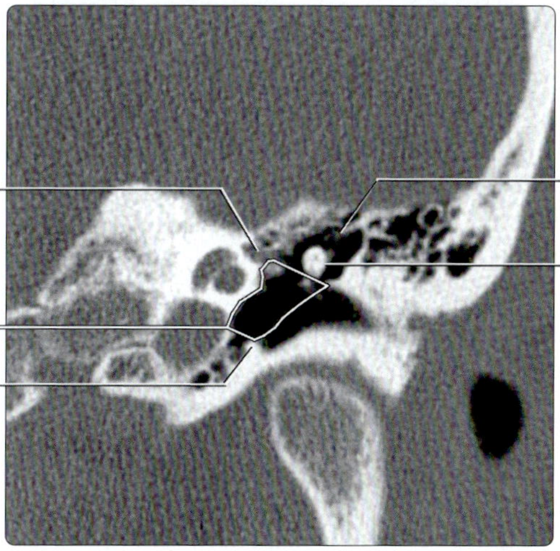

(Top) *In this image through the anterior tympanic cavity, the tendon of the tensor tympani muscle is seen turning 90° in the cochleariform process, then projecting over to the manubrium of the malleus.* **(Middle)** *The lateral process of the malleus and the umbo are both embedded in the medial surface of the TM. The tendon of the tensor tympani muscle inserts on the medial surface of the manubrium of the malleus.* **(Bottom)** *In this image, the head of the malleus can be seen in the anterior epitympanum. The mesotympanum can be defined as the middle ear cavity below the line connecting the tympanic segment of the facial nerve and the inferior tip of the scutum and above the line connecting the superior tip of the tympanic annulus and the inferior margin of the cochlear promontory.*

PART I
SECTION 4

Base of Skull

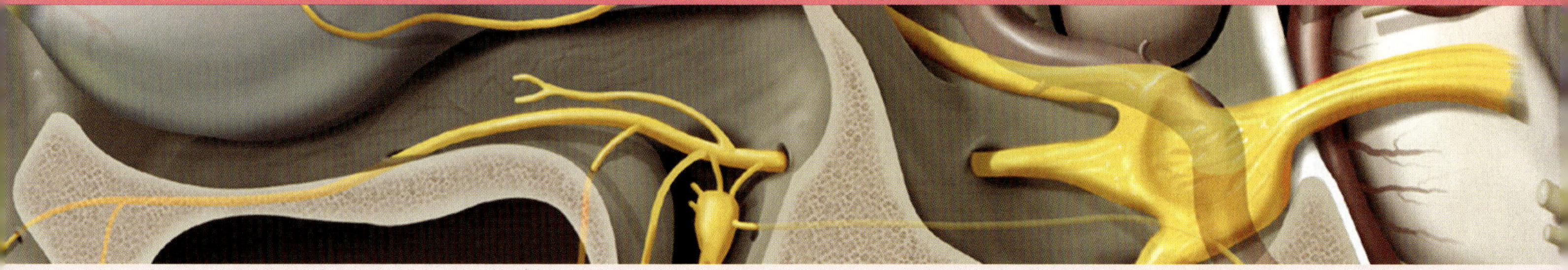

Anterior Skull Base	**98**
Central Skull Base	**104**
Posterior Skull Base	**110**
Styloid Process and Stylohyoid Ligament	**118**

Anterior Skull Base

TERMINOLOGY

Abbreviations

- Anterior skull base (ASB)

Definitions

- Skull base (SB) anterior to lesser wing of sphenoid (LWS) & planum sphenoidale

IMAGING ANATOMY

Overview

- ASB is floor of anterior cranial fossa and roof of nose, ethmoid sinuses, & orbits
- Bones forming ASB
  - Cribriform plate & ethmoid sinus roof of ethmoid bone centrally
  - Orbital plate of frontal bone laterally
  - Planum sphenoidale & LWS posteriorly
- Boundaries of ASB
  - Anterolaterally: Frontal bone
  - Posteriorly: LWS & planum sphenoidale
- Relationships of ASB
  - Superior: Frontal lobes, CNI
  - Inferior: Nasal vault & ethmoid sinus medially, orbit laterally

Bony Landmarks of Anterior Skull Base

- **Frontal crest**: Anterior midline ridge between frontal bones; falx cerebri attaches here
- **Crista galli**: Midline upward triangular process of ethmoid; anteroinferior falx cerebri attaches here
- **Anterior clinoid processes**: Medial aspect of LWS; free edge of tentorium cerebelli attaches here
- **Lesser wing of sphenoid**: Forms sphenoid ridge; separates ASB from central skull base
- **Planum sphenoidale**: Sphenoid bone superomedial plate anterior to tuberculum sellae

Foramina and Fissures of Anterior Skull Base

- **Foramen cecum**
  - Transmits: Variably transmits small emissary vein from nasal mucosa to superior sagittal sinus
  - Location: In margin between posterior aspect of frontal bone & anterior aspect of ethmoid
  - Relationships: Small midline pit found immediately anterior to crista galli
- **Anterior ethmoid foramen**
  - Transmits: Anterior ethmoid artery, vein, nerve
  - Location: Slit between ethmoid and frontal bones
  - Relationships: Just anterior to cribriform foramina
- **Posterior ethmoid foramen**
  - Transmits: Posterior ethmoid artery, vein, nerve
  - Location: Found at seam between sphenoid and ethmoid bones
  - Relationships: Just posterior to cribriform foramina
- **Foramina of cribriform plate**
  - Transmits: Afferent fibers from nasal mucosa to olfactory bulbs (CNI)
  - Location: ~ 20 perforations within cephalad ethmoid bone plate
  - Relationships: Medial aspect of ethmoid, supports olfactory bulbs

Development of Anterior Skull Base

- **Overview**
  - SB originates largely from cartilaginous precursors
    - Minimal contribution from membranous bone
  - > 100 ossification centers in SB development
  - Ossifies posterior to anterior & lateral to medial
  - Ossification is orderly & constant in first 2 years
    - However, does not correspond to exact age
- **Birth**: ASB develops primarily from cartilage with limited ossification at birth
  - Early ethmoid air cells may be seen, but unossified crista galli is faint
- **1 month**: Ossification begins from ethmoid labyrinth & turbinates; proceeds medially
- **3 months**: Roof of nasal cavity & tip of crista galli begin to ossify
  - Ethmoid air cells still inferior to cribriform plate
- **6 months**: Nasal roof is well ossified; > 90% of patients have partial ossification of nasal roof on every coronal CT image
  - Perpendicular plate of ethmoid begins to ossify
  - Ethmoid sinus extends above cribriform plate plane
- **12 months**: Crista galli is well ossified; > 70% of patients have ossified posterior cribriform plate
- **18 months**: Ethmoid air cells now extend above plane of cribriform plate, and orbital plates of frontal bones help form early fovea ethmoidalis
- **24 months**: Fovea ethmoidalis achieves more mature appearance; perpendicular plate of ethmoid begins to fuse with ossified vomer; most patients still have a gap between nasal & ethmoid bones
- **> 24 months**
  - ASB nearly completely ossified; small gaps persist in nasal roof until early 3rd year
  - Foramen cecum ossifies as late as 5 years
  - Majority of cribriform plate & at least some of crista galli should be ossified

ANATOMY IMAGING ISSUES

Questions

- ASB ossification constant but variable in first 5 years
- Understanding of normal development will avoid confusion or misdiagnoses
- Anterior neuropore closes in 4th gestational week

Imaging Recommendations

- MR to search for anterior neuropore anomalies

Imaging Approaches

- Bone CT viewed at wide windows (> 2,000 HU)
- Reformat at least 2 orthogonal planes

Imaging Pitfalls

- Apparent small gaps in ASB under age 3 are normal
- Do not confuse nonossified foramen cecum for anterior neuropore anomaly
- Be aware that fatty marrow in crista galli or ossified falx cerebri is not pathology

GRAPHICS

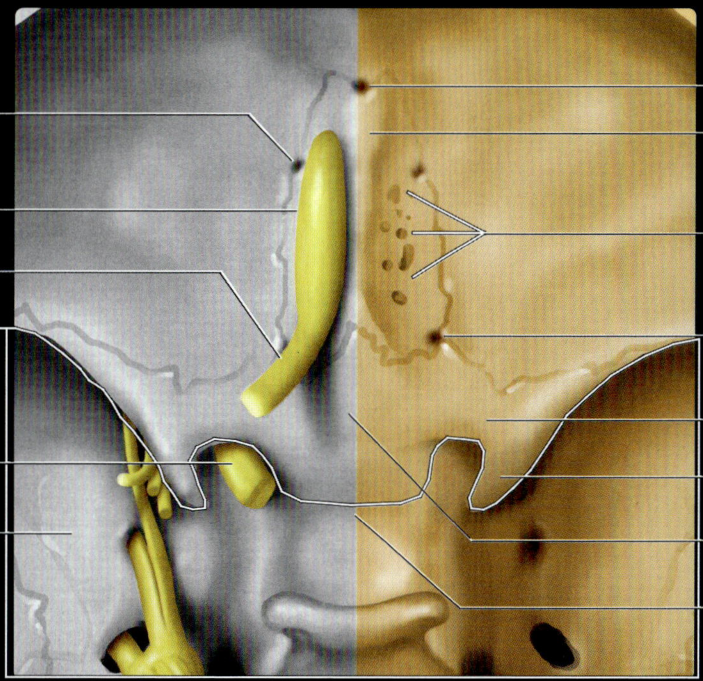

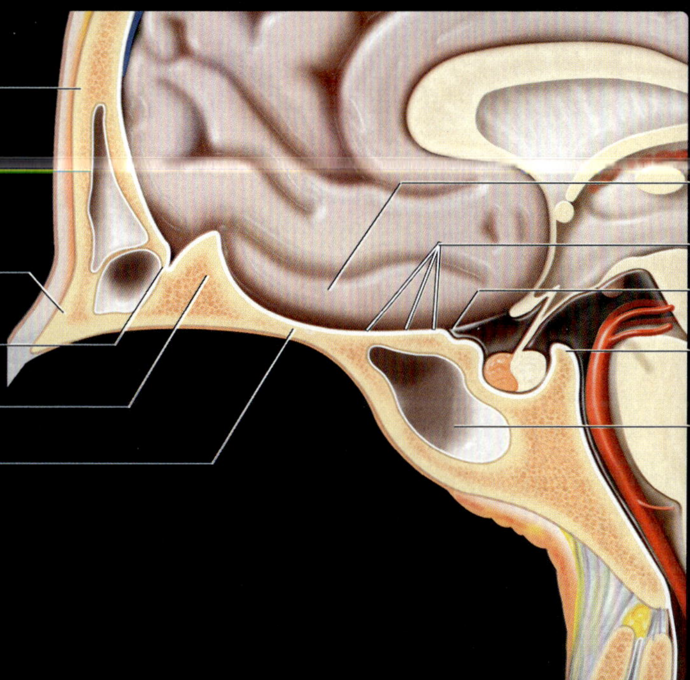

(Top) *Graphic of anterior skull base (ASB) seen from above shows olfactory bulb of CNI lying on cribriform plate. Neural structures have been removed on the right, allowing visualization of numerous perforations in the cribriform plate through which afferent fibers from olfactory mucosa pass to form the olfactory bulb. Note the foramen cecum, a small pit anterior to the crista galli, bounded anteriorly by frontal bone, posteriorly by ethmoid bone. The posterior margin of the ASB is formed by the lesser wing of the sphenoid & planum sphenoidale.* **(Bottom)** *Sagittal graphic of ASB shows midline vertical crista galli. Anterior to crista galli is foramen cecum remnant. Posterolateral to crista galli is horizontal cribriform plate. The planum sphenoidale is the posteromedial anterior skull base.*

GRAPHICS

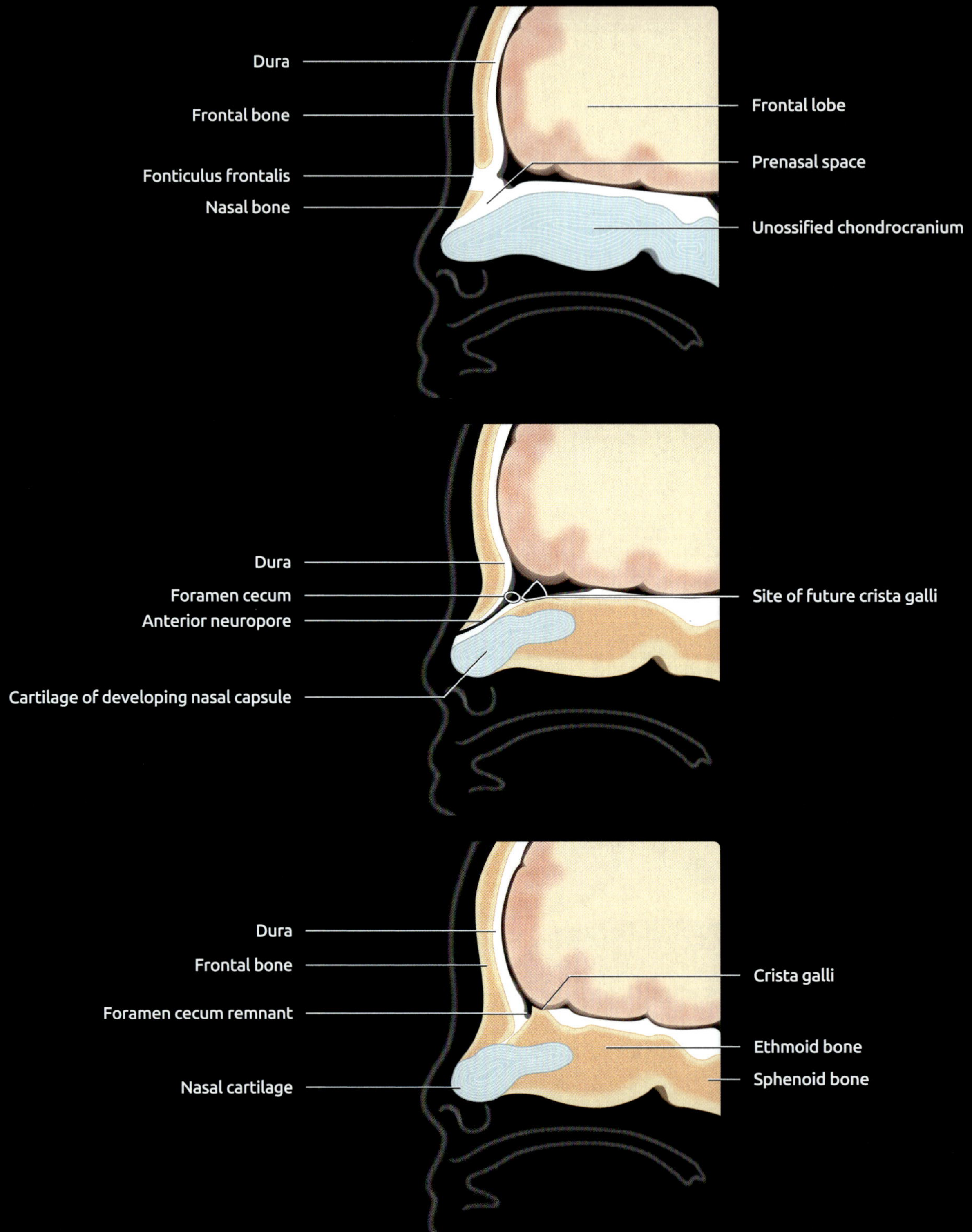

(Top) *Sagittal graphic shows normal ASB development. Fonticulus frontalis, a small ASB fontanelle, is a normal cartilaginous gap between developing partially ossified frontal and nasal bones. Prenasal space is also present at this time as a dura-filled space between developing nasal bones and cartilage of developing nasal capsule. Both sites can become the location of a cephalocele.* **(Middle)** *Sagittal graphic shows ASB slightly later in development. The fonticulus frontalis has closed, and ossification of chondrocranium has proceeded from posterior to anterior. Prenasal space is now encased in bone and becomes foramen cecum. A normal stalk of dura extends through foramen cecum to skin (anterior neuropore).* **(Bottom)** *Sagittal graphic shows ASB even later in development. Anterior neuropore has regressed. Foramen cecum will completely fuse by age 5.*

AXIAL BONE CT

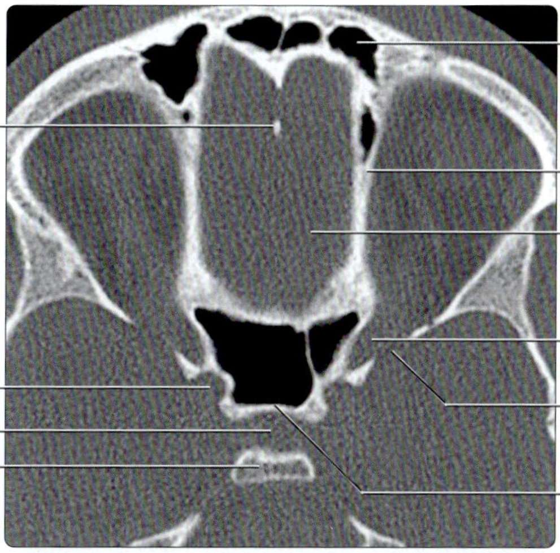

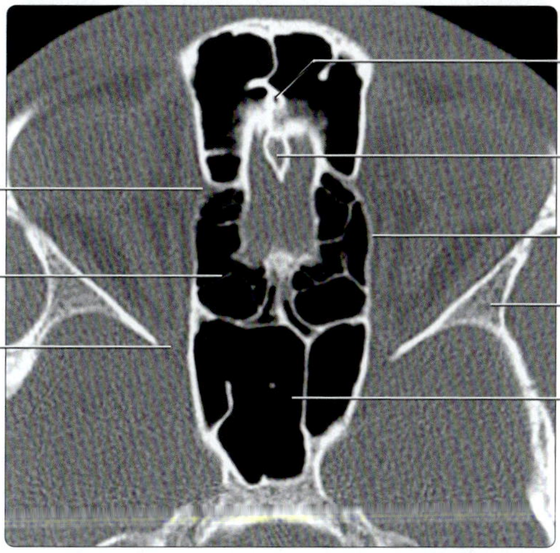

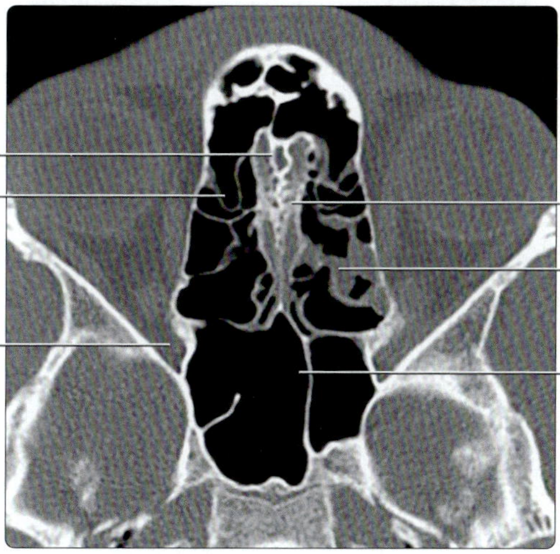

(Top) *This is the 1st of 3 axial bone CT images of the anterior skull base. In this image, the cephalad tip of crista galli is seen in the midline where it and the frontal crest give attachment to the falx cerebri. Superior orbital fissure and optic canal are both visible.* **(Middle)** *In this image, the ethmoid air cells are laterally bounded by the lamina papyracea, the paper-thin medial wall of the orbit. The anterior ethmoid foramen can also be seen bilaterally along the lateral wall of the ethmoid sinuses. This foramen contains the anterior ethmoid artery, vein, and nerve.* **(Bottom)** *The cribriform plate has a variable relationship to the roof of the ethmoid sinuses (fovea ethmoidalis).*

CORONAL BONE CT

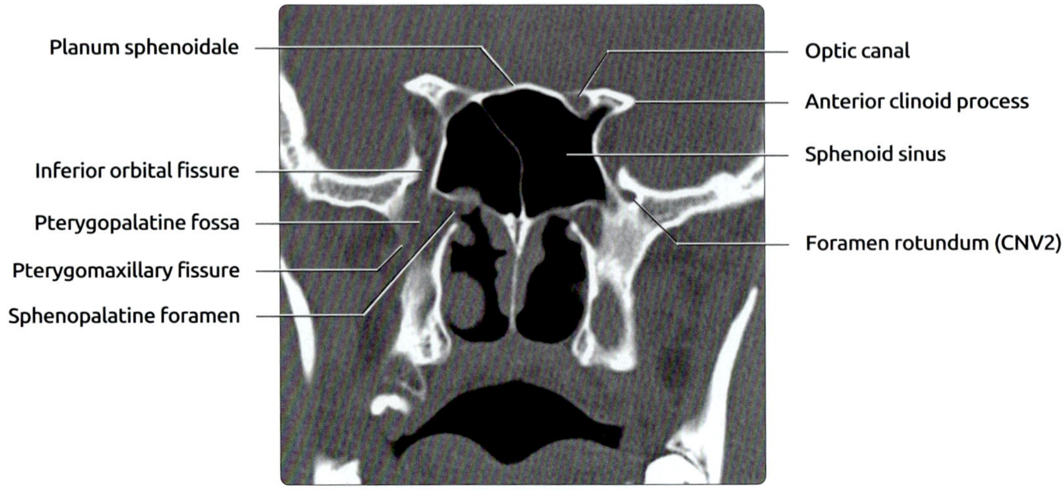

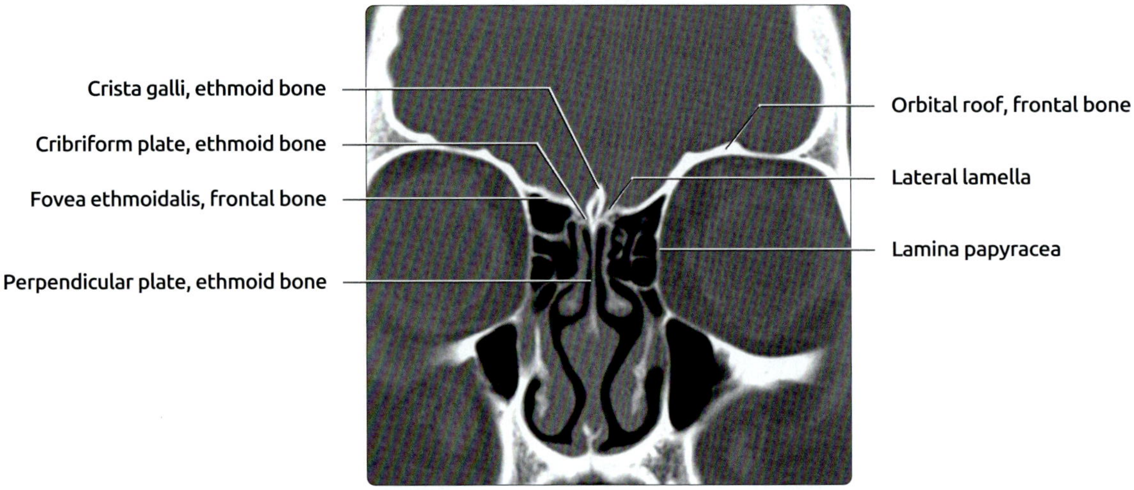

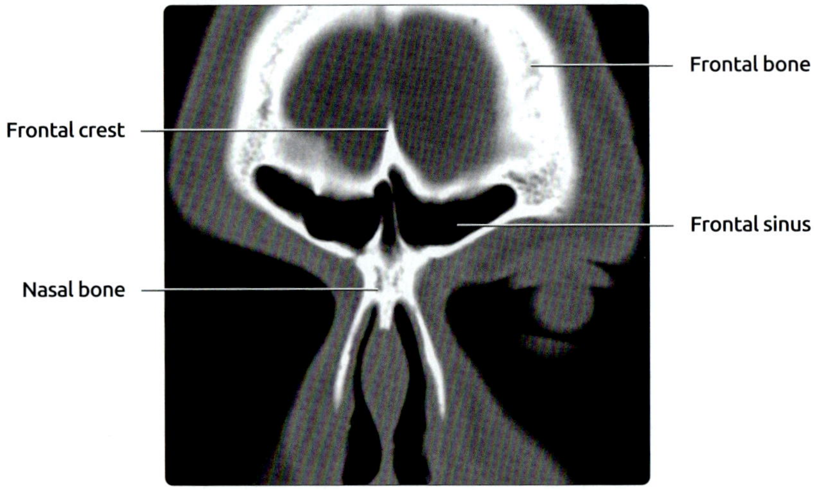

(Top) *First of 3 coronal bone CT images through the ASB shows the transition from central skull base to ASB. Notice the optic canal medial to the anterior clinoid processes. The inferior orbital fissure is seen inferolateral to the optic canal. The planum sphenoidale is the posterior sphenoid sinus roof.* **(Middle)** *More anteriorly at the level of the crista galli, it is possible to see the multiple pieces of the ethmoid bone. The crista galli is the most cephalad portion of the ethmoid bone, extending directly inferiorly into the perpendicular plate of the ethmoid bone. Just lateral to the base of the crista galli are the cribriform plates, lateral lamellae, & fovea ethmoidalis (ethmoid sinus roof) portions of the frontal bone. The more inferior to fovea ethmoidalis the cribriform plate is found, the larger the dimension of the lateral lamella and the more easily a sinus surgery complication may occur.* **(Bottom)** *In this image, the frontal crest of the frontal bones is seen. Do not confuse the more anterosuperior frontal crest with the crista galli (part of ethmoid), which is not seen on this image.*

AXIAL BONE CT DEVELOPMENT

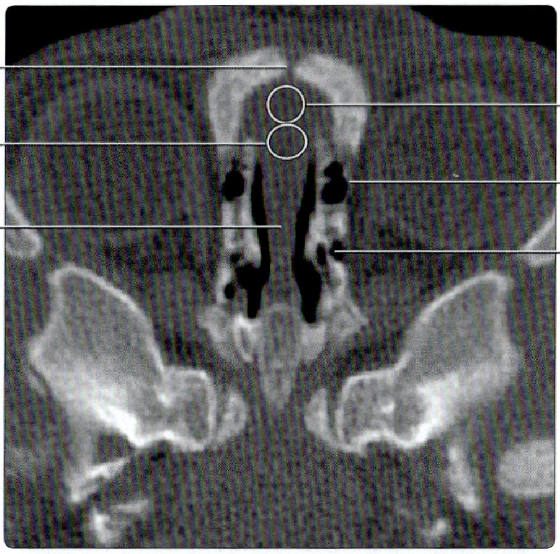

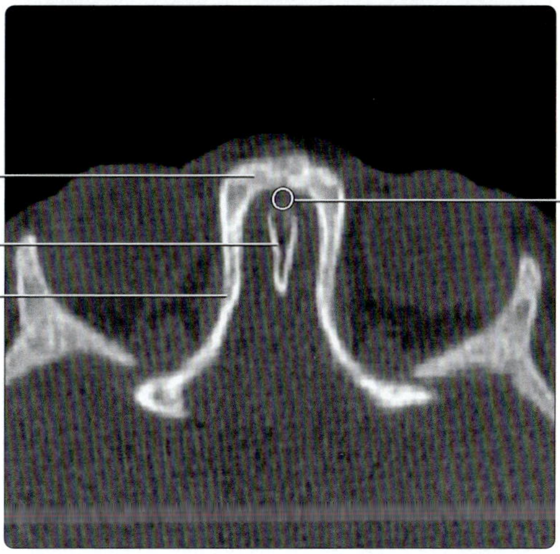

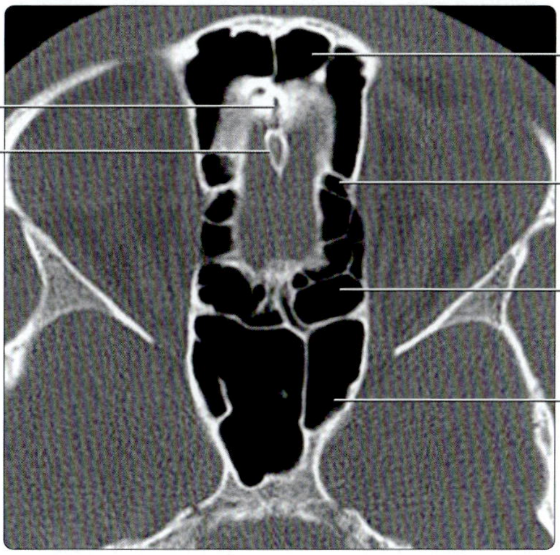

(Top) *Axial bone CT through the ASB in a newborn is shown. The unossified gap between the nasal and frontal bones normally contains dura at this age and represents the regressing anterior neuropore. The area of the foramen cecum, crista galli, cribriform plate, and perpendicular plate of the ethmoid bone are all normally unossified in the newborn.* **(Middle)** *Axial bone CT through the ASB at 12 months is shown. Crista galli is now well ossified. The foramen cecum area is still not ossified. The foramen cecum is still open, but the margins cannot be defined.* **(Bottom)** *Axial bone CT through the ASB in an adult is shown. The ethmoid air cells now extend far above the horizontal plane of the cribriform plate. Crista galli is thickened and heavily ossified. Although closed, the foramen cecum still demonstrates a small remnant pit.*

TERMINOLOGY

Abbreviations

- Central skull base (CSB)

Definitions

- CSB: Skull base (SB) posterior to lesser wings of sphenoid (LWS)/planum sphenoidale & anterior to petrous ridge/dorsum sellae

IMAGING ANATOMY

Overview

- CSB is floor of middle cranial fossa & roof of sphenoid sinus & greater wings of sphenoid (GWS)
- Bones forming CSB
  - Sphenoid bone, basisphenoid, & GWS
  - Temporal bone anterior to petrous ridge
- Boundaries of CSB
  - Anterior boundary: Planum sphenoidale posterior margin (tuberculum sellae) medially & LWS laterally
  - Posterior boundary: Dorsum sellae medially & petrous ridges laterally
- Relationships of CSB
  - Superior: Temporal lobes, pituitary, cavernous sinus, Meckel cave, CNI-IV, CNVI, CNV1-3
  - Inferior: Anterior roof of pharyngeal mucosal, masticator, parotid, & parapharyngeal spaces

Bony Landmarks of Central Skull Base

- **Sella turcica**: Contains pituitary gland
- **Anterior clinoid processes**: Extend posteromedially off LWS
- **Posterior clinoid processes**: Extend posterolaterally off dorsum sellae; provide attachment for tentorium cerebelli
- **Chiasmatic sulcus**: Just posteroinferior from posterior margin of planum sphenoidale; optic chiasm is located here
- **Tuberculum sellae**: Anterosuperior margin of sella turcica

Foramina & Fissures of Central Skull Base

- **Optic canal**
  - Transmits: CNII with dura, arachnoid & pia, CSF & ophthalmic artery
  - Formed by LWS, superomedially to superior orbital fissure
- **Superior orbital fissure**
  - Transmits: CNIII, CNIV, CNV1, & CNVI & superior ophthalmic vein
  - Formed by cleft between LWS & GWS
- **Inferior orbital fissure**
  - Transmits: Infraorbital artery, vein, & nerve
  - Formed by cleft between body of maxilla & GWS
- **Carotid canal**
  - Transmits: Internal carotid artery & sympathetic plexus
  - Formed by GWS & temporal bone
- **Foramen rotundum**
  - Transmits: CNV2, artery of foramen rotundum, & emissary veins
  - Completely within sphenoid bone; superolateral to vidian canal
  - Provides direct connection to pterygopalatine fossa
- **Foramen ovale**
  - Transmits: CNV3, lesser petrosal nerve, accessory meningeal branch of maxillary artery, & emissary vein
  - Completely within GWS
  - Provides direct connection to masticator space
- **Foramen spinosum**
  - Transmits: Middle meningeal artery & vein, meningeal branch of CNV3
  - Within GWS, posterolateral to foramen ovale
- **Foramen lacerum**
  - Not true foramen
  - Between temporal & sphenoid bones
  - Cartilaginous floor of medial part of horizontal petrous internal carotid artery canal
- **Vidian canal**
  - Transmits: Vidian artery & nerve
  - Formed by sphenoid bone, inferomedial to foramen rotundum

Development of Central Skull Base

- CSB formed by > 25 ossification centers
- Ossification occurs from posterior to anterior
- **Important ossification centers**: Orbitosphenoids, alisphenoids, pre- & postsphenoid, basiocciput
  - **Orbitosphenoids** → LWS, **alisphenoids** → GWS
  - **Presphenoid** & **postsphenoid** fuse at ~ 3 months
  - **Postsphenoid** & **basiocciput** fuse → clivus
- **Sphenooccipital synchondrosis**
  - Between postsphenoid & basiocciput
  - Responsible for most of postnatal SB growth
  - One of last sutures of SB to fuse
  - Open until 14 years, fuses by ~ 16 years in girls & ~ 18 years in boys

Variant Anatomy

- **Persistent craniopharyngeal canal**
  - Remnant of Rathke pouch
  - Vertical cleft in sphenoid body at site of fusion of pre- & postsphenoid; just posterior to tuberculum sellae area in adult
  - Extends from sella turcica to nasopharynx
- **Extensive pneumatization of sphenoid sinus**
  - Can cause endosinal vidian canals & foramen rotundum
  - Pneumatized clinoid processes
- **Canaliculus innominatus**
  - Variant canal for lesser superficial petrosal nerve, medial to foramen spinosum
- **Foramen of Vesalius**
  - Transmits emissary vein from cavernous sinus to pterygoid plexus
  - Anterior to foramen ovale

ANATOMY IMAGING ISSUES

Imaging Pitfalls

- Beware sphenoid MR signal changes
  - Sphenoid sinus: Low-signal cartilage until 2 years → high-signal fat until 6 years → low-signal air (adult)
  - Clivus low signal until 25 years, then high-signal fat
- Do not confuse pneumatized clinoid processes with vascular flow voids on MR or focal mass lesions

CENTRAL SKULL BASE GRAPHICS

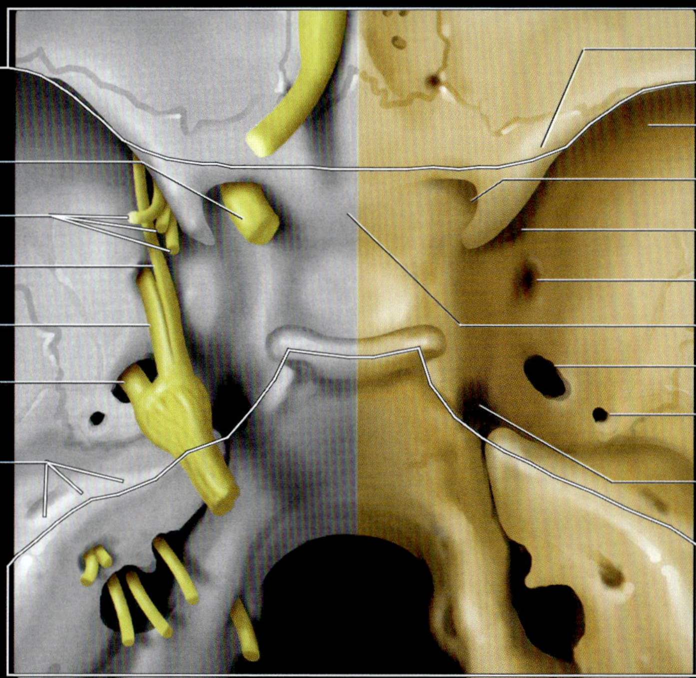

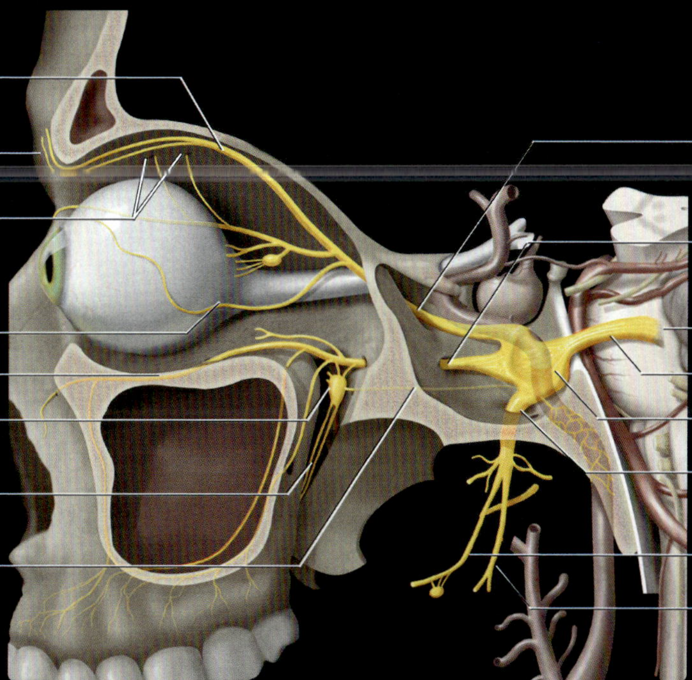

(Top) *Graphic of central skull base from above shows important nerves on the left. The numerous fissures & foramina of the central skull base are shown on the right. The greater wing of the sphenoid forms the anterior wall of the middle cranial fossa. The posterior limit of the central skull base is the dorsum sellae medially & the petrous ridge laterally.* **(Bottom)** *Sagittal graphic through central & anterior skull base depicts trigeminal nerve branches & exiting foramina. Ophthalmic division of CNV exits into the orbit via the superior orbital fissure. Maxillary division of CNV exits via foramen rotundum to become the infraorbital nerve as well as drops the greater & lesser palatine nerves inferiorly to provide sensation for the hard & soft palates. Mandibular division of CNV exits through foramen ovale, then divides into 2 main trunks: the lingual & inferior alveolar nerves. Note the vidian nerve in vidian canal.*

CENTRAL SKULL BASE GRAPHICS

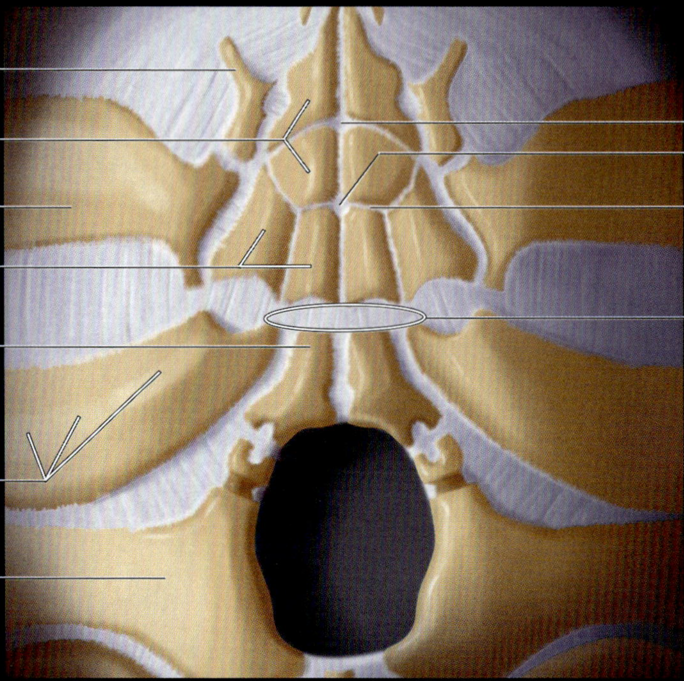

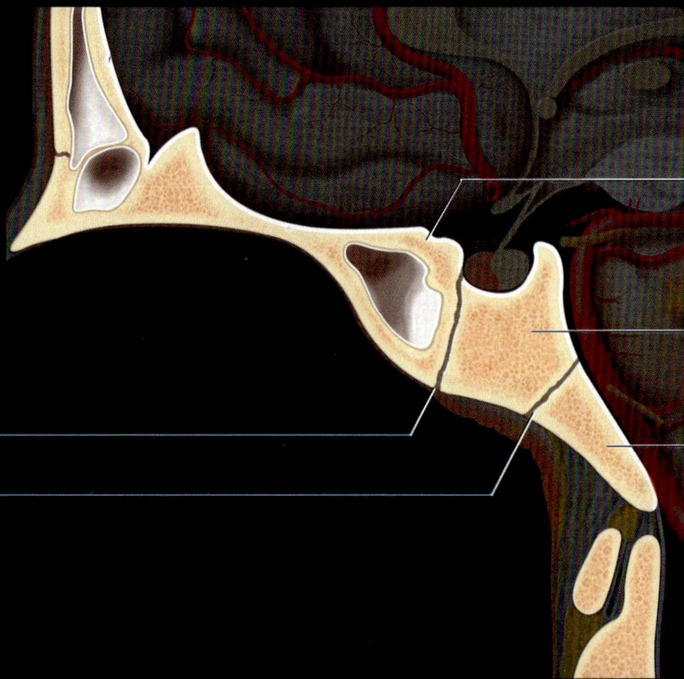

(Top) *Schematic graphic of central skull base from above shows its many ossification centers. Between ossification centers of presphenoid is a cartilaginous gap called olivary eminence, obliterated shortly after birth. A persistent cleft, called craniopharyngeal canal, can also be variably seen in intersphenoid synchondrosis. Do not confuse these variants with pathology.* **(Bottom)** *Lateral graphic of central skull base shows major ossification centers & the location of sutures. Intersphenoidal suture closes at around 3 months of age. At about age 2 years, presphenoid begins to demineralize & become pneumatized. Sphenoid sinus pneumatization progresses posteriorly into postsphenoid until about age 20. Sphenooccipital synchondrosis is one of the last sutures to fuse at about age 20-25. It is the suture most responsible for growth of the skull base.*

AXIAL BONE CT

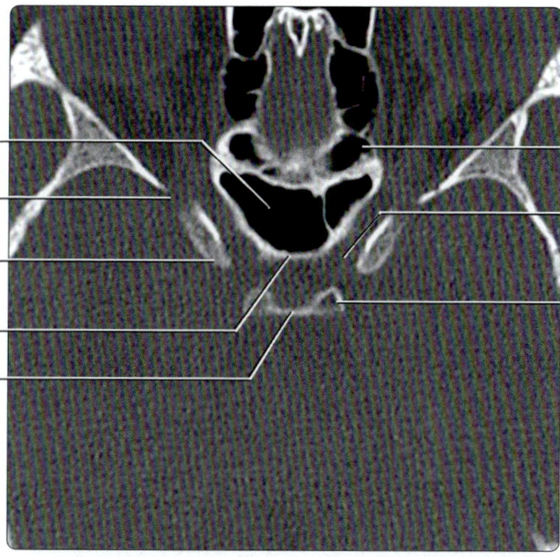

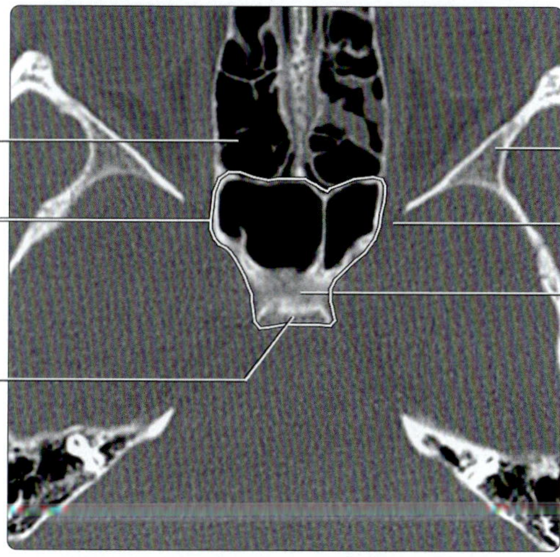

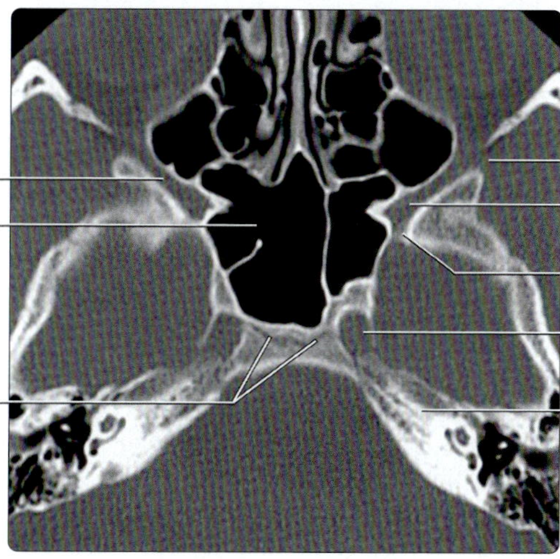

(Top) *This is the 1st of 6 axial bone CT images of the central skull base presented from superior to inferior. Note that the posterior clinoids merge with the dorsum sellae. The optic canal is bound by the sphenoid sinus medially & the anterior clinoid process laterally. Inferolateral to the optic canal is the superior orbital fissure.* **(Middle)** *The body of the sphenoid bone (basisphenoid) is seen to be made up of the sphenoid sinus, sella turcica, & the dorsum sellae. Anterior to the sphenoid bone is the ethmoid bone.* **(Bottom)** *This image shows pneumatization of sphenoid extending up to the sphenooccipital synchondrosis, which is partly unfused in this young adult. Note that the foramen rotundum empties anteriorly into the pterygopalatine fossa, which connects laterally with the masticator space through the pterygomaxillary fissure.*

AXIAL BONE CT

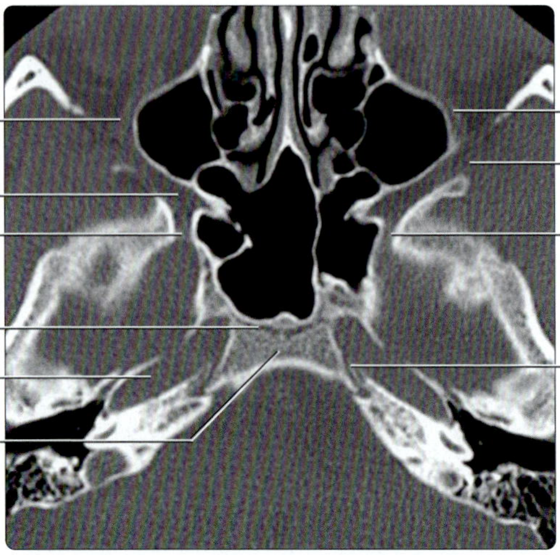

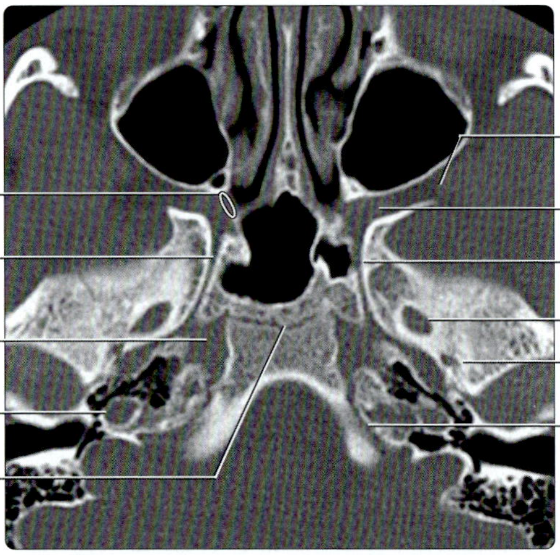

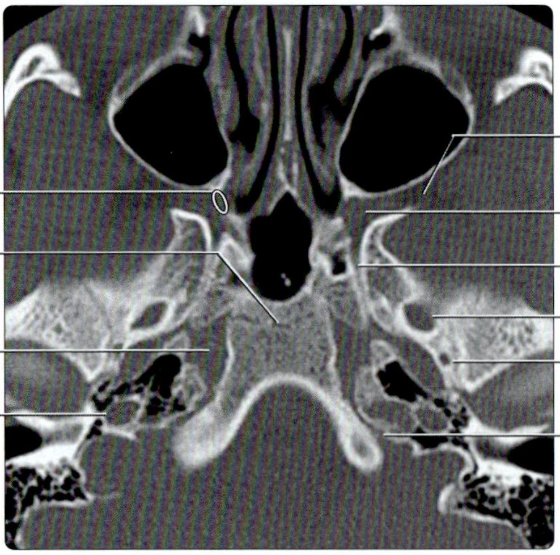

(Top) *At the level of foramen rotundum, both pterygopalatine fossae are visible. The maxillary division of the trigeminal nerve (CNV2) exits the skull base through the foramen rotundum & continues as the infraorbital nerve into the orbit via inferior orbital fissure. Malignant tumors of the cheek skin, orbit, & sinonasal area may all use CNV2 as a perineural route to gain intracranial access.* **(Middle)** *The vidian canal is visible connecting the pterygopalatine fossa anteriorly to the carotid canal floor (foramen lacerum) posteriorly. A malignant tumor that has accessed the pterygopalatine fossa may reach the carotid canal of the skull base via perineural spread on the vidian nerve in the vidian canal. The medial connection between the pterygopalatine fossa & nose is the sphenopalatine foramen.* **(Bottom)** *Note the foramen ovale is located in the greater wing of the sphenoid bone. Extracranial perineural malignancy on CNV3 enters the intracranial area via foramen ovale.*

CORONAL BONE CT

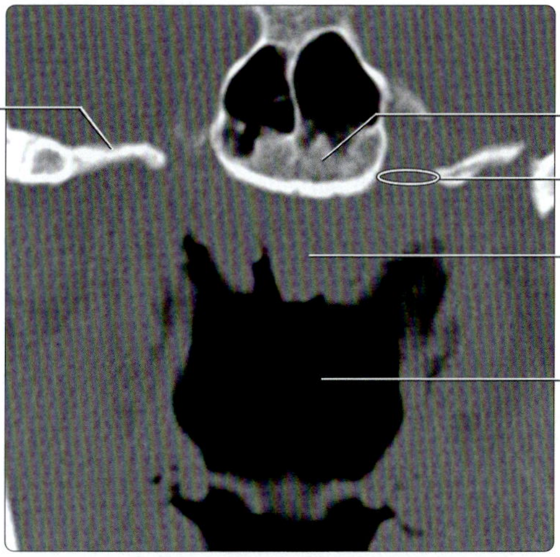

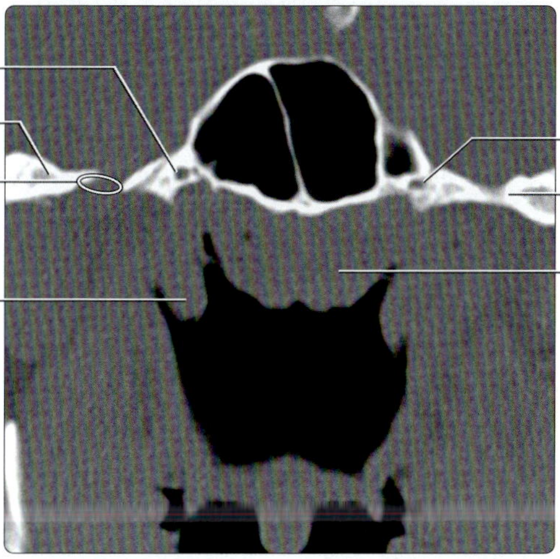

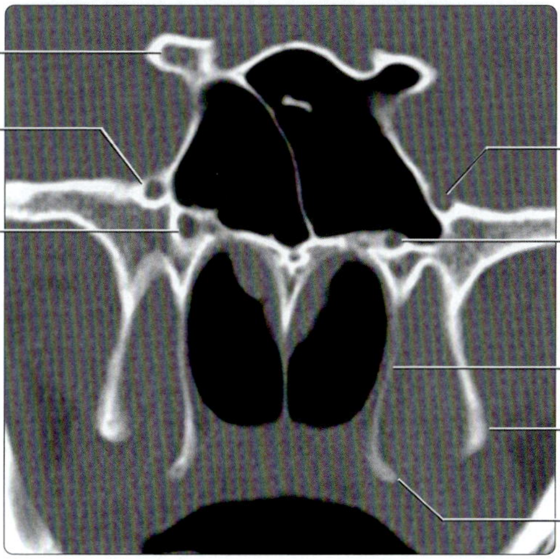

(Top) *This is the 1st of 3 coronal bone CT images of the central skull base presented from posterior to anterior. The foramen lacerum is seen as a large defect between the greater wing of the sphenoid bone & the sphenoid body. Foramen lacerum is not a true foramen; it represents the cartilaginous floor of the anteromedial horizontal segment of the petrous internal carotid artery canal.* **(Middle)** *The foramen ovale is evident lateral to the vidian canal & anterolateral to the foramen lacerum. The foramen ovale transmits CNV3 from the middle cranial fossa to the masticator space. CNV3 provides motor innervation to the muscles of mastication & sensory innervation to the jaw.* **(Bottom)** *More anteriorly, foramen rotundum & vidian canal are both seen running in the transverse plane. Both foramen rotundum & vidian canal open into the pterygopalatine fossa. Also note the pterygoid plates inferiorly. Remember the foramen rotundum contains CNV2, which provides sensory innervation to the cheek.*

TERMINOLOGY

Abbreviations

- Posterior skull base (PSB)

Definitions

- Skull base (SB) posterior to dorsum sella and petrous ridges

IMAGING ANATOMY

Overview

- Made up of posterior temporal bones and occipital bone and transmits CNVII-XII, medulla oblongata, and jugular vein
- Bones of PSB
  - Temporal bones posterior to petrous ridges
  - **Occipital bone** (3 parts)
    - **Basilar part** (basiocciput): Quadrilateral part anterior to foramen magnum
    - **Condylar part** (exoccipital): Occipital condyles here; lateral to foramen magnum
    - **Squamous part**: Large bony plate posterosuperior to foramen magnum
- Boundaries of PSB
  - Anterior boundary: Dorsum sella medially and petrous ridges laterally
  - Posterior boundary: Occipital bone
- Relationships of PSB
  - Inferior relationships: Posterior roof of pharyngeal mucosal space, carotid, parotid, retropharyngeal, perivertebral spaces, and cervical spine
  - Superior relationships: Brainstem, cerebellum, CNVII-VIII, CNIX-XII, transverse-sigmoid sinuses

Bony Landmarks of Posterior Skull Base

- **Petrous ridge of temporal bone (TB)**
  - Divides central skull base (CSB) from PSB
  - Attachment for fixed edge of tentorium cerebelli
- **Jugular tubercle**
  - Roof of hypoglossal canal seen well on coronal imaging
  - "Eagle's head" on coronal images is jugular tubercle

Foramina and Fissures of Posterior Skull Base

- **Internal acoustic meatus**
  - Transmits: CNVII-VIII, labyrinthine artery
  - Opening in posterior wall TB superior to jugular foramen (JF)
  - Porus acusticus: Internal opening of internal acoustic meatus
- **JF**
  - 2 parts: Pars nervosa and pars vascularis partially divided by jugular spine
  - Between temporal and occipital bones
  - Carotid space extends directly up to JF
  - **Pars nervosa**
    - Transmits CNIX, Jacobson nerve, and inferior petrosal sinus
    - Anteromedial but contiguous with pars vascularis
  - **Pars vascularis**
    - Transmits CNX, Arnold nerve, CNXI, jugular bulb, and posterior meningeal artery
    - Larger than pars nervosa
- **Groove for sigmoid sinus**
  - Groove in medial mastoid temporal bone; cradles sigmoid sinus
- **Hypoglossal canal**
  - Transmits: CNXII
  - Formed in condylar occipital bone
  - Inferomedial to JF
- **Foramen magnum**
  - Transmits: CNXI (cephalad component), vertebral arteries, and medulla oblongata
  - Formed completely by occipital bone
- **Stylomastoid foramen**
  - Transmits: CNVII
  - Found in exocranial skull base surface between mastoid tip and styloid process
  - Extends directly into parotid space

Development of Posterior Skull Base

- Occipital bone has 4 major ossification centers around foramen magnum
  - **Supraoccipital**, **basioccipital**, and paired **exoccipital**
- PSB is nearly completely ossified by birth
- **Sutures of PSB** remain unfused until 2nd decade
  - Intraoccipital sutures fuses between 8-16 years
  - Petrooccipital and occipitomastoid sutures are among last to close (15-17 years)

Variant Anatomy of Posterior Skull Base

- **Posterior condylar canal**
  - Inconstant canal for emissary vein and meningeal branch of ascending pharyngeal artery
  - One of largest emissary foramina of SB
- **Asymmetric petrous apices**
  - Can contain high-signal fat or low-signal air
- **Mastoid foramen**
  - Variably transmits emissary vein from sigmoid sinus

ANATOMY IMAGING ISSUES

Questions

- PSB is largely ossified at birth but PSB sutures are last in SB to fuse
- PSB is intimately related to carotid and parotid spaces

Imaging Recommendations

- Bone CT with edge enhancement algorithm and wide windows (> 2,000 HU)
- Use coronal imaging to examine normal "double eagles" of hypoglossal canal and JF area

Imaging Pitfalls

- Watch for asymmetric petrous apex air &/or fat
- Beware of JF pseudolesion from MR flow phenomenon
- Beware open synchondroses/suture as pseudofracture

GRAPHICS

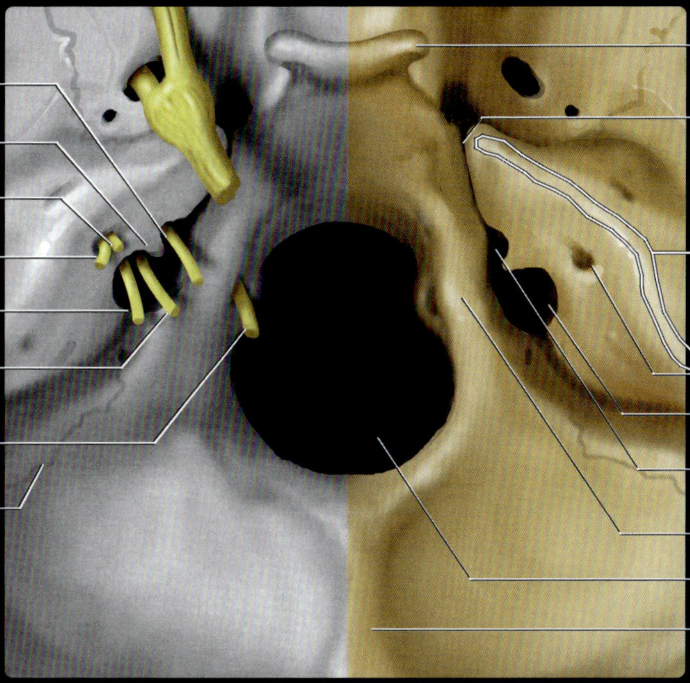

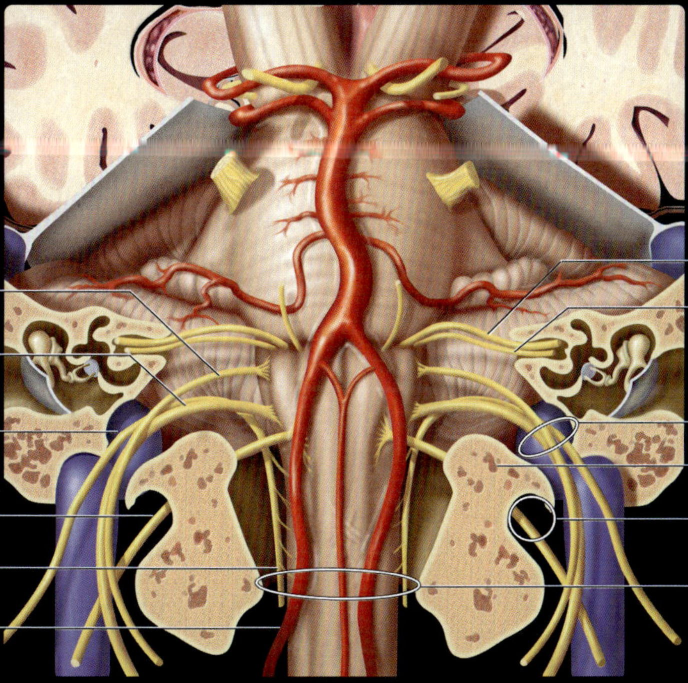

(Top) *Graphic of posterior skull base as seen from above is shown. Neural structures are shown on the left and bony landmarks on the right. Anterior boundary of posterior skull base is clivus medially and petrous ridge laterally. The major foramina are the foramen magnum, porus acusticus, jugular foramen, and hypoglossal canal. Notice that the jugular foramen connects anteriorly with the petrooccipital fissure.* **(Bottom)** *Coronal graphic of posterior skull base viewed from the front shows the classic double eagle appearance in the area of the hypoglossal canal. The jugular tubercle (eagle's head and beak) separates the inferomedial hypoglossal canal from the jugular foramen. The hypoglossal nerve is found in the hypoglossal canal, while CNIX-XI traverse the skull base in the jugular foramen.*

GRAPHIC AND MR OF DURAL SINUSES

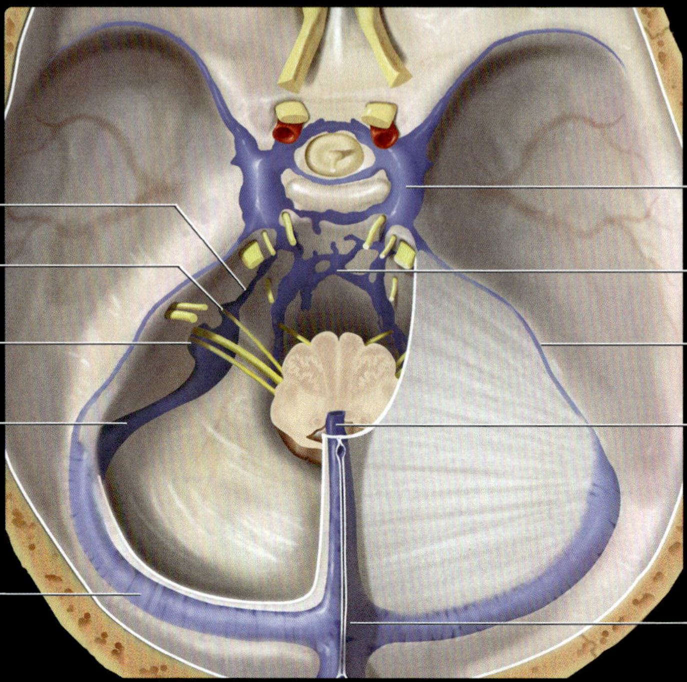

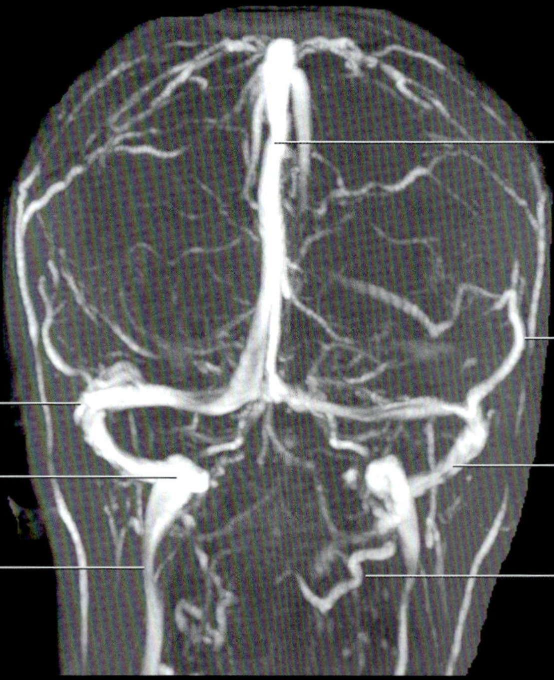

(Top) *Graphic of major dural venous sinuses and jugular foramen as seen from top down is shown. The midbrain and pons, as well as the left 1/2 of the tentorium cerebelli, have been removed. Notice the transverse sinus is in the wall of the occipital bone, while the sigmoid sinus is in the medial wall of the temporal bone. The 2 portions of the jugular foramen are also visible. The anterior pars nervosa receives the glossopharyngeal nerve (CNIX) with the pars vascularis and has the vagus (CNX) and accessory (CNXI) nerves passing through it.* **(Bottom)** *Coronal view of MR venogram shows the transverse sinuses feeding through the sigmoid sinuses into the jugular foramen. The jugular bulb connects inferiorly with the internal jugular vein of the carotid space. The slight asymmetry of transverse sinuses is normal.*

AXIAL BONE CT

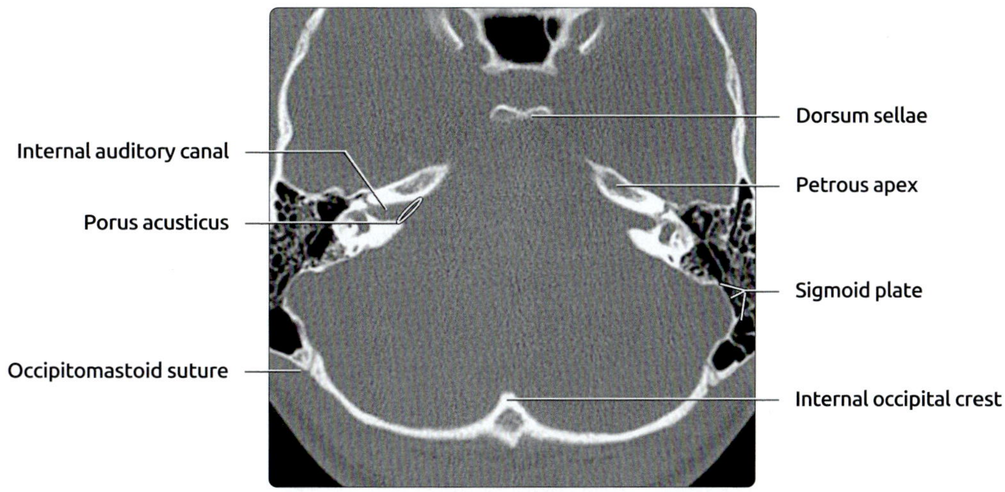

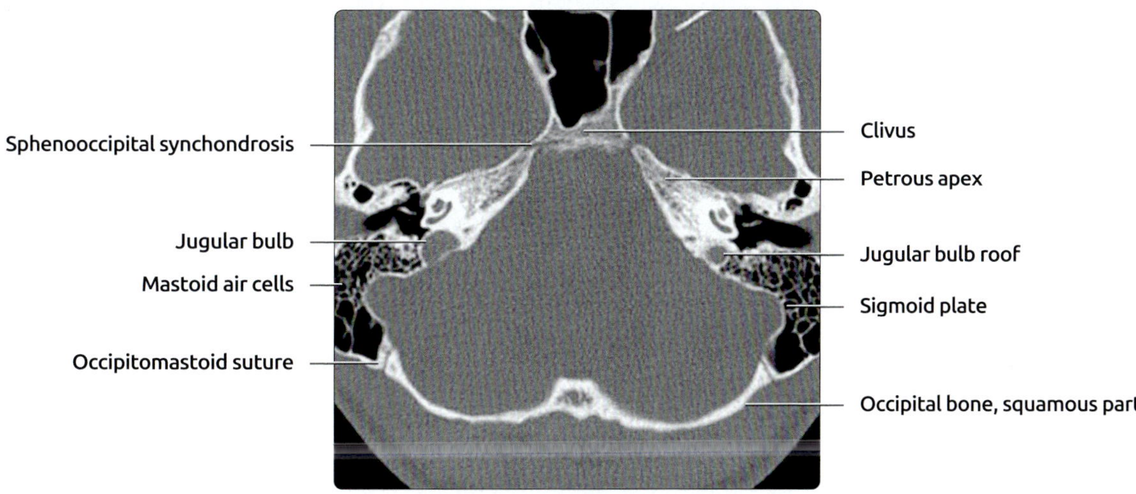

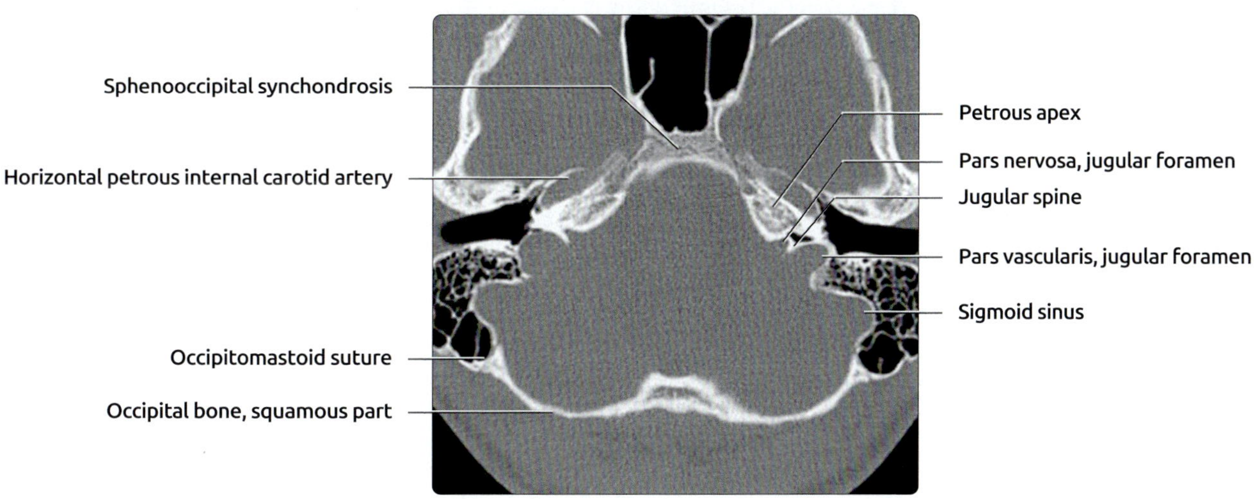

(Top) *First of 9 axial bone CTs presented from superior to inferior shows the dorsum sella and the petrous temporal bone as the anterior margin of the posterior skull base. Posteriorly, the midline is demarcated by the bony internal occipital crest, which provides an attachment for the falx cerebelli. Porus acusticus is the most superior foramen of the posterior skull base and transmits CNVII and VIII.* **(Middle)** *At the level of mid cochlea, the posterior cranial fossa is completely divided from the middle cranial fossa by the clivus and petrous temporal bone. Laterally, the sigmoid plate separates the mastoid air cells from the sigmoid sinus. The jugular bulbs are visible bilaterally.* **(Bottom)** *Note the smaller anteromedial pars nervosa (CNIX, Jacobsen nerve, inferior petrosal sinus) and larger pars vascularis (jugular bulb, Arnold nerve, CNX and XI) at the level of the midjugular foramen.*

AXIAL BONE CT

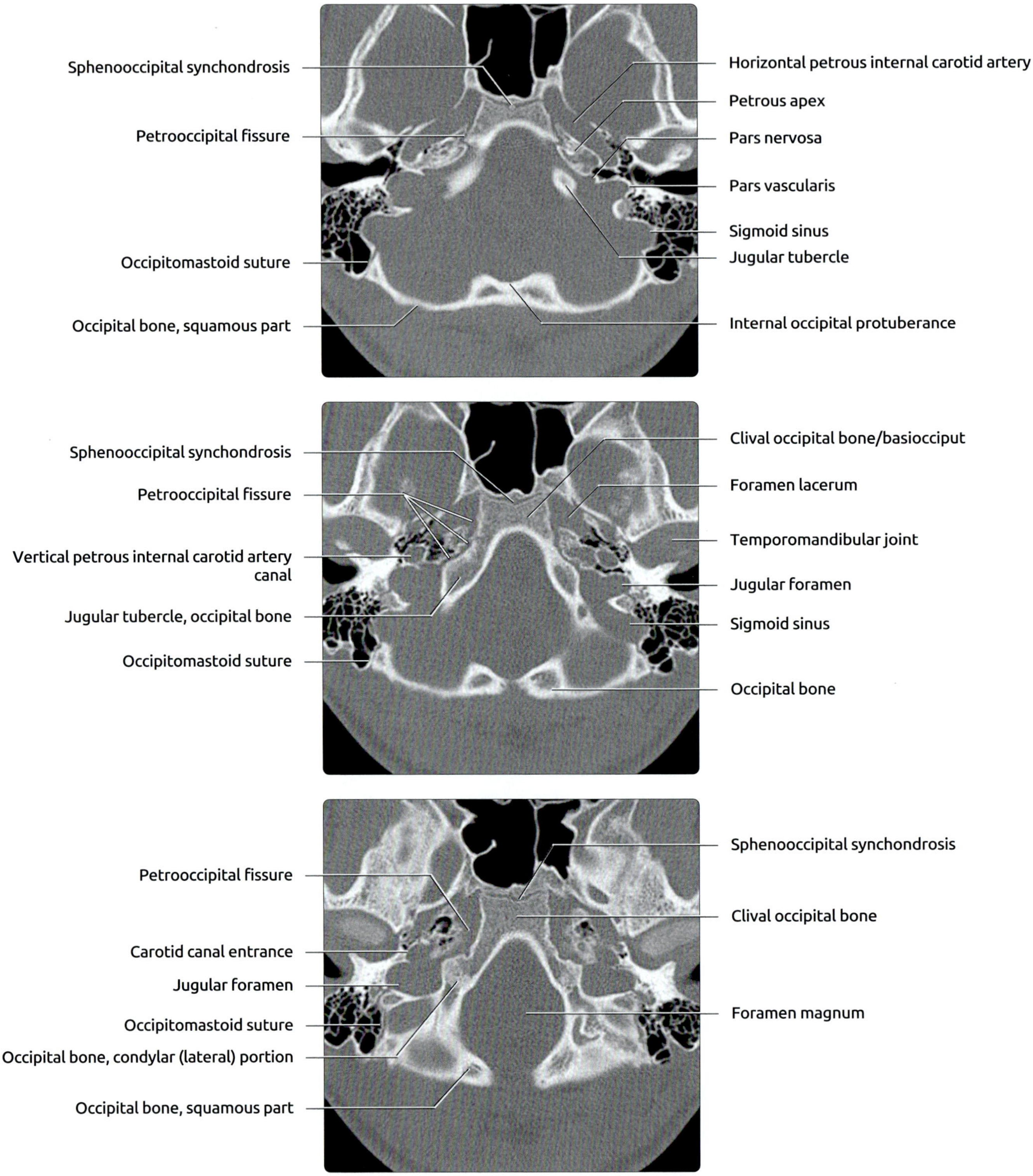

(Top) *CT of the posterior skull base shows the sphenooccipital synchondrosis, the petrooccipital fissure, and the occipitomastoid suture all in the same plane. The sphenooccipital synchondrosis has not yet fused in this adolescent.* **(Middle)** *CT through the jugular tubercle and the clivus is made up almost completely of anterior occipital bone. The upper 1/3 of the clivus is above the sphenooccipital synchondrosis and is therefore part of the sphenoid bone.* **(Bottom)** *In this CT, the lower clivus (below the sphenooccipital synchondrosis) is clearly made up of occipital bone. The petrooccipital fissure separates the temporal bone from the occipital bone. The occipitomastoid suture separates the mastoid sinus from the squamosal portion of the occipital bone.*

AXIAL BONE CT

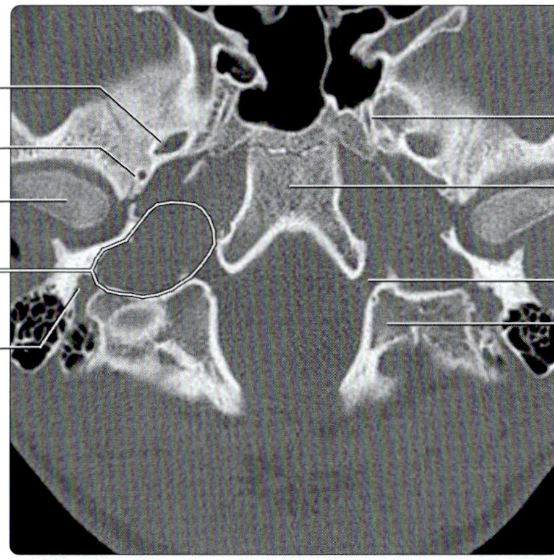

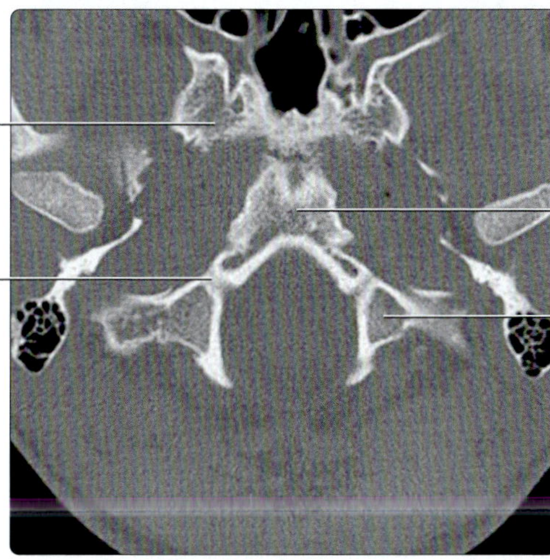

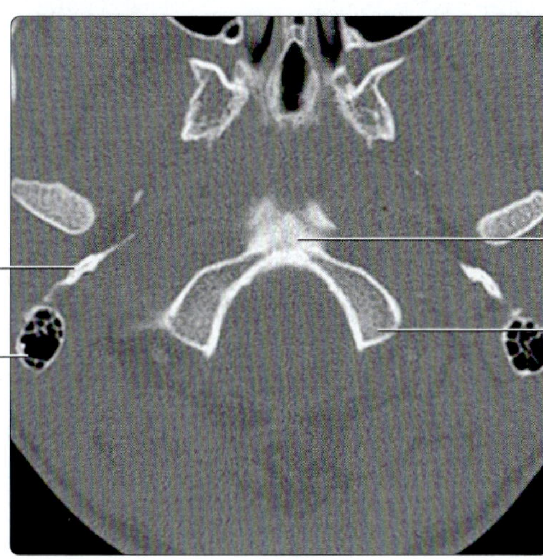

(Top) *CT passes directly through the hypoglossal canal and stylomastoid foramen. This canal transmits only the hypoglossal nerve. Notice that as soon as the nerve exits the hypoglossal canal, it immediately enters the nasopharyngeal carotid space to join the glossopharyngeal (CNIX), vagus (CNX), and accessory (CNXI) cranial nerves.* **(Middle)** *In this CT, the inferior margin of the hypoglossal canal runs within occipital bone, between the basilar (clival) and condylar portions. The inferior surface of the portion of the condylar occipital bone are the occipital condyles.* **(Bottom)** *In this CT through the occipital condyle, the inferior-most junction of the basilar (clival) occipital bone and the condylar occipital bone is visible. The occipital condyles rest the cranium upon the lateral masses of atlas (C1 vertebral body).*

CORONAL BONE CT

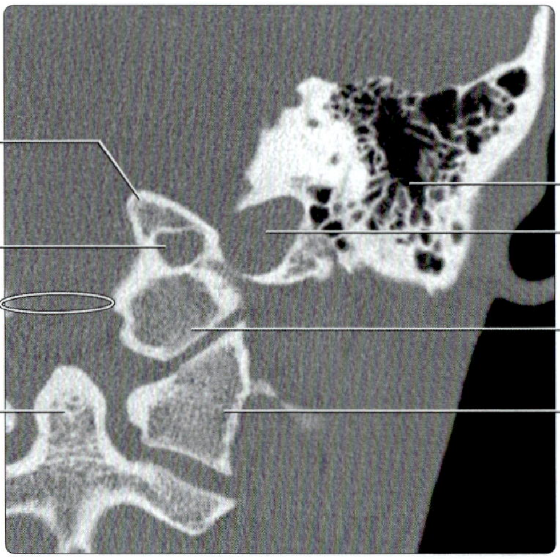

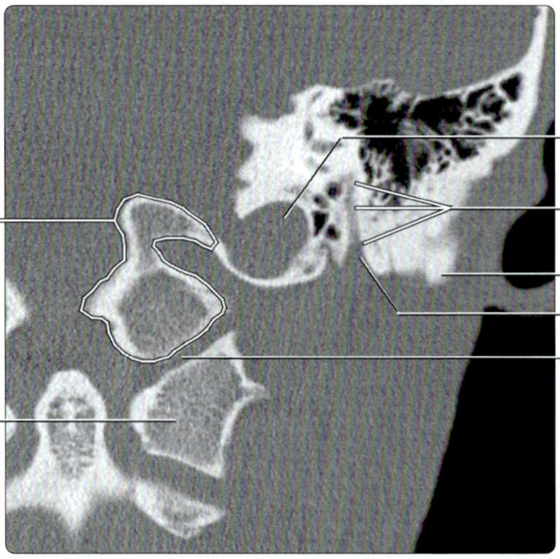

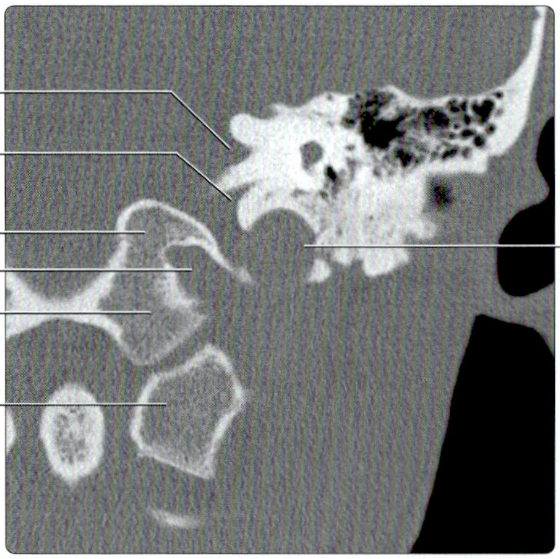

(Top) *The 1st of 6 coronal bone CTs of the left posterior skull base, presented from posterior to anterior, is shown. The hypoglossal canal passes through the condylar (lateral) portion of the occipital bone. In the coronal plane with both sides visible, this area has been referred to as the double eagle. Notice that the eagle's head and beak are the jugular tubercle.* **(Middle)** *In this CT through the mastoid (descending) portion of intratemporal facial nerve canal, the condylar part of the occipital bone is outlined.* **(Bottom)** *This CT shows the classic "eagle" of the posterior skull base with the "beak" of the jugular tubercle separating the jugular foramen from the hypoglossal canal. Lesions of the hypoglossal canal affect the undersurface of the beak, while lesions of the jugular foramen affect the external surface of the beak.*

CORONAL BONE CT

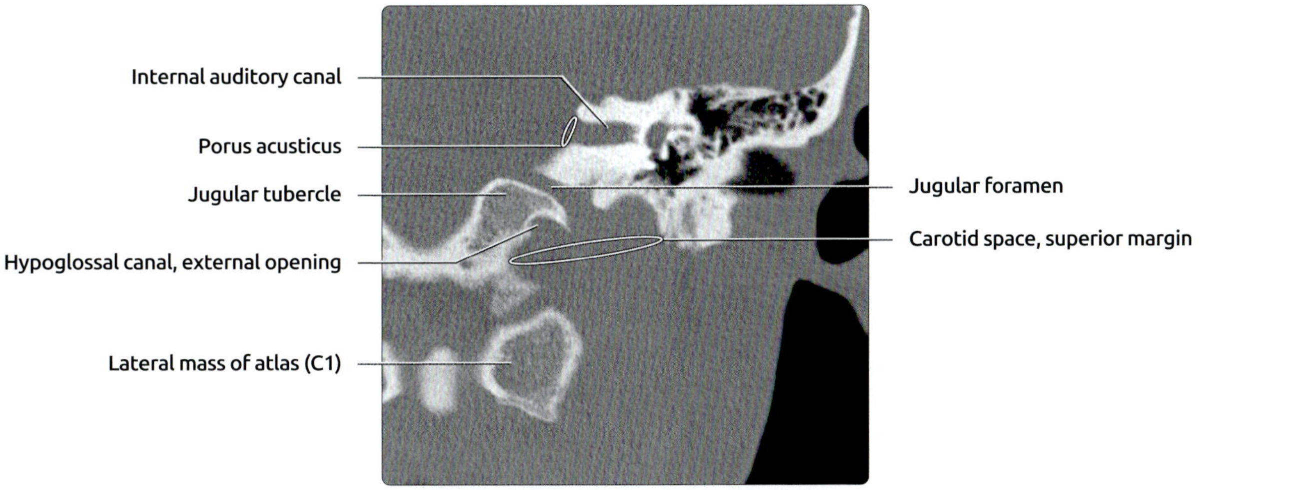

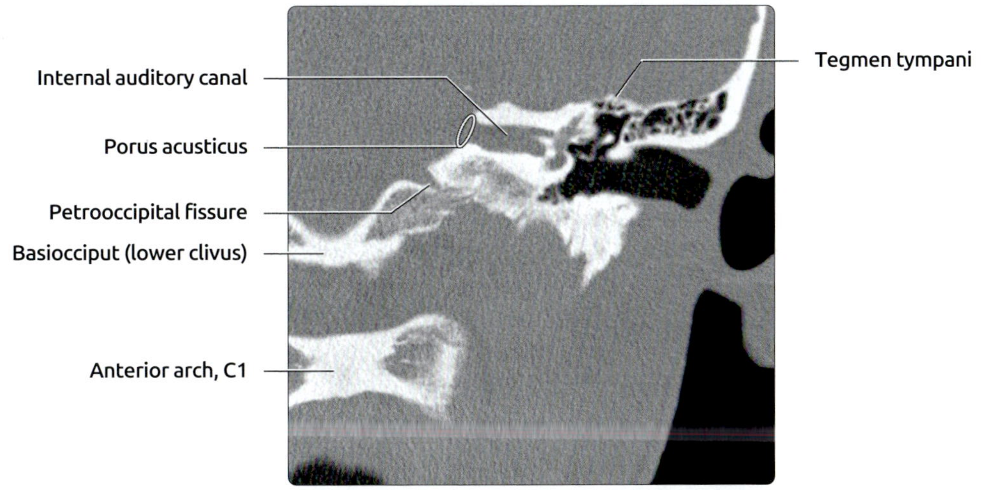

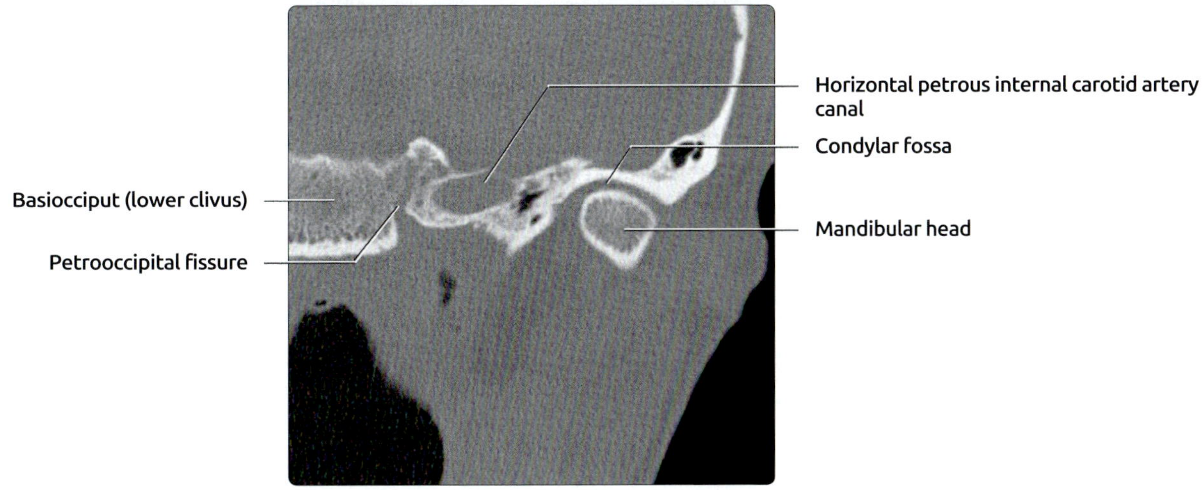

(Top) *In this CT of the left skull base and temporal bone, notice both the hypoglossal canal and the jugular foramen "empty" into the cephalad carotid space. The upper carotid space therefore contains CNIX-XII as well as the internal jugular vein.* **(Middle)** *In this CT through the mid internal auditory canal, the petrooccipital fissure is visible, separating the basioccipital portion of the occipital bone from the temporal bone.* **(Bottom)** *In this CT through the condylar fossa of the temporomandibular joint, the petrooccipital fissure is seen between the basiocciput and the temporal bone. The basiocciput is a large quadrilateral portion of the occipital bone that extends anterosuperiorly from the anterior margin of the foramen magnum to reach the sphenoid bone ~ 2/3 of the way up the clivus.*

TERMINOLOGY

Definitions

- **Styloid process**
  - Thin, elongated, and pointed process of temporal bone extending inferiorly from skull base
- **Stylohyoid ligament**
  - Fibrous band between tip of styloid process to lesser horn of hyoid bone
- Styloid process, stylohyoid ligament, and lesser horn of hyoid form **stylohyoid chain**

IMAGING ANATOMY

Overview

- Styloid process and stylohyoid ligament derive from Reichert cartilage of 2nd branchial arch
  - 4 segments give rise to stylohyoid chain
  - Upper 2 segments form styloid process (tympanohyal and stylohyal)
    - Failure of these to fuse leads to short styloid
  - Lower segment forms lesser horn of hyoid (hypohyal)
  - Stylohyoid ligament formed from segment in between (ceratohyal)
    - Often retains small central cartilaginous remnant
    - Ossification may occur
- Styloid process **normally < 3 cm** in length
  - Located medial to mastoid process and external auditory meatus, anterior to stylomastoid foramen
  - Its proximal part is ensheathed by vaginal process
  - Serves as attachment for ligaments and muscles
    - Stylohyoid ligament
    - Stylomandibular ligament
    - Stylohyoid muscle
    - Styloglossus muscle
    - Stylopharyngeus muscle
  - Located between internal and external carotid arteries and internal jugular vein
  - In close relation to cranial nerves V, VII, IX, X, and XII

Clinical Issues

- **Elongated styloid process and Eagle syndrome**
  - Normal length of styloid process varies significantly
  - Elongation present in 4% of population
  - More rarely do symptoms arise due to impingement of neighboring structures (cranial nerves and vessels)
  - M < F
  - 30+ years of age
- **Clinical symptoms**
  - **Classic syndrome**
    - Facial pain, ear pain
    - Dysphagia
    - Foreign body sensation in pharynx
    - Painful trismus and mandibular excursion
    - Neck mobility limitations
    - Pain on palpation of tonsillar fossa
    - **May mimic temporomandibular joint pain**
  - **Stylocarotid artery syndrome**
    - Neck, eye, infraorbital, or parietal pain
    - Syncopal episodes
    - Visual disturbance
    - Most commonly with neck palpation or head turning; **may mimic headache/migraine**
- Symptoms vary depending on angulation and size of process or ossified ligament
- Rarely cerebrovascular complications may develop
  - Transient or prolonged ischemia due to carotid compression
- Relief from symptoms with local anesthetic infiltration into tonsillar fossa helps confirm diagnosis

Etiology

- Classic syndrome
  - Linked to tonsillectomy or neck trauma, but this is not consistent
  - Granulation tissue and fibrosis may entrap and irritate nerves
  - Fracture of ossified stylohyoid ligament with subsequent nonunion hypothesized
  - Tendinitis at insertion of ligament to hyoid bone
- Stylocarotid syndrome
  - Irritation of carotid sympathetic plexus or compression of artery by tip of styloid process
  - Often due to deviation of process medially

Treatment

- Conservative
  - Steroid and anesthetic injections
- Surgical
  - Extraoral or intraoral shortening of stylohyoid chain

ANATOMY IMAGING ISSUES

Imaging Recommendations

- Imaging of styloid process is usually incidental
- If Eagle syndrome is suspected, use panoramic radiograph
  - Elongated styloid process or ossified stylohyoid ligament is well visualized
  - Examination of lateral portions of film will reveal elongated styloid process originating inferior and posterior to temporomandibular joint and extending anteriorly and inferiorly towards submandibular region
  - May be superimposed over angle of mandible or with other structures in neck
- Bone CT or CBCT also clearly depict these changes and allow accurate measurement
  - 3D CT helps visualize position, angulation, and size
  - CT angiogram to assess cases of vascular compression
- **Different patterns of ossification** may be seen
  - Single, continuous radiopaque band of variable thickness
    - Ossification might extend right to hyoid bone
  - Partial ossification with separate foci of radiopacity: **Segmented**
  - Segments may abut one another with appearance of **pseudoarticulation**

SELECTED REFERENCES

1. Radak D et al: Bilateral Eagle syndrome with associated internal carotid artery kinking and significant stenosis. Ann Vasc Surg. 34:271.e15-8, 2016
2. Elimairi I et al: Eagle's syndrome. Head Neck Pathol. 9(4):492-5, 2015
3. Kent DT et al: Conventional and 3-dimensional computerized tomography in Eagle's syndrome, glossopharyngeal neuralgia, and asymptomatic controls. Otolaryngol Head Neck Surg. 153(1):41-7, 2015

Styloid Process and Stylohyoid Ligament

GRAPHICS

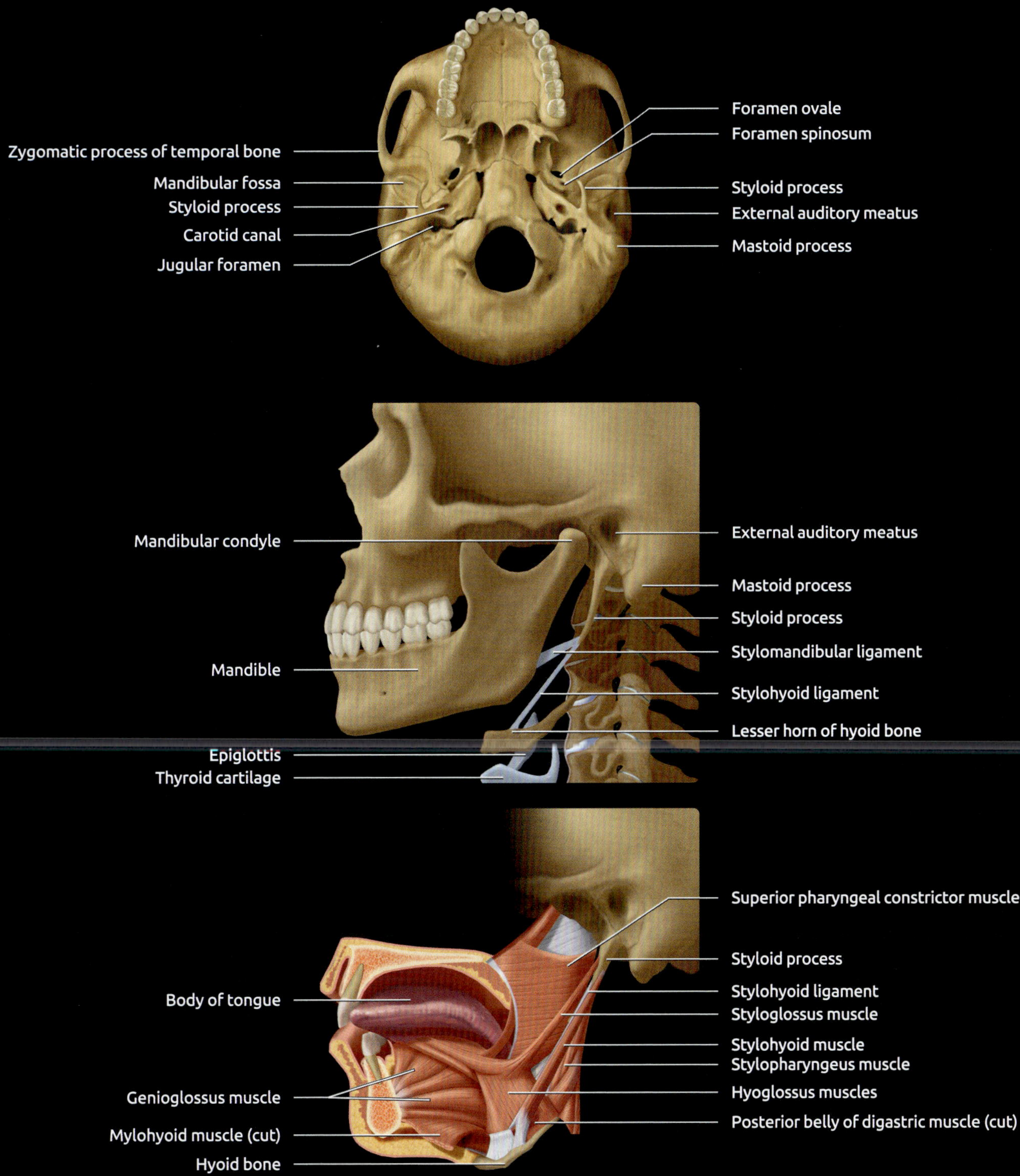

(Top) *Graphic depicts an inferior view of the skull base. The styloid processes are seen as bilateral, thin, tapering projections of the temporal bone. They sit posterior and medial to the mandibular fossae and anterior and medial to the mastoid processes.* **(Middle)** *Lateral graphic shows the attachment of the stylomandibular and stylohyoid ligaments to the styloid process. The stylohyoid ligament may ossify to varying degrees, which can be seen incidentally on imaging studies involving the neck.* **(Bottom)** *Graphic depicts the muscle attachments to the styloid process. These include the styloglossus, stylohyoid, and stylopharyngeus.*

3D CT, PANORAMIC

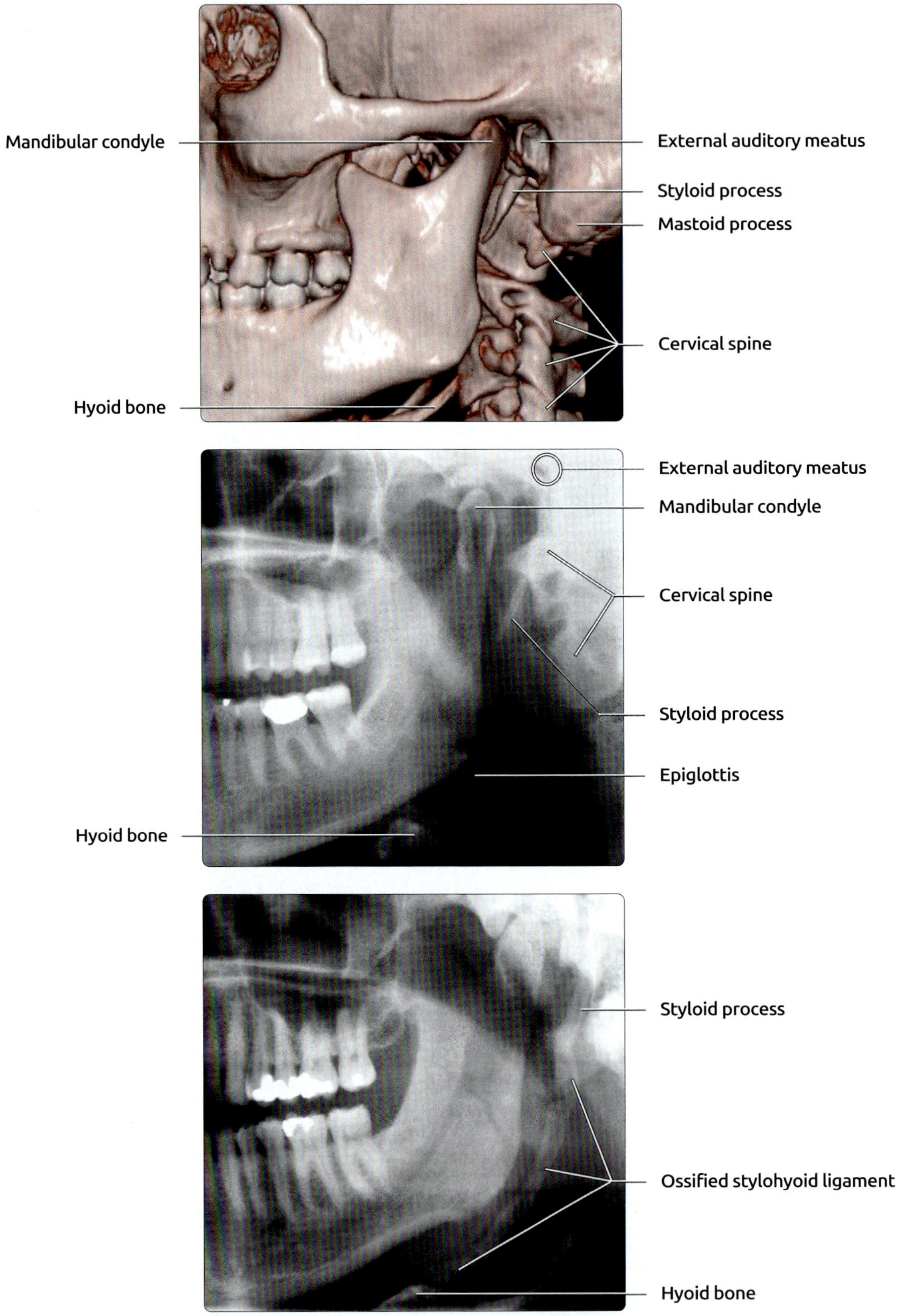

(Top) *3D surface rendering of a CT volume shows a normal styloid process and its position deep to the temporomandibular joint, external auditory meatus, and mastoid process.* **(Middle)** *Cropped panoramic radiograph shows a normal styloid process located posterior to the ramus of the mandible. It is superimposed by the shadows of the upper cervical spine and external ear.* **(Bottom)** *Cropped panoramic radiograph shows a heavily ossified stylohyoid chain. Note its segmented or pseudoarticulated appearance. The inferior aspect of the ossified stylohyoid ligament is seen attaching to the lesser horn of the hyoid bone, inferior to the mandibular body. This was an incidental finding in an asymptomatic patient.*

PANORAMIC, CBCT

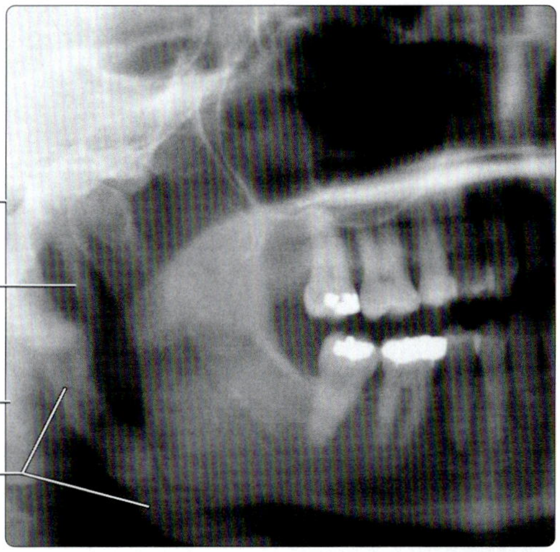

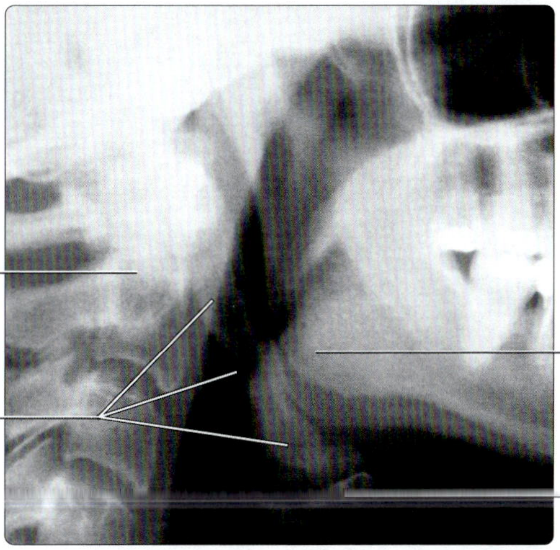

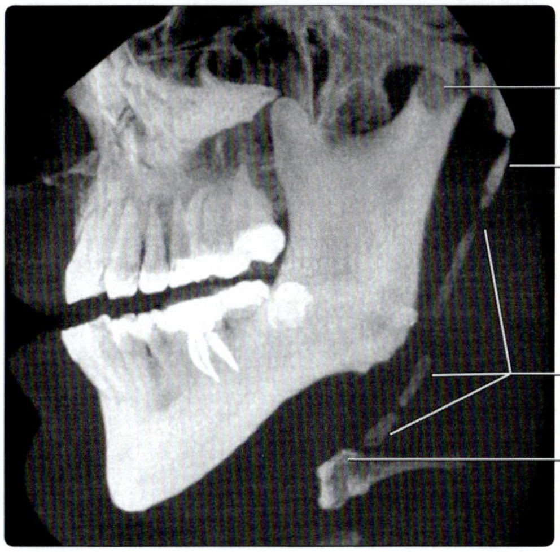

(Top) *Cropped panoramic radiograph of a patient complaining of neck pain, limited neck mobility, and pain on swallowing shows there is pronounced ossification with nodular enlargements of the stylohyoid ligament seen posterior to the mandible. This presentation is highly suggestive of Eagle syndrome.* **(Middle)** *Cropped lateral skull view of the same patient shows the highly thickened ossified stylohyoid ligament.* **(Bottom)** *CBCT MIP reconstruction shows a partially ossified stylohyoid ligament that has a segmented appearance. This was an incidental finding.*

PART I
SECTION 5

Cranial Nerves

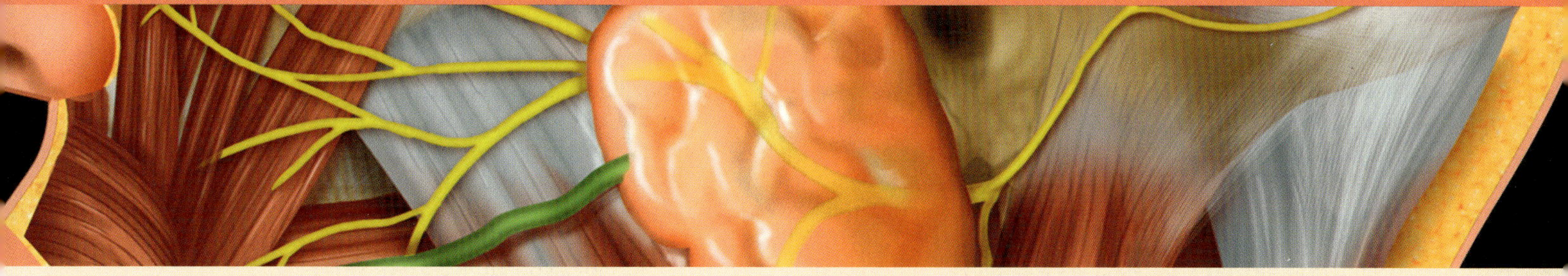

Cranial Nerve V 124
Cranial Nerve VII 138

TERMINOLOGY

Abbreviations

- Cranial nerve V (CNV)

Synonyms

- 5th cranial nerve, trigeminal nerve

Definitions

- CNV
  - Great sensory cranial nerve of head and face
  - Motor nerve for muscles of mastication
- Divisions
  - Ophthalmic division, trigeminal nerve: CNV1
  - Maxillary division, trigeminal nerve: CNV2
  - Mandibular division, trigeminal nerve: CNV3

IMAGING ANATOMY

Overview

- Mixed nerve
  - Both sensory and motor components
- 4 segments: Intraaxial, cisternal, interdural, and extracranial

Intraaxial Segment

- 4 nuclei: 3 sensory, 1 motor
- Located in brainstem, upper cervical cord
  - **Mesencephalic nucleus of CNV**
    - Afferent fibers for **facial proprioception** (teeth, hard palate, and temporomandibular joint)
    - Sickle-shaped mesencephalic tract descends to motor nucleus, conveys impulses that **control mastication and bite force**
  - **Main sensory nucleus of CNV**
    - Provides **facial tactile sensation**
  - **Motor nucleus of CNV**
    - Supplies **muscles of mastication** (medial/lateral pterygoids, masseter, temporalis), tensor palatini, tensor tympani, mylohyoid, and anterior belly of digastric
  - **Spinal nucleus of CNV**
    - Conveys **facial pain, temperature**

Cisternal (Preganglionic) Segment

- 2 roots: Smaller motor, larger sensory
- Emerges from lateral pons at **root entry zone** (REZ)
  - Arterial vascular loop compressing CNV in REZ is principal cause of trigeminal neuralgia
- Enters middle cranial fossa by passing beneath tentorium at apex of petrous temporal bone
- Passes through opening in dura matter called **porus trigeminus** to enter Meckel cave

Interdural Segment

- **Meckel cave** formed by meningeal layer of dura lined by arachnoid
  - Cave is filled with cerebrospinal fluid (CSF) (90%) and continuous with prepontine subarachnoid space
- Pia covers CNV in Meckel cave
- Preganglionic CNV ends at **trigeminal ganglion** (TG)
  - TG located in inferior aspect of Meckel cave
  - TG synonyms: Gasserian or semilunar ganglion

Divisions (Postganglionic) of CNV

- **Ophthalmic nerve (CNV1)**
  - Courses in lateral cavernous sinus wall below CNIV
  - Exits skull through superior orbital fissure
  - Enters orbit, divides into lacrimal, frontal, and nasociliary nerves
    - **Sensory** innervation **scalp, forehead, nose, globe**
- **Maxillary nerve (CNV2)**
  - Courses in cavernous sinus lateral wall below CNV1
  - Exits skull through **foramen rotundum**
  - Traverses roof of pterygopalatine fossa where **pterygopalatine ganglion** is suspended
    - Branches from ganglion supply **nasal fossa, palate,** and **nasopharynx**
  - **Greater and lesser palatine nerves** pass to palate
    - Sensory to **posterior palatal mucosa**
  - **Nasopalatine nerve** courses on nasal septum and through incisive canal in anterior midline
    - Sensory to **anterior palatal mucosa**
  - **Posterior superior alveolar nerve** pierces posterior maxilla
    - Sensory to maxillary **molars, sinus, and buccal gingiva**
  - CNV2 continues anteriorly as **infraorbital nerve** in floor of orbit
  - **Middle and anterior superior alveolar nerves** descend on lateral sinus wall
    - Sensory to maxillary **premolar and anterior teeth, sinus, and buccal gingiva**
  - **Infraorbital nerve** exits via infraorbital foramen
    - Sensory to **lower eyelid, lateral nose, and upper lip**
- **Mandibular nerve (CNV3)**
  - Does **not** pass through cavernous sinus
  - Exits directly from Meckel cave, passing inferiorly through **foramen ovale** into masticator space
  - Has small motor and large sensory components
    - Motor root bypasses trigeminal ganglion, joins CNV3 as it exits through foramen ovale
  - Gives branches from stem and from anterior and posterior divisions
  - **Motor supply to muscles of mastication**
    - Nerve to **medial pterygoid** from stem of CNV3
    - **Medial pterygoid muscle**
      - **Origin**: Larger **deep head** from pterygoid fossa between lateral and medial pterygoid plates, medial surface of lateral pterygoid plate
      - **Origin**: Smaller **superficial head** from pyramidal process of palatine bone, maxillary tuberosity
      - **Insertion**: Angle and medial ramus of mandible
    - Branches to **masseter, temporalis, and lateral pterygoid** from anterior division of CNV3
    - **Masseter muscle**
      - **Origin: Superficial head** from inferior border of anterior 2/3 of zygomatic arch, zygomatic process of maxilla
      - **Insertion**: Angle and lateral inferior ramus of mandible
      - **Origin: Deep head** from inferior border of posterior 1/3 and medial surface of zygomatic arch
      - **Insertion**: Lateral superior ramus and coronoid process

- Temporalis muscle
  - **Origin**: Inferior temporal line of skull, temporal fossa
  - **Insertion**: Coronoid process tip and medial surface, anterior border of ramus
- **Lateral pterygoid muscle**
  - **Origin: Superior head** from infratemporal surface of greater wing of sphenoid
  - **Insertion**: TMJ capsule and disc, pterygoid fovea of condylar neck
  - **Origin: Inferior head** from lateral surface of lateral pterygoid plate
  - **Insertion**: Pterygoid fovea of condylar neck

- Motor branches to **tensor tympani** and **tensor veli palatini** muscles also come from stem
- **Mylohyoid nerve** branches off from posterior division of CNV3 at mandibular foramen
  - Mylohyoid nerve supplies motor innervation to **anterior belly of digastric and mylohyoid muscles**
- Main sensory branches include inferior alveolar, lingual, and auriculotemporal nerves (from posterior division)
- **Inferior alveolar nerve** enters **mandibular foramen**, located on medial mid ramus of mandible
- Inferior alveolar nerve runs through **mandibular canal** (inferior alveolar canal) below apices of teeth
  - Sensory to **mandibular teeth**
- Mental nerve branches off inferior alveolar nerve and exits mandible at **mental foramen**, buccal to apices of premolar teeth
  - Sensory to **lower lip, chin, and anterior labial gingiva**
- Anterior to mental foramen, inferior alveolar nerve becomes **incisive nerve**, supplies **anterior teeth**
- **Lingual nerve** is sensory to **anterior tongue, floor of mouth**, and **lingual gingiva**
  - Lingual nerve also carries afferent taste fibers from anterior 2/3 of tongue via chorda tympani (CNVII)
- Branch of lingual nerve enters **lingual foramen** in midline of mandible, between genial tubercles
  - Anatomy of lingual foramen is highly variable
  - May see multiple
  - Also transmits vessels from lingual artery and vein
- **Auriculotemporal nerve** is sensory to **TMJ, external auditory meatus**, and **temporal skin**
- **Meningeal branch** also arises from stem and returns through skull via **foramen spinosum**
  - Sensory to **dura** of middle cranial fossa

ANATOMY IMAGING ISSUES

Imaging Recommendations

- CT best for skull base and bony foramina
- MR for intraaxial, cisternal, and intradural segments
  - Thin-section T2 in axial and coronal planes best demonstrates cisternal and Meckel cave CNV
- T1 C+ fat-saturated MR of entire extracranial course
  - Delineates CNV perineural tumor best

Imaging Pitfalls

- Trigeminal ganglion is small crescent of tissue found in anteroinferior Meckel cave
  - Lacks blood-nerve barrier; therefore, normally enhances with contrast

CLINICAL IMPLICATIONS

Clinical Importance

- **Anesthesia to teeth and surrounding structures**
  - Anesthesia to maxillary teeth by buccal or labial infiltration of CNV2 branches
  - Palatal anesthesia by greater palatine or incisive nerve blocks
  - Anesthesia to mandibular teeth and surrounding gingiva by inferior alveolar nerve block
    - Injection aimed at lingula: Small bony protuberance partially covering mandibular foramen
- Shared innervation and proximity of posterior maxillary teeth and sinus may result in referred pain between them
  - Intraoral dental radiography and clinical exam to rule out dental cause
  - CT to rule out sinus disease
- Injury to inferior alveolar or mental nerve during extraction, surgery, or by neoplasm may lead to paraesthesia of lip and chin
- **Perineural tumor (PNT) spread along CNV**
  - CNV1: PNT seen on T1 C+ fat-saturated MR as slightly enlarged, enhancing CNV1 in superior orbit
    - Most common cause: Invasive skin squamous cell carcinoma (SCCa) from nose or forehead
  - CNV2: PNT seen on T1 C+ fat-saturated MR as slightly enlarged infraorbital nerve → pterygopalatine fossa → foramen rotundum → cavernous sinus → Meckel cave → REZ
    - Most common causes: Invasive skin SCCa from cheek, orbital or maxillary sinus malignancy, maxillary ridge SCCa
  - CNV3: PNT seen on T1 C+ fat-saturated MR as slightly enlarged, enhancing inferior alveolar nerve → CNV3 → foramen ovale → Meckel cave → REZ
    - Most common causes: Invasive skin SCCa from jaw area; mandibular malignancy; mandibular alveolar ridge SCCa; masticator space malignancy
  - To diagnose PNT on bone CT, look for widening or destruction of any canals or foramina
    - Mental foramen may be widened in lesions extending antegrade along inferior alveolar nerve canal or from posterior extension of lip or skin SCCa
    - Spread from minor salivary gland tumor of palate (i.e., adenoid cystic carcinoma) may be seen as widening of greater/lesser palatine canals, pterygopalatine fossa, or foramen rotundum
    - Malignant infiltration of inferior alveolar nerve canal may also lead to widening & destruction
- Motor (CNV3 only): Weakness in chewing
  - Proximal CNV3 injury (proximal to foramen ovale) causes motor atrophy of masticator muscles within 6 weeks to 3 months
  - Distal CNV3 injury (above mylohyoid nerve branch) affects only anterior belly of digastric & mylohyoid
    - Muscles of mastication spared in distal CNV3 injury
- **Tic douloureux** (trigeminal neuralgia)
  - Sharp, excruciating unilateral pain in CNV2-3 distributions
  - Look for arterial loop vascular compression at REZ (on high-resolution T2, CISS, or FIESTA MR)

CNV GRAPHICS

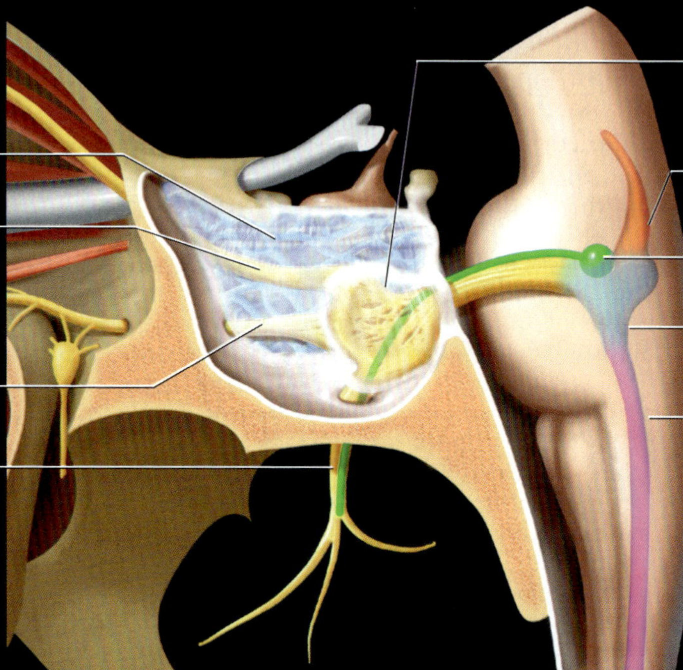

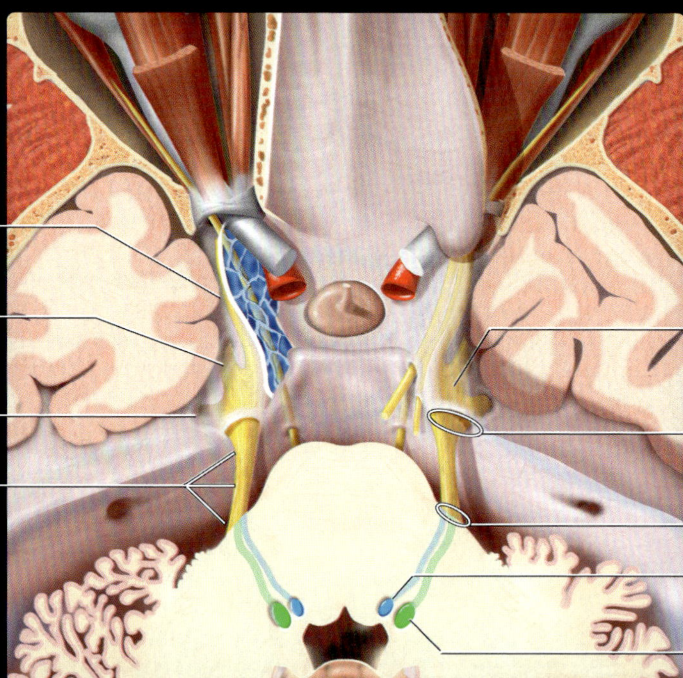

(Top) *Sagittal graphic focuses on the 4 nuclei of the trigeminal nerve. From superior to inferior, note the mesencephalic nucleus in the midbrain, the motor nucleus and main sensory nucleus in the pons, and the spinal nucleus extending from the lower pons into the upper cervical spinal cord. The motor root of CNV sends fibers along the mandibular division only. From Meckel cave, the ophthalmic and maxillary divisions of CNV pass anteriorly through the cavernous sinus while the mandibular division exits inferiorly to foramen ovale.* **(Bottom)** *Axial graphic depicts the course of the trigeminal nerve from its pontine nuclei (main sensory and motor nuclei) to its main 3 branches (CNV1, CNV2, CNV3). Notice the large preganglionic segment exiting the lateral pons at the root entry zone. It then enters Meckel cave through the porus trigeminus to become the trigeminal ganglion. Vascular loop irritation of the root entry zone is the most common cause of trigeminal neuralgia.*

CNV GRAPHICS

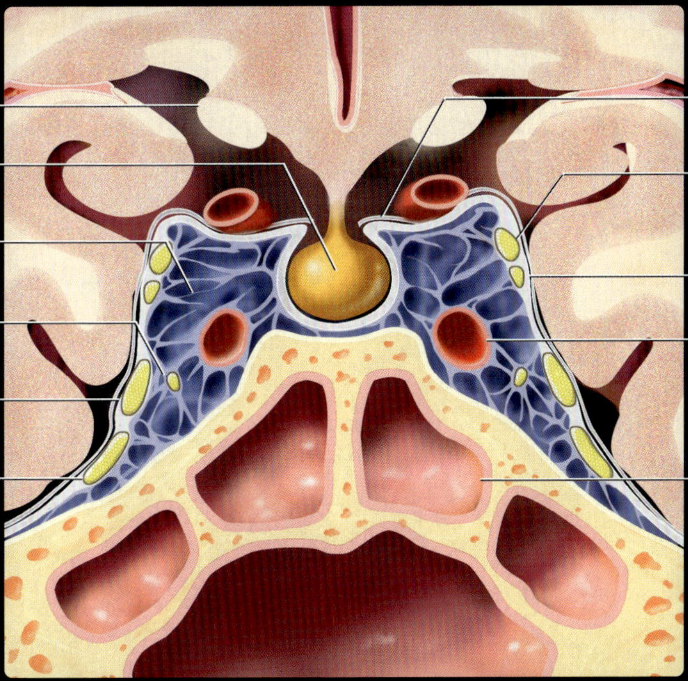

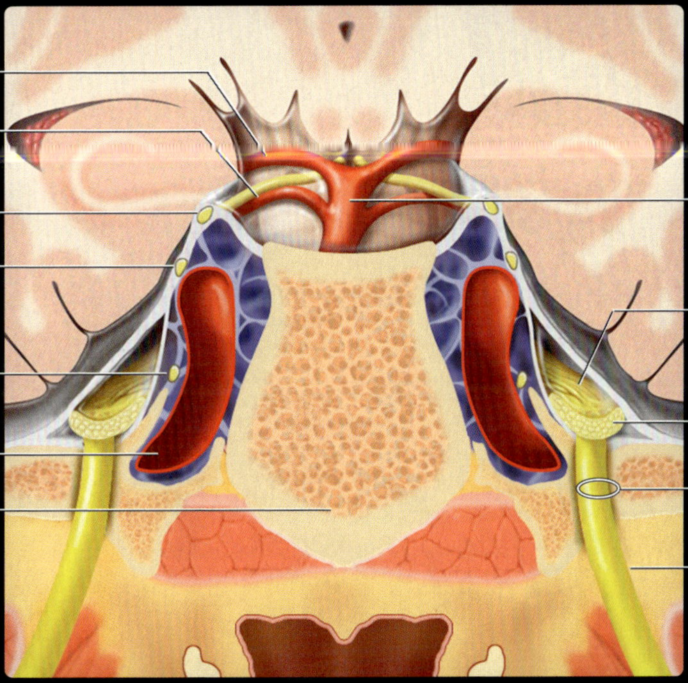

(Top) *Coronal graphic through the cavernous sinus shows that CNV2 is in the lateral wall of the cavernous sinus just inferior to CNV1. CNV1 is also embedded in the lateral wall of the cavernous sinus, as are CNIII and CNIV. The only centrally located intracavernous cranial nerve is the abducens nerve (CNVI).* **(Bottom)** *Coronal graphic depicting the fact that the mandibular division of the trigeminal nerve (CNV3) never enters the cavernous sinus. Instead, CNV3 exits directly from Meckel cave, passing inferiorly through foramen ovale into the nasopharyngeal masticator space. Meckel cave is actually a "pseudopod" of the lateral prepontine cistern, containing both the trigeminal nerve rootlets and the trigeminal ganglion. Remember, it is CNV3 that possesses the motor fibers of the trigeminal nerve.*

CNV GRAPHICS

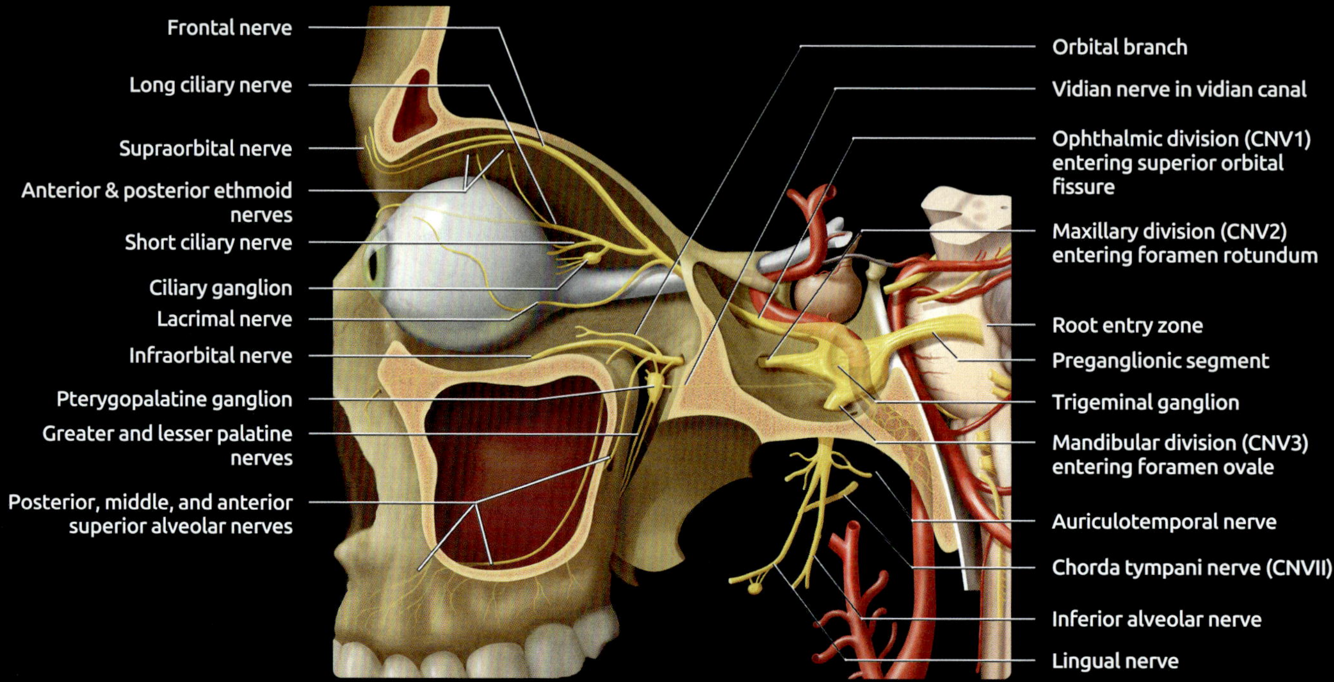

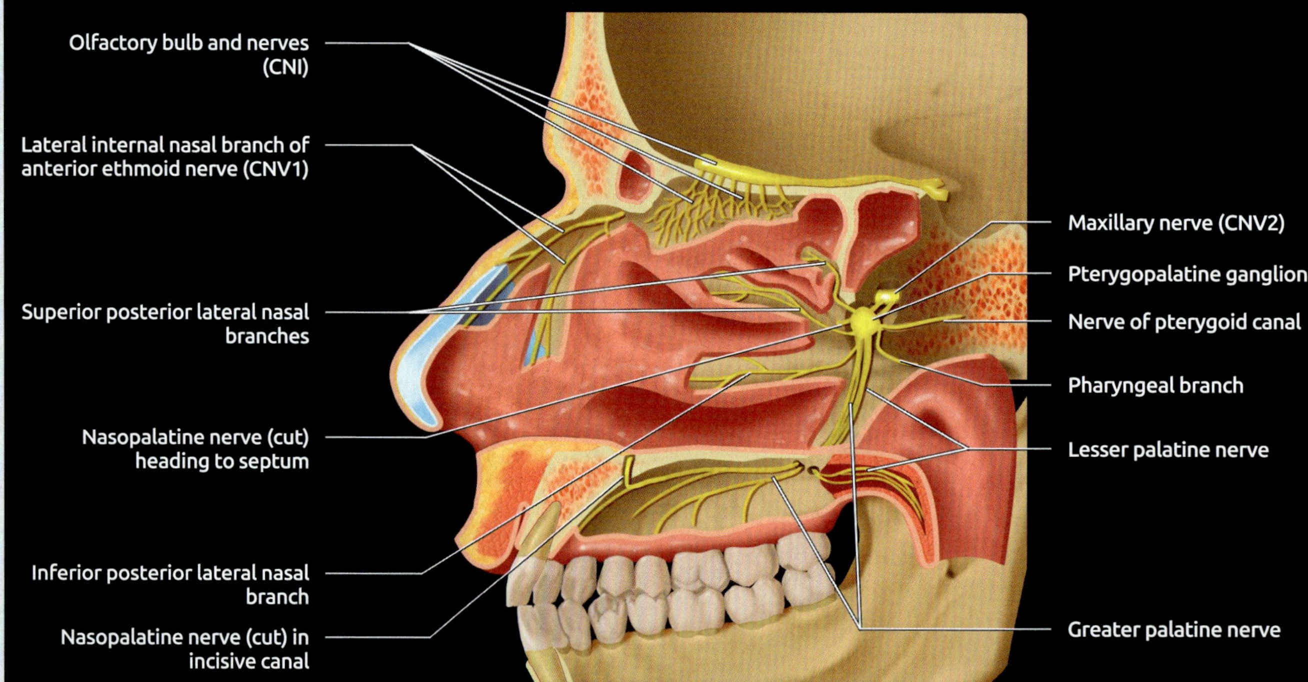

(Top) *Sagittal graphic of the trigeminal nerve shows the major branches and exiting foramina. The ophthalmic division of CNV enters into the orbit via the superior orbital fissure where it divides into frontal, ciliary, and lacrimal branches. The maxillary division of CNV exits via foramen rotundum to become the infraorbital nerve, as well as to drop the greater and lesser palatine nerves inferiorly to provide sensation for the hard and soft palates. The superior alveolar nerves also descend to supply the maxillary teeth. The mandibular division exits through foramen ovale where motor and sensory branches are then given off.* **(Bottom)** *Sagittal graphic shows the lateral nasal wall with the pterygopalatine ganglion of CNV2 exposed. The branches of the pterygopalatine ganglion, which carry sensory, parasympathetic, and sympathetic innervation to the nasal, palatal, and pharyngeal mucosa, are shown.*

CNV GRAPHICS

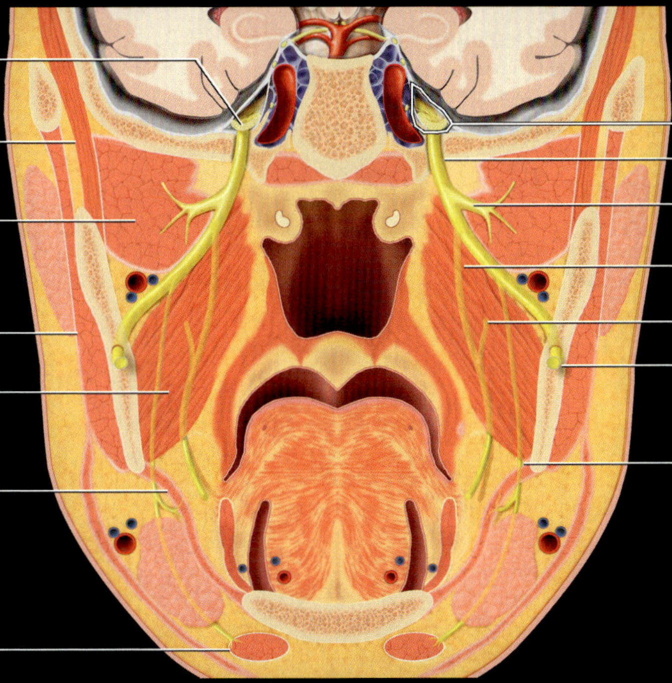

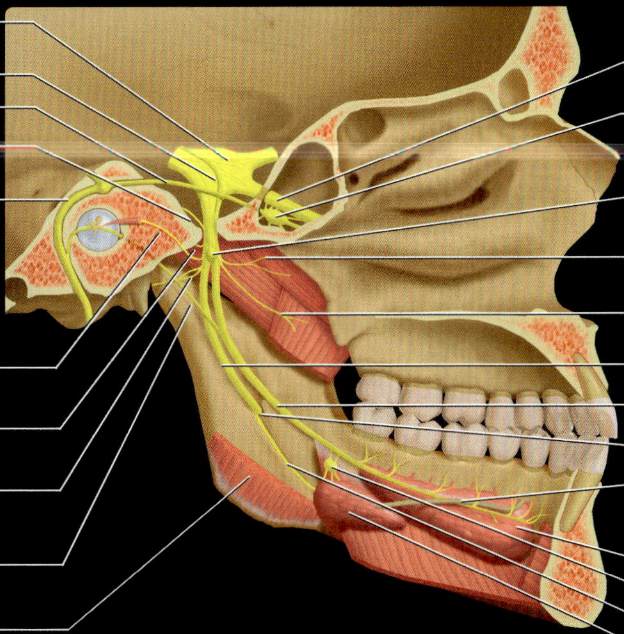

(Top) *Coronal graphic shows the mandibular division of CNV where it exits the skull base through foramen ovale from Meckel cave. The motor nerves arise from the motor root of CNV, which joins the mandibular division as it exits the skull base. In this graphic, the mylohyoid nerve is seen supplying the mylohyoid and anterior belly of digastric muscles.* **(Bottom)** *Sagittal graphic shows the mandibular nerve at foramen ovale. The otic ganglion is seen from this perspective. Parasympathetic fibers from CNIX, via the lesser petrosal nerve, synapse in the otic ganglion, then travel with the auriculotemporal nerve to supply the parotid gland. Chorda tympani is seen leaving CNVII to join the lingual nerve. The lingual nerve travels to the floor of the mouth to provide sensory innervation. The chorda tympani provides taste sensation to anterior tongue & parasympathetic innervation to the submandibular and sublingual glands. Mandibular nerve motor branches are seen supplying medial pterygoid, tensor veli palatini, & tensor tympani muscles.*

CNV GRAPHICS

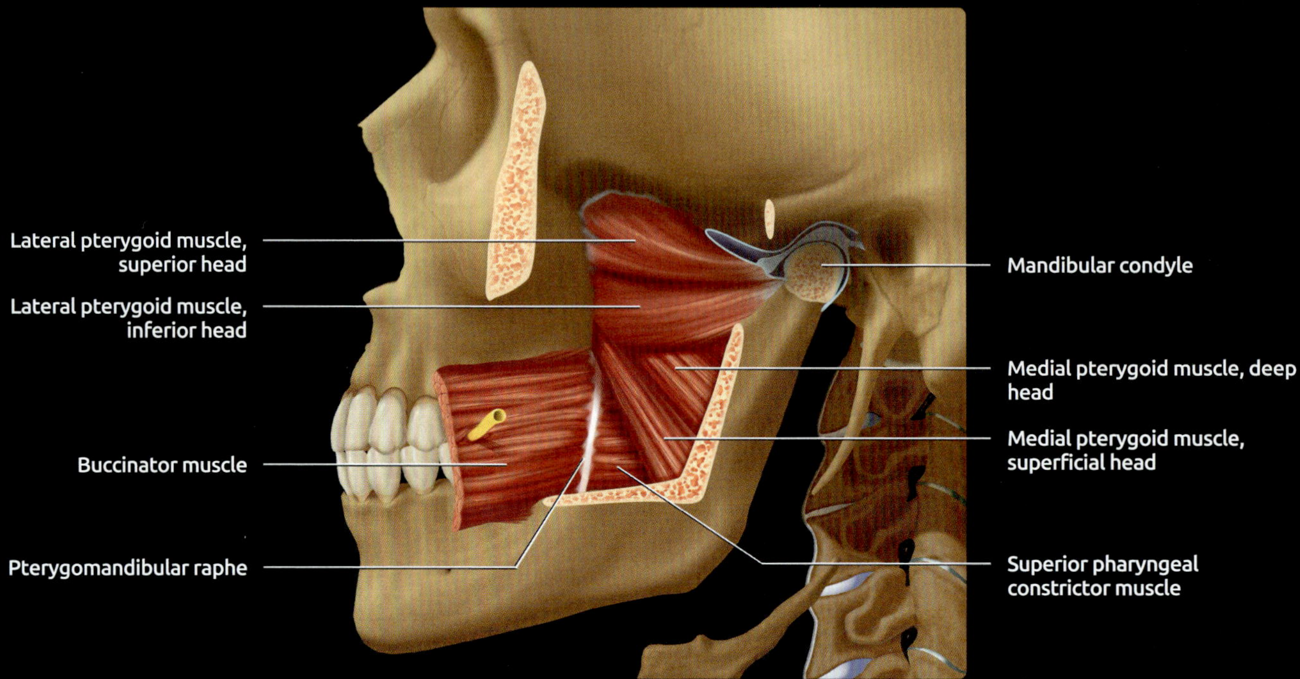

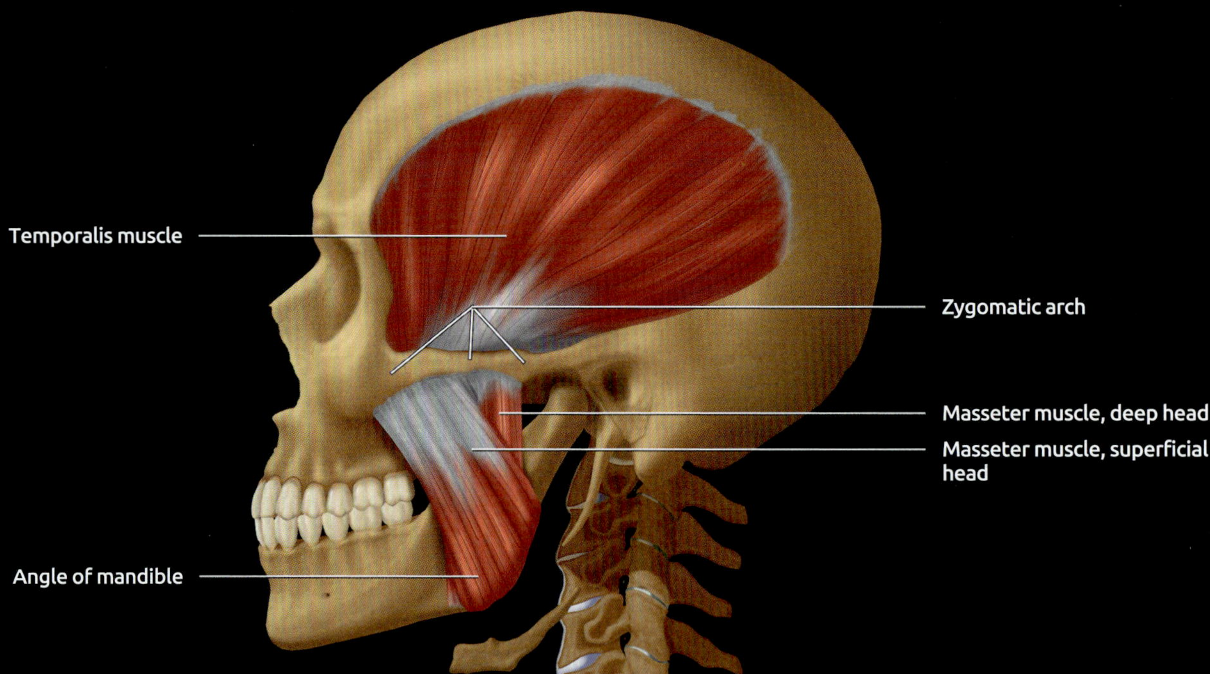

(Top) *Lateral graphic shows part of the ramus and zygomatic arch removed to show the lateral and medial pterygoid muscles. These are 2 of the muscles of mastication, which are innervated by CNV3.* **(Bottom)** *Lateral graphic shows 2 more superficial muscles of mastication: The temporalis and the masseter. Motor innervation to these muscles is provided by CNV3.*

CNV GRAPHICS

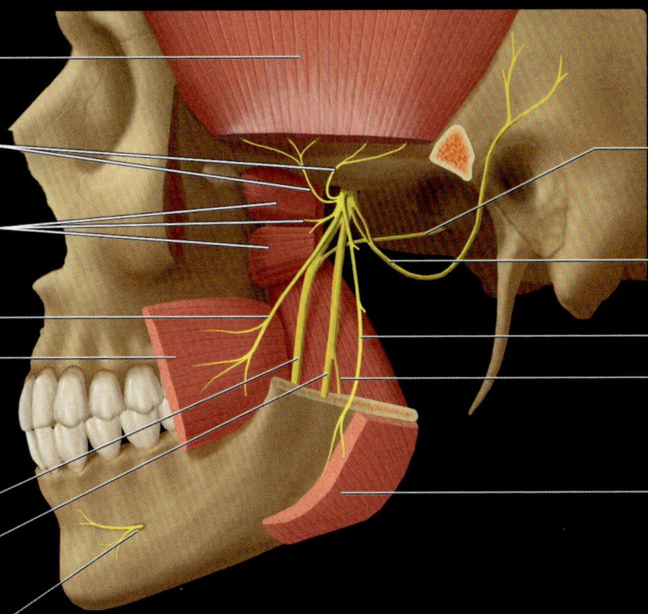

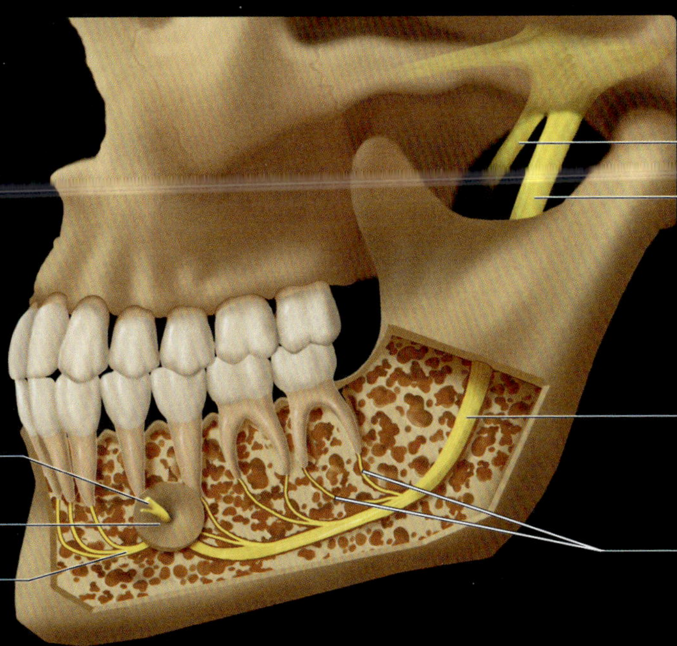

(Top) *Lateral view shows the mandibular nerve and its motor branches to the muscles of mastication. Branches to the temporalis, masseter, and lateral pterygoid muscles arise from the anterior division. The buccal branch is sensory to the cheek and gingiva, buccal to the mandibular molars.* **(Bottom)** *Lateral graphic of the mandible shows the course of the inferior alveolar nerve (IAN) through the mandible. The IAN enters the mandible through the mandibular foramen and travels below the apices of the teeth in the mandibular canal. Small branches travel through the apices of the teeth to supply innervation to the dental pulps. The mental nerve branches off from the IAN and exits through the mental foramen, between the apices of the premolars. The IAN continues anteriorly as the incisive nerve to supply the anterior teeth. The location of the mental foramen is variable, ranging from the mesial of the 1st molar to the mesial of the 1st premolar.*

AXIAL T2 MR

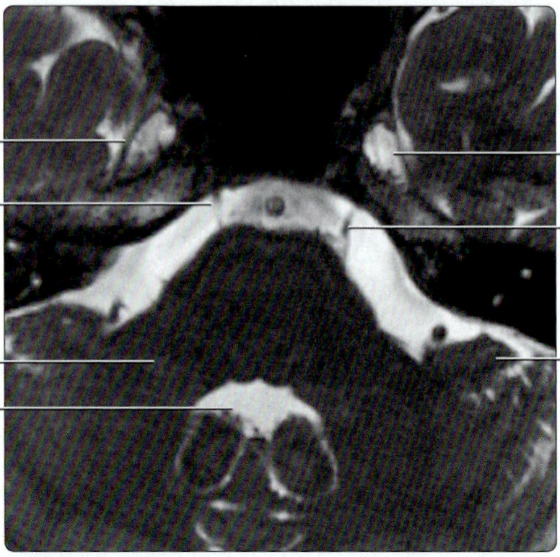

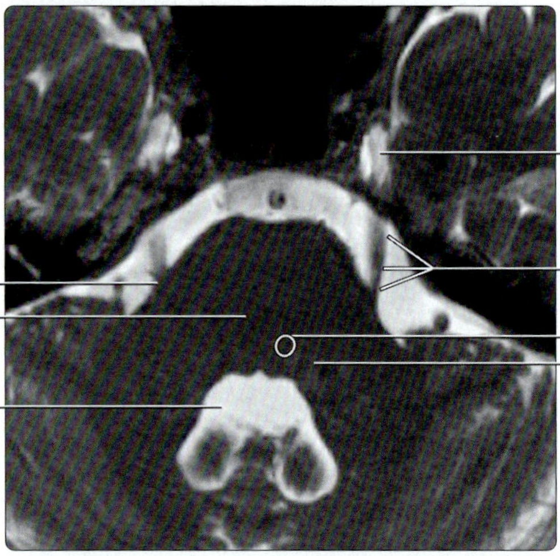

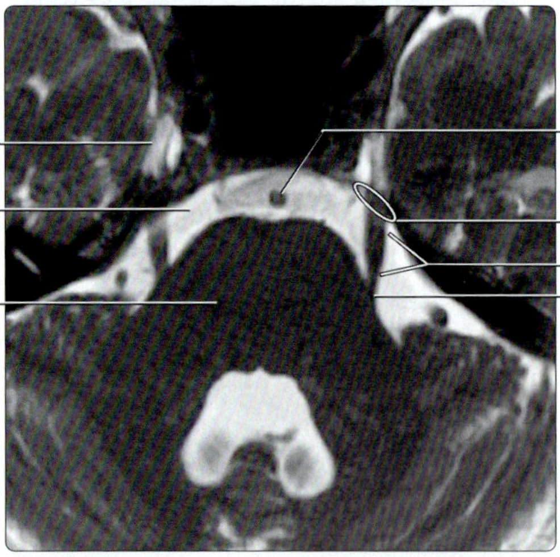

(Top) *First of 3 axial T2 MRs through the trigeminal nerve and Meckel cave presented from inferior to superior demonstrates a layer of hypointense dura mater forming the lateral wall and roof of Meckel cave. The right abducens nerve is seen penetrating dura to enter Dorello canal. Trigeminal nerve fascicles can be seen with the cerebrospinal fluid of Meckel cave.* **(Middle)** *Preganglionic fascicles of CNV are seen within Meckel cave. Meckel cave is an arachnoid lined, dural diverticulum protruding from the lateral aspect of the prepontine cistern. It contains cerebrospinal fluid, trigeminal fascicles, and trigeminal ganglion. Note the approximate location of the main sensory and motor nuclei of CNV.* **(Bottom)** *In this axial T2 MR, the preganglionic segment of CNV is seen spanning the distance between the root entry zone on the lateral pons and the porus trigeminus of Meckel cave.*

AXIAL & CORONAL T2 MR

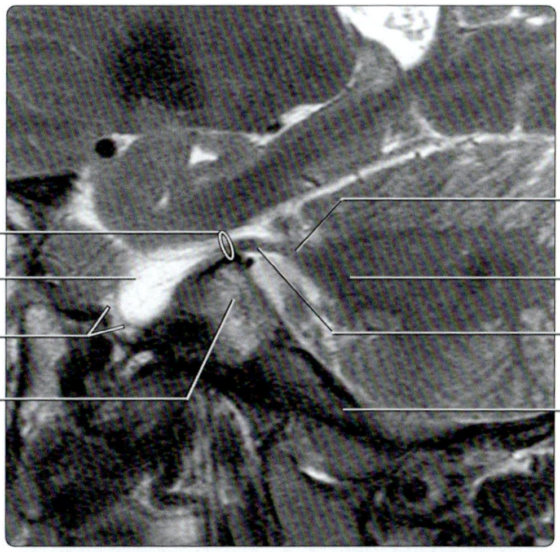

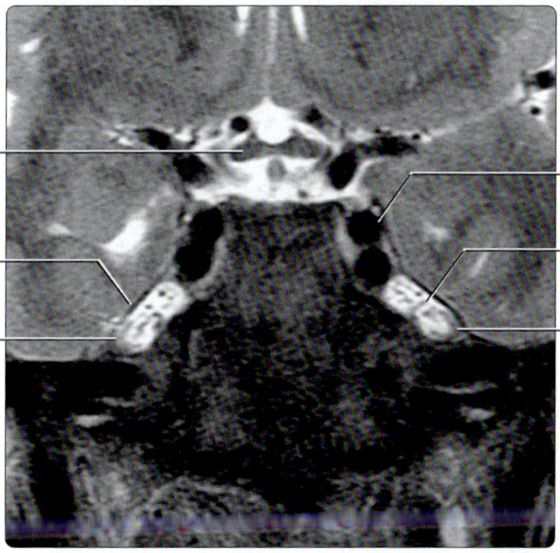

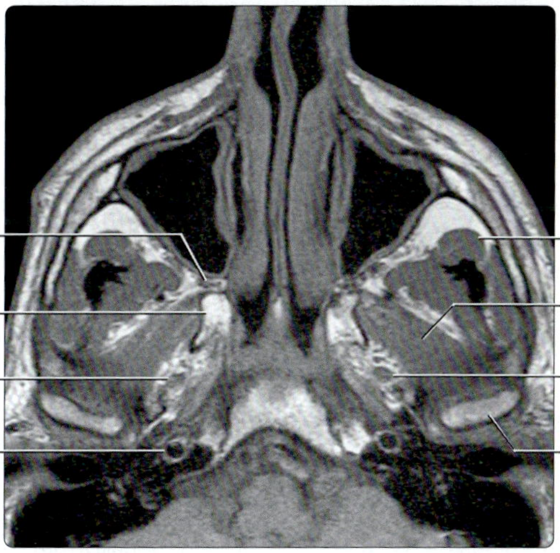

(Top) *Sagittal T2 MR along the line of the proximal trigeminal nerve shows the preganglionic segment between the root entry zone in the lateral pons and the trigeminal ganglion in the anteroinferior Meckel cave. The cerebrospinal fluid within the Meckel cave communicates with prepontine cistern through the porus trigeminus.* **(Middle)** *Coronal T2 MR through Meckel cave delineates the trigeminal fascicles of the preganglionic trigeminal nerve. The trigeminal ganglion is visible bilaterally as a semilunar structure in the floor of Meckel cave.* **(Bottom)** *Axial T1 MR just under the skull base shows both of the mandibular nerves entering the medial portion of the upper masticator space. It is at this level that the mandibular nerve gives off the masticator nerve, which is the motor branch to muscles of mastication. The auriculotemporal nerve branches posterolaterally at this level.*

AXIAL BONE CT

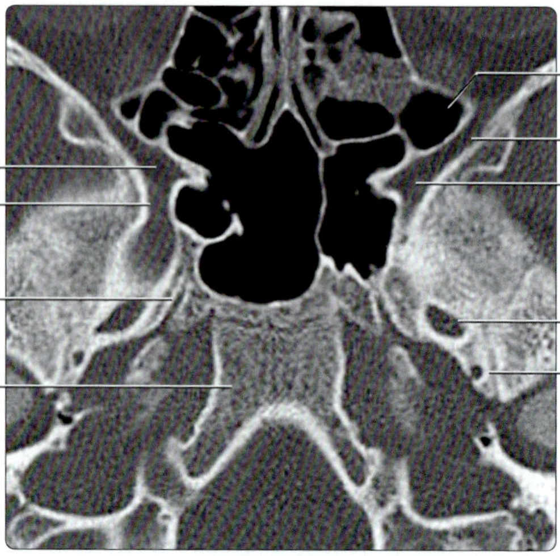

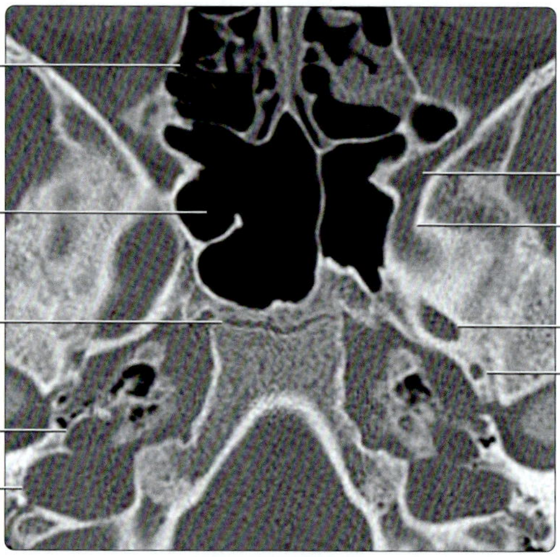

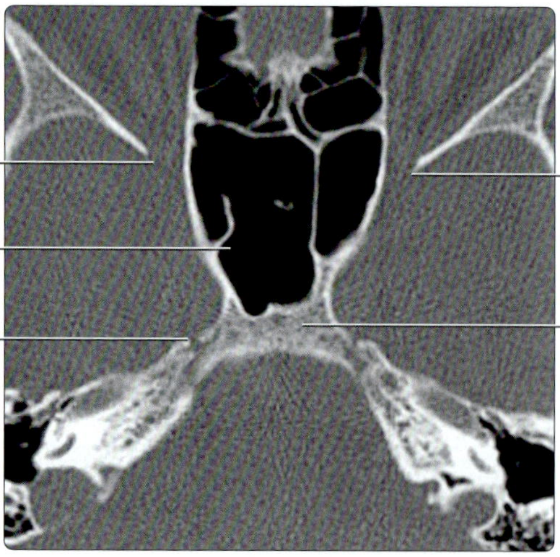

(Top) *The 1st of 3 axial bone CT images presented from inferior to superior through the central skull base is shown. CNV2 exits the skull base through the foramen rotundum to enter the superior margin of the pterygopalatine fossa. CNV3 exits via the foramen ovale to enter the masticator space, where it supplies motor innervation to the muscles of mastication and sensory branches to inferior alveolar, lingual, and auriculotemporal nerves.* **(Middle)** *In this image, the foramen ovale (CNV3) and foramen rotundum (CNV2) are now best seen on the patient's left. Notice that the left foramen rotundum is seen opening into the superior pterygopalatine fossa.* **(Bottom)** *The superior orbital fissure transmits the ophthalmic division of the trigeminal nerve from cranium to orbit. Other structures that pass through the superior orbital fissure include the oculomotor nerve (CNIII), trochlear nerve (CNIV), abducens nerve (CNVI), and the superior ophthalmic vein.*

CBCT REFORMATS

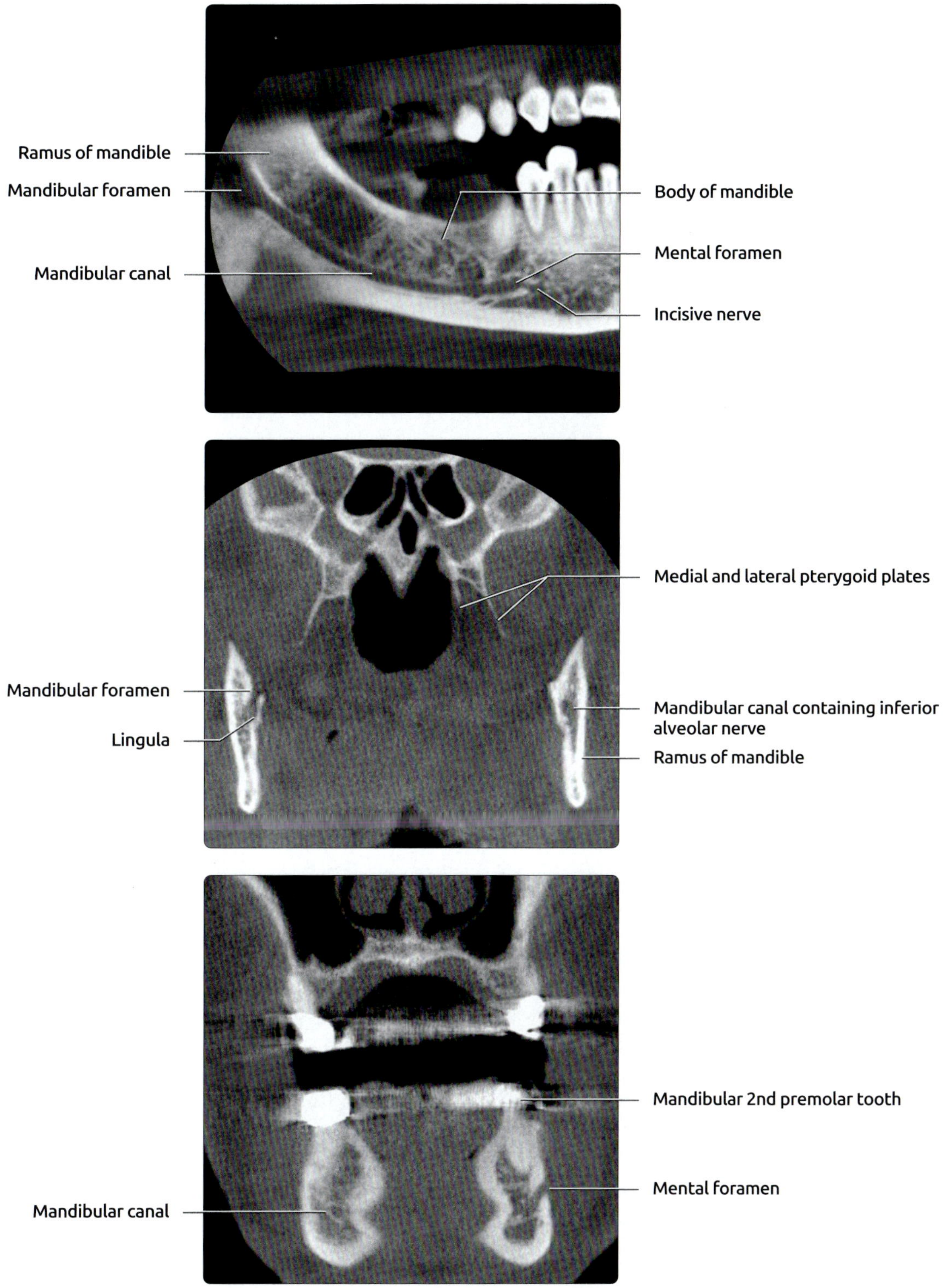

(Top) *Panoramic reformat of the mandible demonstrates the path of the IAN through the lower jaw in the mandibular canal. The canal begins at the mandibular foramen in the ramus and ends at the mental foramen. A small part of the incisive branch, the anterior continuation of the IAN, is also seen in this image.* **(Middle)** *Coronal CBCT slice shows the mandibular foramen opening on the medial aspect of the ramus. The lingula is a thin bony projection partially covering the foramen. This landmark is the target for inferior alveolar nerve block injections, commonly performed to achieve mandibular dental anesthesia.* **(Bottom)** *A more anterior coronal CBCT slice shows the mental foramen exiting the buccal surface of the left mandible. Note that it has an upward-angled course. Damage to the mental or inferior alveolar nerves during surgery can lead to paresthesia of the lip and chin on the ipsilateral side.*

CORONAL CBCT

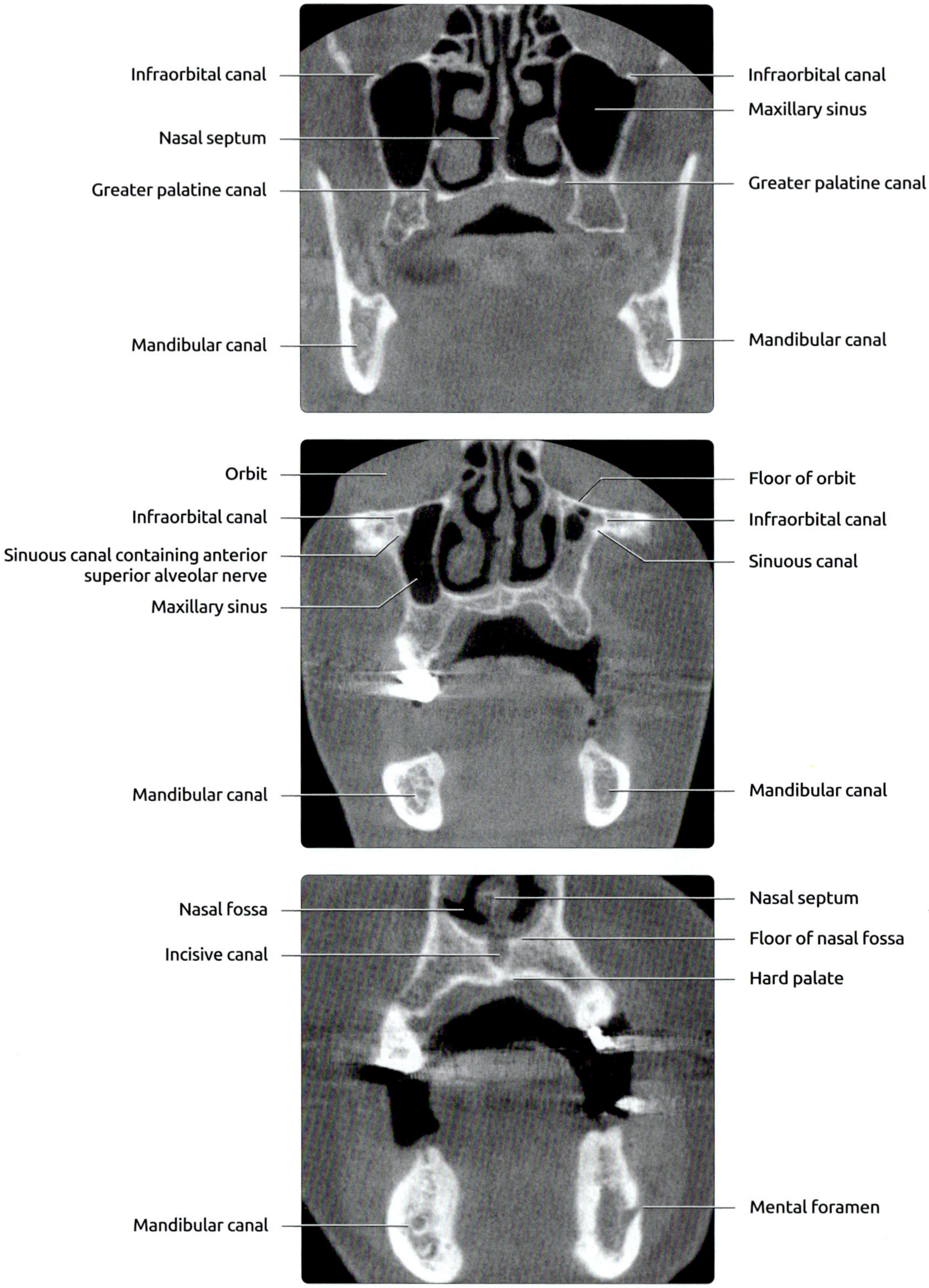

(Top) *The 1st of 3 coronal CBCT slices presented from posterior to anterior is shown. The right and left greater palatine canals are seen opening onto the hard palate, medial to the alveolar process and posterior to the 2nd molars. The greater palatine nerve, which extends from the pterygopalatine ganglion, supplies sensory innervation to the posterior palate and gingiva. The infraorbital canals, running along the floors of the orbits, are also seen.* **(Middle)** *In this more anterior image, the infraorbital canals are in the superior and lateral aspects of the maxillary sinuses. Inferiorly, the small canals carrying the anterior superior alveolar nerves are seen. These nerves will innervate the anterior maxillary teeth.* **(Bottom)** *A coronal section through the anterior maxilla shows the incisive, or nasopalatine, canal where it begins at the floor of the nasal fossa in the midline. This canal carries the nasopalatine nerves, which extend from the pterygopalatine fossa and across the nasal septum.*

SAGITTAL CBCT

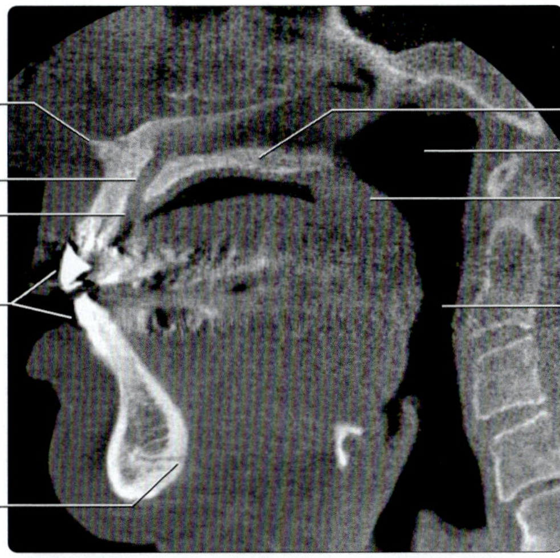

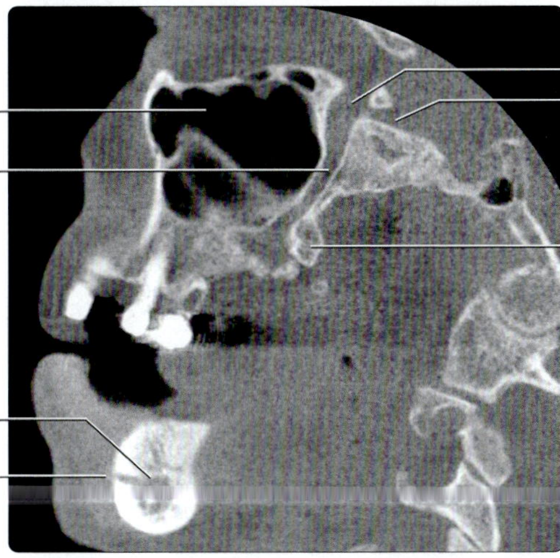

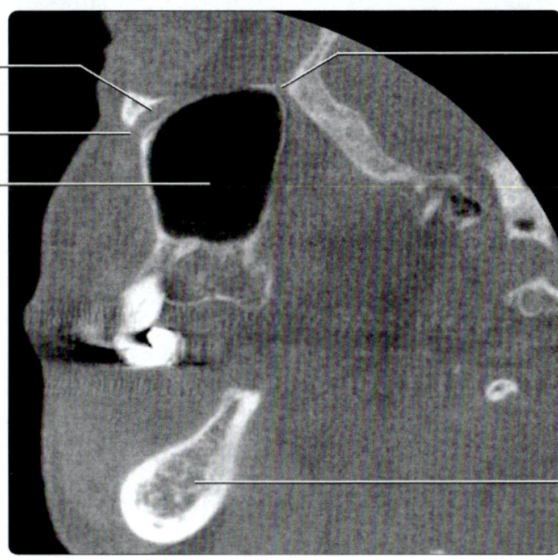

(Top) *The 1st of 3 sagittal CBCT sections extending from the midline laterally shows the entire course of the incisive/nasopalatine canal in the maxillary midline. The canal contains the nasopalatine nerve (CNV2) and opens as the incisive foramen on the palatal aspect of the central incisor teeth. This canal is the site of development of the nasopalatine duct cyst. The lingual foramen is also seen on the posterior surface of the mandibular midline. There may be great variation in the appearance of this structure.* **(Middle)** *This more lateral image shows the superior-inferior path of the greater palatine canal extending between the pterygopalatine fossa to the lateral hard palate. The foramen rotundum, which carries the maxillary branch of CN from the trigeminal ganglion, is also seen opening into the pterygopalatine fossa.* **(Bottom)** *Sagittal image in the midorbital region shows the infraorbital canal (infraorbital nerve CNV2) along the floor of the orbit and opening on the anterior surface of the maxilla. The inferior orbital fissure is also seen posteriorly.*

TERMINOLOGY

Abbreviations

- Cranial nerve VII (CNVII)

Synonyms

- Facial nerve

Definitions

- CNVII: Cranial nerve carrying
  - Motor nerves to muscles of facial expression
  - Parasympathetic nerves to lacrimal, submandibular, and sublingual glands
  - Taste sensation from anterior 2/3 of tongue

IMAGING ANATOMY

Overview

- Mixed nerve: Motor, parasympathetic, and special sensory (taste)
- 2 roots
  - Motor
  - Sensory (nervus intermedius)
    - Nervus intermedius exits lateral brainstem between motor root of facial and vestibulocochlear nerves, hence its name
- 4 segments
  - Intraaxial
  - Cisternal
  - Intratemporal
  - Extracranial (parotid)

Intraaxial Segment

- 3 nuclei (1 motor, 2 sensory)
- **Motor nucleus of facial nerve**
  - Located in ventrolateral pontine tegmentum
  - Efferent fibers loop dorsally around CNVI nucleus in floor of 4th ventricle, forming **facial colliculus**
  - Fibers then course anterolaterally to exit lateral brainstem at pontomedullary junction
- **Superior salivatory nucleus**
  - Located lateral to CNVII motor nucleus in pons
  - Efferent **parasympathetic fibers** exit brainstem posterior to CNVII as nervus intermedius
    - To submandibular, sublingual, and lacrimal glands
- **Solitarius tract nucleus**
  - Termination of taste sensation fibers from anterior 2/3 of tongue
  - **Cell bodies** of these fibers in **geniculate ganglion**
  - Fibers travel within nervus intermedius

Cisternal Segment

- 2 roots in cisternal CNVII
  - Larger motor root anteriorly
  - Smaller sensory nervus intermedius posteriorly
- Emerge from lateral brainstem at **root exit zone** in pontomedullary junction to enter cerebellopontine angle (CPA) cistern
  - CNVIII exits brainstem posterior to CNVII
- 2 roots join together & pass anterolaterally through CPA cistern with CNVIII to internal auditory canal (IAC)

Intratemporal Segment

- CNVII further divided in temporal bone into 4 segments: IAC, labyrinthine, tympanic, and mastoid
- **IAC segment**
  - Porus acusticus to IAC fundus
  - Anterosuperior position above crista falciformis
  - No branches
- **Labyrinthine segment**
  - Connects fundal CNVII to geniculate ganglion (anterior genu)
  - Courses anterolaterally from IAC
  - Passes through bony labyrinth superior to cochlea
- **Geniculate ganglion (anterior genu)**
  - Abrupt turn (genu = Latin for knee)
  - Greater superficial petrosal nerve given off
- **Tympanic segment**
  - After abrupt turn at anterior genu to course posterolaterally
  - Connects anterior genu to posterior genu, passing under lateral semicircular canal
- **Posterior genu**
  - 2nd bend located at posterior wall of middle ear
- **Mastoid segment**
  - After abrupt turn at posterior genu to course inferiorly
  - Through mastoid process to stylomastoid foramen
  - Nerve to stapedius muscle and chorda tympani nerve branch along this segment

Extracranial Segment

- CNVII exits skull base through **stylomastoid foramen** to enter parotid space
- Parotid CNVII passes lateral to retromandibular vein
- Ramifies within parotid, passes anteriorly to innervate **muscles of facial expression**

CNVII Branches

- **Greater superficial petrosal nerve**
  - Arises at geniculate ganglion
  - Passes anteromedially
  - Exits temporal bone via facial hiatus
  - Passes to pterygopalatine fossa via pterygoid canal
  - Enters pterygopalatine ganglion
  - Outgoing fibers travel with sensory fibers of maxillary branch of trigeminal nerve
    - **Parasympathetic** to **lacrimal gland** and **minor glands of nose, sinuses, pharynx, and palate**
- **Stapedius nerve**
  - Arises from high mastoid segment of CNVII
  - Provides **motor** innervation to **stapedius muscle**
- **Chorda tympani nerve**
  - Arises from lower mastoid segment of CNVII
  - Travels anterosuperiorly through thin bony channel
  - Courses across middle ear (tympanic segment)
  - Exits anterior wall of middle ear to enter petrotympanic fissure
    - **Located medial to temporomandibular joint**
  - Exits anterior temporal bone at petrotympanic fissure
  - Fibers then hitchhike with lingual branch of mandibular division of trigeminal nerve
    - Carries **taste** fibers from **anterior 2/3 tongue**

- Carries **parasympathetic** innervation to **submandibular** and **sublingual salivary glands**

- **Terminal motor branches**
  - Posterior auricular nerve
  - Nerve to **posterior belly of digastric muscle**
  - Nerve to **stylohyoid muscle**
  - Nerves to muscles of facial expression
    - Temporal
    - Zygomatic
    - Buccal
    - Mandibular
    - Cervical

Muscles of Facial Expression

- Forehead
  - **Frontal belly of occipitofrontalis**
    - Raises eyebrows; wrinkles forehead
  - **Procerus**
    - Draws medial angles of eyebrows down; horizontal wrinkling of bridge of nose
  - **Corrugator supercilii**
    - Draws eyebrows down and medially; vertical wrinkling of bridge of nose
- Eye
  - **Orbicularis oculi**
    - Encircles orbit; closes eye
- Nose
  - **Nasalis**
    - Compresses and dilates nostrils
  - **Depressor septi nasi**
    - Pulls down on septum and ala
- Cheek
  - **Buccinator**
    - Compresses cheeks against teeth; assists in mastication by pushing food toward occlusal surfaces; blowing and sucking
    - Arises from pterygomandibular raphe and lateral surfaces of maxillary and mandibular alveolar processes in molar region
    - Inserts into **modiolus**; fibromuscular structure at corners of the mouth where multiple muscles converge
- Mouth
  - **Orbicularis oris**
    - Encircles oral orifice; closes mouth; purses lips; "kissing"
  - **Levator anguli oris**
    - Elevates corner of mouth; "smiling"
  - **Depressor anguli oris**
    - Pulls corner of mouth downward; "frowning"
  - **Levator labii superioris**
    - 3 parts; elevates upper lip; dilates nostril
      - Levator labii superioris alaeque nasi
      - Infraorbital head
      - Zygomaticus minor
  - **Depressor labii inferioris**
    - Pulls lower lip downward
  - **Zygomaticus major**
    - Pulls corner of mouth back and up; "sincere smile"
  - **Risorius**
    - Pulls corner of mouth back; "fake smile"
- Chin
  - **Mentalis**
    - Elevates chin; protrudes lower lip; "pout"
    - In patient with retruded mandible (class II malocclusion), mentalis muscles become hyperactive in attempt to produce lip competence and cause wrinkling of the chin
- Neck
  - **Platysma**
    - Pulls skin of neck up; pulls corner of mouth back and down; "grimace"

ANATOMY IMAGING ISSUES

Imaging Recommendations

- Bone CT best for intratemporal segment of CNVII
- MR for intraaxial, cisternal, IAC, and extracranial segments
- Do not image routine Bell palsy

Imaging Sweet Spots

- Include brainstem, CPA cistern, IAC, temporal bone, and **parotid** when MR completed for CNVII palsy

Imaging Pitfalls

- Mild enhancement of labyrinthine segment, geniculate ganglion, and proximal tympanic segments of CNVII can be normal on postcontrast T1 MR
  - Secondary to circumneural arteriovenous plexus
- Always check parotid in peripheral CNVII paralysis

Clinical Issues

- Facial nerve paralysis can be central or peripheral
  - **Central**: Supranuclear injury resulting in paralysis of contralateral muscles of facial expression with forehead sparing
  - **Peripheral**: Injury to CNVII from brainstem nucleus peripherally, resulting in paralysis of all ipsilateral muscles of facial expression
    - If lesion proximal to geniculate ganglion, lacrimation, sound dampening, and taste affected
    - If CNVII involved, check pons for lesion
    - If CNVIII involved, check CPA-IAC for lesion
    - If lacrimation, sound dampening, and taste are variably affected, temporal bone lesion possible
    - If lacrimation, sound dampening, and taste are spared, extracranial CNVII implicated
- **Temporary facial nerve paralysis** can be induced by accidental injection of local anesthetic into parotid gland if inferior alveolar nerve block is delivered too far posteriorly
- When evaluating CBCT volume of patient with clinical presentation of facial paralysis or clinically detectable malignancy of face along distribution of facial nerve
  - Evaluate stylomastoid foramen and intratemporal course of CNVII for abnormal widening or asymmetry
  - If detected, have high suspicion for primary tumor or perineural spread of tumor along CNVII

CNVII GRAPHICS

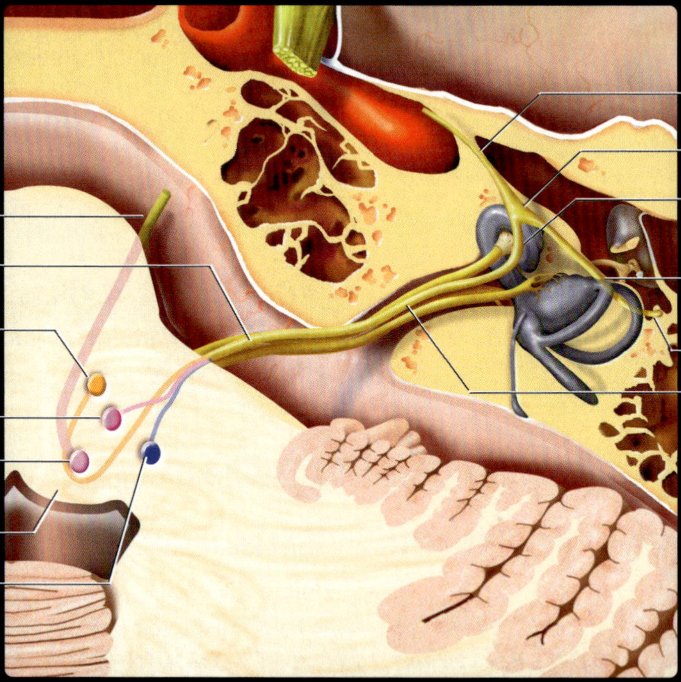

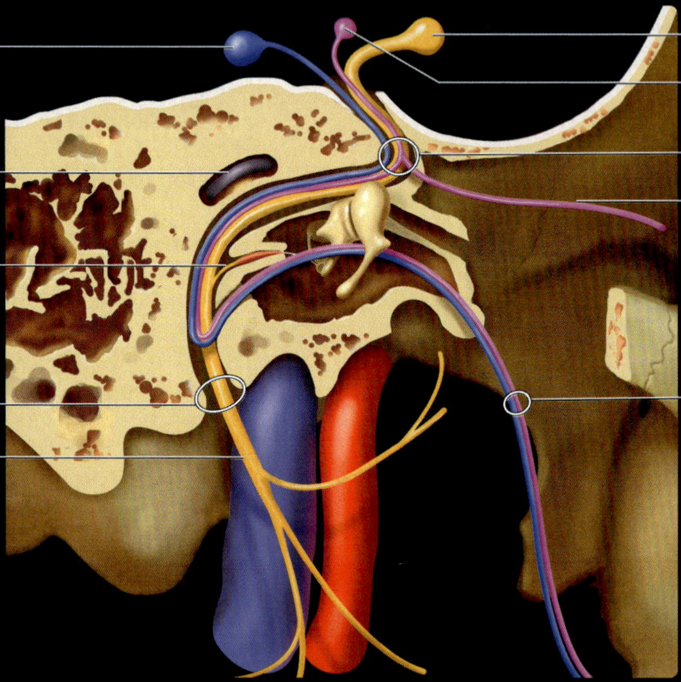

(Top) *Axial graphic of CNVII nuclei shows the motor nucleus sending out its fibers to circle the CNVI nucleus before reaching the root exit zone at the pontomedullary junction. The superior salivatory nucleus sends parasympathetic secretomotor fibers to lacrimal, submandibular, and sublingual glands. The solitary tract nucleus receives the anterior 2/3 of tongue taste information.* **(Bottom)** *Sagittal graphic depicts CNVII within the temporal bone. Motor fibers pass through the temporal bone, dropping the stapedius nerve to the stapedius muscle, then exit via the stylomastoid foramen to become extracranial CNVII (entirely motor). Parasympathetic fibers from the superior salivatory nucleus reach lacrimal gland and minor glands of the oral cavity via the greater (superficial) petrosal nerve and submandibular-sublingual glands via the chorda tympani nerve. The anterior 2/3 of tongue taste fibers comes via the chorda tympani nerve.*

CNVII GRAPHICS

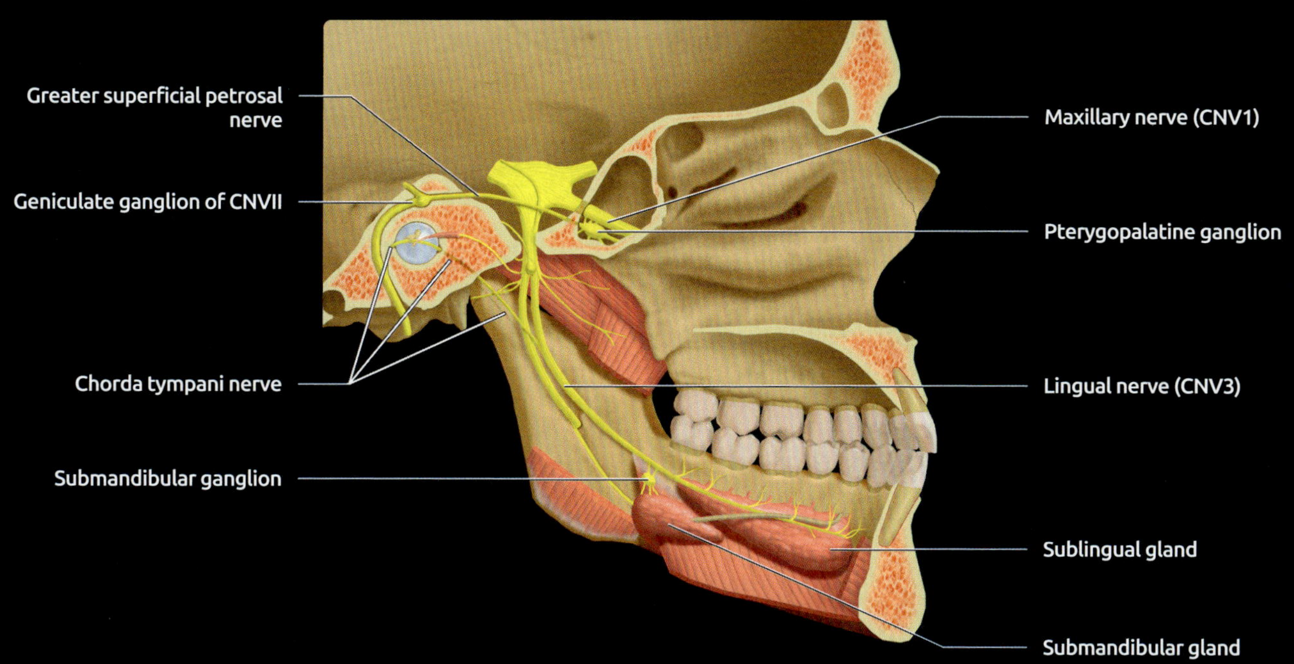

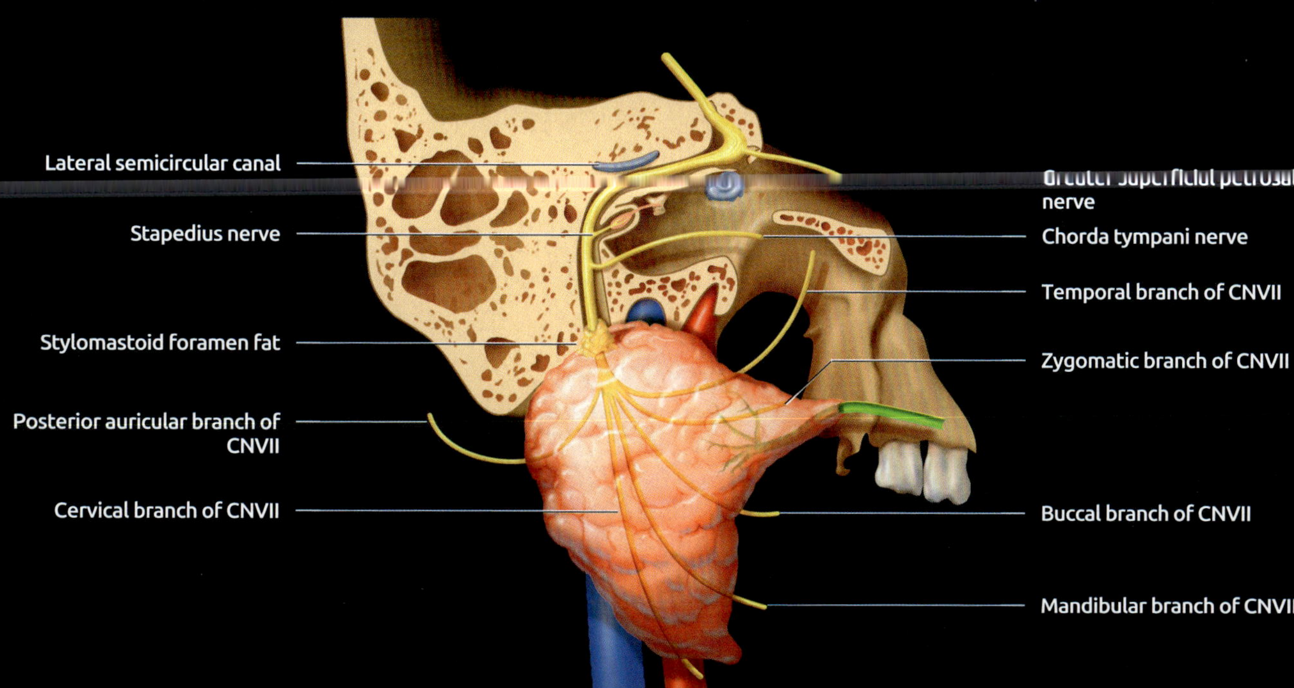

(Top) *Medial view graphic shows the relationship of branches of the facial nerve to CNV. The greater (superficial) petrosal nerve leaves the facial nerve at geniculate ganglion (anterior genu) and crosses the middle cranial fossa. It then passes through the pterygoid canal to enter the pterygopalatine ganglion within the pterygopalatine fossa. Via the many branches of the maxillary nerve from the ganglion, this nerve supplies parasympathetic innervation to the minor glands of the nose, sinuses, palate, and superior pharynx, as well as to the lacrimal gland in the orbit. The chorda tympani nerve also arises from CNVII, and after crossing the middle ear, it exits the petrotympanic fissure. It joins with the lingual nerve to supply parasympathetic innervation to the submandibular and sublingual glands and taste sensation from the anterior tongue.* **(Bottom)** *Sagittal graphic depicts extracranial motor branches of the facial nerve and their relationship to the parotid gland.*

CNVII GRAPHICS

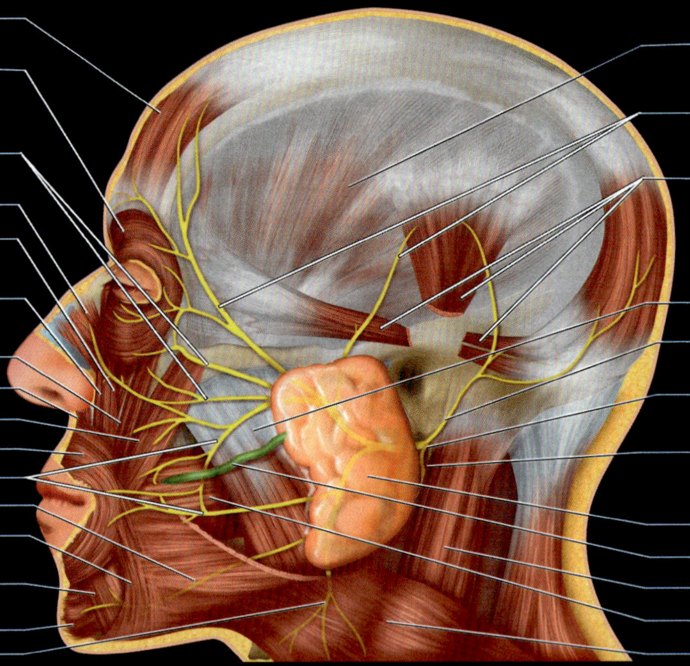

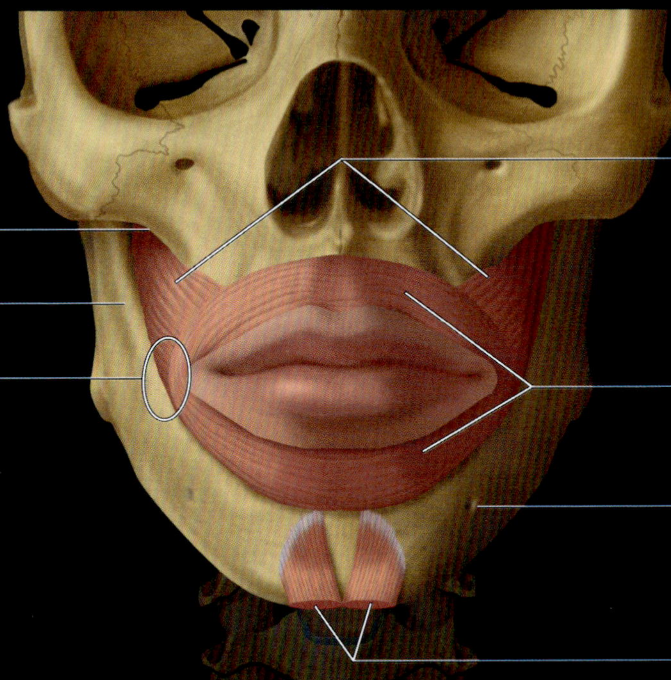

(Top) *Lateral graphic depicts details of the extracranial motor branches of CNVII after the main trunk exits the stylomastoid foramen. The anterior branches are seen traveling through the parotid gland and supplying the muscles of facial expression.* **(Bottom)** *Frontal graphic of 3 of the muscles of facial expression, which are innervated by CNVII, is shown. The orbicularis oris muscles encircle the mouth and acts to close the oral orifice and press the lips against the teeth. The mentalis muscles attach to the mandibular body and the overlying mental soft tissue (cut fibers). The buccinator muscles are seen tucked in between the maxilla and the ramus of the mandible posteriorly. Fibers of the buccinator muscle decussate with fibers of orbicularis oris anteriorly, at the modiolus. Several other muscles also converge at this point but are not shown in this image.*

AXIAL BONE CT

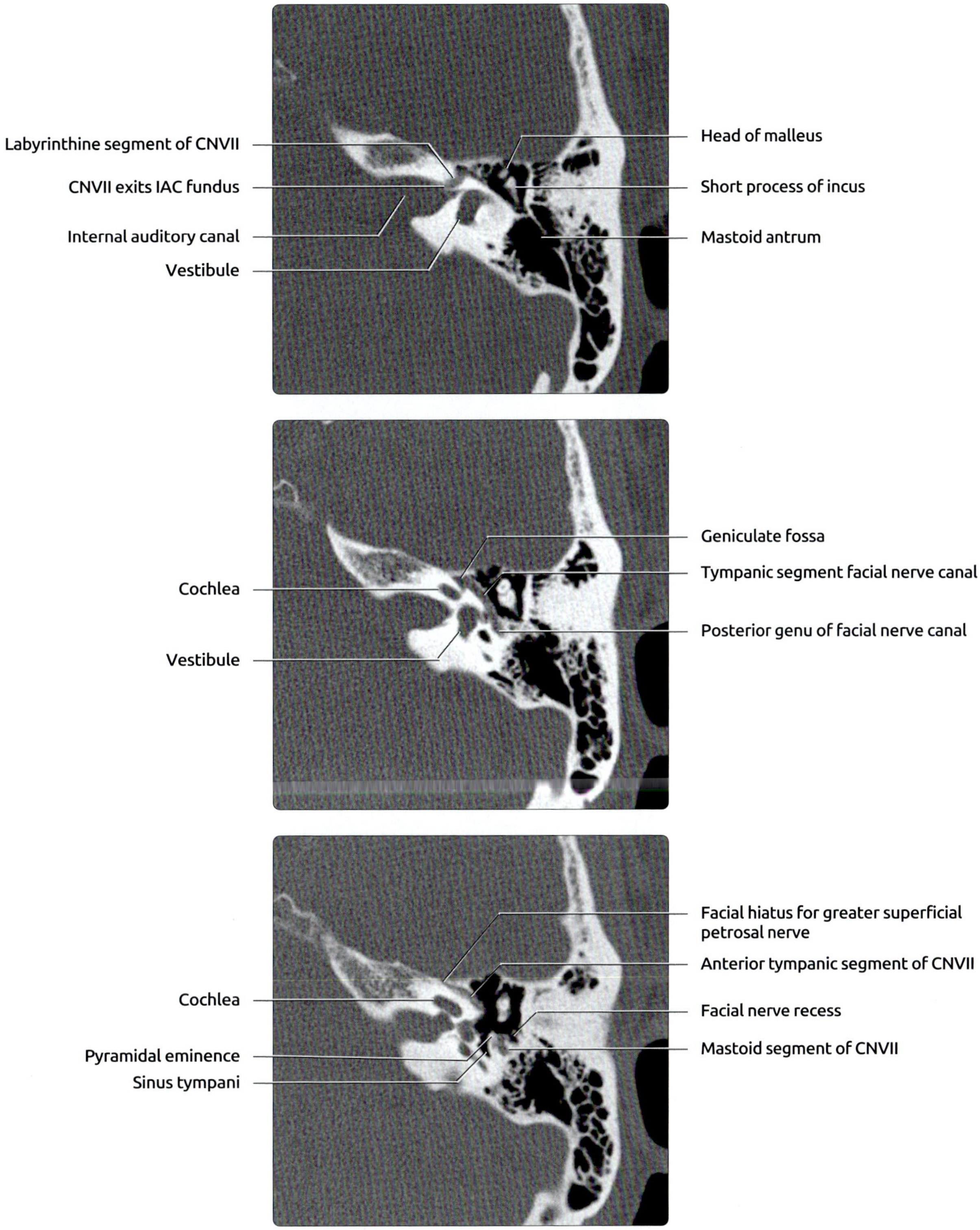

(Top) *The 1st of 6 axial bone CT images of the left temporal bone, presented from superior to inferior, shows the labyrinthine segment of the facial nerve canal as a C-shaped structure arching anterolaterally over the top of the cochlea.* **(Middle)** *In this image, the labyrinthine segment CNVII canal terminates in the geniculate fossa. The facial nerve canal turns abruptly at the geniculate fossa (anterior genu). The tympanic segment arises from the geniculate fossa, coursing posterolaterally in the axial plane and running under the lateral semicircular canal before turning 90° inferiorly at the posterior genu to become the mastoid segment.* **(Bottom)** *At the level of the oval window, the mastoid segment is visible deep to the facial nerve recess. Notice the more medial pyramidal eminence and sinus tympani.*

AXIAL BONE CT

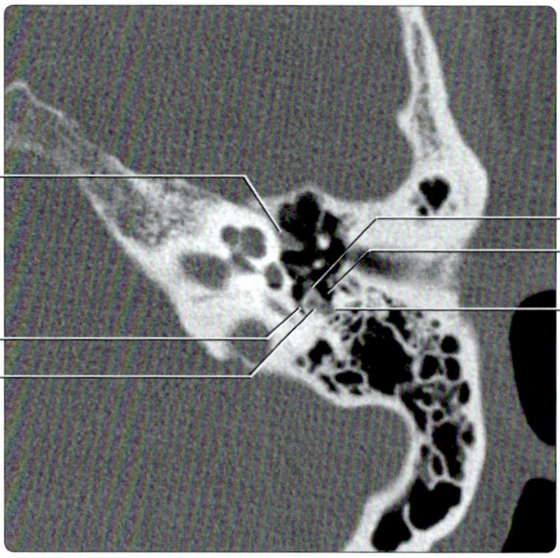

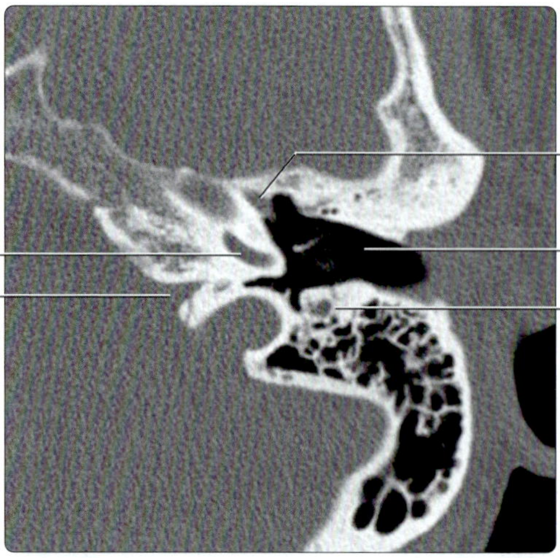

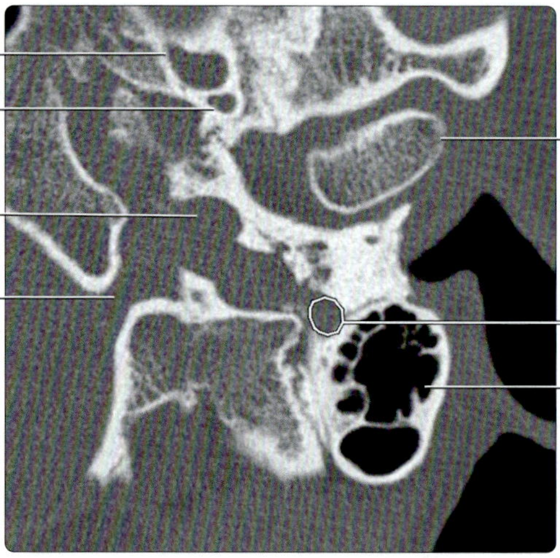

(Top) *The mastoid segment extends ~ 13 mm from the posterior genu to the stylomastoid foramen, coursing inferiorly within the posterior wall of the middle ear cavity. The mastoid segment is related anteriorly to the facial nerve recess and medially to the stapedius muscle within the pyramidal eminence on the posterior wall of the middle ear cavity.* **(Middle)** *At the level of the basal turn of the cochlea, the mastoid segment of CNVII is still visible. Both the nerve to the stapedius muscle proximally and the chorda tympani distally branch off the mastoid segment of CNVII.* **(Bottom)** *Image at the level of the stylomastoid foramen shows the "bell" of the stylomastoid foramen just anteromedial to the mastoid tip. The mastoid tip protects the facial nerve from traumatic injury as it exits the skull base.*

CORONAL BONE CT

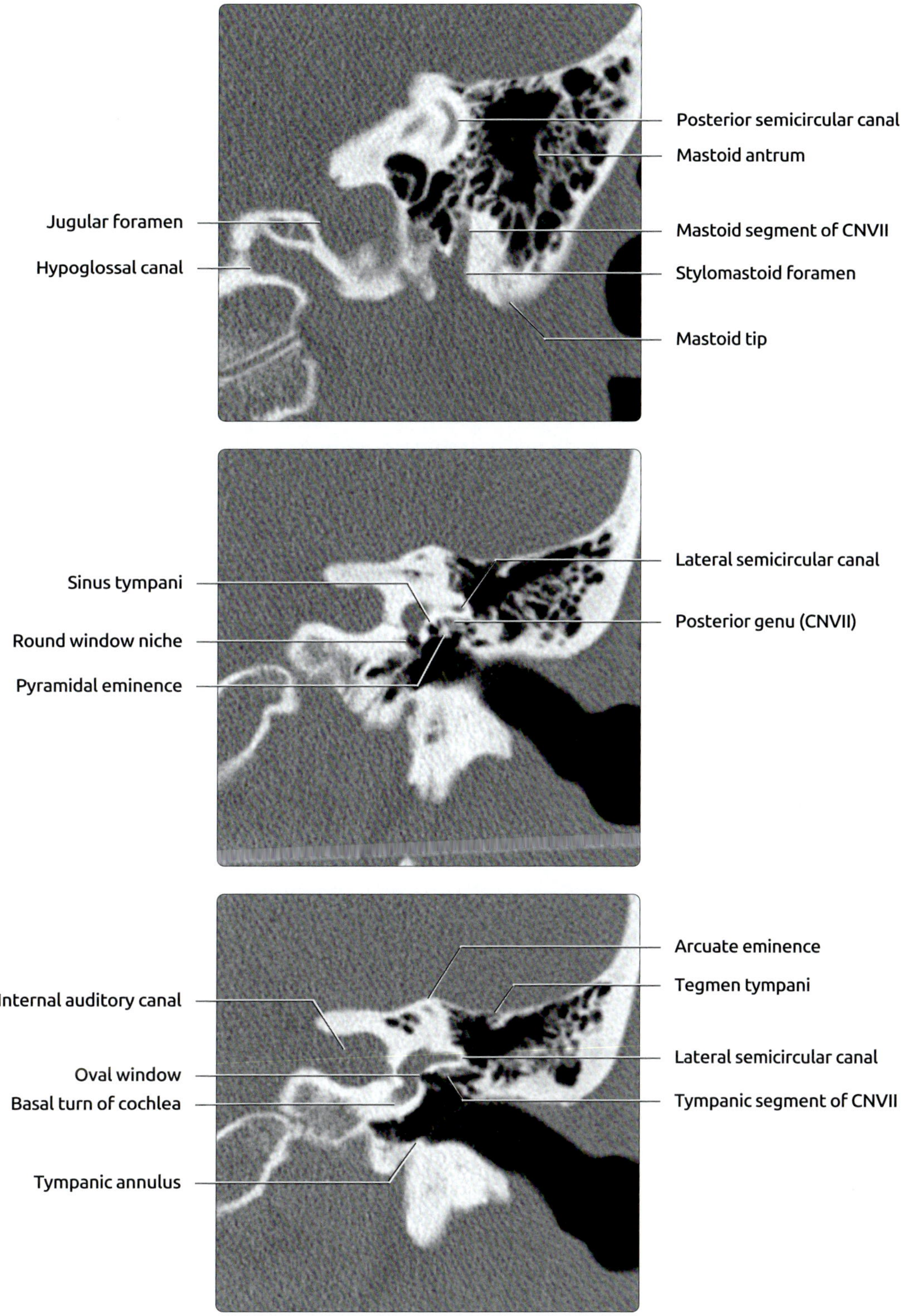

(Top) *The 1st of 6 coronal bone CT images of the left temporal bone, presented from posterior to anterior, shows the lower mastoid segment of the facial nerve (CNVII) and stylomastoid foramen.* **(Middle)** *At the level of the round window, the posterior genu of the facial nerve can be seen just lateral to the pyramidal eminence. Notice the sinus tympani is medial to the pyramidal eminence.* **(Bottom)** *At the level of the oval window, the tympanic segment of the facial nerve can be seen coursing under the lateral semicircular canal. Notice the fine bony covering (thin white line) surrounding the facial nerve. Also note the location relative to the upper margin of the oval window. In patients with oval window atresia, the facial nerve is found near or within the oval window niche.*

CORONAL BONE CT

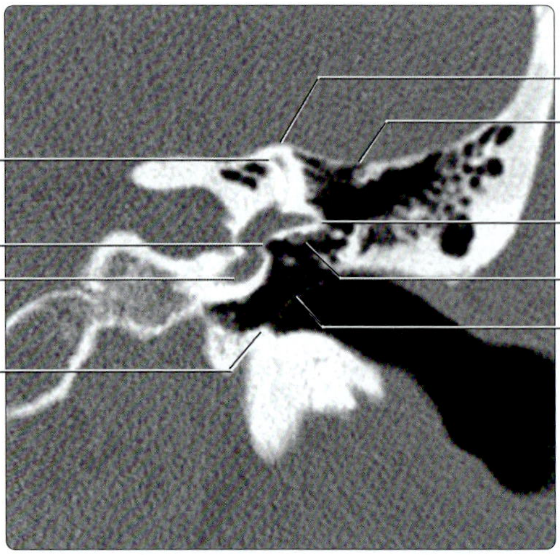

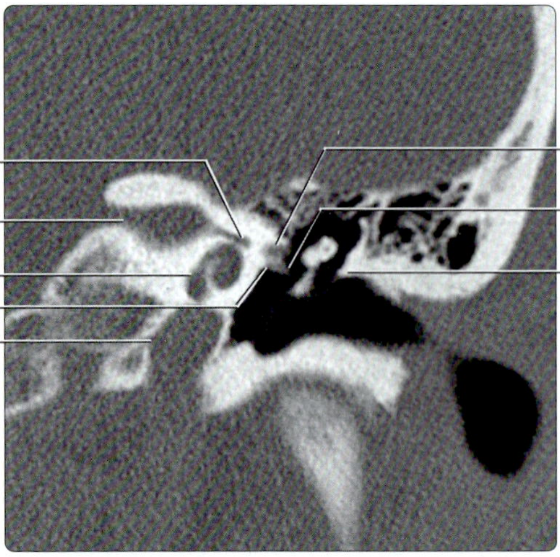

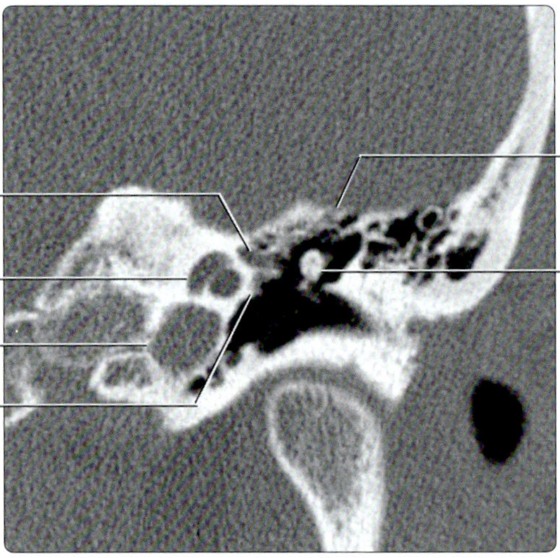

(Top) *At the level of the anterior margin of the oval window, the tympanic segment of CNVII can be seen under the lateral semicircular canal. Notice that the fine, bony covering (thin white line) surrounding the CNVII is now not seen. The facial nerve canal bony covering in this area is normally incomplete.* **(Middle)** *In the anterior middle ear cavity, the labyrinthine segment of CNVII can be seen exiting the internal auditory canal over the top of the cochlea. The anterior tympanic segment of CNVII is also visible. Do not confuse the muscle-tendon of the tensor tympani in the cochleariform process with CNVII.* **(Bottom)** *In the most anterior portion of the middle ear cavity (where both the carotid and the cochlea are visible), the geniculate ganglion is seen within the geniculate fossa as an ovoid structure just above the cochlea.*

T2 & T1 MR

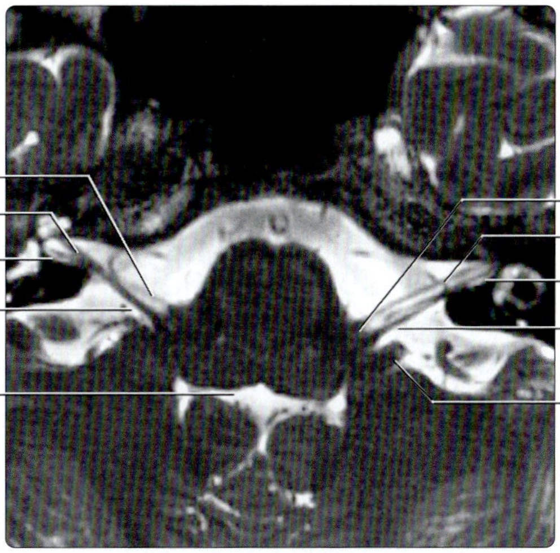

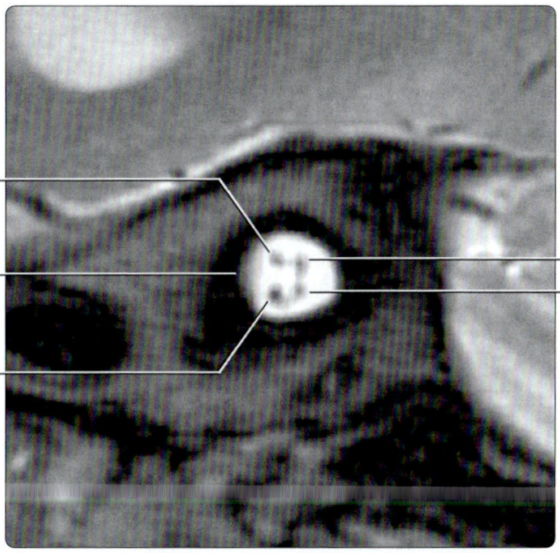

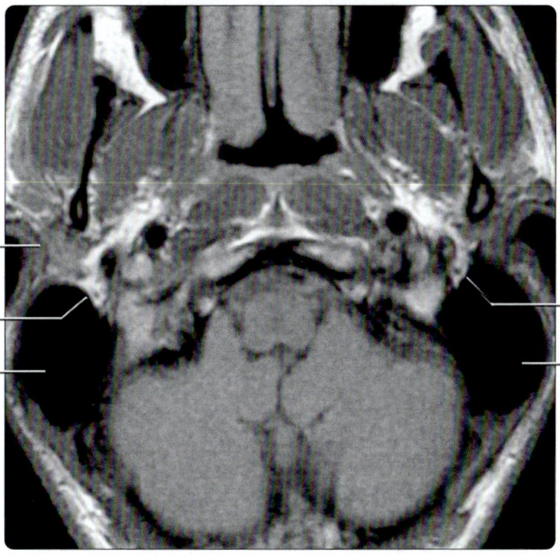

(Top) *Axial high-resolution T2 MR through the cerebellopontine angle cistern and internal auditory canal shows the facial nerve root exit zone anterior to the vestibulocochlear nerve in the pontomedullary junction bilaterally. Notice the facial nerve maintains an anterior relationship with the vestibulocochlear nerve as it crosses through the cerebellopontine angle cistern.* **(Middle)** *Oblique sagittal T2 MR through the mid internal auditory canal shows 4 nerves that are clearly identified. CNVII is anterosuperior. The superior and inferior vestibular and cochlear nerves are divisions of CNVIII.* **(Bottom)** *Axial T1 MR image at the level of the stylomastoid foramen shows the exiting low signal CNVII surrounded by high signal fat in the "bell" of the stylomastoid foramen. If perineural parotid malignancy is present, the fat in this area is obscured.*

PART I
SECTION 6
Cervical Spine

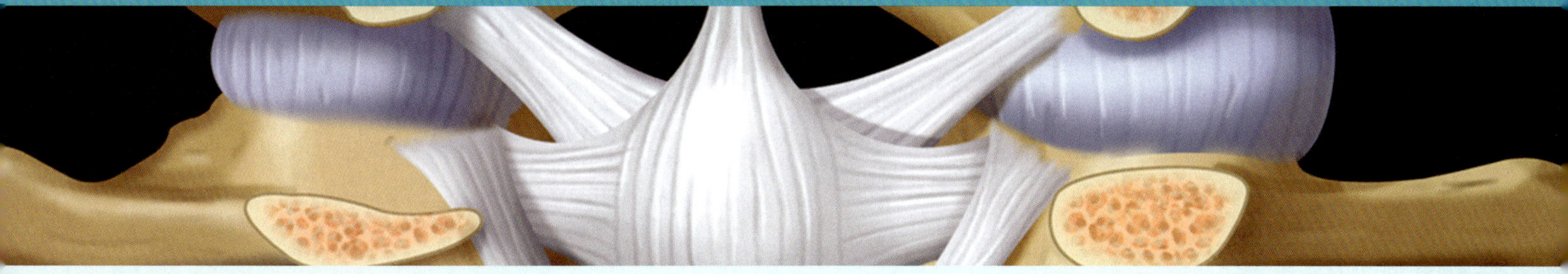

Craniocervical Junction 150

TERMINOLOGY

Abbreviations

- Craniocervical junction (CCJ)

Definitions

- CCJ = C1, C2, & articulation with skull base

GROSS ANATOMY

Overview

- CCJ comprises occiput, atlas, axis, their articulations, ligaments

Components of Craniocervical Junction

- **Bones**
  - **Occipital bone**
    - Occipital condyles are paired, oval-shaped, inferior prominences of lateral exoccipital portion of occipital bone: Articular facet projects laterally
  - **C1 (atlas)**
    - Composed of anterior & posterior arches, no body
    - Paired lateral masses with their superior & inferior articular facets
    - Large transverse processes with transverse foramen
  - **C2 (axis)**
    - Large body & superiorly projecting odontoid process (dens)
    - Superior articulating facet surface is convex & directed laterally
    - Inferior articular process + facet surface is typical of lower cervical vertebrae
    - Superior facet is positioned relatively anteriorly; inferior facet is posterior with elongated pars interarticularis
- **Joints**
  - **Atlantooccipital joints**
    - Inferior articular facet of occipital condyle: Oval, convex surface, projects laterally
    - Superior articular facet of C1: Oval, concave anteroposteriorly, projects medially
  - **Median atlantoaxial joints**
    - Pivot-type joint between dens + ring formed by anterior arch + transverse ligament of C1
    - Synovial cavities between transverse ligament/odontoid & atlas/odontoid articulations
  - **Lateral atlantoaxial joints**
    - Inferior articular facet of C1 is concave mediolaterally & projects medially in coronal plane; superior articular facet of C2 has convex surface & projects laterally
- **Ligaments** (from anterior to posterior)
  - **Anterior atlantooccipital membrane**: Connects anterior arch of C1 with anterior margin of foramen magnum
  - **Odontoid ligaments**
    - Apical ligament: Small fibrous band extending from dens tip to basion
    - Alar ligaments: Thick, horizontally directed ligaments extending from lateral surface of dens tip to anteromedial occipital condyles
  - **Cruciate ligament**
    - Transverse ligament: Strong horizontal component between lateral masses of C1, passes behind dens
    - Craniocaudal component: Fibrous band running from transverse ligament superiorly to foramen magnum & inferiorly to C2
  - **Tectorial membrane**: Continuation of posterior longitudinal ligament; attaches to anterior rim of foramen magnum (posterior clivus)
  - **Posterior atlantooccipital membrane**
    - Posterior arch C1 to margin of foramen magnum
    - Deficit laterally where vertebral artery enters on superior surface of C1
- **Biomechanics**
  - Atlantooccipital joint: 50% cervical flexion/extension & limited lateral motion
  - Atlantoaxial joint: 50% cervical rotation

IMAGING ANATOMY

Overview

- **Lateral assessment of CCJ**
  - **C1-2 interspinous space**: ≤ 10 mm
  - **Atlantodental interval**: Adults < 3 mm, children < 5 mm in flexion
  - **Pseudosubluxation**
    - Physiologic anterior displacement seen in 40% at C2-3 level & 14% at C3-4 level to age 8
    - Anterior displacement of C2 on C3 up to 4 mm
  - **Posterior cervical line**: Line is drawn from anterior aspect of C1-3 spinous processes; anterior C2 spinous process should be within 2 mm of this line
  - **Wackenheim line**
    - Posterior surface of clivus; posterior odontoid tip should lie immediately inferior
    - Relationship does not change in flexion/extension
  - **Welcher basal angle**
    - Angle between lines drawn along plane of sphenoid bone & posterior clivus
    - Normal < 140°, average: 132°
  - **Chamberlain line**
    - Between hard palate & opisthion
    - Odontoid tip ≥ 5 mm above line abnormal
  - **McGregor line**
    - Between hard palate to base of occipital bone
    - Odontoid tip ≥ 7 mm above line abnormal
  - **Redlund-Johnell line**
    - From base of C2 to McGregor line
    - Lower limits 34 mm (men), 29 mm (women)
  - **Clivus canal angle**
    - Junction of Wackenheim line & posterior vertebral body line
    - 180° extension, 150° flexion, < 150° abnormal
  - **McRae line**
    - Drawn between basion & opisthion
    - Normal 35-mm diameter
- **Frontal assessment of CCJ**
  - Lateral masses of C1 & C2 should align
    - Overlapping lateral masses can be normal variant in children
  - **Atlantooccipital joint angle**
    - Angle formed at junction of lines traversing joints
    - 125-130° normal, < 124° may reflect occipital condyle hypoplasia

GRAPHICS

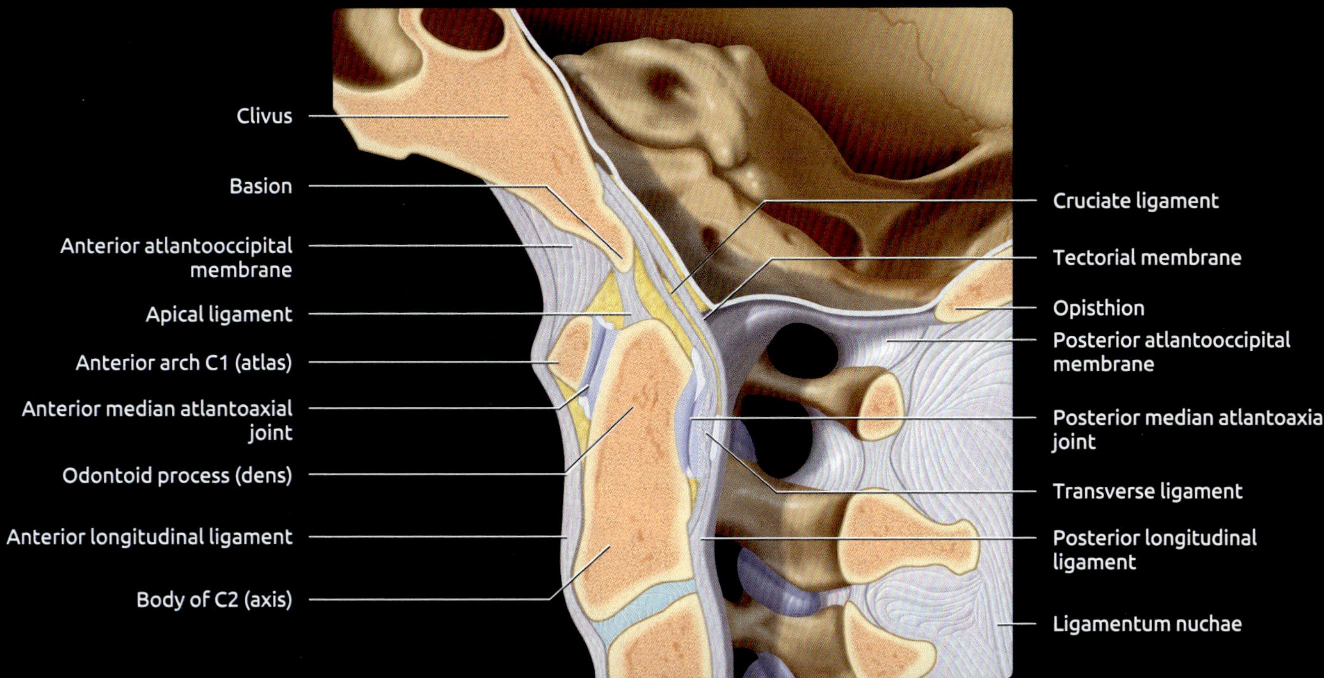

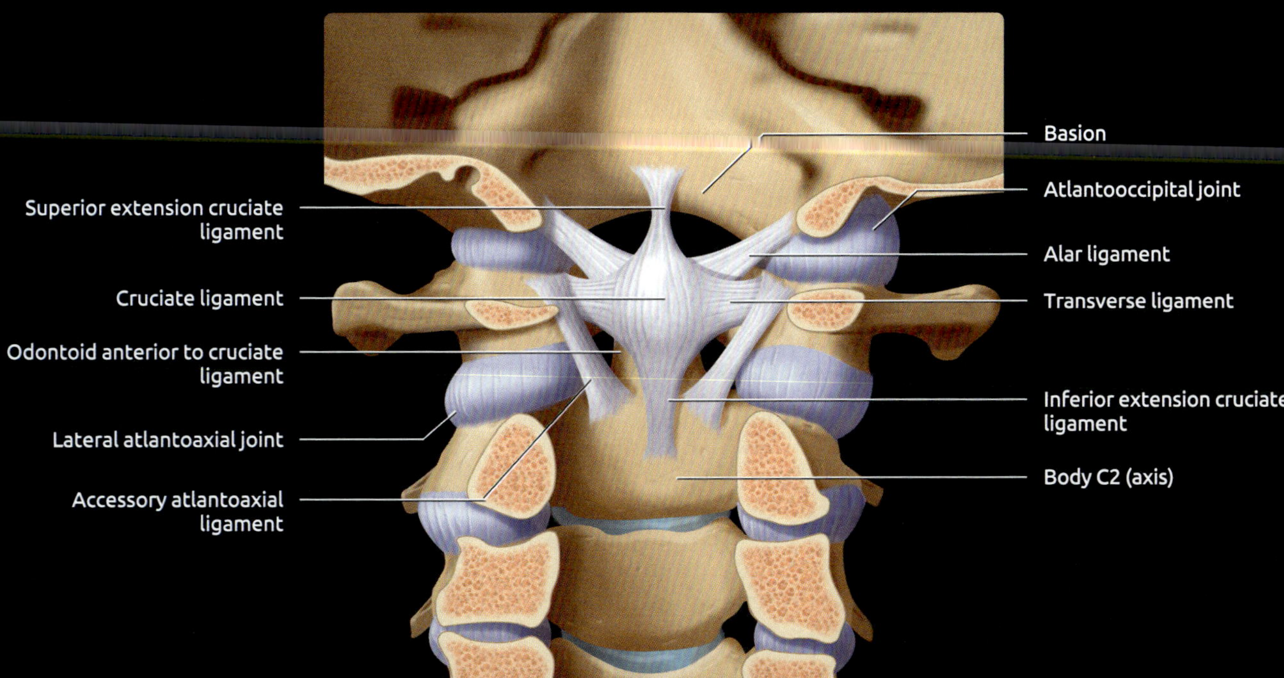

(Top) *The midline atlantoaxial articulations consist of anterior & posterior median atlantoaxial joints. The anterior joint is between the posterior aspect of the anterior C1 arch & the ventral aspect of the odontoid process (dens). The posterior joint is between the dorsal aspect of the odontoid process & the cruciate ligament. The midline view shows a series of ligamentous connections to the skull base, including the anterior atlantooccipital membrane, apical ligament, superior component of cruciate ligament, tectorial membrane, & posterior atlantooccipital membrane.* **(Bottom)** *Posterior view shows the craniocervical junction with posterior elements cut away to define the components of the cruciate ligament & alar ligaments.*

C1 GRAPHICS

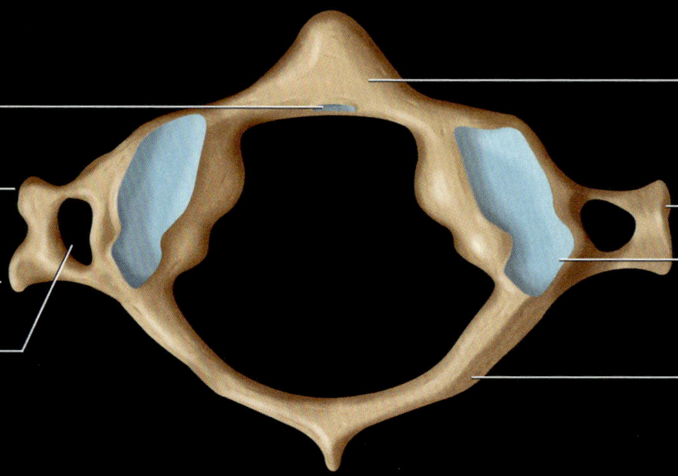

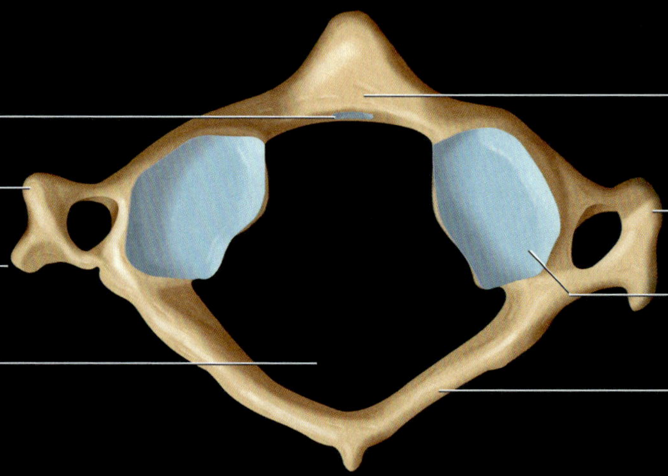

(Top) *Axial graphic view of atlas viewed from above shows the characteristic ring shape, composed of anterior & posterior arches & paired large lateral masses. The superior articular facet is concave anteroposteriorly & projects medially for articulation with the convex surface of the occipital condyle at the atlantooccipital joint. The anterior arch articulates with the odontoid process at the anterior median atlantoaxial joint.* **(Bottom)** *Atlas viewed from below shows that the large inferior facet surface is concave mediolaterally & projects medially for articulation with the convex surface of the superior articular facet of C2. The canal of the atlas measures ~ 3 cm in AP diameter: Spinal cord, odontoid process, & free space for the cord are each ~ 1 cm in diameter. The size of the anterior midline tubercle of the anterior arch & spinous process of posterior arch are quite variable.*

C2 GRAPHICS

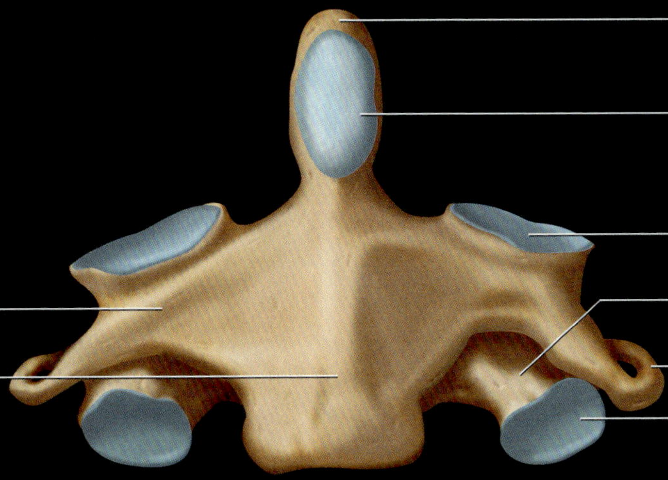

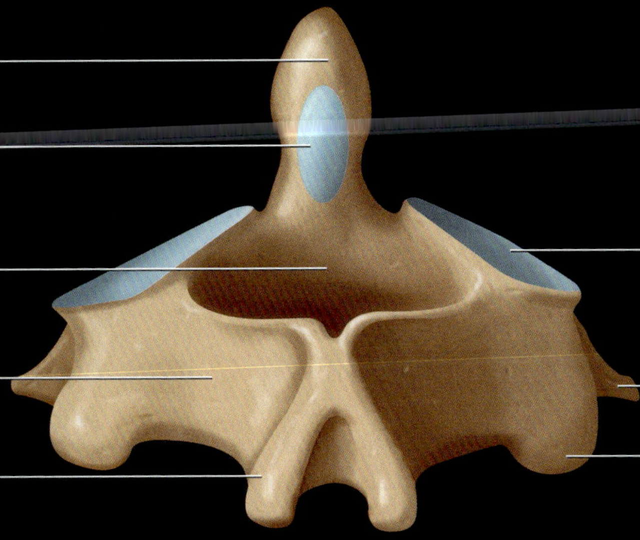

(Top) *Axis viewed from anterior perspective shows the odontoid process is the "purloined" embryologic centrum of C1 that is incorporated into C2, giving C2 its unique morphology. The C2 body laterally is defined by large lateral masses for articulation with the inferior facet of C1. The elongated pars interarticularis of C2 ends with the inferior articular facet for articulation with the superior articular facet of C3.* **(Bottom)** *Axis viewed from posterior perspective shows the odontoid process has anterior & posterior joints for articulation with C1. The anterior median joint articulates with the C1 arch, while the posterior median joint (shown here) involves the transverse ligament.*

CRANIOMETRY GRAPHICS

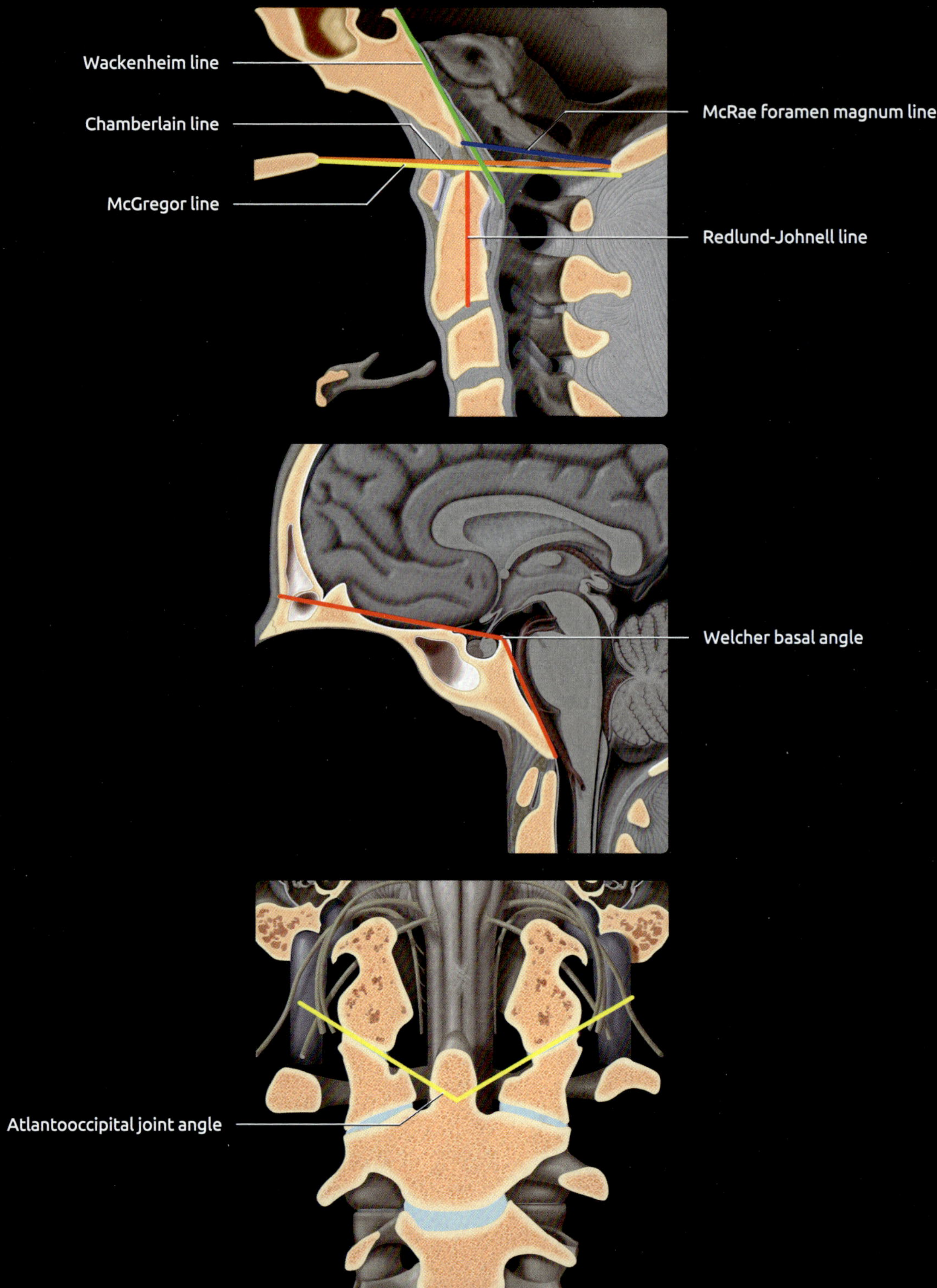

(Top) *Sagittal graphic shows important skull base craniometry. Orange: Chamberlain line is drawn between hard palate & opisthion. Yellow: McGregor line is drawn between hard palate to caudal point of occipital bone (base of occipital bone). Green: Wackenheim line is drawn along posterior surface of clivus. Blue: McRae foramen magnum line is drawn between basion & opisthion. Red: Redlund-Johnell line is drawn from base of C2 to McGregor line.* **(Middle)** *Sagittal midline graphic shows Welcher basal angle, defined by angle between lines drawn along plane of sphenoid bone & along clivus (nasion to sella, sella along posterior clivus to basion). Normal < 140°, platybasia if > 140°.* **(Bottom)** *Coronal graphic of craniocervical junction shows lines drawn along atlantooccipital joints to measure the atlantooccipital joint angle. Normal 125-130°, < 124° may reflect occipital condyle hypoplasia.*

BONE CT & T1 MR CRANIOMETRY

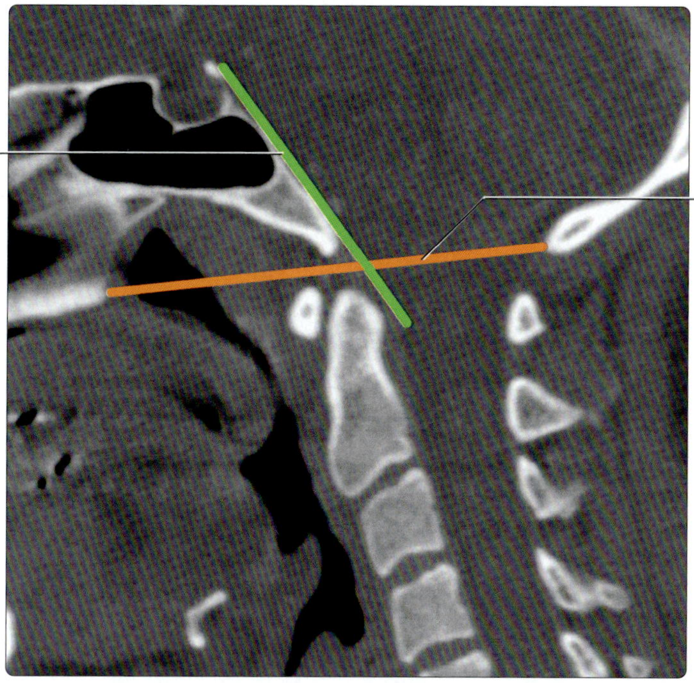

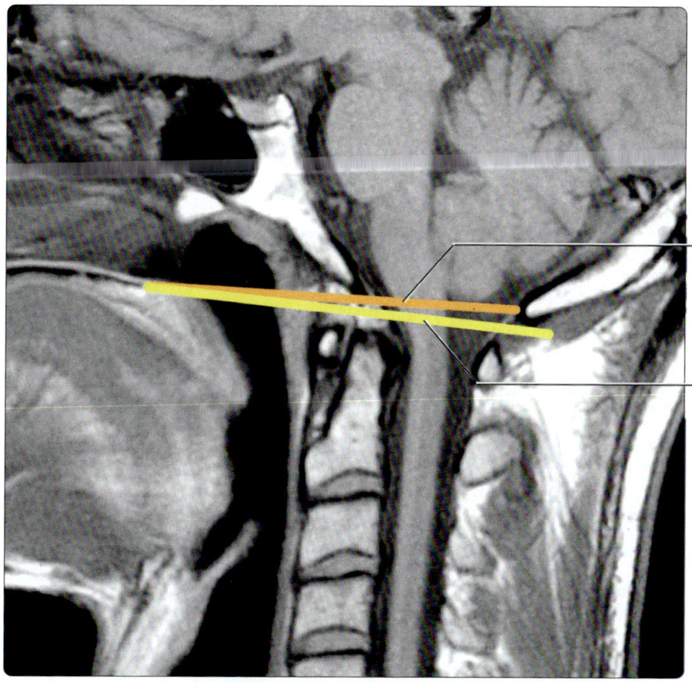

(Top) *Sagittal CT reformat in the midline shows Chamberlain line in orange extending from the hard palate to the opisthion. Projection of up to 1/3 of dens (5 mm) above this line is normal. Wackenheim line is shown in green along the clivus. The dens should lie immediately inferior to this line, & any intersection is considered abnormal.* **(Bottom)** *Sagittal T1 MR shows Chamberlain line in orange. Odontoid tip 5 mm or more above the line defines basilar impression. The McGregor line is shown in yellow. This line has the same significance as the Chamberlain line, with the odontoid tip 7 mm or more above the line defining basilar impression.*

AXIAL BONE CT

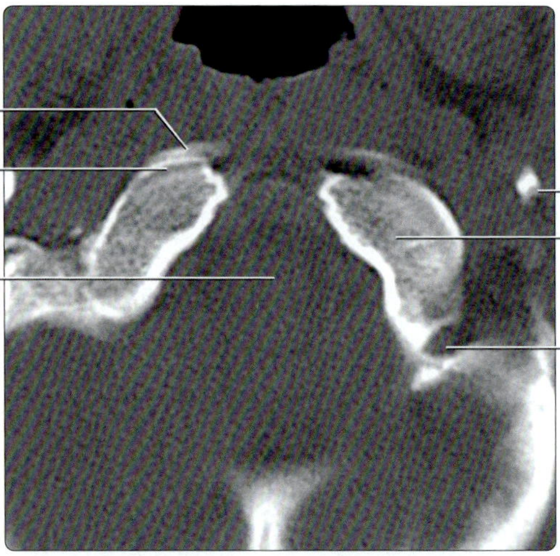

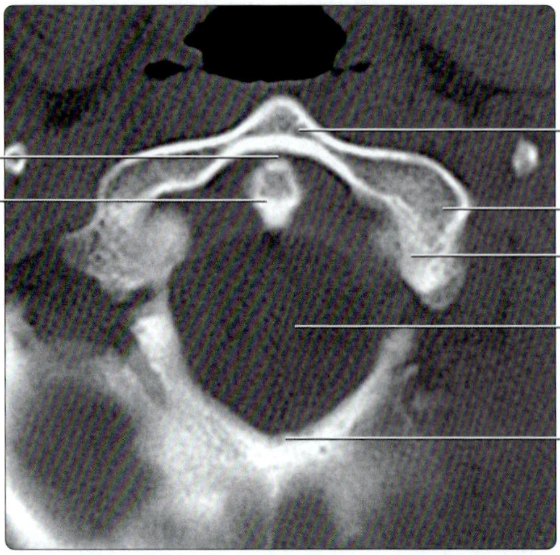

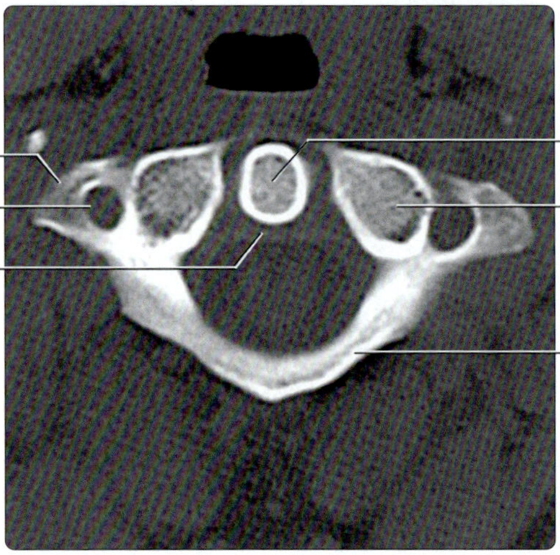

(Top) *This is the 1st of 6 axial bone CT images through the craniocervical junction presented from superior to inferior. The anterolateral margin of the foramen magnum is formed by the prominent occipital condyles that articulate with the superior articular facets of the C1 lateral masses.* **(Middle)** *More inferior image of the craniocervical junction shows that the anterior arch of C1 is now well defined, with the odontoid process of C2 coming into the imaging plane. The atlantooccipital joint is seen in oblique section & therefore has poorly defined margins. The odontoid is tightly applied to the posterior margin of the C1 anterior arch, held in place by the strong transverse component of the cruciate ligament.* **(Bottom)** *In this image at level of atlas, the unique morphology of the C1 body is defined by its large transverse process with transverse foramen & ring shape.*

AXIAL BONE CT

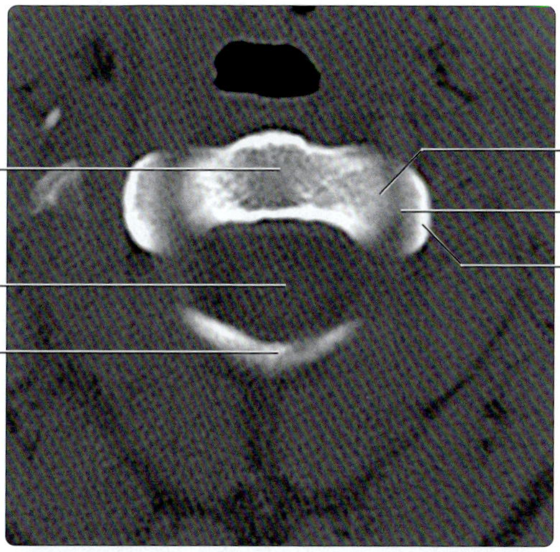

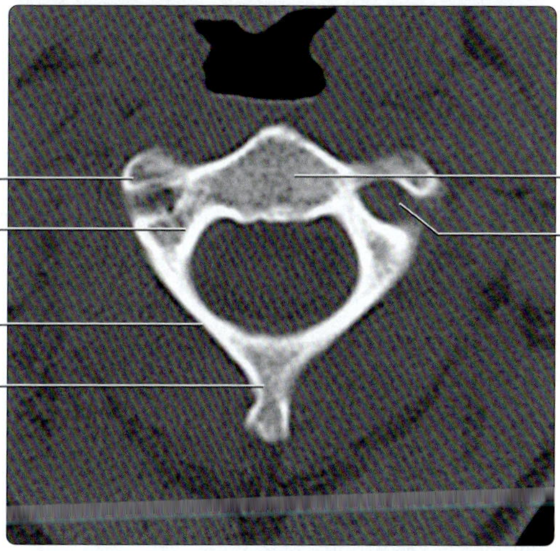

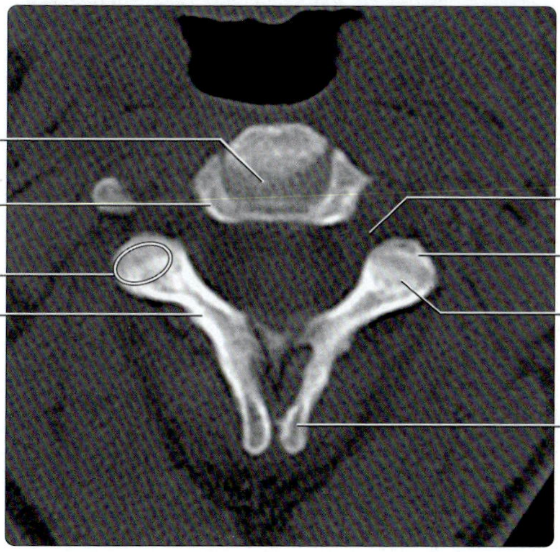

(Top) *Image through lateral atlantoaxial joints is shown. This section defines the junction of the odontoid process with the body of C2. The obliquely oriented atlantoaxial joints are partially seen, with the C1 component lateral to the joint space & the C2 component medial.* **(Middle)** *Image through inferior C2 body level shows large C2 vertebral body & vertebral arch formed by gracile pedicles & laminae.* **(Bottom)** *Image through C2-3 intervertebral disc level is shown. The C2-3 neural foramen is well defined, with the posterior margin formed by the superior articular process of C3. The spinous process of C2 is large & typically bifid. The C2-3 intervertebral disc assumes the characteristic cervical, cup-shaped morphology bounded by the uncinate processes.*

CORONAL BONE CT

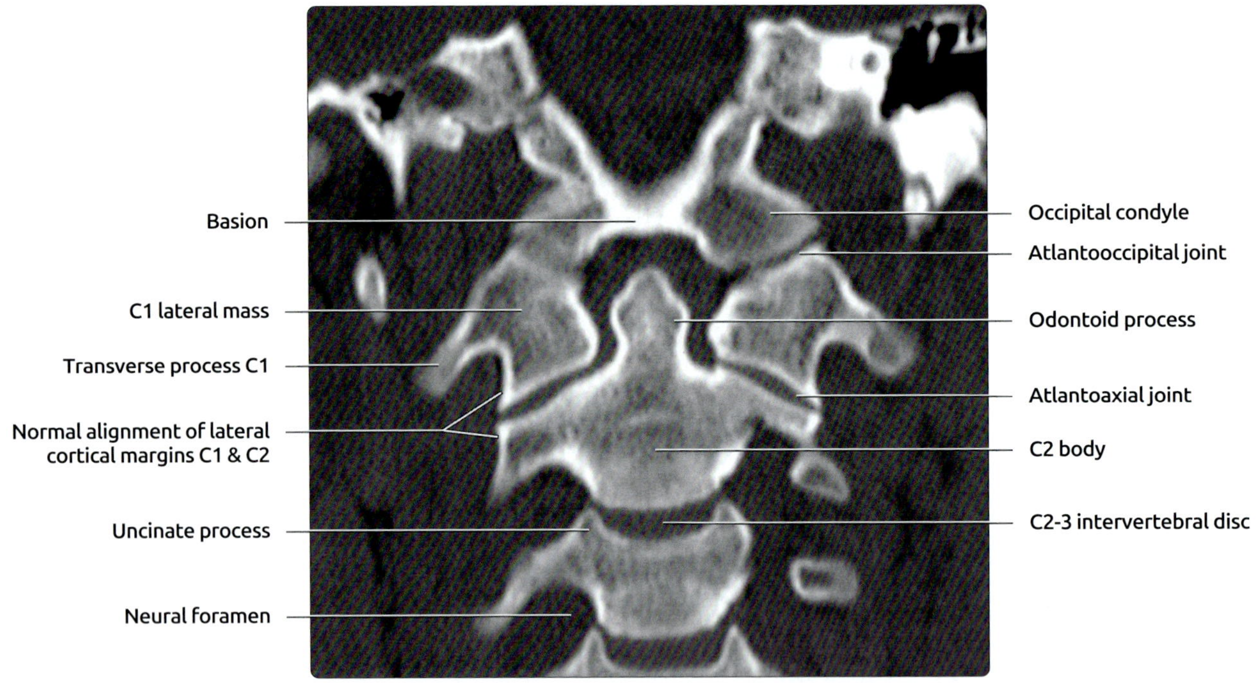

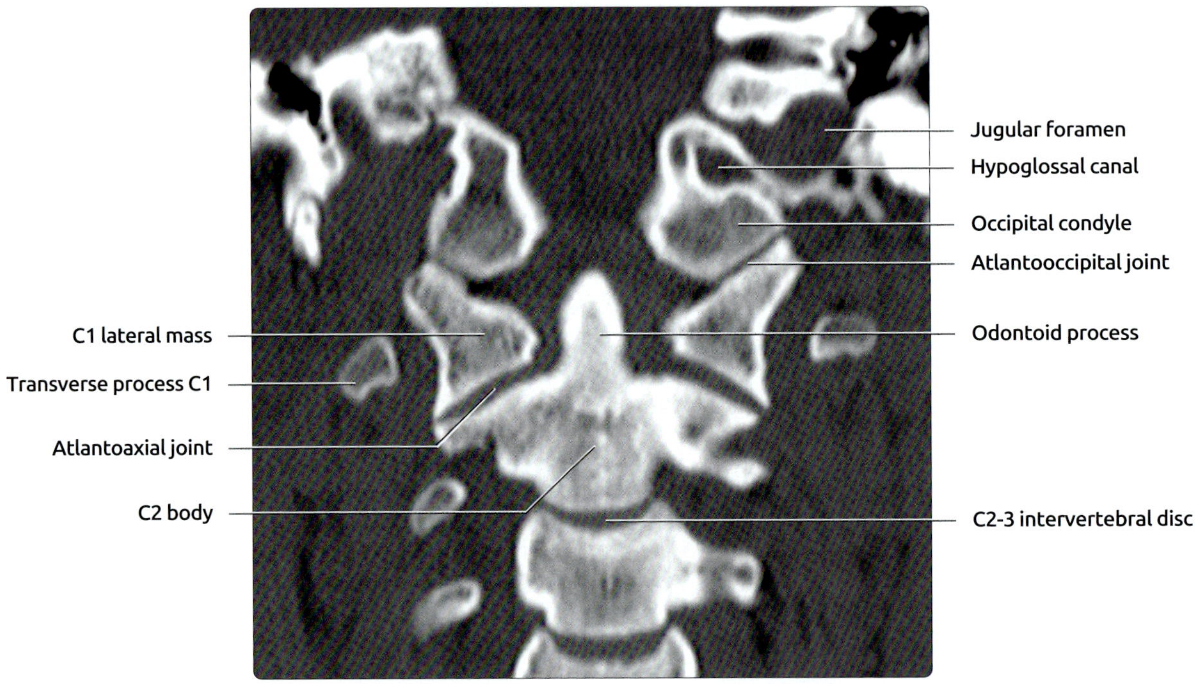

(Top) *First of 2 coronal bone CT reconstructions of the craniocervical junction are presented from anterior to posterior. The odontoid process is visualized in the midline as a sharply corticated bony peg with symmetrically placed lateral C1 masses on either side. The lateral cortical margins of the C1 lateral masses & the C2 lateral masses should align. The atlantooccipital & atlantoaxial joints are visible bilaterally with even joint margins & sharp cortical margins.* **(Bottom)** *A more posterior view of the craniocervical junction shows that both atlantooccipital joints are now well defined with smooth cortical margins sloping superolateral to inferomedial. The atlantoaxial joints are smoothly sloping inferolateral to superomedial.*

SAGITTAL CT & MR

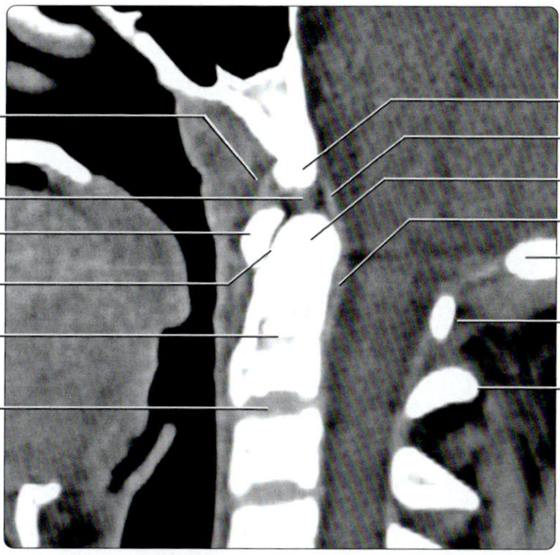

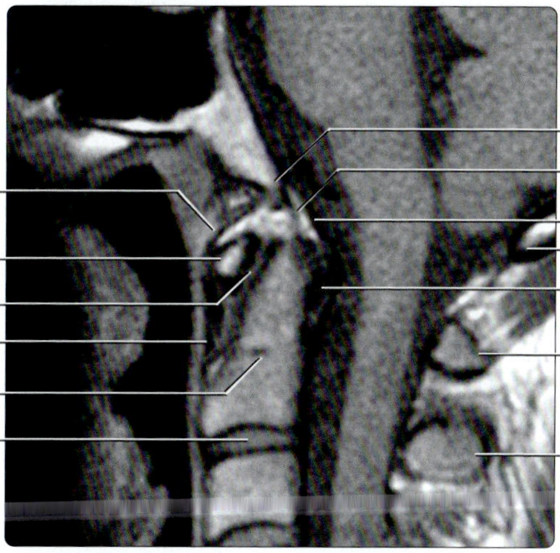

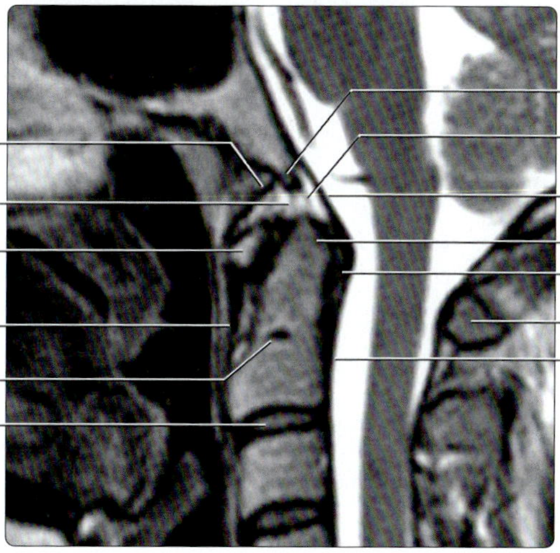

(Top) *Sagittal midline CT reformat shows the ligamentous structures visible at the craniocervical junction. The apical ligament is visible as a linear band between the odontoid tip & clivus. The tectorial membrane is the superior extension of the posterior longitudinal ligament. The anterior atlantooccipital membrane is the extension of the anterior longitudinal ligament.* **(Middle)** *Sagittal T1 MR midline image shows the craniocervical junction. The atlantodental interval is well defined by the adjacent low-signal cortical margins of C1 anterior arch & the odontoid process. The cruciate ligament is a low-signal band dorsal to the odontoid.* **(Bottom)** *Sagittal T2 MR shows the craniocervical junction. The tectorial membrane, superior extension of cruciate ligament, apical ligament, & anterior atlantooccipital membranes are evident.*

PART I
SECTION 7

Suprahyoid Neck

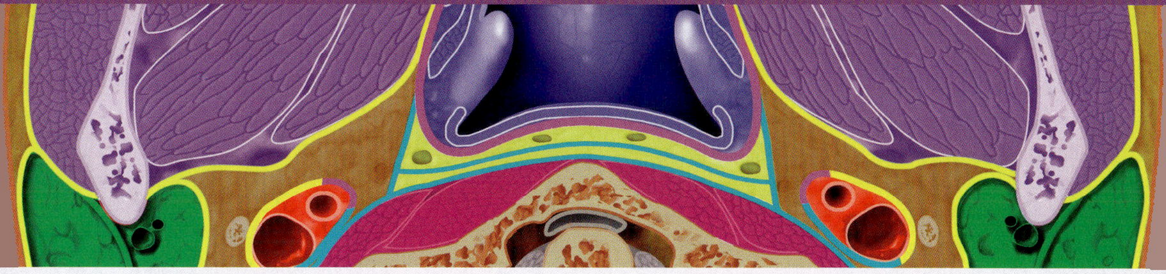

Suprahyoid Neck Overview	**162**
Parapharyngeal Space	**168**
Nasopharynx and Oropharynx	**172**
Masticator Space	**180**
Parotid Space	**184**
Carotid Space	**188**
Retropharyngeal Space	**192**
Perivertebral Space	**196**
Lymph Nodes	**200**
External and Internal Carotid Arteries	**204**

TERMINOLOGY

Abbreviations

- Suprahyoid neck (SHN)
- Infrahyoid neck (IHN)

Definitions

- SHN: Spaces from skull base to hyoid bone (excluding orbit, sinuses, & oral cavity), including parapharyngeal (PPS), pharyngeal mucosal (PMS), masticator (MS), parotid (PS), carotid (CS), buccal, retropharyngeal (RPS), & perivertebral (PVS) spaces
- IHN: Spaces below hyoid bone with some continuing into mediastinum, including visceral space (VS), posterior cervical space (PCS), anterior cervical space, CS, RPS, & PVS

IMAGING ANATOMY

Overview

- **Key** to understanding SHN & IHN spaces is **fascia**
- 3 layers of deep cervical fascia cleave neck into spaces
  - **Superficial layer, deep cervical fascia (SL-DCF)**
    - SHN: Around MS & PS; part of carotid sheath
    - IHN: Invests neck by surrounding strap, sternocleidomastoid, & trapezius muscles
  - **Middle layer, deep cervical fascia (ML-DCF)**
    - SHN: ML-DCF defines PMS deep margin; contributes to carotid sheath
    - IHN: Circumscribes VS; part of carotid sheath
  - **Deep layer, deep cervical fascia (DL-DCF)**
    - SHN & IHN: Surrounds PVS
    - SHN & IHN: Contributes to carotid sheath
    - SHN & IHN: **Alar fascia** is slip of DL-DCF providing lateral wall to RPS & danger space (DS); also posterior wall to RPS separating RPS from DS

Spaces of Suprahyoid & Infrahyoid Neck

- **Parapharyngeal space**
  - Location: SHN from skull base to posterior submandibular space
  - Contents: Fat & pterygoid venous plexus
  - Importance: Pattern of displacement helps define SHN mass space of origin
- **Pharyngeal mucosal space**
  - Location: SHN space medial to PPS, anterior to RPS
  - Contents: Mucosa, minor salivary glands, PMS lymphatic ring, constrictor muscles
    - Nasopharyngeal, oropharyngeal, & hypopharyngeal mucosal surfaces
    - PMS of nasopharynx: Torus tubarius, adenoids, superior constrictor, & levator palatini muscles
    - PMS of oropharynx: Anterior & posterior tonsillar pillars, palatine & lingual tonsils, soft palate
  - Fascia: PMS on airway side of ML-DCF
  - Importance: Squamous cell carcinoma & non-Hodgkin lymphoma here
- **Masticator space**
  - Location: Anterolateral to PPS in SHN
  - Contents: Ramus & condyle of mandible, CNV3, masseter, medial & lateral pterygoid & temporalis muscles, pterygoid venous plexus
  - Fascia: MS surrounded by SL-DCF
  - Importance: Perineural tumor on CNV3; primary tumor in MS is sarcoma
- **Parotid space**
  - Location: Lateral to PPS in SHN
  - Contents: Parotid gland, extracranial CNVII, nodes, retromandibular vein, external carotid artery
  - Fascia: PS surrounded by SL-DCF
  - Importance: Intraparotid CNVII; parotid nodes; perineural tumor on CNVII
- **Carotid space**
  - Location: Posterior to PPS in SHN; lateral to VS & RPS in IHN
    - Begins at inferior jugular foramen & carotid canal of skull base; extends to aortic arch
  - Contents: CNIX-XII, internal jugular vein, carotid artery
  - Fascia: All 3 layers, deep cervical fascia
  - Importance: CNX & carotid here; squamous cell carcinoma nodes along superficial margin
- **Retropharyngeal space**
  - Location: Posterior to PMS in SHN & VS in IHN
    - Begins at clivus; traverses SHN-IHN to T3 level
  - Contents: Nodes & fat in SHN; no nodes in IHN
  - Fascia: Anterior fascia is ML-DCF, lateral & posterior fascia is DL-DCF (alar fascia)
  - Importance: Inferior communication with DS allows infection access to mediastinum
- **Danger space**
  - Posterior to RPS in SHN & IHN; continues inferiorly into mediastinum
- **Perivertebral space**
  - Location: Behind RPS & around spine in SHN & IHN
  - Contents: Prevertebral & paraspinal components
    - Prevertebral: Vertebral body, veins & arteries, prevertebral & scalene muscles, brachial plexus, & phrenic nerve
    - Paraspinal: Posterior elements of vertebra, levator scapulae, & paraspinal muscles
  - Fascia: Surrounded by DL-DCF
  - Importance: PVS malignancy may be epidural
- **Visceral space**
  - Location: IHN only; extends into mediastinum
  - Contents: Thyroid & parathyroids, paratracheal nodes, esophagus, trachea, recurrent laryngeal nerve
  - Fascia: VS surrounded by ML-DCF
  - Importance: Trachea & esophagus traverse VS
- **Posterior cervical space**
  - Location: SHN PCS begins at mastoid tip, extends to clavicle; most PCS volume in IHN
  - Contents: Fat, CNXII, spinal accessory nodes
  - Fascia: Between SL- & DL-DCF
  - Importance: Spinal accessory nodal diseases

Key Spatial Relationships

- **SHN spaces surrounding PPS**
  - Medial is PMS: PMS mass displaces PPS laterally
  - Anterior is MS: MS mass displaces PPS posteriorly
  - Lateral is PS: PS mass displaces PPS medially
  - Posterior is CS: CS mass displaces PPS anteriorly
  - Posteromedial is lateral RPS: Lateral RPS nodal mass displaces PPS anterolaterally

AXIAL NASOPHARYNX & OROPHARYNX SPACE GRAPHICS

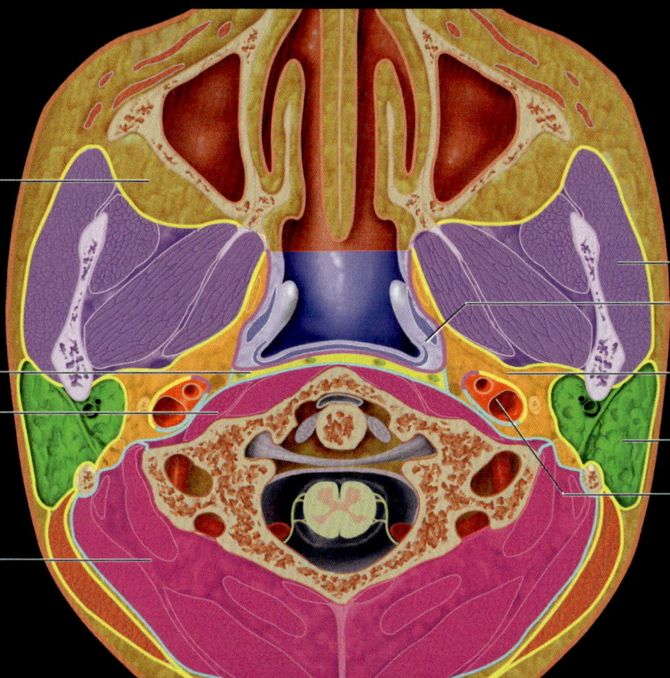

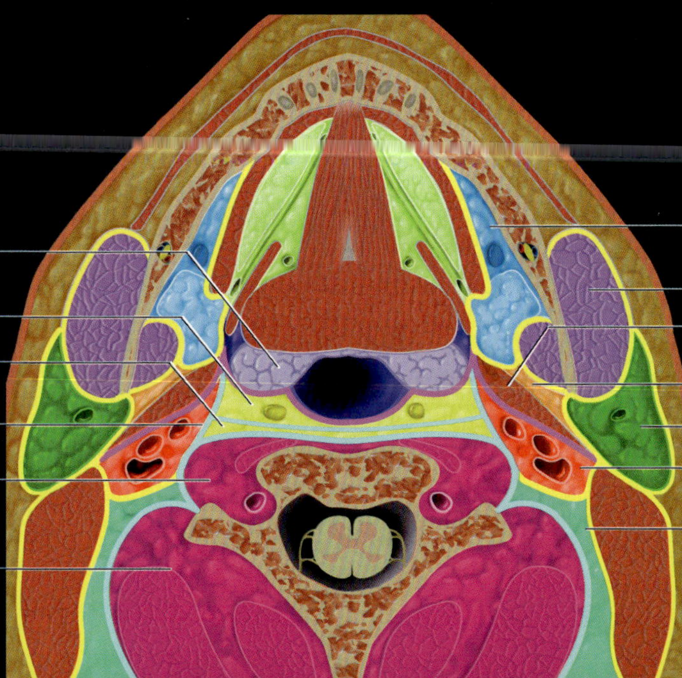

(Top) *Axial graphic depicts the spaces of the suprahyoid neck. Surrounding the paired, fat-filled parapharyngeal spaces are the 4 critical paired spaces of this region: Pharyngeal mucosal, masticator, parotid, and carotid spaces. The retropharyngeal and perivertebral spaces are the midline nonpaired spaces. A Pharyngeal mucosal space mass pushes the parapharyngeal space laterally, masticator space mass pushes parapharyngeal space posteriorly, parotid space mass pushes parapharyngeal space medially, and carotid space mass pushes parapharyngeal space anteriorly.* **(Bottom)** *Axial graphic shows the suprahyoid neck spaces at the level of the oropharynx. The superficial (yellow line), middle (pink line), and deep (turquoise line) layers of deep cervical fascia outline the suprahyoid neck spaces. Notice the lateral borders of the retropharyngeal and danger spaces are called the alar fascia and represents a slip of the deep layer of deep cervical fascia.*

AXIAL & CORONAL SKULL BASE-SPACE INTERACTION GRAPHICS

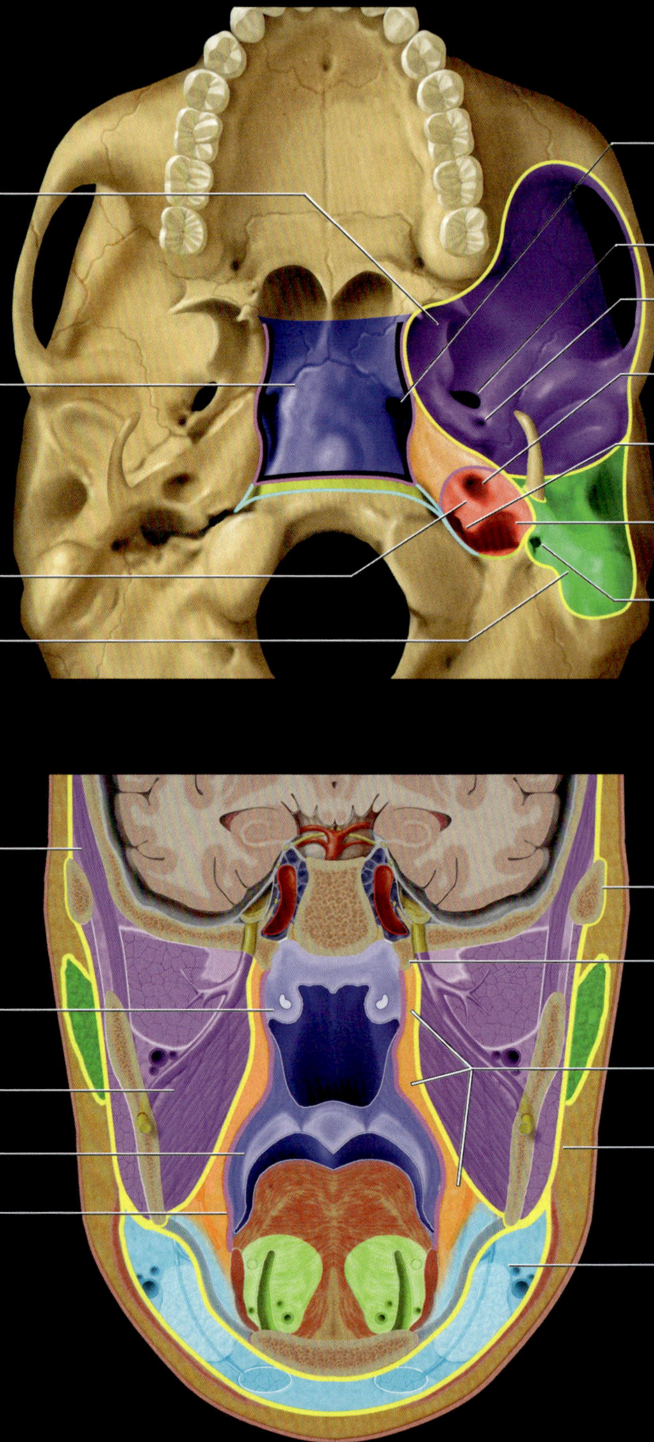

(Top) *Graphic of skull base from below shows spaces of suprahyoid neck relationships to skull base. Four spaces have key interactions with skull base: Masticator, parotid, carotid, and pharyngeal mucosal spaces. Parotid space (green) malignancy can follow CNVII into stylomastoid foramen. Masticator space (purple) receives CNV3 while CNIX-XII enter the carotid space (red). The pharyngeal mucosal space abuts the foramen lacerum, which is covered by fibrocartilage in life. Also note that the superficial layer of deep cervical fascia (yellow line) surrounds the masticator and parotid spaces and middle layer is on nonairway side of the pharyngeal mucosal space (pink line).* **(Bottom)** *Coronal graphic shows the suprahyoid neck spaces and their skull base relationships. The pharyngeal mucosal space abuts the basisphenoid of the skull base with the foramen lacerum within this area of the skull base. The parapharyngeal spaces touch the skull base in an area with no vital structures. The masticator space broadly interacts with the skull base with the foramen ovale/CNV3 and foramen spinosum/middle meningeal artery within this area.*

SAGITTAL & 3D LONGITUDINAL SPATIAL RELATIONSHIPS GRAPHICS

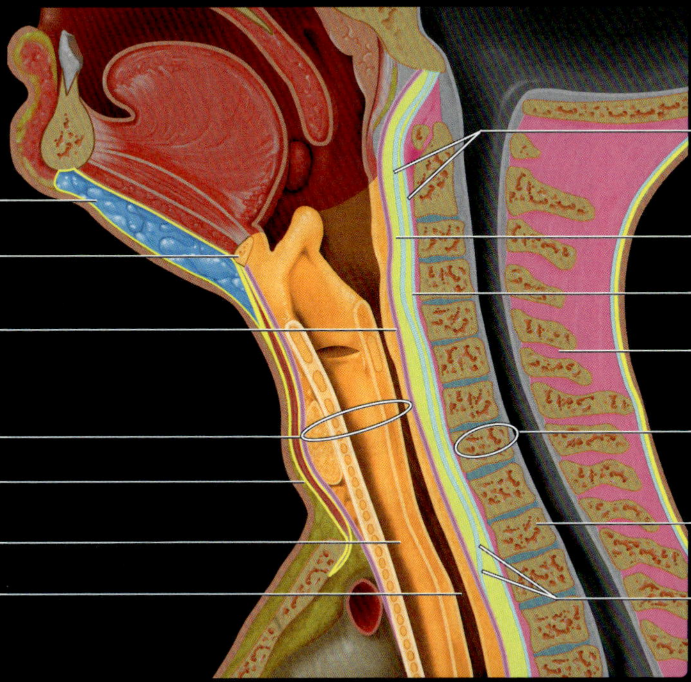

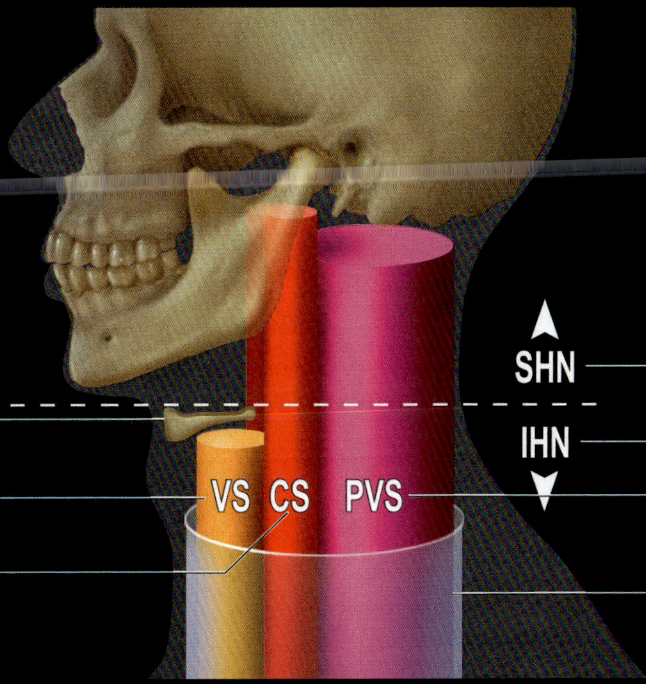

(Top) *Sagittal graphic depicts longitudinal spatial relationships of the neck. Anteriorly, the visceral space is seen surrounded by middle layer of deep cervical fascia. Just anterior to the vertebral column the retropharyngeal and danger spaces run inferiorly toward the mediastinum. Notice the fascial "trap door" found at the approximate level of T3 vertebral body that serves as a conduit from the retropharyngeal to the danger space. Retropharyngeal space infection or tumor may access the mediastinum via this route of spread.* **(Bottom)** *Lateral graphic of extracranial head and neck shows the spaces as "tubes" as they traverse the area. This is particularly true of the carotid spaces, which reach from the skull base to the aortic arch. Both the visceral and perivertebral spaces continue inferiorly into the thorax.*

AXIAL CECT IMAGES OF NORMAL SUPRAHYOID NECK

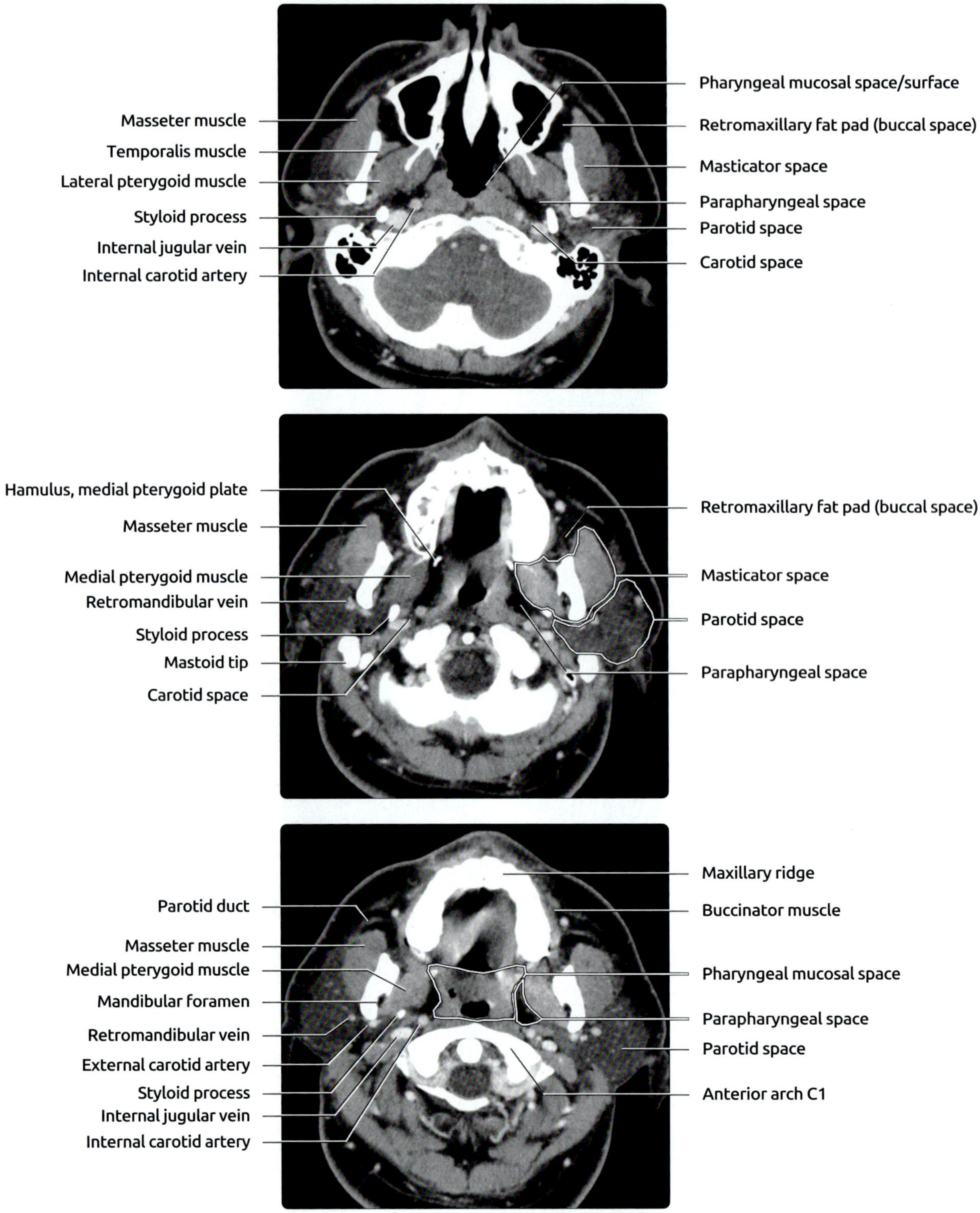

(Top) *First of 6 axial CECT images of both the suprahyoid and infrahyoid aspects of the extracranial head and neck presented from superior to inferior. This image at the level of the nasopharynx shows the 4 key spaces surrounding the parapharyngeal space: Pharyngeal mucosal, masticator, parotid, and carotid spaces.* **(Middle)** *In this CECT at the level of inferior maxillary sinus, the styloid process is seen anterolateral to the carotid space. The superficial layer of deep cervical fascia defines the masticator and parotid spaces. The more anterior buccal space has no fascial definition.* **(Bottom)** *At the level of the maxillary ridge, the area of the pharyngeal mucosal space is outlined between the paired fat-filled parapharyngeal spaces. Posterior to the pharyngeal mucosal space are the tightly packed retropharyngeal and perivertebral spaces.*

AXIAL CECT IMAGES OF NORMAL SUPRAHYOID NECK

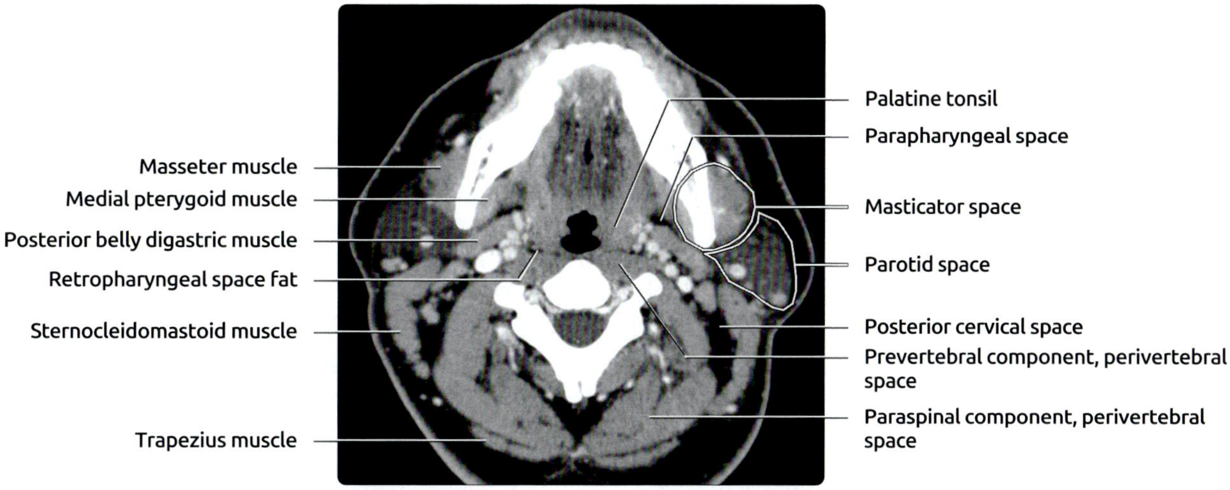

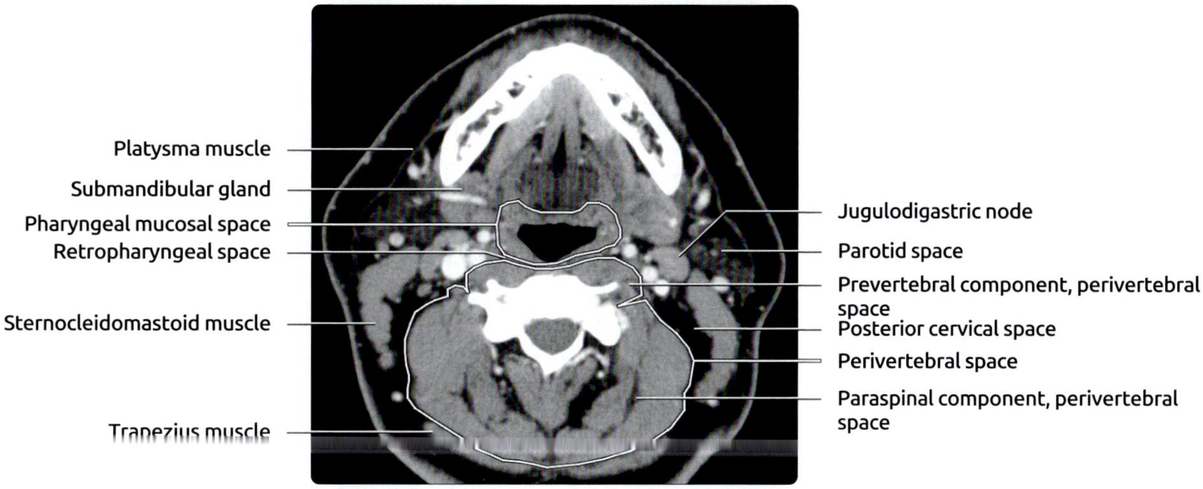

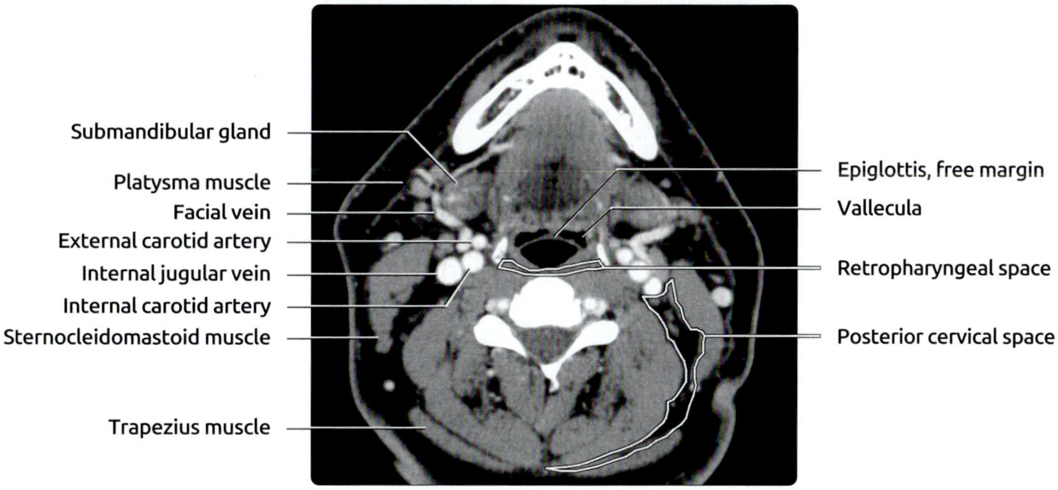

(Top) *In this image at the level of the mandibular body, the posterior belly of the digastric muscle can be seen dividing the parotid tail from the carotid space. The direction of displacement of this muscle can define whether a lesion is in the parotid space (posteromedial displacement) or in the carotid space (anterolateral displacement).* **(Middle)** *In this image through the low oropharynx, the pharyngeal mucosal space has been outlined anterior to the perivertebral space. The space between the 2 is the retropharyngeal space. The alar fascia that makes up the lateral borders of the retropharyngeal space is not shown.* **(Bottom)** *At the level of the free margin of the epiglottis, the retropharyngeal space is outlined behind the pharyngeal mucosal space. The posterior cervical space contains fat, the accessory cranial nerve (CNXI), and the spinal accessory nodal chain (level 5 nodes).*

TERMINOLOGY

Abbreviations

- Parapharyngeal space (PPS)

Synonyms

- PPS has been called "prestyloid parapharyngeal space"
  - Carotid space called "poststyloid parapharyngeal space" in this alterative terminology
  - "Carotid space" preferred terminology

Definitions

- **Parapharyngeal space**: Central, fat-filled spaces in lateral suprahyoid neck (SHN) around which most of important spaces are located
  - These surrounding important spaces are pharyngeal mucosal space (PMS), masticator space (MS), parotid space (PS), and carotid space (CS)

IMAGING ANATOMY

Overview

- PPS contents are limited, therefore few lesions actually begin in this location
  - Diseases of PPS usually arise in adjacent spaces (PMS, MS, PS, CS), spreading secondarily into PPS
- Importance of PPS is its conspicuity on CT and MR as well as its direction of displacement by mass lesions of surrounding spaces
  - **PPS displacement pattern helps define actual space of origin**
    - PMS mass lesion pushes PPS laterally
    - MS mass lesion pushes PPS posteriorly
    - PS mass lesion pushes PPS medially
    - CS mass lesion pushes PPS anteriorly
    - Lateral retropharyngeal space mass (nodal) pushes PPS anterolaterally
  - Combining center of mass lesion with displacement direction of PPS yields strong impression of "space of origin" of SHN mass lesion

Extent

- Crescent-shaped fat-filled space in craniocaudal dimension extends from skull base above to superior cornu of hyoid bone inferiorly

Anatomy Relationships

- As fatty tube separating other SHN spaces from one another, PPS functions as "elevator shaft" through which infection and tumor from these adjacent spaces may travel from skull base to hyoid bone
- Inferiorly there is **no fascia** separating inferior PPS from submandibular space (SMS)
  - Open communication between inferior PPS and posterior SMS therefore exists
- Superiorly PPS interacts with skull base in bland triangular area on inferior surface of petrous apex
  - **No exiting skull base foramina** are found in this area of attachment
- Surrounding spaces include
  - PMS medially
  - MS anterolaterally
  - PS laterally
  - CS posteriorly
  - RPS posteromedially

Internal Contents

- PPS has **no** mucosa, muscle, bone, nodes, or major salivary gland tissue within its boundaries
  - Consequently, few things primarily begin in PPS
- **Critical PPS contents**
  - **Fat**: Key constituent making PPS easily identifiable even with larger SHN mass lesions
  - Minor salivary glands (ectopic, rare)
  - Internal maxillary artery
  - Ascending pharyngeal artery
  - Pterygoid venous plexus (small portion, mostly MS)

Fascial of Parapharyngeal Space

- Fascial margins of PPS are complex; made up of different layers of deep cervical fascia
  - Medial fascial margin of PPS
    - Made up of middle layer, deep cervical fascia as it curves around lateral margin of PMS
  - Lateral fascial margin of PPS
    - Formed by medial slip of superficial layer of deep cervical fascia along deep border of MS & PS
  - Posterior fascial margin of PPS
    - Formed by deep layer of deep cervical fascia on anterolateral margin of retropharyngeal space and anterior part of carotid sheath (made up of components of all 3 layers of deep cervical fascia)

ANATOMY IMAGING ISSUES

Questions

- Because of limited normal anatomic contents of PPS, few lesions primarily arise in PPS
  - Rare lesions found in PPS include benign mixed tumor (from minor salivary gland rests in PPS), lipoma, and atypical 2nd branchial cleft cyst
  - To say lesion is primary to PPS, it must be completely surrounded by PPS fat
  - In most cases where lesion is thought to be primary to PPS, careful observation will find connection to one of surrounding spaces (usually PS)
- **PPS fat displacement** is **key imaging relationship** used in evaluation of SHN mass lesions

Imaging Recommendations

- MR better delineates skull base, meningeal & perineural lesions
  - Fat-saturated contrast-enhanced T1 MR may make PPS fat difficult to see

Imaging Pitfalls

- Remember most lesions of PPS arise from adjacent SHN spaces

CLINICAL IMPLICATIONS

Clinical Importance

- Since PPS empties inferiorly into SMS, PPS lesion may present as "angle of mandible" mass

NORMAL AXIAL & CORONAL PARAPHARYNGEAL SPACE

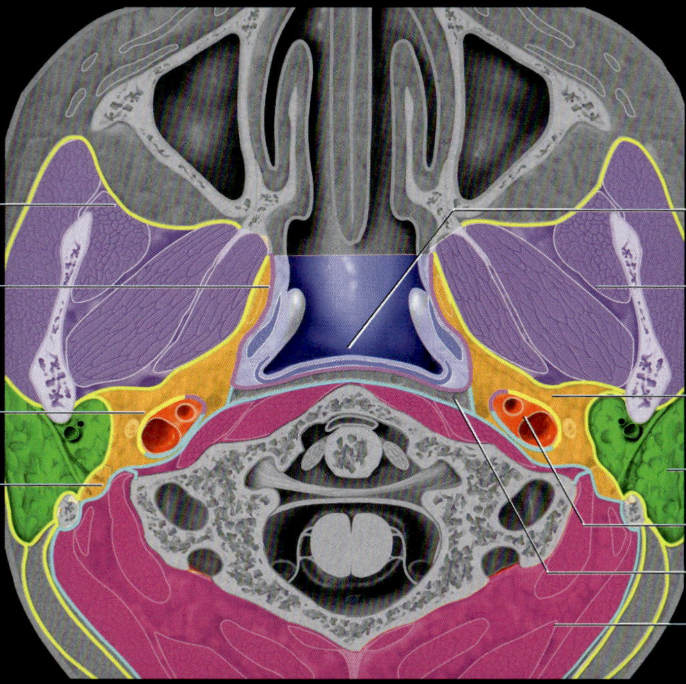

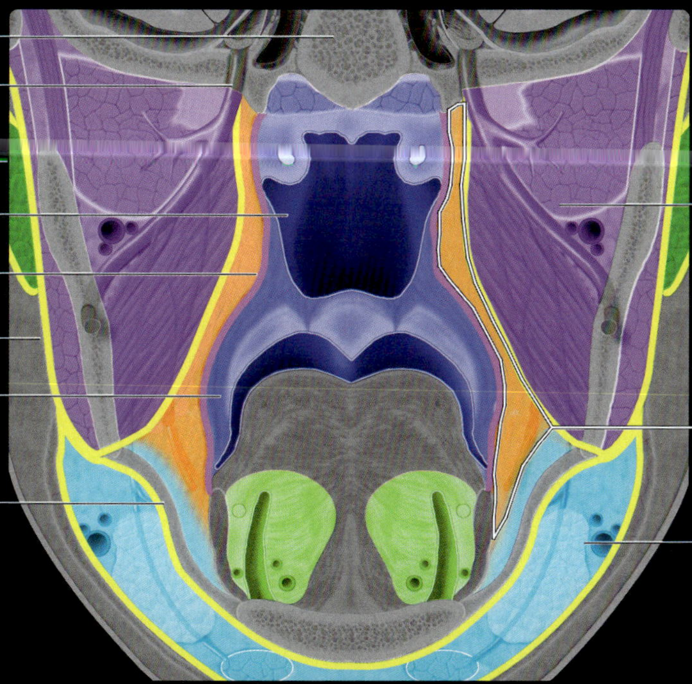

(Top) *Axial graphic of the normal parapharyngeal space at the level of the nasopharynx demonstrates the complex fascial margins and the fat-only contents. The surrounding pharyngeal mucosal, masticator, parotid, and carotid spaces when affected by mass lesions push into the parapharyngeal space. The resulting displacement pattern of the parapharyngeal space may be helpful in defining the space of origin of a mass in the suprahyoid neck.* **(Bottom)** *Coronal graphic shows suprahyoid neck spaces as they interact with the skull base superiorly and the submandibular space inferiorly. The parapharyngeal space interacts with no critical structures as it abuts the skull base. Inferiorly it "empties" into the posterior submandibular space along the posterior margin of the mylohyoid muscle. As a consequence of this anatomic arrangement, it is possible for an infection or a malignant tumor that breaks into the parapharyngeal space to present inferiorly as an "angle of mandible" mass.*

PPS SKULL BASE INTERACTION; NORMAL AXIAL PARAPHARYNGEAL SPACE

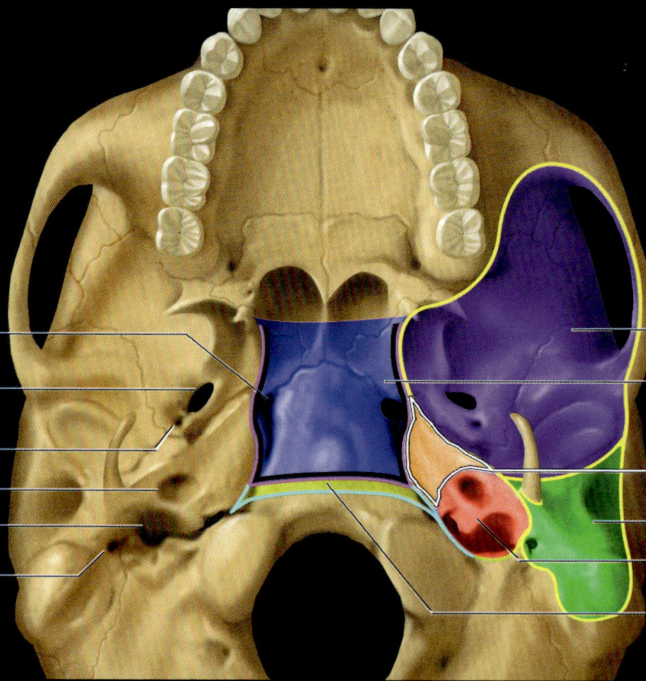

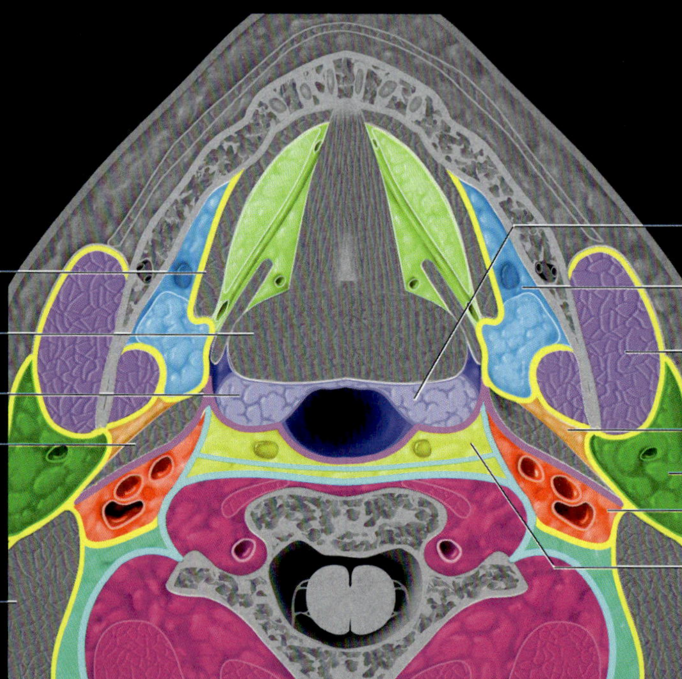

(Top) *Axial graphic of the suprahyoid neck spaces interaction with the skull base highlighting the parapharyngeal space. Notice that the parapharyngeal space abuts the inferior surface of the skull base in an area with no critical structures.* **(Bottom)** *Axial graphic at the level of the low oropharynx shows the slip of parapharyngeal space fat is just anterolateral to the posterior belly of the digastric muscle. Inferior to this level, the parapharyngeal space communicates anteriorly with the submandibular space. Yellow lines in the drawing represent superficial layer, pink lines represent middle, and aquamarine lines represent the deep layer of deep cervical fascia.*

AXIAL CECT & CORONAL T1 MR IMAGES OF NORMAL PARAPHARYNGEAL SPACE

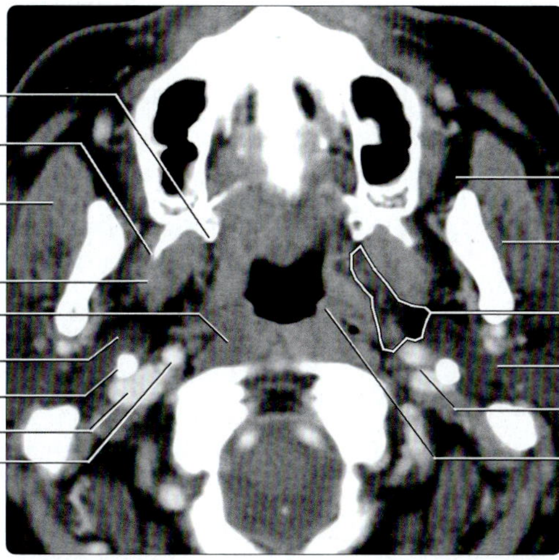

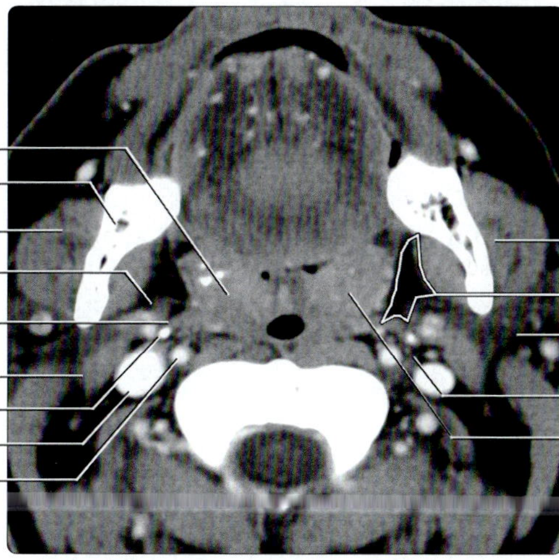

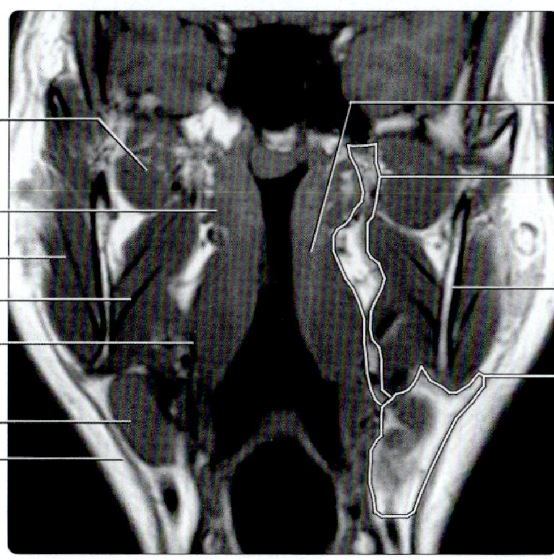

(Top) *Axial contrast-enhanced CT (CECT) at the level of the inferior maxillary sinus shows the complex shape of the parapharyngeal space. Notice the lateral margin of the parapharyngeal space is the deep lobe of the parotid gland.* **(Middle)** *In this axial CECT, the parapharyngeal space points anteriorly toward the submandibular space. On more inferior images it will communicate with the posterosuperior submandibular space in this area. Notice the stylopharyngeus and styloglossus muscle on the posterior margin of the parapharyngeal space.* **(Bottom)** *In this coronal T1 MR, the parapharyngeal space is visible from its superior area of skull base abutment to its inferior merging with the submandibular space. Note the site of abutment with the skull base contains no vital structures. Remember there is no fascia present between the inferior parapharyngeal space and the posterior submandibular space.*

TERMINOLOGY

Definitions

- **Nasopharynx**: Superior part of pharynx connecting nasal cavity to oropharynx
- **Oropharynx**: Middle level of pharynx between nasopharynx and hypopharynx, posterior to oral cavity
- **Pharyngeal mucosal space/surface (PMS)**: Superficial space between middle layer of deep cervical fascia and nasopharyngeal, oropharyngeal, & hypopharyngeal airways

IMAGING ANATOMY

Overview

- Important passage for air (naso- and oropharynx) and food (oropharynx)
- PMS is conceptual construct to complete map of spaces of suprahyoid neck
- There is **no fascia on surface of PMS**, so it is not true fascia-enclosed space

Extent

- Nasopharynx: Extends from base of skull to upper surface of soft palate, posterior to nasal choanae
- Oropharynx: Extends from uvula to epiglottis; includes base of tongue
- PMS is continuous mucosal sheet defined from nasopharynx to hypopharynx (includes soft palate)

Anatomy Relationships

- Posterior to PMS is retropharyngeal space
- Lateral to PMS is parapharyngeal space (PPS)
- Skull base relationship to PMS
  - Broad area of attachment to skull base is present
  - Attachment area includes posterior basisphenoid (sphenoid sinus floor), anterior basiocciput (anterior clivus)
  - Also includes **foramen lacerum**
    - Foramen lacerum: Cartilaginous floor of anterior horizontal petrous internal carotid artery
    - Represents perivascular route for nasopharyngeal carcinoma to access intracranial structures
- Mandibular position affects pharynx volume: Retruded mandible → compressed airway

Internal Contents

- **Mucosal surface of pharynx**
- **Lymphatic tissue**: Forms ring of tissue; normally hyperplastic in youth and declines in size with age
  - Synonym: **Waldeyer** ring
  - Nasopharynx: **Adenoids**
  - Oropharynx, lateral wall: **Palatine (faucial) tonsil**
  - Oropharynx, base of tongue: **Lingual tonsil**
- **Minor salivary glands**
  - Soft palate mucosa has highest concentration
- **Pharyngobasilar fascia**
  - Tough aponeurosis that connects superior constrictor muscle to skull base
  - Posterosuperior margin notch = **sinus of Morgagni**
    - Levator palatini muscle & eustachian tube pass through this notch on way from skull base to PMS
- **Pharyngeal mucosal space muscles**
  - Superior, middle, & inferior constrictor muscles
  - Salpingopharyngeus muscle
  - Levator palatini muscle, distal end
- **Torus tubarius**: Cartilaginous end of eustachian tube extends into nasopharynx
- **Lateral pharyngeal recess/fossa of Rosenmüller**: Posterior to torus tubarius

Fascia of Pharyngeal Mucosal Space

- **Middle layer, deep cervical fascia** (ML-DCF) represents deep margin of PMS

ANATOMY IMAGING ISSUES

Questions

- What imaging findings define lesion as primary to pharyngeal mucosal space?
  - Lesion is designated primary to PMS under following circumstances
    - Lesion center is **medial to parapharyngeal space**
    - PMS mass **pushes PPS fat from medial to lateral**
    - PMS mass **disrupts normal PMS mucosal & submucosal architecture**

Imaging Recommendations

- CECT or MR can both successfully image PMS
- If skull base invasion or perineural tumor suspected, T1 C+ fat-saturated MR best
- Bone CT may then be added to delineate skull base bone changes & tumor matrix
- CBCT useful in evaluating airway volume in cases of suspected airway restriction

Imaging Pitfalls

- Most common error in interpreting images of PMS is labeling normal asymmetry as tumor
- Lateral pharyngeal recess is notoriously asymmetric & may have fluid within it
- Variable amounts of lymphoid tissue can also create misimpression of tumor
  - Enlarged tonsillar tissue is normal finding in children
- Radiolucent shadows created by superimposition of nasopharyngeal and oropharyngeal airway on panoramic radiographs may be mistaken for pathology

CLINICAL IMPLICATIONS

Clinical Importance

- Severely enlarged adenoids or tonsils in adolescents can impede nasal breathing, leading to mouth breathing and altered facial growth
  - Airway obstruction by tonsils is also associated with **sleep apnea**
- Most common lesion of PMS is **squamous cell carcinoma (SCCa)**
- If not obviously SCCa, **differential diagnosis of PMS mass** relies heavily on normal PMS contents
  - From mucosa: SCCa
  - From lymphoid tissue: Non-Hodgkin lymphoma
  - From minor salivary glands: Minor salivary gland malignancies (uncommon)
  - From constrictor or levator palatini muscles: Rhabdomyosarcoma (rare)

GRAPHICS OF NORMAL AXIAL NASOPHARYNX AND PMS MASS

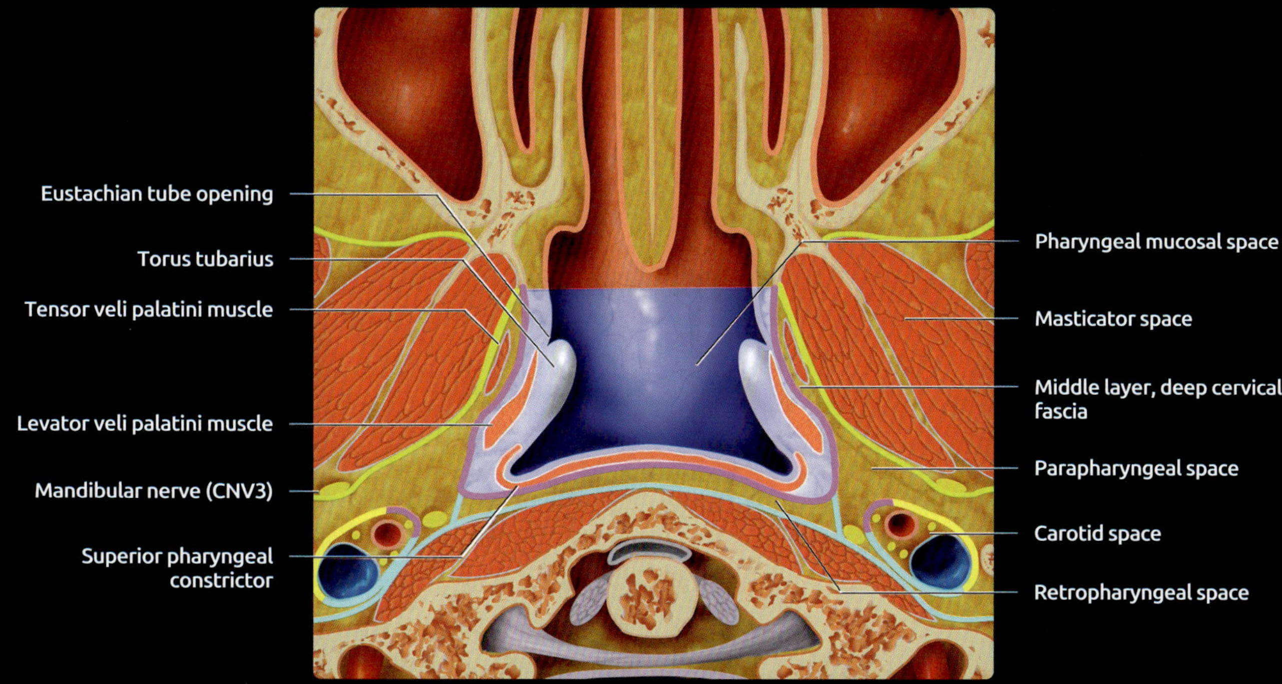

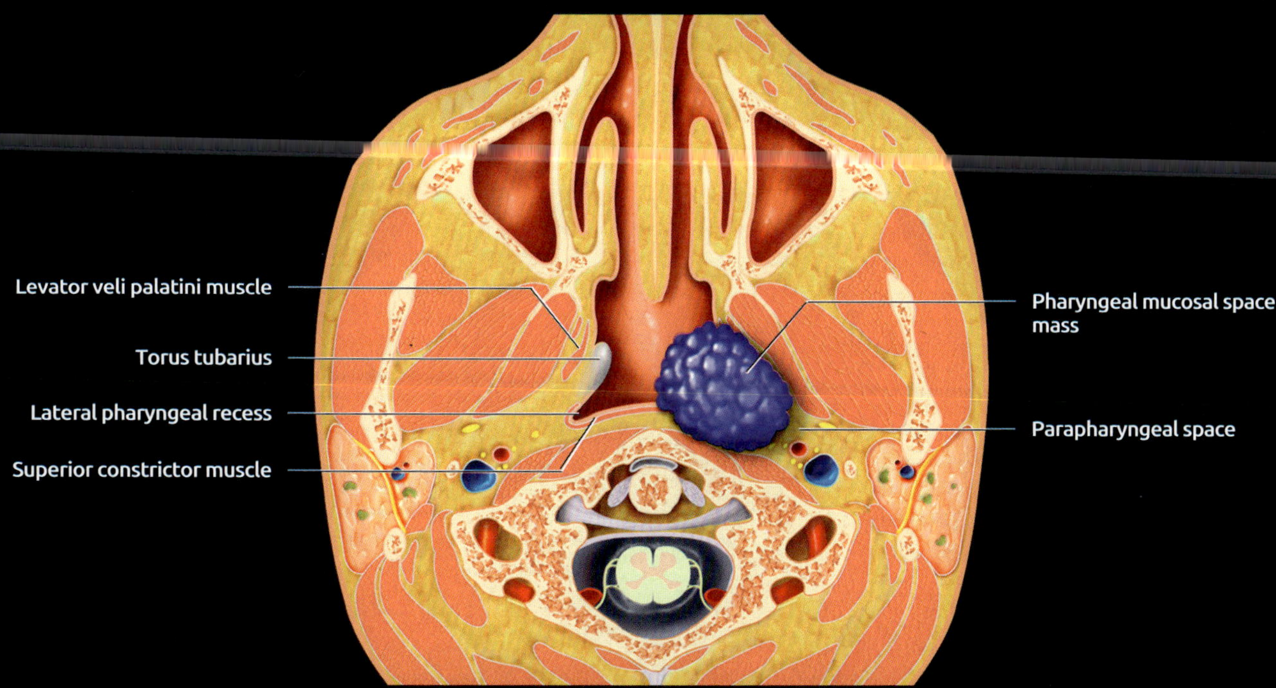

(Top) *Axial graphic of the nasopharyngeal mucosal space (in blue) shows the superior pharyngeal constrictor and levator veli palatini muscles are within the space. The middle layer of deep cervical fascia provides a deep margin to the space. The retropharyngeal space is behind and the parapharyngeal space is lateral to the pharyngeal mucosal space.* **(Bottom)** *Axial graphic of a generic pharyngeal mucosal space mass demonstrates the disruption of the normal architecture of the surface of the pharynx with bulging of the mass into the pharyngeal airway. Also notice the deep margin of the mass displacing the parapharyngeal space fat from medial to lateral.*

GRAPHICS OF SKULL BASE INTERACTIONS AND AXIAL OROPHARYNX

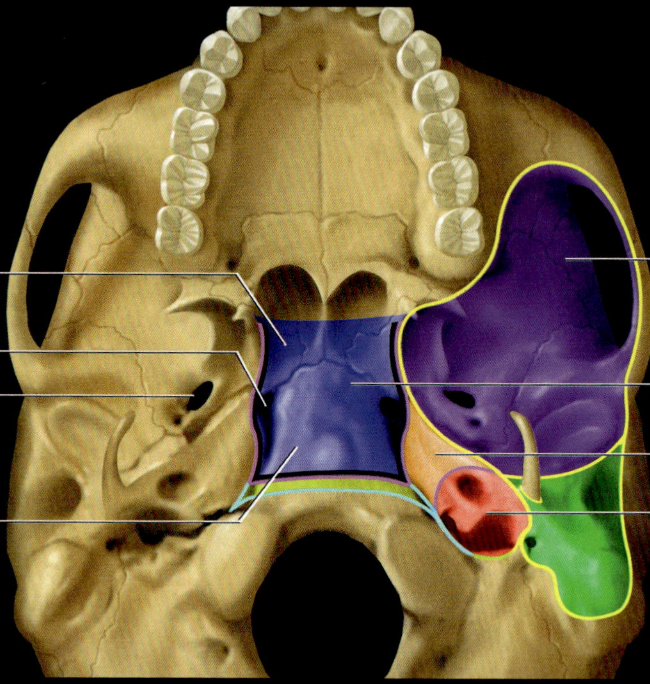

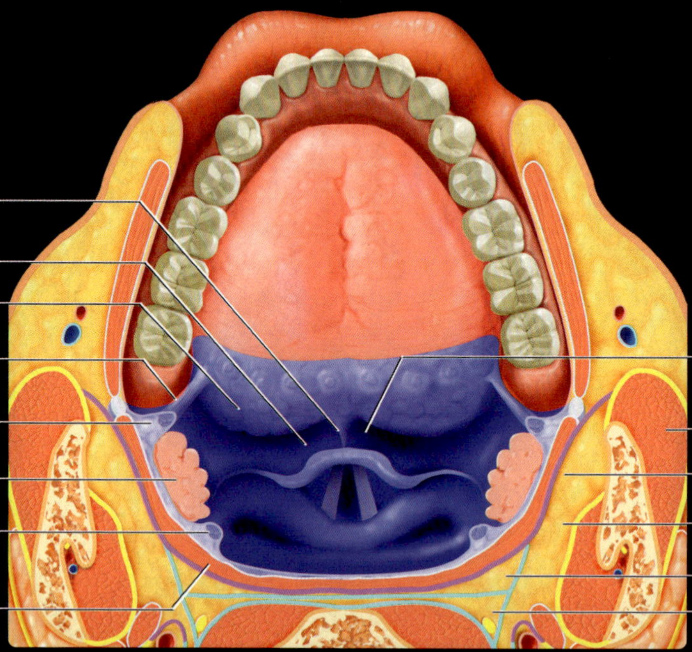

(Top) *Graphic of skull base from below shows spaces of suprahyoid neck relationships to the skull base with emphasis on the pharyngeal mucosal space. Notice the pharyngeal mucosal space abuts a broad area of the sphenoid and occipital bones. The foramen lacerum is within this abutment area. Malignant tumors of the nasopharyngeal mucosal space can access the intracranial compartment via the foramen lacerum.* **(Bottom)** *Axial graphic of the oropharyngeal mucosal space (in blue) viewed from above reveals that the superior pharyngeal constrictor, tonsillar pillars, and palatine and lingual tonsils are all occupants of this space. The middle layer of deep cervical fascia provides a deep margin to the space. The retropharyngeal space is behind, and the parapharyngeal space is lateral to the pharyngeal mucosal space.*

GRAPHICS OF CORONAL NASOPHARYNX AND OROPHARYNX

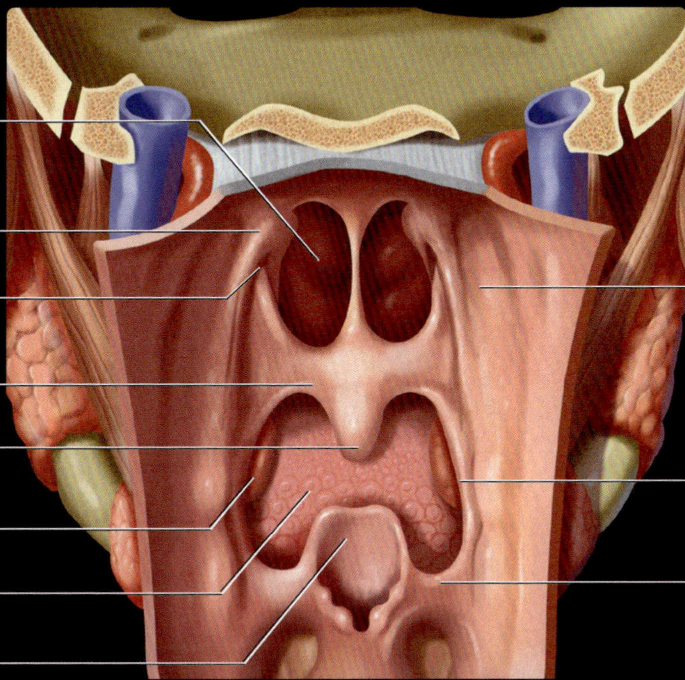

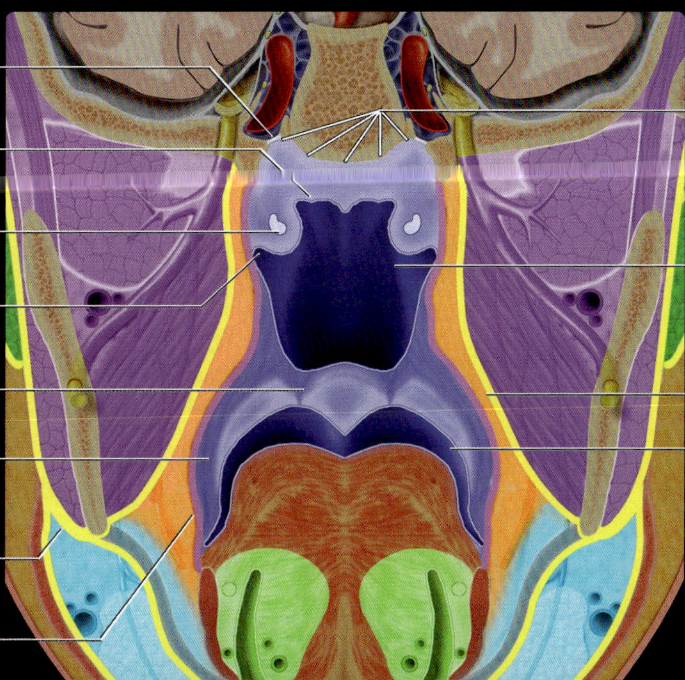

(Top) *Graphic of the pharyngeal mucosal space/surface seen from behind shows the nasopharyngeal and oropharyngeal areas. The lymphatic ring of the pharyngeal mucosal space contains the nasopharyngeal adenoids and the oropharyngeal palatine and lingual tonsils.* **(Bottom)** *Coronal graphic shows nasopharyngeal and oropharyngeal mucosal space. Notice the middle layer of deep cervical fascia defining the lateral margin of the pharyngeal mucosal space. The parapharyngeal spaces are paired fatty spaces lateral to the pharyngeal mucosal space.*

LATERAL CEPHALOMETRIC AND PANORAMIC OF NASOPHARYNX AND OROPHARYNX

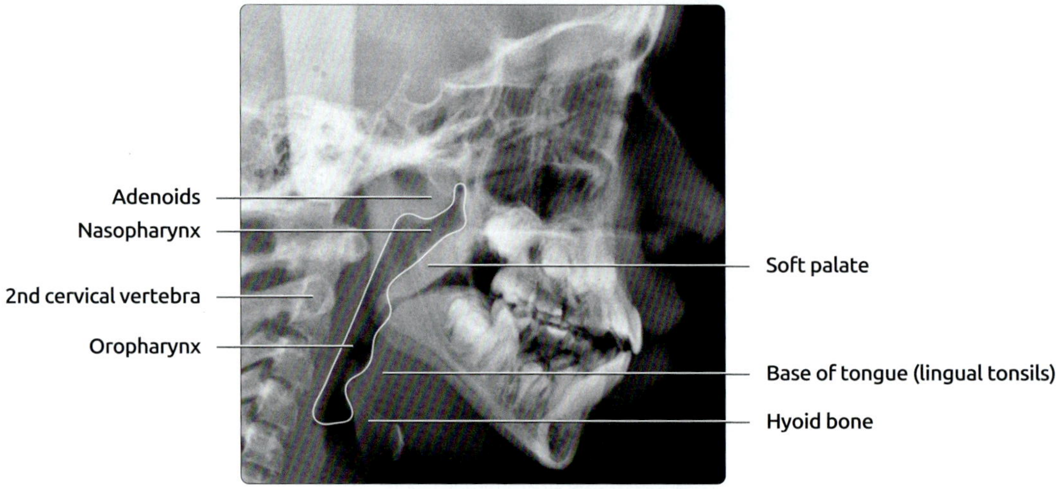

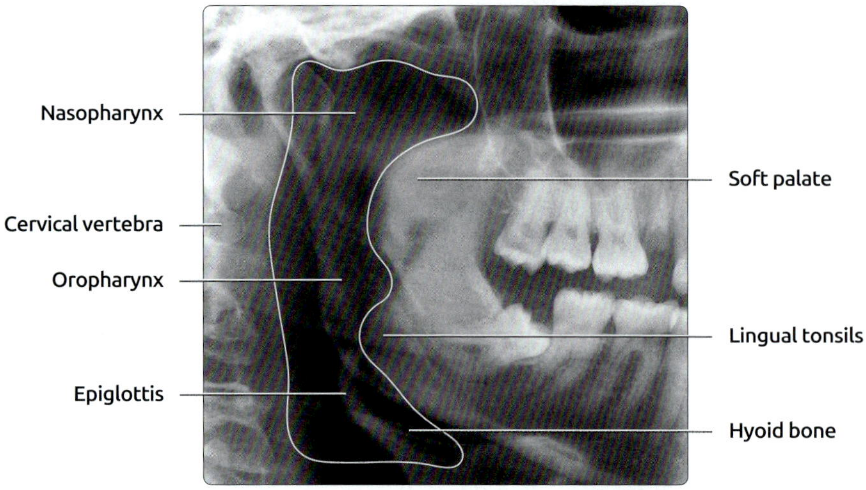

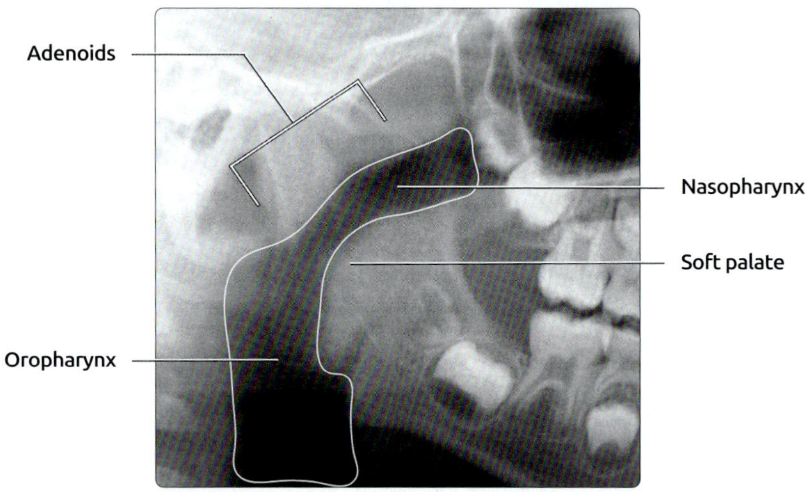

(Top) *The 1st of 3 images with the nasopharynx and oropharynx traced is shown. On this lateral cephalometric radiograph, the hyperplastic adenoids bulge into the nasopharynx. This is a normal anatomic feature in young patients but severe hyperplasia may limit nasal breathing.* **(Middle)** *Cropped panoramic radiograph shows visualization of the nasopharynx and oropharynx is analogous to the lateral view. The dark shadow created by these air-filled spaces is superimposed along the posterior borders of a panoramic radiograph and may obscure visualization of the mandible or mimic pathology. A rounded soft tissue bulge of the lingual tonsils is seen extending from the base of the tongue. The soft palate also creates a soft tissue shadow forming the anterior border of the nasopharynx.* **(Bottom)** *Cropped panoramic radiograph demonstrates the nasopharynx and oropharynx seen as a dark shadow superimposed over the posterior mandible. Decreased size of the nasopharyngeal air space due to hyperplasia of the adenoids can be appreciated in this child.*

CBCT OF NASOPHARYNX AND OROPHARYNX

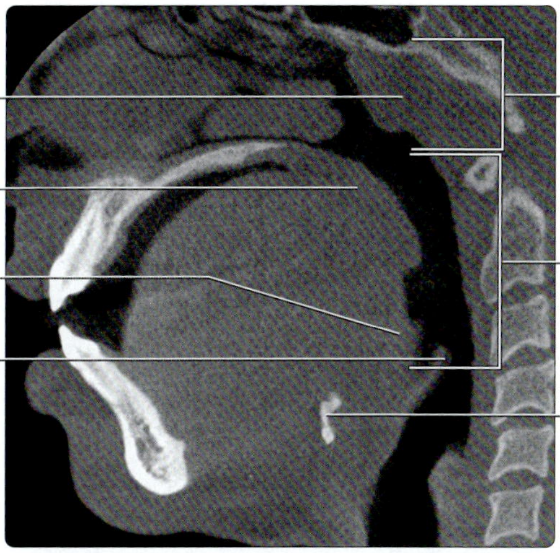

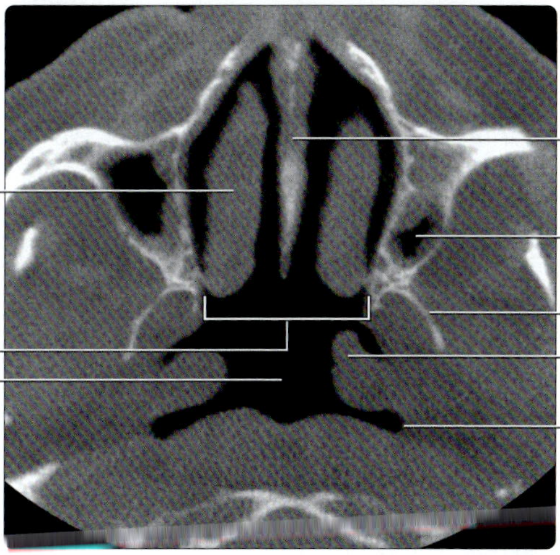

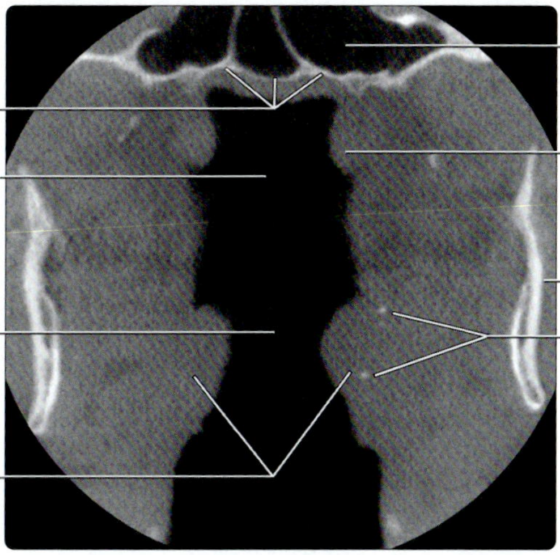

(Top) *This is the 1st of 3 images showing CBCT sections through the nasopharynx and oropharynx. The airway is well visualized in this modality, and abnormalities of the tissues surrounding the airway may compromise its patency. This sagittal image shows mild hyperplasia of the adenoids as a bulbous prominence in the posterior and superior nasopharyngeal wall.* **(Middle)** *Axial CBCT slice of the nasopharynx shows normal anatomic landmarks.* **(Bottom)** *Coronal CBCT slice of the nasopharynx and oropharynx shows enlargement of the palatine tonsils. Small radiopacities are seen in the left tonsil, consistent with tonsilloliths. These are a common incidental finding and represent dystrophic calcification within the tonsil crypts. Tonsilloliths may be associated with halitosis.*

NORMAL AXIAL AND CORONAL MR OF NASOPHARYNX AND OROPHARYNX

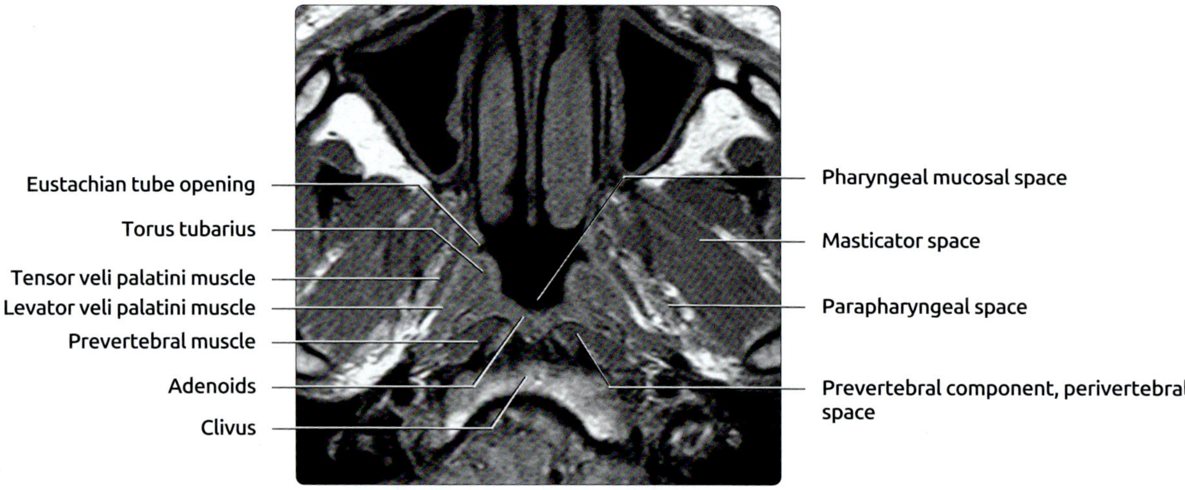

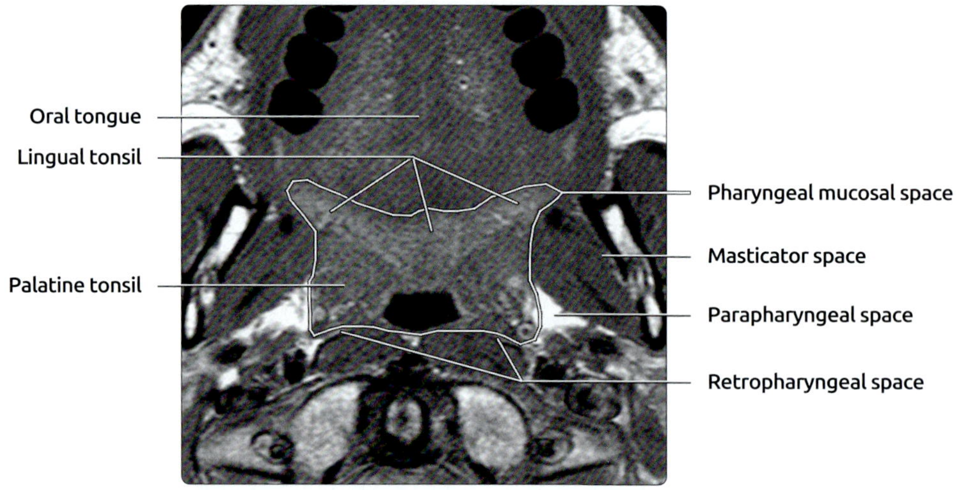

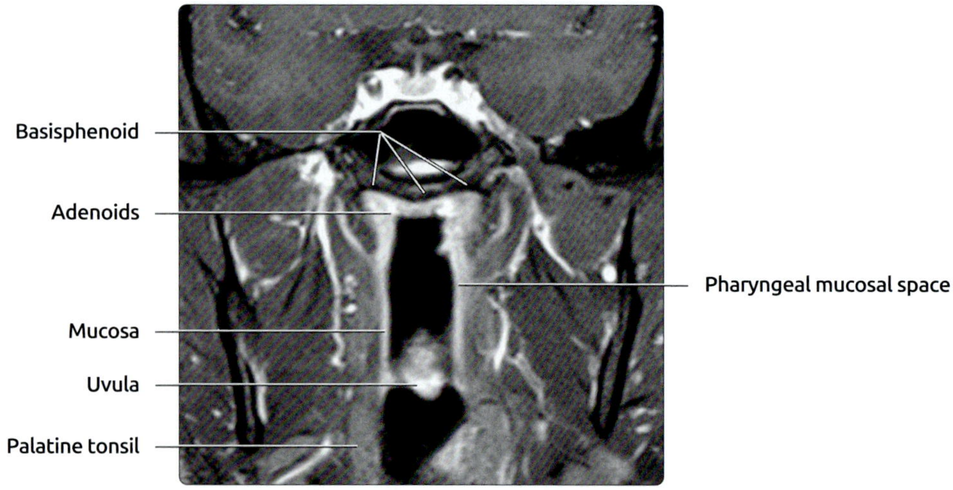

(Top) *Axial T1 unenhanced MR at the level of the nasopharynx shows the pharyngeal mucosal space. Notice the torus tubarius (distal cartilaginous eustachian tube) & nasopharyngeal adenoids. The lateral pharyngeal recess is collapsed & therefore not visible on imaging.* **(Middle)** *Axial T1 unenhanced MR through the mid oropharynx reveals the lingual and palatine tonsils of the pharyngeal mucosal space. Notice the Waldeyer lymphatic ring fills the pharyngeal mucosal space at the level of the oropharynx.* **(Bottom)** *Coronal enhanced fat-saturated T1 MR shows that the normal pharyngeal mucosal space surface enhances. Notice the roof of the nasopharyngeal mucosal space abuts the basisphenoid. Remember that a nasopharyngeal carcinoma that begins in the roof of the nasopharynx will often have invaded the sphenoid sinus at the time of presentation.*

CBCT AIRWAY ANALYSIS

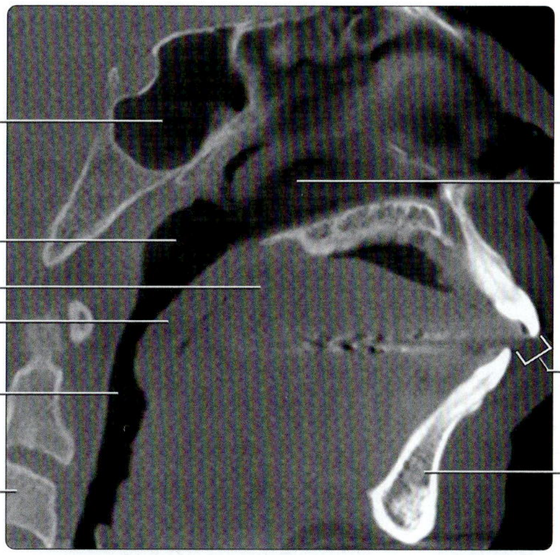

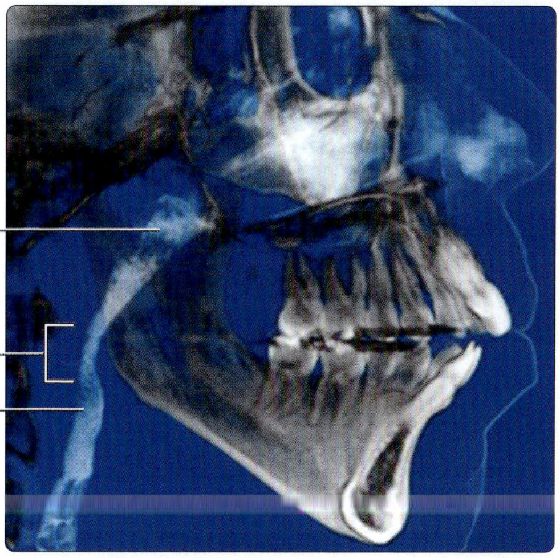

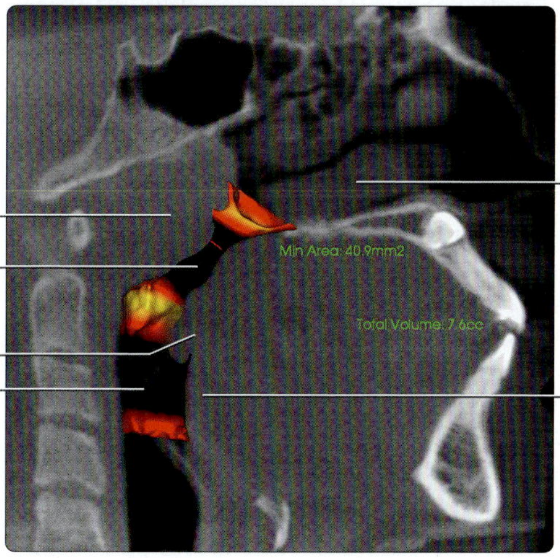

(Top) *This is the 1st of 2 images of a CBCT study demonstrating a restricted airway due to a retruded mandibular position. Arthritis of the temporomandibular joints has led to a downward and backward rotation of the mandible and an anterior open bite. As a result, the soft palate and tongue are displaced posteriorly, partially obstructing the upper airway.* **(Middle)** *3D CBCT reconstruction of the same patient shows the air passages in white. The narrowing of the pharynx is clearly visualized posterior to the angle of the mandible. The anterior open bite is also appreciated.* **(Bottom)** *Sagittal CBCT airway analysis shows enlarged adenoids and tonsils. Software programs can identify the location of and calculate the value of the minimum cross section area as well as determining the airway volume. These values are given in green text in this image. These can then be compared to average population values. Color-coding is used to help visualize areas of greatest restriction.*

TERMINOLOGY

Abbreviations

- Masticator space (MS)

Definitions

- Large, paired anterolateral spaces of suprahyoid neck (SHN) containing muscles of mastication, posterior body & ramus of mandible, & CNV3
- Surgical terms
  - Infratemporal fossa: MS area deep to zygomatic arch, superficial to pterygomaxillary fissure
  - Temporal fossa: Suprazygomatic MS

IMAGING ANATOMY

Overview

- MS is large SHN space spanning area from high parietal calvarium (suprazygomatic MS) above to mandibular angle below
- **Suprazygomatic MS**: Contains only belly of temporalis muscle
- **Infrazygomatic MS**: MS "proper," containing masseter, medial & lateral pterygoids, CNV3, & ramus/posterior body of mandible

Extent

- Craniocaudal extent of MS is more extensive than commonly recognized
- On its cephalad margin, MS reaches high on parietal calvarium at top of suprazygomatic MS

Anatomy Relationships

- Abuts skull base with **foramen ovale** & **foramen spinosum** included

Internal Contents

- **Muscles of mastication**
  - **Masseter**: Originates from zygomatic arch; inserts on lateral surface of ramus/angle of mandible
  - **Temporalis**: Originates from suprazygomatic MS; inserts on medial surface of coronoid process & anterior surface of mandibular ramus
  - **Medial pterygoid**: Originates from medial surface lateral pterygoid plate & palatine bone pyramidal process; inserts on medial surface mandibular ramus
  - **Lateral pterygoid**: Originates from greater wing of sphenoid (superior head) & lateral surface of lateral pterygoid plate (inferior head); inserts on capsule & articular disk of TMJ (superior head) & neck of mandible (inferior head)
- **Mandibular division, trigeminal nerve (V3)**
  - **Masticator nerve branch** (proximal V3 motor to muscles of mastication)
  - **Mylohyoid nerve branch** (motor to anterior belly of digastric & mylohyoid muscles)
  - **Inferior alveolar nerve branch** (V3 sensory to mandible & chin)
  - **Lingual nerve** (V3 sensory to anterior 2/3 tongue, floor of mouth)
  - **Auriculotemporal nerve** (V3 sensory to external auditory canal/TMJ)
- **Ramus and posterior body of mandible**
  - Coronoid process: Temporalis muscle inserts here
  - Condylar process: Mandibular condyle neck & head
  - Temporomandibular joint is within MS but considered separately
- **Pterygoid venous plexus** along posterior border of lateral pterygoid muscle & parapharyngeal space

Fascia of Masticator Space

- **Superficial layer, deep cervical fascia** (SL-DCF) splits along inferior mandible, creating "sling" enclosing MS
  - **Medial fascial slip** runs along deep surface of pterygoid muscles
    - This slip of SL-DCF inserts on undersurface of skull base, just medial to foramen ovale
  - **Lateral slip SL-DCF** covers surface of masseter muscle, attaching to zygomatic arch
    - Slip continues cephalad over surface of temporalis muscle to top of suprazygomatic MS
  - **No horizontal fascia** exists deep to zygomatic arch
    - MS lesions pass freely in cranial-caudal directions under zygomatic arch

ANATOMY IMAGING ISSUES

Questions

- What imaging features define lesion as primary to MS
  - Center of MS lesion must be in muscles of mastication-mandibular ramus
  - MS lesions displace parapharyngeal space from anterior to posterior

Imaging Recommendations

- CECT or MR can both easily image MS
- Enhanced multiplanar MR better for **perineural V3 spread** & intracranial disease manifestations
- If lesion affects skull base or mandible, add bone CT to delineate bony involvement & tumor matrix

Imaging Approaches

- When MS tumor is identified, imaging must include entire course of **CNV3** in search of perineural tumor
- Image distal to mental foramen of mandible & proximal to lateral pons, including mandibular foramen, foramen ovale, & Meckel cave

Imaging Pitfalls

- MS pseudolesions
  - Pterygoid venous plexus asymmetry may appear as infiltrating, enhancing "lesion"
  - V3 motor atrophy of muscles of mastication makes normal contralateral MS look like lesion
  - Asymmetric accessory parotid gland may appear as unilateral "mass" over surface of masseter muscle

CLINICAL IMPLICATIONS

Clinical Importance

- **Trismus** (jaw spasm from masticator muscle spasm) is primary symptom of MS tumor or infection
- Primary MS tumor is **sarcoma**
- Remember to look for perineural V3 tumor whenever MS mass is identified

NORMAL MASTICATOR SPACE; MASTICATOR SPACE MASS

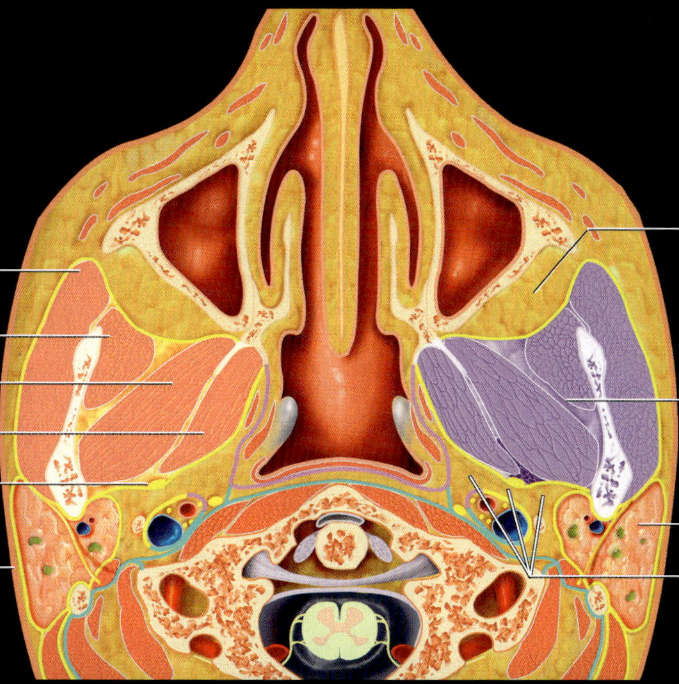

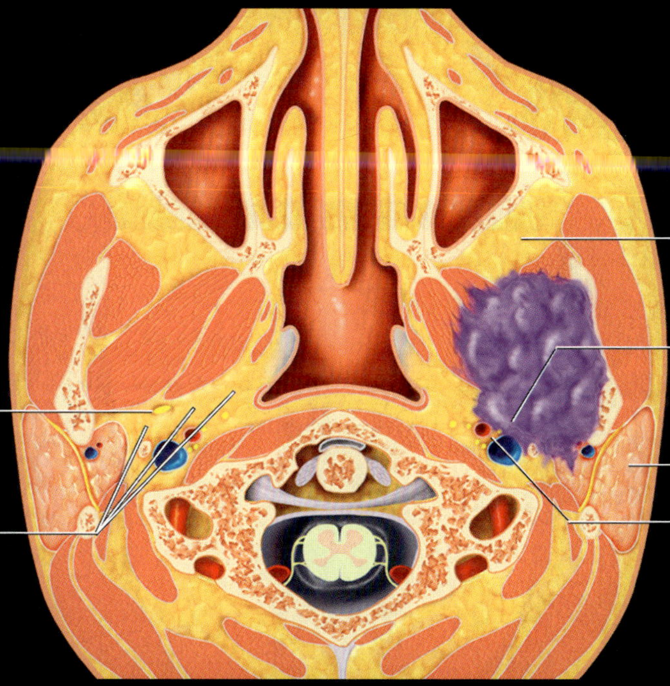

(Top) *Axial graphic shows the masticator space enclosed by the superficial layer of deep cervical fascia (yellow line). The muscles of mastication from medial to lateral are the medial and lateral pterygoid, temporalis, and masseter muscles. Note that the mandibular nerve (CNV3 main trunk) lies just posterior to medial pterygoid muscle inside the superficial layer of deep cervical fascia. The buccal space is anterior, while the parapharyngeal and parotid space are posterior to the masticator space.* **(Bottom)** *Axial graphic at the level of the low nasopharynx demonstrates a generic masticator space mass invading the parapharyngeal space from anterior to posterior. Notice the mandibular nerve is engulfed by the tumor. Masticator space masses invade the masticator muscles and erode the posterior body, ramus, or condylar process of the mandible.*

MASTICATOR SPACE SKULL BASE INTERACTIONS, CNV3, PERINEURAL TUMOR

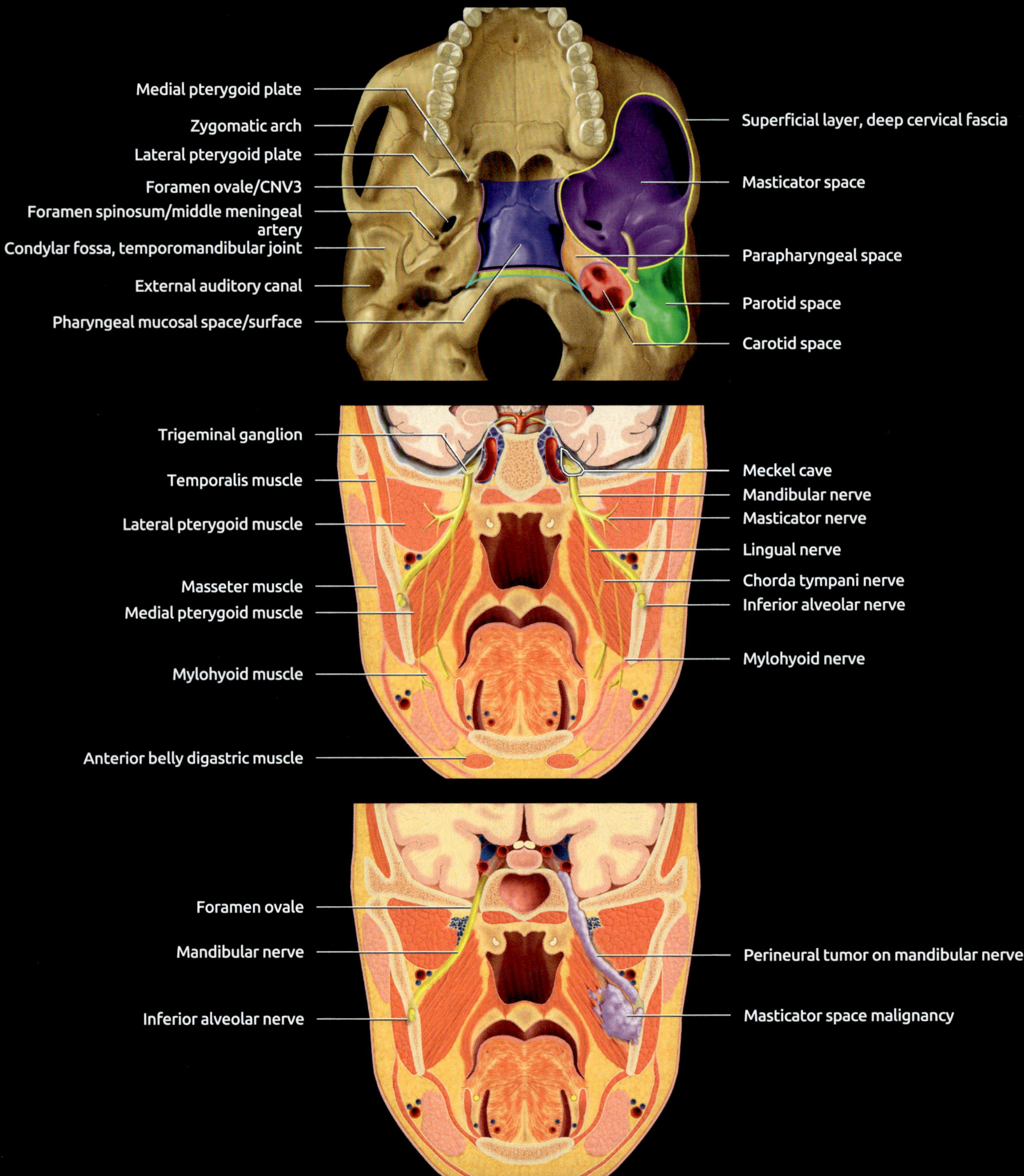

(Top) *Graphic of the skull base viewed from below shows the masticator space abutting the sphenoid and temporal bones. The masticator space (purple) has a broad abutment with the skull base. CNV3 enters the masticator space through the foramen ovale, while the foramen spinosum conveys the middle meningeal artery to the intracranial compartment. Note the temporomandibular joint is within the masticator space confines.* **(Middle)** *Coronal graphic shows mandibular division of the trigeminal nerve. Note CNV3 exits skull base without entering the cavernous sinus.* **(Bottom)** *Coronal graphic of the suprahyoid neck shows the masticator space and the mandibular nerve. In this drawing, a generic masticator space malignancy is visible invading the lower masticator space, invading the adjacent mandible, and spreading via a perineural route up the mandibular nerve through the foramen ovale into the intracranial compartment. Both primary masticator space malignancy and squamous cell carcinoma of the oral cavity can access the intracranial compartment in this manner.*

NORMAL AXIAL CECT OF MASTICATOR SPACE

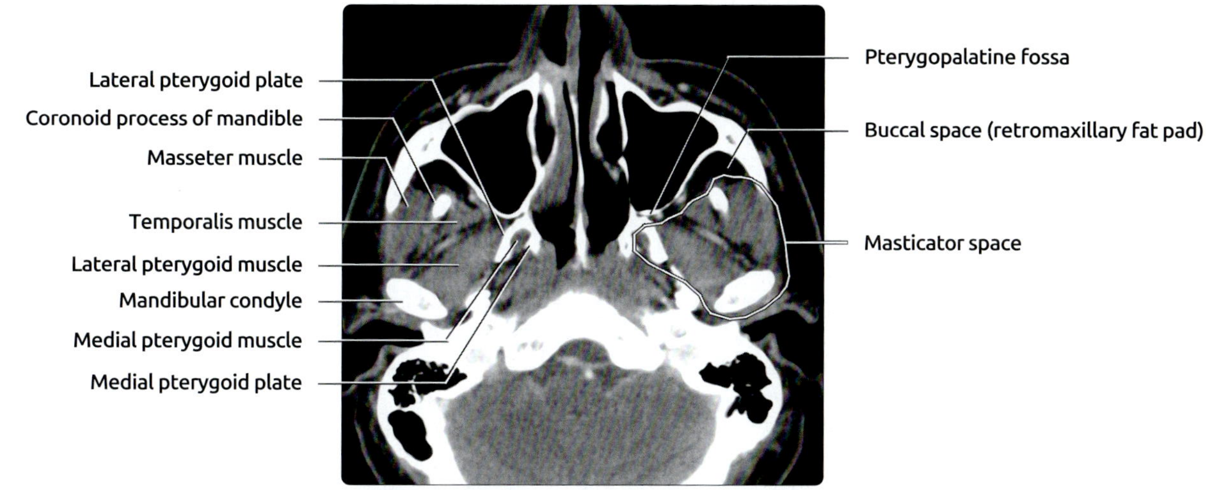

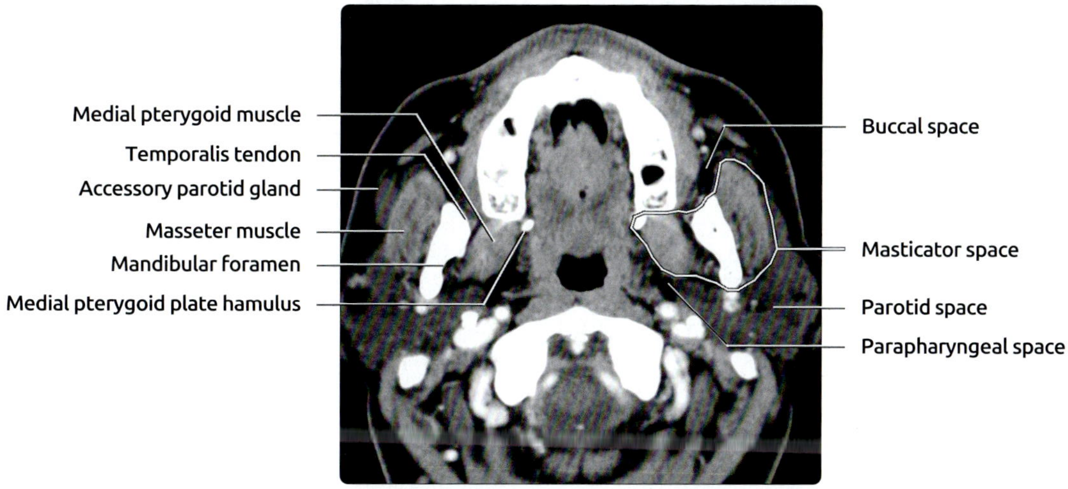

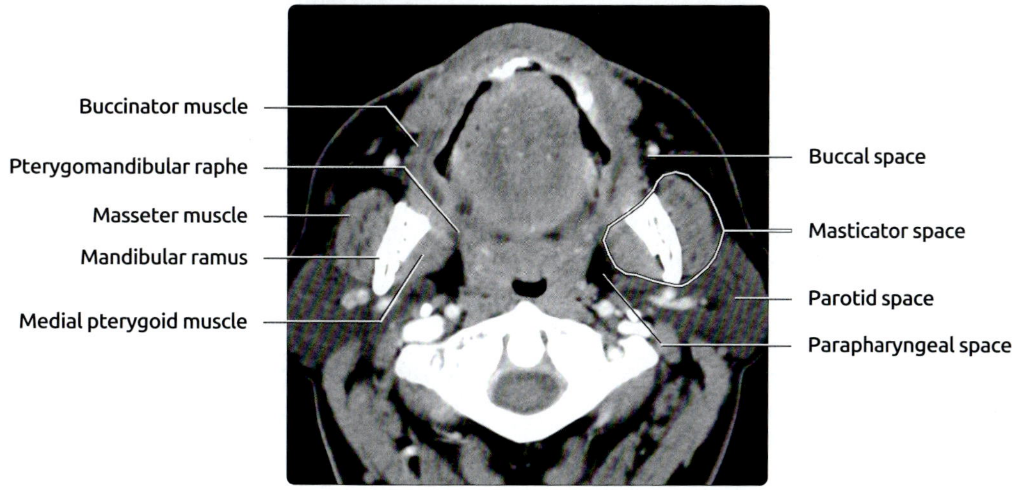

(Top) *This is the 1st of 3 axial CECT images of the masticator space. At the level of the mandibular condyles, the masticator space contains the muscles of mastication and temporomandibular joint. Note the inferior head of the lateral pterygoid muscle arising from the lateral surface of the lateral pterygoid plate. The medial pterygoid muscle arises from the medial surface of the lateral pterygoid plate.* **(Middle)** *In this axial CECT, through the maxillary alveolar process, the mandibular foramen is seen. The inferior alveolar nerve enters the mandible in this location. Note the hamulus of the medial pterygoid plate, which acts as a pulley for the tendon of the tensor veli palatini muscle and is the site of superior attachment of pterygomandibular raphe.* **(Bottom)** *In this axial CECT, the attachment of the medial pterygoid is visible along the medial ramus. Remember, the pterygomandibular raphe is the tendinous point of junction between the buccinator muscle and the superior constrictor muscle.*

TERMINOLOGY

Abbreviations

- Parotid space (PS)

Definitions

- Paired lateral suprahyoid neck spaces enclosed by superficial layer deep cervical fascia containing parotid glands, nodes, & extracranial facial nerve branches

IMAGING ANATOMY

Extent

- PS extends from external auditory canal (EAC) & mastoid tip superiorly to below angle of mandible (parotid tail)
  - Parotid tail inserts inferiorly between platysma & sternocleidomastoid muscles in area of posterior submandibular space

Anatomy Relationships

- Parapharyngeal space (PPS) is directly medial to PS
- Masticator space is anterior to PS
- Carotid space is separated from upper PS by posterior belly digastric muscle

Internal Contents

- **Parotid gland**
  - Superficial lobe represents ~ 2/3 of PS
  - Deep lobe projects into lateral PPS
- **Extracranial facial nerve (CNVII)**
  - Exits stylomastoid foramen as single trunk; ramifies within PS lateral to retromandibular vein
  - Ramifying intraparotid facial nerve creates surgical plane between superficial & deep lobes
  - Intraparotid facial nerve **not visible** with CT or MR except proximally with high-resolution 3T MR
- **External carotid artery**
  - Medial, smaller of 2 vessels seen just behind mandibular ramus in PS
- **Retromandibular vein**
  - Lateral, larger of 2 vessels seen just behind mandibular ramus in parotid
  - Intraparotid facial nerve branches course just lateral to retromandibular vein
- **Intraparotid lymph nodes**
  - ~ 20 lymph nodes found in each parotid gland
  - Parotid nodes are 1st-order drainage for EAC, pinna, & surrounding scalp
- **Parotid duct**
  - Emerges from anterior PS, runs along surface of masseter muscle
  - Duct then arches through buccal space to pierce buccinator muscle at level of upper 2nd molar
- **Accessory parotid glands**
  - Project over surface of masseter muscles
  - Present in ~ 20% of normal anatomic dissections

Fascia of Parotid Space

- Superficial layer of deep cervical fascia surrounds PS

ANATOMY IMAGING ISSUES

Questions

- What imaging features define **primary PS lesion**
  - Center of lesion is within parotid gland
  - If larger mass lesion of deep lobe, mass displaces PPS from lateral to medial with widening of stylomandibular gap

Imaging Recommendations

- CECT or MR can both readily image PS
- T1 C+ fat-saturated axial & coronal MR better for perineural CNVII spread

Imaging Approaches

- Small, superficial lobe PS lesions need no imaging
  - Needle aspiration to confirm benign mixed tumor with superficial parotidectomy sufficient
- If inflammation-infection of PS suspected, CECT best
  - Angle gantry to avoid dental amalgam & visualize parotid duct looking for cause of obstruction
  - 2- to 3-mm CT slice thickness recommended
- If tumor suspected, T1 C+ fat-saturated MR best
  - Look for perineural facial nerve tumor along intratemporal segments CNVII
  - Temporal bone CT helps define associated bony changes

Imaging Pitfalls

- Parotid gland becomes progressively more fatty with advancing age
  - Parotid glands appear similar to soft tissue in children
- Parotid tail mass must be identified as intraparotid or excision may injure facial nerve
  - Parotid tail area defined by superficial platysma, deep sternocleidomastoid & carotid spaces
- Facial nerve plane in parotid can only be estimated

CLINICAL IMPLICATIONS

Clinical Importance

- Intraparotid facial nerve, although invisible to imager, is key PS structure
- Try to assess relationship of mass lesion to estimated facial nerve plane (lateral to retromandibular vein)
  - Superficial, deep, or in plane of intraparotid CNVII?
  - Evidence of perineural tumor affecting CNVII?
- Parotid tumors: Benign mixed tumor (75%), Warthin tumor (5%), adenoid cystic carcinoma (5%), mucoepidermoid carcinoma (5%), other (10%)

EMBRYOLOGY

Embryologic Events

- PS undergoes **late encapsulation** in embryogenesis

Practical Implications

- Late encapsulation results in intraparotid lymph nodes
- Parotid nodes are 1st-order drainage for malignancies of adjacent scalp, EAC, & deep face

NORMAL PAROTID SPACE; DEEP LOBE MASS

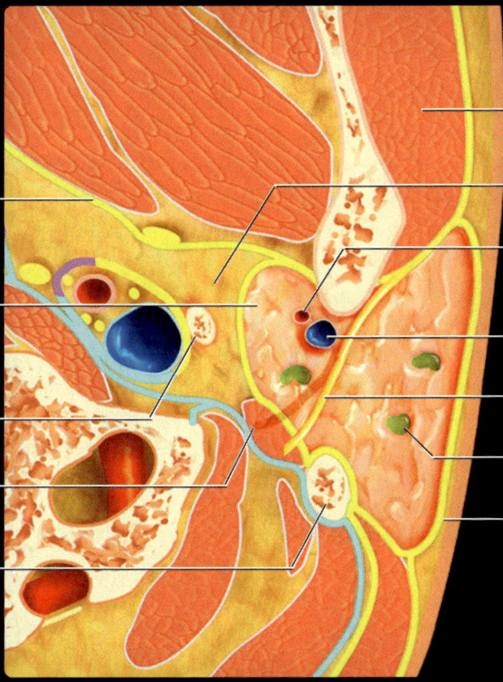

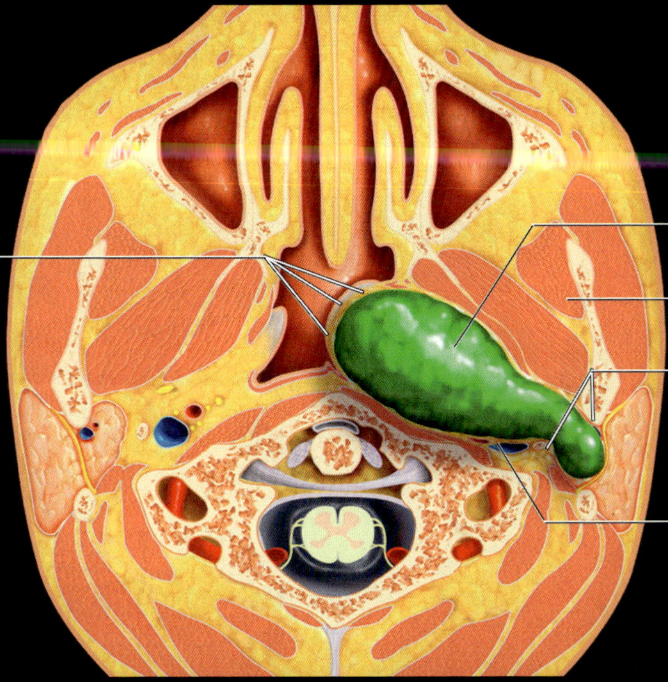

(Top) *Axial graphic of the parotid space (PS) at the level of C1 vertebral body shows the superficial layer of deep cervical fascia circumscribes the PS completely. The intraparotid facial nerve (CNVII) extends from just medial to the mastoid tip to a position just lateral to the retromandibular vein. The intraparotid CNVII divides the gland into deep and superficial lobes. Late embryologic encapsulation of the parotid gland accounts for the intraparotid lymph nodes, which serve as 1st-order drainage for malignancies of the deep face, scalp, and external ear. The normal PS contains ~ 20 nodes. The distal external carotid artery and retromandibular vein are also intraparotid.* **(Bottom)** *Axial graphic of generic deep lobe of parotid gland mass demonstrates medial displacement of the parapharyngeal space fat. Notice also the slight enlargement of the stylomandibular gap. Smaller lesions of the superficial lobe of the parotid gland are easily identified as intraparotid. Larger deep lobe lesions may be more difficult to identify as PS in origin.*

PAROTID SPACE: SKULL BASE INTERACTION, FACIAL NERVE, PERINEURAL TUMOR

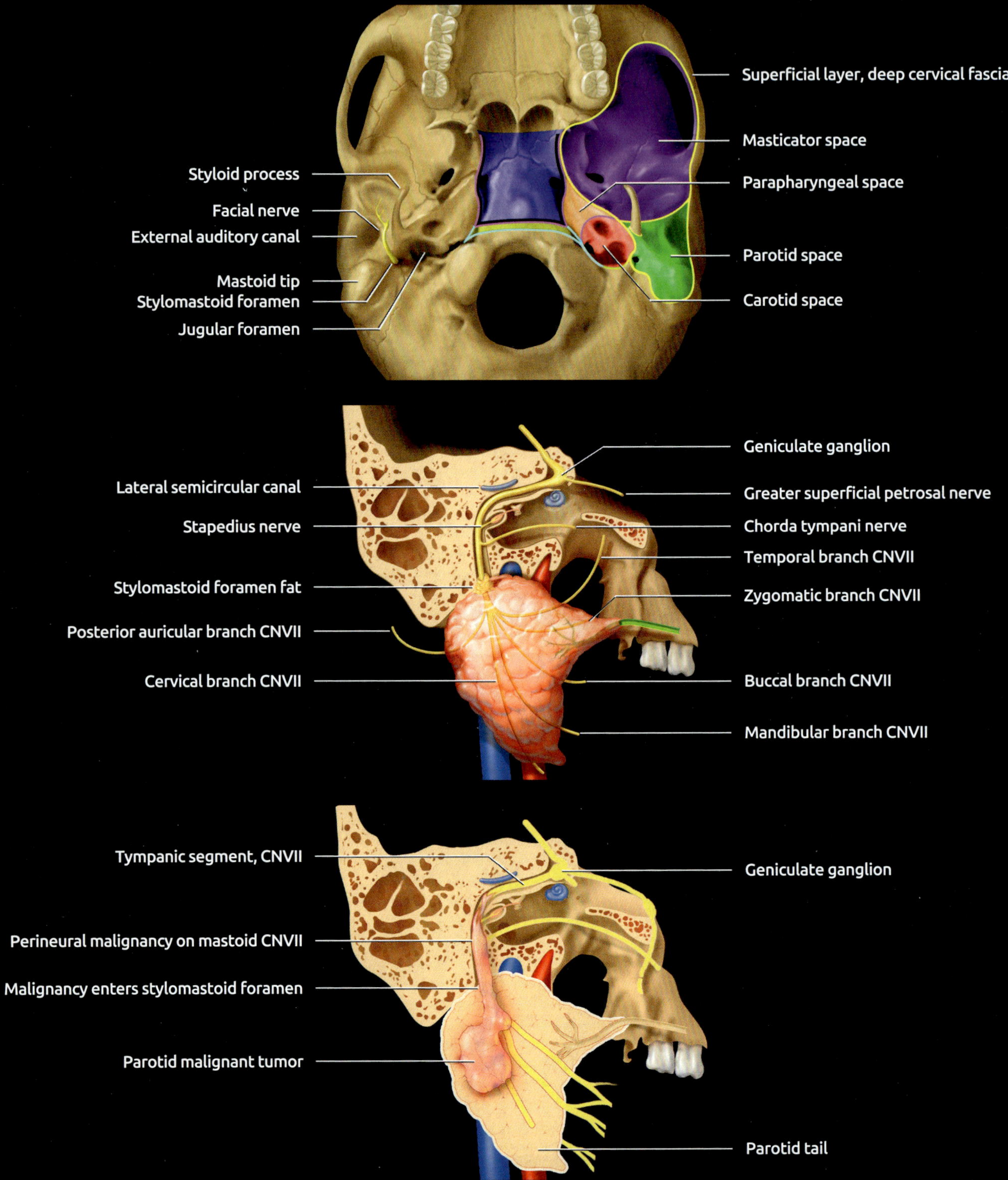

(Top) *Axial graphic of the skull base viewed from below illustrates the interaction between the PS and skull base. CNVII exits through the stylomastoid foramen, just posterior to the styloid process and lateral to the jugular foramen. The PS is the most lateral space in the nasopharyngeal and oropharyngeal area, extending from the external auditory canal above to the level of the mandibular angle below.* **(Middle)** *Sagittal graphic shows the parotid gland and CNVII. CNVII exits the skull base at the stylomastoid foramen, then enters the PS where it has 6 major branches. The plane of the facial nerve branches within the parotid gland defines the superficial and deep lobe of the parotid surgically but not radiographically.* **(Bottom)** *Sagittal graphic shows a parotid malignancy affecting intraparotid CNVII. The tumor spreads along CNVII through the stylomastoid foramen to the proximal mastoid segment within the temporal bone. If left untreated, perineural tumor will access the intracranial compartment via the internal auditory canal.*

NORMAL AXIAL PAROTID SPACE CECT

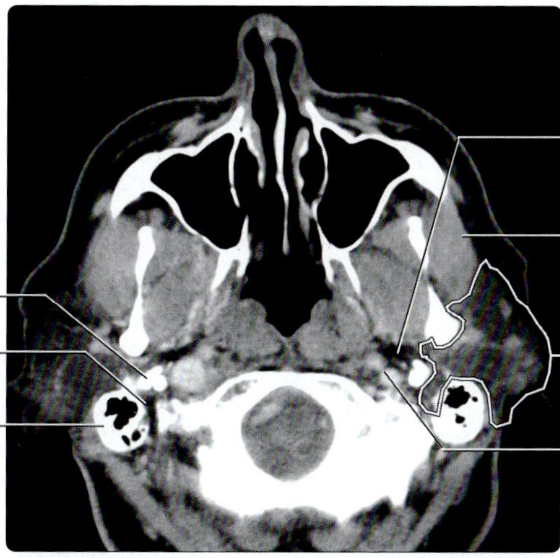

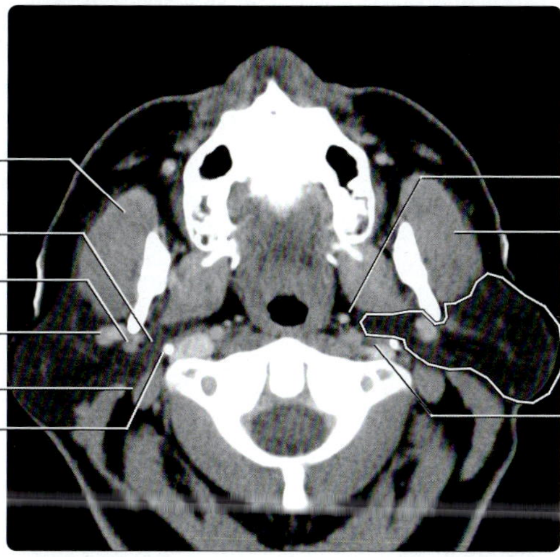

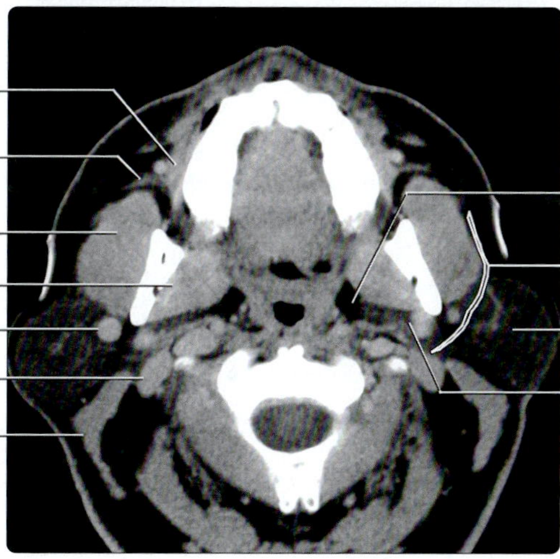

(Top) *First of 3 axial CECT images (presented superior to inferior) shows the right stylomastoid foramen with low-attenuation fat contained within. The facial nerve is not visualized on CT images unless diseased. If a perineural tumor is present, stylomastoid foramen fat will be replaced by tumor.* **(Middle)** *In this axial CECT, the deep lobe of the parotid gland can be seen projecting through the stylomandibular gap to abut the parapharyngeal space. Note the medial external carotid artery and more lateral retromandibular vein. Remember the facial nerve plane passes just lateral to the retromandibular vein but cannot be seen.* **(Bottom)** *In this axial CECT, the parotid duct is seen piercing the buccinator muscle just lateral to the 2nd maxillary molar. The projected course of the extracranial CNVII lateral to the retromandibular vein and over the surface of the masseter muscle is drawn. Note the large size of the superficial lobe compared to the deep lobe of the parotid.*

TERMINOLOGY

Abbreviations

- Carotid space (CS)
- Suprahyoid neck (SHN) and infrahyoid neck (IHN)

Definitions

- Paired tubular spaces surrounded by carotid sheath that contain carotid arteries, internal jugular veins (IJVs), **cranial nerves (CN) IX-XII (SHN) and CNX (IHN)**

IMAGING ANATOMY

Overview

- CS travels from inferior margins of jugular foramen-carotid canal above to aortic arch below
- SHN CS contains CNIX-XII, internal carotid artery (ICA), and IJV
- IHN CS contains CNX only, common carotid artery (CCA), IJV
  - Internal jugular nodal chain is closely associated with CS outer fascial layers

Extent

- CS defined from skull base (carotid canal and jugular foramen) to aortic arch below
- CS can be divided into its major segments
  - Nasopharyngeal, oropharyngeal, cervical, and mediastinal segments

Anatomy Relationships

- **SHN CS adjacent spaces**
  - Retropharyngeal space (RPS) medial
  - Perivertebral space posterior
  - Parotid space lateral
  - Parapharyngeal space (PPS) anterior
- **IHN CS adjacent spaces**
  - Visceral space and RPS medial
  - Perivertebral space posterior
  - Anterior cervical space anterior
  - Posterior cervical space lateral

Internal Contents

- **SHN CS**
  - **ICA**
  - **IJV**
  - **CNIX-XII in nasopharyngeal CS**
  - Only CNX remains in CS from oropharyngeal CS inferiorly
  - CNX located in posterior notch formed by ICA and IJV
  - **Sympathetic plexus** between medial CS and lateral RPS
- **IHN CS**
  - **CCA**
  - **IJV**
  - **Vagus nerve**
  - Internal jugular nodal chain closely associated but **not** in CS from midoropharynx to clavicle

Fascia of Carotid Space

- **Carotid sheath** made from components of **all 3 layers of deep cervical fascia**
  - Suprahyoid CS: Carotid sheath incomplete or less substantial
  - Infrahyoid CS: Carotid sheath well defined, tenacious fascia

ANATOMY IMAGING ISSUES

Questions

- What imaging features define lesion as primary to CS
  - **Lesion in SHN CS**
    - Center of lesion is within area of ICA-IJV, posterior to PPS
    - Lesion displaces PPS fat **anteriorly**
    - Pushes posterior belly of digastric muscle laterally
    - If in nasopharyngeal CS, pushes styloid process anterolaterally
    - If in oropharyngeal CS, pushes posterior belly of digastric anterolateral
    - When mass begins in posterior SHN CS (vagal schwannoma, neurofibroma, paraganglioma), ICA is pushed anteriorly as mass enlarges
  - **Lesion in IHN CS**
    - May engulf CCA and IJV or push them apart
    - May splay external carotid artery and ICA (carotid body paraganglioma)
- What are statistically common lesions found in CS
  - Paraganglioma, schwannoma, IJV thrombosis, and carotid artery dissection/pseudoaneurysm

Imaging Recommendations

- Either CECT or MR can easily identify normal CS anatomy and CS lesions
- If using MR, remember to acquire unenhanced T1 (to look for high-velocity flow voids of paraganglioma)
- MRA and MRV may be helpful in defining normal and diseased vessels of CS (ICA dissection, pseudoaneurysm, IJV thrombosis)

Imaging Approaches

- Remember that CS runs from jugular foramen-carotid canal of skull base above to aortic arch below
- If imaging CS because of **left** vagal neuropathy, must reach aortopulmonic window inferiorly

Imaging Pitfalls

- Normal vascular flow phenomenon of IJV may mimic schwannoma or thrombosis

CLINICAL IMPLICATIONS

Clinical Importance

- **CNIX-XII** and **carotid artery** are vital structures in CS

Function Dysfunction

- **Injury to nasopharyngeal CS** may result in complex cranial neuropathy involving some combination of **CNIX-XII**
- **Vagus nerve injury**: Vocal cord paralysis
- Carotid artery proximity to internal jugular nodal chain makes injury from squamous cell carcinoma extranodal tumor likely

SUPRAHYOID NECK; CAROTID SPACE

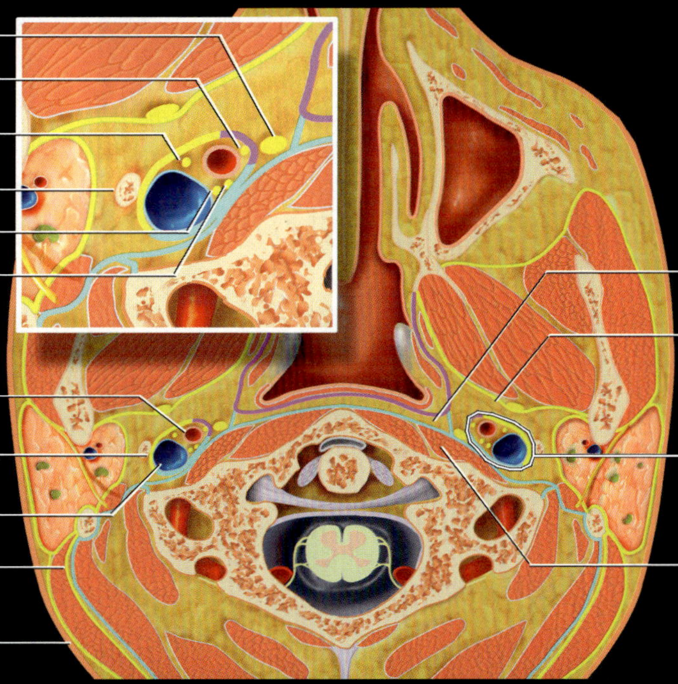

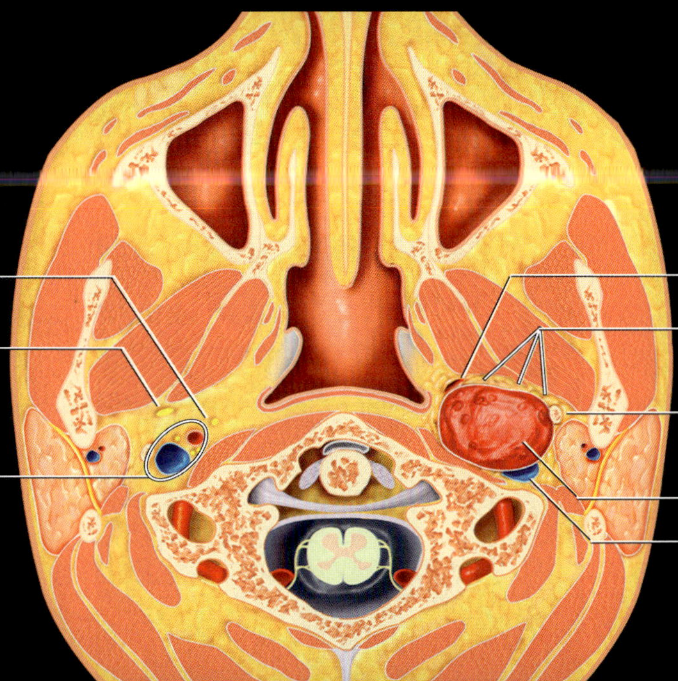

(Top) *Axial graphic shows the suprahyoid neck at the level of C1 vertebral body with insert showing the magnified carotid space (CS). The suprahyoid CS contains CNIX-XII, the internal carotid artery, and the internal jugular vein. The carotid sheath is made up of components of all 3 layers of deep cervical fascia (tricolor line around the CS). In the suprahyoid neck, the carotid sheath is less substantial than in the infrahyoid neck. The sympathetic trunk runs just medial to the CS. Remember that glomus bodies are also normally found in the CS at the carotid bifurcation and nodose ganglion of the vagus nerve.* **(Bottom)** *Axial graphic shows a generic CS mass. A CS mass displaces the parapharyngeal space fat anteriorly as well as lifts the styloid process anterolaterally. Notice that the internal carotid in this example is displaced anteromedially, while the internal jugular vein is displaced posterolaterally. Only a CS lesion could create this displacement pattern.*

CAROTID SPACE SKULL BASE, ANGIOGRAPHY, CT VENOGRAPHY

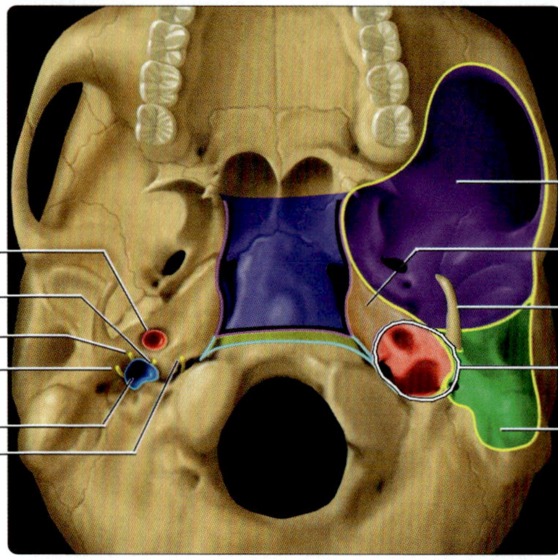

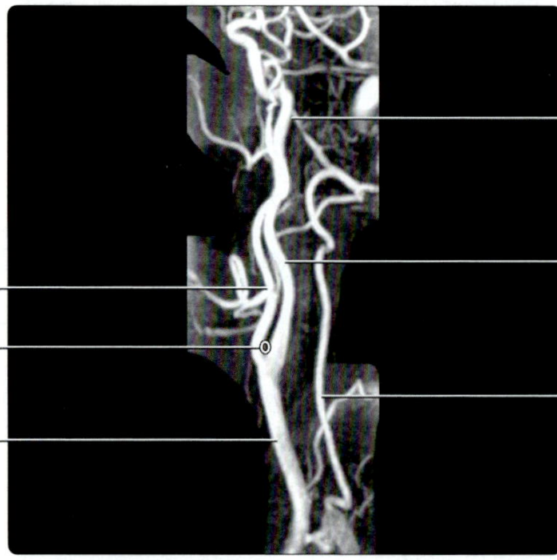

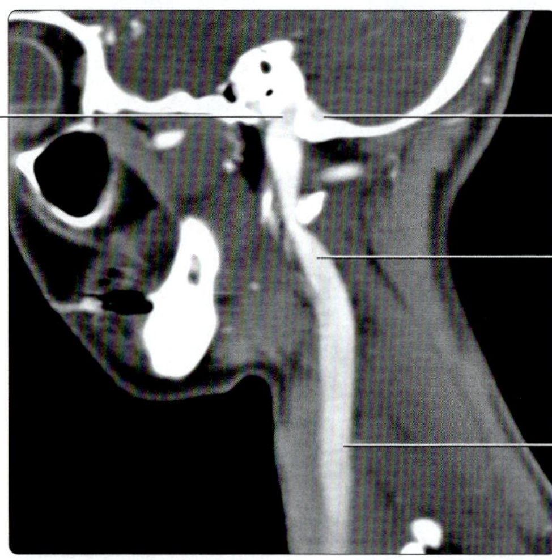

(Top) *Axial graphic shows the skull base viewed from below, illustrating the interaction between the CS and the skull base. The nasopharyngeal CS is the inferior continuation of the carotid canal, jugular foramen, and hypoglossal canal. The internal carotid artery, internal jugular vein, and CNIX-XII are found within the CS. The carotid sheath is depicted as a tricolor line because it is formed from all 3 layers of deep cervical fascia.* **(Middle)** *Lateral view of an extracranial MRA shows the carotid artery from the arch below to the supraclinoid area above. Remember that the carotid artery extends in the CS throughout this entire extracranial H&N. Note the location of the carotid body in the carotid bifurcation; carotid body paraganglioma occurs here.* **(Bottom)** *Sagittal reformation of CECT of the extracranial H&N shows the internal jugular vein from its emergence from the jugular foramen above to the clavicle level below. Glomus jugulare paraganglioma can spread into the nasopharyngeal CS via the internal jugular vein lumen.*

SUPRAHYOID CAROTID SPACE ON CECT

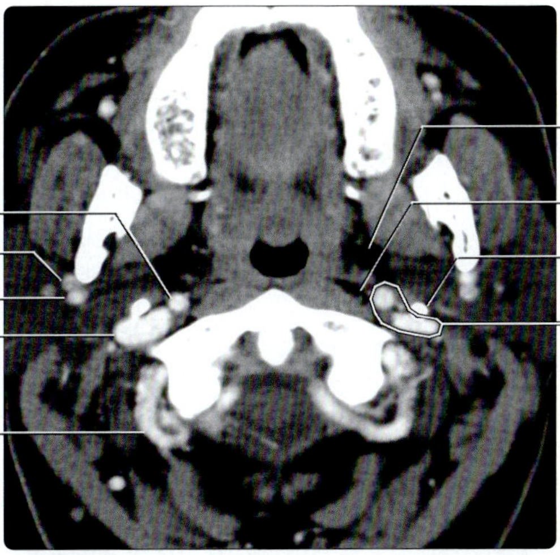

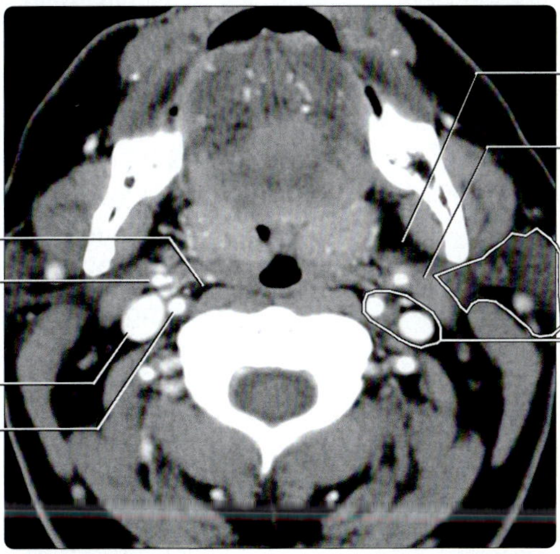

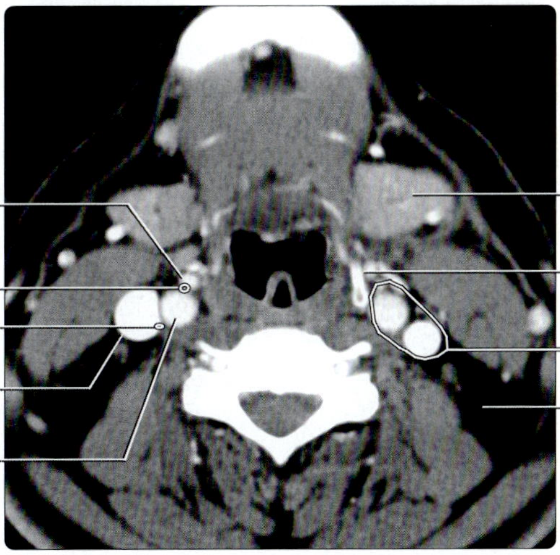

(Top) *First of 3 axial CECT images (presented from superior to inferior) shows that at the level of C1 vertebral body, the nasopharyngeal CS contains the internal carotid artery, internal jugular vein, and CNIX-XII. Notice that the CS is posterior to the styloid process. At the level of the nasopharynx, a CS mass will push from posterior to anterior into the parapharyngeal space and displace the styloid process anterolaterally.* **(Middle)** *In this CECT at the level of the midoropharynx, the posterior belly of the digastric muscle is visible anterolateral to the CS, dividing the CS from the parotid space. A CS mass here would push this muscle anterolaterally and the parapharyngeal space anteriorly.* **(Bottom)** *At the level of the hyoid bone, the common carotid artery and carotid bifurcation can be seen. At this level, only the vagus nerve is left within the CS. The normal carotid body and vagus nerve locations have been marked on the patient's right.*

TERMINOLOGY

Abbreviations

- Retropharyngeal space (RPS)

Definitions

- Midline space just posterior to pharynx & cervical esophagus running from skull base to T3 vertebral level in mediastinum

IMAGING ANATOMY

Overview

- RPS is fat-filled space in posterior midline of neck that can be identified on imaging from skull base to upper mediastinum
- Uppermost RPS (nasopharyngeal portion) is "tight"
  - In RPS abscess, path of least resistance is inferiorly
- **RPS nodes only found in suprahyoid neck (SHN) RPS**

Extent

- Skull base to T3 vertebral body level in upper mediastinum

Anatomy Relationships

- **SHN RPS**
  - Pharyngeal mucosal space (PMS) is anterior
  - Danger space (DS) is directly posterior to RPS
  - Carotid space (CS) is lateral to RPS
- **Infrahyoid neck (IHN) RPS**
  - Hypopharynx & cervical esophagus are anterior
  - DS is directly posterior to RPS
    - RPS empties via "fascial trap door" into DS inferiorly at ~ T3 level
  - CS is lateral to RPS

Internal Contents

- **SHN RPS** (skull base to hyoid bone)
  - Fat is primary occupant of SHN RPS
  - **RPS lymph nodes**
    - **Lateral group**: Also called nodes of Rouvière
    - **Medial group**: Less often visible on imaging
- **IHN RPS** (hyoid bone to T3 vertebral body in mediastinum)
  - **Fat only** in IHN RPS
  - No RPS nodes below hyoid bone

Fascia of Retropharyngeal Space

- RPS has complex fascial margins
- Anterior wall fascia: Middle layer, deep cervical fascia
  - Fascia is just behind constrictor muscle of PMS
- Posterior wall fascia: Deep layer, deep cervical fascia
  - Fascia is just anterior to prevertebral muscles of perivertebral space
  - 2 slips present with DS between
- Lateral fascial wall: Slip of deep layer, deep cervical fascia called **alar fascia**
- **Median raphe** divides RPS into 2 halves
  - Relatively weak fascial slip that is present more consistently in superior RPS

ANATOMY IMAGING ISSUES

Questions

- What radiologic findings define lesion as primary to RPS
  - **Unilateral-nodal SHN mass**
    - Centered posteromedial to parapharyngeal space (PPS) & directly medial to CS
    - Encroaches on PPS from posteromedial to anterolateral (mimics CS mass)
  - **"Extranodal" mass in SHN or IHN** (pus or tumor filling RPS)
    - Rectangular-shaped mass centered behind PMS
    - Mass anterior to prevertebral muscles
    - Mass flattens & remains anterior to prevertebral muscles as it enlarges
    - Contrast with perivertebral space mass, which elevates prevertebral muscles as it enlarges
- **SHN RPS lesion imaging appearances**
  - Lesion begins most commonly in RPS nodes
  - Seen on CT or MR as unilateral RPS mass
  - If extranodal disease (edema, infection, or tumor), will fill RPS from side to side
- **IHN RPS lesion imaging appearances**
  - Originates in SHN RPS, spreads inferiorly into IHN
  - Fills entire IHN RPS from side to side
  - Remember to look at SHN RPS if you find IHN RPS disease

Imaging Approaches

- **CECT best** imaging tool in evaluation of **RPS infection**
- **MR imaging** far more sensitive to presence of **RPS tumor adenopathy**

Imaging Pitfalls

- RPS & DS are indistinguishable on CT or MR imaging
  - Best to consider DS as conduit for RPS disease into mediastinum only
    - Otherwise, describe lesions in RPS only & ignore DS from imaging perspective
- Lateral RPS nodal mass may mimic CS mass
  - Look for mass medial to CS
  - Mass displacement of CS is posterolaterally
  - Both RPS & CS displace PPS anteriorly
- Not all fluid in RPS is abscess
  - Internal jugular vein thrombosis & longus colli tendonitis can both cause RPS edema
  - Nonabscess fluid: No enhancement of wall; minimal mass effect

CLINICAL IMPLICATIONS

Clinical Importance

- RPS nodes are seeded by pharyngitis
  - Once seeded they react, suppurate, & eventually rupture to create RPS abscess
- Squamous cell carcinoma of nasopharynx & posterior wall of oropharynx & hypopharynx drain into RPS nodal chain

NORMAL RETROPHARYNGEAL SPACE; RETROPHARYNGEAL SPACE MASS

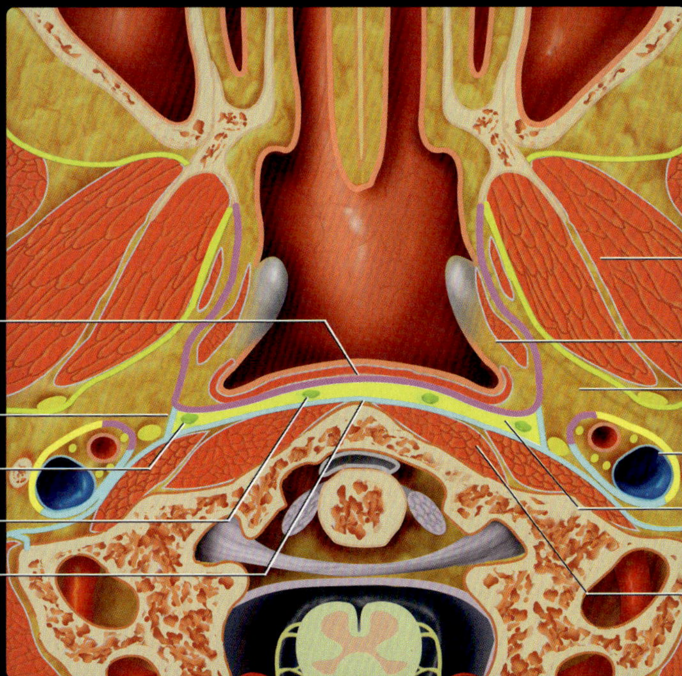

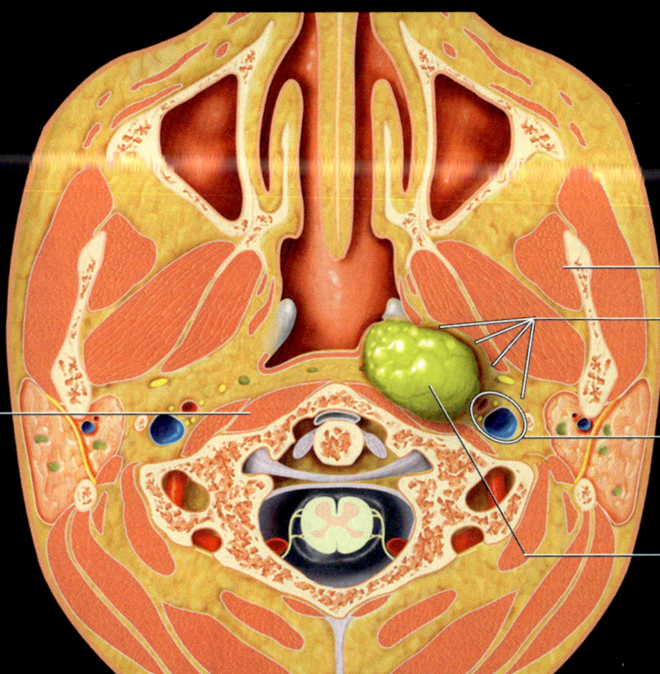

(Top) *Axial graphic shows that the retropharyngeal space (RPS) in the suprahyoid neck has medial and lateral retropharyngeal nodes. Notice that the middle layer of deep cervical fascia is the anterior border of the RPS, while the deep layer of deep cervical fascia is the posterior border. The lateral wall is a slip of the deep layer called the alar fascia.* **(Bottom)** *Axial graphic depicts a generic mass beginning in the lateral retropharyngeal nodal group of the suprahyoid RPS. Notice that the lateral RPS mass displaces the carotid space posterolaterally and the parapharyngeal space anteriorly. This mass lesion can be mistaken for a carotid space mass if the imager is not cognizant of its more medial location.*

RETROPHARYNGEAL SPACE: SKULL BASE GRAPHIC; SAGITTAL RPS GRAPHIC

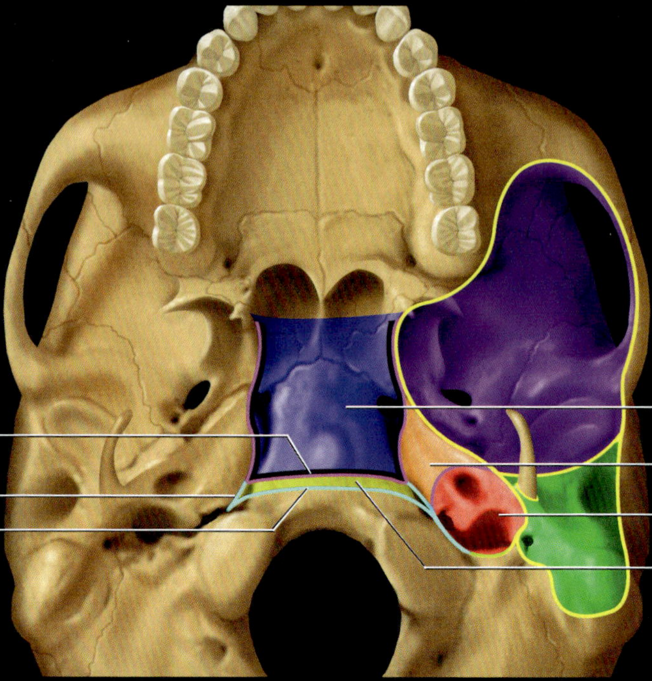

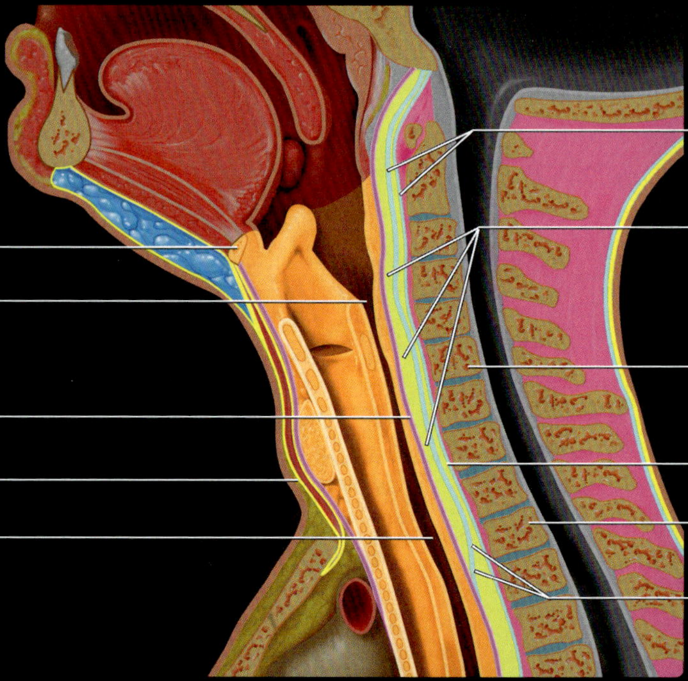

(Top) *Axial graphic of the skull base from below shows the abutment of the RPS with the skull base. Notice that the RPS abuts the external surface of the basiocciput in an area where there are no critical structures (nerves or arteries).* **(Bottom)** *Sagittal graphic depicts longitudinal spatial relationships of the neck with emphasis on the retropharyngeal and danger spaces. Seen just anterior to the vertebral column, the retropharyngeal and danger spaces run inferiorly from the skull base toward the mediastinum. Notice the fascial "trap door" found at the approximate level of T3 vertebral body that serves as a conduit from the retropharyngeal to the danger space. RPS infection or tumor may access the mediastinum via this route of spread.*

NORMAL AXIAL T2 MR, T1 MR, & BONE CT

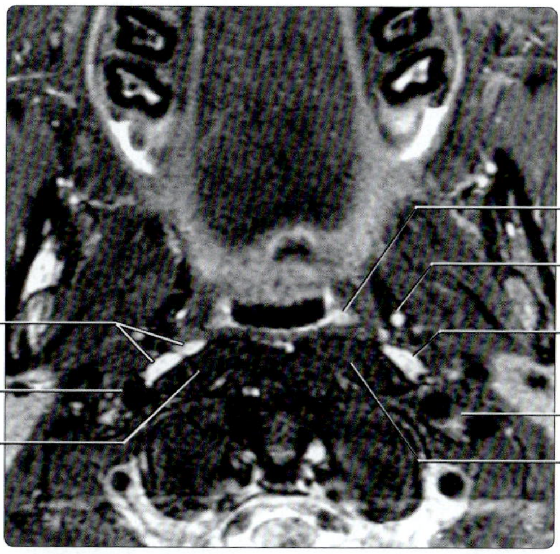

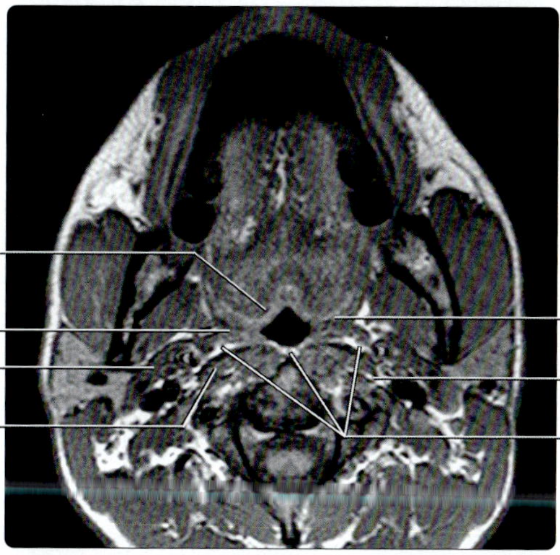

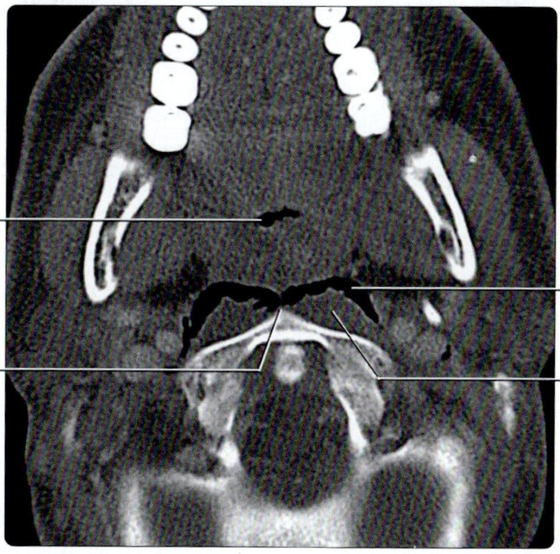

(Top) *Axial fat-saturated T2 MR through the low nasopharynx in a young adolescent reveals normal lateral RPS nodes bilaterally. Notice these nodes are positioned just medial to the internal carotid artery and posteromedial to the fat-saturated parapharyngeal space.* **(Middle)** *Axial T1 MR of the extracranial head and neck at the level of the oropharynx shows a thin stripe of high-signal fat behind the pharyngeal mucosal space that represents the RPS. Posterior to the RPS is the prevertebral portion of the perivertebral space.* **(Bottom)** *Axial bone CT through the midoropharynx in a trauma patient shows air has collected in the RPS, allowing the median raphe to be seen. The median raphe functions as an attachment of the constrictor muscles. In addition, it provides an initial barrier to spread of disease from side to side in the RPS.*

TERMINOLOGY

Abbreviations

- Perivertebral space (PVS)

Synonyms

- Prevertebral space
  - Historically, term "prevertebral space" includes soft tissues behind vertebral column
  - "PVS" terminology adopted to include all tissues under deep layer of deep cervical fascia (DL-DCF), both in front of & behind vertebral column

Definitions

- Cylindrical space surrounding vertebral column extending from skull base to upper mediastinum bounded by deep layer, deep cervical fascia subdivided into prevertebral & paraspinal components
- PVS: Peri (Greek for around) vertebra

IMAGING ANATOMY

Extent

- From skull base above to T4 in posterior mediastinum
- Some anatomists describe PVS as discrete anatomic space to level of coccyx

Anatomy Relationships

- **Consists of 2 major components**
  - Prevertebral portion or space
  - Paraspinal portion or space
- **Prevertebral-PVS** sits directly behind retropharyngeal space throughout extracranial H&N
  - Anterolateral to prevertebral-PVS is carotid space
  - Lateral to prevertebral-PVS is anterior aspect of posterior cervical space
- **Paraspinal-PVS** is deep to posterior cervical space & posterior to transverse processes of cervical spine

Internal Contents

- **Prevertebral-PVS or prevertebral space**
  - Prevertebral muscles (longus colli & capitis)
  - Scalene muscles (anterior, middle, & posterior)
  - Brachial plexus (BP) roots
  - Phrenic nerve (C3-C5)
  - Vertebral artery & vein
  - Vertebral body
- **Paraspinal-PVS or prevertebral space**
  - Paraspinal muscles
  - Posterior elements, vertebral column
- **BP**, proximal aspect
  - BP has complex spatial anatomy
  - C5-T1 roots leave cervical neural foramina, pass between anterior & middle scalene of prevertebral-PVS
  - BP roots pass through opening in DL-DCF, pass into posterior cervical space on their way to axilla

Fascia of Perivertebral Space

- **DL-DCF completely circumscribes PVS**
  - Anterior portion arches from cervical spine transverse process across prevertebral muscles to opposite transverse process
    - Anterior DL-DCF called "**the carpet**" by surgeons
    - Pharynx slides up & down on this smooth, carpet-like surface
    - "Carpet" is tenacious, with infection or tumor of PVS redirected into **epidural space** by this fascia
    - Pharyngeal malignancy blocked from accessing PVS by this tough fascia
  - Posterior portion DL-DCF arches over surface of paraspinal muscles to attach to nuchal ligament of spinous process of vertebral body

ANATOMY IMAGING ISSUES

Questions

- What imaging findings define mass lesion as primary to prevertebral-PVS
  - Mass is centered within prevertebral muscles or corpus of vertebral body
  - Mass lifts prevertebral muscles anteriorly (retropharyngeal space mass pushes them posteriorly)

Imaging Approaches

- Lateral 2D imaging
  - Quick check on prevertebral soft tissue swelling & integrity of cervical vertebral bodies
- CECT with soft tissue & bone algorithm & sagittal reformation
  - Best exam to look at cervical soft tissue & bones
- Cervical spine MR best to assess epidural disease

Imaging Pitfalls

- **Hypertrophic levator scapulae muscle** (LSM): Mistaken for enhancing mass or recurrent tumor
  - Secondary to CNXI injury (during neck dissection)
    - Sternocleidomastoid (SCM) & trapezius atrophy
    - LSM hypertrophies to help lift arm
  - Imaging findings
    - LSM enlarges, may enhance
    - SCM & trapezius small, fatty infiltrated

CLINICAL IMPLICATIONS

Clinical Importance

- Prevertebral-PVS contains important structures
  - Proximal BP, phrenic nerve, vertebral arteries
- Most PVS lesions originate in vertebral body (infection or metastatic tumor)
  - Vertebral body is usually diseased when PVS lesion is found
- Prevertebral-PVS disease may involve epidural space
  - If infection or malignancy breaks out of cervical vertebral body into prevertebral-PVS, 1st obstruction to spread is DL-DCF
  - Path of least resistance of spreading pus or tumor is deep through neural foramen into epidural space
  - When prevertebral PVS disease is found on imaging, **always check for epidural space extension**

AXIAL PERIVERTEBRAL SPACE; SAGITTAL PERIVERTEBRAL SPACE

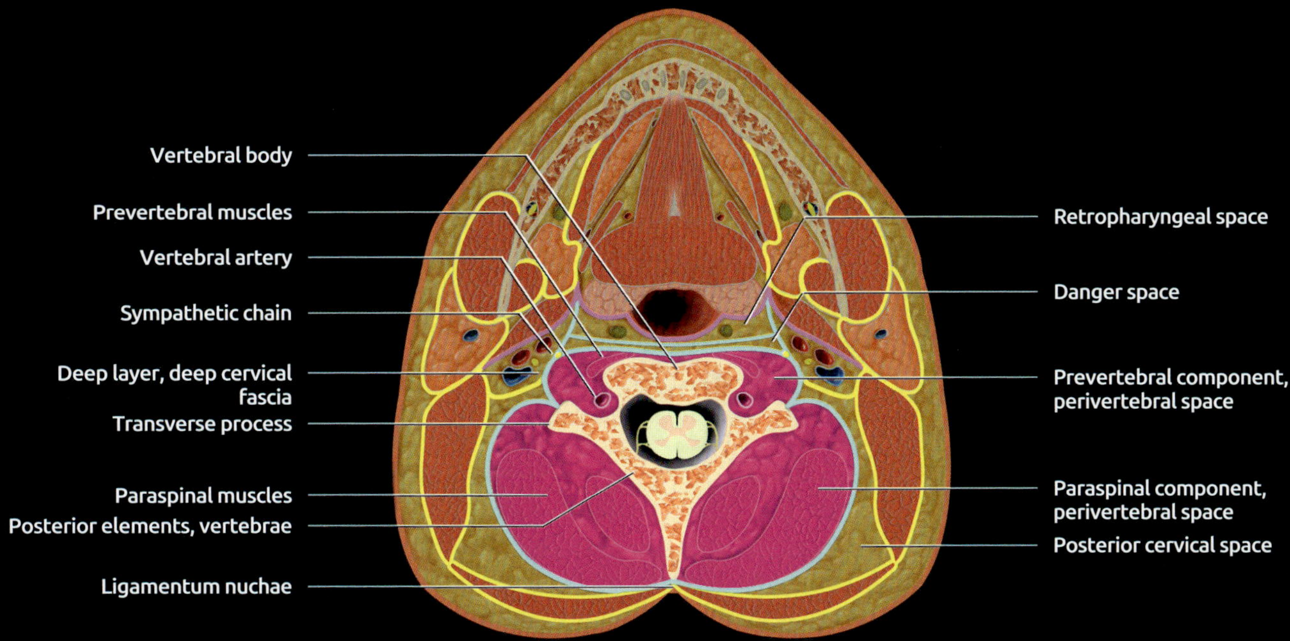

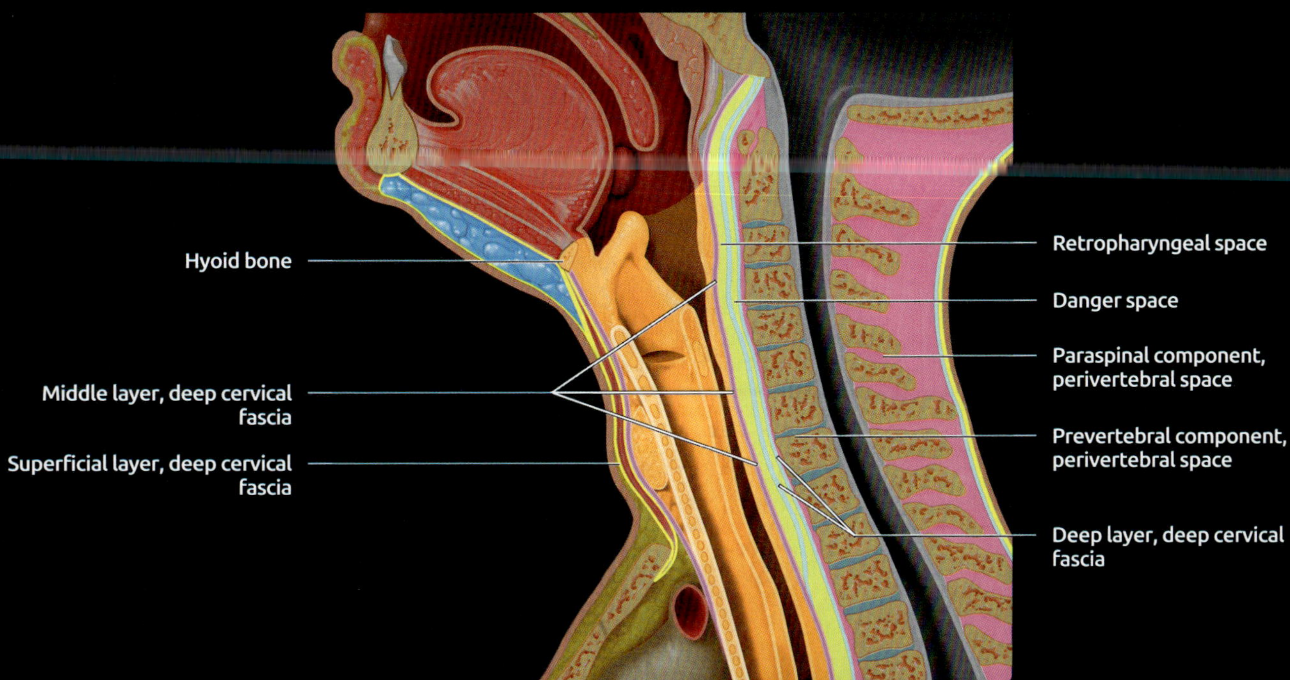

(Top) *Axial graphic through the level of the oropharynx shows prevertebral and paraspinal components of the perivertebral space beneath the deep layer of deep cervical fascia. Notice this fascia curves medially to touch the transverse processes of the vertebrae, dividing the perivertebral space into prevertebral and paraspinal components. The danger and retropharyngeal spaces are anterior to the perivertebral space, while the posterior cervical space is lateral and posterior.* **(Bottom)** *Sagittal graphic depicts midline longitudinal spatial relationships of the neck. In the midline, only the vertebral body is seen in the prevertebral component of the perivertebral space. Just anterior to the vertebral column, the retropharyngeal and danger spaces run inferiorly toward the mediastinum. In the midline paraspinal component of the perivertebral space, only the spinous processes are visible.*

GENERIC PERIVERTEBRAL SPACE MASS; AXIAL T1 MR PERIVERTEBRAL SPACE TUMOR

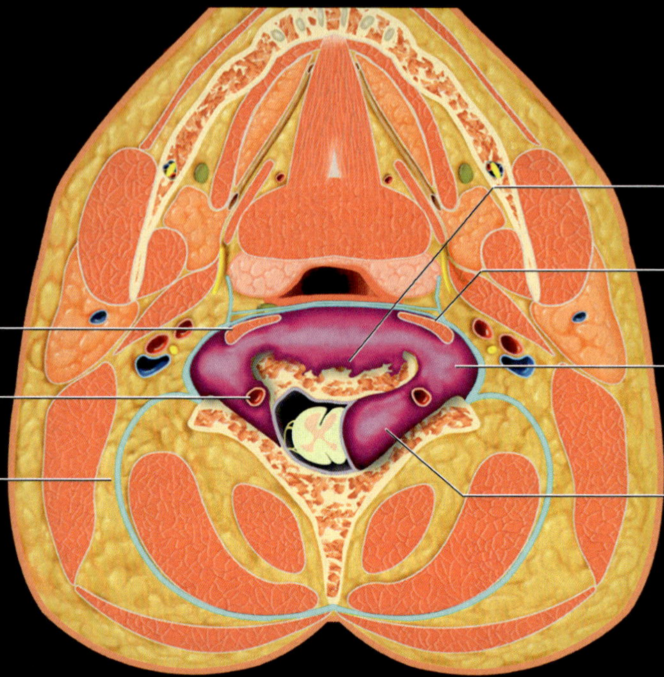

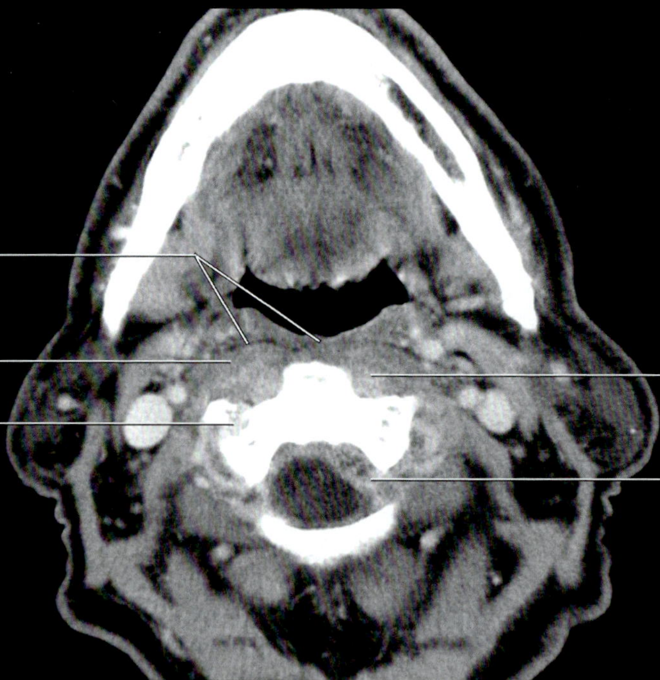

(Top) *Axial graphic through the oropharynx reveals a generic suprahyoid neck perivertebral space mass involving the vertebral body. Notice the vertebral body destruction and the elevation of the prevertebral muscles. The vertebral arteries are engulfed by the tumor. In addition, the tumor is confined by the deep layer of deep cervical fascia, forcing it centrally into the epidural space where it is causing spinal cord compression.* **(Bottom)** *Axial contrast-enhanced CT demonstrates an enhancing malignant tumor involving the prevertebral component of the perivertebral space. The tumor remains confined to the perivertebral space by the deep layer of the deep cervical fascia. Consequently, the tumor has spread centrally into the epidural space where it may cause cord compression.*

NORMAL AXIAL CECT PREVERTEBRAL SPACE

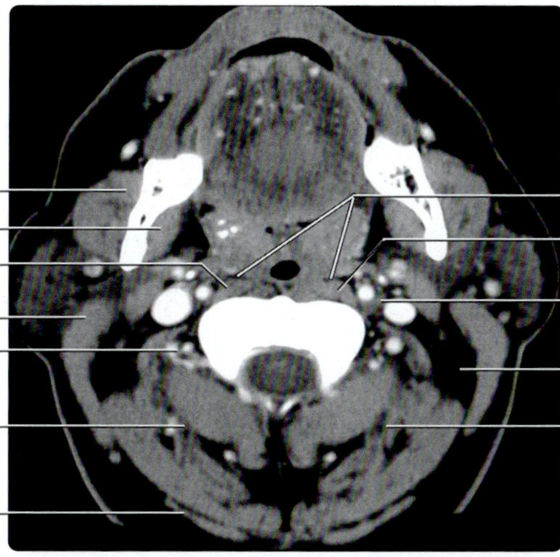

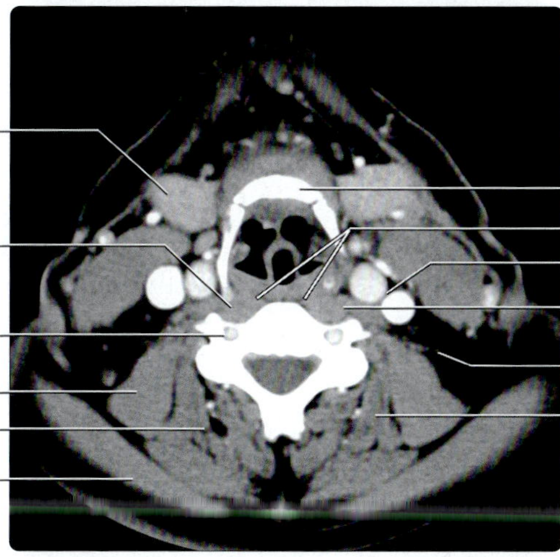

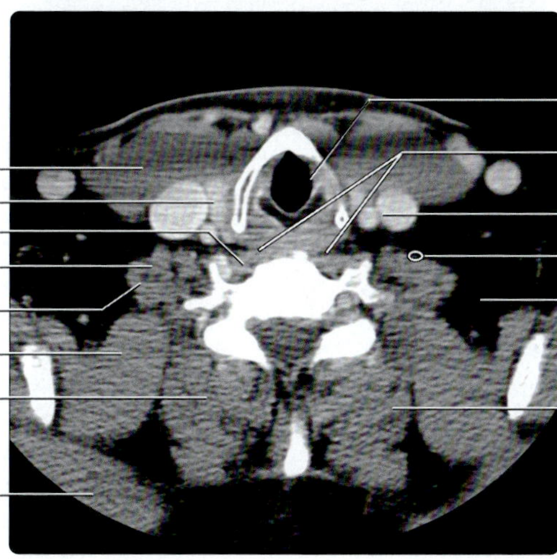

(Top) *This is the 1st of 3 axial CECT images through the extracranial head and neck chosen to highlight the normal features of the perivertebral space. This image at the level of the C2 vertebral body shows that the prevertebral component of the perivertebral space contains the prevertebral muscles, vertebral body, and vertebral artery only. The retropharyngeal space fat stripe is visible anteriorly.* **(Middle)** *In this image at the level of the hyoid bone, the levator scapulae muscles and the paraspinal muscles, along with the posterior elements of the vertebral body, are the principal occupants of the paraspinal component of the perivertebral space.* **(Bottom)** *At the level of the cricoid cartilage, the scalene muscles are visible. The phrenic nerve location is marked on the patient's left to remind the imager of its presence even though it is not visible on imaging.*

TERMINOLOGY

Abbreviations

- Internal jugular chain (IJC)
- Spinal accessory chain (SAC)

Synonyms

- Internal jugular chain: Deep cervical chain
- Spinal accessory chain: Posterior triangle chain

Definitions

- **Jugulodigastric node**: "Sentinel" (highest) node, found at apex of IJC at angle of mandible
- **"Signal" (Virchow) node**: Node found at bottom of IJC in supraclavicular fossa

IMAGING ANATOMY

Overview

- Differentiation between benign or "reactive" nodes vs. pathological nodes
  - Morphology: Oval nodes with central fatty hila
  - Size criteria
    - < 1.5 cm for IJC nodes near angle of mandible
    - < 0.8 mm for retropharyngeal nodes
    - < 1 cm for all other nodal groups
  - PET/CT criteria
    - Intense metabolic activity in any node of neck in setting of squamous cell carcinoma considered malignant node until proven otherwise

Internal Contents

- **Imaging-based nodal classification**
  - **Level I: Submental & submandibular nodes**
    - Level IA: Submental nodes: Found between anterior bellies of digastric muscles
    - Level IB: Submandibular nodes: Found around submandibular glands in submandibular space
  - **Level II: Upper IJC nodes** from posterior belly of digastric muscle to hyoid bone
    - Level IIA: Level II node anterior, medial, lateral, or posterior to internal jugular vein (IJV); if posterior to IJV, node must be inseparable from IJV; this level contains jugulodigastric nodal group
    - Level IIB: Level II node posterior to IJV with fat plane visible between node & IJV
  - **Level III: Mid IJC nodes** from hyoid bone to inferior margin of cricoid cartilage
  - **Level IV: Low IJC nodes** from inferior cricoid margin to clavicle
  - **Level V: Nodes of posterior cervical space (SAC)**
    - SAC nodes lie posteriorly to back margin of sternocleidomastoid muscle
    - Level VA: Upper SAC nodes from skull base to bottom of cricoid cartilage
    - Level VB: Lower SAC nodes from cricoid to clavicle
  - **Level VI: Nodes of visceral space** found from hyoid bone above to top of manubrium below
    - Includes prelaryngeal, pretracheal, and **paratracheal** subgroups
  - **Level VII: Superior mediastinal nodes** found between carotid arteries from top of manubrium above to innominate vein below
- Other nodal groups not included in standard imaging-based nodal classification
  - **Parotid nodal group**: Intraglandular or extraglandular
    - Both intraglandular & extraglandular nodes are within fascia circumscribing parotid space
    - Drains into upper IJC nodes (level II)
    - Most common tumors to involve this group are skin SCCa, melanoma, & parotid malignancy
  - **Retropharyngeal (RPS) nodal group**: 2 subgroups
    - Medial RPS nodes: Found in paramedian RPS in suprahyoid neck (SHN)
    - Lateral RPS nodes: Found in lateral RPS in SHN, lateral to prevertebral muscles, medial to ICA
    - Drainage pattern: Receive drainage from posterior pharynx; drains into high IJC
  - **Facial nodal group**
    - Mandibular nodes: Found along external mandibular surface
    - Buccinator nodes: In buccal space
    - Infraorbital nodes: In nasolabial fold
    - Malar nodes: On malar eminence
    - Retrozygomatic nodes: Deep to zygomatic arch

ANATOMY IMAGING ISSUES

Imaging Approaches

- SCCa nodal staging: CECT or T1 C+ MR
  - Scan extent: Skull base to clavicles
- PET/CT utility in H&N SCCa nodal work-up
  - Small active malignant node identification & treatment planning
- Differentiated thyroid carcinoma: MR preferred
  - Scan extent: Skull base to **carina**

CLINICAL IMPLICATIONS

Clinical Importance

- Presence of malignant SCCa nodes in staging associated with 50% ↓ in long-term survival
  - If extranodal spread present, further 50% ↓
- IJC is final common pathway for all lymphatics of upper aerodigestive tract & neck
  - Since IJC empties into subclavian vein, IJV, or thoracic duct, SCCa does not normally drain directly into mediastinum
  - Neck imaging to stage SCCa: Skull base to clavicles
- **Retropharyngeal space nodal group**
  - Reactive appearing RPS nodes commonly seen in younger patients on brain MR exam
  - Important when identified on imaging in SCCa setting, as often clinically silent
- When **"signal" node** (lowest IJC) found on imaging without upper neck nodes, primary is not in neck
- **Parotid nodal group**
  - Receives lymph drainage from external auditory canal, eustachian tube, skin of lateral forehead & temporal region, posterior cheek, gums & buccal mucous membrane (especially due to skin SCCa & melanoma)

GRAPHICS

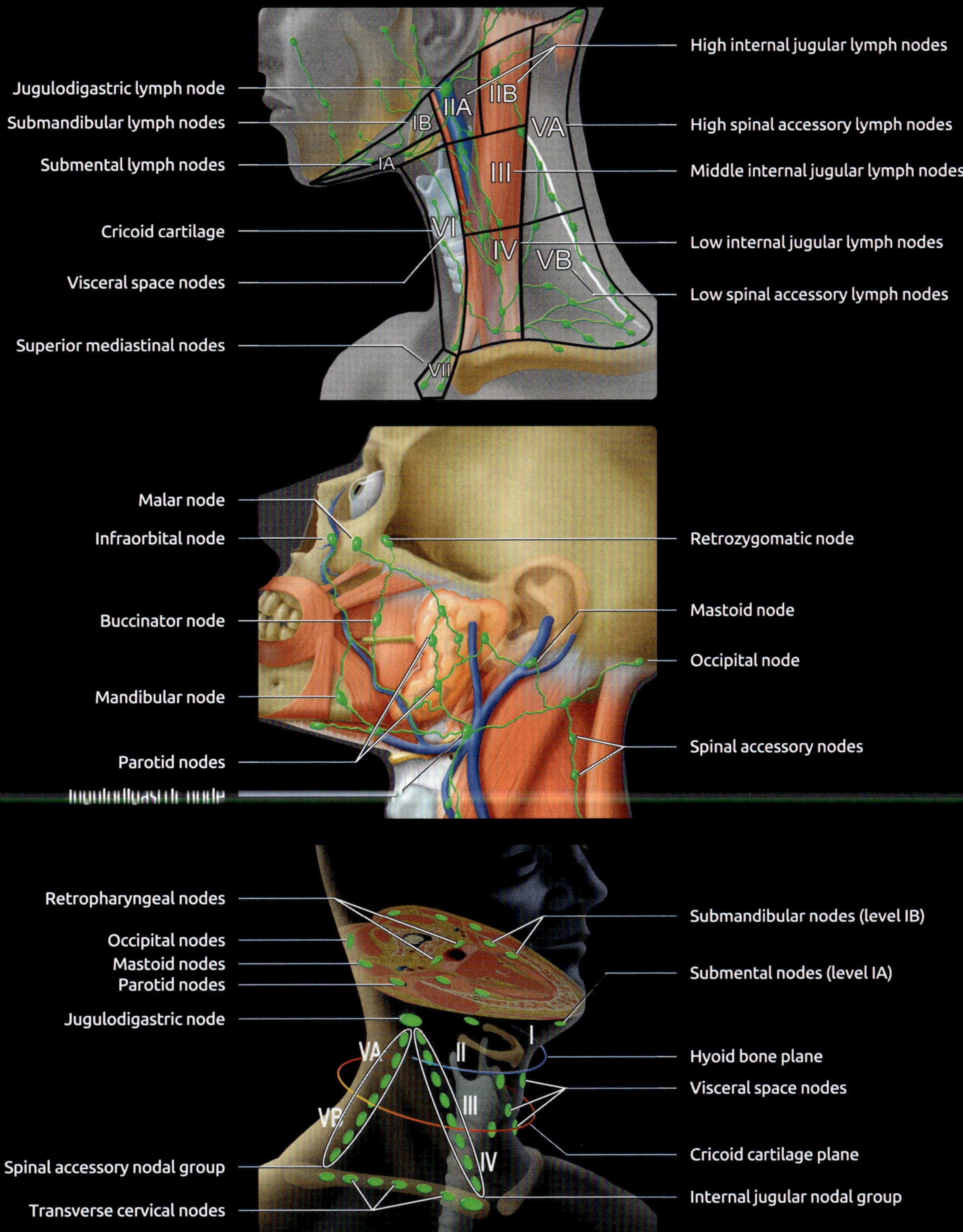

(Top) *Lateral oblique graphic of the neck shows the anatomic locations for the major nodal groups of the neck. Division of the internal jugular nodal chain into high, middle, and low regions is defined by the level of the hyoid bone and cricoid cartilage. Similarly, the spinal accessory nodal chain is divided into high & low regions by the level of the cricoid cartilage.* **(Middle)** *Lateral view shows facial nodes plus parotid nodes. None of these nodes bear level numbers but instead must be described by their anatomic location.* **(Bottom)** *Lateral oblique graphic of cervical neck depicts an axial slice through the suprahyoid neck. Note the retropharyngeal nodes behind the pharynx are often clinically occult. The hyoid bone (blue arc) & cricoid cartilage (orange circle) planes are highlighted as they serve to subdivide the internal jugular & spinal accessory nodal group levels.*

AXIAL CECT

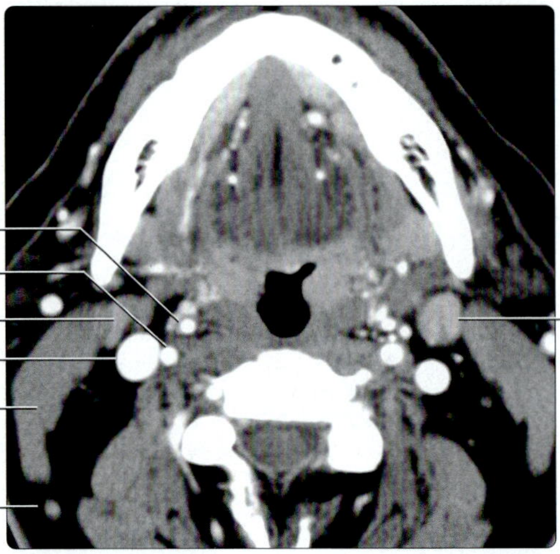

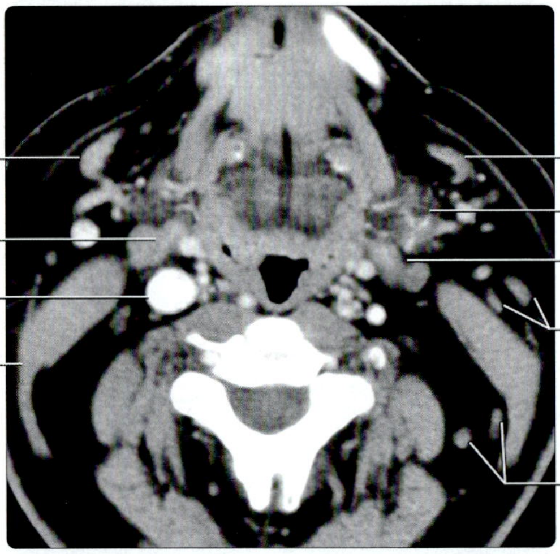

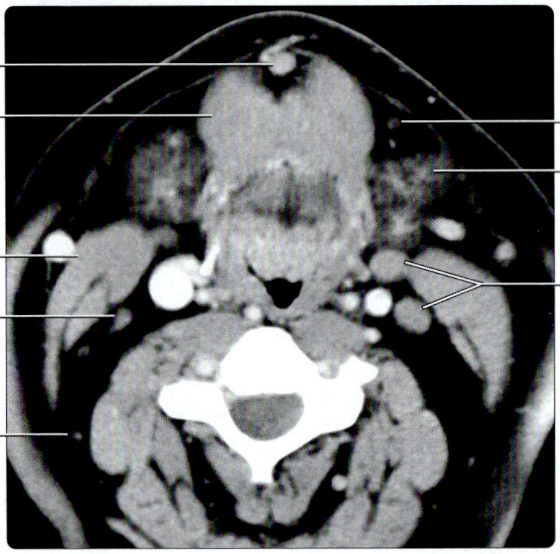

(Top) *First of 3 axial CECT images of the suprahyoid neck presented from superior to inferior demonstrates lymph nodes in the internal jugular (level II) and spinal accessory chains (level V). The jugulodigastric node is the highest or "sentinel" node of the internal jugular chain (deep cervical chain).* **(Middle)** *The internal jugular & spinal accessory lymph nodes are seen along with submandibular nodes (level IA) anterolateral to the submandibular glands in the submandibular space. Note the internal jugular nodes are closely applied to the carotid space while the spinal accessory nodes are in the posterior cervical space.* **(Bottom)** *Just above the hyoid bone, a submental (level IA) node is seen between the anterior bellies of the digastric muscles. Note also the submandibular (level IB), high internal jugular (levels IIA & IIB), & spinal accessory (level VA) nodes.*

AXIAL T1 & T2 MR

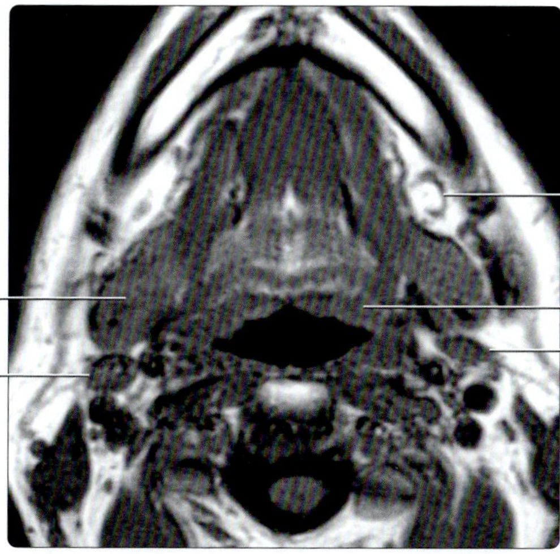

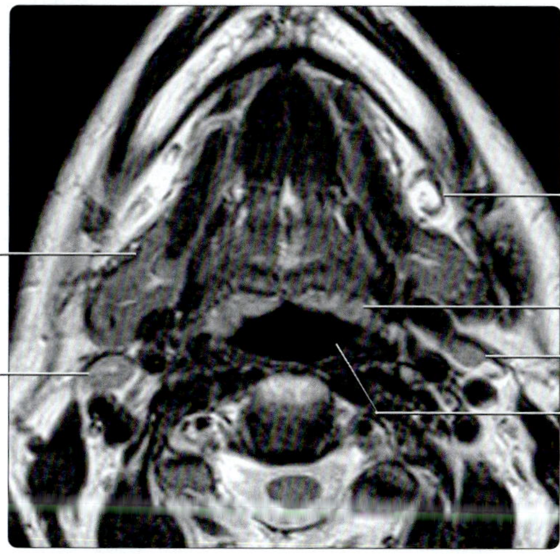

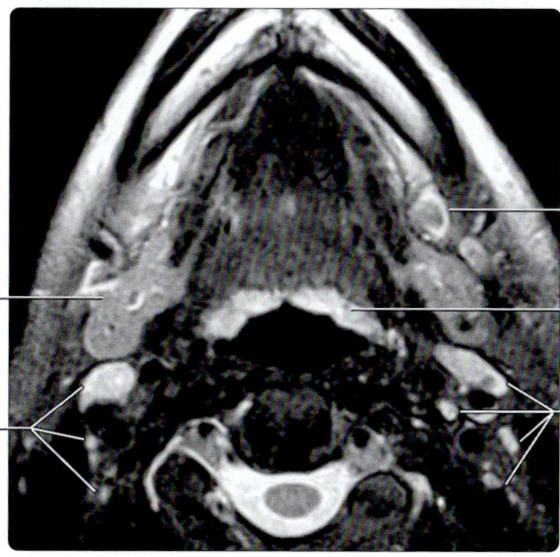

(Top) *Axial T1 MR through low oropharynx shows characteristic low T1 signal of lymph nodes. A prominent submandibular node with a fatty hilum is seen on the left. Level IIA internal jugular nodes are observed bilaterally.* **(Middle)** *Axial T2 MR at level of the low oropharynx shows bilateral high internal jugular nodes as intermediate signal intensity.* **(Bottom)** *Axial T2 MR with fat saturation creates increased conspicuity of lymph nodes. The smaller high internal jugular nodes surrounding the carotid space are easily identified on this fat-saturated T2 image. STIR MR sequences create the same level of nodal conspicuity. Lingual tonsil tissue is also made more conspicuous with the fat-saturation T2 sequence.*

TERMINOLOGY

Abbreviations

- Aortic arch (AA), brachiocephalic trunk (BCT)
- Common (CCA), internal (ICA), and external (ECA) carotid arteries; ophthalmic artery (OA)
- Vertebral artery (VA), basilar artery (BA)
- Cavernous sinus (CS)

IMAGING ANATOMY

Overview

- CCAs terminate by dividing into ECA, ICA
- ECA is smaller of 2 terminal branches
  - Supplies most of head, neck (except eye, brain)
  - Has numerous anastomoses with ICA, VA (may become important source of collateral blood flow)
- Cervical ICA (C1) has no normal extracranial branches
- ICA has 6 intracranial segments (C2-C7)

Cervical Carotid Arteries

- **CCAs**
  - Right CCA originates from BCT; left CCA from AA
  - Course superiorly in carotid space, anteromedial to internal jugular vein (IJV)
  - Divide into ECA, ICA at approximately C3-4 level
- **Cervical ICAs (C1)**
  - 90% arise posterolateral to ECA
  - Carotid "bulb": Focal dilation of ICA at CCA
  - Ascending cervical segment
    - Courses superiorly within carotid space: Enters carotid canal of skull base (petrous temporal bone)
- **ECAs** have 8 major branches
- **Superior thyroid artery**
  - 1st ECA branch (may arise from CCA bifurcation): Arises anteriorly, courses inferiorly to thyroid apex
- **Ascending pharyngeal artery**
  - Arises from posterior ECA (or CCA bifurcation)
  - Courses superiorly between ECA, ICA
  - Visceral branches supply nasopharynx, oropharynx, eustachian tube
- **Lingual artery**
  - 2nd anterior ECA branch
  - Loops anteroinferiorly, then superiorly to tongue
  - Supplies tongue, oral cavity, submandibular gland
  - Common origin with facial artery in 10-20% of cases
- **Facial artery**
  - Originates just above lingual artery
  - Curves around mandible, then passes anterosuperiorly to supply face, palate, lip, cheek
  - **Anastomoses with ophthalmic artery (ICA branch), other ECA branches**
- **Occipital artery**
  - Originates from posterior aspect of ECA
  - Courses posterosuperiorly between occiput and C1
- **Posterior auricular artery**
  - Arises from posterior ECA above occipital artery
  - Courses superiorly to supply pinna, scalp, external auditory canal, chorda tympani
- **Superficial temporal artery**
  - Smaller of 2 terminal ECA branches
  - Runs superiorly behind mandibular condyle, across zygoma
- **Maxillary artery**
  - Larger of 2 terminal ECA branches
  - Arises within parotid gland, behind condylar neck
  - Gives off middle meningeal artery
  - Runs anteromedially in masticator space
  - Within pterygopalatine fossa, sends off terminal branches to deep face, nose
  - Potential major source of collateral flow via inferolateral trunk of cavernous ICA, ophthalmic, and recurrent meningeal arteries
- **Cervical VAs**
  - Originate from subclavian arteries; pass upward in transverse foramina

Intracranial ICAs

- **Petrous (C2) segment**
  - Contained within carotid canal of temporal bone
  - 2 subsegments of C2 joined at genu (knee)
    - Short vertical segment (anterior to IJV)
    - "Genu" (where petrous ICA turns anteromedially)
    - Longer horizontal segment
  - Exits carotid canal at petrous apex
  - Branches: Vidian artery (artery of pterygoid canal) anastomoses with external carotid artery
- **Lacerum (C3) segment**
  - Small segment that extends from petrous apex above foramen lacerum, curving upward toward CS
- **Cavernous (C4) segment**
  - 3 subsegments joined by 2 genus
    - Posterior vertical (ascending) portion
    - Posterior (more medial) genu
    - Horizontal segment
    - Anterior (more lateral) genu
    - Anterior vertical (subclinoid) segment
  - Major branches: Inferolateral trunk arises from horizontal segment, supplies cavernous sinus dura/cranial nerves; **anastomoses with ECA branches through foramen rotundum, spinosum, ovale**
- **Clinoid (C5) segment**
  - Between proximal, distal dural rings of CS
  - Ends as ICA enters subarachnoid space near anterior clinoid process
- **Ophthalmic (C6) segment**
  - From distal dural ring at superior clinoid to just below posterior communicating artery (PCoA) origin
  - 2 important branches: OA, superior hypophyseal artery
- **Communicating (C7) segment**
  - Extends from below PCoA to terminal ICA bifurcation into anterior cerebral artery & middle cerebral artery

Normal Variants, Anomalies

- CCA bifurcation can be from T2 to C2: Medial (not lateral) origin of ICA from CCA in 10-15%

ANATOMY IMAGING ISSUES

Imaging Pitfalls

- Coronal CBCT: Anterior clinoid processes similar to calcified atheromas; differentiate from more superior and medial C5 segment and more inferior C4 segment

GRAPHICS

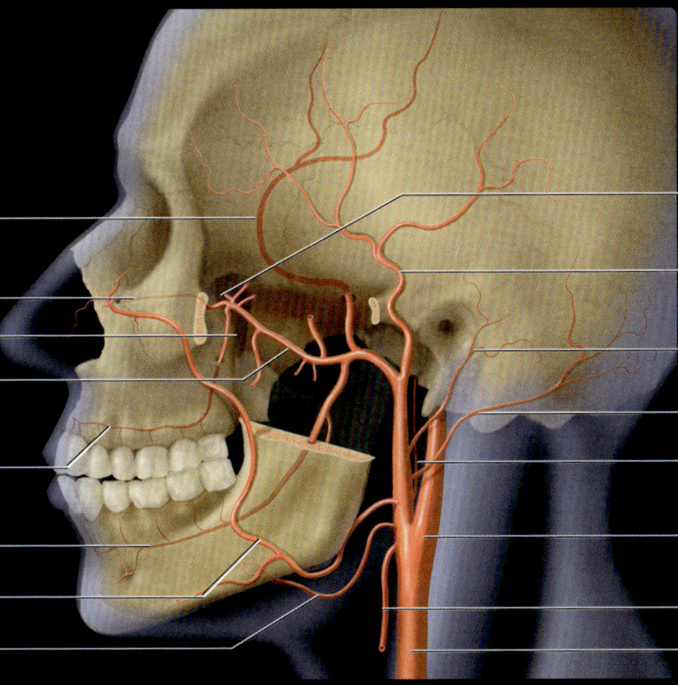

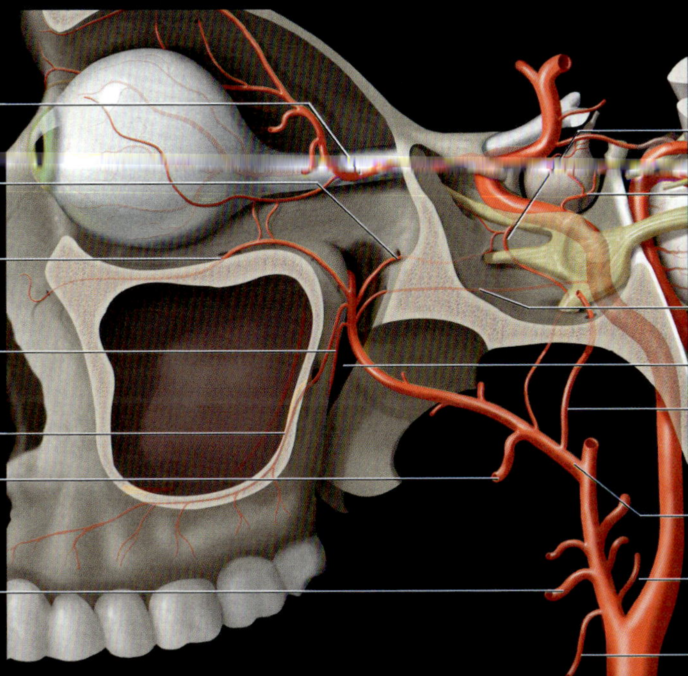

(Top) *Lateral graphic depicts common carotid artery and its 2 terminal branches: External and internal carotid arteries. Scalp and superficial facial structures are removed to show deep ECA branches. ECA terminates by dividing into superficial temporal and internal maxillary arteries (IMA). Within the pterygopalatine fossa, the IMA divides into numerous deep branches. Its distal termination is the sphenopalatine artery, which passes medially into the nasal cavity. Numerous anastomoses between ECA branches (e.g., between the facial and maxillary arteries) as well as between the ECA and orbital and cavernous branches of the ICA provide potential sources for collateral blood flow.* **(Bottom)** *Close-up view shows the deep ECA branches and their numerous anastomoses with branches from the ICA. The maxillary artery terminal branches arise deep within the pterygopalatine fossa.*

GRAPHICS

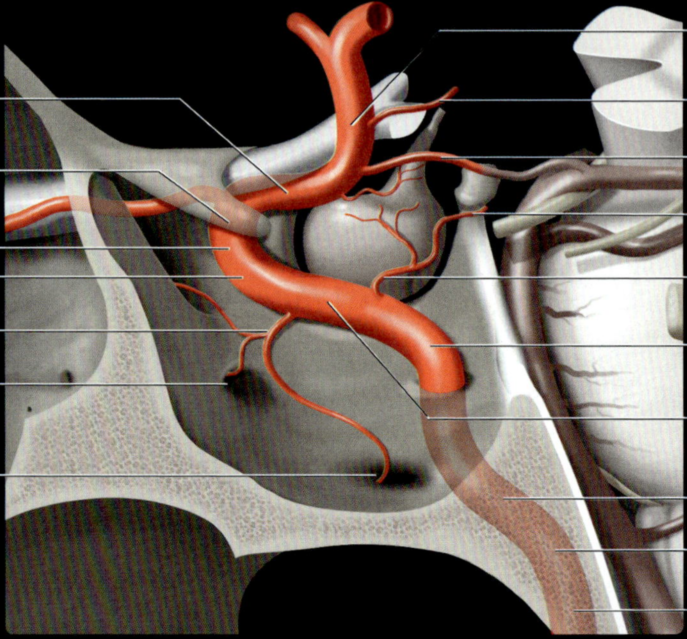

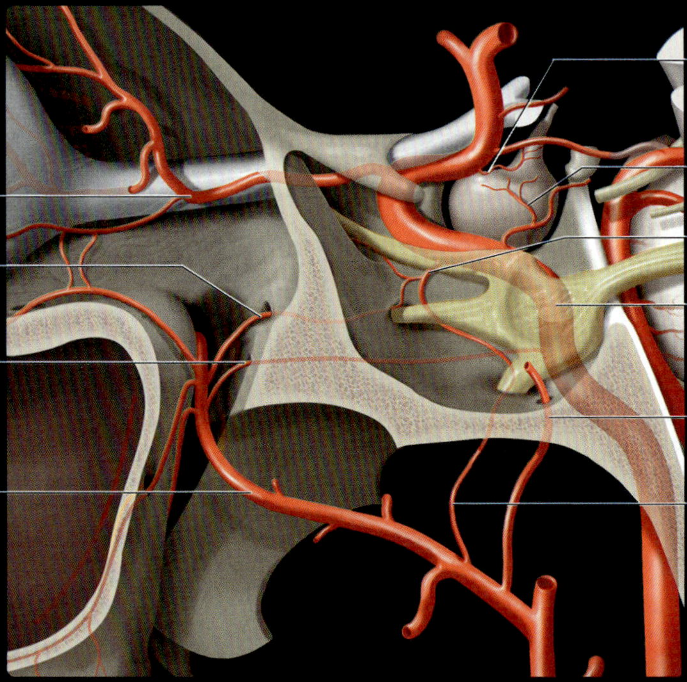

(Top) *Graphic shows the various segments of the intracranial carotid artery. Major branches of the cavernous ICA (C4) segment are depicted with their numerous anastomoses with ECA branches (e.g., arteries of foramen ovale, rotundum).* **(Bottom)** *The lacerum (C3) ICA segment is a short segment that begins where the petrous carotid canal ends. It passes above (not through) the foramen lacerum and is covered by the trigeminal ganglion.There are numerous ICA to ECA anastomoses through cavernous and deep facial branches of the 2 arteries, respectively. A small artery, the vidian artery, is an anastomosis between the IMA and the petrous ICA segment. Numerous anastomoses in and around the orbit are also present. The accessory meningeal artery is a small but important branch that enters the skull through the foramen ovale. It may supply part of the trigeminal ganglion and anastomose with the inferolateral trunk of the cavernous ICA.*

AXIAL NECT

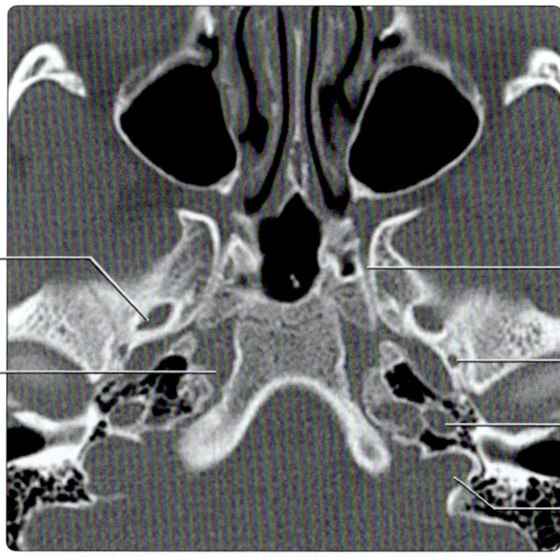

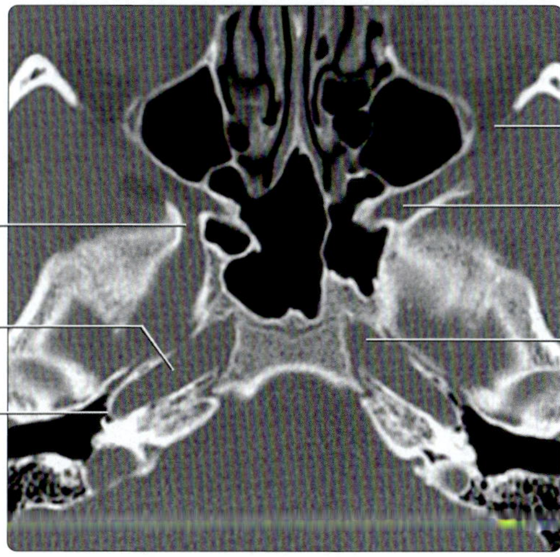

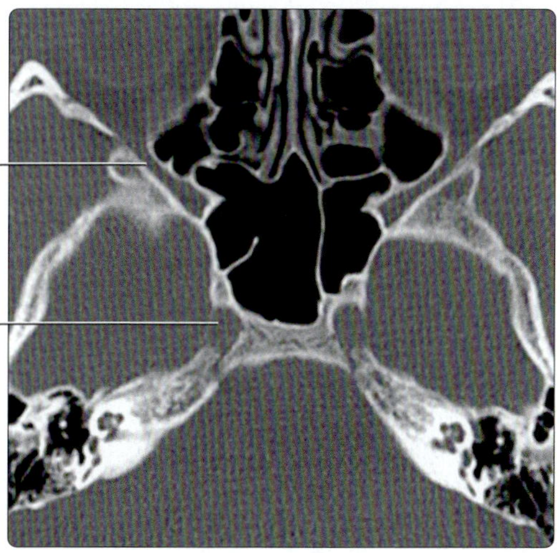

(Top) *Series of 6 axial NECT scans from inferior to superior with bone windows show the major basilar foramina. The ICA follows a complex course through the petrous temporal bone. The C2 or petrous ICA enters the skull base at the exocranial opening of the carotid canal, ascending in front of the internal jugular vein. The petrous ICA has a short vertical and a longer horizontal segment.* **(Middle)** *Slightly more cephalad, the vertical petrous ICA abruptly turns anteromedially and forms the genu of the petrous ICA. The petrous genu is below and slightly in front of the cochlea and middle ear cavity. The long, horizontal petrous segment then courses anteromedially from the genu toward the cavernous sinus.* **(Bottom)** *Section just below the cavernous sinus proper shows the posterior genu of the cavernous (C4) ICA as it curves anteromedially into the cavernous sinus.*

AXIAL NECT

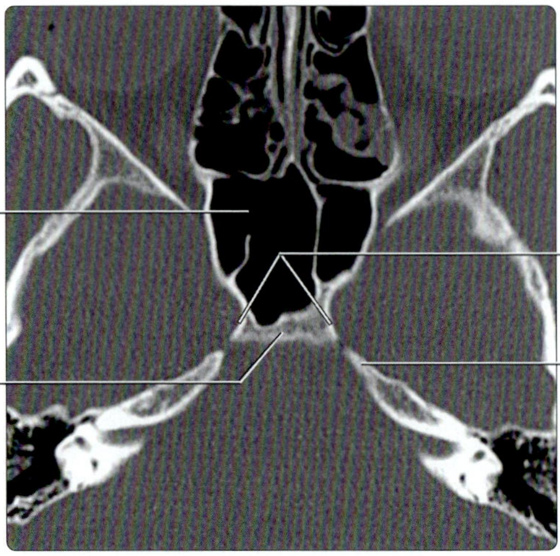

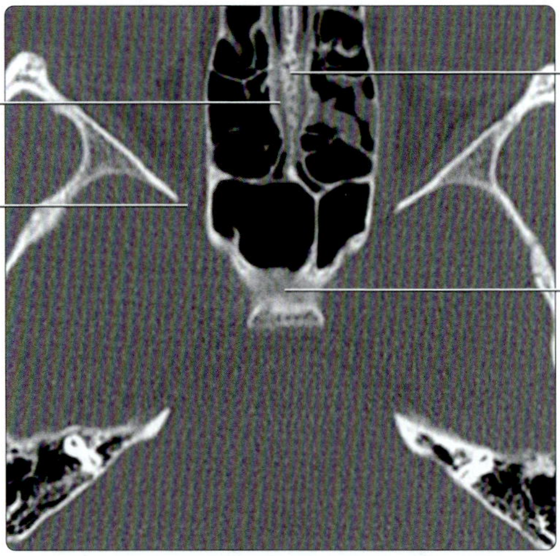

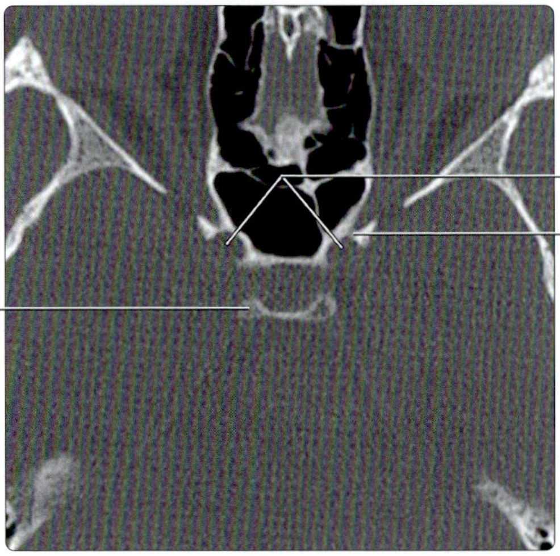

(Top) *Section through the middle of the cavernous sinus shows the bony grooves of the carotid sulcus along the basisphenoid bone. The cavernous (C4) ICA segment courses along the sulcus.* **(Middle)** *At this level, the cavernous internal carotid artery courses through the cavernous sinus proper and then turns superiorly toward the anterior clinoid process.* **(Bottom)** *The 2 cavernous carotid arteries form bony grooves just under the anterior clinoid processes, as seen on this section. This represents the anterior genu of the cavernous ICAs as they curve upward toward the dural ring, where they will enter the cranial subarachnoid space. This represents the very short C5 (clinoid) ICA segment. The C6 (ophthalmic segment) begins at the distal dural ring of the cavernous sinus. The ophthalmic artery originates here and passes anteriorly through the optic canal.*

ARTERIAL CALCIFICATIONS ON PANORAMIC AND CBCT

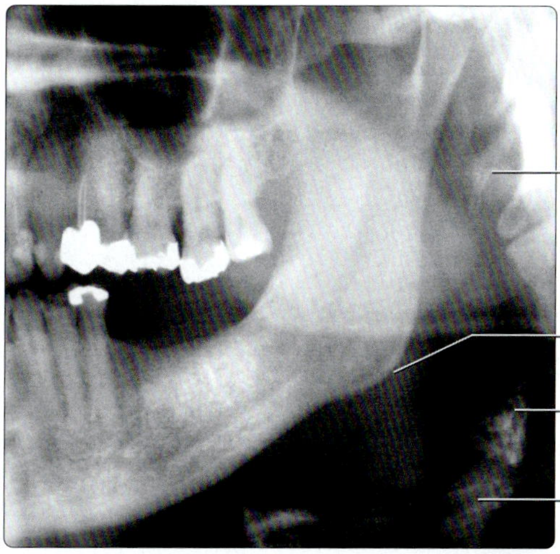

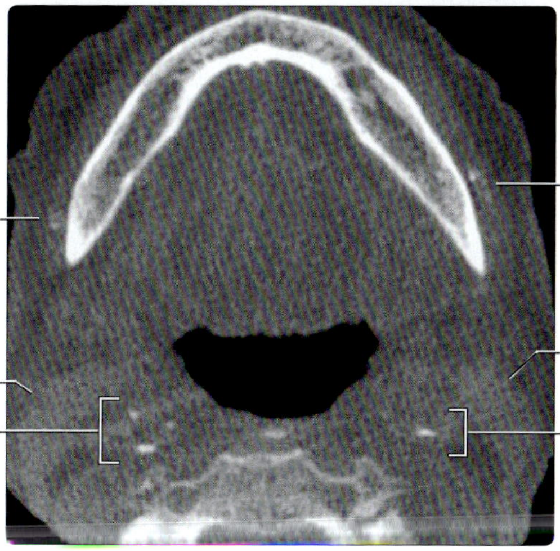

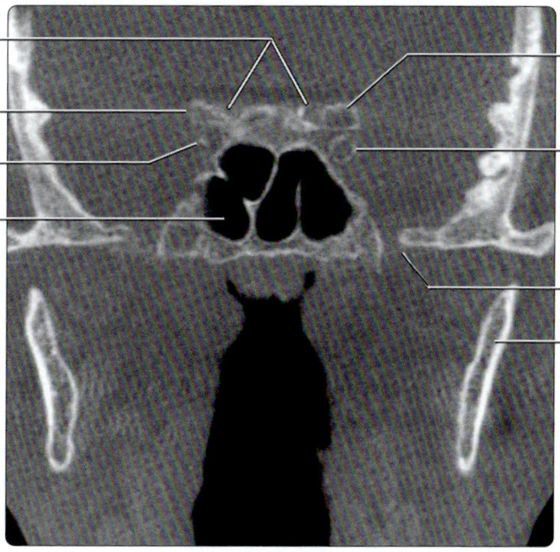

(Top) *Panoramic radiograph shows diffuse calcifications in left carotid. Calcified atheromas are usually found adjacent to C3/C4 at normal location of carotid bifurcation. Calcifications are inferior & posterior to the angle of the mandible. Dental imaging is not diagnostic for the severity of arterial stenosis, & the patient should be referred for Doppler US.* **(Middle)** *Axial CBCT shows calcification of carotid & facial arteries. The facial artery curves around mandible (seen in cross section on patient's right) & then passes anterosuperiorly (seen in longitudinal section on patient's left) to supply the face, palate, lip, & cheek. Calcification of the carotid is seen medially to the faint soft tissue outline of sternocleidomastoid muscle, which lies laterally.* **(Bottom)** *Coronal CBCT shows calcified atheromas (left greater than right) in horizontal segment of cavernous (C4) & ophthalmic (C6) segment. Horizontal segment is posterior & inferior to the anterior genu of C4, where carotid directs superiorly & makes a U-turn anterior to anterior clinoid process, progressing to the clinoid (C5) & posteriorly directed C6 segments.*

PART II

SECTION 1

Teeth

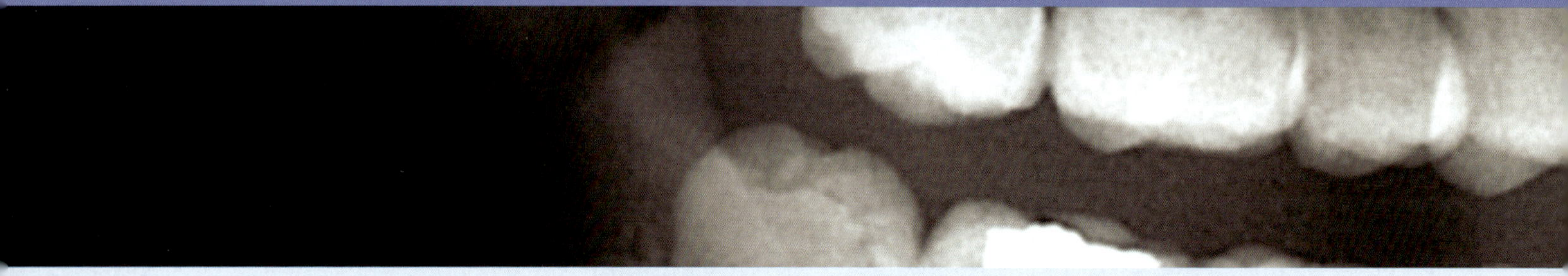

Developmental Alterations in Size and Shape of Teeth

Hypodontia 212

Hyperdontia 214

Macrodontia, Gemination, and Fusion 216

Microdontia 218

Concrescence 219

Talon Cusp 220

Dens Invaginatus 221

Enamel Pearls 222

Taurodontism 223

Dilaceration 224

Supernumerary Roots 225

Developmental Alterations in Structure of Teeth

Amelogenesis Imperfecta 226

Dentinogenesis Imperfecta 230

Dentin Dysplasia 232

Regional Odontodysplasia 233

Segmental Odontomaxillary Dysplasia 234

Acquired Alterations of Teeth and Supporting Structures

Attrition 236

Abrasion 238

Erosion 239

Abfraction 240

Turner Dysplasia 241

Internal and External Resorption 242

Hypercementosis 248

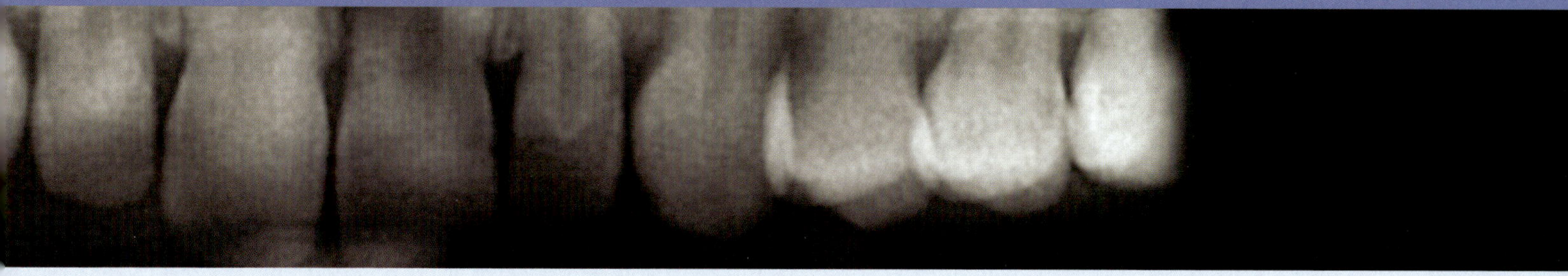

Trauma

Concussion 249

Luxation 250

Dentoalveolar Fractures 254

Infection/Inflammation

Dental Caries 260

Periapical Rarefying Osteitis 264

Periapical Sclerosing Osteitis 268

Periodontal Disease 270

Miscellaneous

Gubernaculum Dentis 276

Hypodontia

KEY FACTS

TERMINOLOGY

- Synonyms: Anodontia, oligodontia
- Definitions
  - **Hypodontia**: Lack of development of 1 or more teeth
  - **Anodontia**: Total lack of development of teeth
  - **Oligodontia**: Lack of development of 6 or more teeth

IMAGING

- Absence of erupted tooth or dental follicle without history of extraction
- Retained primary tooth without evidence of permanent tooth
- Most commonly affects last or most distal of series of teeth decreasing in incidence from posterior to anterior
  - **3rd molars** > 2nd premolars > lateral incisors

TOP DIFFERENTIAL DIAGNOSES

- **Ectodermal dysplasia**
- Basal cell nevus syndrome
- Rieger syndrome
- Focal dermal hypoplasia
- Isolated occurrence

PATHOLOGY

- **Strong genetic correlation with multifactorial nature**
  - Autosomal dominant with incomplete penetrance
- Environmental factors may damage dental lamina
  - **Trauma**, **infection**, radiation, endocrine disturbances

CLINICAL ISSUES

- Uncommon in primary dentition; if present, usually involves mandibular incisors
- Common sequela of failure of development of 2nd mandibular premolar is ankylosis of 2nd deciduous molar

DIAGNOSTIC CHECKLIST

- **Consider hereditary syndromes** when stable teeth (maxillary central incisors or 1st molars) involved or when 6 or more teeth missing

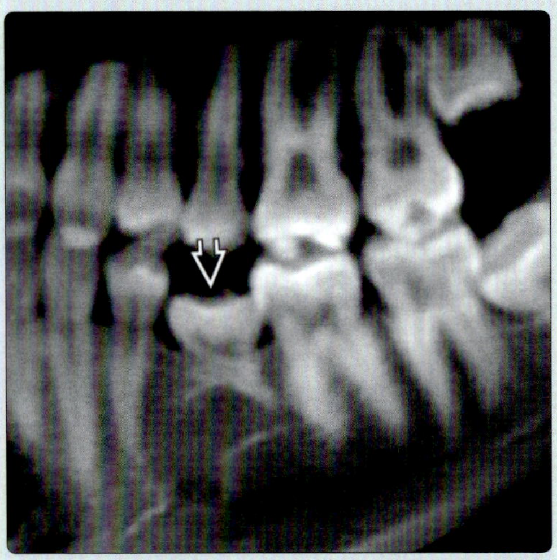
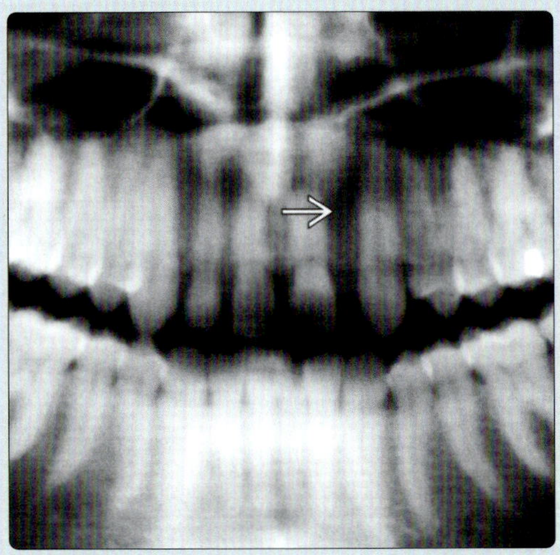

(Left) *CBCT panoramic reformat shows a retained mandibular left deciduous 2nd molar ➡. The succedaneous 2nd premolar is missing and the deciduous tooth is submerged and ankylosed, which is a common sequela.* **(Right)** *Cropped panoramic image demonstrates the absence of the left maxillary lateral incisor ➡. The lateral incisor is a commonly missing tooth.*

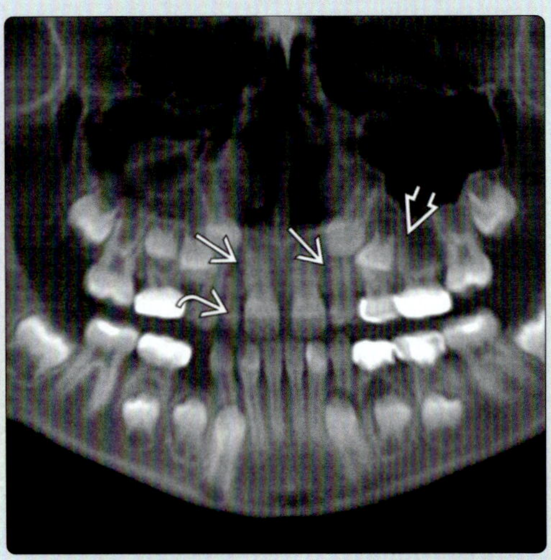
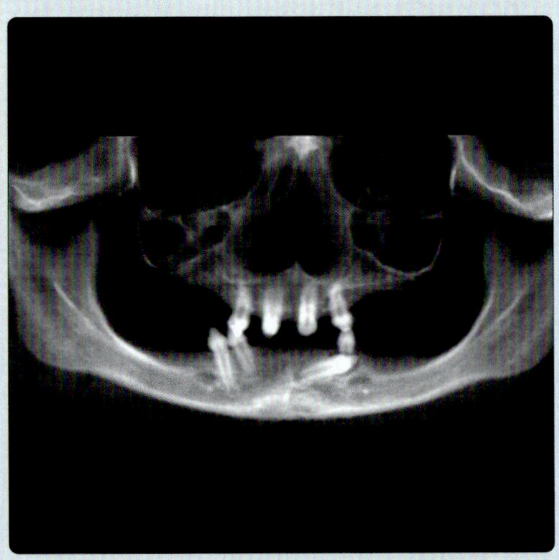

(Left) *CBCT panoramic reformat of an 8-year-old child with mixed dentition shows that the permanent maxillary lateral incisors ➡ and left maxillary 2nd premolar ➡ are missing, and there is no evidence of their developing follicles. Note retained deciduous lateral incisor ➡.* **(Right)** *CBCT panoramic reformat of a 12-year-old girl with ectodermal dysplasia shows oligodontia with characteristic "pointed" teeth. The patient also lacked sweat glands and had abnormal hair.*

TERMINOLOGY

Synonyms

- Anodontia, oligodontia

Definitions

- **Hypodontia**: Lack of development of 1 or more teeth
- **Anodontia**: Total lack of development of teeth
- **Oligodontia**: Lack of development of 6 or more teeth

IMAGING

General Features

- Best diagnostic clue
  - Absence of erupted tooth or dental follicle without history of extraction
  - Retained primary tooth without evidence of permanent tooth
- Location
  - Most commonly affects last or most distal series of teeth decreasing in incidence from posterior to anterior
    - **3rd molars** > 2nd premolars > lateral incisors

Radiographic Findings

- Absence of erupted tooth or dental follicle
- Retained primary tooth without evidence of permanent tooth

Imaging Recommendations

- Best imaging tool
  - Periapical or panoramic images

DIFFERENTIAL DIAGNOSIS

Ectodermal Dysplasia

- Decreased number of sweat glands
- Sparse hair, eyelashes, eyebrows
- **Hypodontia** with abnormal crown shape in teeth that are present

Basal Cell Nevus Syndrome (Gorlin-Goltz Syndrome)

- Multiple basal cell carcinomas
- Odontogenic keratocysts
- Calcification of falx cerebri
- Rib and vertebral anomalies
- **Hypodontia** reported in some cases

Rieger Syndrome

- Abnormalities of iris, cornea
- Glaucoma
- **Hypodontia**

Focal Dermal Hypoplasia

- Skin abnormalities, such as erythematous reticulations, telangiectasia, hypo- or hyperpigmentation, multiple papillomas
- Sparse hair, eyelashes, eyebrows
- Skeletal abnormalities
- Abnormalities of eyes
- **Hypodontia**, abnormalities of palate

Isolated Occurrence

- More common than syndromic association
- May be familial or sporadic
- Association with distinctive craniofacial characteristics such as class III malocclusions and loss of posterior facial height

PATHOLOGY

General Features

- Etiology
  - Absence of dental lamina
  - Environmental factors that may damage dental lamina prior to tooth formation
    - **Trauma**
    - **Infection**
    - Radiation, chemotherapy, or combined treatment
    - Endocrine disturbances
- Genetics
  - **Strong familial link with multifactorial nature**
  - Some cases autosomal dominant with incomplete penetrance and variable expressivity
  - Some cases autosomal recessive or sex-linked pattern
- Associated abnormalities
  - **Associated with numerous hereditary syndromes**

CLINICAL ISSUES

Presentation

- Most common signs/symptoms
  - Absence of 1 or more teeth
- Other signs/symptoms
  - Uncommon in primary dentition; if present, usually involves mandibular incisors
  - Associated with microdontia, reduced development of alveolus, increased freeway space, delayed eruption, ectopic eruption, taurodontism

Demographics

- Gender
  - Slight female predominance (F:M = 3:2)

Natural History & Prognosis

- Common sequela of failure of development of 2nd mandibular premolar is ankylosis of 2nd deciduous molar

Treatment

- Depends on severity
- Ranges from no treatment (absence of 3rd molars) to prosthetic replacement

DIAGNOSTIC CHECKLIST

Consider

- **Hereditary syndromes when stable teeth (maxillary central incisors or 1st molars) involved** or when multiple teeth missing

SELECTED REFERENCES

1. Vucic S et al: Craniofacial characteristics of children with mild hypodontia. Am J Orthod Dentofacial Orthop. 150(4):611-619, 2016
2. Doğan MS et al: An evaluation of clinical, radiological and three-dimensional dental tomography findings in ectodermal dysplasia cases. Med Oral Patol Oral Cir Bucal. 20(3):e340-6, 2015
3. Rakhshan V: Congenitally missing teeth (hypodontia): A review of the literature concerning the etiology, prevalence, risk factors, patterns and treatment. Dent Res J (Isfahan). 12(1):1-13, 2015

Hyperdontia

KEY FACTS

TERMINOLOGY

- Synonyms: Supernumerary tooth or teeth
  - 2nd most common dental anomaly following microdontia
- Definitions: Presence of extra (supernumerary) erupted or unerupted teeth
  - **Mesiodens**: Supernumerary tooth in maxillary incisor region
  - **Distodens** or distomolar: 4th molar
  - **Paramolar**: Supernumerary tooth facial or lingual to molar
  - **Peridens**: Erupted supernumerary tooth located buccal or lingual to normal arch

IMAGING

- Presence of extra erupted or unerupted tooth or teeth
- Supernumerary tooth may be completely formed or still in developmental stage when discovered
- Most common single supernumerary tooth is **mesiodens** or **distodens**
- Multiple supernumerary teeth most commonly found in mandibular premolar region
- Periapical or panoramic images for isolated supernumerary
- CBCT for multiple unerupted supernumeraries

TOP DIFFERENTIAL DIAGNOSES

- Cleidocranial dysplasia
- Gardner syndrome
- Compound odontoma

PATHOLOGY

- Development of excess dental lamina leading to additional tooth buds
- Cleft lip and palate associated

DIAGNOSTIC CHECKLIST

- Consider **Gardner syndrome** or **cleidocranial dysplasia** when multiple unerupted supernumerary teeth are present

(Left) *Periapical radiograph shows a small, unerupted supernumerary tooth ➔ (mesiodens) near the lateral incisor. This is a common location for supernumerary teeth.* **(Right)** *Panoramic image shows the presence of a supernumerary (4th) maxillary molar ➔. This tooth is also referred to as a distodens or distomolar; it is the 2nd most commonly occurring supernumerary tooth after the mesiodens. Supernumerary teeth may be an isolated finding or associated with syndromes, such as cleidocranial dysplasia.*

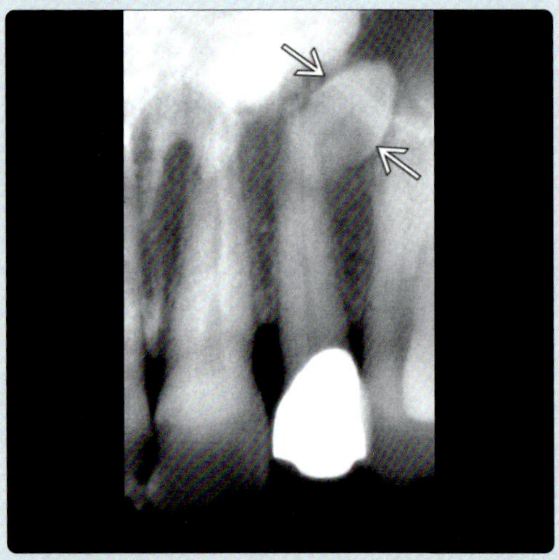

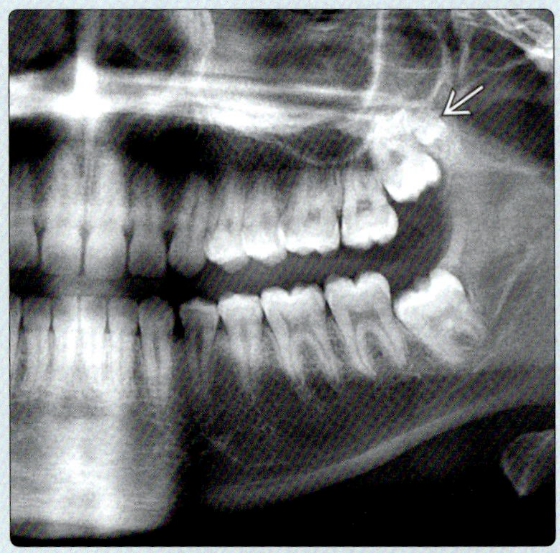

(Left) *Axial CBCT 3D reconstruction of the maxilla in a patient with cleidocranial dysplasia is shown. There are numerous unerupted permanent and supernumerary teeth, some of which have unusual crown ➔ and root ➔ shapes.* **(Right)** *Panoramic reformat CBCT in the same patient shows the hyperdontia seen in both jaws. Note retained deciduous molars ➔ and 3 developing premolars ➔. Patients with cleidocranial dysplasia may also present with absence of, or hypoplastic, clavicles.*

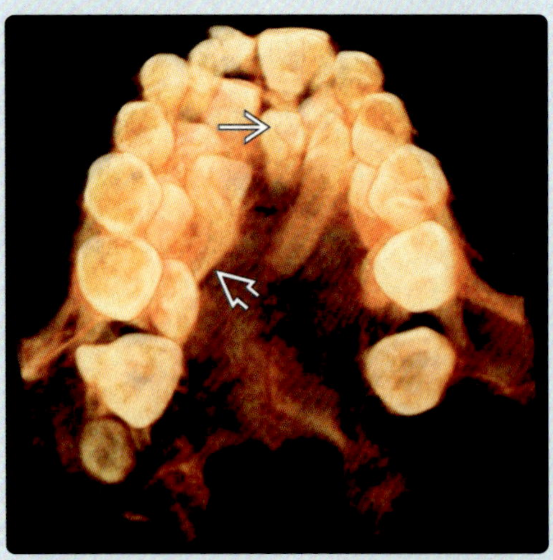

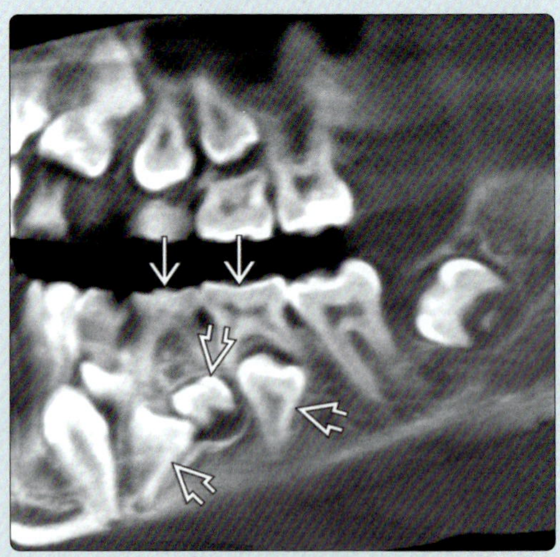

TERMINOLOGY

Synonyms

- Supernumerary tooth or teeth
  - 2nd most common dental anomaly following microdontia

Definitions

- Hyperdontia: Presence of extra (supernumerary) erupted or unerupted teeth
- **Mesiodens**: Supernumerary tooth in maxillary incisor region
- Distodens or distomolar: Supernumerary (4th) molar
- Paramolar: Supernumerary tooth located buccal or lingual to molar
- Peridens: Erupted supernumerary tooth located buccal or lingual to normal arch

IMAGING

General Features

- Best diagnostic clue
  - Presence of additional erupted or unerupted tooth or teeth
  - Supernumerary tooth/teeth may be completely formed or still in developmental stage when discovered
- Location
  - Single supernumerary tooth
    - Most common in permanent maxillary incisor region **(mesiodens)**, 4th molars of either jaw
    - Other sites include premolars, canines, lateral incisors
  - Multiple supernumerary teeth
    - Most common in mandibular premolar region
    - Other sites include molar and anterior regions

Radiographic Findings

- Erupted supernumerary teeth may be in alignment in dental arch or may be situated to facial or lingual of other teeth
- Fully developed unerupted supernumerary teeth have dental follicle around crown
- Immature unerupted supernumerary teeth seen as tooth buds at various stages of development

Imaging Recommendations

- Best imaging tool
  - Periapical or panoramic images for isolated supernumerary
  - CBCT for multiple unerupted supernumeraries
    - 3D rendering and tooth segmentation can help in identifying and visualizing teeth
    - Crucial for determining which tooth is more favorable for extraction and which has better prognosis if retained

DIFFERENTIAL DIAGNOSIS

Cleidocranial Dysplasia

- Absent or hypoplastic clavicles
- High palate, cleft palate
- Open cranial sutures
- **Multiple unerupted supernumerary teeth**

Gardner Syndrome

- Variant of familial adenomatous polyposis
- Osteomas
- Epidermoid cysts of skin
- **Multiple supernumerary teeth**

Compound Odontoma

- Benign mixed odontogenic tumor
- Multiple microdontic teeth with enamel, dentin, and pulpal formation
- Possible common origin has been suggested with supernumerary teeth
- Less prevalent than supernumerary teeth

PATHOLOGY

General Features

- Etiology
  - Development of excess dental lamina leading to additional tooth buds
- Genetics
  - Familial tendency, often autosomal recessive
- Associated abnormalities
  - Cleft lip or palate unrelated to any syndrome
    - Disturbances in craniofacial development may disrupt dental lamina formation, resulting in supernumerary teeth

CLINICAL ISSUES

Presentation

- Most common signs/symptoms
  - Presence of supernumerary teeth may result in delayed eruption, impaction, or ectopic eruption of other teeth

Natural History & Prognosis

- Supernumerary teeth may develop pericoronal pathology
  - Dentigerous cyst: Follicular space enlarged; > 3 mm

Treatment

- Removal of supernumerary teeth to reduce likelihood of complications, such as
  - Resorption of adjacent teeth
  - Crowding, malocclusion
  - Periodontal problems
  - Development of pathology (e.g., dentigerous cyst)

DIAGNOSTIC CHECKLIST

Consider

- When multiple supernumerary teeth are present, consider hereditary conditions: **Gardner syndrome** and **cleidocranial dysplasia**

SELECTED REFERENCES

1. Lubinsky M et al: Syndromes with supernumerary teeth. Am J Med Genet A. 170(10):2611-6, 2016
2. Dhingra S et al: Teeth in rare locations with rare complications: an overview. Indian J Otolaryngol Head Neck Surg. 67(4):438-43, 2015
3. Haque S et al: Common dental anomalies in cleft lip and palate patients. Malays J Med Sci. 22(2):55-60, 2015
4. Menditti D et al: Kissing molars: report of three cases and new prospective on aetiopathogenetic theories. Int J Clin Exp Pathol. 8(12):15708-18, 2015

Macrodontia, Gemination, and Fusion

KEY FACTS

TERMINOLOGY

- **Synonyms**: Megalodontia, megadontia (macrodontia); twinning, double tooth, schizodontia (fusion and gemination)
- **Definitions**
  - **Macrodont/macrodontia**: Tooth/teeth that are larger than usual
  - **Fusion**: Single enlarged or joined tooth; fewer than normal number of teeth
  - **Gemination**: Single enlarged or joined tooth; normal number of teeth

IMAGING

- Most macrodonts are result of fusion or gemination
- Single enlarged crown ± clefting or bifid crown
- Large root with 1 or 2 canals or 2 separate roots
- Single large or partially divided pulp chamber
- Fusion and gemination
  - Both primary and permanent dentitions
  - Anterior areas: Maxilla > mandible

TOP DIFFERENTIAL DIAGNOSES

- KBG syndrome
- Ekman-Westborg and Julin trait

CLINICAL ISSUES

- Treatment: Recontouring/restoration for esthetics
  - Correction of malocclusion or periodontal problems caused by crowding, malalignment

DIAGNOSTIC CHECKLIST

- Tooth count is best way to differentiate fusion from gemination
- Consider KBG syndrome or Ekman-Westborg and Julin trait if multiple macrodonts are seen without fusion or gemination
- Consider oculofaciocardiodental syndrome if radiculomegaly is present

(Left) *Periapical radiograph shows fusion of 2 mandibular incisors in a primary dentition ➡. The crown appears as a macrodont with a central incisal groove ↶. Note the single large pulp chamber and canal ⇨.* **(Right)** *Periapical radiograph shows bilateral gemination of 2 permanent maxillary central incisors. Note that the left anomaly has a single large pulp chamber ➡ but that the patient's right central incisor appears to have 2 pulp chambers ⇨ that join into a single wide pulp canal ➡.*

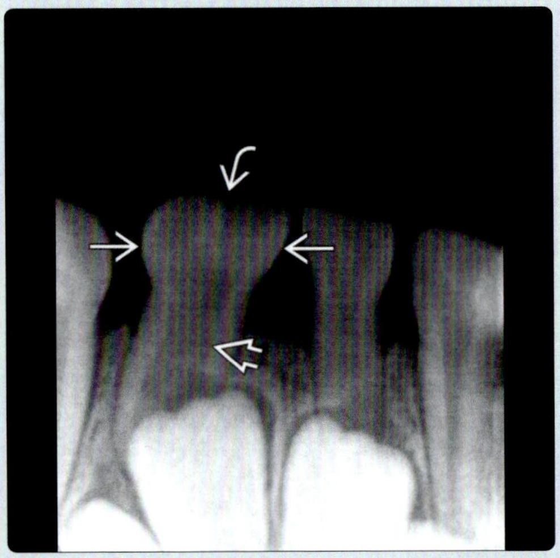

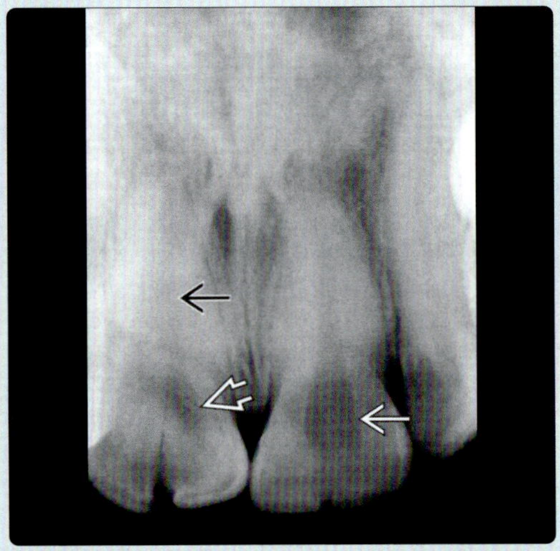

(Left) *Periapical radiograph shows fusion of a permanent mandibular canine and lateral incisor ⇨. The crown appears as a single large tooth (macrodont) with a central incisal groove ↶. Note single pulp chamber and canal. The round radiopacity seen at the midroot of the macrodont ➡ represents a mandibular torus.* **(Right)** *Volume-rendered CBCT shows multiple teeth with excessive root length ➡ and open apices ↶. These findings of radiculomegaly are characteristic of oculofaciocardiodental syndrome.*

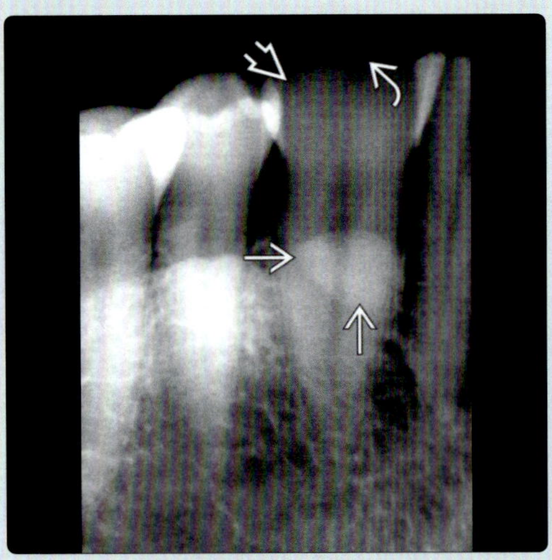

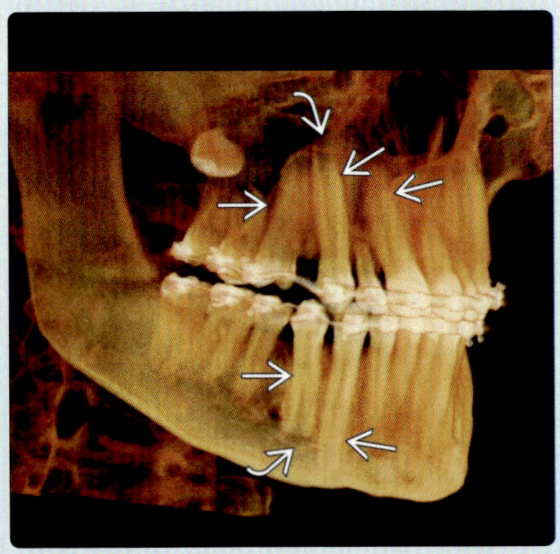

TERMINOLOGY

Synonyms

- Macrodontia
  - Megalodontia
  - Megadontia
- Fusion
  - Double tooth
- Gemination
  - Twinning
  - Double tooth
  - Schizodontia

Definitions

- **Macrodont/macrodontia**: Tooth/teeth that are larger than usual
- **Fusion**
  - Currently considered to be single enlarged or joined tooth in dentition that is missing 1 tooth; anomaly counts as 1 tooth
    - **Fewer than normal number of teeth** present in arch
- **Gemination**
  - Considered to be partial division of single tooth bud with resulting bifid crown and common root and canal
    - **Normal number of teeth** present in arch
  - **Twinning**: Complete division of single tooth bud
    - **Greater than normal number of teeth** present in arch

IMAGING

General Features

- Best diagnostic clue
  - Presence of unusually large tooth or teeth
  - Majority of macrodonts are result of fusion or gemination
    - Macrodonts common with certain syndromes
- Location
  - Fusion and gemination occur most frequently in anterior areas
    - Maxilla > mandible
  - Fusion and gemination occur in both primary and permanent dentitions
- Morphology
  - Single bifid crown often seen with fusion, gemination
    - Central groove may be evident
  - Single large root with 1 or 2 canals
    - In fusion, 2 separate roots may be evident

Radiographic Findings

- Enlarged crown; evidence of clefting may or may not be present
- Single large or partially divided pulp chamber
- Single large root or separate roots

Imaging Recommendations

- Best imaging tool
  - Periapical or panoramic images
  - CBCT useful in complex cases

DIFFERENTIAL DIAGNOSIS

KBG Syndrome

- Named after individuals 1st described with traits
- Rare
- Macrodontia of maxillary central incisors
- Costovertebral anomalies, short stature, ocular and otic abnormalities
- Decreased mental capacity seen in some cases

Ekman-Westborg and Julin Trait

- Sometimes known as multiple **macrodontic multituberculism** (extra tubercles or cusps present on crowns)
- Not syndrome but collection of dental anomalies that may include the following
  - Multiple macrodonts with multituberculism in posterior teeth
  - Single conical molar roots
  - Pulp invaginations and evaginations in premolars

Oculofaciocardiodental Syndrome

- Radiculomegaly, especially canines and premolars
- Delayed eruption
- Oligodontia
- Congenital cataracts, secondary glaucoma, cardiac defects

CLINICAL ISSUES

Treatment

- Recontouring/restoration if esthetics is of concern
- Treatment of malocclusion or periodontal problems caused by crowding, malalignment

DIAGNOSTIC CHECKLIST

Consider

- Consider KBG syndrome or Ekman-Westborg and Julin trait if multiple macrodonts seen without fusion or gemination
- **Tooth count is best way to differentiate** fusion from gemination
- Consider oculofaciocardiodental syndrome if radiculomegaly is present

SELECTED REFERENCES

1. Larhant M et al: Giant canine with dentine anomalies in oculo-facio-cardio-dental syndrome. J Craniomaxillofac Surg. 42(4):321-4, 2014
2. Kumar H et al: KBG syndrome: review of the literature and findings of 5 affected patients. Oral Surg Oral Med Oral Pathol Oral Radiol Endod. 108(3):e72-9, 2009
3. Lucey S et al: Case report: Cone-beam ct imaging in the management of a double tooth. Eur Arch Paediatr Dent. 10 Suppl 1:49-53, 2009
4. Peker I et al: A case of Ekman-Westborg-Julin trait: endodontic treatment of a macrodontic incisor. Oral Surg Oral Med Oral Pathol Oral Radiol Endod. 107(5):e89-92, 2009
5. Veeraiyan DN et al: Dental fusion: a case report of esthetic conservative management. Quintessence Int. 40(10):801-3, 2009
6. Guimarães Cabral LA et al: Double teeth in primary dentition: report of two clinical cases. Med Oral Patol Oral Cir Bucal. 13(1):E77-80, 2008
7. Ezoddini AF et al: Prevalence of dental developmental anomalies: a radiographic study. Community Dent Health. 24(3):140-4, 2007
8. Brancati F et al: KBG syndrome. Orphanet J Rare Dis. 1:50, 2006
9. Nemes JA et al: The Ekman-Westborg and Julin trait: report of a case. Oral Surg Oral Med Oral Pathol Oral Radiol Endod. 102(5):659-62, 2006
10. Favalli O et al: Bilateral twinning: report of case. ASDC J Dent Child. 65(4):268-71, 230, 1998

Microdontia

KEY FACTS

TERMINOLOGY

- Definitions
  - Microdontia: Presence of unusually small tooth or teeth
  - Microdont: Unusually small tooth

IMAGING

- **Maxillary lateral incisor (peg lateral), 3rd molars** most frequently affected
- Presence of abnormally small tooth or teeth
- Panoramic or CBCT will best view 4th molar (supernumerary) microdonts

TOP DIFFERENTIAL DIAGNOSES

- **Down syndrome**
  - Facial features flattened, high-arched palate
  - Prognathism with open bite and macroglossia
  - Dental malformations, including enamel hypoplasia and **microdontia**
- **Pituitary dwarfism**
  - Diminutive stature; sparse, fine hair
  - Delayed eruption &/or shedding of teeth
  - Small jaws with **microdontia** seen in some cases
- **Ectodermal dysplasia**
  - Multiple microdontic teeth with conical crown forms

PATHOLOGY

- Familial
- Local environmental factors may be associated, particularly chemotherapy and radiation at time of development
- **Supernumerary teeth often smaller** than usual
- Presence of peg lateral appears to be autosomal dominant with incomplete penetrance

CLINICAL ISSUES

- **Females have higher frequency** of microdontia
- **Peg lateral**: Maxillary lateral incisor with short, tapering crown
- Restorative or prosthetic treatment for esthetics

(Left) *Periapical radiograph shows a diminutive maxillary lateral incisor ➔. The root is short and tapered, as is the crown. This is the typical appearance of a peg lateral, one of the more common types of microdonts.* **(Right)** *Periapical radiograph shows another maxillary peg lateral ➔. In this example, the root length is normal, but the crown demonstrates the typical conical shape of this type of microdont. Peg lateral is thought to be genetically inherited as an autosomal dominant trait.*

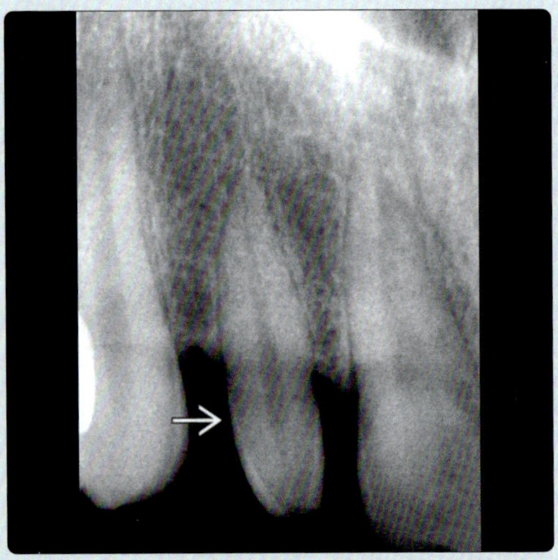

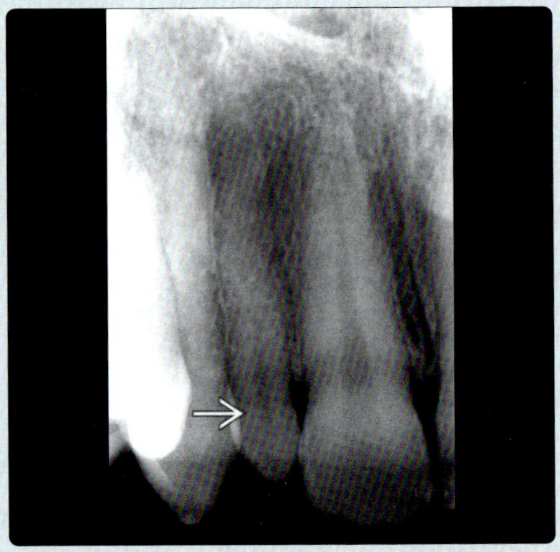

(Left) *Periapical radiograph shows an erupted microdont in the place of the maxillary right 3rd molar ➔. The most distal tooth of a particular type (incisor, premolar, molar) is more likely to be a microdont than the other teeth of that type.* **(Right)** *Sagittal CBCT of the microdontic maxillary 3rd molar is shown. The root exhibits dilaceration superiorly ➔, and there is external root resorption on the maxillary 2nd molar ➔.*

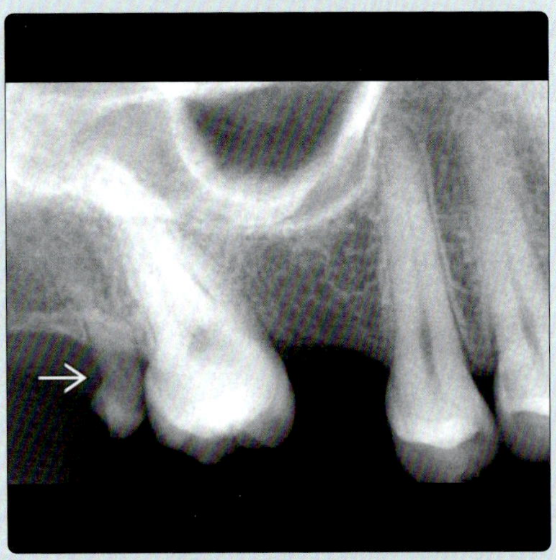

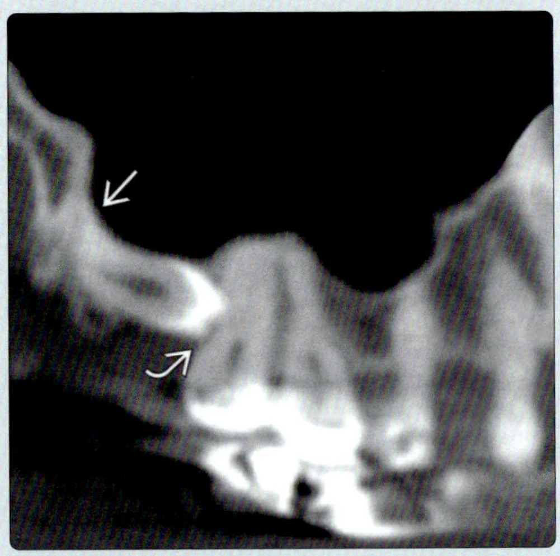

Concrescence

KEY FACTS

TERMINOLOGY

- Definition: Union of 2 or more fully formed teeth by cementum without confluence of dentin

IMAGING

- Difficult to distinguish from teeth that are merely in close proximity
- Obtain **additional 2D projections** at different angles
- CBCT will best show cementum connection
- **Maxilla** > mandible; **posterior** > anterior
- **2nd** and **3rd** molars; **3rd molar** and **supernumerary tooth**
- May involve deciduous or permanent teeth

TOP DIFFERENTIAL DIAGNOSES

- **Fusion**: Union of 2 tooth buds; confluence of dentin
  - Often results in **fusion of roots**
- **Gemination**: Splitting of 1 tooth bud into 2
  - Incomplete separation may result in **joined roots** or single root

PATHOLOGY

- Thought to be result of reparative cementum following inflammation
- Other potential contributing factors
  - Localized trauma
  - Excessive occlusal forces
  - May occur **during** or **following** tooth formation

CLINICAL ISSUES

- May affect treatment planning
  - Extractions: May require surgical extraction
  - Periodontal therapy: Complicates scaling and root planing and exacerbates periodontitis
  - Endodontic treatment: Fused roots often have unusual shapes or curvature
  - Orthodontic treatment: Fused teeth are difficult to move through bone
- Asymptomatic, incidental finding
- Associated tooth may be unerupted

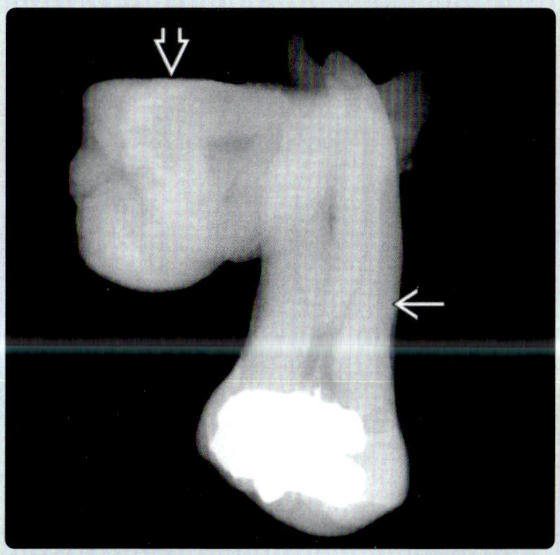
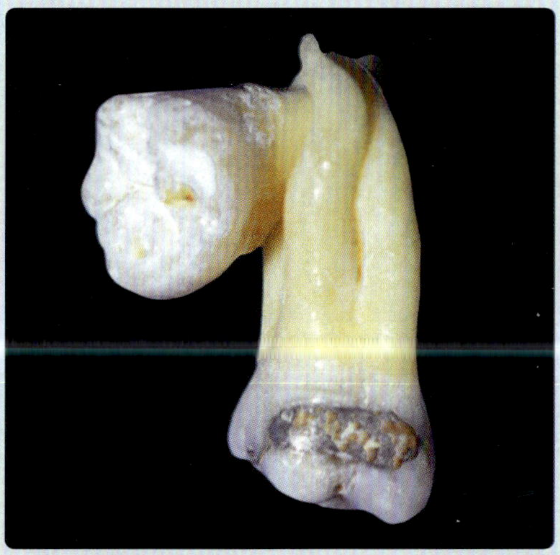

(Left) *Periapical radiograph shows concrescence between a maxillary 2nd molar ➔ and a 3rd molar ➔. The 2nd molar was functional; the 3rd molar was not erupted. From the 2D radiograph alone, concrescence would not necessarily be diagnosed.* **(Right)** *Clinical photograph shows the roots of the 2nd and 3rd maxillary molars fused by cementum. The surgeon was obviously very skilled to remove these 2 teeth as a unit.*

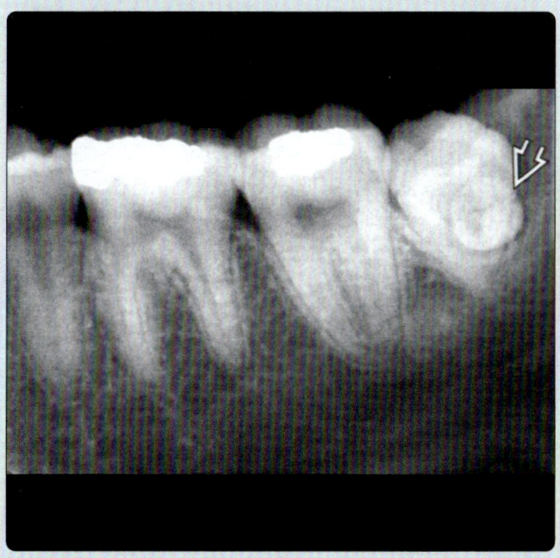
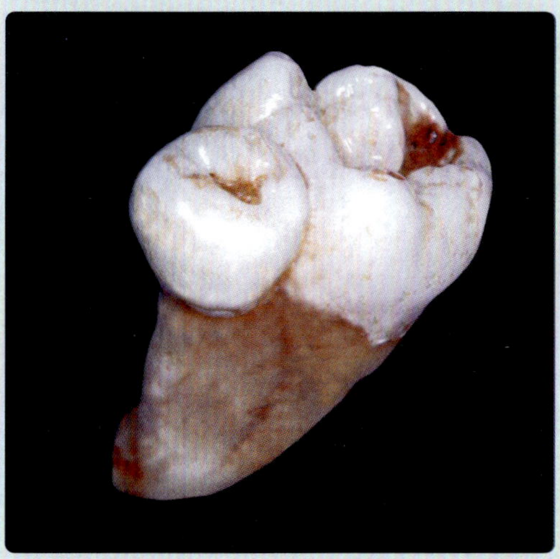

(Left) *Periapical radiograph shows impacted mandibular left 3rd molar with superimposed crown of supernumerary tooth ➔. From this 2D image, it is not possible to determine the exact location of the supernumerary tooth in relation to the 3rd molar or the extent of development of its root.* **(Right)** *Clinical photograph of the extracted tooth from the same patient shows the fully formed supernumerary tooth fused to the 3rd molar by cementum.*

Talon Cusp

KEY FACTS

TERMINOLOGY

- Synonym: Hyperplastic cingulum
- Definition: Well-formed **supernumerary cusp on lingual surface of anterior tooth** extending at least 1/2 distance from cementoenamel junction to incisal edge
    - Said to resemble eagle talon
    - Rare occurrences of facial talon cusps have been reported
    - Classification system is sometimes used

IMAGING

- Superimposition of cusp over other tooth structure
- Smooth outline with **normal enamel and dentin**
- Seen on intraoral, panoramic, or CBCT images
- Pulp extension may not be visible radiographically

CLINICAL ISSUES

- **More common in permanent teeth** than in primary teeth (3:1)
- Prevalence ranges 1-8% in various populations
- **Maxillary laterals incisors (55%)** > maxillary central incisors (33%) > mandibular incisors > maxillary canines
- Often seen in association with other dental anomalies
    - Supernumerary teeth
    - Peg-shaped lateral incisors
    - Impacted teeth
    - Odontomas
    - Dens Invaginatus
- Deep developmental groove may be present between talon cusp and underlying tooth structure
    - May contain pulp extension
    - May require prophylactic treatment (sealant) to prevent dental caries
- Often creates occlusal interference
    - **May expose pulp horn** if removed

(Left) *Periapical radiograph of a maxillary left lateral incisor exhibits a talon cusp ➡ and dens invaginatus ⬅. There is also a prominent lingual cingulum on the maxillary central incisor ⇨. The permanent maxillary lateral incisor is the most commonly affected tooth.* **(Right)** *Sagittal reformat CBCT demonstrates a talon cusp on the left maxillary central incisor ➡. This extra cusp may be creating an occlusal interference. Such cusps must be removed with caution as they may contain a pulpal extension that will be exposed.*

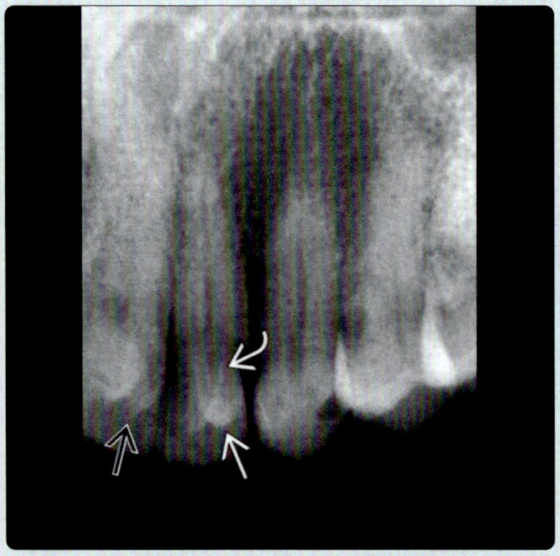

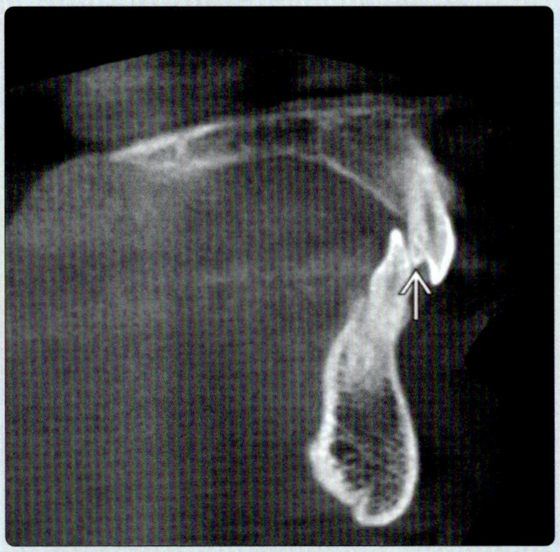

(Left) *3D CBCT of the anterior maxilla viewed from the palatal aspect shows a prominent talon cusp ⇨ on the maxillary left lateral incisor. The dentist had informed the patient that this was a supernumerary tooth.* **(Right)** *Cross section CBCT in the same patient shows the talon cusp contains a pulp canal ➡ that joins the main canal at the level of the cervical margin of the tooth. This presents a challenge for aesthetic recontouring or prosthetic replacement of the crown and endodontic therapy.*

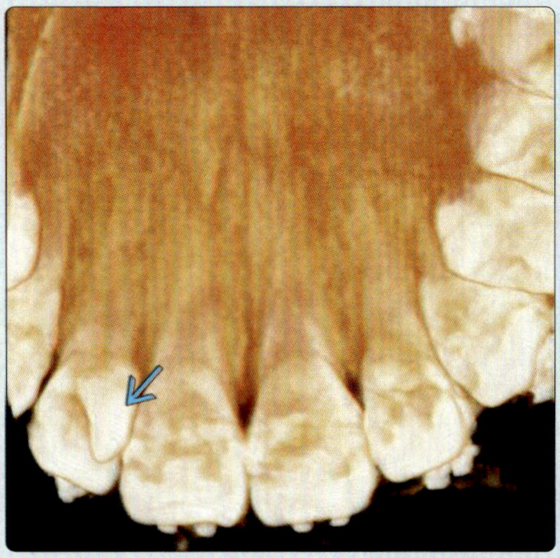

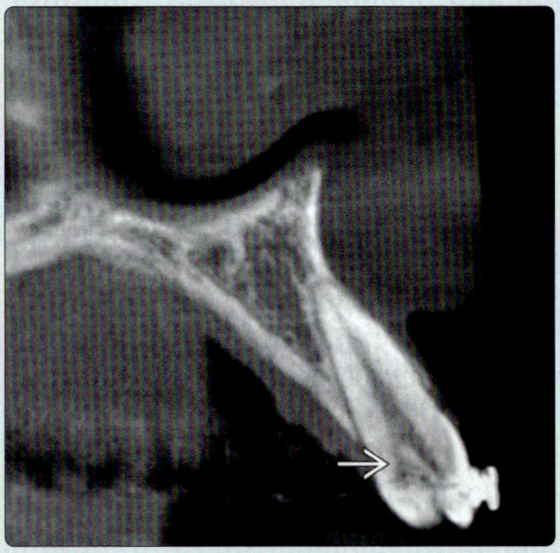

Dens Invaginatus

KEY FACTS

TERMINOLOGY

- Synonym: **Dens in dente** (tooth in tooth)
- Definition: Deep invagination **lined by enamel** in tooth crown or root

IMAGING

- Infolded enamel lining that is more radiopaque than surrounding dental tissues
- Most common in **maxillary lateral incisors** followed by **maxillary central incisors**
- Also seen in **premolars** > **canines** > **molars**
- Ranges from deep cingulum pit to long infolding that extends into root
- **Apical/periradicular radiolucency** sometimes seen
  - Result of inflammatory &/or necrotic changes from carious penetration of deep pit into pulp

PATHOLOGY

- High degree of **familial tendency**
- No specific mode of inheritance identified
- 3 major types (Oehlers classification)
  - **Type I**: Confined to crown
  - **Type II**: Extends apical to cementoenamel junction, ending in blind sac that may or may not communicate with pulp
  - **Type IIIa**: Extends through root and perforates root laterally exhibiting communication with periodontal ligament space
  - **Type IIIb**: Extends through root and communicates with periodontal ligament space at apical foramen

CLINICAL ISSUES

- Prevalence ranges from < 1-10% of all patients
  - White = Asians; uncommon in blacks
- Found incidentally
- Usually asymptomatic unless pulp tissue involved
- Treatment: **Prophylactic sealing or restoration** of deep pit for prevention of caries, root canal therapy, or extraction

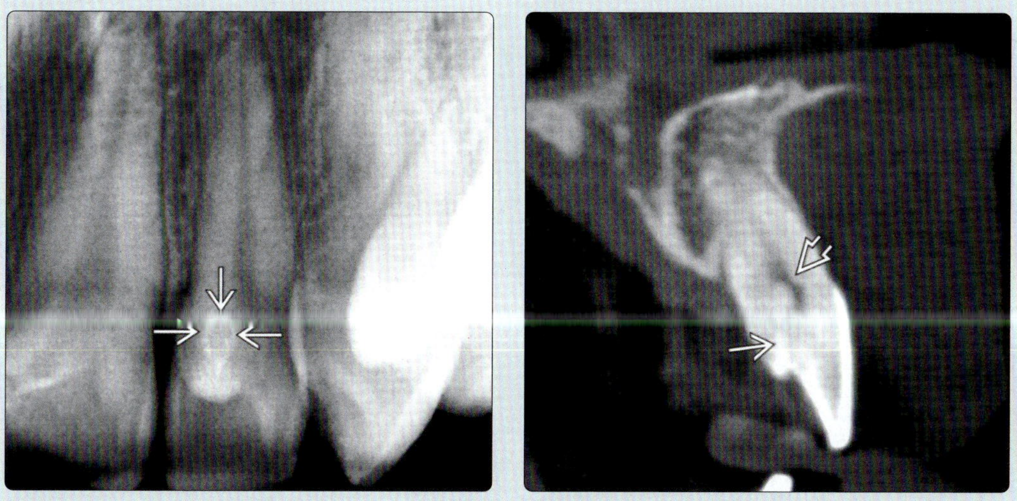

(Left) *Periapical radiograph shows a dens invaginatus presenting as an enamel-lined invagination under the enlarged cingulum of the left lateral incisor. The lateral incisor is the most common location for dens invaginatus.* **(Right)** *CBCT cross-sectional image shows a maxillary central incisor exhibiting dens invaginatus type II. The enamel-lined cavity extends from the pronounced cingulum on the lingual surface superiorly into the pulp chamber.*

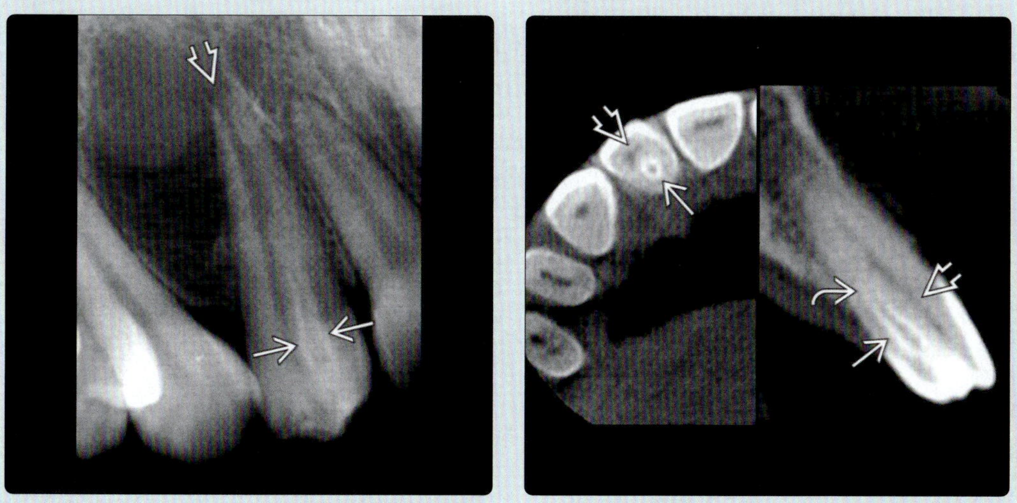

(Left) *Periapical radiograph shows dens invaginatus in the right maxillary lateral incisor. The apex is open, and there is an associated large radiolucency.* **(Right)** *Axial (L) and cross-sectional (R) CBCT images in the same patient show the dens invaginatus located palatally to the normal pulp chamber and canal. The invagination extends radiographically to the midpoint of the root, but clinically, the canal within extended to the apex, making this a type IIIb.*

Enamel Pearls

KEY FACTS

TERMINOLOGY

- Synonyms: Enamel drop, enamel nodule, enamel globule
- Definition: Presence of rounded, 1- to 3-mm **ectopic enamel globule** on **root surface**

IMAGING

- Seen most often on roots of molars: Maxillary > mandibular
  - Permanent molars > primary molars
- Found in furcation or near cementoenamel junction
- Small, well-defined radiopaque nodule

TOP DIFFERENTIAL DIAGNOSES

- Calculus
- Pulp stones
- Supernumerary microdont

PATHOLOGY

- Hertwig epithelial root sheath fails to detach, resulting in ameloblastic differentiation and ectopic enamel formation
- May contain dentin and pulp tissue

CLINICAL ISSUES

- Usually **asymptomatic**
- Prevalence highest in Asians
- Seen in 1-9% of all patients
- Prevents normal periodontal attachment
  - Creates hygiene problems and plaque retention
  - Patients predisposed for localized vertical bone loss
- Can be removed if necessary; if pulp tissue is present, endodontic treatment may be required

DIAGNOSTIC CHECKLIST

- **Calculus** and **pulp stones are less dense**: Compare density to enamel on crown of tooth
  - Changing image angulation will move enamel pearl away from pulp chamber
  - Calculus large enough to be seen on radiograph will be clinically detectable

(Left) *Periapical radiograph shows an enamel pearl ➡ in the furcation of an unerupted left mandibular 3rd molar. It is less common to see a pearl in the mandible than in the maxilla.* **(Right)** *3D reconstructed CBCT of the right mandible viewed from the lingual shows an enamel pearl ➡ in the lingual furcation of the unerupted 3rd molar. The crown exhibits external resorption ⇨.*

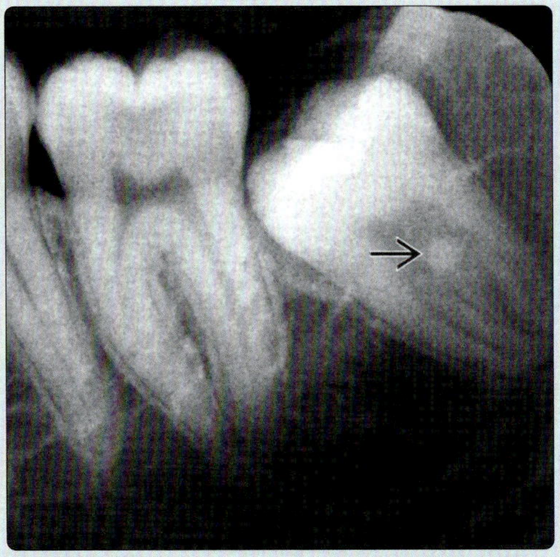

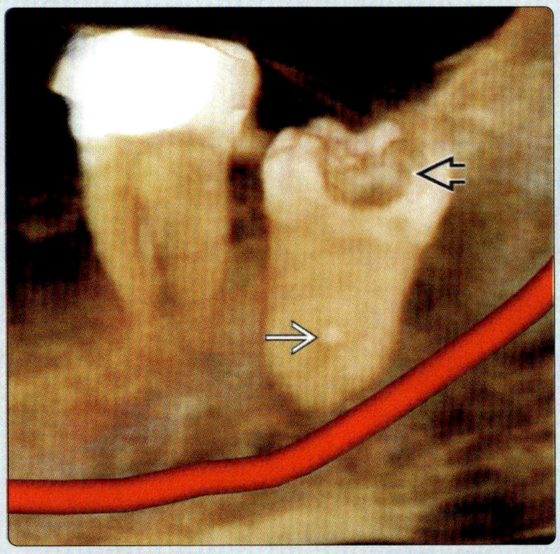

(Left) *Sagittal reformat CBCT shows 2 enamel pearls ➡ in the furcations of a maxillary 1st molar. Note the increased density of the pearl compared to the surrounding dentin and the similarity to the enamel on the crown ⇨.* **(Right)** *Axial CBCT in the same patient shows the 2 enamel pearls ➡ located in the furcations, where the roots stem from the crown of the tooth. This is one of the most common locations to find enamel pearls, which can cause periodontal problems as they prevent normal periodontal attachment.*

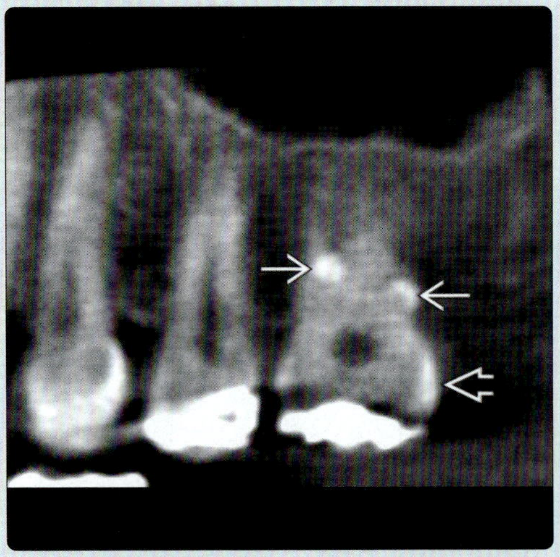

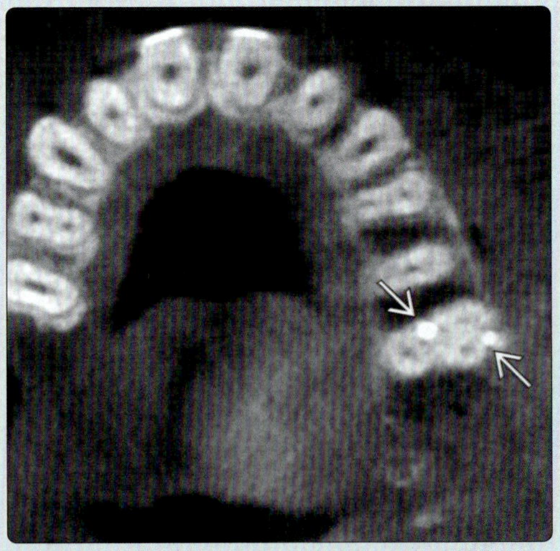

KEY FACTS

TERMINOLOGY

- Definition: **Elongation of pulp chamber** in multirooted tooth with apical displacement of pulpal floor
- **Taurodont** derives from "**bull tooth**"
  - Morphology resembles teeth in ungulates, particularly bulls

IMAGING

- May be unilateral or bilateral
- **Molars** affected more often than premolars
  - **2nd and 3rd molars** often affected more severely than 1st molars
- **Increased distance from cementoenamel junction to root furcation**
- **Short roots**
- Pulp chamber appears **elongated and rectangular**
- 3 classifications of severity of pulpal distortion
  - Hypotaurodontism: Mild
  - Mesotaurodontism: Moderate
  - Hypertaurodontism: Severe
- Elongated pulp chamber + short roots resembling horns is diagnostic

PATHOLOGY

- May occur as **isolated trait** or **in conjunction with syndromes**
- Increased incidence in patients with **cleft palate or lip**
- Failure of Hertwig epithelial sheath to invaginate
- Linked to aberration of *WNT10A* expression

CLINICAL ISSUES

- Clinical **crown appears normal**
- No gender predilection
- ~ 2-3% prevalence in USA
- No specific treatment required
- Locating and obturating pulp canals may be difficult if endodontic treatment is needed
- Asymptomatic

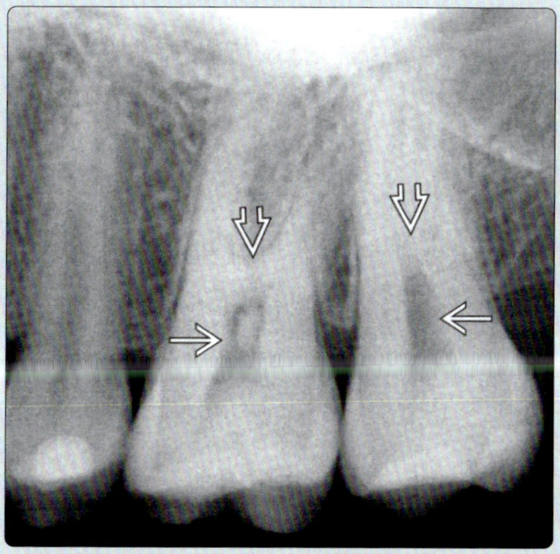

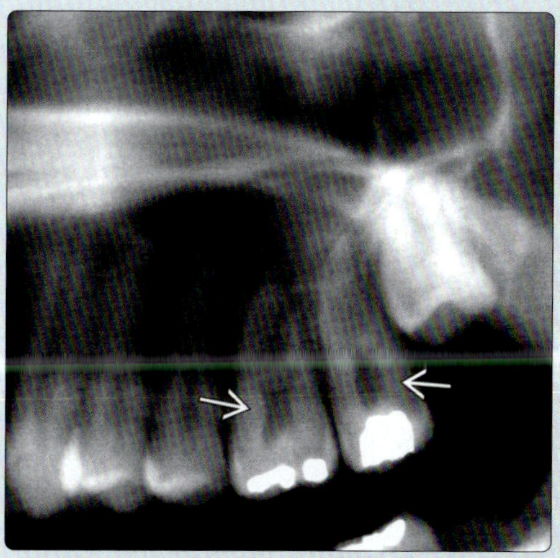

(Left) *Periapical radiograph shows maxillary molar taurodonts with elongated pulp chambers ➡. The root lengths appear relatively normal, but the pulpal floor is positioned more apically than expected ➡. This is an example of hypotaurodontism, the mild form of taurodontism.* **(Right)** *Cropped panoramic image of a 16-year-old male patient exhibits hypotaurodontism of the maxillary molars ➡. There are elongated pulp chambers without typical cervical constriction.*

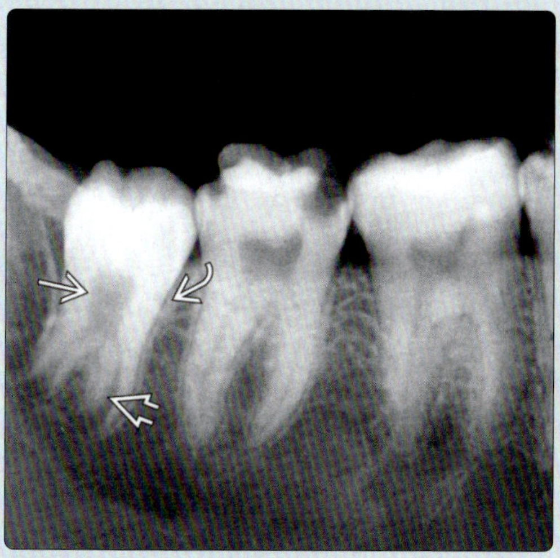

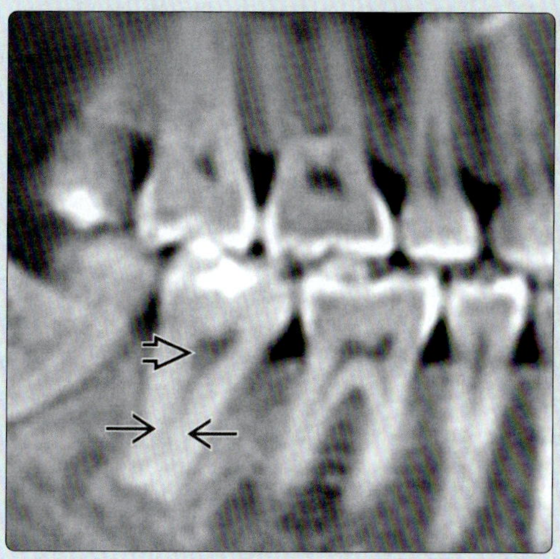

(Left) *Periapical radiograph shows an elongated, rectangular pulp chamber ➡ and short roots in this developing 3rd molar taurodont. Second and 3rd molars are more frequently affected than 1st molars. Note the increased distance between furcation ➡ and cementoenamel junction ➡ compared to the normal 2nd molar.* **(Right)** *Sagittal reformat CBCT shows an elongated pulp chamber ⇨ and very short roots in this 2nd mandibular molar taurodont. Root canals are correspondingly short ⇨.*

Dilaceration

KEY FACTS

TERMINOLOGY

- **Abnormal bend or curve** in tooth root or, less commonly, in crown

IMAGING

- **Root dilaceration** may occur anywhere in dentition
  - Most frequently seen in **permanent maxillary premolar area**
    - Wide range of prevalence (0.42-92%) reported
  - Bend occurs most often in **apical 1/2 of root**
  - Does not affect eruption or tooth function
- **Crown dilaceration** most frequently seen in permanent maxillary incisors followed by permanent mandibular incisors
  - May prevent eruption of tooth
  - Those that erupt are often in labial or lingual position

PATHOLOGY

- **Trauma or injury** to calcified portion of tooth germ
- Frequently follows injury to overlying primary tooth, especially in anterior teeth
  - Usually this type of injury occurs in 4-5 year range
    - Coronal portions of teeth have fully formed
  - Develops secondary to presence of cyst, tumor, or supernumerary tooth
- Some cases appear to be idiopathic

CLINICAL ISSUES

- Root dilaceration is not detected clinically
- Crown dilaceration seen as angular distortion
- Dilacerated root may complicate extraction, endodontic treatment, orthodontic treatment, or preclude use as abutment
- Dilacerated crown may be restored with full-coverage crown to improve esthetics and function
- Grossly deformed teeth may require extraction

(Left) *Periapical radiograph shows the dilacerated roots ⇨ of this permanent mandibular 1st molar. This tooth would pose a challenge for the clinician if root canal treatment or extraction was needed. Note that the crown is clinically normal.* **(Right)** *Periapical radiograph shows a gentle mesial curve ➡ in the apical 1/2 of the root of the maxillary 2nd premolar. It is common to see root curvature but is most often in the distal direction. A mesial curvature such as this is more unusual.*

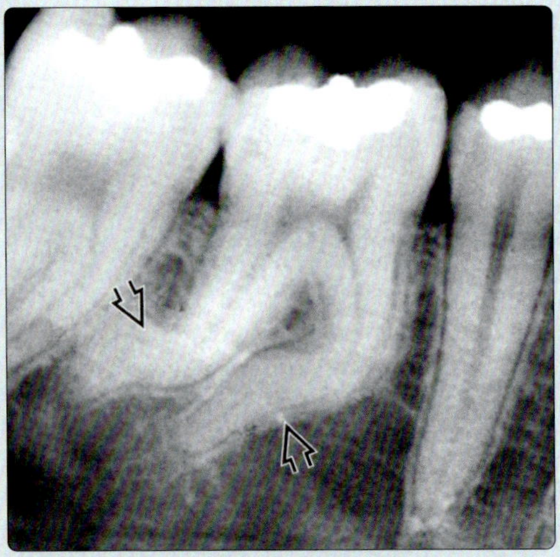

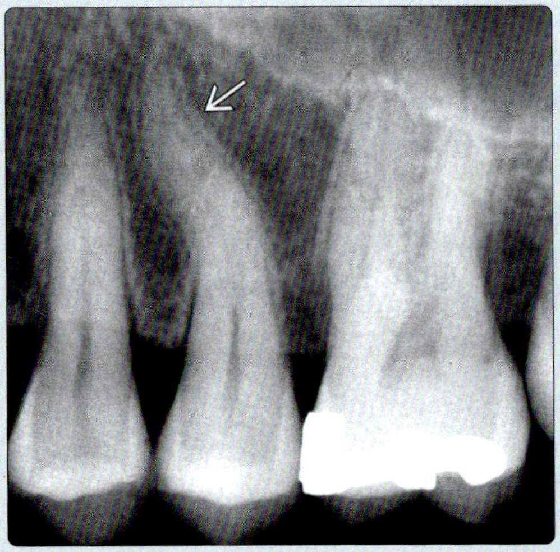

(Left) *Coronal CBCT image shows dilaceration of a maxillary right canine ➡. The dilacerated tip of the canine engaging the lateral cortical wall of the nasal fossa creates a "lock" that makes orthodontic realignment challenging.* **(Right)** *3D lateral CBCT shows acute dilaceration ➡ of the buccal root of the maxillary left first premolar in a young male with history of prior trauma. Note the occlusal table is visible ➡ indicating the crown is also dilacerated. The crown of the second premolar exhibits hypoplastic defects ⇨.*

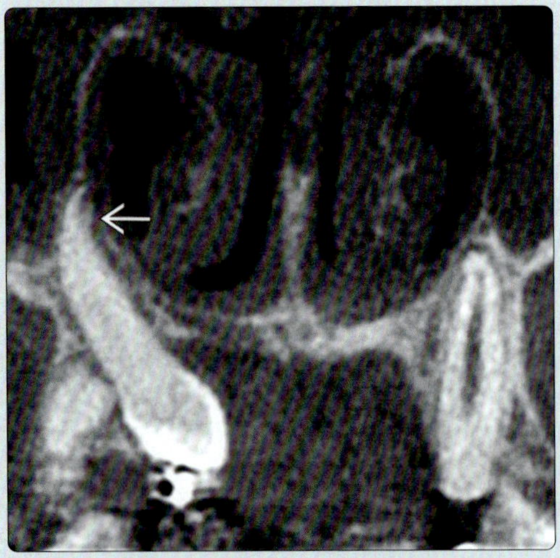

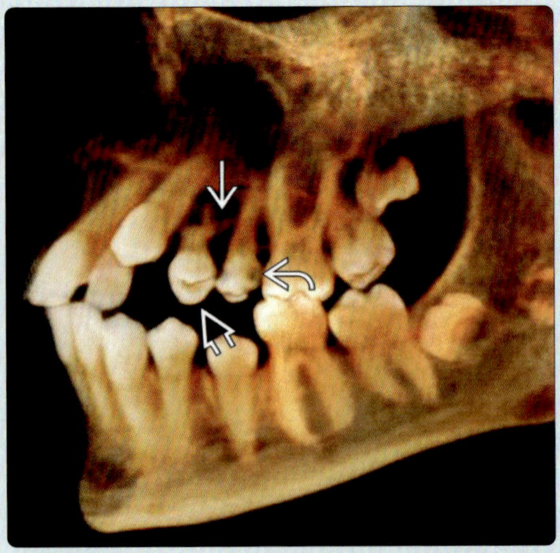

Supernumerary Roots

KEY FACTS

TERMINOLOGY

- Definition: **Increased number of roots** compared to usual anatomic number
  - Radix entomolaris is extra lingual root on mandibular molars
  - Radix paramolaris is extra buccal root on mandibular molars

IMAGING

- May affect any tooth
- Commonly affected teeth: Mandibular canines, mandibular and maxillary premolars, mandibular molars
  - Mandibular 1st premolar affected more often than 2nd premolar (13:1)
  - Incidence of 3rd root on mandibular molars reported to range from 3-40%
    - Radix entomolaris significantly more common
- Extra roots may be fully developed or smaller than normal
- Extra root may be fused to other roots
- Single root may bifurcate at apical 1/2-1/3 of root

TOP DIFFERENTIAL DIAGNOSES

- Hypercementosis
  - Periodontal ligament (PDL) space **continuous around radiopacity**
- Condensing osteitis
  - **Widened PDL space** separates radiopacity from **nonvital** tooth
- Idiopathic osteosclerosis
  - Separated from **vital** tooth by **normal PDL space**

CLINICAL ISSUES

- Clinical crown normal
- Condition detected by imaging
- 3-rooted mandibular 1st molars seen more often in Asians and Native Americans compared to Caucasians
- Presence of supernumerary roots may affect treatment: Orthodontics, endodontics, extractions

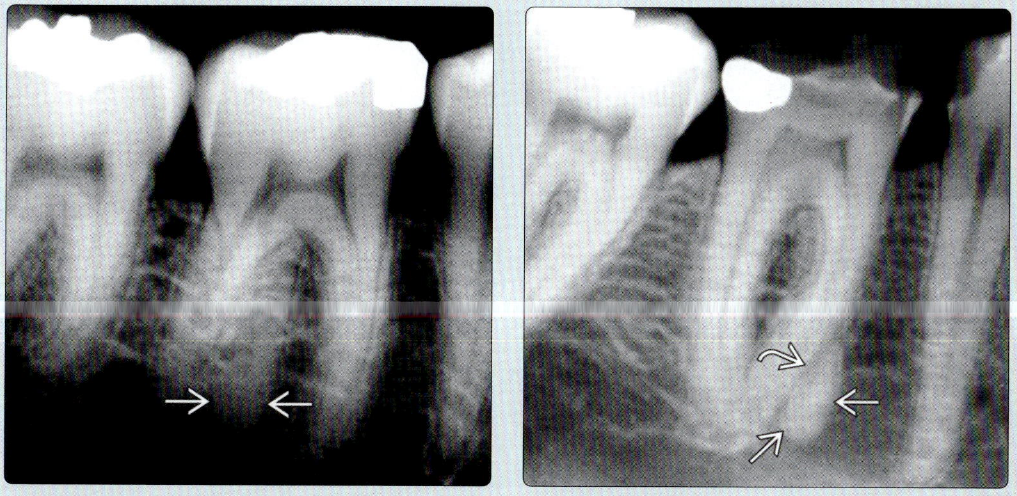

(Left) *Periapical radiograph shows a supernumerary root on this mandibular 1st molar seen between the mesial and distal roots* ➡. **(Right)** *Periapical radiograph shows an extra mesial root* ➡ *on this mandibular 1st molar. Presence of periodontal ligament space* ➡ *on normal mesial root rules out hypercementosis. Periodontal ligament space around radiopacity rules out condensing osteitis and idiopathic osteosclerosis.*

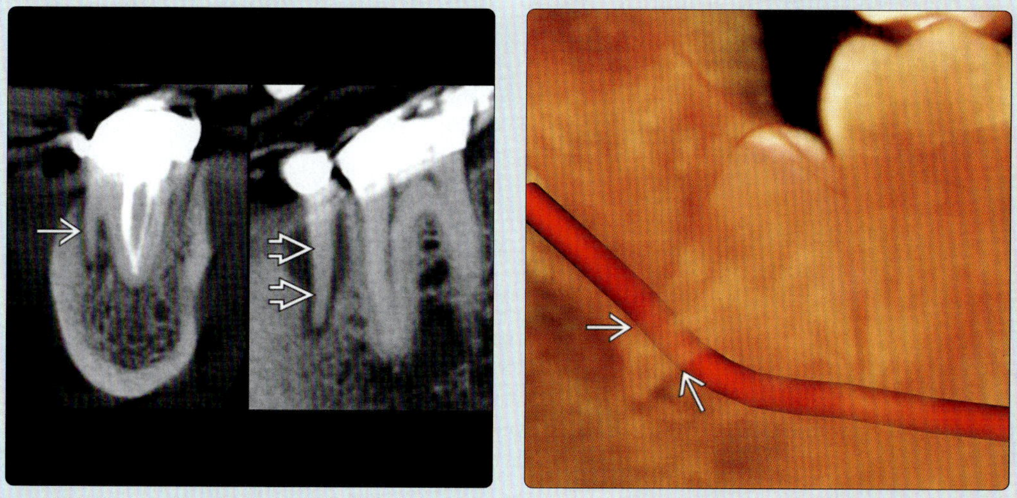

(Left) *Cross section CBCT (L) shows a supernumerary mesial buccal root* ➡ *(radix paramolaris) on a mandibular right 2nd molar, which remained symptomatic following endodontic therapy. Sagittal CBCT (R) shows the slender supernumerary root with evidence of a canal* ➡. **(Right)** *3D CBCT shows a supernumerary lingual root on the mandibular left 3rd molar. The inferior alveolar canal passes between the supernumerary root* ➡ *and the mesial and distal roots, significantly complicating extraction.*

Amelogenesis Imperfecta

KEY FACTS

TERMINOLOGY

- **Definition**: Group of conditions with developmental alterations of enamel structure

IMAGING

- **Hypoplastic types**: Thin radiopaque enamel
- **Hypomaturation types**: Enamel has same radiodensity as dentin
- **Hypomineralized types**: Enamel has same radiodensity as dentin
- **Hypoplastic-hypomaturation types**: Enamel normal to slightly greater density as dentin

TOP DIFFERENTIAL DIAGNOSES

- Environmental defects of enamel
- Dental fluorosis
- Trichodentoosseous syndrome
- Morquio syndrome

PATHOLOGY

- **Hypoplastic types**
  - Generalized or localized pitting
  - Diffuse smooth or rough type
  - Enamel agenesis
- **Hypomaturation types**
  - Enamel soft enough to be punctured with explorer
  - Mottled brown appearance to **snow-capped** patterns
- **Hypomineralized types**
  - Normally shaped teeth with yellow/brown enamel
  - Enamel soft and easily lost
- **Hypomaturation/hypoplastic types**
  - Combination of both forms, may see **large pulp chambers** and varying degrees of **taurodontism**

CLINICAL ISSUES

- Discolored, thin, &/or pitted enamel present **throughout dentition**
- Full crown coverage advisable as soon as practical

(Left) *Cropped panoramic radiograph demonstrates the lack of radiopaque enamel on the teeth. The tapered appearance of the crowns as well as the lack of proximal contacts is due to the relative lack of enamel in this hypoplastic form of amelogenesis imperfecta. This morphology has been likened to the appearance of teeth that have been prepared for prosthetic crowns.* **(Right)** *Bitewing radiograph shows only a very thin layer of radiodense enamel ➡ on the teeth in this hypoplastic form of amelogenesis imperfecta.*

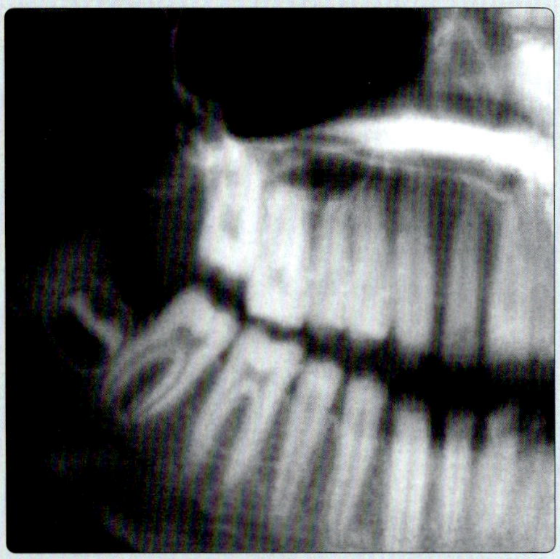

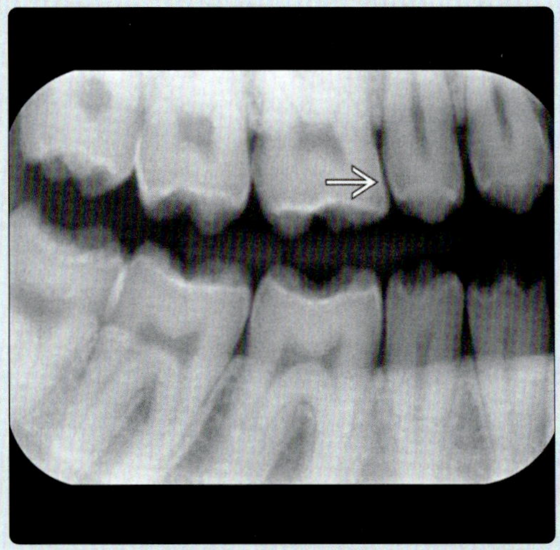

(Left) *Cropped panoramic radiograph demonstrates an anterior open bite associated with the hypomineralized type of amelogenesis imperfecta. The hypomineralized form is characterized by yellow-brown enamel that is easily lost in the most coronal portions of the crown. Loss of enamel is seen on several teeth ➡. Cervical enamel is sometimes retained.* **(Right)** *Periapical radiograph shows mandibular anterior teeth with pitted and irregular enamel ➡ in a patient with the hypomineralized type of amelogenesis imperfecta.*

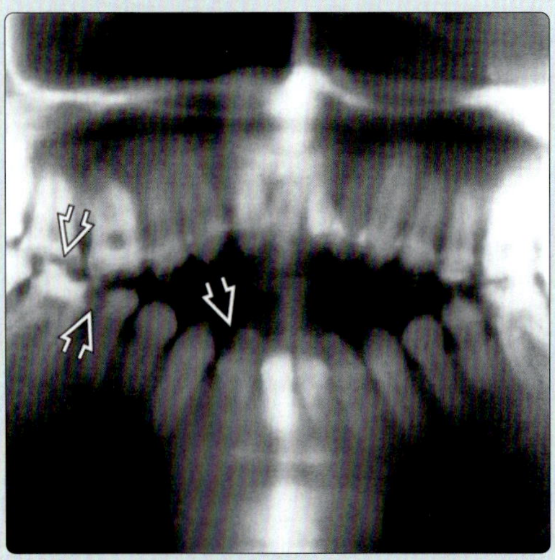

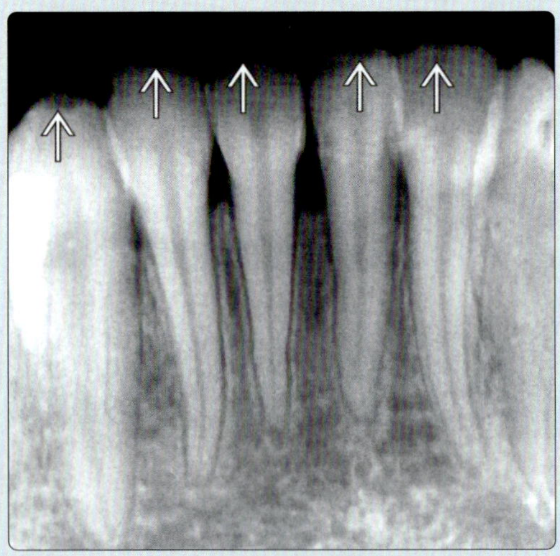

TERMINOLOGY

Definitions

- **Amelogenesis imperfecta**: Group of conditions with developmental alterations of enamel structure
  - **Hypoplastic amelogenesis imperfecta (type I)**: Inadequate deposition of enamel matrix
  - **Hypomaturation amelogenesis imperfecta (type II)**: Defective maturation of normal enamel matrix
  - **Hypomineralized amelogenesis imperfecta (type III)**: Defective mineralization of normal enamel matrix
  - **Hypomaturation/hypoplastic amelogenesis imperfecta (type IV)**: Combination of inadequate deposition and defective maturation of enamel matrix, often with taurodontism

IMAGING

General Features

- Best diagnostic clue
  - Thin enamel
  - Enamel with same radiodensity as dentin
- Morphology
  - **Hypoplastic types**
    - Thin periphery of radiopaque enamel
    - Open contacts: Spaces between teeth
      - Teeth look like they have been **"prepped for crowns"** (dental procedure in which coronal tooth structure is removed in preparation for replacement crown)
    - Unerupted teeth often exhibit resorption
  - Enamel agenesis: No radiopaque enamel overlying dentin
  - **Hypomaturation types**: Enamel has same radiodensity as dentin
  - **Hypomineralized types**
    - Enamel has same radiodensity as dentin
    - Presence of unerupted teeth
    - Worn-down enamel irregular on occlusal surfaces
  - **Hypomaturation/hypoplastic types**
    - Enamel thin but radiopaque **or**
    - Enamel of normal thickness but same radiodensity as dentin
    - Taurodontism sometimes seen

Imaging Recommendations

- Best imaging tool
  - Intraoral imaging: Periapical and bitewing views
    - Best show detail of enamel and dentin
  - Panoramic imaging
    - Demonstrates generalized condition
    - Will show occlusal discrepancies: Anterior open bite
  - CBCT
    - Difficult to discern fine detail: Artifact from metallic restorations may interfere with interpretation

DIFFERENTIAL DIAGNOSIS

Environmental Defects of Enamel

- Hypoplasia
  - Pits or grooves
  - **Large areas of missing enamel**
- Diffuse opacities
  - Normal thickness of enamel
  - Increased opacity with no clear boundary with adjacent enamel
- Demarcated opacities
  - Normal thickness of enamel
  - Increased opacity with distinct boundary with adjacent enamel
- Symmetric distribution corresponding to time of insult
  - First 2 years of life: Seen on anterior teeth and 1st molars
  - 4-5 years of age: Seen on cuspids, premolars, 2nd molars
- Numerous causes
  - Trauma
  - Chemicals or drugs
  - Infectious agents

Dental Fluorosis

- **Hypomineralized enamel**
- White, chalky appearance with possible pitting
- Bilateral, symmetric distribution corresponding to time of exposure

Trichodentoosseous Syndrome

- Autosomal dominant disorder
- Osteosclerosis of base of skull and mastoid process
- Mandible with shortened ramus and obtuse angle
- Kinky hair, brittle nails
- **Thin enamel with same radiodensity as dentin**
- Large pulp chambers, taurodontism

Morquio Syndrome

- Mucopolysaccharidosis type IV
- Patients present frequently with mental disabilities, multiple dysostosis, cardiovascular issues, ocular abnormalities, and dermal thickening
- Dental changes include **generalized enamel hypoplasia** mimicking amelogenesis imperfecta

PATHOLOGY

General Features

- Genetics
  - Majority are autosomal dominant
  - Autosomal recessive: 1 form each of hypocalcified, hypomaturation, hypoplastic types
  - X-linked dominant: 1 form of hypoplastic type
  - X-linked recessive: 1 form of hypomaturation type

Staging, Grading, & Classification

- **Hypoplastic types**
  - Generalized pitted pattern
    - Pinpoint- to pinhead-sized pits scattered across tooth surfaces
    - Does not correlate with pattern of environmental damage
    - Nonpitted enamel is normal
  - Localized pitted pattern
    - Horizontal rows of pits, linear groove, or 1 large area of hypoplastic enamel surrounded by zone of hypocalcification
    - Located in middle 1/3 of buccal surfaces

- Incisal/occlusal areas not affected
  - May affect primary dentition only or both dentitions
  - May affect all teeth in dentition or only isolated teeth
- Diffuse smooth type
  - Smooth, hard, thin layer of enamel on all teeth
  - Small tapered teeth, resulting in open contacts
  - Tooth color ranges from opaque white to translucent brown
- X-linked dominant diffuse smooth type
  - Males: Thin, smooth, shiny enamel on all teeth in both dentitions
  - Females: Vertical grooves of thin enamel alternating with bands of normal enamel
- Diffuse rough type
  - Thin, hard, rough enamel on all teeth
  - Enamel denser than in smooth patterns
  - Small tapered teeth with open contacts
- Enamel agenesis
  - Rare; autosomal recessive
  - Total lack of enamel formation
  - Teeth have shape and color of dentin

- **Hypomaturation types**
  - Pigmented pattern
    - Mottled brown appearance
    - Enamel soft enough to be punctured with explorer
  - X-linked pattern
    - Males
      - Primary teeth are opaque white with translucent mottling
      - Permanent teeth are opaque yellow-white and darken with age
      - Enamel chips off easily and may be pierced with explorer point
    - Females
      - Similar pattern in both dentitions
      - Random asymmetric bands of opaque white enamel and normal translucent enamel
      - May not be obvious under regular lighting; requires transillumination
      - Not apparent on radiographs
  - Snow-capped patterns
    - White opaque enamel on incisal or occlusal 1/4 to 1/3 of crown
    - Both dentitions affected
- **Hypomineralized types**
  - Normally shaped teeth with yellow-orange enamel that becomes stained brown
  - Enamel soft and easily lost
  - Rapid calculus apposition
- **Hypomaturation-hypoplastic types**
  - Hypomaturation-hypoplastic pattern
    - Mottled yellowish enamel of normal thickness
    - Buccal pitting
    - Large pulp chambers
    - Varying degrees of taurodontism
  - Hypoplastic-hypomaturation pattern
    - Thin layer of enamel
    - May see large pulp chambers
    - Varying degrees of taurodontism

CLINICAL ISSUES

Presentation

- Most common signs/symptoms
  - Discolored, thin, &/or pitted enamel present throughout dentition
- Other signs/symptoms
  - Significant wearing of incisal and occlusal surfaces

Demographics

- Epidemiology
  - Frequency reported to range from 1:700 to 1:14,000

Treatment

- Problems include
  - Esthetics
  - Tooth sensitivity
  - Loss of vertical dimension
  - Increased prevalence of caries
  - Anterior open bite
  - Unerupted teeth
- Full crown coverage advisable as soon as practical
- Dentures or overdentures in cases of significant wear or tooth loss
- Esthetic treatment (bonding, veneers) for less severe cases

SELECTED REFERENCES

1. de Santana Sarmento DJ et al: Mucopolysaccharidosis: radiographic findings in a series of 16 cases. Oral Surg Oral Med Oral Pathol Oral Radiol. 120(6):e240-6, 2015
2. Hegde S: Multiple unerupted teeth with amelogenesis imperfecta in siblings. N Am J Med Sci. 4(5):235-7, 2012
3. Atar M et al: Systemic disorders and their influence on the development of dental hard tissues: a literature review. J Dent. 38(4):296-306, 2010
4. Bronckers AL et al: The impact of fluoride on ameloblasts and the mechanisms of enamel fluorosis. J Dent Res. 88(10):877-93, 2009
5. Hart TC et al: Genetic studies of craniofacial anomalies: clinical implications and applications. Orthod Craniofac Res. 12(3):212-20, 2009
6. Ng FK et al: Dental management of amelogenesis imperfecta patients: a primer on genotype-phenotype correlations. Pediatr Dent. 31(1):20-30, 2009
7. Bailleul-Forestier I et al: The genetic basis of inherited anomalies of the teeth. Part 1: clinical and molecular aspects of non-syndromic dental disorders. Eur J Med Genet. 51(4):273-91, 2008
8. Bailleul-Forestier I et al: The genetic basis of inherited anomalies of the teeth. Part 2: syndromes with significant dental involvement. Eur J Med Genet. 51(5):383-408, 2008
9. Barron MJ et al: Hereditary dentine disorders: dentinogenesis imperfecta and dentine dysplasia. Orphanet J Rare Dis. 3:31, 2008
10. Ismail AI et al: Fluoride supplements, dental caries and fluorosis: a systematic review. J Am Dent Assoc. 139(11):1457-68, 2008
11. Poulsen S et al: Amelogenesis imperfecta - a systematic literature review of associated dental and oro-facial abnormalities and their impact on patients. Acta Odontol Scand. 66(4):193-9, 2008
12. Crawford PJ et al: Amelogenesis imperfecta. Orphanet J Rare Dis. 2:17, 2007
13. Hu JC et al: Enamel formation and amelogenesis imperfecta. Cells Tissues Organs. 186(1):78-85, 2007
14. Pemberton TJ et al: Inherited dental anomalies: a review and prospects for the future role of clinicians. J Calif Dent Assoc. 35(5):324-6, 328-33, 2007
15. Santos MC et al: The genetics of amelogenesis imperfecta: a review of the literature. J Appl Oral Sci. 13(3):212-7, 2005
16. Ayers KM et al: Amelogenesis imperfecta–multidisciplinary management from eruption to adulthood. Review and case report. N Z Dent J. 100(4):101-4, 2004
17. Aldred MJ et al: Amelogenesis imperfecta: a classification and catalogue for the 21st century. Oral Dis. 9(1):19-23, 2003

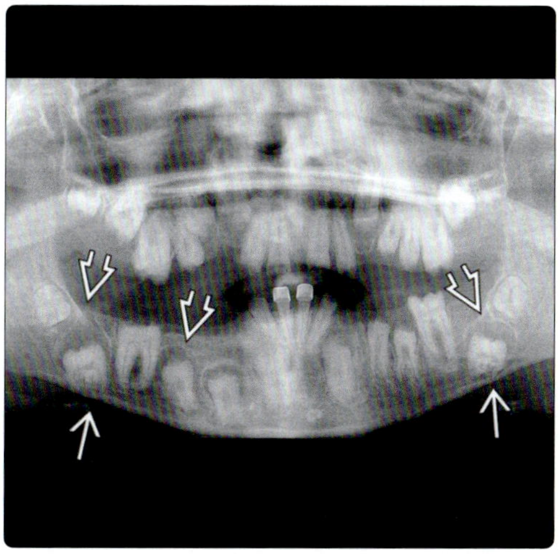

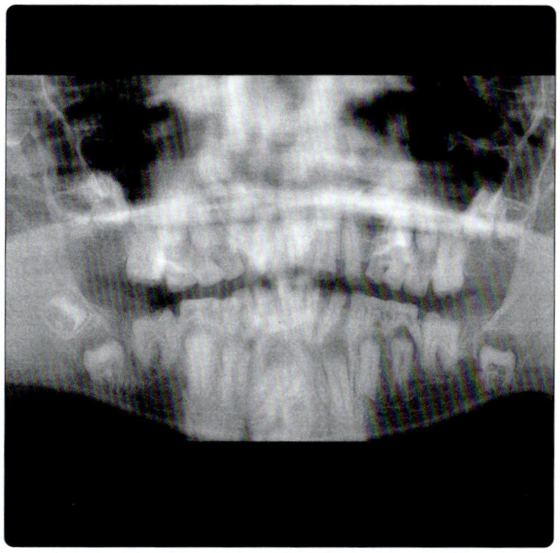

(Left) *Cropped panoramic image of a young male patient shows the hypoplastic variant of amelogenesis imperfecta. There are multiple unerupted teeth with anomalous root formation ➡. Additionally, several of the teeth follicles are mildly enlarged ➡.* **(Right)** *Cropped panoramic image shows the hypoplastic variant of amelogenesis imperfecta in the sister of the previous patient. Both primary and permanent dentition are affected with similar coexisting anomalies.*

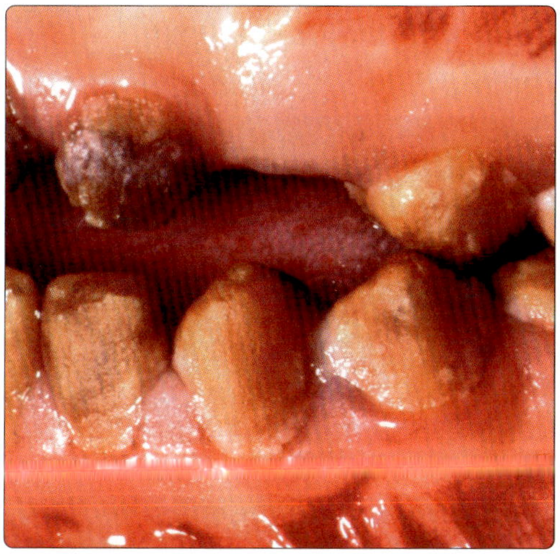

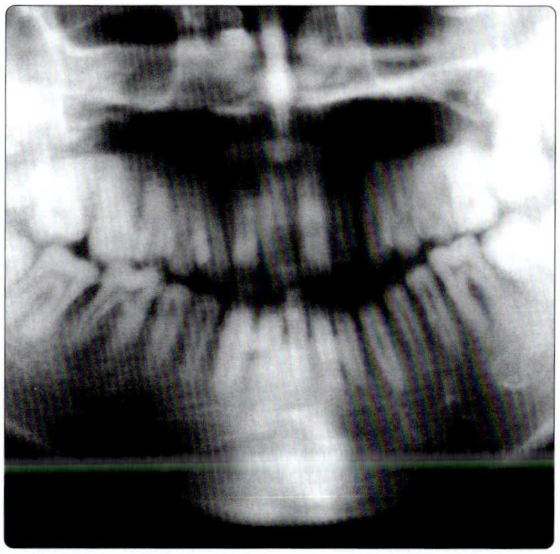

(Left) *Clinical photograph shows the thin, brown, rough surface of the remaining enamel in this patient with hypomineralized amelogenesis imperfecta. Note the anterior open bite.* **(Right)** *Cropped panoramic radiograph shows thin enamel that is the same radiodensity as the adjacent dentin. This feature is seen in both the hypomineralized and hypomaturation types. Teeth appear tapered with loss of proximal contacts.*

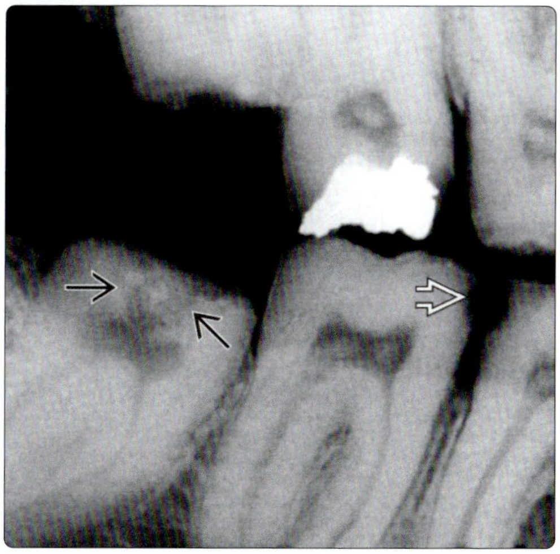

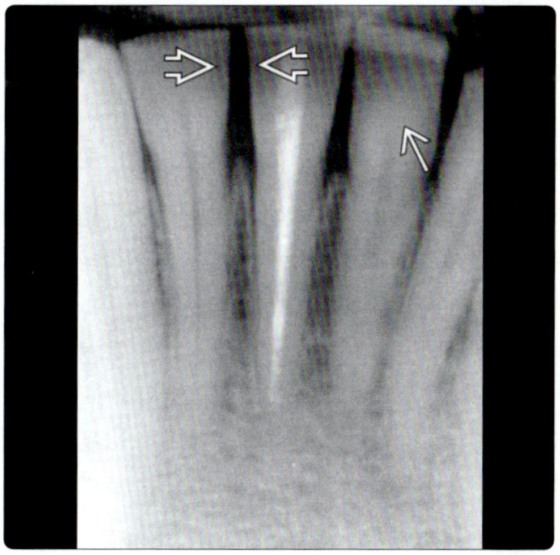

(Left) *Bitewing radiograph shows virtually no remaining enamel on the teeth. Note carious lesions ➡ and apparent resorption of the occlusal surface ⇨ of the partially erupted 3rd molar. Resorption of unerupted teeth is seen in the hypoplastic form of amelogenesis imperfecta.* **(Right)** *Periapical radiograph of the mandibular incisors shows very thin enamel ➡ typically seen in the hypoplastic type of amelogenesis imperfecta. Note the open contacts and square appearance of the left lateral incisor ➡.*

Dentinogenesis Imperfecta

KEY FACTS

TERMINOLOGY

- **Definition**: Hereditary developmental disturbance of dentin **without** accompanying systemic disorder
- **Synonym**: Hereditary opalescent dentin

IMAGING

- Bulbous crowns
- Cervical constrictions
- Thin roots
- **Obliteration of pulp chambers** and root canals
- Shell teeth
  - Rare variant
  - Normal thickness of enamel with extremely thin dentin
  - Very large pulps and canals

TOP DIFFERENTIAL DIAGNOSES

- Osteogenesis imperfecta
- Dentin dysplasia (type II)

PATHOLOGY

- Autosomal dominant
- Occurs in 1:6,000-8,000 whites in USA

CLINICAL ISSUES

- Seen in both dentitions
- Translucent blue to brown teeth
- Enamel separates easily from dentin due to **faulty dentinoenamel junction**
- Most enamel is normal
  - 1/3 of patients also have hypoplastic or hypomineralized enamel
- **Accelerated attrition**
- Periapical inflammatory lesions may result from microexposures of pulp tissue
- Crowning teeth not successful due to cervical fractures
- Overlay dentures successful in some cases

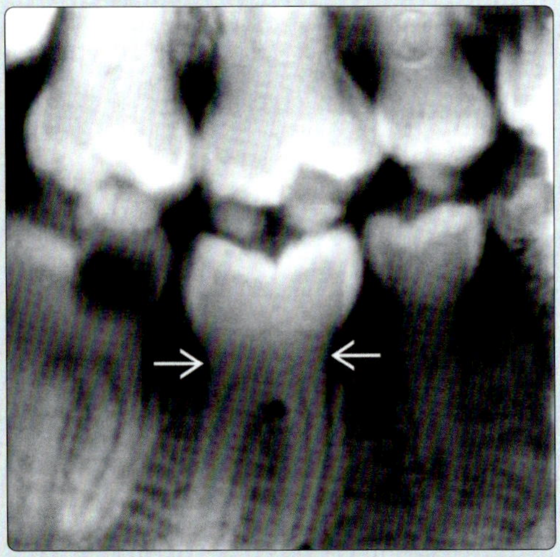
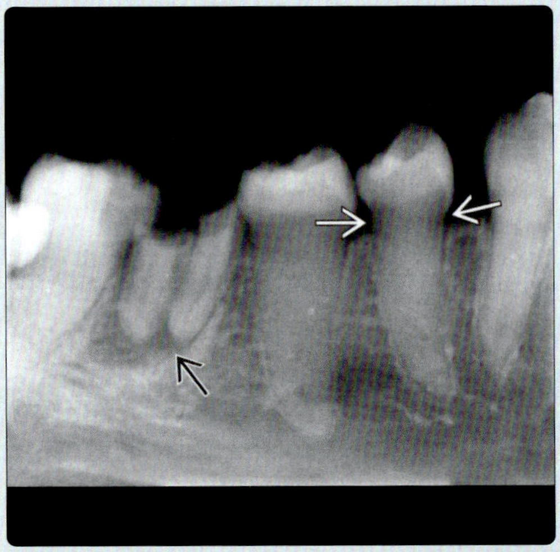

(Left) *Bitewing radiograph shows constricted cervical areas ➡ and short, bulbous crowns in an adolescent with opalescent teeth. Note absence of pulp chambers; however, root canals are visible in the mandibular molars.* **(Right)** *Intraoral periapical image shows a 29-year-old woman with dentinogenesis imperfecta. The mandibular right premolars exhibit constriction of the cervical aspects of the roots ➡ and calcified pulps. The mandibular right molar has unrelated severe caries with apical periodontitis ⇨.*

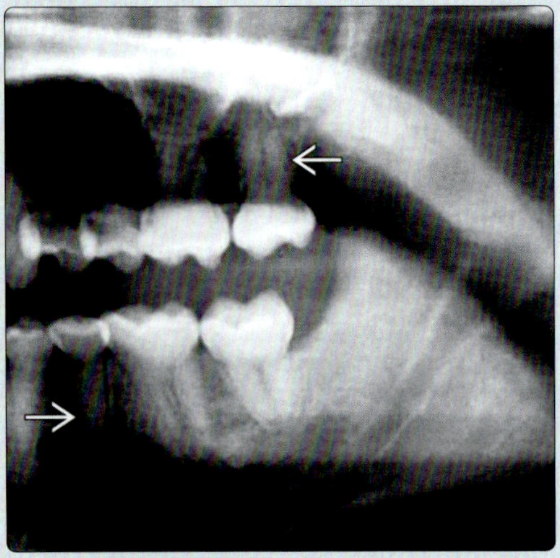
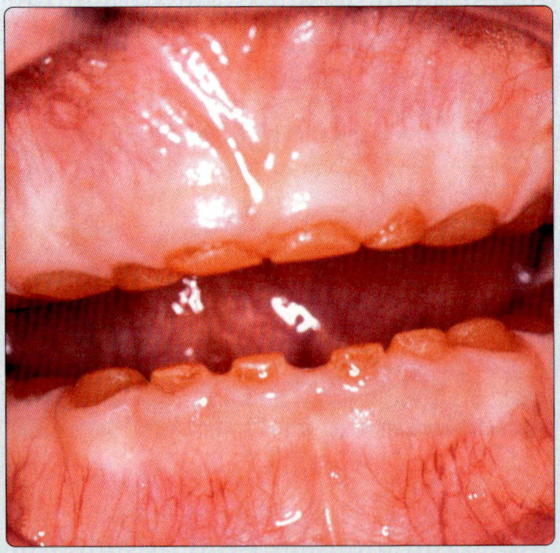

(Left) *Cropped panoramic radiograph shows the bulbous crown shape and absence of pulp chambers and canals typical of dentinogenesis imperfecta. Roots are thin and tapered ➡.* **(Right)** *Clinical photograph shows the translucent brown hue of the remaining teeth in this 6-year-old patient with dentinogenesis imperfecta. Because the enamel is lost due to the faulty dentinoenamel junction, the teeth are subject to pronounced attrition, even at this young age.*

TERMINOLOGY

Synonyms

- Hereditary opalescent dentin

Definitions

- Hereditary developmental disturbance of dentin **without** accompanying systemic disorder

IMAGING

General Features

- Best diagnostic clue
  - Bulbous crowns
  - Cervical constrictions
  - Thin roots
  - **Obliteration of pulp chambers and root canals**
- Morphology
  - Shell teeth
    - Rare variant
    - Normal thickness of enamel with extremely thin dentin
    - Very large pulps and canals
    - Seen more often in primary dentition

DIFFERENTIAL DIAGNOSIS

Osteogenesis Imperfecta

- Inherited disorder of impaired collagen maturation
- Deformities in long bones
- Multiple fractures
- Blue sclera
- Opalescent teeth
- Multiple clinical types depending on clinical presentation and phenotypic characteristics

Dentin Dysplasia (Type II Primarily)

- Affected **primary teeth** resemble dentinogenesis imperfecta
  - Opalescent dentin
  - Bulbous crowns with cervical constriction
  - Thin roots
  - Early obliteration of pulp chamber
- **Permanent teeth** with dentin dysplasia appear **clinically normal**

Tetracycline Staining

- Yellow to dark brown or blue appearance of teeth
- Fluoresce yellow in ultraviolet light
- Severity depends on timing, dose, and duration of drug use

PATHOLOGY

General Features

- Genetics
  - Autosomal dominant
  - Occurs in 1:6,000-8,000 whites in USA
  - Defects linked to *DSPP* gene (4q22.1)
- Histology
  - Short, misshapen dentin tubules throughout dentin
  - Dentin normal near enamel junction

Staging, Grading, & Classification

- **Type I (Shields)**: Defects associated with osteogenesis imperfecta
- **Type II (Shields)**: Defects **not** associated with osteogenesis imperfecta
- **Type III (Shields)**: "Brandywine" type
  - Found in people originating from southern Maryland
  - Opalescent appearance in both dentitions
  - Enamel often pitted
  - Permanent teeth exhibit bulbous crowns
  - Multiple pulp exposures in primary teeth
    - Larger than normal pulps vs. obliterated pulps
  - Variations in tooth appearance within individuals
- Alternate Online Mendelian Inheritance in Man (OMIM) classification system is also used

CLINICAL ISSUES

Presentation

- Most common signs/symptoms
  - Seen in both dentitions
    - Primary dentition may be more severely affected than permanent
  - Translucent blue to brown discoloration
  - Enamel separates easily from dentin
    - Most enamel is normal
    - **Dentinoenamel junction is faulty**
    - 1/3 of patients also have hypoplastic or hypomineralized enamel
- Other signs/symptoms
  - Accelerated attrition
  - Periapical inflammatory lesions from microexposures of pulp tissue
  - Low susceptibility to dental caries

Demographics

- Ethnicity
  - Whites with English or French ancestry
  - Stems from communities near English Channel

Treatment

- Entire dentition at risk
- Full crown coverage may not be successful due to cervical fractures
- Overlay dentures successful in some cases

SELECTED REFERENCES

1. Kawashima N et al: Odontoblasts: Specialized hard-tissue-forming cells in the dentin-pulp complex. Congenit Anom (Kyoto). 56(4):144-53, 2016
2. de La Dure-Molla M et al: Isolated dentinogenesis imperfecta and dentin dysplasia: revision of the classification. Eur J Hum Genet. 23(4):445-51, 2015
3. Barron MJ et al: Hereditary dentine disorders: dentinogenesis imperfecta and dentine dysplasia. Orphanet J Rare Dis. 3:31, 2008
4. Hart PS et al: Disorders of human dentin. Cells Tissues Organs. 186(1):70-7, 2007
5. Kim JW et al: Hereditary dentin defects. J Dent Res. 86(5):392-9, 2007
6. Beattie ML et al: Phenotypic variation in dentinogenesis imperfecta/dentin dysplasia linked to 4q21. J Dent Res. 85(4):329-33, 2006
7. Sánchez AR et al: Tetracycline and other tetracycline-derivative staining of the teeth and oral cavity. Int J Dermatol. 43(10):709-15, 2004
8. Malmgren B et al: Assessment of dysplastic dentin in osteogenesis imperfecta and dentinogenesis imperfecta. Acta Odontol Scand. 61(2):72-80, 2003

Dentin Dysplasia

KEY FACTS

TERMINOLOGY

- **Definition**: Autosomal dominant disorder characterized by normal enamel but atypical dentin and pulpal dysmorphology

IMAGING

- **Type I**
  - Ranges from no pulp chambers to crescent- or chevron-shaped
  - Short roots
  - No apparent root canals
  - 20% have associated periapical radiolucencies **without evident caries**
- **Type II**
  - Enlarged pulp chambers (thistle tube appearance)
  - Multiple **pulp stones**
  - In milder forms stones in canals may give appearance of water-over-rocks
  - Thin root canals

TOP DIFFERENTIAL DIAGNOSES

- Dentinogenesis imperfecta
- Fibrous dysplasia of dentin (rare)
- Pulpal dysplasia (rare)
- Radiation therapy-induced changes

CLINICAL ISSUES

- **Type I** ("rootless teeth")
  - Clinically normal teeth
  - Both dentitions affected; prevalence is 1:100,000
  - Reduced strength of roots leading to root fracture
- **Type II**
  - Normal root lengths
  - Primary dentition resembles dentinogenesis imperfecta
  - Permanent teeth normal clinically
- **Treatment**
  - Good oral hygiene to prevent bone loss in type I
  - Aggressive caries prevention

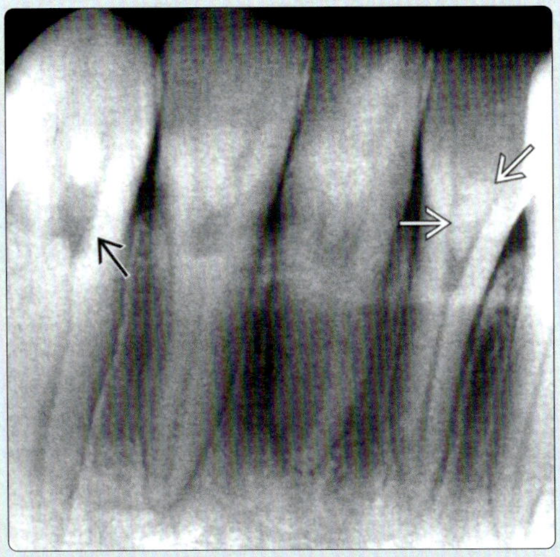

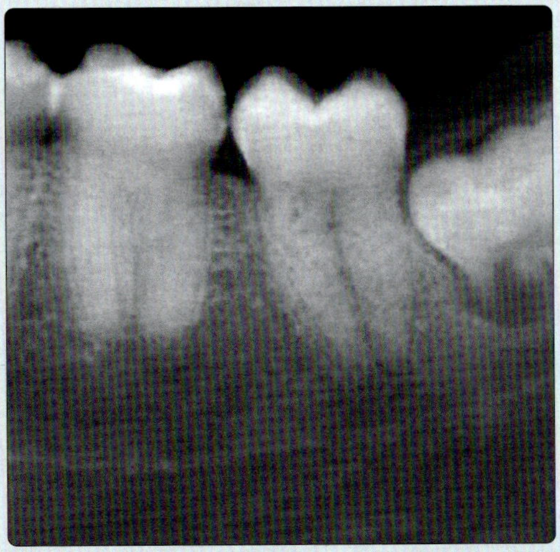

(Left) *Periapical radiograph demonstrates the enlarged pulp chambers ⇨ with multiple pulp stones ➡ in a patient with type II dentin dysplasia. Both father and son have the disorder.* **(Right)** *Periapical radiograph of a 16-year-old boy with dentin dysplasia type I is shown. Note that the pulp chambers and canals are severely diminished if not totally absent in the 1st and 2nd mandibular molars, as was the case in all of his dentition.*

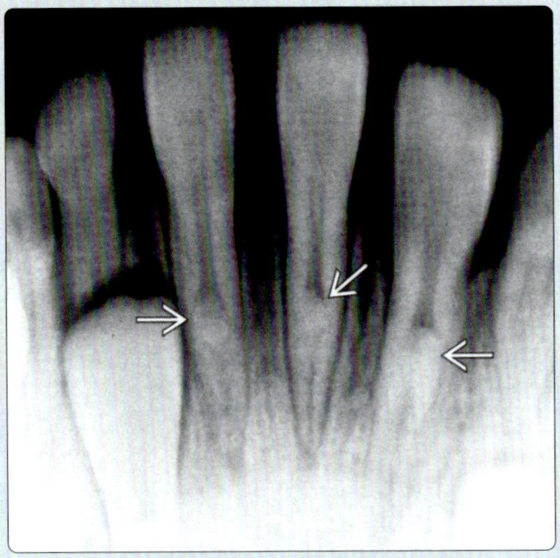

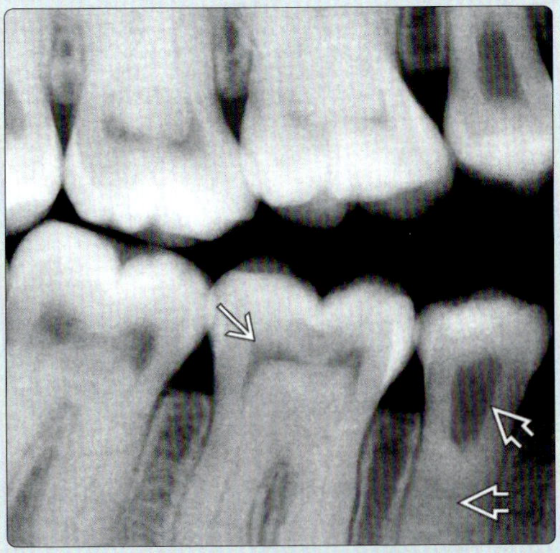

(Left) *Periapical radiograph shows a primary dentition with stone-like formations in the root canals ➡, giving the water-over-rocks appearance seen in milder forms of type II dentin dysplasia.* **(Right)** *Bitewing radiograph shows chevron-shaped pulp chambers in the molars ➡ often associated with type I, but the premolar has an enlarged chamber with a thin canal ➡ creating the so-called thistle tube appearance of type II dentin dysplasia. Root length was normal.*

Regional Odontodysplasia

KEY FACTS

TERMINOLOGY

- Definition: **Localized**, noninherited developmental abnormality of enamel, dentin, and pulp
- Synonym: **Ghost teeth**

IMAGING

- Extremely thin enamel and dentin surrounding enlarged pulp
- **Lack of radiographic contrast between enamel and dentin**
- Short roots, open apices
- Surrounding alveolar bone often less dense than other areas

TOP DIFFERENTIAL DIAGNOSES

- Compound odontoma prior to complete mineralization
- Dentinogenesis imperfecta, dentin dysplasia types I and II, rickets, amelogenesis imperfecta, ectodermal dysplasia, hypophosphatasia, and segmental odontomaxilla dysplasia

PATHOLOGY

- Primarily idiopathic
- Occasionally associated with other pathoses, such as ectodermal dysplasia, hypophosphatasia, neurofibromatosis, vascular nevi of head and neck

CLINICAL ISSUES

- Focal area with several adjacent teeth affected
- Involvement of more than 1 quadrant is rare
- Discovered at 2-4 and 7-11 years of age
- Slight female predilection of 1.4:1
- Maxilla > mandible (2.5:1), anterior > posterior
- Teeth often fail to erupt
- If erupted, crowns are small, irregular, rough, yellow-brown
- Seen in either primary or permanent dentitions
- Treatment
    - Retention of teeth to preserve alveolar ridge
    - Unsalvageable and unerupted teeth extracted after skeletal growth completed

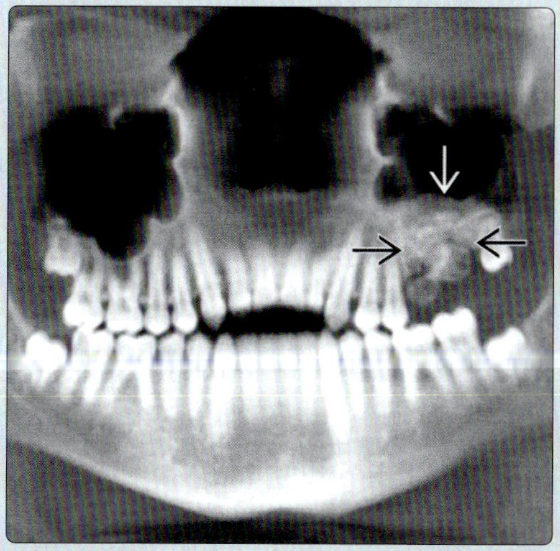

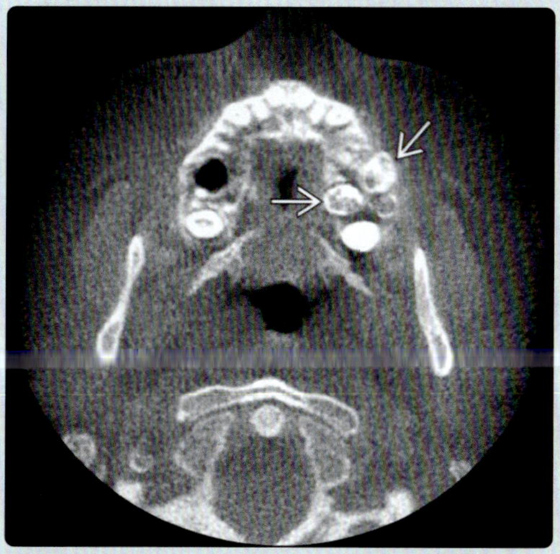

(Left) *Panoramic reformat CBCT shows regional odontodysplasia in the left maxillary molar region ⇨. Note the teeth appear indistinct with little radiodensity compared to their normal counterparts. The antral mucosa is thickened in the area of the affected teeth ➡. (Courtesy E. Parks, DDS.)* **(Right)** *Axial CBCT of the same patient demonstrates the thin enamel and dentin in the affected teeth ➡. (Courtesy E. Parks, DDS.)*

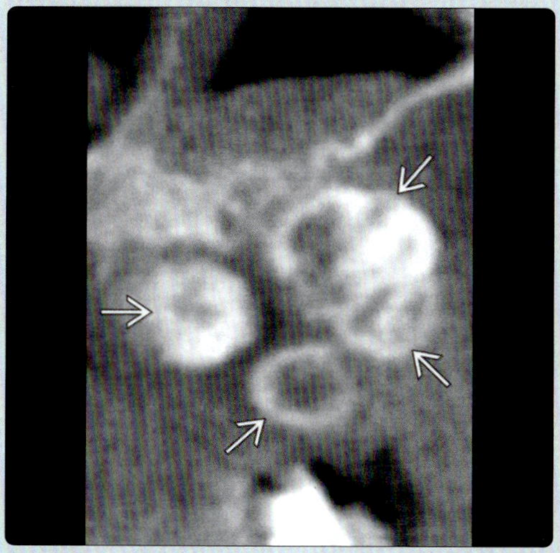

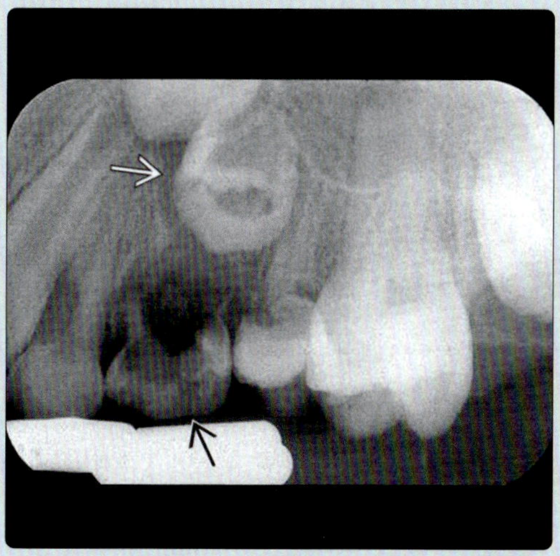

(Left) *Coronal CBCT in the same patient shows that there also appear to be supernumerary teeth that are similarly affected. Four crowns can be counted in an area where there should only be 2 ➡. (Courtesy E. Parks, DDS.)* **(Right)** *Periapical radiograph shows regional odontodysplasia of the maxillary left premolars. The contralateral premolars exhibited normal coronal and root development. Note the shell-like appearance of the 1st premolar ➡. The primary 1st molar has severe caries involvement ⇨.*

Segmental Odontomaxillary Dysplasia

KEY FACTS

TERMINOLOGY

- Segmental odontomaxillary dysplasia: Developmental abnormality of bone of unknown etiology, unilaterally affecting maxilla, teeth, and associated gingiva
- Synonym: Hemimaxillofacial dysplasia

IMAGING

- Localized, unilateral enlargement of maxilla with teeth abnormalities and vertically oriented trabeculae
- Increased density of maxillary alveolar bone with vertically oriented coarse trabeculae; bone may appear as ground-glass
- Teeth may be missing (frequently premolars) or have abnormal or delayed root development
- Thin, vertical radiolucencies may represent nutrient canals

TOP DIFFERENTIAL DIAGNOSES

- Fibrous dysplasia
- Regional odontodysplasia
- Segmental hemifacial hyperplasia
- Gingival fibromatosis

CLINICAL ISSUES

- Asymptomatic unilateral enlargement of maxilla with absent premolars and retained deciduous teeth
- Facial cutaneous lesions: Becker nevus, hypo- and hyperpigmentation
- Facial hypertrichosis, facial asymmetry
- 5-27 years; usually diagnosed in 1st decade
- M > F; some report M = F
- Removal of nonrestorable teeth; orthodontic treatment &/or prosthetic recontouring of teeth to restore form and function
- Nonprogressive; prognosis excellent

DIAGNOSTIC CHECKLIST

- Consider: Definitive treatment should be delayed until end of somatic growth

(Left) *Sagittal CBCT reformat in an 8-year-old girl shows ↑ density of the left maxilla with linear radiolucencies →, possibly representing nutrient canals, and abnormal resorption of the deciduous canine → and 1st molar →. Features are consistent with segmental odontomaxillary dysplasia (SOD).* **(Right)** *Coronal CBCT in same patient shows ↑ width of left maxilla →. Developing 1st premolar → is displaced palatally and is smaller than right →. 2nd premolar was missing. Left 1st deciduous molar → is larger than right →.*

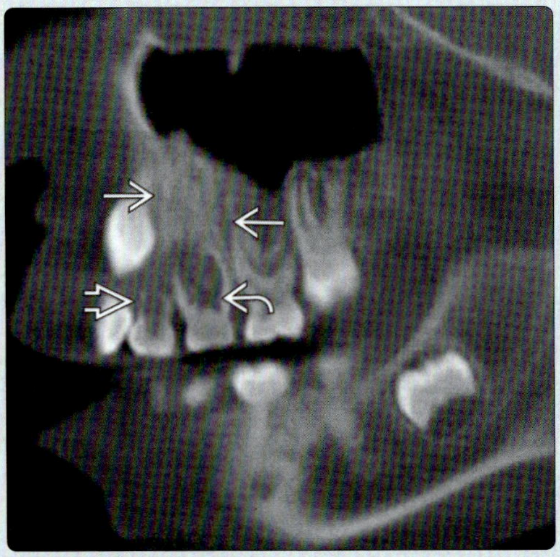

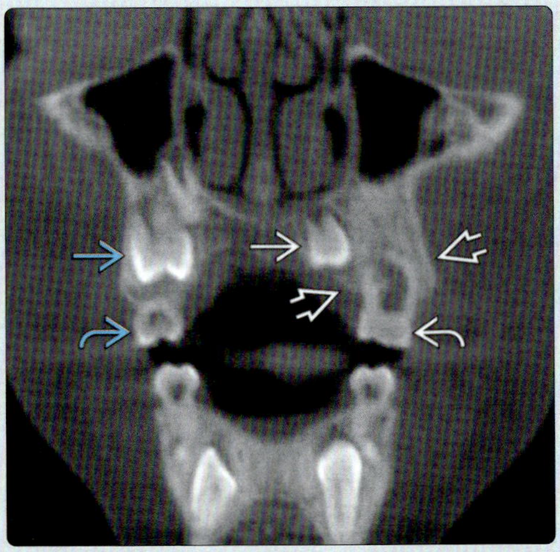

(Left) *Cropped panoramic radiograph in a 26-year-old woman shows increased density → of the alveolar bone in the right maxillary premolar area. There is a radiolucency → between the deciduous 1st molar and the canine suggestive of a cleft. Clefting has been reported in other cases. Both premolar teeth are missing.* **(Right)** *Photograph of the same patient shows commissural lip clefting → and facial hyperpigmentation →, which are frequently associated with SOD. Hypertrichosis was also present.*

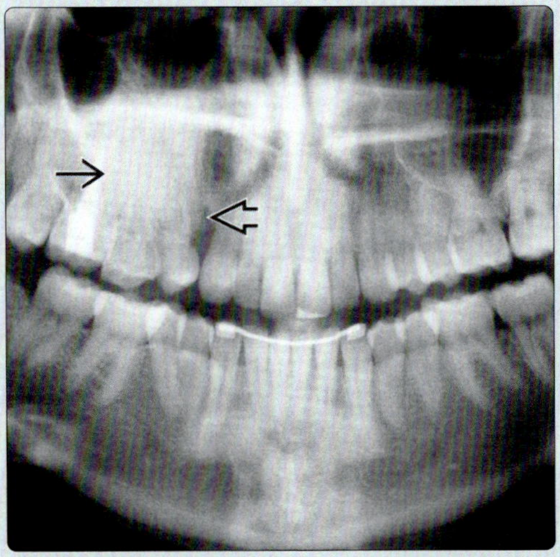

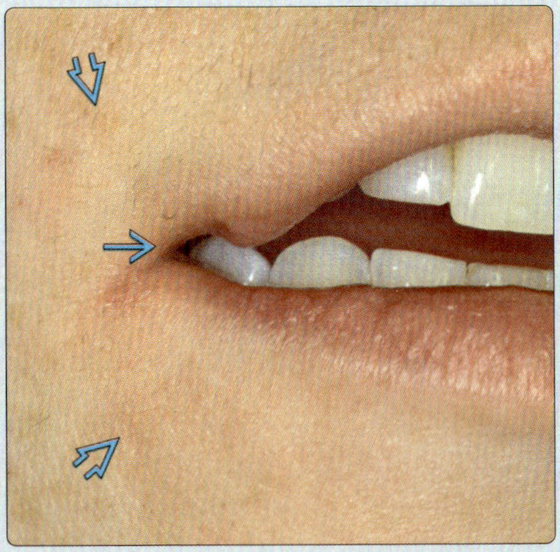

TERMINOLOGY

Abbreviations

- Segmental odontomaxillary dysplasia (SOD)

Synonyms

- Hemimaxillofacial dysplasia
- **HATS**: **H**emimaxillofacial enlargement, **a**symmetry of face, **t**eeth abnormalities, **s**kin findings

Definitions

- Developmental abnormality of bone of unknown etiology, unilaterally affecting maxilla, teeth, and associated gingiva

IMAGING

General Features

- Best diagnostic clue
  - Unilateral enlargement of maxilla with teeth abnormalities and vertically oriented trabeculae
- Location
  - Maxilla: Unilateral; right and left side equally affected
  - May extend from canine eminence to tuberosity

Radiographic Findings

- Intraoral plain film
  - Increased density of maxillary alveolar bone with vertically oriented, coarse trabeculae; bone may appear as ground-glass
  - Thin, vertical radiolucencies may be seen within dense bone, possibly representing nutrient canals
  - Teeth may be missing (frequently premolars) or have abnormal or delayed root development
  - Deciduous teeth may be significantly or abnormally resorbed and larger than contralateral side

CT Findings

- CBCT
  - Buccal and palatal expansion well demonstrated
  - May see decrease in size of maxillary sinus

DIFFERENTIAL DIAGNOSIS

Fibrous Dysplasia

- Unilateral bony expansion of maxilla or mandible
- Bone may appear as ground-glass
- Teeth not usually affected or missing
- Expansion is progressive

Regional Odontodysplasia

- Localized disturbance of teeth which appear ghost-like
- Associated bone not affected or expanded

Segmental Hemifacial Hyperplasia

- Not associated with dense bone or vertically oriented trabeculae
- Teeth may be enlarged, and deciduous teeth may prematurely exfoliate

Gingival Fibromatosis

- Overgrowth (hyperplasia) of gingiva ± syndromes
- Usually generalized
- Associated bone not affected or expanded

PATHOLOGY

General Features

- Etiology
  - Unknown but several theories
    - Developmental disturbance in utero, developmental defect of 1st and 2nd branchial arches, viral or bacterial infection of maxillary division of CNV

Staging, Grading, & Classification

- Classification into 2 major types suggested
  - **Type I** (classic): Dentoalveolar and gingival presentation without facial involvement
  - **Type II** (cutaneous): Dentoalveolar and gingival presentation with facial involvement
    - Further subdivided into 4 categories: Hypertrichotic, pigmentory, erythematous, and commissural defect

Gross Pathologic & Surgical Features

- Thick, coarse trabeculae of immature woven bone; absence of lamellar bone and osteoblastic/osteoclastic rimming
- Fibrous enlargement of pulps of deciduous teeth

CLINICAL ISSUES

Presentation

- Most common signs/symptoms
  - Asymptomatic unilateral enlargement of maxilla with absent premolars and retained deciduous teeth
- Other signs/symptoms
  - Facial cutaneous lesions: Becker nevus, hypo- and hyperpigmentation
  - Facial hypertrichosis and asymmetry; cheek depression
  - Commissural lip clefting
  - Clefting between deciduous 1st molars and canines
  - Hyperlinear palms reported; association not confirmed

Demographics

- 5-27 years; usually diagnosed in first decade
- M > F; some report M = F

Natural History & Prognosis

- Nonprogressive; prognosis excellent

Treatment

- Removal of nonrestorable teeth; orthodontic treatment &/or prosthetic recontouring of teeth to restore form and function
- Implants have been placed successfully in altered bone, but results cannot be guaranteed

DIAGNOSTIC CHECKLIST

Consider

- Delay definitive treatment until end of somatic growth

SELECTED REFERENCES

1. Agrawal A et al: Segmental odontomaxillary dysplasia. J Indian Soc Pedod Prev Dent. 32(1):83-6, 2014
2. Rai S et al: Unilateral segmental odontomaxillary dysplasia: a rare entity of 3 cases and review. Indian J Dent Res. 25(1):102-6, 2014
3. González-Arriagada WA et al: Segmental odontomaxillary dysplasia: report of 3 cases and literature review. Head Neck Pathol. 6(2):171-7, 2012

Attrition

KEY FACTS

TERMINOLOGY

- Synonyms: Functional or **parafunctional tooth wear**, physiologic tooth wear
- Definition: **Loss of tooth structure due to tooth-tooth contact** during occlusion and mastication

IMAGING

- Loss of enamel on **functional surfaces** of teeth (incisal or occlusal)
- Decrease in tooth crown vertical height
- Narrowing or obliteration of pulp canal and chamber
- Best imaging tool: Periapical radiography to determine periodontal status, pulpal involvement

TOP DIFFERENTIAL DIAGNOSES

- Abrasion
- Erosion
- Tooth fracture

CLINICAL ISSUES

- Large, flat, shiny wear facets corresponding to areas of occlusion
- **Parafunctional grinding can exacerbate**
- Temporomandibular joint disorders may or may not be present
- Hypercementosis may develop on roots
- Treatment: Mild wear requires no treatment
  - If excessive tooth structure is lost, restoration of tooth by fillings or crowns may be indicated
  - May involve full-mouth rehabilitation and TMJ evaluation and treatment

DIAGNOSTIC CHECKLIST

- Mention **condition of periodontium**
- Note patency of pulp
- Examine root outline for irregularity (hypercementosis)
- Check TMJs for remodeling or degenerative joint disease

(Left) *Sagittal CBCT shows incisal wear of enamel on the maxillary and mandibular incisors →. Edge-to-edge incisal relationship is seen. Pulpal narrowing is often noted with more extensive attrition.* **(Right)** *Sagittal CBCT shows wear of the lingual (functional) aspect of the maxillary incisor. Note that the outline of the wear follows the contour of the opposing tooth ↪.*

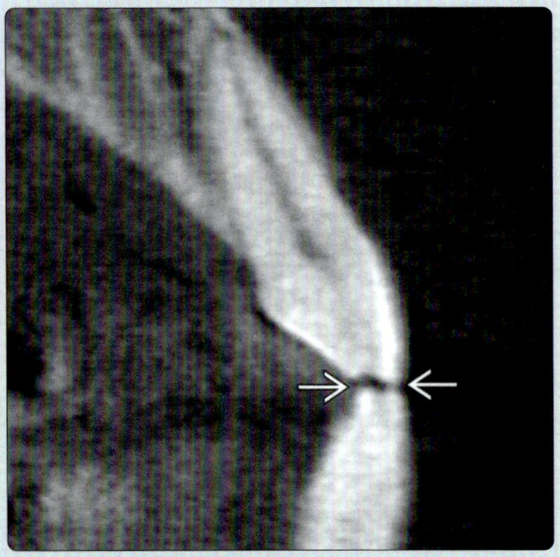

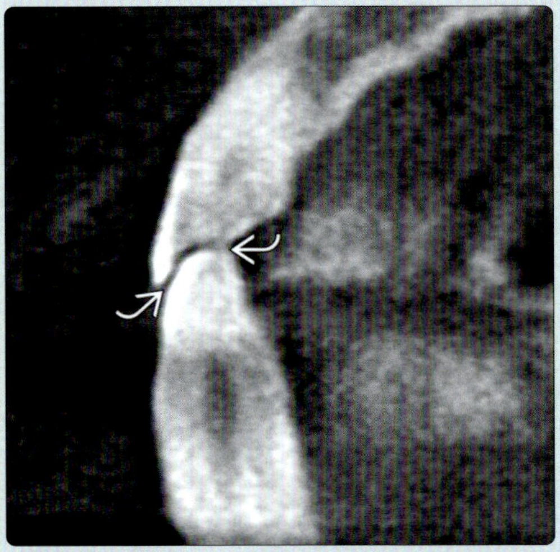

(Left) *Periapical radiograph shows wear of enamel and dentin on the incisal edges (functional surfaces) of the maxillary incisors ↪. Slight dental floss abrasion is noted on the cervical aspect (nonfunctional surface) of the central incisors ↪.* **(Right)** *Bitewing radiograph shows the loss of enamel on the mandibular right 1st molar ↪ and functional cusps of the premolars →.*

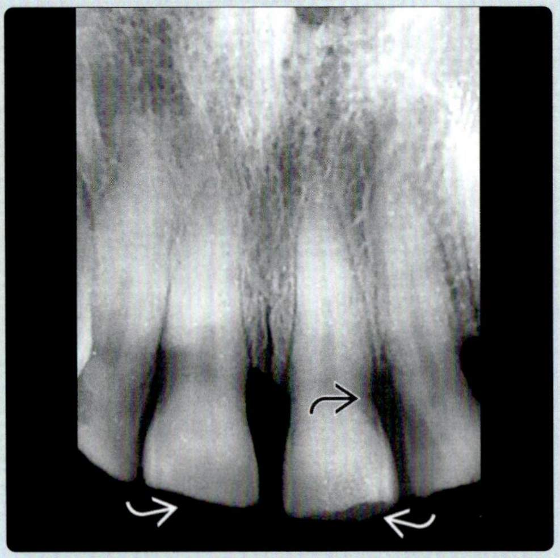

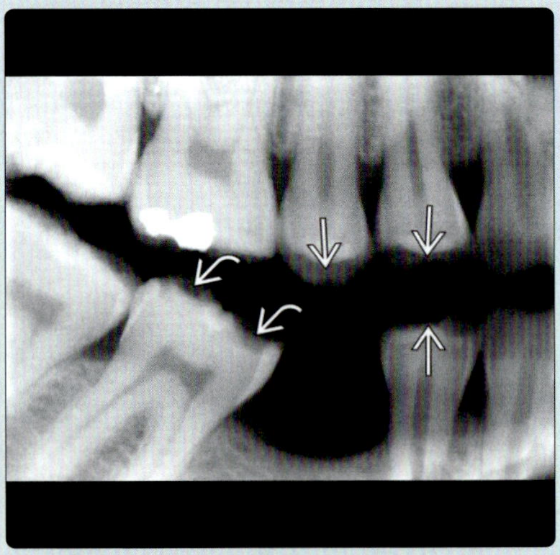

TERMINOLOGY

Synonyms

- Functional or **parafunctional tooth wear**, physiologic tooth wear

Definitions

- **Loss of tooth structure** due to tooth-tooth contact during occlusion and mastication

IMAGING

General Features

- Best diagnostic clue
  - **Loss of enamel** on incisal surfaces of anterior teeth
  - Loss of enamel on occlusal surfaces of posterior teeth
- Location
  - **Functional surfaces** of teeth
    - Incisal edges of anterior teeth
    - Facial surface of mandibular anterior teeth
    - Lingual surface of maxillary anterior teeth
    - Occlusal surfaces of posterior teeth
- Size
  - Varies depending on severity of function or parafunction
    - Mild: Thinned enamel
    - Moderate: Loss of enamel
    - Severe: Loss of enamel and part of dentin

Radiographic Findings

- Intraoral plain film
  - Loss of enamel on incisal &/or occlusal surfaces of teeth
  - May involve loss of dentin if severe
  - Decrease in tooth crown vertical height
  - Narrowing or obliteration of pulp canal and chamber by secondary dentin can occur
  - Periodontal ligament space widening if tooth is clinically mobile
  - **Hypercementosis** of root(s) can be associated

Imaging Recommendations

- Best imaging tool
  - Imaging generally not necessary
  - Periapical radiography to determine periodontal status and pulpal involvement if needed

DIFFERENTIAL DIAGNOSIS

Abrasion

- Usually on **facial or cervical surfaces** of tooth
- Due to mechanical wear, like toothbrush or dental floss overuse
- Can appear on incisal edge as notching due to oral habits involving hard objects, such as cracking pumpkin seeds or holding smoking pipe

Erosion

- Usually on **lingual surfaces** of tooth
- Caused by chemical demineralization (e.g., bulimia-induced vomiting)
- Can be seen on labial surfaces as with citrus sucking

Tooth Fracture

- **Irregular edge**
- Localized to 1 tooth or group of teeth in same location
- History of trauma

CLINICAL ISSUES

Presentation

- Most common signs/symptoms
  - Loss of tooth structure on surfaces of teeth in contact with opposing dentition
  - Large, flat, shiny wear facets corresponding to areas of occlusion
  - Interproximal contacts flattened due to vertical motion during grinding
  - Interproximal contact loss can cause teeth to drift
- Other signs/symptoms
  - Temporomandibular joint disorders may be present
  - Hypercementosis may develop on roots
    - Postulated to be response of tooth to changing occlusion

Natural History & Prognosis

- Tooth-tooth contact can cause wearing of tooth structure over time
- Tooth wear is more noticeable with age
- Premature occlusal contacts (edge-to-edge occlusion or "high" filling or crown) can predispose
- **Parafunctional grinding can exacerbate**

Treatment

- Mild wear requires no treatment
- If excessive tooth structure is lost, restoration of tooth by fillings or crowns may be indicated
- Parafunctional grinding must be addressed prior to restoration
- May involve full mouth rehabilitation and TMJ evaluation and treatment

DIAGNOSTIC CHECKLIST

Consider

- Tooth crown fracture
- Tooth crown preparation for dental filling or crown/onlay

Reporting Tips

- **Mention condition of periodontium**
- Note patency of pulp
- Examine root outline for irregularity (hypercementosis)
- Check TMJs for remodeling or degenerative joint disease

SELECTED REFERENCES

1. Neville B et al: Abnormalities of teeth. In: Oral and Maxillofacial Pathology. 4th ed. St. Louis: Elsevier, 2016
2. Wetselaar P et al: The tooth wear evaluation system: a modular clinical guideline for the diagnosis and management planning of worn dentitions. J Oral Rehabil. 43(1):69-80, 2016
3. Jonsgar C et al: Sleep bruxism in individuals with and without attrition-type tooth wear: an exploratory matched case-control electromyographic study. J Dent. 43(12):1504-10, 2015
4. Kontaxopoulou I et al: Risk Assessment for tooth wear. Prim Dent J. 4(3):25-9, 2015
5. Yule PL et al: Worn down by toothwear? aetiology, diagnosis and management revisited. Dent Update. 42(6):525-6, 529-30, 532, 2015
6. Hotta TH et al: Tooth wear and loss: symptomatological and rehabilitating treatments. Braz Dent J. 11(2):147-52, 2000

Abrasion

KEY FACTS

TERMINOLOGY

- Synonyms
  - Tooth brush injury
  - Dental floss injury
- Definition
  - Pathologic wearing away of tooth structure **due to mechanical action from external source** (e.g., toothbrushing, dental floss, toothpicks, etc.)

IMAGING

- Location
  - Surface of tooth crown exposed to long-term mechanical action
  - **Tooth brush injury**: Facial aspect of cervical portions of maxillary incisors, canines, and premolars
  - More severe on **opposite side to dominant hand**
- Shape
  - Depends on mechanical movement and causative agent
  - Toothbrush: **Horizontal notches on facial aspect of cervical portion** of tooth
  - Dental floss: **Narrow, semilunar lucency in interproximal surfaces of cervical portion** of tooth
  - Toothpicks, denture clasps, cutting thread, opening bobby pins, holding sewing needles or pins, cracking pumpkin/sunflower seeds, or holding tobacco pipe with teeth: **Takes shape of causative agent**
- Imaging
  - Usually evident clinically
  - Periapical radiography can show depth of abrasion lesions if located on proximal surfaces
  - CBCT can show depth of facial abrasion lesions, but **not indicated as diagnostic tool for these lesions**

TOP DIFFERENTIAL DIAGNOSES

- **Caries**
  - Class V caries involves **demineralization and softening** of enamel and dentin
  - Varying degrees of density at lesion/tooth interface
- **Cavity preparation**
  - When restoration lost, cavity preparation may appear similar
  - Usually more **symmetrical** and **sharply defined**
- **Abfraction**
  - Thought to result from flexural forces on teeth
  - **Deep, narrow, wedge-shaped** defects
  - Often affects facial surface of **single posterior tooth**
  - More prevalent in **bruxism** patients
- **Erosion**
  - **Shallow, saucer-shaped defects**
  - History of acidic intake or reflux
- **Attrition**
  - Compare to pipe holding or holding other foreign objects between teeth
  - Usually more **generalized and uniform** on incisal aspects of teeth

CLINICAL ISSUES

- Etiology
  - Long-term use of hard objects to clean teeth or use of teeth to hold hard objects
  - Toothbrushing injury is due to improper **back-and-forth motion of hard toothbrush with heavy pressure**
  - Abrasive toothpaste may exacerbate
  - Dental floss injury is due to excessive or improper use of dental floss; causes **deeper distal lesions** (more pressure) than mesial lesions
  - Enamel limits coronal extent of abrasion
- Symptoms
  - **Sensitivity** as dentin becomes exposed
  - Secondary dentin is laid down, so **pulp exposure is rare**
- Treatment
  - Cessation of causative habit
  - Restoration of abrasion lesions with dental restorative materials

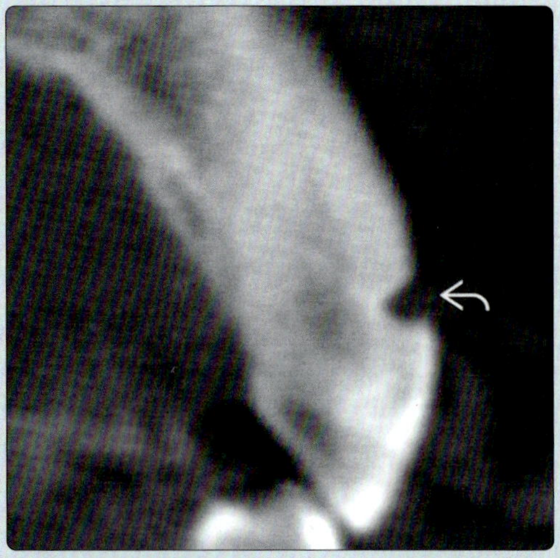

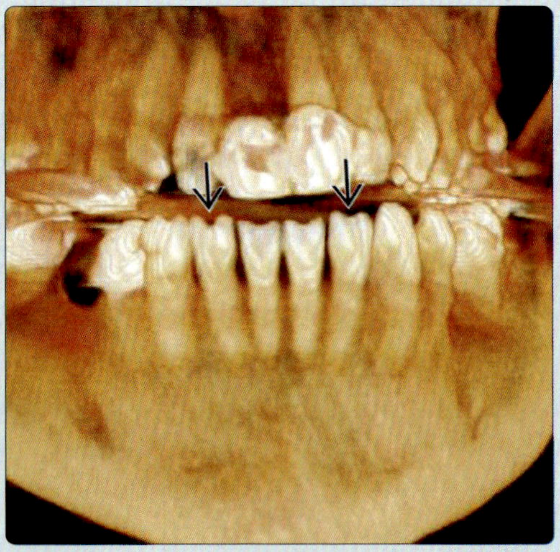

(Left) *Sagittal CBCT shows a facial abrasion lesion ➡ at the cervical portion of the maxillary canine. This is most likely caused by improper toothbrushing.* **(Right)** *3D CBCT in a 42 year-old female shows notch-like abrasion defects ➡ on the mandibular anterior teeth. The patient admitted to the habit of cracking water melon seeds with her teeth since a young child. Note the crowns on the maxillary anterior teeth which were probably restored for esthetic reasons due to similar defects.*

KEY FACTS

TERMINOLOGY

- **Synonyms**
  - Dental corrosion, chemical tooth wear
- **Definition**
  - Loss of tooth structure due to **nonbacterial chemical process** (e.g., bulimia-induced vomiting, citrus fruit sucking, excessive at-home bleaching)

IMAGING

- **CT or CBCT**
  - **Shallow, spoon-shaped tooth structure loss** on 1 or several tooth surfaces
  - Facial &/or lingual surfaces of maxillary anterior teeth
  - Occlusal and facial surfaces of mandibular posterior teeth
  - If associated with dietary acidic intake: Localized to area of habit, usually facial of maxillary anterior teeth
  - If associated with acid reflux of vomiting: Localized to lingual surfaces of teeth
  - Loss or marked thinning of enamel on 1 surface of tooth
  - Dentin may be partially lost
  - Can extend to area of pulp chamber, with calcification of pulp (secondary dentin)
- **Intraoral radiography**
  - Loss of tooth density
  - **Rounded radiolucent defects on crown of tooth**
  - Depth is not well visualized, as it appears on facial and lingual aspects of tooth
- **Imaging recommendation**
  - Periapical radiograph if symptomatic to rule out pulpal and periapical involvement

TOP DIFFERENTIAL DIAGNOSES

- **Abrasion**
  - Facial location if caused by aggressive tooth brushing
  - Margins are sharper; can appear V-shaped
- **Cervical (class V) caries**
  - Irregular borders
  - Usually localized to 1 tooth but can affect > 1 tooth
  - Clinically, dentin is soft and penetrable
- **External resorption**
  - Occurs on root surfaces within alveolar bone
  - May involve crown of unerupted tooth
  - Localized to 1 tooth, less commonly to multiple teeth

CLINICAL ISSUES

- **Location**
  - Facial or lingual surfaces of maxillary incisors
  - Buccal &/or occlusal surfaces of mandibular posterior teeth
  - Involving multiple teeth
- **Appearance**
  - **Lesions are smooth, spoon-shaped depressions**
  - Loss of enamel
  - **Perimolysis**: Loss of enamel around filling (amalgam) so that filling appears higher than tooth
  - May involve dentinal loss
  - Pulp may show through dentin or become exposed
- **Clinical history as correlates to location**
  - Chronic excessive vomiting (e.g., acid reflux/bulimia) → lingual erosion
  - High dietary acidic intake (carbonated beverages, citrus fruits, acidic foods) → facial erosion
- **Treatment**
  - Removal of causative agent (acidic foods)
  - Psychiatric analysis may be needed for bulimic patients
  - Daily fluoride rinse
  - Restoration of defect

DIAGNOSTIC CHECKLIST

- **Examine periapical area for signs of pulpal involvement**
  - Widening of periodontal ligament → rarefying osteitis
  - Sclerosis of bone → sclerosing osteitis
- Check history for causative factors and refer to physician for evaluation if eating disorder suspected

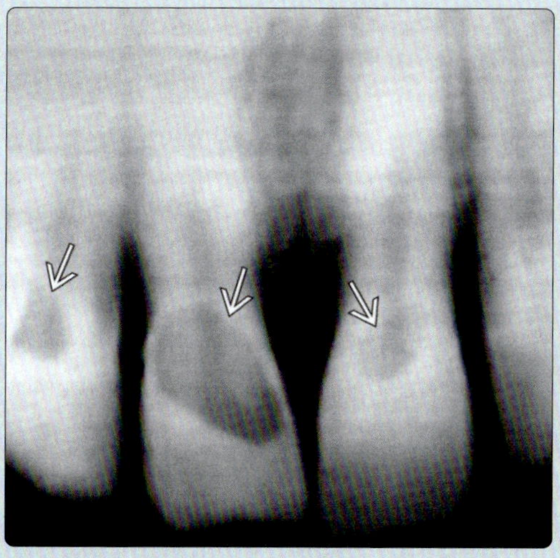

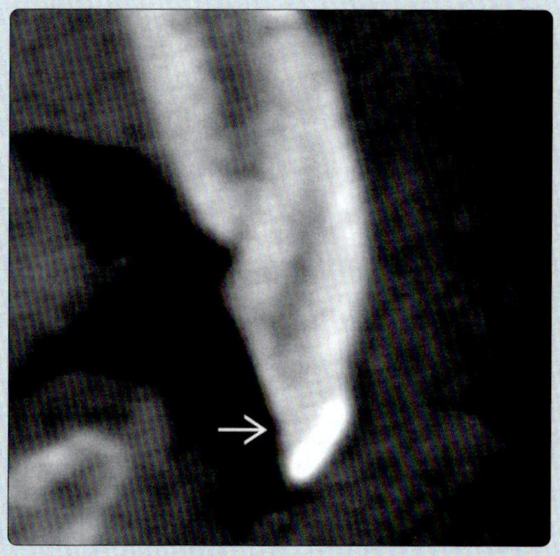

(Left) *Periapical radiograph shows the rounded lesions ➡ typically seen in dental erosion. These lesions are on the lingual (palatal) surface of the teeth. (Courtesy B. Friedland, BDS.)* **(Right)** *CBCT cross section of the maxillary central incisor shows marked loss of enamel and dentin on the lingual (palatal) surface of the tooth with slight rounding at the incisal aspect of the lesion ➡. Note that there is no opposing tooth. This patient was bulimic.*

Abfraction

KEY FACTS

TERMINOLOGY

- Definition
  - Loss of tooth structure due to **occlusal stresses that create repeated tooth flexion**
  - Failure of enamel and dentin integrity occurs at location away from point of loading

IMAGING

- Localized to 1 tooth
- Deep, narrow, wedge-shaped defects
- **Base is too narrow for toothbrush bristles to reach and contact it**
- Location
  - Facial aspect of cervical 3rd of tooth crown
  - Premolars and molars more affected
  - Single tooth with adjacent unaffected teeth
  - Some lesions are subgingival: Area where abrasion does not occur
- Imaging appearance
  - **Radiographic imaging** to investigate this entity is **not recommended** unless pulp exposure is suspected
  - Pulp exposure is unlikely, but if it occurs, periapical radiographic examination is recommended to rule out periapical pathology
  - Clinical examination should show lesions sufficiently
  - On CBCT **dental cross sections**, abfraction lesions may become apparent on **facial aspects** of teeth

TOP DIFFERENTIAL DIAGNOSES

- **Abrasion**
  - Wider, v-shaped lesion
  - Due to mechanical wear from improper toothbrush use
  - Involves > 1 tooth
  - Lesions bigger on contralateral side to dominant hand
- **Erosion**
  - Shallow, saucer-shaped lesion with rounded edges
  - History of high acid intake or reflux
- **Class V (cervical) caries**
  - Irregular borders
  - Wide base
  - May extend to pulp, causing pulpitis and pulp death
- **Class V (cervical) cavity preparation (no restoration)**
  - Box-like defect (prepared by dentist)
  - Wide base
- **External resorption**
  - Occurs **beneath soft tissue or bone coverage** (needs vascular supply for osteoclastic recruitment)
  - Larger irregular defects

CLINICAL ISSUES

- History of **bruxism** is often present
- Symptoms
  - **Hypersensitivity** of teeth may be present
  - Teeth usually vital unless other disease present
- **Progression**
  - Abfraction lesions **progress slowly**
  - Lesions thought to be produced by **disruption of enamel crystals** at cervical 1/3 of tooth crown due to eccentric occlusal forces
  - Occlusal forces thought to create flexure of tooth around cervical portion
  - **Cracked enamel** becomes more susceptible to **displacement by tooth brushing**
  - **Secondary or tertiary dentin** deposition in pulp chamber **prevents pulp exposure**
- **Treatment**
  - Reduction of occlusal stresses
  - Restoration with **dental restorative materials**
  - Application of desensitizing solutions
  - Use of desensitizing toothpaste

DIAGNOSTIC CHECKLIST

- Consider: Some older, tooth-colored restorative materials are radiolucent and will not show radiographically
- Existence of abfraction as separate entity from abrasion is controversial

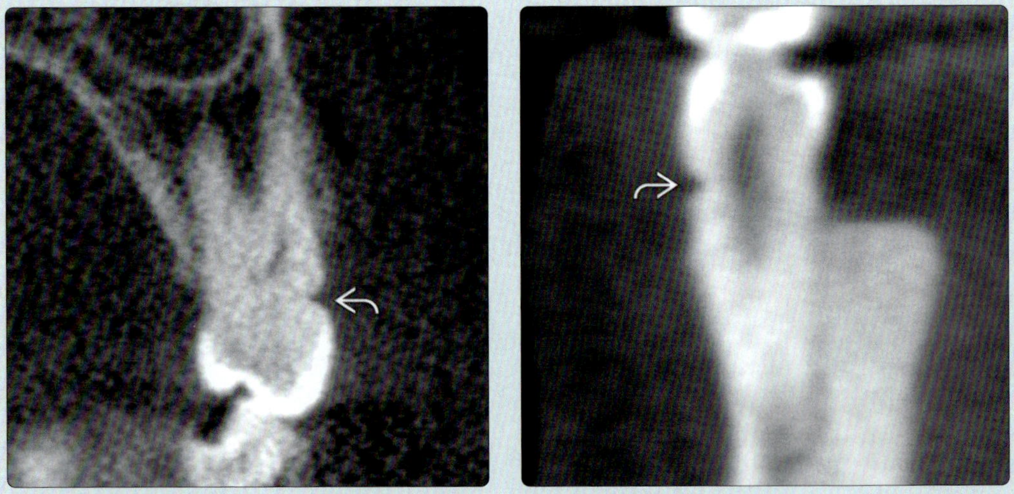

(Left) *Cross section CBCT of a maxillary premolar shows a narrow, wedge-shaped defect ➡ on the facial aspect of the cervical 1/3 of the tooth. This is an isolated tooth with a single, narrow facial lesion. This tooth can be restored with a dental restorative material, such as glass ionomer cement.* **(Right)** *Cross section CBCT of a mandibular premolar shows a single, isolated abfraction lesion ➡ at the facial cervical margin. None of the adjacent teeth had cervical defects.*

Turner Dysplasia

KEY FACTS

TERMINOLOGY

- Synonyms
  - Turner hypoplasia, Turner tooth
- Definition
  - Enamel defect in permanent teeth **caused by odontogenic inflammation or trauma to primary predecessor tooth**

IMAGING

- Best diagnostic clue
  - Lack of significant enamel and irregularity of dentin surface in **isolated tooth**
- Location
  - Most common in premolars, less frequent in anterior teeth
  - **Never occurs in permanent molars** (no predecessors)
- **In posterior tooth**
  - Deformed tooth crown with lack of significant enamel
  - Irregularity of dentin surface
- **In anterior tooth**
  - Horizontal, low-density **band of hypoplasia** across tooth crown
  - Often associated with trauma
- Best imaging tool
  - **Periapical radiography**
  - Check for possible **widening of apical periodontal ligament space, rarefying osteitis, or condensing osteitis** due to susceptibility to caries and subsequent development of pulpal pathology

TOP DIFFERENTIAL DIAGNOSES

- **Amelogenesis imperfecta**
  - Genetic anomaly
  - **Affects all or almost all teeth** in both dentitions
  - Square crown; thin or absent enamel
  - Open contact between teeth: **Picket fence** appearance
- **Environmental enamel hypoplasia**
  - Occurs on **multiple teeth**
  - Usually tied to recognizable event: **Drug ingestion, nutrition deficit, radiation therapy**
  - Affects tooth crown at specific point of development at time insult occurs
- **Crown preparation**
  - Iatrogenic
  - Tooth may have been previously prepared to receive crown or dental filling
  - Filling or crown may have fallen out or never been placed
  - **History should clarify**

CLINICAL ISSUES

- Most common clinical presentation
  - **Tooth defects vary** from focal areas of white, yellow, and brown to extensive hypoplasia involving entire crown
- Natural history
  - Primary tooth is affected by **inflammation or trauma**
  - Insult transfers to underlying developing permanent tooth
  - Developing enamel and dentin are affected
  - Severity depends on severity of insult and on stage of development of permanent tooth
  - May disturb enamel matrix formation or calcification causing **localized hypoplastic or hypomineralized defect**
  - More severe insult may result in **pitting of crown** or severe deformity
- **Treatment**: If root is sound and tooth is fully erupted, **tooth may be restored**
  - Restoration of small defect: Composite restoration
  - Restoration of large defect: Prosthetic crown with root canal therapy and post and core if periapical pathology is present

DIAGNOSTIC CHECKLIST

- Examine rest of dentition for defects
- Check clinical history for possible contributing event

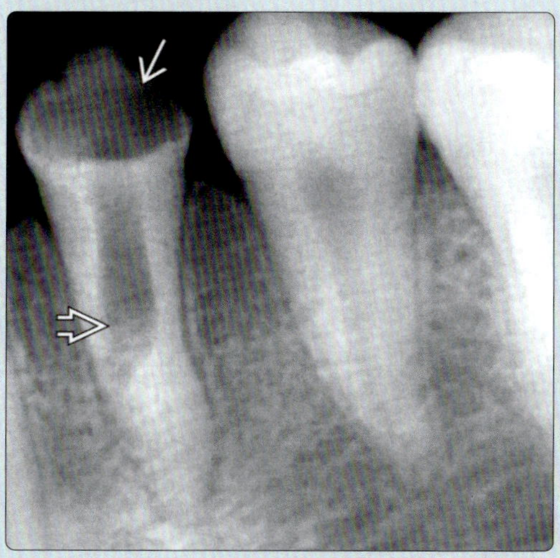

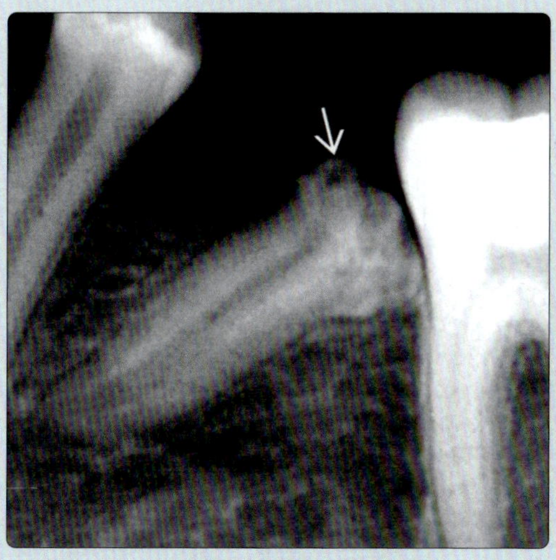

(Left) *Periapical radiograph shows loss of crown structure ➔ of the mandibular left 1st premolar affected by Turner dysplasia. The widening of the pulp canal ➔ may be due to either internal resorption or excessive instrumentation during root canal treatment. (Courtesy B. Friedland, DDS.)* **(Right)** *Periapical radiograph shows an impacted mandibular left 2nd premolar affected by Turner dysplasia. Note the irregular appearance of the crown enamel and dentin ➔. (Courtesy M. Ahmad, DDS.)*

Internal and External Resorption

KEY FACTS

TERMINOLOGY

- Definition: Resorption of tooth structure on internal or external surfaces of root by odontoclasts

IMAGING

- Irregular loss of tooth structure on **internal (pulpal) surface** or **external (periodontal) surface of parts of tooth beneath bone or soft tissue**
- Size varies according to progression of lesion
- Late stages of resorption may pose diagnostic dilemma as to whether resorption is internal or external
- Periapical radiography with application of **SLOB rule** if surface localization necessary
- CBCT: Can show facial and lingual lesions

TOP DIFFERENTIAL DIAGNOSES

- Large pulp chamber in young permanent teeth
- Overinstrumentation of pulp canal
- Caries
- Volume averaging artifact
- Abrasion and erosion
- Normal external resorption of primary teeth

CLINICAL ISSUES

- **Treatment of internal resorption**
  - If tooth is not weakened: Root canal therapy to stop resorption
  - Small perforations of root may be surgically exposed and retrofilled
  - Nonrestorable tooth: Extraction
- **Treatment of external resorption**
  - Examination of cause of resorption and removal of cause
  - Cervical lesions can be filled
  - Extraction if tooth is nonrestorable
- **Treatment of invasive cervical resorption**
  - Inactivation of all resorbing tissue and reconstitution of resorptive defect

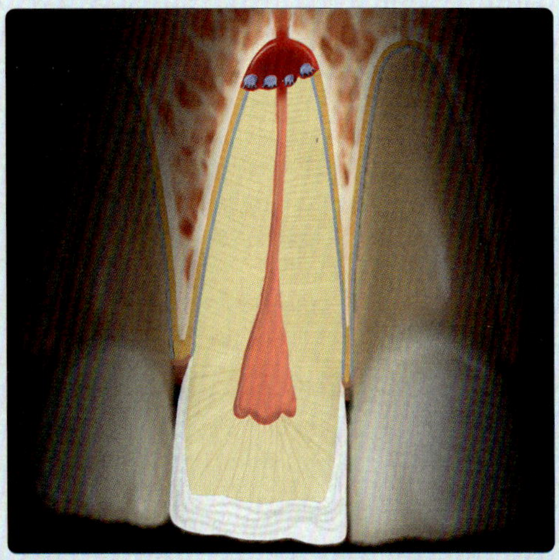

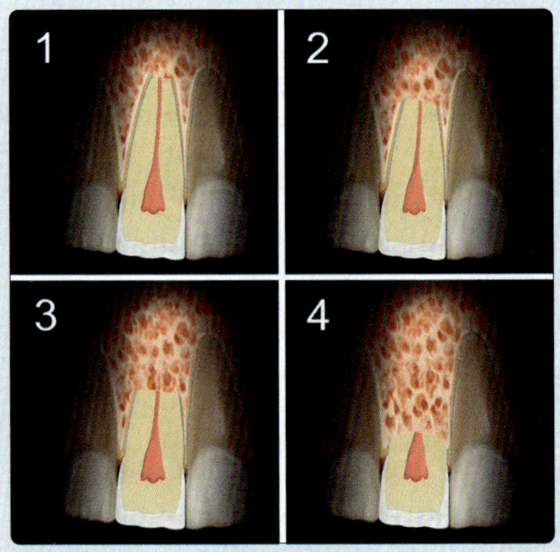

(Left) *Graphic shows external resorption of the apex of a tooth. This pattern of resorption presents as blunting of the apex of the root and is often associated with high orthodontic forces.* **(Right)** *Anterior view of the maxillary incisors shows sequential blunting (1) and external resorption of the apical (2), middle (3), and coronal (4) thirds of the root. The greater the root resorption, the worse the prognosis of the tooth. This can be associated with increased mechanical (orthodontic) forces.*

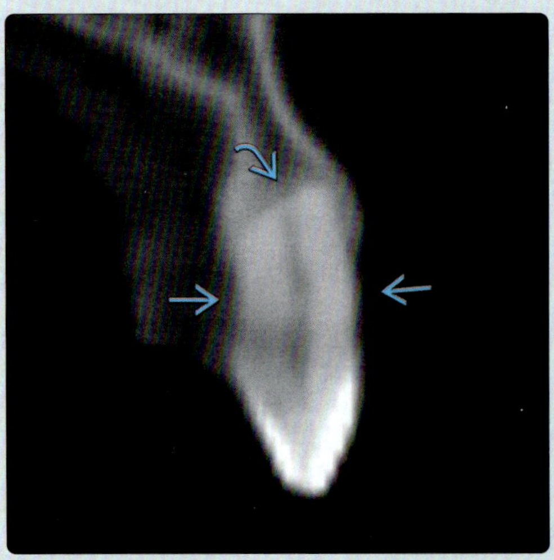

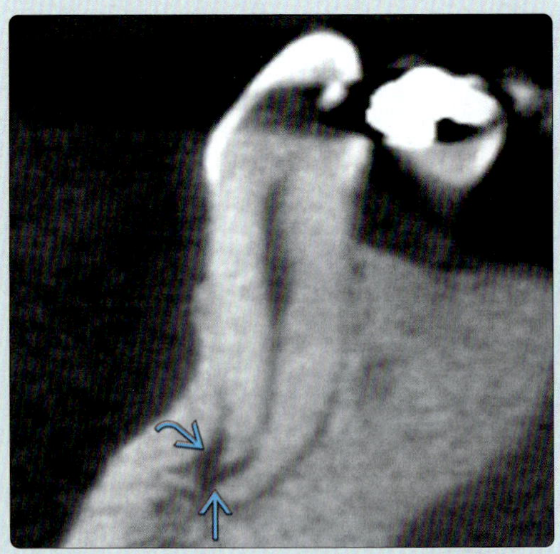

(Left) *Sagittal CBCT shows a maxillary central incisor with blunting of the apical 1/3 of the root. When combined with periodontal bone loss, this can worsen the prognosis of the tooth. (Courtesy M. Noujeim, DDS.)* **(Right)** *Custom cross section of a mandibular canine shows periapical periodontal ligament space widening with surrounding sclerosis, suggestive of periapical inflammation. The apical foramen is widened due to inflammatory resorption of the root. Tooth structure can resorb with chronic inflammation.*

TERMINOLOGY

Definitions

- Resorption of tooth structure on internal or external surfaces of root by odontoclasts
- **Internal resorption**
  - Destruction of **internal surface** of root caused by dentinoclastic cells **within pulp chamber or canal**
- **External resorption**
  - Destruction of **external surface** of root caused by dentinoclastic cells **in periodontal ligament (PDL)**
- **Invasive cervical resorption**
  - Relatively uncommon form of external root resorption

IMAGING

General Features

- Best diagnostic clue
  - Irregular loss of tooth structure on **internal (pulpal) surface** or **external (periodontal) surface of parts of tooth beneath bone or soft tissue**
  - **Internal resorption**
    - Irregular widening of pulp chamber or canal that **does not follow external contour of dentin**
    - **Completely radiolucent with no calcification**
    - Tends to be **localized** to 1 area of pulp chamber or canal
    - Can expand entire pulp uniformly
    - Can be balloon-like, oval, or slightly scalloped
  - **External resorption**
    - **Apical** aspect of root
      - Blunting of apices of teeth with normal PDL space and lamina dura
      - Lamina dura may be lost if inflammation present
      - **Pulp canal opening at apex is wide**
    - **Lateral** aspect of root
      - Irregular lesions, "moth-eaten," may involve 1 or more teeth
      - May be due to **adjacent unerupted tooth** or **pathology pressing against affected tooth**
    - **Facial or lingual** aspect of root
      - Radiolucency will superimpose over pulp chamber; however, normal **outline of pulp chamber will be evident through radiolucency**
      - Even when extensive, thin outline of pulp canal tends to be preserved
    - Entire tooth
      - Longstanding impacted teeth may undergo **external/internal resorption**
  - **Invasive cervical resorption**
    - Cervical location and origin point small and often punctate
    - Resorption invasive and leads to progressive and usually destructive loss of tooth structure
- Location
  - Primary or permanent teeth; permanent teeth more common
  - **Internal resorption**
    - Central incisors, 1st and 2nd molars most common
  - **External resorption**
    - More prevalent in mandible but can occur anywhere
    - Central incisors, canine, and premolars
    - Commonly seen in **apical or cervical** regions of tooth
    - Can occur in enamel if tooth unerupted
- Size
  - Varies according to progression of lesion
  - Internal
    - **Early**: May be slight irregularity in outline
    - **Late**: May extend to external surface of tooth
  - External
    - **Early**: Slight irregularity of external surface of root
    - **Late**: May extend to pulp chamber
  - Late stages of resorption may pose diagnostic dilemma as to whether resorption internal or external

Imaging Recommendations

- Best imaging tool
  - Periapical radiography with application of **SLOB rule** (**s**ame **l**ingual, **o**pposite **b**uccal) if necessary
  - CBCT
    - Shows facial & lingual lesions; their extent & depth
    - Can show relationship with adjacent unerupted tooth or pathology that may cause external resorption
    - Custom cross sections can demonstrate invasive cervical resorption origin and extent
- Protocol advice
  - If only periapical radiography is available and differentiating external from internal resorption cannot be done, or if facial or lingual location of lesion needs to be determined, **use SLOB rule**
  - SLOB rule for object localization
    - 2 projections taken at different angles
    - If lesion moves in **same** direction as radiation source, then it is on **lingual**
    - If it moves in **opposite** direction, it is **buccal**

DIFFERENTIAL DIAGNOSIS

Large Pulp Chamber in Young Permanent Teeth

- **Follows outline of dentinoenamel junction**
- Diminishes in size with age as dentin is laid down

Overinstrumentation of Pulp Canal

- History of endodontic treatment or presence of access
- **Takes shape of instrument used**, such as large round bur

Caries

- Starts from external surface of tooth **exposed to oral cavity**
- **Cemental/root caries** occurs on cervical surfaces of tooth **exposed to oral cavity** due to loss of periodontal attachment
  - Occurs above bone level

Volume Averaging Artifact

- Occurs in presence of high-density structures, such as **metallic restorations**
- Appears as low-density area in close contact with high-density material
- Examine entire tooth and adjacent teeth with similar restorations for similar "lesions"

Abrasion and Erosion

- Occur on tooth surfaces **exposed to oral cavity**

- **Can be visualized clinically**
- Need to be differentiated from internal resorption on periapical radiography as may appear similar
- Clearly originating from external surface of tooth when viewed on CBCT

Normal External Resorption of Primary Teeth

- Primary teeth roots resorb as their successors start to erupt beneath them
- When roots are lost, primary tooth exfoliates
- Abnormal or **irregular resorption** (1 root but not the rest) **should be reported**

Idiopathic Cervical Resorption

- Resorption of cervical portion of teeth with no known cause
- Occurs on surfaces of tooth above **and** below bone
  - Extension of radiolucency below bone differentiates from caries
- Can affect all teeth, causing loss of teeth

PATHOLOGY

General Features

- Etiology
  - **Internal resorption**
    - Physical trauma
    - Inflammatory pulpitis due to caries
    - Direct and indirect pulp capping for acute pulp exposures during cavity preparation
    - Pulpotomy
    - Incomplete pulp extirpation or root canal therapy
    - Dens-in-dente (dens invaginatus)
  - **External resorption**
    - **Resorptive pressure** due to cysts, benign tumors, adjacent impacted teeth, orthodontic forces
    - Dental trauma
    - Localized inflammatory lesions
    - Reimplantation of avulsed teeth
    - Excessive occlusal forces
    - Paget disease of bone
    - Intracoronal bleaching of pulpless tooth
    - Hormonal imbalances
      - Evaluation by primary care physician recommended if no other etiologic factors can be determined
  - **Invasive cervical resorption**
    - Etiology unknown; localized fibrous in-growth seen

CLINICAL ISSUES

Presentation

- Most common signs/symptoms
  - **Internal resorption**
    - **Usually asymptomatic**
    - Pain may be reported if associated with significant pulpitis
    - If affects coronal pulp, pink discoloration of tooth may be noted **(pink tooth of Mummery)**
  - **External resorption**
    - Usually not recognized clinically; incidental finding on imaging
    - **No signs or symptoms**; no tooth mobility noted
  - **Invasive cervical resorption**
    - Can resemble "pink tooth" seen in internal resorption if large

Natural History & Prognosis

- **Internal resorption**
  - Relatively rare; may affect primary or permanent teeth; **more common in permanent**
  - Occurs after injury to pulpal tissues, such as trauma or inflammatory pulpitis
  - **May continue as long as vital pulp tissue remains**
  - May result in communication of pulp with PDL
  - May repair with reparative dentin (appears mixed in density)
- **External resorption**
  - Common; not self-limiting; may continue until lesion reaches pulp or until fracture of tooth occurs
  - Resorption defect may fill with bone = inostosis and ankylosis
- **Invasive cervical resorption**
  - Starts at point on supragingival cervical margin; spreads longitudinally along length of dentin
  - Progressive and destructive

Treatment

- Internal resorption
  - If tooth is not weakened: **Root canal therapy to stop resorption**
  - **Small perforations** of root may be **surgically exposed and retrofilled**
  - Nonrestorable tooth: **Extraction**
- External resorption
  - Determination of and **removal of cause**
  - Cervical lesions can be filled
  - Extraction if tooth nonrestorable
- **Invasive cervical resorption**
  - Inactivation of all resorbing tissue and reconstitution of resorptive defect
  - Treatment may be ineffective → loss of teeth

DIAGNOSTIC CHECKLIST

Image Interpretation Pearls

- **Lesions should be located in area where odontoclasts present**
  - External: Beneath bone or soft tissue
  - Internal: Within pulp chamber
- Resorption **can extend to involve entire width of dentin**: Differentiating internal or external resorption may be difficult

Reporting Tips

- History of orthodontic treatment may contribute to blunting of apices in absence of all other etiologic factors

SELECTED REFERENCES

1. Ucar FI et al: Effects of impacted maxillary canines on root resorption of lateral incisors: a cone beam computed tomography study. J Orofac Orthop. ePub, 2017
2. Vaz de Souza D et al: External cervical resorption: a comparison of the diagnostic efficacy using 2 different cone-beam computed tomographic units and periapical radiographs. J Endod. 43(1):121-125, 2017

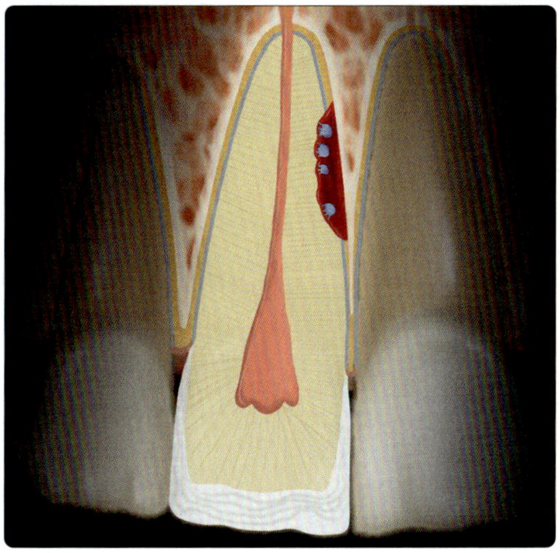

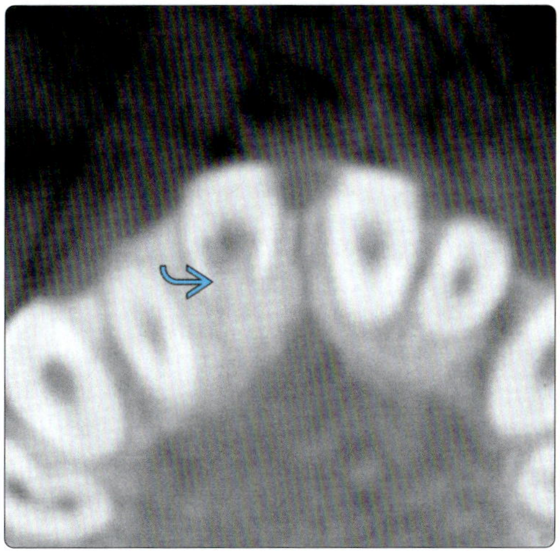

(Left) *Graphic shows external resorption of the lateral aspect of the root. This can occur due to inflammatory resorption, pressure resorption, trauma, or idiopathic origin.* **(Right)** *Axial CBCT shows external resorption of a root, which was previously traumatized. The resorption has extended to the pulp, and bone has grown into the defect ⤻ (inostosis), causing the tooth to be ankylosed.*

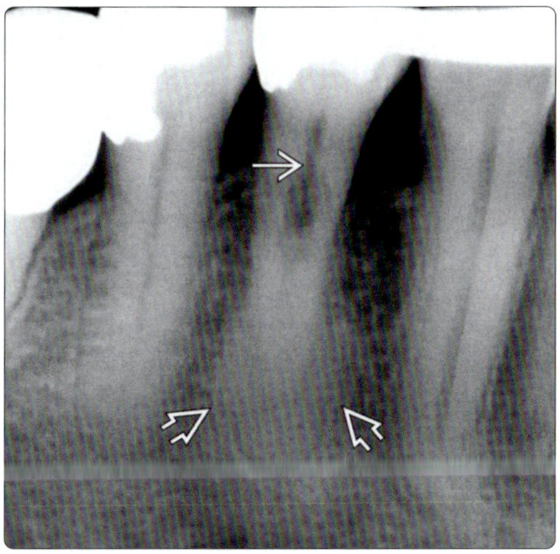

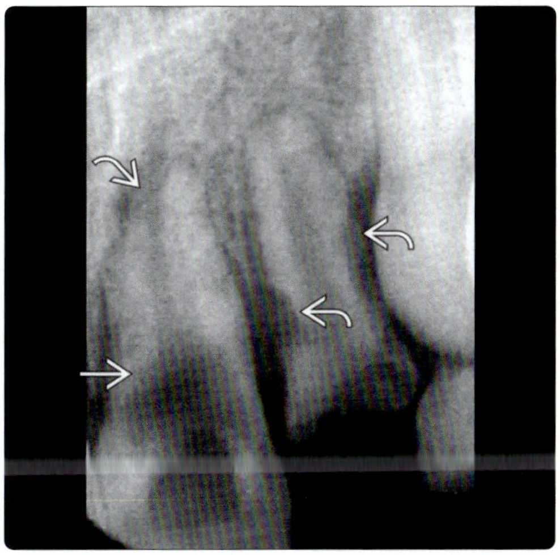

(Left) *Periapical radiograph shows external resorption superimposing on the pulp. The outline of the pulp chamber is clearly seen →, differentiating it from internal resorption. Note hypercementosis on apex of root ⇨.* **(Right)** *Periapical radiograph shows maxillary left central and lateral incisors with prior history of trauma and pulp removal. Root canal therapy was not completed, and internal → and external ⤺ resorption has occurred. (Courtesy H. Needleman, DDS.)*

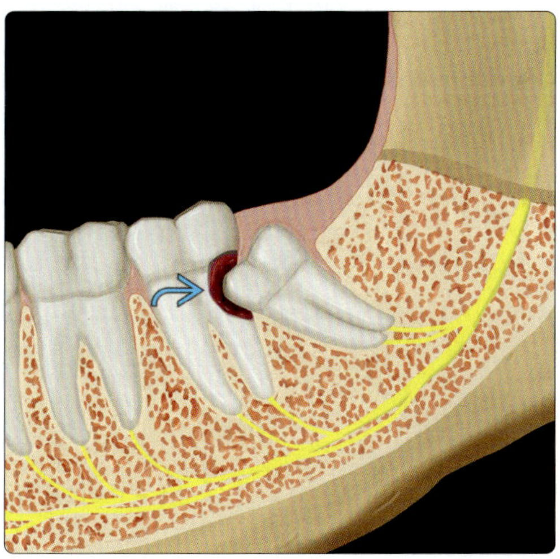

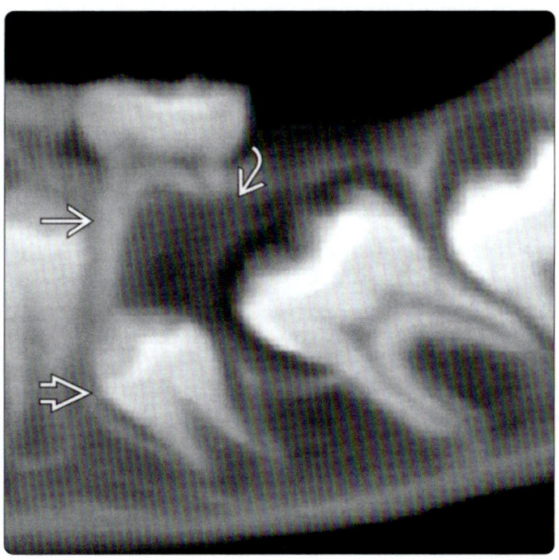

(Left) *Graphic demonstrates pressure resorption ⤻ of the 2nd molar tooth due to the ectopic eruption of the impacted 3rd molar.* **(Right)** *Panoramic radiograph shows ameloblastic fibroma pericoronal to the mandibular left 1st permanent molar. This is causing resorption of the distal root of the primary 2nd molar ⤻ as well as displacement of the 2nd premolar ⇨. Mesial root → is of normal length. Benign tumors can cause external resorption of adjacent teeth. (Courtesy M. Noujeim, DDS.)*

(Left) *Sagittal CBCT shows external resorption of a maxillary central incisor* ➡*due to pressure from an impacted canine* ➡*. Teeth in relation to impacted teeth should always be scrutinized for this type of resorption.* **(Right)** *Sagittal CBCT shows an impacted maxillary 3rd molar resorbing the distal root of the adjacent 2nd molar* ➡*. The 3rd molar should also be evaluated for the presence of coronal pathology that may also contribute to pressure resorption.*

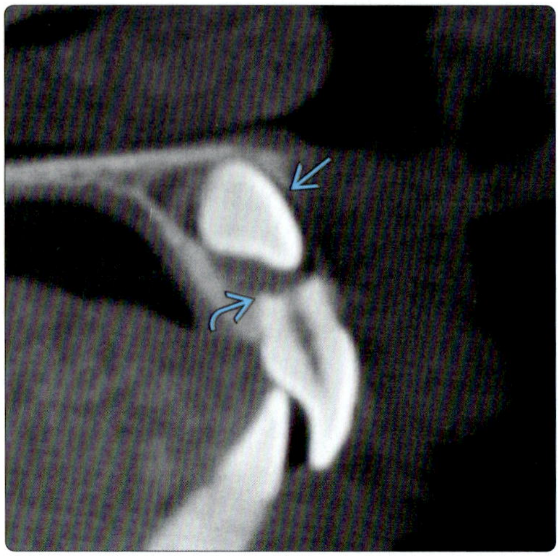

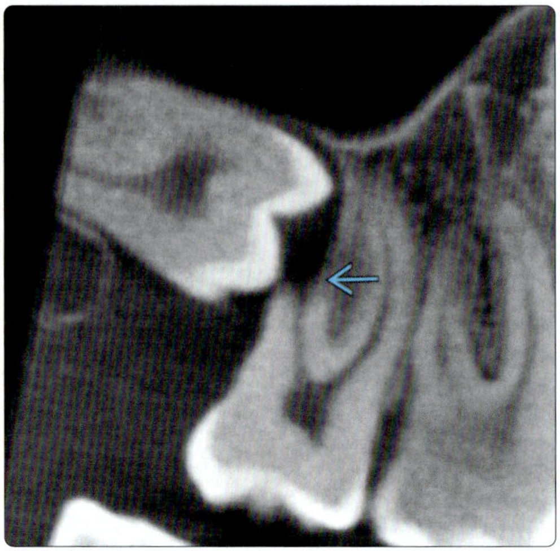

(Left) *Graphic shows a pure internal resorption of a tooth. This presents radiographically as fusiform widening of the pulp canal or chamber. Large lesions may communicate with the external surface of the root.* **(Right)** *Cross-section CBCT shows internal resorption of a mandibular lateral incisor. The pulp chamber is nonuniformly expanded with possible communication with the periodontal ligament* ➡*.*

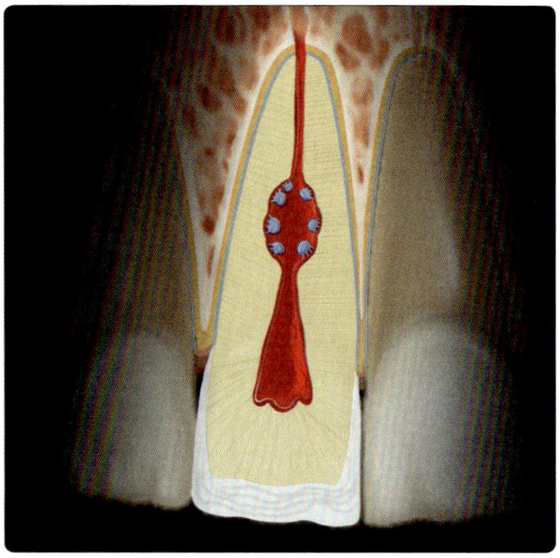

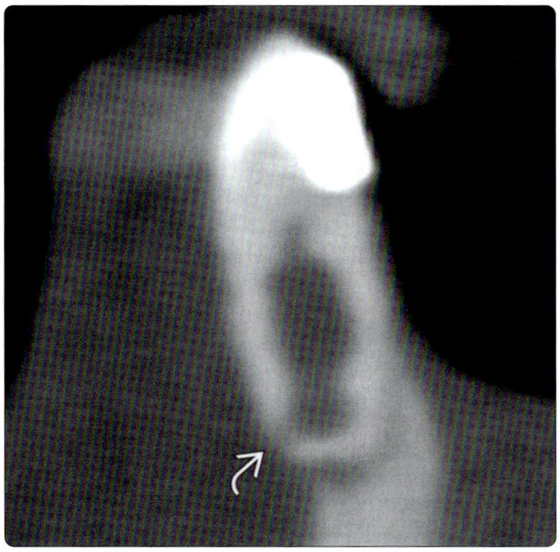

(Left) *Axial CBCT shows internal resorption of the mandibular left lateral incisor* ➡*. When evaluating the teeth in the axial plane, look for any abnormal, asymmetrical low densities within a single tooth. Comparing to the tooth pulp size on the contralateral side may aid in evaluation.* **(Right)** *Axial CBCT shows 2 chronically impacted supernumerary teeth* ➡*. These teeth have undergone internal resorption, and the follicle spaces have diminished. Such teeth are usually left alone unless they develop pathology.*

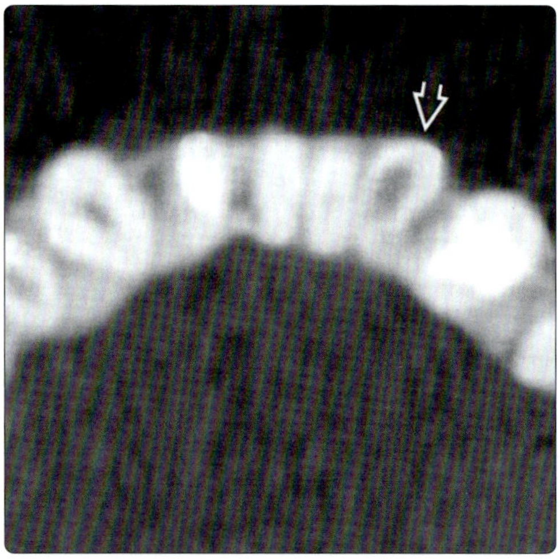

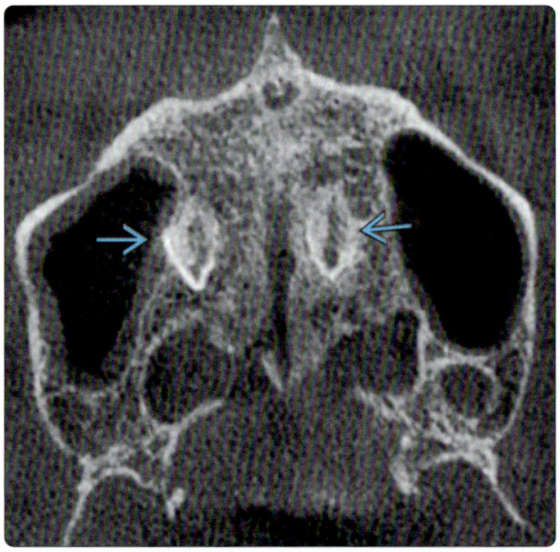

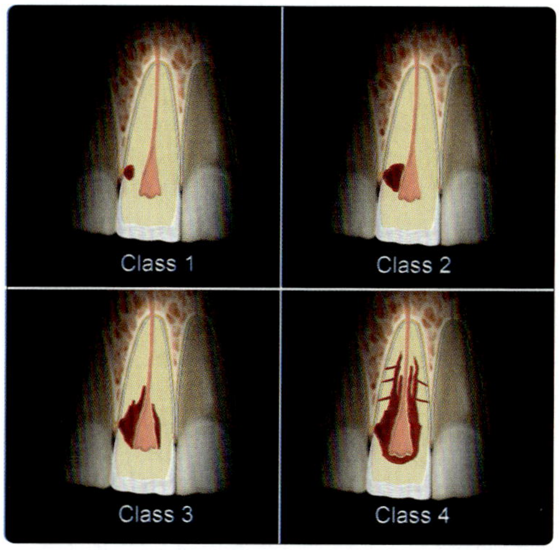

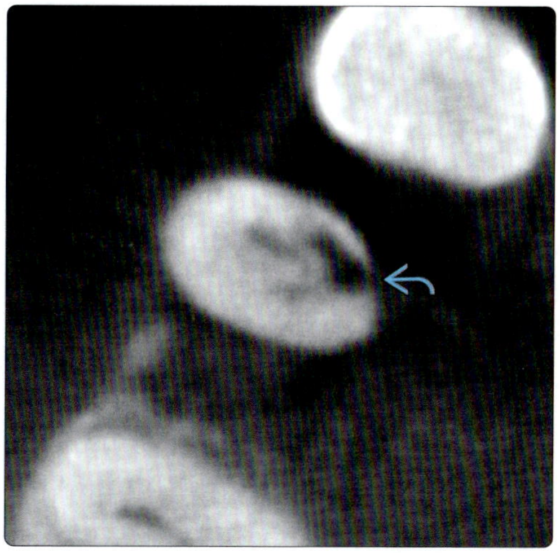

(Left) *Graphic representation of the classes of invasive cervical resorption reported in the literature is shown. These lesions originate from a small punctate point in the cervical portion of the root. Resorption is invasive and leads to progressive and usually destructive loss of tooth structure.* **(Right)** *Axial CBCT shows class 2 or 3 invasive cervical resorption. The punctate origin point can be visualized on the mesiolingual aspect of the root. (Courtesy M. Noujeim DDS.)*

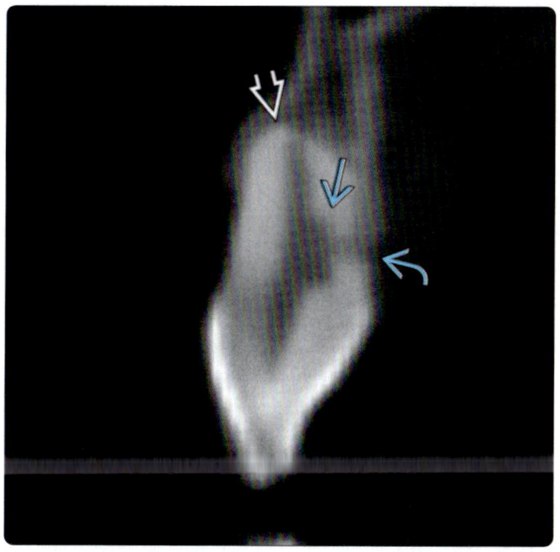

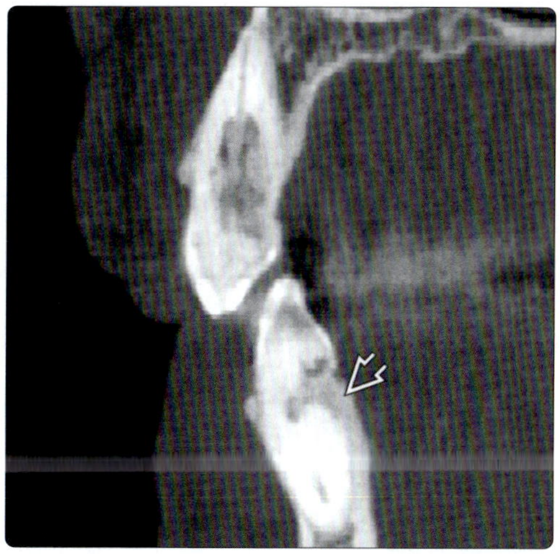

(Left) *Sagittal CBCT of a maxillary central incisor shows class 2 invasive cervical resorption. The origin can be seen on the lingual aspect. Localization of the origin is best done using custom cross sections. There is also apical external resorption. (Courtesy M. Noujeim, DDS.)* **(Right)** *Cross-section CBCT reformation shows classes 3 & 4 invasive cervical resorption of opposing teeth. The mandibular canine shows a lesion that is communicating with the external surface of the root with bony ingrowth (inostosis).*

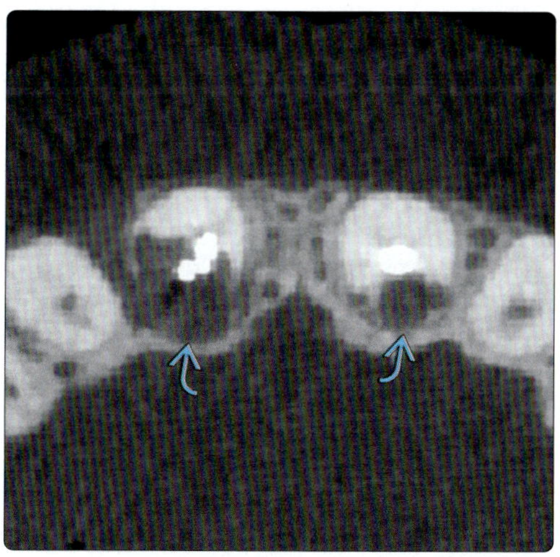

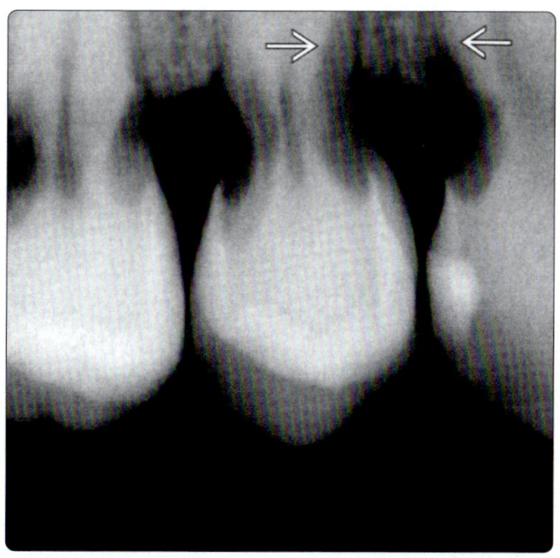

(Left) *Axial CBCT shows root canal-treated maxillary incisor teeth with extensive invasive cervical resorption. The etiology of this form of tooth resorption is unknown. These lesions can lead to loss of the teeth.* **(Right)** *Bitewing radiograph shows generalized idiopathic cervical resorption extending below the alveolar crestal bone, differentiating it from cemental caries. Opposing mandibular teeth have been lost due to this process.*

KEY FACTS

TERMINOLOGY

- **Definition**
  - **Excessive** deposition of **cementum** on tooth roots

IMAGING

- **Radiographic appearance**
  - Excessive buildup of tooth density material (cementum) around all or parts of tooth root
  - Difference in density between dentin and cementum (not usually apparent) becomes evident when hypercementosis is present
  - May be irregular or smooth
  - Bulbous enlargement of root is noted
- **Location**
  - Can be confined to apical 3rd or can extend along entire length of tooth root
  - **Mandible** affected twice as often
  - **Molars** followed by **premolars** more affected
- **Imaging modality of choice**
  - Periapical radiography: **Periodontal ligament (PDL) space and lamina dura relationship can be better evaluated**

TOP DIFFERENTIAL DIAGNOSES

- **Cementoblastoma**
  - True benign tumor of cementum attached to tooth
  - May cause root resorption: Apex of tooth seems to disappear into lesion
  - More rounded with peripheral radiolucency
- **Dilacerated tooth root**
  - Tooth root uniformly wide but bent like arc or at 90°
  - Small bends in apical 3rd of root may be most difficult to differentiate from hypercementosis
  - Pulp canal follows bends of root
- **Mature periapical osseous dysplasia**
  - Normal tooth root morphology
  - Uniform PDL space is not present
  - Radiopacity more irregular
- **Idiopathic osteosclerosis/enostosis/dense bone island**
  - May occur near root apex
  - Separated from tooth by normal-appearing PDL space
- **Sclerosing osteitis**
  - Separated from tooth by **widened PDL space**
  - Sclerotic reaction of bone due to inflammatory process at apex of tooth caused by pupal pathology
  - Tooth is **nonvital**

PATHOLOGY

- **Etiology**
  - Unknown but theorized to be response of tooth to unstable or changing occlusion
  - Sometimes appears on **supererupted tooth** as it erupts into space of missing opposing tooth
  - **Inflammation** may cause deposition on apical root surfaces
  - **Traumatic occlusion** may cause hypercementosis
  - **Fractured vital teeth** may develop hypercementosis in area of fracture, like **callus**
- Gross appearance
  - Extracted tooth root surface looks irregular with loss of cervicoapical tapering

CLINICAL ISSUES

- **Signs and symptoms**
  - No clinical signs or symptoms; tooth is vital
- **Related conditions**
  - Paget disease (strongest association)
  - Hyperpituitarism (acromegaly and gigantism)
  - Drug-induced osteonecrosis, arthritis, calcinosis, thyroid goiter, Gardner syndrome, florid osseous dysplasia
- **Treatment**
  - Requires no treatment
- **Clinical considerations**
  - May pose problem if extraction of tooth is planned
  - Surgical tooth removal if hypercementosis severe

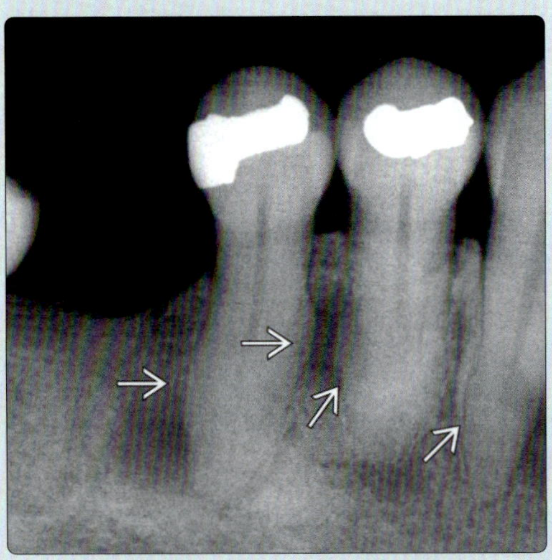

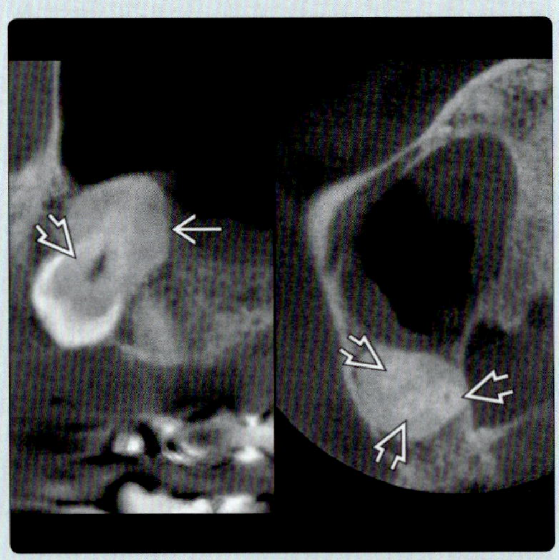

(Left) *Periapical radiograph shows mandibular teeth with hypercementosis of the middle and apical 3rds of the roots ➡. The cementum is located within a normal-appearing periodontal ligament space and lamina dura. The hypercementosis is associated with florid osseous dysplasia.* **(Right)** *Sagittal (left) and axial (right) CBCT shows an impacted right maxillary third molar with hypercementosis ➡. Note that the normal higher density dentin of the roots ➡ can be seen within the lower density cementum.*

Concussion

KEY FACTS

TERMINOLOGY

- **Synonym**
  - Dental concussion
- **Definition**
  - **Crush injury** to vascular structures at root apex and periodontal ligament (PDL) resulting in inflammatory edema
  - **No displacement** and only minimal loosening of tooth

IMAGING

- Imaging modality of choice
  - **Periapical radiography**
- Radiographic appearance
  - **No radiographic changes** or **slight widening** of PDL space
- Location
  - Maxillary anterior teeth more affected
  - **Apical PDL space**

TOP DIFFERENTIAL DIAGNOSES

- **Extrusive luxation**
  - Tooth is displaced
  - Radiolucency is seen at apex representing vacated socket due to tooth displacement
- **Rarefying osteitis**
  - Pulp is dead or dying
  - Usually caused by coronal pathology (caries or fracture) that has penetrated to pulp
  - Recent history of trauma and tenderness to touch indicates dental concussion
  - May occur few months or years after traumatic injury

CLINICAL ISSUES

- **Signs and symptoms**
  - Tooth tender to touch
  - Horizontal or vertical percussion of tooth yields **sensitivity**
  - Tooth may be sensitive to biting forces
  - Vitality testing may be normal or unreliable initially
  - Retest for vitality after several weeks
- **Natural history and prognosis**
  - Pulpal blood supply is more likely to return to normal than other traumatic injuries
  - Regular clinical and radiographic monitoring recommended
  - **Reduction** in size of **pulp** chamber and root canals may develop in **months or years after trauma**
  - Pulp may become necrotic with time
  - Necrotic pulps do not have viable odontoblasts, and secondary dentin may not be deposited
  - Rarefying osteitis may occur
  - Internal root resorption rare but has been documented
- **Treatment**
  - **Usually conservative** unless tooth becomes nonvital
  - Defer definitive treatment (root canal therapy) for ~ 6 weeks: Retest for vitality
  - Slight adjustment and grinding of opposing teeth
  - Nonrigid splint application
  - Patient may be instructed to not bite on tooth
  - Dental arch wire can be fixed to teeth with composite filling material to splint and stabilize teeth
  - Regular clinical and radiographic monitoring are recommended

DIAGNOSTIC CHECKLIST

- **Consider**
  - Luxation
  - Rarefying osteitis
- **Reporting tips**
  - Examine all teeth and alveolar bone for fractures
  - Do not forget opposing teeth
  - If examining few months or years after trauma to tooth, examine for internal resorption or signs of pulp death
  - Examine for **calcific metamorphosis**: Narrowing of pulp chamber and canal

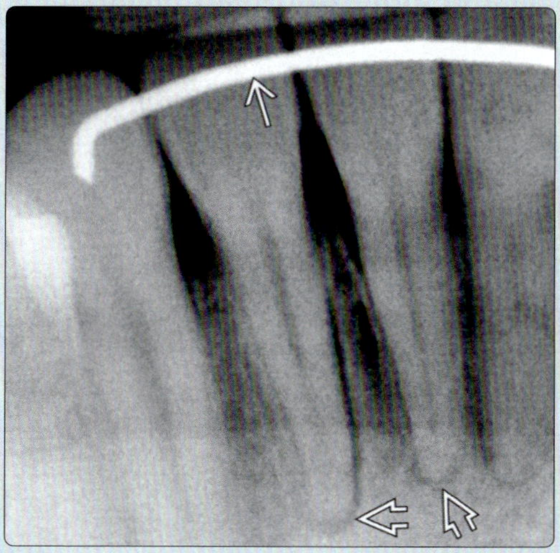

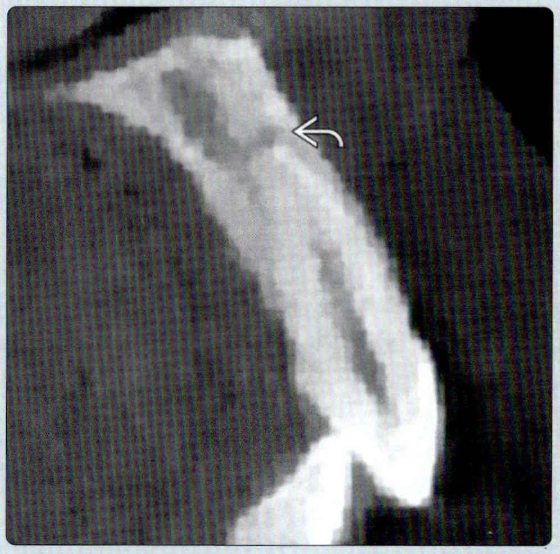

(Left) *Periapical radiograph shows slight widening of the periapical periodontal ligament (PDL) spaces ➡ of the mandibular central incisors after a dental concussion. Stabilization with a dental archwire ➡ was performed. (Courtesy T. Sawisch, DDS.)* **(Right)** *Sagittal CBCT shows the widening of the periapical PDL space ➡ of a maxillary central incisor following traumatic injury to the tooth. No clinical mobility was noted. (Courtesy T. Sawisch, DDS.)*

Luxation

KEY FACTS

TERMINOLOGY

- Definition
  - Dislocation of tooth from its socket with **tooth still attached**

IMAGING

- CBCT
  - Usually maxillary anterior teeth
  - **Extrusive**: Tooth displaced **coronally** or **lingually** with root-form low-density area representing socket
  - **Intrusive**: Tooth displaced **apically** with loss of periodontal ligament (PDL) space
  - **Lateral**: Tooth moved to one side with **PDL widened on side of impact**

TOP DIFFERENTIAL DIAGNOSES

- **Concussion**
  - No radiographic change or slight widening of periapical PDL space may be present
- **Subluxation**
  - Normal-appearing PDL
  - Abnormal mobility of tooth
- **Malocclusion**
  - Abnormal positioning of teeth
  - No history of trauma

CLINICAL ISSUES

- Intruded primary tooth **may damage permanent successor** tooth follicle

DIAGNOSTIC CHECKLIST

- Evaluate position of tooth in arch
- Rule out fractures of tooth structure
- Evaluate adjacent teeth for traumatic injury
- Evaluate condition of alveolar bone

(Left) *Sagittal reformat CBCT shows the lingual tilt of the crown of the primary lateral incisor ➡ and extrusion of the root through the facial cortex of the alveolar process ➡. The tooth socket can be seen ➡ between the primary tooth root and the follicle of the permanent tooth.* **(Right)** *Axial CBCT in the same patient shows the extrusion of the apices of the primary left lateral incisor ➡ and canine ➡ through the facial cortex of the alveolar process.*

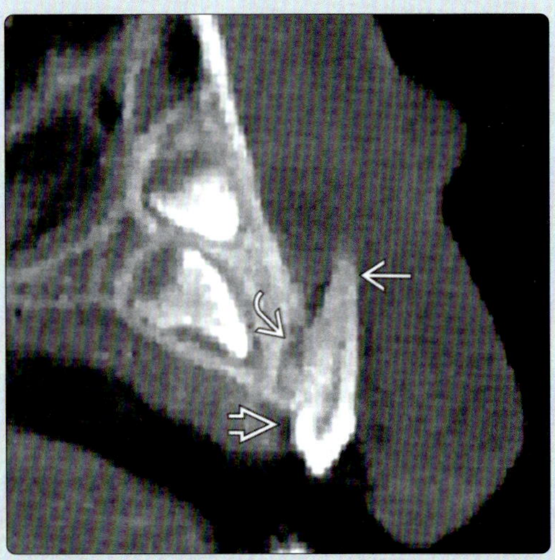

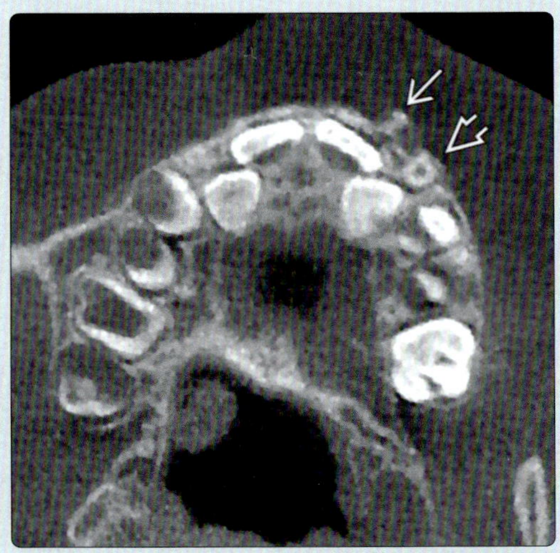

(Left) *A clinical photograph shows the appearance of the intruded maxillary left central incisor ➡. Enamel-dentin fracture is seen on the maxillary right central incisor ➡. (Courtesy H. Needleman, DDS.)* **(Right)** *Periapical radiograph of the same patient shows intrusion of the maxillary left central incisor ➡. Note apex located superiorly ➡ to right central incisor apex ➡. The fracture on the right central incisor has been restored with composite filling ➡. (Courtesy H. Needleman, DDS.)*

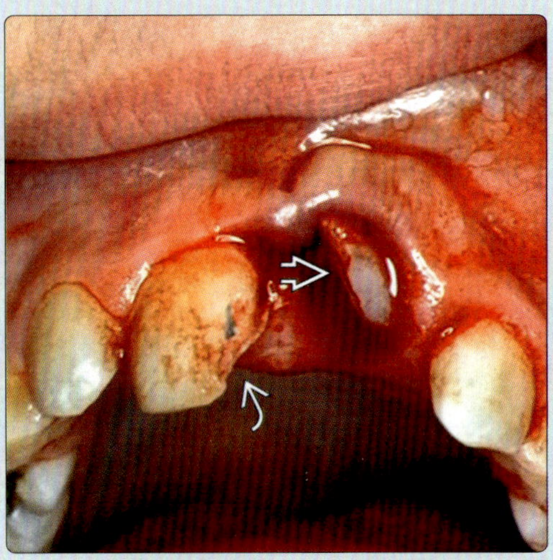

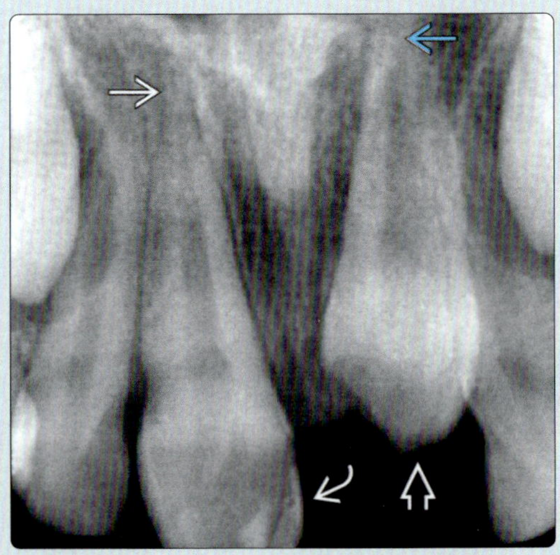

TERMINOLOGY

Synonyms

- **Extrusion**, extrusive luxation, **intrusion**, intrusive luxation, **lateral luxation**

Definitions

- Dislocation of tooth from its socket with **tooth still attached**

IMAGING

General Features

- Best diagnostic clue
  - **Extrusive**: Tooth displaced **coronally** or **lingually** with root-form low-density socket apparent
  - **Intrusive**: Tooth displaced **apically** with loss of periodontal ligament (PDL) space
  - **Lateral**: Tooth moved to one side with **PDL widened on side of impact**
- Location
  - Usually **maxillary anterior teeth**
  - Rarely in mandibular anterior teeth

CT Findings

- CBCT
  - **Extrusive**
    - Seen in **permanent** and **primary** dentitions
    - Sagittal plane
      - Tooth crown displaced **lingually** and **coronally**
      - Tooth root displaced facially, usually through facial cortex
  - **Intrusive**
    - Seen more commonly in **primary** teeth
    - Tooth is displaced **apically**
    - Apex is higher than that of contralateral tooth
    - Periapical PDL space is partially or totally obliterated
    - Possible impingement of intruded primary tooth on permanent tooth follicle
  - **Lateral**
    - Seen in **permanent** and **primary** dentitions
    - Displacement depends on direction of trauma
    - **PDL space is widened on side of impact**

Imaging Recommendations

- Best imaging tool
  - CBCT
    - 3D evaluation of condition and position of tooth and surrounding structures can be achieved
    - If not available: Combination of periapical and occlusal radiographs at right angles to each other

DIFFERENTIAL DIAGNOSIS

Concussion

- No radiographic change or slight widening of periapical PDL space may be present
- Possible reduction in size of pulp chamber or internal resorption in months/years to follow

Subluxation

- Clinically: Abnormal mobility of tooth with radiographically normal PDL

Malocclusion

- Abnormal positioning of teeth
- No history of trauma
- No widening of PDL space unless affected by odontogenic inflammation

CLINICAL ISSUES

Presentation

- Most common signs/symptoms
  - History of trauma, usually an emergency dental visit
  - **Abnormal tooth position**
    - **Extrusive**: Tooth is inferior to incisal edge of adjacent teeth
    - **Intrusive**: Tooth is superior to incisal edge of adjacent teeth; can be pushed all the way into alveolar process
    - **Lateral**: Tooth is pushed laterally
      - Differentiate from malocclusion by presence of widened PDL on impact side
  - Bleeding from gingival crevices
  - Very tender to percussion and mastication
  - Response to pulp vitality testing may be negative or decreased

Natural History & Prognosis

- **Intruded primary tooth may damage permanent successor tooth follicle**
- Tooth vitality may return in weeks or months
- Tooth may undergo external &/or internal resorption

Treatment

- **Deciduous**
  - Evaluation for damage to permanent tooth follicle
  - Extraction if possible damage is detected
  - Reposition tooth if such damage is not present; follow up regularly for discomfort or discoloration
  - Extraction can be considered if pain or inflammation ensue
- **Permanent**
  - Reposition tooth to normal alignment in arch using fingers
  - Slight grinding/reduction of opposing teeth to minimize discomfort
  - Splinting using a flexible splint may be considered
  - Bone fragments should be repositioned by digital pressure

DIAGNOSTIC CHECKLIST

Reporting Tips

- Evaluate position of tooth in arch
- Rule out fractures of tooth structure
- Evaluate adjacent teeth for traumatic injury
- If intruded tooth is primary: Evaluate for damage to underlying permanent tooth
- Evaluate condition of alveolar bone
- Look for bony fragments in adjacent soft tissue

SELECTED REFERENCES

1. Chafaie A: Partial and total luxations of permanent teeth in children: Clinical management. Int Orthod. 14(1):32-47, 2016

(Left) *Clinical photograph shows labial luxation (a form of lateral luxation) of the maxillary left central incisor.* **(Right)** *Periapical radiograph of the same patient shows that no changes can be seen in this radiographic plane because the tooth was moved labially. CBCT could have shown the widening of the periodontal ligament (PDL) space lingually but was not available. This tooth was repositioned manually and splinted. (Courtesy H. Needleman, DDS.)*

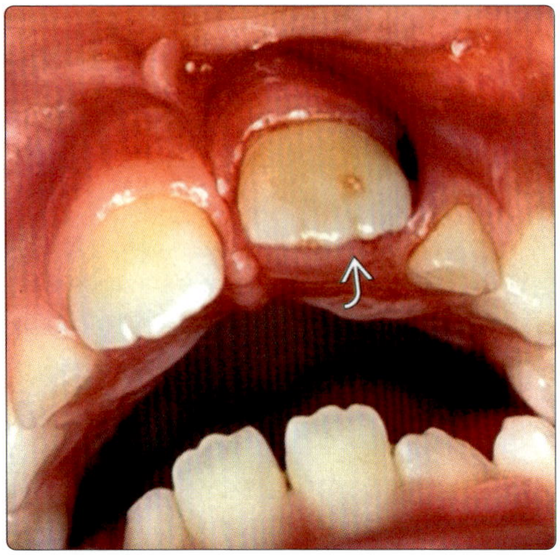

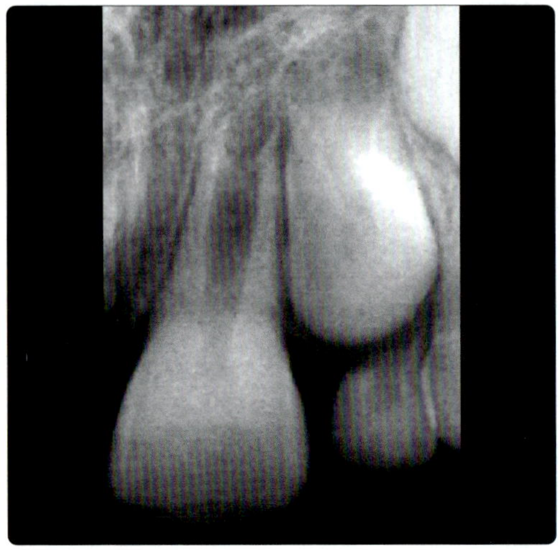

(Left) *Periapical radiograph in the same patient 10 years post trauma shows that the tooth apex has closed, and no root canal treatment was needed. The pulp of the affected tooth has calcified, most likely in response to the trauma. (Courtesy H. Needleman, DDS.)* **(Right)** *Periapical radiograph shows intrusion and incisal fracture of the maxillary left central and lateral incisors. Note the absence of the PDL space at the apex of the central incisor. (Courtesy H. Needleman, DDS.)*

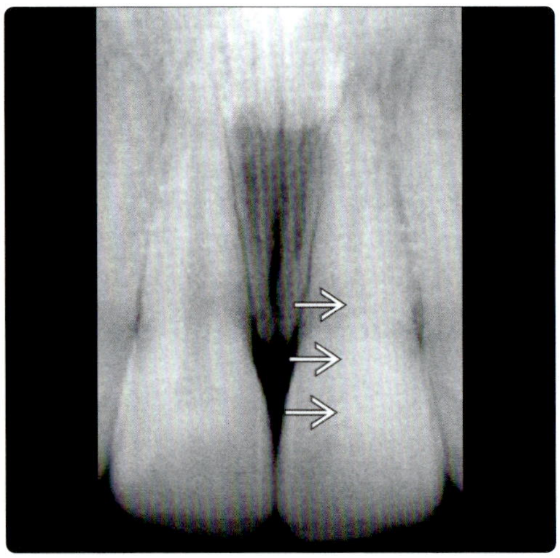

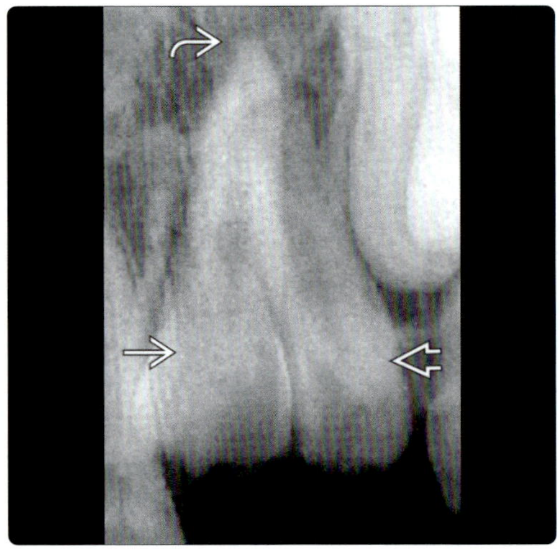

(Left) *Periapical radiograph shows the repositioning and stabilization of the intruded central and lateral incisors with a wire and composite splint. Note the development of rarefying osteitis at the apex of the lateral incisor. (Courtesy H. Needleman, DDS.)* **(Right)** *A follow-up periapical radiograph in the same patient shows internal and external resorption of the teeth, as root canal treatment was initialized but never completed. (Courtesy H. Needleman, DDS.)*

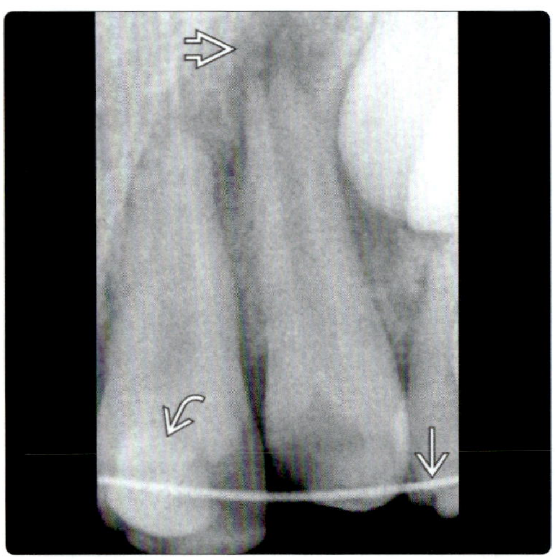

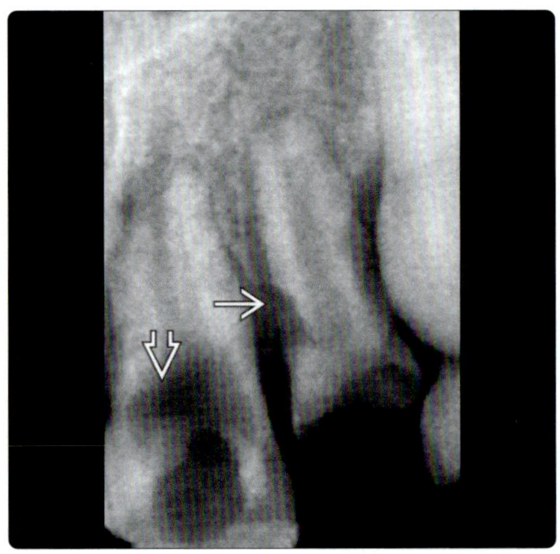

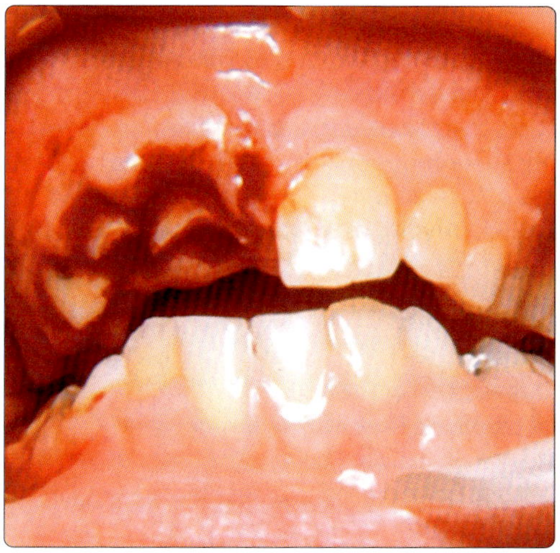

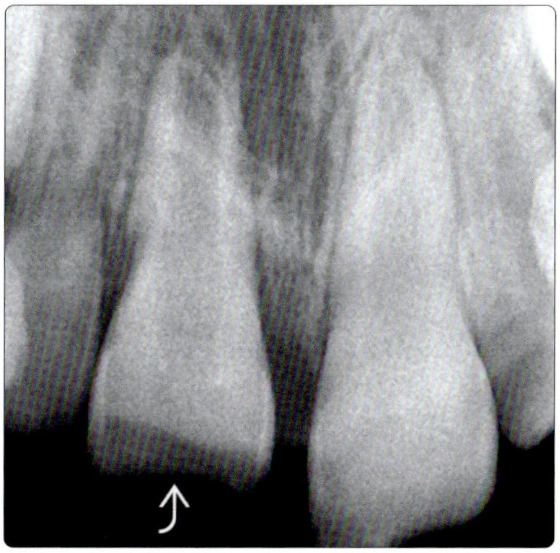

(Left) *Clinical photograph shows intrusion of the maxillary right central and lateral incisors. Note the blood oozing from the gingival crevice, indicative of acute trauma. (Courtesy H. Needleman, DDS.)* **(Right)** *Periapical radiograph in the same patient shows fracture of the incisal edge ➔. (Courtesy H. Needleman, DDS.)*

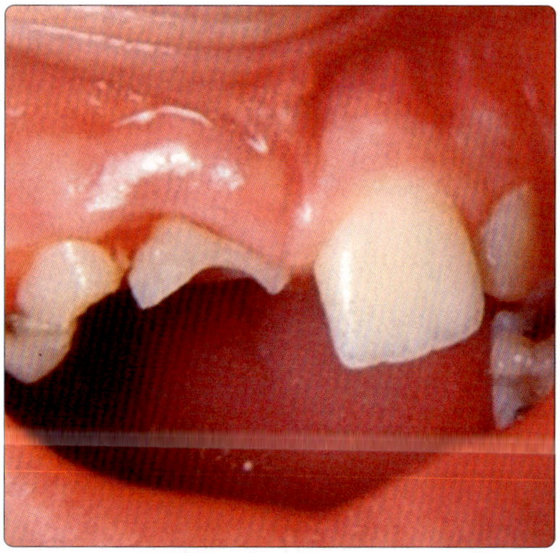

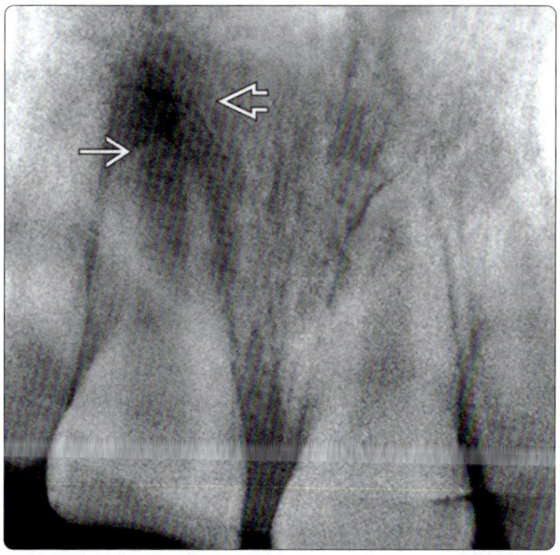

(Left) *Clinical photograph in the same patient demonstrates gradual spontaneous reeruption of the teeth and healing of the periodontium. (Courtesy H. Needleman, DDS.)* **(Right)** *Periapical radiograph in the same patient shows rarefying osteitis ➔ apical to the maxillary central incisor. Treatment by root canal therapy is recommended. Note that the death of the pulp occurred prior to the closing of the apex of the tooth, resulting in an open apex ➔. (Courtesy H. Needleman, DDS.)*

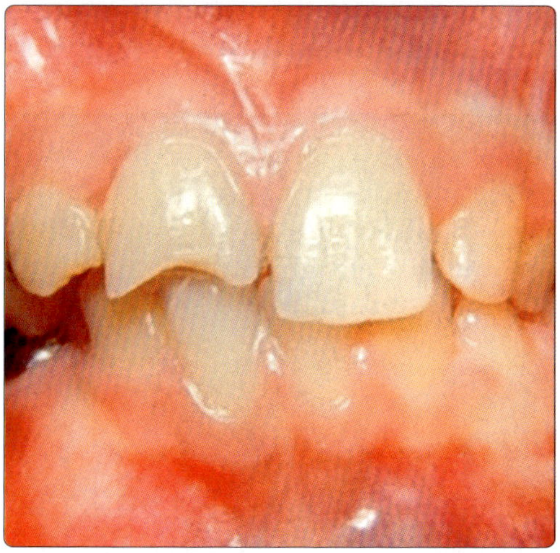

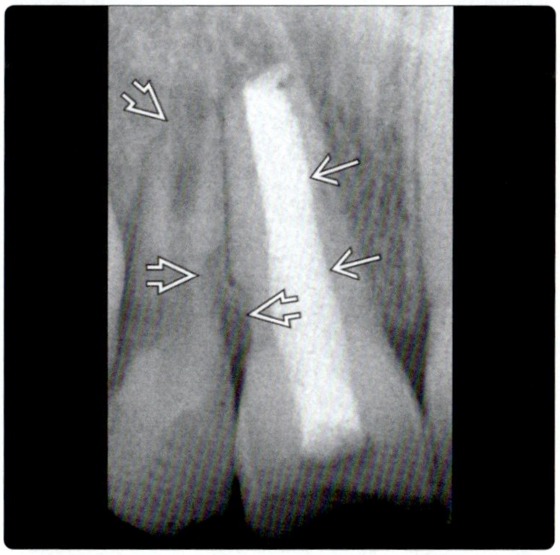

(Left) *Clinical photograph in the same patient shows full spontaneous reeruption of the intruded teeth. The fractured incisal edges can be repaired by composite restoration. (Courtesy H. Needleman, DDS.)* **(Right)** *Periapical radiograph in the same patient shows the root canal treatment and obturation of the pulp canal by gutta percha ➔. Note the external resorption ➔ of the root of both incisors. (Courtesy H. Needleman, DDS.)*

Dentoalveolar Fractures

KEY FACTS

TERMINOLOGY

- Abbreviation: Fracture (fx)
- **Definition**: Fx of tooth structure &/or alveolar bone

IMAGING

- **Thin radiolucent line** running partially or fully through tooth structure
- **Horizontal fx**: Most common in maxillary anterior teeth due to trauma
  - Root fx is visualized if x-ray beam passes through fx line
  - May see 2 lines corresponding to buccal and lingual margins of fx: Lines join at margins of root
- **Vertical fx**: Teeth with complex restorative procedures, such as root canal treatment and intraradicular post retention (post and core)
  - Difficult to diagnose if nondisplaced
  - May be difficult to visualize on CT due to metal artifact from intraradicular filling and restoration

TOP DIFFERENTIAL DIAGNOSES

- Fxs of alveolar process
  - 2D imaging: May see superimposition of image of alveolar fx on root surface
- Superimposition of soft tissue structures
  - 2D imaging: Superimposition of image of lip, ala of nose, or nasolabial fold over root
  - Outline extends **beyond root margins**

CLINICAL ISSUES

- Mobile or displaced teeth
- Mild pain on biting
- Treatment: Depends on type of fx
  - **Horizontal crown fx**: Restoration or root canal treatment
  - **Horizontal root fx**: Leave alone unless mobile → splint, then follow up to determine vitality of tooth
  - **Vertical fx**: Extraction or root amputation

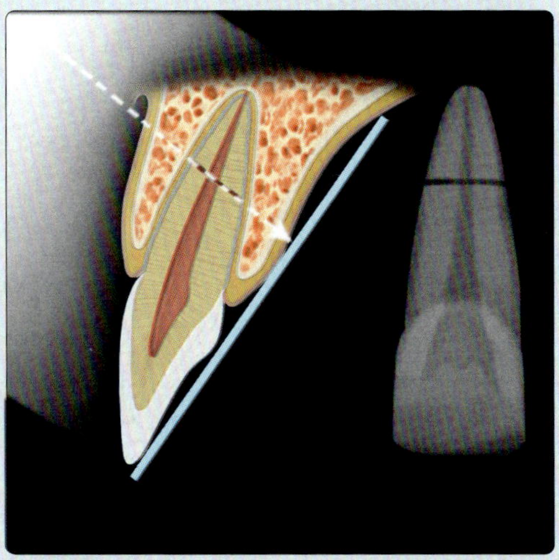

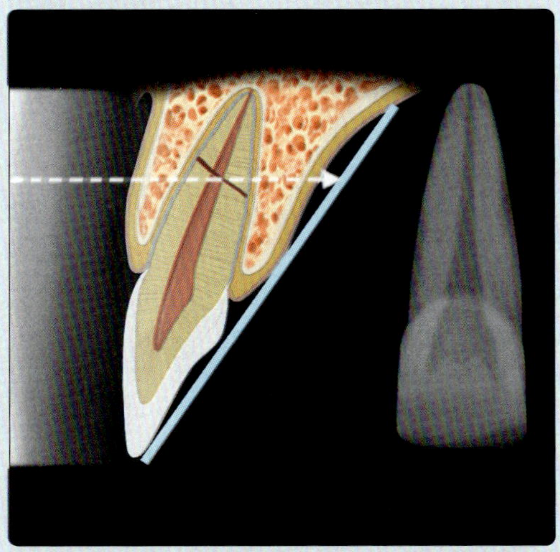

(Left) *Graphic drawing demonstrates the correct vertical angulation of the x-ray beam to pass through the horizontal root fracture line in order for the fracture to be visible on the image. This drawing shows the use of this technique with the bisecting angle periapical radiographic technique but can be used with the paralleling technique as well.* **(Right)** *This graphic shows that an incorrectly vertically angulated x-ray beam may lead to the superimposition of the fragments on the fracture line, reducing visibility.*

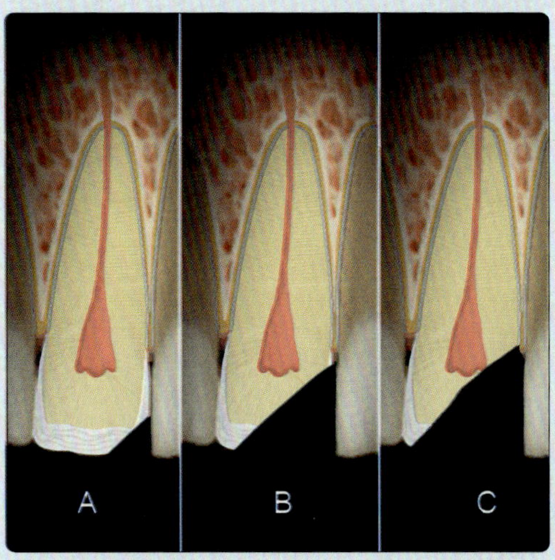

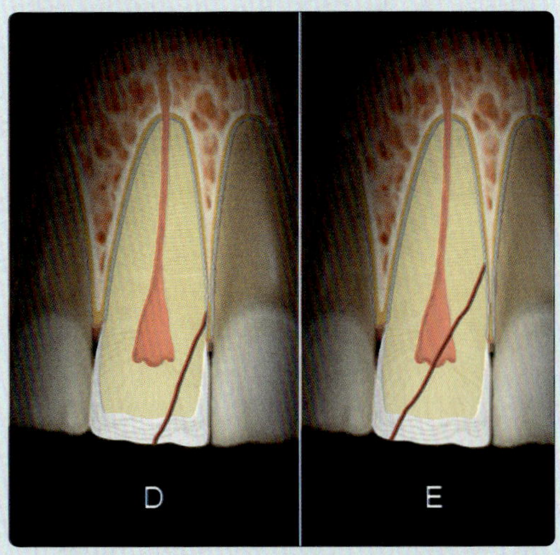

(Left) *This graphic shows supracrestal oblique coronal fractures with the cervical fracture margin above the alveolar bone crest involving enamel only (A), enamel and dentin (B), and enamel, dentin, and pulp (C).* **(Right)** *Graphic drawing shows subcrestal oblique coronal fractures. These may involve the enamel and dentin (D) or enamel, dentin, and pulp (E) but have the cervical fracture margin under the crest of the alveolar bone, which complicates treatment and prognosis.*

TERMINOLOGY

Abbreviations

- Fracture (fx)

Synonyms

- **Horizontal fx** = crown-root fx = transverse fx
- **Vertical fx** = longitudinal fx

Definitions

- Fx of tooth structure &/or supporting alveolar process

IMAGING

General Features

- Best diagnostic clue
  - **Thin radiolucent line running through tooth structure &/or alveolar process**
- Location
  - **Horizontal fx**
    - Most common in **maxillary anterior teeth** (trauma)
  - **Vertical fx**
    - Teeth with complex restorative procedures, such as **root canal treatment** and intraradicular post retention (**post and core**)
    - Located in **facial-lingual plane of tooth**
  - **Oblique fx**
    - Oblique fx can involve
      - Enamel only, enamel and dentin, or enamel, dentin and pulp
      - Can be supracrestal and subcrestal
  - **Cemental fx**
    - Teeth with high occlusal forces with hypercementosis may show fx limited to cementum
    - May predispose to periodontal infection

Radiographic Findings

- Intraoral plain film
  - Horizontal root fx is visualized **if x-ray beam passes through fx line**
    - May be missed if central beam direction is not parallel or close to parallel to fx line
    - Steep vertical angulation (**foreshortening**) exposure and parallel technique exposure will detect many fxs, especially apical 3rd fx
    - May see **2 radiolucent lines** corresponding to buccal and lingual margins of fx
      - **Lines join** at lateral margins of root
  - Vertical fx
    - Nondisplaced fx difficult to diagnose
      - Presence of **deep periodontal defect, J-shaped bone loss** and bone resorption can be tip-off
    - Displaced fx shows splitting of root

CT Findings

- CBCT
  - **Use custom cross sections**
  - Follow course of lucent line and describe direction
  - Tooth pieces may not be displaced, confounding dx
  - **Vertical fx**: Examine facial and lingual surfaces of root
    - May be difficult to visualize due to **metal artifact from intraradicular filling and restoration**

Imaging Recommendations

- Protocol advice
  - Periapicals
    - Multiple exposures at **different vertical angulations** to reveal fx not in line with x-ray beam when using conventional paralleling technique
  - CBCT
    - Use custom cross sections to evaluate all surfaces of tooth ("pan around tooth")

DIFFERENTIAL DIAGNOSIS

Fractures of Alveolar Process

- 2D imaging: May see superimposition of image of alveolar fx on root surface

Superimposition of Soft Tissue Structures

- 2D imaging: Superimposition of image of lip, ala of nose, or nasolabial fold over root
  - Outline extends **beyond root margins**

CLINICAL ISSUES

Presentation

- Most common signs/symptoms
  - Mobile or displaced teeth and mild pain on biting

Treatment

- **Horizontal crown fx**
  - Treatment depends on involved dental tissue
    - Enamel and dentin only: Composite restoration
    - Enamel, dentin, and pulp: Root canal treatment
- **Horizontal root fx**: Divide root into thirds
  - **Apical**
    - Leave alone; may heal spontaneously or after splinting
      Root canal treatment if rarefying osteitis occurs
  - **Middle**
    - If coronal segment of tooth is not mobile, leave alone
    - If coronal segment is mobile, stabilize by splinting with orthodontic archwire and light-cured resin
    - Root canal: Treat if becomes necrotic
  - **Coronal**
    - Poorest prognosis; tooth pulp most likely to necrose
    - Reposition crown and stabilize with splinting for up to 12 weeks to allow repair of periodontium
    - **If no rarefying osteitis** noted when repair occurs, **no root canal treatment necessary**
- **Vertical fx**
  - Dx difficult, but treatment simple: Extraction
  - Root amputation or hemisection **(bicuspidization)** for multirooted teeth
- **Oblique fx**
  - Subcrestal crown fx: May need crown lengthening procedure or extraction
- Monitor: Traumatized teeth at risk for resorption/ankylosis

SELECTED REFERENCES

1. Serra-Pastor B et al: Treatment and restoration of adult dentoalveolar trauma: a clinical case report. J Clin Exp Dent. 8(5):e634-e637, 2016

(Left) *Coronal CBCT of a maxillary premolar shows an oblique crown fracture. The cervical margin is above the crest of the bone (supracrestal). Pulp involvement is sometimes difficult to determine, especially in lower resolution scans. (Courtesy M. Noujeim, DDS.)* **(Right)** *Graphic shows the degree of coronal involvement in horizontal crown fractures. These fragments are usually displaced and lost with the pulp tissue exposed to the oral cavity.*

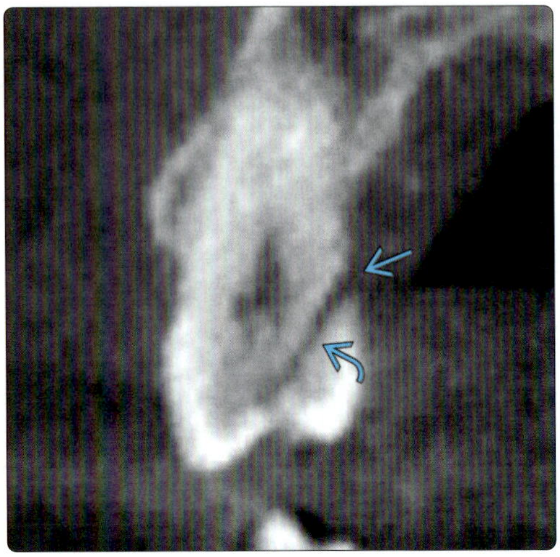

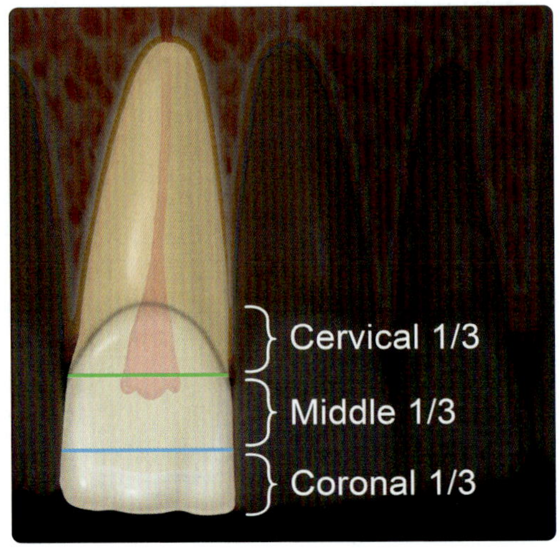

(Left) *CBCT 3D surface rendering shows a horizontal coronal fracture on the maxillary right lateral incisor and a fracture of the coronal 1/3 of the root of the right central incisor. (Courtesy M. Noujeim, DDS.)* **(Right)** *Graphic shows the degrees of root involvement in horizontal root fractures. The apical 1/3 fractures have a better prognosis than the middle 1/3 fractures. The coronal 1/3 fractures have the worst prognosis.*

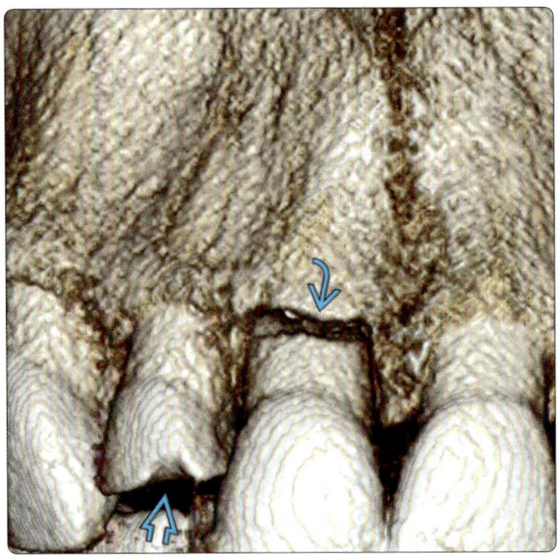

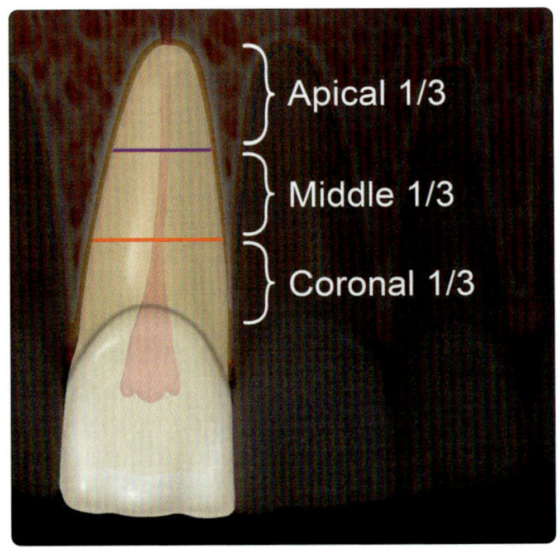

(Left) *Periapical radiograph shows a horizontal fracture in the middle 1/3 of the maxillary left central incisor. Horizontal root fractures may appear as 2 radiolucent lines representing the buccal and lingual margins of the fracture. The lines join at the lateral margins of the root.* **(Right)** *Periapical radiograph shows a horizontal fracture of the apical 1/3 of the root of the maxillary right lateral incisor. Faint, high-density material is noted in the root canal, suggestive of inadequate obturation with root canal filling material.*

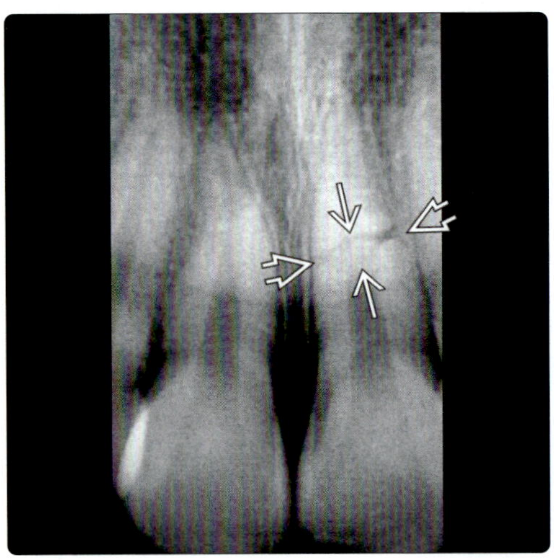

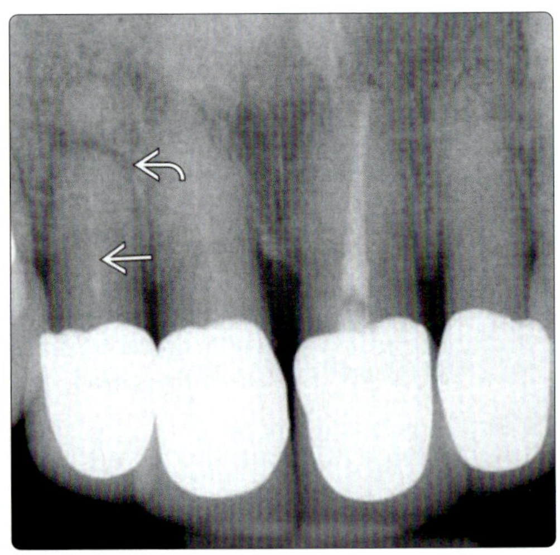

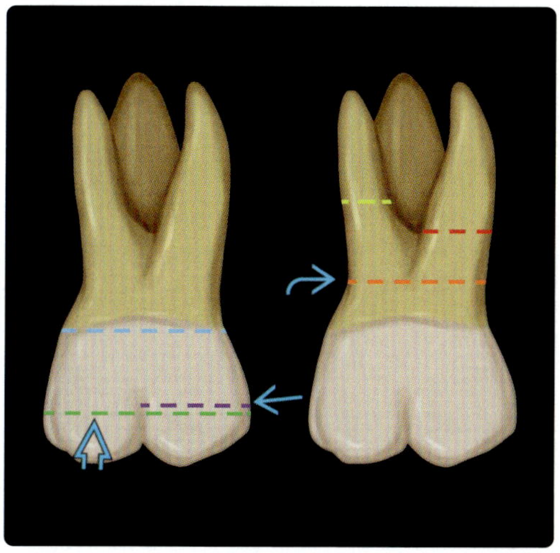

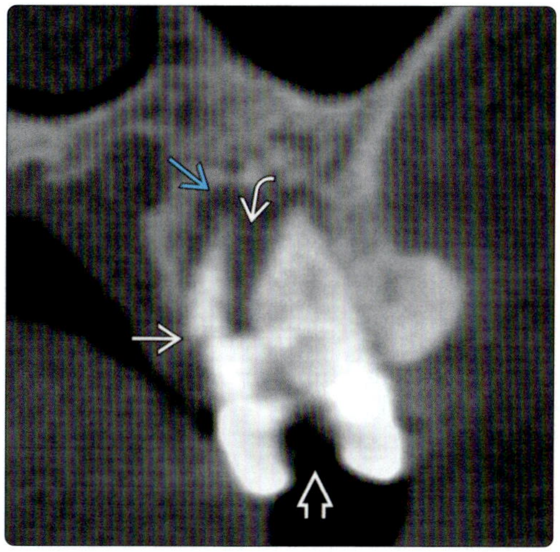

(Left) *Graphic shows the possible horizontal tooth fractures in a posterior tooth. Coronal fractures can involve 1 cusp, 1 side of a tooth (buccal or lingual, often with an oblique component), or the entire crown may be fractured. Root fractures can involve 1 root in the apical, middle, or furcation 1/3 or may be coronal to the furcation.* **(Right)** *Coronal CBCT shows vertical and horizontal root fractures of a left maxillary molar. There is associated bone loss and a missing filling in the crown.*

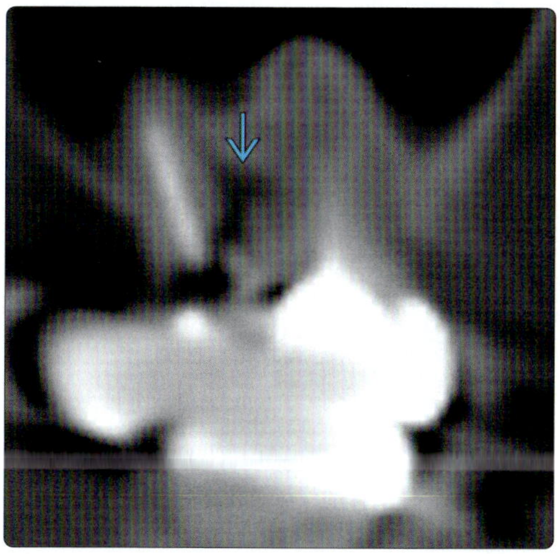

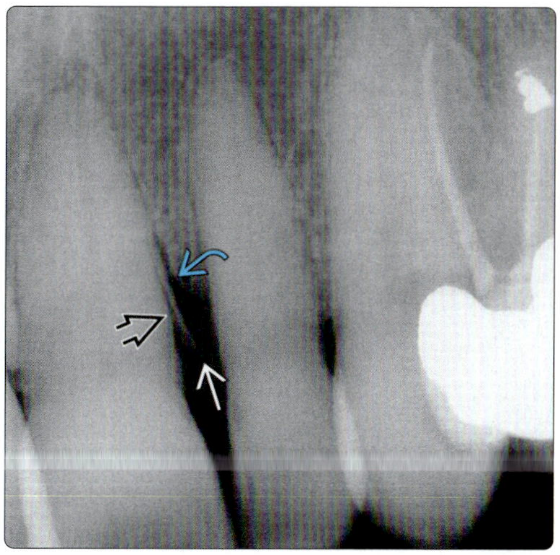

(Left) *Coronal CBCT of a maxillary left 1st molar shows root fracture of the palatal root. The tooth is root canal treated and shows moderate to severe periodontal bone loss in relation to this fracture.* **(Right)** *Periapical radiography shows a cemental fracture on the distal aspect of the left central incisor. These cemental fractures (also called tears) are a separation of the cementum (in hypercementosis) from the root, leading to periodontal bone loss. (Courtesy T. Orazio, DDS.)*

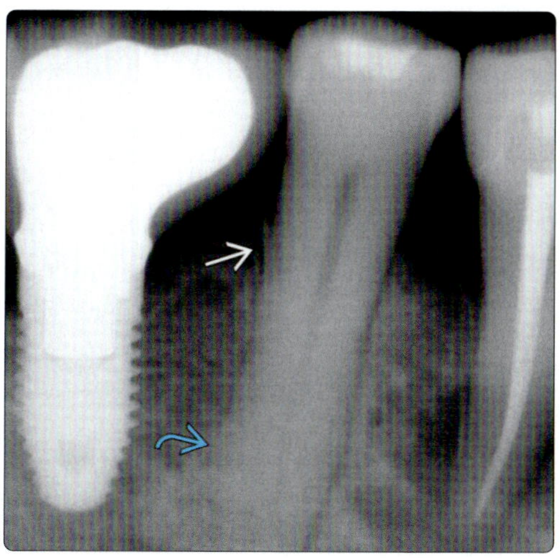

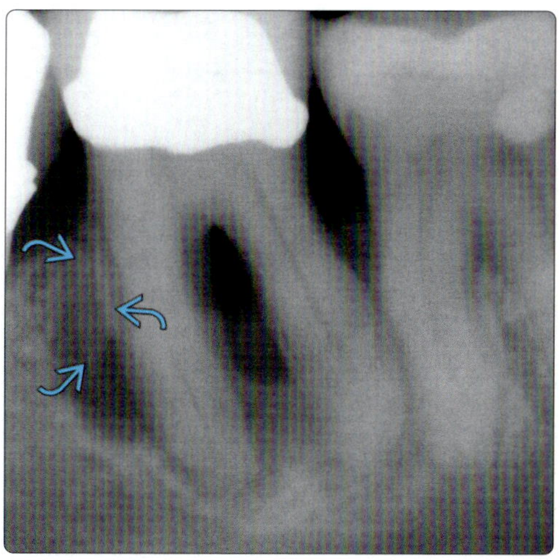

(Left) *Periapical radiograph shows a tooth with a bulbous root (hypercementosis). There is a separation of the cementum from the middle 1/3 of the root. (Courtesy J. Levy, DDS.)* **(Right)** *Periapical radiography (same patient) shows hypercementosis of the roots with severe periodontal bone loss. High-density material is seen separating from the root surface (cemental fracture). Clinically, there was a fistula tracing back to this tooth. (Courtesy J. Levy, DDS.)*

(Left) *CBCT 3D reformation shows a vertical root fracture. This tooth was endodontically treated. These fractures can occur at the time of root canal filling or months or years after treatment.* **(Right)** *Axial CBCT shows a low-density line running from the mesial surface to the distolingual surface of the maxillary right 2nd premolar root. The best tip-off to the presence of a vertical fracture is localized periodontal pockets that may or may not communicate with the crest of the bone.*

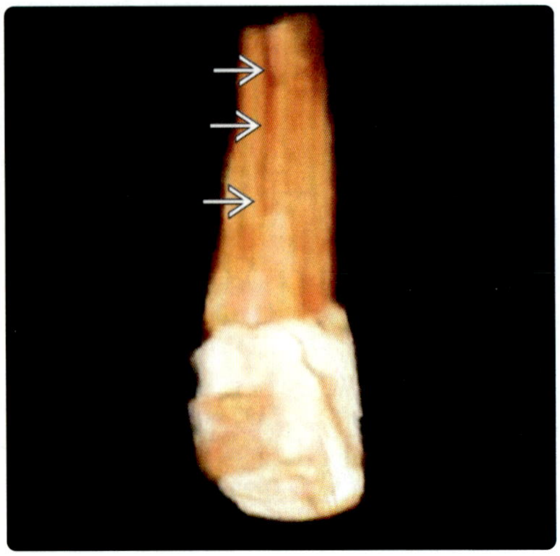

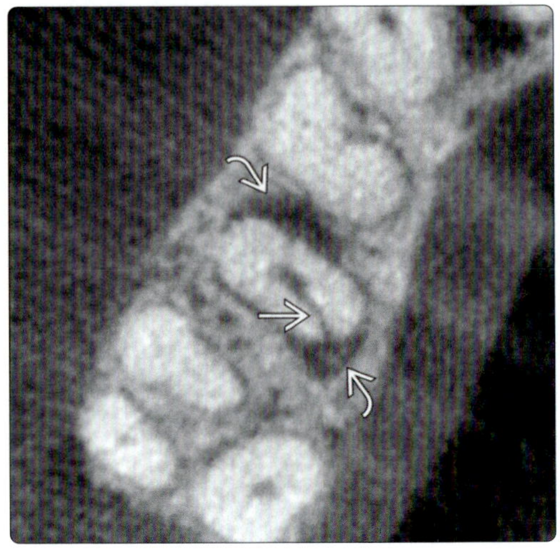

(Left) *Axial CBCT shows a vertical fracture of a maxillary molar with surrounding rarefaction.* **(Right)** *Coronal CBCT of a maxillary right 3rd molar shows a root canal-treated mesiobuccal root. There is a vertical periodontal bone defect along the lingual aspect of the root that extends to the apex of the root, with widening of the periapical periodontal ligament space. These are often indirect signs of vertical root fractures if no displaced fragments are noted.*

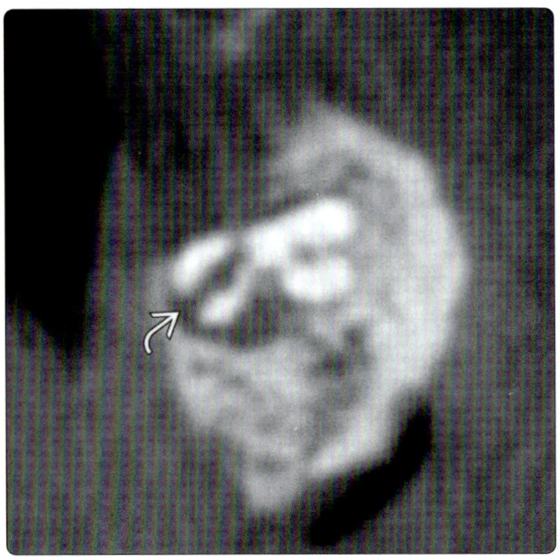

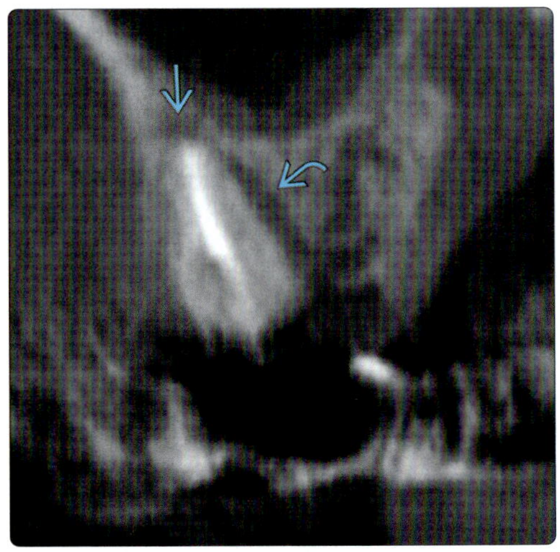

(Left) *Sagittal section shows a vertical fracture of the mesial root of the right mandibular 1st molar. The fractured fragments are displaced, making visualization of the fracture easy. There is periodontal and periapical rarefaction, often seen with these fractures.* **(Right)** *Axial view in the same patient shows the separation of the fractured fragments. This tooth is root canal treated, and fractures are usually difficult to evaluate on root canal-treated teeth due to a metal artifact that mimics fracture lines.*

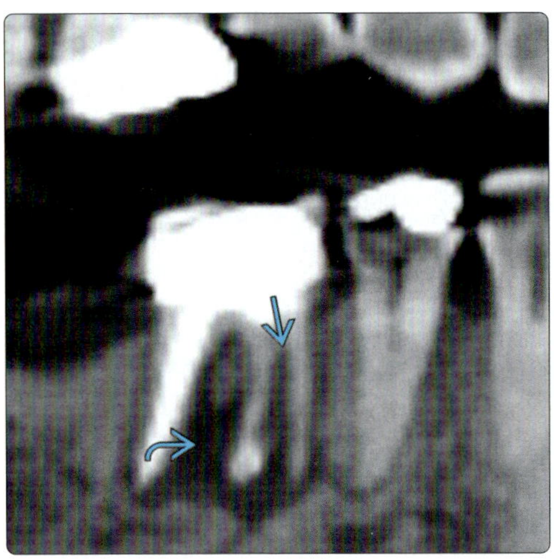

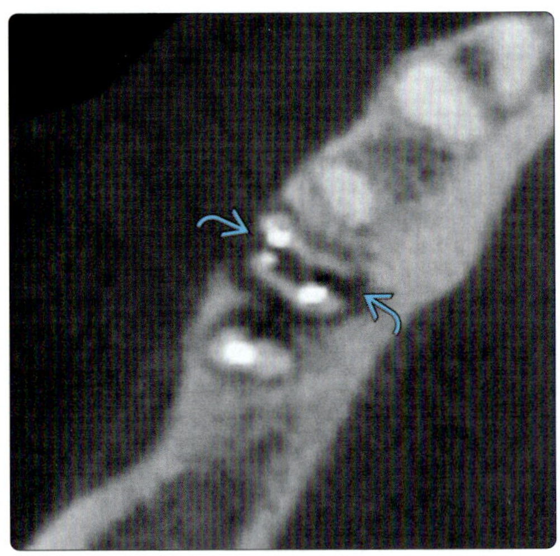

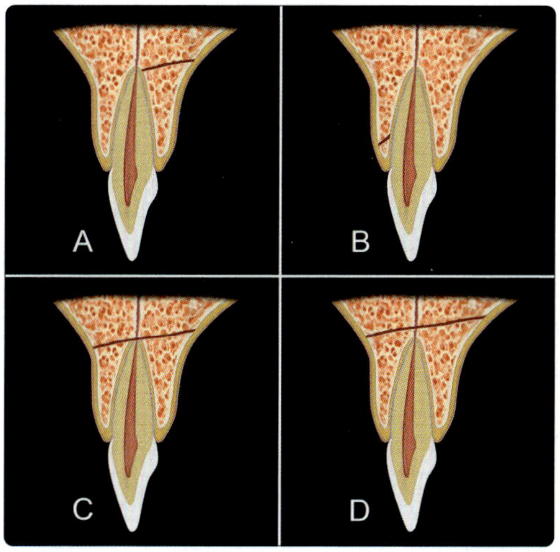

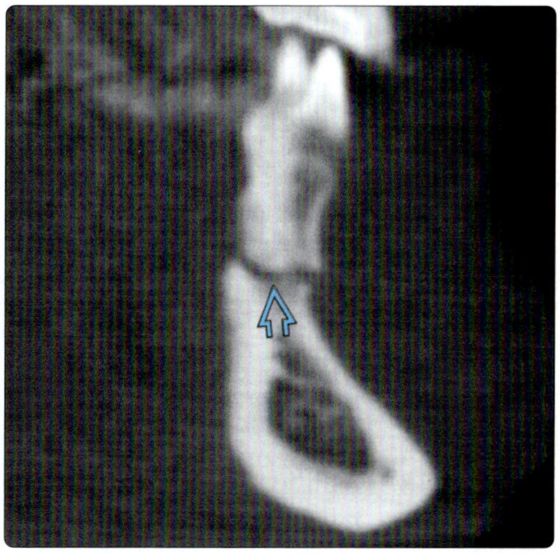

(Left) *Graphic drawing shows the different types of horizontal alveolar bone fractures encountered that do not involve fractures of the tooth structure. The facial or lingual plates can be involved separately and at different levels in relation to the tooth structure (A, B) or can run across the bone at the level of the tooth apex (C) or separate from it (D).* **(Right)** *Sagittal CBCT of the mandibular anterior alveolar process shows a horizontal fracture of the bone at the level of the apices of the teeth without fracture of the root.*

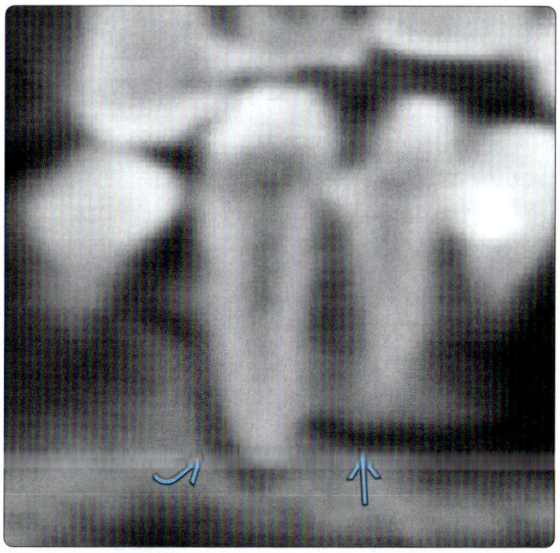

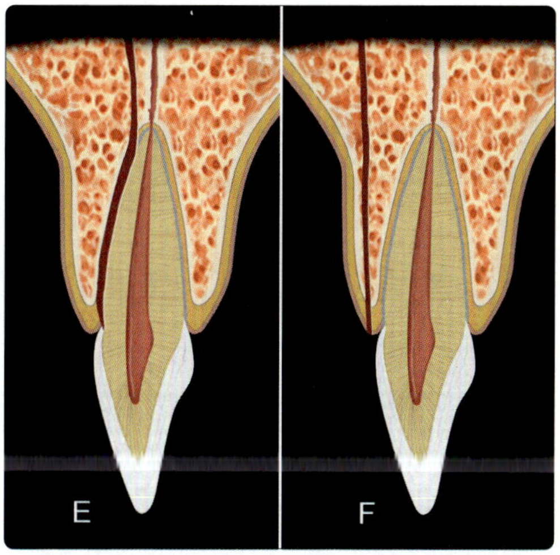

(Left) *Coronal oblique CBCT shows a horizontal alveolar bone fracture that involves the periodontal ligament space of the mandibular right canine. The periodontal ligament space is widened.* **(Right)** *Graphic shows the different types of vertical alveolar bone fractures, those involving the periodontal ligament space (E) and those that do not (F).*

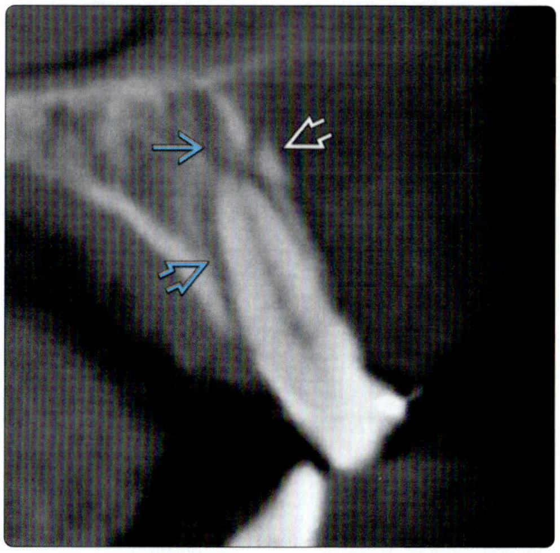

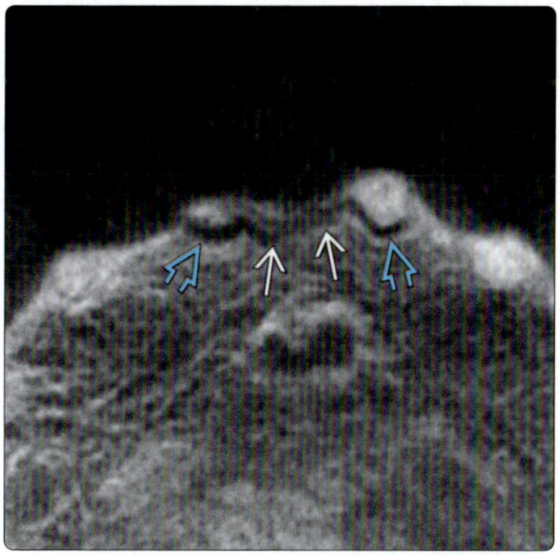

(Left) *Sagittal CBCT shows a vertical alveolar fracture involving a maxillary lateral incisor. There is a vertical low-density fracture line in the alveolus associated with the periodontal ligament of the tooth. The tooth is displaced facially (lateral luxation), and a small fractured fragment of the bone cortex is noted. (Courtesy M. Noujeim, DDS.)* **(Right)** *Axial CBCT shows a vertical alveolar bone fracture involving the periodontal ligament spaces of the maxillary central incisors. (Courtesy M. Noujeim, DDS.)*

Dental Caries

KEY FACTS

TERMINOLOGY

- Definition: **Infectious disease** caused by lactic acid secretion from *Streptococcus mutans* that causes **demineralization of tooth structure**

IMAGING

- Can affect any surface of tooth
- Size depends on severity
- **Bitewing radiography** for posterior teeth
- Transillumination (clinical) and **periapical radiography** for anterior teeth
- **CBCT should not be used** for evaluation or diagnosis of caries

TOP DIFFERENTIAL DIAGNOSES

- Unfilled cavity preparations
- Radiolucent fillings
- Cervical burnout
- Idiopathic cervical resorption
- Dental anomalies
- Tooth wear
- Mach band effect

CLINICAL ISSUES

- Sensitivity to hot, cold, or air; pain
- Small lesions: Fluoride application and diet modification
- Larger lesions: Caries excavation and restoration of tooth structure ± root canal therapy
- If tooth is nonrestorable → extraction

DIAGNOSTIC CHECKLIST

- Clinical caries bigger than appears radiographically
- Radiation caries is due to destruction of salivary gland tissue causing **xerostomia**, not direct effect of radiation on tooth structure

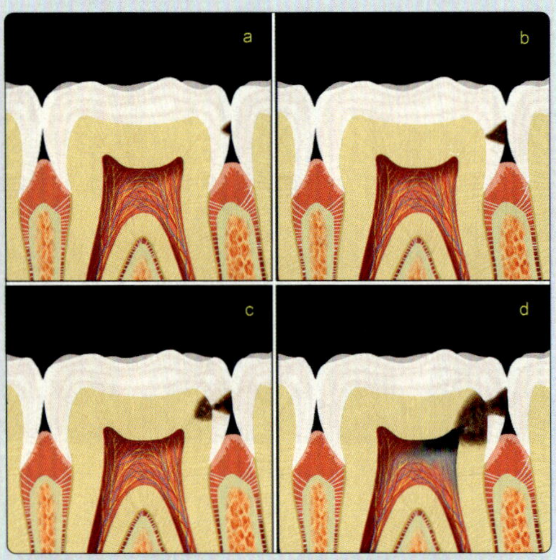

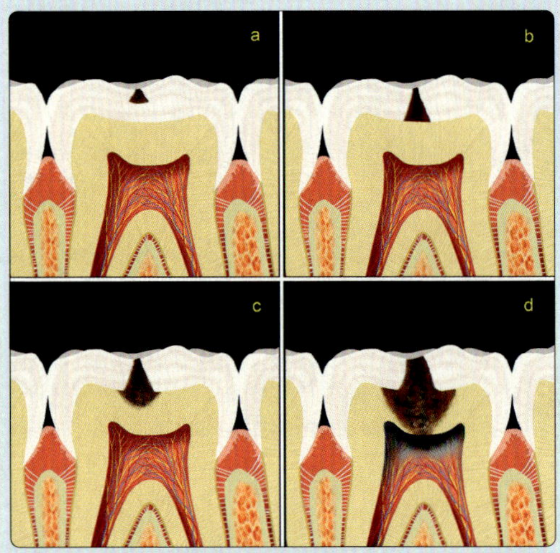

(Left) *Graphic representation shows the progression of proximal caries: (a) Incipient, (b) moderate, (c) advanced, and (d) severe. Note that the enamel caries triangle tip is at the dentinoenamel junction (DEJ) and the base is at the enamel surface under the contact point.* **(Right)** *Graphic representation shows the progression of occlusal caries. The stages of progression are the same as for proximal caries, but the base of the enamel caries triangle is at the DEJ. Clinically, caries is always larger than it appears radiographically.*

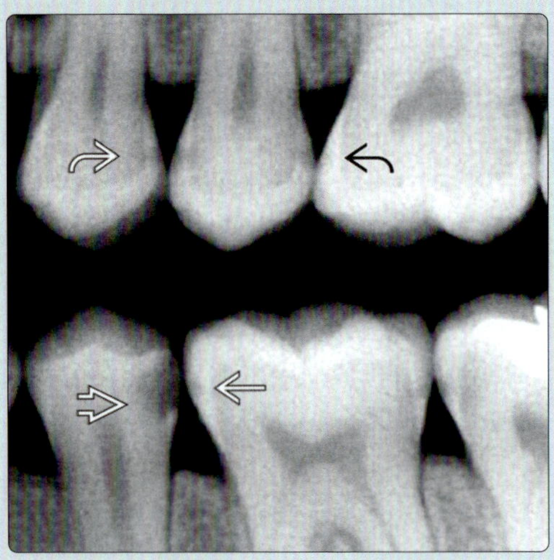

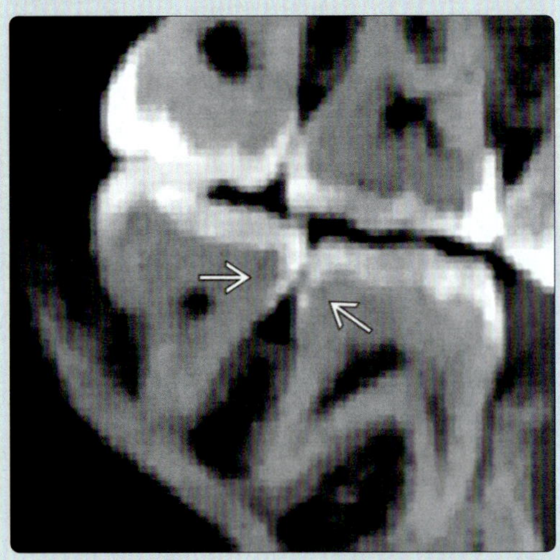

(Left) *Bitewing (BW) radiograph shows incipient , moderate , advanced , and severe class II carious lesions. BWs have higher resolution than CBCT. Lesions limited to enamel will not appear until 30-40% demineralization has occurred. (Courtesy B. Friedland, BDS.)* **(Right)** *Sagittal CBCT shows proximal caries of the mandibular molars. CBCT is suboptimal for evaluation and diagnosis of these lesions and should be preceded or followed by bitewing radiography if caries is suspected in the oral cavity.*

TERMINOLOGY

Synonyms

- Dental decay, cavities (layperson's term)

Definitions

- Infectious disease caused by lactic acid secretion from *Streptococcus mutans* that causes demineralization of tooth structure

IMAGING

General Features

- Location
  - Any surface of tooth
    - Occlusal and pits = **class I** caries
    - Posterior proximal = **class II** caries
    - Anterior proximal = **class III** caries
    - Anterior proximal and incisal = **class IV** caries
    - Cervical 1/3 of crown = **class V** caries
    - Root = **root** caries, senile caries, or cemental caries
    - Adjacent to restorations = **recurrent** caries
    - All teeth (severe destruction) = **rampant** caries
- Size
  - Depending on severity
    - **Incipient**: In enamel only; less than halfway from outer surface to dentinoenamel junction (DEJ)
    - **Moderate**: In enamel only, up to **DEJ**
    - **Advanced**: Spreads along DEJ in dentin but does not reach more than halfway from DEJ to pulp
    - **Severe**: More than halfway from DEJ to pulp (pulp may be breached)
  - **Radiographic lesion smaller than clinical lesion**, as 40% decalcification required before evident on intraoral imaging
- Morphology
  - Occlusal caries
    - Enamel: Radiolucent triangle with apex directed toward outer surface of enamel and base toward DEJ; **not seen radiographically**
    - Dentin: Radiolucent triangle with broad base at DEJ and apex directed toward pulp; base of enamel triangle meets base of dentin triangle at DEJ
  - Interproximal caries
    - Enamel: Radiolucent triangle with base at outer surface of enamel and apex directed toward DEJ
    - Dentin: Radiolucent triangle with broad base at DEJ and apex directed toward pulp
  - Cemental caries
    - Lesions appear **"scooped out"** apical to CEJ

Imaging Recommendations

- Best imaging tool
  - **Bitewing** radiography for posterior teeth
  - **Transillumination** (clinical) and **periapical** radiography for anterior teeth
  - Subtraction digital radiography may be used to follow-up for new or recurrent lesions
  - **CBCT should not be used for evaluation or diagnosis of caries**
    - If evident on CBCT, follow-up with appropriate intraoral radiography and clinical examination

DIFFERENTIAL DIAGNOSIS

Unfilled Cavity Preparations

- Cavity preparations are usually sharply marginated unless secondarily affected by caries

Radiolucent Fillings

- Older anterior restorative materials may be completely radiolucent and confused with caries
- "C" shape of cavity preparation helps to distinguish

Cervical Burnout

- Overpenetration of cervical area of tooth due to decrease in mass and density of tooth structure
- Can extend below level of bone; **caries does not**

Idiopathic Cervical Resorption

- External resorption of cervical portions of teeth

Dental Anomalies

- Irregularities and hypoplasias may mimic caries

Tooth Wear

- Physiologic wear (attrition) or nonphysiologic wear (abrasion & erosion) will result in low-density areas that may mimic caries

Mach Band Effect

- Optical illusion producing radiolucency along DEJ

PATHOLOGY

General Features

- Etiology
  - Combination of organisms (*S. mutans*), appropriate substrate (dietary sugars), and tooth morphology (deep pits and fissures)
    - Risk factors include xerostomia (**medications**, XRT) and high sugar intake (e.g., soda)

CLINICAL ISSUES

Presentation

- Most common signs/symptoms
  - Sensitivity to hot, cold, or air as lesion traverses DEJ
  - Pain if lesion reaches pulp and causes pulpitis

Treatment

- Small lesions: Fluoride application and diet modification
- Larger lesions: Caries excavation and restoration of tooth structure ± root canal therapy
  - If tooth is nonrestorable → extraction

DIAGNOSTIC CHECKLIST

Image Interpretation Pearls

- Clinical caries bigger than appears radiographically
- Radiation caries is due to destruction of salivary gland tissue causing **xerostomia**, not direct effect of radiation on tooth structure

SELECTED REFERENCES

1. Gaalaas L et al: Ex vivo evaluation of new 2D and 3D dental radiographic technology for detecting caries. Dentomaxillofac Radiol. 45(3):20150281, 2016

(Left) *BW radiograph shows recurrent caries* → *under the distal filling of the mandibular left 1st molar. Adjacent caries* → *appears in enamel as a triangle with its tip at the DEJ. The caries spreads along the DEJ to form a radiolucent triangle base in dentin. (Courtesy B. Friedland, BDS.)* **(Right)** *BW radiograph of the mixed dentition shows multiple proximal carious lesions* →*. Caries in the primary dentition invades enamel and dentin faster as the rods and tubules are wider.*

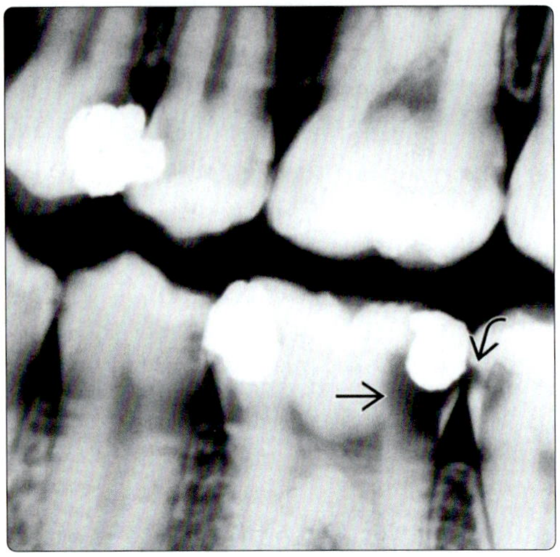

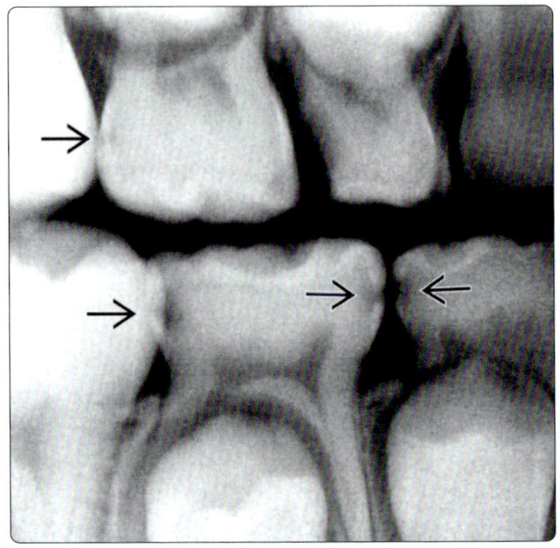

(Left) *BW radiograph shows the classic appearance of proximal caries: An enamel triangle with its base at the surface and its tip at the DEJ and a dentin triangle with its base at the DEJ and its tip directed pulpally* →. **(Right)** *Periapical radiograph shows demineralization beneath the occlusal aspect of the DEJ of the molars* →*. The overlying enamel appears intact radiographically. These lesions can be detected clinically with a dental explorer. Note incipient lesion on mesial of 1st molar* →.

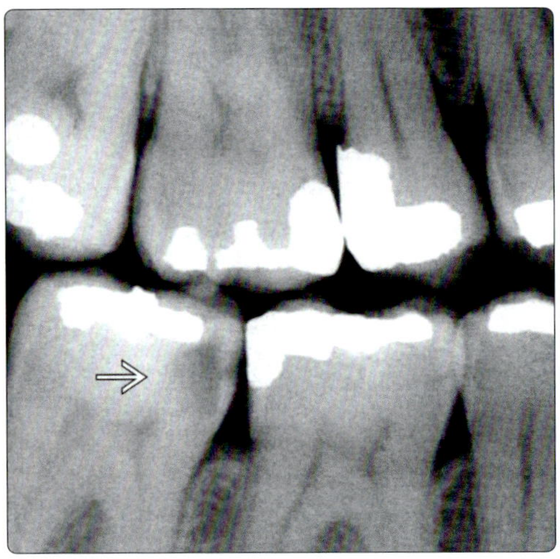

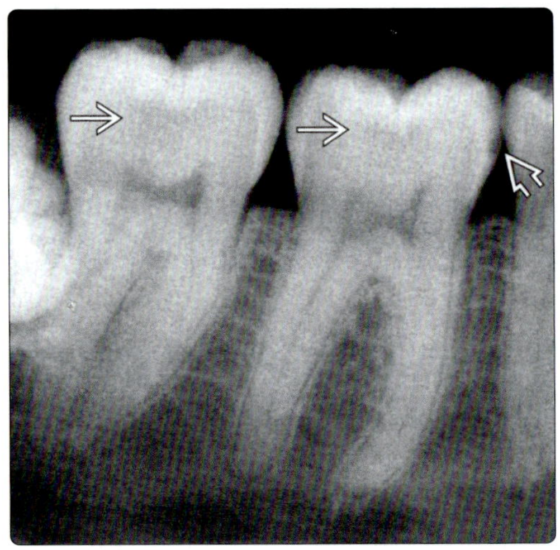

(Left) *Periapical radiograph of anterior teeth shows an advanced class III carious lesion* → *on the distal surface of the right lateral incisor. It is common for the adjacent tooth to also develop a carious lesion (kissing lesions).* **(Right)** *Periapical radiograph shows an advanced/severe class III carious lesion* →*. Note progression of caries through enamel and dentin is same as in posterior lesions. Compare to composite radiolucent restoration with radiopaque liner* → *in the adjacent tooth. (Courtesy B. Friedland, BDS.)*

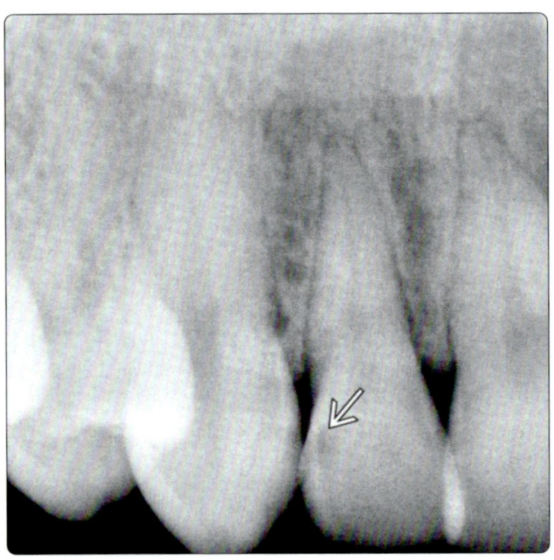

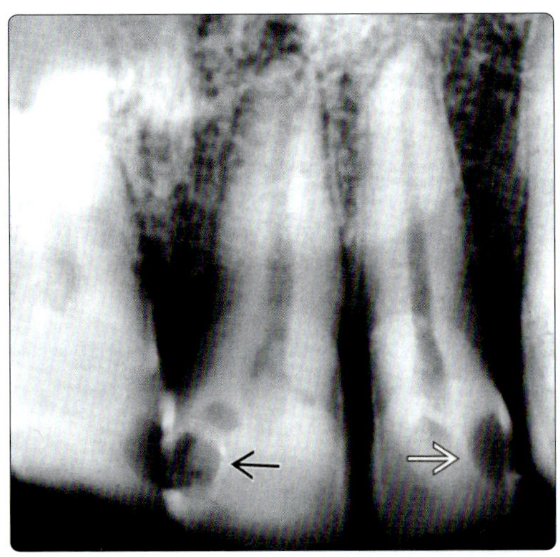

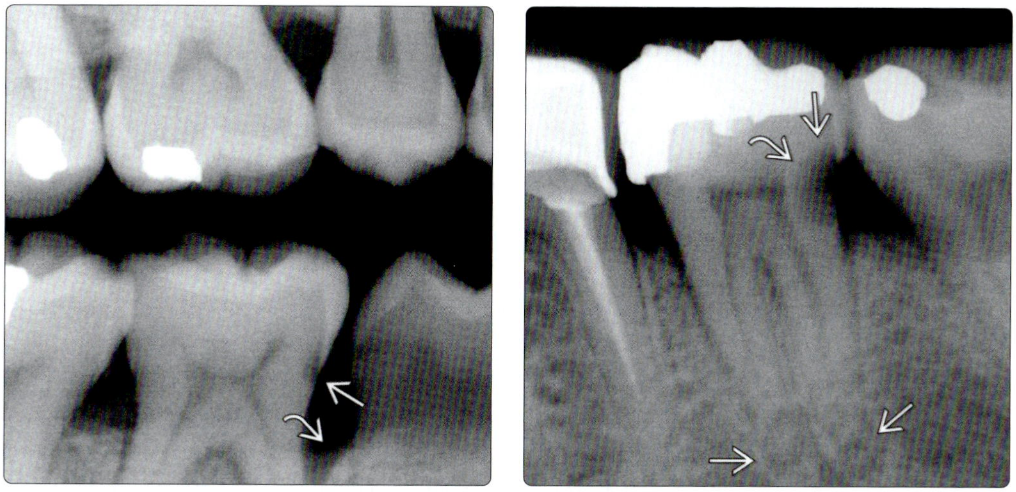

(Left) *BW radiograph shows periodontal recession → on the mesial surface of the mandibular 1st molar. Mesial cemental caries is evident at the cementoenamel junction →.* **(Right)** *Periapical radiograph shows advanced cemental caries → on the distal surface of the mandibular left 2nd molar. The presence of a thin band of dentin does not discount microbial invasion of the pulp, as there is evident periapical rarefying osteitis →. The caries remains above the bone.*

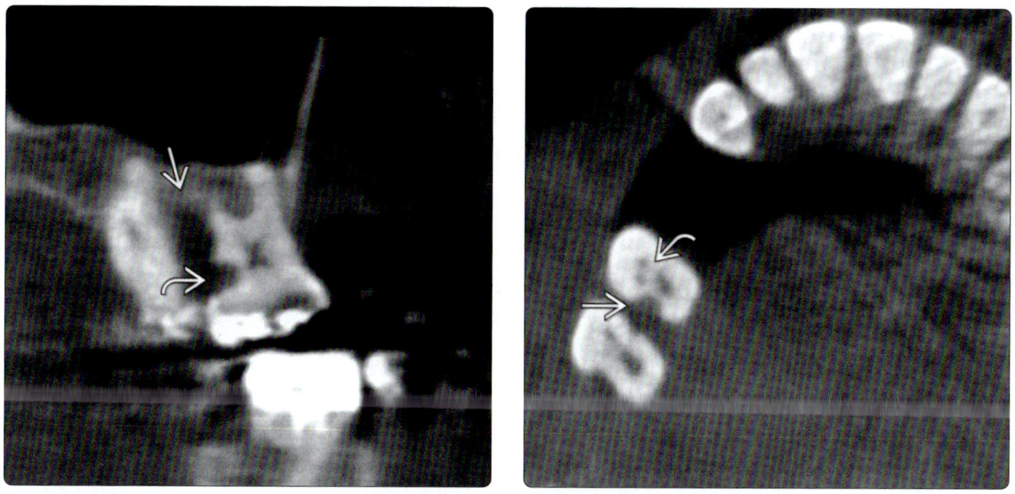

(Left) *Sagittal CBCT shows a severe cemental carious lesion on the distal surface of the maxillary 1st molar →. Note the periodontal bone loss on the distal surface of this tooth →.* **(Right)** *Axial CBCT of the same patient shows the cemental caries → approaching the furcation area of the pulp →. The findings of caries on CBCT are incidental and should not be the main reason for obtaining the scan, as the diagnosis can be made with less radiation and more accuracy with intraoral radiography.*

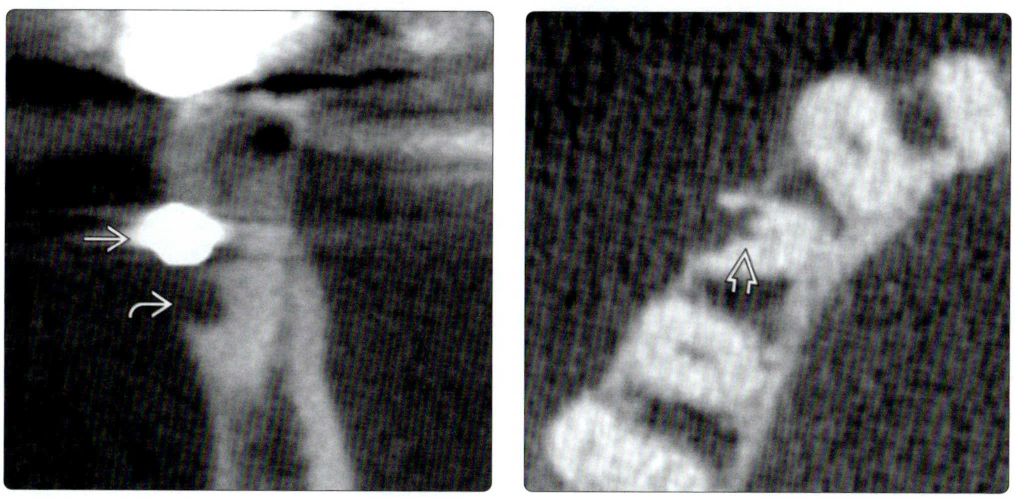

(Left) *Cross-section CBCT shows a mandibular premolar with a class V restoration → and recurrent root caries → on the facial surface of the tooth. Periodontal bone recession is noted on the facial surface.* **(Right)** *Axial CBCT of the same tooth shows the pulpal extent of the root caries lesion →. These lesions may be confused with tooth wear lesions such as abrasion and erosion, but caries is always irregular in outline, whereas tooth wear is usually smooth (erosion) or angular (abrasion).*

Periapical Rarefying Osteitis

KEY FACTS

TERMINOLOGY

- Definition: Loss of bone density surrounding apex of tooth in response to devitalization and necrosis of pulp
- Periapical rarefying osteitis includes periapical abscess, granuloma, and cyst

IMAGING

- Located at apex of **nonvital** tooth
- Early lesions: Widening of apical PDL space
- **Apical lamina dura** is gradually **lost**
- May occur in furcation area of primary molars
- May occur on **lateral surface** of root if inflammation associated with **lateral canal**
- May be **corticated** in case of **radicular cyst**
- May be surrounded by sclerotic bone (sclerosing osteitis)
- **Periapical radiography** is modality of choice

TOP DIFFERENTIAL DIAGNOSES

- Periapical osseous dysplasia
- Periapical scar
- Acute osteomyelitis
- Odontogenic keratocyst
- Malignancy/metastatic disease
- Incompletely formed root apex

CLINICAL ISSUES

- **Vitality testing** should be performed
- May be asymptomatic (chronic)
- Spontaneous or lingering pain (acute)
- May see sinus tract formation and **parulis** (gum boil)
- Endodontic treatment or retreatment ± apicoectomy
- **Extraction** if tooth is nonrestorable

DIAGNOSTIC CHECKLIST

- CT interpretation: Examine apices of teeth in axial plane for low density that signifies widening of PDL
- **May refer pain to surrounding muscles and TMJ; exclude dental pain as source of TMD**

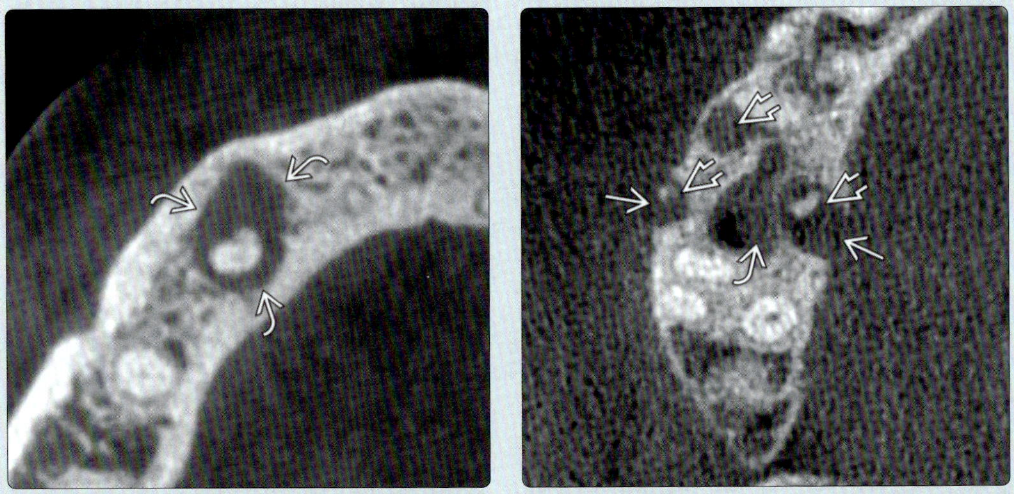

(Left) *Axial CBCT shows periapical rarefying osteitis surrounding the apical 1/3 of the mandibular right canine root. This appears as an irregular low-density halo around the apex of the tooth ➔.* **(Right)** *Axial CBCT of the maxillary right molar area shows rarefying osteitis at the apex of all 3 roots of the 1st molar ➔. Defects are noted in the facial and lingual cortices of the alveolar bone ➔. Mucosal thickening of the maxillary sinus ➔ is noted.*

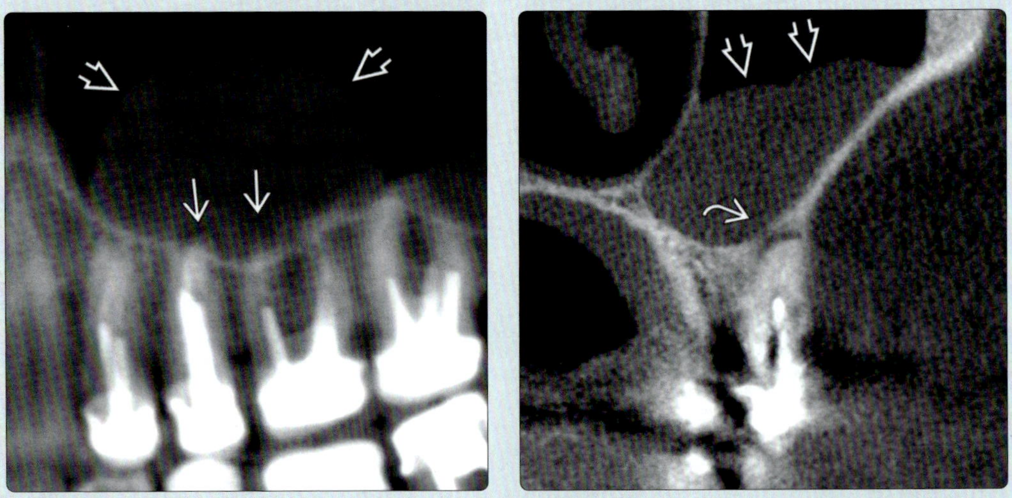

(Left) *Panoramic reformat CBCT shows rarefying osteitis at the apex of the maxillary left 2nd premolar and mesial buccal root of the 1st molar ➔. The teeth are root canal treated and require retreatment or apicoectomies. Note the large mucous retention pseudocyst in sinus ➔.* **(Right)** *Cross-sectional CBCT shows widening of the periapical PDL space in this maxillary molar. Note the loss of the cortical density of the floor of the maxillary sinus ➔ with inflammatory changes ➔ within the sinus that may be odontogenic in origin.*

TERMINOLOGY

Synonyms

- Following terms all fall under description of **periapical rarefying osteitis**
  - Periapical abscess = radicular abscess = acute apical periodontitis
  - Periapical granuloma = radicular granuloma = chronic apical periodontitis
  - Periapical cyst = radicular cyst = apical periodontal cyst

Definitions

- **Loss of bone density surrounding apex of tooth** in response to devitalization and necrosis of pulp

IMAGING

General Features

- Best diagnostic clue
  - Poorly defined **loss of bone density at apex of tooth** with
    - Large carious lesion
    - Large coronal restoration
    - Fracture (traumatic or iatrogenic)
    - Inadequate root canal treatment (overfill, underfill, missed canal, unfilled lateral canal)
- Location
  - At apex of devitalized tooth
  - May occur in **furcation area of primary molars**
  - May occur on **lateral surface** of root if inflammation associated with **lateral canal**
    - Called **lateral radicular** cyst, granuloma, or abscess
- Size
  - Varies from slight widening of periapical periodontal ligament (PDL) space to several centimeters in diameter
  - Corticated lesions **> 1 cm** in diameter are most likely **radicular cysts**
  - "**Endo-perio**" lesion
    - If involves entire length of root and communicates with crest of ridge
    - Etiology is undetermined
      - Inflammation is either originating from root canal (pulpal) or from periodontal disease (periodontal)
- Morphology
  - Loss of bone density surrounding apex of tooth with **gradual transition to normal bone pattern**
  - Trabeculation is more sparse at apex of tooth
  - May be surrounded by sclerotic bone (sclerosing osteitis)
  - May be **corticated** in case of **radicular cyst**

Radiographic Findings

- Intraoral plain film
  - Early lesions may show slight loss of bone density
  - Slight widening of periapical PDL with haziness of lamina dura
  - **Apical lamina dura is gradually lost** as more bone destruction occurs
  - **Bone sclerosis** may be seen surrounding rarefaction (**sclerosing osteitis**)
  - Periosteal reaction may occur in floor of maxillary sinus if lesion abuts sinus
- Extraoral plain film
  - Superior-inferior extent of rarefaction may be appreciated if not completely included in periapical radiograph

CT Findings

- CBCT
  - **Axial**: Loss of bone density surrounding apex of tooth
    - May be minute: Compare to adjacent apices
    - May be large enough to communicate with maxillary sinus lumen
      - Odontogenic sinusitis may ensue
    - May expand alveolar bone cortices
    - May involve > 1 apex but is usually centered around necrotic tooth
  - **Coronal**: If multifocal, relationship to each apex may be observed
    - Sinus changes due to odontogenic sinusitis or mucositis, if present, can be evaluated
    - Lifting of floor of maxillary sinus by radicular cysts as well as destruction of floor of sinus if present
  - **Cross sections**
    - Evaluate possible communication with or destruction of facial or lingual alveolar bone cortices
      - Correlation with clinical finding of sinus tract can be performed by placing gutta percha cone through sinus tract

Imaging Recommendations

- Best imaging tool
  - **Periapical radiography**
    - Best resolution to diagnose early lesions; will show subtle increase in PDL space and early loss of lamina dura
    - Conventionally used for root canal therapy measurements
      - CBCT has recently been adopted for endodontic analysis
    - CT and CBCT may show periapical rarefying osteitis
      - Visualization may be hindered by metal artifact, especially adjacent to implants

DIFFERENTIAL DIAGNOSIS

Periapical Osseous Dysplasia

- Early lesions may appear like rarefying osteitis
- PCD shows gradual calcification with maturation
- Teeth are **vital**

Periapical Scar

- Associated with endodontically treated tooth
- Apical rarefying osteitis heals with fibrous connective tissue instead of mineralizing
- Also seen after root apex amputation (apicoectomy)
  - **Root has blunted apex slanted facially** (appreciated on CBCT sagittal or cross sections) and **retrograde metallic filling**
  - **Facial surface surgical access defect** is usually still present
  - Some metallic fragments may be present in periapical tissues

- Differentiation from periapical pathology based on clinical symptoms

Acute Osteomyelitis

- Early acute osteomyelitis shows slight decrease in trabeculation
- More common in mandible due to poorer vascularity
- Clinical symptoms include rapid onset, pain, swelling, fever, lymphadenopathy, and leukocytosis

Odontogenic Karatocyst

- Differentiate from more well-defined radicular cysts
- Epicenter may be anywhere in bone, not necessarily around apex
- Teeth are vital

Malignancy/Metastatic Disease

- May grow **within PDL space**
- Examination of bone for other foci or destruction is recommended

Incompletely Formed Root Apex

- Teeth at final stages of root development show **periapical radiolucencies** signifying last of dental follicle
- Correlate dental age with chronological age
- Completely formed root has rounded apex; incompletely formed root (open apex) ends with **pointed dentin and funnel-shaped pulp canal** opening
- Correlate to history of trauma, and examine crown for caries or large restoration
  - Developing teeth may become necrotic before apex closes
  - Superimposition of rarefying osteitis on apical dental follicle may occur

Mental Foramen

- Can be superimposed on apices of mandibular premolars in 2D imaging

PATHOLOGY

General Features

- Etiology
  - **Devitalization of tooth may occur due to**
    - Caries
    - Mechanical/chemical/thermal irritation during crown preparation and restoration
    - Trauma
  - Bacterial invasion and toxic byproducts of necrotic pulp travel through pulp canal to periapical tissues
  - Pus may form due to neutrophil reaction (abscess)
  - Granulation tissue may form in effort to heal inflammation (granuloma)
  - Epithelial rests of Malassez may divide and form radicular cyst wall (cyst)

CLINICAL ISSUES

Presentation

- Most common signs/symptoms
  - Acute: Pain localized to tooth or generalized to jaw
    - Spontaneous pain or pain that lingers with hot and cold stimuli indicates irreversible pulpitis
  - Chronic: May not be painful, or dull pain
- Other signs/symptoms
  - Swelling
  - Trismus
  - Sinus pain (if adjacent to maxillary sinus)
  - May refer pain to surrounding muscles and TMJ
  - Sinus tract formation and **parulis** (gum boil) clinically

Treatment

- **Vitality testing** should be performed
  - If tooth is **nonvital**
    - **Root canal** (endodontic) therapy
    - **Extraction** if destruction to tooth is severe and tooth is nonrestorable
  - If tooth is **vital**
    - Consider other noninflammatory lesions
- For "endo-perio" lesions
  - Treatment should involve multifactorial approaches targeting etiology
- If tooth is already **endodontically treated**
  - Root canal retreatment
  - Apicoectomy

DIAGNOSTIC CHECKLIST

Consider

- If periapical rarefying osteitis is suspected but not confirmed on CBCT due to low resolution, **periapical radiographic examination** is recommended

Image Interpretation Pearls

- For CT interpretation
  - Examine apices of teeth as they appear on axial plane for low density that signifies widening of PDL
  - Look for any irregularity in width of PDL or low density surrounding apices of teeth
- **CT and CBCT are not initial imaging modalities of choice** for periapical rarefying osteitis
  - Periapical radiography should be considered 1st if main imaging indication is investigation of periapical rarefying osteitis; radiation dose is significantly lower than CT, and image quality is higher
  - CBCT helpful to determine relationship to vital structures, e.g., maxillary sinus and mandibular canal

Reporting Tips

- Examine and report on patency of root canals for **tertiary dentin and pulp stones** that may complicate root canal therapy

SELECTED REFERENCES

1. Bornstein MM et al: Comparison between radiographic (2-dimensional and 3-dimensional) and histologic findings of periapical lesions treated with apical surgery. J Endod. 41(6):804-11, 2015
2. Giménez-García R et al: Cutaneous sinus tracts of odontogenic origin: two Case reports. J Am Board Fam Med. 28(6):838-40, 2015
3. Okada K et al: Noninvasive differential diagnosis of dental periapical lesions in cone-beam CT scans. Med Phys. 42(4):1653-65, 2015
4. Neville BW et al: Oral and Maxillofacial Pathology. 3rd ed. St. Louis: Saunders Elsevier, 2009
5. White SC et al: Oral Radiology Principles and Interpretation. 7th ed. St. Louis: Mosby Elsevier, 2014
6. Marmary Y et al: The effect of periapical rarefying osteitis on cortical and cancellous bone. A study comparing conventional radiographs with computed tomography. Dentomaxillofac Radiol. 28(5):267-71, 1999

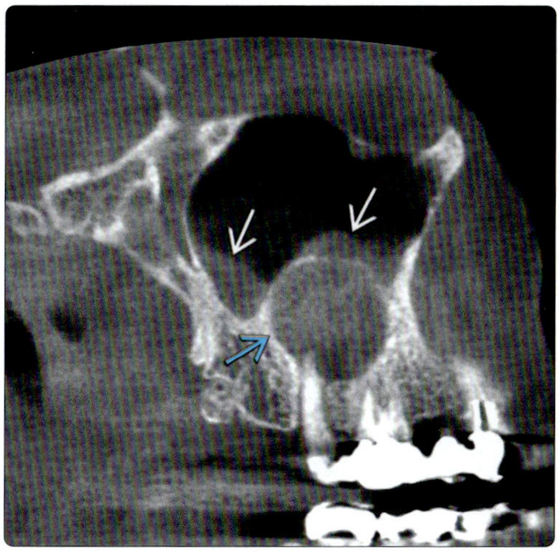

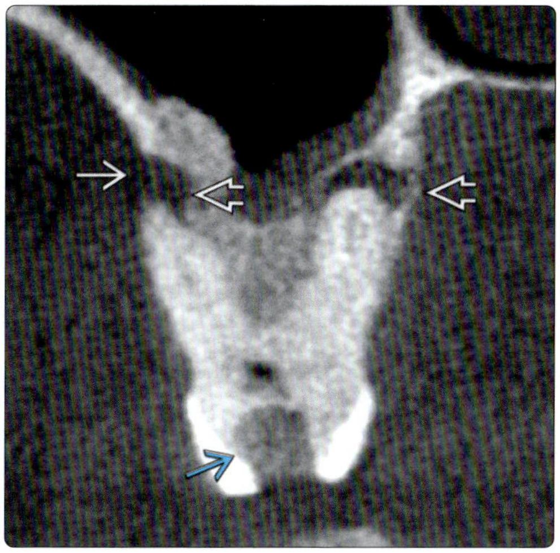

(Left) *Sagittal CBCT shows a large radicular cyst* → *lifting the floor of the maxillary sinus and occupying the inferior 1/3 of the sinus. Note the inflammatory changes within the sinus* →. **(Right)** *Cross-sectional CBCT shows a large carious lesion* → *in a nonvital maxillary molar with 2 periapical abscesses* →. *The lesion on the buccal root has broken through the buccal cortex of the alveolar process* →. *Narrowing of the pulp canals should be noted as a potential complication for root canal treatment.*

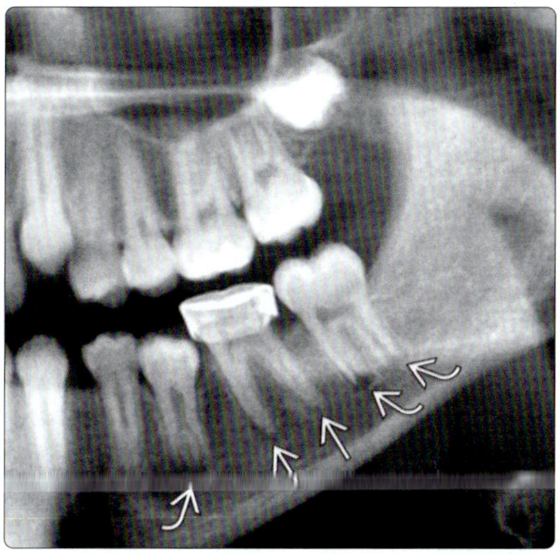

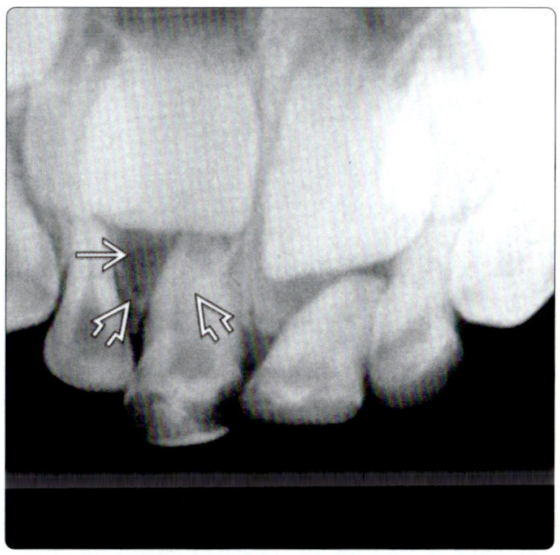

(Left) *Panoramic radiograph shows radiolucencies at the apices of multiple teeth. The 1st molar apices are closed, and the apical radiolucencies represent rarefying osteitis* →. *The 2nd molar and 2nd premolar apices are still developing* →. **(Right)** *Periapical radiograph shows periapical rarefaction* → *surrounding the apical 1/3 of the root of the primary right central incisor. The follicle space* → *of the permanent successor superimposes on this finding. (Courtesy S. Darwish, BDS.)*

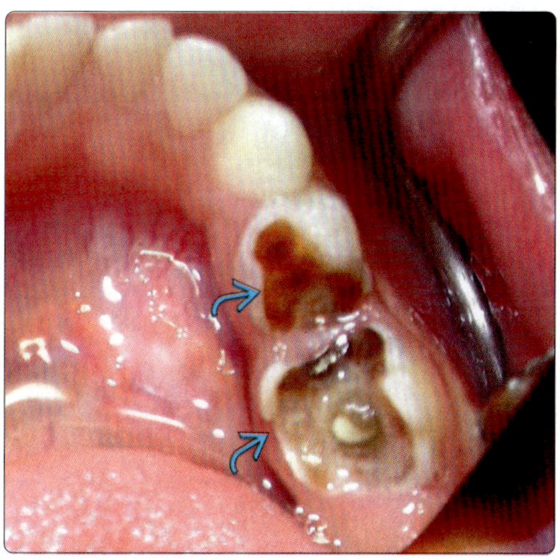

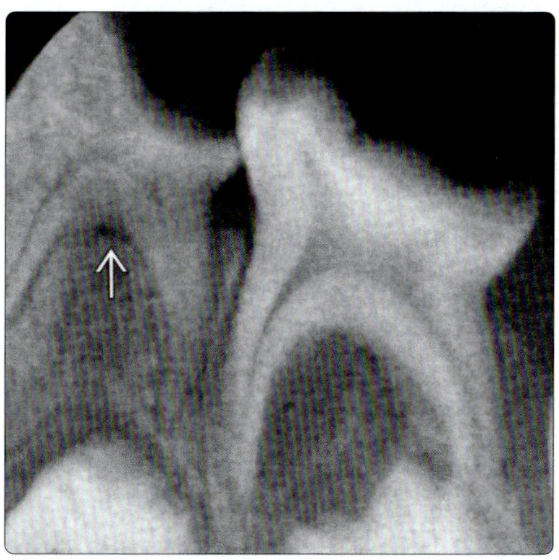

(Left) *Clinical photograph shows severe caries of the primary left 1st and 2nd molars* →. **(Right)** *Periapical radiograph in the same patient shows widening of the furcation area* → *of a necrotic primary molar. In primary molars, rarefying osteitis occurs in the furcation due to the narrow distance between the pulp chamber and the furcal bone. (Courtesy S. Darwish, BDS.)*

Periapical Sclerosing Osteitis

KEY FACTS

TERMINOLOGY

- Most common synonym: **Condensing osteitis**
- Definition: **Sclerosis of bone surrounding apex** of necrotic tooth in response to chronic inflammation

IMAGING

- Dense, hazy bone with increased number of trabeculae and **periapical widening of periodontal ligament (PDL) space**
- Irregular outline
- **Gradual decrease of bone trabeculae** from center of lesion toward normal trabecular bone
- Lamina dura may be indistinguishable from lesion
- Implant analysis of cross sections can show dense bone in area surrounding tooth socket
- **Periapical radiography** is imaging modality of choice: Shows PDL and lamina dura detail

TOP DIFFERENTIAL DIAGNOSES

- Idiopathic osteosclerosis
- Periapical osseous dysplasia
- Cementoblastoma
- Hypercementosis

CLINICAL ISSUES

- Treatment: Extraction or root canal therapy of associated tooth → widened PDL space will resolve, but **sclerotic bone usually remains**

DIAGNOSTIC CHECKLIST

- Consider: **Time since root canal treatment** (if present); if tooth recently treated, lesion may be healing
- If area is considered for implant placement, comment on density of bone
    - Sclerotic bone has **less vascularity** with potential for worse healing after implant placement

(Left) *Panoramic reformat of CBCT data shows an endodontically treated tooth with periodontal bone loss, widening of the periapical PDL space →, and surrounding wide area of sclerosing osteitis →.* **(Right)** *Periapical radiograph shows periapical sclerosing osteitis surrounding the apical and middle thirds of the roots → of the mandibular left 1st molar. Root canal treatment failure is noted with periodontal furcation bone loss and filling material → in the furcation area caused by a perforation of the mesial root.*

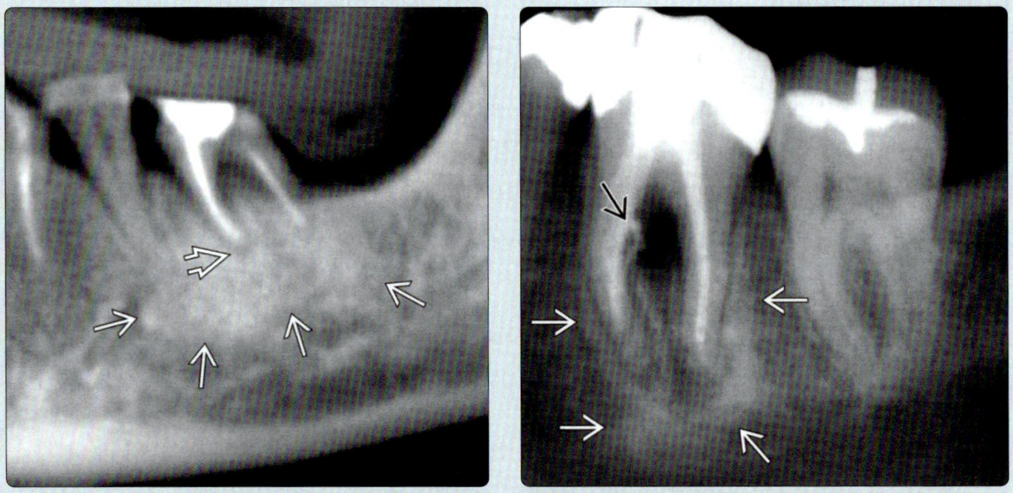

(Left) *Cross-sectional CBCT shows a grafted extraction socket →. The necrotic tooth had caused a marked surrounding sclerosing osteitis →. The sclerosis persisted even though the tooth was removed. The sclerosis blends into the cortices of the mandible and the IAN canal →.* **(Right)** *Panoramic reformat CBCT shows slight periapical sclerosis → surrounding a widened PDL space → at the apex of the tooth. Endodontically treated teeth should show no signs of inflammation prior to restoration with crowns.*

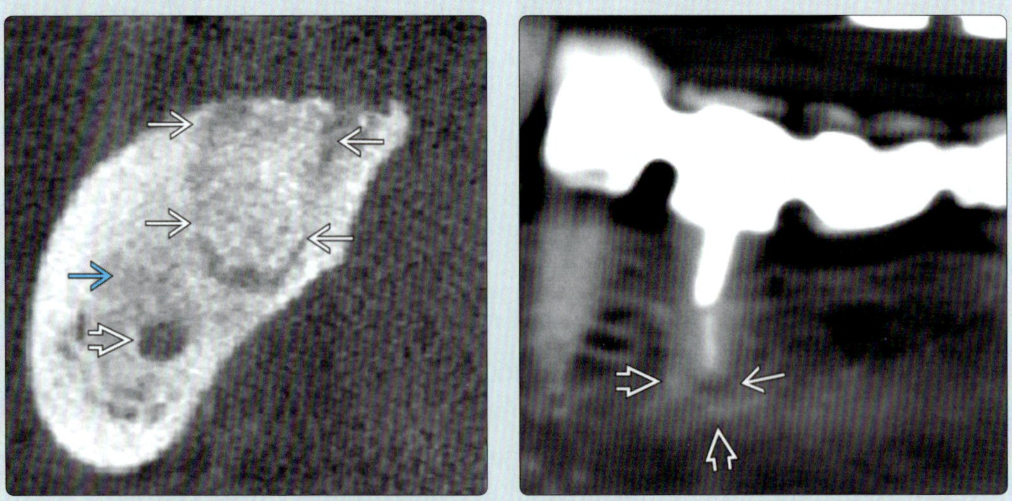

TERMINOLOGY

Synonyms

- **Condensing osteitis**, sclerosing osteitis, focal sclerosing osteomyelitis, focal sclerosing osteitis

Definitions

- **Sclerosis of bone surrounding apex** of necrotic tooth in response to chronic inflammation

IMAGING

General Features

- Best diagnostic clue
  - **Increased density of bone** at apical area of carious tooth, tooth with large restoration, or tooth with root canal treatment that has failed
- Location
  - Surrounds apex of **nonvital tooth**
  - May extend to cortices of alveolar processes and to adjacent structures
- Size
  - Ranges from few mm to involving entire alveolar process in area of tooth
- Morphology
  - Dense lesion with increased number of trabeculae and **periapical widening of periodontal ligament (PDL) space**
  - **Irregular outline**
  - **Gradual decrease of bone trabeculae** away from center of lesion toward normal trabecular bone
  - Lamina dura may be indistinguishable from lesion

CT Findings

- CBCT
  - Implant analysis of cross sections can show dense bone in area surrounding tooth socket
  - Faciolingual extent can be analyzed
    - **Lesion may be indistinguishable from surrounding cortical bone** on cross section
  - May extend to inferior alveolar nerve canal and even surround it
  - External root resorption may be seen

Imaging Recommendations

- Best imaging tool
  - **Periapical radiography**
    - Shows fine detail of PDL morphology and lamina dura integrity

DIFFERENTIAL DIAGNOSIS

Idiopathic Osteosclerosis (Enostosis)

- May occur close to apex of tooth and look similar
- **PDL normal** and lamina dura intact; **tooth is vital**
- Appears similar in trabecular pattern and outline but **does not blend into surrounding trabeculation**

Periapical Osseous Dysplasia

- Mature phase may be completely calcified and dense
- **Thin radiolucent line periphery**
- Teeth are vital
- Most commonly at apices of mandibular anterior teeth

Cementoblastoma

- Mixed density lesion with high-density rim and low-density band within it
- Root **apex is not visible within** lesion

Hypercementosis

- Bulbous excess cementum around root
- Surrounded by **normal PDL space**

CLINICAL ISSUES

Presentation

- Most common signs/symptoms
  - May be asymptomatic with occasional flare-ups
    - **Chronic inflammatory dental lesions may have acute exacerbations**
      - Patient may complain of intermittent pain

Natural History & Prognosis

- Periapical inflammation starts with widening of PDL and rarefying osteitis but becomes more sclerotic as **surrounding bone attempts to wall off inflammation or repair bone** lysed by inflammatory process
- Untreated lesions may progress to osteomyelitis

Treatment

- Removal of cause: Extraction or root canal therapy of associated tooth
  - Widened PDL space will resolve, but **sclerotic bone usually remains**

DIAGNOSTIC CHECKLIST

Consider

- **Time since root canal treatment** (if present)
  - If tooth recently treated → may be healing lesion
  - If tooth treated some time ago → may be new lesion (especially if lucent component is present at apex)
- Malignancies, both primary and metastatic, may cause widened PDL spaces; absence of other malignant radiographic signs should help in differentiation

Image Interpretation Pearls

- Sclerosing osteitis may occur in areas other than apices of teeth
  - In response to periodontal inflammation, inflammation caused by pericoronitis or surrounding infected benign cysts/tumors
  - Most common location is surrounding apices

Reporting Tips

- If area is considered for implant placement, comment on density of bone
  - Sclerotic bone has **less vascularity with potentially worse healing** after implant placement

SELECTED REFERENCES

1. White SC et al: Oral Radiology, Principles and Practice. 7th ed. St. Louis: Mosby Elsevier, 2014
2. Holly D et al: Condensing osteitis in oral region. Bratisl Lek Listy. 110(11):713-5, 2009
3. Kosti E et al: Healing of a radiolucent periradicular lesion with periradicular radiopacity. J Endod. 30(7):548-50, 2004
4. al-Sebaei MO et al: A clinico-pathologic correlation. Condensing osteitis (focal sclerosing osteomyelitis). J Mass Dent Soc. 52(1):52-4, 2003

Periodontal Disease

KEY FACTS

TERMINOLOGY

- Definition: Inflammatory disease of supporting structures of teeth (periodontium)

IMAGING

- **Horizontal bone loss**: Interdental bone (alveolar crest) parallel to imaginary line drawn between cementoenamel junction (CEJ) of adjacent teeth
- **Vertical (angular) bone loss**: Interdental bone slants at angle (not parallel to imaginary CEJ line)
    - 1-, 2-, and 3-walled defects
- **Facial or lingual bone loss**: Seen as multilevel shadow on tooth and interdental bone on intraoral imaging
- **Interdental craters**: Concavities in alveolar crest
- **Furcation bone loss**: Classes II and III radiographically
- **Periodontal abscess**: Blockage of pocket or pus draining from sulcus
- **Imaging of choice**: Bitewings (vertical) and periapical radiographs

TOP DIFFERENTIAL DIAGNOSES

- Primary malignancy
- Metastasis
- Surgical defect
- Langerhans histiocytosis

PATHOLOGY

- Most common etiology: Bacterial plaque accumulation (poor oral hygiene) and calculus

CLINICAL ISSUES

- Treatment: Scaling, root planing, periodontal surgery, chlorhexidine mouthwash

DIAGNOSTIC CHECKLIST

- Look at jaws together to recognize patterns of bone loss (localized or generalized)
- If ill-defined lucency is not localized to alveolar process, suspect malignancy or Langerhans disease

(Left) *Graphic of sagittal cross section of mandibular molar shows the different levels of periodontal bone loss. Early loss ➔ presents as blunting of the crestal bone: A = mild loss (1-2 mm); B = moderate loss (3 mm to mid root); C = severe loss (midroot to apex). If bone is lost between the roots of a tooth, it is called furcation bone loss.* **(Right)** *Periapical radiograph shows loss of density of the alveolar crest ➔ and vertical ➔ and horizontal ➔ periodontal bone loss. (Courtesy B. Friedland, BDS.)*

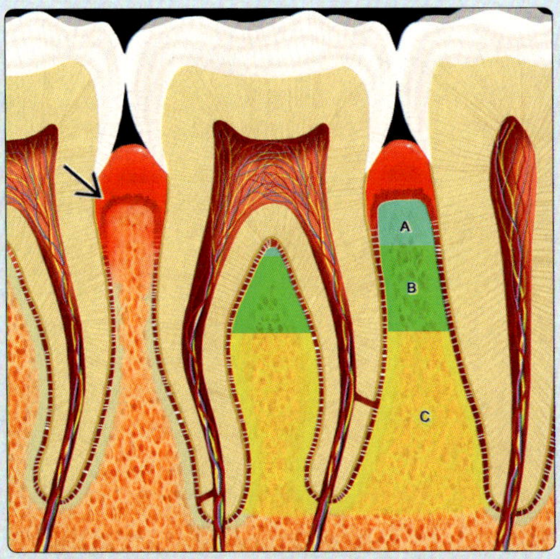

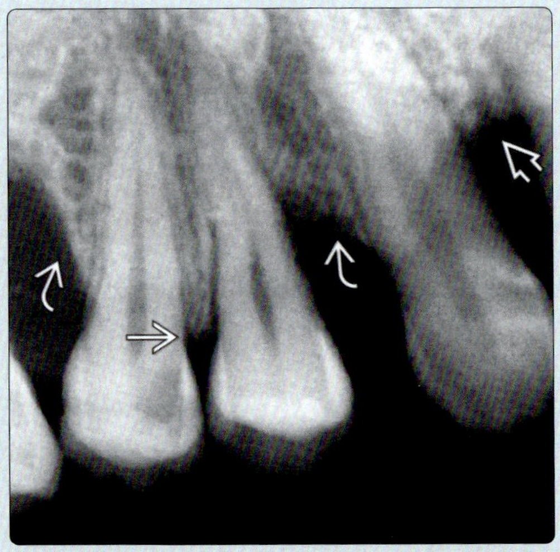

(Left) *Periapical radiograph shows mild horizontal bone loss ➔ as well as severe vertical periodontal bone loss ➔ and a suspected perioendo lesion. (Courtesy B. Friedland, BDS.)* **(Right)** *Periapical radiograph shows severe horizontal ➔ and vertical ➔ periodontal bone loss. An imaginary line is drawn between the cementoenamel junctions (CEJs) of adjacent teeth. If bone is parallel to the line, it is described as horizontal bone loss. If not, it is vertical bone loss. (Courtesy B. Friedland, BDS.)*

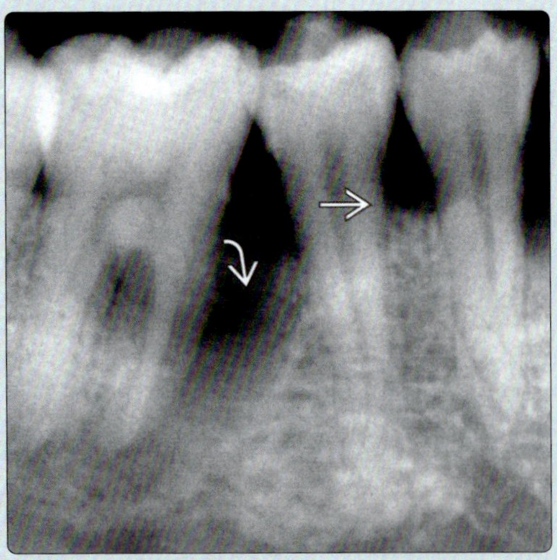

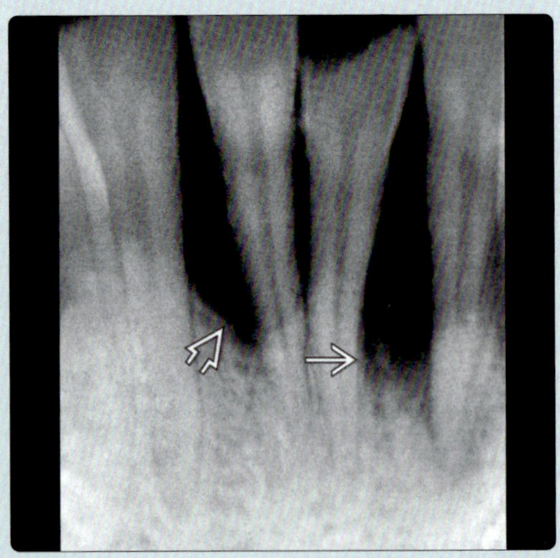

TERMINOLOGY

Synonyms

- **Periodontitis**, gingivitis (not visualized radiographically), gum disease (layperson term)

Definitions

- Inflammatory disease of supporting structures of teeth (periodontium)

IMAGING

General Features

- Best diagnostic clue
  - Loss of bone surrounding teeth
- Location
  - May affect 1 tooth or few teeth (localized) or affect all teeth (generalized)
- Morphology
  - **Horizontal bone loss**: Interdental bone (alveolar crest) parallel and apical to imaginary line drawn between cementoenamel junction (CEJ) of adjacent teeth
  - **Vertical (angular) bone loss**: Interdental bone slants at angle (not parallel to imaginary CEJ line)
  - Sclerosis may be seen in underlying bone

Radiographic Findings

- **Early**: Loss of crestal density, blunting of alveolar crests
  - Alveolar crest is normally located 1-2 mm below CEJ
- **Horizontal bone loss**
  - **Mild**: 1- to 2-mm bone loss
  - **Moderate**: From 2 mm to 1/2 of bone support
  - **Severe**: Past midroot to apex of tooth
- **Vertical bone loss**: Hollowed out trough in bone is left alongside root
  - Named according to number of walls left: **1 walled, 2 walled, and 3 walled**
  - If facial or lingual walls are present, may be difficult to see on intraoral radiographs → clinical, surgical evaluation
  - CBCT axials can show number of walls present, but this usually does not justify increased radiation to patient with this imaging technique
- **Facial or lingual bone loss**
  - Cortical plates along buccal or lingual surfaces of teeth may recede
  - **Intraoral radiography**: Seen as **multilevel shadow** on tooth and in interdental bone
  - **CBCT: Loss of facial or lingual bone** can be appreciated on **cross sections**
- **Interdental craters**
  - **Concavities in crest of interdental bone** confined between facial and lingual plates
  - **Intraoral**: Radiolucent band or trough apical to crest of ridge
  - Can be visualized on CBCT cross sections but may be difficult to see if tooth is not parallel to long axis of cross section
- **Periodontal furcation bone loss**
  - Loss of alveolar bone within furcation area of roots of multirooted tooth
    - Can involve 1 surface (facial or lingual, mesial or distal) or can be through and through (bone loss occurs on both sides of alveolar process)
    - Clinical classification from I-IV
      - **Class I**: Incipient bone loss
      - **Class II**: Bone loss on 1 side of furcation
      - **Class III**: Through-and-through bone loss
      - **Class IV**: Through-and-through bone loss with gingival recession
    - Intraoral radiographs can show facial and lingual single surface and through-and-through lesions
    - CBCT can show all **single surface furcation bone loss** on sagittal series as well as class III lesions
  - **Enamel pearls** (dental anomaly) in furcation can lead to periodontal furcation bone loss
- **Perioendo lesions**
  - Severe periodontal defects that involve tooth apex
  - Etiology may be pulpal, periodontal, or combination of both
- **Periodontal abscess**
  - Caused by **foreign material** in periodontal pocket or **blockage of pocket**
  - Pain, swelling, sinus tract formation, or pus draining from sulcus may be noted
- **Aggressive periodontitis**
  - Localized: Limited to 1st molars and anterior teeth
    - May see arc-shaped defects
  - Generalized: Involving at least 3 teeth and not confined to 1st molars and anteriors
  - Most common cause: *Actinobacillus actinomycetemcomitans*
- **Acute necrotizing ulcerative periodontitis**
  - Progression of acute necrotizing ulcerative gingivitis, a.k.a. trench mouth
  - Foul odor is present
  - Immune dysfunction may predispose

CT Findings

- CBCT
  - **Not imaging technique of choice for periodontal evaluation** as intraoral radiography and clinical probing can provide same information with less radiation to patient
  - Mesial and distal furcation bone loss can be detected on sagittal and coronal series
  - 1-, 2-, and 3-walled defects can be visualized
  - Early lesions cannot be detected
  - **False-positive lesions can be seen in area of metal restorations and implants due to metal artifact**

Imaging Recommendations

- Best imaging tool
  - **Intraoral radiography**
    - Bitewings (horizontal or vertical); interproximal alveolar bone must be visible
    - Periapicals: To see crown:root ratio, root shape, and periapical area
- Protocol advice
  - Horizontal bitewings: If periodontal bone loss < 3 mm
  - Vertical bitewings: If bone loss > 3 mm in both arches

DIFFERENTIAL DIAGNOSIS

Primary Malignancy

- Primary malignancy in bone or soft tissues surrounding teeth may give appearance of bone destruction similar to periodontal bone loss
- Ill-defined bone loss; may or may not be adjacent to tooth
- **Teeth floating in air** appearance
- Asymmetric widening of periodontal ligament (PDL) space may be seen in **non-Hodgkin lymphoma, leukemia, and osteosarcoma**
- Biopsy of any surgical tissues to rule out malignancy

Metastasis

- Secondary malignancy may show patterns similar to periodontal bone loss
- **Irregular widening of PDL space** may be noted if tumor seeds there

Surgical Defect

- Incomplete bone remodeling after surgical intervention, leading to appearance of defect adjacent to teeth
- Patient history helpful
- With periodontal disease, soft tissues usually inflamed and bleeding

Langerhans Histiocytosis

- Destroys alveolar bone and **leaves teeth floating in space**
- Alveolar process lesions are usually multiple
- Circular in shape; when crest of bone is destroyed, defect appears **scooped out**
- When in doubt, biopsy

Orthodontic Movement

- Teeth undergoing active orthodontic treatment can show **widening of PDL** on surface of tooth **opposite to direction of tooth movement**

PATHOLOGY

General Features

- Etiology
  - **Microbial**
    - Chronic accumulation of bacterial plaque due to
      - □ Poor oral hygiene
      - □ Overcontoured or overhanging restorations
      - □ Open contacts between teeth and restorations
      - □ Malalignment of teeth
      - □ Tipping of teeth (mesial or distal drift after extraction of adjacent tooth)
  - **Mechanical**
    - Overhanging restorations that impinge on gingival tissues
    - Dental anomalies, such as enamel pearls
    - **Calculus** build-up (calcification of plaque)
    - Chronic injury, such as habitual toothpick insertion and aggressive toothbrushing
    - Tooth grinding/traumatic occlusion (controversial)
  - Stress may predispose
  - Radiation therapy to jaws may hinder periodontium's ability to regenerate and remodel, making it more susceptible to infection
- Associated abnormalities
  - Genetic and hereditary disease that may predispose
    - Papillon-Lefèvre syndrome (hyperkeratosis palmoplantaris), Down syndrome, hypophosphatemia, Chédiak-Higashi syndrome

CLINICAL ISSUES

Presentation

- Most common signs/symptoms
  - Red, swollen, bleeding, and receding gums, loose teeth, halitosis

Demographics

- Older adults (with exception of aggressive periodontitis)
- Diabetes, hematologic disorders, and HIV can predispose due to interference with immune system
- **Smoking**
- Low socioeconomic level
- Poor oral hygiene
- Incidence may increase in times of hormonal changes, such as pregnancy, puberty, and menopause

Treatment

- **Periodontal therapy**: Scaling, root planing, periodontal surgery, chlorhexidine mouthwash
- Follow-up to periodontal therapy
  - Subtraction digital radiography can be used to assess regeneration of bone if present
  - Bone grafting material may appear as granular opacity adjacent to tooth
- Bone regeneration not possible even with treatment, but reestablishment of crestal cortex is sign of health

DIAGNOSTIC CHECKLIST

Consider

- **Aggressive periodontitis** if patient < 30 years old and disease progresses rapidly
- **Acute necrotizing ulcerative periodontitis** if very foul odor and immune dysfunction are present

Image Interpretation Pearls

- **Look for calculus**
  - Areas of **roughness** on supraalveolar root surface
  - **Triangle-shaped** calcifications on surfaces of root
  - Bands of radiopaque material on cervical portion of tooth
  - Not always calcified enough to be visualized on radiographs → clinical examination with explorer

Reporting Tips

- **Step back and get big picture**
  - Look at jaws together to recognize patterns of bone loss (localized or generalized)
  - If ill-defined lucency is not localized to alveolar process, suspect malignancy or Langerhans histiocytosis
  - Determine age of patient to assess if aggressive periodontitis

SELECTED REFERENCES

1. Goodarzi Pour D et al: Accuracy of cone beam computed tomography for detection of bone loss. J Dent (Tehran). 12(7):513-23, 2015

TERMINOLOGY

Synonyms

- Gubernacular cord
- Gubernacular canal

Definitions

- **Band of connective tissue and dental lamina epithelium (cord)**, lying in bony canal, connecting dental follicle of permanent teeth to overlying mucoperiosteum

IMAGING

General Features

- Best diagnostic clue
  - **Well-defined, mostly corticated, radiolucent tract or band**
- Location
  - Contiguous with and extends from superior aspect of impacted permanent tooth follicle to normal site of eruption on alveolar crest
  - For permanent teeth with deciduous predecessors, cord passes **lingual** to deciduous tooth
- Size
  - Size varies from tooth to tooth and with tooth development
- Morphology
  - Uniform tract of varying length

Radiographic Findings

- Intraoral plain film
  - Well-defined, mostly corticated, radiolucent tract extending from crown of impacted tooth to location of normal eruption site at alveolar crest

CT Findings

- CBCT
  - **Corticated tract of low density (radiolucency)** contiguous with dental follicle of impacted tooth and extending to alveolar crest

Imaging Recommendations

- Best imaging tool
  - Periapical radiographs
  - **CBCT imaging**

DIFFERENTIAL DIAGNOSIS

Sinus Tract

- Drainage pathway for infection
- Takes path of least resistance
- Can be traced back to source of infection
  - Usually apical area of tooth, **not** crown

Accessory Mandibular Canal

- Extension of canal beyond normal boundary
  - In posterior, accessory canal may exit main canal close to mandibular foramen
  - In anterior, canal may extend beyond mental foramen
- Nutrient canals are sometimes seen extending upward from canal to molar teeth
- Traces back to mandibular canal
- **Not associated with impacted tooth**

PATHOLOGY

General Features

- Etiology
  - Failure of normal eruption of permanent tooth, resulting in retention of gubernacular cord
  - Cord acts as guide or pathway for eruption rather than actual stimulus
    - Loss of gubernacular cord does **not** cause failure of eruption
- Associated abnormalities
  - Retained deciduous tooth
  - Recent reports have associated pericoronal form of adenomatoid odontogenic tumor (AOT) with gubernacular cord
    - Theory: AOT arises from dental lamina epithelium in cord near crown of developing tooth and may move along canal with tooth during eruption

Microscopic Features

- Centrally oriented ribbon of dental lamina epithelium surrounded by fibrous connective tissue
- Connective tissue continuous superiorly with subcutaneous connective tissue of oral mucosa and inferiorly with connective tissue of dental sac of developing tooth
- Expresses type IV collagen α chains; E-cadherin and β-catenin also thought to be involved with tooth morphogenesis and cytodifferentiation

CLINICAL ISSUES

Presentation

- Most common signs/symptoms
  - Failure of eruption of permanent tooth
- Other signs/symptoms
  - If permanent tooth has deciduous predecessor, deciduous tooth may be retained
  - Potential for communication with oral cavity and hence infection

Treatment

- No treatment required unless infected
- Impacted tooth may or may not be removed or uncovered depending on location and association with vital structures

SELECTED REFERENCES

1. Philipsen HP et al: The adenomatoid odontogenic tumour: an update of selected issues. J Oral Pathol Med. 45(6):394-8, 2016
2. Ide F et al: Development and growth of adenomatoid odontogenic tumor related to formation and eruption of teeth. Head Neck Pathol. 5(2):123-32, 2011
3. Nagai N et al: Localization of type IV collagen a 1 to a 6 chains in basement membrane during mouse molar germ development. Int J Dev Biol. 45(7):827-31, 2001
4. Fausser JL et al: Localization of antigens associated with adherens junctions, desmosomes, and hemidesmosomes during murine molar morphogenesis. Differentiation. 63(1):1-11, 1998
5. Cahill DR et al: Tooth eruption: evidence for the central role of the dental follicle. J Oral Pathol. 9(4):189-200, 1980
6. Carollo DA et al: Histology and function of the dental gubernacular cord. Angle Orthod. 41(4):300-7, 1971
7. Hodson JJ: The gubernaculum dentis. Dent Pract Dent Rec. 21(12):423-8, 1971

PART II
SECTION 2
Oral Cavity

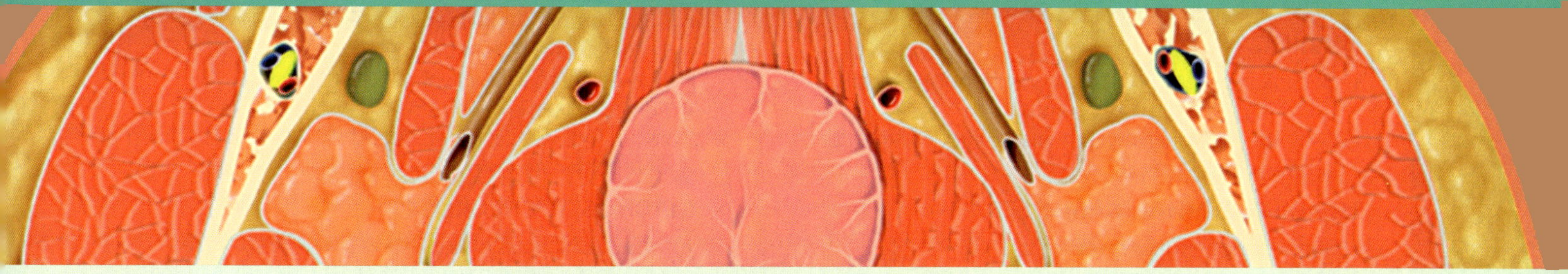

Congenital/Genetic

Submandibular Space Accessory Salivary Tissue 280
Lingual Thyroid 282
Dermoid and Epidermoid 284
Submandibular Gland Aplasia-Hypoplasia 288
Foregut Duplication Cyst in Tongue 290

Infection

Oral Cavity Soft Tissue Infections 292

Inflammation

Ranula 296
Submandibular Gland Sialadenitis 300
Oral Cavity Sialocele 302
Submandibular Gland Mucocele 304

Neoplasm, Benign

Sublingual Gland Benign Mixed Tumor 306
Submandibular Gland Benign Mixed Tumor 308
Palate Benign Mixed Tumor 310

Neoplasm, Malignant

Oral Cavity Minor Salivary Gland Malignancy 312
Sublingual Gland Carcinoma 314
Submandibular Gland Carcinoma 316
Submandibular Space Nodal Non-Hodgkin Lymphoma 318
Oral Tongue Squamous Cell Carcinoma 320
Floor of Mouth Squamous Cell Carcinoma 324
Gingival Squamous Cell Carcinoma 326
Retromolar Trigone Squamous Cell Carcinoma 328
Submandibular Space Nodal Squamous Cell Carcinoma 330
Buccal Mucosa Squamous Cell Carcinoma 332
Hard Palate Squamous Cell Carcinoma 334

Miscellaneous/Idiopathic

Motor Denervation CNXII 336
Submandibular Sialoliths 338

Submandibular Space Accessory Salivary Tissue

KEY FACTS

TERMINOLOGY

- Accessory salivary tissue in mylohyoid boutonnière
- Normal salivary tissue in abnormal position within submandibular space (SMS)

IMAGING

- Benign-appearing SMS mass, with density/intensity following normal salivary glands
- SMS; inferior to mylohyoid, most commonly anterior to submandibular gland

TOP DIFFERENTIAL DIAGNOSES

- SMS reactive nodal disease
- SMS lymphatic malformation
- SMS abscess
- Diving ranula
- Submandibular gland mucocele

PATHOLOGY

- Ectopic sublingual or submandibular gland tissue in SMS

CLINICAL ISSUES

- Most commonly **incidental** & discovered on imaging for unrelated indications
- May occasionally present as SMS mass
- Subject to same spectrum of disease as other salivary tissue, including sialadenitis and sialolithiasis, though these occur only rarely

DIAGNOSTIC CHECKLIST

- Include diagnosis of accessory salivary tissue when evaluating submandibular masses
- Accessory SMS salivary tissue focus, when discovered, is "leave alone" lesion
- Look for density/intensity that follows normal submandibular gland parenchyma

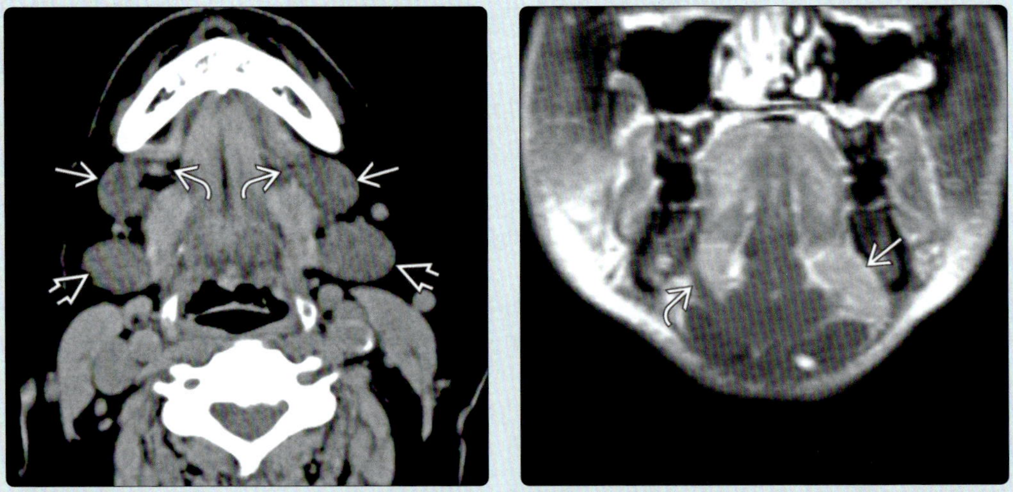

(Left) *Axial NECT demonstrates bilateral accessory salivary gland tissue in the submandibular space ➡. Bilateral mylohyoid dehiscence is evident ➡. Note density of the accessory salivary gland tissue is identical to that of the native submandibular glands ➡.* **(Right)** *Coronal T1 postcontrast MR reveals the left sublingual gland ➡ extending into the submandibular space through a defect in the left mylohyoid muscle. The right mylohyoid muscle is intact ➡.*

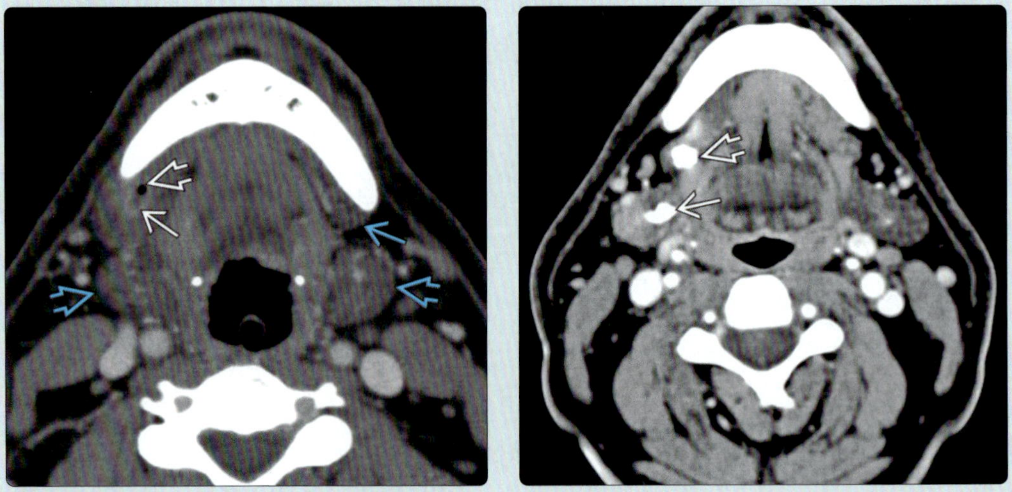

(Left) *Axial CECT image shows relative enhancement of inflamed right accessory salivary tissue, particularly of its duct ➡, which contains gas ➡. Compare to the normal density of the left accessory tissue ➡. Note normal submandibular glands ➡.* **(Right)** *Axial CECT shows a calcified mass in hyperdense right submandibular gland ➡. Accessory salivary tissue is present anteriorly & medially with an additional stone ➡. This appearance is consistent with sialolithiasis within both native & accessory salivary tissue.*

TERMINOLOGY

Synonyms

- Accessory salivary tissue in mylohyoid boutonnière

Definitions

- Normal salivary tissue in abnormal position in submandibular space (SMS)

IMAGING

General Features

- Best diagnostic clue
  - Benign-appearing SMS mass, with density/intensity following normal salivary glands
- Location
  - SMS; inferior to mylohyoid, most commonly anterior to submandibular gland (SMG)
- Size
  - Variable, usually small, < 2 cm
- Morphology
  - Ovoid to lobulated
  - Pear-shaped when projects into mylohyoid defect

CT Findings

- NECT
  - SMS mass with density similar to normal SMG
  - Mylohyoid defect may be visible
- CECT
  - Enhances similar to normal SMG
    - Increased density common, indicative of inflammation

MR Findings

- T1WI
  - SMS mass with signal similar to SMG
- T2WI
  - Signal parallels SMG
- T1WI C+
  - Enhancement similar to SMG

Imaging Recommendations

- Best imaging tool
  - CECT
- Protocol advice
  - Thin sections with multiplanar reformations, especially coronal

DIFFERENTIAL DIAGNOSIS

Submandibular Space Reactive Nodal Disease

- SMS mass distinct from SMG
  - Nodal morphology will vary based on underlying disease

Submandibular Space Abscess

- Rim-enhancing cystic mass with extensive cellulitis

Diving Ranula

- Comet-shaped unilocular mass with tail in collapsed sublingual space (tail sign) & head in posterior SMS
- May dive through mylohyoid defect

Submandibular Space Lymphatic Malformation

- Multilocular transspatial cystic mass

Submandibular Gland Mucocele

- Well-circumscribed SMG cystic mass

PATHOLOGY

General Features

- Etiology
  - Ectopic sublingual or SMG tissue in SMS
    - Present in ~ 1/3 of individuals
  - Occurs in association with congenital defect in mylohyoid boutonnière
    - Defects occur in ~ 75% of individuals
      - May contain fat, blood vessels, salivary tissue
    - Occasionally, entire sublingual glands may herniate through defect & lie completely below mylohyoid

Gross Pathologic & Surgical Features

- Normal salivary gland parenchyma

Microscopic Features

- Normal salivary gland cellular makeup

CLINICAL ISSUES

Presentation

- Most common signs/symptoms
  - Most commonly **incidental imaging finding**
  - Other signs/symptoms
    - May occasionally present as SMS mass

Treatment

- Imaging diagnosis allows avoidance of intervention
- When accessory tissue involved with salivary disease, treatment is determined by pathological process

DIAGNOSTIC CHECKLIST

Consider

- Include diagnosis of accessory salivary tissue when evaluating submandibular masses
- Accessory SMS salivary tissue focus, when discovered, is "leave alone" lesion

Image Interpretation Pearls

- Look for density/intensity that follows normal SMG parenchyma
- Susceptible to same pathology as orthotopic glands

SELECTED REFERENCES

1. Sanchez Barrueco A et al: Sialolithiasis in an accessory submandibular gland identified by magnetic resonance sialography. Ann Otol Rhinol Laryngol. ePub, 2016
2. Desai RS et al: Pleomorphic adenoma of an accessory submandibular salivary gland: a rare entity. Br J Oral Maxillofac Surg. 53(8):e33-5, 2015
3. Bryan S et al: Pleomorphic adenoma occurring outside the submandibular gland: a case report of an accessory submandibular gland. J Oral Maxillofac Surg. 71(10):1703-5, 2013
4. Harrison JD et al: Postmortem investigation of mylohyoid hiatus and hernia: aetiological factors of plunging ranula. Clin Anat. 26(6):693-9, 2013
5. Kiesler K et al: Incidence and clinical relevance of herniation of the mylohyoid muscle with penetration of the sublingual gland. Eur Arch Otorhinolaryngol. 264(9):1071-4, 2007
6. du Toit DF et al: Salivary glands: applied anatomy and clinical correlates. SADJ. 59(2):65-6, 69-71, 73-4, 2004
7. Hopp E et al: Mylohyoid herniation of the sublingual gland diagnosed by magnetic resonance imaging. Dentomaxillofac Radiol. 33(5):351-3, 2004

Lingual Thyroid

KEY FACTS

TERMINOLOGY

- Definition: Thyroid tissue in abnormal location in base of tongue or floor of mouth
- Synonym: Ectopic thyroid tissue

IMAGING

- Well-circumscribed, rounded, midline base of tongue mass
  - Usually at site of foramen cecum
- Less commonly in sublingual space or tongue root
- Imaging features similar to normal thyroid tissue
- **High density on NECT due to iodine content**
- Usually avid homogeneous enhancement
- Tc-99m pertechnetate or radioiodine scan confirms diagnosis & determines other sites of thyroid tissue

TOP DIFFERENTIAL DIAGNOSES

- Venous malformation
- Hemangioma, upper airway
- Tonsillar tissue, prominent/asymmetric
- Non-Hodgkin lymphoma, lingual tonsil

PATHOLOGY

- Arrest of thyroid precursor descent in 1st trimester

CLINICAL ISSUES

- Often incidental finding
- May present with dysphagia, dysphonia, dyspnea, obstructive sleep apnea
- Most common location of ectopic thyroid (90%)
- In 75%, lingual thyroid is only functioning tissue
- Lingual thyroid may expand rapidly during puberty
- Lingual thyroid carcinoma is rare
- Treatment: Levothyroxine, surgery, radioiodine ablation

DIAGNOSTIC CHECKLIST

- Diagnosis suggested by well-defined, ovoid, or round mass in base of tongue or floor of mouth
- Intrinsic high density on CT characteristic
- Must **check for additional cervical thyroid** tissue

(Left) *Axial graphic depicts lingual thyroid ➡ in posterior midline of tongue, just deep to location of foramen cecum. Sharply defined contour and midline location in floor of mouth or tongue base are typical of lingual thyroid.* **(Right)** *Axial CECT shows round, well-delineated enhancing mass in midline of tongue base ➡ with minimal distortion of genioglossus muscles ➡. Lingual thyroid is markedly hyperdense relative to minimally enhancing lingual tonsil ➡.*

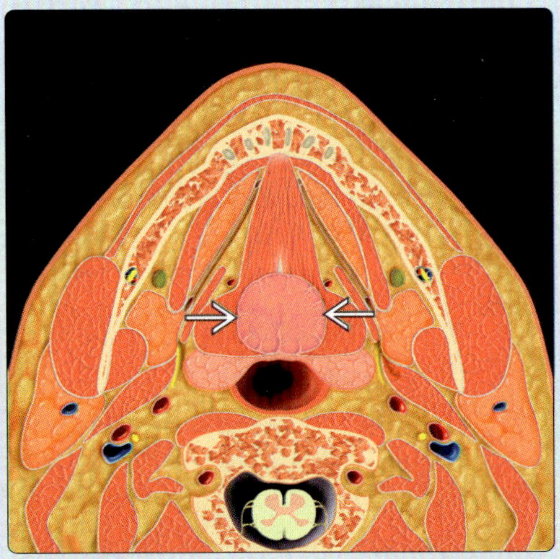

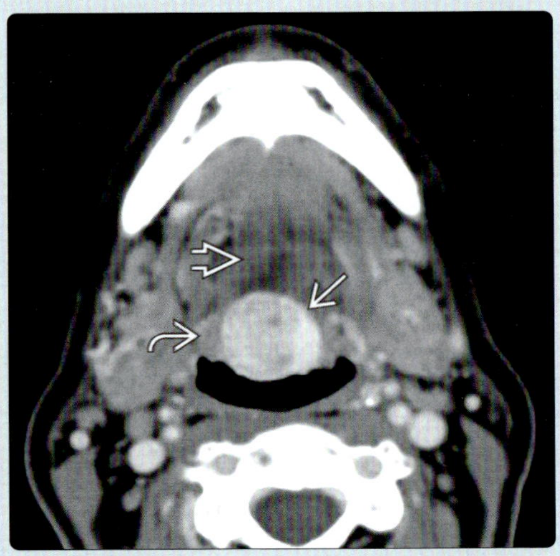

(Left) *Axial CECT demonstrates a sharply defined mass ➡ in the midline floor of mouth. This ectopic thyroid tissue is heterogeneous in density, compatible with early goitrous change.* **(Right)** *Midline sagittal STIR MR reveals a well-demarcated heterogeneously hyperintense mass within base of tongue, filling the valleculae ➡. In this case, the lingual thyroid is producing significant narrowing of the oropharyngeal airway ➡ and displaces the epiglottis posteroinferiorly ➡.*

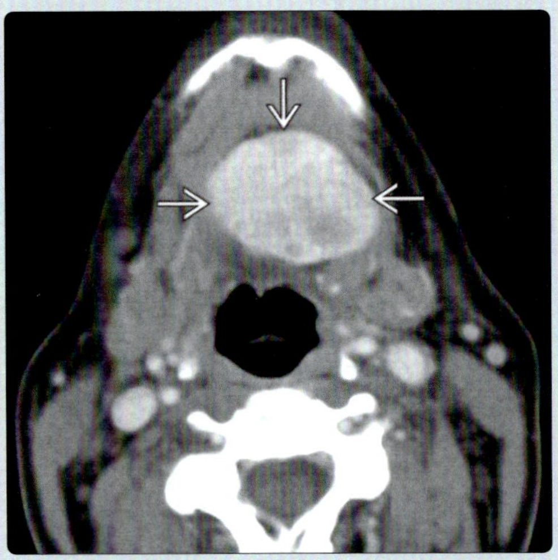

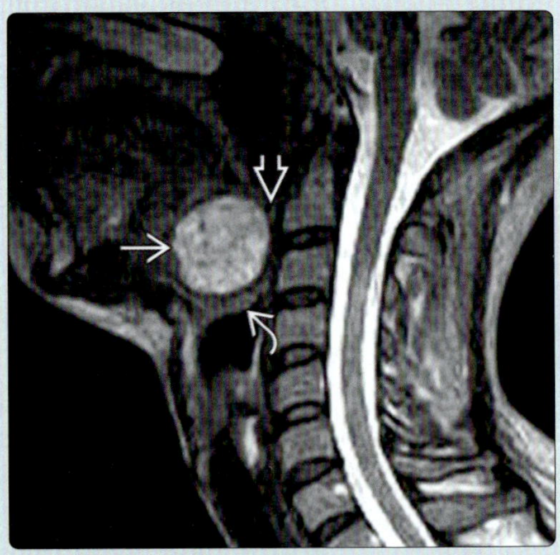

Lingual Thyroid

TERMINOLOGY

Synonyms

- Ectopic thyroid tissue

Definitions

- Thyroid tissue in abnormal location in base of tongue or floor of mouth

IMAGING

General Features

- Best diagnostic clue
  - Well-circumscribed midline base of tongue mass
  - Imaging characteristics similar to normal thyroid
- Location
  - Midline base of tongue at level of foramen cecum
  - Less commonly in sublingual space or tongue root
- Size
  - 1-3 cm
- Morphology
  - Well circumscribed, round, or ovoid

CT Findings

- NECT
  - Sharply marginated rounded mass
  - High density secondary to iodine accumulation
- CECT
  - Avid homogeneous enhancement

MR Findings

- T1WI
  - Isointense to mildly hyperintense relative to tongue
- T2WI
  - Mildly to strikingly hyperintense relative to tongue
- T1WI C+
  - Variable; most often homogeneous enhancement greater than tongue

Nuclear Medicine Findings

- Tc-99m pertechnetate or radioiodine scan to confirm diagnosis

Imaging Recommendations

- Best imaging tool
  - NECT: High-density rounded mass characteristic
- Protocol advice
  - Continue imaging through neck to determine if thyroid tissue is also present in normal location

DIFFERENTIAL DIAGNOSIS

Venous Malformation

- Vasoformative anomaly demonstrates prominent T2 hyperintensity & contrast enhancement

Hemangioma, Upper Airway

- Cavernous more common than capillary (infantile)

Tonsillar Tissue, Prominent/Asymmetric

- Hypertrophic lingual tonsil demonstrates imaging features similar to other lymphoid structures

Non-Hodgkin Lymphoma, Lingual Tonsil

- Isolated or in association with nodal or tonsillar lymphoma

PATHOLOGY

General Features

- Etiology
  - Arrest of thyroid anlage migration within tongue base between 3rd & 7th week of gestation
    - Complete arrest: No cervical thyroid (75%)
    - Partial arrest: High cervical thyroid (25%)
- Associated abnormalities
  - May occur in association with other thyroid migration anomalies, such as thyroglossal duct cyst

CLINICAL ISSUES

Presentation

- Often incidental finding
- Most common signs/symptoms
  - Dysphagia, dysphonia, dyspnea, obstructive sleep apnea
  - Most patients hypothyroid (60%) or euthyroid
- Other signs/symptoms
  - 25% of infants with congenital hypothyroidism will have ectopic gland

Demographics

- Gender
  - Females more often than males (F:M = 4:1)
- Epidemiology
  - Most common site of ectopic thyroid (90%)
  - Estimated incidence: 1:100,000 to 1:300,000

Natural History & Prognosis

- Lingual thyroid may expand rapidly during puberty
- Lingual thyroid goiter has been reported
- Carcinoma of lingual thyroid rare
  - Most often papillary thyroid carcinoma

Treatment

- Suppressive dose of levothyroxine
- Surgical if persistent obstructive symptoms
- Some advocate radioiodine ablation

DIAGNOSTIC CHECKLIST

Consider

- When lingual thyroid identified, must comment on status of cervical thyroid tissue
  - Only functioning thyroid tissue in 75%

Image Interpretation Pearls

- Well-defined midline tongue base mass with intrinsic high density is highly suggestive

SELECTED REFERENCES

1. Fiaschetti V et al: Diagnostic evaluation of a case of lingual thyroid ectopia. Radiol Case Rep. 11(3):165-70, 2016
2. Gandhi A et al: Lingual thyroid ectopia: diagnostic SPECT/CT imaging and radioactive iodine treatment. Thyroid. 26(4):573-9, 2016
3. Guerra G et al: Morphological, diagnostic and surgical features of ectopic thyroid gland: a review of literature. Int J Surg. 12 Suppl 1:S3-11, 2014
4. Gupta M et al: Lingual thyroid. Ear Nose Throat J. 88(6):E1, 2009
5. Arekapudi SR et al: Lingual thyroid. Pediatr Radiol. 37(9):940, 2007

Dermoid and Epidermoid

KEY FACTS

TERMINOLOGY

- Definition: Cystic mass resulting from **congenital** epithelial inclusion or rest
  - Epidermoid: Epithelial elements only
  - Dermoid: Epithelial elements + dermal substructure, including dermal appendages

IMAGING

- Epidermoid: Cystic, well-demarcated mass with **fluid contents** only
- Dermoid: Cystic, well-demarcated mass with **fatty, fluid, or mixed contents**
- Location
  - Oral cavity: Submandibular space, sublingual space, or root of tongue
  - Anterior neck, usually midline
  - Orbit: Adjacent to frontozygomatic suture > frontolacrimal suture
  - Nasal cyst in association with nasal dermal sinus (NDS) ± intracranial extension
- Scalloping or remodeling of bone common
- Subtle rim enhancement of wall sometimes seen
- Dermoid & epidermoid cysts may see **restricted diffusion**
- Protocol advice
  - Routine CECT of cervical soft tissues
  - MR: T1 precontrast & use fat saturation postcontrast for orbit, neck, & oral cavity lesions
  - High-resolution anterior skull base MR in NDS; image from tip of nose to posterior to crista galli
  - Sagittal to define tract: Nose → anterior skull base

DIAGNOSTIC CHECKLIST

- Complex lesion with fat, consider dermoid cyst
- Simple lesion (may be proteinaceous fluid) = epidermoid or dermoid cyst

(Left) *Sagittal CT reconstruction in a 10-year-old child following cleft palate repair shows a large nasal dermoid ➡ with nasal dermal sinus tract ➡ extending toward the cribriform plate.* **(Right)** *Sagittal T2WI MR in an 8-month-old girl shows a hyperintense sinus tract ➡ extending from the dermoid at the tip of the nose ➡ toward the cribriform plate. Notice there is no evidence for intracranial dermoid or epidermoid.*

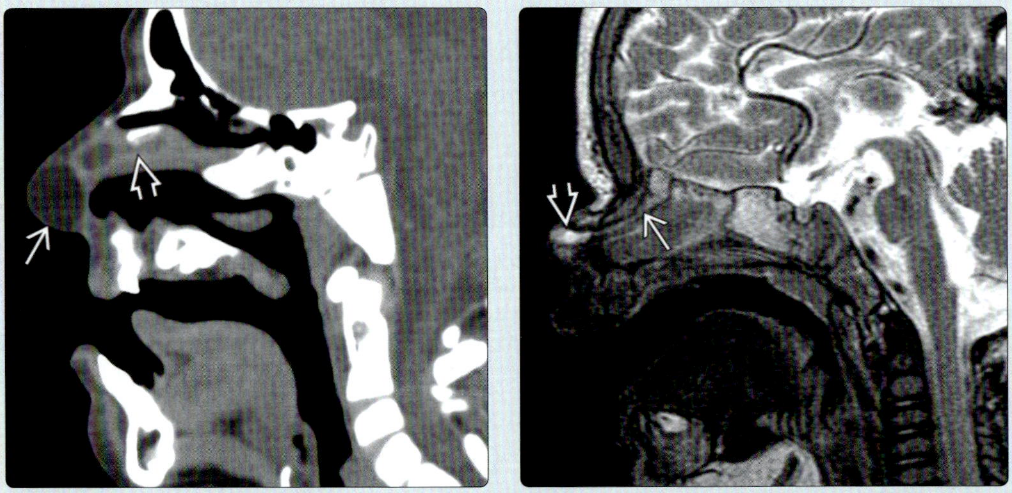

(Left) *Longitudinal ultrasound in a 14-year-old boy shows a submental mass with heterogeneous echotexture and minimal increase through transmission. One hyperechoic focus ➡ has posterior acoustical shadowing ➡, consistent with calcification in a dermoid.* **(Right)** *Coronal CECT in the same patient shows a low-density mass ➡ with a few calcifications ➡ within the oral cavity. Inferior displacement of the mylohyoid muscle ➡ indicates this dermoid is in the sublingual space.*

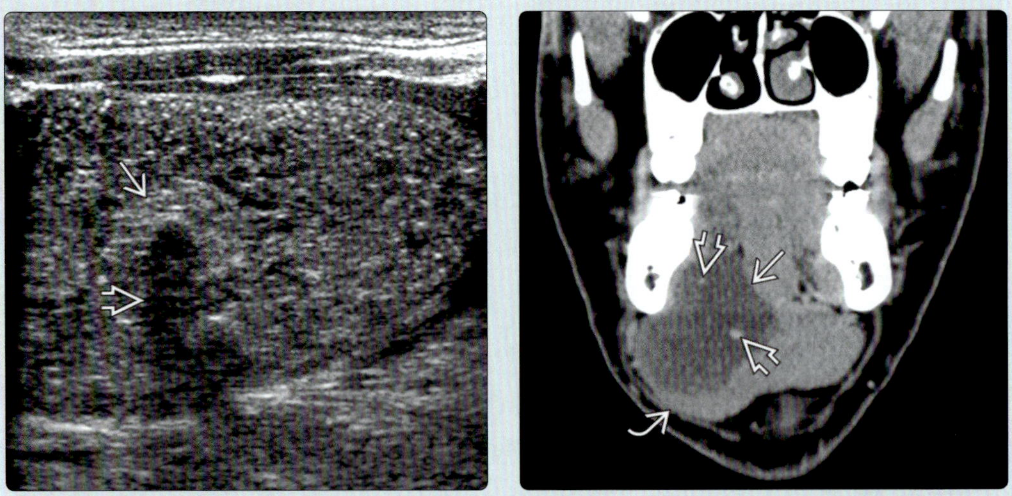

TERMINOLOGY

Synonyms

- Developmental cyst, ectodermal inclusion cyst, dermoid cyst

Definitions

- **Congenital** epithelial inclusion or rest → cystic mass
  - **Epidermoid**: Epithelial elements only
  - **Dermoid**: Epithelial elements + dermal substructure, including dermal appendages

IMAGING

General Features

- Best diagnostic clue
  - Epidermoid: Cystic, well-demarcated mass with **fluid contents** only
  - Dermoid: Cystic, well-demarcated mass with **fatty, fluid, or mixed contents**
- Location
  - Epidermoid & dermoid lesions
    - Oral cavity (OC): Submandibular space (SMS), sublingual space (SLS), or root of tongue
    - Anterior neck, usually midline
    - Orbit: Adjacent to frontozygomatic suture > frontolacrimal suture
    - Nasal cyst + nasal dermal sinus (NDS) ± intracranial extension
      - Tract or cyst nasal bridge to crista galli
      - Large foramen cecum with **bifid or deformed crista galli** or cribriform plate clue to intracranial extension
- Morphology
  - Ovoid or tubular

CT Findings

- NECT
  - Low-density, well-circumscribed cystic mass
    - Epidermoid: Fluid density material inside lesion without complex features
    - Dermoid: Fatty internal material, mixed density fluid, calcification (< 50%) all possible
      - When fluid density without complex features, indistinguishable from epidermoid
  - Scalloping or remodeling of bone common
- CECT
  - Lesion wall may be imperceptible
  - Subtle rim enhancement of wall sometimes seen

MR Findings

- T1WI
  - Epidermoid: Well-circumscribed mass with homogeneous fluid signal
    - **Diffuse ↑ signal** if **high protein** fluid
  - Dermoid: Well-circumscribed mass with complex fluid signal
    - If **fatty** elements, **focal or diffuse ↑ signal**
- T2WI
  - Epidermoid: Homogeneous high signal
  - Dermoid: Heterogeneous high signal
    - Intermediate signal if fat
    - Focal areas of low signal if calcifications
- DWI
  - Dermoid & epidermoid cysts ± **restricted diffusion**
- T1WI C+
  - Thin rim enhancement or none
  - If fat saturation used, fat will be low signal in dermoid

Ultrasonographic Findings

- Epidermoid: **Pseudosolid** appearance with uniform internal echoes
  - Cellular material in cyst → pseudosolid appearance
  - Posterior wall echo enhancement = cystic lesion
- Dermoid: Mixed internal echoes from fat with echogenic foci & dense shadowing if calcifications

Imaging Recommendations

- Best imaging tool
  - CECT is best imaging tool for OC lesions (unless obscured by dental amalgam, then MR best)
  - CECT or MR for neck lesions
  - MR for orbit lesions
  - MR for NDS to better evaluate intracranial extent
    - CT to evaluate skull base & crista galli deformity
- Protocol advice
  - Routine CECT of cervical soft tissues
  - MR: Include T1 precontrast, & use fat saturation techniques postcontrast for orbit, neck, & OC lesions
  - High-resolution anterior skull base MR in NDS; image from **tip of nose to posterior to crista galli**
    - Sagittal to define tract: Nose → anterior skull base
    - DWI hyperintensity may diagnose epidermoid

DIFFERENTIAL DIAGNOSIS

Pediatric SLS, SMS, or Neck Lesions

- Thyroglossal duct cyst
  - Midline unilocular cystic mass between hyoid bone & foramen cecum
  - No fat or calcifications
- Lymphatic malformation
  - Unilocular or multilocular, transspatial common
  - Fluid-fluid levels common
- Ranula
  - Simple: Unilateral low-density/signal mass in SLS with thin, nonenhancing wall
  - Diving: Comet-shaped unilocular mass with tail in collapsed SLS (tail sign) & head in posterior SMS
- Abscess
  - Clinical: Fever, erythema, elevated white blood cell count
  - Imaging: Rim-enhancing cyst often with soft tissue cellulitis, edema, & adenopathy

Pediatric Orbital Lesions

- Orbital Langerhans cell histiocytosis
  - Enhancing soft tissue mass with smoothly marginated lytic bone lesion
- Rhabdomyosarcoma
  - Moderately enhancing mass frequently inseparable from extraocular muscle
  - Frequently without bone erosion when in orbit
- Orbital infantile hemangioma

  - Significant contrast enhancement, no bone erosion, & presents in infancy
- Orbital lymphatic malformation
  - Nonenhancing, fluid-fluid levels common
- Orbital venous malformation
  - Moderate enhancement
  - Calcifications/phleboliths common
- Orbital idiopathic inflammatory pseudotumor
  - Painful proptosis common
  - Moderately enhancing mass, any area of orbit

Pediatric Nasal Lesions

- Normal fatty marrow in crista galli
  - No mass or pit on nose
- Nonossified foramen cecum
  - Ossifies postnatally in first 5 years of life
- Frontoethmoidal cephalocele
- Nasal glioma (nasal glial heterotopia)
  - Most commonly projects extranasally onto paramedian bridge of nose

PATHOLOGY

General Features

- Etiology
  - Congenital inclusion of dermal elements at site of embryonic fusion
    - Sequestration of trapped surface ectoderm

Staging, Grading, & Classification

- Meyer classification dysontogenetic cysts floor of mouth
  - **Epidermoid cyst**: Lined with simple squamous epithelium & surrounding connective tissue
  - **Dermoid cyst**: Epithelium-lined cyst that contains skin appendages
  - **Teratoid cyst**: Epithelium-lined cyst that contains mesodermal or endodermal elements, such as muscle, bones, teeth, & mucous membranes

Gross Pathologic & Surgical Features

- Oily or cheesy material, tan, yellow, or white
- Cyst wall = fibrous capsule; 2-6 mm in thickness

Microscopic Features

- Epidermoid
  - Simple squamous cell epithelium with fibrous wall
- Dermoid
  - Contains dermal structures, including sebaceous glands, hair follicles, blood vessels, fat ± collagen
    - Lined by keratinizing squamous epithelium
- Teratoid cysts (rare lesion)
  - Contain elements from all 3 germ cell layers

CLINICAL ISSUES

Presentation

- Most common signs/symptoms
  - Painless mass in floor of mouth, anterior neck, orbit, or nasoglabellar region
- Other signs/symptoms
  - OC lesions: Dysphagia, globus oral sensation, airway encroachment when large
  - Orbit lesions: Proptosis, diplopia
  - Nasal lesions: Pit on skin of nasal bridge ± protruding hair, recurrent meningitis, intermittent sebaceous material discharged from pit

Demographics

- Age
  - OC lesions: Mean age in late teens to 20s
    - Most dermoid cysts of floor of mouth present at 5-50 years
    - Average age = 30 years
  - Orbit lesions: Children or early adulthood
  - Nasal lesions: Newborn to 5 years
    - Mean age: 32 months
- Epidemiology
  - Present from birth; spontaneous occurrence
  - Dermoid/epidermoid are least common of all congenital neck lesions
  - Orbit most common dermoid of H&N
  - OC dermoids account for < 25% of all H&N dermoids

Natural History & Prognosis

- Benign lesion, very slow growth
  - Present during childhood but small & dormant
  - Symptomatic during rapid growth phase in young adult
- Sudden growth or change following rupture
  - Significant inflammation & increased size (rare complication)

Treatment

- Surgical resection is curative
  - Entire cyst must be removed to prevent recurrence
  - OC lesions: Surgical approach may be decided by lesion position relative to mylohyoid muscle
    - SLS: Intraoral approach
    - SMS: Submandibular approach

DIAGNOSTIC CHECKLIST

Image Interpretation Pearls

- Complex lesion with fat density or signal intensity, consider dermoid cyst
- Simple lesion (may be proteinaceous fluid) = epidermoid or dermoid cyst
- If dermal sinus tract reaches dura of anterior cranial fossa, crista galli may be bifid & foramen cecum large

SELECTED REFERENCES

1. Moses MA et al: The management of midline frontonasal dermoids: a review of 55 cases at a tertiary referral center and a protocol for treatment. Plast Reconstr Surg. 135(1):187-96, 2015
2. Paradis J et al: Pediatric teratoma and dermoid cysts. Otolaryngol Clin North Am. 48(1):121-36, 2015
3. Papadogeorgakis N et al: Surgical management of a large median dermoid cyst of the neck causing airway obstruction. A case report. Oral Maxillofac Surg. 13(3):181-4, 2009
4. Lee SS et al: Refinement in technique for pediatric dermoid cyst excision: technical note. Plast Reconstr Surg. 122(4):1059-61, 2008
5. Suzuki C et al: Apparent diffusion coefficient of subcutaneous epidermal cysts in the head and neck comparison with intracranial epidermoid cysts. Acad Radiol. 14(9):1020-8, 2007
6. Hedlund G: Congenital frontonasal masses: developmental anatomy, malformations, and MR imaging. Pediatr Radiol. 36(7):647-62; quiz 726-7, 2006
7. Charrier JB et al: Craniofacial dermoids: an embryological theory unifying nasal dermoid sinus cysts. Cleft Palate Craniofac J. 42(1):51-7, 2005

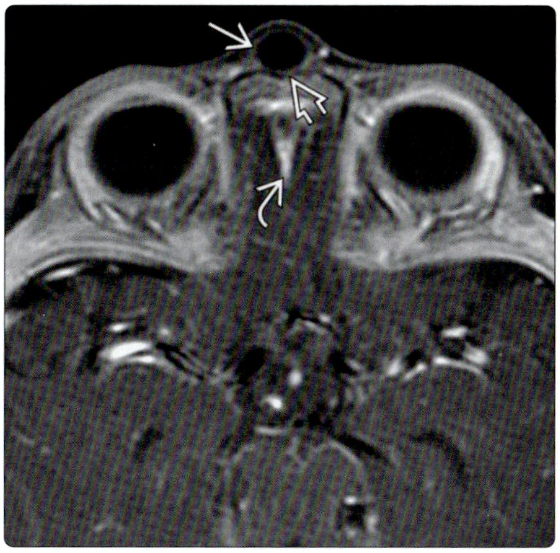

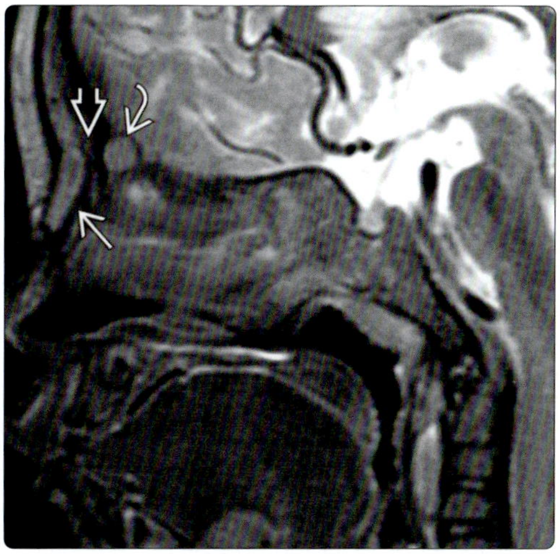

(Left) *Axial T1 C+ FS MR in a 6-month-old infant shows a typical nasal glabella dermoid, well defined and nonenhancing, with adjacent osseous remodeling. Notice the normal appearance of the crista galli.* **(Right)** *Sagittal T2 MR in an 18-month-old infant shows oblong midline dermoid remodeling the underlying frontal bone. Deep to the thin but intact frontal bone is a noncontiguous intracranial dermoid at the foramen cecum.*

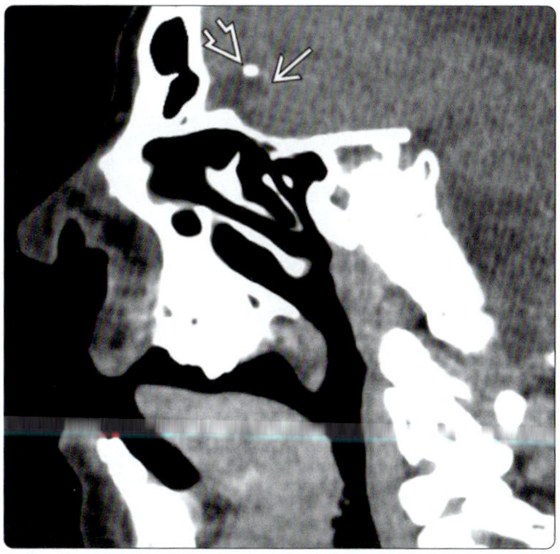

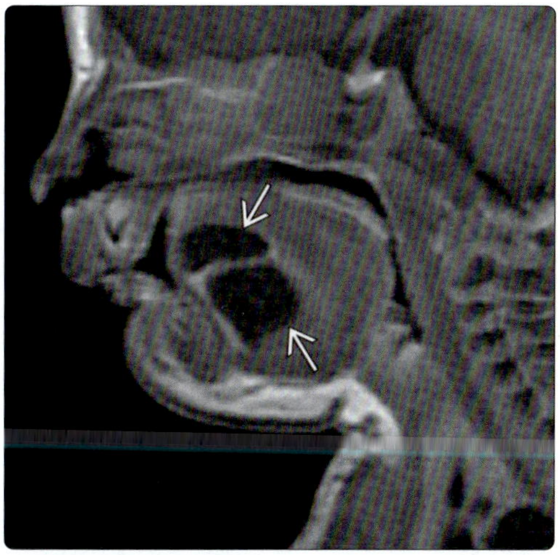

(Left) *Sagittal CT reconstruction shows intracranial extension of a dermoid cyst in a 10-year-old child with nasal dermal sinus. Note the calcification in the superior margin of the dermoid cyst.* **(Right)** *Sagittal T1 C+ FS MR in a 4-day-old infant with floor of mouth mass demonstrates a multiloculated midline mass, histologically proven to be a dermoid cyst. Differential diagnosis would include epidermoid cyst and lymphatic malformation.*

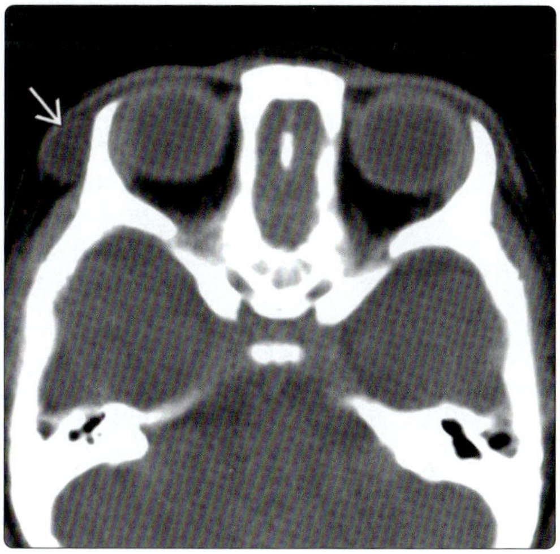

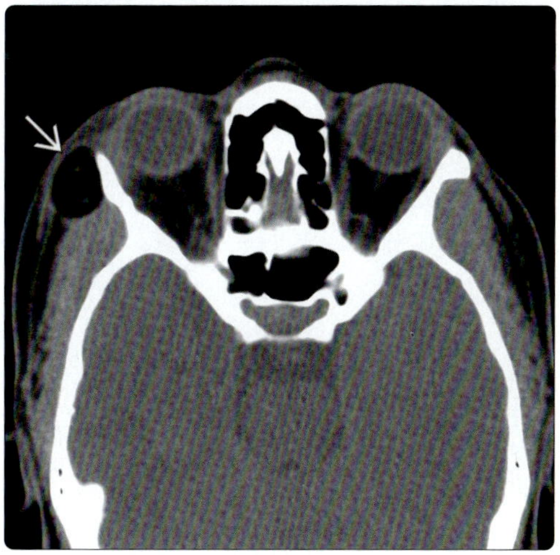

(Left) *Axial NECT in a 4-year-old girl shows a well-defined, low-attenuation mass lateral to the right lateral orbital wall without fat or calcific attenuation; therefore, differential diagnosis would include epidermoid and dermoid cysts. Histologically, this lesion contained skin appendages and therefore represents a dermoid cyst.* **(Right)** *Axial NECT in a child with longstanding history of palpable periorbital mass demonstrates a well-defined fat-containing dermoid with flattening of the adjacent lateral orbital wall.*

Submandibular Gland Aplasia-Hypoplasia

KEY FACTS

TERMINOLOGY

- Definition: Underdeveloped or absent submandibular gland (SMG) at expected location

IMAGING

- In aplasia, submandibular **fossa may be filled with fat and lymphatic tissue**
- SMG smaller than typical (28 mm x 18 mm ± 5 mm in axial plane) or absent

PATHOLOGY

- May be congenital (autosomal dominant)
- May be associated with developmental anomalies
  - Ectodermal dysplasia
  - Lacrimo-auriculo-dento-digital (LADD) syndrome; atresia/absence of lacrimal puncta
  - Hemifacial microsomia
  - Mandibulofacial dysostosis (Treacher-Collins syndrome)
  - Feature in 1st and 2nd branchial arch anomalies
  - Congenital malformations of temporomandibular component
  - Melkersson-Rosenthal syndrome

CLINICAL ISSUES

- **May be completely asymptomatic** and diagnosed by chance
- **Xerostomia**, dental caries, and dysphagia
- Irritable eyes, recurrent eye infections, and epiphora (constant tearing) with LADD

DIAGNOSTIC CHECKLIST

- CT/MR/US: Asymmetry may confuse presentation
- Associated with hypertrophy of contralateral SMG (unilateral aplasia) or sublingual gland, which may prolapse/herniate through mylohyoid boutonnière
- **Sialolithiasis** associated with SMG hypoplasia reported
- **Wharton duct ± sialolithiasis may be present,** even in aplasia

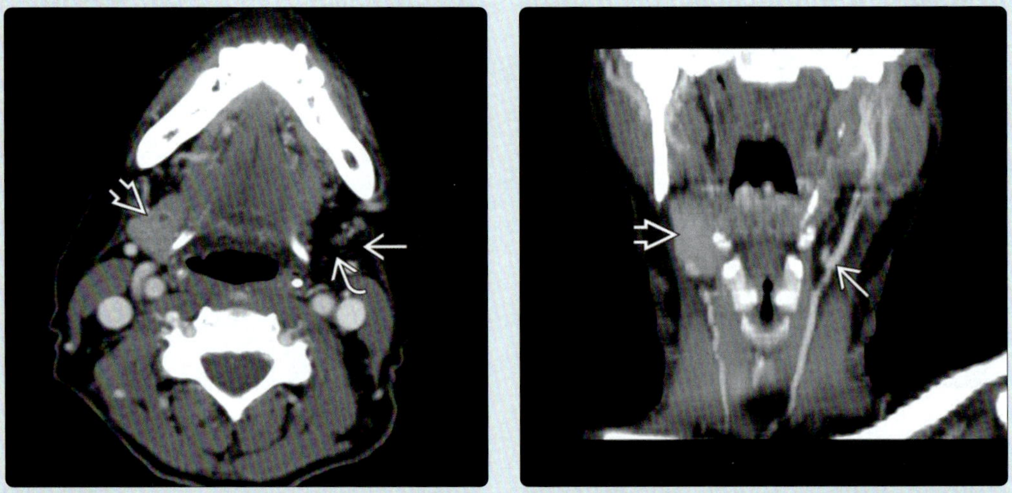

(Left) *Axial CECT through the neck shows unilateral aplasia of the submandibular gland. The left submandibular gland ➔ is absent, but there is a normal, though slightly enlarged, right submandibular gland ➔. The left fossa is filled with fat, small lymph nodes, and facial veins ➔.* **(Right)** *Coronal CECT in the same patient shows aplasia of the left submandibular gland ➔ and a slightly enlarged right submandibular gland ➔.*

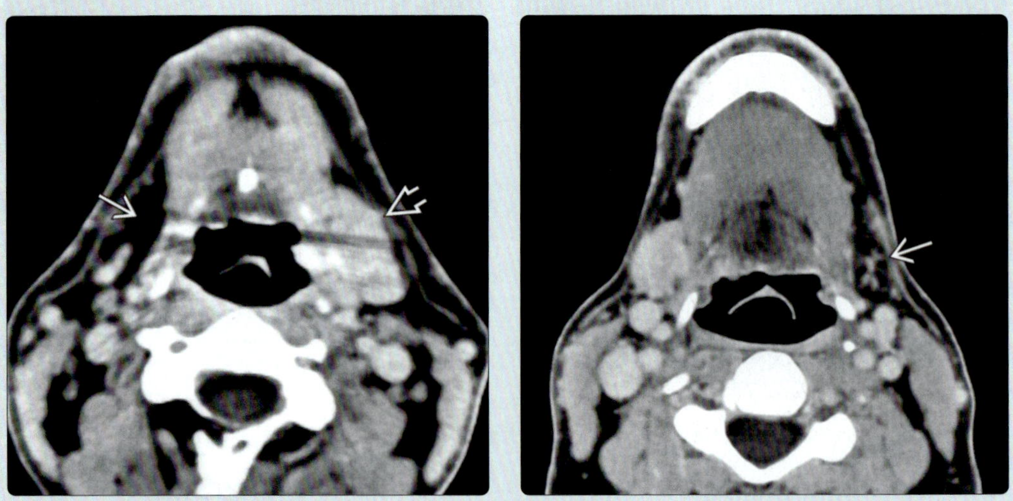

(Left) *Axial CECT shows absence of the right submandibular gland ➔. The left submandibular gland is slightly hypertrophic ➔.* **(Right)** *Axial CECT shows fatty atrophy of the left submandibular gland ➔ as a consequence of a sialolith in the Wharton duct, which is not visualized in this slice. Even in aplasia, Wharton duct may still be present.*

TERMINOLOGY

Abbreviations

- Submandibular gland (SMG) aplasia/hypoplasia

Definitions

- Underdeveloped or absent SMG

IMAGING

General Features

- Best diagnostic clue
  - Confirm aplastic SMG by evaluating normal anatomy
    - Close relationship of SMG to facial artery and vein
    - SMG wraps around posterior margin of mylohyoid muscle, resulting in superficial and deep portion of gland
  - Compensatory hypertrophy of ipsilateral sublingual gland (SLG) &/or contralateral SMG, which may present as masses
  - In aplasia, submandibular **fossa may be filled with fat, blood vessels, and lymphatic tissue**
- Location
  - Submandibular fossa
- Size
  - SMG smaller than typical (28 mm x 18 mm ± 5 mm in axial plane) or absent

Imaging Recommendations

- Best imaging tool
  - CT, MR, US, scintigraphy
- Protocol advice
  - Soft tissue NECT may serve as initial single procedure for definitive diagnosis

PATHOLOGY

General Features

- Etiology
  - Aplasia: Likely due to arrest in organogenesis and seen in combination with congenital anomalies
  - Hypoplasia: May be secondary to infection, ductal obstruction, diet, or pharmaceuticals; may be associated with Melkersson-Rosenthal syndrome
- Genetics
  - Familial cases reported, generally with autosomal dominant pattern of inheritance
- Associated abnormalities
  - May be isolated or **associated with multiple other developmental anomalies**, particularly of face
    - Ectodermal dysplasia
    - Lacrimo-auriculo-dento-digital (LADD) syndrome; atresia/absence of lacrimal puncta
    - Hemifacial microstomia
    - Mandibulofacial dysostosis (Treacher-Collins syndrome)
    - Congenital malformations of temporomandibular component
    - May be feature in 1st and 2nd branchial arch anomalies
    - Melkersson-Rosenthal syndrome
  - Parotid hypoplasia
  - Sialolithiasis
- Isolated unilateral SMG is rare

CLINICAL ISSUES

Presentation

- Most common signs/symptoms
  - **May be completely asymptomatic** and diagnosed by chance
  - **Xerostomia** if total salivary flow decreased by > 50% with oral burning sensation, taste alterations, dry lips, and smooth surface dental caries
  - Dysphagia
  - Irritable eyes, recurrent eye infections, and epiphora (constant tearing) if associated with LADD

Demographics

- Gender
  - No predilection
- Epidemiology
  - Congenital or developmental

Natural History & Prognosis

- Good with treatment

Treatment

- Treat only if symptoms or side effects present
  - Sialogogue agents such as pilocarpine or cevimeline and sugarless chewing gum/sour candy to stimulate remaining salivary flow
  - Fluoridated toothpastes/mouthwashes, dental sealants, alkaline mouth rinses, and meticulous oral home care to minimize dental caries secondary to xerostomia

DIAGNOSTIC CHECKLIST

Image Interpretation Pearls

- CT/MR/US: Asymmetry may confuse presentation
  - Aplasia: Absence of SMG at expected location
    - May be associated with hypertrophy of contralateral SMG (with unilateral aplasia) or ipsilateral SLG
  - Hypoplasia: SMG smaller than typical (28 mm x 18 mm ± 5 mm in axial plane)
  - **Wharton duct may be present**, even in aplasia
    - Sialolithiasis reported

Reporting Tips

- May be mistaken for Sjögren syndrome
  - Rule out by minor salivary gland biopsy and serology

SELECTED REFERENCES

1. Kara M et al: Agenesis of submandibular glands: a report of two cases with review of literature. Case Rep Otolaryngol. 2014:569026, 2014
2. Berta E et al: Complete agenesis of major salivary glands. Int J Pediatr Otorhinolaryngol. 77(10):1782-5, 2013
3. Haktanir A: CT and MR findings of bilateral submandibular gland aplasia associated with hypertrophied symmetrical sublingual glands herniated through mylohyoid defects. Dentomaxillofac Radiol. 41(1):79-83, 2012
4. Taji SS et al: Congenital aplasia of the major salivary glands: literature review and case report. Pediatr Dent. 33(2):113-8, 2011
5. García-Consuegra L et al: Unilateral absence of submandibular gland secondary to stones. Aplasia versus early atrophy. Med Oral Patol Oral Cir Bucal. 15(5):e752-4, 2010
6. Yilmaz MD et al: Unilateral aplasia of the submandibular gland. Eur Arch Otorhinolaryngol. 259(10):554-6, 2002

Foregut Duplication Cyst in Tongue

KEY FACTS

TERMINOLOGY

- Synonyms
  - Enteric duplication cyst
  - Gastrointestinal cyst
  - Choristomatic cyst
- Definition
  - **Choristoma containing heterotopic islands of gastrointestinal mucosa**

IMAGING

- Final diagnosis made only with excisional biopsy
- CECT
  - Circumscribed, **nonenhancing cystic mass**
  - Well-defined, thick, **enhancing wall** (thinly rim enhancing)
- MR
  - Isointense to muscle on short T1 inversion recovery images; hyperintense if proteinaceous fluid/blood products present
  - Uniformly hyperintense on short T2
- Ultrasound
  - Bowel wall signature

TOP DIFFERENTIAL DIAGNOSES

- Dermoid cyst
- Ranula
- Cystic hygroma/lymphangioma
- Suprahyoid thyroglossal duct cyst

CLINICAL ISSUES

- **Infancy** but more rare in adults where it is manifested as asymptomatic swelling
- May be diagnosed antenatally

DIAGNOSTIC CHECKLIST

- **Cystic lesion between genioglossus muscles**
- Frequently indistinguishable from dermoid cyst due to proteinaceous contents
- **Biopsy required for final diagnosis**

(Left) *Sagittal T2WI FS MR shows a separated foregut duplication cyst ➡ at the base of the tongue. The homogeneous thick wall ➡ is a diagnostic feature to distinguish from thyroglossal duct cyst or epidermoid cyst.* **(Right)** *Sagittal T1WI MR shows the tongue elevated to the roof of mouth ➡. Variable signal intensity on T1 images ➡ is related to presence of variable amounts of proteinaceous contents.*

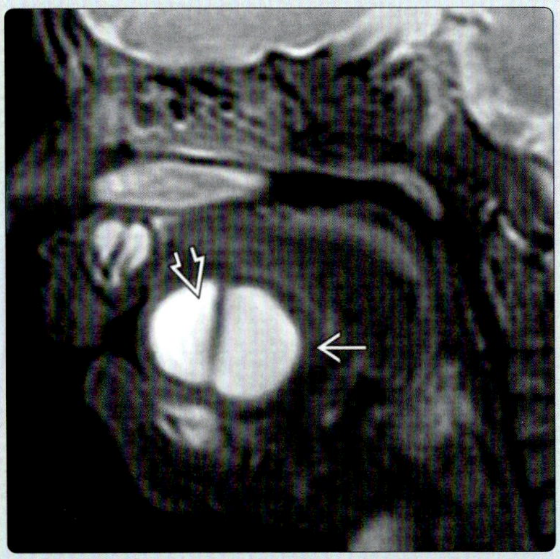

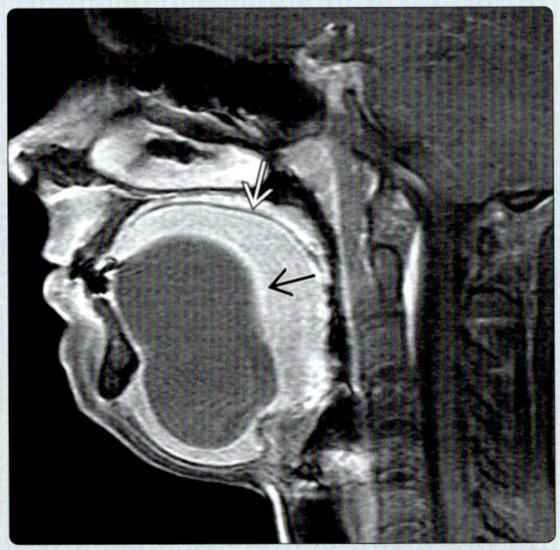

(Left) *Coronal T1WI MR of 10-week-old boy shows a low-signal expansile lesion ➡ at the base of the tongue. The lesion on the ventral surface of the tongue was present since birth. The homogeneous thick wall ➡ suggests a foregut duplication cyst.* **(Right)** *Sagittal T2WI MR of the same patient shows a high-signal fluid-filled cystic lesion ➡ of the base of the tongue.*

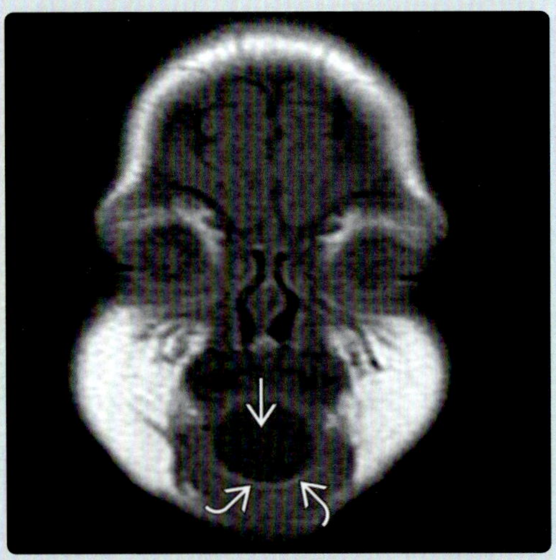

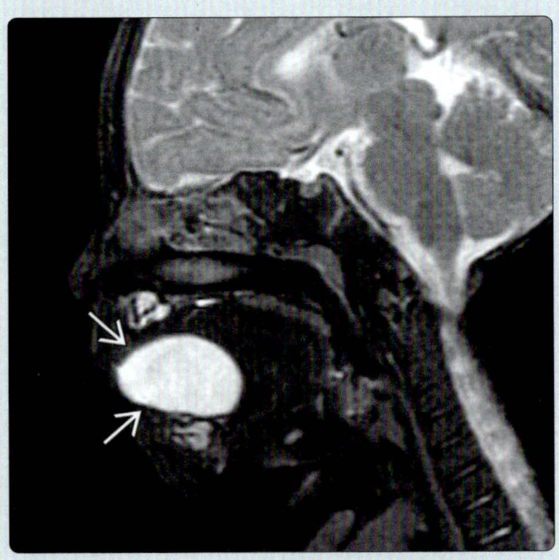

TERMINOLOGY

Synonyms

- Enteric duplication cyst
- Gastrointestinal cyst
- Choristomatic cyst

Definitions

- **Choristoma containing heterotopic islands of gastrointestinal mucosa**

IMAGING

General Features

- Best diagnostic clue
  - **Thick wall**
- Location
  - **Cystic lesion between genioglossus muscles**
  - May occur on ventral and dorsum of tongue, anterior 2/3 of tongue, and hard palate

Imaging Recommendations

- Best imaging tool
  - MR due to lack of ionizing radiation and superior soft tissue resolution
  - Ultrasound helpful in antenatal diagnosis
- Protocol advice
  - Final diagnosis is made only with excisional biopsy

CT Findings

- CECT
  - Circumscribed, **nonenhancing cystic mass**
  - Well-defined, thick, **enhancing wall** (thinly rim enhancing)

MR Findings

- T1WI
  - Variable intensity due to presence and amount of proteinaceous contents
    - Isointense to muscle on short T1 inversion recovery images
    - Hyperintense if proteinaceous fluid/blood products present
- T2WI
  - Uniformly hyperintense on short T2

DIFFERENTIAL DIAGNOSIS

Dermoid Cyst

- Cystic form of teratoma
- **Indistinguishable from foregut duplication cyst**
- May contain dental structures and present with corresponding high-density areas
- Homogeneous thick wall not present

Cystic Hygroma/Lymphangioma

- Fluid-fluid level often seen within multiple compartments
- Imperceptible wall; homogeneous **thick wall not present**

Suprahyoid Thyroglossal Duct Cyst

- Homogeneous **thick wall not present**
- Midline unilocular lesion between hyoid and foramen cecum

Ranula

- Obstruction and enlargement of Wharton duct
- Associated with sublingual gland
- Well-circumscribed, water density mass
- **Tail sign and comet-shaped in diving ranula**

PATHOLOGY

General Features

- Etiology
  - Uncommon congenital anomaly

Gross Pathologic & Surgical Features

- Choristoma containing gastric or intestinal mucosa ectopic to site of origin

Microscopic Features

- Lined with alimentary tract epithelium

CLINICAL ISSUES

Presentation

- Most common signs/symptoms
  - Most are diagnosed in asymptomatic infants
  - Feeding difficulty in infants
  - Respiratory distress when large

Demographics

- Age
  - **Infancy** but more rare in adults where it is manifested as asymptomatic swelling
  - May be diagnosed antenatally
- Epidemiology
  - 0.3% of all enteric duplications
  - Rare lesion

Treatment

- Options, risks, complications
  - Incomplete removal of functional mucosal lining may allow continued secretion of mucus and acid with risk of ulceration and bleeding
  - In infants, may lead to failure to thrive, respiratory difficulty, and more extensive future surgery
- Definitive surgical excision with removal of mucosal lining

DIAGNOSTIC CHECKLIST

Image Interpretation Pearls

- **Cystic lesion between genioglossus muscles**
- Thick wall
- Indistinguishable from dermoid cyst

SELECTED REFERENCES

1. Hambarde S et al: Foregut duplication cyst presenting as lingual swelling: case report and review of literature. Natl J Maxillofac Surg. 2(1):2-5, 2011
2. Houshmand G et al: Prenatal magnetic resonance imaging (MRI) findings of a foregut duplication cyst of the tongue: value of real-time MRI evaluation of the fetal swallowing mechanism. J Ultrasound Med. 30(6):843-50, 2011
3. Patel P et al: Lingual foregut duplication in a middle-aged adult. AJNR Am J Neuroradiol. 32(3):E40-1, 2011
4. Puvaneswary M et al: Magnetic resonance imaging findings of a foregut duplication cyst of the floor of the mouth in a fetus. Australas Radiol. 49(1):66-8, 2005

Oral Cavity Soft Tissue Infections

KEY FACTS

TERMINOLOGY

- Definition: Oral cavity soft tissue abscess: Focal collection of pus within oral cavity soft tissue space(s)
    - May be in 1 or more contiguous soft tissue spaces (transspatial)

IMAGING

- CECT to evaluate extent of soft tissue abscess
    - Abscess: Rim-enhancing fluid collection
    - Found within anatomic spaces [sublingual space (SLS), submandibular space (SMS), or root of tongue (ROT)]
    - Phlegmon: Enhancing inflammatory tissue without focal fluid/pus
    - Cellulitis: Adjacent soft tissue stranding ± dermal thickening
    - Reactive/suppurative nodes
- Intraoral/panoramic radiograph or CBCT for evaluating mandible and dental sources of infection

TOP DIFFERENTIAL DIAGNOSES

- Oral cavity dermoid and epidermoid cyst
- Simple or diving ranula
- Sialolithiasis/sialodochitis/sialocele
- Oral tongue squamous cell carcinoma (SCCa)

CLINICAL ISSUES

- Sublingual, submandibular, or vestibular swelling
- Painful tongue with dysphagia, dysphonia

DIAGNOSTIC CHECKLIST

- Consider abscess mimics: Primary oral cavity SCCa, ranula, epidermoid, sialocele
- Define space(s) with abscess: SLS, SMS, ROT
- Find underlying cause: Tooth abscess ± mandibular osteomyelitis; Wharton duct sialolithiasis; pharyngitis + suppurative node
- Report both abscess location(s) and probable origin of infection

(Left) *Panoramic radiograph shows a deep dental restoration ➡ and a periapical inflammatory lesion ➡, which may be an abscess. If associated with a clinical cellulitis or soft tissue swelling, this suggests a dental origin.* **(Right)** *Sagittal CECT through the midline demonstrates an unusual oral cavity soft tissue abscess with fluid tracking both superior ➡ and inferior ➡ to the mylohyoid muscle ➡. This patient had an infected dental extraction site.*

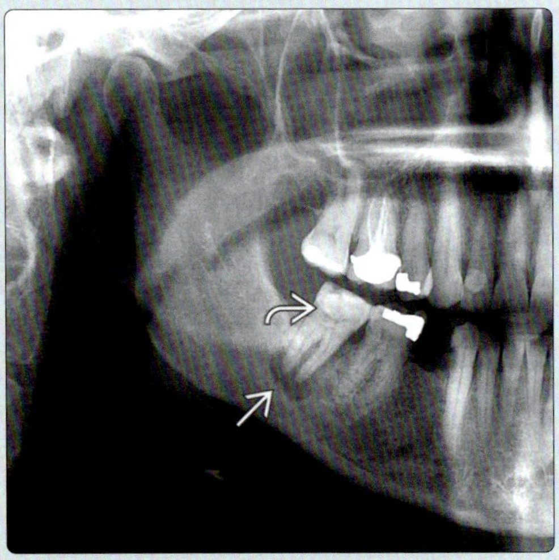

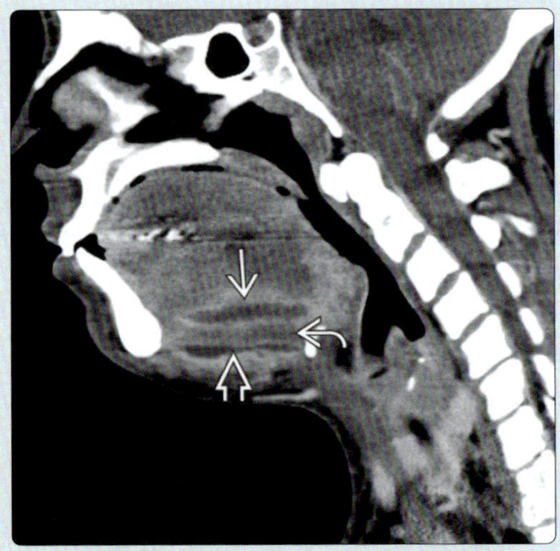

(Left) *Axial graphic depicts a bilateral sublingual space abscess ➡. The walled-off infected fluid collection is seen superomedial to the mylohyoid muscles and has a characteristic midline isthmus ➡ anteriorly.* **(Right)** *Axial CECT shows a horseshoe-shaped bilateral sublingual space abscess ➡ manifesting as a fluid collection with surrounding enhancement connected by anterior isthmus ➡. The sublingual spaces connect anteriorly under the frenulum of the tongue. Small submandibular space abscess pockets also seen ➡.*

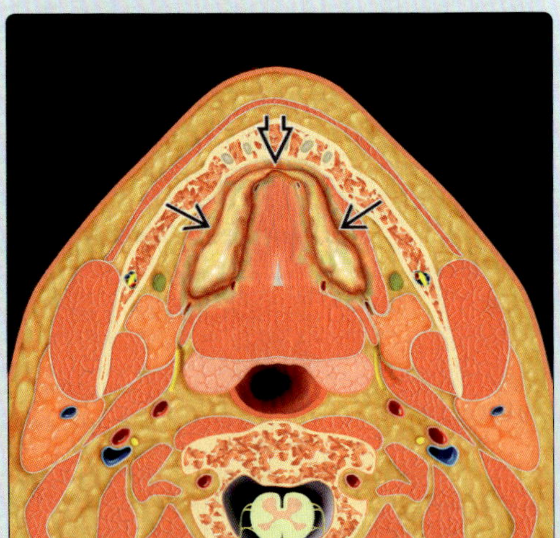

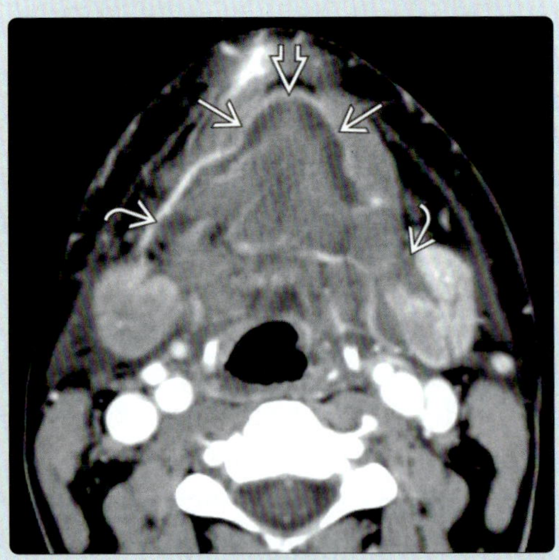

Oral Cavity Soft Tissue Infections

TERMINOLOGY

Definitions

- Oral cavity soft tissue abscess: Focal collection of pus within oral cavity soft tissue space(s)
  - May be in 1 or more contiguous soft tissue spaces (transspatial)

IMAGING

General Features

- Best diagnostic clue
  - CECT shows rim-enhancing, focal fluid collection in oral cavity space(s)
- Location
  - Oral cavity space(s): Sublingual space (SLS), submandibular space (SMS), or root of tongue (ROT) in lingual septum between genioglossus muscles
- Size
  - May become large in deep oral cavity spaces
- Morphology
  - Conforms to surrounding anatomic landscape/spaces (mandible, SMS, SLS, ROT)

Radiographic Findings

- Radiograph may show soft tissue swelling
- Intraoral or panoramic radiographs
  - Periapical dental abscess or other inflammatory lesion
  - Mandibular cortex dehiscence secondary to pus draining from tooth

CT Findings

- CECT
  - **Abscess**: Rim-enhancing fluid collection
  - **SLS abscess**
    - Unilateral: Fluid collection superomedial to mylohyoid muscle
    - Bilateral: **Horseshoe-shaped** fluid collection with anterior "isthmus"
  - **SMS abscess**: Fluid collection inferolateral to mylohyoid muscle
  - **ROT abscess**: Midline fluid collection between genioglossus muscles in low lingual septum
  - Associated phlegmon, cellulitis, or myositis
    - Phlegmon: Enhancing inflammatory tissue without focal fluid/pus
    - Cellulitis: Adjacent soft tissue stranding
      - ± dermal thickening
    - Myositis: Enhancing, enlarged muscle
  - Submandibular, high internal jugular chain reactive or suppurative adenopathy
- Bone CT/CBCT
  - Underlying **odontogenic infection** usually secondary to dental caries or trauma
    - Tooth with abscess of other periapical inflammatory lesion
    - Focal mandibular cortex dehiscence possible
  - **Mandibular osteomyelitis**
    - Permeative mandibular bone changes
    - Focal bone destruction possible
    - Periosteal reaction common

MR Findings

- T1WI
  - Low signal in fatty marrow of alveolar bone at site of infected tooth
- T2WI
  - Abscess: High-signal focal fluid collection
- T1WI C+
  - Rim-enhancing fluid collection(s)
  - Coronal plane helps define SLS (superomedial to mylohyoid muscle) from SMS (inferolateral to mylohyoid muscle) abscesses

Ultrasonographic Findings

- Hypoechoic collection within oral cavity musculature is diagnostic in septic clinical setting
- Needle aspiration for diagnosis done simultaneously

Nuclear Medicine Findings

- Bone scan
  - Increased uptake in regions of mandibular osteomyelitis
  - 3-phase bone scan very sensitive for osteomyelitis

Imaging Recommendations

- Best imaging tool
  - CECT to assess soft tissue extent of abscess
  - Intraoral or panoramic radiograph ± CBCT to assess potential dental origin and periosteal reactions
  - CECT/MR/conventional sialography to assess salivary origin
- Protocol advice
  - CECT is study of choice to assess soft tissue extent of abscesses in oral cavity
    - Soft tissue windows: Identify abscess location
    - Bone window: Identify dental inflammatory lesions, osteomyelitis, or sialolithiasis
    - Artifacts from metallic dental materials may obscure abscess and dental caries
  - Intraoral/panoramic radiograph or CBCT often helpful in evaluating mandible and possible dental sources of infection
    - CBCT may be reformatted as pseudopanoramic or alveolar cross sections
    - Intraoral radiographs have superior resolution but are limited by 2D image format

DIFFERENTIAL DIAGNOSIS

Oral Cavity Dermoid and Epidermoid Cyst

- Clinical: Slowly expanding soft tissue mass in floor of mouth or SMS
- CT findings
  - Epidermoid: Unilateral, low-density, nonenhancing SMS or SLS mass
  - Dermoid: Unilateral fluid ± fat density, nonenhancing SMS or SLS mass
  - No associated cellulitis/edema with either
- MR findings
  - Epidermoid: Low T1, high T2, DWI hyperintensity
  - Dermoid: If fat macroscopic, high T1 within mass

Simple or Diving Ranula

- Clinical

- Simple ranula: Sublingual bluish translucent mass
- Diving ranula: Compressible angle of mandible mass
- CT/MR findings
  - Simple ranula: Nonenhancing low T1/high T2 SLS lesion
    - May mimic SLS epidermoid on imaging
  - Diving ranula: Nonenhancing low T1/high T2 SMS lesion with SLS "tail"

Dilation of Submandibular Duct

- True sialocele: Enlarged proximal Wharton duct ± obstructing sialolith
- False sialocele: Fluid collection adjacent to duct in SLS without enhancing wall
- Both sialoceles are noninflammatory in nature

Oral Tongue Squamous Cell Carcinoma

- Clinical: Mucosal squamous cell carcinoma (SCCa) lesion usually obvious
- CT/MR findings
  - Enhancing invasive oral tongue mass
  - Cystic-necrotic neoplasm may mimic oral cavity soft tissue abscess

PATHOLOGY

General Features

- Etiology
  - Most common cause: Advanced dental caries with periapical dental abscess leading to mandibular osteomyelitis
    - SLS abscess: Dental root abscess drains superiorly to mylohyoid line of medial mandible with pus then walled off in SLS
    - SMS abscess: Dental abscess drains inferiorly to mylohyoid line of medial mandible with pus then walled off in SMS
  - Other causes of oral cavity soft tissue abscess
    - Sialolithiasis/sialadenitis
      - Submandibular gland: SLS abscess
    - Pharyngitis + suppurative SMS nodes: SMS abscess
    - Penetrating trauma: SLS, SMS, or ROT abscess
  - Up to 20% of deep neck infections have no identifiable source

Gross Pathologic & Surgical Features

- Putrid-smelling abscess pocket entered with surgical drain

Microscopic Features

- Oral flora predominate: *Streptococcus*, *Staphylococcus*
- Abscess is mixed culture of aerobic and anaerobic organisms
- Many oral, acid-producing, aerobic and anaerobic bacteria are capable of initiating tooth abscess
  - *Streptococcus mutans*, *Actinomyces viscosus*, and *Lactobacillus acidophilus*
- Some specific organisms predominate in dentoalveolar abscesses
  - *Fusobacterium*, *Prevotella*, *Porphyromonas*, and *Peptostreptococcus*

CLINICAL ISSUES

Presentation

- Most common signs/symptoms
  - Sublingual, submandibular, or vestibular swelling
- Other signs/symptoms
  - Painful tongue with dysphagia, dysphonia
  - Elevation and backward displacement of tongue may compromise airway
  - History of recent oral antibiotic treatment common
  - Difficulty opening mouth
- Clinical profile
  - Older patients with poor dentitions

Treatment

- Extraction of infected tooth (if present)
- Endodontic therapy
- Surgical drainage of abscess cavity
- Intravenous antibiotics
  - Penicillin or amoxicillin effective against most aerobic and anaerobic bacteria
  - When penicillin-resistant organisms present
    - Use amoxicillin-clavulanate, clindamycin, or combination of metronidazole plus amoxicillin or macrolide

DIAGNOSTIC CHECKLIST

Consider

- Lesions mimicking soft tissue abscesses in oral cavity
  - Cystic-necrotic oral cavity primary SCCa
  - Ranula, epidermoid: No inflammatory changes
  - False sialocele: May be superinfected

Image Interpretation Pearls

- 1st define abscess space(s): SLS, SMS, or ROT
- Comment on unilateral or bilateral, uni- or transspatial nature of abscess
- Search for underlying cause
  - Review mandible in bone window images for **dental abscess ± osteomyelitis**
  - If teeth appear normal, check for **sialolithiasis**
  - In children, look for **pharyngitis with suppurative SMS node**

SELECTED REFERENCES

1. Chapman MN et al: Periapical lucency around the tooth: radiologic evaluation and differential diagnosis. Radiographics. 33(1):E15-32, 2013
2. Rana RS et al: Head and neck infection and inflammation. Radiol Clin North Am. 49(1):165-82, 2011
3. Boon M et al: Lingual abscess from a grill cleaning brush bristle. Laryngoscope. 119(1):79-81, 2009
4. Nicolas J et al: Thrombophlebitis of the sigmoid sinus after tongue piercing: a case report. J Oral Maxillofac Surg. 65(6):1232-4, 2007
5. Kim HJ et al: Tongue abscess mimicking neoplasia. AJNR Am J Neuroradiol. 27(10):2202-3, 2006
6. Ozturk M et al: Tongue abscesses: MR imaging findings. AJNR Am J Neuroradiol. 27(6):1300-3, 2006
7. Balatsouras DG et al: Lingual abscess: diagnosis and treatment. Head Neck. 26(6):550-4, 2004
8. Eviatar E et al: Lingual abscess: secondary to follicular tonsillitis. Otolaryngol Head Neck Surg. 131(4):558-9, 2004
9. Branstetter BF 4th et al: Infection of the facial area, oral cavity, oropharynx, and retropharynx. Neuroimaging Clin N Am. 13(3):393-410, ix, 2003

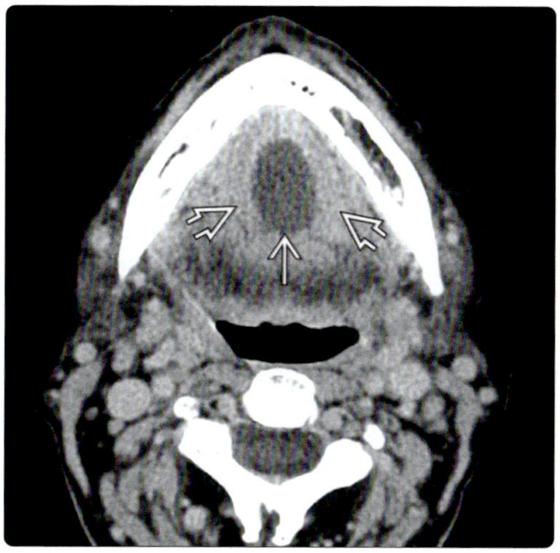

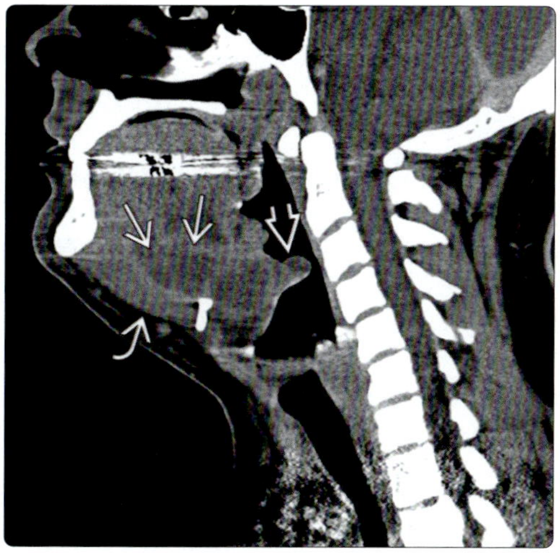

(Left) *Axial CECT shows a midline oral cavity abscess as an oval fluid-density collection* → *located centrally within the root of the tongue, bowing the genioglossus muscles* → *laterally.* **(Right)** *Sagittal CECT in a similar case shows a multiseptated peripherally enhancing fluid collection within the posterior root of the tongue* → *with posterior extension into the epiglottis* → *displacing the geniohyoid musculature* → *inferiorly.*

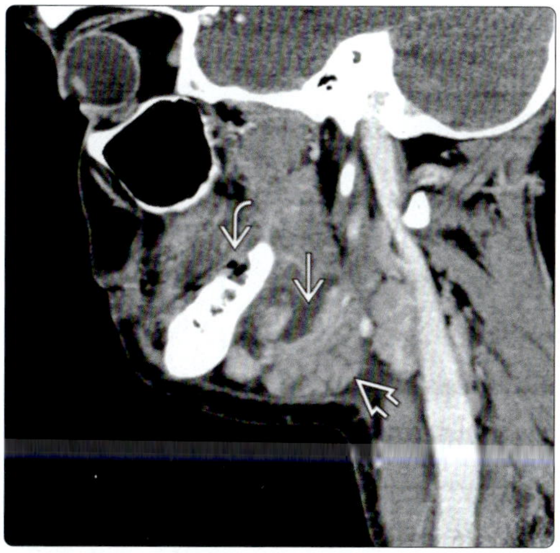

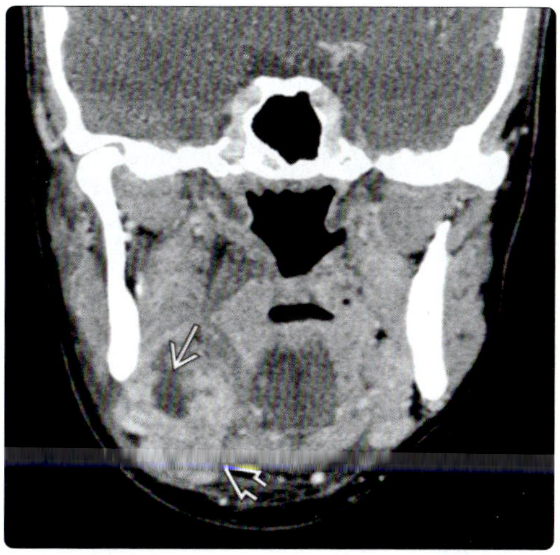

(Left) *Sagittal CECT reveals an infected mandibular tooth socket* → *with pus* → *extending inferiorly into the submandibular space. The inflamed submandibular gland* → *is displaced inferiorly by the abscess.* **(Right)** *Coronal CECT in the same patient shows the posterior submandibular space abscess* → *displacing the enlarged, inflamed submandibular gland* → *inferiorly. Sialadenitis in this case is secondary to the adjacent infected extraction socket and abscess.*

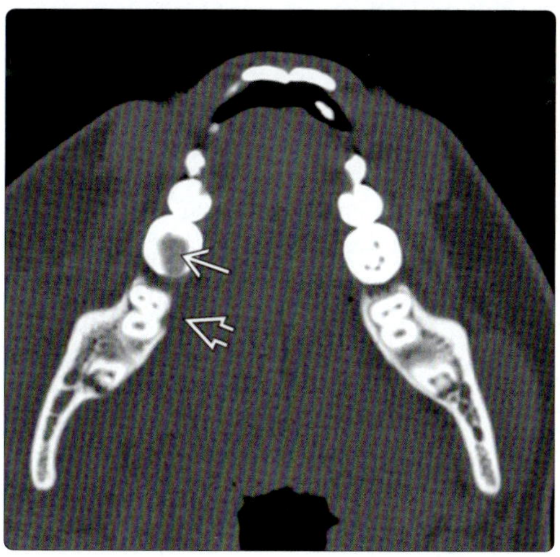

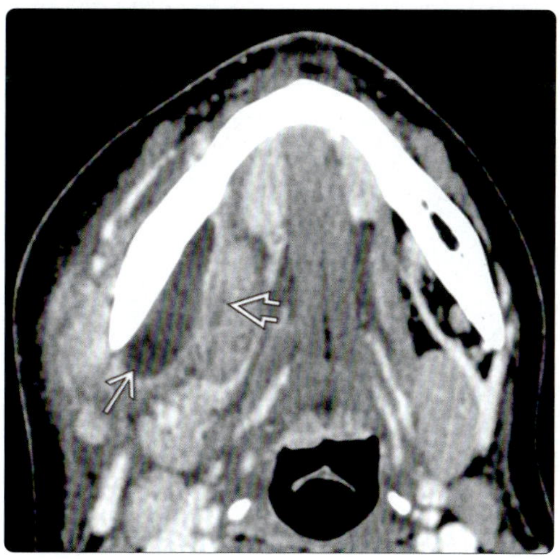

(Left) *Axial bone CT through the mandibular teeth shows demineralization of the coronal tooth structure suggestive of severe dental caries* → *with mandibular lingual cortex loss* →*, suggesting an abscess drainage pathway and communication of odontogenic infection with the soft tissues.* **(Right)** *Axial CECT in the same patient shows that the pus has drained inferiorly into the subjacent submandibular space. The submandibular space abscess* → *displaces the mylohyoid muscle* → *medially as a result.*

Ranula

KEY FACTS

TERMINOLOGY

- Synonyms: Simple ranula (SR), diving ranula (DR)
- Definition: Sublingual gland or sublingual space (SLS) minor salivary gland retention cyst
- SR = true cyst confined to SLS
- DR = SR ruptured to submandibular space (SMS)

IMAGING

- SR: Unilocular SLS cyst
  - Unilateral oval or bilateral horseshoe shape
- DR: Comet-shaped unilocular cyst
  - "Body" in SMS and "tail" in SLS
- **Tail sign** = collapsed SLS portion
- Posterior: Tail medial to mylohyoid, body medial to submandibular gland (SMG)
- Lateral: Tail in anterior SLS and body anterior to SMG
- CECT: Unilocular cyst, thin wall enhancement
- MR C+: Signal intensity follows CSF

TOP DIFFERENTIAL DIAGNOSES

- Oral cavity lymphatic malformation
- Oral cavity dermoid and epidermoid
- 2nd branchial cleft anomaly
- Suppurative lymph nodes

PATHOLOGY

- Retention cyst resulting from trauma or inflammation of SLG or SLS minor salivary gland

CLINICAL ISSUES

- Simple more common than DR
- Posterior DR more common than lateral DR

DIAGNOSTIC CHECKLIST

- Many imaging and clinical mimics
- "Tail" is key to determining DR
  - T2 FS MR best delineates subtle tail sign

(Left) Axial graphic depicts diving ranula (DR) herniating posteriorly from the sublingual space (SLS) into the submandibular space (SMS) ➡. Tail sign ⇨ is the collapsed portion of cyst in SLS. ***(Right)*** *Axial CECT demonstrates a rounded, cystic mass ➡ in SMS abutting posterior margin of mylohyoid muscle and displacing submandibular gland (SMG) ➡ posterolaterally. Linear low-density "tail" ⇨ extends anteriorly within left SLS, representing tail sign of collapsed ranula cyst.*

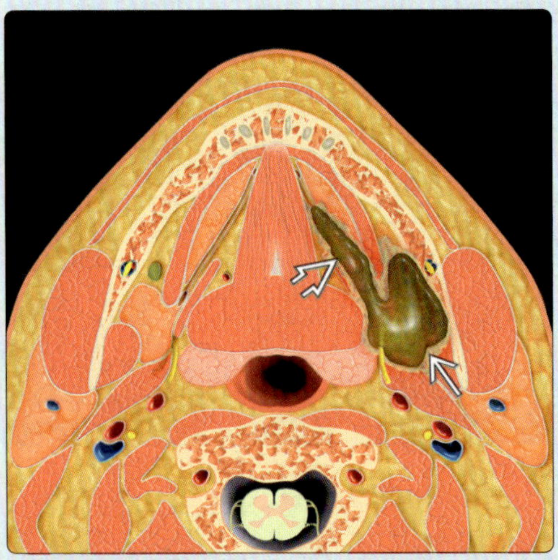

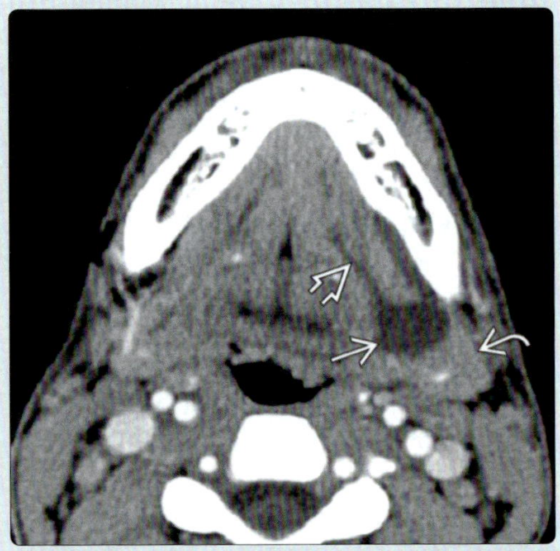

(Left) *Axial CECT shows simple unilateral ranula as an ovoid, low-density lesion in the left anterior SLS ➡. There is no perceptible thickening or enhancement of wall. Mylohyoid is displaced posterolaterally ⇨, and genioglossus ➡ is bowed medially.* ***(Right)*** *Axial CECT demonstrates a cystic, horseshoe-shaped lesion ➡ in the anterior SLS, curving around and above genioglossus muscle ⇨ insertion on mandible, characteristic of a simple ranula (SR) involving both sides of SLS.*

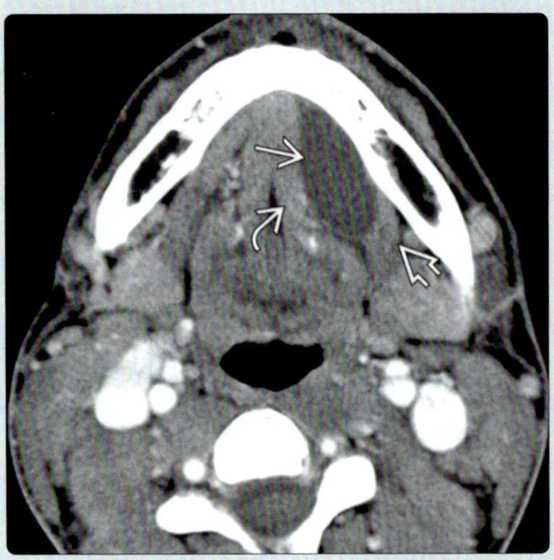

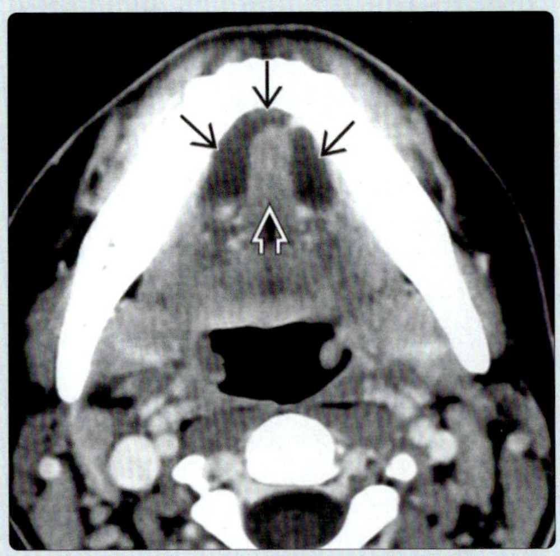

TERMINOLOGY

Abbreviations

- Simple ranula (SR)
- Diving ranula (DR)

Synonyms

- **SR** = sublingual gland (SLG) mucocele, SLG mucous retention cyst
- **DR** = plunging ranula

Definitions

- SLG or minor salivary gland retention cyst
  - SR: True cyst confined to sublingual space (SLS)
  - DR: Extravasation pseudocyst; ruptured SR extending into submandibular space (SMS)

IMAGING

General Features

- Best diagnostic clue
  - SR: Well-defined, thin-walled SLS cyst
  - DR: Thin-walled SMS pseudocyst with SLS "tail"
- Location
  - SR: SLS (i.e., above mylohyoid muscle)
  - DR: SMS and SLS
- Size
  - SR: < 3 cm as limited to SLS
  - DR: ≤ 10 cm; may be giant
- Morphology
  - SR
    - Unilateral, oval or lenticular, unilocular SLS cyst
    - Bilateral, horseshoe-shaped, unilocular SLS cyst
  - DR
    - Comet-shaped, unilocular SMS pseudocyst, "tail" in SLS
    - If large, may involve parapharyngeal space

CT Findings

- CECT
  - SR
    - Unilocular, low-density SLS cystic mass with subtle linear wall enhancement
    - May extend to contralateral SLS (horseshoe shape)
  - DR
    - **Tail sign** = collapsed SLS portion
    - **Posteriorly** over back of mylohyoid: Tail medial to mylohyoid and body often medial to submandibular gland (SMG)
    - **Laterally** through mylohyoid muscle defect: Tail in anterior SLS and body often anterior to SMG
  - Infected ranula (current or recent)
    - Distended cyst with thick, enhancing wall

MR Findings

- T1WI
  - Diffuse low signal intensity = CSF
- T2WI
  - Markedly high signal intensity = CSF
- T1WI C+
  - Thin, linear enhancement of wall
  - Current or recent infection → thicker wall; may alter T1 and T2 signal also

Ultrasonographic Findings

- Hypoechoic, well-defined mass within SLS ± SMS if diving

Imaging Recommendations

- Best imaging tool
  - CECT is best study for defining extent of ranula
- Protocol advice
  - CT multiplanar reformats aid delineation of diving component
  - T2 FS MR best sequence for demonstrating subtle tail sign

DIFFERENTIAL DIAGNOSIS

Oral Cavity Lymphatic Malformation

- Multilocular transspatial cystic mass
- Lobulation, septation, and heterogeneity suggest lymphatic malformation (LM)
- LM typically does not involve SLS

Oral Cavity Dermoid and Epidermoid

- Unilateral low-density/signal mass in SLS with thin, nonenhancing wall
- In SLS, epidermoid looks identical to SR
- Fat density (CT) or high signal (T1 MR) diagnostic of dermoid

2nd Branchial Cleft Anomaly

- Ovoid, unilocular mass in posterior SMS
- No tail sign to SLS
- Tends to displace SMG anteriorly, not laterally

Suppurative Lymph Nodes

- Multiple cystic-appearing SMS nodes
- Separate suppurative/reactive nodes suggest diagnosis
- Associated inflammation and clinical history are key

Oral Cavity Abscess

- Patient usually septic with tender oral cavity
- Single or multiple collections with enhancing wall(s)
- Associated inflammatory changes in fat

Submandibular Gland Mucocele

- Cyst "bubbles" off margin of SMG
- No tail sign to SLS

Oral Cavity Sialocele

- True sialocele: Distended submandibular duct
- False sialocele: Extravasated saliva contained within fibrous pseudocapsule

PATHOLOGY

General Features

- Etiology
  - Retention cyst resulting from trauma or inflammation of SLG or SLS minor salivary gland
  - Congenital ranula from imperforate salivary duct or ostial adhesion
  - SR ruptures → pseudocyst without epithelial lining (DR)

- Ruptures posteriorly over posterior margin of mylohyoid to posterior SMS
- Ruptures laterally through boutonnière defect, anterior to SMG
- Extension to parapharyngeal space in < 10%

Staging, Grading, & Classification

- SR develops 1st in SLS
  - May enlarge to fill entire unilateral SLS
  - May extend to contralateral SLS above mandibular insertion of genioglossus muscle
- DR secondary to rupture of SR
  - Rupture of retention cyst into subjacent SMS

Gross Pathologic & Surgical Features

- SR: Fluctuant sublingual mass, often with bluish color
- DR: Fluctuant mass of extravasated mucus

Microscopic Features

- SR has squamous, cuboidal, or columnar epithelial lining
  - Cyst contains mucus-saliva
- DR is pseudocyst with no epithelial lining but has fibrous and granulation tissue, dense connective tissue, and chronic inflammatory cells
  - Contains mucus pools

CLINICAL ISSUES

Presentation

- Most common signs/symptoms
  - Painless swelling of floor of mouth (SR)
  - DR typically present as submandibular mass, which is displaced SMG
    - Displaced SMG may have partially obstructed duct ± inflammatory changes
  - Either can present as waxing and waning masses
- Other signs/symptoms
  - 50% have history of prior neck or oral cavity trauma
- Clinical profile
  - 30-year-old man with painless floor of mouth mass

Demographics

- Age
  - Pediatric to adults; median: 30 years
  - Congenital ranula in infant
- Gender
  - M slightly > F
- Ethnicity
  - Increased incidence of DR in Maori and Pacific Islanders
- Epidemiology
  - SR more common than DR
  - Posterior more common than lateral DR
  - Congenital ranula is rare

Natural History & Prognosis

- Large SR can fill unilateral SLS; may involve contralateral side
- Children: May spontaneously resolve in 6 months
- Adults: Tend to rupture to SMS as DR
- Recurrence may occur depending on surgical treatment

Treatment

- Controversial: Multiple options described
  - Transoral excision of SLG and evacuation of cyst
    - Fewest complications and lowest recurrence rate
    - Biopsy of pseudocyst wall important to confirm diagnosis
  - Transoral excision of SLG and cyst
  - Transcervical excision of SMG, SLG, and cyst
  - Marsupialization
    - Associated with high recurrence rate
  - Laser excision and vaporization
- Nonsurgical options
  - Sclerotherapy with intracystic OK-432 and bleomycin
  - Cyst aspiration alone; highest recurrence rate

DIAGNOSTIC CHECKLIST

Consider

- Many imaging and clinical mimics

Image Interpretation Pearls

- DR is suspected based on "tail" observation
  - If behind posterior margin of mylohyoid muscle, SMS cyst often medial to SMG
  - If laterally through mylohyoid defect, SMS cystic component often anterior to SMG
- While helpful, direction of SMG displacement not diagnostic of lateral or posterior DR
  - Must demonstrate **"tail"**
- T2 FS MR best sequence and modality for delineating subtle tail sign

SELECTED REFERENCES

1. Brown RE et al: Diagnostic imaging of benign and malignant neck masses in children-a pictorial review. Quant Imaging Med Surg. 6(5):591-604, 2016
2. Lee JY et al: Plunging ranulas revisited: A CT study with emphasis on a defect of the mylohyoid muscle as the primary route of lesion propagation. Korean J Radiol. 17(2):264-70, 2016
3. Margalit I et al: Point-of-care ultrasound to diagnose a simple ranula. West J Emerg Med. 17(6):827-828, 2016
4. Carlson ER: Diagnosis and management of salivary lesions of the neck. Atlas Oral Maxillofac Surg Clin North Am. 23(1):49-61, 2015
5. Chen CJ et al: Recurrent sublingual ranula or saliva leakage from the submandibular gland? Anatomical consideration of the ductal system of the sublingual gland. J Oral Maxillofac Surg. 73(4):675.e1-7, 2015
6. Fontenot TE et al: Swelling of submandibular region. Plunging ranula. JAMA Otolaryngol Head Neck Surg. 139(10):1073-4, 2013
7. McKinstry S et al: Bilateral plunging ranula: two case reports and a review of the literature. N Z Med J. 126(1385):81-6, 2013
8. Kadom N et al: Neck masses in children: current imaging guidelines and imaging findings. Semin Roentgenol. 47(1):7-20, 2012
9. Harrison JD: Modern management and pathophysiology of ranula: literature review. Head Neck. 32(10):1310-20, 2010
10. Clyburn VL 3rd et al: Ascending and plunging ranula in a pediatric patient. Otolaryngol Head Neck Surg. 140(6):948-9, 2009
11. Patel MR et al: Oral and plunging ranulas: What is the most effective treatment? Laryngoscope. 119(8):1501-9, 2009
12. Zhi K et al: Management of the pediatric plunging ranula: results of 15 years' clinical experience. Oral Surg Oral Med Oral Pathol Oral Radiol Endod. 107(4):499-502, 2009
13. Rosa PA et al: Congenital neck masses. Oral Maxillofac Surg Clin North Am. 20(3):339-52, 2008
14. Haberal I et al: Surgical management of pediatric ranula. Int J Pediatr Otorhinolaryngol. 68(2):161-3, 2004
15. Choi TW et al: Hydrodissection for complete removal of a ranula. Ear Nose Throat J. 82(12):946-7, 951, 2003
16. Fukase S et al: Treatment of ranula wth intracystic injection of the streptococcal preparation OK-432. Ann Otol Rhinol Laryngol. 112(3):214-20, 2003
17. Macdonald AJ et al: Giant ranula of the neck: differentiation from cystic hygroma. AJNR Am J Neuroradiol. 24(4):757-61, 2003

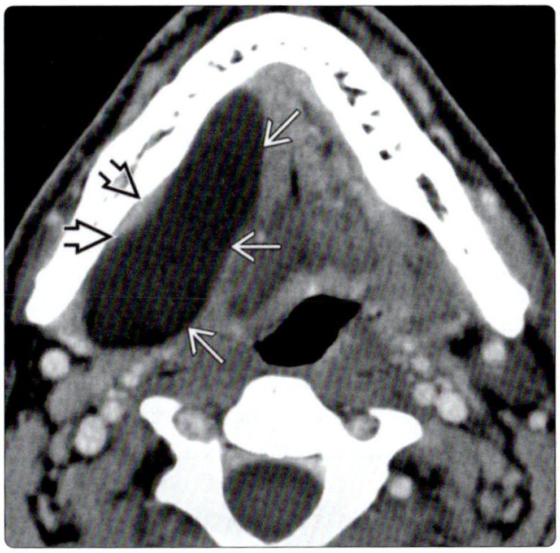

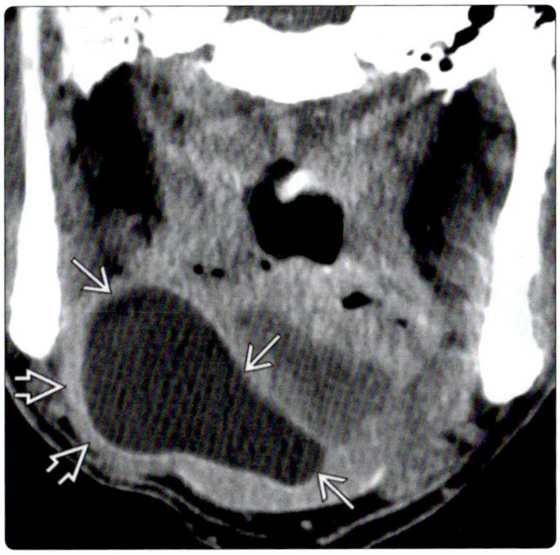

(Left) *Axial CECT shows large SR distending the right SLS and bowing the mylohyoid muscle laterally. There is no appreciable enhancement or thickening of cyst wall or adjacent inflammatory changes.* **(Right)** *Coronal delayed CECT in the same patient shows inferolateral bowing of the mylohyoid muscle by a large, thin-walled, unilocular cyst. SR appears identical to SLS epidermoid, and definitive diagnosis requires pathology or clear congenital history.*

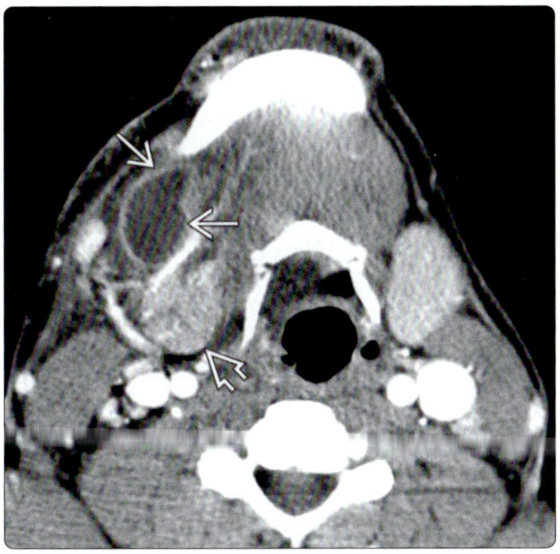

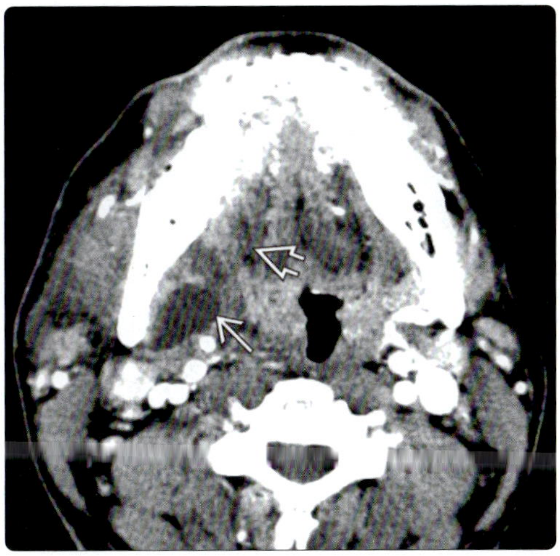

(Left) *Axial CECT in a young adult with marked pain and swelling shows a rim-enhancing, low-density mass in the right SMS anterolateral to the SMG with extensive adjacent inflammatory changes.* **(Right)** *Axial CECT in the same patient shows the posterosuperior aspect of lesion extending toward posterior margin of mylohyoid muscle, suggesting diagnosis of DR, which has become acutely secondarily infected. Note swelling of right floor of mouth.*

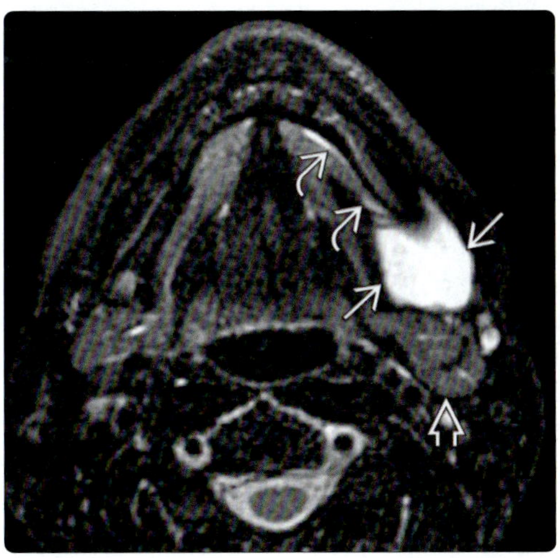

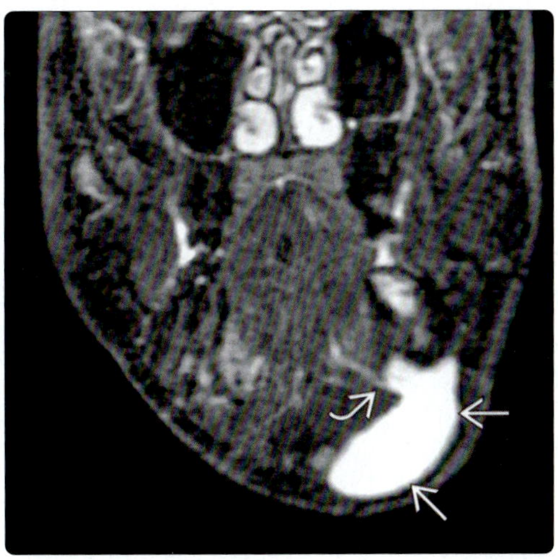

(Left) *Axial T2WI FS MR in a young adult with recurrent submandibular mass and 2 prior cyst aspirations shows a well-defined, markedly hyperintense mass anterior to the SMG and lateral to mylohyoid muscle. T2 FS best shows subtle tail sign from less common laterally DR.* **(Right)** *Coronal T2WI FS MR in the same patient shows laterally DR as a large SMS cystic mass and subtle tail sign through boutonnière defect of mylohyoid muscle.*

Submandibular Gland Sialadenitis

KEY FACTS

TERMINOLOGY

- Inflammation of submandibular gland (SMG)

IMAGING

- Most often **acute inflammation** + obstructed duct
  - **Duct calculus** or stenosis, floor of mouth tumor
  - 90% calculi opaque on occlusal image
  - Submandibular sialography rarely used
- CECT recommended to evaluate gland ± calculus
  - Ductal dilation ± calculus, stenosis, or tumor
  - Ipsilateral enlarged SMG + cellulitis
- NECT unnecessary; calculus & vessel densities differ
- **Chronic recurrent sialadenitis** less common
  - Ipsilateral atrophic SMG, ± fatty change
- **Autoimmune** disease (Sjögren) uncommon
- **Fibroinflammatory** disease (Küttner tumor) rare
- MR more sensitive for gland parenchymal changes

TOP DIFFERENTIAL DIAGNOSES

- Dental infection
- Squamous cell carcinoma nodal metastases
- SMG carcinoma
- SMG gland benign mixed tumor

CLINICAL ISSUES

- SMG calculi more often within duct than gland
- SMG sialadenitis comprises only 10% of major gland sialadenitis
- Most calculus disease: 30-60 years

DIAGNOSTIC CHECKLIST

- Most often results from ductal calculus or stenosis
- Determine where in duct stones are located
- Look carefully for obstructing floor of mouth tumor
- If no calculi, consider duct stenosis or gland disease

(Left) *Axial graphic depicts submandibular duct calculus in distal duct just proximal to papilla. Proximal duct and tertiary ducts are enlarged. Submandibular gland (SMG) is inflamed and enlarged.* **(Right)** *Axial CECT demonstrates asymmetrically enhancing, enlarged left SMG compared to right. Calculus is evident in distal submandibular duct at level of ductal papilla. Only mild prominence of duct at hilum is evident. Prominent vessel in floor of mouth is also noted.*

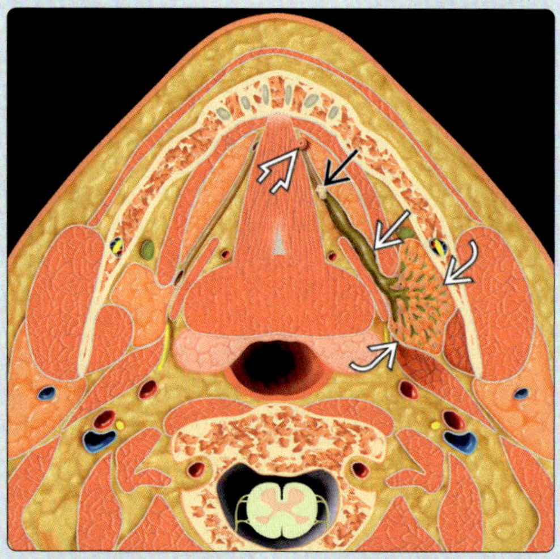

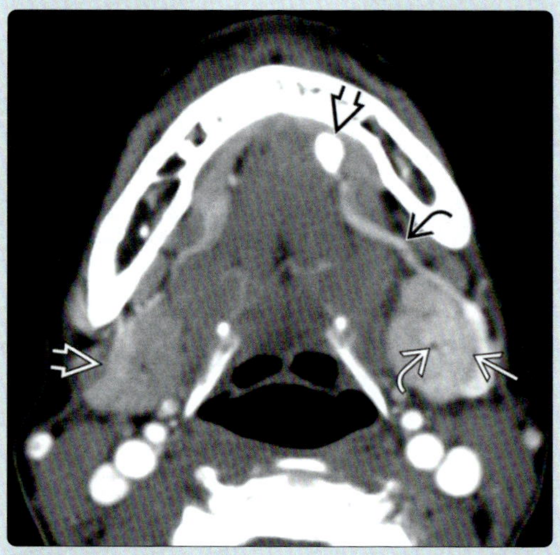

(Left) *Axial T2WI FS MR demonstrates well-circumscribed mass in left floor of mouth in patient with mucosal SCCa. Mass is obstructing left submandibular duct, and there is secondary inflammation of left SMG, which is hyperintense.* **(Right)** *Axial CECT through floor of mouth in patient with right submandibular "mass" shows dense calculus in proximal duct at left SMG hilus. Note marked fatty atrophy with left chronic sialadenitis. Right "mass" was normal SMG.*

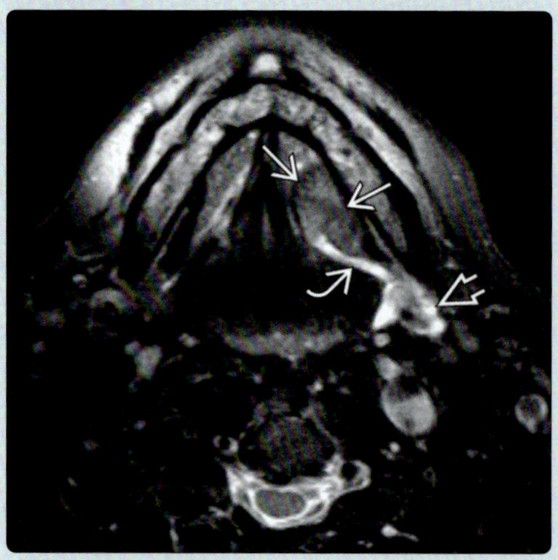

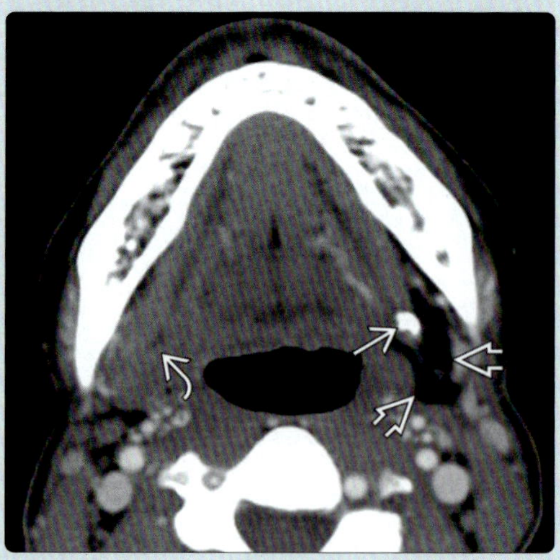

TERMINOLOGY

Abbreviations

- Submandibular gland (SMG) sialadenitis

Definitions

- Inflammation of SMG of any cause
- **Acute sialadenitis**: Usually with duct calculus
- **Chronic sialadenitis**: Recurrent SMG inflammation with reduced saliva flow
- **Secondary SMG sialadenitis**: Ductal obstruction from floor of mouth squamous cell carcinoma
- **Sialolithiasis**: Concretions within SMG ductal system
- **Autoimmune sialadenitis**: Sjögren syndrome
- **Chronic sclerosing sialadenitis**: Küttner tumor
- **Sialadenosis**: Noninflammatory SMG swelling
  - Causes include: Diabetes, cirrhosis, hypothyroidism

IMAGING

General Features

- Best diagnostic clue
  - Ductal dilation ± calculus or stenosis
    - Acute: Ipsilateral enlarged SMG + cellulitis
    - Chronic: Ipsilateral atrophic SMG
- Location
  - SMG stones can be divided by location
    - Distal: Ductal opening in anterior floor of mouth
    - Proximal: Toward SMG hilum
  - Calculi typically within duct, not SMG parenchyma
- Size
  - Acute-subacute inflammation: SMG enlarged
  - Chronic: SMG small, ± fatty replacement

Radiographic Findings

- Radiography
  - Occlusal views: 90% calculi radiopaque

CT Findings

- CECT
  - Acute sialadenitis secondary to **calculus**
    - Duct calculus with dilated duct and enlarged, enhancing SMG
    - Reactive nodes, ± floor of mouth cellulitis
  - Chronic sialadenitis ± calculus
    - SMG small, fatty infiltrated ± intraductal calculus
  - **Secondary SMG sialadenitis**
    - Anterior floor of mouth invasive, enhancing mass
    - Dilated SMG duct and enlarged, enhancing SMG
    - Look for erosion of mandible

MR Findings

- MR typically not obtained in acute inflammation
  - MR sialography may show calculus as low signal
- Chronic sialadenitis including autoimmune disease
  - Heterogeneous gland, prominent T2 intense ducts
  - May have fatty gland with T1 & T2 hyperintensity

Ultrasonographic Findings

- With calculus: Duct dilation in enlarged gland
  - Ability to visualize calculus is operator dependent

Imaging Recommendations

- Best imaging tool
  - CECT to evaluate gland ± calculus
  - NECT unnecessary: Calculus & vessel densities differ

DIFFERENTIAL DIAGNOSIS

Dental Infection

- Spreads from jaw to masticator space/oral cavity
- Bone CT shows periapical lucency

Squamous Cell Carcinoma Nodal Metastases

- Submandibular space (SMS) mass distinct from SMG

Submandibular Gland Carcinoma

- Infiltrating mass arising in SMG

Submandibular Gland Benign Mixed Tumor

- Well-circumscribed SMG mass, ± calcifications

PATHOLOGY

General Features

- Etiology
  - Most commonly SMG duct (Wharton) obstruction
    - Calculi, duct stenosis, rarely floor of mouth tumor
  - Less common: Chronic recurrent inflammation
  - Rarely: Primary gland inflammation
    - Sjögren syndrome, chronic sclerosing sialadenitis, sialadenosis, bacterial or viral infection

CLINICAL ISSUES

Presentation

- Other signs/symptoms
  - 30% of calculi present with painless mass
  - 80% of painful SMS masses due to calculus disease

Demographics

- Epidemiology
  - Gland calculi: 85% SMG ducts, 15% parotid
  - SMG comprises only 10% of major gland sialadenitis

Treatment

- Treatment focused on causative factors
  - Inflammation but no ductal dilation → antibiotics
  - Unrelenting obstructive sialadenitis: Resect SMG

DIAGNOSTIC CHECKLIST

Consider

- **Most common cause is ductal calculus or stenosis**

Reporting Tips

- Determine where in duct stones are located
  - Beware: Calculi may be obscured by dental amalgam
- Look carefully for obstructing floor of mouth tumor
- If no calculi, may be duct stenosis or **gland disease**
  - Sjögren, chronic sclerosing sialadenitis, sialadenosis

SELECTED REFERENCES

1. Abdel Razek AA et al: Imaging of sialadenitis. Neuroradiol J. 1971400916682752, 2017

Oral Cavity Sialocele

KEY FACTS

TERMINOLOGY

- Sialocele definition: Ruptured submandibular duct (SMD) extravasates saliva into sublingual space (SLS)

IMAGING

- CECT findings
  - SLS fluid density lesion ± enhancing adjacent inflammatory soft tissues
  - Rarely extends into posterior submandibular space (SMS)
  - If associated with SMD calculus, SMD enlargement with enhancing, enlarged submandibular gland
  - Fluid collection is distinct from SMD
- CECT best delineates sialocele & calculus if present

TOP DIFFERENTIAL DIAGNOSES

- Ranula
- SLS epidermoid
- SLS abscess
- SLS lymphatic malformation

PATHOLOGY

- Etiology: **Submandibular duct injury** with leakage of saliva into SLS
  - SMD calculus with rupture > > rupture from trauma or surgery
- Saliva outside SMD but contained within **fibrous pseudocapsule**

CLINICAL ISSUES

- Common presentation: Fluctuant, soft, painless SLS mass
  - Patient with SMD stone or recent oral cavity surgery or trauma presents with new SLS mass
- Sialocele location: Parotid space > > SLS > SMS

DIAGNOSTIC CHECKLIST

- Consider: Simple ranula, SLS epidermoid, & sialocele without SMD calculus have similar appearances
- When cystic SLS lesion is identified, look closely for possible obstructing calculi

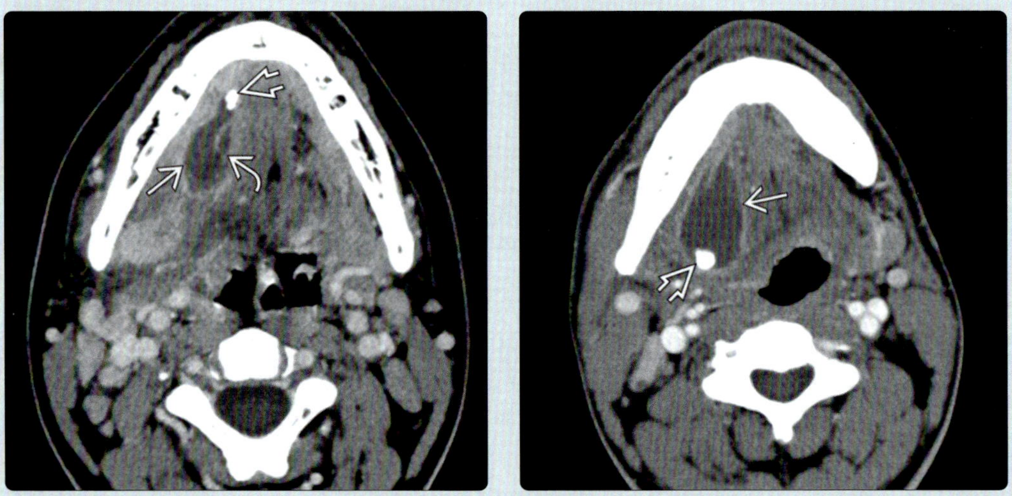

(Left) *Axial CECT shows a calculus obstructing the submandibular duct ➡ at the terminal papilla, causing the submandibular duct to dilate ➡. Duct rupture has occurred with sialocele ➡ visible in the medial sublingual space.* **(Right)** *Axial CECT reveals an ovoid cystic lesion in the right sublingual space ➡. Dependent calculus is seen posteriorly ➡. This patient most likely began with a sialolith-obstructing submandibular duct. When duct ruptured, the sialolith fell into the sialocele.*

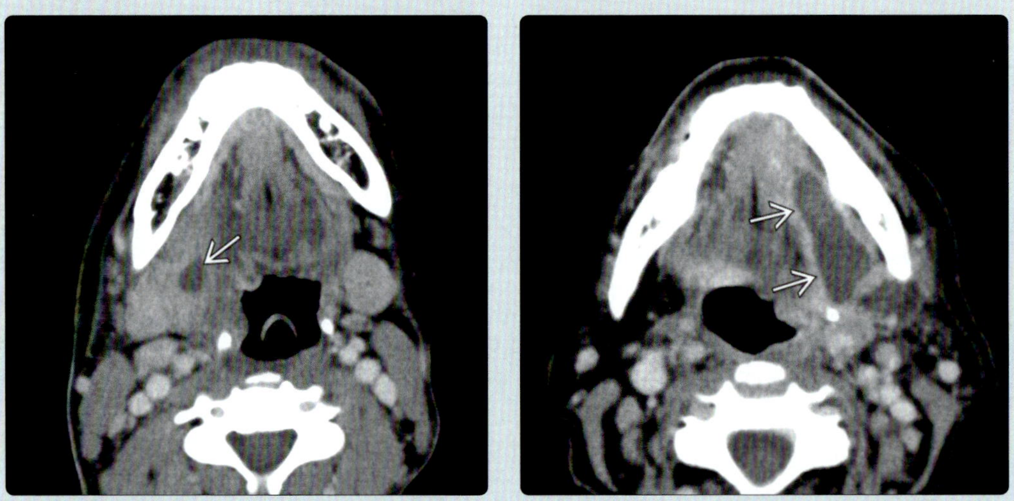

(Left) *Axial CECT demonstrates a small cystic mass in the posterior sublingual space ➡. Ranula, sialocele, and epidermoid were all considered. At surgery, a small pocket of saliva with a fibrous pseudocapsule was found.* **(Right)** *Axial CECT in a patient with history of facial trauma and floor of mouth swelling shows a cystic lesion in the left sublingual space ➡. Both ranula and sialocele were considered; sialocele was found at surgery. History of facial trauma supported sialocele diagnosis.*

Oral Cavity Sialocele

TERMINOLOGY

Abbreviations

- Oral cavity (OC) sialocele

Synonyms

- Floor of mouth sialocele, sublingual sialocele, submandibular duct (SMD) sialocele

Definitions

- Ruptured SMD extravasates saliva into sublingual space (SLS)

IMAGING

General Features

- Best diagnostic clue
    - Cystic SLS lesion along course of SMD
- Location
    - Sublingual space ± submandibular space (SMS)
- Size
    - Variable, usually < 3 cm
- Morphology
    - Ovoid to lenticular

CT Findings

- CECT
    - SLS fluid density lesion ± enhancing adjacent inflammatory soft tissues
        - Rarely extends into posterior SMS
    - If associated with SMD calculus, SMD enlargement with enhancing and enlarged submandibular gland (SMG)
    - Fluid collection is distinct from SMD
        - SMD may or may not be dilated

MR Findings

- T1WI
    - Low-signal lesion in SLS ± dilated SMD
- T2WI
    - High-signal lesion in SLS ± dilated SMD
- T1WI C+
    - Rim-enhancing fluid signal lesion

Imaging Recommendations

- Best imaging tool
    - CECT best delineates sialocele & calculus if present
- Protocol advice
    - Multislice CT scanners can reformat volumetric data sets in oblique planes

DIFFERENTIAL DIAGNOSIS

Ranula

- Unilateral fluid collection in SLS; no calculus

Sublingual Space Epidermoid

- Ovoid fluid collection in SLS
- DWI shows restricted diffusion

Oral Cavity Abscess in Sublingual Space

- Rim-enhancing SLS fluid collection

Sublingual Space Lymphatic Malformation

- SLS-SMS multilocular transspatial cystic lesion
- No perceptible wall visible

PATHOLOGY

General Features

- Etiology
    - **Submandibular duct injury** with leakage of saliva into SLS
        - SMD calculus with rupture > > rupture from trauma or surgery

Gross Pathologic & Surgical Features

- Saliva outside SMD but contained within **fibrous pseudocapsule**

Microscopic Features

- Fibrous granulation tissue capsule surrounding saliva pocket

CLINICAL ISSUES

Presentation

- Most common signs/symptoms
    - Fluctuant, soft, painless sublingual mass
- Clinical profile
    - Patient with SMD sialolith or recent oral cavity surgery or trauma presents with new SLS mass

Demographics

- Epidemiology
    - Obstructing SMD calculus > > posttraumatic or postoperative
    - Parotid space sialocele > > SLS sialocele > SMS sialocele

Natural History & Prognosis

- If left alone, sialocele may continue to enlarge

Treatment

- Multiple aspirations, pressure dressings, & antisialagogic agents often successful
- Surgery
- Local injection of botulinum toxin type A (30-50 U)
    - Used for parotid sialoceles

DIAGNOSTIC CHECKLIST

Consider

- When cystic SLS lesion is identified, look closely for possible obstructing calculi
- Simple ranula, SLS epidermoid, & sialocele without SMD calculus have similar appearances
    - Simple ranula: Ovoid SLS retention cyst
    - SLS epidermoid: DWI shows restricted diffusion
    - SLS sialocele: Saliva-filled cystic SLS collection
        - History of oral cavity surgery, trauma, or SMD calculus

SELECTED REFERENCES

1. Witt RL: The incidence and management of siaolocele after parotidectomy. Otolaryngol Head Neck Surg. 140(6):871-4, 2009
2. Capaccio P et al: Comparative ultrasonographic, magnetic resonance sialographic, and videoendoscopic assessment of salivary duct disorders. Ann Otol Rhinol Laryngol. 117(4):245-52, 2008
3. Ang AH et al: Idiopathic submandibular sialoceles in the neck. Otolaryngol Head Neck Surg. 132(3):517-9, 2005

Submandibular Gland Mucocele

KEY FACTS

TERMINOLOGY

- Synonyms
  - Submandibular gland (SMG) retention cyst
  - Sialocele
- Definition: Mucus/salivary **extravasation phenomenon** of ductal components of SMG

IMAGING

- **Homogeneous unilocular circumscribed mass** immediately adjacent to or within SMG
- Floor of mouth or neck
- CT: Fluid density cystic structure: Density greater than water but less than surrounding tissues
- MR: Homogeneous cystic signal (low T1, high T2)
- Well-defined, benign appearance: **Enhancing rim often seen**
- **No evidence of tail sign**, which suggests ranula (SLG origin)

TOP DIFFERENTIAL DIAGNOSES

- **Ranula**
- Lymphangioma/cystic hygroma
- Cystic submandibular lymph node

PATHOLOGY

- **May be secondary to trauma**, surgical transection of duct, or ductal obstruction (sialolith associated)

CLINICAL ISSUES

- **Swelling in floor of mouth** and neck

DIAGNOSTIC CHECKLIST

- Consider lymphangioma if subadult
- Consider ranula if mucocele extends inferiorly to mylohyoid muscle &/or appearance of **tail sign**
- Consider cystic lymph node if facial vein is not displaced posteriorly or laterally
- Look for possible ductal obstruction: **Sialolith**

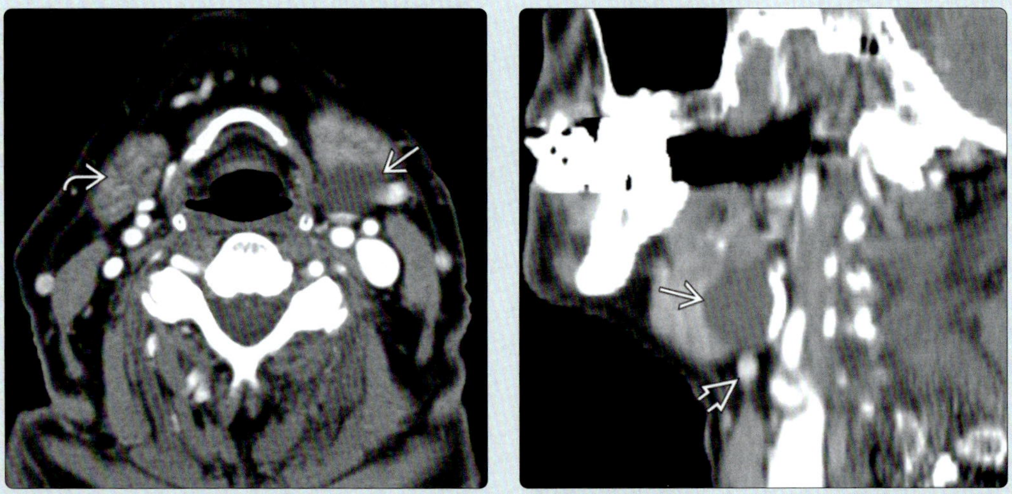

(Left) *Axial CECT shows an oval fluid-filled (low-density) mass → emerging from the left posterior submandibular gland, which is not separated from the adjacent submandibular gland. The right submandibular gland is normal →.* **(Right)** *Sagittal CECT of the same patient shows the mucocele bulging from the posterior margin of the submandibular gland →. Notice the left facial vein → is directly along the lateral margin of the mucocele, excluding the possible diagnosis of a cystic submandibular node.*

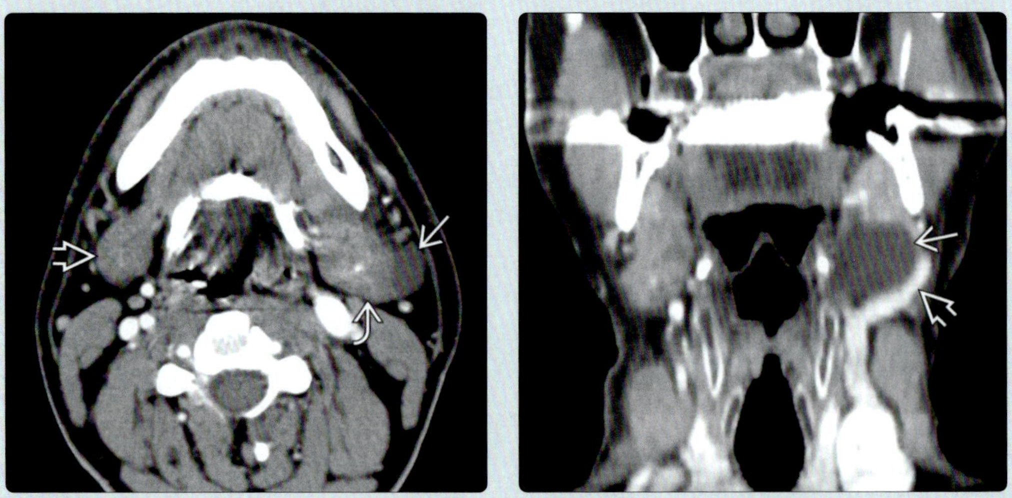

(Left) *Axial CECT demonstrates an unusual appearance of the left submandibular gland. There is an eccentric low density → that is inseparable from the gland →, which is otherwise only slightly enlarged compared to the right submandibular gland →. There is no ductal dilation.* **(Right)** *Coronal CECT shows a typical case of submandibular gland mucocele. An oval fluid density mass → is evident. Note the facial vein → curving around lateral margin of lesion.*

TERMINOLOGY

Abbreviations

- Submandibular gland (SMG) benign mixed tumor (BMT)

Synonyms

- Pleomorphic adenoma

Definitions

- Benign heterogeneous salivary gland primary tumor

IMAGING

General Features

- Best diagnostic clue
  - Enlarged SMG with focal or diffuse heterogeneous mass ± calcification
- Location
  - Submandibular space (SMS)
- Size
  - Variable: 1-4 cm
- Morphology
  - Small: Ovoid, well-demarcated SMG mass
  - Large: Lobulated, heterogeneous mass ± calcification

CT Findings

- CECT
  - Small lesion, usually well defined; may deform external contour
  - Large lesion better illustrates heterogeneous density & texture
  - ± calcification, cystic changes in larger lesions
  - Mild to moderate enhancement

MR Findings

- Findings again largely determined by BMT size
  - **Small lesion**: Low T1, high T2 intensity, homogeneous enhancement
  - **Large lesion**: More heterogeneous, ± focal areas of very high T2 signal, signal loss with calcification
  - ± low T2 intensity "capsule"
  - Enhancement more heterogeneous with large BMT

Ultrasonographic Findings

- Grayscale ultrasound
  - Well-defined, solid, intraglandular lesion
  - Large lesion may show focal cysts, calcification

Nuclear Medicine Findings

- Marked FDG avidity on PET/CT

Imaging Recommendations

- Best imaging tool
  - Either CECT or MR; however, be aware that SMG lesions may be subtle or occult on CECT
  - **US affords excellent SMG evaluation**

DIFFERENTIAL DIAGNOSIS

Submandibular Gland Sialadenitis

- Acute: Enlarged gland that completely enhances
- Chronic: Atrophic gland with little enhancement

Submandibular Gland Mucocele

- Fluid collection within SMG

Submandibular Gland Carcinoma

- Enhancing, invasive mass emanating from SMG

Reactive Lymph Nodes

- Ovoid mass with fat plane separating it from SMG

Nodal SSCa in Submandibular Space

- Nodal mass separate from SMG, ± necrosis

PATHOLOGY

Gross Pathologic & Surgical Features

- Encased in fibrous capsule or well demarcated

Microscopic Features

- Interspersed epithelial, myoepithelial, & stromal cells
  - Calcification, hyalinization, & rarely ossification

CLINICAL ISSUES

Presentation

- Most common signs/symptoms
  - Slow-growing, painless SMS mass

Demographics

- Age
  - Most commonly present in patients > 40 years
- Epidemiology
  - BMT is most common tumor of SMG

Natural History & Prognosis

- Untreated, 10-25% degenerate to malignant tumor

Treatment

- Complete excision of intact gland & tumor
- Operative rupture of BMT capsule seeds surgical bed
  - Results in multifocal recurrence; surgically challenging

DIAGNOSTIC CHECKLIST

Consider

- Fine-needle aspiration has variable success
  - Sampling & interpretation errors common

Image Interpretation Pearls

- If patient presents with submandibular mass
  - Determine if mass is in SMG or extrinsic to it
  - BMT often well-demarcated; however, so are low-grade malignancies
  - If no mass found on CECT, recommend US or MR
    - **Beware** of subtle or occult SMG tumors

Reporting Tips

- Well-defined lesion within gland is favored to be benign; however, pathology is only definitive study
  - Similarly, calcification favors BMT but may be present in malignant mixed tumor

SELECTED REFERENCES

1. Knight J et al: Metastasising pleomorphic adenoma of the submandibular salivary gland presenting with spinal cord compression: case report and review of cases with CNS involvement. Br J Neurosurg. 1-3, 2016

Palate Benign Mixed Tumor

KEY FACTS

TERMINOLOGY

- Abbreviation: Palate benign mixed tumor (BMT)
- Synonym: Palate pleomorphic adenoma
- Benign tumor arising from minor salivary glands within palate arising from epithelial & mesenchymal tissues

IMAGING

- General imaging findings
  - Most commonly found at soft-hard palate junction
  - Small BMT: Well-defined palatal mass with homogeneous avid enhancement
  - Large BMT: Lobulated with heterogeneous enhancement
- Bone CT: Larger BMT remodels bony hard palate
- MR findings
  - Intermediate to high T2 signal ovoid palatal mass
  - Very **high T2 signal suggests BMT**
  - Homogeneous (small) to heterogeneous (large) enhancement
  - Larger BMT often with inhomogeneous signal (necrosis, blood products, calcification)

TOP DIFFERENTIAL DIAGNOSES

- Hard palate squamous cell carcinoma
- Palatal minor salivary gland malignancy
- Nasopalatine duct cyst
- Palatal torus
- Palatal abscess

PATHOLOGY

- Arises in minor salivary glands of palate
- Interspersed epithelial, myoepithelial, & stromal cellular components must be identified to diagnose BMT

CLINICAL ISSUES

- Presentation: Slow-growing, painless palatal mass
- Complete surgical resection of encapsulated mass
- Reconstruction not needed without erosion of hard palate

(Left) *Coronal CBCT shows mucosal asymmetry in the right posterior aspect of the hard palate ➡. Remodeling of the palate and the greater palatine groove can be appreciated ⇨. The mucosal thickening seen in the floor of the right maxillary sinus is an incidental finding not related to the lesion.* **(Right)** *Axial CECT demonstrates a well-circumscribed, somewhat heterogeneous, mildly enhancing soft tissue mass ➡ in the soft palate. Surgical pathology revealed this to be a benign mixed tumor (BMT).*

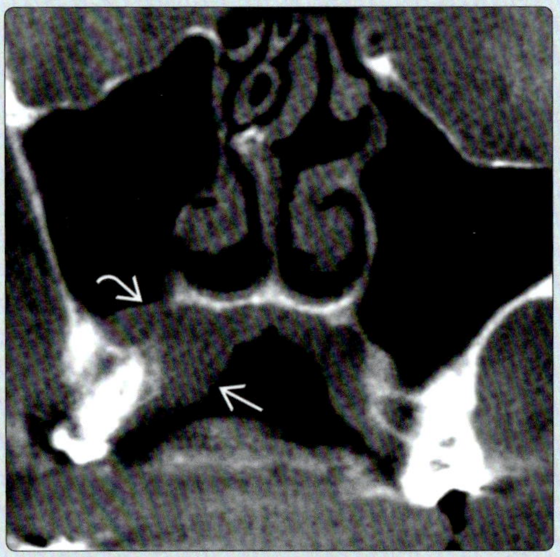

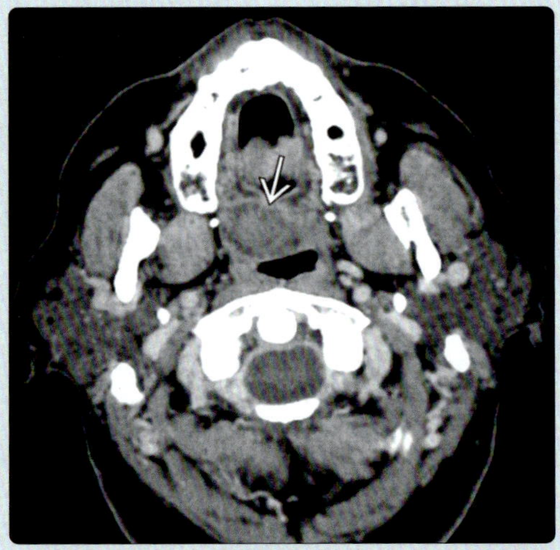

(Left) *Axial T1WI C+ FS MR reveals a subtle heterogeneously enhancing mass ➡ at the hard palate-soft palate junction on the left. Margins were worrisome for malignancy, but surgical pathology revealed it to be BMT.* **(Right)** *Coronal T1 C+ FS MR on the same patient shows uniform enhancement ➡. Comment: Imaging findings are nonspecific, although well-defined margins and smooth bony remodeling favor a benign or low-grade tumor. After complete resection, this was shown to be a pleomorphic adenoma.*

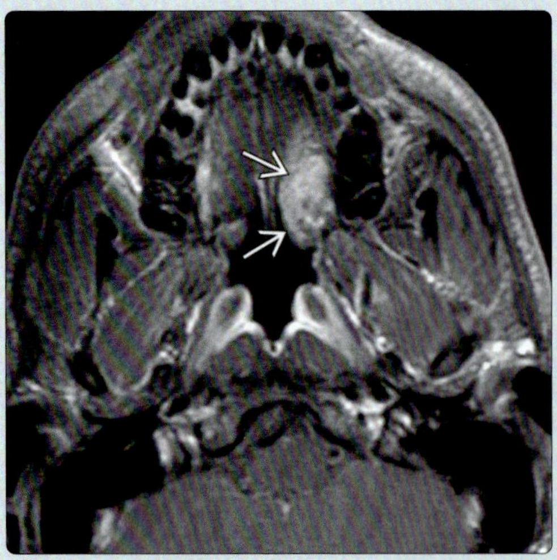

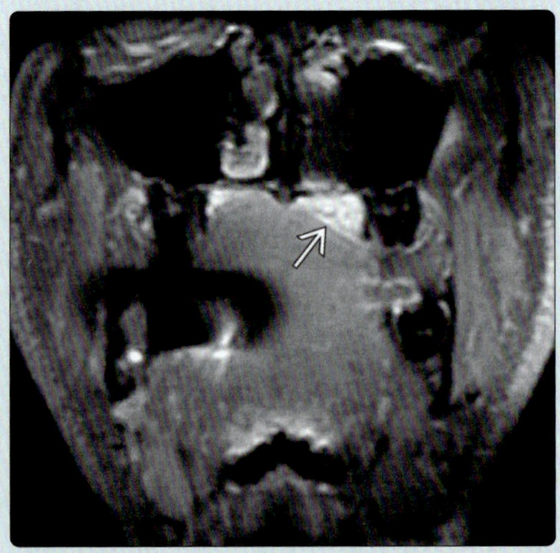

Palate Benign Mixed Tumor

TERMINOLOGY

Abbreviations

- Palate benign mixed tumor (BMT)

Synonyms

- Palate pleomorphic adenoma

Definitions

- Benign tumor arising from minor salivary glands within palate arising from epithelial & mesenchymal tissues

IMAGING

General Features

- Best diagnostic clue
  - Small lesion: Well-defined palatal mass with **avid enhancement**
  - Large lesion: Often lobulated mass with **heterogeneous enhancement**
- Location
  - Junction of soft & hard palate
- Morphology
  - Round or oval lesion
- Size: Variable; usually < 2 cm

CT Findings

- CECT
  - Small palate BMT: Well-defined, homogeneously enhancing, ovoid mass
  - Large palate BMT: Lobulated mass with heterogeneous enhancement
    - Dystrophic calcifications uncommon
    - Low-attenuation areas of degenerative necrosis
    - Old blood products possible
- CBCT & bone CT
  - Larger lesions cause remodeling of hard palate

MR Findings

- T1WI
  - Small BMT: Homogeneous low- to intermediate-signal mass
  - Large BMT: Lobulated heterogeneous mass
    - Hyperintense signal foci if blood products
    - Hypointense signal areas if focal necrosis present
- T2WI
  - Small BMT: Uniform intermediate- to high-signal mass
  - Large BMT: Heterogeneous high-signal mass
    - Low-signal tumor capsule often visible
  - **Very high T2 signal** suggests **BMT**
- STIR
  - High signal may be more conspicuous than on T2
- DWI
  - May have ↑ ADC values compared to malignant tumor
    - DWI signal intensity nonspecific
- T1WI C+
  - Variable heterogeneous or avid homogeneous enhancement

Imaging Recommendations

- Best imaging tool
  - Enhanced MR with thin sections through palate
  - Bone CT or CBCT helps define tumor bony margins
- Protocol advice
  - Axial & coronal T2 & T1 C+ FS MR sequences key

DIFFERENTIAL DIAGNOSIS

Hard Palate Squamous Cell Carcinoma

- Aggressive tumor + **osseous destruction**
- May mimic palatal BMT when small

Palatal Minor Salivary Gland Malignancy

- Invasive tumor with **osseous destruction**
- Perineural tumor spread along CNV2 likely

Nasopalatine Duct Cyst

- Central midline cyst in anterior hard plate
- Sharp osseous cortical margins

Palatal Torus

- Osseous benign overgrowth in hard palate midline
- Normal overlying mucosa

Palatal Abscess

- May be dental periapical or periodontal in origin
- Soft tissue enlargement; usually nonmidline

PATHOLOGY

General Features

- Etiology
  - Benign tumor arising from minor salivary gland tissue

Microscopic Features

- Interspersed epithelial, myoepithelial, & stromal cellular components must be identified to diagnose BMT
- May have components of calcification, necrosis, blood products, & hyalinization

CLINICAL ISSUES

Presentation

- Most common signs/symptoms
  - Asymptomatic palatal mass
  - Palatal neuropathy suggests malignancy

Demographics

- Age range: 30-60 years with slight F > M

Natural History & Prognosis

- Slow-growing, painless palatal mass
  - Rapid enlargement of lesion is concerning for **malignant degeneration to carcinoma ex pleomorphic adenoma**

Treatment

- Complete surgical resection of encapsulated mass
  - Critical to include adequate soft tissue margin to avoid cellular "spillage" & future seeding
- Reconstruction not needed without erosion of hard palate

SELECTED REFERENCES

1. Wu YC et al: Clinicopathological study of 74 palatal pleomorphic adenomas. J Formos Med Assoc. 115(1):25-30, 2016
2. Sahoo NK et al: Pleomorphic adenoma palate: major tumor in a minor gland. Ann Maxillofac Surg. 3(2):195-7, 2013

Oral Cavity Minor Salivary Gland Malignancy

KEY FACTS

TERMINOLOGY

- Abbreviation: Minor salivary gland malignancy (MSGM)
- Most common MSGM: Adenoid cystic carcinoma (ACCa) & mucoepidermoid carcinoma (MECa)

IMAGING

- MSGM location: Submucosa of upper aerodigestive tract
  - Hard-soft palate junction > > buccal mucosa
- Oral cavity well defined, smooth submucosal mass
- Bone CT findings
  - Bone erosion: Palate, mandible
  - Greater and lesser palatine foramen enlargement
- MR findings
  - T1: Low signal tumor replaces hard palate marrow fat
  - T1 C+ FS for perineural tumor spread (PNTS)
- PET imaging best for staging/restaging

TOP DIFFERENTIAL DIAGNOSES

- Squamous cell carcinoma
- Benign mixed tumor of palate
- Dermoid & epidermoid cysts
- Dentigerous cyst
- Nasopalatine duct cyst

PATHOLOGY

- Prognosis depends on **stage > histologic grade**

CLINICAL ISSUES

- **ACCa**: Tendency for **PNTS**, lung metastases
- **MECa**: Tendency for regional malignant **nodes**
- Treatment: Surgical resection ± postoperative radiation

DIAGNOSTIC CHECKLIST

- Long-term (> 10 year) imaging follow-up recommended given **tendency to recur late**
- Check for PNTS in MSGM
- Remove FS on T1 C+ MR if susceptibility obscures anatomy
- Noncontrast T1 MR may offer best inherent contrast

(Left) *Axial CECT shows classic example of an adenoid cystic carcinoma (ACCa) in the right hard palate invading adjacent bone & thus gaining access to the greater palatine nerve in the greater palatine canal.* **(Right)** *Axial bone CT shows widening of the right greater palatine canal, indicating perineural tumor spread along the greater palatine nerve. Note normal left canal. Tumor can now spread to the pterygopalatine fossa giving access to V2, vidian nerve, orbit, nasal cavity, & infratemporal fossa.*

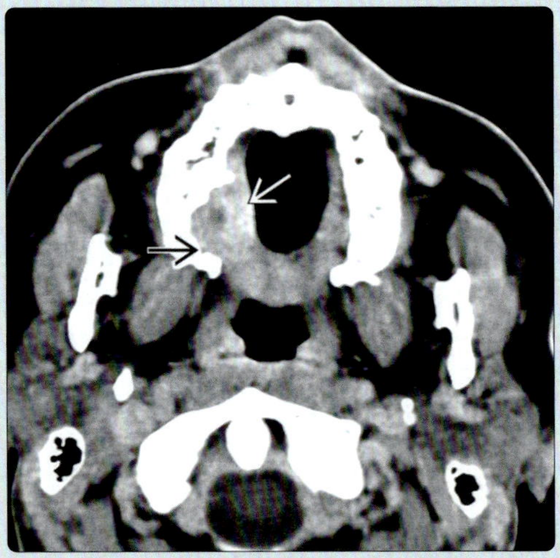

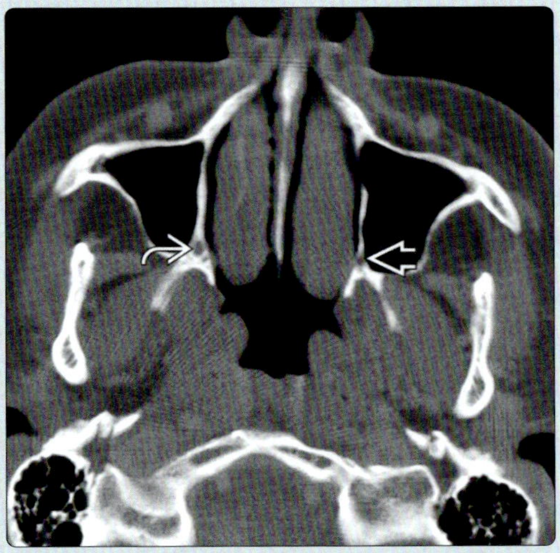

(Left) *Coronal T1WI MR shows dark tumor infiltration of the hard palate marrow in this patient with ACCa. Note normal fat signal in the contralateral hard palate. Noncontrast T1 MR may offer better inherent tumor contrast in areas with fat.* **(Right)** *Axial T1 C+ MR in a patient with hard palate ACCa shows perineural tumor along the maxillary division of trigeminal nerve (V2) in foramen rotundum and cavernous sinus, from contiguous greater palatine nerve and pterygopalatine fossa involvement (not shown).*

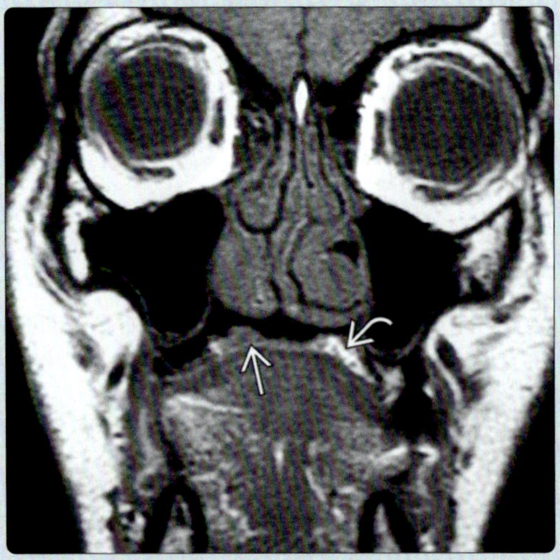

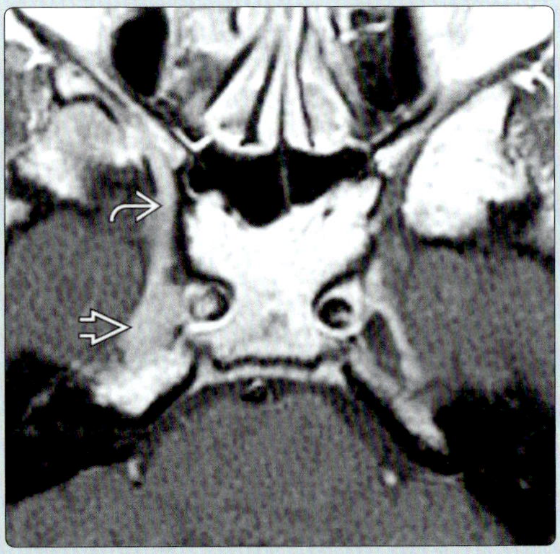

TERMINOLOGY

Abbreviations

- Oral cavity minor salivary gland malignancy (MSGM)

Definitions

- Primary minor salivary gland malignancy
  - Located in submucosa upper aerodigestive tract

IMAGING

General Features

- Best diagnostic clue
  - Oral cavity well-defined, smooth submucosal mass
- Location
  - Hard palate > > buccal mucosa > other oral cavity sites
- Size
  - Small (< 2 cm), visible on physical exam

CT Findings

- CECT
  - Homogeneously enhancing mass
- Bone CT
  - Bone erosion (palate, mandible)
  - Greater & lesser palatine foramen enlargement

MR Findings

- T1WI
  - Tumor isointense to muscle
  - Excellent inherent contrast
- T2WI
  - High-signal lesion compared to muscle
- T1WI C+
  - Homogeneously enhancing tumor
  - Best delineates perineural tumor spread (PNTS)

Nuclear Medicine Findings

- PET imaging best for staging/restaging

Imaging Recommendations

- Best imaging tool
  - MR less affected by dental amalgam artifacts than CT
    - T1 C+ FS MR visualizes PNTS best
      - Remove FS if susceptibility obscures anatomy

DIFFERENTIAL DIAGNOSIS

Squamous Cell Carcinoma

- May mimic minor salivary gland malignancy

Benign Mixed Tumor of Palate

- Well-circumscribed oral mucosal mass

Dermoid or Epidermoid Cysts

- Well-defined oral cavity mass with fatty ± fluid contents

Dentigerous Cyst

- Well-defined cystic lesion around crown of unerupted or impacted tooth; usually canine or 3rd molar

Nasopalatine Duct Cyst

- Well-defined cystic lesion in midline anterior palate

PATHOLOGY

General Features

- Etiology
  - Mucoepidermoid carcinoma (MECa): Associated with radiation exposure

Staging, Grading, & Classification

- MSGM uses same TNM staging as squamous cell carcinoma in each anatomic site
- TNM staging system
  - T1: ≤ 2 cm
  - T2: > 2 & ≤ 4 cm
  - T3: Tumor > 4 cm
  - T4a: Cortical bone, CNV3, extrinsic tongue muscles, skin
  - T4b: Masticator space, pterygoid plates, or skull base, ± encases internal carotid artery
- Prognosis depends on stage > histologic grade

Microscopic Features

- Adenoid cystic carcinoma (ACCa): Unencapsulated neoplasm with varied growth patterns (cribriform, tubular, & solid)
- MECa: Epidermoid, intermediate, & mucus-secreting cells

CLINICAL ISSUES

Presentation

- Most common signs/symptoms
  - Painless, slowly enlarging submucosal mass
    - MSGM in adults unless proven otherwise
  - Other signs/symptoms
    - Facial numbness signifies PNTS along CNV2

Demographics

- Age
  - 30-60 years old
- Epidemiology
  - MSGM: 0.5-1.5% of all H&N carcinoma
    - **ACCa** = **40%** of malignancies in MSG

Natural History & Prognosis

- **ACCa**: Tendency for **PNTS** + lung metastases
- **MECa**: Tendency for regional malignant **nodes**

Treatment

- Tumor resection, including perineural extension
- Postoperative radiotherapy for high grade/high stage

DIAGNOSTIC CHECKLIST

Consider

- Long-term (> 10 year) imaging follow-up recommended given **tendency to recur late**

Image Interpretation Pearls

- Hard palate MSGM: Check for CNV PNTS
- Remove FS on T1 C+ MR if susceptibility obscures anatomy
- Noncontrast T1 MR may offer better inherent contrast

SELECTED REFERENCES

1. Aydil U et al: Neoplasms of the hard palate. J Oral Maxillofac Surg. 72(3):619-26, 2014

Sublingual Gland Carcinoma

KEY FACTS

TERMINOLOGY

- Abbreviation: Sublingual gland (SLG)
- Definition: Primary salivary malignancy of SLG

IMAGING

- CT: Well-defined or invasive mass in anterolateral floor of mouth
  - Mild to moderately enhancing; may be subtle
  - Look for evidence of **mandible erosion**
- MR: Variable signal & contrast enhancement
  - Well-differentiated tumors may have high T2 signal
- PET: Generally low FDG avidity unless high grade

TOP DIFFERENTIAL DIAGNOSES

- Floor of mouth squamous cell carcinoma
- Ranula
- Oral cavity abscess
- Oral cavity lymphatic malformation

CLINICAL ISSUES

- Painless, hard sublingual space mass on bimanual palpation
- **80% of SLG masses are malignant**
- Prognosis depends on stage > histologic grade
- Treatment primarily surgical ± radiotherapy
- Natural History & Prognosis
  - Adenoid cystic carcinoma (ACCa)
    - Strong propensity for **perineural tumor spread**
    - Tends to hematogenously spread to lungs
    - Slow growing; may **metastasize many years later**
  - Mucoepidermoid carcinoma (MECa)
    - Tends to spread to lymph nodes
  - Malignant degeneration of benign mixed tumor (BMT)

DIAGNOSTIC CHECKLIST

- Look for bone invasion & perineural tumor spread, especially with ACCa

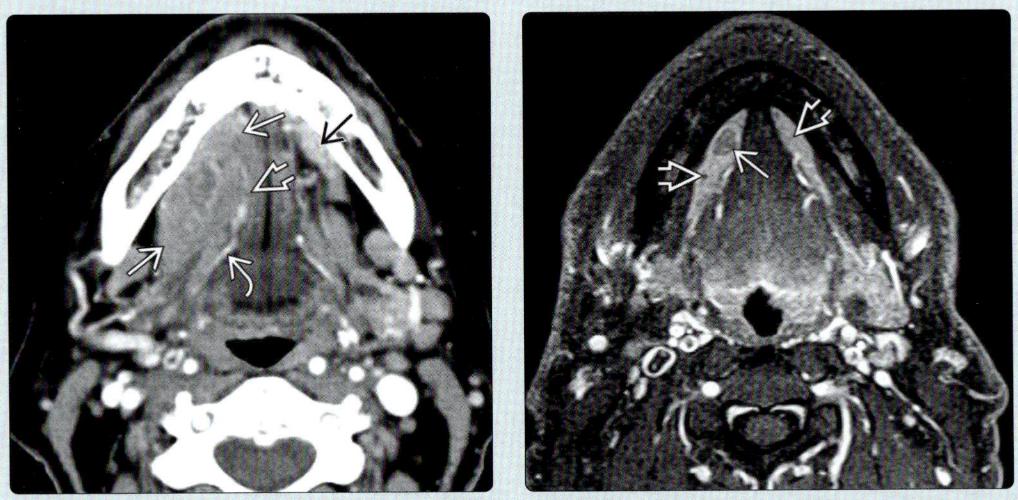

(Left) *Axial CECT shows asymmetric floor of mouth from large infiltrative ACCa ➡ in right sublingual gland (SLG). Tumor extends into genioglossus muscle ➡ & neurovascular bundle ➡, allowing ready access to CNV3 and CNXII. Note the normal left SLG ⇨.* **(Right)** *Axial T1WI C+ FS MR shows a well-defined small mass ➡ in the right SLG representing early MECa. Tumor is hypointense to normal SLG ➡ but can have variable enhancing characteristics. There is no evidence of infiltration to mandible.*

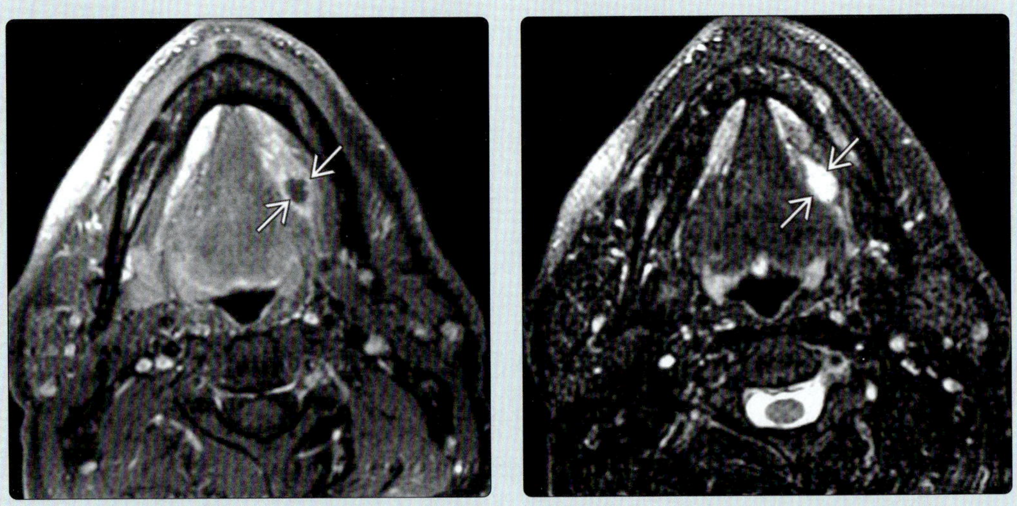

(Left) *Axial T1WI C+ FS MR demonstrates small, heterogeneous, left SLG lesion ➡ with ill-defined borders. Contours suggest this mass may be malignant; however, even well-defined lesions are statistically more likely to be malignant in the SLG.* **(Right)** *Axial T2WI FS MR in the same patient shows lesion ➡ to be markedly hyperintense. More differentiated salivary malignancies produce fluid/mucin & have high signal. Margins are again irregular. This was found to be mucoepidermoid carcinoma.*

TERMINOLOGY

Abbreviations

- Sublingual gland (SLG)

Definitions

- Primary salivary malignancy in SLG
  - Adenoid cystic carcinoma (ACCa), mucoepidermoid carcinoma (MECa), malignant degeneration of benign mixed tumor (BMT)

IMAGING

General Features

- Best diagnostic clue
  - Well-defined or invasive mass in anterolateral floor of mouth
- Location
  - Sublingual space (SLS): Potential space superomedial to mylohyoid muscle
- Size
  - Usually < 2 cm

CT Findings

- CECT
  - Mild to moderately enhancing SLS mass
  - May be subtle lesion on imaging
- CBCT & bone CT
  - Look for evidence of mandible erosion

MR Findings

- T1WI
  - Isointense to muscle
- T2WI
  - Variable: Well differentiated, may be high signal
- T1WI C+
  - Variable contrast enhancement

Nuclear Medicine Findings

- PET
  - Generally low FDG avidity unless high grade

Imaging Recommendations

- Best imaging tool
  - CECT is 1st-line tool, but if hampered by dental amalgam artifact, use MR
- Protocol advice
  - Thin-section CECT with bone & soft tissue algorithm

DIFFERENTIAL DIAGNOSIS

Floor of Mouth Squamous Cell Carcinoma

- Not able to distinguish from SLG carcinoma

Ranula

- Unilocular fluid-filled lesion without enhancement

Oral Cavity Abscess

- Rim-enhancing cystic mass with cellulitis

Oral Cavity Lymphatic Malformation

- Multilocular nonenhancing cystic mass

PATHOLOGY

General Features

- Etiology
  - MECa associated with radiation exposure

Staging, Grading, & Classification

- Adapted from 7th edition AJCC Staging Forms (2010)
  - **T1**: ≤ 2 cm without extraparenchymal extension
  - **T2**: > 2 & ≤ 4 cm, no extraparenchymal extension
  - **T3**: > 4 cm &/or extraparenchymal extension
  - **T4a**: Invades mandible or skin
  - **T4b**: Invades skull base, pterygoid plates, & encases carotid

Microscopic Features

- **ACCa**
  - Unencapsulated; cribriform, tubular, & solid variants
- **MECa**
  - Epidermoid, intermediate, & mucous-secreting cells
- **Malignant degeneration of BMT**
  - Metastasizing BMT; carcinoma ex pleomorphic adenoma (malignant mixed tumor); carcinosarcoma
  - All extremely rare in SLG

CLINICAL ISSUES

Presentation

- Most common signs/symptoms
  - Painless, hard SLS mass on bimanual palpation
- Other signs/symptoms
  - Numbness suggests lingual nerve perineural tumor

Demographics

- Age
  - 30-60 years
- Epidemiology
  - 80% of SLG masses are malignant

Natural History & Prognosis

- ACCa: Slow-growing tumor
  - Strong propensity for perineural tumor spread
  - Does not tend to metastasize to nodes
  - Metastasizes to lungs; may be delayed (> 10 years)
- MECa: Less indolent tumor
  - Greater likelihood of node metastases
- Prognosis depends on **stage > histologic grade**

Treatment

- En bloc resection of anterior floor of mouth
- Postoperative radiotherapy for high stage, high grade

DIAGNOSTIC CHECKLIST

Reporting Tips

- Look for bone invasion & perineural tumor spread, especially with ACCa

SELECTED REFERENCES

1. Lee RJ et al: Malignant sublingual gland tumors: demographics, prognostic factors, and treatment outcomes. Oral Surg Oral Med Oral Pathol Oral Radiol. 121(2):180-7, 2016

Submandibular Gland Carcinoma

KEY FACTS

TERMINOLOGY

- Definition: Primary malignancy arising in submandibular gland (SMG)
- Most commonly: **Adenoid cystic** (ACCa), mucoepidermoid (MECa), adenocarcinoma (AdCa)

IMAGING

- Either focal mass within SMG or irregular mass centered on SMG invading adjacent tissues
- CECT: Asymmetric &/or heterogeneous SMG
  - Well-defined or ill-defined mass
  - Gland may be focally or diffusely hypodense
  - Mild to moderate enhancing SMG mass
- MR: Intermediate to high mixed T2 signal
  - T1W1 C+: Variable contrast enhancement
- PET/CT: Low FDG avidity, unless high grade
- US: Ill-defined, hypoechoic lesion

TOP DIFFERENTIAL DIAGNOSES

- SMG sialadenitis
- SMG mucocele
- SMG benign mixed tumor
- Reactive lymph nodes
- Nodal squamous cell carcinoma in submandibular space

CLINICAL ISSUES

- Painless submandibular swelling or focal mass
- **45%** SMG tumors are **malignant**
- ACCa: Spreads via nerves, also to lungs
- MECa & AdCa: Nodal & hematogenous spread

DIAGNOSTIC CHECKLIST

- If clinical mass, determine if within SMG or if nodal
- If none found on CECT, recommend US or MR
- **Beware** of subtle or occult SMG mass on CECT

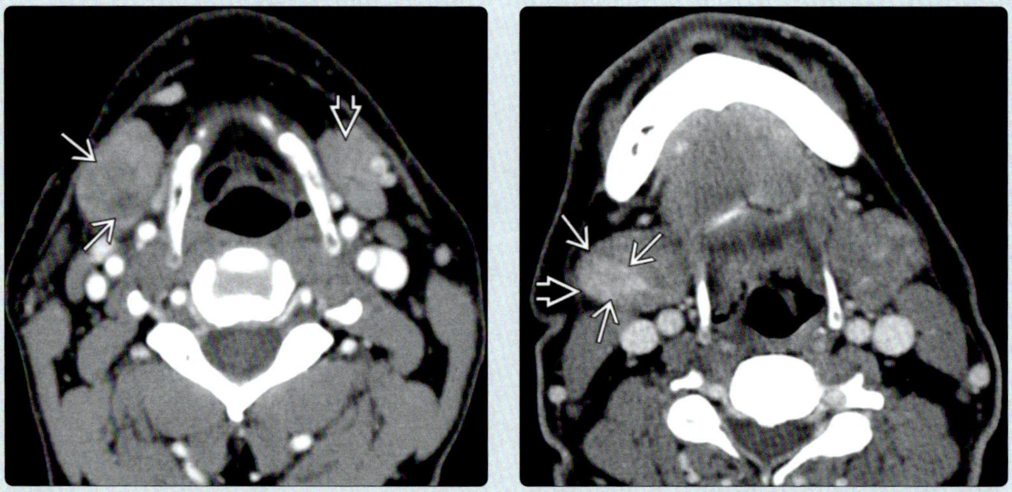

(Left) *Axial CECT shows asymmetric enlargement of the right submandibular gland (SMG) compared to the left ➔ with a hypodense, ill-defined mass ➔ in posterior aspect. On resection, mass was found to be AdCa confined to SMG.* **(Right)** *Axial CECT in an adult with fluctuating neck fullness shows asymmetric fullness ➔ & poorly marginated enhancement ➔ of lateral aspect right SMG. Image was originally interpreted as vascular malformation, but patient age & MR did not support this. Fine-needle aspiration revealed ACCa.*

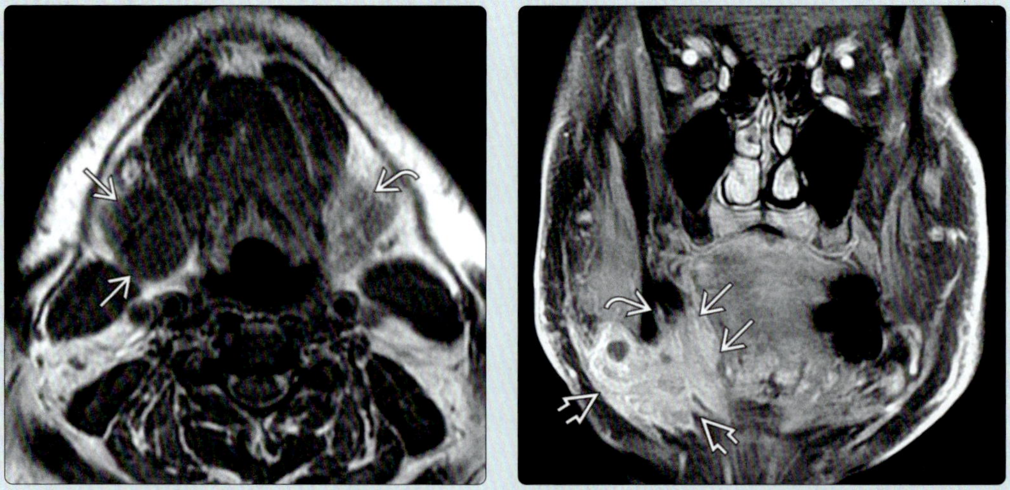

(Left) *Axial T1WI MR demonstrates subtly fuller & more hypointense right SMG ➔ compared to left ➔ in a patient presenting with palpable fullness, interpreted as "asymmetry of SMG but no mass." No adenopathy was seen.* **(Right)** *Coronal T1WI C+ FS MR in the same patient 2 years later reveals ill-defined, heterogeneous right SMG ➔ with infiltration of tumor medially through mylohyoid muscle ➔. Note involvement of mandible & inferior alveolar nerve ➔. Tumor was found to be AdCa with metastatic nodes.*

Submandibular Gland Carcinoma

TERMINOLOGY

Abbreviations

- Submandibular gland (SMG) carcinoma

Definitions

- Primary malignancy arising in SMG

IMAGING

General Features

- Best diagnostic clue
  - Well-defined or invasive mass arising from SMG
- Location
  - Most often superficial aspect of SMG in submandibular space (SMS)
    - Inferolateral to mylohyoid muscle
- Size
  - Usually < 3 cm
- Morphology
  - Well-defined or invasive SMG mass
  - May have homogeneous, enlarged SMG

CT Findings

- CECT
  - Asymmetric &/or heterogeneous SMG
  - Mild to moderately enhancing SMG mass
- Bone CT
  - Bone erosion uncommon, best in coronal plane

MR Findings

- T1WI
  - Isointense to muscle, hypointense to gland
- T2WI
  - Intermediate to high mixed signal intensity
  - **High grade** tends to be **intermediate to low signal**
- T1WI C+
  - Variable contrast enhancement

Nuclear Medicine Findings

- PET/CT
  - Generally low FDG avidity unless high grade

Ultrasonographic Findings

- Grayscale ultrasound
  - Typically ill-defined, hypoechoic lesion

Imaging Recommendations

- Best imaging tool
  - Multiplanar CECT often 1st-line tool
  - US: Excellent for superficial portion SMG
  - MR offers best delineation of contours
- Protocol advice
  - Thin-section CECT: Bone & soft tissue algorithm
  - MR: Use fat saturation on T2 & postcontrast T1

DIFFERENTIAL DIAGNOSIS

Submandibular Gland Sialadenitis

- Enlarged, diffusely enhancing SMG ± sialolith
- Chronic disease leads to atrophic SMG

Submandibular Gland Mucocele

- Unilocular, fluid-filled intraglandular lesion
- Usually no enhancement

Submandibular Gland Benign Mixed Tumor

- Well-demarcated, ovoid SMG mass

Reactive Lymph Nodes

- Ovoid lesion adjacent to normal SMG

Nodal Squamous Cell Carcinoma in Submandibular Space

- Enlarged node adjacent to SMG

PATHOLOGY

Staging, Grading, & Classification

- American Joint Committee on Cancer (2010)
  - **T1**: ≤ 2 cm without extraparenchymal extension
  - **T2**: > 2 & ≤ 4 cm, no extraparenchymal extension
  - **T3**: > 4 cm &/or extraparenchymal extension
  - **T4a**: Invades skin, mandible, ear canal, ± facial nerve
  - **T4b**: Invades skull base ± pterygoid plates ± encasing carotid artery

Microscopic Features

- 3 main pathologies: **ACCa, MECa, AdCa**

CLINICAL ISSUES

Presentation

- Most common signs/symptoms
  - Painless submandibular swelling or focal mass
- Other signs/symptoms
  - Chin or lower lip numbness suggests infiltration of mandible & inferior alveolar nerve
  - Lower lip weakness suggests facial nerve branches

Demographics

- Age
  - 40-70 years old
- Epidemiology
  - **45%** of SMG tumors are **malignant**
  - **40%** of malignant SMG tumors are **ACCa**

Treatment

- En bloc complete resection of tumor
- Postoperative radiotherapy for high stage, high grade

DIAGNOSTIC CHECKLIST

Image Interpretation Pearls

- **If presentation of mass or fullness**
  - 1st determine whether mass is **within gland or extrinsic**, such as node
  - If **no mass or subtle asymmetry on CECT**, recommend **further imaging with US or MR**
    - May be very subtle or **occult** on CECT

SELECTED REFERENCES

1. Gill I et al: Unexpected case of sclerosing mucoepidermoid carcinoma of the submandibular salivary gland. Br J Oral Maxillofac Surg. ePub, 2017

Submandibular Space Nodal Non-Hodgkin Lymphoma

KEY FACTS

TERMINOLOGY

- Submandibular space (SMS) nodal non-Hodgkin lymphoma (NHL)
- NHL develops in lymphoreticular system

IMAGING

- CECT findings
  - Multiple, bilateral, nonnecrotic enlarged level I SMS nodes
  - May see only dominant, single large node
  - Usually large, solid, round nodes
  - Necrosis/extranodal spread indicate aggressive NHL
- PET/CT increasingly used to determine disease extent

TOP DIFFERENTIAL DIAGNOSES

- Reactive lymph nodes
- Nodal squamous cell carcinoma of SMS
- Nodal metastases from systemic primary
- Sarcoidosis lymph nodes
- Tuberculosis lymph nodes

PATHOLOGY

- Unregulated malignant monoclonal lymphocytes in lymphoreticular system
- Multiple different NHL subtypes
  - Most common (> 30%) diffuse large B-cell lymphoma
  - Multiple other subtypes

CLINICAL ISSUES

- Presentation: Painless multiple SMS masses
- Treatment: Radiotherapy, chemotherapy, or both
- 5% of all H&N cancers
- Prognosis
  - 5-year survival: Stage I-II (85%), stage III-IV (50%)

DIAGNOSTIC CHECKLIST

- Consider NHL if imaging reveals multiple 1- to 3-cm cervical nodes in multiple nodal chains, especially if nonnecrotic

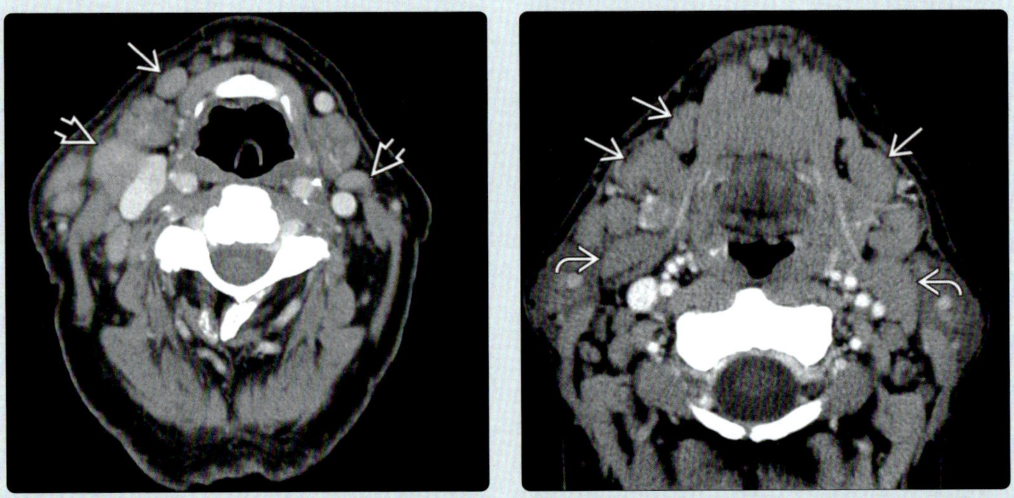

(Left) *Axial CECT at the level of the hyoid bone in a patient with non-Hodgkin lymphoma (NHL) demonstrates diffuse adenopathy in the upper neck, with a prominent right submandibular IB node ➡ and bilateral level II nodes ➡.* **(Right)** *Axial CECT reveals multiple smoothly marginated, enlarged level IB nodes in the submandibular space bilaterally ➡ along with large, solid level II nodes ➡ in a patient with NHL.*

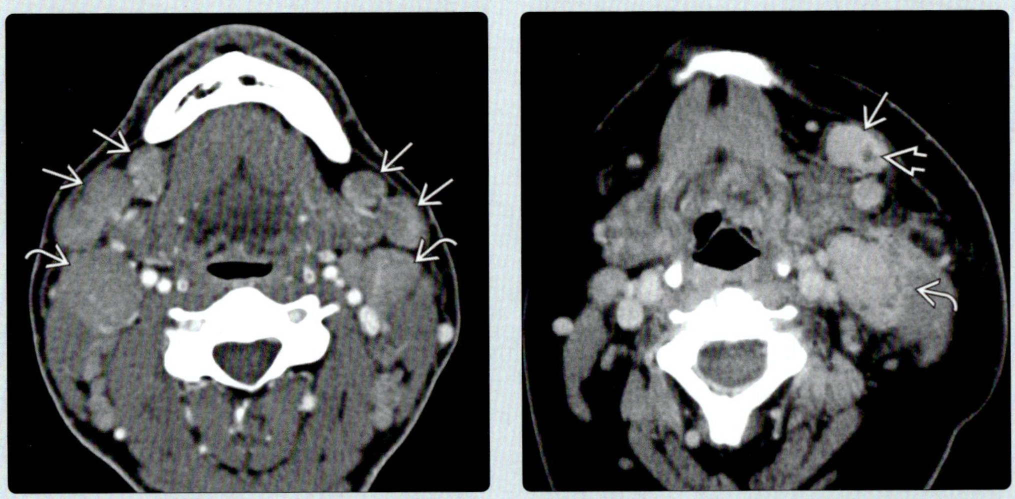

(Left) *Axial CECT at the level of the inferior mandible shows large nonnecrotic NHL nodes in the level IB submandibular chain ➡ and bilateral level II jugulodigastric group ➡.* **(Right)** *Axial CECT in this HIV(+) patient with NHL shows a prominent left level IB submandibular space node ➡ with a small focus of cystic change ➡. A larger level II jugulodigastric node appears to invade the adjacent sternocleidomastoid muscle ➡. Nodal necrosis and extranodal NHL spread usually indicate a high-grade NHL is present.*

Submandibular Space Nodal Non-Hodgkin Lymphoma

TERMINOLOGY

Abbreviations

- Submandibular space (SMS) nodal non-Hodgkin lymphoma (NHL)

Definitions

- NHL = lymphoreticular system malignancy, postulated to arise from lymphocytes & derivatives

IMAGING

General Features

- Best diagnostic clue
  - Multiple, bilateral, large nodes involving multiple nodal chains
- Location
  - Any nodal chain may be affected, including level I
- Size
  - Multiple 1- to 3-cm nodes common
  - Dominant node may reach 3-5 cm in size
- Morphology
  - Nodes round or oval, typically solid

CT Findings

- CECT
  - Multiple bilateral round nodes; multiple nodal chains
  - Enhancement pattern variable
    - From isodense to muscle to diffuse enhancement

MR Findings

- T1WI
  - Nodes isointense to muscle
- T2WI
  - Nodes iso- or slightly hyperintense to muscle
- T1WI C+
  - Mild homogeneous nodal enhancement
  - Necrotic nodes enhance peripherally

Imaging Recommendations

- Best imaging tool
  - CECT usually initial imaging exam
- Protocol advice
  - PET/CT increasingly used to determine disease extent

DIFFERENTIAL DIAGNOSIS

Reactive Lymph Nodes

- Patient < 20-30 years with viral infection
- Diffuse, nonnecrotic nodes; usually < 2 cm

Nodal Squamous Cell Carcinoma of SMS

- Known oral cavity, anterior face or skin squamous cell carcinoma
- Level IA & IB nodes > 1.5 cm ± central nodal necrosis

Nodal Metastases From Systemic Primary

- Known primary tumor (lung, breast, etc.)
- Often unilateral

Sarcoidosis Lymph Nodes

- Diffuse cervical nodes may exactly mimic NHL
- Calcifications may be seen

Tuberculosis Lymph Nodes

- Systemically ill patient with strongly positive purified protein derivative (PPD) test + abnormal chest x-ray
- Diffuse heterogeneously enhancing nodes

PATHOLOGY

General Features

- Etiology
  - Unregulated malignant monoclonal lymphocytes in lymphoreticular system
  - Evidence suggests viral cause but yet to be proven
- Associated abnormalities
  - Often associated with AIDS in children & adults
    - 2nd most common cancer in AIDS patients
- Multiple different NHL subtypes
  - Most common (> 30%) diffuse large B-cell lymphoma

Microscopic Features

- Microscopic features depend on cell of origin
  - B- & T-cell lymphomas composed of precursor (lymphoblastic) cells or mature lymphocytes

CLINICAL ISSUES

Presentation

- Most common signs/symptoms
  - Painless multiple small rubbery SMS masses
- Other signs/symptoms
  - Systemic symptoms include night sweats, recurrent fevers, weight loss, fatigue, rash

Demographics

- Age
  - Median: 50-55 years
- Epidemiology
  - NHL incidence ↑ with age; ↑ in immunocompromised patients
  - 5% of all H&N cancers

Natural History & Prognosis

- May be indolent, progressive but not curable, or aggressive but curable
- Predictors of poorer prognosis
  - Age > 60 years, > 1 extranodal site, stage III or IV, AIDS related

Treatment

- Depends on cell type, stage, & patient age
- Usually treated with XRT ± chemotherapy
  - Stage I and II: H&N NHL, XRT alone
  - Stage III and IV: Disseminated NHL, chemotherapy ± XRT

DIAGNOSTIC CHECKLIST

Consider

- NHL: If imaging reveals multiple 1- to 3-cm cervical nodes in multiple nodal chains, especially if nonnecrotic

SELECTED REFERENCES

1. Walter C et al: Malignant lymphomas in the head and neck region–a retrospective, single-center study over 41 years. Int J Med Sci. 12(2):141-5, 2015

Oral Tongue Squamous Cell Carcinoma

KEY FACTS

TERMINOLOGY

- Oral tongue squamous cell carcinoma (SCCa) definition: Oral cavity mucosal malignancy arising from anterior 2/3 of tongue

IMAGING

- Imaging used to define deep extent and nodes
- Lateral margin > undersurface > > tip of tongue
- CECT/MR: Variably enhancing invasive lesion
- Superficial lesion may be occult to imaging
- MR better evaluates extent of primary than CT
- MR less affected by dental amalgam artifact

TOP DIFFERENTIAL DIAGNOSES

- Lingual tonsil SCCa
- Tongue schwannoma
- Venous malformation of tongue
- Oral cavity abscess
- Alveolar soft part sarcoma of tongue

PATHOLOGY

- Strong association with tobacco and alcohol
- Clinical assessment more accurate than imaging for mucosal size (T1-T3)
- Imaging important for deep extent and nodes
- 1st-order nodal drainage: Submandibular (IB), then jugulodigastric group (IIA)
- Beware of skip nodes where anterior tongue tumors drain directly to levels III or IV
- Up to 35% have ≥ N1 disease at diagnosis
- 30% N0 necks have microscopic nodal metastases

CLINICAL ISSUES

- Painful nonhealing ulcer of oral tongue
- Median age: 61 years; M:F = 4:1
- Treatment: Primarily surgical resection ± radiation
- Overall 5-year survival: 60%

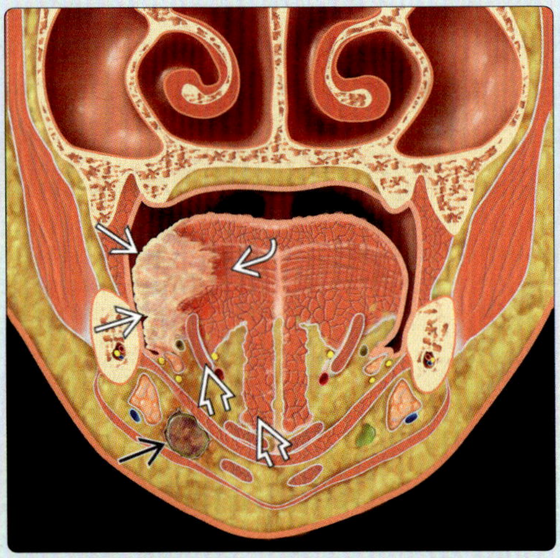

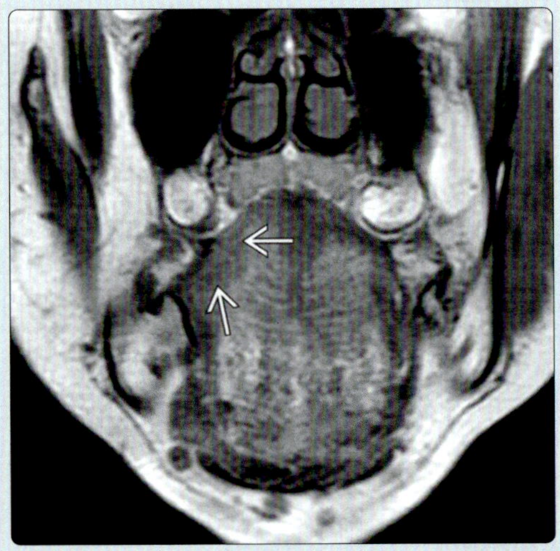

(Left) *Coronal graphic illustrates lateral oral tongue squamous cell carcinoma (SCCa) → infiltrating intrinsic tongue muscles →. Coronal plane allows scrutiny of extrinsic tongue muscles →, infiltration of which designates the tumor as T4a. Ipsilateral 1B node is also shown →.* **(Right)** *Coronal T1WI MR in a woman with a painful right tongue ulcer shows subtle low signal intensity at the lateral tongue margin →. There is no evidence of involvement of extrinsic muscles or contralateral tumor spread.*

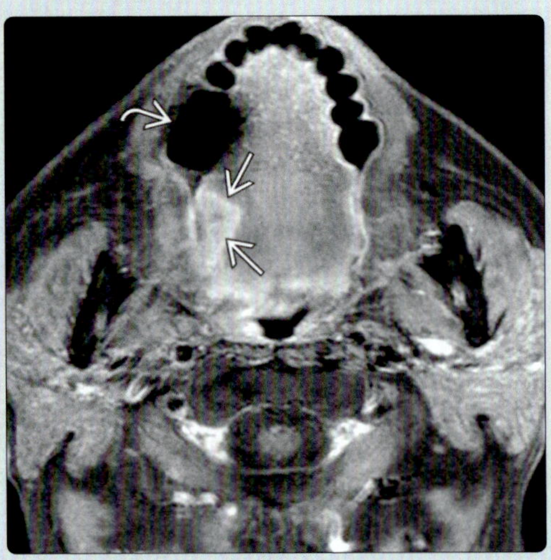

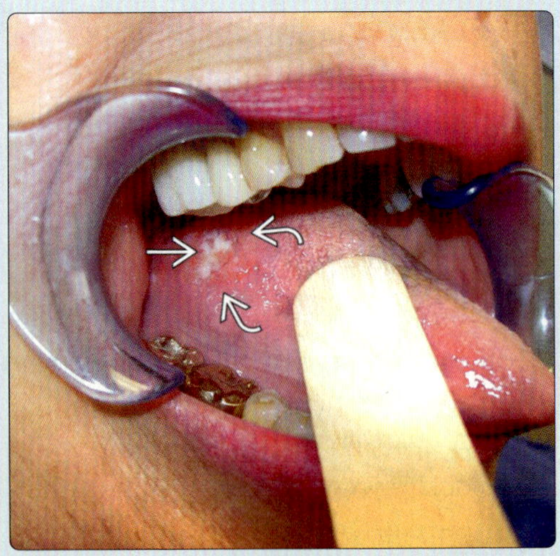

(Left) *Axial T1WI C+ FS MR in the same patient shows marked enhancement of a wedge-shaped ulcer at posterolateral tongue surface →. No enlarged neck nodes are present. Note that despite amalgam →, the tumor is still well seen.* **(Right)** *Clinical photograph demonstrates a lateral tongue ulcer → with indurated adjacent tissue →. Tumor was staged as T2N0 by clinical exam and imaging and treated by hemiglossectomy with ipsilateral selective neck dissection (SND) (I-III). Final pathology concurred: pT2N0 SCCa, stage II.*

Oral Tongue Squamous Cell Carcinoma

TERMINOLOGY

Abbreviations

- Oral tongue squamous cell carcinoma (SCCa)

Definitions

- Oral cavity (OC) mucosal malignancy arising from anterior 2/3 of tongue
  - Distinct from base of tongue (oropharyngeal SCCa)

IMAGING

General Features

- Best diagnostic clue
  - Asymmetric enhancement ± ulcer of lateral aspect tongue
- Location
  - Oral tongue defined as freely mobile portion
    - Tip, lateral borders, dorsum, and undersurface
  - Most commonly arises from **lateral margin**
    - Next most common is undersurface
- Size
  - Variable, both in superficial and deep extent
    - Mucosal size best determined clinically
- Morphology
  - Irregular ulcer with variable deep invasion

CT Findings

- CECT
  - Variably enhancing oral tongue mucosal lesion
  - Superficial lesion may be occult to imaging
- Bone CT
  - If deep infiltration to floor of mouth, may invade mandible

MR Findings

- T1WI
  - Low signal intensity compared to tongue tissues
- T2WI
  - Typically increased signal intensity
  - Most readily observed with fat saturation
- T1WI C+
  - Variable enhancement, mild to moderate
  - Large tumors show ulceration with rim enhancement

Nuclear Medicine Findings

- PET/CT
  - SCCa is reliably FDG avid
  - Modality not often employed unless large primary or extensive nodal metastases

Imaging Recommendations

- Best imaging tool
  - MR preferred imaging modality in OC
    - Superior tissue contrast to identify primary and deep or contralateral extent of tumor
    - Less affected by dental amalgam artifact than CT
- Protocol advice
  - Fat saturation helps with tissue contrast for T2WI and T1WI C+
  - If CECT obtained, thin slices allow coronal reformats, which aid in evaluating deep extent

DIFFERENTIAL DIAGNOSIS

Lingual Tonsil SCCa

- Invasive tongue base tumor may extend into oral tongue
- More commonly invades floor of mouth, tongue root

Tongue Schwannoma

- Well-circumscribed mass within oral tongue
- Homogeneous enhancement

Venous Malformation of Tongue

- Congenital vascular lesion
- Calcified phleboliths virtually diagnostic

Oral Cavity Abscess

- Rim-enhancing cystic mass often with extensive cellulitis
- Typically associated with dental disease

Alveolar Soft Part Sarcoma of Tongue

- Aggressive enhancing tumor may involve body of tongue
- Typically women < 35 years

PATHOLOGY

General Features

- Etiology
  - Strong link with smoking, chewing tobacco, and alcohol
    - Also, chewing betel nut, paan
  - Conflicting evidence for alcohol-containing mouthwash and OC cancer
    - Some advise use of mouthwash without alcohol
  - Fruit and vegetable consumption appears to reduce risk of OC SCCa
- Genetics
  - Squamous cell carcinoma-related oncogene (*DCUN1D1*)
    - May play role in pathogenesis of oral tongue SCCa through amplification of chromosome 3q26
    - May be predictor of regional metastases and marker for aggressiveness and outcome

Staging, Grading, & Classification

- **American Joint Committee on Cancer (AJCC) staging forms (2010)**
- Note that clinical assessment is more accurate than imaging for mucosal size
- Imaging is important for determination of **deep extent: Must look for features that make tumor T4**
  - T4a: Tumor invades through cortical bone, deep muscles of tongue, maxillary sinus, skin of face
  - T4b: Tumor invades masticator space, pterygoid plates, skull base, or encases carotid
  - Contralateral spread important for surgical resection
- Anterior tongue SCCa
  - More often involves floor of mouth
- **Malignant nodes common at presentation**
  - Up to 35% have ≥ N1 disease preoperatively
  - 30% N0 necks have microscopic nodal metastases
- 1st-order nodal drainage: Submandibular (IB), then jugulodigastric group (IIA)
  - Occasionally, anterior tumors drain directly to midjugular (III) or low jugular (IV): **Skip nodes**
  - Midline tumor more likely to have **bilateral** nodes

AJCC Oral Cavity Staging (2010)

Tumor (T): Clinical assessment of mucosal extent more accurate than imaging	Nodal stage (N)
Tis: Carcinoma in situ	**N1**: Ipsilateral node ≤ 3 cm
T1: Tumor ≤ 2 cm	**N2a**: Ipsilateral node > 3 cm, ≤ 6 cm
T2: Tumor > 2 & ≤ 4 cm	**N2b**: Multiple ipsilateral nodes ≤ 6 cm
T3: Tumor > 4 cm	**N2c**: Bilateral or contralateral ≤ 6 cm
T4a: Tumor invades deep tongue muscles (genioglossus, hyoglossus, palatoglossus, styloglossus), maxillary sinus, skin of face, through cortical bone	**N3**: Nodal mass > 6 cm
T4b: Tumor invades masticator space, pterygoid plates, skull base, or encases carotid	**Distant metastasis (M)**
	M0: No distant metastasis
	M1: Distant metastasis
Adapted from 7th edition AJCC Staging Forms.	

T = tumor, N = nodal, M = metastasis.

- Tongue tip tumors may drain to submental (I)
- Lower nodes more likely to have distant mets
  - Lungs > bones or liver

Gross Pathologic & Surgical Features

- Red or red and white well-demarcated areas of roughness and induration
- Ulcerated areas clearly indurated, hard on palpation with pain

Microscopic Features

- Squamous differentiation with intracellular bridges or keratinization, ± keratin pearls
- Further classified by amount of differentiation
  - Well, moderately, poorly, or undifferentiated

CLINICAL ISSUES

Presentation

- Most common signs/symptoms
  - Pain; occurs with smaller size than many OC tumors
  - Nonhealing ulcer of oral tongue mucosa
    - Ulcer older than 3 weeks is suspicious
- Other signs/symptoms
  - Tongue mass + neck masses from regional nodes
  - Bleeding

Demographics

- Age
  - Median: 61 years
- Gender
  - M:F = 4:1
- Epidemiology
  - > 90% of OC malignancies are SCCa
    - Most common sites: Tongue and floor of mouth
  - Rising incidence of tongue SCCa

Natural History & Prognosis

- Survival significantly impacted by ongoing tobacco and alcohol abuse
- Invasion of adjacent structures significantly reduces prognosis
- **Overall 5-year survival: 60%**
  - If no nodal metastases: ~ 77%

Treatment

- Primarily surgical resection ± radiation
  - Local resection
  - Hemiglossectomy
    - If large tumor not crossing midline
    - Midline determined by fatty lingual septum
  - Total glossectomy
    - Rarely performed, high morbidity
- To minimize recurrence, 1.5- to 2-cm margin required
  - Hence preoperative (imaging) determination of **deep** extent may be **crucial** to surgeon
- Some programs advocate elective selective neck dissection for OC SCCa due to high risk of occult nodal metastases

DIAGNOSTIC CHECKLIST

Consider

- Clinical assessment of **mucosal extent** more accurate than imaging
  - Superficial lesion may be occult on MR/CECT
- Imaging evaluation of **deep extent and nodes** better than clinical
  - MR typically evaluates extent better than CECT
  - Nodes frequently present, often occult to clinical exam and imaging

Reporting Tips

- Determine if tumor crosses to contralateral side, as this prohibits hemiglossectomy
- Look for deeply invasive features that upstage tumor to T4a/b
- Evaluate for ipsilateral and contralateral IB and IIA nodes
- Beware skip nodes (III or IV without higher levels), especially with anterior tongue tumors

SELECTED REFERENCES

1. Mücke T et al: Tumor thickness and risk of lymph node metastasis in patients with squamous cell carcinoma of the tongue. Oral Oncol. 53:80-4, 2016
2. Seki M et al: Histologic assessment of tumor budding in preoperative biopsies to predict nodal metastasis in squamous cell carcinoma of the tongue and floor of the mouth. Head Neck. 38 Suppl 1:E1582-90, 2016
3. Madana J et al: Computerized tomography based tumor-thickness measurement is useful to predict postoperative pathological tumor thickness in oral tongue squamous cell carcinoma. J Otolaryngol Head Neck Surg. 44:49, 2015

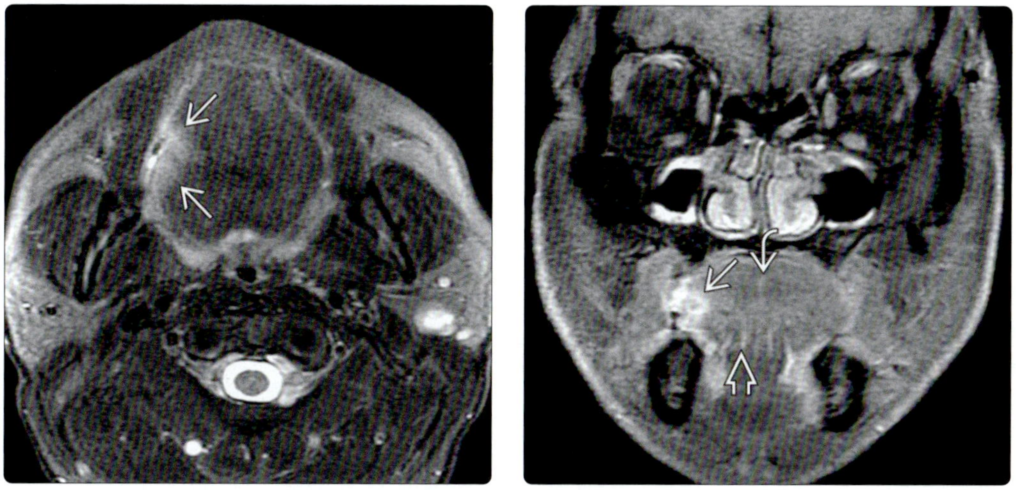

(Left) *Axial T2WI FS MR demonstrates a small right lateral tongue tumor, subtly evident as lenticular region of increased signal intensity ➔. Ill-defined margins are typical. The lesion does not approach the midline.* **(Right)** *Coronal T1WI C+ FS MR in the same patient demonstrates enhancement of lateral tongue ulcer ➔. The lesion does not extend inferiorly to genioglossus ➔ or other extrinsic tongue muscles and does not reach the midline lingual septum ➔. Hemiglossectomy and SND showed T1N0 SCCa, stage I.*

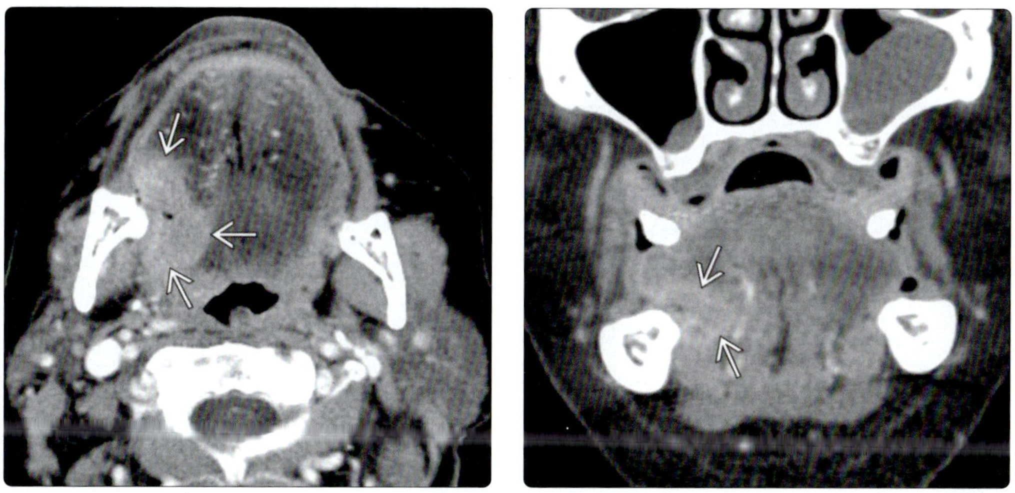

(Left) *Axial CECT in a 59-year-old smoker with a 5-month history of painful tongue lesion demonstrates avidly enhancing irregular ulcerative mass ➔ arising from lateral posterior margin of tongue. Single level II node is evident on inferior CT images.* **(Right)** *Coronal CECT reformatted image shows irregular enhancement of ulcer ➔. There is no evidence of deep infiltration of extrinsic tongue muscles, and tumor did not approach midline. Right hemiglossectomy and modified neck dissection revealed T2N1 SCCa, stage III.*

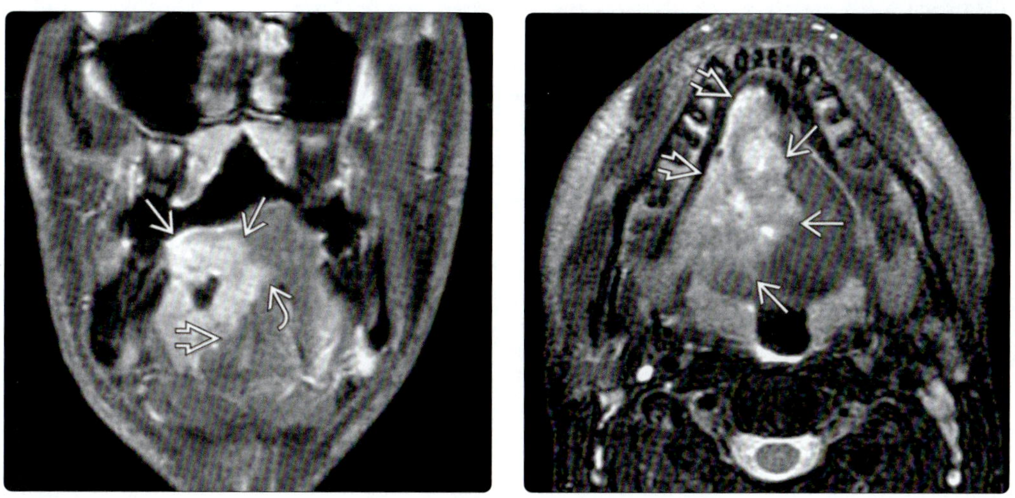

(Left) *Coronal T1WI C+ FS MR demonstrates a large, enhancing, but centrally necrotic irregular mass ➔ arising in the right lateral tongue, invading genioglossus ➔, & extending across the midline ➔.* **(Right)** *Axial T2WI FS MR through the floor of mouth (same patient) better illustrates tumor infiltration ➔ & extension up to the right mandible ➔, although no evidence of bone infiltration is present. Total glossectomy & floor of mouth resection was performed, as patient was only 31 years old; T4aN2b SCCa, stage IVA was proven.*

Floor of Mouth Squamous Cell Carcinoma

KEY FACTS

TERMINOLOGY

- Floor of mouth (FOM) squamous cell carcinoma (SCCa)
  - FOM mucosa overlies mylohyoid and hyoglossus muscles and body of tongue rests on it

IMAGING

- CECT: Irregular mild to moderately enhancing mass
- MR: Loss of normal FOM anatomical planes on T1
  - Increased T2 signal intensity and enhancement
- SCCa reliably FDG avid; increasing role in current practice
- May exactly mimic sublingual gland carcinoma

TOP DIFFERENTIAL DIAGNOSES

- Sublingual gland carcinoma
- Oral tongue SCCa
- Venolymphatic malformation
- Ranula
- Oral cavity abscess

PATHOLOGY

- Strongly associated with tobacco (smoking and chewing) and alcohol abuse
- ≤ 35% have nodes at presentation: Levels I, II
- High incidence of occult nodal metastases

CLINICAL ISSUES

- Most commonly 50-70 years; M:F = 2:1
- Painful hard ulcer/lesion, ± loose teeth
- Overall 5-year survival = 60%

DIAGNOSTIC CHECKLIST

- May present as submandibular gland obstructive sialadenitis
- Clinical mucosal size more accurate than imaging
- Imaging important for deep extent and nodes
  - Genioglossus, mylohyoid, base of tongue
  - Cortical bone erosion, marrow infiltration

(Left) *Graphic illustrates the most common location of floor of mouth (FOM) squamous cell carcinoma within 2 cm of midline anterior FOM. It is important at imaging to evaluate for invasion inferiorly to genioglossus & mylohyoid muscles, posteriorly to tongue base, & mandibular involvement anteriorly or laterally. This may require both MR & CT. Second aim of imaging is evaluation of nodal disease.* **(Right)** *Sagittal T1WI MR demonstrates mass of low intensity compared to tongue muscles, abutting midline mandible.*

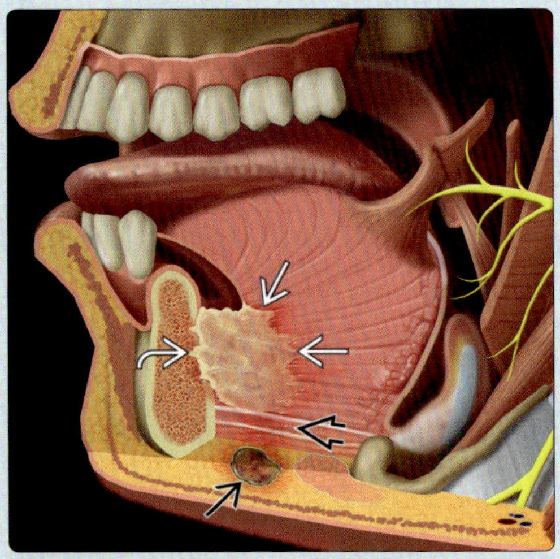

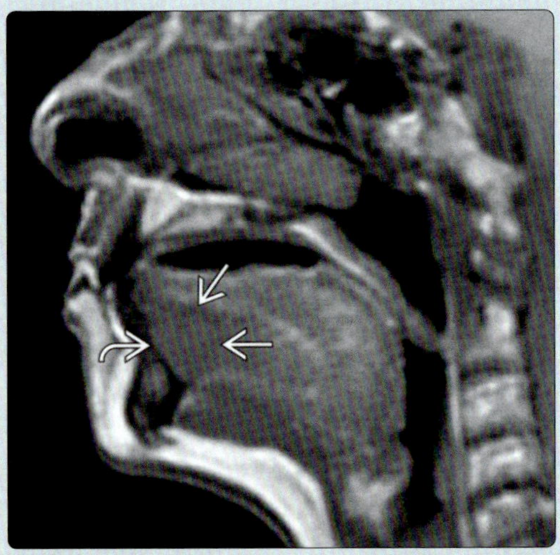

(Left) *Axial T1WI C+ FS MR in the same patient shows a subtle anterior midline FOM lesion that involves the anterior aspect of the right sublingual gland (SLG). Note the loss of low-intensity cortex of the adjacent mandible. This was confirmed on bone CT. No abnormal nodes were found.* **(Right)** *Clinical photograph in same patient reveals a tumor in anterior FOM and shows relation to SLG. Composite resection and bilateral selective neck dissection (I-III) confirmed T4aN0 disease (mandible involvement).*

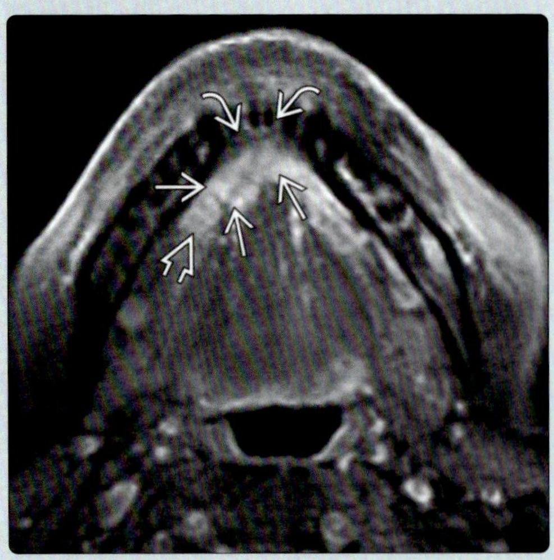

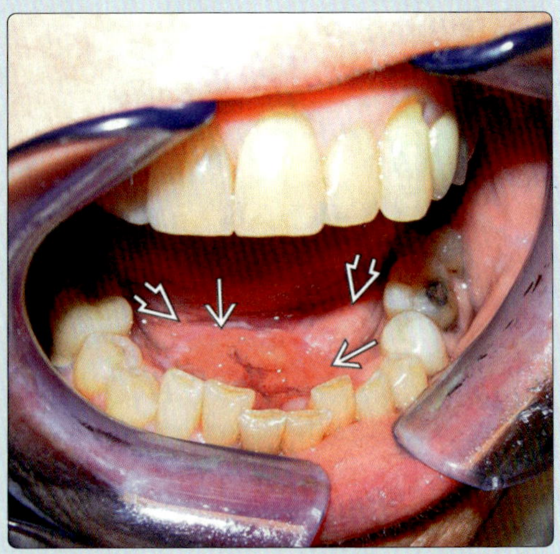

TERMINOLOGY

Abbreviations

- Floor of mouth (FOM) squamous cell carcinoma (SCCa)

Definitions

- Oral cavity mucosal malignancy arising from FOM
  - Inner surface of mandibular alveolar ridges to undersurface of tongue

IMAGING

General Features

- Best diagnostic clue
  - Irregular enhancing mass in anterior FOM
- Location
  - Most within 2 cm of anterior midline FOM
- Size
  - Variable: Several mm to several cm

CT Findings

- CECT
  - Mild to moderately enhancing irregular FOM mass
  - May exactly mimic sublingual gland carcinoma
  - May obstruct drainage of 1 or both submandibular gland (SMG) ducts → sialadenitis
- Bone CT
  - Must evaluate carefully for cortical erosion

MR Findings

- T1WI
  - Low-signal mass in relation to FOM tissues
    - **Subtle loss of normal anatomical contours**
- T2WI
  - Increased signal intensity
    - Often easier to identify with fat saturation
- T1WI C+
  - Variable enhancement: Mild to moderate
  - Tumor infiltrating marrow typically enhances

Nuclear Medicine Findings

- PET/CT
  - SCCa reliably FDG avid; increasing role in current practice

Imaging Recommendations

- Best imaging tool
  - MR best for determining tumor extent
  - Bone CT important when tumor abuts mandible
  - Expanding role of PET/CT; highest sensitivity
- Protocol advice
  - CECT: Soft tissue and bone algorithm in 2 planes
    - Puffed cheek scan improves mucosal assessment

DIFFERENTIAL DIAGNOSIS

Sublingual Gland Carcinoma

- May be impossible to distinguish by imaging

Oral Tongue Squamous Cell Carcinoma

- Anterior &/or large lesions may invade FOM

Venolymphatic Malformation

- Heterogeneous moderate to marked enhancement
- Calcified phleboliths essentially diagnostic

Ranula

- Rim-enhancing fluid mass in FOM

Oral Cavity Abscess

- Rim-enhancing collection(s) + FOM cellulitis

PATHOLOGY

General Features

- Etiology
  - Strongly associated with tobacco (smoking and chewing) and alcohol abuse
    - Chewing betel nut, paan in parts of Asia

Staging, Grading, & Classification

- American Joint Committee on Cancer (AJCC) (2010)
- Same classification for all oral cavity tumors
  - T1: ≤ 2 cm in greatest diameter
  - T2: > 2 & ≤ 4 cm in greatest diameter
  - T3: > 4 cm in greatest diameter
  - T4a: Tumor invades through cortical bone into extrinsic tongue muscles, skin of face
  - T4b: Tumor invades masticator space, pterygoid plates, skull base, or encases carotid
- Clinical **mucosal extent** more accurate than imaging
- Imaging important for **deep extent: Look for features that make tumor T4**
- Nodal staging: AJCC follows oropharyngeal and laryngeal nodal staging
- 1st-order drainage is **level I, then level II**
  - **Up to 35%** have nodes found at presentation
  - **30% occult nodal metastases** in oral cavity SCCa
- Metastatic disease: Absent = M0, present = M1
  - Lung metastases more common than bone and liver

CLINICAL ISSUES

Presentation

- Most common signs/symptoms
  - Painful hard ulcer/lesion in FOM
- Other signs/symptoms
  - Invasion of mandible may lead to loose teeth

Demographics

- Age
  - Most commonly 50-70 years

Natural History & Prognosis

- **Overall 5-year survival = 60%**

Treatment

- Primary resection ± reconstruction, ± neck dissection
- ± adjuvant radiation
- Future role of superselective intraarterial chemotherapy

SELECTED REFERENCES

1. Arya S et al: Oral cavity squamous cell carcinoma: role of pretreatment imaging and its influence on management. Clin Radiol. 69(9):916-30, 2014
2. Hong HR et al: Clinical values of (18) F-FDG PET/CT in oral cavity cancer with dental artifacts on CT or MRI. J Surg Oncol. 110(6):696-701, 2014
3. American Joint Committee on Cancer: AJCC Cancer Staging Manual. 7th ed. New York: Springer, 2010

Gingival Squamous Cell Carcinoma

KEY FACTS

TERMINOLOGY

- Definition: Invasive malignant neoplasm of squamous epithelium arising in gingiva, often spreads to underlying bone

IMAGING

- Small lesions confined to gingiva may be occult to imaging
- Larger lesions: **Enhancing, infiltrating jaw mass ± bone destruction**
- CBCT & bone CT: Cortical destruction ± enlarged nerve canal, widened periodontal ligament spaces
- MR: Marrow signal enhancement similar to tumor

TOP DIFFERENTIAL DIAGNOSES

- Osteomyelitis
- Osteoradionecrosis
- Osteonecrosis
- Metastasis
- Osteosarcoma

CLINICAL ISSUES

- **10-30%** of oral cavity squamous cell carcinoma
- Nonhealing ulcer of gingiva, swelling, bleeding
- Nonulcerated mass also common & easily mistaken for benign gingival lesion
- Can resemble periodontal lesion or periapical disease
- Recent tooth extraction: Nonhealing site or soft tissue mass arising from socket
- Overall 5-year survival ~ 60%

DIAGNOSTIC CHECKLIST

- Evaluate local spread, bone infiltration, nodes
- Mandible: Buccal space, masticator space, floor of mouth
- Maxilla: Nasal cavity, maxillary sinus, palate, infratemporal fossa
- Gingival mucosa attached to bone; allows early marrow infiltration: T4a
- If in bone, evaluate for perineural tumor spread
- Metastatic spread favors facial, level I & II nodes

(Left) *Graphic illustrates SCCa arising from mandibular gingiva and invading the mandible body, making it T4a. Note involvement of inferior alveolar nerve, which is important for complete resection.* **(Right)** *Axial CECT shows heterogeneous mass with destruction of left mandibular body. Mass extends laterally to involve the gingivobuccal sulcus and cheek and medially to involve the floor of the mouth. The lesion was T4aN1 and completely excised with reconstruction by composite flap.*

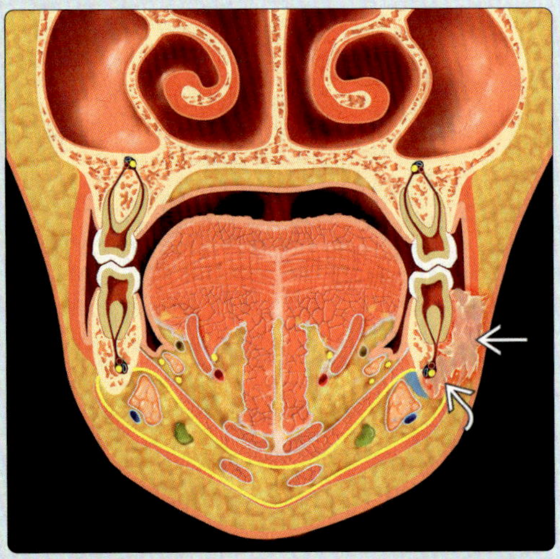

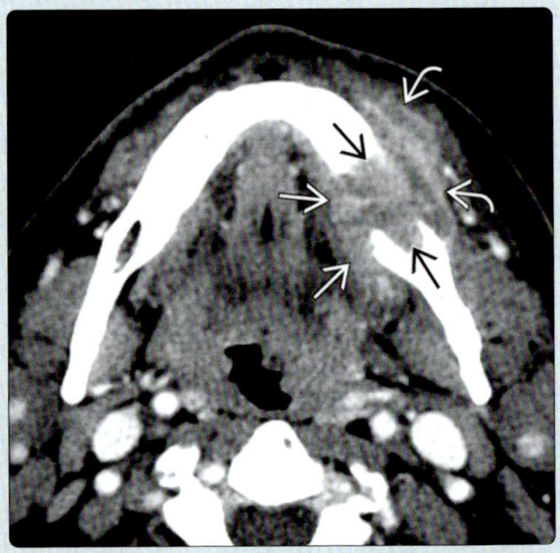

(Left) *Clinical intraoral photograph of a 66-year-old man depicts irregular, red, indurated, ulcerated lesion of left maxillary buccal gingiva in 1st premolar to molar area. Biopsy revealed invasive SCCa.* **(Right)** *Axial T1WI MR in the same patient shows subtle soft tissue fullness lateral to the maxillary alveolus with loss of normal fat planes compared to contralateral side. No convincing marrow infiltration is illustrated by imaging.*

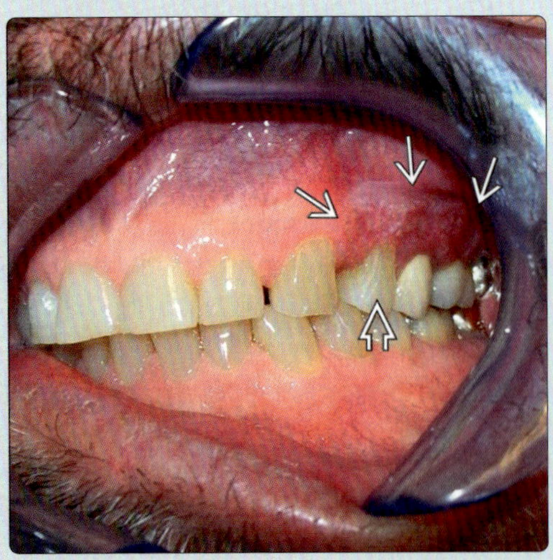

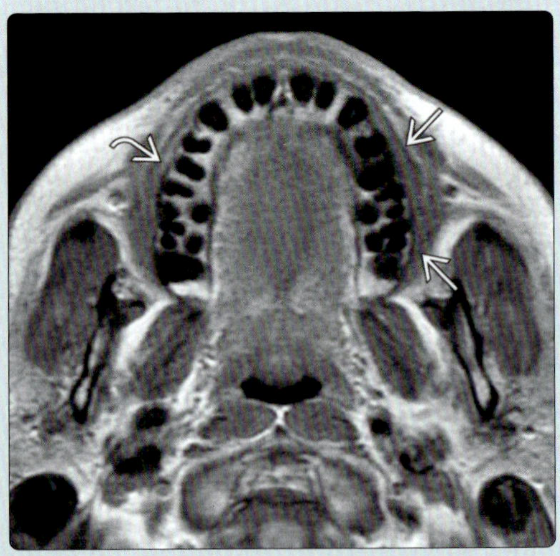

TERMINOLOGY

Abbreviations

- Squamous cell carcinoma (SCCa)

Definitions

- Invasive malignant neoplasm of squamous epithelium arising in gingiva
    - Because gingiva is ≤ 2-3 mm thick, strong predilection for bone invasion to underlying alveolus

IMAGING

General Features

- Best diagnostic clue
    - No imaging findings in lesions confined to gingiva
    - **Enhancing, infiltrating jaw mass** with underlying **bone destruction** if spreads to adjacent bone
- Location
    - Mandibular or maxillary gingiva; more common in mandible, posterior to premolars
- Size
    - Varies from mm to several cm
- Morphology
    - Poorly marginated mass

CT Findings

- CECT
    - Irregular, mild to moderately enhancing lesion
    - Small lesions may be occult to imaging
    - Perineural spread: Loss of normal fat density or excessive enhancement in foramina
- CBCT or bone CT
    - Destruction of alveolar bone of mandible/maxilla, widened periodontal ligament spaces

MR Findings

- T1WI
    - Isointense to muscle
    - Bone infiltration suggested by loss of high signal
- T1WI C+
    - Moderately enhancing mass of jaw
    - Marrow enhancement suggests invasion
        - Evaluate entire length of nerve to brainstem

Imaging Recommendations

- Best imaging tool
    - MR preferred for complete tumor extent
    - Bone CT or CBCT used for bone invasion
- Protocol advice
    - MR: Axial & coronal planes, fat saturation on T1 C+
    - CECT: Bone & soft tissue algorithm; axial, cross-sectional, & coronal planes, **thin sections**

Radiographic Findings

- Radiography
    - Widened periodontal ligament spaces, lamina dura destruction

DIFFERENTIAL DIAGNOSIS

Mandible-Maxilla Osteomyelitis

- Destructive focus ± adjacent soft tissue abscess

Mandible-Maxilla Osteoradionecrosis

- Destructive mandibular focus, prior XRT

Mandible-Maxilla Osteonecrosis

- Most commonly seen now with bisphosphonate use

Mandible-Maxilla Metastasis

- Aggressive mandibular mass, known primary

Mandible-Maxilla Osteosarcoma

- Aggressive mandibular lesion with periosteal reaction

PATHOLOGY

General Features

- Etiology
    - Alcohol & tobacco use with epithelial metaplasia → neoplasia

Staging, Grading, & Classification

- TNM staging is same for all oral cavity malignancies
- **Imaging is critical for determination of bone invasion**

CLINICAL ISSUES

Presentation

- Most common signs/symptoms
    - Nonhealing painless gingival ulcer is classic presentation
        - Nonulcerated mass also common and easily mistaken for benign lesion
    - Recent tooth extraction: Nonhealing site or soft tissue mass arising from socket
    - Can resemble periodontal lesion or periapical disease

Demographics

- Age
    - Mean age: 65 years
- Gender
    - M:F = 2:1

Natural History & Prognosis

- Gingival SCCa spreads locally to underlying bone and adjacent spaces
- **Overall 5-year survival** ~ **60%**
    - Cervical lymph node metastasis is most significant independent prognostic factor & decreases survival by almost 50%

Treatment

- Surgical resection ± reconstruction
    - ± adjuvant radiation, ± neck dissection depending on T stage

DIAGNOSTIC CHECKLIST

Consider

- Gingival mucosa attached to bone; allows early marrow infiltration: T4a

SELECTED REFERENCES

1. Yang X et al: Clinicopathological characteristics and outcome predictors in squamous cell carcinoma of the maxillary gingiva and hard palate. J Oral Maxillofac Surg. 73(7):1429-36, 2015

Retromolar Trigone Squamous Cell Carcinoma

KEY FACTS

TERMINOLOGY

- Retromolar trigone (RMT) squamous cell carcinoma (SCCa)
- RMT has complex shape: Mucosa over mandibular body & ramus posterior to molars, ascending to maxillary tuberosity

IMAGING

- RMT contiguous with anterior tonsillar pillar, buccal mucosa, & alveolar ridge mucosa
  - SCCa primary site may be difficult to determine
- CECT: Mildly enhancing mass, may be occult if small
  - Look for asymmetry of fat planes
  - Puffed-cheek technique may improve visualization of mucosal space tumor in RMT
  - Dental amalgam artifact may obscure primary tumor or tumor spreading via pterygomandibular raphe
- MR: Allows most accurate delineation of primary tumor, marrow infiltration, perineural & perifascial tumor
  - Less affected by dental amalgam artifact
- SCCa reliably FDG avid on PET/CT
  - Not often used unless extensive nodal disease

TOP DIFFERENTIAL DIAGNOSES

- Masticator space abscess
- Buccal mucosa SCCa
- Oral minor salivary gland malignancy

CLINICAL ISSUES

- Tumor often indolent with late presentation
- Bone/masticator muscle involvement → pain, trismus
  - Both indicate T4 disease; poorest prognosis
  - **Imaging key for determination of T4 disease**

DIAGNOSTIC CHECKLIST

- RMT site results in complex tumor spread patterns
  - Buccal & masticator spaces, oral cavity, & oropharynx
  - Mandible, maxilla, inferior alveolar nerve
  - Via **pterygomandibular raphe** to pterygoid plate
- Must evaluate for all potential spread sites

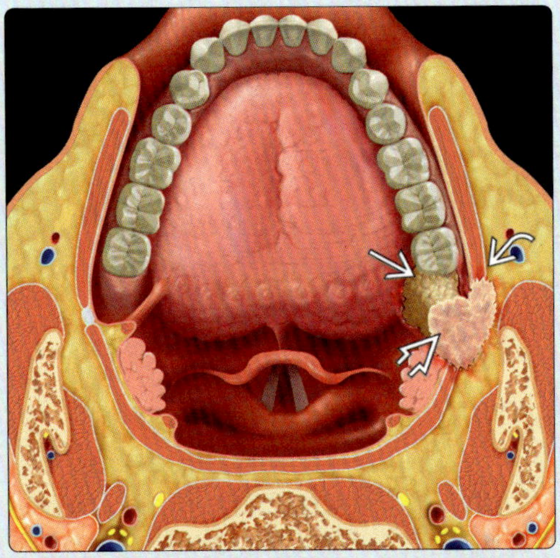

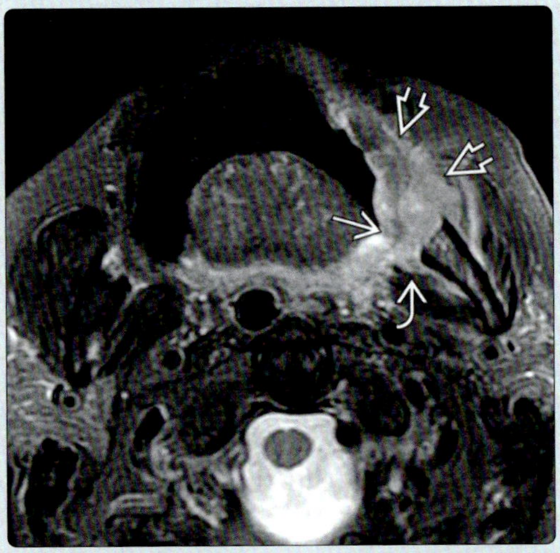

(Left) *Graphic illustrates squamous cell carcinoma (SCCa) ➔ arising posterior to the 3rd molar and extending superiorly along the pterygomandibular raphe and laterally onto the buccinator ➔. Tumor encroaches on the anterior tonsillar pillar ➔ of oropharynx.* **(Right)** *Axial T2WI FS MR in a patient with poorly healing socket following tooth extraction shows a mildly hyperintense soft tissue mass ➔ from RMT, which infiltrates to medial pterygoid ➔ (T4b disease). SCCa also infiltrates laterally to masseter and cheek ➔ along buccinator.*

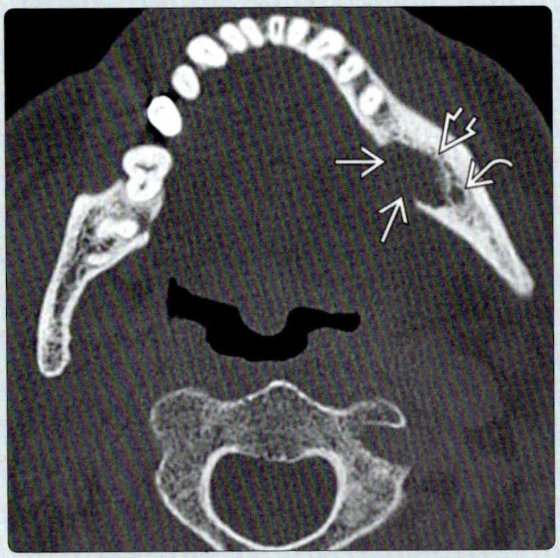

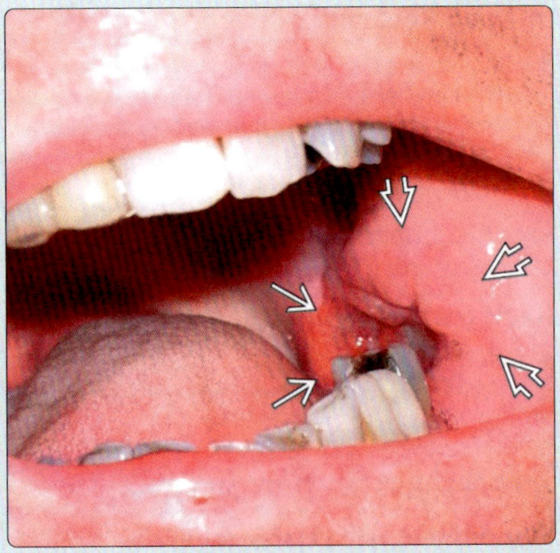

(Left) *Axial bone CT in the same patient shows a large lytic defect ➔ in the left mandible with an ill-defined lateral margin ➔. Note the proximity of the defect to the inferior alveolar canal ➔. Imaging features stage this as T4b.* **(Right)** *Clinical photograph in the same patient shows mucosal well-differentiated SCCa ➔ in the RMT. Note fullness of the left cheek ➔, indicating submucosal infiltration of the tumor and correlating with MR findings.*

TERMINOLOGY

Abbreviations

- Retromolar trigone (RMT) squamous cell carcinoma (SCCa)

Definitions

- Oral cavity mucosal malignancy
- RMT: Mucosa overlying ascending ramus of mandible posterior to molars, extending superiorly to maxillary tuberosity

IMAGING

General Features

- Best diagnostic clue
  - Focal enhancing lesion centered in RMT ± mandible or maxilla invasion
- Location
  - Mandibular angle, posterior to molars
  - RMT contiguous with anterior tonsillar pillar, buccal mucosa, & alveolar ridge mucosa, so primary site may be difficult to determine
- Size
  - Variable: < 2 cm (T1) to large mass infiltrating cheek & oropharynx

CT Findings

- CECT
  - Mildly enhancing infiltrative mass
- Bone CT
  - Important for cortical disruption, marrow infiltration

MR Findings

- T1WI
  - Isointense to muscle
    - Look for loss of marrow intensity
- T2WI
  - Hyperintense as compared to muscle
- T1WI C+ FS
  - Mild to moderately enhancing infiltrating mass
  - Evaluate for perineural tumor if mandible invaded

Nuclear Medicine Findings

- PET/CT
  - SCCa reliably FDG avid

Imaging Recommendations

- Best imaging tool
  - MR gives best delineation of tumor extent, marrow infiltration, perineural tumor
    - Small lesion may be occult on CECT
    - MR less affected by dental amalgam artifact
- Protocol advice
  - If CECT obtained, reformat in coronal plane as well
    - Bone & soft tissue algorithm postprocessing

DIFFERENTIAL DIAGNOSIS

Masticator Space Abscess

- Heterogeneous enhancement, cellulitis

Buccal Mucosa Squamous Cell Carcinoma

- Lesion arising from inner surface of cheeks or lips

Oral Minor Salivary Gland Malignancy

- Often more focal mass but has perineural spread

PATHOLOGY

Staging, Grading, & Classification

- American Joint Committee on Cancer (AJCC) 2010
  - **T1**: ≤ 2 cm in greatest diameter
  - **T2**: > 2 & ≤ 4 cm in greatest diameter
  - **T3**: > 4 cm in greatest diameter
  - **T4a**: Tumor invades through cortical bone & into extrinsic tongue muscles, skin of face
  - **T4b**: Tumor invades masticator space, pterygoid plates, skull base, or encases carotid
- Clinical mucosal extent more accurate than imaging
- **Imaging key for determination of T4 disease**

CLINICAL ISSUES

Presentation

- Most common signs/symptoms
  - Often indolent: Late presentation, high T stage
  - Bone/masticator muscle involvement results in pain, trismus

Demographics

- Age
  - Mean: 67 years
- Epidemiology
  - 7% of oral cavity tumors

Natural History & Prognosis

- Site of RMT allows for **unique tumor spread patterns**
  - Anterolaterally to buccinator muscle & cheek
  - Posterolaterally to buccal fat & masticator space
  - Posteromedially to tongue
  - Posteriorly to anterior tonsillar pillar & oropharynx
  - Superiorly to maxilla via **pterygomandibular raphe**
  - Inferiorly into mandible ± inferior alveolar nerve (IAN)
  - Presence of retromolar foramen may ↑ access to IAN
- Poor prognosis if bone or masticator space invasion
- 30% have nodal metastasis at diagnosis
- **Overall 5-year survival: ~ 60%**

Treatment

- Typically surgical resection ± adjuvant radiation
  - Surgery + radiation = best 5-year survival
- Some advocate primary radiation for low T-stage

DIAGNOSTIC CHECKLIST

Reporting Tips

- Tumor has **complex potential spread patterns**; important that imaging studies evaluated for all

SELECTED REFERENCES

1. Hitchcock KE et al: Retromolar trigone squamous cell carcinoma treated with radiotherapy alone or combined with surgery: a 10-year update. Am J Otolaryngol. 36(2):140-5, 2015
2. Mazziotti S et al: Diagnostic approach to retromolar trigone cancer by multiplanar computed tomography reconstructions. Can Assoc Radiol J. 65(4):335-44, 2014

Submandibular Space Nodal Squamous Cell Carcinoma

KEY FACTS

TERMINOLOGY

- Submandibular space (SMS), nodal squamous cell carcinoma (SCCa)

IMAGING

- SMS level IA & IB nodes
  - Level IA: Suprahyoid node(s) between anterior belly of digastric muscles
  - Level IB: Suprahyoid node(s) located lateral, & immediately anterior to a line tangent to posterior border of submandibular glands
- CECT or MR findings
  - CECT generally preferred over MR for nodal staging
  - CECT improves N staging accuracy over clinical staging
  - SMS nodes **> 1.5 cm** considered malignant in context of H&N SCCa
  - **Central nodal necrosis** considered sign of malignant involvement in any size node
  - Irregular enhancing margin invades adjacent soft tissues implies **extracapsular spread**
- PET/CT
  - Superior to CT/MR in clinical N0 neck
- Ultrasonographic findings
  - Round node with loss of hilar echogenicity
  - Main limitation is some nodes are inaccessible

TOP DIFFERENTIAL DIAGNOSES

- Suppurative lymph nodes
- Nodal non-Hodgkin lymphoma

CLINICAL ISSUES

- Treatment: Primary tumor resection vs. chemoradiotherapy ± nodal dissection
- Prognostic implication of malignant adenopathy
  - Single unilateral node ↓ prognosis by 50%
  - Bilateral nodes ↓ prognosis by 75%
  - Extracapsular spread ↓ prognosis by further 50%

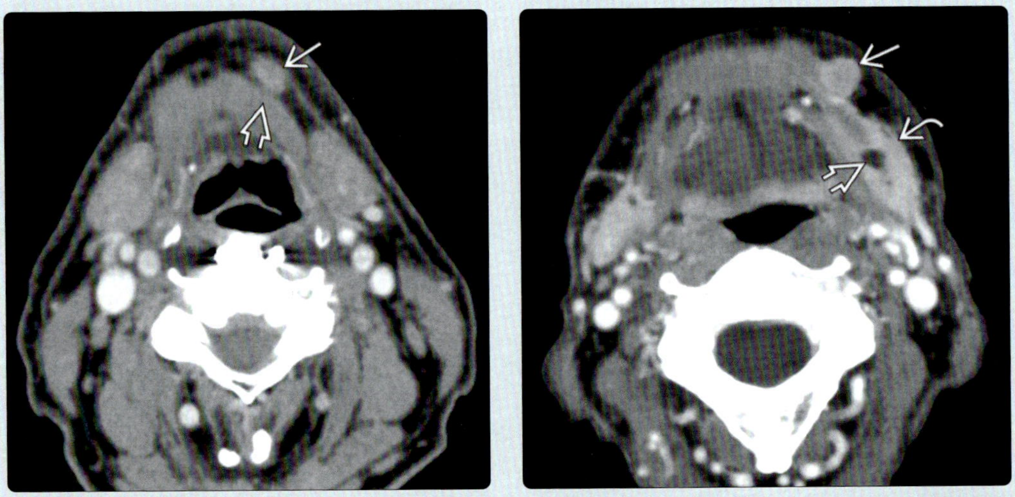

(Left) *Axial CECT in a patient with a lower lip squamous cell carcinoma (SCCa) shows a single pathologic (subtle low-density center) SMS node. The node is lateral to the anterior belly of the digastric muscle, making it a level IB node.* **(Right)** *Axial CECT through the suprahyoid neck reveals an enlarged, round, enhancing metastatic level IB SCCa node. The left submandibular gland (SMG) is enlarged & enhancing with dilated hilar duct. Anterior floor of mouth SCCa (not shown) has obstructed the submandibular duct.*

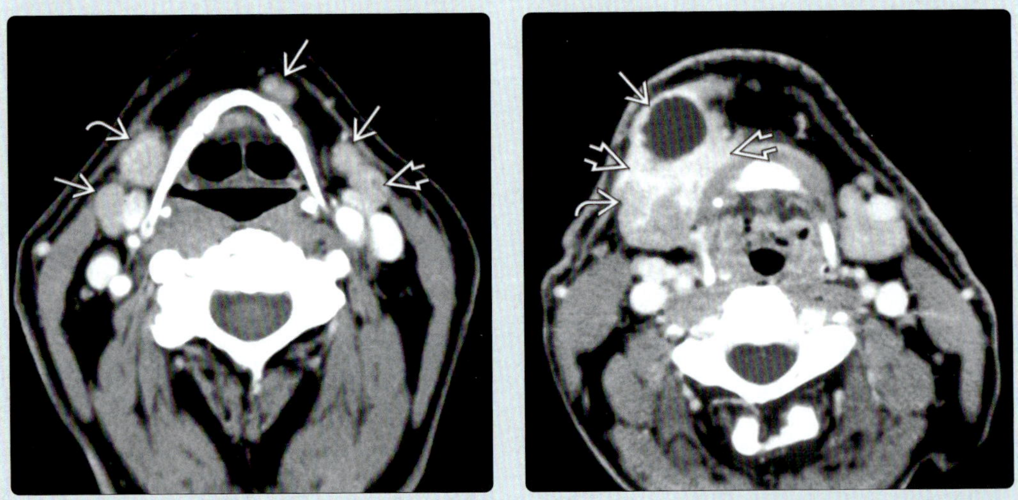

(Left) *Axial CECT in a patient with anterior floor of mouth primary SCCa shows multiple level IB nodes. A few enhance, but not all are malignant by CT criteria. Two nodes meet criteria for malignancy: 1 on right based on size > 1.5 cm, and 1 on left due to central low density.* **(Right)** *Axial CECT reveals a large cystic level IB SMS nodal mass in a patient with lateral tongue SCCa. Enhancing spreading nodal margins inseparable from surrounding tissues suggest extracapsular extension. The SMG is engulfed by spreading tumor.*

TERMINOLOGY

Abbreviations

- Submandibular space (SMS), squamous cell carcinoma (SCCa)

Definitions

- Submandibular level I nodal metastasis from primary H&N SCCa

IMAGING

General Features

- Best diagnostic clue
  - Enlarged (> 1.5 cm), abnormally rounded, or centrally necrotic SMS node(s)
- Location
  - SMS level IA & IB nodes
    - Level IA nodes: Between anterior bellies of digastric muscles
    - Level IB nodes: Anterior, lateral, & anterior to posterior border of submandibular glands
- Size
  - SMS nodes > 1.5 cm considered malignant in context of H&N SCCa
    - Central nodal necrosis in any size node considered pathologic
- Morphology
  - Round contour + loss of fatty hilum: Suspicious for malignant involvement
  - Node with enhancing, irregular margins: Suspicious for extracapsular tumor spread

CT Findings

- CECT
  - Enhancing level IA or IB nodal mass > 1.5 cm ± central necrosis
  - Irregular enhancing margin invades adjacent soft tissues: Extranodal spread
  - High prevalence of positive nodes in clinically N0 necks in oral cavity SCCa, especially tongue

MR Findings

- T1WI C+
  - Enhancing level IA or IB nodal mass > 1.5 cm ± central low signal

Ultrasonographic Findings

- Grayscale ultrasound
  - Round node with loss of hilar echogenicity
  - Main limitation is nodes too deep for visualization (e.g., retropharyngeal nodes)

Nuclear Medicine Findings

- PET/CT
  - FDG: Focal areas of ↑ uptake matching SMS node indicates malignant nature
    - Superior to CT/MR in clinically N0 neck

DIFFERENTIAL DIAGNOSIS

Suppurative Lymph Nodes

- Sick or septic patient
- Central fluid density within nodes
- Can mimic SCCa nodes

Nodal Non-Hodgkin Lymphoma of SMS

- Multiple bilateral, large, usually nonnecrotic nodes
- No primary SCCa on clinical exam

PATHOLOGY

General Features

- Etiology
  - Lymphatic spread of primary SCCa to SMS nodes
  - Common drainage pathways for SCCa SMS nodes
    - All oral cavity sites
    - Anterior facial structures, lips, and skin
    - Oropharynx & hypopharynx SCCa can spread to SMS nodes if N2 disease (1 or more nodes in levels II-IV already involved)

Microscopic Features

- Metastases 1st lodge in subcapsular sinus → spread through node
- Characterized by squamous differentiation frequently with keratinizing morphology
- Necrosis, edema, or tumor cells in nodes may appear as nodal low density on CECT

CLINICAL ISSUES

Presentation

- Most common signs/symptoms
  - Painless, firm SMS mass
    - May be fixed to mandible ± adjacent tissues

Demographics

- Age
  - Most commonly > 40 yr

Natural History & Prognosis

- **Nodal metastasis** is single **most important prognostic factor** for H&N SCCa
  - Single unilateral node ↓ prognosis by 50%
  - Bilateral nodes reduce prognosis by 75%
  - Extranodal spread reduces prognosis by further 50%
    - Risk of recurrence ↑ 10x

Treatment

- Surgical resection ± chemoradiotherapy ± node dissection

DIAGNOSTIC CHECKLIST

Consider

- Nodal size (> 1.5 cm) or parenchymal inhomogeneity key to labeling malignant based on imaging

SELECTED REFERENCES

1. Brockhoff HC 2nd et al: Correlating the depth of invasion at specific anatomic locations with the risk for regional metastatic disease to lymph nodes in the neck for oral squamous cell carcinoma. Head Neck. ePub, 2017
2. Furukawa M et al: The prevalence of lymph node metastases in clinically N0 necks with oral cavity squamous cell carcinoma: is CT good enough for nodal staging? Acta Radiol. 55(5):570-8, 2014
3. King AD et al: Necrosis in metastatic neck nodes: diagnostic accuracy of CT, MR imaging, and US. Radiology. 230(3):720-6, 2004

Buccal Mucosa Squamous Cell Carcinoma

KEY FACTS

TERMINOLOGY

- Buccal mucosa squamous cell carcinoma (SCCa)
- Oral cavity mucosal malignancy arising from inner lining of cheek and lips

IMAGING

- Typically difficult to identify with routine imaging
- Mild to moderately enhancing irregular lesion
- Look for asymmetrically infiltrated buccal fat
- CECT: Puffed cheek method works well to separate mucosal surfaces and see site of origin
- MR: Hypointense gauze padding works similarly and often better tolerated with long MR sequences
- FDG avid (reserved for advanced nodal disease)
  - Nodes are important prognostic factor

TOP DIFFERENTIAL DIAGNOSES

- Oral cavity infection
- Oral cavity minor salivary gland malignancy

PATHOLOGY

- Traditionally poorest prognosis of oral cavity SCCa
  - Recent studies suggest similar prognosis to cancers in other oral cavity sites once age at diagnosis, tumor stage, treatment, and race are taken into consideration
- Strong association with tobacco, alcohol, betel nut, & paan
- All oral cavity tumors use same TNM classification
- Imaging important for deep extent
  - Identifying buccal space invasion & T4 features
  - T4a: Tumor invades skin of face, through cortical bone, into extrinsic tongue muscles
  - T4b: Tumor invades masticator space, pterygoid plates, skull base, or encases carotid

DIAGNOSTIC CHECKLIST

- Clinical history indicating site of lesion important
- Look for infiltration of buccal space fat
  - If present, evaluate for masticator space infiltration
- 1st-order node drainage: Buccal & level I, II nodes

(Left) *Coronal graphic depicts T2 (2-4 cm) buccal mucosal squamous cell carcinoma (SCCa) that has invaded the underlying buccinator muscle & subcutaneous fat. If the lesion had involved the cheek skin, it would be staged as T4. Note the normal left buccinator.* **(Right)** *Coronal T1WI MR performed with a patient using the puffed cheek method shows the cheek displaced from gingival mucosa and subtle nodularity of the right buccal mucosa, representing SCCa. No evidence of deep infiltration is seen.*

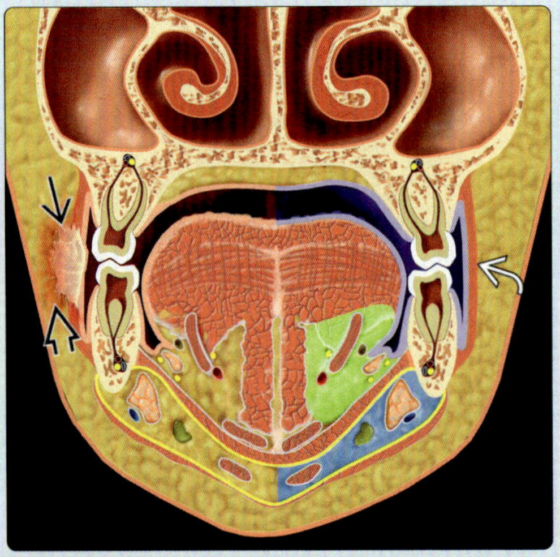

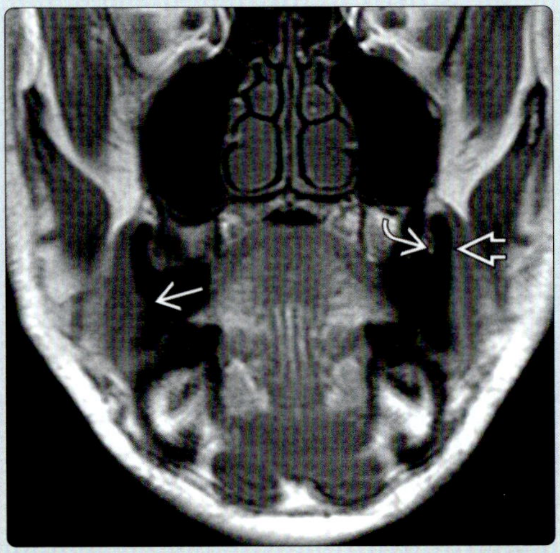

(Left) *Axial T1WI MR demonstrates an ill-defined tissue filling the buccal fat pad from deep infiltration of buccal mucosal malignancy. Note the smooth contours on the contralateral side and the clean buccal fat. Without a clear history of the primary site, buccal fat infiltration may only be a subtle imaging finding.* **(Right)** *Clinical photograph in the same patient shows buccal mucosal primary SCCa along the posterior aspect of the inner cheek, extending to the posterior margin maxillary (edentulous) alveolus.*

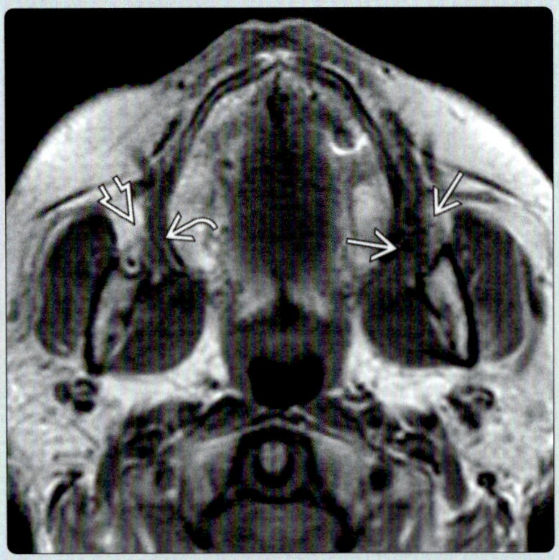

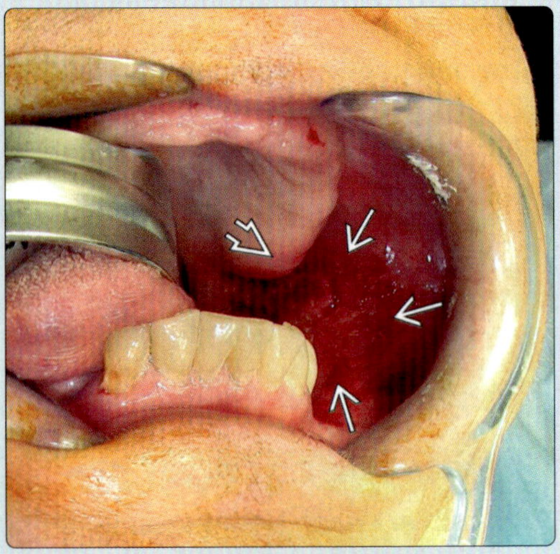

TERMINOLOGY

Abbreviations

- Buccal mucosa squamous cell carcinoma (SCCa)

Definitions

- Mucosal malignancy arising from inner lining of cheek, lips

IMAGING

General Features

- Best diagnostic clue
  - May be very subtle, even when infiltrating buccal fat
- Location
  - Most often inner aspect of cheek
- Size
  - Variable: Several mm to several cm

CT Findings

- CECT
  - Often extremely difficult to see on routine imaging
  - Look for subtle asymmetry of buccal fat
  - Mild to moderately enhancing irregular lesion

MR Findings

- Hard to see primary lesion without clinical history
  - Isointense on T1, slightly hyperintense on T2
  - Look for infiltration of buccal fat
- Variable enhancement: Mild to moderate

Nuclear Medicine Findings

- PET/CT
  - SCCa reliably FDG avid

Imaging Recommendations

- Best imaging tool
  - MR generally preferred in oral cavity with better tissue contrast for delineation of tumor extent
- Protocol advice
  - CECT: Soft tissue and bone algorithm in 2 planes
    - **Puffed cheek method** works well to separate opposed mucosal surfaces
  - MR: Puffed cheek method not often successful because of sequence time
    - Consider use of **gauze padding** in cheek instead

DIFFERENTIAL DIAGNOSIS

Oral Cavity Infection

- Superinfected traumatic ulcer may result in local inflammation ± cellulitis
- May have reactive buccal adenopathy

Oral Cavity Minor Salivary Gland Malignancy

- Uncommonly arises from buccal mucosa
- Indistinguishable from SCCa

PATHOLOGY

General Features

- Etiology
  - Strongly associated with tobacco (smoking and chewing) and alcohol abuse
    - In oral cavity, the association with tobacco is strongest for floor of mouth and buccal mucosa
  - In central and Southeast Asia, associated with chewing betel nut and paan (tobacco + nut + lime)

Staging, Grading, & Classification

- American Joint Committee on Cancer (AJCC) 2010
- **Same classification for all oral cavity tumors**
  - T1: ≤ 2 cm in greatest diameter
  - T2: > 2 & ≤ 4 cm in greatest diameter
  - T3: > 4 cm in greatest diameter
  - T4a: Tumor invades skin of face, through cortical bone, into extrinsic tongue muscles
  - T4b: Tumor invades masticator space, pterygoid plates, skull base, or encases carotid
- **Nodal staging**: AJCC, follows oropharyngeal and laryngeal nodal staging
- **Metastatic disease**: Absent = M0, present = M1

CLINICAL ISSUES

Presentation

- Most common signs/symptoms
  - Mild discomfort; may "catch" in teeth

Demographics

- Age
  - Mean: 50-70 years
- Gender
  - M > F
- Epidemiology
  - In North America, represents 10% of oral malignancies
  - In Taiwan, represents up to 37% from chewing betel nut and paan

Natural History & Prognosis

- Tendency for submucosal spread, then laterally to skin
- Generally poor prognosis because of high recurrence rate and invasive spread
  - Overall prognosis: Up to 60% 5-year survival
- Poor prognostic factors: Positive surgical margin, **cervical nodal metastasis (especially if extracapsular spread)**, advanced tumor stage, tumor thickness > 7 mm

Treatment

- Surgical: Resection ± reconstruction ± nodal dissection
- ± adjuvant radiation

DIAGNOSTIC CHECKLIST

Image Interpretation Pearls

- Clinical history indicating site of lesion important
- Look for infiltration of buccal fat
  - If present, evaluate for masticator space infiltration
- Look for buccal and level I, II nodes

SELECTED REFERENCES

1. Camilon PR et al: Does buccal cancer have worse prognosis than other oral cavity cancers? Laryngoscope. 124(6):1386-91, 2014
2. Erdogan N et al: Puffed-cheek computed tomography: a dynamic maneuver for imaging oral cavity tumors. Ear Nose Throat J. 91(9):383-4, 386, 2012
3. Dillon JK et al: Gauze padding: a simple technique to delineate small oral cavity tumors. AJNR Am J Neuroradiol. 32(5):934-7, 2011

Hard Palate Squamous Cell Carcinoma

KEY FACTS

TERMINOLOGY

- Hard palate squamous cell carcinoma (SCCa)
- Oral cavity mucosal malignancy of roof of mouth

IMAGING

- Often extremely subtle, may be occult to imaging
- Variable size from several mm to several cm
- **Coronal plane** imaging **key** for either CT or MR
- CECT: Mild to moderately enhancing ill-defined lesion with associated bone erosion
  - Both soft tissue and bone algorithm important
- MR: Low T1 tumor signal contrasts against hyperintense palate marrow and mucosa
  - T1 C+ FS and T2 FS aid tumor delineation
  - Look at **greater palatine canal** and **pterygopalatine fossa** for CNV2 perineural tumor spread

TOP DIFFERENTIAL DIAGNOSES

- Hard palate minor salivary gland carcinoma
- Palate benign mixed tumor
- Invasive sinonasal SCCa

CLINICAL ISSUES

- Ulcer ± mass on roof of mouth; often painful
- Clinically obvious lesion may be subtle on CT or MR
- Rare tumor; least common oral cavity site
- In this location, SCCa is less common than minor salivary malignancies
- Overall 5-year survival ~ 60%
- Treatment: Surgical resection ± neck dissection ± XRT
  - Elective neck dissection associated with lower recurrence rate, better overall survival

DIAGNOSTIC CHECKLIST

- Must evaluate bone for erosion ± infiltration
- MR better evaluates **greater palatine canal** and **pterygopalatine fossa** for CNV2 perineural tumor spread
- Evaluate carefully for nodal metastases

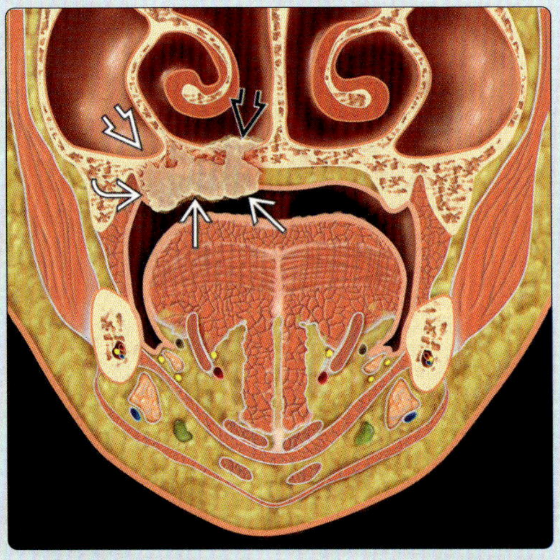

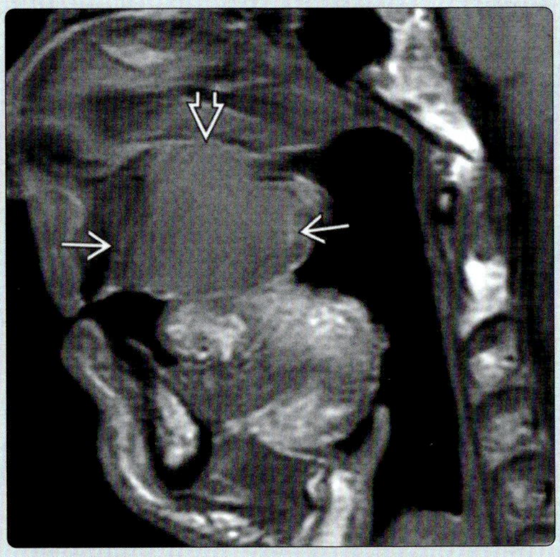

(Left) *Coronal graphic illustrates oral cavity SCCa ➔ arising from mucosa of the hard palate and infiltrating underlying bone. The tumor may extend through palatine portion of maxilla ➔ to floor of the nasal cavity or through the alveolar bone ➔ to the maxillary sinus ➔. Perineural tumor spread may occur along the 2nd division of trigeminal nerve, V2.* **(Right)** *Sagittal T1WI MR shows a patient with prior retromolar trigone SCCa and a new large oral cavity SCCa ➔ that destroys the hard palate and extends into the nasal cavity ➔.*

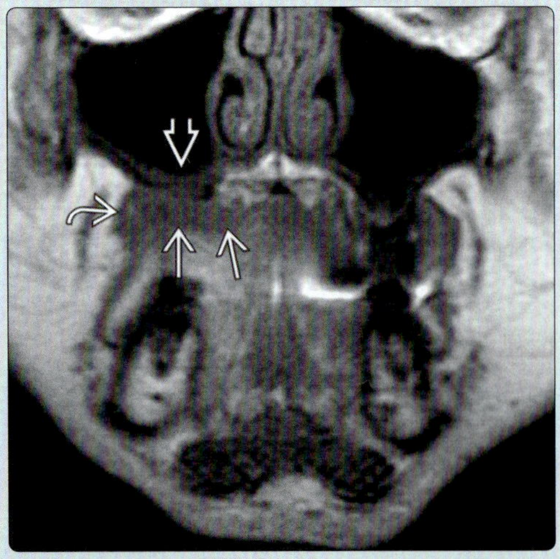

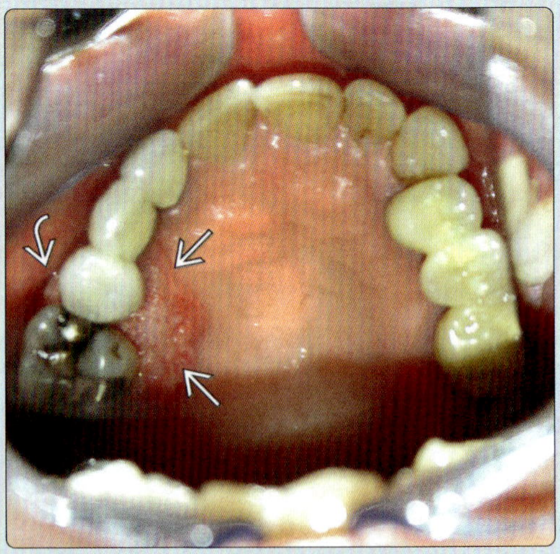

(Left) *Coronal T1WI MR demonstrates subtle mucosal lesion ➔ of hard palate that extends through maxillary alveolus to both buccal mucosa ➔ and the maxillary sinus floor ➔. The tumor is T4aN0, stage IVA disease. Palatal lesions are often best seen on T1 precontrast and in coronal plane.* **(Right)** *Clinical photograph taken with an oral mirror demonstrates a clinically obvious maxillary mass involving the palatal mucosa ➔. The tumor was extremely subtle on imaging. Extension through to buccal surface is also evident ➔.*

TERMINOLOGY

Abbreviations

- Hard palate squamous cell carcinoma (SCCa)

Definitions

- Oral cavity malignancy arising from mucosa overlying hard palate

IMAGING

General Features

- Location
  - Hard palate (best known as roof of mouth)
- Size
  - Variable: Several mm to several cm

CT Findings

- CECT
  - Often extremely subtle or occult to imaging
  - Mild to moderate enhancement
- Bone CT
  - Erosion of bone often found

MR Findings

- Low T1 signal contrasts against bright palate marrow
- Mild to moderate enhancement

Imaging Recommendations

- Best imaging tool
  - MR allows evaluation of marrow and perineural tumor spread along palatine canals
- Protocol advice
  - Coronal plane essential for either CT or MR
  - CECT: Obtain soft tissue and bone algorithm

DIFFERENTIAL DIAGNOSIS

Hard Palate Minor Salivary Gland Carcinoma

- Mucoepidermoid and adenoid cystic carcinoma most frequent and much more common than SCCa
- May be smooth bone erosion or aggressive destruction
- Perineural tumor spread frequently found

Palate Benign Mixed Tumor

- Well-circumscribed T2 intense round mass
- Typically smooth erosion of bone

Sinonasal Squamous Cell Carcinoma

- Maxillary sinus tumor may extend into palate
- Clinically presents as submucosal mass

PATHOLOGY

General Features

- Etiology
  - Associated with tobacco and alcohol abuse but not as strong association as other oral cavity SCCa sites
  - Fruits and vegetables appear to have protective effect

Staging, Grading, & Classification

- American Joint Committee on Cancer (AJCC) 2010
- All oral cavity malignancies use same TNM staging
- **T1**: ≤ 2 cm in greatest diameter
- **T2**: > 2 & ≤ 4 cm
- **T3**: > 4 cm
- **T4a**: Tumor invades maxillary sinus, skin of face, through cortical bone, deep tongue muscles
- **T4b**: Tumor invades masticator space, pterygoid plates, skull base, or encases carotid
- Size of mucosal component best evaluated clinically

Gross Pathologic & Surgical Features

- Red and white well-demarcated areas of induration
- Ulcerated areas indurated, tender upon palpation

Microscopic Features

- Squamous differentiation with intracellular bridges or keratinization, ± keratin pearls
- Further classified by degree of differentiation

CLINICAL ISSUES

Presentation

- Most common signs/symptoms
  - Painful ulcer on roof of mouth
- Other signs/symptoms
  - Bleeding, ill-fitting dentures, loose teeth
  - Facial tingling/pain → **V2 perineural tumor spread**

Demographics

- Age
  - Mean: 70 years
- Gender
  - M > F

Natural History & Prognosis

- Survival strongly correlates with T stage
  - Mean survival: T1 = 8 years, T4 ~ 4 years
- Nodal metastasis significantly impacts survival
  - **Levels I, II** are 1st-order drainage sites
- Overall 5-year survival ~ 60%

Treatment

- Surgical resection ± neck dissection ± adjuvant radiation

DIAGNOSTIC CHECKLIST

Consider

- Often very subtle lesion at imaging, though typically clinically apparent

Image Interpretation Pearls

- Coronal plane imaging is key for either CT or MR

Reporting Tips

- Must evaluate bone for erosion &/or infiltration
- MR better evaluates palatine canals for greater palatine nerve (CNV2) perineural tumor
- Evaluate carefully for nodal metastases

SELECTED REFERENCES

1. Givi B et al: Impact of elective neck dissection on the outcome of oral squamous cell carcinomas arising in the maxillary alveolus and hard palate. Head Neck. 38 Suppl 1:E1688-94, 2016
2. Arya S et al: Oral cavity squamous cell carcinoma: role of pretreatment imaging and its influence on management. Clin Radiol. 69(9):916-30, 2014
3. Kato H et al: CT and MR imaging findings of palatal tumors. Eur J Radiol. 83(3):e137-46, 2014

Motor Denervation CNXII

KEY FACTS

TERMINOLOGY

- Abbreviation: Hypoglossal nerve (CNXII)
- Definition: Loss of nerve supply to muscles in 1/2 of tongue

IMAGING

- Asymmetry of tongue appearance with linear demarcation of abnormality; varies over time
- CT density and MR signal intensity vary over time
- Acute (typically < 1 month)
  - 1/2 of tongue initially **swollen**, then atrophies
  - Enhancement variable
- Subacute (typically 1-20 months)
  - Loss of volume and **fatty change** of half of tongue
  - Decreasing enhancement
- Chronic (typically > 20 months)
  - **Fatty atrophy**, no enhancement
- Image course of **CNXII from skull base to hyoid**

TOP DIFFERENTIAL DIAGNOSES

- Lingual tonsil squamous cell carcinoma
- Oral tongue squamous cell carcinoma
- Oral cavity lymphatic malformation
- Oral cavity venous malformation

PATHOLOGY

- Many causes; may be isolated or with CNIX-XI

DIAGNOSTIC CHECKLIST

- Consider: Frequent source of mistaken identity
  - Flaccid 1/2 of tongue hangs posteriorly into oropharynx; mistaken for tongue base tumor
  - Contralateral larger 1/2 of tongue may be mistaken for tongue tumor
  - Loss of FDG uptake may be mistaken for contralateral tumor
- **Sharp line** delineating unilateral changes **is key**

(Left) *Axial T2WI MR shows acute stage of tongue denervation with swollen left hemitongue and markedly increased T2 signal from edema ➡. Note sharp delineation of abnormality. Denervation was due to perineural tumor spread along CNXII.* **(Right)** *Coronal T1WI C+ FS MR shows subacute denervation changes with heterogeneous enhancement of unilateral left tongue musculature ➡. Note again sharp demarcation of changes. Finding was secondary to skull base metastatic focus involving hypoglossal canal.*

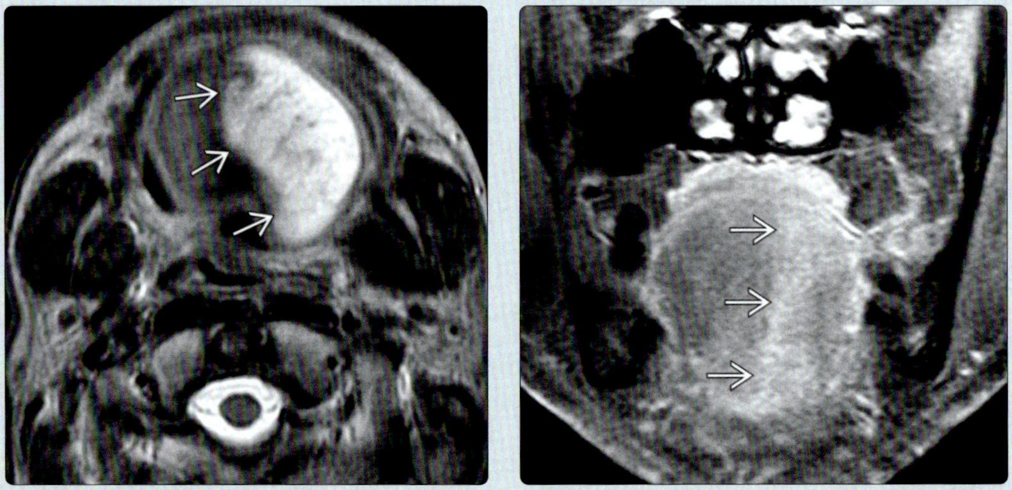

(Left) *Axial T1WI MR shows chronic changes of tongue denervation with markedly increased signal ➡ in left hemitongue, consistent with fatty replacement. Hypoglossal denervation was due to jugular foramen paraganglioma (not shown).* **(Right)** *Axial CECT shows fatty atrophy from chronic left hypoglossal nerve denervation ➡. Right 1/2 of tongue appears larger than left and can be mistaken for tongue tumor. Denervation was found to be secondary to destructive bone lesion at hypoglossal canal.*

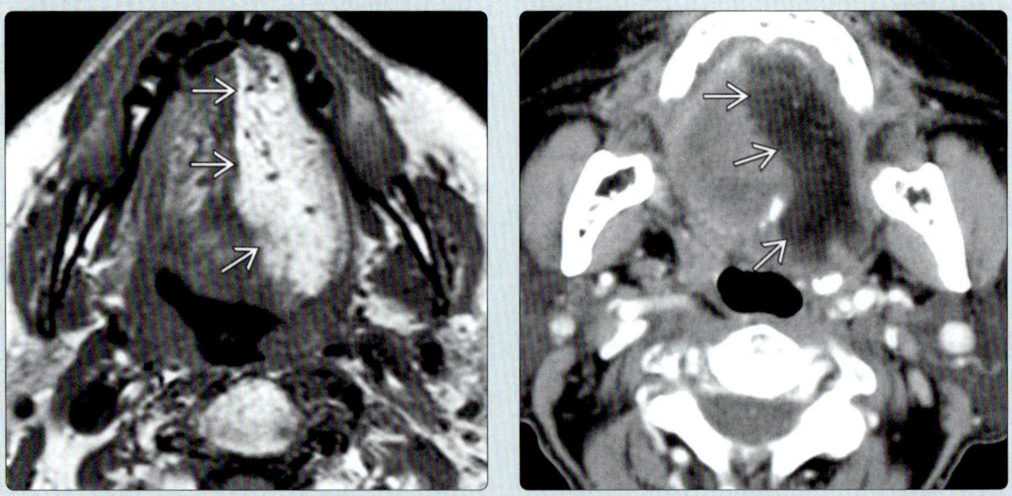

TERMINOLOGY

Synonyms

- Hypoglossal nerve (CNXII) palsy, hypoglossal nerve paralysis, tongue denervation

Definitions

- Loss of nerve supply to muscles in 1/2 of tongue
  - Note palatoglossus supplied by CNX

IMAGING

General Features

- Best diagnostic clue
  - Asymmetry of tongue appearance with linear demarcation of abnormality
- Location
  - Unilateral tongue musculature
- Morphology
  - Varies over time
    - Initially swollen then atrophies
    - Flaccidity of ipsilateral tongue muscles

CT Findings

- CECT
  - Initial: Unilateral swelling of tongue
    - Ipsilateral tongue flaccidity
  - Later: Loss of volume and decreased density of 1/2 of tongue

MR Findings

- Signal intensity varies over time following denervation
- Acute (typically < 1 month)
  - **Tongue swollen**, flaccid
  - Increased T2 intensity of 1/2 of tongue; subtly decreased T1 signal
  - Enhancement variable in acute phase
- Subacute (typically 1-20 months)
  - **Swelling resolves**, fatty atrophy
  - Increasing T1 intensity, decreasing enhancement
- Chronic (typically > 20 months)
  - **Atrophy** of hemitongue
  - Marked T1 intensity, enhancement resolves

Nuclear Medicine Findings

- PET/CT
  - Denervated 1/2 of tongue has loss of FDG uptake

Imaging Recommendations

- Best imaging tool
  - Either CECT or MR evaluates CNXII course well
- Protocol advice
  - **Must image from skull base to hyoid along course of CNXII**

DIFFERENTIAL DIAGNOSIS

Lingual Tonsil Squamous Cell Carcinoma

- Enhancing tumor at base of tongue

Oral Tongue Squamous Cell Carcinoma

- Enhancing lesion most commonly arising from lateral margin

Oral Cavity Lymphatic Malformation

- Multiloculated septated transspatial lesion

Oral Cavity Venous Malformation

- Enhancing, irregular lesion involving multiple spaces

PATHOLOGY

General Features

- Etiology
  - Lesion along course of CNXII
  - If isolated, CNXII neuropathy most commonly due to skull base lesion
    - Bone lesion: Metastasis or direct tumor invasion, osteomyelitis
    - Postoperative: Injury at endarterectomy, neck dissection
    - Vascular: Carotid dissection, vascular malformation
    - Post radiation: Fibrosis
    - Rarely brainstem or cerebellopontine angle lesion
  - With other cranial nerves: CNIX-XI
    - Upper carotid sheath lesion; skull base lesion to jugular foramen

CLINICAL ISSUES

Presentation

- Most common signs/symptoms
  - Tongue **deviation to side of denervation** on protrusion
  - Tongue paralysis, fasciculations, loss of tone
- Other signs/symptoms
  - Other cranial nerves may be involved: CNIX-XI
- Clinical profile
  - Most often older patient with skull base lesion or head and neck tumor

DIAGNOSTIC CHECKLIST

Consider

- Frequent source of mistaken identity
  - Flaccid 1/2 of tongue hangs posteriorly into oropharynx, mimicking tongue base tumor
  - Contralateral tongue may be mistaken as abnormally enlarged secondary to tongue tumor
  - Loss of FDG uptake may be mistaken for contralateral tumor on PET/CT

Image Interpretation Pearls

- Key imaging feature is **sharp line** delineating unilateral tongue changes

Reporting Tips

- Carefully review from low cerebellopontine angle along course of CNXII to find cause

SELECTED REFERENCES

1. Nestola DF et al: Isolated hypoglossal nerve palsy mimicking a base of tongue tumor. J Craniofac Surg. 28(1):e78-e80, 2017
2. Stino AM et al: Hypoglossal nerve palsy: 245 cases. Muscle Nerve. 54(6):1050-1054, 2016
3. Junquera L et al: Images in clinical medicine. Denervation atrophy of the tongue after hypoglossal-nerve injury. N Engl J Med. 367(2):156, 2012

Submandibular Sialoliths

KEY FACTS

TERMINOLOGY

- Synonyms: Salivary stone, salivary calculus, mucus plug

IMAGING

- Imaging protocol
  - Intraoral (occlusal) and panoramic radiographs, consider US
  - Conventional sialography or MR sialography is appropriate for minimally calcified sialoliths (mucus plugs)
  - Begin with intraoral (occlusal) and panoramic radiographs: If further localization is required, CBCT or CECT is appropriate
- Appearance and location
  - Ovoid, concentrically calcified radiopaque mass medial/lingual to posterior mandible in area of submandibular gland and Wharton duct
  - May be associated with sialodochitis from retrograde ductal infection

TOP DIFFERENTIAL DIAGNOSES

- Calcified lymph node
- Phlebolith
- Idiopathic osteosclerosis/enostosis

PATHOLOGY

- **Submandibular gland is most common site** for sialoliths due to high mucous viscosity of submandibular saliva
- 30% of submandibular sialoliths are at hilum or in **proximal portion of Wharton duct**

CLINICAL ISSUES

- May be multiple
- Swelling and **discomfort, particularly at meal times**, but may be asymptomatic
- Intermittent ductal dilation and stricture from retrograde infection is commonly present (sialodochitis)
- Treatment: Surgical retrieval of sialolith or excision of entire gland

(Left) *Cropped panoramic radiograph shows a right submandibular gland sialolith* ➡ *imaged adjacent to the inferior mandibular border. Submandibular sialoliths may mimic focal idiopathic osteosclerosis when superimposed over the mandible.* **(Right)** *Occlusal radiograph of the right mandible shows an oblong-shaped sialolith* ➡ *in the Wharton duct of the submandibular gland. Thirty percent of submandibular sialoliths are at the hilum or in the proximal portion of the Wharton duct.*

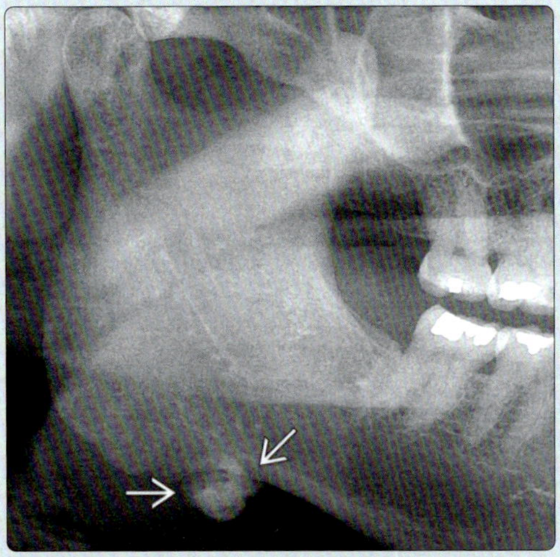

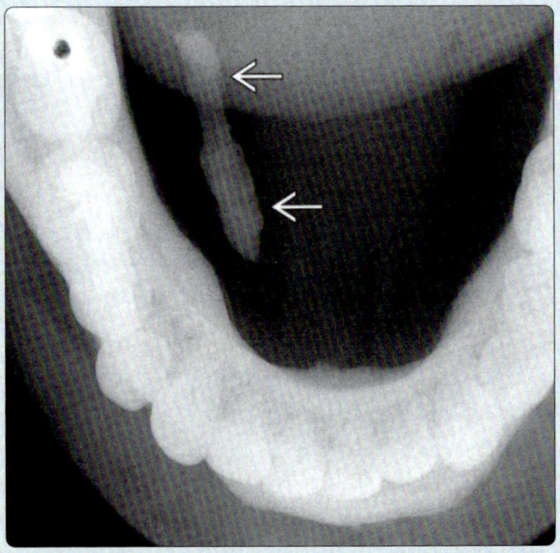

(Left) *Coronal CBCT shows a submandibular sialolith* ➡ *located in the left Wharton duct. Note the variable calcification layers and ovoid morphology.* **(Right)** *Conventional sialography demonstrates radiopaque* ➡ *and radiolucent* ➡ *sialoliths with the classic ductal dilation and stricture (sausage-link) pattern of secondary sialodochitis. Twenty percent of submandibular sialoliths are poorly calcified and will appear as a filling void or radiolucency.*

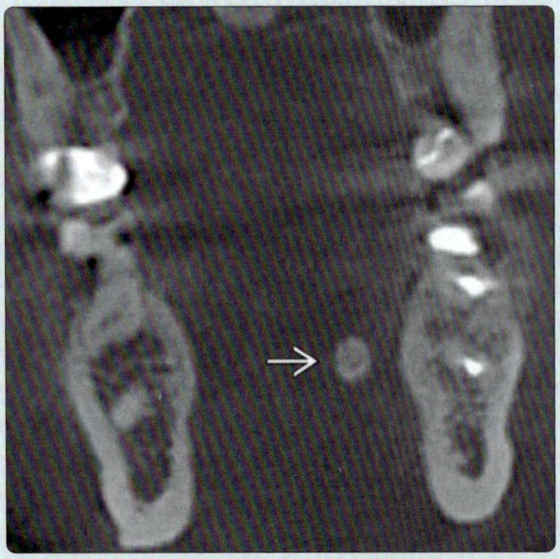

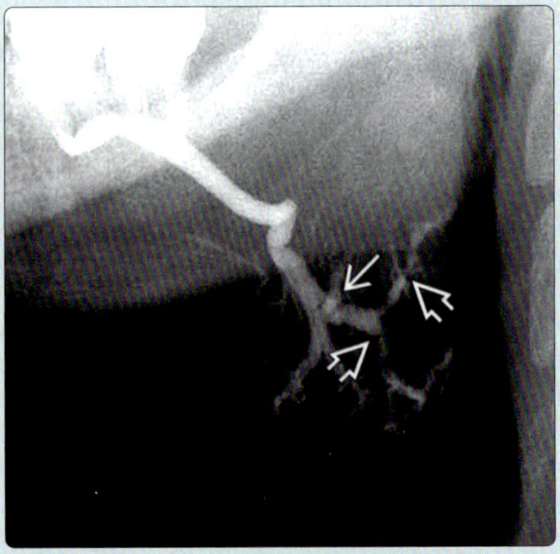

TERMINOLOGY

Synonyms

- Salivary stone/calculus, mucus plug, sialolithiasis

Definitions

- Calcified ductal obstruction within submandibular gland

IMAGING

General Features

- Best diagnostic clue
  - Typically single or multiple ovoid radiopaque masses
  - Some are not significantly calcified (mucus plugs)
  - Duct proximal to obstruction may demonstrate intermittent dilation/stricture on sialography
- Location
  - Submandibular gland is most common site of sialoliths
  - Often incidental finding below inferior border of mandible on panoramic radiograph
- Morphology
  - Somewhat smooth and ovoid, possibly with concentric calcification, but can be oblong-shaped

Radiographic Findings

- Intraoral and panoramic radiography and sialography
  - Round, oval or oblong-shaped radiopacity; ± lamination
  - Radiopaque mass or radiolucent ductal filling void on conventional sialography
  - Intermittent dilation and stricture of duct from secondary ductal infection on conventional sialography

CT Findings

- CECT
  - Density along path of Wharton duct if sialolith is significantly calcified
- CBCT
  - Visualized only if significantly calcified

MR Findings

- T2WI
  - Low-signal void in Wharton duct or at hilum surrounded by high signal of saliva
  - Difficult to visualize if poor salivary flow is present

Ultrasonographic Findings

- Ductile, highly mineralized sialoliths > 1.5 mm imaged with 99% accuracy

Imaging Recommendations

- Best imaging tool
  - Intraoral (occlusal) and panoramic radiographs, ultrasound
  - Conventional sialography or MR sialography for minimally calcified sialoliths (mucus plugs)
- Protocol advice
  - Begin with intraoral (occlusal) and panoramic images
  - Use 50% decreased exposure for occlusal to improve visualization of calcification within soft tissue
  - If further localization is required, CBCT or CECT is appropriate; consider US
  - CT or MR if sialolith not visualized on plain images or if conventional sialography not available or contraindicated

DIFFERENTIAL DIAGNOSIS

Dystrophic Calcification of Lymph Nodes

- Typical multilobular or **cauliflower** appearance
- Rule out scrofula/chronic tuberculosis, especially if patient has been in developing country

Phlebolith

- Concentric, laminated, oval radiopacities in soft tissue associated with vascular malformations

Idiopathic Osteosclerosis/Enostosis

- Well-defined **intraosseous** radiopacity directly blending into normal bone trabecular pattern
- Sialolith superimposed over mandible can mimic enostosis

PATHOLOGY

General Features

- 30% of submandibular sialoliths are at hilum or in proximal portion of Wharton duct
- **Submandibular gland is most common site** for sialoliths due to high mucous viscosity of submandibular saliva
- Mean size: 7.3 mm but can be as large as 7 cm

CLINICAL ISSUES

Presentation

- Most common signs/symptoms
  - Swelling and **discomfort, particularly at meal times**
- Other signs/symptoms
  - May be asymptomatic
  - May result in salivary stasis, sialodochitis, &/or sialadenitis

Treatment

- Facilitate discharge with sialogogues
- Surgical removal of sialolith if in favorable location
- Surgical excision of entire gland as last resort

DIAGNOSTIC CHECKLIST

Consider

- Often multiple and associated with sialadenitis
- Intermittent ductal dilation and stricture from retrograde infection is commonly present (sialodochitis)
- Minimally calcified sialoliths may not be visualized, especially on intraoral and panoramic radiographs

Image Interpretation Pearls

- 20% of submandibular sialoliths are poorly calcified and may appear as mucus plugs (filling voids on sialography)

SELECTED REFERENCES

1. Rauso R et al: A case of a giant submandibular gland calculus perforating the floor of the mouth. Ear Nose Throat J. 91(6):E25-7, 2012
2. Eun YG et al: Advantages of intraoral removal over submandibular gland resection for proximal submandibular stones: a prospective randomized study. Laryngoscope. 120(11):2189-92, 2010
3. Hasson O: Modern sialography for screening of salivary gland obstruction. J Oral Maxillofac Surg. 68(2):276-80, 2010
4. Su YX et al: Sialoliths or phleboliths? Laryngoscope. 119(7):1344-7, 2009
5. Capaccio P et al: Modern management of obstructive salivary diseases. Acta Otorhinolaryngol Ital. 27(4):161-72, 2007
6. Langlais RP et al: Sialolithiasis: the radiolucent ones. Oral Surg Oral Med Oral Pathol. 40(5):686-90, 1975

PART II
SECTION 3
Mandible and Maxilla

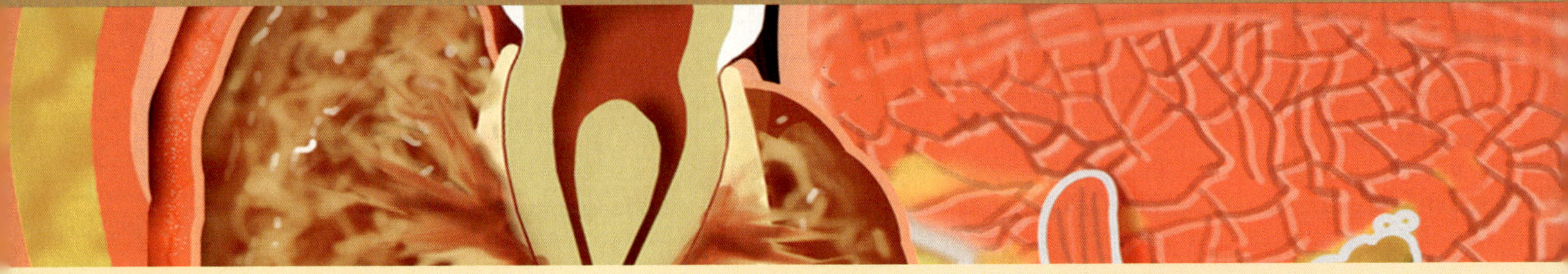

Normal Variants

Buccal and Palatal Exostoses 342
Mandibular Torus 344
Palatal Torus 346
Accessory Mandibular Canal 348
Mandibular Salivary Gland Defect (Stafne) 350
Mandible-Maxilla Idiopathic Osteosclerosis 354

Congenital/Genetic

Clefts 356
Cherubism 358
Basal Cell Nevus Syndrome 362
Cleidocranial Dysplasia 364
Pierre Robin Sequence 366
Treacher Collins Syndrome 368

Trauma

Mandible Fracture 370
Nasoethmoid Complex Fracture 374
Complex Midfacial Fracture 376
Zygomaticomaxillary Complex Fracture 378
Transfacial Fracture (Le Fort) 380

Infection/Inflammation

Mandible-Maxilla Osteomyelitis 384
Mandible-Maxilla Osteoradionecrosis 388
Mandible-Maxilla Osteonecrosis 392

Cysts, Odontogenic

Dentigerous Cyst 396
Odontogenic Keratocyst 400
Lateral Periodontal Cyst 404
Residual Cyst 406
Buccal Bifurcation Cyst 408
Calcifying Odontogenic Cyst 412

Cysts, Nonodontogenic

Mandible-Maxilla Aneurysmal Bone Cyst 414
Nasopalatine Duct Cyst 418
Nasolabial Cyst 422
Mandible-Maxilla Simple (Traumatic) Bone Cyst 424

Fibroosseous Lesions

Periapical Osseous Dysplasia 428
Florid Osseous Dysplasia 432
Ossifying Fibroma 436
Mandible-Maxilla Fibrous Dysplasia 440

Metabolic/Systemic

Paget Disease 446

Neoplasm, Benign, Odontogenic

Odontoma 450
Adenomatoid Odontogenic Tumor 454
Ameloblastoma 456
Ameloblastic Fibroma 460
Ameloblastic Fibroodontoma 464
Calcifying Epithelial Odontogenic Tumor 466
Cementoblastoma 468
Odontogenic Myxoma 470
Central Odontogenic Fibroma 472

Neoplasm, Benign, Nonodontogenic

Central Hemangioma 474
Osteoid Osteoma 476
Osteoblastoma 478
Mandible-Maxilla Osteoma 480
Nerve Sheath Tumor 482
Neurofibromatosis Type 1 486
Desmoplastic Fibroma 490

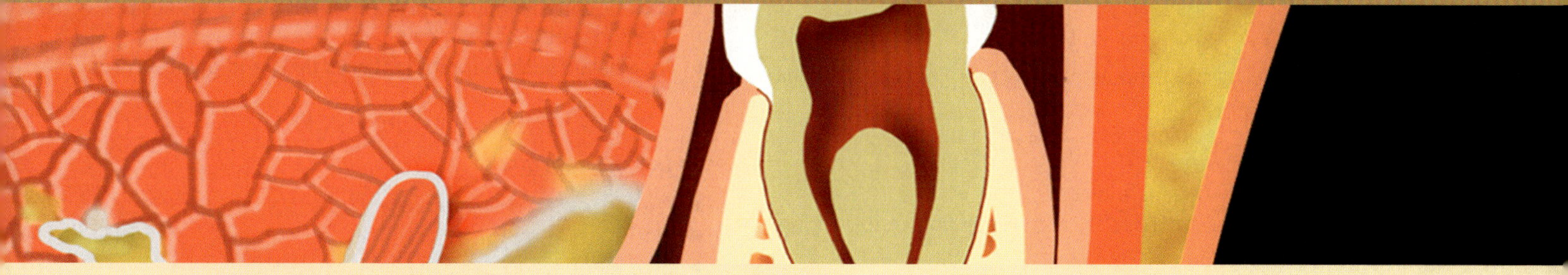

Neoplasm, Malignant, Odontogenic

Malignant Ameloblastoma and Ameloblastic Carcinoma **492**

Neoplasm, Malignant, Nonodontogenic

Mandible-Maxilla Metastasis **494**
Mandible-Maxilla Osteosarcoma **500**
Mandible-Maxilla Chondrosarcoma **504**
Primary Intraosseous Squamous Cell Carcinoma **508**
Central Mucoepidermoid Carcinoma **510**
Burkitt Lymphoma **512**
Non-Hodgkin Lymphoma of Pharyngeal Mucosal Space **516**
Multiple Myeloma **520**
Ewing Sarcoma **524**
Leukemia **528**

Tumor-Like Lesions

Mandible-Maxilla Central Giant Cell Granuloma **530**
Langerhans Histiocytosis **534**

Buccal and Palatal Exostoses

KEY FACTS

TERMINOLOGY

- Synonyms: **Hyperostoses**; tori maxillaris; buccal lipping
- Definition: Hyperplastic protuberances of normal cortical and cancellous bone

IMAGING

- Varies from small cervical marginal prominences to larger exophytic nodules
- More common in maxilla: ~ 10% occur palatally in 1st molar to tuberosity area
- Intraoral 2D imaging findings
  - Well-defined radiopacity **without radiolucent periphery**
- CBCT findings
  - Exophytic high-density lesions
  - Maxillary and mandibular **buccal alveolar processes** in molar and premolar areas

TOP DIFFERENTIAL DIAGNOSES

- Idiopathic osteosclerosis (2D imaging)
- Mandibular torus or palatal torus
- Osteoma

PATHOLOGY

- Genetic with overlay of environmental factors: Occlusal stress, parafunctional habits
- **Associated with mandibular torus (MT) and palatal torus (PT)**
  - Greatest occurrence in subjects with both MT and PT

CLINICAL ISSUES

- Prevalence increases with age
- M > F
- Excellent prognosis; no malignant potential
- No treatment required: Removed if traumatized or interfere with function or fabrication of prostheses

DIAGNOSTIC CHECKLIST

- Consider **Gardner syndrome** if not in expected location for exostoses

(Left) *Periapical radiograph shows subtle radiopacities along the cervical margins of the anterior teeth ➡. These protuberances are known as buccal lipping and are more common in the mandible. Clinically, they appear as small bumps under normal mucosa.* **(Right)** *Axial 3D CBCT demonstrates multiple buccal maxillary exostoses in the molar and premolar areas ➡. Prolific exostoses such as these may interfere with function and be removed. Buccal lipping is evident in the anterior maxilla ➡.*

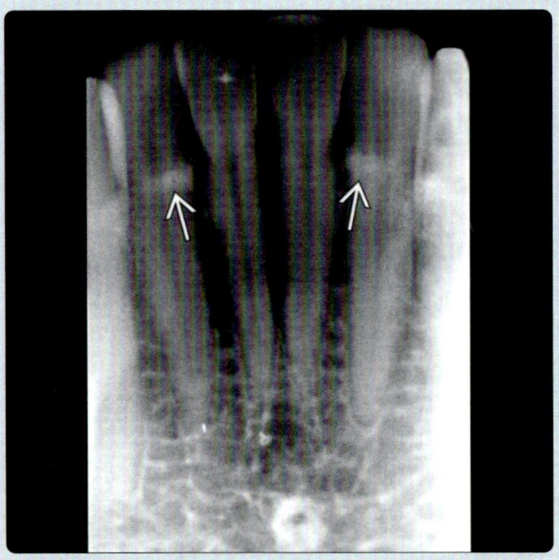

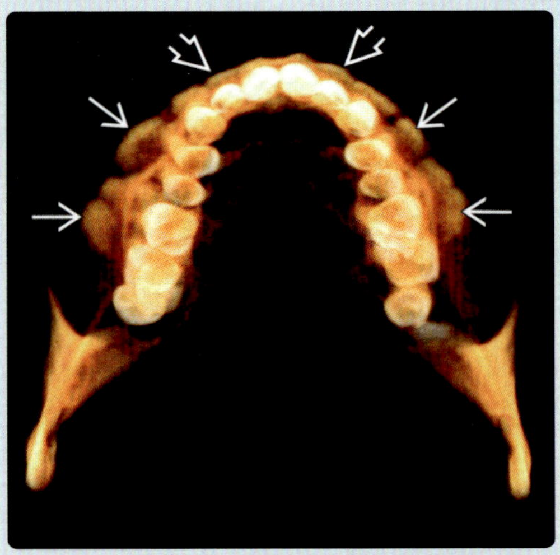

(Left) *Coronal CBCT demonstrates buccal ➡ and palatal ➡ exostoses in the posterior maxilla. A palatal exostosis is sometimes referred to as a torus maxillaris. Note the presence of a small palatal torus ➡, which often appears concurrently with exostoses.* **(Right)** *Axial CBCT shows multiple buccal exostoses in premolar areas of the mandible ➡. Prominent mandibular tori are also present ➡. Occurrence of exostoses is greatest when both mandibular tori and palatal torus are present.*

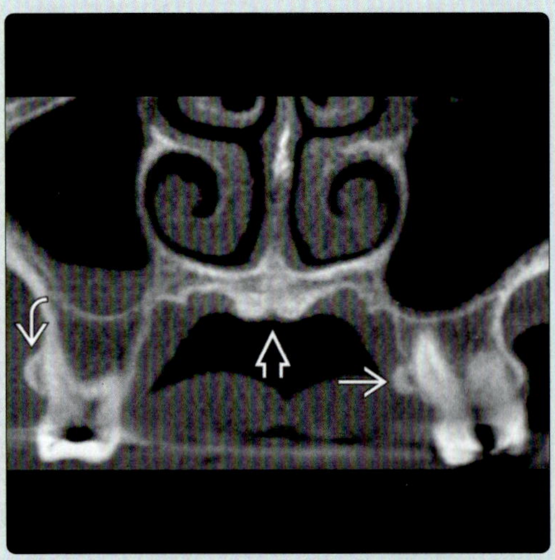

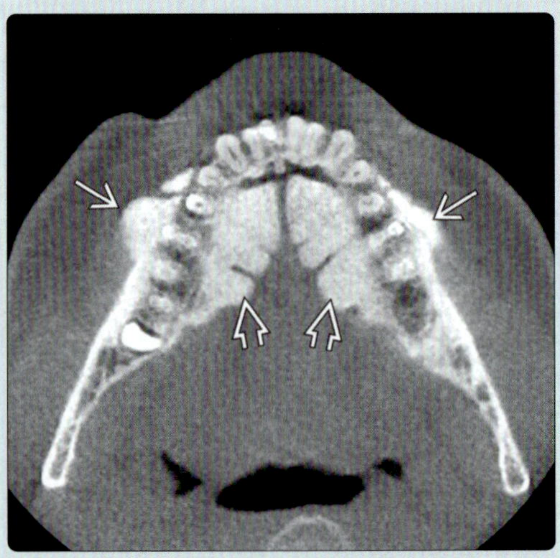

TERMINOLOGY

Synonyms

- **Hyperostoses**; palatal exostoses (a.k.a. tori maxillaris); buccal lipping

Definitions

- Hyperplastic protuberances of normal cortical and cancellous bone

IMAGING

General Features

- Best diagnostic clue
  - Well-defined radiopacity **without** radiolucent periphery on intraoral images
- Location
  - Maxillary and mandibular **buccal alveolar processes in molar and premolar areas**
  - More common in maxilla: ~ 10% occur palatally in 1st molar to tuberosity area
  - Prominences at buccal cervical margin (buccal lipping) more common in anterior mandible
- Size
  - Varies from small cervical marginal prominences to larger exophytic nodules
- Morphology
  - Round, nodular, flat, or pedunculated

Imaging Recommendations

- Best imaging tool
  - Occlusal views will demonstrate exophytic nature
  - CBCT imaging

Radiographic Findings

- Intraoral plain film
  - Well-defined, smooth radiopacity **without radiolucent periphery** in alveolar processes

CT Findings

- CBCT
  - Exophytic areas of normal-appearing bone located close to alveolar crest

DIFFERENTIAL DIAGNOSIS

Idiopathic Osteosclerosis

- 2D imaging: May look similar
  - Periphery more irregular
  - Occurs in locations other than alveolar processes
- CBCT: High-density areas **within confines of alveolar cortices**

Mandibular Torus

- CBCT: Bony protuberances of lingual mandible in premolar area

Palatal Torus

- CBCT: Bony excrescence comes off central hard palate

Osteoma

- Exophytic, often pedunculated, bony protuberance
- More common in ramus and inferior border of mandible
- Multiple osteomas may signify Gardner syndrome

PATHOLOGY

General Features

- Etiology
  - Recent study shows dominant genetic influence
  - Most likely multifactorial with overlay of environmental factors: Occlusal stress, parafunctional habits, free gingival graft procedures
- Genetics
  - Possibly autosomal dominant or X-linked
- Associated abnormalities
  - **Associated with mandibular torus (MT) and palatal torus (PT)**
    - Greatest occurrence (42%) in subjects with both MT and PT
  - Possible association with dermatofibromas

Microscopic Features

- Dense bone with lacunae and normal osteocytes

CLINICAL ISSUES

Presentation

- Most common signs/symptoms
  - Asymptomatic unless traumatized
- Other signs/symptoms
  - Attrition of teeth may be evident, supporting theory that occlusal stress stimulates formation of exostoses

Demographics

- Age
  - Prevalence increases with age
  - Highest occurrence in patients ≥ 55 years
- Gender
  - M > F
- Epidemiology
  - More often in Asians, blacks

Natural History & Prognosis

- Excellent prognosis; no malignant potential

Treatment

- No treatment required unless traumatized or interfere with function or fabrication of prostheses

DIAGNOSTIC CHECKLIST

Consider

- **Gardner syndrome** if not in expected location for exostoses

SELECTED REFERENCES

1. Auškalnis A et al: Oral bony outgrowths: prevalence and genetic factor influence. Study of twins. Medicina (Kaunas). 51(4):228-32, 2015
2. Medsinge SV et al: Buccal exostosis: a rare entity. J Int Oral Health. 7(5):62-4, 2015
3. Gedik R et al: Multiple lesions in the upper jaw. West Indian Med J. 63(7):796-8, 2014
4. Bansal M et al: Multiple mandibular exostoses: a rare case report. J Clin Diagn Res. 7(8):1802-3, 2013
5. Ruiz LP et al: Craniomaxillofacial features in hereditary multiple exostosis. J Craniofac Surg. 23(4):e336-8, 2012
6. Jainkittivong A et al: Buccal and palatal exostoses: prevalence and concurrence with tori. Oral Surg Oral Med Oral Pathol Oral Radiol Endod. 90(1):48-53, 2000

Mandibular Torus

KEY FACTS

TERMINOLOGY

- Synonyms: Torus mandibularis
- Definition: Exophytic proliferation of cortical and trabecular bone on lingual aspect of mandible in premolar areas

IMAGING

- Round or nodular, well-defined, can be multiple
- 2D imaging findings
  - Bilateral radiopacities **without radiolucent halo**
  - Occasionally unilateral
- CBCT findings
  - Bilateral, exophytic, high-density areas lingual to mandibular premolars ± molar and canine areas

TOP DIFFERENTIAL DIAGNOSES

- Idiopathic osteosclerosis
- Sialolith in Wharton duct
- Buccal exostosis
- Osteoma

PATHOLOGY

- Up to 36% associated with buccal or palatal exostoses
- Up to 50% associated with palatal torus
- Hereditary with overlay of environmental influence: Occlusal stress, parafunctional habits
- Recently associated with square-shaped mandible, which favors stress concentration

CLINICAL ISSUES

- M > F
- Rare before 1st decade, usually 4th decade
- May slowly increase in size
- Prognosis excellent; no malignant potential
- Tori are removed when consistently traumatized or interfere with function

DIAGNOSTIC CHECKLIST

- Consider **Gardner syndrome** if radiopacities not in expected location for tori

(Left) *Periapical radiograph of left premolar area demonstrates well-defined radiopacity* ➡ *at midroot of the premolars. This is the normal location for mandibular tori, although large tori may extend posteriorly to the molars or anteriorly to the incisors. Note there is no radiolucent periphery. The smooth, regular outline helps to differentiate from idiopathic osteosclerosis.* **(Right)** *This mandibular central incisor periapical radiograph displays the typical appearance of bilateral mandibular tori* ➡*.*

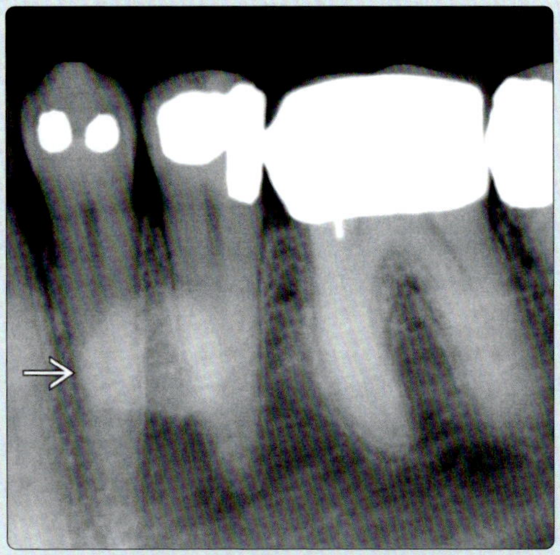

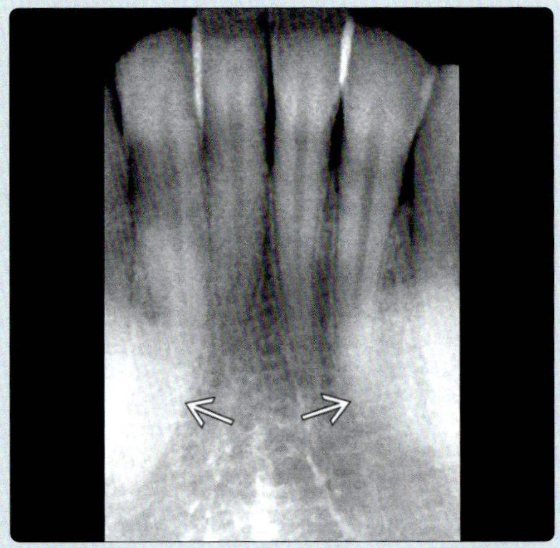

(Left) *Axial CBCT shows large, bilateral, multilobed radiopacities* ➡ *representing exuberant mandibular tori.* **(Right)** *Coronal CBCT demonstrates constriction of tongue space* ➡ *by extremely large mandibular tori. Tori are covered with a thin layer of overlying mucosa, which may become traumatized. Tori that are chronically irritated or interfere with function are removed. Note maxillary* ➡ *and mandibular* ➡ *buccal exostoses, which frequently occur concurrently with mandibular tori.*

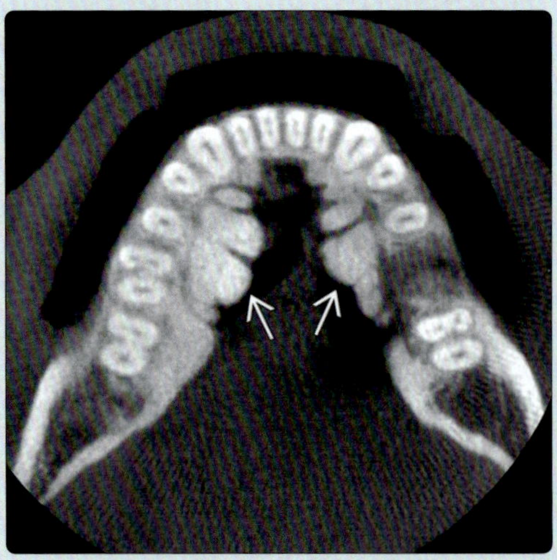

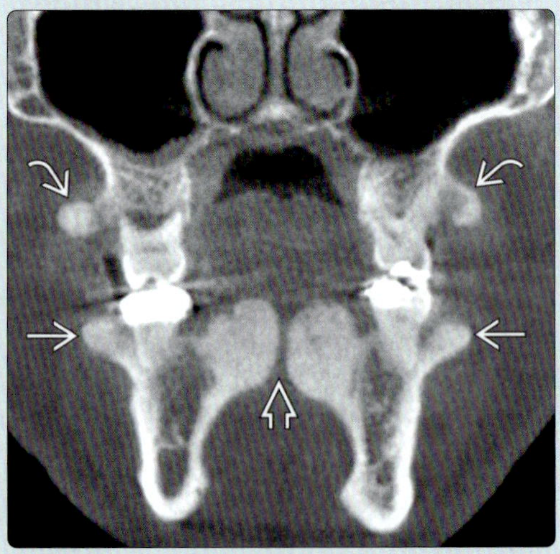

Mandibular Torus

TERMINOLOGY

Synonyms

- Torus mandibularis

Definitions

- Exophytic proliferation of cortical and trabecular bone located on lingual aspect of mandible, usually in premolar areas

IMAGING

General Features

- Best diagnostic clue
  - Bilateral, well-defined radiopacities **without radiolucent halo** on intraoral films
- Location
  - Lingual of mandible in premolar area; may extend posteriorly to molars or anteriorly to canine
  - Above mylohyoid ridge
  - Occasionally unilateral
- Size
  - Variable from very small (< 2 mm) to extremely large
  - Size may be increased by long-term use of phenytoin, which functions as osteogenic agent
- Morphology
  - Round or nodular, well-defined, can be multiple

Imaging Recommendations

- Best imaging tool
  - Periapical or occlusal views; CBCT imaging

Radiographic Findings

- Intraoral plain film
  - Bilateral, well-defined radiopacities at midroot of mandibular premolars

CT Findings

- CBCT
  - Bilateral, exophytic, high-density areas lingual to mandibular premolars

DIFFERENTIAL DIAGNOSIS

Idiopathic Osteosclerosis (Enostosis)

- 2D imaging
  - Dense sclerotic bone with irregular outline
  - Occurs in locations other than mandibular premolar
- CBCT: High-density areas **within confines of buccal and alveolar cortices**

Sialolith in Wharton Duct

- 2D imaging: Calcifications in Wharton duct may appear similar to tori
- CBCT: Calcifications **lingual and separate from mandible**

Buccal Exostosis

- 2D imaging: Well-defined radiopacity on buccal alveolar bone more cervical than tori
- CBCT: Exophytic bony protuberances **on buccal alveolar processes**

Osteoma

- Exophytic nodules **more common on ramus and inferior border of mandible**
- May be multiple; consider Gardner syndrome

PATHOLOGY

General Features

- Etiology
  - Hereditary with overlay of environmental influence: Occlusal stress, parafunctional habits
    - Recently associated with square-shaped mandible, which favors stress concentration
- Genetics
  - Autosomal dominant
- Associated abnormalities
  - Up to 36% associated with buccal or palatal exostoses; up to 50% associated with palatal torus

Microscopic Features

- Hyperplasia of mature cortical and trabecular bone

CLINICAL ISSUES

Presentation

- Most common signs/symptoms
  - Asymptomatic unless traumatized
- Other signs/symptoms
  - Large tori may cause difficulty eating and speaking

Demographics

- Age
  - Rare before 1st decade, usually 4th decade
- Gender
  - M > F
- Epidemiology
  - Occurrence may be higher in certain ethnic groups: Mongols, Eskimos

Natural History & Prognosis

- May slowly increase in size
- Prognosis excellent; no malignant potential

Treatment

- Tori are removed when consistently traumatized or interfere with function or fabrication of prostheses

DIAGNOSTIC CHECKLIST

Consider

- Consider Gardner syndrome if radiopacities not in expected location for tori

SELECTED REFERENCES

1. Maduakor SN et al: Prevalence of mandibular and palatine tori among the Ibos in Enugu, South-East Nigeria. Niger J Clin Pract. 20(1):57-60, 2017
2. Scott GR et al: Northern exposure: Mandibular torus in the Greenlandic Norse and the whole wide world. Am J Phys Anthropol. 161(3):513-521, 2016
3. Auškalnis A et al: Oral bony outgrowths: prevalence and genetic factor influence. Study of twins. Medicina (Kaunas). 51(4):228-32, 2015
4. Cortes AR et al: Mandibular tori are associated with mechanical stress and mandibular shape. J Oral Maxillofac Surg. 72(11):2115-25, 2014
5. García-García AS et al: Current status of the torus palatinus and torus mandibularis. Med Oral Patol Oral Cir Bucal. 15(2):e353-60, 2010

Palatal Torus

KEY FACTS

TERMINOLOGY

- Synonym: Torus palatinus
- Definition: Exophytic proliferation of normal cortical and cancellous bone in midline of hard palate

IMAGING

- Size varies from very small nodule to large, multilobed protuberances
- Flat, nodular, multilobed, or spindle-shaped
- Intraoral imaging: Well-defined radiopacities that may superimpose on maxillary sinus in posterior periapical views
- CBCT: **Exophytic high-density areas in middle of hard palate**

TOP DIFFERENTIAL DIAGNOSES

- Exostoses
- Osteoma

PATHOLOGY

- Genetic with overlay of environmental influences: Parafunctional activity
- Possibly X-linked, accounting for higher incidence in women
- Associated with **buccal and palatal exostoses** and **mandibular tori**

CLINICAL ISSUES

- **F > M**
- More common in some ethnic groups: Mongols and Eskimos
- Prognosis excellent; no malignant potential
- Tori are removed when consistently traumatized or interfere with function

DIAGNOSTIC CHECKLIST

- Consider: Osteoma/**Gardner syndrome** if not in expected location for tori

(Left) *Periapical radiograph of right edentulous maxilla shows well-defined radiopacities ➡ in the superior aspect of the maxillary sinus. These represent a multilobed palatal torus. The sickle-shaped radiopacity ➡ is the zygomatic process of the maxilla, and the radiopacity extending posteriorly ➡ is the inferior border of the zygoma.* **(Right)** *Coronal CBCT shows small palatal torus ➡ in the midline of the palate. Note palatal exostosis ➡. Exostoses often occur concurrently with palatal tori.*

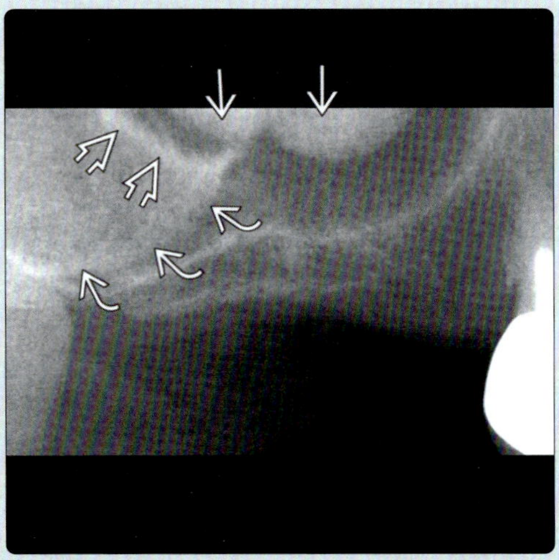

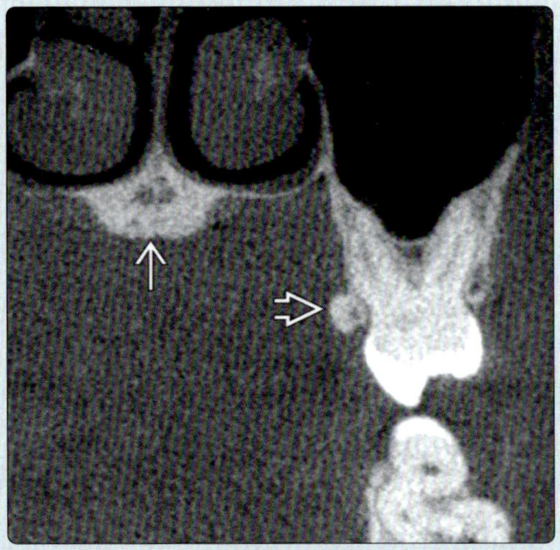

(Left) *Coronal CBCT shows large, bilobed palatal torus ➡. Tori this large may interfere with function and are often chronically traumatized, requiring removal. The overlying mucosa is usually thin. (Courtesy M. Ahmad, DDS.)* **(Right)** *Axial CBCT in the same patient reveals the multilobed nature of the palatal torus ➡. Note the overall symmetric enlargement and smooth borders, indicating benign growth characteristics. (Courtesy M. Ahmad, DDS.)*

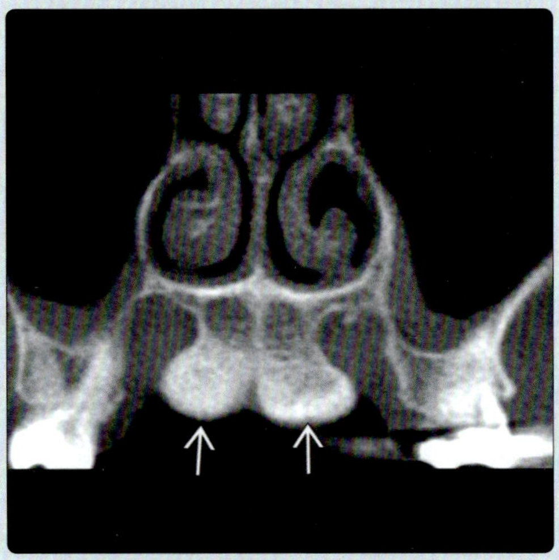

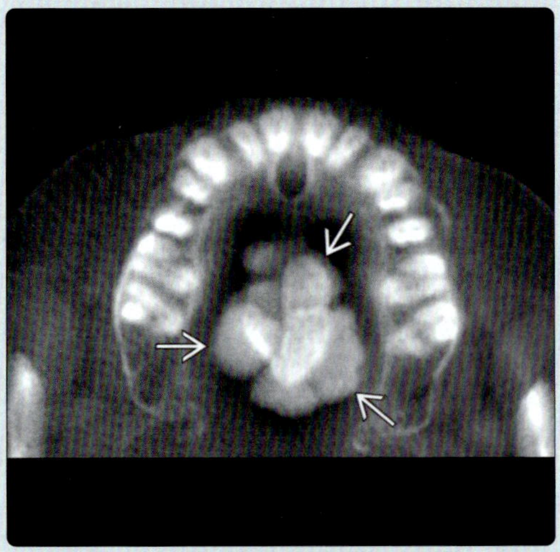

TERMINOLOGY

Abbreviations

- Patalal torus (PT)

Synonyms

- Torus palatinus

Definitions

- Exophytic proliferation of normal cortical and cancellous bone in midline of hard palate

IMAGING

General Features

- Location
  - Midline of hard palate
- Size
  - Varies from very small nodule to large, multilobed protuberances
- Morphology
  - Flat, nodular, multilobed, or spindle-shaped

Radiographic Findings

- Intraoral plain film
  - Well-defined radiopacities that may superimpose on maxillary sinus in posterior periapical views

CT Findings

- CBCT
  - Exophytic high-density areas in middle of hard palate

DIFFERENTIAL DIAGNOSIS

Exostoses

- 2D imaging: Well-defined radiopacity usually more cervical than PT
- CBCT: Exophytic bony protuberances on **buccal or palatal alveolar processes**

Osteoma

- Exophytic nodules more common on **ramus and inferior border of mandible**
- May be multiple: Gardner syndrome

PATHOLOGY

General Features

- Etiology
  - Genetic with overlay of environmental influences: Parafunctional activity
- Genetics
  - Possibly X-linked, accounting for higher incidence in women
- Associated abnormalities
  - Buccal and palatal exostoses
  - Mandibular tori

Microscopic Features

- Dense cancellous bone with rim of cortical bone of various thickness
- Bone from torus has been used successfully in grafting for alveolar ridge reconstruction

CLINICAL ISSUES

Presentation

- Most common signs/symptoms
  - Asymptomatic unless traumatized
- Other signs/symptoms
  - Large tori may cause difficulty eating and speaking
  - Large tori may be chronically traumatized during mastication
  - Osteonecrosis has been reported following trauma to palatal torus in patients with long-term oral bisphosphonate use

Demographics

- Age
  - Usually develops before 30 years
- Gender
  - F > M
- Epidemiology
  - More common in some ethnic groups: Mongols and Eskimos
  - Studies have shown that postmenopausal women with large PT have higher mean bone density than their peers and much younger women

Natural History & Prognosis

- May slowly increase in size
- Prognosis excellent; no malignant potential

Treatment

- No treatment required
- Tori are removed when consistently traumatized or interfere with function or fabrication of prostheses to replace missing teeth

DIAGNOSTIC CHECKLIST

Consider

- Osteoma/**Gardner syndrome** if not in expected location for tori

SELECTED REFERENCES

1. AlZarea BK: Prevalence and pattern of torus palatinus and torus mandibularis among edentulous patients of Saudi Arabia. Clin Interv Aging. 11:209-13, 2016
2. Ryan JL et al: Osteonecrosis of the torus palatinus in the setting of long-term oral bisphosphonate use–a case report. S D Med. 69(1):23-5, 2016
3. Scrieciu M et al: Morphological and clinical characteristics of the torus palatinus and torus mandibularis in a sample of young and adults' Romanian people. Rom J Morphol Embryol. 57(1):139-44, 2016
4. Kaneko K et al: Bisphosphonate-related osteonecrosis of the palatal torus. ORL J Otorhinolaryngol Relat Spec. 76(6):353-6, 2014
5. Godinho M et al: Torus palatinus osteonecrosis related to bisphosphonate: a case report. Case Rep Dermatol. 5(1):120-5, 2013
6. Nogueira AS et al: Clinical, tomographic aspects and relevance of torus palatinus: case report of two sisters. Surg Radiol Anat. 35(9):867-71, 2013
7. Beena JP: Torus palatinus in an infant: a case report. J Dent Child (Chic). 79(3):181-4, 2012
8. Cantín M et al: A proposed explanation for the development of the torus palatinus. Clin Anat. 24(6):789-90, 2011
9. García-García AS et al: Current status of the torus palatinus and torus mandibularis. Med Oral Patol Oral Cir Bucal. 15(2):e353-60, 2010
10. Moraes Junior EF et al: Torus palatinus: a graft option for alveolar ridge reconstruction. Int J Periodontics Restorative Dent. 30(3):283-9, 2010
11. Belsky JL et al: Torus palatinus: a new anatomical correlation with bone density in postmenopausal women. J Clin Endocrinol Metab. 88(5):2081-6, 2003

Accessory Mandibular Canal

KEY FACTS

TERMINOLOGY

- Synonyms
    - Accessory inferior alveolar canal (IAC)
    - Bifid mandibular canal
    - Duplication/division of mandibular canal

IMAGING

- Well-defined, mostly **corticated radiolucent tract** arising from main mandibular canal or foramen
- Mostly posterior area
- Mandibular canal may continue anteriorly beyond mental foramen
- Best imaging modality: CBCT
    - Studies show higher incidence (15%) of bifid mandibular canals observed on CBCT images than on panoramic images (only 8%)
    - **CBCT can detect canals that orient in buccal-lingual direction**

TOP DIFFERENTIAL DIAGNOSES

- Sinus tract
- Gubernaculum dentis

PATHOLOGY

- Associated anomalies
    - Accessory or duplicated mandibular, mental, or lingual foramina
    - Lingual bony canals

CLINICAL ISSUES

- Complications for **tooth extraction, implant placement, & bone harvesting**
    - Difficulty in obtaining anesthesia
    - Excessive bleeding
    - Paresthesia
    - Traumatic neuroma
- Accessory canals & foramina may provide **route for tumor invasion or perineural tumor spread**

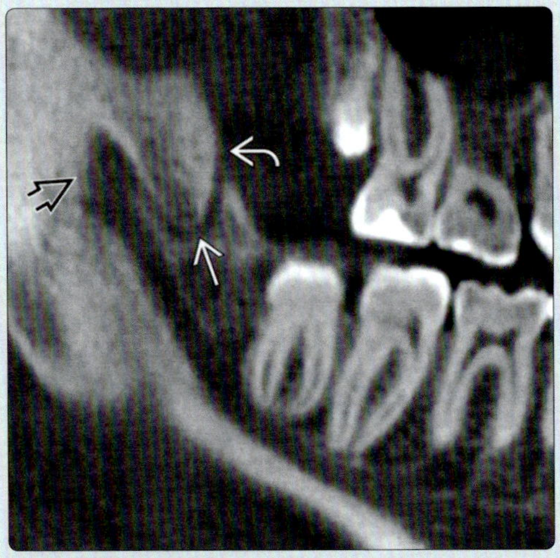
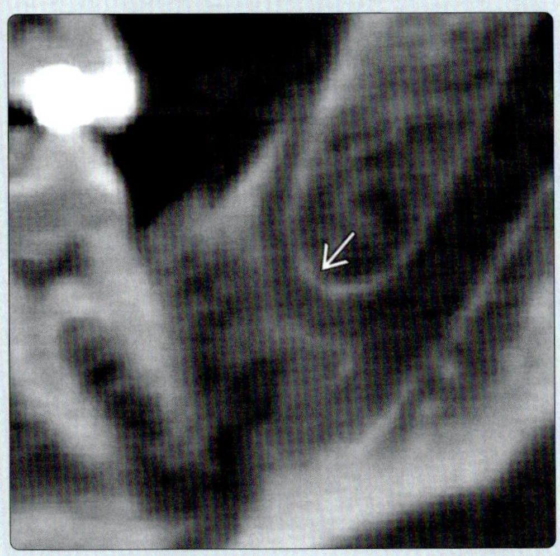

(Left) *Panoramic reformat CBCT shows accessory mandibular canal arising from the large mandibular foramen and exiting in the retromolar region as a retromolar foramen. These canals may provide route for perineural tumor spread from retromolar trigone carcinomas.* **(Right)** *Panoramic reformat CBCT shows accessory canal exiting from main canal in 3rd molar area. Canals exiting in the retromolar region present problems for 3rd molar removal and bone block harvesting.*

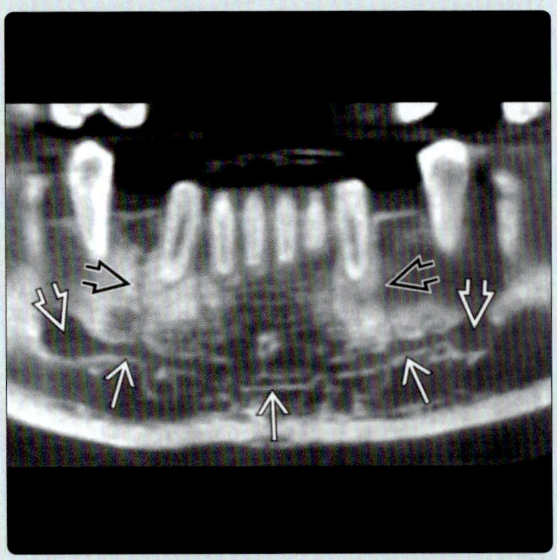
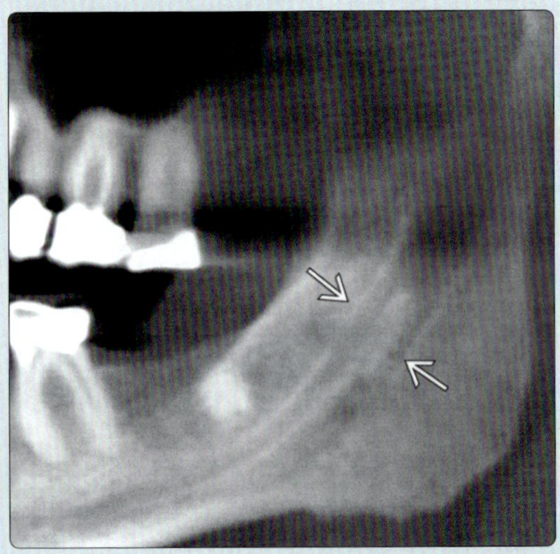

(Left) *Panoramic reformat CBCT shows extension of the mandibular canal beyond the mental foramen bilaterally. The canal on the left crosses the midline and may communicate with the anterior extension from the right. Note smaller accessory canals (nutrient canals) arising from these anterior branches. Identification of these variants is important for implant planning.* **(Right)** *Panoramic reformat CBCT image shows 2 distinct canals arising from 1 large main canal.*

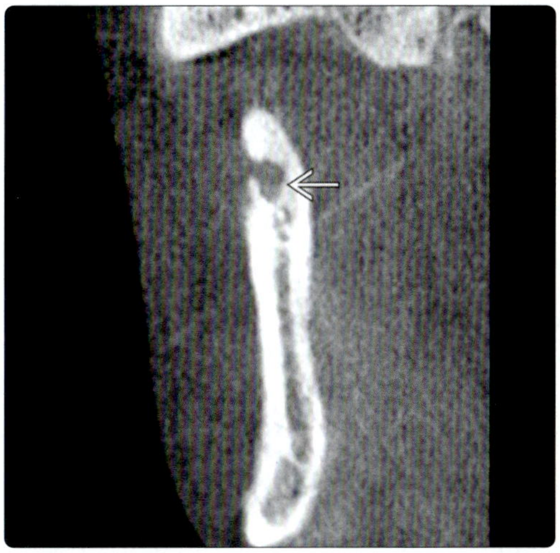
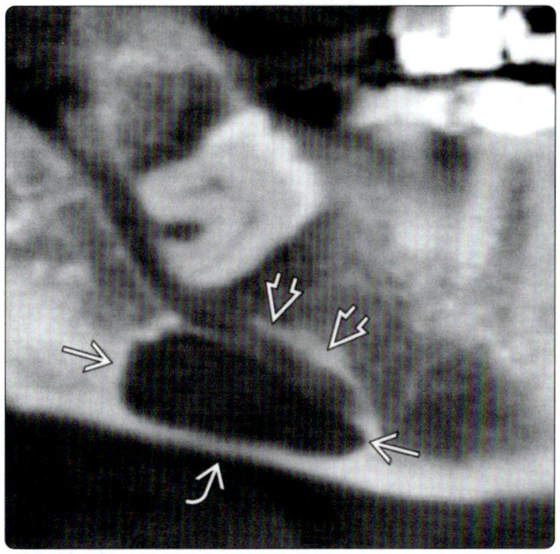

(Left) *Coronal CBCT through posterior right ramus shows a very rare parotid gland defect on the buccal aspect of the ramus. Most parotid gland defects occur on the lingual aspect of the ramus close to the condylar neck. (Courtesy M. Noujeim, DDS.)* **(Right)** *Panoramic reformat CBCT shows large, oval, mandibular salivary gland defect inferior to the impacted right mandibular 3rd molar. The mandibular canal appears to have been deflected superiorly. Note the inferior cortex is thinned but intact .*

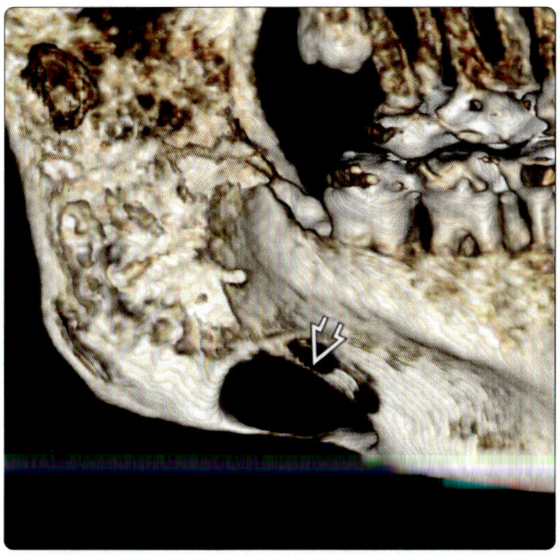
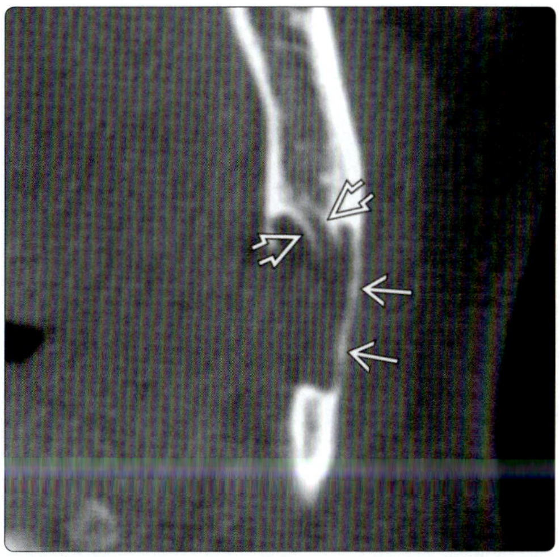

(Left) *Lateral 3D CBCT reformation in the same patient shows the mandibular salivary gland defect on the lingual aspect of the mandible. The intact inferior border of the mandibular canal can be seen.* **(Right)** *Axial CBCT in the same patient shows the extent of the defect. Only a thin margin of buccal cortex remains. The mandibular canal can be seen coursing forward in the anterior aspect of the defect.*

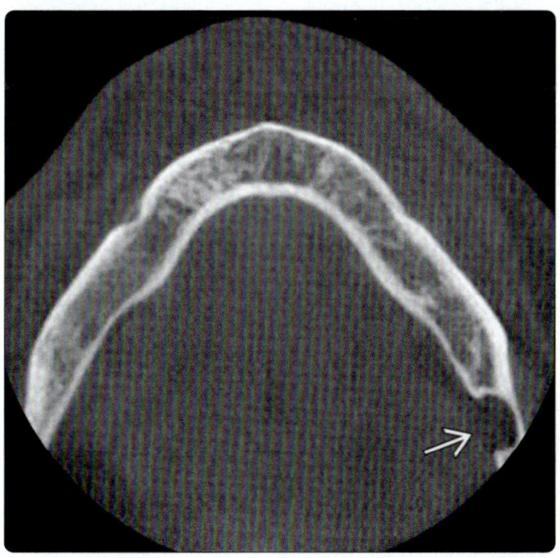
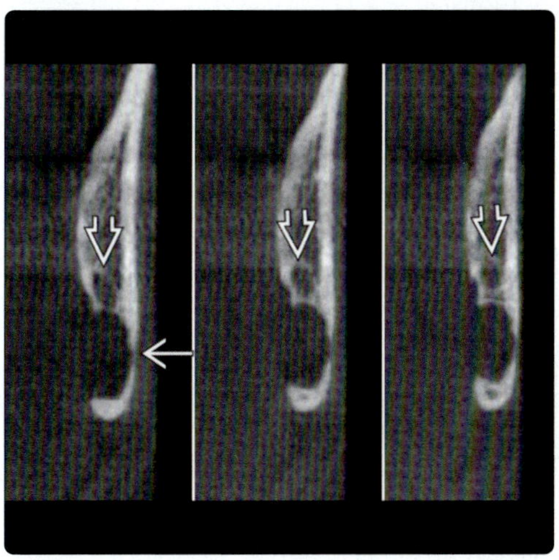

(Left) *Axial CBCT shows a well-defined invagination on the lingual aspect of the left mandible. This Stafne defect was an incidental finding on a CBCT taken for implant planning.* **(Right)** *Sequential coronal CBCT images through the posterior mandible in the same patient show the defect extends to the buccal cortex , which is thinned. The mandibular canal can be seen at the superior margin of the defect. The defect may contain submandibular gland tissue or just fat.*

Mandible-Maxilla Idiopathic Osteosclerosis

KEY FACTS

TERMINOLOGY

- Synonyms: Dense bone island, bone scar, bone whorl, bone eburnation, enostosis, focal osteopetrosis
- Definition: Localized area of increased radiodensity (radiopacity) of unknown cause and **without association to inflammatory, dysplastic, or neoplastic process**

IMAGING

- Well-defined, **nonexpansile**, homogeneous radiopacity **without radiolucent periphery**
- Location: Mandible > > maxilla, premolar/molar area
  - **Within confines of buccal and lingual cortices**
- Size: Varies from 1 mm to 2 cm; average: ~ 5 mm
  - **Giant dense bone island** (> 2 cm) is thought to be just larger variant
- May have radiolucent areas within

TOP DIFFERENTIAL DIAGNOSES

- Sclerosing osteitis (condensing osteitis)
- Periapical osseous dysplasia
- Hypercementosis
- Complex odontoma
- Mandibular torus
- Gardner syndrome

CLINICAL ISSUES

- Asymptomatic
- F ≥ M
- May increase in size in young patients
- Rarely may cause ectopic eruption or root resorption
- Implant placement at sites of osteosclerosis questionable
- No treatment necessary

DIAGNOSTIC CHECKLIST

- Consider **Gardner** syndrome if multiple lesions
- When in close proximity to teeth, look for presence of **normal periodontal ligament space** to rule out sclerosing osteitis caused by pulpal inflammation

(Left) *Periapical radiograph shows area of idiopathic osteosclerosis (IO) ➡ at apex of mandibular right canine. Note area of decreased density ➡, which may cause confusion with sclerosing osteitis. The normal apical PDL space ➡ and absence of coronal pathology helps differentiate.* **(Right)** *Mandibular right periapical radiograph shows socket sclerosis ➡ following extraction. Compare to root fragment from 2nd deciduous molar ➡, which has a thin radiolucent periphery representing the PDL space.*

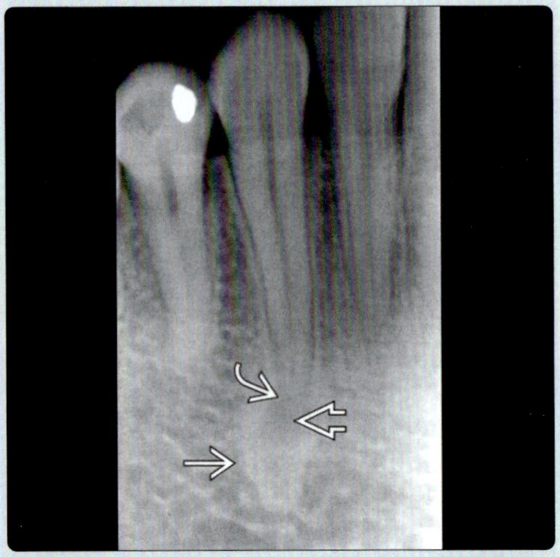

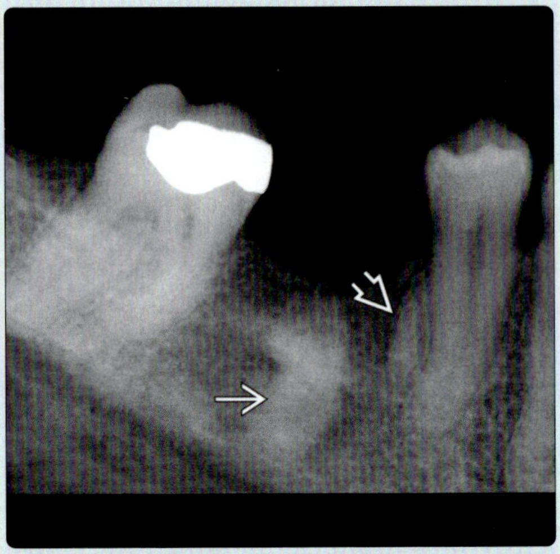

(Left) *Axial (left) and sagittal (right) CBCT images show a well-defined, homogeneously dense area of IO between the left mandibular 1st and 2nd molars. Note the continuity with the buccal cortex ➡. Areas of IO often exhibit contiguity with either the buccal or lingual cortex.* **(Right)** *Axial (left) and coronal (right) CBCT images show a rare example of IO ➡ in the maxillary left premolar area. Note the well-defined margins and absence of a peripheral zone of radiolucency.*

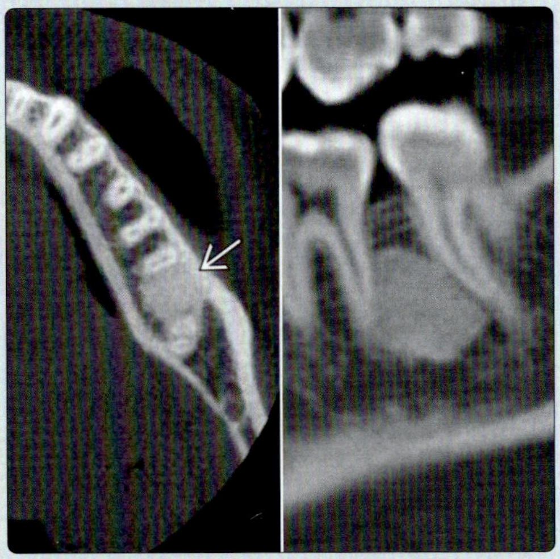

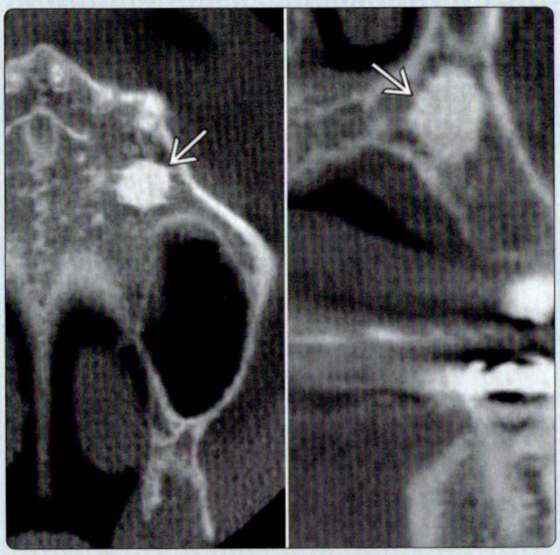

TERMINOLOGY

Synonyms

- Dense bone island, bone scar, bone whorl, bone eburnation, enostosis, focal osteopetrosis

Definitions

- Localized area of increased radiodensity (radiopacity) of unknown cause and **without association to inflammatory, dysplastic, or neoplastic process**

IMAGING

General Features

- Best diagnostic clue
  - Well-defined, **nonexpansile**, homogeneous radiopacity **without radiolucent periphery**
- Location
  - Mandible > > maxilla
    - Premolar/molar area
    - **Within confines of buccal and lingual cortices**
- Size
  - Varies from 1 mm to 2 cm
    - Average size: ~ 5 mm
  - **Giant dense bone island** (> 2 cm) is thought to be just larger variant
    - Nonexpansile and same location predilection: Mandibular molar-premolar area
- Morphology
  - Varies: Round, elliptical, irregular

Radiographic Findings

- Intraoral plain film
  - Well-defined radiopacity
    - Usually homogeneously radiopaque but may have areas of low density (radiolucency) within
  - May be in close proximity to apex and roots of teeth
    - Differentiate from sclerosing osteitis (condensing osteitis) by absence of inflammatory process and **normal periodontal ligament (PDL) space**

CT Findings

- CBCT
  - Nonexpansile area of **high density** within confines of buccal and lingual cortical plates
  - May be contiguous with buccal or lingual cortex

DIFFERENTIAL DIAGNOSIS

Sclerosing Osteitis (Condensing Osteitis)

- Inflammatory process producing dense reactive bone **at apex** of pulpally involved tooth (dead or dying)
- Widened PDL space: **Thin radiolucency between tooth root and radiopacity**
- Associated coronal etiology, such as caries, fractured tooth, or large restoration

Periapical Osseous Dysplasia

- Nonneoplastic replacement of normal bone at tooth apex by dysplastic cementum &/or abnormal bone
- Radiopacity is **surrounded by radiolucency**

Hypercementosis

- Excessive production of cementum, primarily around apical area of tooth root
- PDL space is continuous around bulbous cementum, giving **radiolucent periphery**

Complex Odontoma

- Irregular radiopaque mass with **radiolucent periphery**
- Density of tooth structure (enamel and dentin)
- May be associated with tooth crown

Mandibular Torus

- **Exophytic** hyperplastic normal bone on lingual of mandible
- Usually midroot of mandibular premolar teeth
- May look similar on intraoral radiographs
  - CBCT imaging, occlusal view, or clinical examination will demonstrate exophytic nature

Gardner Syndrome

- Multiple osteomas
- Usually **exophytic** in ramus and inferior border of mandible

CLINICAL ISSUES

Presentation

- Most common signs/symptoms
  - Asymptomatic

Demographics

- Age
  - Develops in early adolescence
- Gender
  - F ≥ M

Natural History & Prognosis

- May increase in size in young patients
  - Usually stable in adults but ↑ or ↓ in size reported
- Rarely may cause ectopic eruption or root resorption
- May form in tooth sockets following extraction
- Implant placement into sites of osteosclerosis is questionable

Treatment

- No treatment necessary

DIAGNOSTIC CHECKLIST

Consider

- **Gardner** syndrome if multiple lesions

Image Interpretation Pearls

- If close to apex of tooth, look for normal PDL space to **rule out sclerosing osteitis**

SELECTED REFERENCES

1. Mainville GN et al: Asymptomatic, nonexpansile radiopacity of the jaw associated with external root resorption: a diagnostic dilemma. Gen Dent. 64(1):32-5, 2016
2. Moshfeghi M et al: Radiologic assessment and frequency of idiopathic osteosclerosis of jawbones: an interpopulation comparison. Acta Radiol. 55(10):1239-44, 2014
3. Tolentino Ede S et al: Idiopathic osteosclerosis of the jaw in a Brazilian population: a retrospective study. Acta Stomatol Croat. 48(3):183-92, 2014
4. Sisman Y et al: The frequency and distribution of idiopathic osteosclerosis of the jaw. Eur J Dent. 5(4):409-14, 2011

Clefts

KEY FACTS

TERMINOLOGY

- Cleft: Developmental disturbance resulting in failure of proper fusion of various orofacial tissues
  - **Cleft lip (CL)**: Defective fusion of median nasal process with maxillary process
  - **Cleft palate (CP)**: Fusion failure of primary palatal shelves

IMAGING

- Clefts of alveolus usually between lateral incisor and canine
- Often accompanied by missing teeth (lateral incisor) or supernumerary teeth
- Defect often extends into nasal cavity
  - Resulting asymmetry of nasal cavity floor

TOP DIFFERENTIAL DIAGNOSES

- Fracture
  - History of trauma

PATHOLOGY

- Isolated CL and CL + CP thought to be related etiologically
  - May be related to number of genes &/or environmental factors
- > 250 syndromes associated with CL ± CP
  - Account for 3-8% of orofacial clefts

CLINICAL ISSUES

- Most common major congenital defect in humans
- CL and CP occur together in 45% of cases
- 80% of CL cases unilateral
- Gender
  - CL ± CP = M > F; CP = F > M
- Ethnicity
  - Native Americans > Asians > whites > blacks
- Treatment: Sequence of surgical repairs with multidisciplinary approach

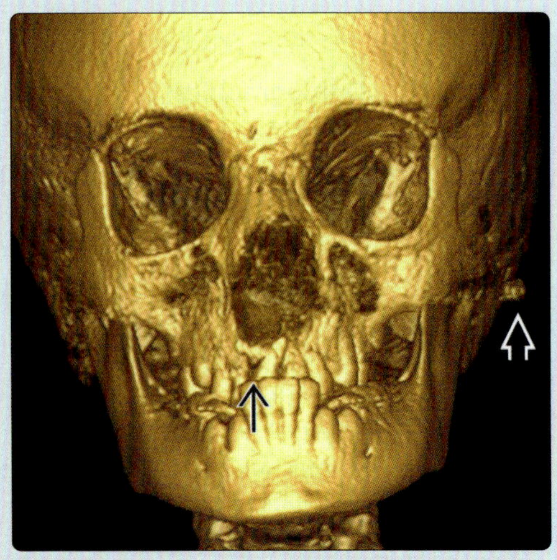

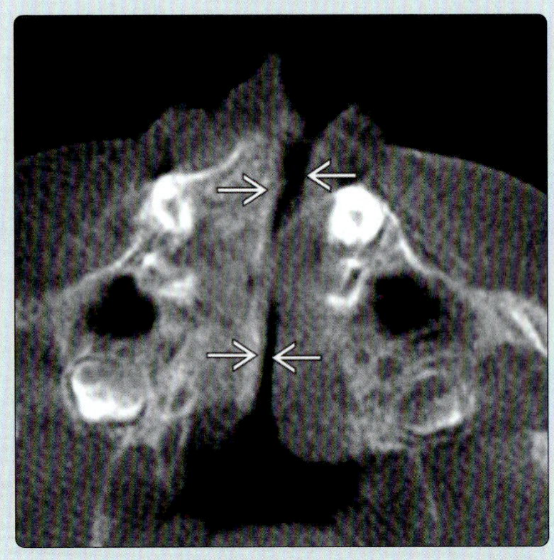

(Left) *3D CBCT reformation shows a child with multiple craniofacial and dental defects but not a recognized syndrome. Note the cleft in the maxilla, the missing right lateral incisor and canine, and the asymmetry of the nasal cavity. The round device on the left side of the head is a portion of a hearing aid. The patient had auditory canal defects as well.* **(Right)** *Axial CBCT shows a distinct defect in the maxilla consistent with a cleft. The defect involves both the primary and secondary palatal shelves.*

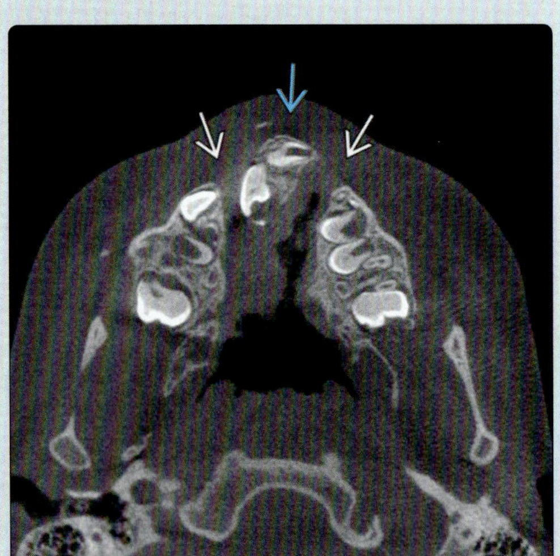

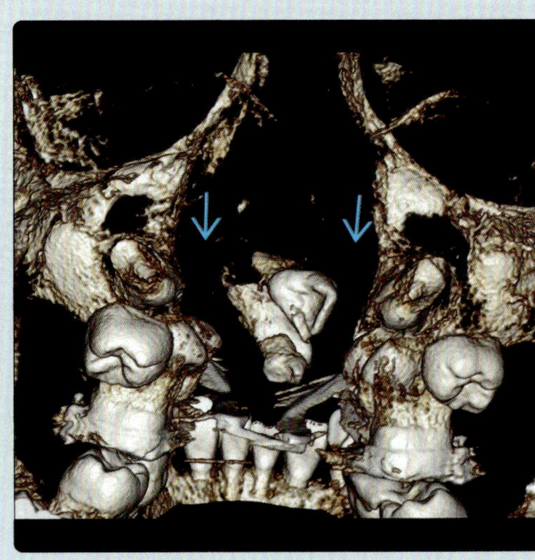

(Left) *Axial CBCT of an 8-year-old girl shows bilateral clefts of the palate. The patient did not have any known syndromes, and there are no clefts of the upper lip. A midline bony island contains a maxillary central incisor, lateral incisor, and what appears to be a supernumerary tooth.* **(Right)** *3D CBCT rendering shows the same patient as viewed from posterior to anterior. The complete bilateral clefts into the nasal fossa are clearly seen. Note the 3 isolated teeth in the midline.*

Clefts

TERMINOLOGY

Definitions

- Developmental disturbance resulting in failure of proper fusion of various orofacial tissues
    - Common clefts
        - **Cleft lip (CL)**: Defective fusion of median nasal process with maxillary process
        - **Cleft palate (CP)**: Fusion failure of primary palatal shelves
    - Uncommon clefts
        - **Lateral facial cleft**: Lack of fusion of maxillary and mandibular processes
            - Extends from commissure toward ear
        - **Oblique facial cleft**: Failure of fusion of lateral nasal process with maxillary process
            - Extends from upper lip to eye
        - **Median cleft of upper lip**: Failure of fusion of medial nasal processes
        - **Median maxillary anterior alveolar cleft**: Failure of fusion of secondary palatal shelves

IMAGING

General Features

- Location
    - Clefts of alveolus usually between lateral incisor and canine
    - Often accompanied by **missing teeth** (lateral incisor) or supernumerary teeth
    - Defect often extends into nasal cavity
        - Resulting asymmetry of nasal cavity floor, nasal cavity contents

Imaging Recommendations

- Best imaging tool
    - Panoramic for general overview
    - CT in multiplanar format, including CBCT, with 3D reconstruction

DIFFERENTIAL DIAGNOSIS

Fracture

- History of trauma

PATHOLOGY

General Features

- Etiology
    - Isolated CL and CL + CP thought to be related etiologically
        - Exact cause still unknown
        - May be related to a number of genes &/or environmental factors
            - Environmental factors include maternal age, maternal use of certain medications, smoking, alcohol use during pregnancy
    - > 250 syndromes associated with CL ± CP
        - Account for 3-8% of orofacial clefts
- Genetics
    - Single gene defects
        - Autosomal dominant
        - Autosomal recessive
        - X-linked
    - Chromosome anomalies (includes deletion 22q11, trisomy 21, trisomy 13)
    - Idiopathic
- Associated abnormalities
    - Pierre Robin sequence (most common association)
        - CP
        - Mandibular micrognathia and glossoptosis

CLINICAL ISSUES

Presentation

- Clinical profile
    - CL and CP **occur together in 45%** of cases
        - Isolated CP in 30% of cases
        - Isolated CL in 25% of cases
    - Reported prevalence
        - CL ± CP 9.92 per 10,000

Demographics

- Gender
    - M > F for CL ± CP
        - Isolated CL ratio: 1.5:1
        - CL + CP ratio: 2:1
    - F > M for isolated CP (2:1)
- Ethnicity
    - CL ± CP
        - Native Americans: 3.6/1,000 births
        - Asians: 1.5x higher than whites
        - Whites: 1/700-1,000 births
        - Blacks: 0.4/1,000 births
    - Isolated CP: 0.4/1,000 in whites and blacks
- Epidemiology
    - CL/CP most common major congenital defect in humans
        - 80% of CL cases unilateral
            - 70% of unilateral CL occurs on left side
    - Uncommon clefts
        - Lateral facial cleft: 0.3% of orofacial clefts
            - Isolated defect or associated with mandibulofacial dysostosis (Treacher Collins syndrome)
        - Oblique facial cleft: 1/1,300 clefts

Treatment

- **Multidisciplinary approach** ideal
    - Pediatrician, pediatric dentist, oral and maxillofacial surgeon, orthodontist
    - Otolaryngologist, plastic surgeon, speech pathologist, geneticist
- Sequence of surgical repairs
- Genetic counseling
    - Risk for sibling/offspring of patient: 3-5%
    - Risk up to 20% for sibling/offspring of patient if other 1st-degree relatives affected

SELECTED REFERENCES

1. Phan M et al: Tooth agenesis and orofacial clefting: genetic brothers in arms? Hum Genet. 135(12):1299-1327, 2016
2. IPDTOC Working Group.: Prevalence at birth of cleft lip with or without cleft palate: data from the International Perinatal Database of Typical Oral Clefts (IPDTOC). Cleft Palate Craniofac J. 48(1):66-81, 2011

KEY FACTS

TERMINOLOGY

- Definition: Rare nonneoplastic hereditary disease related to genetic mutations characterized by bilateral jaw enlargement in childhood
- Name derives from round face and lower eyelid retraction that leads to **"eyes raised to heaven"** or cherub-like appearance

IMAGING

- Bilateral expansile multilocular mandibular radiolucencies
- Posterior mandible: Angle, ramus, retromolar region
- Maxilla: Tuberosity affected initially, later infraorbital area, orbital floor, and anterior maxilla
- Because lesions originate in posterior areas, teeth often displaced anteriorly
- Teeth may exhibit significant displacement, malformation, ectopic eruption or failure to erupt

TOP DIFFERENTIAL DIAGNOSES

- Nevoid basal cell carcinoma syndrome
- Fibrous dysplasia
- Central giant cell granuloma
- Brown tumor of hyperparathyroidism
- McCune-Albright syndrome

CLINICAL ISSUES

- Painless, firm, bilateral, symmetric enlargement of lower face
- Self-limiting, and lesions usually regress after puberty
- Clinical swelling usually abates by 3rd decade
- Radiolucent lesions replaced by sclerotic or granular-appearing bone that undergoes progressive remodeling to essentially normal appearance and morphology
- **Many cases do not require treatment** because they regress; conservative surgery for cosmetic or functional purposes

(Left) *Panoramic radiograph shows cherubism in the right mandible that appears as a scalloping multilocular radiolucency occupying the right ramus and body →. The permanent 1st molar tooth is tipped →, and the developing premolars are malposed →. (Courtesy M. Noujeim, DDS.)* **(Right)** *Panoramic radiograph in the same patient shows cherubism affecting the left side. The 2nd mandibular premolar tooth is displaced anteriorly →, and the 1st molar is tipped distally →. (Courtesy M. Noujeim, DDS.)*

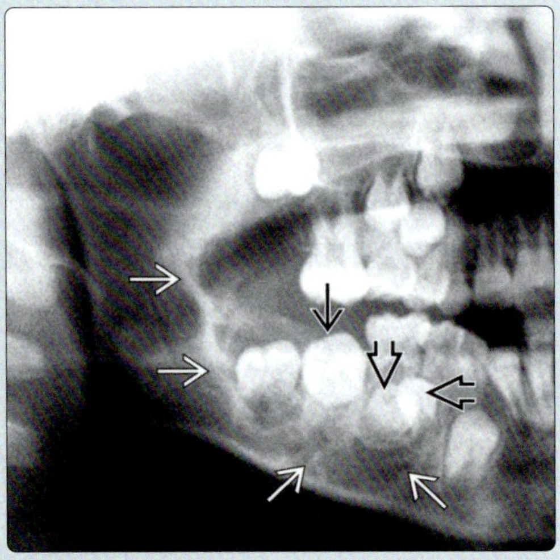

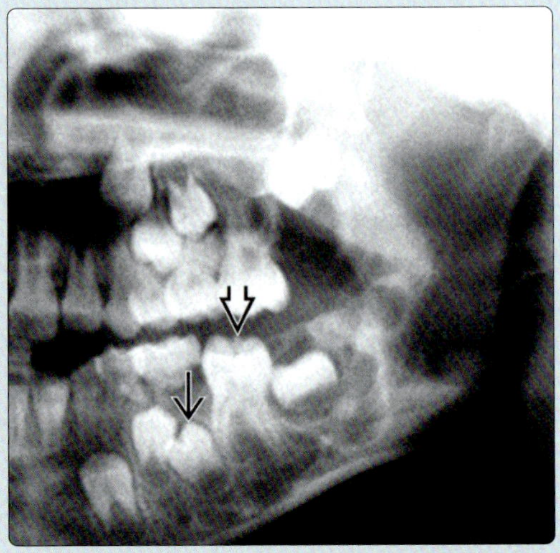

(Left) *PA radiograph in the same patient shows cherubism presenting as symmetrical involvement of the mandible with mild expansion →. (Courtesy M. Noujeim, DDS.)* **(Right)** *Panoramic radiograph shows cherubism in the right mandible of a young adult. The lesion in the ramus → is starting to regress and has a granular internal appearance. The portion of the lesion apical to the molar teeth still has a multilocular cystic appearance →. (Courtesy G. Packota, DMD.)*

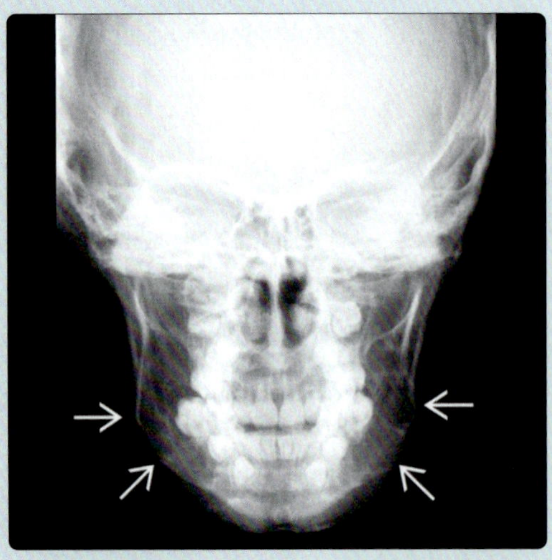

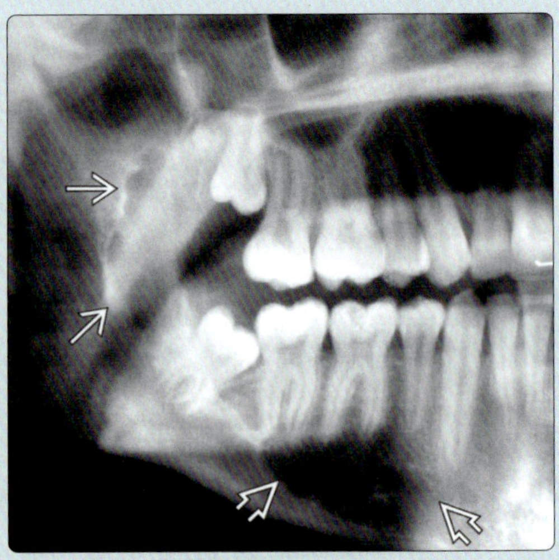

TERMINOLOGY

Synonyms

- Familial fibrous dysplasia (FD)
- Familial multilocular cystic disease of jaw, familial benign giant cell tumor of jaw

Definitions

- Rare nonneoplastic hereditary disease characterized by bilateral jaw enlargement in childhood
  - Related to genetic mutations
  - Genetically distinct from FD
- Round face and lower eyelid retraction that leads to **"eyes raised to heaven"** or cherub-like appearance

IMAGING

General Features

- Best diagnostic clue
  - **Bilateral expansile multilocular mandibular radiolucencies**
    - Unilateral cases reported
    - Often also submandibular lymph node enlargement
- Location
  - Mandible > maxilla
    - Lesions originate in **posterior regions**
    - Mandible: Angle, ramus, retromolar region
    - Coronoid process may be involved
    - Condyles usually spared but condylar lesions reported
    - Maxilla: Tuberosity affected 1st, later infraorbital area, orbital floor, and anterior maxilla
      - If maxilla involved, mandible always involved
  - Can affect other bones: Humerus, ribs, femoral necks
- Size
  - Ranges from mild mandibular involvement to extensive involvement of both jaws with massive deformity
- Morphology
  - Bilateral symmetric cystic multilocular radiolucencies

Imaging Recommendations

- Best imaging tool
  - Panoramic radiograph good for initial diagnosis
  - Bone CT or CBCT to determine local extent of lesions in all planes and localize impacted teeth

Radiographic Findings

- **Bilateral multilocular well-defined expansile radiolucencies**
- Lesions usually **symmetrical** on both sides
- Because lesions originate in posterior areas, **teeth** often **displaced anteriorly**
  - Tooth roots **deformed** or **resorbed**
  - Tooth buds may be **destroyed**
  - Some permanent teeth missing or malformed, especially **mandibular 1st and 2nd molars**
  - Primary teeth may prematurely erupt or **exfoliate**
- Mandibular canal displaced inferiorly

CT Findings

- Multilocular expansile radiolucencies displacing teeth
  - Cortical thinning and **expansion** but no periosteal reaction

MR Findings

- Hypointense or intermediate T1 signal
- Variable T2 signal: Hypo-, hyper-, or intermediate signal intensity
  - May show areas of hyperintensity that are normal on CT

DIFFERENTIAL DIAGNOSIS

Nevoid Basal Cell Carcinoma Syndrome

- Multiple odontogenic keratocysts
- May present as bilateral multilocular radiolucencies
- Less expansile

Fibrous Dysplasia

- Normal medullary bone replaced by mixture of fibrous tissue & immature bone
- Sclerotic ground-glass, mixed cystic & sclerotic, and cystic variants
- Most cases of FD are **unilateral** and **monostotic**
- Cheeks not symmetrically swollen
- No (or minor) tooth displacement in FD
- Later onset in FD
- Lesions stabilize rather than regress in adulthood

Central Giant Cell Granuloma

- Expansile multilocular radiolucency with granular wispy trabeculae
- Most common in anterior mandible; cherubism originates in ramus
- Not bilateral, usually unilateral
- Does not regress in adulthood

Brown Tumor of Hyperparathyroidism

- Occurs in both mandible and maxilla but later onset
- Increased serum Ca, phosphorus, alkaline phosphatase vs. normal levels in cherubism

McCune-Albright Syndrome

- Subtype of polyostotic FD
- Multiple jaw lesions may mimic cherubism
- Classic triad of polyostotic FD, precocious puberty, and cutaneous hyperpigmentation

PATHOLOGY

General Features

- Genetics
  - **Autosomal dominant**
    - 100% penetrance in male patients and 50-70% penetrance in female patients
  - Heterozygous mutation in *SH3BP2* gene, gene map locus 4p16.3
- Associated abnormalities
  - Noonan syndrome: Ocular hypertelorism, ptosis, downward slanting palpebral fissures, broad neck, and cryptorchidism
  - Ramon syndrome: Short stature, mental retardation, gingival fibromatosis, and epilepsy
  - Neurofibromatosis type 1

Staging, Grading, & Classification

- Arnott grading system based on radiographic location and lesion severity

- Grade 1: Posterior mandible involvement only
- Grade 2: Full mandibular involvement and minimal maxillary involvement
- Grade 3: Both jaws diffusely affected
- Grade 4: All classical features of disease present but exceed grade 3

- Grade can change depending on findings at follow-up examination
- Some clinicians do not use grading system and instead gauge disease severity based on rate of lesion growth, size, cortical bone perforation or thinning, tooth displacement, and functional deficits
- Other grading systems are based on lesion location with presence/absence of root resorption &/or extragnathic involvement (Motamedi)
  - Raposo-Amaral system subdivides grades based on solitary vs. multiple lesions of involved jaw sites

Microscopic Features

- Osteolytic stage: Proliferating vascular fibrous connective tissue with abundant multinucleated giant cells
  - Similar to brown tumor of hyperparathyroidism, giant cell tumor, and central giant cell granuloma
- Repair stage: Well-vascularized nodules with highly active fibroblasts
- Bone restoration stage: Osteogenesis

CLINICAL ISSUES

Presentation

- Most common signs/symptoms
  - Painless, firm, bilateral, symmetric enlargement of lower face
    - May affect only mandible or both jaws
    - Maxillary enlargement usually not as severe as mandibular enlargement
      - Mandibular enlargement usually symmetric, whereas maxillary involvement can be asymmetric
- Other signs/symptoms
  - Premature exfoliation of primary and permanent teeth, especially mandibular 1st and 2nd molars
  - Teeth: Displacement, malformation, agenesis, ectopic, unerupted
    - Impact on development and eruption of teeth varies depending on time of disease onset and severity of expansile lesions
  - If maxilla also involved: Problems with speech, respiration, swallowing, and mastication
  - Proptosis, upward displacement of globes
    - Lid retraction, diplopia, visual loss due to optic atrophy
    - Lower eyelid retraction ("eyes raised to heaven"); cherub-like appearance
- Clinical profile
  - Young child with nontender bilateral jaw enlargement

Demographics

- Age
  - Develops between 2-7 years old with rapid progression until puberty
- Gender
  - M:F = 2:1, although some reports of M = F

Natural History & Prognosis

- Self-limiting, and lesions usually regress after puberty
  - Clinical swelling usually abates by 3rd decade
  - Aggressive form in which enlargement continues and lesions do not involute in adulthood
- With regression
  - Radiolucent lesions replaced by **sclerotic or granular-appearing bone**
  - New bone undergoes progressive remodeling to essentially **normal trabecular appearance and morphology**
  - Jaws may appear normal in adulthood

Treatment

- Usually only observation because lesions regress
- May need conservative surgery for cosmetic or functional purposes
  - Surgery to uncover unerupted, displaced teeth
  - Orthodontics to treat malocclusion

DIAGNOSTIC CHECKLIST

Consider

- If bilateral painless facial swelling in young child, think cherubism
- Several or all of following may point to cherubism
  - Family history
  - Characteristic facial appearance
  - Early extensive bilateral mandibular swelling
  - Absence of other bone pathology
  - Submandibular lymphadenopathy
  - Impacted or congenitally missing permanent molars

Reporting Tips

- At follow-up examinations, check for following
  - Lesion progression
  - Effects on unerupted teeth to assess need for surgical procedures to uncover or remove impacted teeth
  - Maxillary and orbital involvement if it was not previously present
  - Lesion regression in older patients

SELECTED REFERENCES

1. Jiao Y et al: Cherubism misdiagnosed as giant cell tumor: a case report and review of literature. Int J Clin Exp Med. 8(3):4656-63, 2015
2. Kömerik N et al: Cherubism. Head Neck Pathol. 8(2):164-7, 2014
3. Pinheiro LR et al: Clinical and imagiological findings of central giant cell lesion and cherubism. Braz Dent J. 24(1):74-9, 2013
4. Redfors M et al: Cherubism: panoramic and CT features in adults. Dentomaxillofac Radiol. 42(10):20130034, 2013
5. Papadaki ME et al: Cherubism: best clinical practice. Orphanet J Rare Dis. 7 Suppl 1:S6, 2012
6. Roginsky VV et al: Familial cherubism: the experience of the Moscow Central Institute for Stomatology and Maxillo-Facial Surgery. Int J Oral Maxillofac Surg. 38(3):218-23, 2009
7. Carvalho Silva E et al: Cherubism: clinicoradiographic features, treatment, and long-term follow-up of 8 cases. J Oral Maxillofac Surg. 65(3):517-22, 2007
8. Pontes FS et al: Aggressive case of cherubism: 17-year follow-up. Int J Pediatr Otorhinolaryngol. 71(5):831-5, 2007
9. Jain V et al: Radiographic, CT and MRI features of cherubism. Pediatr Radiol. 36(10):1099-104, 2006

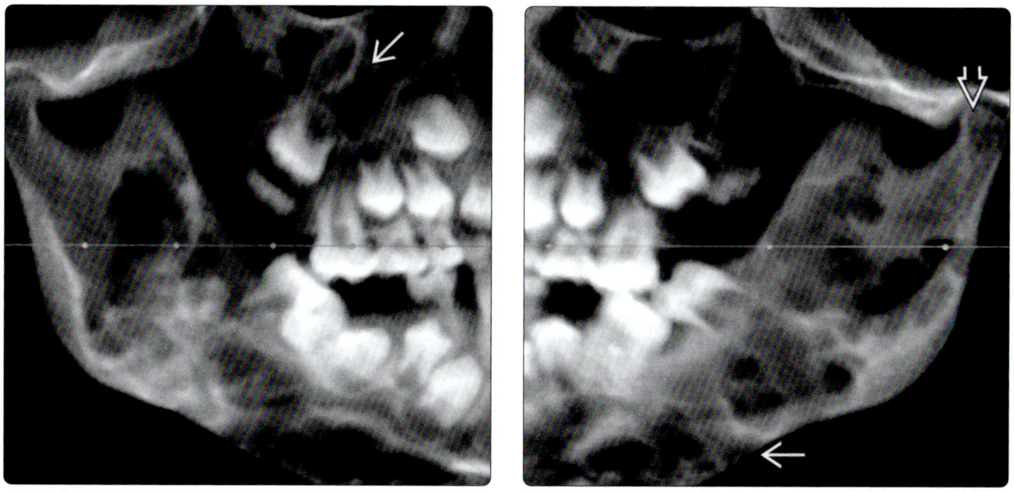

(Left) *Panoramic reformat CBCT shows cherubism in the right maxilla and mandible. The lesion has a typical scalloped multilocular appearance. Note the anterior displacement of the unerupted mandibular teeth and obliteration of the maxillary sinus* ➡. **(Right)** *Panoramic reformat CBCT in the same patient shows symmetrical and similar changes on the left side of the jaws. Note involvement of the entire ramus and mandibular body, with a thinned and expanded inferior mandibular border* ➡. *The condyle is spared* ➡.

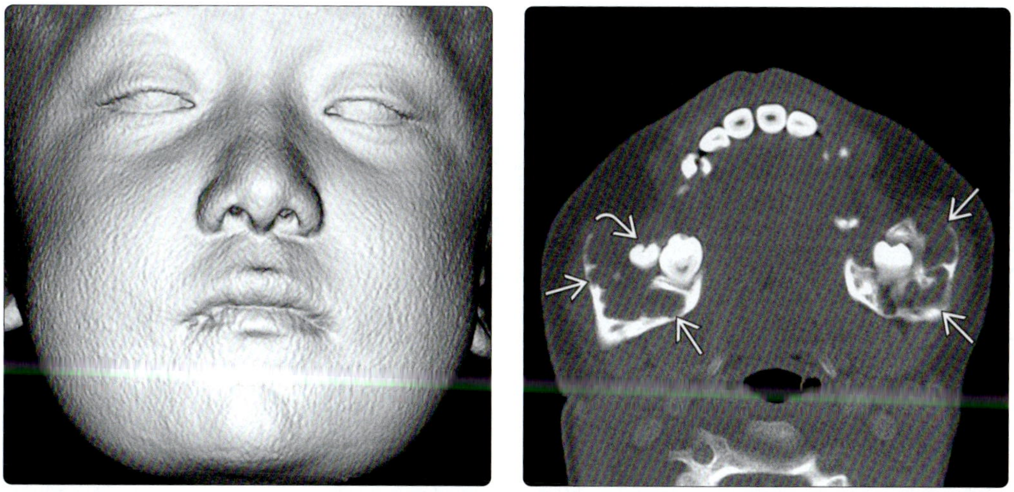

(Left) *Soft tissue rendering CBCT in the same patient shows the characteristic fullness of cheeks and mandible typically seen in cherubism.* **(Right)** *Axial bone CT shows bilateral multilocular cystic lesions in the mandible* ➡ *with several areas of diffuse cortical thinning without aggressive bone destruction or periosteal reaction, typical of cherubism. Note the anterior displacement of the molar tooth on the right side* ➡ *and the relative bilateral symmetry of the lesions. (Courtesy J. Curé, MD.)*

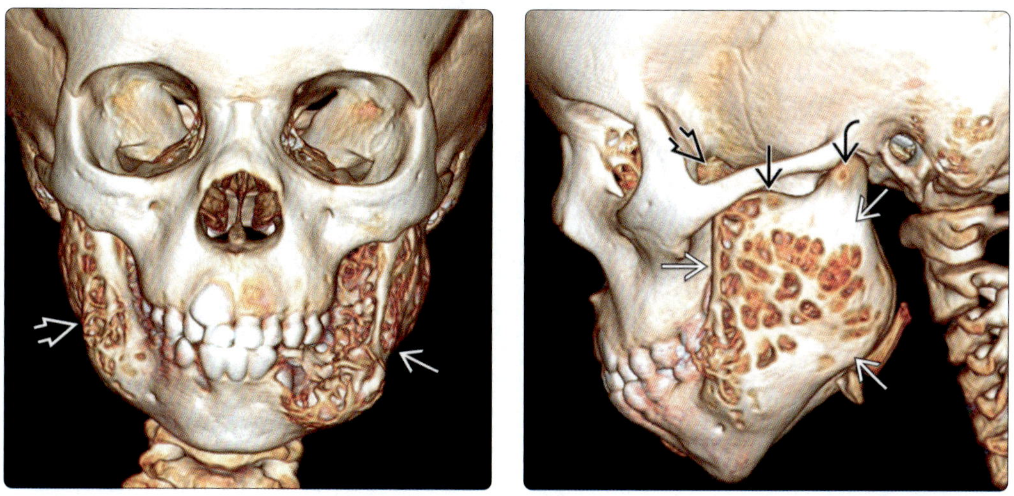

(Left) *3D reconstruction image shows the deformity with left* ➡ *greater than right* ➡ *enlargement of the mandible due to the expansile multilocular lesions of cherubism. Maxillary involvement is not evident in this case. (Courtesy J. Curé, MD.)* **(Right)** *Lateral 3D reconstruction in the same patient shows diffuse expansion of the left mandible* ➡. *Note involvement of the coronoid process* ➡, *expansion of the coronoid notch* ➡, *and early condylar involvement* ➡. *(Courtesy J. Curé, MD.)*

Basal Cell Nevus Syndrome

KEY FACTS

TERMINOLOGY

- Basal cell nevus syndrome (BCNS): **Autosomal dominant** disorder with multiple odontogenic keratocysts (OKC), basal cell carcinomas (BCCa), and other skeletal and craniofacial abnormalities
- Synonyms: Gorlin syndrome, **Gorlin-Goltz syndrome**, nevoid basal cell carcinoma syndrome

IMAGING

- Multiple cyst-like lesions in mandible and maxilla
- Radiolucent with well-defined, corticated periphery
- **Displacement of developing and erupted teeth**

TOP DIFFERENTIAL DIAGNOSES

- OKC (nonsyndromic)
- Multiple dentigerous cysts
- Cherubism
- Langerhans cell histiocytosis

PATHOLOGY

- Jaw lesions histologically identical to OKCs
- Associated abnormalities
  - Multiple **basal cell carcinomas**
  - Marked **calcification of falx cerebri**
  - **Rib and vertebral abnormalities**
  - Frontal and parietal bossing, macrocephaly, hypertelorism
  - Medulloblastoma

CLINICAL ISSUES

- Lesions may cause delayed eruption, malocclusion, or swelling
- OKCs in BCNS develop at earlier age than nonsyndromic OKCs (~ 15 years)
- High recurrence rate of jaw lesions
- Regular **radiographic monitoring for recurrence and new lesions** essential
  - Panoramic, CBCT modalities of choice

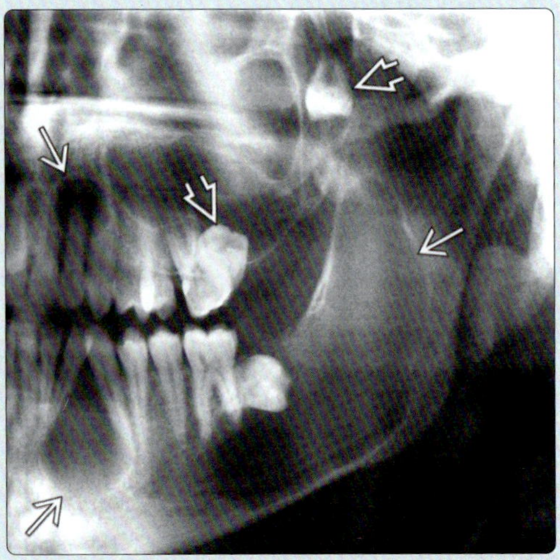

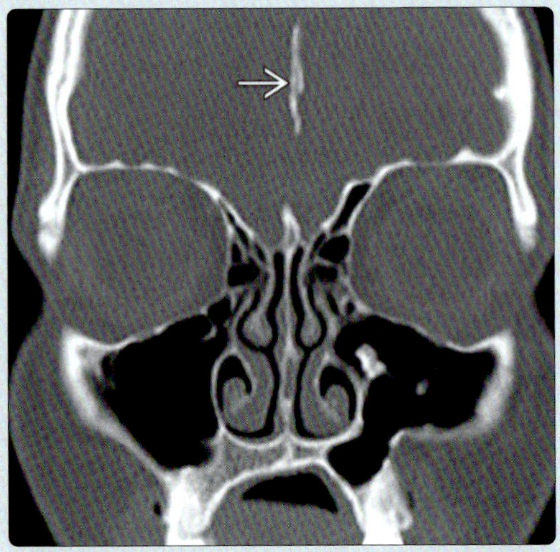

(Left) *Cropped panoramic radiograph shows at least 4 cystic lesions present in the left side of the jaws ➡. In the posterior maxilla, the displaced molars ➡ are more clearly seen than the lesion itself. Multiple cyst-like lesions in the jaws raise suspicion of basal cell nevus syndrome (BCNS).* **(Right)** *Coronal bone CT of a patient with BCNS demonstrates calcification of the falx cerebri ➡. Though this may occur in the normal population, it is evident at a much earlier age in patients with this syndrome.*

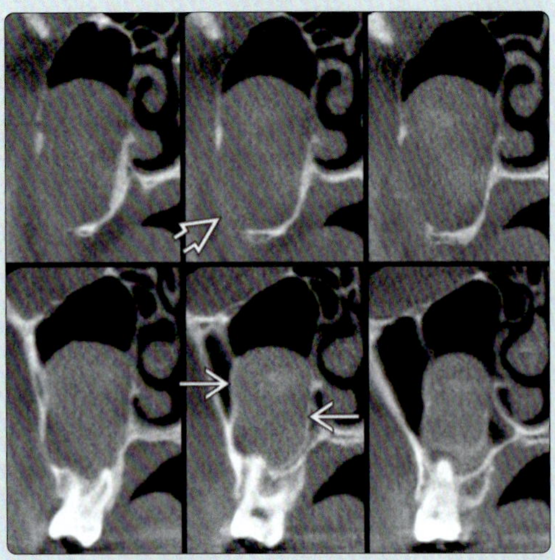

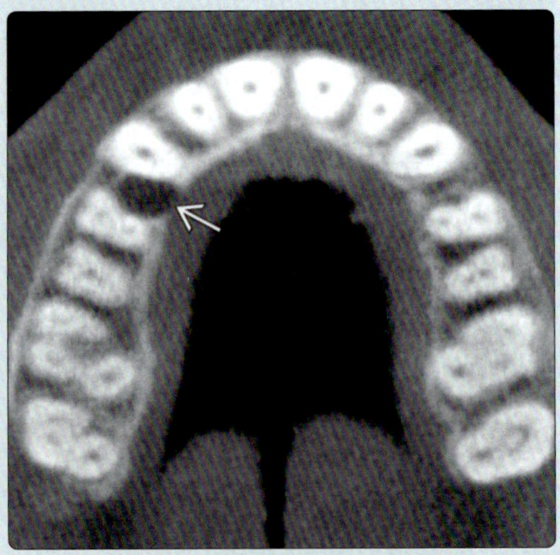

(Left) *CBCT cross sections of the posterior right maxilla in a patient with BCNS show a cyst-like lesion in the 3rd molar region extending into the maxillary sinus. The cortication around the periphery ➡ indicates the lesion originated outside the sinus. The lateral wall of the maxilla is perforated ➡.* **(Right)** *Axial CBCT of the same patient shows a small developing lesion in the right maxilla ➡. This was an incidental finding and highlights the importance of thoroughly examining patients for additional lesions.*

TERMINOLOGY

Abbreviations

- Basal cell nevus syndrome (BCNS)

Synonyms

- **Gorlin-Goltz syndrome**, Gorlin syndrome, nevoid basal cell carcinoma syndrome, bifid rib syndrome

Definitions

- **Autosomal dominant** disorder with multiple odontogenic keratocysts (OKC), basal cell carcinomas (BCCa), and other skeletal and craniofacial abnormalities

IMAGING

General Features

- Best diagnostic clue
  - Multiple cyst-like lesions in jaws of young patient with displacement of teeth
  - Lesion characteristics same as OKC
- Location
  - Mandible > maxilla
  - Often involving follicle of developing teeth
- Morphology
  - Most lesions rounded, unilocular

Radiographic Findings

- Radiography
  - Radiolucent with well-defined, corticated periphery
  - **Displacement of developing and erupted teeth**

CT Findings

- Low-density internal structure
- Periphery may scallop and thin cortices
- Tendency to grow along bone ± expansion
- May detect small lesions unseen on plain radiography
  - **Essential to examine both jaws thoroughly**

MR Findings

- Low to intermediate T1, high T2 signal

Imaging Recommendations

- Best imaging tool
  - MDCT: If extension into soft tissues suspected
  - CBCT: Lower dose = advantage since multiple follow-up studies needed
  - Panoramic: For follow-up

DIFFERENTIAL DIAGNOSIS

Multiple Odontogenic Keratocysts (Nonsyndromic)

- 5% of OKCs may be multiple
- Rule out other features of BCNS

Multiple Dentigerous Cysts

- Always around crowns of unerupted teeth with symmetrical enlargement of follicles

Cherubism

- Also multiple lesions in children but more posteriorly
- Lesions are multilocular, **highly expansile**

Langerhans Cell Histiocytosis

- Multiple lesions in young patient
- Lesions are noncorticated, do not displace teeth

PATHOLOGY

General Features

- Etiology
  - OKC arises from remnants of dental lamina
  - UV radiation strong risk factor for BCCa
- Genetics
  - **Autosomal dominant**
  - Mutations of *PTCH1* gene (hedgehog pathway tumor suppressor)
  - 50% of cases are new mutations
- Associated abnormalities
  - Multiple **basal cell carcinomas**: Face, neck, and thorax
  - **Palmar and plantar pitting**
  - Marked **calcification of falx**, dura, bridged sella
  - **Rib abnormalities**: Bifid, fused, splayed
  - Frontal and parietal bossing, macrocephaly, hypertelorism
  - Kyphoscoliosis and vertebral abnormalities
  - Medulloblastomas: Very early age (0-2 years)

Microscopic Features

- Jaw lesions identical to OKCs

CLINICAL ISSUES

Presentation

- Most common signs/symptoms
  - Asymptomatic, delayed eruption, malocclusion, or swelling
  - Pain is present occasionally

Demographics

- Age
  - OKC in BCNS develop earlier than nonsyndromic OKC
- Gender
  - M = F

Natural History & Prognosis

- **High recurrence rate** of OKC (60%)
- BCCa ↑ proliferation after puberty but rarely invasive

Treatment

- OKC: Enucleation or marsupialization with curettage and Carnoy solution, en block resection
- Vismodegib (hedgehog pathway inhibitor) shows promise in reducing size of OKCs
- Regular **radiographic monitoring for recurrence and new lesions** essential

DIAGNOSTIC CHECKLIST

Reporting Tips

- Examine jaws for additional developing lesions

SELECTED REFERENCES

1. Tang JY et al: Inhibition of the hedgehog pathway in patients with basal-cell nevus syndrome: final results from the multicentre, randomised, double-blind, placebo-controlled, phase 2 trial. Lancet Oncol. ePub, 2016

Cleidocranial Dysplasia

KEY FACTS

TERMINOLOGY

- Formerly known as **cleidocranial dysostosis**

IMAGING

- Numerous unerupted, **supernumerary teeth**
- Dense, coarse trabecular pattern
- Hypoplastic maxilla
- Small or absent maxillary sinuses
- High arched palate
- Open mandibular symphysis
- Delayed closure of sutures
- Secondary centers of ossification in sutures
- Wormian bones
- Brachycephaly

TOP DIFFERENTIAL DIAGNOSES

- **Gardner syndrome**
- **Pycnodysostosis**

PATHOLOGY

- Autosomal-dominant pattern; 40% spontaneous mutations
- Incidence: 1:1,000,000
- **Absence of cellular cementum** plus dense bone thought to **hinder tooth eruption**

CLINICAL ISSUES

- Short stature
- Large head with pronounced frontal and parietal bossing
- Hypoplastic &/or malformed clavicles
  - Absent clavicles in 10% of cases (unilateral or bilateral)
  - In some patients, shoulders may approximate in midline
- Prolonged retention of primary teeth
- Delayed or failed eruption of permanent teeth
- Treatment
  - Often no treatment required for skeletal abnormalities
  - Removal of primary and supernumerary teeth
  - Orthodontic extrusion of permanent teeth
  - Prosthodontic replacement

(Left) *Cropped panoramic image of 28-year-old woman exhibits multiple supernumerary teeth* ➔*, retained primary teeth* ➔*, anomalous tooth formation* ➔*, and missing teeth* ➔*.* **(Right)** *Panoramic radiograph shows multiple unerupted (impacted) teeth in an 80-year-old woman whose concern was a tooth coming in under her denture. Note the development of pathology between the right mandibular molars* ➔*, which caused eruption of the 2nd molar into the oral cavity.*

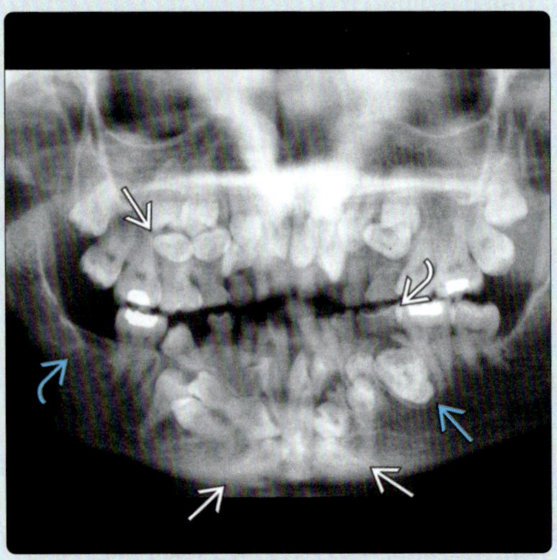

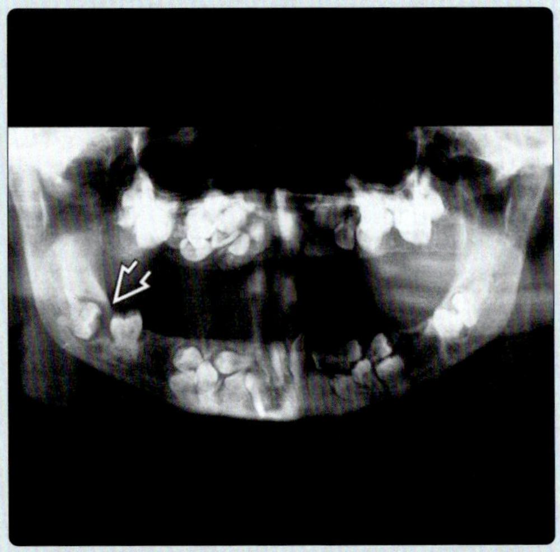

(Left) *Sagittal reformat CBCT demonstrates several unerupted permanent teeth* ➔ *and supernumerary teeth* ➔ *in a young girl with cleidocranial dysplasia.* **(Right)** *3D reformatted CBCT in the same patient shows the multiple unerupted permanent and supernumerary teeth in the maxilla. Treatment of these individuals should ideally involve a multidisciplinary approach including an oral surgeon, orthodontist, pediatric dentist, and possibly a prosthodontic specialist.*

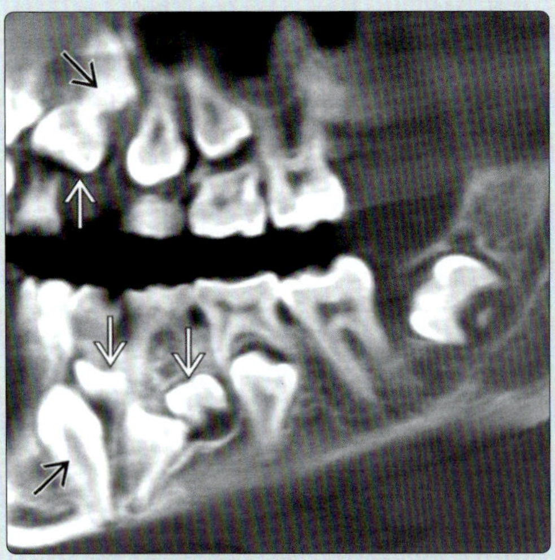

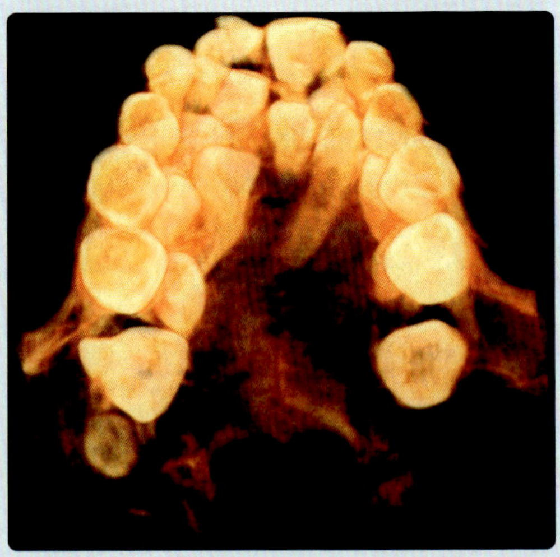

TERMINOLOGY

Synonyms

- Formerly known as **cleidocranial dysostosis**
- Scheuthauer-Marie-Sainton syndrome

Definitions

- Developmental defect with skeletal and dental abnormalities

IMAGING

General Features

- Best diagnostic clue
  - Brachycephaly
  - Clavicular abnormalities
  - Multiple unerupted permanent and supernumerary teeth

Radiographic Findings

- Craniofacial complex
  - Multiple **supernumerary teeth**
  - Numerous unerupted permanent teeth, retained primary teeth
  - Dense, coarse trabecular pattern in jaws
  - Short, narrow ascending mandibular rami, slender pointed coronoid process
  - High arched palate
  - Thin zygomatic arch
  - Small or absent maxillary sinuses
  - Open mandibular symphysis
    - 3% of adults
    - 64% of children
- Skull
  - Delayed closure of sutures
  - Secondary centers of ossification in sutures
  - Wormian bones

Imaging Recommendations

- Best imaging tool
  - Lateral and PA skull views
  - Panoramic images
  - CBCT or medical CT

DIFFERENTIAL DIAGNOSIS

Gardner Syndrome

- Familial colorectal polyposis
- Multiple osteomas: In jaws, most commonly on ramus and inferior border of mandible
- **Supernumerary teeth**
- Epidermoid cysts

Pycnodysostosis

- Short stature
- Dense, brittle bones
- Open sutures
- Hypoplastic maxilla
- Delayed dental eruption
- **Supernumerary teeth**

PATHOLOGY

General Features

- Etiology
  - Defect in *RUNX2* gene on chromosome 6p21
  - Gene codes for osteoblast-specific transcription factor
  - Initially thought to affect only membranous bones (clavicle, flat bones)
  - Now thought to be generalized disorder affecting endochondral ossification
- Genetics
  - Autosomal-dominant pattern
  - 40% spontaneous mutations
  - Incidence: 1:1 million
  - Variable expressivity

Gross Pathologic & Surgical Features

- Little to no cellular cementum on erupted or unerupted teeth
- **Absence of cementum** plus dense bone thought to **hinder tooth eruption**

CLINICAL ISSUES

Presentation

- Most common signs/symptoms
  - Hypoplastic &/or **malformed clavicles**
  - Absent clavicles in 10% of cases (unilateral or bilateral)
  - Narrow, drooping shoulders
    - In some patients, shoulders nearly approximate each other in front of chest
  - Narrow, high arched palate
  - Increased prevalence of cleft palate
  - Prolonged retention of primary teeth
  - Delayed or failed eruption of permanent teeth
  - Hypoplastic maxilla
- Other signs/symptoms
  - Short stature
  - Large head with pronounced frontal and parietal bossing
  - Ocular hypertelorism
  - Broad nose base
  - Depressed nasal bridge

Treatment

- Often no treatment required for skeletal abnormalities
- Dental problems
  - Pronounced malocclusion is result of crowding, disorganized dentition
  - Team approach ideal
    - Removal of primary and supernumerary teeth
    - Orthodontic extrusion of permanent teeth

SELECTED REFERENCES

1. Lubinsky M et al: Syndromes with supernumerary teeth. Am J Med Genet A. 170(10):2611-6, 2016
2. Yamasaki S et al: Generation of cleidocranial dysplasia-specific human induced pluripotent stem cells in completely serum-, feeder-, and integration-free culture. In Vitro Cell Dev Biol Anim. 52(2):252-64, 2016
3. Schnutenhaus S et al: Histological examination and clinical evaluation of the jawbone of an adult patient with cleidocranial dysplasia: a case report. Int J Clin Exp Pathol. 8(7):8521-31, 2015

Pierre Robin Sequence

KEY FACTS

TERMINOLOGY

- Pierre Robin sequence (PRS)
- Micrognathia or retrognathia, glossoptosis, respiratory distress, ± posterior U-shaped cleft palate

IMAGING

- Bilateral symmetric micrognathia
- Elevated, posteriorly displaced tongue
- Posterior U-shaped cleft palate
- Additional features depend on syndromic etiology

TOP DIFFERENTIAL DIAGNOSES

- Stickler & related syndromes (18% of PRS)
- Velocardiofacial syndrome (VCFS) (7% of PRS)
- Treacher Collins syndrome (5% of PRS)

PATHOLOGY

- Collagen (COL) gene mutations: Stickler syndromes
- 22q11.2 deletion: Velocardiofacial syndrome
- 17q24; *SOX9* regulatory mutations: PRS locus
- Primary micrognathia → glossoptosis → failure of palatal shelf elevation ± fusion

CLINICAL ISSUES

- Feeding & breathing difficulties, failure to thrive
- Stickler: Progressive myopia, joint degeneration
- VCFS: Cardiac anomalies, adenoid hypoplasia, velopharyngeal insufficiency, learning difficulties
- Neonatal treatment: Prone position, respiratory & nutritional support, mandibular distraction osteogenesis

DIAGNOSTIC CHECKLIST

- Consider Stickler syndrome: Familial myopia, premature joint degeneration
- Consider VCFS: Adenoid hypoplasia, medial deviation of cervical internal carotid arteries

(Left) *Lateral 3D reformation of a 3-week-old girl with Pierre Robin sequence (PRS) shows moderate, symmetric micrognathia. Note that the zygomatic arch and external auditory canal are present.* **(Right)** *Sagittal CT reconstruction in the same patient reveals a shortened hard palate and glossoptosis (abnormal inferior or posterior displacement of the tongue). The tongue protrudes above and behind the palate and obstructs the oropharynx. Retrusion of the mandible is also noted.*

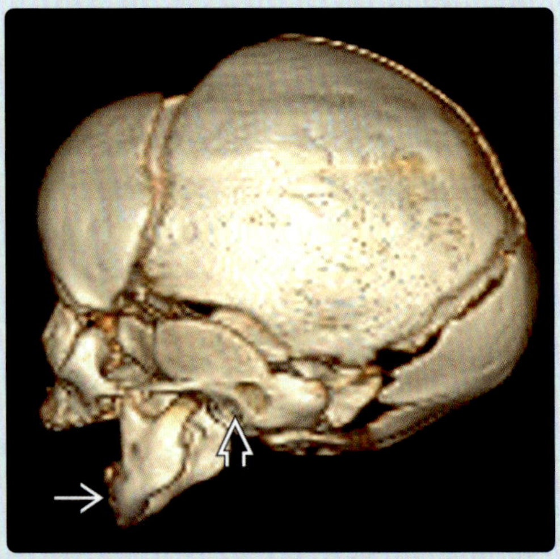

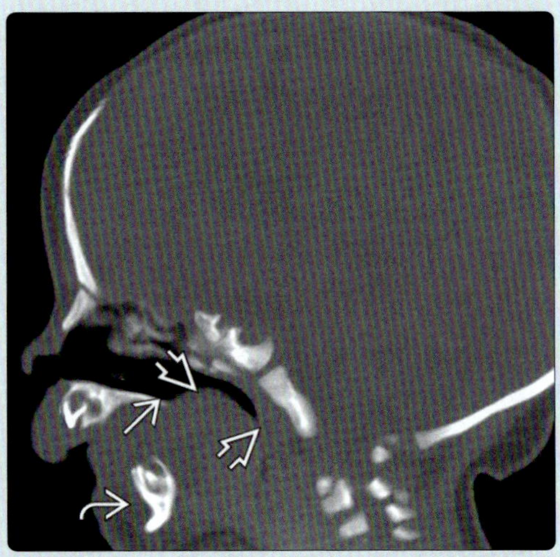

(Left) *Axial bone CT in the same patient shows a U-shaped cleft palate caused by micrognathia, glossoptosis, and failure of development and migration of the palatal shelves. Crowding of teeth is common due to micrognathia.* **(Right)** *Lateral NECT scout view shows the mandibular distraction osteogenesis apparatus used to lengthen the micrognathic mandible in a patient with PRS. Relationship of the apparatus to the developing tooth buds and the inferior alveolar nerve canal should be examined.*

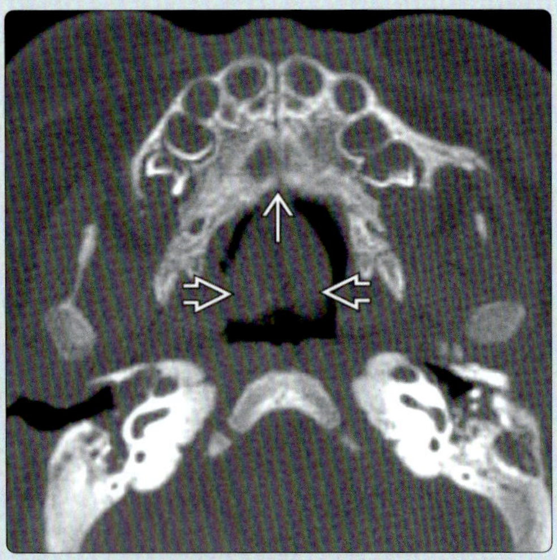

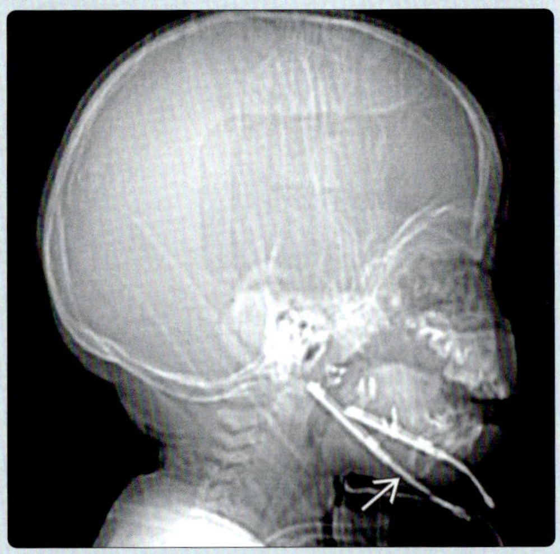

TERMINOLOGY

Abbreviations

- Pierre Robin sequence (PRS)

Synonyms

- Robin sequence

Definitions

- Micrognathia or retrognathia, glossoptosis, respiratory distress, ± posterior U-shaped cleft palate
- Developmental sequence: Malformation → subsequent derived structural changes

IMAGING

General Features

- Best diagnostic clue
  - Bilateral symmetric micrognathia, posterior cleft palate
- Location
  - Mandible, palate, tongue

CT Findings

- Bone CT
  - Bilateral symmetric micrognathia
  - Elevated, posteriorly displaced tongue
  - Posterior **U-shaped cleft palate**
  - Additional features depend on syndromic etiology

MR Findings

- Micrognathia
- Elevated, posteriorly displaced tongue
- Posterior U-shaped cleft palate
- Velocardiofacial syndrome: Medial deviation of internal carotid arteries (ICAs), polymicrogyria (occasional)

Imaging Recommendations

- Best imaging tool
  - CT or MR as required

DIFFERENTIAL DIAGNOSIS

Stickler and Related Syndromes

- Most common syndromes with PRS

Velocardiofacial Syndrome

- Relatively common syndrome with PRS

Treacher Collins Syndrome

- Ear anomalies & zygomatic hypoplasia distinguish from PRS

PATHOLOGY

General Features

- Genetics
  - Identifiable syndrome ~ 46%
  - Collagen (COL) gene mutations: Stickler & related syndromes
    - Most forms autosomal dominant
  - 22q11.2 deletion; *TBX1* gene: Velocardiofacial syndrome (VCFS)
    - Autosomal dominant
  - 17q24; loss-of-function *SOX9* mutation: Camptomelic dysplasia
  - 17q24; putative *SOX9* regulatory mutations: PRS locus

Gross Pathologic & Surgical Features

- Primary micrognathia → glossoptosis → failure of palatal shelf elevation ± fusion

CLINICAL ISSUES

Presentation

- Most common signs/symptoms
  - PRS: 1 per 2,000-10,000 neonates
  - Feeding & breathing difficulties, failure to thrive
  - Cardiac anomalies
- Other signs/symptoms
  - **Stickler syndrome**
    - Progressive myopia, retinal detachment, & blindness
    - Premature joint degeneration, joint laxity
    - Hearing loss
  - **Velocardiofacial syndrome**
    - Characteristic facial dysmorphism
    - Learning disabilities, schizophrenia/psychiatric illness
    - Cardiac anomalies
    - Adenoid hypoplasia
    - Velopharyngeal insufficiency
    - Hypernasal speech
    - Slender hands & digits
  - Camptomelic dysplasia: Bowing & angulation of long bones

Natural History & Prognosis

- Varies with severity & etiology

Treatment

- Airway support: Prone position, intubation, tracheotomy
- Nutritional support
- Palatal repair
- Mandibular distraction osteogenesis
- Pharyngeal surgery for velopharyngeal insufficiency

DIAGNOSTIC CHECKLIST

Consider

- Stickler syndrome if + familial myopia
- VCFS if adenoid hypoplasia, medial deviation of ICAs

Image Interpretation Pearls

- Look for medial deviation of cervical ICAs in VCFS

SELECTED REFERENCES

1. Acke FR et al: Cephalometrics in Stickler syndrome: objectification of the typical facial appearance. J Craniomaxillofac Surg. 44(7):848-53, 2016
2. Collares MV et al: Neonatal mandibular distraction osteogenesis reduces cleft palate width and lengthens soft palate, influencing palatoplasty in patients with Pierre Robin sequence. J Craniofac Surg. ePub, 2016
3. Pasetti M et al: Temporomandibular joint ankylosis as part of the clinical spectrum of Carey-Fineman-Ziter syndrome? Am J Med Genet A. ePub, 2016
4. Ryan G et al: Airway compromise in the fetus and neonate: prenatal assessment and perinatal management. Semin Fetal Neonatal Med. ePub, 2016
5. Yang AS et al: Klippel-Feil syndrome associated with Pierre Robin sequence and mandibular duplication. J Plast Reconstr Aesthet Surg. ePub, 2016
6. Benko S et al: Highly conserved non-coding elements on either side of SOX9 associated with Pierre Robin sequence. Nat Genet. 41(3):359-64, 2009
7. Evans AK et al: Robin sequence: a retrospective review of 115 patients. Int J Pediatr Otorhinolaryngol. 70(6):973-80, 2006

Treacher Collins Syndrome

KEY FACTS

TERMINOLOGY

- Treacher Collins syndrome (TCS), a.k.a. Treacher Collins-Franceschetti syndrome

IMAGING

- External auditory canal (EAC) stenosis/atresia
- Hypoplastic/atretic middle ear space
- Malformed, fused, or absent ossicles
- Oval window stenosis/atresia
- Decreased/absent mastoid pneumatization
- Symmetric micrognathia, zygomatic/malar hypoplasia
- Hypoplasia of condyles & coronoid processes
- Prominent antegonial notching

TOP DIFFERENTIAL DIAGNOSES

- Bilateral facial microsomia
- Nager syndrome
- Congenital external ear dysplasia
- Branchiootorenal syndrome
- X-linked maxillofacial dysostosis

PATHOLOGY

- Autosomal dominant, phenotypic variability
- Gene map locus: 5q32-q33.1
- *TCOF1*, *POLR1C*, or *POLR1D* gene mutations
  - Results in defect in nucleolar trafficking protein required during craniofacial development
- Incidence: 1/25,000-50,000 births

CLINICAL ISSUES

- Airway obstruction/hypoplasia of airways
- **Downslanting** palpebral fissures (100%)
- Lower eyelid coloboma in 75% of patients
- Micrognathia with retruded chin
- EAC stenosis/atresia, conductive hearing loss
- Cleft palate in 1/3 of patients
- Treatment: Airway support, reconstructive surgery, hearing aids, developmental support

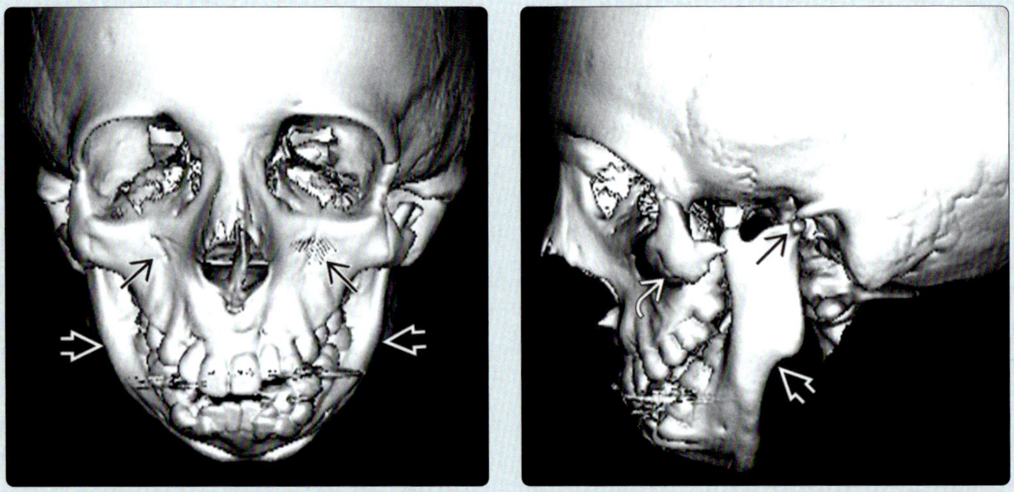

(Left) *Anteroposterior 3D CT in a 13-year-old girl with Treacher Collins syndrome (TCS) demonstrates bilateral symmetric malar concavity* ⇨ *& micrognathia* ➡. **(Right)** *Lateral 3D CT in the same patient shows a small mandibular condyle* → *& an obtuse mandibular angle with antegonial notching* ➡. *There is marked hypoplasia of the zygomatic complex* ➡, *& the zygomatic arch fails to meet the calvarium posteriorly. There is also atresia of the external auditory meatus.*

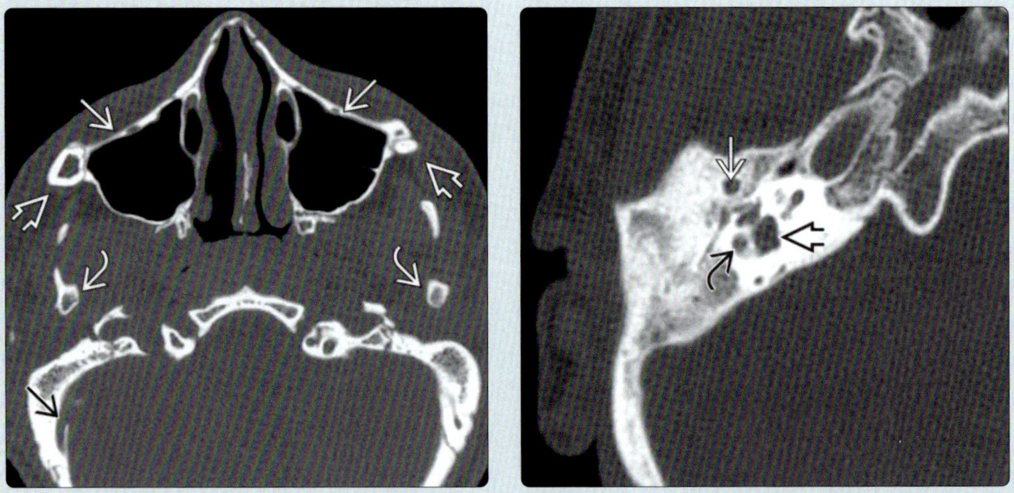

(Left) *Axial bone CT in the same patient shows zygomatic complex hypoplasia with posteriorly slanted maxilla* ➡, *absent zygomatic arches* ➡, *& hypoplastic mandibular condyles* ➡. *Note external auditory canal (EAC) atresia, absent mastoid pneumatization, & enlarged mastoid emissary vein* →. **(Right)** *Axial bone CT in a 16-year-old girl with TCS shows EAC atresia, absent middle ear space & ossicles, ventrally placed descending CNVII canal* ➡, *prominent vestibule* ⇨, *& a malformed horizontal semicircular canal* ↷.

TERMINOLOGY

Abbreviations

- Treacher Collins syndrome (TCS)

Synonyms

- Treacher Collins-Franceschetti syndrome
- Mandibulofacial dysostosis (MFD1)

Definitions

- Craniofacial malformation: Downslanting palpebral fissures, micrognathia, zygomatic & malar hypoplasia, microtia, macrostomia, coloboma

IMAGING

General Features

- Best diagnostic clue
  - Symmetric micrognathia
  - Zygomatic complex hypoplasia
  - Bilateral external auditory canal (EAC) atresia
- Location
  - Mandible, face, ears

Imaging Recommendations

- Best imaging tool
  - High-resolution bone CT
- Protocol advice
  - Bone CT with multiplanar & 3D reformats: Maxilla, mandible, temporal bones (T-bones)

CT Findings

- Bone CT
  - T-bone findings
    - EAC stenosis/atresia
    - Decreased/absent mastoid pneumatization
    - Hypoplastic/atretic middle ear space
    - Malformed, fused, or absent ossicles
    - Oval window stenosis/atresia
    - Normal or malformed cochlea (flattened turns)
    - Normal or malformed horizontal semicircular canal
  - Symmetric micrognathia
  - Zygomatic complex hypoplasia
  - Hypoplasia of condyles & coronoid processes
  - Prominent antegonial notching
  - Variable cleft palate

DIFFERENTIAL DIAGNOSIS

Bilateral Facial Microsomia

- Oculoauriculovertebral spectrum

Preaxial Acrofacial Dysostosis (Nager Syndrome)

- Similar to TCS + limb anomalies

Congenital External Ear Dysplasia

- EAC dysplasia + ossicle deformity
- No mandible or maxillary deformity

Branchiootorenal Syndrome

- T-bone anomalies, branchial cleft cyst, renal cysts

X-Linked Maxillofacial Dysostosis

- Micrognathia, midface hypoplasia, ear abnormalities, & palpebral fissures

PATHOLOGY

General Features

- Genetics
  - Autosomal dominant, phenotypic variability
  - Incidence: 1/25,000-50,000 births
  - Gene map locus: 5q32-q33.1
  - *TCOF1*, *POLR1C*, or *POLR1D* gene mutations
  - Results in defect in nucleolar trafficking protein required during craniofacial development

CLINICAL ISSUES

Presentation

- Most common signs/symptoms
  - **Downslanting** palpebral fissures (100%)
  - Hypoplasia mandible/zygomatic complex
  - Micrognathia with retruded chin
  - Lower eyelid coloboma in 75% of patients
  - Microtia, EAC stenosis/atresia, conductive hearing loss
  - Airway obstruction/hypoplasia of airways
- Other signs/symptoms
  - Cleft palate in 1/3 of cases
  - Delayed motor/speech development
  - Hypoplastic or absent parotid salivary glands

Treatment

- Airway support
- Reconstructive surgery
- Hearing aids
- Developmental support
- Early intervention

DIAGNOSTIC CHECKLIST

Consider

- TCS as cause of symmetric micrognathia, zygomatic complex hypoplasia, external ear anomalies
- TCS-like + limb deformities = Nager syndrome

Image Interpretation Pearls

- Absent zygomatic arches & posteriorly slanted anterior wall of maxilla

Reporting Tips

- Look for ocular coloboma

SELECTED REFERENCES

1. Ibrahim A et al: Combined soft and skeletal tissue modelling of normal and dysmorphic midface postnatal development. J Craniomaxillofac Surg. 44(11):1777-1785, 2016
2. Plomp RG et al: Treacher Collins syndrome: A systematic review of evidence-based treatment and recommendations. Plast Reconstr Surg. 137(1):191-204, 2016
3. Tse WK: Treacher Collins syndrome: New insights from animal models. Int J Biochem Cell Biol. 81(Pt A):44-47, 2016
4. Robson CD: Congenital hearing impairment. Pediatr Radiol. 36(4):309-24, 2006
5. Teber OA et al: Genotyping in 46 patients with tentative diagnosis of Treacher Collins syndrome revealed unexpected phenotypic variation. Eur J Hum Genet. 12(11):879-90, 2004

Mandible Fracture

KEY FACTS

IMAGING

- Best diagnostic clue: Discontinuity in mandibular osseous structure
- Panoramic radiograph best initial evaluation, followed by CBCT (max 0.4 mm voxel) or thin-slice axial bone CT with coronal and 3D reformat
- CBCT/bone CT appearance
  - Radiolucent, noncorticated lines with variable diastasis, angulation, & comminution
  - Condylar fx: **Condylar head pulled medially and inferiorly** by lateral pterygoid muscle ("unfavorable fx")
- Intraoral periapical or CBCT if alveolar or dental fx suspected
- Mandible simulates bony "ring": **2 breaks** common (50%)
  - Parasymphyseal fx often associated with contralateral angle/body or subcondylar fx
  - Bilateral subcondylar fractures after direct impact to symphysis

TOP DIFFERENTIAL DIAGNOSES

- Pseudofractures
  - Nutrient canal
  - Inferior alveolar nerve canal/accessory canals
  - Mental foramen
  - Palatoglossal airway space on panoramic images

PATHOLOGY

- Causes of mandibular fracture: Motor vehicle crashes (40%), assault (40%), fall (10%), sports (5%)
- 15% have ≥ 1 other facial bone fx

CLINICAL ISSUES

- Presentation: Jaw pain, abnormal mobility, malocclusion
- Mandibular fracture frequencies
  - Condylar process (36%), body (21%), angle (20%), symphyseal/parasymphyseal (15%), ramus (3%), alveolar (3%), coronoid process (2%)

(Left) *CBCT 3D reformation shows an unfavorable fracture of the mandible. The fracture is displaced (unfavorable) with a step sign at the inferior mandibular cortex. Fixation wires are seen in the premolar regions. 3D reformatted images are often helpful for surgical planning.* **(Right)** *Axial bone CT through the retromolar pad shows a displaced fracture through anterior ramus. The mandibular canal appears disrupted, suggesting possible clinical paresthesia. Air inclusions are noted in the adjacent soft tissue.*

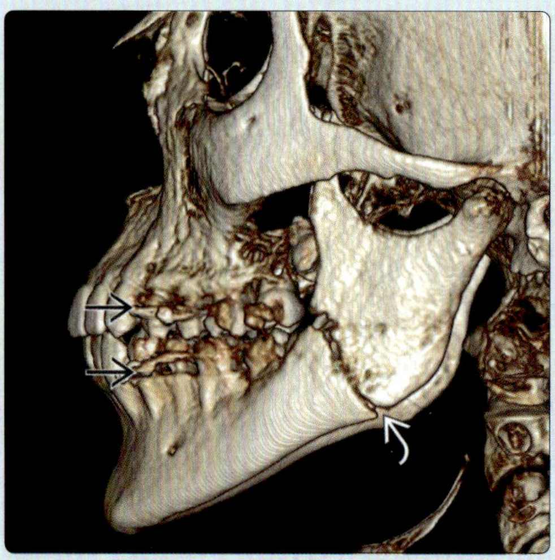

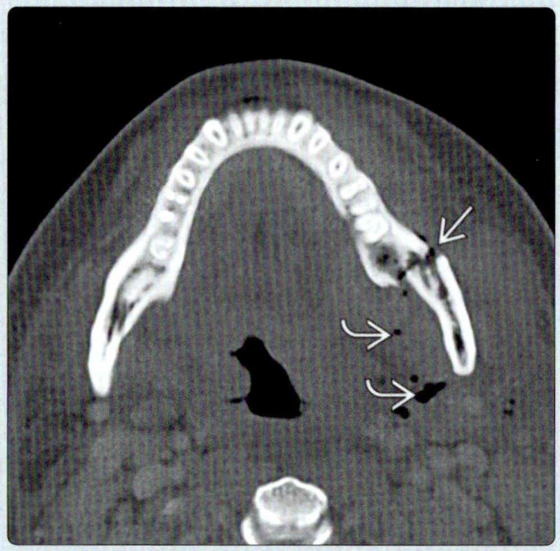

(Left) *Axial bone CT shows displaced mandibular fractures of the right angle and left parasymphysis. Contralateral fractures are commonly seen in the mandible. Extensive lacerations were responsible for the associated soft tissue emphysema.* **(Right)** *Panoramic radiograph of right mandibular body fracture shows step sign and separation sign. Note enlarged soft palate/uvula.*

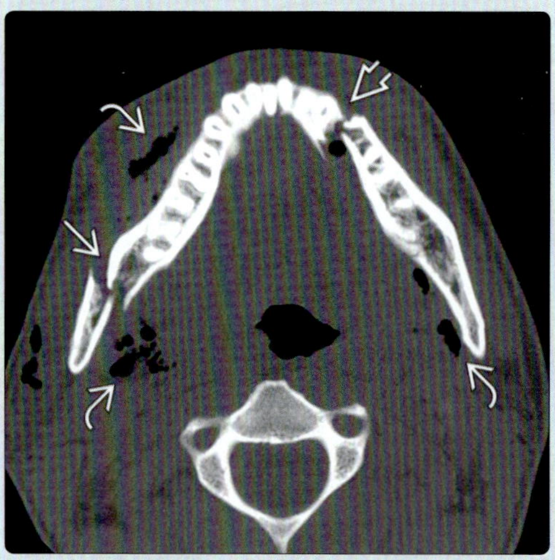

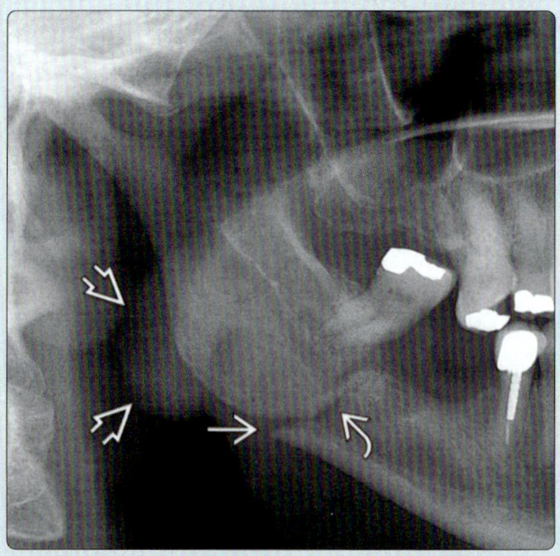

TERMINOLOGY

Abbreviations

- Fracture (fx)

Definitions

- Traumatic break in mandibular osseous structure

IMAGING

General Features

- Best diagnostic clue
    - Discontinuity in mandibular osseous structure
- Location
    - Mandible simulates bony ring
        - **2 breaks in "ring" common** (50%): Bilateral fx
            - Parasymphyseal fx on 1 side often associated with contralateral angle/body or **subcondylar fx**
            - Bilateral subcondylar fractures after direct impact to symphysis
        - Alternatively, unilateral mandibular fx may occur with **contralateral temporomandibular joint (TMJ) dislocation**

Radiographic Findings

- Radiography
    - Panoramic is best initial image
        - Fx appears as linear radiolucency overlying mandible (separation sign), linear radiopacity (overlap sign), or morphologic displacement (step sign)
    - Intraoral periapical or CBCT if alveolar or dental fx suspected
    - CT/CBCT has largely replaced 2D imaging evaluation of facial trauma, but not for mandibular trauma

CT Findings

- Bone CT
    - Radiolucent, noncorticated fx lines with variable diastasis, angulation, and comminution
    - Condylar neck fx: **Condyle may be pulled medially and inferiorly** by lateral pterygoid muscle ("unfavorable fx")

MR Findings

- T1WI
    - ↓ marrow signal intensity from edema
    - Well-defined hypointense fx line
    - Hypointense joint effusion if TMJ affected
    - Hyperintense blood products may also be seen
- T2WI
    - Hypointense fracture line
    - ↑ signal from surrounding soft tissue edema

Imaging Recommendations

- Best imaging tool
    - Panoramic best initial evaluation; intraoral periapical if alveolar fracture suspected
    - Thin-slice axial bone algorithm CT or CBCT (max 0.4-mm voxel) through mandible & TMJs
    - Postoperative cases with **significant hardware** may be better evaluated with **panoramic** views

DIFFERENTIAL DIAGNOSIS

Nutrient/Neurovascular Canal

- Radiolucent channels may mimic fx (pseudofracture)

Inferior Alveolar (Mandibular) Canal

- Usually located inferior & medial within mandible
- Accessory canals from main mandibular canal may mimic fx

Mental Foramen

- Oval foramen at anterolateral mandible, where mental nerve and vessels emerge

Mandibular Lingula

- Tongue-shaped bony projection extending from medial mandible to cover mandibular foramen

Palatoglossal Airway

- On panoramic images, superimposed linear/curved radiolucency over mandibular ramus

PATHOLOGY

General Features

- Etiology
    - Fx causes
        - Motor vehicle accidents (40%), assault (40%), fall (10%), sports (5%)
- Associated abnormalities
    - 15% of cases with mandibular fx have ≥ 1 other facial bone fx

CLINICAL ISSUES

Presentation

- Most common signs/symptoms
    - Jaw pain, abnormal mobility upon palpation, malocclusion

Demographics

- Epidemiology
    - Mandibular fracture frequencies
        - Condylar process (36%), body (21%), angle (20%), symphyseal/parasymphyseal (15%), ramus (3%), alveolar (3%), coronoid process (2%)

Treatment

- Goals of treatment are restoration of normal occlusion & complete bony union

SELECTED REFERENCES

1. Kaeppler G et al: Diagnostic efficacy of cone-beam computed tomography for mandibular fractures. Oral Surg Oral Med Oral Pathol Oral Radiol. 116(1):98-104, 2013
2. Winegar BA et al: Spectrum of critical imaging findings in complex facial skeletal trauma. Radiographics. 33(1):3-19, 2013
3. Ogura I et al: Characterization of mandibular fractures using 64-slice multidetector CT. Dentomaxillofac Radiol. 41(5):392-5, 2012
4. Rudderman RH et al: The biophysics of mandibular fractures: an evolution toward understanding. Plast Reconstr Surg. 121(2):596-607, 2008
5. Ellis E 3rd et al: Fractures of the mandible: a technical perspective. Plast Reconstr Surg. 120(7 Suppl 2):76S-89S, 2007
6. Hobbs DL et al: Trauma radiography of the mandible. Radiol Technol. 78(4):265-8, 2007

(Left) *Axial bone CT shows an oblique fracture line* ➔ *to the right of the midline of the mandible. Note adjacent abnormal air* ➔ *along the inner symphyseal cortex.* **(Right)** *Panoramic radiograph shows a nondisplaced parasymphyseal fracture through the buccal and lingual cortices* ➔*. Note the palatoglossal airway* ➔ *simulating a fracture through the mandibular angle.*

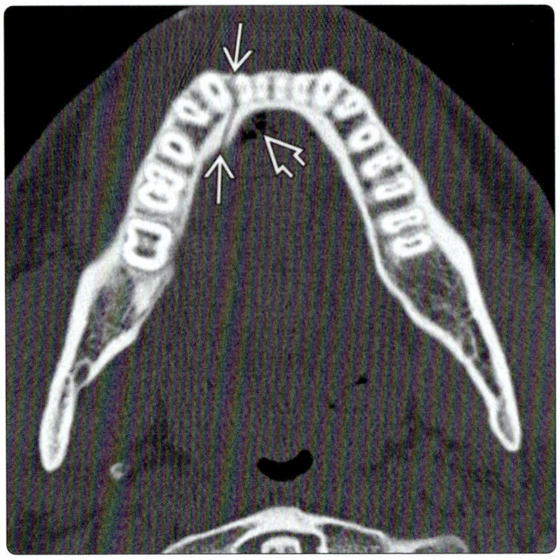

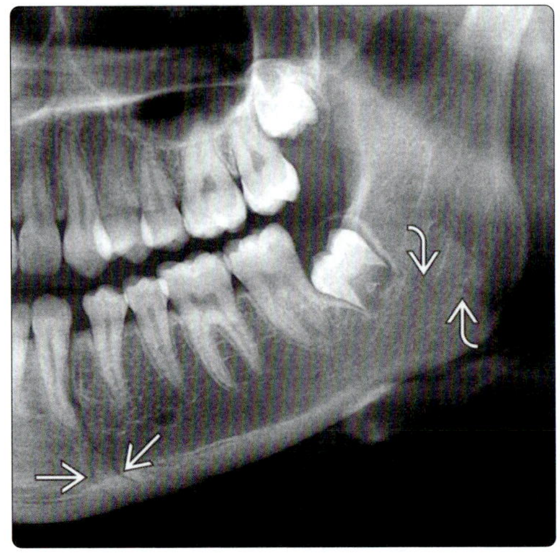

(Left) *Panoramic radiograph shows a fracture through both the buccal and lingual cortices of the right mandibular angle* ➔*. A surgical plate with multiple screws* ➔ *was used to reduce the fracture. A bony callus* ➔ *is seen on the inferior aspect of the mandible. Note the palatoglossal airway space* ➔*.* **(Right)** *Axial bone CT shows a comminuted fracture of the left body of the mandible, with multiple fracture fragments extending into the overlying subcutaneous tissues* ➔*.*

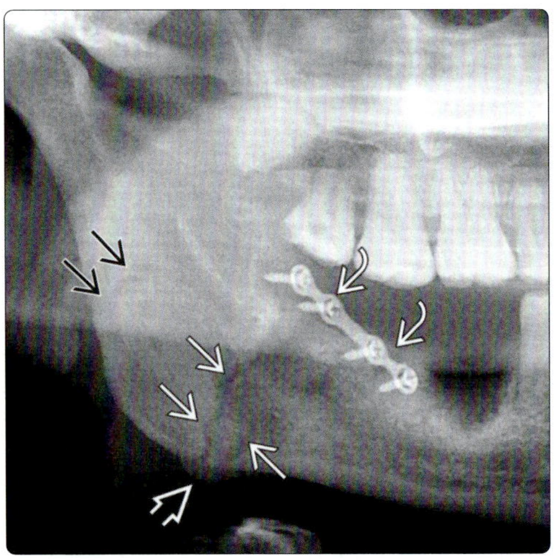

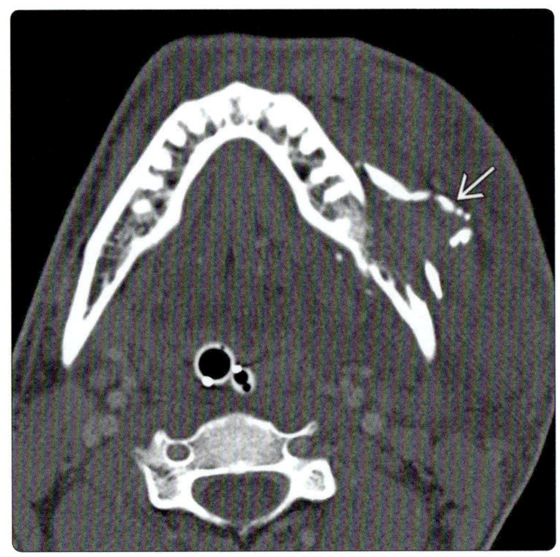

(Left) *Maximum intensity projection (MIP) generated from CBCT shows a pathologic fracture at the mesial extent of bone graft* ➔ *secondary to squamous cell carcinoma. The distal portion* ➔ *of the graft does not appear significantly displaced and is asymptomatic. Note metallic vascular clips* ➔*.* **(Right)** *Panoramic radiograph shows oblique displaced fracture of the right condyle* ➔*. The vertical height of the ramus was much less on the side of the fracture compared to the contralateral side.*

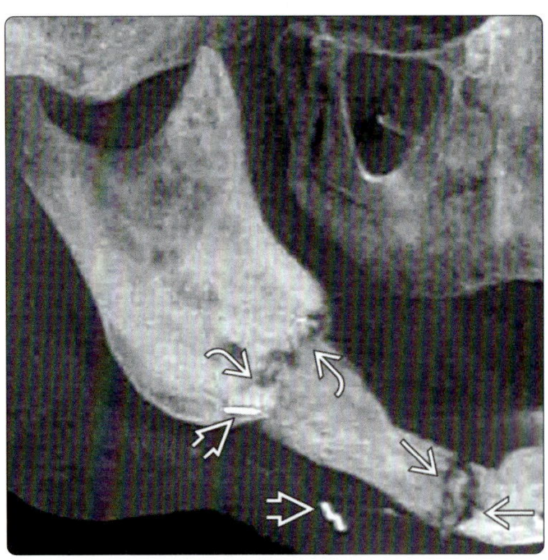

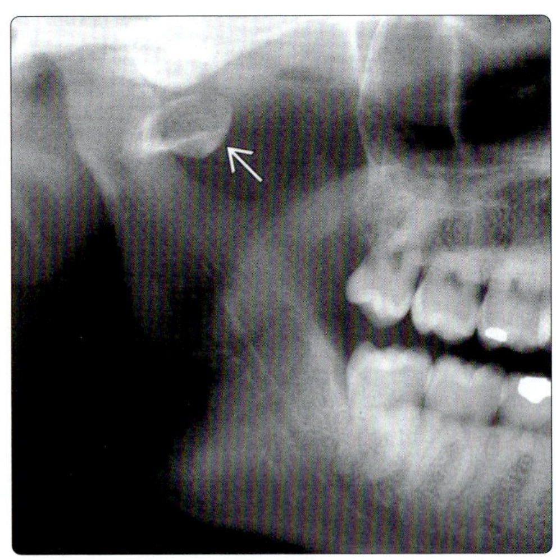

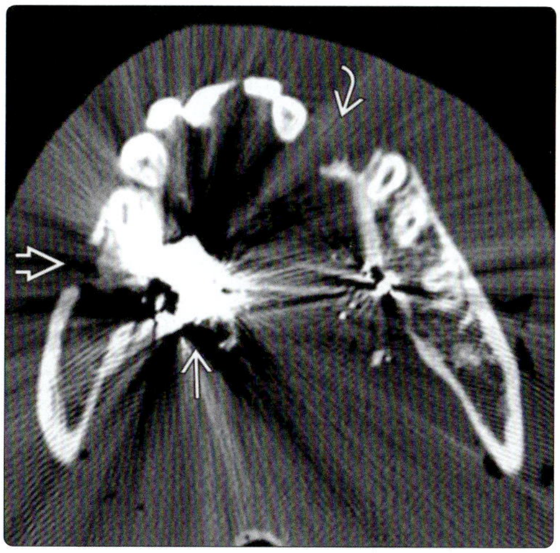

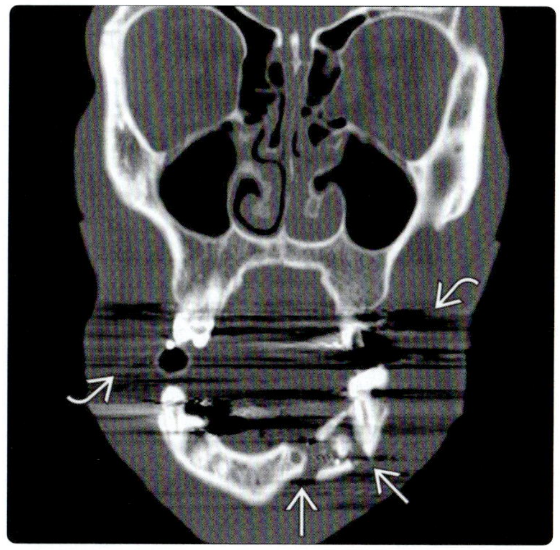

(Left) *Axial bone CT shows markedly comminuted fractures of anterior mandible secondary to gunshot injury. Artifact from metallic bullet fragment is scattered among the fracture fragments with the largest located in the right floor of mouth. Main fracture lines involve right mandibular body and left parasymphysis.* **(Right)** *Coronal bone CT of comminuted fractures in the same patient shows parasymphyseal fractures. Note axial artifact from metallic fragments and dental restorations.*

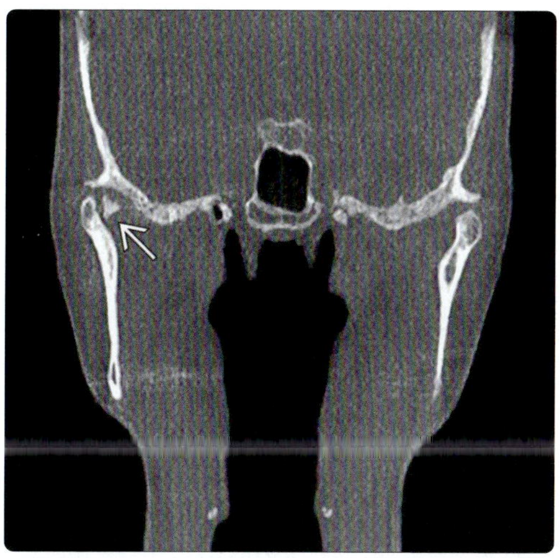

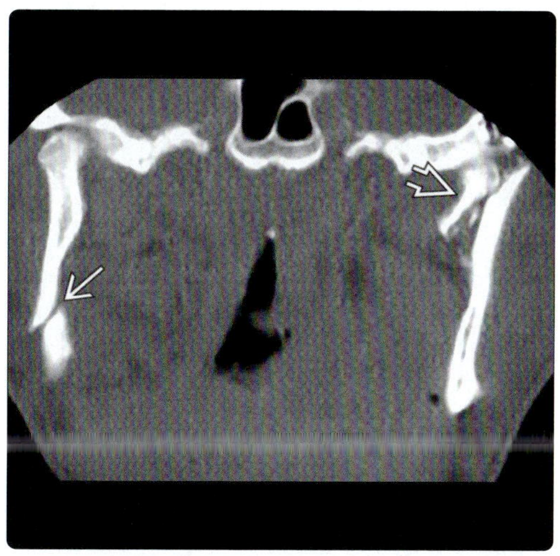

(Left) *Coronal CBCT reformation shows an oblique fracture through the right condyle. The medial segment is separated and displaced from contraction of lateral pterygoid muscle.* **(Right)** *Coronal bone CT shows 2 fractures of the mandibular "ring." A right ramus fracture is present with a left condylar neck fracture. Note that the left condylar head is displaced medially and inferiorly by the lateral pterygoid. This is a typical presentation from direct forceful trauma to the right mandible.*

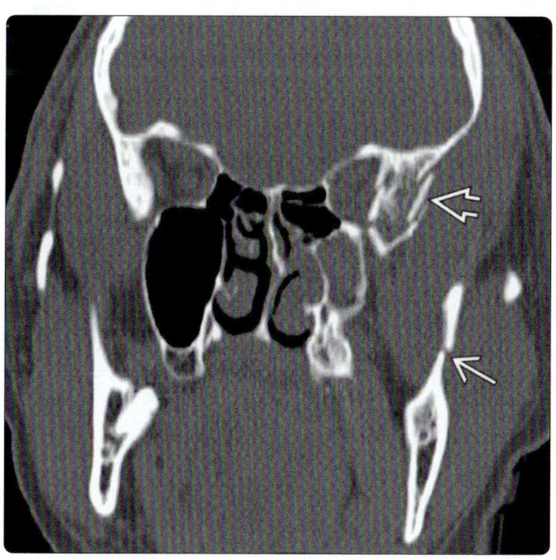

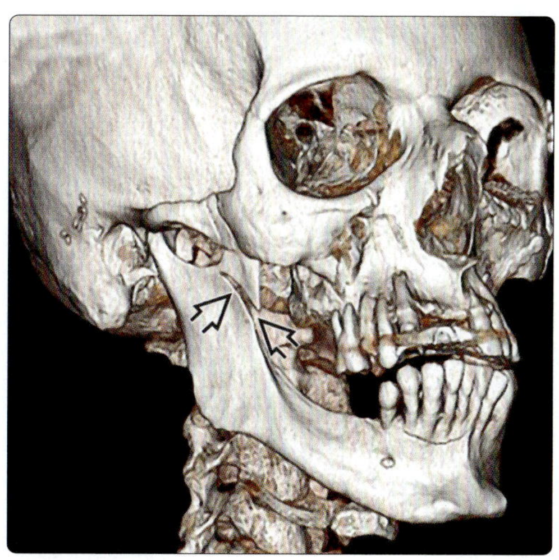

(Left) *Coronal bone CT reveals fractures of the mandibular coronoid process and a comminuted lateral orbital wall fracture. About 15% of mandibular fractures have associated facial bone fractures.* **(Right)** *3D reformation shows an obliquely oriented fracture through the coronoid process of the mandible on the right. The ramus, angle, body, and symphysis are intact. 3D reformatted images are often helpful for surgical planning for treatment of facial fractures.*

Nasoethmoid Complex Fracture

KEY FACTS

TERMINOLOGY

- Definition: **Central upper midface fracture** (fx) involving confluence of medial & upper maxillary buttresses & their posterior extensions; disruption of medial canthal regions, ethmoids, & medial orbital walls distinguishes it from simple nasal fx

IMAGING

- Bone CT/CBCT: Nasal bone fx in combination with fxs of medial orbital wall & frontal process of maxilla

TOP DIFFERENTIAL DIAGNOSES

- Complex midfacial fx
- Nasal bone fx
- Medial orbital blowout fx

PATHOLOGY

- Force transmitted through nasal bones & involves ethmoid sinuses & medial orbits
- May involve frontal recess resulting in impaired frontal sinus drainage
- May involve cribriform plate resulting in CSF leak, meningoencephalocele, intracranial infection, olfactory bulb injury
- Manson classification
  - Type I: Medial canthal insertion on large fx fragment
  - Type II: Canthal tendon attached to small bone fragment
  - Type III: Complete avulsion of medial canthal tendon
- Fx through lacrimal duct resulting in dacryocystitis & dacryocystocele formation

CLINICAL ISSUES

- Symptoms & signs
  - Loss of normal pyramidal nasal projection in profile & increased intercanthal distance (telecanthus)
- Nasoorbitalethmoid fxs can be one of most difficult facial fx patterns to accurately reduce

(Left) *Axial bone CT shows markedly comminuted fractures (fxs) involving the nasoorbitalethmoid (NOE) complex. Multiple small fx fragments are noted in the medial canthal regions ➡, and there is a degree of telecanthus. Soft tissue swelling, emphysema, and a lateral orbital fx ➡ are noted.* **(Right)** *Axial bone CT in the same patient inferior to the previous image shows that the fxs involve both nasolacrimal ducts ➡. In such a patient, epiphora would be an expected complication of the injury.*

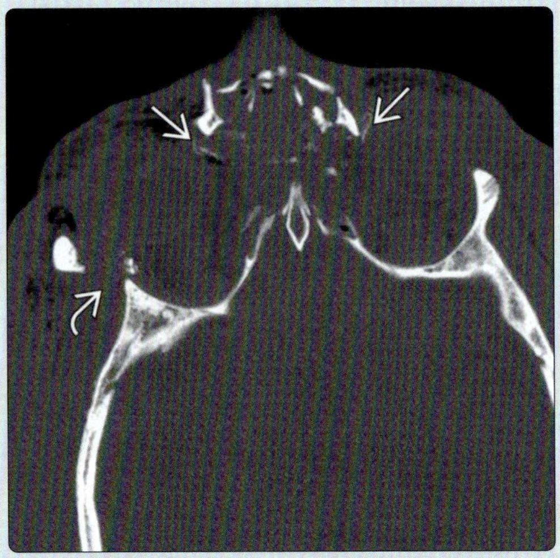

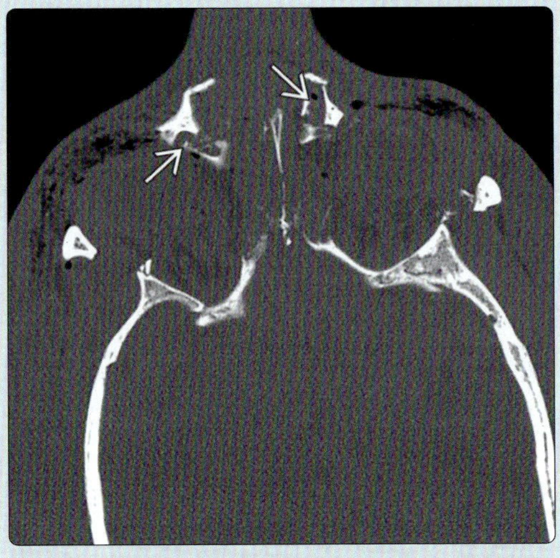

(Left) *This 3D CT reconstruction demonstrates NOE fxs ➡ at the nasal bridge. The lateral orbital fxs ➡ and maxillary fxs ➡ can be seen in patients with Le Fort III and Le Fort II fxs, respectively. It is not uncommon to see components of more than 1 fx pattern in severe facial trauma.* **(Right)** *Axial bone CT shows dominant medial orbital fx fragments ➡ to which the medial canthal tendons are attached. This NOE fx would be a Manson type I with the best postsurgical prognosis.*

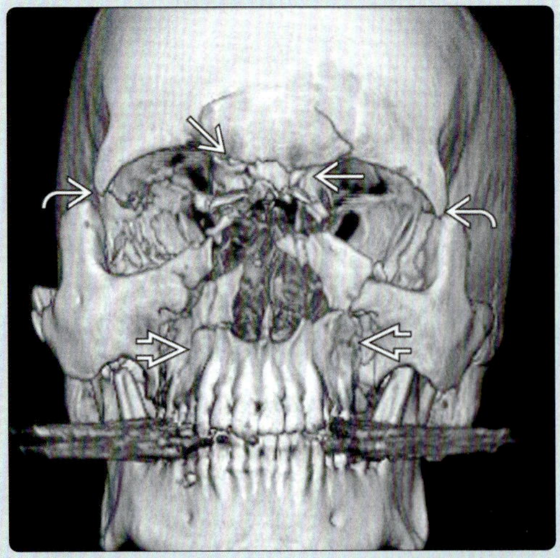

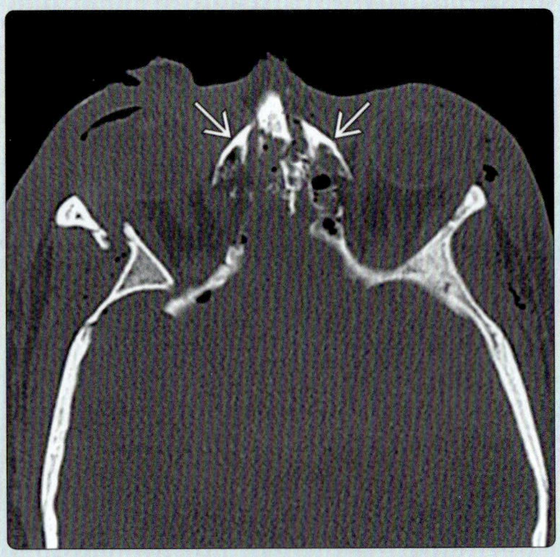

TERMINOLOGY

Abbreviations

- Nasoorbitalethmoid fracture (NOE fx)

Definitions

- **Central upper midface fx** involving confluence of medial & upper maxillary buttresses & their posterior extensions along medial orbital wall & floor
    - Distinguished from simple nasal fxs by posterior disruption of medial canthal regions, ethmoids, & medial orbital walls
    - Uncommon

IMAGING

General Features

- Best diagnostic clue
    - **Nasal bone** fx in combination with fxs of **medial orbital wall** & **frontal process** of maxilla/orbital rim

Imaging Recommendations

- Best imaging tool
    - Thin-section bone algorithm CT or CBCT
- Protocol advice
    - 0.60- to 1.25-mm axials; coronal & 3D reformatted images helpful for evaluating medial canthal tendon attachment

CT Findings

- Bone CT
    - Nasal bone fxs in combination with fxs of medial orbital wall & frontal process of maxilla
    - Frontal recess involvement likely if displaced anterior table fx medial to supraorbital notch involving frontal sinus floor

DIFFERENTIAL DIAGNOSIS

Complex Midfacial Fracture

- Severe injury with fx pattern not falling into other classification
- Highly comminuted & involves bones of lower central midface

Nasal Bone Fracture

- Impact to nasal dorsum
- Intact medial orbital walls & frontal process of maxilla

Medial Orbital Blowout Fracture

- Direct impact to globe with orbital rims spared
- Enophthalmos without telecanthus

PATHOLOGY

General Features

- Etiology
    - NOE: Facial unit composed of nasal bones, medial orbital walls, & frontal process of maxillary bones
    - **High-force trauma** transmitted through nasal bones to involve underlying ethmoid sinuses & orbits
        - Thin nasal bones, ethmoid sinus walls, & medial orbits act as "crumple zone," allowing traumatic force to be dissipated
        - Critical structures (brain & optic nerve) lie in stronger bone posteriorly & are relatively protected
- Associated abnormalities
    - Fxs through **frontal recess** with disruption of frontal sinus drainage
    - Associated fxs of **cribriform plate/anterior skull base** resulting in CSF leak, meningoencephalocele, intracranial infection, olfactory bulb injury
    - Severe **ocular injuries** including hyphema, vitreous hemorrhage, lens dislocation, & globe rupture
    - Fx through **nasolacrimal duct** resulting in dacryocystitis & dacryocystocele formation

Staging, Grading, & Classification

- Manson classification system (3 major subsets based upon degree of injury to medial canthal attachment)
    - Type I: Single-segment fxs of medial orbital rim without comminution
    - Type II: Comminution of medial orbital rim, but tendon remains attached
    - Type III: Comminution of bone at site of tendon attachment or tendon avulsion
        - Diagnosis is made clinically, not with imaging

CLINICAL ISSUES

Presentation

- Most common signs/symptoms
    - Loss of normal nasal pyramidal projection in profile
    - Increased distance between inner corners of eyes (telecanthus)

Treatment

- NOE fxs can be one of most difficult fx patterns to accurately reduce
- Incomplete surgical reduction results in telecanthus

DIAGNOSTIC CHECKLIST

Reporting Tips

- Imaging description should include
    - **Degree of comminution** of medial vertical maxillary buttress in region of medial canthal tendon attachment
    - **Distance between lacrimal fossae** in coronal plane
    - Involvement of **frontal sinus drainage pathway & orbit**
    - **Frontal lobe contusion**
- Also report degree of comminution of surrounding nasal, maxillary, & orbital walls for surgical planning purposes

SELECTED REFERENCES

1. Baril SE et al: Naso-orbito-ethmoidal (NOE) fractures: a review. Int Ophthalmol Clin. 53(4):149-55, 2013
2. Winegar BA et al: Spectrum of critical imaging findings in complex facial skeletal trauma. Radiographics. 33(1):3-19, 2013
3. Kim JJ et al: Maxillofacial (midface) fractures. Neuroimaging Clin N Am. 20(4):581-96, 2010
4. Papadopoulos H et al: Management of naso-orbital-ethmoidal fractures. Oral Maxillofac Surg Clin North Am. 21(2):221-5, vi, 2009
5. Fraioli RE et al: Facial fractures: beyond Le Fort. Otolaryngol Clin North Am. 41(1):51-76, vi, 2008
6. Hopper RA et al: Diagnosis of midface fractures with CT: what the surgeon needs to know. Radiographics. 26(3):783-93, 2006
7. Remmler D et al: Role of three-dimensional computed tomography in the assessment of nasoorbitoethmoidal fractures. Ann Plast Surg. 44(5):553-62; discussion 562-3, 2000

Complex Midfacial Fracture

KEY FACTS

TERMINOLOGY

- Synonyms: Facial "smash" injury; panfacial fracture
- No widely accepted definition
  - Severely comminuted fractures involving multiple facial bones
  - Does not follow pattern described for traditional transfacial (Le Fort) fracture

IMAGING

- Best diagnostic clue
  - Numerous markedly comminuted fractures from high-energy impact that cannot be classified as traditional transfacial types
- Thin-section axial bone CT or CBCT with multiplanar reconstruction is modality of choice
  - 3D CT reformatted images improve appreciation of disrupted facial architecture for surgical planning
- Fractures may involve frontal, nasoethmoid, midfacial, or craniofacial regions
  - May also involve mandible
- CTA may be necessary to exclude carotid artery injury
- May involve frontal, nasoethmoid, midfacial, or craniofacial regions

TOP DIFFERENTIAL DIAGNOSES

- Transfacial (Le Fort) fracture
- Zygomaticomaxillary complex fracture (ZMC)
- Naso-orbital-ethmoid fracture

PATHOLOGY

- High association with intracranial injuries

CLINICAL ISSUES

- Soft tissue injuries & loss of bone structure may lead to malocclusion, "dish" face deformity, & enophthalmos
- Treatment often delayed because of other life-threatening injuries
- Reconstruction often performed in multiple stages

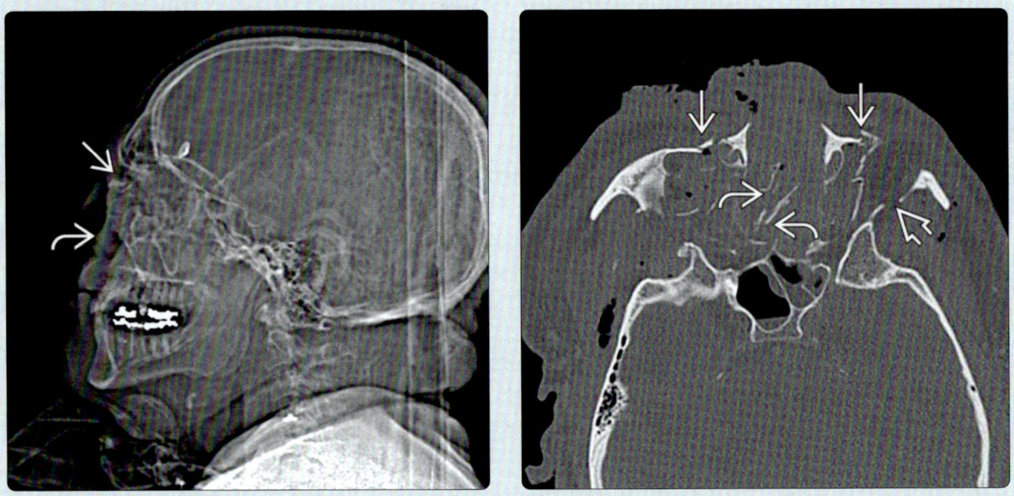

(Left) *Lateral CT scout image in a patient status post high-force blunt facial trauma demonstrates flattening of facial projection involving the nasal dorsum ➡ and midface ➡ ("dish" face).* **(Right)** *Axial bone CT in the same patient demonstrates significant injuries to the facial soft tissues and underlying facial skeleton. Lacerations with soft tissue emphysema are seen. Severely comminuted fractures involve the maxillae ➡, orbital wall ➡, and nasal septum ➡. The entire face is depressed.*

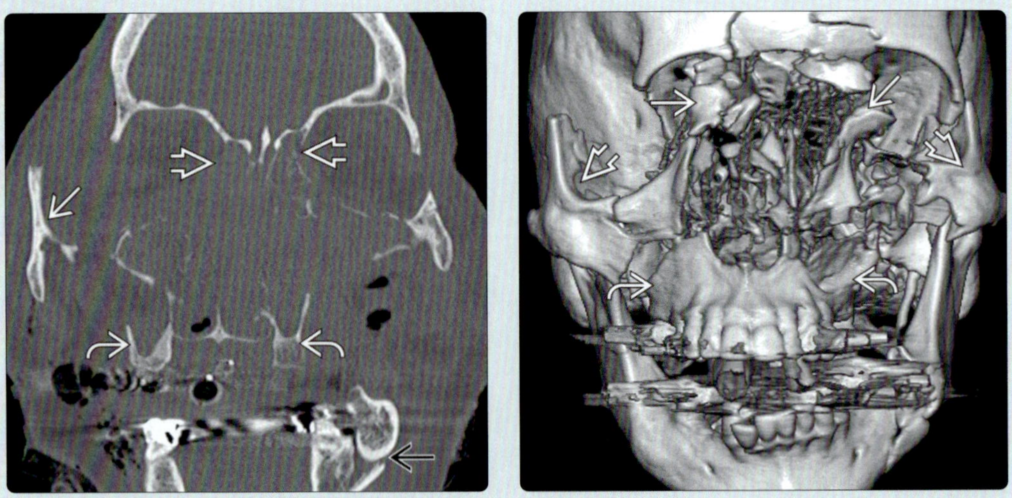

(Left) *Coronal bone CT image shows diffuse widening of the midface, with lateral displacement of the right malar eminence ➡, rightward displacement of the maxillary alveolar ridges and palate ➡ with respect to the remaining midface, fx of the medial orbital walls ➡, and left mandibular body fx ➡.* **(Right)** *Frontal 3D reformation in same patient better delineates the relationship of the extensive fractures. There are components of naso-orbital-ethmoid complex fx ➡, LeFort 1 injury ➡, and bilateral ZMC injury ➡.*

TERMINOLOGY

Abbreviations

- Complex facial fracture (CFFx)

Synonyms

- Facial "smash" injury; panfacial fracture

Definitions

- No widely accepted definition of CFFx or panfacial fracture
  - "Pure" bilateral Le Fort, naso-orbito-ethmoid, and zygomatic complex fractures uncommon
- Definitions include
  - Severely comminuted fractures involving multiple facial bones that do not follow pattern described for traditional transfacial (Le Fort) fracture
  - Fracture patterns involving midface & mandible
  - Fractures involving upper, middle, & lower face (naso-orbito-ethmoid, zygomatic complex, central midface, & mandible)

IMAGING

General Features

- Best diagnostic clue
  - **Numerous markedly comminuted** fractures from high-energy impact that cannot be classified as traditional transfacial types
- Location
  - May involve frontal, nasoethmoid, midfacial, or craniofacial regions
  - May also involve mandible

Imaging Recommendations

- Best imaging tool
  - Thin-section axial bone CT or CBCT with multiplanar reconstruction
- Protocol advice
  - 3D CT reformatted images improve appreciation of disrupted facial architecture for surgical planning
  - CTA may be necessary to exclude carotid artery injury
  - MR helpful to assess associated intracranial & orbital injuries

CT Findings

- Bone CT and CBCT
  - Multiple severely comminuted fractures
  - Fractures do not conform to classic pattern of facial trauma

DIFFERENTIAL DIAGNOSIS

Transfacial (Le Fort) Fractures

- Fxs occur on 3 lines of weakness in facial skeleton
- Bilateral pterygoid plate fractures required

Zygomaticomaxillary Complex Fracture

- Lateral midface fracture complex from blunt trauma to malar eminence
- Fractures involve anterior and lateral walls of maxillary sinus, zygomatic arch, & lateral orbital wall
- Orbital floor frequently involved

Naso-Orbital-Ethmoid Fracture

- Comminuted fractures from high-impact force to nasal bridge
- Frequently involve frontal recess, cribriform plate, nasolacrimal duct, & medial canthal tendon

PATHOLOGY

General Features

- Etiology
  - High-energy impact to face
- Associated abnormalities
  - High association with intracranial injuries
  - CFFx involving frontal & nasoethmoid regions have ↑ incidence of dural tears
  - CFFx of nasoethmoid region may have associated injuries to lacrimal apparatus, medial canthal tendon, frontal recess, & cribriform plate

Staging, Grading, & Classification

- No widely accepted definition or classification of CFFx
  - Some describe as involving both midface & mandible
  - Others describe them as involving upper, middle, & lower face (naso-orbito-ethmoid, zygomatic complex, central midface, & mandible)
  - Still others divide panfacial ("smash") fxs into 4 types: Frontal, nasoethmoid, central midface, and craniofacial

CLINICAL ISSUES

Presentation

- Most common signs/symptoms
  - Gross facial deformity
- Other signs/symptoms
  - Telecanthus, CSF leak, visual loss

Natural History & Prognosis

- Soft tissue injuries & loss of bone structure may lead to malocclusion, "dish" face deformity, & enophthalmos
- Difficult to completely reduce; patients often left with cosmetic deformity & functional deficits

Treatment

- Goal → restore preinjury function & contours
- Life-threatening injuries may delay treatment

SELECTED REFERENCES

1. Kochhar A et al: Surgical management of complex midfacial fractures. Otolaryngol Clin North Am. 46(5):759-78, 2013
2. Buchanan EP et al: Zygomaticomaxillary complex fractures and their association with naso-orbito-ethmoid fractures: a 5-year review. Plast Reconstr Surg. 130(6):1296-304, 2012
3. Patel R et al: Multidetector computed tomography of maxillofacial fractures: the key to high-impact radiological reporting. Semin Ultrasound CT MR. 33(5):410-7, 2012
4. Canter HI et al: Use of rigid external distraction device in treatment of complex maxillofacial fractures. J Craniofac Surg. 19(2):306-12, 2008
5. Sargent LA: Nasoethmoid orbital fractures: diagnosis and treatment. Plast Reconstr Surg. 120(7 Suppl 2):16S-31S, 2007
6. Saigal K et al: Use of three-dimensional computerized tomography reconstruction in complex facial trauma. Facial Plast Surg. 21(3):214-20, 2005
7. Buitrago-Téllez CH et al: A comprehensive classification of craniofacial fractures: postmortem and clinical studies with two- and three-dimensional computed tomography. Injury. 33(8):651-68, 2002

Zygomaticomaxillary Complex Fracture

KEY FACTS

TERMINOLOGY

- Definition: Fracture complex with fracture lines involving zygomatic arch, lateral orbital wall, anterior & lateral walls of maxillary sinus, & orbital floor
- Synonym: Commonly called **trimalar** or **tripod** fracture; **zygomaticomaxillary complex fracture** or "**quadripod fracture**" is more accurate terminology as fracture involves orbital floor

IMAGING

- Fracture lines **surround malar eminence**
- Imaging modality of choice
  - Thin-slice axial bone algorithm CT or CBCT
  - CBCT ≤ 0.4-mm voxel size
  - Can be reformatted in coronal plane
  - 3D & MIP reformatted images very helpful for demonstrating degree of fracture displacement & angulation

TOP DIFFERENTIAL DIAGNOSES

- Complex midfacial fracture
- Transfacial (Le Fort) fractures
- Zygomatic arch fracture
- Prominent zygomatic sutures

PATHOLOGY

- Most commonly occurs after direct blow to cheek (malar eminence/zygomatic arch)
- Classification systems not often used to plan treatment since advent of miniplates & microplates

CLINICAL ISSUES

- Signs & symptoms
  - Loss of cheek projection with ↑ facial width
  - Impaired sensation/anesthesia of cheek/upper lip
- Excellent prognosis for restored cosmetics after surgical fixation

(Left) *Axial bone CT shows a right zygomaticomaxillary complex (ZMC) fracture. There is premaxillary soft tissue swelling. Fractures of the anterior ➡ and lateral ➡ right maxillary sinus walls are noted, in addition to a right zygomatic arch fracture ➡. Note the opacification of the maxillary sinus from bleeding as an indirect fracture sign ⇨.* **(Right)** *Axial bone CT through the orbits shows a displaced lateral orbital wall fracture ➡ as a feature of a ZMC fracture. The bone fragment protrudes into the extraconal fat near the lateral rectus muscle.*

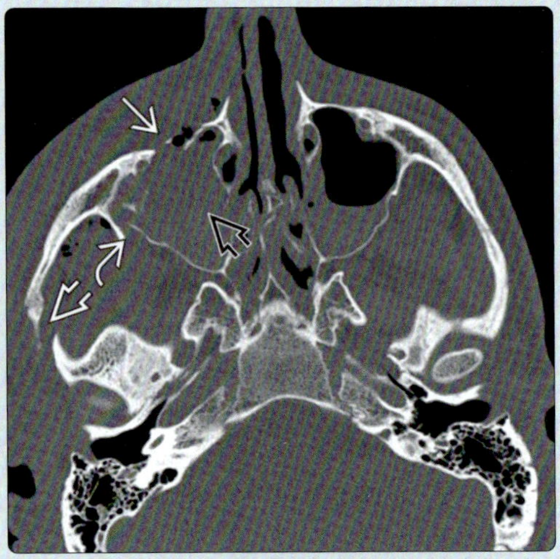

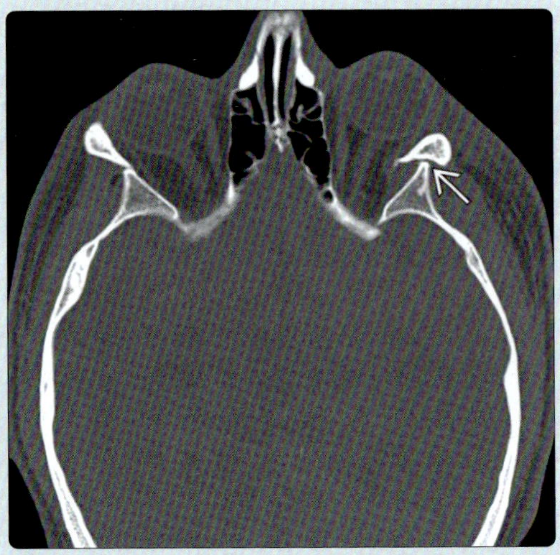

(Left) *Axial CBCT shows a left ZMC fracture. Fractures of the anterior ➡ and lateral ➡ antral walls are noted. There is a minimal depressed fracture of the zygomatic arch ➡. The left maxillary sinus is opacified ⇨ due to bleeding.* **(Right)** *CBCT MIP is shown. This is a typical example of a ZMC fracture through the zygomaticofrontal ➡, zygomaticomaxillary ➡, and zygomaticotemporal ➡ sutures. Separation of the zygomaticosphenoid suture is not visualized on this image.*

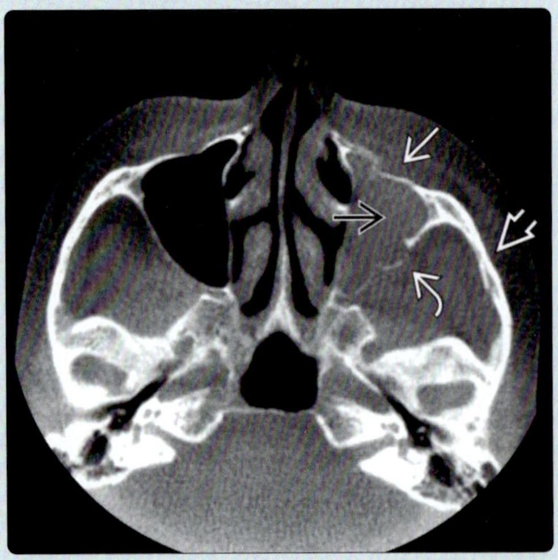

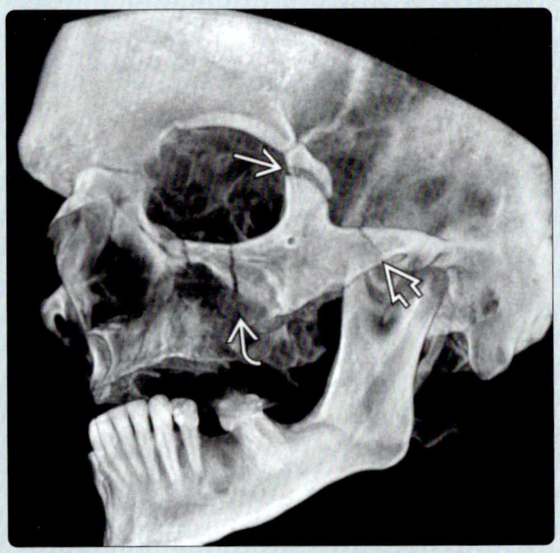

TERMINOLOGY

Abbreviations

- Zygomaticomaxillary complex (ZMC)

Synonyms

- Quadripod or quadramalar fracture, displaced ZMC fracture = trimalar or tripod fracture (old terminology)
- **ZMC fracture is more accurate terminology** as this fracture also involves orbital floor

Definitions

- Complex fracture involving the zygomaticotemporal, zygomaticomaxillary, zygomaticofrontal, and zygomaticosphenoid sutures

IMAGING

General Features

- Best diagnostic clue
  - Fracture complex with fracture lines involving zygomatic arch, lateral orbital wall, anterior & lateral walls of maxillary sinus, & orbital floor
- Location
  - Fracture lines **surround malar eminence**

CT Findings

- Bone CT
  - Radiolucent fracture line locations
    - Along lateral orbital wall (**zygomaticofrontal & zygomaticosphenoid sutures**)
    - From inferior orbital fissure to orbital floor (**near infraorbital canal**)
    - Down anterior maxilla (**near zygomaticomaxillary suture**)
    - Up posterior maxillary wall to inferior orbital fissure
    - Also fracture through **zygomatic arch**

Imaging Recommendations

- Best imaging tool
  - Thin-slice (0.6-1.0 mm) axial bone algorithm CT
  - CBCT ≤ 0.4-mm voxel size
- Protocol advice
  - 3D & MIP reformatted images very helpful for demonstrating degree of fracture displacement & angulation

DIFFERENTIAL DIAGNOSIS

Complex Midfacial Fracture

- Multiple markedly comminuted fractures not fitting into classification
- Bilateral

Transfacial (Le Fort) Fractures

- Common to all 3 types are fractures involving pterygoid processes
- Le Fort III is only type involving zygomatic arch

Zygomatic Arch Fracture

- Isolated zygomatic arch fracture(s) without maxillary wall or lateral orbital wall involvement
- Decreased projection of lateral cheek (malar eminence/zygomatic arch)

Inferior Orbital (Blowout) Fracture

- Fractures involve orbital floor ± inferior orbital rim
- Sparing of zygomatic arch, lateral orbital wall, maxillary sinus walls

Prominent Zygomatic Sutures

- Zygomaticotemporal, zygomaticomaxillary, zygomaticofrontal, zygomaticosphenoid sutures
- Wide sutures with no displacement

PATHOLOGY

General Features

- Etiology
  - Most commonly occurs after **direct blow to cheek** (malar eminence)
  - Paired zygomas each have 2 attachments to cranium & 2 to maxilla, creating large portions of orbital floors & lateral orbital walls
    - These complexes are referred to as "ZMCs"

Staging, Grading, & Classification

- Classification systems not often used to plan treatment since advent of miniplates & microplates
- One of more complete classification systems based upon type, frequency, & postreduction stability of malar fractures

CLINICAL ISSUES

Presentation

- Most common signs/symptoms
  - Loss of cheek projection with increased facial width
  - **Impaired sensation** or anesthesia of cheek/upper lip
    - Infraorbital nerve injury in orbital floor (**> 90% of cases**)

Demographics

- Epidemiology
  - Zygomatic fractures are **2nd most common facial fractures** after nasal bone trauma

Natural History & Prognosis

- Surgical results depend somewhat upon degree of comminution, fracture displacement, & angulation

Treatment

- Surgical exposure indicated if angulated or severely comminuted
  - Rigid plate & screw fixation of involved buttresses to reapproximate & restore facial symmetry & orbital volume

SELECTED REFERENCES

1. Winegar BA et al: Spectrum of critical imaging findings in complex facial skeletal trauma. Radiographics. 33(1):3-19, 2013
2. Meslemani D et al: Zygomaticomaxillary complex fractures. Arch Facial Plast Surg. 14(1):62-6, 2012
3. Avery LL et al: Multidetector and three-dimensional CT evaluation of the patient with maxillofacial injury. Radiol Clin North Am. 49(1):183-203, 2011
4. Fraioli RE et al: Facial fractures: beyond Le Fort. Otolaryngol Clin North Am. 41(1):51-76, vi, 2008
5. Hopper RA et al: Diagnosis of midface fractures with CT: what the surgeon needs to know. Radiographics. 26(3):783-93, 2006

Transfacial Fracture (Le Fort)

KEY FACTS

TERMINOLOGY

- Definition: Fractures disrupting pterygomaxillary junction, pterygoid processes/plates, & disjoining portions of face (maxilla) from skull
- **Le Fort type I**: Guérin fracture; **"floating palate"**
- **Le Fort type II**: **Pyramidal fracture** (fx), separates midface from skull
- **Le Fort type III**: **Craniofacial dissociation**

IMAGING

- Best diagnostic clue: Pterygoid process & pterygoid plate fxs in patient with **clinically mobile facial skeleton**
- Best imaging tool: Thin-section (≤ 1 mm) bone CT or CBCT (≤ 0.4-mm voxel)
  - **3D reconstructions** greatly facilitate fx analysis & assist in surgical planning
- **Le Fort I**: Pterygomaxillary disjunction + fx of inferior medial and lateral maxillary buttress
  - Unique finding: Fracture of lateral margin of nasal fossa
  - Clue: Best seen in coronal plane
- **Le Fort II**: Pterygomaxillary disjunction + superior medial maxillary buttress + inferior lateral maxillary buttress
  - Unique finding: Fracture of inferior orbital rim
  - Clue: Spares medial wall of maxillary sinus, unlike Le Fort I
  - Most common Le Fort fracture type
- **Le Fort III**: Pterygomaxillary disjunction + zygomatic arch + superior lateral & medial maxillary buttress
  - Unique finding: Fracture of zygomatic arch
  - Clue: Distinguish from zygomaticomaxillary complex fracture by medial orbital and pterygoid plate fractures
  - Least common Le Fort fracture type (in isolated form)

TOP DIFFERENTIAL DIAGNOSES

- Zygomaticomaxillary complex fracture
- Nasoorbitalethmoid fracture
- Complex facial fracture
- Pterygoid plate avulsion

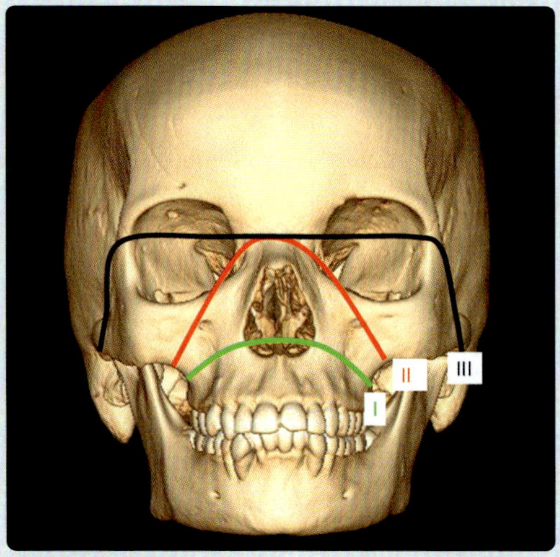

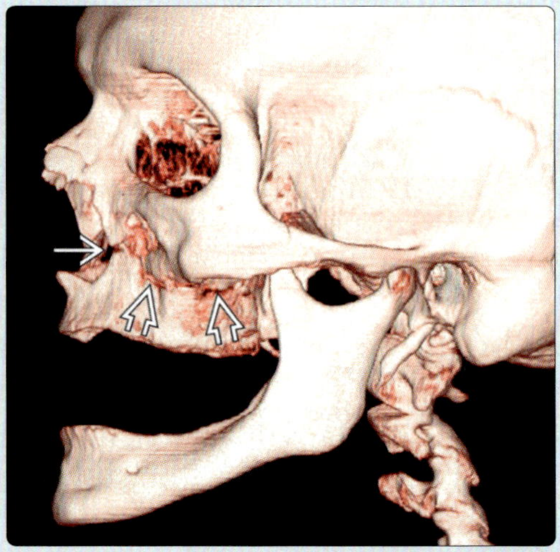

(Left) *Coronal graphic shows lines defining the 3 types of Le Fort fractures (fxs). Le Fort I (green) involves the nasal aperture, Le Fort II (red) traverses the inferior orbital rim, and Le Fort III (black) extends through the zygomatic arches.* **(Right)** *Lateral 3D CT reformation shows a horizontal Le Fort I fx ➔ separating the maxillary alveolus from the midface. Note the involvement of the nasal aperture ➔ but intact inferior orbital rim and zygomatic arch.*

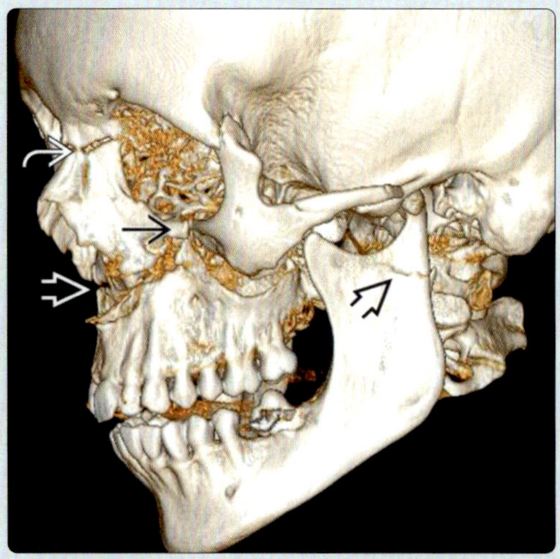

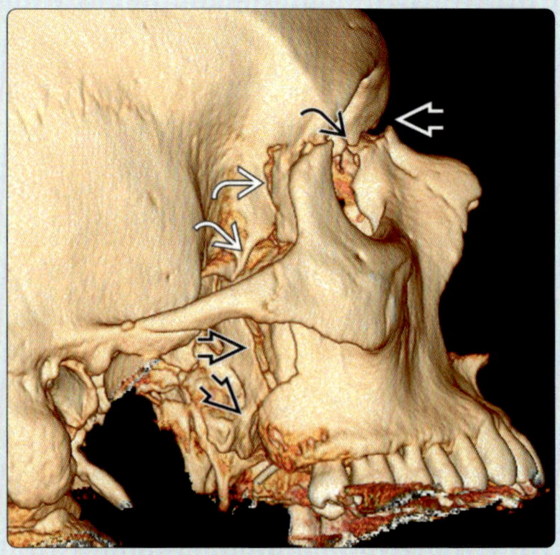

(Left) *Lateral 3D CT reformation shows a Le Fort II fx with a fx through the nasofrontal junction ➔ and extending obliquely through the inferior orbital rim ➔. There is also an associated Le Fort I fx ➔ and a fx through the subcondylar region of the mandible ➔.* **(Right)** *Lateral 3D CT reformation of a right Le Fort III fx shows frontonasal diastasis ➔, medial ➔ and lateral ➔ orbital wall fxs, & pterygoid plate fxs ➔ with sparing of inferior orbital rim.*

TERMINOLOGY

Abbreviations

- Le Fort (LF), fracture (fx)

Definitions

- Fractures disrupting pterygomaxillary junction, fracturing pterygoid processes/plates, & **disjoining portions of face (maxilla) from skull**

IMAGING

General Features

- Best diagnostic clue
  - **Pterygoid process & pterygoid plate fractures** in patients with clinically mobile facial skeleton

Imaging Recommendations

- Best imaging tool
  - Thin-section bone CT or CBCT
- Protocol advice
  - Noncontrast axial helical CT (slice thickness ≤ 1 mm) or CBCT (voxel size ≤ 0.4 mm) with bone algorithm, coronal, and 3D reconstructions

CT Findings

- Bone CT
  - **LF I**: Pterygomaxillary disjunction + fx of inferior medial & lateral maxillary buttress
    - Fx involving pyriform rim + medial & lateral walls of maxillary sinus/alveolus + pterygoid plates + nasal septum
  - **LF II**: Pterygomaxillary disjunction + superior medial maxillary buttress + inferior lateral maxillary buttress
    - Fx of superior medial maxillary buttress = [illegible] junction & inferior orbital rim
    - Fx of inferior lateral maxillary buttress = zygomaticomaxillary suture
  - **LF III**: Pterygomaxillary disjunction + zygomatic arch + superior lateral & medial maxillary buttress
    - Fx of upper transverse maxillary buttress = zygomatic arch
    - Fx of zygomaticofrontal, zygomaticosphenoid sutures, orbital floor, nasofrontal junction
  - **Sinus opacification** from bleeding is indirect sign of fracture

DIFFERENTIAL DIAGNOSIS

Zygomaticomaxillary Complex Fracture

- Associated with blow to malar eminence
- Spares pterygoid process/plates
- Involves zygomaticofrontal, zygomaticomaxillary, zygomaticosphenoid, & zygomaticotemporal sutures

Nasoorbitalethmoid Fracture

- Associated with focal blow over nasal bridge
- Spare pterygoid processes/plates
- Depression of nasal pyramid ± telecanthus due to displacement of medial canthal ligament

Complex Facial Fracture

- Highly comminuted midface fx
- In "pure form" spares pterygoid processes/plates, but frequently coexists with LF fxs

Pterygoid Plate Avulsion

- Associated with violent trauma to mandible
- Lateral pterygoid plate typically involved; pterygoid process usually spared

PATHOLOGY

General Features

- Etiology
  - Most cases due to trauma from motor vehicle accidents, assaults, or falls

CLINICAL ISSUES

Presentation

- Most common signs/symptoms
  - "Mobile face" (maxillary alveolus & hard palate, midface, or entire face)
  - Midface depression (retrusion), also called "dish face"

Natural History & Prognosis

- Long-term complications may include facial deformity, breathing difficulty, malocclusion, telecanthus, visual changes, diplopia, epiphora, anosmia, facial numbness, & headaches

Treatment

- Surgical reduction & fixation starts with frontal bar (attached to thickened frontal bone above frontonasal sutures & superior orbital rims); other facial bones are "suspended" from frontal bar

DIAGNOSTIC CHECKLIST

Image Interpretation Pearls

- Remember components that are unique to each LF fx type
  - LF I: Lateral margin of nasal aperture
  - LF II: Inferior orbital rim
  - LF III: Zygomatic arch

SELECTED REFERENCES

1. Kim JJ et al: Maxillofacial (midface) fractures. Neuroimaging Clin N Am. 20(4):581-96, 2010
2. Back CP et al: The conservative management of facial fractures: indications and outcomes. J Plast Reconstr Aesthet Surg. 60(2):146-51, 2007
3. Hopper RA et al: Diagnosis of midface fractures with CT: what the surgeon needs to know. Radiographics. 26(3):783-93, 2006
4. Zimmermann CE et al: Pediatric facial fractures: recent advances in prevention, diagnosis and management. Int J Oral Maxillofac Surg. 35(1):2-13, 2006
5. Connor SE et al: Computed tomography pseudofractures of the mid face and skull base. Clin Radiol. 60(12):1268-79, 2005
6. Rhea JT et al: How to simplify the CT diagnosis of Le Fort fractures. AJR Am J Roentgenol. 184(5):1700-5, 2005
7. Linnau KF et al: Imaging of high-energy midfacial trauma: what the surgeon needs to know. Eur J Radiol. 48(1):17-32, 2003
8. Linnau KF et al: Orbital apex injury: trauma at the junction between the face and the cranium. Eur J Radiol. 48(1):5-16, 2003
9. Salvolini U: Traumatic injuries: imaging of facial injuries. Eur Radiol. 12(6):1253-61, 2002

(Left) *Coronal planar reconstruction from axial helical CT shows bilateral fxs through the pterygoid processes, the sine qua non of Le Fort fxs, and is seen in types I, II, and III.* **(Right)** *Coronal CBCT reformatted image shows fxs through the medial facial buttress as a component of the Le Fort I pattern. Note that the vertical medial maxillary buttress is intact. Axial scatter artifact from metallic dental restorations is present.*

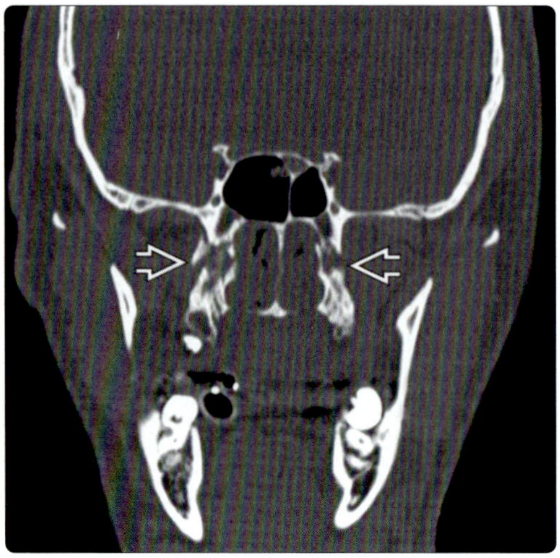

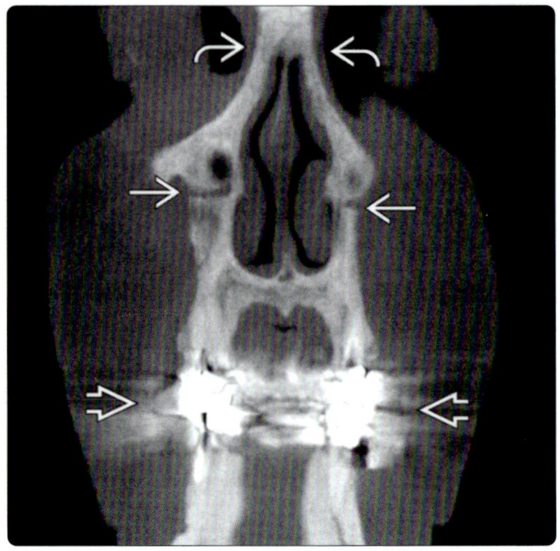

(Left) *Coronal bone CT shows fxs involving the inferomedial orbital walls extending from the nasofrontal junction. There are fxs through the upper transverse maxillary buttress (orbital rim and floors) and inferior medial and lateral maxillary buttresses (Le Fort II and I, respectively).* **(Right)** *Axial bone CT shows bilateral pterygoid plate fxs in a patient with a Le Fort type I fx. Opacification of the maxillary sinuses suggests bleeding, a common indirect sign of midfacial fracture.*

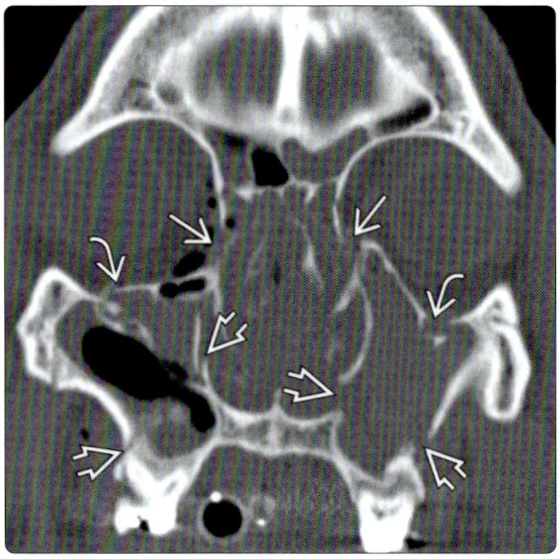

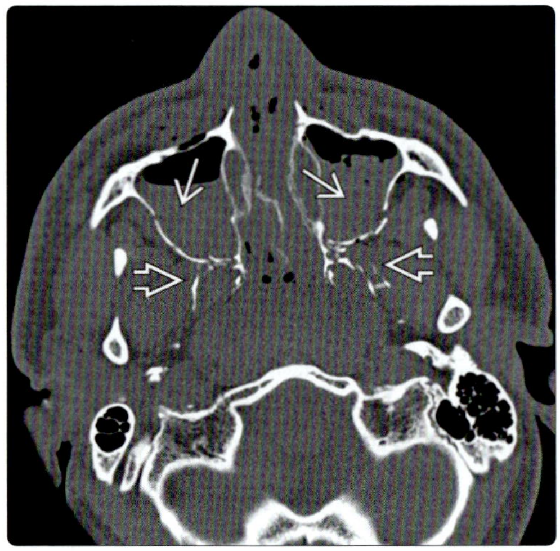

(Left) *Coronal bone CT shows fx through the nasofrontal junction common to Le Fort II and III patterns. This fracture site is at the confluence of the vertical (medial maxillary) & transverse (upper transverse maxillary) buttresses, forming the anterior point of midfacial or craniofacial disjunction.* **(Right)** *Coronal bone CT shows fx of the upper transverse buttresses and zygomaticofrontal suture in the Le Fort II and III pattern. Note the right Le Fort I fracture.*

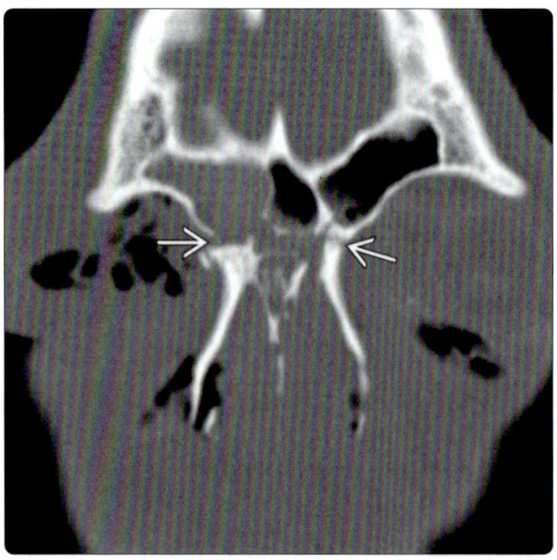

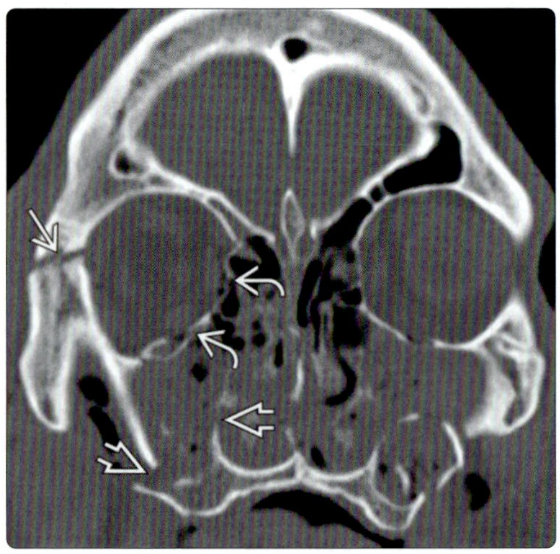

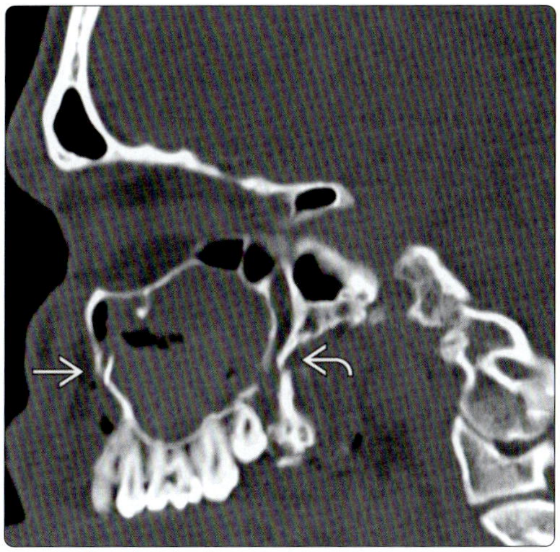

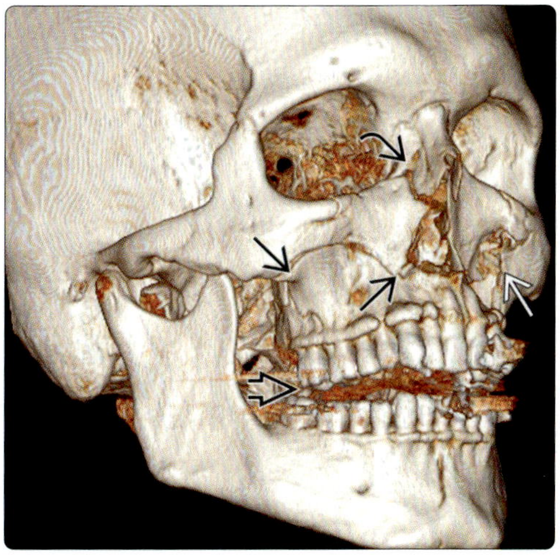

(Left) *Sagittal CT reconstruction shows the utility of sagittal reformats for demonstrating the maxillary disjunction of a Le Fort I with fx extending from the lateral aspect of the nasal aperture through the pterygoid plate.* **(Right)** *Oblique 3D CT reformation shows a right Le Fort I fx mobilizing the right hemimaxilla, which is rotated inferiorly. In addition, there are multiple nasal bone fxs and comminuted left maxillary fxs.*

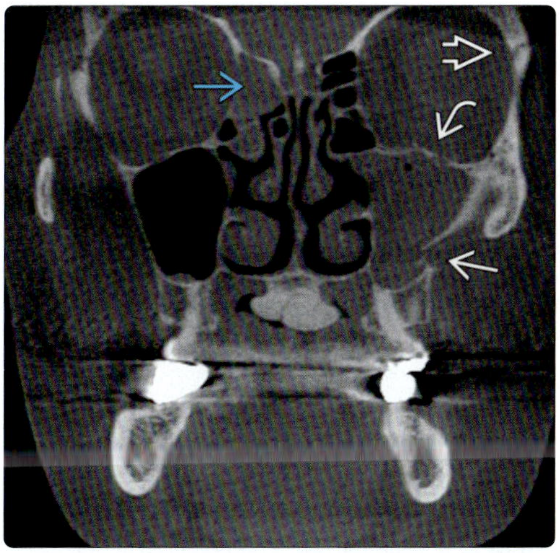

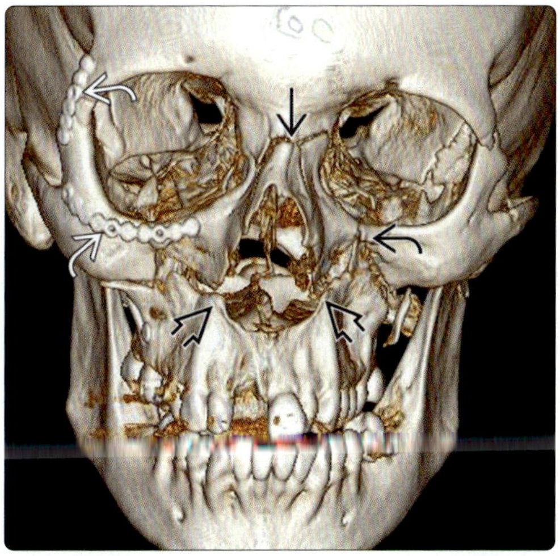

(Left) *Coronal CBCT shows fxs of left antral wall, orbital rim and floor, and separation of the zygomaticofrontal suture. Bleeding into the ethmoid sinus is an indirect sign of nasofrontal separation, which was visualized in other views. This is the Le Fort II and III patterns.* **(Right)** *Anteroposterior 3D CT reformation shows a fx through the ethmoid complex and anteroinferiorly to the orbital rim. Note the bilateral Le Fort I fxs and bone plates from an old zygomaticomaxillary fx.*

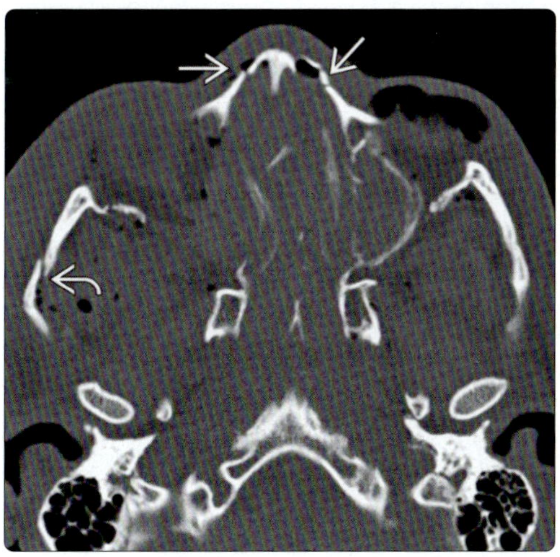

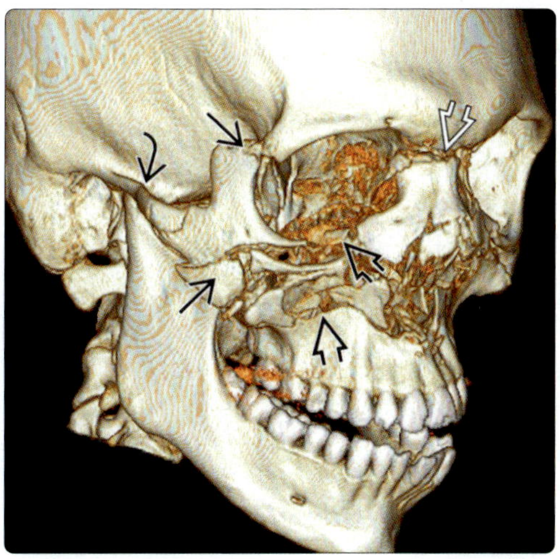

(Left) *Axial bone CT of right Le Fort III shows bilateral nasal bone fxs and a right zygomatic arch fx. A combination of nasoethmoid and zygoma fxs should prompt a search for Le Fort III.* **(Right)** *Oblique 3D CT reformation of an impure right Le Fort III fx shows the craniofacial disjunction as a depressed nasal fx, zygoma fxs, and depressed zygomatic arch fx. Note the accompanying comminuted orbital and maxillary smash fxs.*

Mandible-Maxilla Osteomyelitis

KEY FACTS

TERMINOLOGY

- Definition: Polymicrobial bacterial **infection of bone**

IMAGING

- **Mandible** > > maxilla
- **Odontogenic source** most common (i.e., nonvital tooth)
  - Periapical radiolucency related to carious, fractured, or periodontally involved tooth
- Hallmarks are **sequestra** and laminated/**onion skin** periosteal new bone
- **Mixed sclerosis and bone destruction** most common presentation
- CT most useful for identifying bone changes
- MR depicts soft tissue alterations
- MR sensitive for identifying full extent of marrow involvement
  - See loss of normal T1 fat signal
- Nuclear bone scan identifies early and multifocal lesions
  - i.e., in SAPHO syndrome

TOP DIFFERENTIAL DIAGNOSES

- **Infiltrative neoplasm** invading mandible
  - Alveolar ridge or other perimandibular SCCa
  - Osteosarcoma
  - Mandibular metastasis
    - Look for soft tissue mass, irregular periodontal ligament space widening
- Fibrous dysplasia
- Medication-related osteonecrosis
- Osteoradionecrosis

DIAGNOSTIC CHECKLIST

- Identify source of infection
- Rule out malignancy: Biopsy may be necessary
- Examine soft tissues of masticator and submandibular spaces for abscess and sinus tract
- **Pearl**: Periosteal new bone parallel to original cortex (may be fragmented but still visible) + sequestra most suggestive of osteomyelitis

(Left) *Panoramic radiograph of the left mandible shows osteomyelitis originating from a partially impacted 3rd molar. There is generalized sclerosis, evident by the relative prominence of the mandibular canal ➡. Regions of destruction along the inferior border are also seen ➡.* **(Right)** *Axial bone CT of the same patient shows sclerosis ➡ and destructive changes of the cortex ➡. There is also periosteal new bone formation ➡ with evidence of the original cortex now forming a sequestrum ➡.*

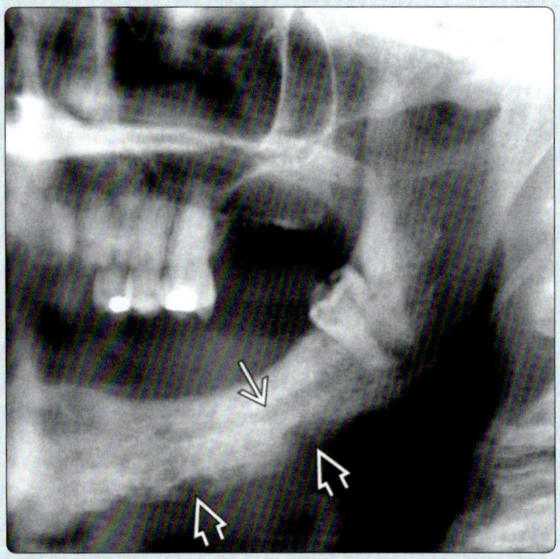

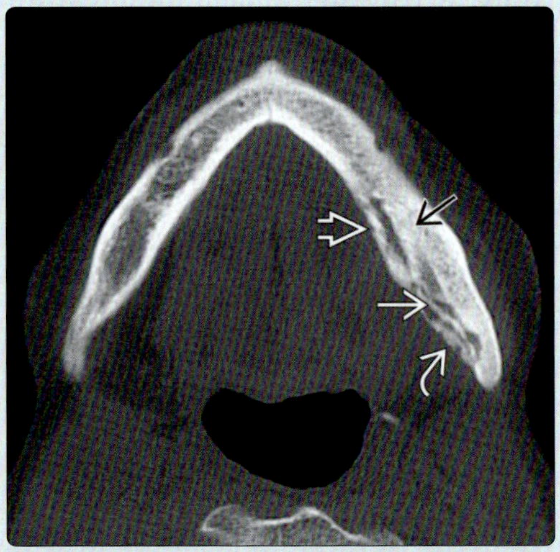

(Left) *Coronal CBCT shows a periapical radiolucency ➡, consistent with infection, related to the mandibular left 3rd molar. The infection has drained through the buccal cortex ➡ and led to significant periosteal new bone formation ➡.* **(Right)** *Axial CBCT of the same patient shows reactive bone sclerosis ➡ around the mandibular canal and the periosteal new bone formed on the buccal aspect of the posterior mandible ➡, consistent with osteomyelitis.*

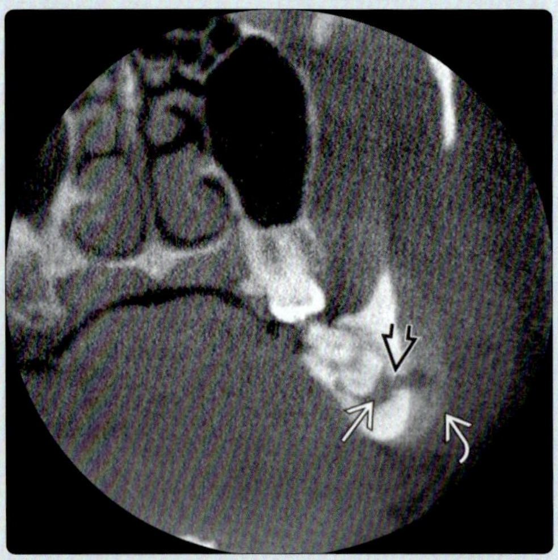

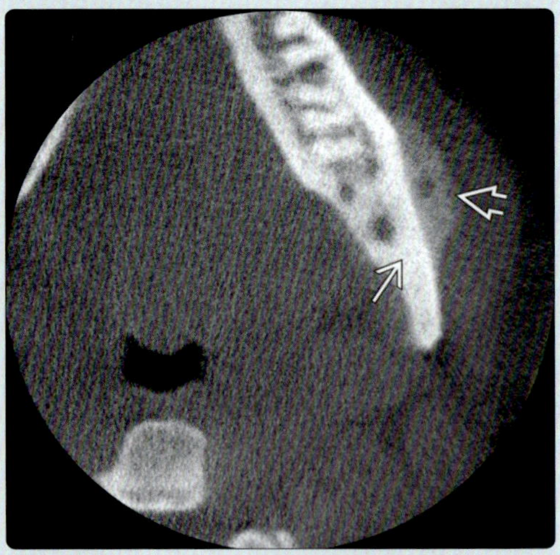

TERMINOLOGY

Synonyms

- Acute suppurative osteomyelitis, chronic sclerosing osteomyelitis, proliferative periostitis

Definitions

- Inflammation of bone and bone marrow
- Most commonly due to bacterial infection
  - Noninfectious osteomyelitis is separate condition in children

IMAGING

General Features

- Best diagnostic clue
  - Mixed lytic and sclerotic bone changes with **sequestra and laminated periosteal new bone** formation
  - Source of infection identified (odontogenic, surgical, trauma)
  - Inflammatory soft tissue changes
- Location
  - Mandible > > maxilla
    - Less vascular, denser bone
  - Molar region most common
  - Uncontrolled infection may spread to TMJ (septic arthritis), ear, and mastoids
  - May have associated soft tissue inflammation
- Size
  - Variable from localized → entire jaw bilaterally
- Morphology
  - Ill-defined, permeative or blending periphery
    - May appear **moth-eaten**
  - Jaw becomes enlarged with extensive periosteal bone formation

Imaging Recommendations

- Best imaging tool
  - CECT: Use both soft tissue and bone algorithms
    - CT best able to demonstrate sequestra and periosteal new bone
  - Panoramic radiograph useful for monitoring response to treatment
- Protocol advice
  - Consider angled CT as additional series to avoid dental amalgam artifacts

Radiographic Findings

- Acute: Ill-defined lucency of bone
- Chronic: ↑ **sclerosis** of trabecular bone; may have ground-glass pattern
  - With profound sclerosis, mandibular nerve canal seen prominently
  - Also lose contrast of inferior cortex of mandible
- **Sequestra**: Radiopaque island of bone surrounded by radiolucent region of bone destruction
- **Periosteal new bone** runs parallel to original cortex
  - Multiple parallel laminations create **onion skin** appearance
  - More exuberant in younger patients
- Radiolucent **sinus tract** through cortex
- **Odontogenic source** (i.e., nonvital tooth)
  - Periapical radiolucency related to carious, fractured, or periodontally involved tooth
  - Loss of lamina dura around tooth apex

CT Findings

- Bone CT/CBCT
  - Mixed, irregular **bone destruction and sclerosis**
    - Acute: Predominantly lysis of cancellous bone with fragmentation of cortices
    - Chronic: Greater sclerosis of trabecular bone
  - Sequestra more clearly visualized with CT
  - Periosteal new bone deposited parallel to original cortex
    - **Enlargement of jaw** may confuse with other conditions
      - Identifying fragments of original cortex helps confirm periosteal origin of change
- CECT
  - Soft tissue inflammatory changes (fat streaking, skin thickening, lymphadenopathy)
  - Visualize submandibular, sublingual, or masticator space abscess when present

MR Findings

- T1WI
  - **Loss of T1 signal** as marrow fat replaced by exudate (acute) or fibrosis/sclerosis (chronic)
- STIR
  - Acute: Marked hyperintensity of marrow due to edema or hyperemia
  - Chronic: Variable, depending on degree of fibrosis and sclerosis
  - Inflammation in surrounding soft tissues detected by high signal
- T1WI C+ FS
  - Acute: Marked marrow space enhancement
  - Chronic: Variable enhancement
  - Enhancement of surrounding soft tissues, particularly masseter muscle

Nuclear Medicine Findings

- Tc-99m MDP bone scan sensitive but not specific
  - Able to detect early lesions before radiographic evidence is seen
  - Useful if multifocal disease is suspected [SAPHO (**s**ynovitis, **a**cne, **p**ustulitis, **h**yperostosis, **o**steitis) syndrome]
  - SPECT aids in localizing affected bone
- Ga-67 citrate helps distinguish inflammatory disease from other bone abnormalities

DIFFERENTIAL DIAGNOSIS

Squamous Cell Carcinoma

- Purely lytic changes; no periosteal reaction
- **Soft tissue mass** or infiltration
- Superimposed infection may complicate appearance

Osteosarcoma

- Combination of bone destruction and formation may mimic osteomyelitis
- Look for more centric enlargement of bone, suggesting tumor-type growth

- Periosteal new bone creates **sun-ray pattern** with thin linear new bone extending from central origin

Metastasis

- Prostate or breast may be osteoblastic
  - Sclerotic changes mimic inflammatory reaction
  - **Hair on end pattern** of periosteal new bone in prostate mets
- Irregular widening of periodontal ligament spaces suggests malignant infiltration

Fibrous Dysplasia

- Increased bone density and expansion may mimic chronic osteomyelitis
- **Expanded cortex is intact** rather than permeated and not surrounded by new periosteal bone
- No clinical symptoms of infection

Medication-Related Osteonecrosis

- Bone changes in patient with history of **antiresorptive or antiangiogenic drug use**
- Usually associated with exposed bone clinically

Osteoradionecrosis

- Bone lysis and sclerosis in patient with history of **radiation therapy**

PATHOLOGY

General Features

- Etiology
  - Most cases are **odontogenic**: Periapical or periodontal lesion or pericoronitis
    - Carious tooth → central pulp infection → periapical abscess → marrow space extension → cancellous and cortical destruction
  - Nonodontogenic: Trauma, postsurgical, hematogenous
  - No single dominant microbial agent responsible: Mixed bacterial species found on culture
- Associated abnormalities
  - Abnormalities in bone metabolism lead to increased risk: Paget disease, osteopetrosis
  - Lesions of **cementoosseous dysplasia may become secondarily infected** and lead to osteomyelitis
    - Avascular, cementum-like masses act as sequestra and nidi for infection

Staging, Grading, & Classification

- Acute < 4 weeks
- Many names and classifications suggested
  - Primary vs. secondary chronic; focal vs. diffuse sclerosing; suppurative vs. nonsuppurative; proliferative periostitis
  - Variable presentations of same inflammatory condition
- Osteomyelitis with SAPHO syndrome has multifocal involvement
- Chronic recurrent multifocal osteomyelitis is separate disorder in children, rarely involving jaws; symptoms of osteomyelitis without infection

Microscopic Features

- Acute: Necrotic bone with no osteocytes present; inflammatory cell infiltrate, including neutrophils; necrotic debris and bone resorption
- Chronic: Marrow fibrosis, lymphocytes, plasma cells
  - Osteoblastic activity and new bone formation indicates attempt at repair and corresponds to granular or sclerotic patterns seen radiographically

CLINICAL ISSUES

Presentation

- Most common signs/symptoms
  - Pain and swelling around jaw; lymphadenopathy
- Other signs/symptoms
  - Fistula formation with purulent discharge
  - Trismus if infection spreads to masticator muscles
  - Unilateral mandibular/chin hypesthesia or anesthesia if mandibular nerve canal involved

Demographics

- Age
  - All ages affected
- Epidemiology
  - Increased risk in immune-compromised patients: Diabetes, malnutrition, anemia
  - Alcohol and tobacco abuse also linked to higher risk

Natural History & Prognosis

- Acute disease may progress to chronic if not treated adequately
- Chronic disease difficult to manage

Treatment

- Control source of infection: Extraction or endodontic therapy of causative tooth, removal of foreign object
- **Long-term oral ± IV antibiotics**, ideally based on deep tissue culture
- Surgical debridement: Decortication and sequestra removal
- Hyperbaric oxygen therapy may help improve vascularity in refractory cases

DIAGNOSTIC CHECKLIST

Consider

- Consider malignancy if persistent soft tissue lesion with bone destruction
  - Biopsy required to rule out aggressive lesion
- Serial exams often necessary to confirm osteomyelitis and document positive clinical response

Image Interpretation Pearls

- Periosteal new bone parallel to original cortex (may be fragmented but still visible) + sequestra most suggestive of osteomyelitis

Reporting Tips

- Identify source (i.e., offending tooth) where applicable
- Identify location of sequestra to allow surgical treatment planning

SELECTED REFERENCES

1. Koorbusch GF et al: How can we diagnose and treat osteomyelitis of the jaws as early as possible? Oral Maxillofac Surg Clin North Am. 23(4):557-67, vii, 2011
2. Tanaka R et al: Computed tomography findings of chronic osteomyelitis involving the mandible: correlation to histopathological findings. Dentomaxillofac Radiol. 37(2):94-103, 2008

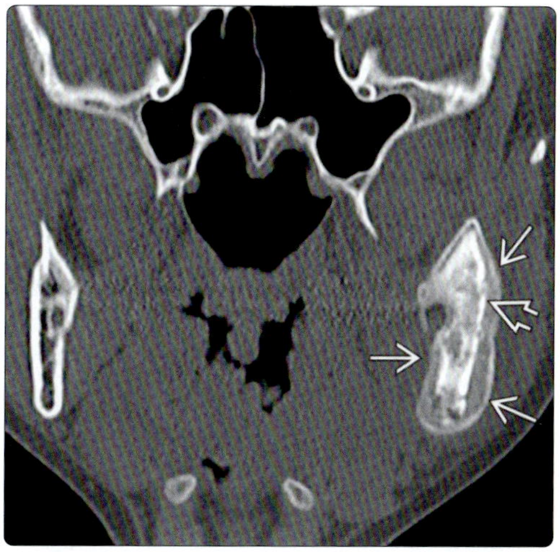

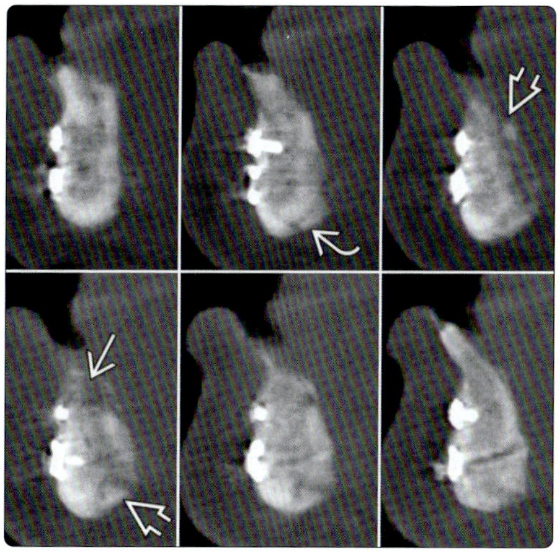

(Left) *Coronal bone CT in a young patient shows profound periosteal new bone formation encircling the entire left ramus. The original mandibular cortex is still visible, though partially resorbed. Destructive and sclerotic changes are also seen in the trabecular bone.* **(Right)** *CBCT cross sections in a patient with mandibular fracture with nonunion and osteomyelitis are shown. Rarefaction and sequestra of the lingual cortex are seen. There is periosteal new bone formation at the inferior border.*

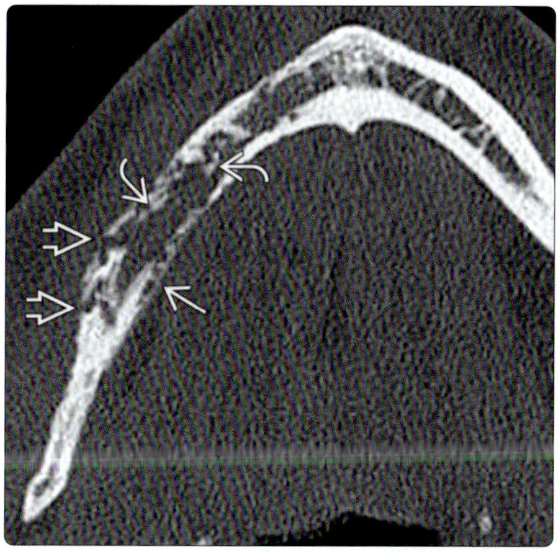

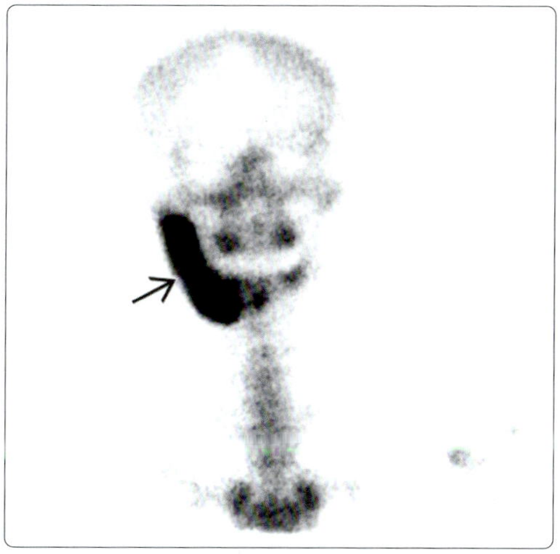

(Left) *Axial bone CT shows the ill-defined, moth-eaten appearance of the right mandible in a male patient with osteomyelitis. The cortex is destroyed in some areas. Note periosteal new bone formation on lingual and evidence of sequestra, which helps to differentiate from malignancy. There are no apparent soft tissue changes in this patient. (Courtesy P. Hawkins, DDS.)* **(Right)** *Anterior Tc-99m MDP bone scan of a patient with osteomyelitis of the right mandible shows profound uptake of the tracer.*

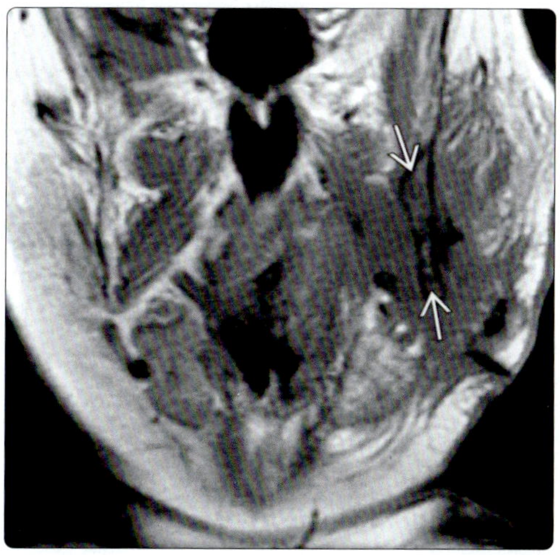

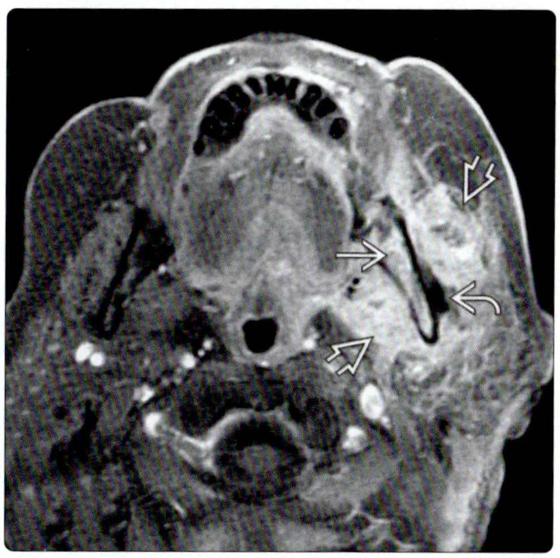

(Left) *Coronal T1WI MR shows a 79 year old with recurrent masticator space abscess 12 weeks following initial diagnosis and previous drainage. Normal high-signal marrow fat has been completely replaced in left mandible, consistent with osteomyelitis.* **(Right)** *Axial T1WI C+ fat-saturated MR in the same patient reveals diffuse enhancement of the left marrow space with masticator space enhancement (phlegmon) and small lateral compartment abscess.*

Mandible-Maxilla Osteoradionecrosis

KEY FACTS

TERMINOLOGY

- Osteoradionecrosis (ORN)
- Bone death resulting from exposure to therapeutic radiation and not related to tumor recurrence

IMAGING

- Progressive, ill-defined, lytic bone changes in mandible of patient with **previous radiation therapy**
- Sclerosis, **sequestra,** and pathologic fracture are also seen
- **Posterior mandible** is most commonly affected
    - Mandible:maxilla = 24:1 due to less vascularity
- **Nonhealing** extraction or mandibulotomy site
- Soft tissue thickening adjacent to bone changes
- CT provides detailed view of bone changes, establishes extent of disease, and helps **rule out recurrence of malignancy**
- T1WI: Low signal in marrow
- T2WI: Hyperintense with inflammation

TOP DIFFERENTIAL DIAGNOSES

- Malignancy recurrence
    - ORN especially difficult to differentiate from local recurrence of original tumor
    - **Soft tissue mass** seen in malignancy recurrence
- Osteonecrosis (medication related)
- Osteomyelitis

CLINICAL ISSUES

- **Dehiscence of overlying skin or mucosa** with underlying bone exposure for > 3 months
- **Site of previous trauma** (dental extraction, mucosal ulceration from denture injury)
- **Preradiation dental management is key** to avoiding need for postradiation extractions

DIAGNOSTIC CHECKLIST

- **Progressive bone destruction** with sclerosis in radiated field is suggestive of ORN

(Left) *Panoramic radiograph shows osteoradionecrosis (ORN) in the posterior right mandible causing lytic bone destruction. Sclerosis of the surrounding bone and sequestra are noted. The periodontal ligament space widening on the 1st molar represents a common postradiation change.* **(Right)** *Cropped panoramic radiograph shows ORN in a mandibulotomy site. Note the resorption along the surgical site and destruction of the inferior cortex. There is also fracture of the surgical plate.*

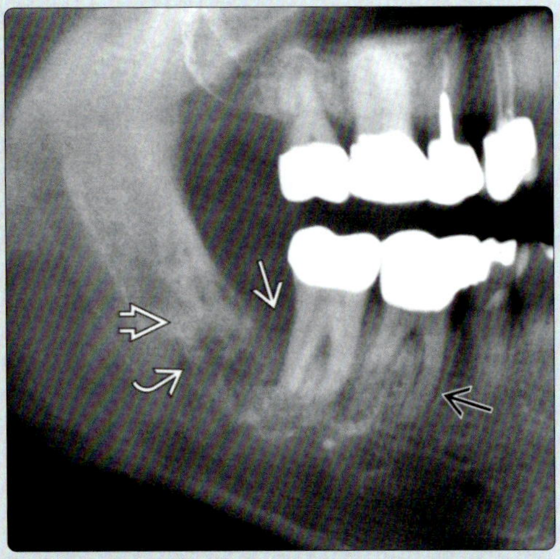

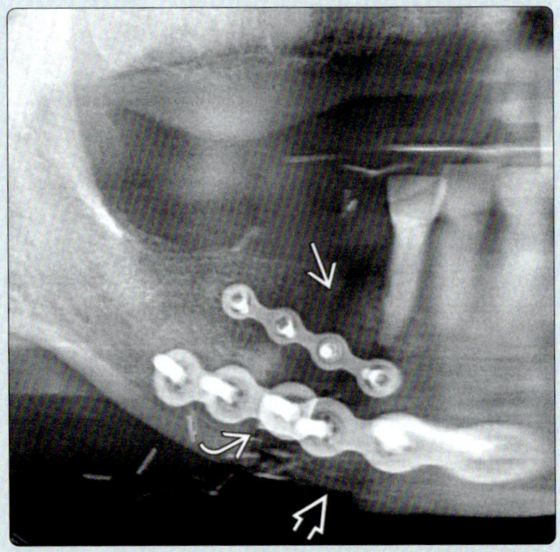

(Left) *Axial CBCT shows ORN around the left mandibular 1st molar. There is destruction of the lingual cortex with formation of sequestra. Resorption of trabecular bone is also seen. Note the fixation plate on the contralateral side.* **(Right)** *Coronal CBCT of the same patient shows early sequestrum formation in the buccal cortex seen as a central island of bone surrounded by a radiolucent rim of resorption. There is also destruction of the lingual alveolar crest.*

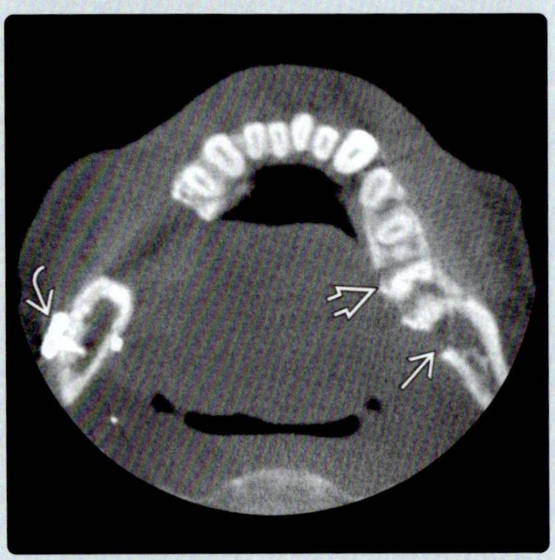

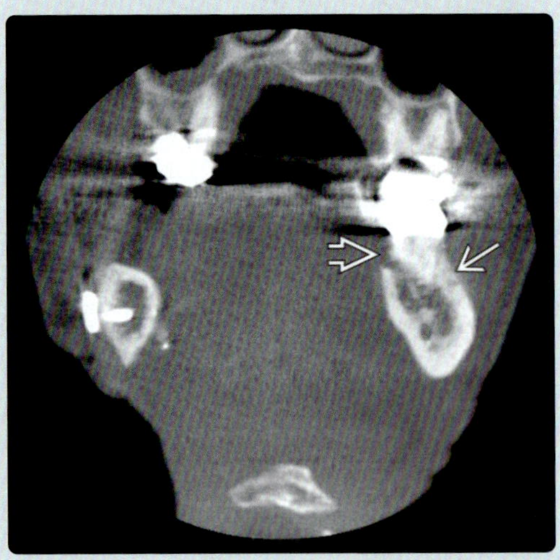

TERMINOLOGY

Abbreviations

- Osteoradionecrosis (ORN)

Synonyms

- Radiation necrosis, radiation osteitis

Definitions

- Bone death resulting from exposure to therapeutic radiation and not related to tumor recurrence

IMAGING

General Features

- Best diagnostic clue
  - Progressive, ill-defined, lytic bone changes in patient with **previous radiation therapy**
- Location
  - Mandible:maxilla = 24:1; often **posterior mandible**
  - Site of **previous trauma** (dental extraction, mucosal ulceration from dentures)

Radiographic Findings

- Mixed lytic bone destruction and sclerosis
- **Nonhealing** extraction or mandibulotomy site
- Destruction of cortices and **pathologic fracture**
- May see radiologic signs without overlying ulceration
- Widening of periodontal ligament spaces post irradiation change: May indicate bone "at risk"

CT Findings

- Localizes **lytic changes** and erosion of cortices
- Associated **sclerosis** seen around bone loss
- **Sequestra** and fracture more clearly identified
- May see soft tissue thickening adjacent to bone changes, especially if inflammation present
- Periosteal new bone not common

MR Findings

- T1WI
  - Homogeneous low marrow signal due to fibrosis
- T2WI
  - May see variable high signal in marrow with inflammation
  - Neighboring muscles may show hyperintense signal
- T1WI C+ FS
  - Mild to avid irregular enhancement seen in affected bone and soft tissues

Imaging Recommendations

- Best imaging tool
  - Panoramic radiographs are efficient for monitoring patients post radiation therapy
  - CT best for assessment of bony changes
    - Necessary to **rule out recurrence of malignancy**

DIFFERENTIAL DIAGNOSIS

Malignancy Recurrence

- More likely to see **soft tissue mass, sclerosis less likely**
- Bone changes **away from primary tumor site** but in radiation field helps rule out recurrence of malignancy

Osteonecrosis (Medication Related)

- **History of antiresorptive drug use** (bisphosphonate, denosumab) rather than radiation therapy

Osteomyelitis

- Lack of patient history of radiation therapy
- Clinical: Fever, lymphadenopathy, no exposed bone

PATHOLOGY

General Features

- Etiology
  - Fibroatrophic theory: Fibrosis, inflammatory cascade, and impaired healing

Microscopic Features

- Necrotic bone with lacunae void of osteocytes, absence of osteoblasts or new osteoid

CLINICAL ISSUES

Presentation

- Most common signs/symptoms
  - **Dehiscence of overlying skin or mucosa** with underlying bone exposure for > 3 months
  - Pain is common but not invariably present
  - Secondary infection with purulent discharge, extraoral fistulation possible

Demographics

- Epidemiology
  - 2-15% of patients receiving H&N radiation therapy

Natural History & Prognosis

- Onset commonly 4 months to 3 years post radiation
- Risk factors
  - **Treatment factors**: Dose (> 60 Gy), dose rate, field size, radiation modality (IMRT = ↓ risk)
  - **Tumor factors**: Size, location, involvement of bone
  - **Patient factors**: Infectious dental disease, trauma, alcohol or tobacco abuse, immunocompromised

Treatment

- **Preradiation dental management is key** to avoiding need for postradiation extractions
- **Conservative**: Debridement, antibiotics, irrigation
- **Surgical**: Sequestrectomy, complete resection and reconstruction required in refractory cases
- Hyperbaric oxygen therapy and antifibrotic, antioxidant, and bisphosphonate drugs under study

DIAGNOSTIC CHECKLIST

Image Interpretation Pearls

- **Progressive bone destruction** with sclerosis in radiated field is suggestive of ORN

Reporting Tips

- Recurrence of **malignancy must be ruled out**

SELECTED REFERENCES

1. Obinata K et al: Image findings of bisphosphonate related osteonecrosis of jaws comparing with osteoradionecrosis. Dentomaxillofac Radiol. 20160281, 2017

(Left) *Cropped panoramic radiograph shows ORN in the site of a previous 3rd molar extraction. There is a mixed lytic and sclerotic bone pattern. Sequestra are seen internally. A step defect of the inferior cortex suggests the presence of a pathologic fracture.* **(Right)** *Axial bone window CECT of the same patient shows more clearly the osseous changes in the right mandible. Loss of trabecular bone and destruction of cortical plates are seen. Remnants of the cortices are also sequestered.*

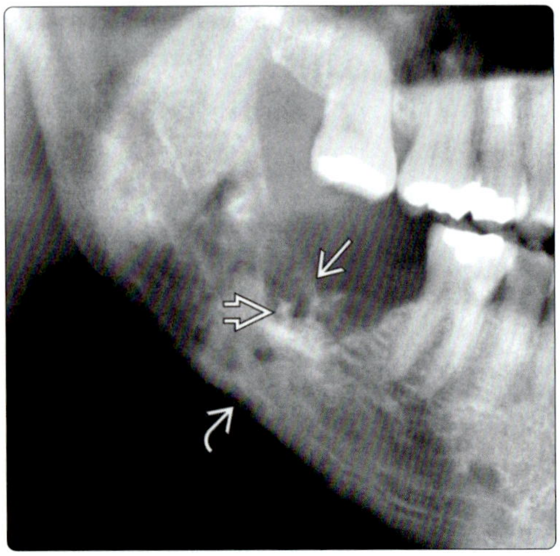

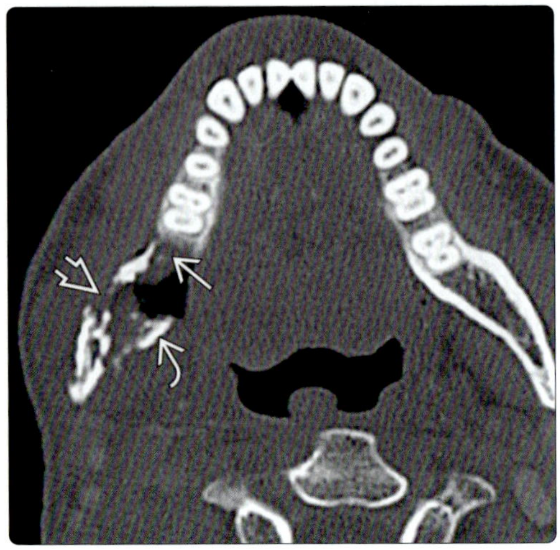

(Left) *Coronal bone CT of the same patient clearly demonstrates fragmentation of the buccal and lingual cortical plates and loss of trabecular bone in the right mandible. Sclerosis of the residual cancellous bone is also seen.* **(Right)** *Axial bone CT of the same patient in a more superior position shows more mild changes of ORN. There is loss of the buccal cortex at the level of the mandibular foramen.*

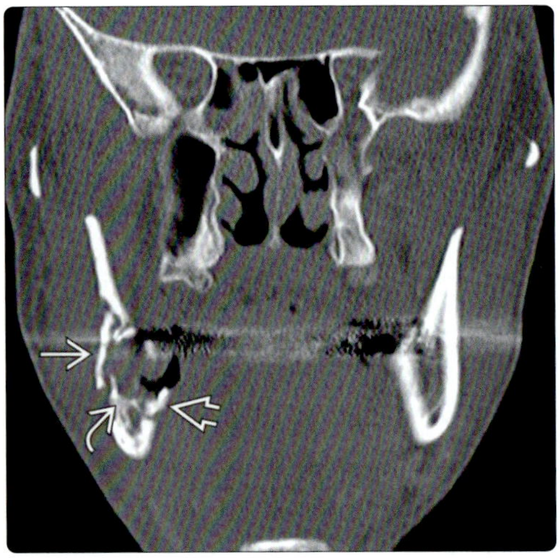

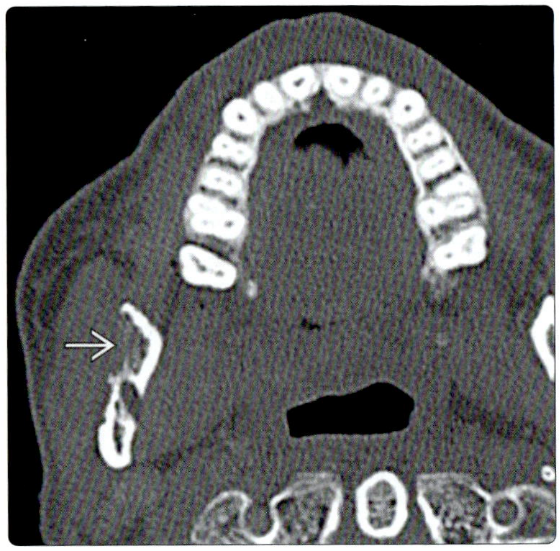

(Left) *Axial CECT of the same patient demonstrates minimal soft tissue enlargement. The streaking of the subcutaneous fat, thickening of the skin, and increased attenuation of the fat planes in the region are consistent with postirradiation changes.* **(Right)** *Cropped panoramic radiograph shows the same patient after complete resection and reconstruction of the right mandible. This is an example of radical treatment performed for ORN.*

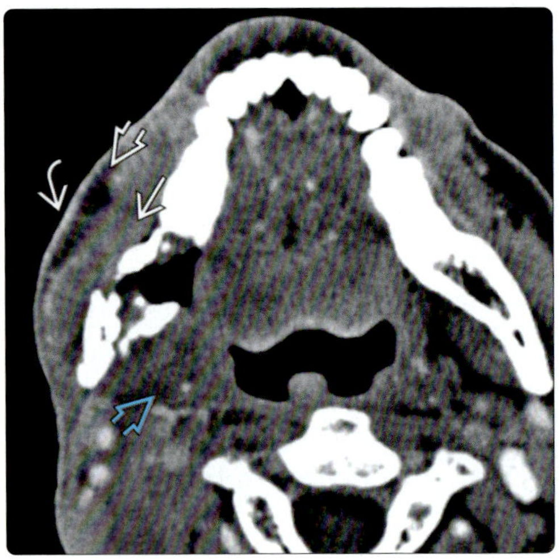

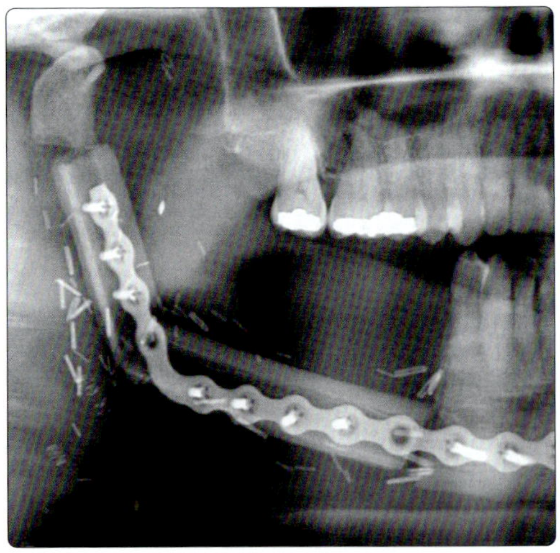

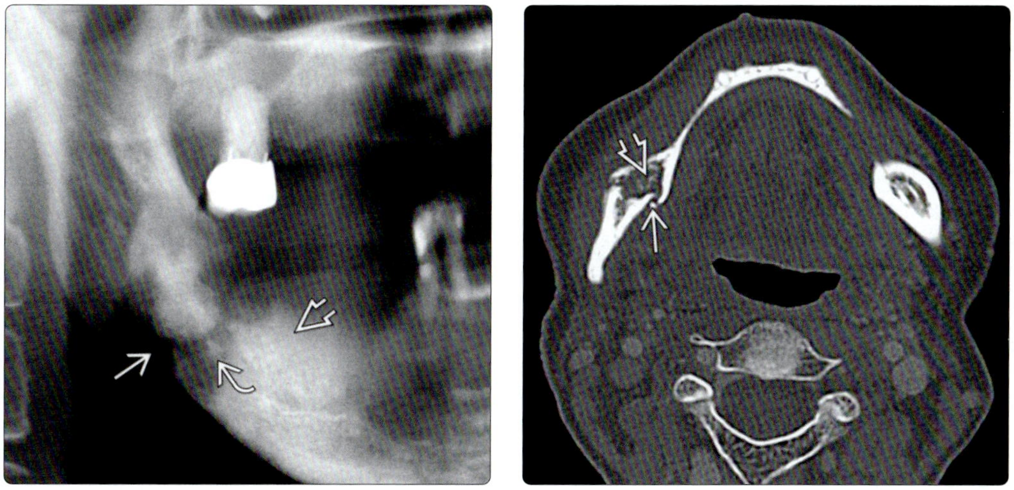

(Left) *Cropped panoramic radiograph shows ORN in the posterior right mandible after extraction of a molar. There has been significant bone destruction with a resultant pathologic fracture ➡. Sclerosis of the surrounding bone ➡ and sequestra ➡ are also appreciated.* **(Right)** *Axial bone window CECT of the same patient demonstrates a pathologic fracture of the right mandible with telescoping of the fragments secondary to ORN ➡. Small sequestra are also seen within the cancellous bone ➡.*

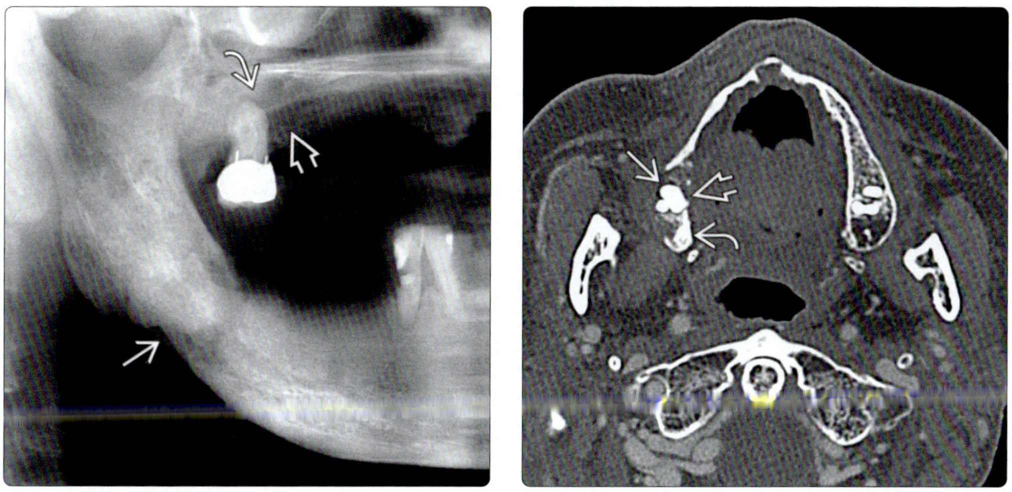

(Left) *Cropped panoramic radiograph shows the same patient 14 months later. The mandibular lesion is resolving ➡. There is bone resorption mesial to the maxillary molar ➡ with loss of the sinus floor ➡, suggestive of ORN.* **(Right)** *Axial bone window CECT in the same patient shows ORN also affecting the right maxilla. Destruction of the buccal ➡ and palatal ➡ cortices and sclerosis of the maxillary tuberosity ➡ are seen.*

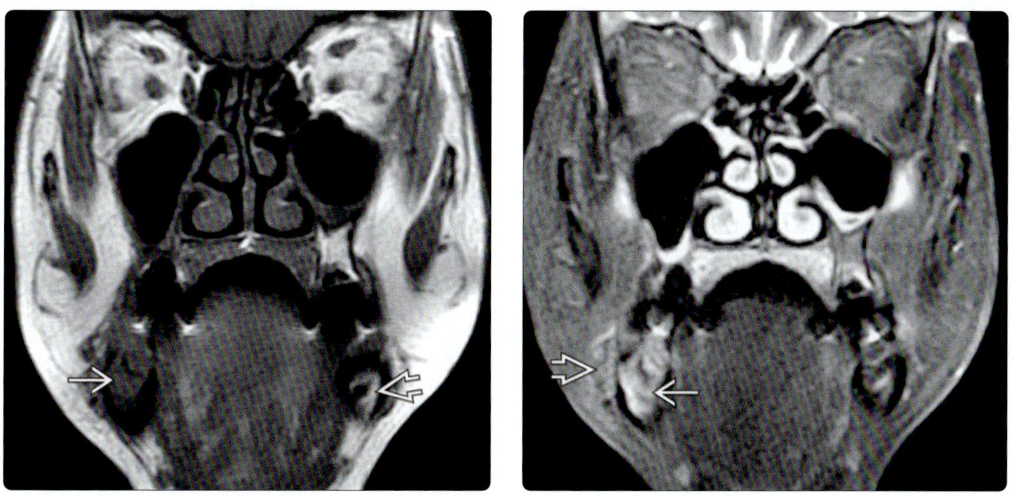

(Left) *Coronal T1WI MR of the same patient demonstrates low signal in the marrow of the right mandible due to fibrosis associated with ORN ➡. Note the normal fatty marrow signal in the left mandible ➡.* **(Right)** *Coronal T2WI FSE MR of the same patient shows a moderately bright signal in the marrow of the right mandibular region affected by ORN ➡. There is also slight increase in signal of the surrounding soft tissues ➡. These changes are due to secondary inflammation.*

Mandible-Maxilla Osteonecrosis

KEY FACTS

TERMINOLOGY

- Definition: Necrosis of mandible or maxilla associated with **antiresorptive/antiangiogenic drug** use
  - i.e., bisphosphonates, denosumab
  - Exposed bone, not healed in 8 weeks, in patient **without history of radiation** to jaws
  - Symptoms & radiologic changes may be present without exposed bone

IMAGING

- Lytic bone destruction with **sclerosis & sequestra**
- **Mandible** > maxilla (2:1)
- Persistent, **nonhealing extraction sockets**
- Pathologic **fracture** in severe cases
- CT: Better able to delineate extent of bone involvement & details of changes
  - Associated thickening & edema of soft tissues may be seen, especially with secondary infection
- MR: **Low T1 signal intensity** of trabecular bone
  - ↑ T2 signal due to inflammation & ↑ vascularity
  - **Enhancement** in bone & surrounding soft tissues

TOP DIFFERENTIAL DIAGNOSES

- Osteomyelitis
- Osteoradionecrosis
- Metastasis

CLINICAL ISSUES

- Commonly at site of previous dental extraction
- **Exposed bone**, pain, swelling
- Loosened teeth, intraoral or extraoral fistula ± suppuration, neurosensory alteration
- **Females** > males
- **Thorough dental work-up** indicated prior to commencement of IV bisphosphonates

DIAGNOSTIC CHECKLIST

- Metastasis is often differential of greatest concern: Sequestra & periosteal new bone help to rule out

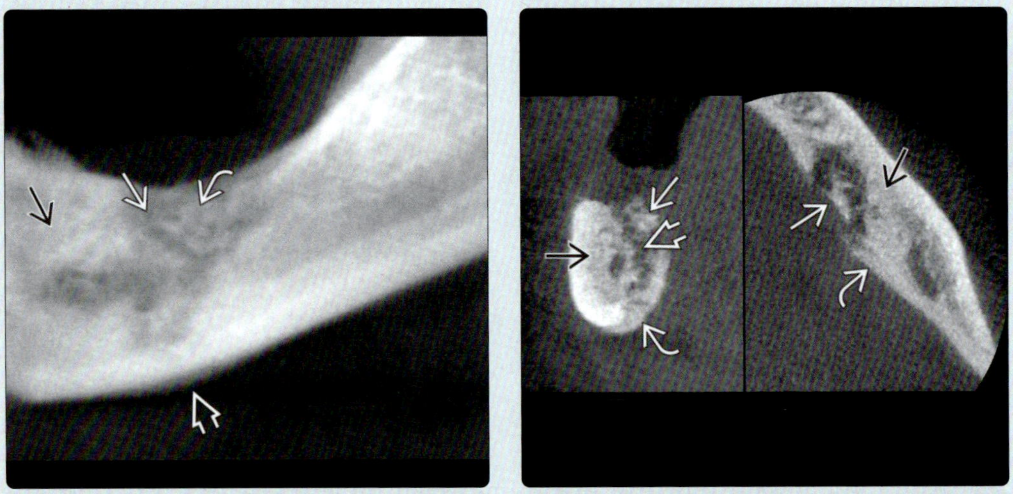

(Left) *CBCT reconstruction shows a patient on oral bisphosphonates for 5 years who developed pain, swelling, and a parulis. Note lytic ➡ and sclerotic ⇨ changes and evidence of sequestrum ➡ and periosteal new bone formation ➡ consistent with osteonecrosis.* **(Right)** *Coronal (left) and axial (right) CBCT reconstructions in the same patient confirm sequestrum ➡ and show fragmentation of the lingual cortex ➡ and adjacent periosteal bone formation ➡. There is profound sclerosis of the adjacent bone ⇨.*

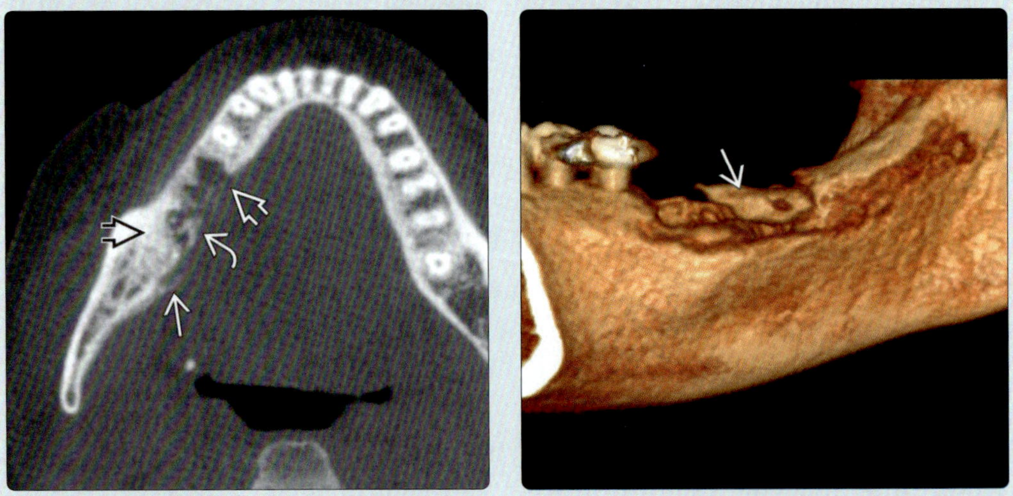

(Left) *Axial CBCT shows a failed dental implant site in the right mandible of a patient with a history of bisphosphonate use. There is lysis of the trabecular bone and lingual cortex ➡ with surrounding sclerosis ⇨. Sequestra ➡ and periosteal new bone ➡, consistent with osteonecrosis, are also appreciated. (Courtesy M. Ahmad, DDS.)* **(Right)** *CBCT 3D reformation of the same patient demonstrates the sequestration of the alveolar crest at the previous implant site ➡. (Courtesy M. Ahmad, DDS.)*

Mandible-Maxilla Osteonecrosis

TERMINOLOGY

Synonyms

- Medication-related osteonecrosis of jaws (MRONJ), bisphosphonate-related osteonecrosis of jaws

Definitions

- Necrosis of mandible or maxilla associated with **antiresorptive** (bisphosphonate, denosumab) **or antiangiogenic drug** use
  - Clinically exposed bone has not healed in 8 weeks in patient **without history of radiation** to jaws

IMAGING

General Features

- Best diagnostic clue
  - Mixed bone sclerosis & lysis at nonhealing extraction site
- Location
  - **Mandible** > maxilla (2:1)
  - Areas subjected to trauma (**extraction sites, edentulous ridge, mylohyoid ridge, tori**)

Radiographic Findings

- Radiography
  - Radiolucent bone destruction with sclerosis
  - Persistent, **nonhealing extraction sockets**
  - **Sequestra** indicate necrotic islands of bone
  - Thickened lamina dura
- CBCT & CT findings
  - **Patchy bone lysis** & fragmentation with **sclerosis of surrounding trabecular bone**
  - **Periosteal reaction parallel** to original cortex
  - Pathologic **fracture** in advanced cases
  - Associated thickening & edema of soft tissues

MR Findings

- T1WI
  - **Low signal intensity** of affected trabecular bone
- T2WI & STIR
  - Variable signal changes depending on stage
  - **Often high signal intensity** seen due to inflammation & increased vascularity
- T1WI C+ FS
  - **Enhancement** in bone & surrounding soft tissues
  - Enhancement & **enlargement of muscles** may be confused with malignant involvement

Nuclear Medicine Findings

- Bone scan
  - Increased uptake, even in early lesions
  - Poor specificity: Cannot differentiate from inflammatory or malignant disease

Imaging Recommendations

- Best imaging tool
  - Panoramic for initial examination & follow-up
  - CT better delineates extent & details

DIFFERENTIAL DIAGNOSIS

Osteomyelitis

- Patient **without history of bisphosphonate use**
- **Odontogenic source** nearly always detected

Osteoradionecrosis

- History of **prior radiation therapy** to jaws

Metastasis

- Purely lytic changes more likely to be malignant
- Associated destructive soft tissue mass

PATHOLOGY

General Features

- Etiology
  - Bisphosphonates & denosumab are potent osteoclast inhibitors therefore ↓ bone remodeling
  - Antiangiogenic properties may contribute to necrosis of bone or soft tissues
  - Infection likely important factor in onset & progression

Staging, Grading, & Classification

- American Association of Oral & Maxillofacial Surgery staging system identifies "at risk" & stages 0-3

Microscopic Features

- Necrotic bone lacking cellularity with few vessels

CLINICAL ISSUES

Presentation

- Most common signs/symptoms
  - **Exposed bone**, pain, swelling, ± fistula

Demographics

- Gender: Females > males
- Risk factors
  - Drug factors: **IV > > > oral**; zoledronate ≈ denosumab > pamidronate
  - Increased duration of therapy (> 4 year) = ↑ risk
  - Local factors: Extractions, trauma, dental disease
    - **Dental work-up indicated** before starting IV
    - **Biopsy should be avoided**
  - Systemic factors: Immunocompromised, age

Natural History & Prognosis

- Early detection & management minimizes progression

Treatment

- Pain control, oral antimicrobial rinses, systemic antibiotics
- Removal of sequestra without exposure of vital bone
- Advanced disease: Surgical debridement or resection

DIAGNOSTIC CHECKLIST

Consider

- Metastasis is often differential of greatest concern: Sequestra & periosteal new bone help to rule out

Image Interpretation Pearls

- Bone lysis + sclerosis around nonhealing extraction socket
- Loss of T1 MR signal identifies early involvement

SELECTED REFERENCES

1. Ruggiero SL et al: American Association of Oral and Maxillofacial Surgeons position paper on medication-related osteonecrosis of the jaw–2014 update. J Oral Maxillofac Surg. 72(10):1938-56, 2014

(Left) *Cropped panoramic radiograph shows preextraction appearance of bone. Note the sclerosis of the alveolar crest and lamina dura of the premolar and molar suggestive of bisphosphonate-related changes.* **(Right)** *Axial bone CT in the same patient, 1 year post extraction of decayed 1st molar, shows osteonecrosis of the bone in the extraction site. The bone posteriorly is highly sclerotic. Bone was exposed clinically. Note the thickened lamina dura around the teeth on the right side.*

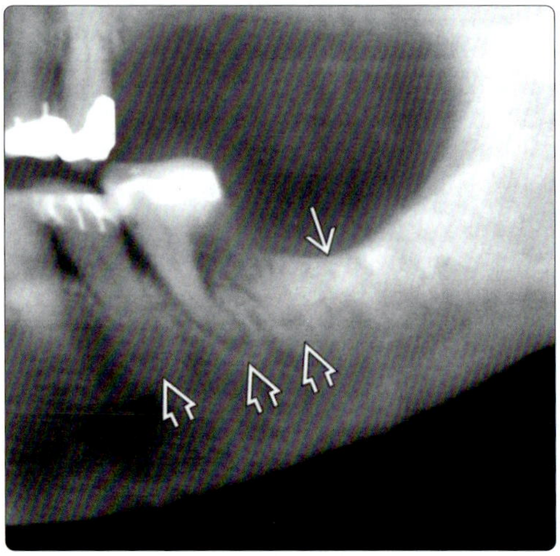

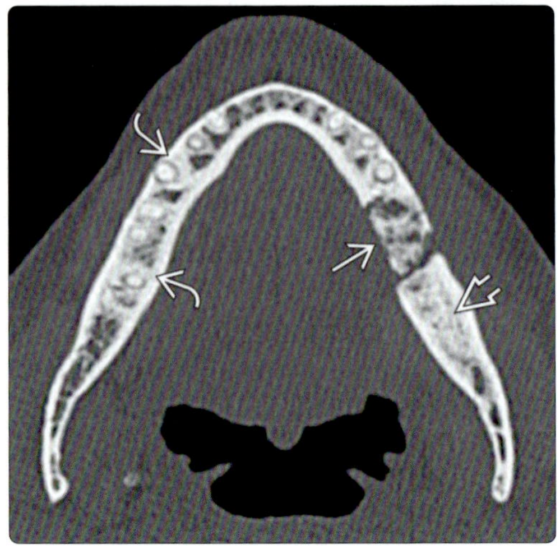

(Left) *Coronal bone CT of the same patient demonstrates the sequestration of the alveolar crest and sclerosis of the body of the mandible on the left. The patient had been taking oral bisphosphonates for 15 years.* **(Right)** *Coronal soft tissue algorithm CT in the same patient shows an associated soft tissue swelling on the buccal aspect of the mandible. There is also streaking and swelling of the subcutaneous fat. Compare to the normal appearance on the right side.*

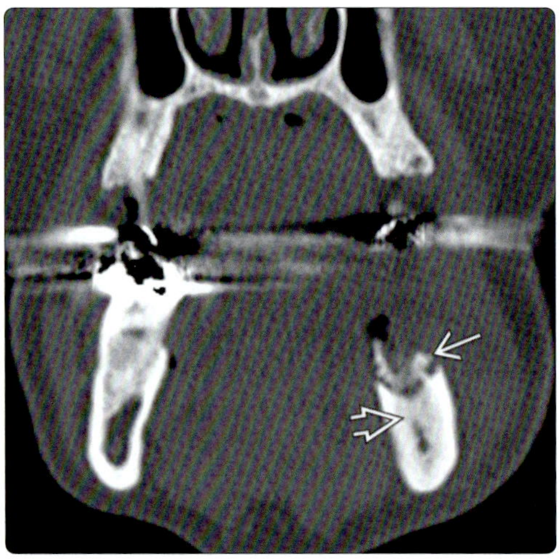

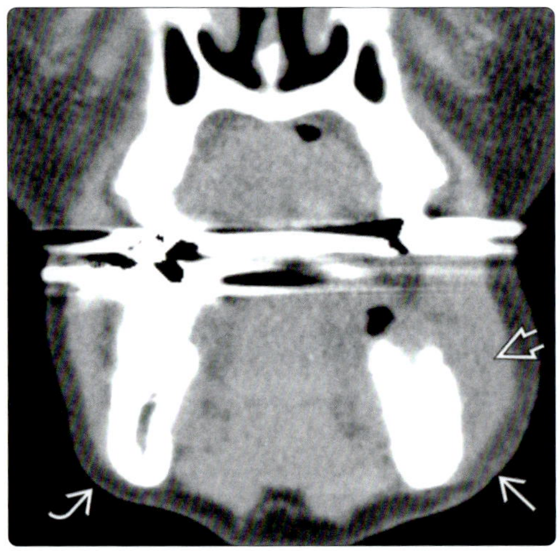

(Left) *Occlusal image of the edentulous anterior maxilla in a female patient taking oral bisphosphonates for 10 years presenting with postextraction pain and swelling with probable bone is shown. Radiologic exam shows sequestration of anterior maxilla with surrounding sclerosis.* **(Right)** *Axial CBCT in the same patient further details the lytic and sclerotic bone patterns in the site of the previously extracted maxillary incisors consistent with osteonecrosis. The sequestered alveolar ridge is more clearly visible.*

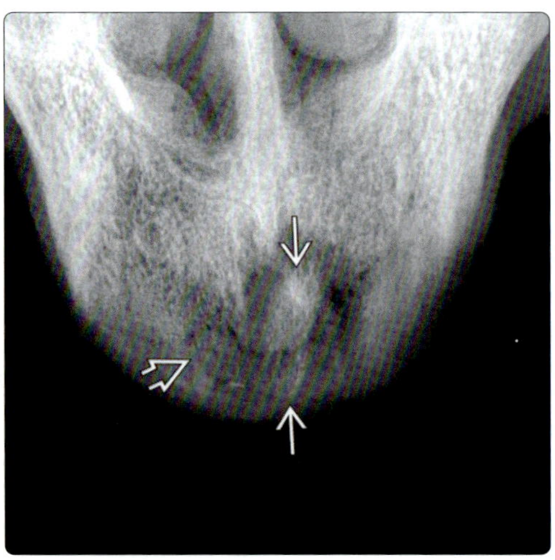

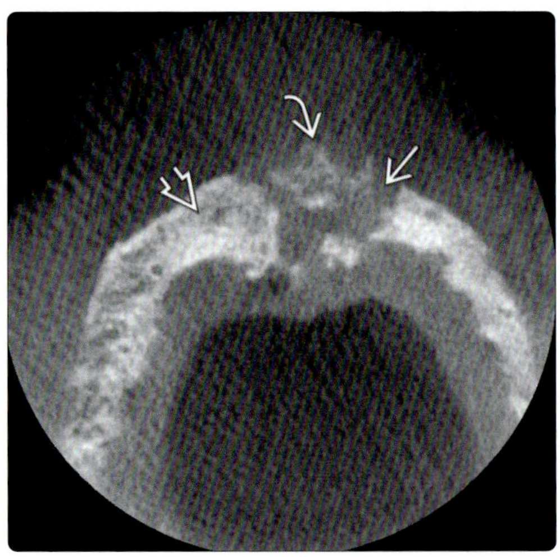

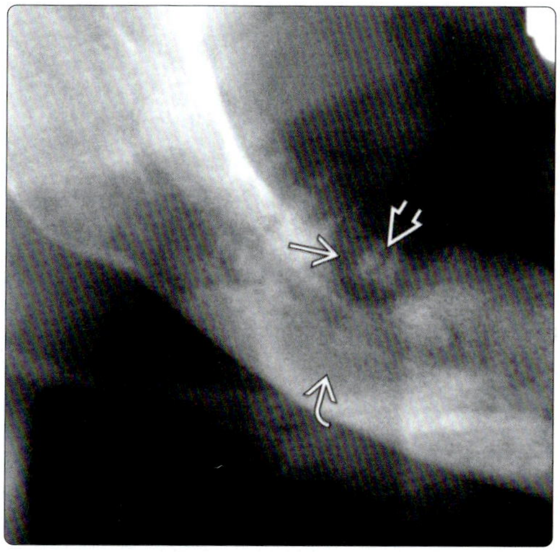
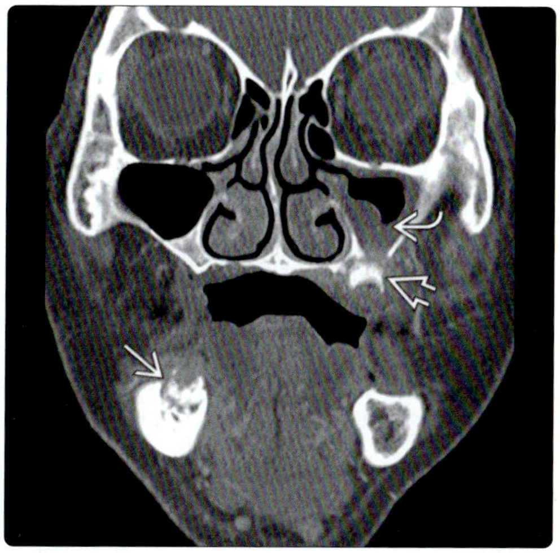

(Left) *Cropped panoramic radiograph of a patient taking oral bisphosphonates, with pain several years after dental extractions, shows incomplete healing of an extraction socket appearing as a radiolucent bone defect ➔. There is a central sequestrum ➔ and peripheral sclerosis ➔.* **(Right)** *Coronal bone-window CECT in the same patient shows the sequestrum ➔ and sclerosis of the mandible. There is also osteonecrosis of the maxilla. The left maxillary alveolar process has sequestered ➔. Secondary sinusitis is also evident ➔.*

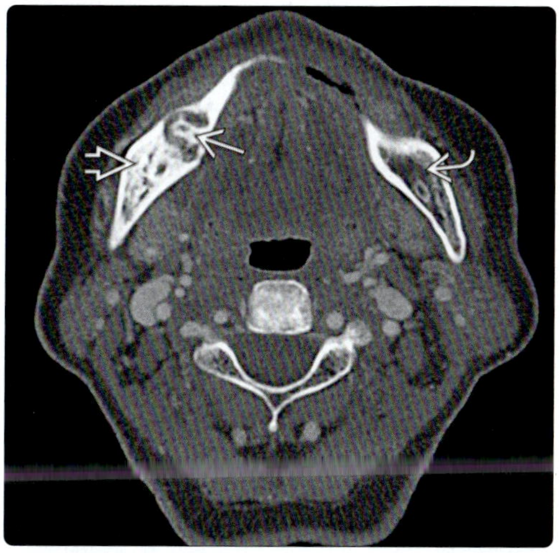
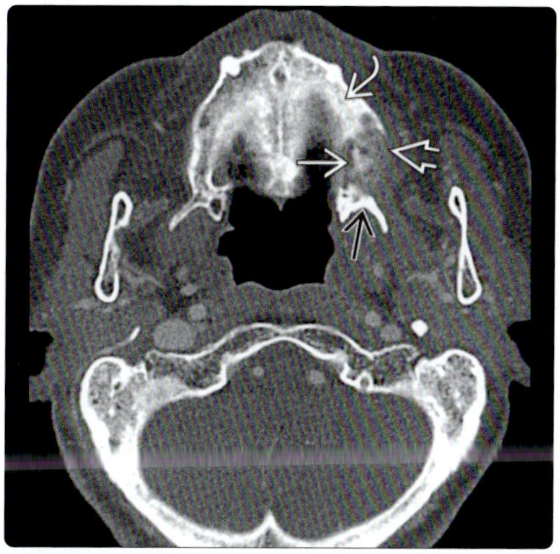

(Left) *Axial bone-window CECT of the same patient shows changes of osteonecrosis in the right mandible. The low-density area of bone loss has a central sequestrum ➔. There is dense sclerosis of the surrounding bone ➔ compared to the normal left side ➔.* **(Right)** *Axial bone-window CECT of the same patient shows bone destruction and central sequestra due to osteonecrosis in the maxilla ➔. The cortical bone is lost ➔, sclerosis is seen in the alveolar process ➔ and in the pterygoid plates ➔.*

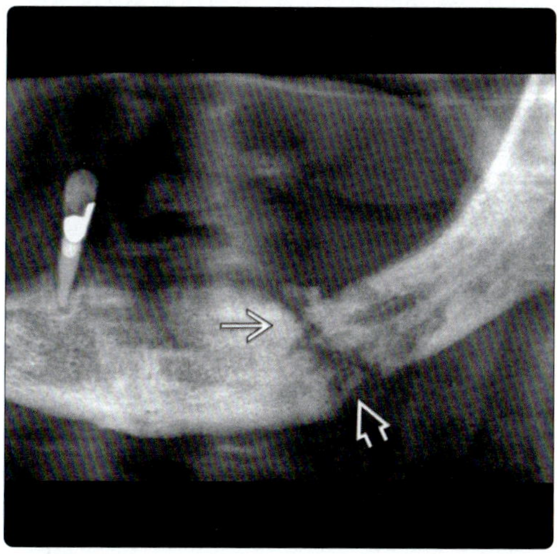
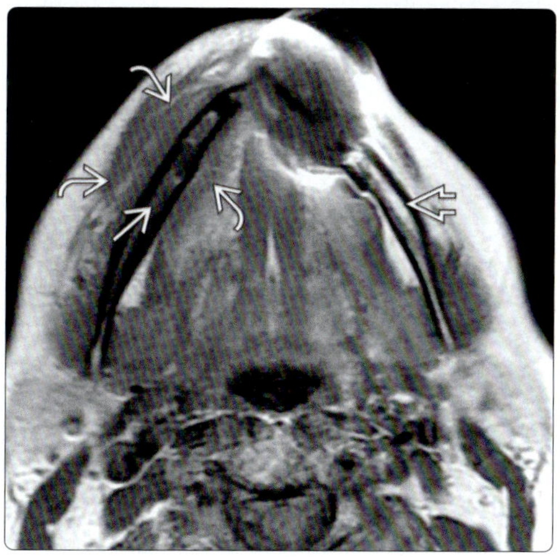

(Left) *Cropped panoramic radiograph shows an elderly female patient treated with bisphosphonates for osteoporosis. Osteonecrosis is seen as ragged bone lysis with surrounding sclerosis ➔. A pathologic fracture and sequestra are also seen ➔. (Courtesy L. Flygare, Odont Dr.)* **(Right)** *Axial T1WI MR in a patient on bisphosphonates for metastatic breast cancer shows replacement of normally hyperintense mandibular marrow ➔ with low signal ➔. Adjacent soft tissue inflammation ➔ is noted.*

Dentigerous Cyst

KEY FACTS

TERMINOLOGY

- Definition: Benign developmental jaw cyst associated with crown of unerupted/impacted tooth
- Synonym: Follicular cyst

IMAGING

- Well-circumscribed, usually corticated, expansile, unilocular, radiolucency surrounding **crown of unerupted or impacted tooth (pericoronal)**
- 75% found in mandible
- Mandibular 3rd molars > maxillary 3rd molars > maxillary canines; supernumerary teeth = 5%
- Size greater than normal follicular space (3 mm)
- May see significant displacement of associated tooth
- Tendency to resorb roots of adjacent teeth

TOP DIFFERENTIAL DIAGNOSES

- Unicystic (mural) ameloblastoma
- Keratocystic odontogenic tumor
- Ameloblastic fibroma
- Immature odontoma

PATHOLOGY

- Multiple cysts found in Maroteaux-Lamy syndrome (mucopolysaccharidosis type VI)

CLINICAL ISSUES

- Delayed eruption of affected tooth
- Mural ameloblastomas, squamous cell carcinoma, & mucoepidermoid carcinoma may develop in lining
- **Biopsy critical** to rule out other pathology

DIAGNOSTIC CHECKLIST

- Consider: Early **pericoronal lesions containing opacities** (e.g., odontoma), which may appear completely radiolucent
- Imaging pearls: Follicular space > 3 mm gives high index of suspicion for development of pathology
  - Loss of corticated border suggests infection or different lesion

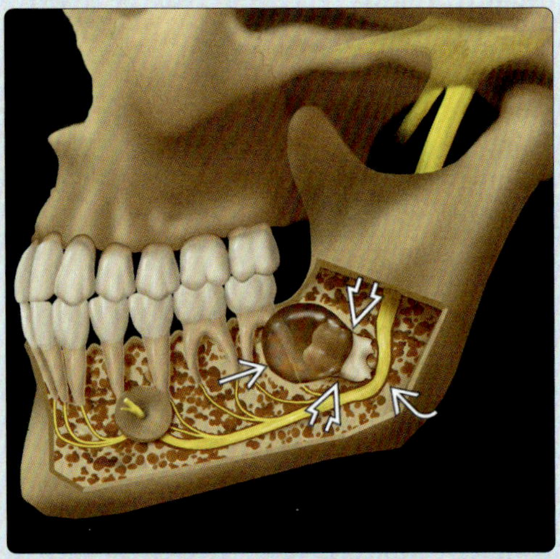

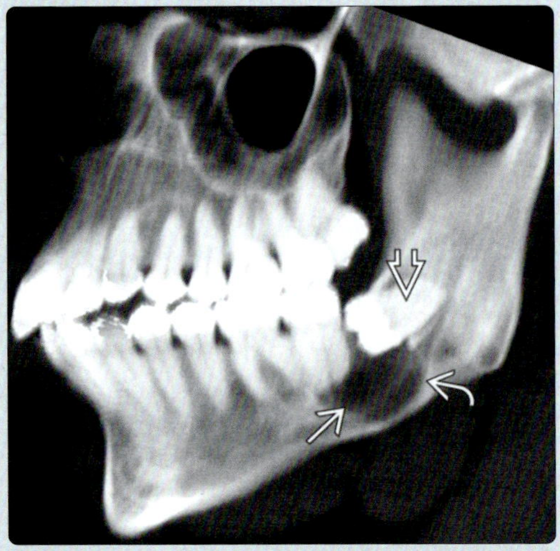

(Left) *Lateral graphic of mandible depicts a unilocular dentigerous cyst ➡ around the crown (pericoronal) of the developing left mandibular 3rd molar. Note attachment at the CEJ ➡ & inferior displacement of the tooth & mandibular canal ➡.* **(Right)** *Ray-sum CT rendering shows the classic appearance of a dentigerous cyst as a well-defined unilocular radiolucency ➡ pericoronal to the impacted mandibular left 3rd molar ➡ in a 38-year-old woman. The mandibular canal ➡ is displaced inferiorly. (Courtesy J. Curé, MD.)*

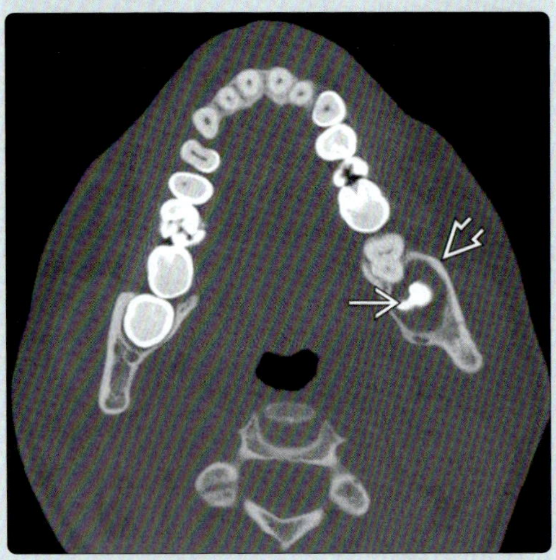

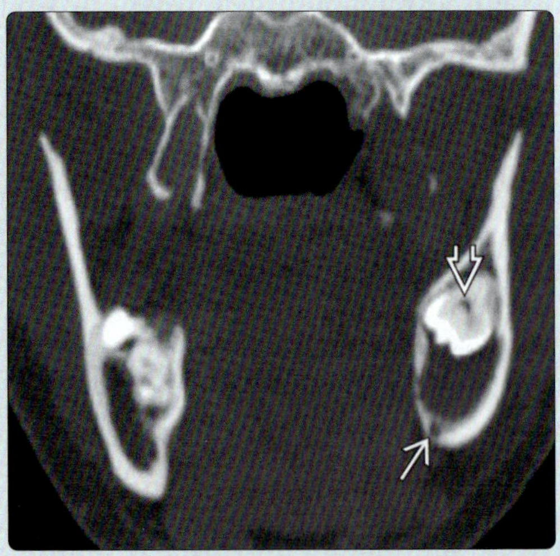

(Left) *Axial bone CT in the same patient shows the impacted mandibular 3rd molar crown ➡ in the center of the dentigerous cyst. The buccal cortex is expanded ➡. (Courtesy J. Curé, MD.)* **(Right)** *Coronal bone CT in the same patient shows that the dentigerous cyst surrounds the crown of the associated tooth ➡. There are no abnormal calcifications or periosteal reactions & no associated soft tissue mass. The mandibular canal is displaced inferiorly ➡. (Courtesy J. Curé, MD.)*

TERMINOLOGY

Synonyms

- Follicular cyst

Definitions

- Benign developmental jaw cyst associated with crown of unerupted/impacted tooth

IMAGING

General Features

- Best diagnostic clue
  - Well-circumscribed, usually corticated, expansile, unilocular radiolucency surrounding **crown of unerupted or impacted tooth (pericoronal)**
- Location
  - **75% found in mandible**
  - Mandibular 3rd molars > maxillary 3rd molars > maxillary canines; supernumerary teeth = 5%
    - Rarely bilateral/multiple & nonsyndromic
- Size
  - > normal follicular space (3 mm), may be very large
- Morphology
  - Unilocular exhibiting hydraulic expansion

Radiographic Findings

- Intraoral & panoramic images
  - Well-defined, unilocular, pericoronal radiolucency
  - May see significant displacement of associated tooth
  - Tendency to resorb roots of adjacent teeth

CT Findings

- CBCT or bone CT
  - Lumen completely radiolucent (no radiopacities)
  - Shows buccal-lingual expansion & association with vital structures: Maxillary sinus & mandibular canal

MR Findings

- T1WI
  - Low to intermediate signal intensity cyst
  - Associated tooth appears as focal absent signal
- T2WI
  - Hyperintense signal of cyst

DIFFERENTIAL DIAGNOSIS

Unicystic (Mural) Ameloblastoma

- Arises in wall of existing cyst: Enhancing nodule
- May be unilocular or multilocular expansile mass
- May see aggressive root resorption

Odontogenic Keratocyst

- Uni- or multilocular: **Not always pericoronal**
- Less expansion & less likely to resorb teeth

Ameloblastic Fibroma

- Unilocular or multilocular
- Mean age: ~ 15 years

Immature Odontoma

- Radiopacities may not be radiographically evident in early lesions

PATHOLOGY

General Features

- Etiology
  - Fluid accumulates between reduced enamel epithelium & surface of crown → pericoronal cyst
- Associated abnormalities
  - Multiple dentigerous cysts found in Maroteaux-Lamy syndrome (mucopolysaccharidosis type VI)
  - May arise in conjunction with odontoma & rarely odontogenic keratocyst & calcifying odontogenic cyst

Microscopic Features

- Nonkeratinized, stratified squamous epithelium
  - Attaches to cementoenamel junction
  - May contain acute or chronic inflammatory cells

CLINICAL ISSUES

Presentation

- Most common signs/symptoms
  - Delayed eruption of affected tooth
- Other signs/symptoms
  - Symptomatic if cyst infection or fracture

Demographics

- Age
  - Most common in 2nd & 3rd decades
- Gender
  - M:F = 3:2
- Epidemiology
  - 2nd most common jaw cyst after radicular cyst
  - Incidence: Whites > blacks or Asians

Natural History & Prognosis

- Epithelium (follicle) has bone-resorbing potential so lesions can become very large; COX-2 expression in epithelium may contribute to proliferation of cells
- Mural ameloblastomas, squamous cell carcinoma, & mucoepidermoid carcinoma may develop in lining
  - Cyst may take on appearance of secondary lesion

Treatment

- Enucleation of cyst & extraction of tooth or marsupialization & orthodontic intervention
- Biopsy critical to rule out other pathology

DIAGNOSTIC CHECKLIST

Consider

- Pericoronal lesions containing opacities (e.g., odontoma), which may appear completely radiolucent initially

Image Interpretation Pearls

- Follicular space > 3 mm gives high index of suspicion for development of pathology
- Loss of corticated border suggests infection or different lesion

SELECTED REFERENCES

1. Alsaegh MA et al: Odontogenic epithelial proliferation is correlated with COX-2 expression in dentigerous cyst and ameloblastoma. Exp Ther Med. 13(1):247-253, 2017

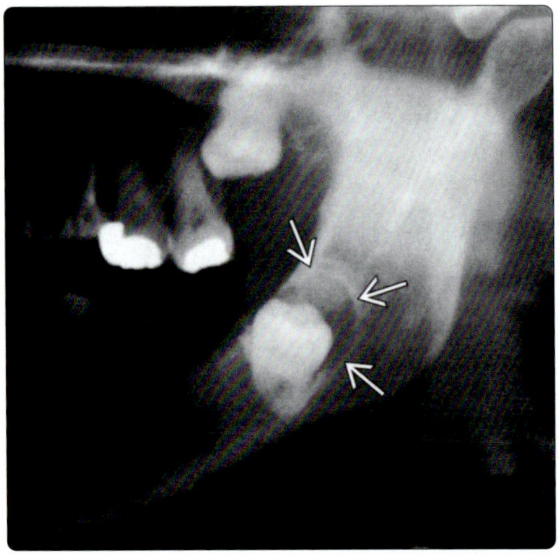

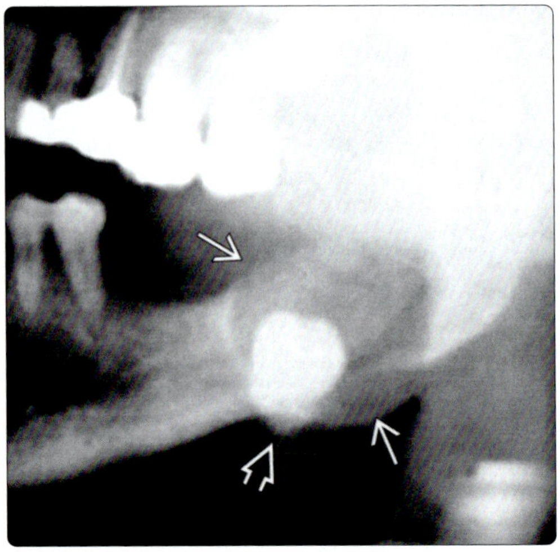

(Left) *Panoramic radiograph shows a well-defined pericoronal radiolucency associated with the crown of the impacted left mandibular 3rd molar. When small, a dentigerous cyst cannot be differentiated from other pericoronal radiolucencies.* **(Right)** *Panoramic radiograph in the same patient 4 years later shows increase in size, a thin corticated margin, & hydraulic expansion characteristic of a dentigerous cyst. Note displacement of the involved 3rd molar roots through the inferior border of the mandible.*

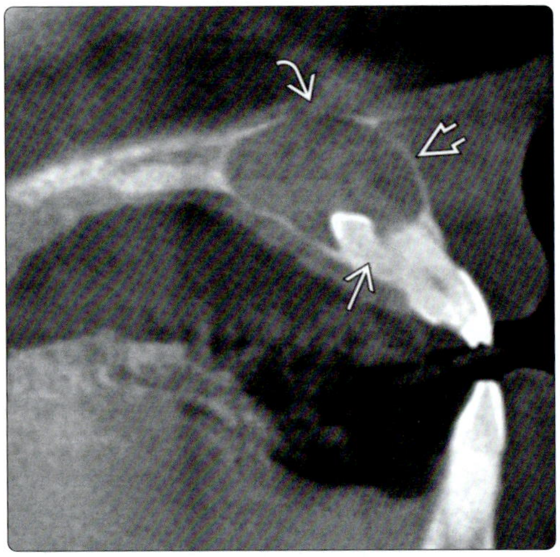

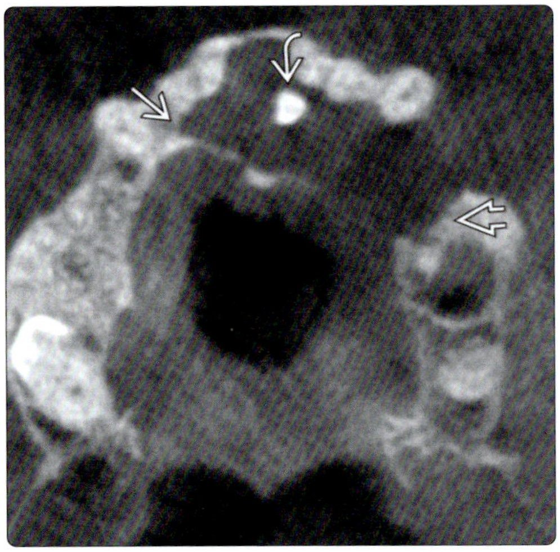

(Left) *Sagittal CBCT shows a large corticated radiolucency around the crown of an inverted mesiodens (supernumerary tooth in anterior maxilla). The lesion has caused slight expansion of the buccal cortex & floor of the nasal cavity. The lesion attaches at the CEJ.* **(Right)** *Axial CBCT in the same patient shows extension of the lesion to the right canine & left maxillary sinus. Note that the lesion is unilocular without calcifications. The tooth is seen as a high density in the center of the lesion.*

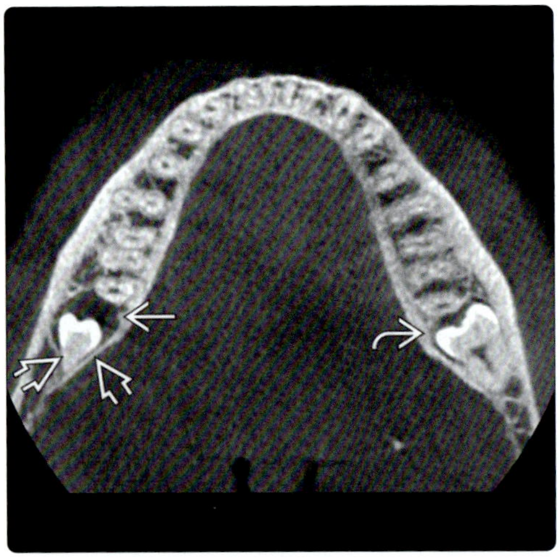

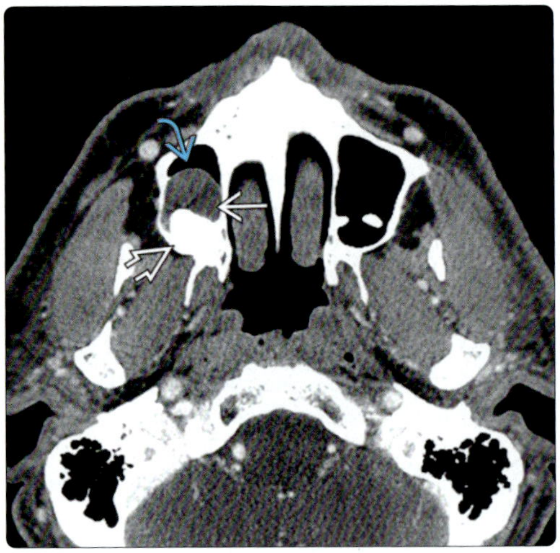

(Left) *Axial CBCT shows impacted mandibular 3rd molars with an enlarged follicular space (> 3 mm) on the right consistent with a dentigerous cyst. Compare to normal left side. The lesion attaches at or near the CEJ.* **(Right)** *Axial CECT, soft tissue window, shows a dentigerous cyst associated with an impacted maxillary right 3rd molar. There is no enhancement within the lesion to suggest a solid neoplasm. Note the corticated border, indicative of a lesion growing into the maxillary sinus. (Courtesy A. Ahuja, MD.)*

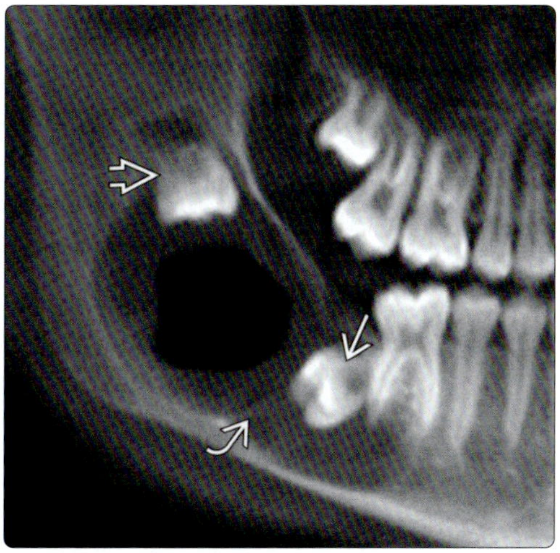
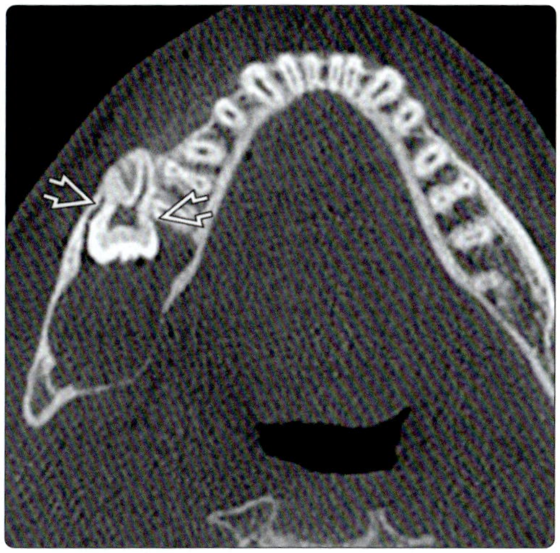

(Left) *Panoramic reformat CBCT shows pericoronal radiolucencies around both the right mandibular 2nd → & 3rd → molars. These proved to be 2 separate lesions: an OKC associated with the 3rd molar & a dentigerous cyst associated with the 2nd molar. Note septum separating the lesions →. (Courtesy M. Noujeim, DDS.)* **(Right)** *Axial CBCT in the same patient shows the 2nd molar displaced buccally with its crown oriented distally. The dentigerous cyst attaches at the CEJ →. (Courtesy M. Noujeim, DDS.)*

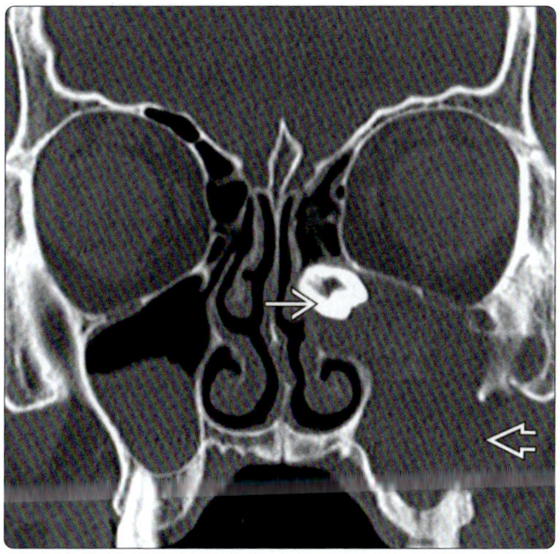
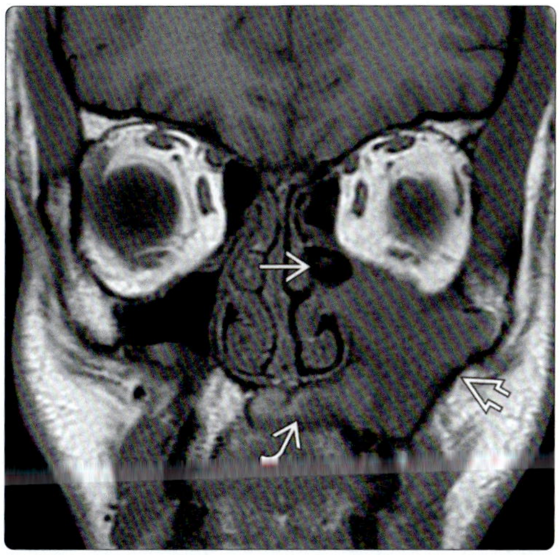

(Left) *Coronal bone CT shows a very large dentigerous cyst associated with the left maxillary 3rd molar →. Significant displacement of the associated tooth is a common feature of dentigerous cysts, particularly in the maxillary sinus. Note loss of lateral wall of sinus →. (Courtesy D. Schatzkes, MD.)* **(Right)** *Coronal T1WI MR in the same patient shows the tooth as a signal void →. The lateral wall of the sinus is preserved →, but the lesion can be seen extending along the palate → in this slice. (Courtesy D. Schatzkes, MD.)*

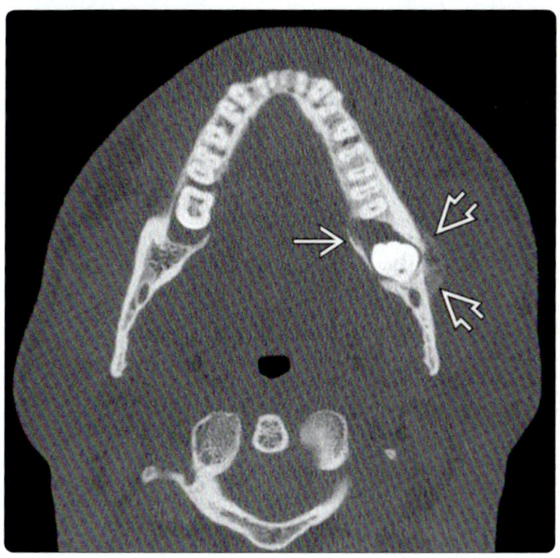
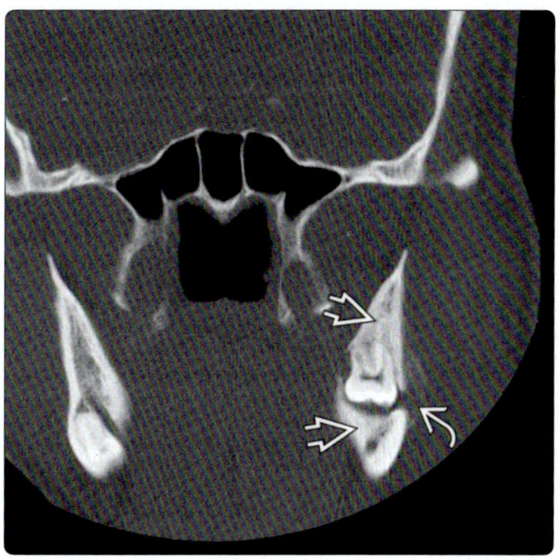

(Left) *Axial bone CT shows a secondarily infected dentigerous cyst associated with the mandibular left 3rd molar. Note buccal → & lingual → periosteal reactions. (Courtesy J. Curé, MD.)* **(Right)** *Coronal bone CT in the same patient shows the discontinuity in the buccal cortex → representing a sinus tract & the buccal periosteal reaction. Note loss of the corticated cyst border suggesting infection or a different lesion. Sclerosis of surrounding bone → indicates an inflammatory response. (Courtesy J. Curé, MD.)*

Odontogenic Keratocyst

KEY FACTS

TERMINOLOGY
- Odontogenic cyst with aggressive behavior & high recurrence rate
  - Previously known as keratocystic odontogenic tumor

IMAGING
- Posterior mandible, 3rd molar region
  - Pericoronal position common
- Corticated periphery
- Well-defined **cystic or scalloping shape**
  - Scalloping of cortices and between teeth
- Large lesions **may appear multilocular**
- Expansion in maxilla and upper ramus
  - More growth along length of bone in body of mandible
- Tooth displacement and root resorption
- CECT: No solid enhancement
- C+ MR: Cystic, thin enhancing rim

TOP DIFFERENTIAL DIAGNOSES
- Dentigerous cyst
- Ameloblastoma
- Radicular cyst
- Simple bone cyst

PATHOLOGY
- Thin-walled, friable cyst containing fluid & debris
- Viscosity of contents depends on keratin debris
  - Straw-colored fluid → pus-like → "cheesy" mass
- Inflammation may destroy histologic characteristics

CLINICAL ISSUES
- Often incidental or may present with jaw swelling
- **High recurrence rate**
  - Long-term follow-up essential

DIAGNOSTIC CHECKLIST
- If multiple, consider **basal cell nevus syndrome**

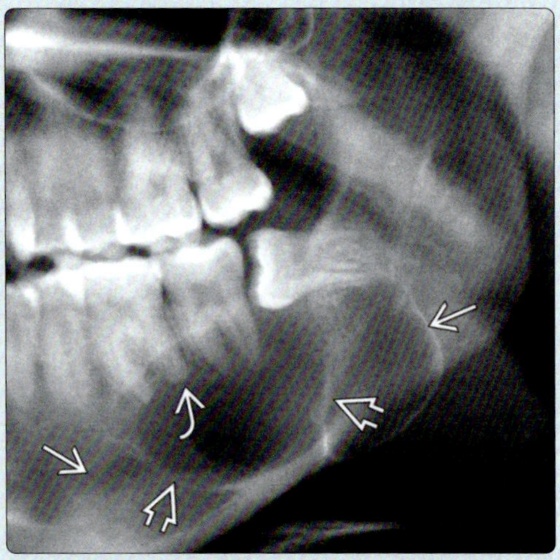
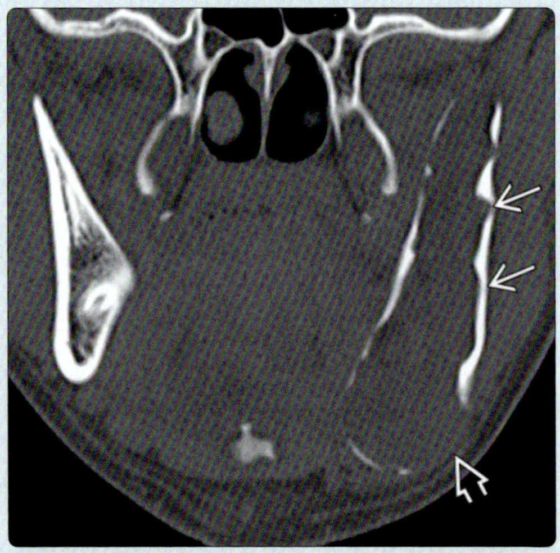

(Left) *Cropped panoramic radiograph shows a well-defined, radiolucent, corticated odontogenic keratocyst (OKC) in the posterior left mandible ➡. Internal septa ➡ create a multilocular appearance. Note mild root resorption ➡ of 1st molar.* **(Right)** *Coronal bone CT shows a large OKC occupying the posterior mandible and ramus of a young female patient. Although there is expansion of the bony cortices, there is greater growth along the bone than mediolaterally. Scalloping ➡ and perforation ➡ of cortices are also seen.*

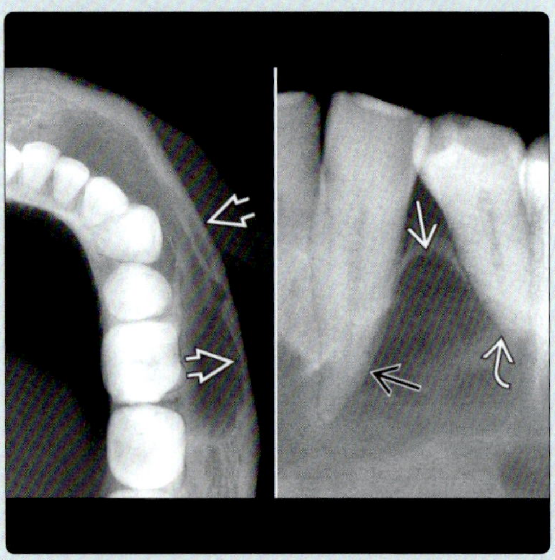
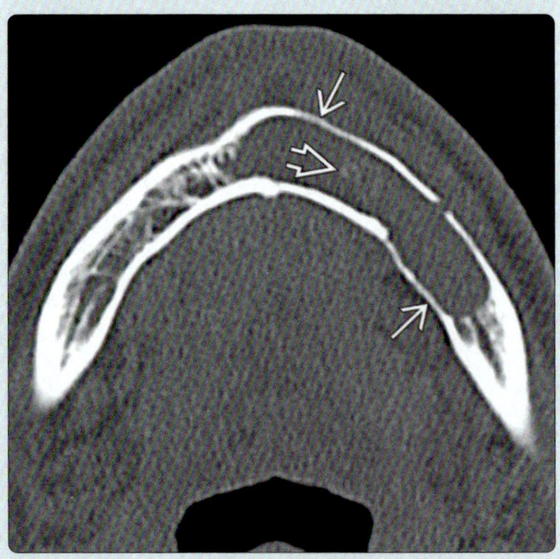

(Left) *Occlusal and periapical radiographs show an OKC scalloping between the teeth ➡ and scooping into the buccal cortex of the mandible ➡. These features are also characteristic of a simple bone cyst; however, displacement of the teeth ➡ and resorption of the lamina dura ⇨ are suggestive of a more aggressive lesion.* **(Right)** *Axial bone CT of the same patient shows the lesion extending along the mandible without causing much expansion ➡. This is characteristic of an OKC. High-attenuation areas are also seen internally ➡.*

TERMINOLOGY

Abbreviations

- Odontogenic keratocyst (OKC)

Synonyms

- Previously know as keratocystic odontogenic tumor

Definitions

- Odontogenic cyst with locally aggressive behavior & high recurrence rate

IMAGING

General Features

- Best diagnostic clue
  - Well-defined, cystic lesion causing minimal expansion relative to its size in posterior mandible
- Location
  - **Mandible:maxilla = 2:1**
    - More common in posterior of both jaws
      - Especially **3rd molar region**
      - Extension into ramus
  - In tooth-bearing regions
    - Epicenter above inferior alveolar nerve canal in mandible
  - Commonly in **pericoronal relationship** to unerupted tooth
- Size
  - From small, unilocular lesion to large, loculated lesion occupying length of mandible and ramus
- Morphology
  - Unilocular lesion most common
  - Multilocular presentation also seen, especially in large lesions
    - Loculations (when present) usually large and few
    - Multilocular appearance often attributable to border scalloping

Radiographic Findings

- Radiography
  - Shape
    - Hydraulic or scalloping
  - Periphery
    - Well-defined, corticated
  - Internally
    - Completely radiolucent
    - Few septa may give multilocular appearance
  - Effects on structures
    - Occasional tooth displacement and root resorption
    - Apical displacement of tooth when in pericoronal position
    - Extension into and filling of maxillary sinus
    - Inferior displacement of mandibular nerve canal

CT Findings

- Bone CT/CBCT
  - Hydraulic expansion in maxilla and upper ramus
    - Less expansion seen in body of mandible
      - Lesion grows along bone
  - **Scalloping of endosteal surface** of cortices
    - Mimics simple bone cyst in this regard
    - Look for additional aggressive signs with OKC
  - Perforation of cortices also seen
    - Possible indication of soft tissue involvement
- Soft tissue algorithm CT
  - High-attenuation areas internally
- CECT
  - No internal enhancement

MR Findings

- T1WI
  - Intermediate signal intensity
    - Due to internal keratinaceous debris
- T2WI
  - Heterogeneous, low to high signal intensity
- DWI
  - Low apparent diffusion coefficient values in cystic space
    - Indicates increased viscosity in lumen
- T1WI C+
  - Thin or no enhancing rim
  - No solid mass

Imaging Recommendations

- Best imaging tool
  - Bone algorithm best delineates periphery
  - CECT determines no solid enhancement
  - MR can help differentiate from other lesions
- Protocol advice
  - Thin-section CT/CBCT with multiplanar reformats

DIFFERENTIAL DIAGNOSIS

Dentigerous Cyst

- **Always around crown of unerupted tooth**
- Pericoronal OKC may mimic dentigerous cyst
- Septa or minimal expansion suggests OKC
- MR: More homogeneous high T2 signal

Ameloblastoma

- Multilocular lesion with more numerous, thicker septa
  - Unicystic ameloblastoma more likely to mimic OKC
- Greater expansion
- More likely to resorb and displace teeth
- MR: Thicker enhancement of walls, solid mass enhancement
- Higher apparent diffusion coefficient values in cystic areas than OKC

Radicular Cyst

- Unilocular cyst
- Epicenter at apex of tooth
- Associated with **nonvital tooth**
  - See carious lesion, large restoration, endodontic treatment
  - Loss of lamina dura at apex of involved tooth

Simple Bone Cyst

- Also has minimal expansion and **scalloping periphery**
  - Both can scallop between roots of teeth
- Periphery is less well corticated
- Does not displace or resorb teeth
  - Lamina dura intact
- Mandibular canal not displaced

PATHOLOGY

General Features

- Etiology
  - Arises from remnants of **dental lamina**
  - Although aberrant cell proliferation suggestive of neoplasm, clinically behaves and treated as cyst
    - Therefore, classified as odontogenic cyst
- Genetics
  - Normal function of *PTCH* tumor suppressor gene lost on chromosome 9q22.3
- Associated abnormalities
  - Multiple OKCs in **basal cell nevus syndrome**
    - ~ 5% of patients with OKCs
    - Other features
      - Multiple basal cell carcinomas
      - Congenital skeletal anomalies
      - Calcification of falx cerebri
      - Palmar and plantar pitting
  - 5% of OKCs multiple and not associated with syndrome

Staging, Grading, & Classification

- OKC considered different entity from orthokeratinized odontogenic cyst

Gross Pathologic & Surgical Features

- Thin, friable cyst containing fluid & keratin debris
  - Internal material on aspiration or enucleation
    - Straw-colored fluid → pus-like → **"cheesy" mass**

Microscopic Features

- Thin, stratified squamous epithelium, 6-8 cells thick
- Corrugated, parakeratinized surface
- Prominent, palisaded basal cell layer
- Flat epithelial-connective tissue wall interface
  - Detachment of epithelium common
- Budding of basal layer and **daughter cysts in wall**
- Inflammation may destroy characteristic architecture and make histologic diagnosis impossible

CLINICAL ISSUES

Presentation

- Most common signs/symptoms
  - Most asymptomatic or with jaw enlargement
- Other signs/symptoms
  - Pain, swelling, or drainage
    - More likely if secondarily infected
    - Radiologic signs of infection
      - Thick, sclerotic periphery around lesion
      - Laminated periosteal new bone formation

Demographics

- Age
  - Wide range
    - Peaks in 2nd to 3rd decade
- Gender
  - M > F
- Epidemiology
  - 5-10% of jaw cysts

Natural History & Prognosis

- **High recurrence rate**
  - Average reported: 30% (up to 60%)
  - Most recur within 5 years but can be later
  - **Long-term follow-up required**
- Recurrence due to
  - Friable epithelial lining left behind
  - Formation of daughter cysts
- Recurrence more likely around teeth
  - Extraction of involved teeth often necessary

Treatment

- Enucleation with peripheral ostectomy or Carnoy solution (chemical fixative) provides more favorable outcome
- En bloc resection
  - More aggressive loss of tissue
    - Disadvantage in young patients
    - Difficult to reconstruct
- Marsupialization (decompression) with subsequent enucleation
  - Surgical exposure of lesion and insertion of drain
  - Requires patient compliance, daily irrigation
  - Imaging after marsupialization important to ensure success of treatment
    - Bone CT/CBCT best
    - See bone fill from periphery of lesion toward center
- **Long-term follow-up for recurrence essential**

DIAGNOSTIC CHECKLIST

Consider

- If multiple OKCs, consider basal cell nevus syndrome
  - Look for dural calcifications (e.g., falx cerebri) on same CT scan

Image Interpretation Pearls

- Well-defined, corticated lesion with few septa and growth along bone (rather than expansion) suggestive of OKC

Reporting Tips

- Identify involved teeth
- Identify cortical perforations
- Describe relationship to mandibular nerve canal

SELECTED REFERENCES

1. Abdi I et al: The effect of ameloblastoma and keratocystic odontogenic tumor on the displacement pattern of inferior alveolar canal in CBCT examinations. J Dent Res Dent Clin Dent Prospects. 10(3):155-61, 2016
2. Gotmare SS et al: Keratocystic odontogenic tumor with ossification and calcification: a case report with unusual histological findings. Indian J Dent Res. 27(4):441-444, 2016
3. Gupta RK et al: A rare simultaneous occurrence of odontogenic keratocyst and unicystic ameloblastoma in mandible: a case report. J Clin Diagn Res. 10(8):ZD01-4, 2016
4. Kaushik R et al: Giant keratocystic odontogenic tumor: a challenging diagnosis. Autops Case Rep. 6(3):41-46, 2016
5. Kakimoto N et al: Contrast-enhanced multidetector computerized tomography for odontogenic cysts and cystic-appearing tumors of the jaws: is it useful? Oral Surg Oral Med Oral Pathol Oral Radiol. 115(1):104-13, 2013

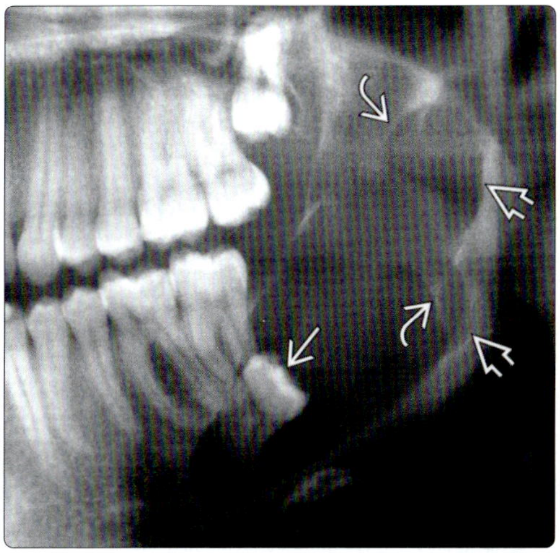

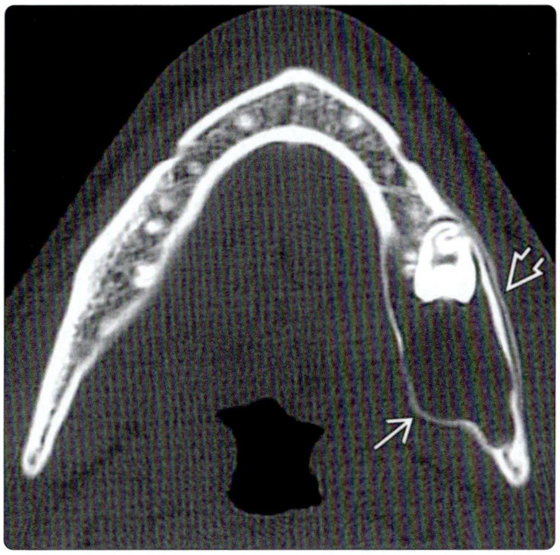

(Left) *Cropped panoramic radiograph shows a large OKC in a pericoronal relationship to the displaced impacted mandibular 3rd molar → and occupying the entire ramus. The periphery is scalloping →, and several small septa are apparent internally →.* **(Right)** *Axial bone CT of the same patient shows a low-attenuation internal structure and expansion of the lingual cortex of the mandible →. There is a periosteal bone reaction parallel to the buccal cortex, indicating secondary infection →.*

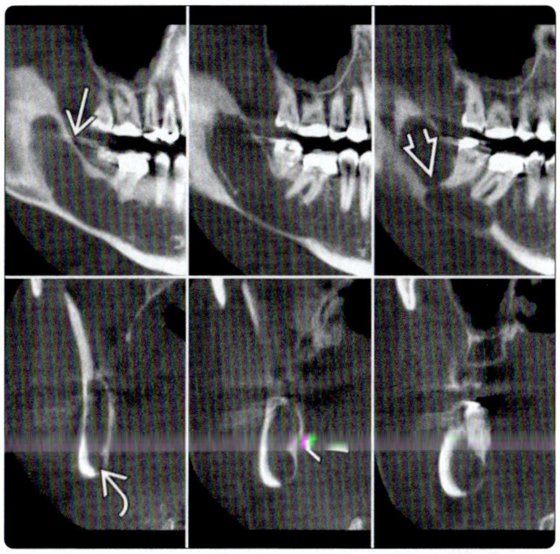

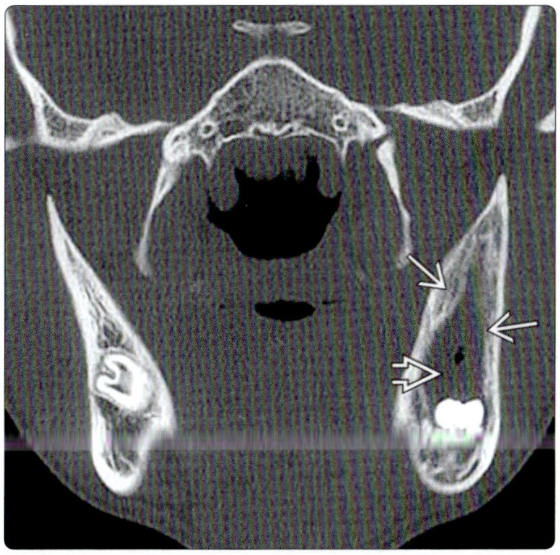

(Left) *Sagittal oblique and cross-sectional CBCT reconstructions of an OKC demonstrate a well-defined, low-attenuation cystic lesion with a scalloping periphery → and a single internal septum →. There is minimal expansion but the mandibular canal is displaced inferiorly →.* **(Right)** *Coronal bone CT shows an OKC that has been marsupialized. There is new bone filling in from the peripheral cortices → where the lesion used to extend to, leaving the existing defect much smaller →.*

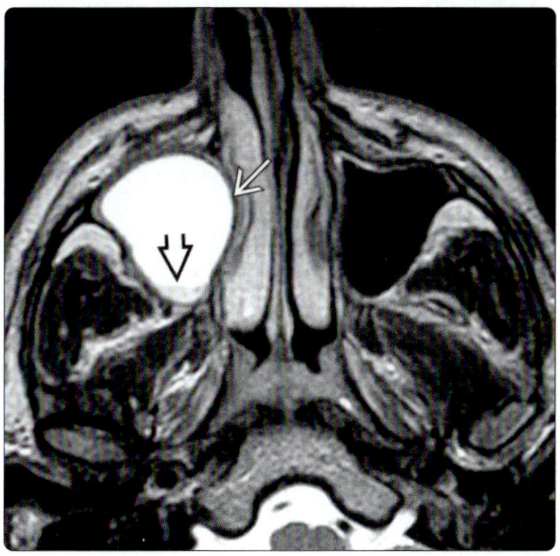

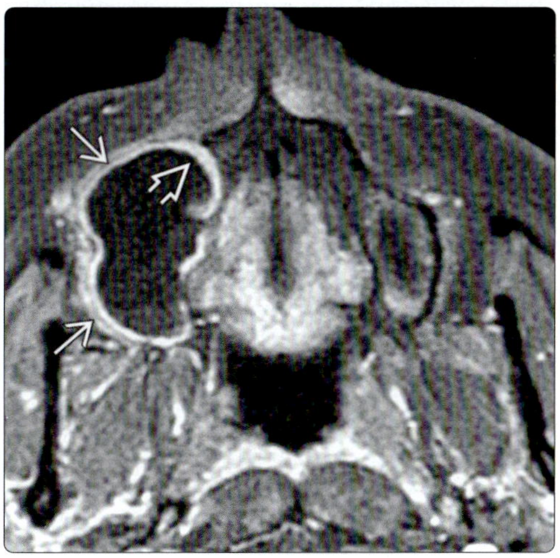

(Left) *Axial T2WI FSE MR shows an OKC filling the right maxillary sinus with displacement of the medial wall →. The lesion has a high signal with a small area of intermediate signal due to internal debris →. The T2 signal of OKC varies depending on the amount of debris within.* **(Right)** *Axial T1WI C+ FS MR of the same patient shows undulating expansion of the alveolar process of the maxilla →. There is low internal signal with a thin, enhancing peripheral rim →. No solid enhancing mass is present.*

Lateral Periodontal Cyst

KEY FACTS

TERMINOLOGY

- Synonyms: **Botryoid odontogenic cyst** is multilocular variant
- Definition: Noninflammatory, developmental odontogenic cyst lateral to erupted **vital tooth**

IMAGING

- Well-defined, **round or teardrop interradicular radiolucency**
- **Mandible** > maxilla; **anterior to molars**
  - Usually < 10 mm
- **Botryoid odontogenic cyst** is **multilocular**

TOP DIFFERENTIAL DIAGNOSES

- Osteoporotic bone marrow defect
- Simple (traumatic) bone cyst
- Odontogenic keratocyst
- Lateral radicular cyst (lateral periapical cyst)
- Ameloblastoma

PATHOLOGY

- Arises from **rests of dental lamina** located buccally
  - Thin, nonkeratinized, cuboidal to stratified squamous epithelium containing **clear cells**

CLINICAL ISSUES

- Usually asymptomatic
- Associated teeth are **vital**
- Wide age range reported (14-85 years)
  - Peak in 6th decade
- M ≥ F
- Insidious slow growth
- Treatment is **enucleation**
  - Recurrence is higher with curettage

DIAGNOSTIC CHECKLIST

- If multilocular, consider ameloblastoma, central giant cell granuloma, or other multilocular lesions

(Left) *Periapical radiograph of the right mandible shows a lateral periodontal cyst ➡ located between the 1st and 2nd premolar teeth. This is the most common location for a lateral periodontal cyst. Note the classic teardrop appearance to the lesion. (Courtesy M. Ahmad, DDS.)* **(Right)** *Sagittal 3D CBCT shows a multilocular lesion ➡ between the mandibular left 1st premolar and canine. Biopsy confirmed the lesion to be a botryoid odontogenic cyst (BOC).*

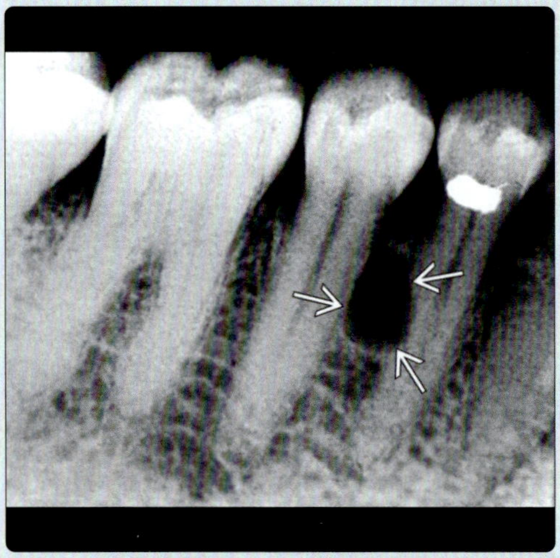

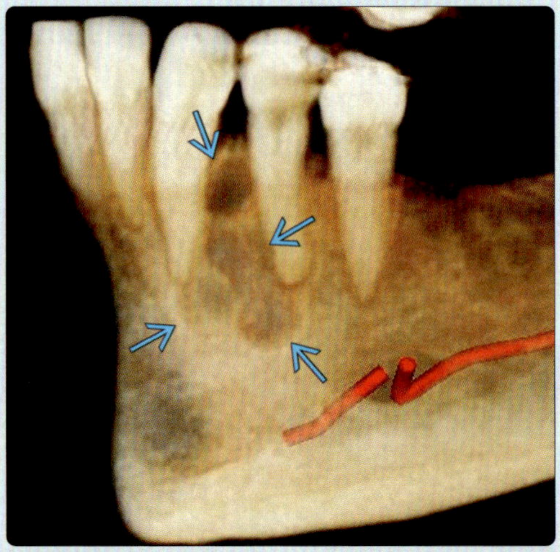

(Left) *Coronal CBCT (left) in the same patient shows small, circular, well-defined, corticated loculations. Cross-section CBCT (right) shows thinning of the buccal cortex ➡ but no expansion, helping to differentiate from ameloblastoma.* **(Right)** *Coronal CBCT (left) in the same patient shows an additional unilocular lesion ➡ in the right anterior mandible. 3D CBCT (right) shows the typical teardrop interradicular appearance ➡ of a lateral periodontal cyst. Lateral periodontal cysts and BOCs can be multifocal.*

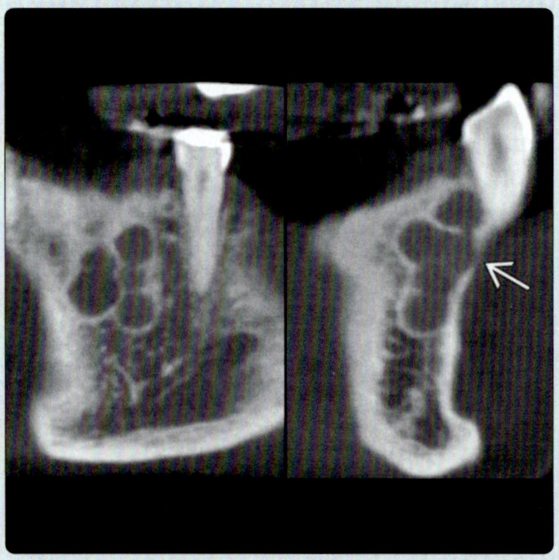

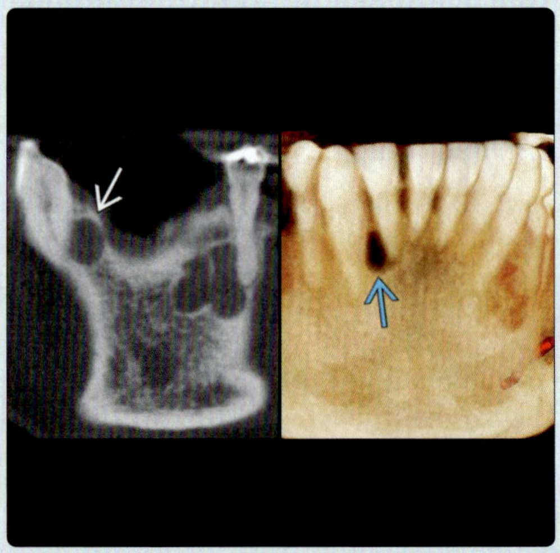

TERMINOLOGY

Abbreviations

- Lateral periodontal cyst (LPC)

Synonyms

- Botryoid odontogenic cyst (BOC) is multilocular variant

Definitions

- Noninflammatory, developmental cyst of odontogenic origin lateral to erupted vital tooth

IMAGING

General Features

- Best diagnostic clue
  - Well-defined, unilocular, **round** or **teardrop interradicular radiolucency**
- Location
  - **Mandible** > maxilla; anterior to molars
  - **Canine/premolar area** lateral to and usually at **midpoint of root** of tooth
- Size
  - Usually < 10 mm
- Morphology
  - **Round or teardrop** shape
  - Botryoid odontogenic cyst is multilocular

Radiographic Findings

- Intraoral plain film
  - Well-defined interradicular radiolucency
  - Usually has **corticated** border

CT Findings

- CBCT
  - Buccal to erupted tooth roots
  - Occasionally buccal expansion; rarely cortical perforation

DIFFERENTIAL DIAGNOSIS

Osteoporotic Bone Marrow Defect

- Large bone marrow space
- Radiographic follow-up shows no change in size or shape

Simple (Traumatic) Bone Cyst

- Primarily young males in bone below apices
- **Endosteal scalloping** common
- **Scallops** upward between roots

Odontogenic Keratocyst

- Benign odontogenic tumor lined with thin para- or orthokeratinized epithelium
- Anteroposterior growth in mandible
- **May be multilocular**

Lateral Radicular Cyst (Lateral Periapical Cyst)

- Inflammatory cyst associated with lateral pulp canal
- Located **closer to apex** rather than midroot
- Teeth are **nonvital**

Ameloblastoma

- Most common benign tumor and multilocular radiolucency
- **Expansion** and root resorption

PATHOLOGY

General Features

- Etiology
  - Arises from **rests of dental lamina**, which are more prolific in buccal alveolar bone compared to rests of Malassez that occur around apices of teeth
  - Multicystic variant (BOC) is thought to be coalescence of several LPCs or cystic transformation of multiple dental lamina rests
  - Development of BOC in epithelial lining of LPC reported

Microscopic Features

- Thin, nonkeratinized, cuboidal to stratified squamous epithelium
- **Clear cells** containing glycogen produce nodules or intraluminal protuberances
- BOC lined with same epithelium containing clear cells; nodules may be more numerous

CLINICAL ISSUES

Presentation

- Most common signs/symptoms
  - Usually asymptomatic
  - Associated teeth are **vital**
- Other signs/symptoms
  - Swelling and drainage

Demographics

- Age
  - Wide range reported (14-85 years)
  - Peak in 6th decade
  - Mean age lower in females
- Gender
  - M ≥ F
- Ethnicity
  - Caucasian > black

Natural History & Prognosis

- Insidious slow growth
- **Recurrence** has been reported and is **higher with multicystic variant**

Treatment

- **Enucleation**
  - Recurrence is higher with curettage

DIAGNOSTIC CHECKLIST

Consider

- If multilocular, consider ameloblastoma, central giant cell granuloma, or other multilocular lesions

SELECTED REFERENCES

1. A A et al: Botryoid odontogenic cyst: a diagnostic chaos. J Clin Diagn Res. 8(12):ZD11-3, 2014
2. Govil S et al: Bilateral lateral periodontal cyst. BMJ Case Rep. 2013
3. Arora P et al: Botryoid odontogenic cyst developing from lateral periodontal cyst: a rare case and review on pathogenesis. Contemp Clin Dent. 3(3):326-9, 2012
4. de Andrade M et al: Lateral periodontal cyst: report of case and review of the literature. Oral Maxillofac Surg. 16(1):83-7, 2012

Residual Cyst

KEY FACTS

TERMINOLOGY

- Definition: Inflammatory odontogenic cyst remaining in bone following extraction of involved nonvital tooth caused by incomplete removal of original radicular cyst

IMAGING

- Unilocular, round, **well-corticated** radiolucency
- **Maxilla** more common than mandible
  - Anterior > posterior
- **Above mandibular canal** in posterior mandible
- **Missing tooth** or teeth

TOP DIFFERENTIAL DIAGNOSES

- Odontogenic keratocyst
- Anterior mandibular salivary gland defect (Stafne)
- Surgical ciliated cyst
- Nasopalatine duct cyst
- Glandular odontogenic cyst

PATHOLOGY

- Lined with simple stratified squamous epithelium

CLINICAL ISSUES

- Asymptomatic: Incidental finding
  - Occasionally pain &/or swelling
  - Symptomatic cysts more common in anterior maxilla and may be less corticated
- Large cysts may cause mandibular fracture
- M > F
- Treatment: Enucleation or marsupialization if large

DIAGNOSTIC CHECKLIST

- Consider
  - Anterior salivary gland defect if in anterior mandible
  - Nasopalatine duct cyst if in anterior maxilla
- Tip: **Tooth** or teeth will be **missing**

(Left) *Panoramic reformat CBCT shows a round, corticated radiolucency ➔ in the left maxilla. This is the typical appearance of a residual cyst. Note expansion into and elevation of the floor ➔ of the left maxillary sinus.* **(Right)** *Axial CBCT in the same patient shows the residual cyst ➔ with a well-defined corticated border ➔ separate from the posterior border of the maxillary sinus ➔. The cortication of the lesion helps differentiate growth from outside the sinus rather than from within.*

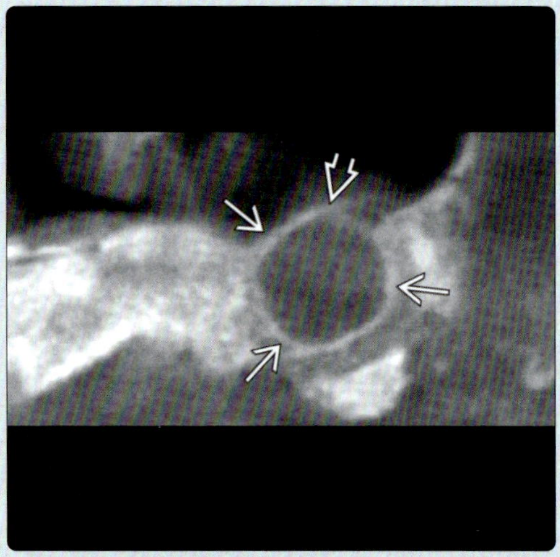

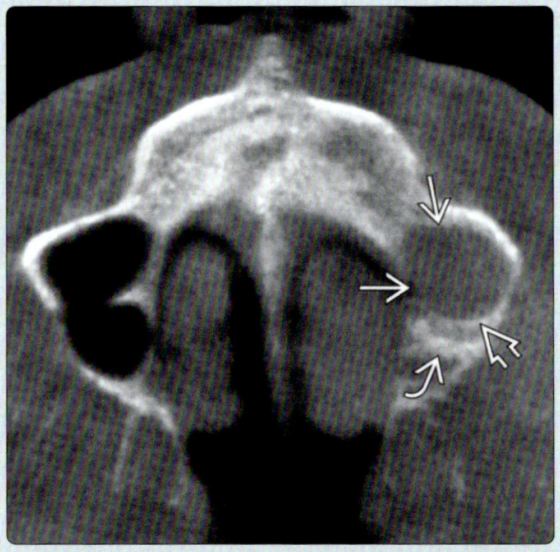

(Left) *Axial CBCT shows a well-defined, round, unilocular radiolucency ➔ in the right maxilla consistent with a residual cyst. The round shape and corticated borders are indicative of typical hydraulic expansion associated with cystic lesions. (Courtesy M. Noujeim, DDS.)* **(Right)** *Axial CBCT shows typical presentation of a residual cyst ➔ in the right posterior maxilla. This was an incidental finding on a scan for implant planning. Residual cysts are more common in the maxilla than mandible.*

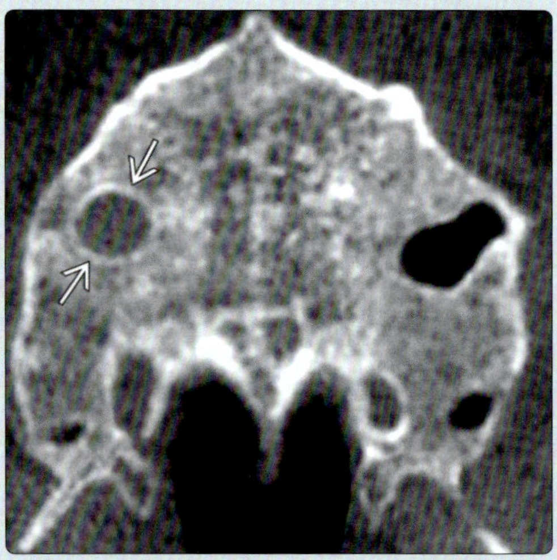

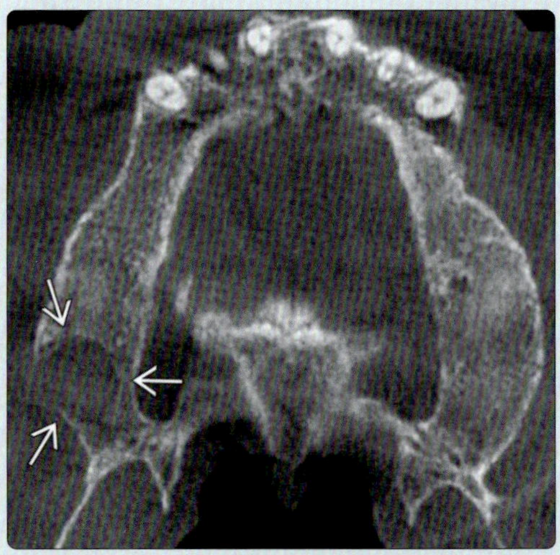

TERMINOLOGY

Definitions

- Inflammatory odontogenic cyst remaining in bone following extraction of involved nonvital tooth caused by incomplete removal of original radicular cyst

IMAGING

General Features

- Best diagnostic clue
  - Unilocular, round, **well-corticated** radiolucency
- Location
  - **Maxilla** more common than mandible
    - Anterior > posterior
  - **Above mandibular canal** in posterior mandible
- Size
  - Varies from very small to very large
    - Symptomatic cysts larger than asymptomatic
- Morphology
  - Round, well-corticated, unilocular lesions
    - Symptomatic lesions may be less corticated

Radiographic Findings

- Intraoral plain film
  - Well-defined, **corticated**, **round radiolucency**
  - **Missing tooth** or teeth
  - May not be able to visualize full extent of lesion

CT Findings

- CBCT
  - Will best demonstrate encroachment on vital structures: Maxillary sinus and mandibular canal

DIFFERENTIAL DIAGNOSIS

Odontogenic Keratocyst

- Benign odontogenic neoplasm lined with thin para- or orthokeratinized epithelium
- Expands in posteroanterior direction in mandible
- Expansion may be more hydraulic and hence **similar to residual cyst in maxilla**
- May be unilocular, multilocular, or pericoronal

Anterior Mandibular Salivary Gland Defect (Stafne)

- Salivary gland depression on lingual aspect of mandible
- Well-defined, unilocular, **round or oval**, **corticated radiolucency**
- Posterior variants are below mandibular canal and can be excluded
- Anterior variants **may mimic residual cyst**

Surgical Ciliated Cyst

- History of surgical procedure; usually Caldwell-Luc
- Develops from trapped respiratory epithelium
- Have also been reported in mandible

Nasopalatine Duct Cyst

- **Midline** anterior maxillary cyst lined with epithelium from nasopalatine duct
- Round or oval, well-defined, **corticated radiolucency**

Glandular Odontogenic Cyst

- Can be uni- or multilocular
- More common in mandible

PATHOLOGY

General Features

- Etiology
  - Incomplete removal of radicular cyst when involved nonvital tooth extracted

Microscopic Features

- Lined with simple stratified squamous epithelium

CLINICAL ISSUES

Presentation

- Most common signs/symptoms
  - Asymptomatic: Incidental finding
- Other signs/symptoms
  - Pain &/or swelling
    - Symptomatic cysts more common in anterior maxilla
    - Symptomatic cysts may be less corticated
  - Large cysts may cause mandibular fracture

Demographics

- Gender
  - M > F

Natural History & Prognosis

- Asymptomatic cysts may slowly decrease in size due to atrophy of epithelium
- Enlargement may be due to persistence of original inflammation or due to trauma of asymptomatic cysts, e.g., pressure from prosthesis
- Primary intraosseous carcinoma and unicystic ameloblastoma arising in residual cyst have been reported

Treatment

- Enucleation
- Marsupialization if large

DIAGNOSTIC CHECKLIST

Consider

- Anterior salivary gland defect if in anterior mandible
- Nasopalatine duct cyst if anterior maxilla

Image Interpretation Pearls

- **Tooth** or teeth will be **missing**

SELECTED REFERENCES

1. Sukegawa S et al: Primary intraosseous squamous cell carcinoma of the maxilla possibly arising from an infected residual cyst: a case report. Oncol Lett. 9(1):131-135, 2015
2. Mahajan AD et al: Unicystic ameloblastoma arising from a residual cyst. BMJ Case Rep. 2014, 2014
3. Sperandio FF et al: Noninvasive treatment choice for an aged down syndrome patient presenting a residual periapical cyst. J Contemp Dent Pract. 15(2):254-7, 2014
4. Sridevi K et al: Residual cyst associated with calcifications in an elderly patient. J Clin Diagn Res. 8(2):246-9, 2014
5. Leung YY et al: Surgical ciliated cysts may mimic radicular cysts or residual cysts of maxilla: report of 3 cases. J Oral Maxillofac Surg. 70(4):e264-9, 2012
6. Galzignato PF et al: Dental implant failure associated with a residual maxillary cyst. Br Dent J. 208(4):153-4, 2010

Buccal Bifurcation Cyst

KEY FACTS

TERMINOLOGY

- Synonyms: Mandibular infected buccal cyst, paradental cyst, inflammatory collateral cyst
- Definition: Cyst in buccal bifurcation area of molar teeth often as consequence of inflammatory process

IMAGING

- Well-defined, often corticated, cystic radiolucency
- Mandibular molars primarily affected
- Maxillary molars rarely affected
- May be **bilateral**
- Tipping of affected tooth and **displacement of apices toward lingual cortex**
  - Occlusal surface tipped buccally
  - Increased **prominence of lingual cusps**
- Best imaging tool: CBCT or CT bone window
  - Expansion of buccal bone and any periosteal reactions well visualized

TOP DIFFERENTIAL DIAGNOSES

- Dentigerous cyst
- Odontogenic keratocyst
- Langerhans cell histiocytosis

CLINICAL ISSUES

- Asymptomatic swelling
- Failure of eruption of affected tooth
- Surgical enucleation
- **Extraction** of tooth **not necessary**

DIAGNOSTIC CHECKLIST

- Consider: Involvement of contralateral or maxillary teeth with unilateral mandibular lesion
- Inflammatory component is nonspecific, so definitive diagnosis is made from radiographic appearance with support of clinical findings
- Displacement of apices of involved tooth toward lingual cortex is diagnostic

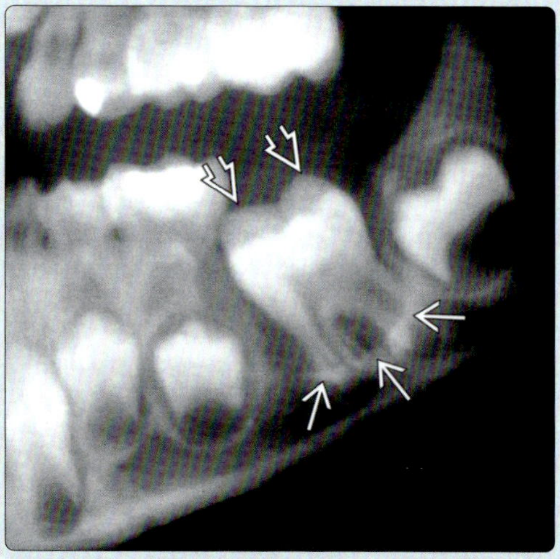

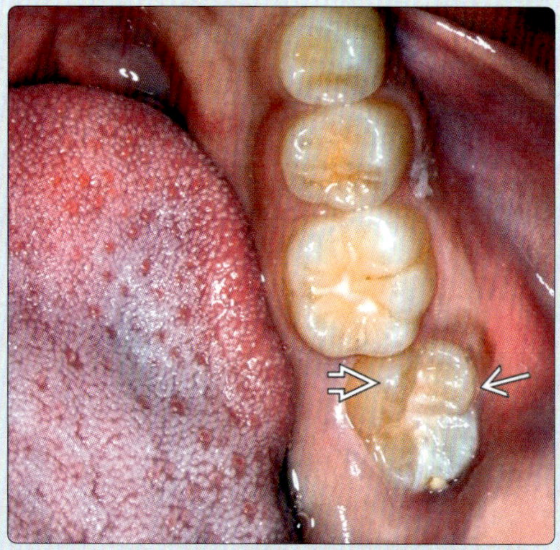

(Left) *Panoramic radiograph shows buccal bifurcation cyst (BBC) associated with the mandibular left 1st permanent molar. The lesion has caused characteristic tipping of the crown and prominence of the lingual cusps* ➡*. Note the more densely corticated border inferiorly* ➡*, suggestive of an inflammatory response. (Courtesy M. Noujeim, DDS.)* **(Right)** *Intraoral photograph shows classic buccal tipping of the crown of a mandibular left 2nd molar* ➡ *by a BBC. Note prominence of the lingual cusps* ➡*.*

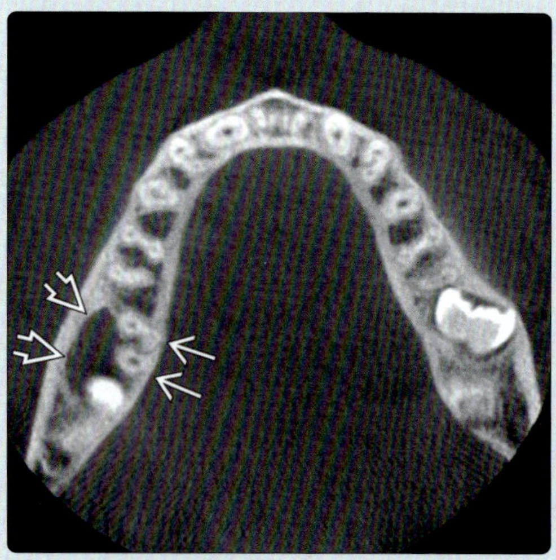

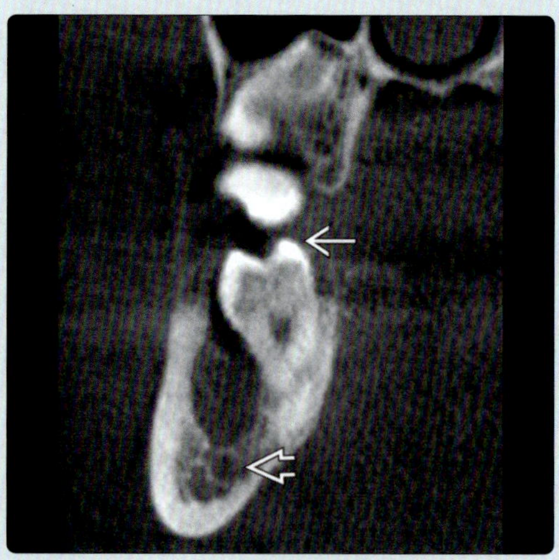

(Left) *Axial CBCT shows well-defined radiolucency* ➡ *centered at the buccal bifurcation of the mandibular right 2nd permanent molar. This was an incidental finding in a 17-year-old boy referred for evaluation of impacted 3rd molars. Note the location of the roots at the lingual cortex* ➡*.* **(Right)** *Cross-section CBCT in the same patient shows tipping of the occlusal table and prominence of the lingual cusps* ➡*. The mandibular canal is located at the inferior border of the lesion* ➡*.*

TERMINOLOGY

Abbreviations

- Buccal bifurcation cyst (BBC)

Synonyms

- Mandibular infected buccal cyst
- Paradental cyst
- Inflammatory paradental cyst
- Inflammatory collateral cyst
- Circumferential dentigerous cyst

Definitions

- Cyst occurring in buccal bifurcation area of molar teeth often as consequence of inflammatory process

IMAGING

General Features

- Best diagnostic clue
  - Well-defined, often corticated, cystic radiolucency with epicenter at buccal bifurcation area of molar teeth
- Location
  - Buccal bifurcation area of permanent molar teeth
    - Can rarely occur in primary teeth
  - Mandibular molars primarily affected
    - 1st molar > 2nd molar > 3rd molar
    - Lesions on 3rd molars may be more distal
  - Maxillary molars rarely affected
  - May be **bilateral**
    - Unilateral lesion should raise suspicion for potential lesion on contralateral side
- Size
  - 0.6-2.5 cm
  - May extend beyond roots
- Morphology
  - Round or oval

Radiographic Findings

- Intraoral plain film
  - Well-defined radiolucency in buccal bifurcation area of affected tooth
  - Superimposed over roots of affected tooth
    - If periphery not well defined, **may be difficult to see small lesions**
  - Lesion causes tipping of tooth by downward extension of cyst
    - Occlusal surface tipped buccally
    - Increased **prominence of lingual cusps**
  - Periodontal ligament space and **lamina dura intact**
  - Teeth of normal structure and caries free
  - Rarely extends to inferior border of mandible
- Extraoral plain film
  - Occlusal views will demonstrate expansion
    - **Periosteal new bone** formation may be seen if lesion secondarily infected
  - Rarely see buccal bone loss
  - Tipping of affected tooth and **displacement of apices toward lingual cortex**

CT Findings

- CBCT
  - Expansion of buccal bone and any periosteal reactions well visualized
  - Apices of teeth displaced to lingual cortex due to tipping of teeth
    - Best visualized on coronal views

MR Findings

- T1WI
  - Low to intermediate signal intensity within cyst
  - Associated tooth may present as focal lack of signal
- T2WI
  - Increased signal intensity within cyst

Imaging Recommendations

- Best imaging tool
  - CBCT or CT
- Protocol advice
  - Bone algorithm thin-section CT of face with axial and coronal sections

DIFFERENTIAL DIAGNOSIS

Dentigerous Cyst

- Accumulation of fluid between reduced enamel epithelium and crown of unerupted tooth
- **Surrounds crown** of tooth (pericoronal)
- Round, well defined
- Expansile

Hyperplastic Dental Follicles

- Enlarged normal follicle
- Surrounds crown of developing tooth
  - Follows general **outline of tooth crown**

Odontogenic Keratocyst

- Benign odontogenic tumor lined with para- or orthokeratinized epithelium
- Can be pericoronal and look like dentigerous cyst in early stages
- May look similar to BBC if located adjacent to roots
- **Little expansion** in mandible

Langerhans Cell Histiocytosis

- Abnormal proliferation of Langerhans cells
- Localized solitary form (eosinophilic granuloma) may present at midroot of teeth
- Usually symptomatic: Pain, soft tissue swelling, bleeding
- Margins may be well defined but **not corticated**
- Bone destruction and **lamina dura not present**

Lateral Radicular Cyst

- Odontogenic inflammatory cyst associated with **nonvital tooth**
- Epicenter located **close to apex**
- Large cysts may extend toward furcation area and be confused with BBC
- Not as expansile as BBC

Lateral Periodontal Cyst

- Odontogenic cyst occurring lateral to tooth roots
- Usually **interradicular** radiolucency
- Mandibular premolar area most common
- Older age group

Squamous Odontogenic Tumor

- Benign epithelial odontogenic tumor
- More common in maxilla lateral-canine area followed by mandibular molar/premolar area
- Triangular or semicircular radiolucency
- Usually **between roots** of teeth (interradicular)

PATHOLOGY

General Features

- Etiology
  - Thought to be inflammatory process occurring in connective tissue as tooth erupts
  - Epithelium may originate from any of following
    - Rests of Malassez
    - Rests of Serres
    - Cells of dental lamina
    - Reduced enamel epithelium remnants
  - Presence of developmental projection of enamel into furcation, as possible etiology has not been corroborated in literature

Microscopic Features

- Lined with nonkeratinized stratified squamous epithelium
  - Edema and neutrophil infiltration common
- Fibrous connective tissue contains extensive acute and chronic inflammatory cell infiltrate
  - Prominent plasma cell component

CLINICAL ISSUES

Presentation

- Most common signs/symptoms
  - Asymptomatic swelling
  - Failure of eruption of affected tooth
- Other signs/symptoms
  - Pain and tenderness if infected
  - Suppuration rare
  - Enlarged palpable lymph nodes
  - Teeth are **always vital**
  - If teeth partially erupted, will see **prominence of lingual cusps**

Demographics

- Age
  - Before or during 3rd decade
  - Mean age in one study: **7.5 years**
    - Related to timing of eruption of mandibular 1st molar
  - Strongly correlated with eruption pattern of involved teeth
- Gender
  - M = F

Natural History & Prognosis

- No recurrence
- No malignant potential
- If unilateral, monitor for development on contralateral side
  - **20% of patients with unilateral lesions develop subsequent lesions** during follow-up period
- Eruption pattern normalized after removal
- Teeth remain **vital**

Treatment

- Surgical enucleation
- Normal regeneration of bone and periodontal healing in most cases
- Extraction of tooth not necessary
  - Extraction more common when 3rd molars involved

DIAGNOSTIC CHECKLIST

Consider

- Involvement of contralateral or maxillary teeth when presented with unilateral mandibular lesion

Image Interpretation Pearls

- Inflammatory component is nonspecific, so definitive diagnosis is made from radiographic appearance with support of clinical findings
- Displacement of apices of involved tooth toward lingual cortex is diagnostic

SELECTED REFERENCES

1. Borgonovo AE et al: Paradental cyst of the first molar: Report of a rare case with bilateral presentation and review of the literature. J Indian Soc Pedod Prev Dent. 30(4):343-8, 2012
2. Ramos LM et al: Bilateral buccal bifurcation cyst: case report and literature review. Head Neck Pathol. 6(4):455-9, 2012
3. Corona-Rodriguez J et al: Bilateral buccal bifurcation cyst: case report and literature review. J Oral Maxillofac Surg. 69(6):1694-6, 2011
4. Iatrou I et al: Intraosseous cystic lesions of the jaws in children: a retrospective analysis of 47 consecutive cases. Oral Surg Oral Med Oral Pathol Oral Radiol Endod. 107(4):485-92, 2009
5. Morimoto Y et al: Inflammatory paradental cyst (IPC) in the mandibular premolar region in children. Oral Surg Oral Med Oral Pathol Oral Radiol Endod. 97(2):286-93, 2004
6. David LA et al: The buccal bifurcation cyst: in non-surgical treatment an option? J Can Dent Assoc. 64(10):712-6, 1998
7. Pompura JR et al: The buccal bifurcation cyst: a prospective study of treatment outcomes in 44 sites. Oral Surg Oral Med Oral Pathol Oral Radiol Endod. 83(2):215-21, 1997
8. Magnusson B et al: The paradental cyst a clinicopathologic study of 26 cases. Swed Dent J. 19(1-2):1-7, 1995
9. Martinez-Conde R et al: Paradental cyst of the second molar: report of a bilateral case. J Oral Maxillofac Surg. 53(10):1212-4, 1995
10. Bossong L et al: Mandibular infected buccal cyst: case report and review of literature. N Y State Dent J. 60(10):22-5, 1994
11. Bohay RN et al: The paradental cyst of the mandibular permanent first molar: report of a bilateral case. ASDC J Dent Child. 59(5):361-5, 1992
12. Ackermann GL et al: Diagnosing the paradental cyst. J Oral Maxillofac Surg. 48(1):100, 1990
13. Packota GV et al: Paradental cysts on mandibular first molars in children: report of five cases. Dentomaxillofac Radiol. 19(3):126-32, 1990
14. Wolf J et al: The mandibular infected buccal cyst (paradental cyst). A radiographic and histological study. Br J Oral Maxillofac Surg. 28(5):322-5, 1990
15. Fowler CB et al: The paradental cyst: a clinicopathologic study of six new cases and review of the literature. J Oral Maxillofac Surg. 47(3):243-8, 1989
16. Vedtofte P et al: Inflammatory paradental cysts in the globulomaxillary region. J Oral Pathol Med. 18(3):125-7, 1989
17. Vedtofte P et al: The inflammatory paradental cyst. Oral Surg Oral Med Oral Pathol. 68(2):182-8, 1989
18. Ackermann G et al: The paradental cyst: a clinicopathologic study of 50 cases. Oral Surg Oral Med Oral Pathol. 64(3):308-12, 1987
19. Berteşteanu A et al: Maxillary paradental cyst appearing 26 years after radical maxilloethmoidal treatment. Rev Chir Oncol Radiol O R L Oftalmol Stomatol Otorinolaringol. 28(2):137-40, 1983
20. Kumazawa Y et al: A case of a paradental cyst near the mandibular wisdom tooth. Shigaku. 71(3):527-31, 1983
21. Stoneman DW et al: The mandibular infected buccal cyst--molar area. Dent Radiogr Photogr. 56(1):1-14, 1983

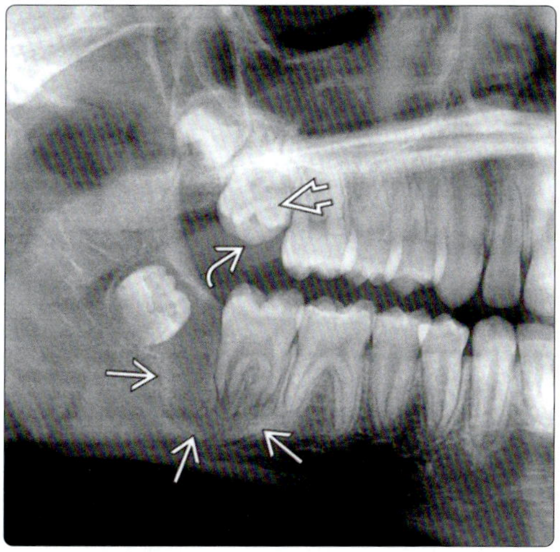

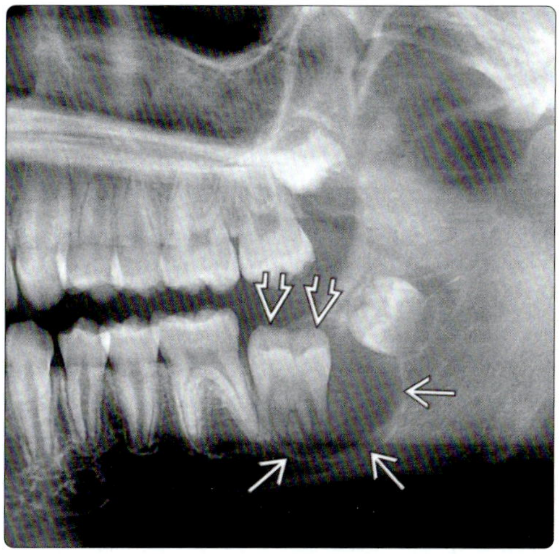

(Left) *Cropped panoramic radiograph shows a well-defined radiolucency associated with the mandibular right 2nd permanent molar in an 11-year-old boy. Note that the maxillary right 2nd permanent molar is not erupted and demonstrates occlusal tipping with prominence of the lingual cusps.* **(Right)** *Cropped panoramic radiograph in the same patient shows a similar well-defined corticated radiolucency associated with the left mandibular 2nd molar. Note the prominence of the lingual cusps.*

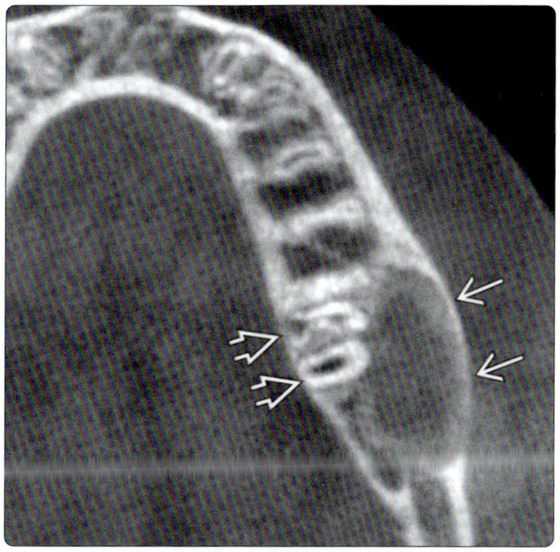

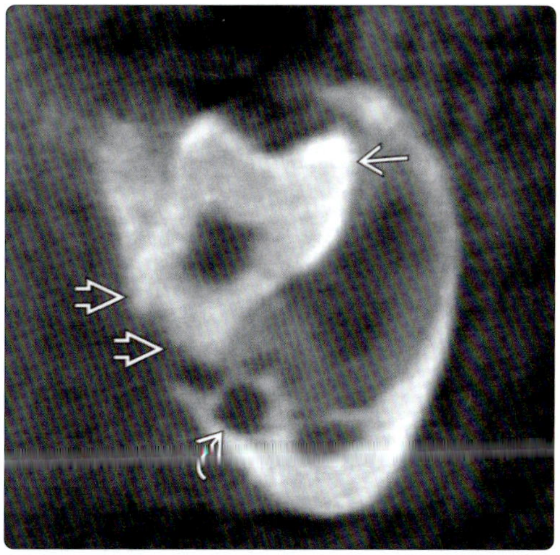

(Left) *Axial CBCT in the same patient shows expansion and thinning of the buccal cortex by the lesion in the left mandible. Note the roots of the 2nd molar are displaced toward the lingual cortex.* **(Right)** *Cross-section CBCT in the same patient shows tipping of the left 2nd molar with the crown inclined toward the buccal and the root apices at the lingual cortex. This radiographic appearance is diagnostic for BBC. Note the proximity to the mandibular canal.*

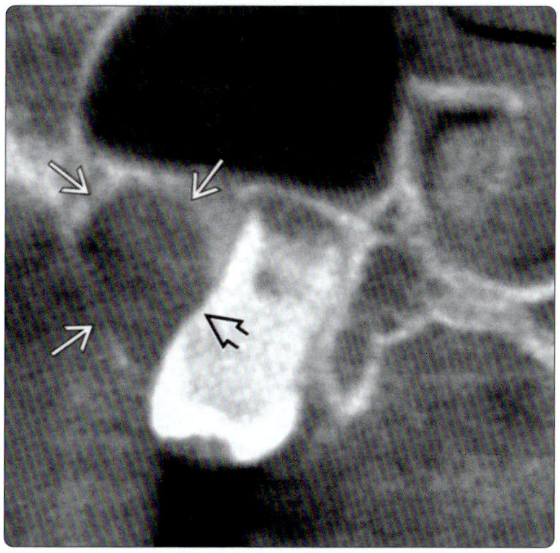

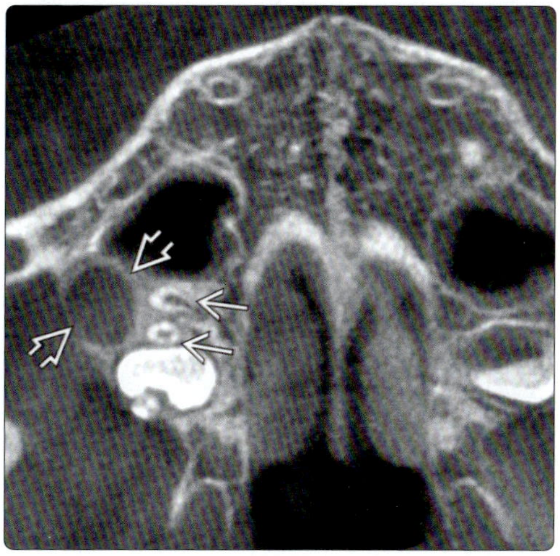

(Left) *Coronal CBCT in the same patient shows a maxillary BBC associated with the right 2nd molar. The epicenter of the lesion is at the buccal bifurcation. Tipping of the tooth is clearly evident.* **(Right)** *Axial CBCT in the same patient shows displacement of the apices of the buccal roots toward the palate. Tipping of the tooth was evident on the original panoramic radiograph, but the radiolucency was not. Consequently, this lesion was missed at initial presentation.*

Calcifying Odontogenic Cyst

KEY FACTS

TERMINOLOGY

- Synonyms: Calcifying cystic odontogenic tumor, calcifying epithelial odontogenic cyst, Gorlin cyst
- Definition: Odontogenic cyst exhibiting both **cystic and neoplastic properties**

IMAGING

- Well-defined radiolucency with **calcifications from small flecks to large masses**
- Maxilla = mandible: Anterior > posterior
- Unilocular, round or oval: **May be pericoronal**
  - Rarely multilocular: 5%
- CBCT or bone CT better to show sparse calcifications

TOP DIFFERENTIAL DIAGNOSES

- Adenomatoid odontogenic tumor
- Ameloblastic fibroodontoma
- Calcifying epithelial odontogenic tumor (Pindborg)

PATHOLOGY

- May occur with odontoma, ameloblastoma, ameloblastic fibroma, ameloblastic fibroodontoma, and orthokeratinized odontogenic cyst
- Epithelial lining exhibits characteristic **ghost cells** with varying degrees of dystrophic calcification

CLINICAL ISSUES

- Asymptomatic, incidental finding or hard swelling
- Recurrence more likely with neoplastic variants
- **Malignant variant reported**: Odontogenic ghost cell carcinoma
- Treatment: Surgical enucleation or removal of lesion and orthodontic realignment of associated tooth
- Radiographic follow-up to monitor for recurrence

DIAGNOSTIC CHECKLIST

- Consider: May mimic dentigerous cyst if pericoronal without radiographic evidence of calcifications

(Left) *Periapical radiograph shows a COC with a corticated border and calcifications at the center of the lesion. There is a peripheral zone of radiolucency resembling an adenomatoid odontogenic tumor, but resorption of the lateral incisor root favors COC. (Courtesy P. Hawkins, DDS.)* **(Right)** *Occlusal radiograph shows a COC associated with an impacted left mandibular canine. The calcifications are clustered around the crown. Note the lingual expansion. (Courtesy M. Noujeim, DDS.)*

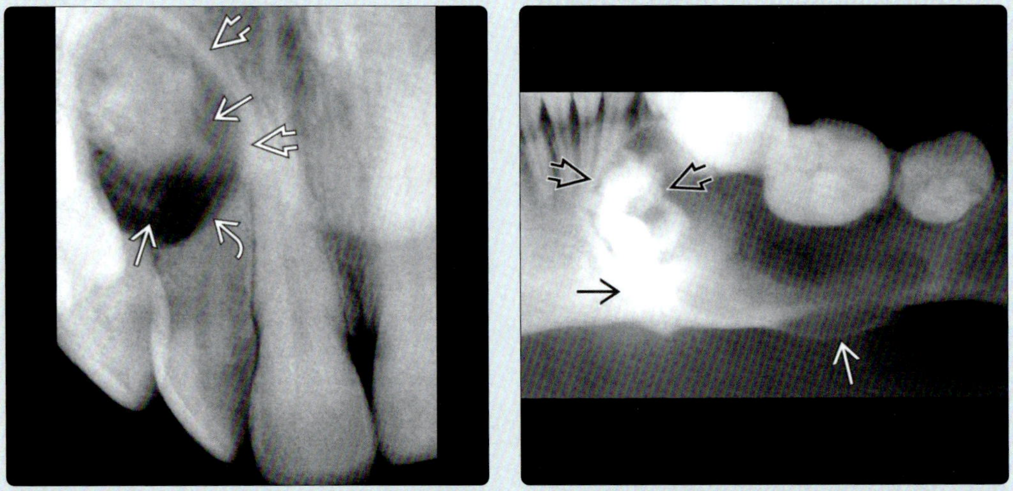

(Left) *Periapical radiograph of the left mandibular canine area shows a COC containing diffuse and discrete radiopacities. The diffuse calcifications resemble the "driven snow" seen in calcifying epithelial odontogenic tumors. (Courtesy R. Langlais, DDS.)* **(Right)** *Occlusal radiograph in the same patient shows that the COC has extended across the midline of the mandible. Note the well-defined corticated superior border. (Courtesy R. Langlais, DDS.)*

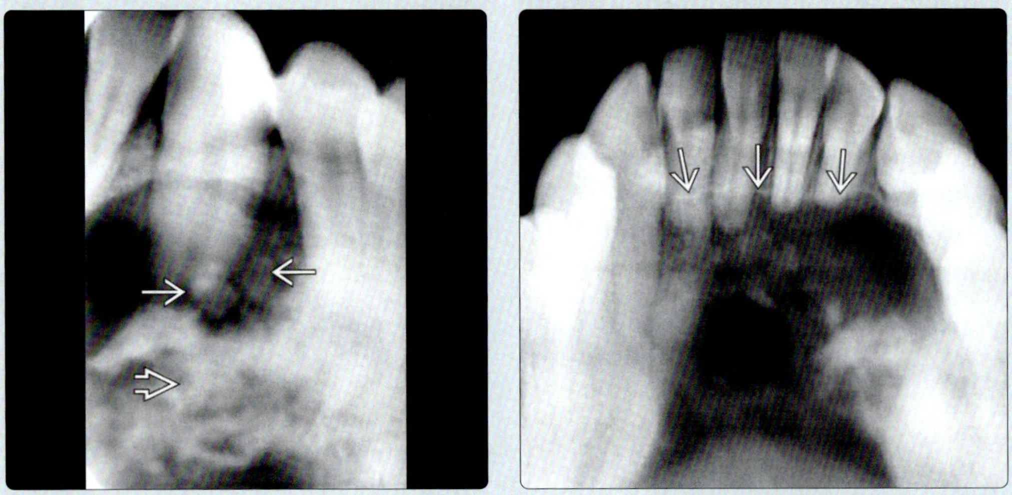

Calcifying Odontogenic Cyst

TERMINOLOGY

Abbreviations

- Calcifying odontogenic cyst (COC)

Synonyms

- Calcifying cystic odontogenic tumor
- Calcifying epithelial odontogenic cyst
- Gorlin cyst

Definitions

- Odontogenic cyst containing variable amounts of calcified tissue and exhibiting both **cystic and neoplastic properties**

IMAGING

General Features

- Best diagnostic clue
  - Well-defined, usually unilocular radiolucency containing varying amounts of calcifications
- Location
  - Maxilla = mandible; anterior > posterior
    - **Pericoronal** presentations tend to be posterior
    - Rare bilateral presentations reported
- Morphology
  - Unilocular, round or oval
  - Rarely multilocular: 5% (usually neoplastic variants)

Radiographic Findings

- Intraoral plain film
  - Unilocular lesion with well-defined, **often corticated** margin containing **varying amounts of calcifications** from small flecks to large masses
  - Calcifications may not be evident radiographically, and lesion appears completely radiolucent
    - If pericoronal, mimics dentigerous cyst

CT Findings

- CBCT or bone CT
  - Better shows sparse calcifications and any expansion
  - Calcifications may orient along periphery of lesion

DIFFERENTIAL DIAGNOSIS

Adenomatoid Odontogenic Tumor

- Well-defined radiolucency with variable amounts of calcification
- May see **peripheral zone of radiolucency** within lesion
- Anterior maxilla: May be pericoronal

Ameloblastic Fibroodontoma

- Well-defined radiolucency with **sparse calcifications**
- Posterior mandible: May be pericoronal

Calcifying Epithelial Odontogenic Tumor (Pindborg)

- Well-defined radiolucency with calcifications clustered near crown of involved tooth
- Calcifications described as "**driven snow**"

Dentigerous Cyst

- Most common **pericoronal** radiolucency
- Indistinguishable from radiolucent pericoronal COC

PATHOLOGY

General Features

- Genetics
  - Mutation on β-catenin gene has been reported
- Associated abnormalities
  - May occur with odontoma (~ 20%), ameloblastoma, ameloblastic fibroma, ameloblastic fibroodontoma, and orthokeratinized odontogenic cyst

Staging, Grading, & Classification

- Cystic nonneoplastic type: Simple unicystic, odontoma-producing, ameloblastomatous proliferating tumor
- Solid neoplastic type: Dentinogenic "ghost cell" tumor, epithelial odontogenic ghost cell tumor
- Cystic and neoplastic nature is likely reflection of pluripotential differentiation properties of odontogenic epithelium

Microscopic Features

- Epithelial lining exhibits characteristic **ghost cells** with varying degrees of dystrophic calcification

CLINICAL ISSUES

Presentation

- Most common signs/symptoms
  - Asymptomatic, incidental finding or hard swelling
- Other signs/symptoms
  - Root resorption or displacement of adjacent teeth

Demographics

- Age
  - 10-30 years: Maxillary lesions in older patients
  - 4th decade; M > F for malignant variant

Natural History & Prognosis

- Recurrence more likely with neoplastic variants
- Malignant variant reported arising in, or as recurrence of, preexisting COC or de novo: **Odontogenic ghost cell carcinoma**
  - More common in maxilla
  - Metastasis to lungs

Treatment

- Surgical enucleation: Orthodontic realignment of associated tooth if pericoronal
- Radiographic follow-up to monitor for recurrence

DIAGNOSTIC CHECKLIST

Consider

- May mimic dentigerous cyst if pericoronal without radiographic evidence of calcifications

SELECTED REFERENCES

1. Dutra SN et al: Immunoexpression of Wnt/β-catenin signaling pathway proteins in ameloblastoma and calcifying cystic odontogenic tumor. J Clin Exp Dent. 9(1):e136-e140, 2017
2. Urs AB et al: Calcifying ghost cell odontogenic tumor (CGCOT) with predominance of clear cells: a case report with important diagnostic considerations. Oral Surg Oral Med Oral Pathol Oral Radiol. 121(2):e32-7, 2016
3. Gadipelly S et al: Bilateral calcifying odontogenic cyst: A rare entity. J Maxillofac Oral Surg. 14(3):826-31, 2015

Mandible-Maxilla Aneurysmal Bone Cyst

KEY FACTS

TERMINOLOGY

- Definition: Benign lesion speculated to be reactive or proliferative vascular response to unknown stimulus
- Term aneurysmal describes radiographic ballooned appearance of cortex

IMAGING

- Best clue: **Fluid-fluid levels** representing sedimentation of red blood cells in blood-filled cavities
- Rare in jaws: Only 1.9% of all aneurysmal bone cysts
    - Mandible:maxilla = 3:1
- Multilocular radiolucency with characteristic **"ballooning" expansion of cortex**
- Loculations: Septa may orient at right angles to cortex & mimic central giant cell granuloma
- Soft tissue CT window may show low-density areas consistent with vascular spaces
- T2WI best shows fluid-fluid levels
- T1WI C+: Solid periphery = intense enhancement
    - Cystic components do not enhance

TOP DIFFERENTIAL DIAGNOSES

- Central giant cell granuloma (CGCG)
- Ameloblastoma
- Giant cell lesion of hyperparathyroidism

PATHOLOGY

- Etiology: Trauma or **altered hemodynamic state**
- In jaws, most commonly associated with CGCG
- Fibrous connective tissue, blood-filled sinusoids or caverns, hemosiderin, & **multinucleated giant cells**

CLINICAL ISSUES

- Age: 2nd decade (mean: 14.3 years)
- M = F; some report female preponderance

DIAGNOSTIC CHECKLIST

- Rapidly expanding, multilocular radiolucency in posterior jaws of young person highly suggestive

(Left) *Axial bone CT in a 16-year-old patient shows an expansile, multilocular lesion of the zygomatic bone exhibiting thin, corticated margins ➔. The lesion, confirmed at biopsy to be an aneurysmal bone cyst (ABC), protrudes into the maxillary sinus ➔. (Courtesy S. Blaser, MD.)* **(Right)** *Axial T1WI MR in the same patient performed 1 month later shows interval growth and mixed increased signal intensity of the lesion with multifocal bright signal foci ➔. (Courtesy S. Blaser, MD.)*

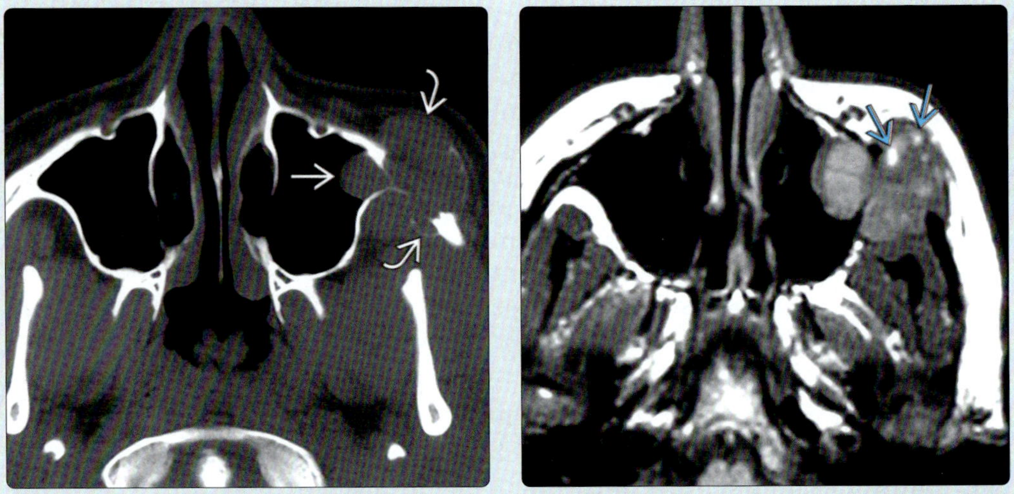

(Left) *Axial T2WI FS MR in the same patient shows fluid-fluid levels ➔ suggestive of ABC. (Courtesy S. Blaser, MD.)* **(Right)** *Axial CECT in the same patient, 3 months following MR, reveals marked expansion of the lesion, which now protrudes beyond the margins of the zygomatic arch into the subcutaneous tissues and obliterates the maxillary sinus. Fluid-fluid levels ➔ are evident. A rapidly expanding, multilocular lesion in a young person is highly suggestive of ABC. (Courtesy S. Blaser, MD.)*

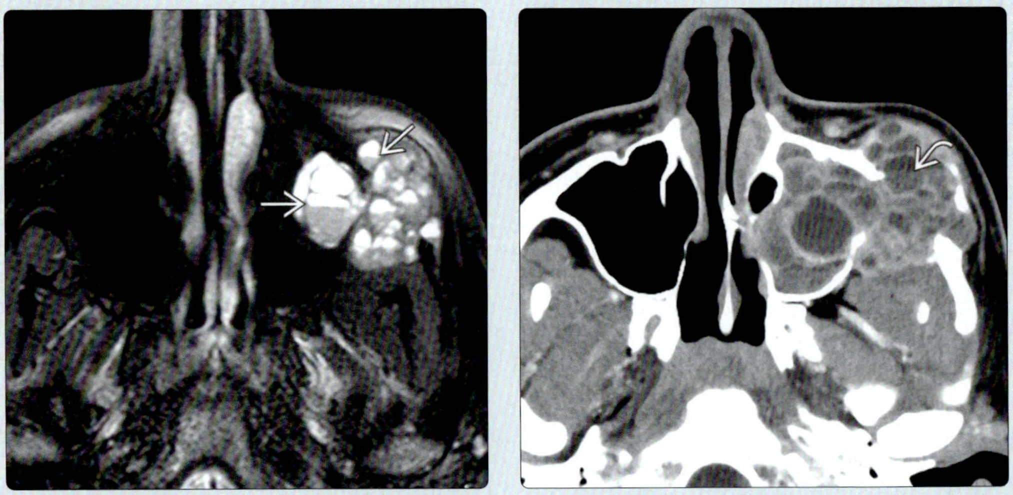

Mandible-Maxilla Aneurysmal Bone Cyst

TERMINOLOGY

Abbreviations

- Aneurysmal bone cyst (ABC)

Definitions

- Benign osseous lesion speculated to be reactive or proliferative vascular response to unknown stimulus
  - Not true cyst as it **lacks epithelial lining** (pseudocyst)
  - Term aneurysmal describes radiographic ballooned appearance of cortex

IMAGING

General Features

- Best diagnostic clue
  - **Fluid-fluid levels** representing sedimentation of red blood cells in blood-filled cavities
- Location
  - More common in long bones and spine
  - Rare in jaws: Only 1.9% of all ABCs
    - Mandible:maxilla = 3:1
      - □ Molar/ramus area most common
      - □ Rarely coronoid process or condyle
- Size
  - Varies; can become very large (> 10 cm)
- Morphology
  - Round, ovoid, unilocular (less expansion) or multilocular (significant expansion)

Radiographic Findings

- Extraoral plain film
  - Multilocular radiolucency with characteristic **"ballooning" expansion of cortex**

CT Findings

- CECT
  - Shows septal uptake and fluid-fluid levels
- NECT & CBCT
  - Loculations: Septa may orient at right angles to cortex & mimic central giant cell granuloma (CGCG)
  - Soft tissue window may show low-density areas consistent with vascular spaces

MR Findings

- T1WI
  - Subacute blood = hyperintense
- T2WI
  - Best shows fluid-fluid levels
- T1WI C+
  - Solid periphery = intense enhancement
  - Cystic components do not enhance

DIFFERENTIAL DIAGNOSIS

Central Giant Cell Granuloma

- Expansile, multilocular radiolucency; **anterior mandible**
- Septa orient at right angles to cortex (T-junction)
  - May be indistinguishable from ABC

Ameloblastoma

- Multilocular ("soap-bubble") expansile lesion
- Posterior mandible in **older age group**

Giant Cell Lesion of Hyperparathyroidism

- Brown tumor histologically similar to CGCG and ABC
- Serum calcium levels ↑ in hyperparathyroidism
- **Women in middle decades**

PATHOLOGY

General Features

- Etiology
  - Trauma; often no history elicited, however
  - **Altered hemodynamic state**
  - Vascular malformation occurring in preexisting lesion (secondary ABC): CGCG, fibrous dysplasia, nonossifying fibroma, hemangioma, osteoblastoma, simple bone cyst, chondroblastoma, osteosarcoma
    - In jaws, associated lesions less frequent; mostly CGCG
    - Unclear if ABCs precede or follow associated lesions as ABCs in most instances occur in younger age group
  - Chromosomal anomalies reported: Band 16q22

Staging, Grading, & Classification

- Solid type (5% of cases): Smaller, often asymptomatic lesion with less swelling and less bleeding at surgery
- Vascular type: Rapidly growing, expansile, destructive lesion with excessive bleeding at surgery
- Mixed type: Possibly represents transition phase

Microscopic Features

- Fibrous connective tissue, blood-filled sinusoids or caverns, hemosiderin, & **multinucleated giant cells**

CLINICAL ISSUES

Presentation

- Most common signs/symptoms
  - Solid type: Slow growing with mild facial deformity
  - Vascular type: Rapidly growing swelling
- Other signs/symptoms
  - Pain or tenderness
  - Aspiration of blood suspicious for ABC: Absence of bruits or pulse rules out hemangioma

Demographics

- Age
  - 2nd decade (mean: 14.3 years)
- Gender
  - M = F; some report female preponderance

Natural History & Prognosis

- Recurrence fairly high: Up to 90% with curettage

Treatment

- Curettage, cryotherapy, excision, block resection and grafting, embolization if vascular type

SELECTED REFERENCES

1. Flores IL et al: Simple and aneurysmal bone cyst: Aspects of jaw pseudocysts based on an experience of Brazilian pathology service during 53 years. Med Oral Patol Oral Cir Bucal. 22(1):e64-e69, 2017
2. Motamedi MH et al: Assessment of 120 maxillofacial aneurysmal bone cysts: a nationwide quest to understand this enigma. J Oral Maxillofac Surg. 72(8):1523-30, 2014
3. Urs AB et al: Aneurysmal bone cyst of the jaws: Clinicopathological study. J Maxillofac Oral Surg. 13(4):458-63, 2014

(Left) *Axial NECT shows a thinly corticated, expansile lesion* ➡ *in the left posterior mandible and ramus of an 11-year-old girl struck by a softball. (Courtesy M. Noujeim, DDS.)* **(Right)** *Coronal bone CT in the same patient shows "ballooning" expansion* ➡ *typical of an ABC. (Courtesy M. Noujeim, DDS.)*

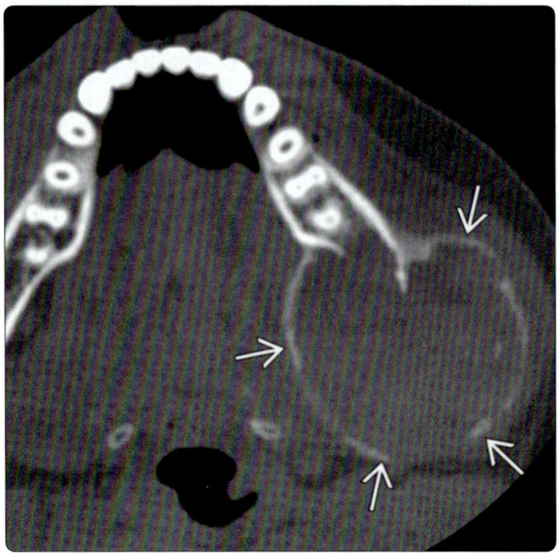

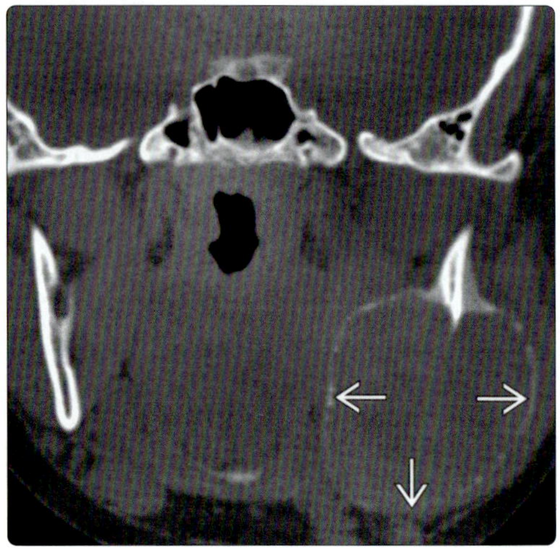

(Left) *Coronal NECT, soft tissue window, in the same patient shows a corticated, expansile lesion of ABC with a small buccal cortical perforation* ⇨*. Areas of low density representing vascular spaces can be seen within the lesion* ➡*. (Courtesy M. Noujeim, DDS.)* **(Right)** *Axial CECT, soft tissue window, in the same patient shows septal uptake* ➡ *within the lesion and differing densities* ➡ *that represent fluid-fluid levels within the loculations of the ABC. (Courtesy M. Noujeim, DDS.)*

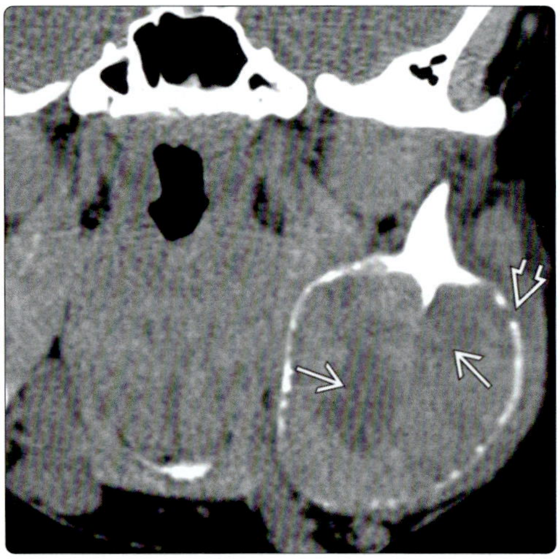

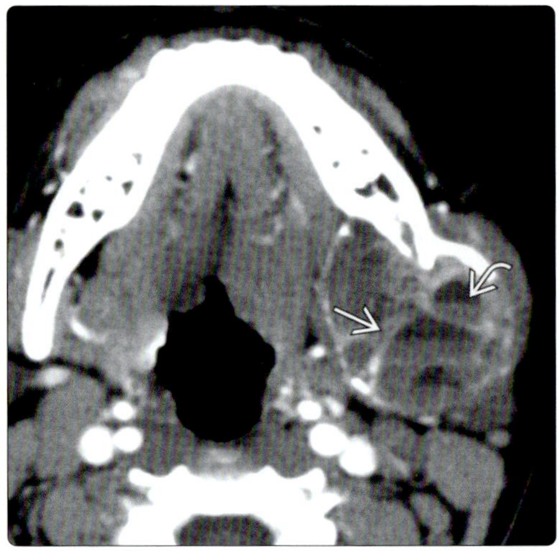

(Left) *Axial T2WI FS MR in the same patient shows high signal and fluid-fluid levels* ➡ *characteristic of ABC. (Courtesy M. Noujeim, DDS.)* **(Right)** *Axial T1WI C+ FS MR in the same patient shows septal contrast enhancement. (Courtesy M. Noujeim, DDS.)*

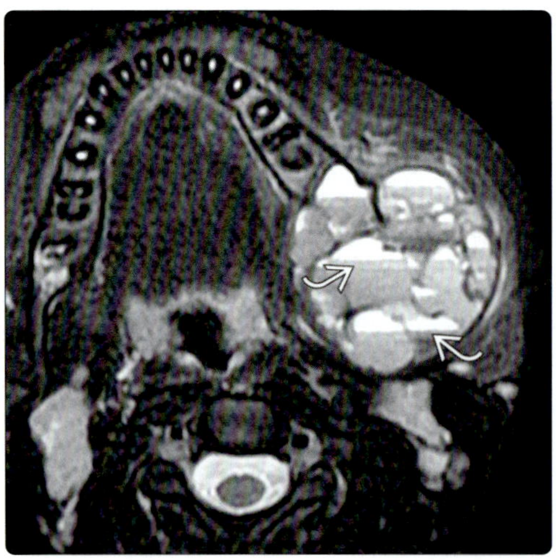

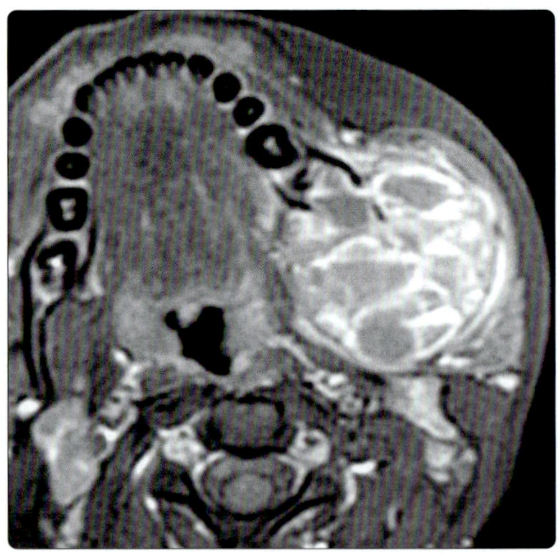

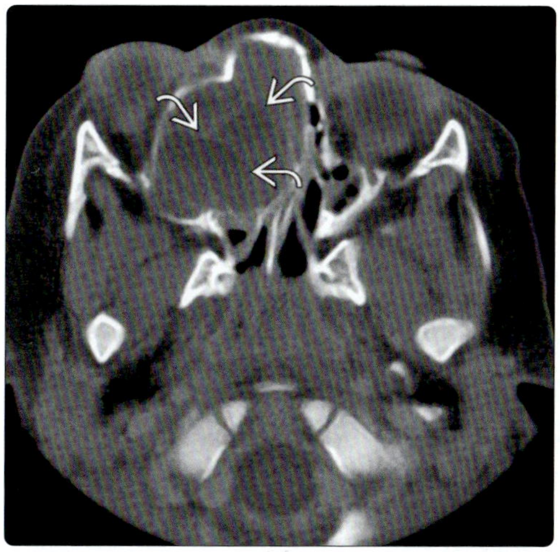

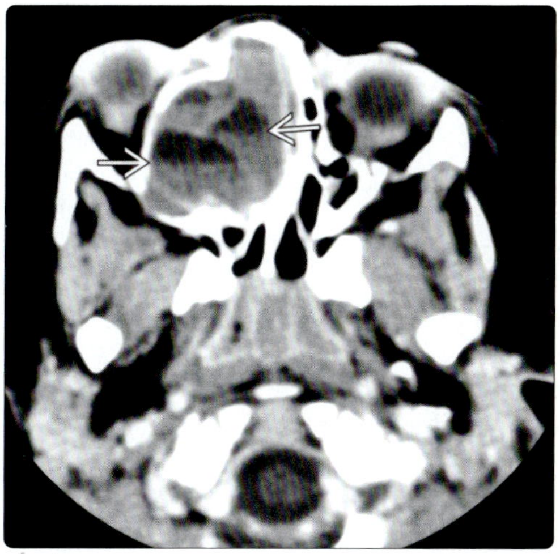

(Left) *Axial bone CT shows an expansile mass involving the nose, ethmoid sinus, and orbit in a 1-year-old child. It is possible to see the different densities within the lesion, although faint, and delicate loculations →.* **(Right)** *Axial CECT in the same patient shows fluid-fluid levels → within the substance of the ABC. ABC and lymphatic malformation are the 2 lesions to consider when a fluid-fluid level is seen within a lesion in a very young child.*

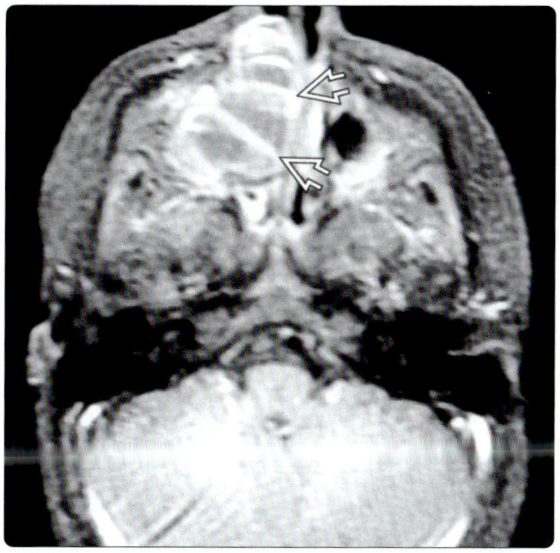

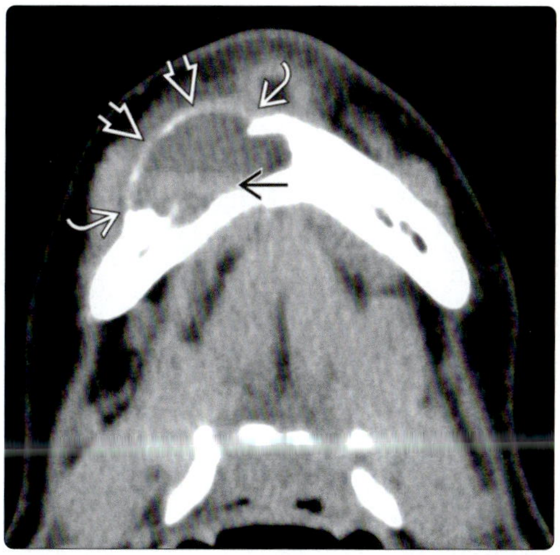

(Left) *Axial T1WI C+ FS MR in the same patient shows rim enhancement → along the margins of the multiple loculations of the ABC.* **(Right)** *Axial NECT shows a balloon-like, expansile lesion within the parasymphyseal mandible. Note the expanded and thinned buccal cortex → and fluid-fluid level with high-density blood product sedimentation on the dependent side →. The ABC makes equal and obtuse angles with the normal cortex → typical of cystic expansion. (Courtesy L. Lowe, MD.)*

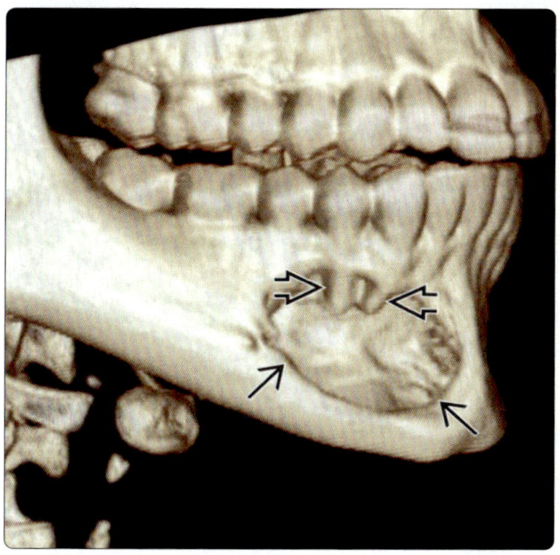

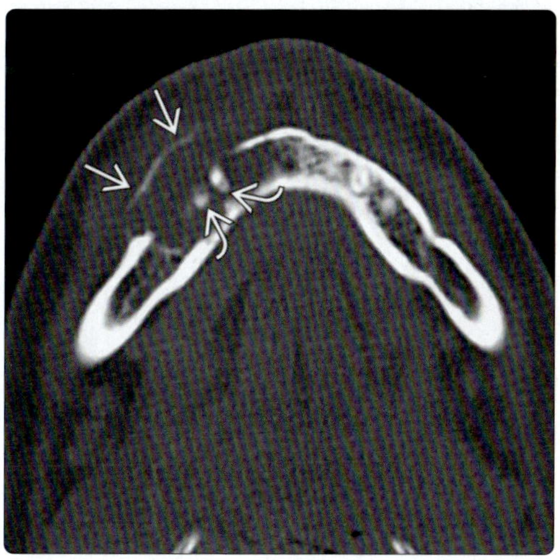

(Left) *Lateral 3D reformation in the same patient shows the benign bony margins → of the ABC. Note the root apices → of the canine and 1st premolar teeth exposed within the lesion. (Courtesy L. Lowe, MD.)* **(Right)** *Axial bone CT in the same patient shows the thin, expanded buccal cortical margin → and apices of the canine and premolar teeth → within the lesion. (Courtesy L. Lowe, MD.)*

Nasopalatine Duct Cyst

KEY FACTS

TERMINOLOGY

- Nasopalatine duct cyst (NPDC): Developmental cyst arising from remnants of nasopalatine duct epithelium

IMAGING

- Intraoral 2D imaging
  - Well-defined, round or oval, **> 1-cm** radiolucency between roots of maxillary central incisors
  - Larger lesions may appear **heart-shaped** due to superimposition of anterior nasal spine
  - Lamina dura of adjacent teeth intact
- CBCT or bone CT findings
  - Axial: Round **corticated expansion** of nasopalatine canal
  - Coronal and sagittal: **Cortication discontinuous at superior and inferior margins** of canal

TOP DIFFERENTIAL DIAGNOSES

- Large nasopalatine foramen
- Periapical (radicular) cyst
- Residual cyst
- Central giant cell granuloma
- Odontogenic keratocyst

CLINICAL ISSUES

- Most common nonodontogenic cyst
- Clinical presentation: Usually asymptomatic incidental finding
  - Less commonly: Pain, swelling of anterior maxilla
  - Patients may complain of **salty** taste
- Treatment: Enucleation, usually palatally
  - Recurrence rate very low
  - Paresthesia in < 10% of cases

DIAGNOSTIC CHECKLIST

- **Check vitality of teeth** to rule out periapical pathology of pulpal origin
- Single rounded, corticated, radiolucent lesion in midline maxilla highly suggestive

(Left) *Periapical radiograph of the anterior maxilla shows a large, well-defined nasopalatine duct cyst (NPDC) ➔. Note the corticated border, > 1 cm, and hydraulic expansion. Superimposition of the anterior nasal spine ➔ gives it the characteristic heart shape seen in larger lesions. (Courtesy M. Ahmad, DDS.)* **(Right)** *Axial CBCT shows a well-defined, corticated area of low density in the anterior maxilla ➔. The NPDC has extended between the maxillary central incisor roots, but the lamina dura ➔ is intact.*

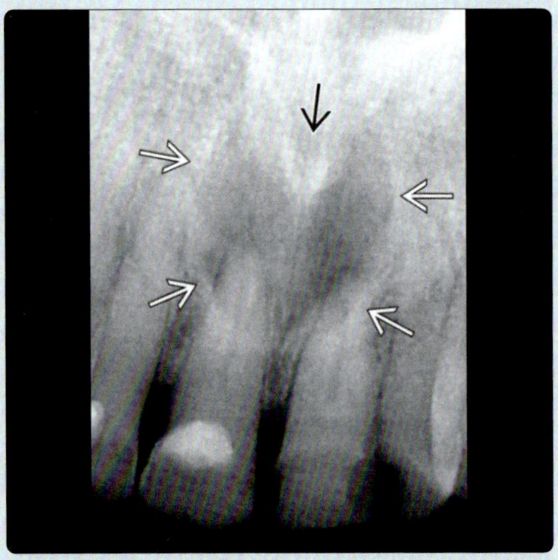

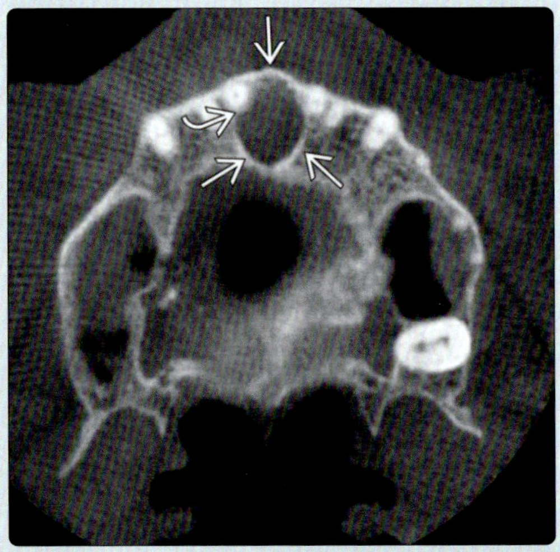

(Left) *Sagittal CBCT in the same patient shows significant buccal-palatal expansion of the nasopalatine canal (> 1 cm).* **(Right)** *Periapical radiograph in the same patient shows the well-defined, corticated borders ➔ of the cyst. Due to foreshortening of the image, the superior foramina of the nasopalatine canal ➔ are superimposed within the superior aspect of the lesion and the anterior nasal spine ➔ is projected inferiorly.*

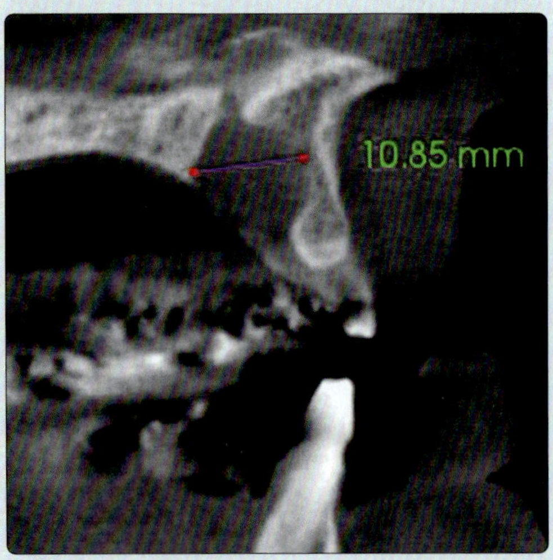

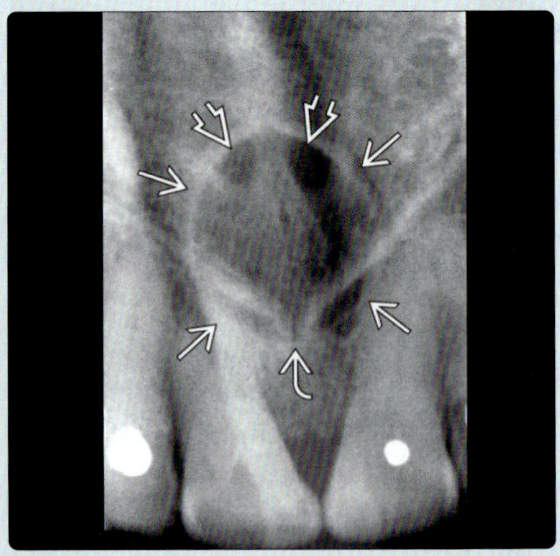

Nasopalatine Duct Cyst

TERMINOLOGY

Abbreviations

- Nasopalatine duct cyst (NPDC)

Synonyms

- Incisive canal cyst
- Anterior middle cyst
- Maxillary midline cyst
- Anterior middle palatine cyst
- Incisor duct cyst

Definitions

- Developmental cyst arising from remnants of nasopalatine duct epithelium
- **Most common** nonodontogenic developmental cyst: 1% of all maxillary cysts

IMAGING

General Features

- Best diagnostic clue
    - Well-circumscribed, rounded enlargement of incisive canal in maxilla
- Location
    - Incisive canal palatal (posterior) to maxillary central incisor teeth
        - Superficial or inferior (caudal) location within canal most common
        - Deep or more nasally oriented lesions less common
    - Bilateral NPDCs reported occurring as 2 distinct cysts in incisive canals (canals of Stensen)
- Size
    - 1 cm or greater
        - Incisive canal with diameter **> 1 cm presumed NPDC**
        - Some reports of normal variants > 1 cm; If doubt monitor carefully
        - Lesions tend to be larger in males
- Morphology
    - Round or oval
    - When large, may appear **heart-shaped** on intraoral images

Imaging Recommendations

- Best imaging tool
    - CBCT or thin-section bone algorithm CT
        - CBCT best demonstrates lesion in relation to lingual aspect of teeth
- Protocol advice
    - Thin-section facial bone CT with axial, coronal, sagittal reformations

Radiographic Findings

- Intraoral plain film
    - Well-defined, rounded or oval radiolucency in anterior maxilla between roots of central incisor teeth
    - Larger lesions may present as **heart-shaped** due to superimposition of anterior nasal spine
    - **Lamina dura** and periodontal ligament (PDL) space of adjacent teeth **intact**

CT Findings

- NECT
    - Lesion is hypodense
- CBCT and bone CT
    - Smooth, rounded **enlargement of incisive canal of > 1 cm**
    - Axial views: **Corticated periphery** representing walls of nasopalatine canal
    - Coronal and sagittal views: **Cortication discontinuous at superior and inferior margins** of canal
        - Cortication at superior and inferior margins of canal infers different lesion
    - May cause thinning and dehiscence of lingual cortex of maxilla
    - Larger lesions will extend to nasal cavity
    - Lamina dura and PDL space of adjacent teeth intact

MR Findings

- T1WI
    - Homogeneously iso- to hyperintense
- T2WI
    - Homogeneous hyperintense T2 signal
- Typically nonenhancing
    - May enhance with inflammatory component

DIFFERENTIAL DIAGNOSIS

Large Nasopalatine Foramen

- Intraoral images: Maintains oval or teardrop shape
    - Noncorticated
- Usually < 1 cm diameter
- Comparison to prior images helpful

Periapical (Radicular) Cyst

- Cyst arising **at apex** of **nonvital** teeth
- Caused by caries or trauma
- **Lamina dura not present at apex of tooth** but contiguous with corticated border of cyst
- **Not centrally located** within incisive canal but may involve it secondarily

Residual Cyst

- Persistent radicular cyst remaining after extraction or loss of infected tooth
- Tooth will be missing
- Adjacent to, **not centrally located** within, incisive canal

Central Giant Cell Granuloma

- Benign reactive lesion of bone
- Anterior > posterior: Mandible most common
- Small, **unilocular lesions may simulate NPDC**
- May see root resorption

Odontogenic Keratocyst

- Varied radiographic appearance ± associated teeth
- When small and unilocular, may simulate NPDC
- When large, expands and **behaves more aggressively** than NPDC
    - May erode maxilla, maxillary sinus floor, and floor of nose
- Typically arises in canine region in maxilla, molars in mandible; rare in midline maxilla

Apical Periodontitis

- Infection (abscess or granuloma) **at apex** of tooth root associated with caries or trauma
- **Loss of lamina dura** and widening of PDL space around root apex
- Diffuse lytic area mm to cm in size: **Noncorticated**
- May extend into incisive canal secondarily

Median Palatal Cyst

- Now thought to be variant of NPDC

Dentigerous (Follicular) Cyst

- Associated with **unerupted or impacted tooth**: Pericoronal
- Mandibular 3rd molar teeth most common
- May look similar to NPDC if associated with **mesiodens** (supernumerary tooth located in anterior maxilla)

PATHOLOGY

General Features

- Etiology
  - Developmental cyst arising from spontaneous proliferation of epithelial remnants of nasopalatine duct between oral & nasal cavities
  - Other possibilities
    - Trauma
    - Ill-fitting dentures
    - Local infection
    - Recent reports have suggested trauma from dental implant placement adjacent to nasopalatine canal may induce NPDC formation
- Associated abnormalities
  - Bacterial rhinitis

Microscopic Features

- Cyst usually lined by stratified squamous epithelium (SSE) &/or combination of SSE and respiratory epithelium
  - Postulated respiratory epithelium (pseudostratified, ciliated columnar) most likely seen if cyst located more nasally
  - Presence of melanin has been reported
- Cyst lumen may contain inflammatory infiltrate secondary to chronic inflammation

CLINICAL ISSUES

Presentation

- Most common signs/symptoms
  - Usually asymptomatic incidental finding
  - Symptoms occur sooner in lesions located more caudally
- Other signs/symptoms
  - Pain and itching
  - Pressure on nasopalatine nerve may cause burning sensation
  - Swelling of anterior maxilla: Usually palatal
    - Rare large nasolabial swelling reported
  - Ulceration
  - Sinus tract with drainage: Patients may complain of **salty** taste
  - **Anterior teeth are vital** unless coincidentally pulpally involved
  - Does not tend to displace teeth or resorb roots unless very large

Demographics

- Age
  - Wide range: 7-84 years
  - Maximum incidence: 40-60 years (mean: 42.5 years)
- Gender
  - M > F = 3:1
- Epidemiology
  - May be more aggressive in adolescent black South Africans

Natural History & Prognosis

- Slow-growing benign lesion
  - If cortex perforated, extraosseous component grows more rapidly
- Recurrence rate very low: < 2% when enucleated
- Metaplasia of cyst wall resulting in squamous cell carcinoma reported
  - Treatment more aggressive and prognosis poorer

Treatment

- Surgical enucleation via palatine or (rarely) buccal approach with careful dissection of neurovascular bundle
- Electrosurgery for control of bleeding
- Palatine plaque placed postoperatively helps prevent formation of submucosal hematoma
- Paresthesia of anterior palate occurs in < 10% of cases

DIAGNOSTIC CHECKLIST

Consider

- Periapical pathology of pulpal origin: **Check vitality of teeth** to rule out

Image Interpretation Pearls

- Single, rounded, corticated, radiolucent lesion in midline maxilla highly suggestive

Reporting Tips

- Comment on any extension to nasal cavity

SELECTED REFERENCES

1. Al-Shamiri HM et al: Development of nasopalatine duct cyst in relation to dental implant placement. N Am J Med Sci. 8(1):13-6, 2016
2. Bains R et al: Nasopalatine duct cyst mimicking an endodontic periapical lesion: a case report. Gen Dent. 64(1):63-6, 2016
3. Gopal D et al: Nasopalatine duct cyst associated with a mesiodens: misdiagnosis or missed diagnosis? J Clin Diagn Res. 9(5):ZD21-2, 2015
4. McCrea SJ: Nasopalatine duct cyst, a delayed complication to successful dental implant placement: diagnosis and surgical management. J Oral Implantol. 40(2):189-95, 2014
5. Sane VD et al: Role of cone-beam computed tomography in diagnosis and management of nasopalatine duct cyst. J Craniofac Surg. 25(1):e92-4, 2014
6. Perumal CJ: An unusually large destructive nasopalatine duct cyst: a case report. J Maxillofac Oral Surg. 12(1):100-4, 2013
7. Shylaja S et al: Nasopalatine duct cyst: report of a case with review of literature. Indian J Otolaryngol Head Neck Surg. 65(4):385-8, 2013
8. Cicciù M et al: Rare bilateral nasopalatine duct cysts: a case report. Open Dent J. 4:8-12, 2010
9. Nelson BL et al: Nasopalatine duct cyst. Head Neck Pathol. 4(2):121-2, 2010
10. Escoda Francolí J et al: Nasopalatine duct cyst: report of 22 cases and review of the literature. Med Oral Patol Oral Cir Bucal. 13(7):E438-43, 2008

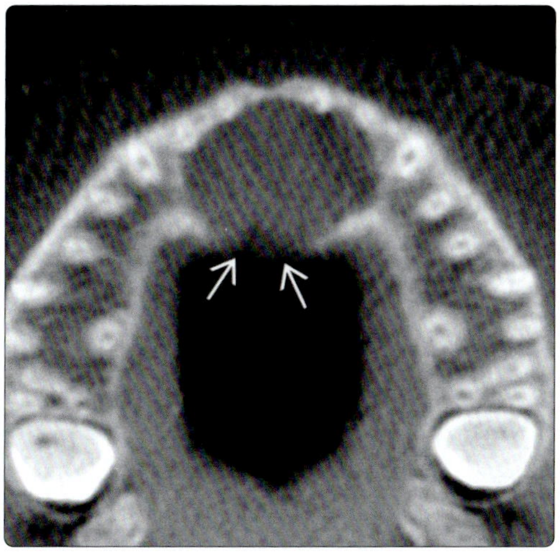

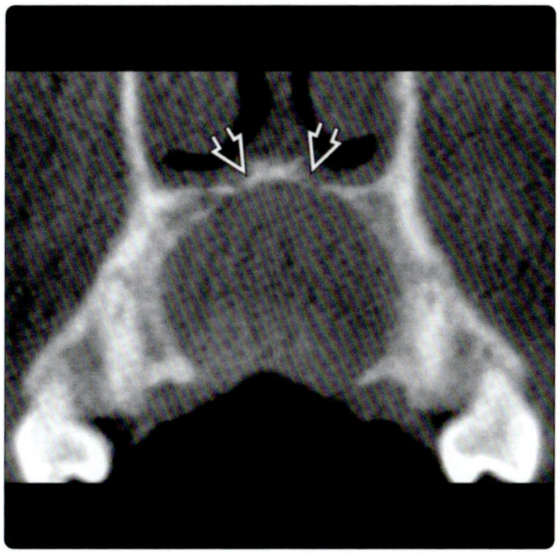

(Left) *Axial CBCT shows a very large NPDC that has caused thinning and dehiscence of the lingual cortical plate* ➡. *(Courtesy M. Ahmad, DDS.)* **(Right)** *Coronal CBCT in the same patient shows symmetric enlargement of the nasopalatine canal by the very large NPDC. The floor of the nose is slightly elevated* ➡ *but remains intact. The superior margin is corticated because the slice is anterior to the nasal opening of the canal. (Courtesy M. Ahmad, DDS.)*

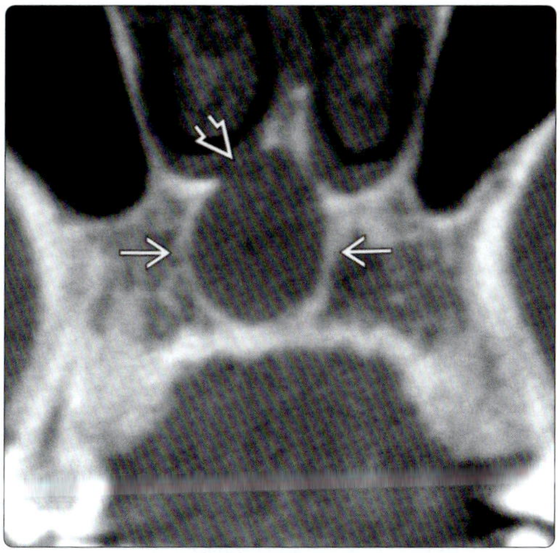

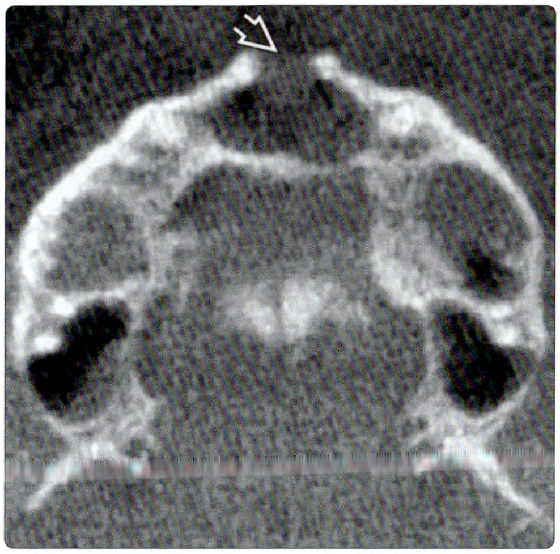

(Left) *Coronal CBCT shows a large NPDC* ➡ *expanding into the floor of the nose. Note thinned but intact corticated border on the superior right side* ➡. **(Right)** *Axial CBCT shows a large NPDC that has expanded and perforated through the buccal cortex* ➡. *This is an unusual presentation as expansion is usually greatest on the palatal aspect.*

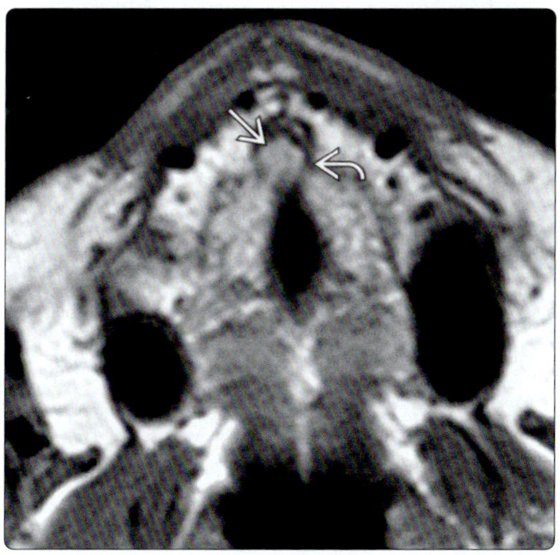

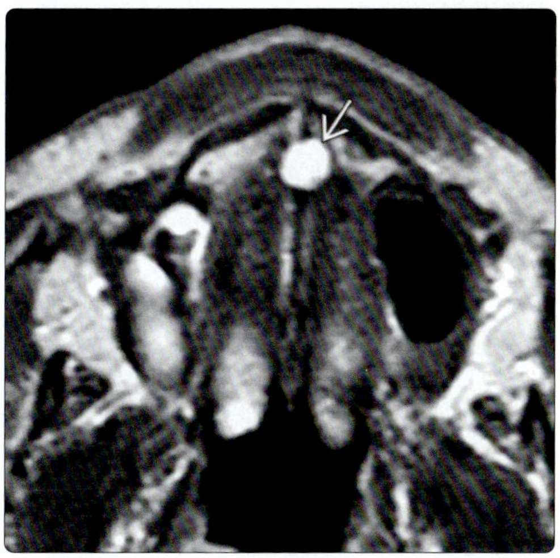

(Left) *Axial T1WI MR shows an intermediate to slightly T1 hyperintense expansion of the incisive canal* ➡ *by a NPDC. Note the thin but preserved cortex* ➡. **(Right)** *Axial T2WI MR shows the classic MR appearance of a NPDC. Note the uniformly round, homogeneously T2-hyperintense area in the midline maxilla* ➡.

KEY FACTS

TERMINOLOGY

- Definition: Rare, benign, developmental cyst in nasal ala between upper lip & nasal vestibule
- Synonyms: Nasoalveolar cyst, Klestadt cyst

IMAGING

- Typically < 2 cm; ≤ 10% bilateral
- Pyriform rim, between upper lip & nasal vestibule
- CT: Nonenhancing, hyperdense ± dense fluid levels
  - May cause bone remodeling of maxilla as enlarges
- MR: T2-hyperintense cyst with variable T1 intensity
  - No contrast enhancement of lesion

TOP DIFFERENTIAL DIAGNOSES

- Nasopalatine duct cyst
- Nasolacrimal duct mucocele
- Periapical (radicular) cyst
- Dermoid & epidermoid cyst of oral cavity

PATHOLOGY

- Developmental; 2 theories of pathogenesis
  - Persistence of anlage of nasolacrimal duct (**favored theory**) or inclusion cyst from formation of facial skeleton

CLINICAL ISSUES

- Mean age: 40 years; F:M = 3:1
- More prevalent in black & Hispanic populations
- Presents as facial swelling ± nasal obstruction
- Smooth fluctuant mass, loss of nasolabial fold
- 30% present with infection: Swelling, pain, erythema
- Surgical excision is definitive treatment

DIAGNOSTIC CHECKLIST

- Extraalveolar origin distinguishes from odontogenic lesions
- Look for bone erosion, extension to turbinate, or nasolacrimal duct obstruction

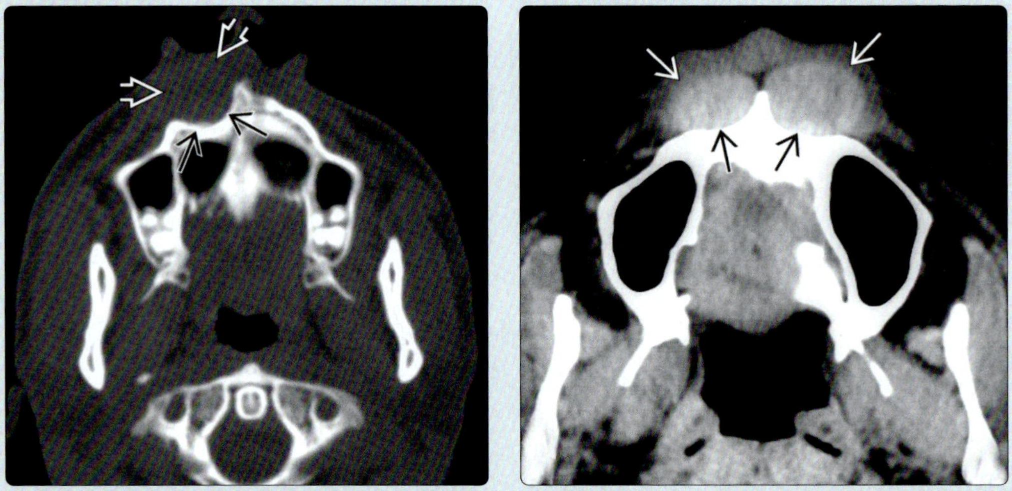

(Left) *Axial bone CT shows remodeling of the right anterior maxilla ⇨ caused by a unilateral nasolabial cyst ➡. (Courtesy T. El-Helw, MD.)* **(Right)** *Axial NECT demonstrates bilateral, well-demarcated, hyperdense, rounded lesions ➡ approximating the anterior maxilla. The lesions have resulted in subtle, left > right, remodeling of anterior maxilla ⇨. Fewer than 10% of nasolabial cyst cases are bilateral.*

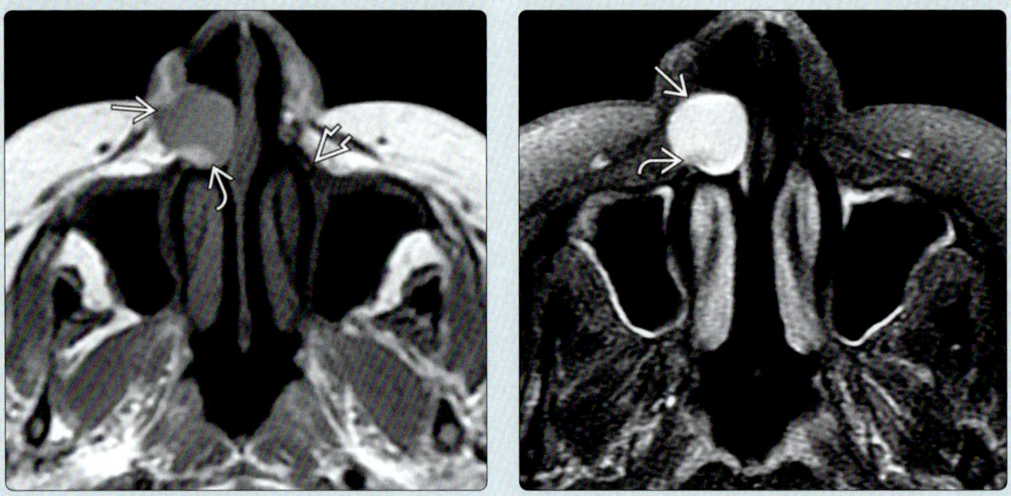

(Left) *Axial T1WI MR shows a well-defined mass ➡ at the pyriform rim that extends into the nasal vestibule. Mass appears slightly increased in signal compared to muscle with more focal hyperintensity ↪, likely reflecting proteinaceous debris. Note the lesion nestles into the maxilla with subtle bone erosion compared to contralateral side ⇨.* **(Right)** *Axial T2WI FS MR same patient reveals typical homogeneous T2 hyperintensity of a nasolabial cyst ➡ with subtly hypointense proteinaceous debris ↪.*

TERMINOLOGY

Synonyms

- Nasoalveolar cyst, Klestadt cyst

Definitions

- Rare, benign, developmental cyst in nasal ala between upper lip & nasal vestibule

IMAGING

General Features

- Best diagnostic clue
  - **Extraosseous** cystic mass in paramedian location at nares
- Location
  - Submucosal, anterior nasal floor
  - Pyriform rim, between upper lip & nasal vestibule
- Size
  - Typically < 2 cm; < 10% bilateral

CT Findings

- CBCT or bone CT
  - May cause bone remodeling of maxilla as enlarges
- CECT
  - Iso- to hyperdense nonenhancing soft tissue mass
  - May have dense-dependent fluid levels from calcium oxalate crystals

MR Findings

- T1WI
  - Slightly **hyperintense** from proteinaceous debris
- T2WI
  - Homogeneously hyperintense
- T1WI C+
  - No contrast enhancement of lesion

Imaging Recommendations

- Best imaging tool
  - CBCT or CT is adequate for delineation of lesion
  - MR for relationship to adjacent soft tissues
- Protocol advice
  - CECT confirms absence of solid component
  - Bone CT for remodeled bone change

DIFFERENTIAL DIAGNOSIS

Nasopalatine Duct Cyst

- Occurs in nasopalatine duct/incisive foramen → intraosseous midline maxillary alveolus lesion
- Uniform corticated expansion of incisive foramen & nasopalatine canal
- Typically no extraalveolar extension to nasolabial unless very large

Nasolacrimal Duct Mucocele

- Failure of canalization of nasolacrimal duct
- Typically appear in infancy
- Usually accompanying dacryocystitis, epiphora, or intranasal mass

Periapical (Radicular) Cyst

- Intraosseous alveolar location
- Associated with root apex of tooth having caries or periodontal disease

Dermoid and Epidermoid Cyst of Oral Cavity

- Usually presents in infancy, childhood
- Very rare in nasolabial area

PATHOLOGY

General Features

- Etiology
  - Developmental; 2 theories of pathogenesis
    - Persistence of anlage of nasolacrimal duct
      - Favored theory of formation
    - Inclusion cyst from formation of facial skeleton
      - After fusion of medial & lateral nasal processes & maxillary prominence

Gross Pathologic & Surgical Features

- Gray-blue color; thick fibrous capsule
- Contains mucoid or serous fluid

Microscopic Features

- Pseudostratified, stratified, or mixed respiratory & squamous epithelium

CLINICAL ISSUES

Presentation

- Most common signs/symptoms
  - Swelling of nasolabial fold, upper lip
  - ± nasal obstruction

Demographics

- Age
  - Lesions present in adults; mean: 40 years
- Gender
  - F:M = 3:1
- Ethnicity
  - More prevalent in black & Hispanic populations

Natural History & Prognosis

- May grow toward nasolabial fold or vestibule of mouth or nose
- 30% present with infection of cyst

Treatment

- Surgical excision is definitive treatment
  - Sublabial approach; recurrence rare

DIAGNOSTIC CHECKLIST

Image Interpretation Pearls

- **Extraosseous origin** distinguishes from odontogenic lesions
  - Prevents unnecessary maxillary surgical/dental intervention

SELECTED REFERENCES

1. Kadiyoran C et al: Klestadt cyst: magnetic resonance imaging. J Craniofac Surg. ePub, 2017
2. Patil AR et al: Bilateral nasolabial cysts - case report and review of literature. Indian J Radiol Imaging. 26(2):241-4, 2016

Mandible-Maxilla Simple (Traumatic) Bone Cyst

KEY FACTS

TERMINOLOGY

- Definition: Solitary, empty or partially empty, bony cavity
- "Cyst" designation misnomer: Lacks epithelial lining

IMAGING

- **Unilocular corticated radiolucency** in mandible
- **Endosteal scalloping** characteristic & may cause multilocular appearance on plain radiographs
- Typically **nonexpansile**; if present, mild
- Margins uniform; lesion may scallop between teeth
- T2 MR: Hyperintense; no fluid-fluid levels

TOP DIFFERENTIAL DIAGNOSES

- Osteoporotic bone marrow defect
- Odontogenic keratocyst
- Lateral periodontal cyst
- Periapical (radicular) cyst (tooth nonvital)
- Langerhans histiocytosis

PATHOLOGY

- Cystic cavity with connective tissue membrane & **no epithelial lining**: May contain "straw-colored" fluid
- < 1/2 associated with prior trauma
- Frequently seen with **lesions of osseous dysplasia**, less commonly osteomas & hypercementosis

CLINICAL ISSUES

- Incidental finding on imaging
- Most in 2nd decade: Lesions associated with osseous dysplasia are seen in 5th decade
- Low recurrence rate reported
- Treatment: Surgical exploration & curettage to stimulate bleeding & promote healing
- Lesions can spontaneously resolve: Healing bone may appear **granular**
    - Conservative radiographic follow-up may be alternative to surgery in very young patients with small lesions

(Left) *Cropped panoramic radiograph of a 17-year-old boy shows a large radiolucency ➔ in the anterior mandible. Note the periodontal ligament spaces around the involved teeth are prominent due to orthodontic movement.* **(Right)** *Axial CBCT in the same patient shows the lesion is unilocular and exhibits mild expansion. Note the undulating appearance along the inner surface of the buccal cortex ➔ known as endosteal scalloping.*

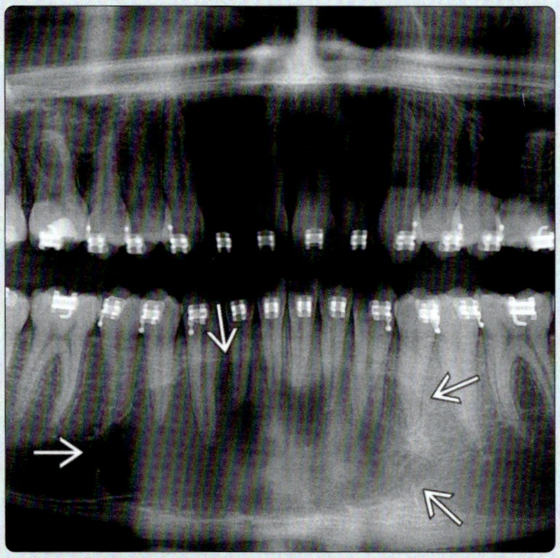

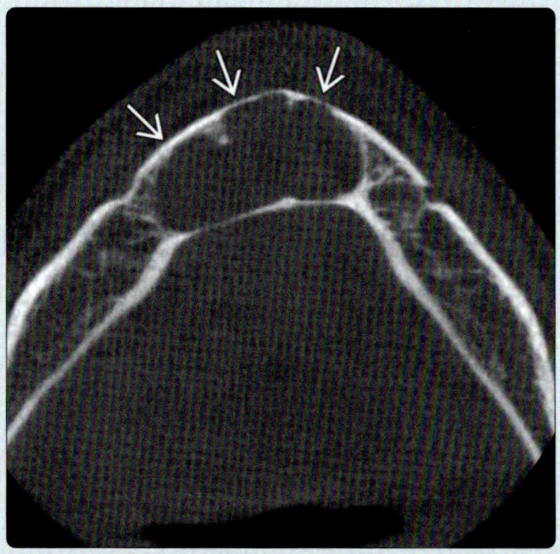

(Left) *Coronal CBCT in the same patient shows the lesion is unilocular and exhibits a scalloped appearance along the inferior cortex ➔.* **(Right)** *Cross section CBCT images in the same patient are shown. Endosteal scalloping ➔ is evident along the lingual cortex (left) in a slice to the left of the mandibular midline. In the midline (right), the lesion shows expansion and thinning of the lingual cortex ➔ and scalloping buccally ➔. Simple bone cysts most commonly occur in the mandible of young patients in their 2nd decade.*

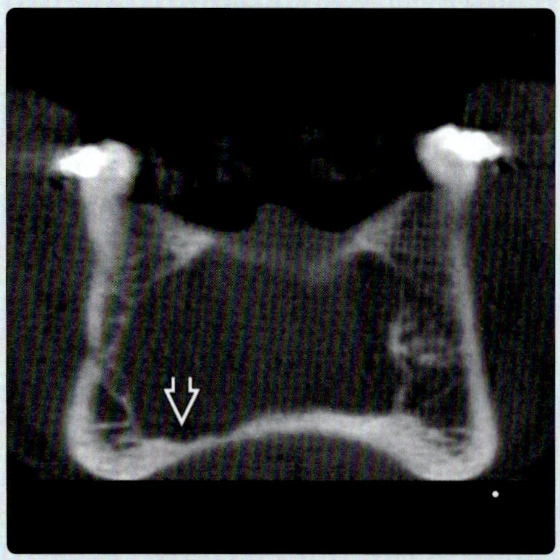

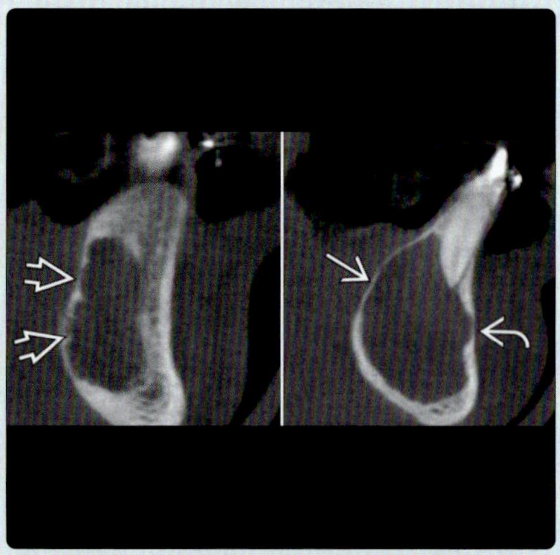

TERMINOLOGY

Abbreviations

- Simple bone cyst (SBC)

Synonyms

- Solitary bone cyst, hemorrhagic bone cyst, idiopathic bone cavity, extravasation cyst, unicameral bone cyst

Definitions

- Solitary, empty or partially empty, bony cavity
  - "Cyst" designation misnomer: Lacks epithelial lining

IMAGING

General Features

- Best diagnostic clue
  - **Unilocular, corticated, radiolucency** in mandible
- Location
  - Anywhere in mandible, including condyle; most common in posterior molar regions, ramus
  - Maxillary lesions rare; more common in females
- Size
  - Typically 1 cm or larger at time of discovery
- Morphology
  - Well defined, unilocular; rarely multilocular

Radiographic Findings

- Intraoral plain film
  - Well-defined radiolucency superimposed over or below root apices; may **scallop** up between teeth
  - May appear multilocular due to **endosteal scalloping**
  - Lamina dura & periodontal ligament space intact; **teeth vital**

CT Findings

- CECT
  - Mildly enhancing at periphery
- CBCT & bone CT
  - Solitary, well-corticated, **unilocular** radiolucency
  - Typically **nonexpansile**; if present, mild
  - Bone margins uniform but may see **endosteal scalloping**

MR Findings

- T2WI
  - Homogeneous hyperintensity without fluid-fluid levels

DIFFERENTIAL DIAGNOSIS

Osteoporotic Bone Marrow Defect

- Large bone marrow space may mimic SBC
- Normal anatomic variant: Middle-aged women

Odontogenic Keratocyst

- Older patients (> 30 years old)
- Little expansion in mandible & may be indistinguishable from SBC if unilocular

Lateral Periodontal Cyst

- Unilocular radiolucency between **vital** teeth
- Lamina dura & periodontal ligament space intact
- Mandibular premolar area: Older males

Periapical (Radicular) Cyst

- Radiolucent lesion at root apex of **nonvital tooth**
- Lamina dura & periodontal ligament space is **lost at apex** of associated tooth

Langerhans Histiocytosis

- Well-defined, unilocular, **punched-out** radiolucency
- Does not have corticated margin

Central Giant Cell Granuloma

- Usually **multilocular** & expansile; anterior mandible

Aneurysmal Bone Cyst

- Fluid-fluid levels on T2WI MR; **very expansile**

PATHOLOGY

General Features

- Etiology
  - Unknown: Previously thought to occur from medullary infarct following trauma but < 1/2 associated with prior trauma
- Associated abnormalities
  - Frequently seen with **lesions of osseous dysplasia**, less commonly with osteomas & hypercementosis

Gross Pathologic & Surgical Features

- Empty/partially empty bone cavity with "straw-colored" fluid or old necrosis

Microscopic Features

- Cystic cavity with connective tissue membrane; **no epithelial lining**

CLINICAL ISSUES

Presentation

- Most common signs/symptoms
  - Incidental finding on imaging
- Other signs/symptoms
  - Pain, swelling if associated with trauma

Demographics

- Age
  - Most in 2nd decade: Lesions associated with florid osseous dysplasia are seen in 5th decade

Natural History & Prognosis

- Lesions can spontaneously resolve: Healing bone may appear **granular**
- Low recurrence rate reported

Treatment

- Surgical exploration & curettage to stimulate bleeding & promote healing
- As lesions may spontaneously heal, conservative radiographic follow-up may be alternative to surgery in very young patients with small lesions

SELECTED REFERENCES

1. Fernandes DT et al: Florid osseous dysplasia associated with multiple simple bone cysts: a patient with 22 years of follow-up. Gen Dent. 64(2):21-5, 2016
2. Xindi J et al: [Simple bone cyst of the jaw: a retrospective study of 11 cases.] Hua Xi Kou Qiang Yi Xue Za Zhi. 34(3):272-6, 2016

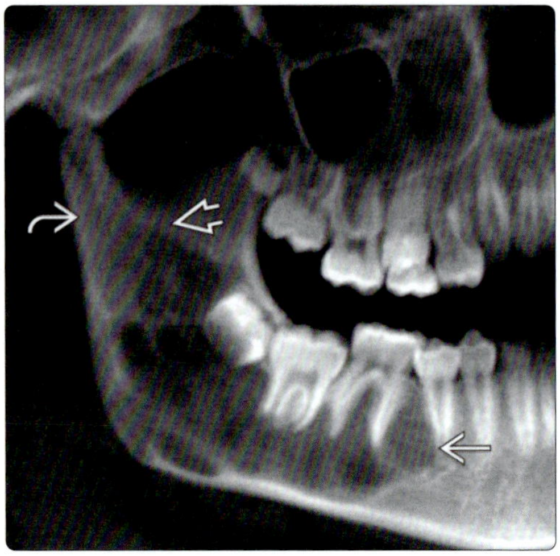

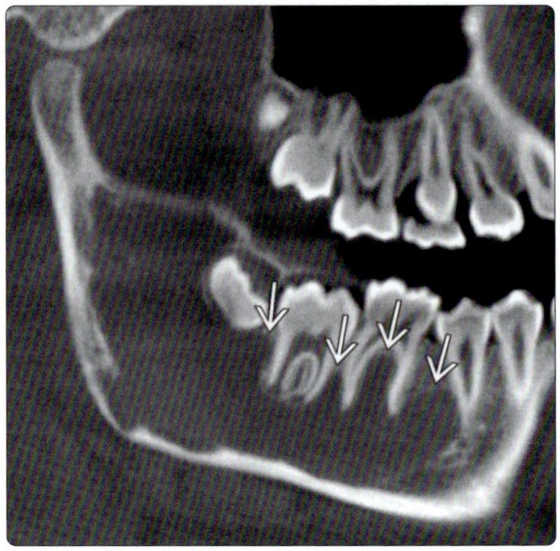

(Left) *Panoramic reformat CBCT in an 11-year-old boy shows what appears to be a large multilocular radiolucency extending from the distal of the right mandibular 2nd premolar posteriorly into the ramus almost to the mandibular notch and condylar neck. (Courtesy P. Hawkins, DDS.)* **(Right)** *Sagittal CBCT slice in the same patient shows the lesion is unilocular with no evidence of septa, typical of a simple bone cyst. Note scalloping between the teeth and roots. (Courtesy P. Hawkins, DDS.)*

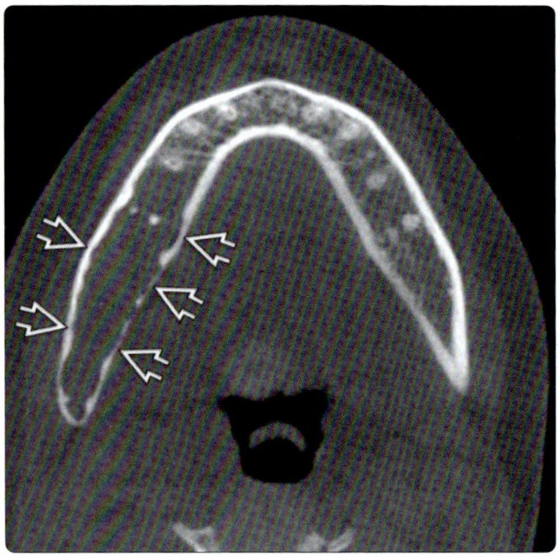

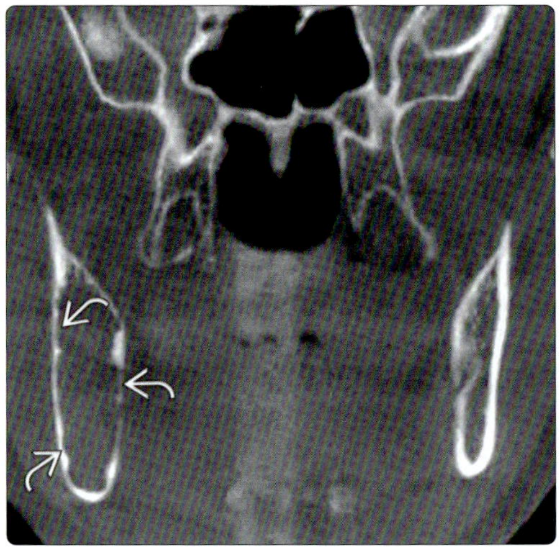

(Left) *Axial CBCT in the same patient shows endosteal scalloping along the buccal and lingual cortices. This may give the appearance of septa on plain radiographs, prompting a differential for multilocular lesions. Note minimal expansion despite size of lesion. (Courtesy P. Hawkins, DDS.)* **(Right)** *Coronal CBCT in the same patient shows the scalloping along the buccal and lingual cortices, which are thinned. The cavity was empty on surgical exploration. (Courtesy P. Hawkins, DDS.)*

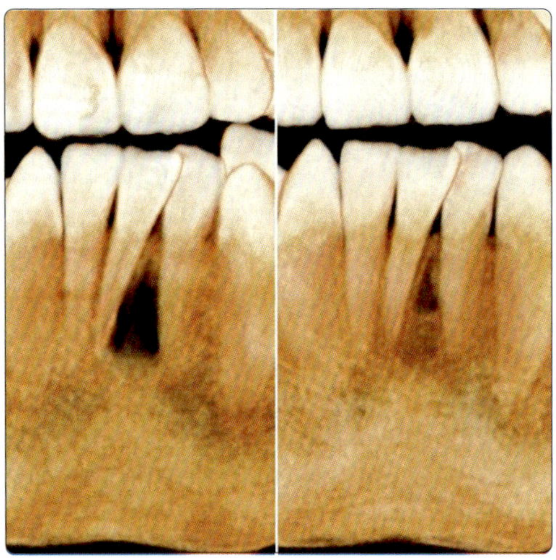

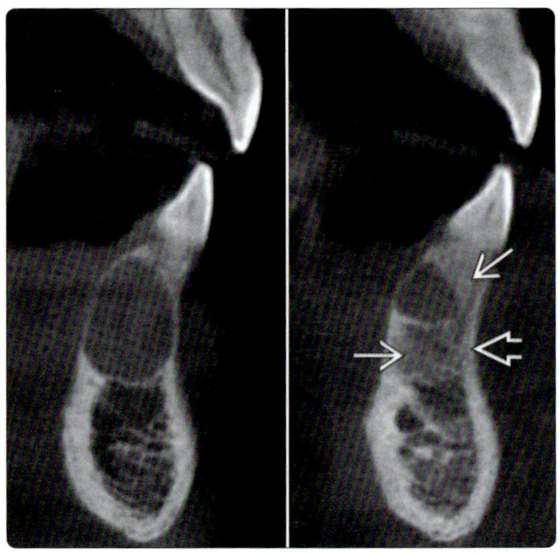

(Left) *Coronal 3D CBCT images show a simple bone cyst in the anterior mandible (left) in an 11-year-old girl. Eight months later, following simple curettage, the lesion has decreased in size (right). (Courtesy W. Pietz, DDS.)* **(Right)** *Cross section CBCT images in the same patient show the initial lesion (left) as a unilocular radiolucency with thin, mildly expanded cortices. The lesion 8 months later (right) shows a granular healing bone pattern and regeneration of the buccal cortex. (Courtesy W. Pietz, DDS.)*

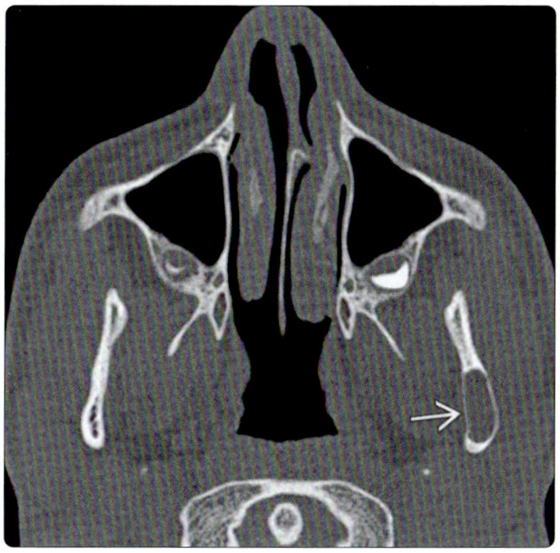
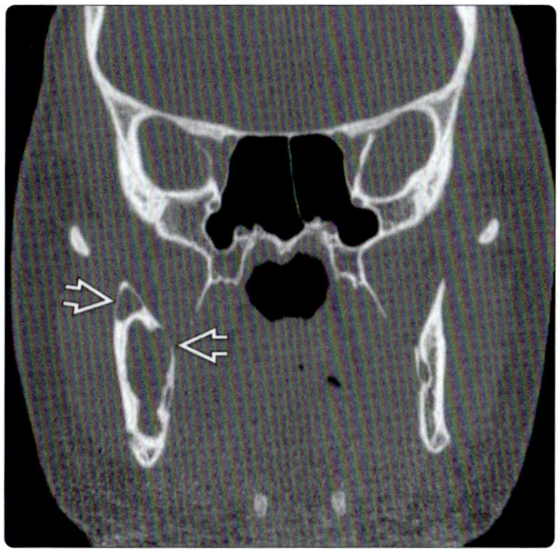

(Left) *Axial bone CT shows a unilocular radiolucency ➔ in the posterosuperior aspect of the left mandibular ramus. The lesion is well defined, and the cortices are thinned and mildly expanded without dehiscence. Surgical exploration demonstrated a simple bone cyst.* **(Right)** *Coronal bone CT demonstrates a simple bone cyst involving and mildly expanding the posterior mandibular right body, angle, and ramus compared to normal contralateral side. The buccal and lingual cortices are thinned ➔.*

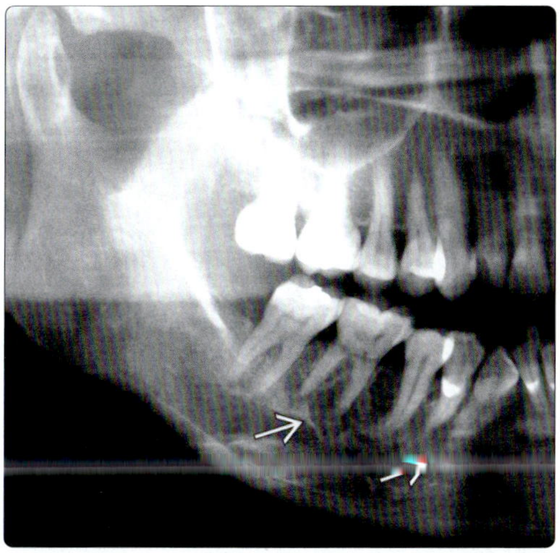
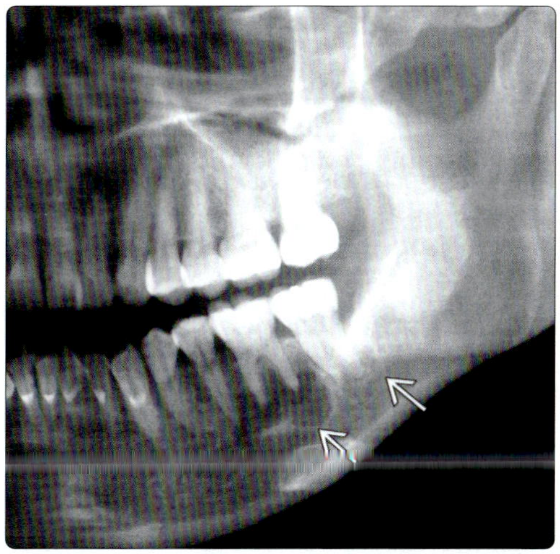

(Left) *Panoramic radiograph shows simple bone cysts ➔ in the right mandible associated with lesions of florid osseous dysplasia (FOD). Patients with FOD are typically middle-aged black women, so these simple bone cysts occur in an older age group than nonassociated lesions. (Courtesy E. Lam, DDS.)* **(Right)** *Panoramic radiograph in the same patient shows similar lesions ➔ of simple bone cyst on the left side of the mandible. (Courtesy E. Lam, DDS.)*

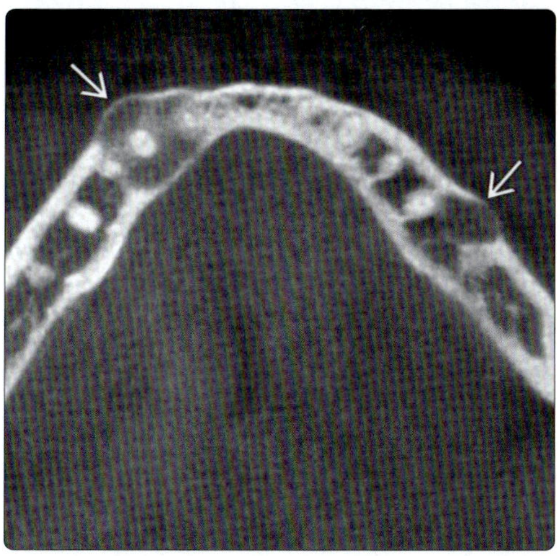
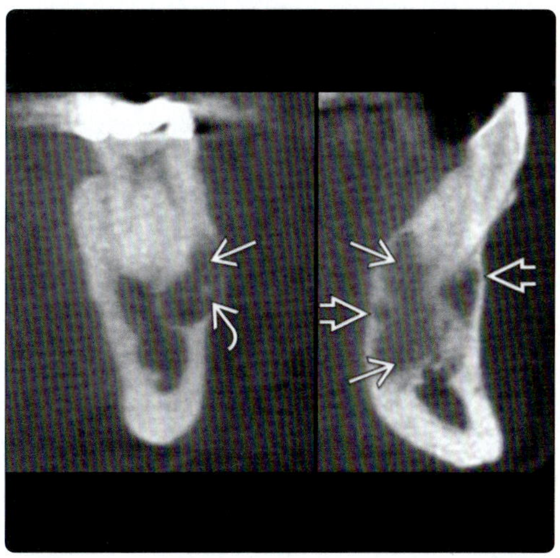

(Left) *Axial CBCT shows 2 lesions of osseous dysplasia with likely associated simple bone cysts. Note mild thinning and expansion ➔ of the buccal cortices.* **(Right)** *Cross section CBCT images in the same patient show the granular appearance ➔ of the lesions possibly representing spontaneous resolution of the simple bone cysts. Note radiopacity ➔ of osseous dysplasia in left mandibular 1st molar lesion (left) and endosteal scalloping ➔ in right mandibular canine lesion (right).*

Periapical Osseous Dysplasia

KEY FACTS

TERMINOLOGY

- Definition: Nonneoplastic localized replacement of normal trabecular bone at tooth apex
- Contains fibrous tissue and cementum-like material &/or abnormal bone

IMAGING

- Most common **at apex** of 1 or more **vital** mandibular incisors (77%) but can form anywhere
- Early stage: Entirely radiolucent
- Intermediate stage: Gradual deposition of **pearl-like** cemental masses within radiolucency
- Late stage: Uniformly radiopaque, sometimes **crescent-shaped** masses cupping apex of tooth
- ± hypercementosis of involved tooth

TOP DIFFERENTIAL DIAGNOSES

- Apical rarefying osteitis
- Florid osseous dysplasia
- Central ossifying fibroma
- Cementoblastoma
- Chronic osteomyelitis

PATHOLOGY

- Simple bone cysts may form in large lesions, can become secondarily infected

CLINICAL ISSUES

- Most common in **4th-5th decades**
- **F:M = 9:1**
- Most common in **blacks** and **Asians**
- Usually asymptomatic
- Tooth is **vital**
- Treatment: **None** unless secondarily infected
- **Biopsy contraindicated** due to risk of infection

DIAGNOSTIC CHECKLIST

- In early stage, consider periapical pulpal inflammatory disease: **Check tooth vitality**

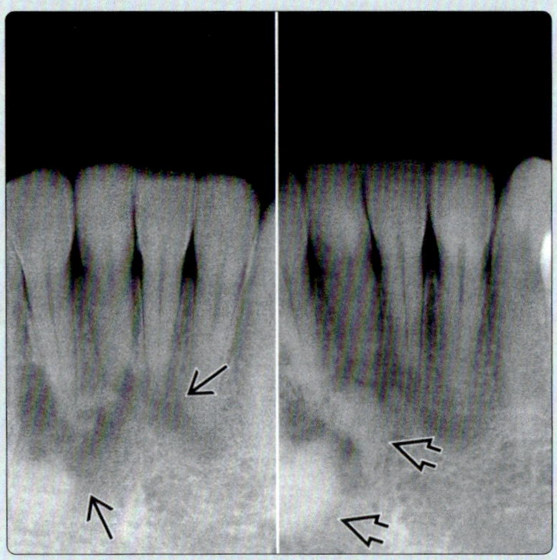

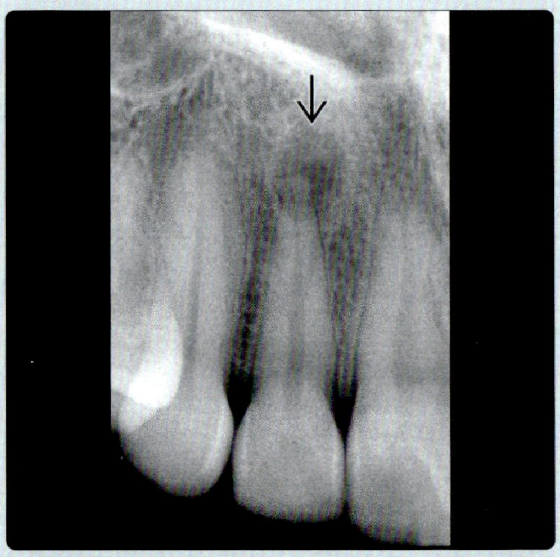

(Left) *Periapical radiographs of the mandibular incisors in the same patient taken 7 years apart show maturation of periapical osseous dysplasia (POD). Well-defined radiolucencies → with a broad sclerotic rim are centered over the apices (early stage). Well-defined radiopaque material ⇨ has formed in the former radiolucent areas over time (intermediate stage).* **(Right)** *Periapical radiograph shows early POD → in a maxillary tooth. The periodontal ligament space is visible, which distinguishes the lesion from a radicular cyst.*

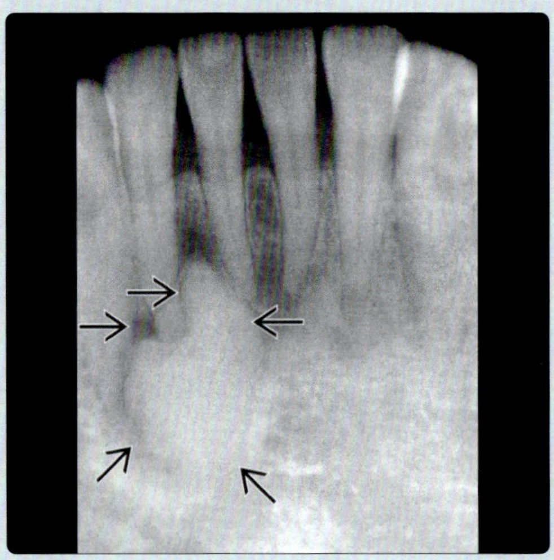

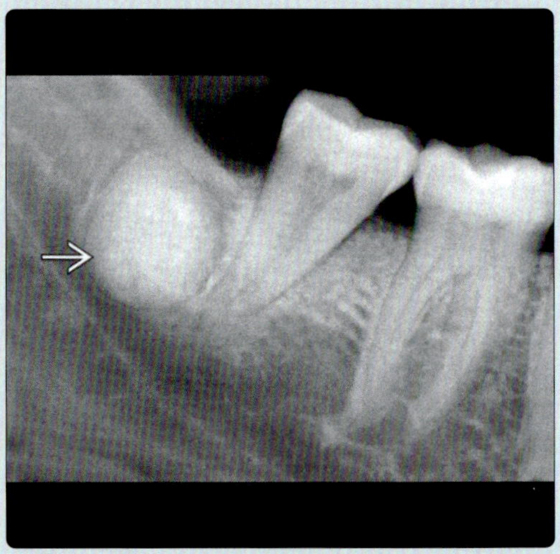

(Left) *Periapical radiograph shows a well-defined radiopaque lesion of mature POD, with a narrow radiolucent border →, at the apex of the mandibular right lateral incisor. The root is distinct from the lesion, which differentiates from cementoblastoma.* **(Right)** *Periapical radiograph shows a well-defined whorled radiopacity surrounded by a narrow radiolucent periphery in the mandibular 3rd molar area representing mature POD ➡. The lesion may have persisted and grown after extraction of the molar.*

TERMINOLOGY

Abbreviations

- Periapical osseous dysplasia (POD)

Synonyms

- Periapical, cemental, or cementoosseous dysplasia, focal cementoosseous dysplasia, cementoma, fibrocementoma, periapical osteofibrosis, sclerosing cementoma, periapical fibroosteoma, periapical fibrous dysplasia

Definitions

- Nonneoplastic localized replacement of normal trabecular bone at tooth apex due to reactive or dysplastic process
- Contains fibrous tissue and cementum-like material &/or abnormal bone

IMAGING

General Features

- Best diagnostic clue
  - Usually well-defined **radiolucency with sclerotic rim**
  - May contain varying amounts of **well-defined radiopaque** material located at **apex** of **vital** tooth
  - Radiologic appearance depends on **stage of lesion maturation**
  - Often **multiple** teeth involved
- Location
  - Most common at apex of 1 or more **mandibular incisors** (77%) but can form in any tooth-bearing area
  - Lesion **centered over apex** of involved tooth
  - Other mandibular teeth less commonly affected
  - Maxillary teeth least commonly affected
    - If maxillary teeth involved, usually also have mandibular lesions
  - May form in alveolus **after tooth extraction**
    - Lesion outline round or ovoid
    - Radiopaque portion often has whorled internal aspect
  - Lesions single or multiple
    - Multiple lesions often bilateral
- Size
  - Most lesions < 1 cm in diameter
    - Adjacent lesions may coalesce to form larger lesions
- Morphology
  - Well defined, occasionally expansile if large

Radiographic Findings

- Radiography
  - Round, oval, or irregular shape
  - Well-defined radiolucent border with band of sclerotic bone of varying width
  - Internal aspect has **varying degree of radiopacity** depending on stage of maturation
  - Lamina dura lost
  - Periodontal ligament space **lost or widened**
  - Root resorption rare, no tooth displacement
  - **± hypercementosis** of involved tooth
  - Small lesions located within cortical borders
  - Large lesions may **expand** jaw
    - Cortices maintained but **thinned**
  - **Early** stage
    - Well-defined **radiolucency** centered over tooth apex
    - Periodontal ligament space may be normal or lost, lamina dura usually intact
  - **Intermediate** stage
    - Radiopacities form within radiolucent area but radiolucent periphery maintained
      - Radiopacities may have round, oval, or irregular shape, will enlarge and coalesce
      - Radiopacities may be well defined and resemble **pearls** or **crescents**
    - Occasionally has **granular** pattern, similar to fibrous dysplasia
  - **Late** stage
    - Internal aspect uniformly **radiopaque** with smooth surface
    - When centered over tooth root, radiopacity often **crescent-shaped** with most convex aspect oriented apically
    - Periodontal ligament space may appear lost or widened
    - May or may not have thin radiolucent margin
    - Presence of prominent radiolucency in involved area indicates formation of **secondary simple bone cyst**
    - Occasional mild expansion with intact but thin cortex
  - May see **various stages** of development in different teeth if multiple teeth involved

CT Findings

- Bone CT
  - Shows extent of involvement
  - May show expansion, which is not evident in dental films

Imaging Recommendations

- Best imaging tool
  - Periapical intraoral radiograph or panoramic radiograph
  - CT recommended if secondary infection to determine extent of involvement

DIFFERENTIAL DIAGNOSIS

Apical Rarefying Osteitis

- Tooth is **nonvital**
- Tooth may have caries or deep restoration
- No radiopacity within radiolucency: Indistinguishable from **early stage** of POD

Florid Osseous Dysplasia

- Similar to POD but larger lesions
- Often involves all **4 quadrants**
- More jaw **expansion** than POD
- Simple bone cysts more often associated

Central Ossifying Fibroma

- Well defined
- Slow expansion around epicenter, greater than POD
- Tooth displacement, root divergence common
- **Solitary**
- Internal radiopaque component fine and evenly distributed

Cementoblastoma

- **Attached** to root surface
- May resorb root or disappear into lesion
- **Solitary**
- Clinical symptoms of pain

Odontoma

- Compound type has **tooth-like** structures
- Radiopacity has density of dentin &/or enamel
- Well defined, corticated
- Uniform, narrow, radiolucent soft tissue capsule
- **Solitary**

Idiopathic Osteosclerosis (Dense Bone Island)

- No radiolucent periphery
- Periphery **irregular**, jagged, or flame-like
- Often blends with buccal or lingual cortex

Chronic Osteomyelitis

- Areas of sclerosis may occur near apex
- Not restricted to tooth-bearing areas
- Symptomatic: Cyclic episodes of pain and swelling

PATHOLOGY

General Features

- Associated abnormalities
  - **Simple bone cysts** may form in large lesions
    - Scalloping radiolucency, which may contain radiopaque portions of POD
    - Often expands jaw
  - **Infection**: After extraction of associated tooth or if cemental mass exposed to oral environment due to trauma or ridge resorption

Staging, Grading, & Classification

- Clinical presentations
  - Periapical: In anterior mandible and involves only few adjacent teeth
  - Focal: Similar to periapical but with limited number of lesions occurring in posterior jaw quadrant

Gross Pathologic & Surgical Features

- Easily fragmented hemorrhagic mass of gritty tissue
- Cannot be shelled out; often removed with difficulty and in fragments

Microscopic Features

- Mixture of bone and cementum-like material in fibrous stroma

CLINICAL ISSUES

Presentation

- Most common signs/symptoms
  - Usually asymptomatic **incidental** finding
  - Tooth is **vital**
- Other signs/symptoms
  - Occasionally painful
  - May expand jaw

Demographics

- Age
  - Most common in **4th-5th decades**, although occasionally seen in younger patients
- Gender
  - **F:M = 9:1**
- Ethnicity
  - Most common in **blacks** and **Asians**

Natural History & Prognosis

- Undergoes maturation stages whereby lesions become more radiopaque with time
- Lesions enlarge over time
- May progress to florid osseous dysplasia
- Simple bone cyst may form in 1 or more areas of involvement
- Occasionally, lesions become **infected** if exposed to oral environment
  - POD acts as sequestrum and must be removed

Treatment

- **None** usually indicated
- If involved tooth extracted or area of POD exposed to oral environment due to trauma or alveolar ridge resorption, removal of associated lesion is advised to prevent secondary infection
- **Biopsy not recommended** due to risk of secondary infection
- Diagnosis usually evident based on radiographic appearance, patient demographics, and tooth vitality test result
- Periodic radiographic follow-up to monitor for development of simple bone cyst
  - If simple bone cyst develops, treatment of cyst and removal of POD recommended, depending on extent of POD involvement

DIAGNOSTIC CHECKLIST

Consider

- Must test tooth vitality, especially in early radiolucent lesions to **differentiate POD from inflammatory disease**
- Differential diagnosis depends on lesion maturation stage and secondary infection or simple bone cyst development may complicate differential diagnosis

Image Interpretation Pearls

- Lesion centered over tooth apex, often multiple teeth involved
- Radiopaque internal cemental masses often have well-defined, round, pearl-like, or crescent shapes
- Look for surrounding thin radiolucent line and broad band of sclerosis

SELECTED REFERENCES

1. Senia ES et al: Periapical cemento-osseous dysplasia: a case report with twelve-year follow-up and review of literature. Int Endod J. 48(11):1086-99, 2015
2. de Noronha Santos Netto J et al: Benign fibro-osseous lesions: clinicopathologic features from 143 cases diagnosed in an oral diagnosis setting. Oral Surg Oral Med Oral Pathol Oral Radiol. 115(5):e56-65, 2013
3. Eskandarloo A et al: CBCT findings of periapical cemento-osseous dysplasia: a case report. Imaging Sci Dent. 43(3):215-8, 2013
4. Alsufyani NA et al: Cemento-osseous dysplasia of the jaw bones: key radiographic features. Dentomaxillofac Radiol. 40(3):141-6, 2011
5. MacDonald-Jankowski DS: Fibro-osseous lesions of the face and jaws. Clin Radiol. 2004 Jan;59(1):11-25. Review. Erratum in: Clin Radiol. 64(1):107, 2009
6. Kawai T et al: Cemento-osseous dysplasia of the jaws in 54 Japanese patients: a radiographic study. Oral Surg Oral Med Oral Pathol Oral Radiol Endod. 87(1):107-14, 1999
7. Su L et al: Distinguishing features of focal cemento-osseous dysplasia and cemento-ossifying fibromas. II. A clinical and radiologic spectrum of 316 cases. Oral Surg Oral Med Oral Pathol Oral Radiol Endod. 84(5):540-9, 1997
8. Waldron CA: Fibro-osseous lesions of the jaws. J Oral Maxillofac Surg. 51(8):828-35, 1993

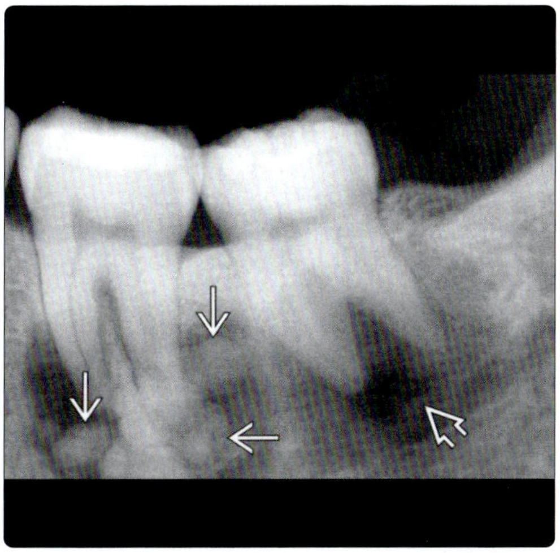

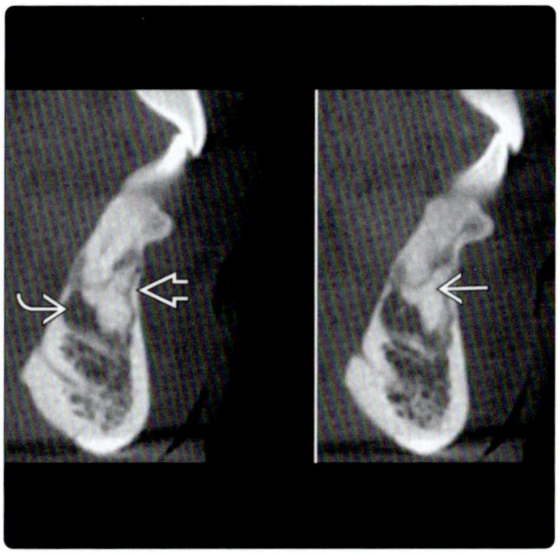

(Left) *Periapical radiograph shows POD at the mandibular 1st and 2nd molar apices. The pearl-like radiopacities represent cemental masses (intermediate-stage POD). The lesion at the apex of the 2nd molar is entirely radiolucent (early-stage POD).* **(Right)** *Cross-section CBCT shows a crescent-shaped, irregular cemental mass at the central incisor apex. Note the thin radiolucent line on the buccal aspect and thinning of the buccal and lingual cortices. The radiolucent area is suggestive of simple bone cyst formation.*

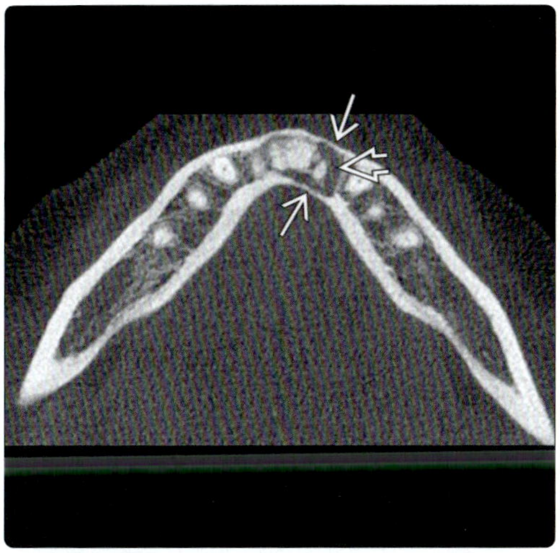

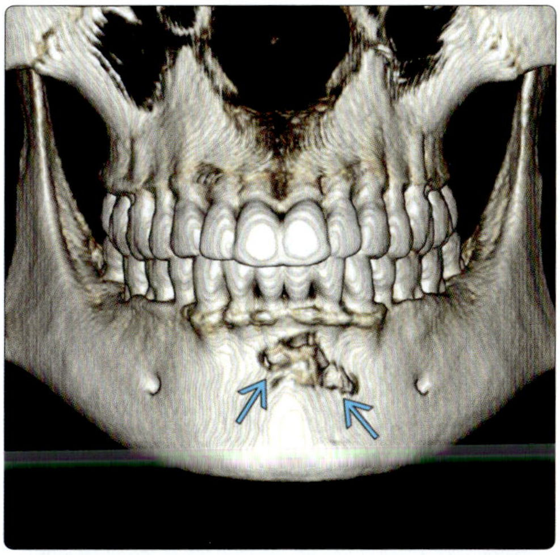

(Left) *Axial CBCT in the same patient shows thinning of the buccal and lingual cortical plates and a broader zone of radiolucency on the distal aspect of the lesion that suggests development of an associated simple bone cyst.* **(Right)** *Frontal CBCT 3D reformat of the same patient shows the extent of POD involvement and irregular lesion outline. An intact buccal cortex is present but the thinned cortex is not visible due to CT volume averaging.*

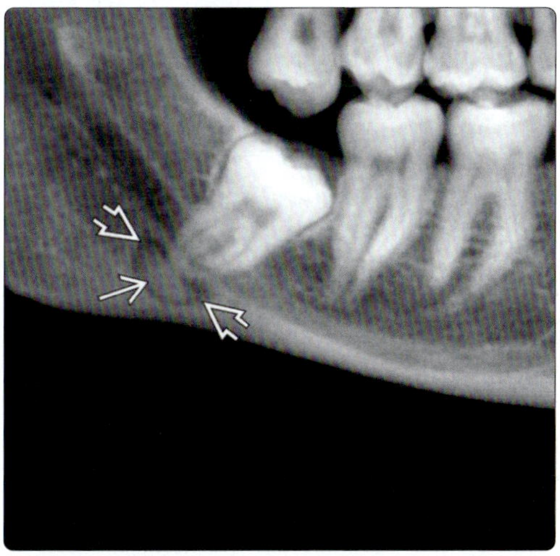

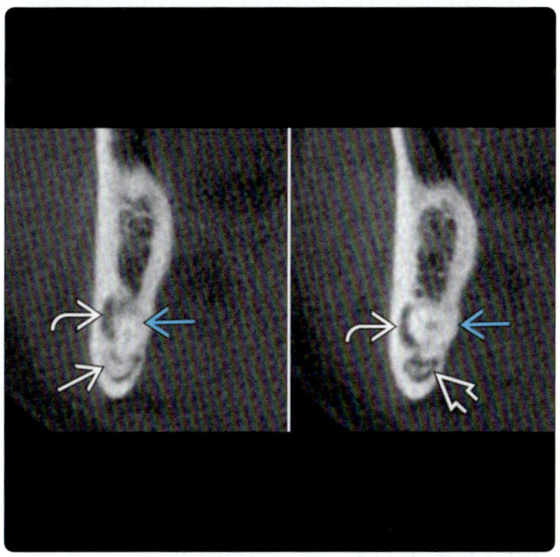

(Left) *Panoramic CBCT reformat shows an impacted mandibular right 3rd molar with a crescent-shaped radiopacity representing a central cemental mass surrounded by a radiolucent line of variable width (intermediate-stage POD) at the apex of the tooth.* **(Right)** *Cross-section CBCT of the same patient shows a typical crescent-shaped central radiopacity at the molar apex surrounded by a thin radiolucent line. The mandibular canal is located buccal to the root apex.*

Florid Osseous Dysplasia

KEY FACTS

TERMINOLOGY

- Definition: Extensive form of **periapical osseous dysplasia (POD) affecting 3 or more quadrants** or widespread involvement in 1 jaw

IMAGING

- Mandible > maxilla if only 1 jaw involved
- Well defined, often expansile
  - Wide radiolucent margins if secondary infection
- Lesions > 1 cm; **above mandibular canal**
- **Densely radiopaque globular masses** with less well-defined areas of radiolucent/radiopaque patterns

TOP DIFFERENTIAL DIAGNOSES

- **POD**
- Paget disease
- Osteomyelitis
- Fibrous dysplasia
- Gardner Syndrome

CLINICAL ISSUES

- **Teeth vital**
- Usually incidental finding unless secondary infection from mucosal irritation, ulceration from prosthesis, periodontal or dental disease
  - Pain, sequestration, fistulous tract, ulceration
- **4th-5th decades**; mean age: 42 years
- **Females** > males; commonly in **blacks** and Asians
- Lesions mature and become larger and more radiopaque with time
- **Simple bone cyst may form** in 1 or more areas

DIAGNOSTIC CHECKLIST

- **Biopsy avoided** due to risk of secondary infection
- Diagnosis based on radiographic appearance, patient demographics, and tooth vitality
- Interpretation pearl: **Multiple widespread involvement in tooth-bearing areas**

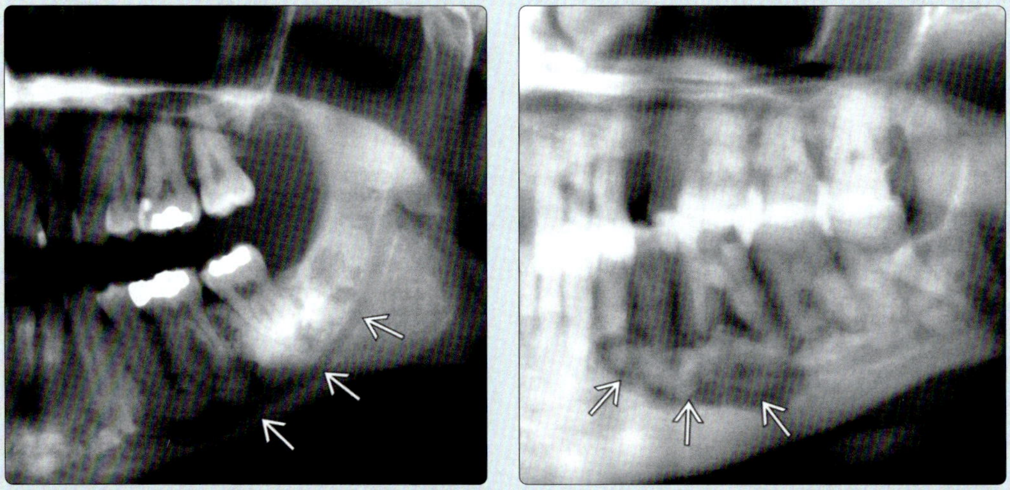

(Left) *Panoramic radiograph shows florid osseous dysplasia (FOD) above the mandibular canal. The right side (not shown) is similarly affected, but the maxilla is spared.* **(Right)** *Panoramic radiograph shows radiopaque foci of FOD in the left mandible. The lesion apical to the mandibular left bicuspids and 1st molar has a broad radiolucent border indicating secondary infection. A possible etiology of the infection is periodontal disease.*

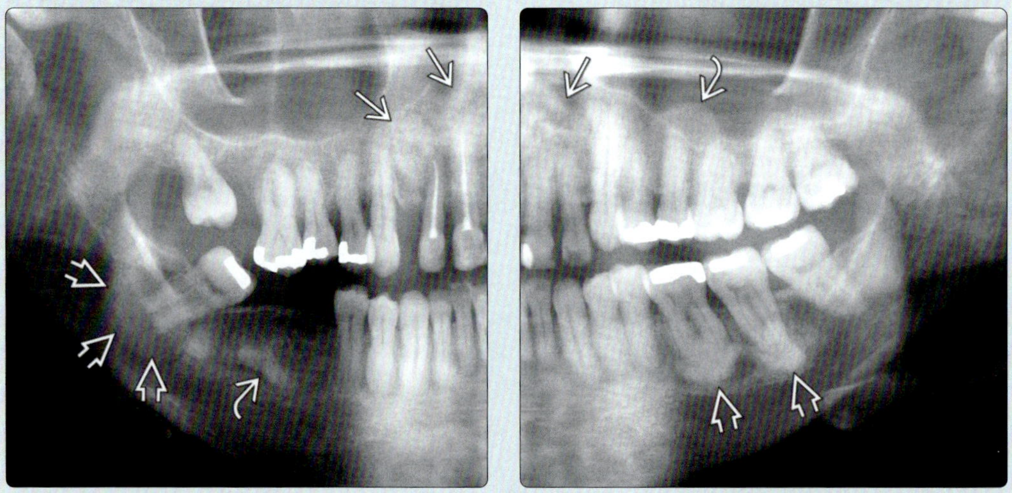

(Left) *Panoramic radiograph of the right side shows mature radiopaque lesions of FOD in the anterior maxilla. Granular pattern is seen apical to the mandibular molar and an irregular radiopacity with a surrounding radiolucent zone is seen in the edentulous area.* **(Right)** *Panoramic radiograph of the left side of the same patient shows the extent of the maxillary lesions. Crescent-shaped radiopacities are apical to the 1st and 2nd mandibular molar roots. Note the mucous retention pseudocyst in the left maxillary sinus.*

TERMINOLOGY

Abbreviations

- Florid osseous dysplasia (FOD)

Synonyms

- Florid cementoosseous dysplasia, florid-ossifying dysplasia, gigantiform cementoma, familial multiple cementomas, multiple periapical osteofibromatosis, familial gigantiform cementoma, sclerotic cemental masses

Definitions

- Extensive form of periapical osseous dysplasia (POD) affecting 3 or more quadrants or widespread involvement in 1 jaw
  - **"Florid" indicates multiquadrant involvement**
- Nonneoplastic process confined to tooth-bearing areas of jaws
- Normal trabecular bone replaced with dense acellular cemental and osseous tissue in fibrous tissue stroma

IMAGING

General Features

- Best diagnostic clue
  - Multiple, often symmetrical jaw involvement
  - Most common presentation: Densely sclerotic globular masses
- Location
  - Usually bilateral, symmetrical
  - Affects both jaws in tooth-bearing areas
    - **Above mandibular canal** in mandible
      - Not seen in ramus
    - **Secondary simple bone cysts** may extend to inferior mandibular cortical border
  - Lesion epicenters at tooth apices
  - Usually affects bicuspid and molar teeth, but all teeth may be involved
  - Mandible most commonly affected if only 1 jaw involved
  - **Can cross midline**
- Size
  - Lesion diameter > 1 cm
- Morphology
  - Well defined, often expansile

Imaging Recommendations

- Best imaging tool
  - Panoramic radiograph
  - Bone algorithm CT or CBCT to examine lesion extent, secondary infection, or development of simple bone cyst
  - CT or **CBCT best to depict expansion** since expansion may be mild

Radiographic Findings

- Radiography
  - Similar appearance to maturation stages of POD
    - Densely **radiopaque globular masses** in association with less well-defined areas of mixed radiolucent/radiopaque patterns
  - Sclerotic border
    - Mature lesions may be ill defined
    - Wide radiolucent margins if secondary infection
  - Lamina dura around affected roots may be lost
  - Inferior displacement of mandibular canal
  - Expansion may be slight or prominent
    - Enlarging, well-defined radiolucency suggests **development of secondary simple bone cyst**
  - Maxillary sinus floor unaffected or elevated but intact

CT Findings

- CBCT
  - Large expansile masses with varying degrees of radiopacity
    - Opaque areas continuous with root apices
  - Roots may have **hypercementosis**
    - Cemental tissue of lesion may fuse with hypercementosis

DIFFERENTIAL DIAGNOSIS

Periapical Cemental Dysplasia

- POD is localized form of FOD
- POD lesions smaller (< 1 cm) and **not expansile**
- Usually anterior mandible in association with **vital incisor teeth**
- Same demographics as FOD
  - Females > males
  - 4th and 5th decades
  - More common in blacks and Asians

Paget Disease

- Systemic bone disease
  - Affects all bones, especially skull
  - **Affects entire mandible or maxilla**; FOD affects only tooth-bearing areas
- Typically described as **cotton wool** radiographic appearance
- Radiopacities not surrounded by radiolucent border
- More common in **white men** in 5th or 6th decade
- Increased serum alkaline phosphatase

Osteomyelitis

- Inflammation of bone marrow
- **Sequestra** are hallmark
  - Cemental masses of FOD may resemble sequestra
  - Wider radiolucent border in infected FOD
- Osteomyelitis usually presents as diffuse radiopacity with ill-defined borders
- Usually only 1 segment of jaw involved; FOD affects multiple quadrants
- FOD lesions may become secondarily infected so will see features of both FOD and osteomyelitis
- Patient is often symptomatic: Febrile, lymphadenopathy, sinus tracts

Fibrous Dysplasia

- Nonneoplastic condition of bone with formation of dysplastic bone in fibrous connective tissue
- Young females
- **Unilateral expansion**
  - FOD is bilateral in older patients
- Fibrous dysplasia **borders blend with surrounding bone**, and internal structure is granular and often described radiographically as **ground glass**

Gardner Syndrome

- Associated with other skeletal changes, skin tumors, and dental abnormalities

PATHOLOGY

General Features

- Etiology
  - Unknown
- Genetics
  - Familial pattern in some cases
  - May be autosomal dominant
  - Sporadic cases without family history are spontaneous mutations
- Associated abnormalities
  - Simple bone cysts

Staging, Grading, & Classification

- Classification of FOD and POD not clear
  - POD and FOD may represent continuum of disease
  - Diagnosis of FOD is made if **3 or more quadrants involved** or extensive involvement in 1 jaw
- Gigantiform cementoma is familial form of FOD
  - Autosomal dominant, occurs in younger patients than FOD
  - Massive multifocal lesions occurring in all 4 jaw quadrants
- Early stage
  - **Well-defined radiolucencies** at apices of multiple teeth
- Intermediate stage
  - **Radiopacities form** within radiolucent areas
  - Radiopacities round, oval, or irregular shape
  - Radiopacities may be well defined and resemble **pearls** or **crescents**
- Late stage
  - Internal aspect **uniformly radiopaque** with smooth surface
- May see various stages of development in different teeth or quadrants

Microscopic Features

- Variations in amount and size of acellular cementum-like material and irregular trabeculae in fibrous tissue stroma, depending on maturation stage
- Relatively avascular
- **Cannot distinguish between FOD and POD** based on microscopic features; clinical and radiographic features important

CLINICAL ISSUES

Presentation

- Most common signs/symptoms
  - Usually asymptomatic incidental finding unless secondary infection
  - Occasional facial swelling or deformity if lesion(s) expansile
  - **Teeth vital**
- Other signs/symptoms
  - Occasionally painful, even without secondary abnormalities
  - **Secondary infection**: Pain, swelling, sequestration, fistulous tract, mucosal ulceration
  - May have pain with secondary simple bone cyst

Demographics

- Age
  - Most common in 4th-5th decades; mean age: **42 years**
- Gender
  - More common in **females**
- Ethnicity
  - More common in **blacks and Asians**

Natural History & Prognosis

- Undergoes maturation stages whereby lesions become larger and more radiopaque with time
  - Mature lesions are relatively avascular and at risk for secondary infection
- **Simple bone cyst may form** in 1 or more areas of involvement
- Secondary infection common, especially if mucosal irritation and ulceration from prosthesis, periodontal or dental disease

Treatment

- None indicated, but **observe radiographically** to monitor for lesion extent and development of simple bone cysts
- Treatment necessary if secondary infection or simple bone cyst develop
  - Cemental masses act as sequestra and must be removed if in area of secondary infection
- **Avoid biopsy** or elective tooth extraction

DIAGNOSTIC CHECKLIST

Consider

- Teeth are vital unless other dental disease present
- Biopsy not recommended due to risk of secondary infection
- Diagnosis based on radiographic appearance, patient demographics, and tooth vitality test result

Image Interpretation Pearls

- **Multiple widespread involvement in tooth-bearing areas**

SELECTED REFERENCES

1. Akbulut S et al: Maxillectomy for cementifying osseous dysplasia of the maxilla: a case report. Acta Medica (Hradec Kralove). 58(1):32-4, 2015
2. Delai D et al: Florid cemento-osseous dysplasia: a case of misdiagnosis. J Endod. 41(11):1923-6, 2015
3. Thorawat A et al: Familial florid cemento-osseous dysplasia - case report and review of literature. Clin Case Rep. 3(12):1034-7, 2015
4. de Noronha Santos Netto J et al: Benign fibro-osseous lesions: clinicopathologic features from 143 cases diagnosed in an oral diagnosis setting. Oral Surg Oral Med Oral Pathol Oral Radiol. 115(5):e56-65, 2013
5. Kutluay Köklü H et al: Florid cemento-osseous dysplasia: Report of a case documented with clinical, radiographic, biochemical and histological findings. J Clin Exp Dent. 5(1):e58-61, 2013
6. Kumar VV et al: Clinicopathologic conference: multiquadrant expansile fibro-osseous lesion in a juvenile. Oral Surg Oral Med Oral Pathol Oral Radiol. 113(3):286-92, 2012
7. Singer SR et al: Florid cemento-osseous dysplasia and chronic diffuse osteomyelitis report of a simultaneous presentation and review of the literature. J Am Dent Assoc. 136(7):927-31, 2005
8. MacDonald-Jankowski DS: Florid cemento-osseous dysplasia: a systematic review. Dentomaxillofac Radiol. 32(3):141-9, 2003
9. Beylouni I et al: Florid cemento-osseous dysplasia: Report of a case documented with computed tomography and 3D imaging. Oral Surg Oral Med Oral Pathol Oral Radiol Endod. 85(6):707-11, 1998

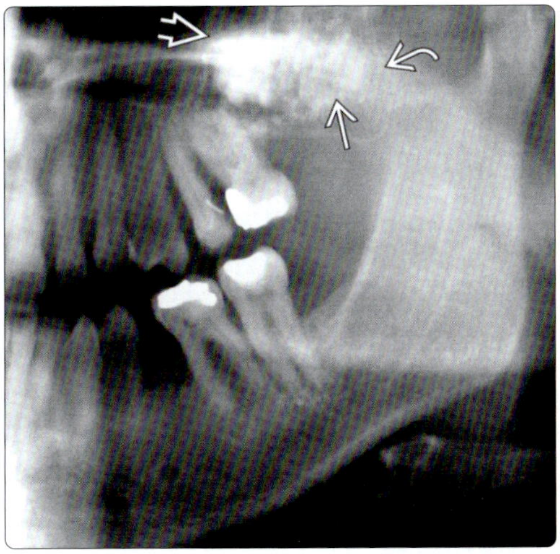

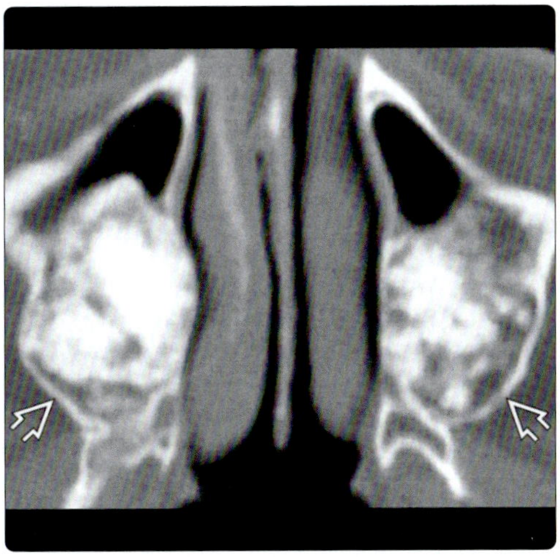

(Left) *Panoramic radiograph shows mature FOD that has expanded the posterior wall of the left maxilla. The lesion has also extended into the maxillary sinus and raised the sinus floor.* **(Right)** *Axial bone CT in the same patient shows bilateral involvement and expansion of the posterior-lateral maxillary sinus borders. The mature radiopaque FOD lesions partially fill the maxillary sinuses, reducing aeration. Note the relative symmetry of the lesions.*

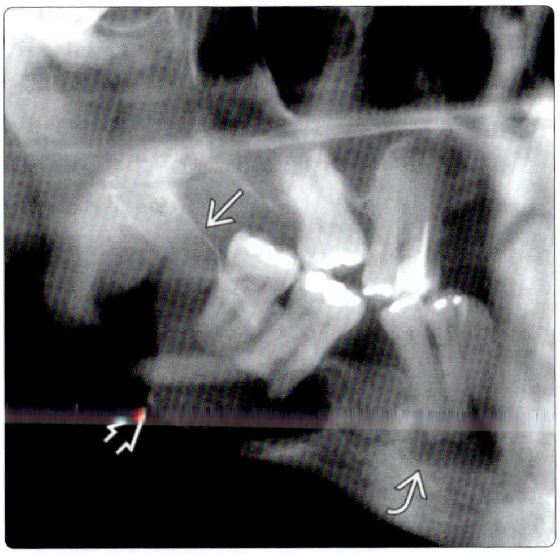

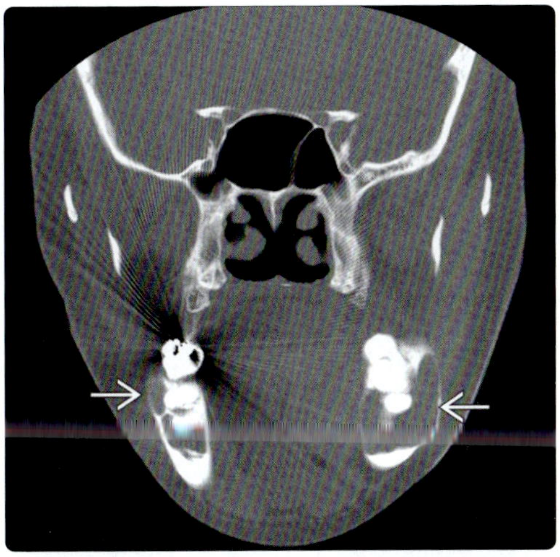

(Left) *Panoramic radiograph shows a large, corticated, scalloping radiolucency in the posterior right mandible, which has expanded the inferior mandibular border and the alveolar crest in the 3rd molar area. A similar, smaller lesion is apical to the bicuspid teeth. These lesions represent simple bone cysts that formed in areas of FOD.* **(Right)** *Coronal bone CT in the same patient shows expansile simple bone cysts affecting both sides of the mandible.*

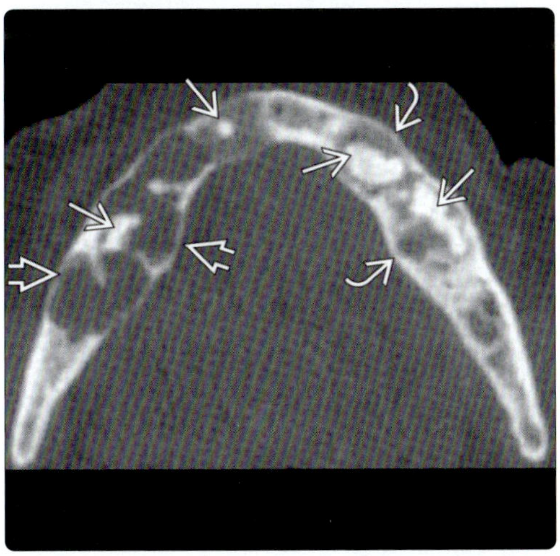

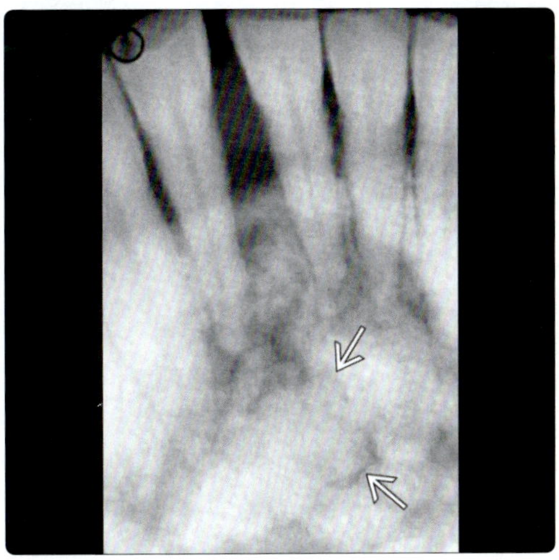

(Left) *Note FOD with bilateral cemental masses. Large radiolucency with thinned & expanded cortical borders indicates secondary simple bone cyst formation on the right side. Widened radiolucent zones with thinned & expanded cortices on the left side indicate additional simple bone cysts.* **(Right)** *Periapical radiograph shows mature FOD in the anterior mandible. Globular radiopacities are surrounded by thin radiolucent lines, which distinguish this from the bone pattern in Paget disease.*

Ossifying Fibroma

KEY FACTS

TERMINOLOGY

- Ossifying fibroma (OF): Encapsulated benign neoplasm composed of varying amounts of bone or cementum-like tissue in fibrous tissue stroma

IMAGING

- Round or oval, well-defined, **expansile** mass with corticated border and variable degree of internal radiopacity
- Most common craniofacial site is mandible (80%)
- Internal aspect can be granular, resembling fibrous dysplasia
- May have **thin, radiolucent periphery** representing fibrous capsule

TOP DIFFERENTIAL DIAGNOSES

- Fibrous dysplasia
- Periapical osseous dysplasia
- Osteogenic sarcoma
- Cementoblastoma

PATHOLOGY

- May be histologically indistinguishable from active form of fibrous dysplasia

CLINICAL ISSUES

- Usually asymptomatic, incidental finding
- Female predominance (70%)
- Any age but most common in 2nd-4th decade
- Slow-growing but occasionally aggressive, especially juvenile subtypes
- Usually **concentric growth**
- Surgical **enucleation or resection**

DIAGNOSTIC CHECKLIST

- Differential diagnosis depends on degree and pattern of internal radiopacity
- Identification of **well-defined margin** helps to **distinguish OF from fibrous dysplasia**

(Left) *Panoramic radiograph shows a large ossifying fibroma (OF) in the left posterior mandible. The inferior border of the mandible is expanded ➡, and the 3rd molar tooth is displaced superiorly ➡. There are large, radiopaque foci ➡ within the lesion.* **(Right)** *Axial bone CT shows a corticated OF in the left mandible. Note the prominent internal radiopacities ➡, symmetrical buccal-lingual expansion, and thin, radiolucent rim ➡ that represents a fibrous tissue capsule.*

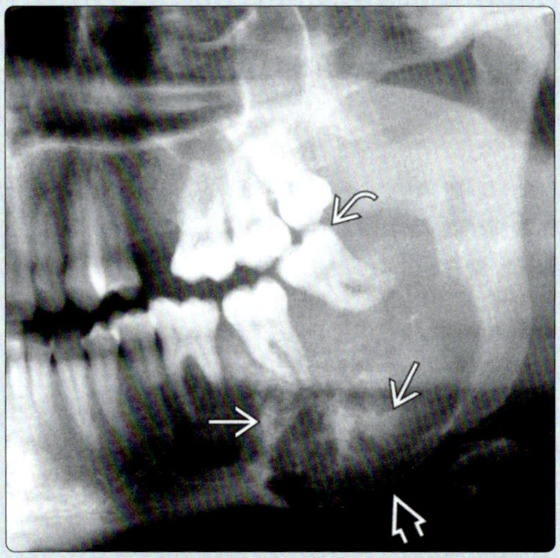

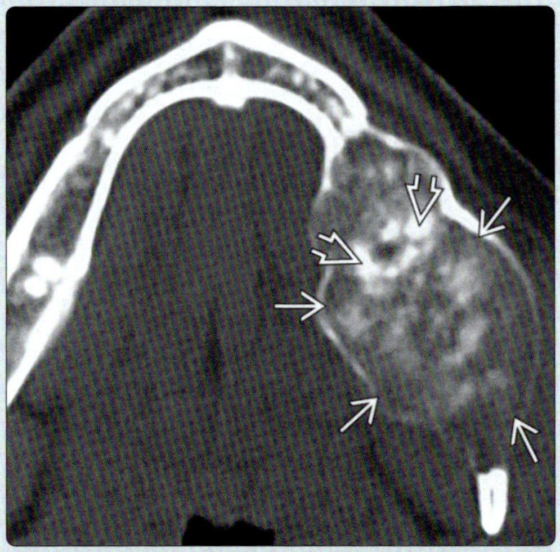

(Left) *Axial bone CT shows a predominantly radiolucent mandibular OF with an undulating border ➡. Air in the central aspect ➡ is a result of a biopsy procedure.* **(Right)** *Occlusal radiograph of the right mandible shows concentric expansion of an OF. The internal aspect is a mixture of granular ➡ and discrete ➡ radiopacities.*

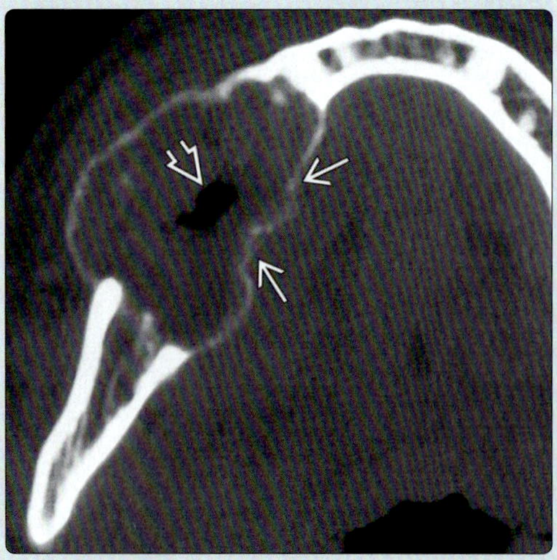

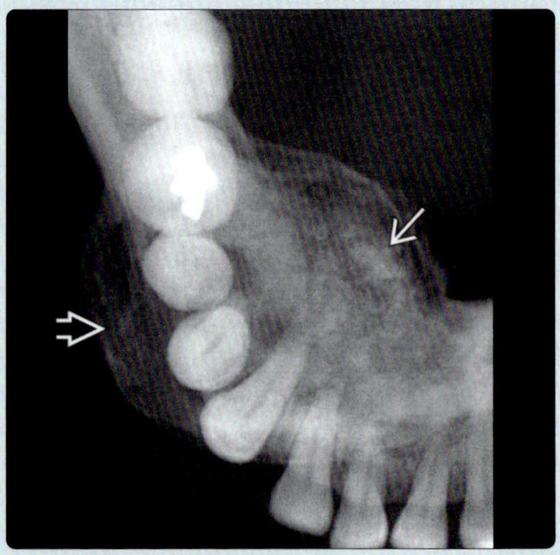

Ossifying Fibroma

TERMINOLOGY

Abbreviations

- Ossifying fibroma (OF)

Synonyms

- Cemento-ossifying fibroma
- Cementifying fibroma
- Fibro-osteoma
- Osteofibroma

Definitions

- Encapsulated, benign neoplasm composed of varying amounts of bone or cementum-like tissue in fibrous tissue stroma

IMAGING

General Features

- Best diagnostic clue
  - Round or oval, well-defined, **expansile mass** with variable degree of internal radiopacity surrounded by **corticated border**
- Location
  - Most common craniofacial site is **mandible** (80%)
    - Mandible: Most common in molar and premolar area
  - Maxilla: Most common in cuspid & zygomatic arch areas
    - Maxillary sinus often involved
  - Other locations: Frontal, ethmoid, sphenoid, temporal, and orbital areas
  - Reports of multiple lesions, sometimes involving both jaws
- Size
  - 0.5-10 cm
- Morphology
  - Round or oval shape, well defined
  - Expansile

Radiographic Findings

- Radiography
  - Often corticated or surrounded by sclerotic bone
    - Cortex thin and eggshell-like in some cases
    - May have **thin, radiolucent periphery** representing fibrous capsule
  - Unilocular more common but may be multilocular
  - Variable degree of radiopacity depending on lesion maturity
    - Ranges from completely radiolucent to radiolucent with scattered, radiopaque foci (most common) to mature, dense internal radiopacity
    - Juvenile psammomatoid subtype: Often has ground-glass bone pattern
    - Juvenile trabecular subtype: Often radiolucent with irregular, scattered calcifications
  - Internal aspect can be granular, resembling fibrous dysplasia
  - Mandibular canal displaced inferiorly
  - Inferior mandibular border often expanded inferiorly and occasionally eroded
  - Maxillary sinus floor displaced superiorly
  - Resorption or displacement of roots
  - Lamina dura of involved teeth missing

CT Findings

- CBCT
  - Well-defined, corticated, expansile, mixed radiopaque-radiolucent lesion

MR Findings

- T1WI
  - Intermediate to low signal throughout tumor
  - Fibrous areas intermediate signal
  - Radiopaque areas hypointense
- T2WI
  - Mixed low and high signal
  - Fibrous areas hyperintense (usually lesion center)
  - Osseous/cemental areas hypointense (usually lesion periphery)
- T1WI C+
  - Moderate **enhancement of outer margin**

Imaging Recommendations

- Best imaging tool
  - Fibroosseous lesions of craniofacial area best studied with bone algorithm CT or CBCT
  - Since OF treated with surgery, T1 C+ FS MR provides best images of affected soft tissues

Nuclear Medicine Findings

- Bone scan
  - Increased uptake in affected area

DIFFERENTIAL DIAGNOSIS

Fibrous Dysplasia

- Replacement of normal bone with fibrous tissue containing foci of immature woven bone
- Poorly defined expansion
- Maintains general **shape of involved bone**
  - OF has tumor-like, concentric expansion
- May be monostotic (70%) or polyostotic (30%)

Periapical Osseous Dysplasia

- Replacement of normal bone with fibrous tissue, cementum, &/or abnormal bone
- Epicenter at **apex of tooth**
- Usually multiple lesions
- No tooth displacement
- If associated simple bone cyst is seen, most likely periapical osseous dysplasia

Osteogenic Sarcoma

- Destructive, aggressive mixed lesion of craniofacial bones
- May see characteristic **"sunray spicules"** periosteal reaction
- More common in males

Cementoblastoma

- True, benign tumor of cementum with capacity for limitless proliferation
- Bulbous, often expansile, growth of cementum **on root of tooth**
- Has similar radiolucent periphery
- Root may be resorbed or disappear into lesion
- Characteristically painful

PATHOLOGY

General Features

- Etiology
  - Thought to arise from mesenchyme of periodontal ligament but not all in dental areas
- Genetics
  - Familial cases described
  - Multiple lesions seen in 30-40% of patients with hyperparathyroidism-jaw tumor syndrome
    - Autosomal dominant, multiple neoplastic syndrome characterized by hyperparathyroidism caused by parathyroid adenoma or adenocarcinoma
- Associated abnormalities
  - Lesions in paranasal sinuses may obstruct sinus drainage pathways and lead to mucocele formation
  - Large lesions may result in cosmetic deformity
    - In maxilla, may cause ocular dysfunction
  - Intracranial extension complicated by tension pneumocephalus has been reported

Staging, Grading, & Classification

- Juvenile subtypes described: Psammomatoid and trabecular
  - Aggressive, higher recurrence rates
  - Most occur in 1st and 2nd decades, but reported range of 3-72 years
  - M = F
  - Psammomatoid subtype occurs more commonly in vicinity of paranasal sinuses
  - Trabecular subtype occurs more commonly in maxilla

Gross Pathologic & Surgical Features

- Specimen usually large and intact because lesion enucleates in 1 piece
- Gritty, gray to white, hard lesion

Microscopic Features

- Encapsulated lesion with highly cellular, predominantly fibrous stroma containing varying amounts of woven bone and cementum-like tissue
- Variable level of expression of fibrous and vascular components
- May be histologically **indistinguishable from active form of fibrous dysplasia**
  - Correct diagnosis may only be achieved when **correlation between clinical, imaging, and pathology findings** completed

CLINICAL ISSUES

Presentation

- Most common signs/symptoms
  - Usually asymptomatic, incidental finding
- Other signs/symptoms
  - Swelling, facial asymmetry
  - Tooth displacement
  - Pain

Demographics

- Age
  - Any age but most common in 2nd-4th decade
- Gender
  - Female predominance (70%)

Natural History & Prognosis

- Slow-growing but occasionally aggressive
- Usually **concentric growth**
- Juvenile varieties have rapid growth, jaw deformity
- Lesions affecting paranasal sinuses more aggressive than lesions affecting mandible
- Prognosis excellent after complete resection
- Recurrence in 12%

Treatment

- Surgical **enucleation or resection**
- Curettage if lesion borders not clear or if complete removal not possible due to large lesion size or lack of surgical access

DIAGNOSTIC CHECKLIST

Consider

- Differential diagnosis depends on degree and pattern of internal radiopacity
- Differential diagnosis may include other benign mixed radiolucent-radiopaque neoplasms; diagnosis determined by clinical and radiographic behavior

Image Interpretation Pearls

- Identification of **well-defined margin helps to distinguish OF from fibrous dysplasia**
- OF lesion enlarges equally in all directions

Reporting Tips

- Must describe position in relation to sinus drainage pathways and whether obstructed secretions present
- Describe mass effect on adjacent structures, such as orbit, neural foramina, intracranial cavity, and mandibular canal

SELECTED REFERENCES

1. Ciniglio Appiani M et al: Ossifying fibromas of the paranasal sinuses: diagnosis and management. Acta Otorhinolaryngol Ital. 35(5):355-61, 2015
2. Gantala R et al: Psammomatoid juvenile ossifying fibroma involving upper jaw: a rare case report. J Clin Diagn Res. 9(7):ZD17-9, 2015
3. Mohanty S et al: Retrospective analysis of ossifying fibroma of jaw bones over a period of 10 years with literature review. J Maxillofac Oral Surg. 13(4):560-7, 2014
4. Wang TT et al: Two cases of multiple ossifying fibromas in the jaws. Diagn Pathol. 9:75, 2014
5. de Andrade M et al: Ossifying fibroma of the jaws: a clinicopathological case series study. Braz Dent J. 24(6):662-6, 2013
6. Osunde O et al: Juvenile aggressive ossifying fibroma of the maxilla: a case report and review of the literature. Ann Med Health Sci Res. 3(2):288-90, 2013
7. Akcam T et al: Synchronous ossifying fibromas of the jaws: a review. Oral Surg Oral Med Oral Pathol Oral Radiol. 114(5 Suppl):S120-5, 2012
8. Hara M et al: Ossifying fibroma of the maxilla: a case report including its imaging features and dynamic magnetic resonance imaging findings. Oral Surg Oral Med Oral Pathol Oral Radiol. 114(4):e139-46, 2012
9. Triantafillidou K et al: Ossifying fibroma of the jaws: a clinical study of 14 cases and review of the literature. Oral Surg Oral Med Oral Pathol Oral Radiol. 114(2):193-9, 2012
10. Liu Y et al: Ossifying fibromas of the jaw bone: 20 cases. Dentomaxillofac Radiol. 39(1):57-63, 2010
11. MacDonald-Jankowski DS: Ossifying fibroma: a systematic review. Dentomaxillofac Radiol. 38(8):495-513, 2009
12. Chang CC et al: Central ossifying fibroma: a clinicopathologic study of 28 cases. J Formos Med Assoc. 107(4):288-94, 2008

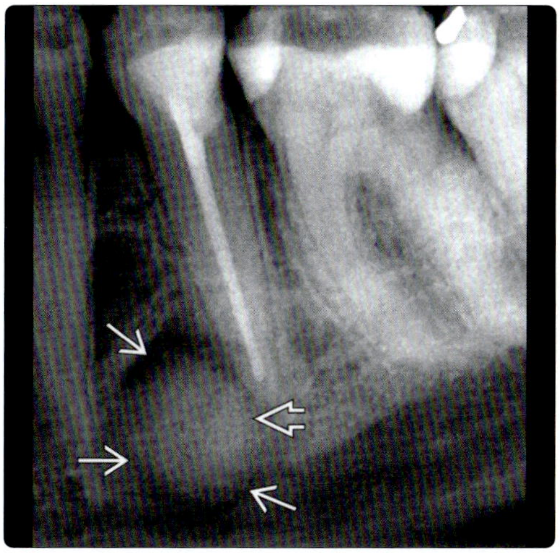

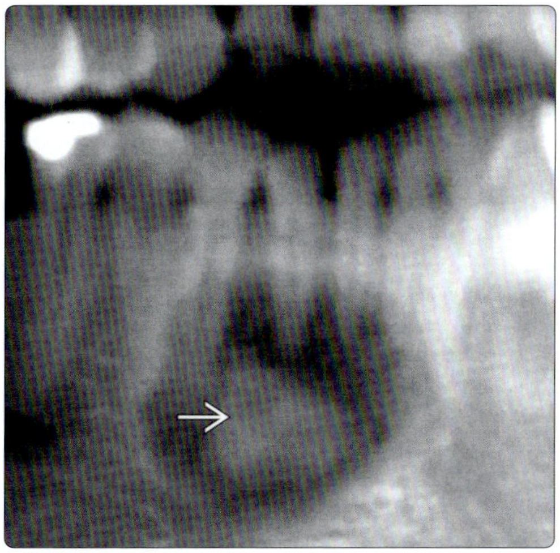

(Left) *Periapical radiograph shows a small OF consisting of a densely radiopaque central aspect with a surrounding zone of radiolucency. This lesion resembles a cementoblastoma but is located at the side of the tooth root and outside the periodontal ligament space.* **(Right)** *Panoramic radiograph of an OF in the anterior mandible shows a large, central radiopacity surrounded by a broad radiolucent zone. Note the concentric shape of the lesion.*

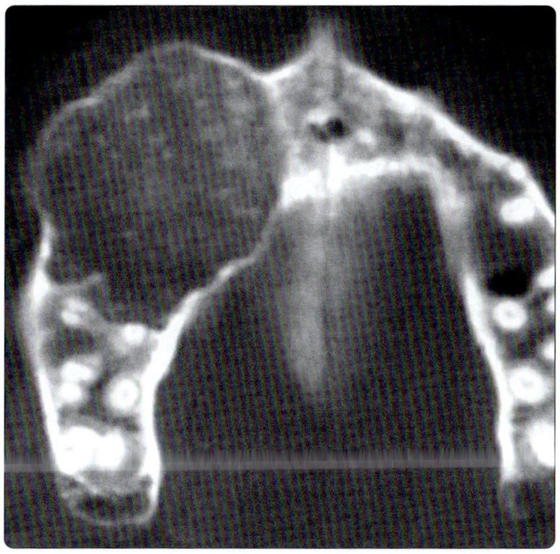

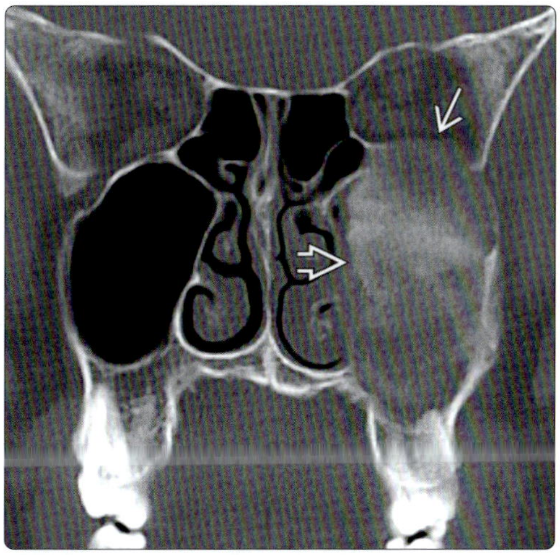

(Left) *Axial bone CT shows concentrically expanding mixed OF in the right maxilla. Note the sparsely speckled internal aspect.* **(Right)** *Coronal bone CT shows a large OF affecting the left maxillary sinus. The lesion has a granular internal aspect, resembling fibrous dysplasia. Note the mass effect on the orbit and resorption of the medial sinus wall.*

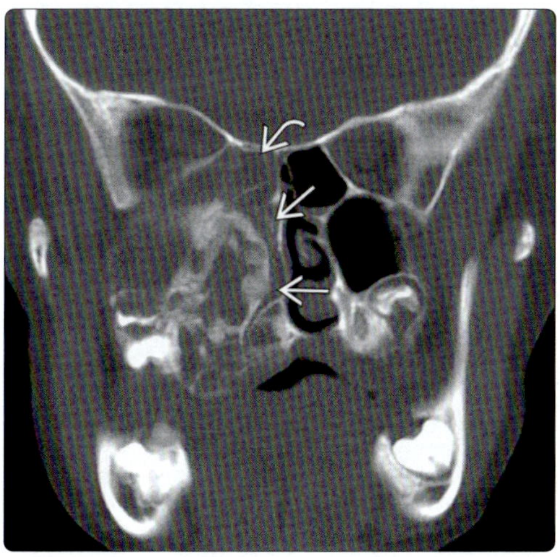

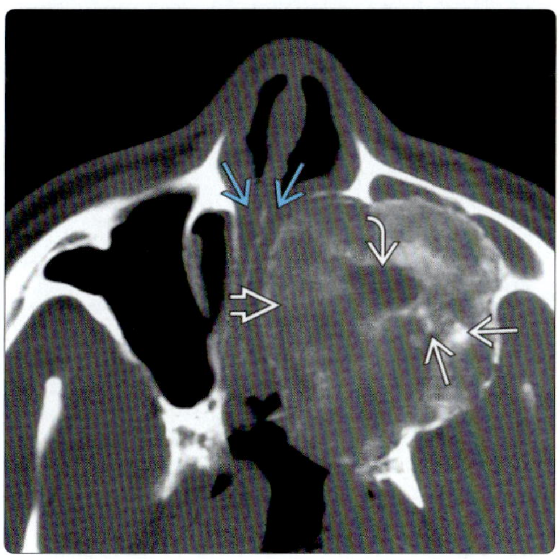

(Left) *Coronal bone CT shows a large, maxillary OF that nearly fills the entire right maxillary sinus. The right nasal airway is obstructed, and there are postobstructive secretions in the right ethmoid sinuses.* **(Right)** *Axial bone CT shows a large, well-demarcated, left maxillary OF obliterating most of the maxillary sinus air space. The internal aspect has radiopaque foci and granular and soft tissue density components. Note obstruction of both sides of the nasal airway.*

Mandible-Maxilla Fibrous Dysplasia

KEY FACTS

TERMINOLOGY

- Definition: Benign fibroosseous disease

IMAGING

- **Superior displacement of mandibular canal pathognomonic** for fibrous dysplasia (FD)
- Maxilla > mandible
    - Posterior areas more common, usually **unilateral**
- Any bone, including skull, skull base, & facial bones
- Expansion: Bone larger but **maintains overall shape**
- Ill defined: Borders gradually blend with surrounding normal bone
- Lesion bone pattern may be granular (ground glass), resemble orange peel, swirling (fingerprint), wispy (cotton wool), or amorphous dense pattern

TOP DIFFERENTIAL DIAGNOSES

- Paget disease
- Osteomyelitis
- Osteosarcoma
- Ossifying fibroma

PATHOLOGY

- Monostotic (80%)
- Cases affecting maxilla often affect contiguous bones, such as zygoma & sphenoid
    - If sphenoid, zygomatic, frontonasal bones, & base of skull affected, termed **craniofacial FD**

CLINICAL ISSUES

- Rare in TMJ condyle
- Often incidental finding or painless facial swelling
- May be discovered at any age, but most are < 30 years old
- Usually stops growing at end of somatic growth
- Recurrence/reactivation (18%)
- Simple bone cyst, central giant cell granuloma, or aneurysmal bone cyst may develop in affected bone
- Malignant transformation rare, particularly in jaws

(Left) *Occlusal radiograph of fibrous dysplasia (FD) in the right maxilla shows the lesion has a ground-glass matrix and blends with adjacent normal trabeculae. The developing 2nd bicuspid is displaced. The laminae dura of the 1st permanent and 2nd primary molars are altered to the new bone pattern, and periodontal ligament spaces are narrowed.* **(Right)** *Periapical radiograph shows FD with an orange peel pattern. The follicular cortex of the developing tooth is altered to the lesion bone pattern.*

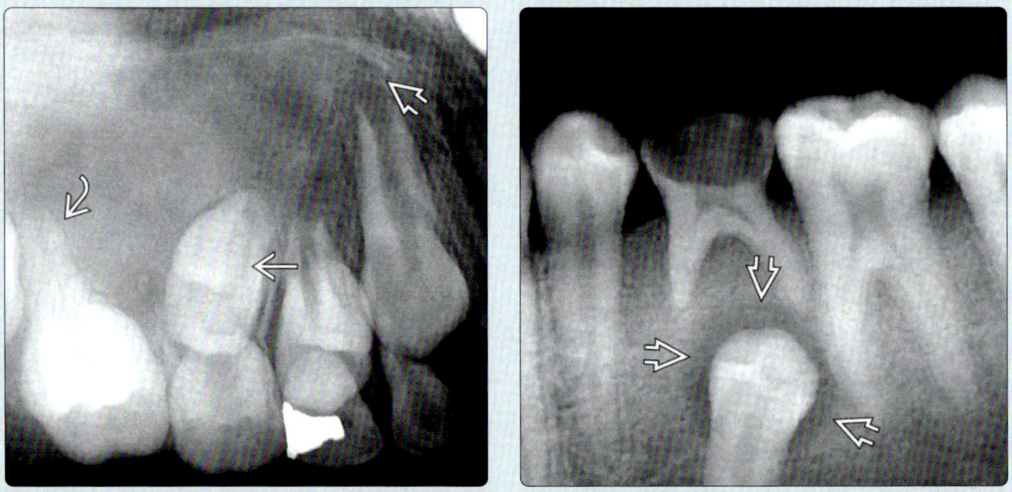

(Left) *Panoramic radiograph shows FD affecting the left mandible. There are numerous cyst-like cavities indicating simple bone cyst formation and expansion of the inferior border. FD may also be associated with aneurysmal bone cyst and central giant-cell granuloma.* **(Right)** *Panoramic radiograph in the same patient 20 years later shows partial healing with bone fill of the cystic areas.*

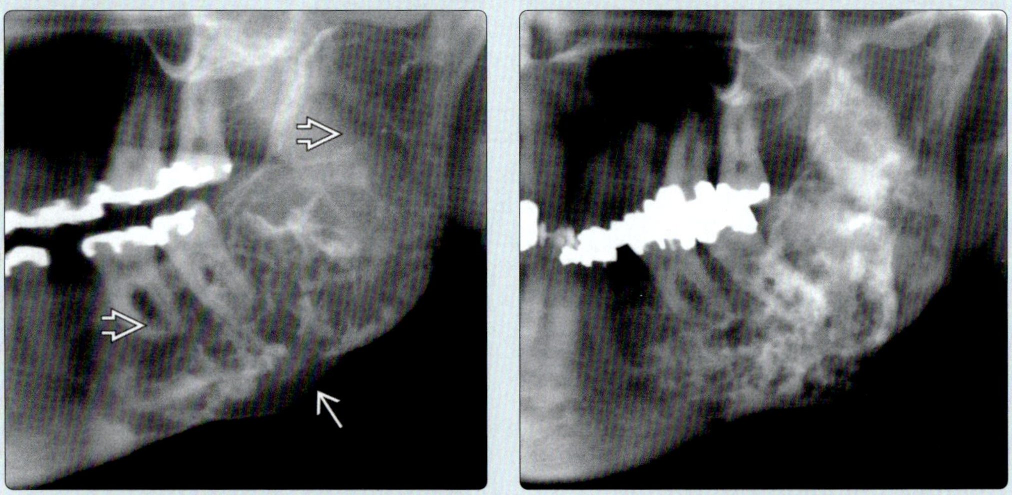

TERMINOLOGY

Abbreviations

- Fibrous dysplasia (FD)

Synonyms

- Osteitis fibrosa, osteodystrophia fibrosa, fibrous osteoma, fibrous osteodysplasia

Definitions

- Benign fibroosseous disease
- Replacement of normal cancellous bone with cellular fibrous tissue containing foci of immature woven bone

IMAGING

General Features

- Best diagnostic clue
  - Expansile lesion with ground-glass matrix in young patient
  - **Superior displacement of mandibular canal pathognomonic** for FD
- Location
  - Maxilla > mandible
    - Posterior areas more common, usually unilateral
  - Affects any bone, including skull, skull base, & facial bones
  - Rare in TMJ condyle
  - If sinus involvement in craniofacial case, sphenoid sinus is most common
- Size
  - Ranges from small nonexpanding subclinical lesion to large facial deformity
- Morphology
  - Expansion: Bone larger but maintains overall shape
  - Ill defined: Borders gradually blend with surrounding normal bone
  - Lesions affecting bones other than jaws or lesions in young patients may have more well-defined borders

Imaging Recommendations

- Best imaging tool
  - Intraoral or panoramic radiograph excellent for evaluating bone pattern & extent of jaw involvement
  - Bone CT or cone beam CT to determine if also craniofacial involvement; to monitor for progression, reactivation, or malignant transformation
  - MR useful for evaluating compression of neurological structures, identifying cystic degeneration or aneurysmal bone cyst formation
  - MR is adjunct to CT when secondary malignancy suspected

Radiographic Findings

- Intraoral plain film
  - Density & trabecular pattern varies depending on lesion maturity & amount of dysplastic bone
    - Early lesions may be more radiolucent than mature lesions
    - Lesion density varies from radiolucent, radiopaque, or mixture of densities
  - Lesion bone pattern may be granular (**ground glass**), resemble orange peel, or show swirling (fingerprint), wispy (cotton wool), or amorphous dense pattern
  - Periodontal ligament spaces may appear narrowed
  - Laminae dura altered to abnormal bone pattern
  - Teeth displaced or impacted
    - Teeth may have hypercementosis
    - Root resorption uncommon
    - May be associated with enamel hypoplasia, dentin dysplasia, taurodontism
- Extraoral plain film
  - Expansion: Cortices thinned or altered to abnormal bone pattern
  - Simple bone cyst may form in mature FD lesion: 1 or more radiolucent areas & increased expansion

CT Findings

- Bone CT
  - Expansile lesion in medullary space with variable attenuation
    - Mixed radiolucency & radiopacity or ground-glass appearance
  - CT patterns may overlap/coexist
    - Depends on prevalence of bony vs. fibrous tissue
  - Cranial cortices may be thickened if involved
  - If paranasal sinuses involved, **overall shape of sinus maintained** but walls thickened

MR Findings

- T1WI
  - Expansile mass with low or intermediate signal in ossified &/or fibrous portions of lesion
- T2WI
  - Expansile mass with low signal due to numerous bony trabeculae
  - Sometimes increased signal intensity in early lesions during bone resorptive phase
  - Heterogeneous signal pattern often in active phase
    - Patchy high signal usually seen in areas that appear radiolucent on bone CT
- T1WI C+
  - Areas of enhancement: Often maximal in areas that appear T2 hyperintense & radiolucent on bone CT
- Signal intensity & extent of contrast enhancement on T1- & T2-weighted images depend on amount & degree of fibrous tissue, bone trabeculae, cellularity, & hemorrhagic phenomena

DIFFERENTIAL DIAGNOSIS

Paget Disease

- Entire bone affected, so it is **bilateral**; FD often unilateral
- Paget disease affects older age group than does FD

Osteomyelitis

- May cause jaw enlargement, but **new bone originates from periosteum** & is deposited on outer surface, so original cortex may still be visible
  - FD expands from trabecular bone & thins or alters cortex to lesion bone pattern
- Osteomyelitis has **sequestra**

Osteosarcoma
- Bone pattern similar to FD but see other **malignant characteristics**
- Osteosarcoma may have characteristic periosteal response

Ossifying Fibroma
- **Tumor-like concentric expansion** & is monostotic
- Well-defined border, often has radiolucent rim

PATHOLOGY

General Features
- Genetics
  - Sporadic *GNAS* gene mutation
    - Gene found on chromosome 20q13
- Associated abnormalities
  - ± endocrine disorders, café au lait spots

Staging, Grading, & Classification
- Monostotic (80%)
  - Type most often affecting jaws
- Polyostotic can be uni- or bilateral
  - Can affect skull, facial bones, pelvis, spine, or shoulder
  - Cases affecting maxilla often affect contiguous bones, such as zygoma & sphenoid
- If sphenoid, zygomatic, frontonasal bones, & base of skull affected, termed **craniofacial FD**
- McCune-Albright syndrome = polyostotic FD with cutaneous pigmentation (**café au lait spots**) & endocrine abnormalities (precocious puberty)
- Mazabraud syndrome = FD with soft tissue myxomas

Gross Pathologic & Surgical Features
- Tan-yellow to white, firm, rubbery, gritty mass

Microscopic Features
- Short, randomly oriented, irregularly shaped trabeculae (**"Chinese characters"**) of woven bone in fibrous connective tissue stroma
- Lesions vary in amount & distribution of bone & in cellularity & vascularity of stroma

CLINICAL ISSUES

Presentation
- Most common signs/symptoms
  - Often incidental finding or painless facial swelling
  - Symptoms depend on FD lesion location
    - Craniofacial FD: Facial enlargement/asymmetry
    - Jaw involvement: Enlarged alveolar process, tooth displacement
- Other signs/symptoms
  - Impingement of nerve foramina in extensive cases leading to nerve deficits
  - Atypical facial pain, headache, sinusitis-like symptoms, occasionally blindness if optic nerve compressed

Demographics
- Age
  - May be discovered at any age but most < 30 years
  - Polyostotic usually found in children (mean: 8 years)
    - More severe skeletal & craniofacial involvement
  - Monostotic often diagnosed between 20-30 years old because usually asymptomatic
- Gender
  - M = F
  - McCune-Albright syndrome: F > M
- Epidemiology
  - Monostotic (75%)

Natural History & Prognosis
- Lesions usually stop growing at end of somatic growth
  - Enlargement may continue, especially in polyostotic cases
  - Recurrence/reactivation (18%)
  - Lesion growth may occur in pregnancy, with use of oral contraceptives, or after surgical treatment in young patients
- Malignant transformation rare (< 1%): May occur ± history of therapeutic radiation
  - Malignant transformation more frequent in polyostotic disease, rare in craniofacial area
- May develop secondary simple bone cyst, central giant cell granuloma, or aneurysmal bone cyst

Treatment
- Ranges from none (monitor patient) to conservative recontouring to radical resection
- Treatment done for cosmetic or functional reasons
- Bisphosphonates used occasionally
- Radiation therapy contraindicated due to risk of malignant transformation

DIAGNOSTIC CHECKLIST

Consider
- Polyostotic FD if ill-defined bone expansion involving > 1 bone

Image Interpretation Pearls
- Expands & widens bone from medullary compartment with thinning of overlying cortical bone
- Check for effect on neural & vascular foramina

Reporting Tips
- If have only jaw radiographs & both jaws involved, suggest bone CT or cone beam CT to determine if extragnathic sites involved

SELECTED REFERENCES

1. Atalar MH et al: CT and MR imaging in a large series of patients with craniofacial fibrous dysplasia. Pol J Radiol. 80:232-40, 2015
2. Wu H et al: Clinical characteristics of craniomaxillofacial fibrous dysplasia. J Craniomaxillofac Surg. 42(7):1450-5, 2014
3. Akintoye SO et al: Dental perspectives in fibrous dysplasia and McCune-Albright syndrome. Oral Surg Oral Med Oral Pathol Oral Radiol. 116(3):e149-55, 2013
4. Cheng J et al: Spontaneous malignant transformation in craniomaxillofacial fibrous dysplasia. J Craniofac Surg. 24(1):141-5, 2013
5. Hanifi B et al: Craniofacial fibrous dysplasia. Clin Imaging. 37(6):1109-15, 2013
6. Menon S et al: Craniofacial fibrous dysplasia: surgery and literature review. Ann Maxillofac Surg. 3(1):66-71, 2013
7. Nadaf A et al: Monostotic fibrous dysplasia with nonspecific cystic degeneration: A case report and review of literature. J Oral Maxillofac Pathol. 17(2):274-80, 2013
8. Sontakke SA et al: Computed tomographic features of fibrous dysplasia of maxillofacial region. Imaging Sci Dent. 41(1):23-8, 2011

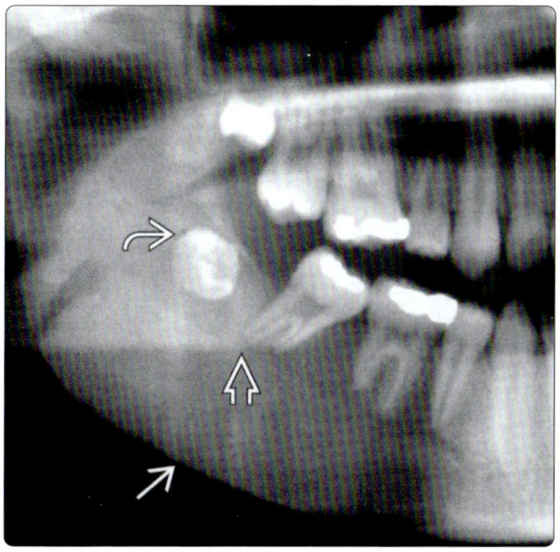

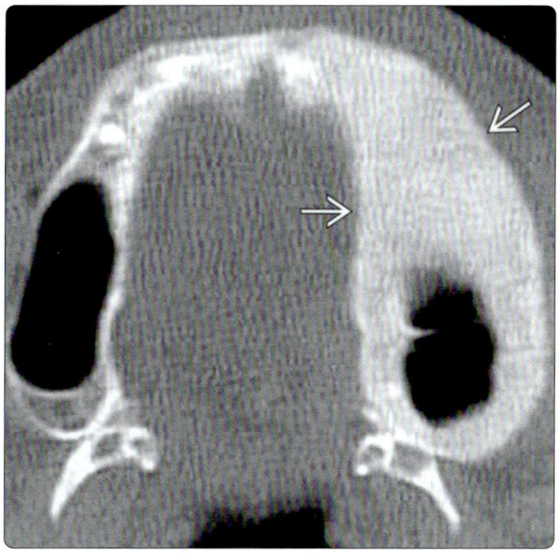

(Left) *Cropped panoramic radiograph shows FD in the right mandible. The mandibular canal is superiorly displaced, a pathognomic feature. The inferior border of the mandible is expanded and the cortex altered to the lesion bone pattern. The developing 3rd molar is displaced posteriorly.* **(Right)** *Axial bone CT shows a ground-glass bone pattern of FD and expansion of the left maxillary alveolus. The buccal and palatal cortices are not distinct. The lesion has not crossed the midline.*

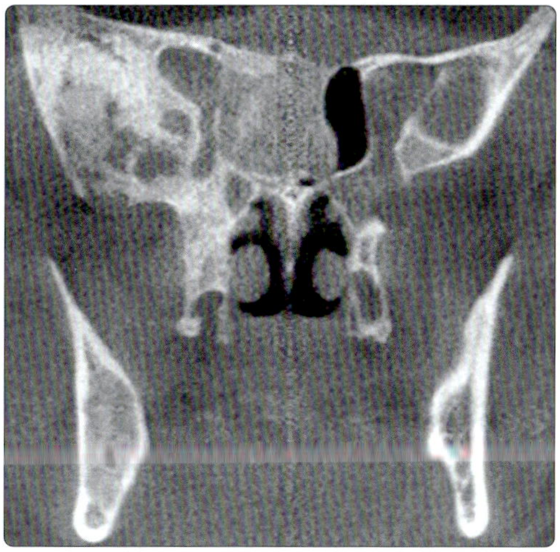

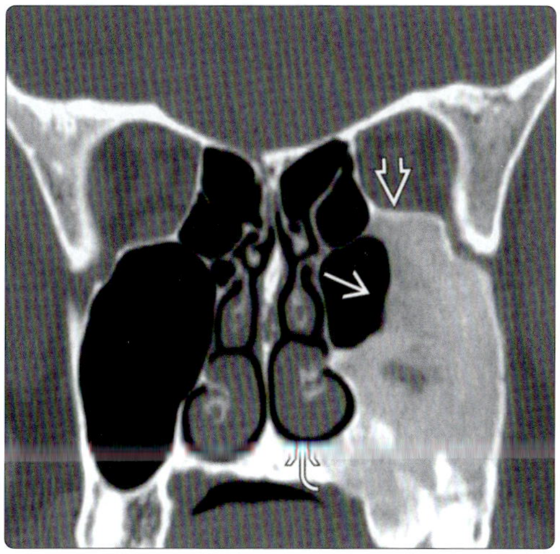

(Left) *Coronal CBCT shows polyostotic FD affecting the right mandible, maxilla, sphenoid, and zygomatic areas. The lesional bone pattern is a mixture of granular and ground glass. There is enlargement of the affected bones with overall maintenance of shape.* **(Right)** *Coronal bone CT shows lesion of FD encroaching on and reducing the size of the left maxillary sinus and elevating the floor of the left nasal fossa. The lesion has also extended superiorly and elevated the orbital floor.*

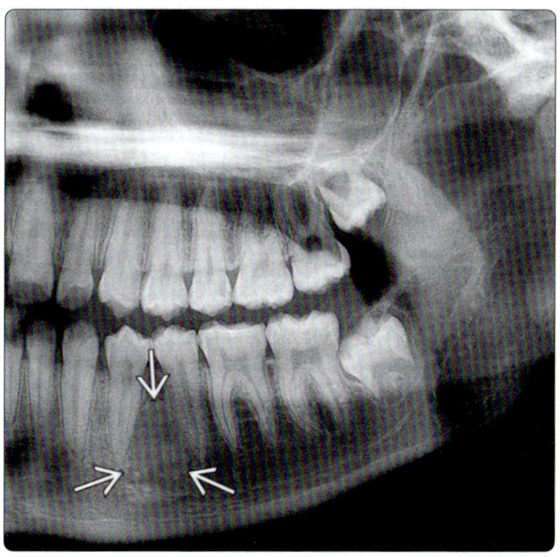

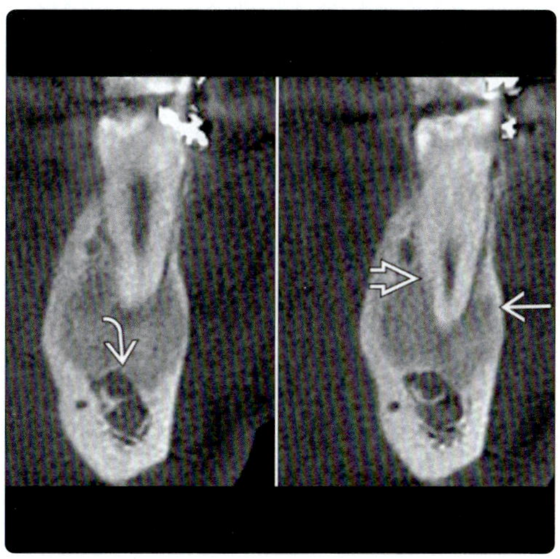

(Left) *Panoramic radiograph shows localized FD between the left mandibular premolar roots with an orange peel internal pattern. The lesion is well defined and has splayed the tooth roots apart.* **(Right)** *Cross-sectional cone beam CT reformats of the same patient show thinning and expansion of the buccal cortex. Note replacement of the lamina dura and superior cortex of the mandibular canal with a lesion bone pattern. The canal is not displaced or compressed by the lesion.*

(Left) *Frontal CBCT 3D reformat of a 49-year-old woman with McCune-Albright syndrome shows enlargement and deformity of the mandible and most of the facial bones. Note relative sparing of the left zygoma ➔ and anterior maxilla ➔ with a large defect and altered bone pattern in the anterior mandible ➔.* **(Right)** *Midline sagittal CBCT reformat in the same patient shows altered bone in the mandible ➔, mandibular incisor root resorption ➔, clivus enlargement ➔, and normal bone in maxillary midline area ➔.*

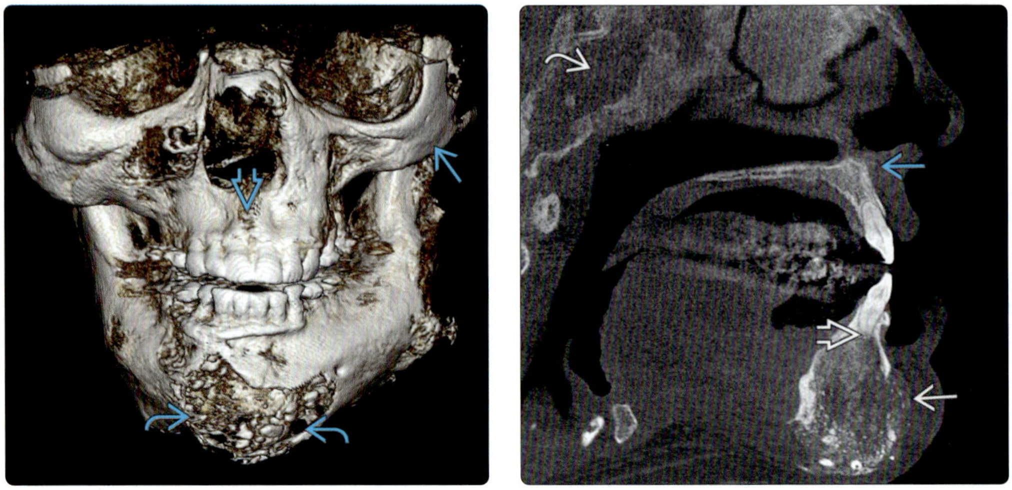

(Left) *Right lateral 3D CBCT reformat in the same patient shows mandibular and zygomatic enlargement with sparing of the right condyle ➔. Note mandibular enlargement but maintenance of normal mandibular shape ➔.* **(Right)** *Left lateral CBCT 3D reformat in the same patient shows a large scalloped mandibular defect ➔ as a result of simple bone cyst formation. Bilateral enlargement and widespread osseous involvement is typical of McCune-Albright syndrome.*

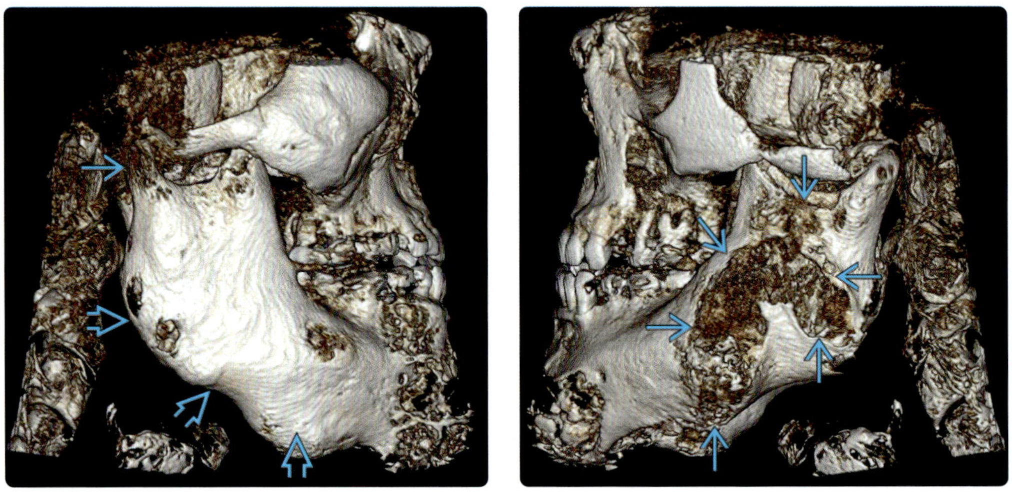

(Left) *Panoramic CBCT reformat in the same patient shows a mixed bone pattern consisting of a granular ➔, radiolucent ➔, and amorphous ➔ bone pattern in the expanded mandible. The radiolucent areas represent simple bone cyst formation. The condyle ➔ is spared.* **(Right)** *Panoramic CBCT reformat in the same patient shows involvement of the left mandible and maxilla. The left condyle and condylar neck have a granular bone pattern ➔. A simple bone cyst ➔ occupies the posterior mandible.*

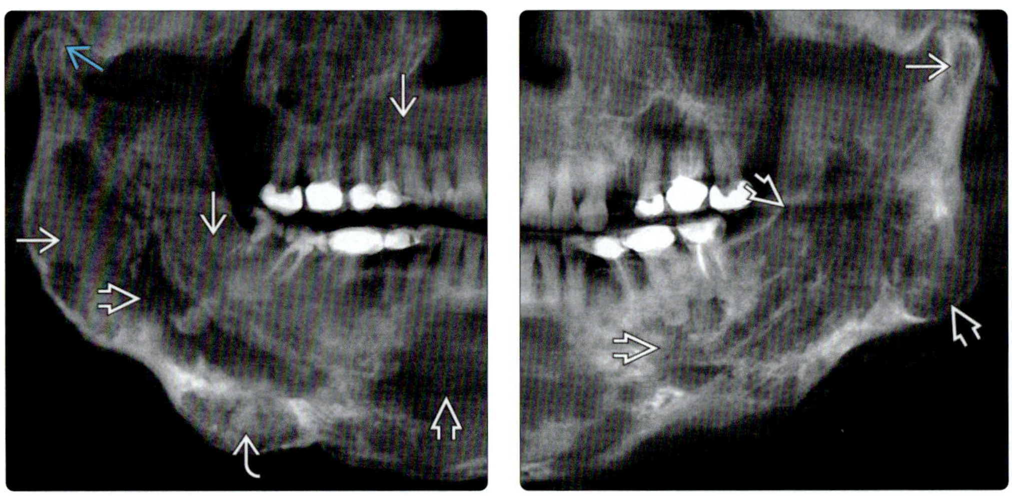

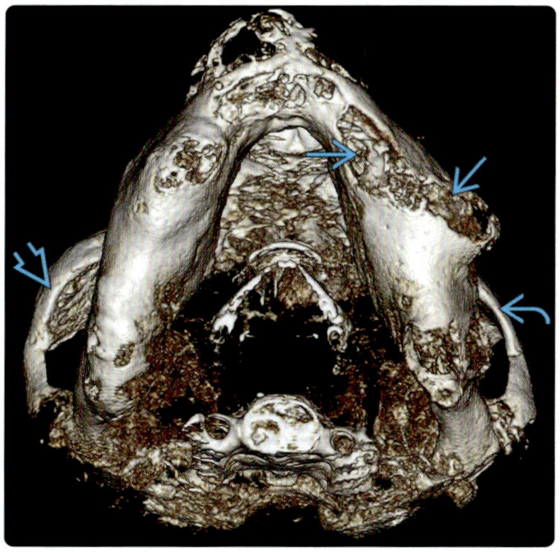

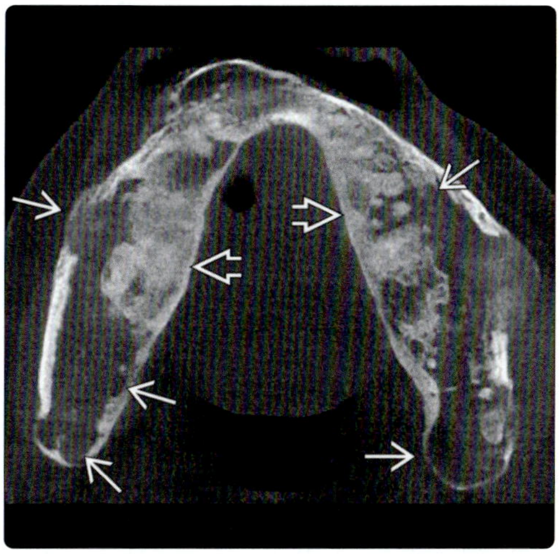

(Left) *Axial CBCT 3D reformat in the same patient shows asymmetric enlargement of the mandible. A simple bone cyst has created a large defect on the left side* ➡*. Note enlargement of the right zygomatic arch* ➡ *compared with the normal contralateral side* ➡*.* **(Right)** *Axial CBCT reformat in the same patient shows the scalloping outline of the simple bone cysts bilaterally* ➡*. Granular bone has replaced normal cortical bone* ➡*.*

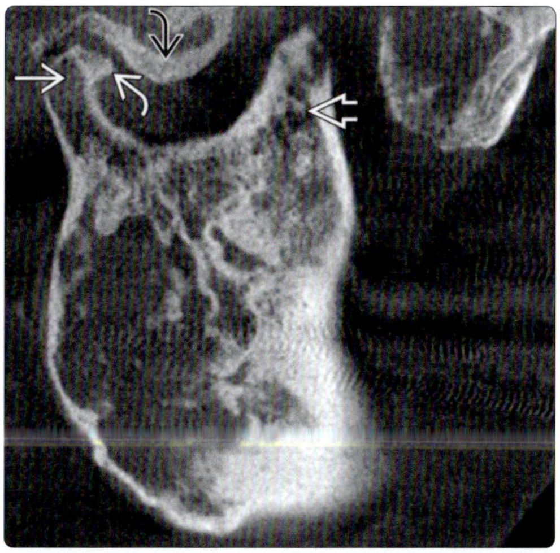

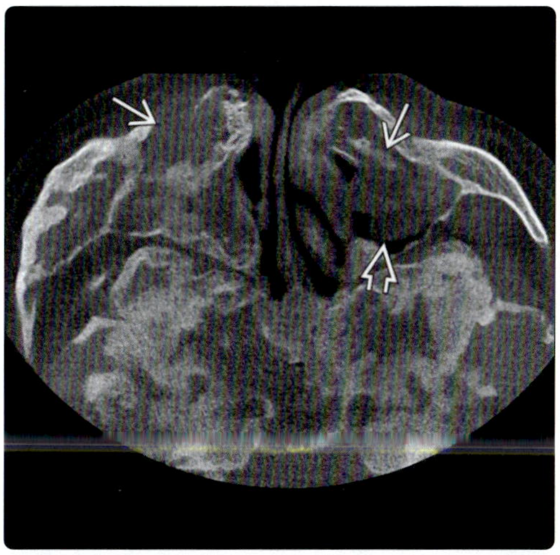

(Left) *Sagittal CBCT reformat in the same patient shows sparing of the right condyle* ➡ *but involvement of the coronoid process* ➡ *and articular eminence* ➡*. An osteophyte* ➡ *extends from the anterior condylar surface due to degenerative joint disease.* **(Right)** *Coronal CBCT reformat in the same patient shows extensive granularity and enlargement of the skull base with bilateral maxillary sinus involvement and reduction in sinus volume* ➡*. There is mucosal thickening at the posterior aspect of the left maxillary sinus* ➡*.*

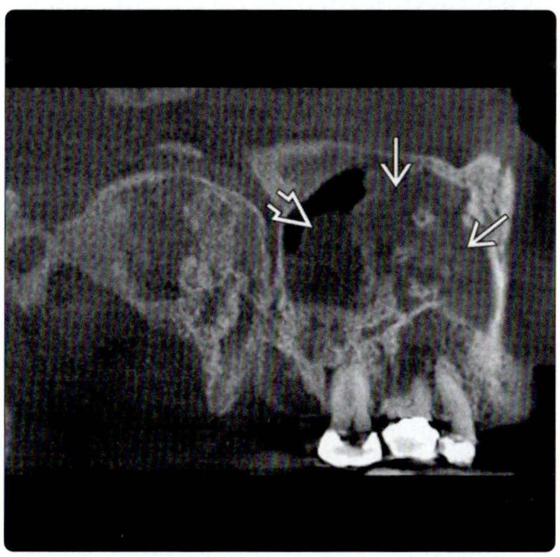

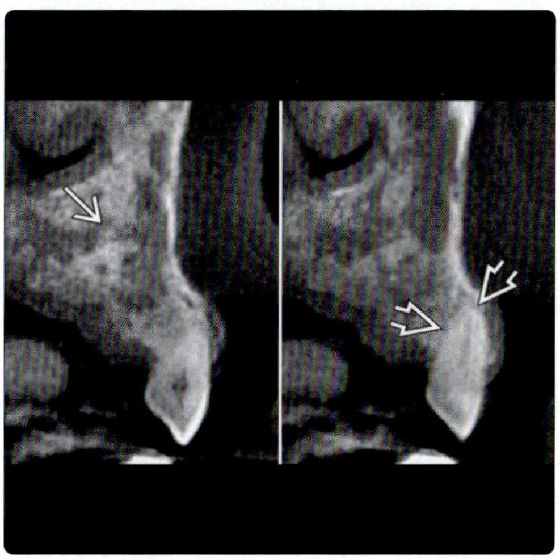

(Left) *Sagittal CBCT reformat in the same patient shows dysplastic bone replacing most of the sinus air space* ➡ *and a soft tissue mass* ➡ *that may be secondary to impaired sinus drainage.* **(Right)** *Cross-sectional CBCT reformats in the same patient show an inhomogeneous ground-glass pattern in the maxillary cuspid area* ➡*. Note loss of lamina dura and narrowed periodontal ligament spaces* ➡*.*

Paget Disease

KEY FACTS

TERMINOLOGY

- Paget disease (PD): Disease of osteoclasts causing disordered and excessive bone remodeling from alternating waves of osteoclastic and osteoblastic activity
- Sites of PD progress at variable rates; may see differing phases in same patient

IMAGING

- Skull: Well-defined radiolucent defect &/or marked cortical thickening with sclerosis
- Jaws: Enlargement affecting entire jaw with trabecular and cortical thickening
- Well-defined lysis; commonly frontal > occipital
- **Laminae dura** not distinct and **altered** to pagetoid bone pattern
- **Hypercementosis** or cemental masses at root apices
- Aggressive osteolysis, cortical destruction, soft tissue mass, without periosteal reaction
- **"Cotton wool" skull**: Focal sclerosis within previous lytic areas
- Platybasia, basilar invagination, frontal bossing

TOP DIFFERENTIAL DIAGNOSES

- Fibrous dysplasia
- Florid osseous dysplasia
- Osteosclerotic or osteolytic metastases

CLINICAL ISSUES

- Asymptomatic in early phase; bone pain and enlargement, deformity, malocclusion in later phases
- > 40 years, M:F = 2:1
- **Sarcomatous transformation** (< 1%)
- Skull/facial giant cell tumor almost always associated

DIAGNOSTIC CHECKLIST

- Trabecular changes, bone enlargement, late onset and ↑ serum alkaline phosphatase suggestive of PD

(Left) *Coronal graphic shows diffuse Paget disease (PD) of the skull with severe diploic widening.* **(Right)** *Lateral skull radiograph shows late-phase PD involving the temporal bone and calvarium. There is some demineralization indicating an acute/subacute phase ⇨ and also diffuse "cotton wool" change ⇨ seen in the chronic phase. This widespread involvement may result in foraminal narrowing, leading to nerve compression and associated neural deficits.*

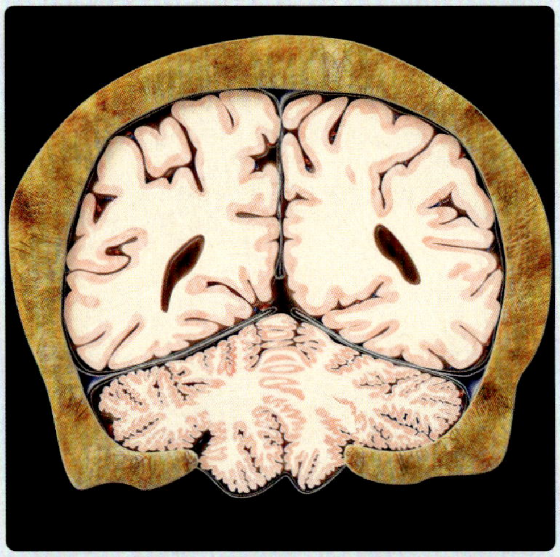

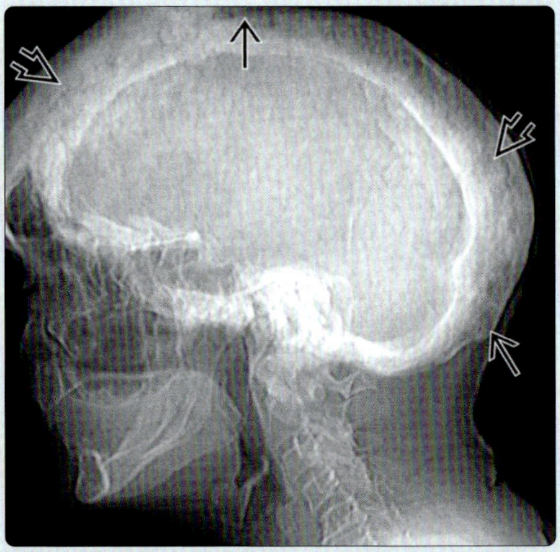

(Left) *Lateral scanogram shows PD of the mandible, which is enlarged. There is a discrepancy in the size of the mandible vs. the maxilla with a resultant anterior crossbite* ➡. **(Right)** *Axial bone CT in the same patient shows the mandible is expanded, especially in the parasymphyseal region. Note that there is no apparent periodontal ligament space around the tooth roots.*

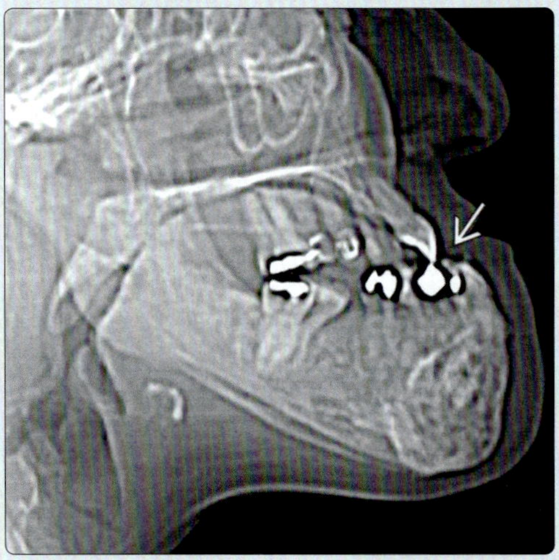

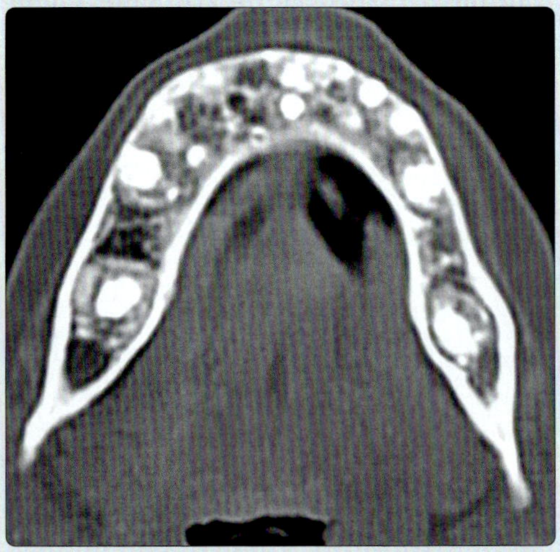

Paget Disease

TERMINOLOGY

Abbreviations

- Paget disease (PD)

Synonyms

- Osteitis deformans

Definitions

- Chronic disease of osteoclasts: Disordered and excessive bone remodeling resulting from alternating waves of osteoclastic and osteoblastic activity
  - Active and quiescent phases
  - Anatomic distribution asymmetric and not all bones may be involved
- Individual sites progress at variable rates; differing phases may be seen within same patient

IMAGING

General Features

- Best diagnostic clue
  - Skull: Well-defined, radiolucent defect &/or marked cortical thickening with sclerosis
  - Jaws: Enlargement affecting entire jaw with trabecular and cortical thickening
- Location
  - Most common sites: Pelvis, lumbosacral spine, femur, skull, and vertebrae
    - Jaws less commonly involved
    - Maxilla:mandible = 2:1
- Morphology
  - Affects entire bone: Usually bilateral although degree of involvement may differ on each side

Radiographic Findings

- Radiography
  - Radiographic appearance depends on disease phase
  - Diploic widening, coarse trabeculae, thick cortices
  - Early destructive phase
    - Well-defined lysis; commonly frontal > occipital
    - Osteoporosis circumscripta (focal osteolytic lesions) affects both skull tables; inner > outer
    - Jaws: Decreased number of trabeculae, altered trabecular shape
      - ± jaw enlargement
  - Intermediate phase
    - Both lytic and blastic lesions
    - Coarsening and thickening of trabeculae and cortices
    - Irregular, spotty areas of increased density
    - Jaws: Granular trabecular pattern
      - **Laminae dura** not distinct and **altered** to pagetoid bone pattern
      - **Hypercementosis** or cemental masses at root apices; possible response to changing occlusion
      - ± ankylosis
  - Late sclerotic phase
    - Blastic lesions, often crossing sutures
    - Uniform increase in density, enlargement
    - "Tam-o' Shanter" skull: Marked widened diploic space, especially inner table, resulting in skull enlargement and appearance similar to Scottish hat
    - **"Cotton wool" skull**: Focal sclerosis within previous lytic areas
    - Platybasia, basilar invagination (BI), frontal bossing
    - Jaws: Linear trabecular pattern or cotton wool pattern
      - Tooth movement due to bone enlargement

CT Findings

- NECT
  - Can use CBCT or NECT
  - Bones: 3 phases of PD same as radiography
  - Sarcomatous transformation
    - Aggressive osteolysis, cortical destruction, soft tissue mass, without periosteal reaction
  - Giant cell tumor (GCT) transformation
    - Lytic lesion without periosteal reaction or mass
    - Marrow replacement distinguishes from PD lysis
    - Cystic and hemorrhagic regions possible
- CECT
  - Enhancement reflects pathologic increase in vascularity
  - Sarcomatous transformation: Mass enhancement, often with central necrosis
  - GCT transformation: Enhancing solid tumor areas

MR Findings

- T1WI
  - Early destructive to early intermediate phase
    - Decreased marrow intensity secondary to marrow replacement
    - Residual normal yellow marrow foci excludes malignant transformation
  - Late sclerotic phase: Marrow hypointensity from sclerosis of coarse trabeculae and cortical thickening
- T2WI
  - Marrow changes with marrow replacement
- T1WI C+
  - Increased enhancement due to increased vascularity
  - Sarcomatous transformation: Mass enhancement, often with central necrosis
  - GCT transformation: Enhancing solid tumor areas

Imaging Recommendations

- Best imaging tool
  - Radiography
  - NECT or CBCT defines detail/extent, especially PD of skull base and jaw involvement
  - MR for imaging PD complications
- Protocol advice
  - MR: Coronal + sagittal sequences for BI; add contrast for malignant transformation work-up

Nuclear Medicine Findings

- Bone scan
  - Increased uptake in all phases of PD
    - Findings may precede radiographic changes
    - Positive uptake is nonspecific so need to rule out metastases, metabolic bone disease, and fibrous dysplasia
  - Can be "cold" or normal in late sclerotic stage due to decreased bone vascularity

DIFFERENTIAL DIAGNOSIS

Fibrous Dysplasia

- Younger age group than PD
- Usually asymmetric, **unilateral, localized**
- Ground-glass trabecular pattern

Florid Osseous Dysplasia

- Limited to jaws in **tooth-bearing regions**
- Often radiolucent fibrous tissue capsule

Osteosclerotic Metastases

- May mimic cotton wool appearance of PD but **no calvarial thickening**
- Usually history of primary tumor

Osteolytic Metastases

- Permeative borders, **no calvarial thickening**
- Usually history of primary tumor

PATHOLOGY

General Features

- Etiology
  - Unknown but may include environmental and genetic factors
  - Viral theory
    - Probable chronic paramyxoviral infection, possibly measles
  - Genetic factors, particularly mutations in SQTM1/p62 gene

Gross Pathologic & Surgical Features

- Abnormally soft new bone causing deformity

Microscopic Features

- Early destructive phase: Giant osteoclasts with numerous nuclei show intense activity and aggressive bone resorption
- Intermediate phase: Repeated osteoclastic and osteoblastic activity; return of yellow marrow gradually occurs
- Late sclerotic phase: High osteoblastic activity leads to sclerotic bone

CLINICAL ISSUES

Presentation

- Most common signs/symptoms
  - Usually asymptomatic in early phase
  - Later phases: Bone pain and enlargement, deformity
  - Jaw pain uncommon
- Other signs/symptoms
  - Malocclusion
  - Neurologic pain due to impingement on nerve foramina
    - Hyperthermia from hypervascularity
  - New pain/swelling = malignant transformation
  - Increased serum alkaline phosphatase and serum/urine hydroxyproline

Demographics

- Age
  - Usually > 55 years; rare prior to 40 years
- Gender
  - M:F = 2:1
- Ethnicity
  - Caucasian/European origin
- Epidemiology
  - Affects 2.5-5.0% of patients > 55 years old
  - Affects 10-15% of elderly patients

Natural History & Prognosis

- 10% develop secondary hyperparathyroidism from hypercalcemia related to aggressive bone remodeling
- Skull base thickening leads to CNS deficit(s) and hearing loss
- BI in up to 30%; more common in women → brainstem compression, syrinx, obstructive hydrocephalus
- Malignant transformation
  - Sarcomatous transformation (< 1%)
    - M:F = 2:1; 55-80 years
    - Most common sites: Pelvis, femur, humerus, skull, and facial bones
    - Osteosarcoma (50-60%), fibrosarcoma/malignant fibrous histiocytoma (20-25%), chondrosarcoma (10%)
    - Rarely lymphoma and angiosarcoma (1-3%)
    - < 10% 3-year survival
    - Metastasizes frequently, most commonly to lung
  - GCT
    - Skull/facial GCT almost always associated with PD
    - M:F = 1.6:1; 32-85 years
    - Solitary or multiple; 91% in polyostotic PD
    - Rarely cause mortality; generally do not metastasize

Treatment

- If asymptomatic, no treatment
- Calcitonin, bisphosphonates, mithramycin
- NSAIDs and acetaminophen for pain
  - Goal: Control, reduction, and alleviation of pain rather than return to normal bone
- Surgery for cosmesis, nerve decompression

DIAGNOSTIC CHECKLIST

Consider

- Extent of bone involvement: PD affects entire bone, other conditions usually localized
- Trabecular changes, bone enlargement, late onset, and ↑ serum alkaline phosphatase suggestive of PD

Image Interpretation Pearls

- Trabecular pattern can vary in enlarged jaw bone: Radiolucent/fewer trabeculae, granular/ground-glass, linear pattern, cotton wool appearance

Reporting Tips

- Check for BI because of risk for associated complications

SELECTED REFERENCES

1. Al-Rashid M et al: Paget disease of bone. Orthop Clin North Am. 46(4):577-85, 2015
2. Bolland MJ et al: Paget's disease of bone: clinical review and update. J Clin Pathol. 66(11):924-7, 2013
3. Hansen MF et al: Osteosarcoma in Paget's disease of bone. J Bone Miner Res. 21 Suppl 2:P58-63, 2006
4. Roodman GD et al: Paget disease of bone. J Clin Invest. 115(2):200-8, 2005
5. Smith SE et al: From the archives of the AFIP. Radiologic spectrum of Paget disease of bone and its complications with pathologic correlation. Radiographics. 22(5):1191-216, 2002

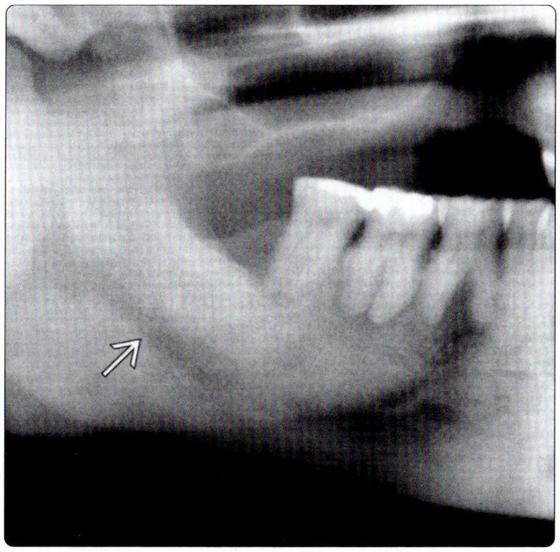
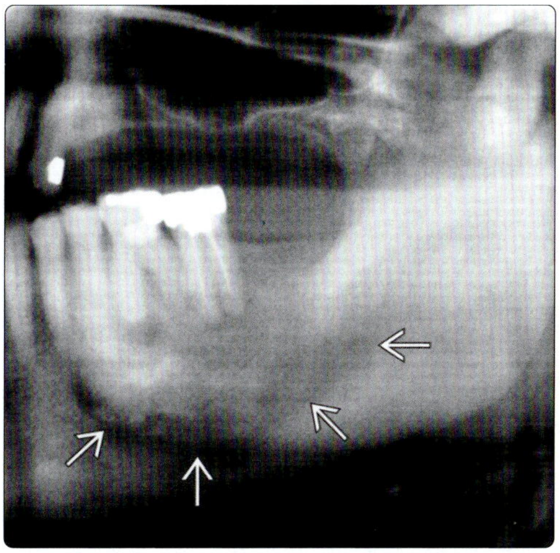

(Left) *Panoramic radiograph shows the late sclerotic phase of PD in the right mandible. The trabecular pattern is coarse and sclerotic, and the inferior cortex cannot be distinguished. The mandibular canal ➡ is easily seen due to the bone sclerosis.* **(Right)** *Panoramic radiograph in the same patient shows involvement of the left mandible. There is a well-defined area of radiolucency in the premolar-molar area ➡ representing an earlier disease phase.*

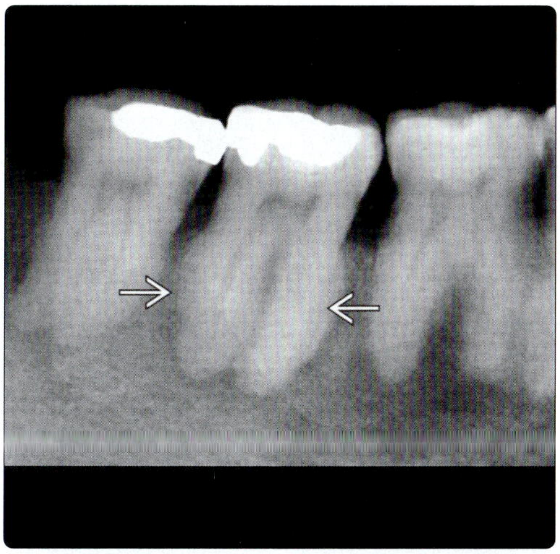
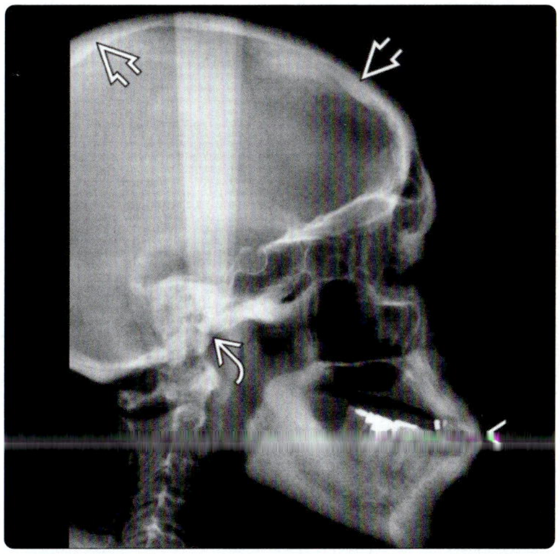

(Left) *Periapical radiograph in the same patient shows hypercementosis of the right 2nd mandibular molar tooth roots ➡ and alteration of laminae dura to the pagetoid bone pattern. The periodontal ligament spaces are narrowed or absent.* **(Right)** *Lateral skull radiograph in the same patient shows thickening of the diploë ➡ and sclerosis of the skull base ➡. The jaw enlargement has caused flaring of the incisor teeth and malocclusion ➡. The maxilla was not involved in this case.*

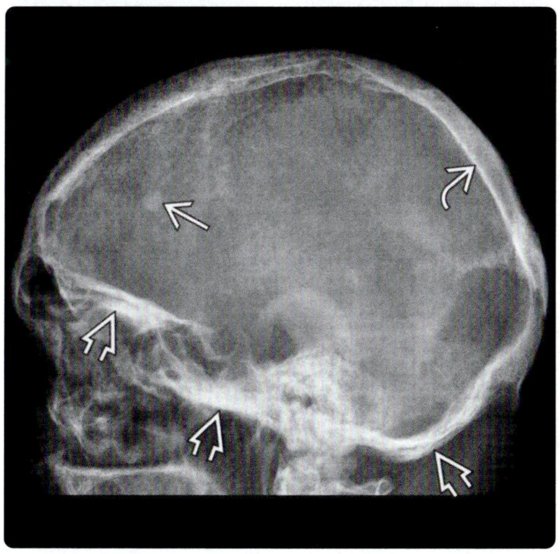
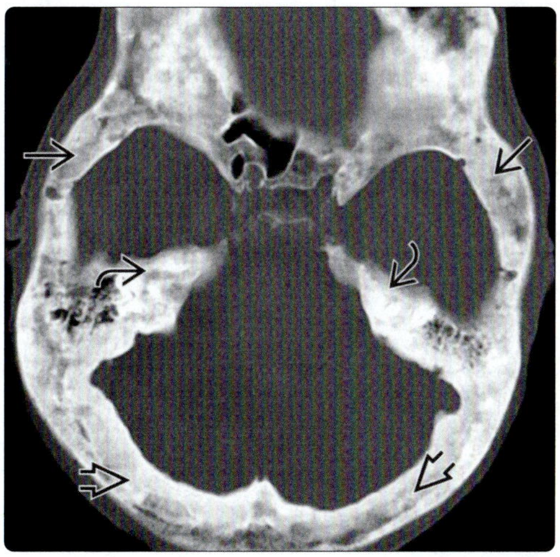

(Left) *Lateral skull radiograph shows PD involving the cranial base and temporal bone. There is dense sclerosis ➡ of the parietal bone and cortical thickening ➡ with a frontal focus having a cotton wool appearance ➡.* **(Right)** *Axial bone CT shows mixed-phase PD involving the entire calvarium and cranial base ➡. There is diffuse cotton wool appearance of the squamous temporal bone ➡ and the occipital bone ➡.*

Odontoma

KEY FACTS

TERMINOLOGY

- Definition: Tumor that produces mature enamel, dentin, cementum, and pulp tissue

IMAGING

- Compound: Small, **tooth-like structures** surrounded by radiolucent (low-density) rim
- Complex: **Amorphous, mineralized (radiopaque) mass** surrounded by radiolucent (low-density) rim
- Location
  - **Tooth-bearing area**: May be **pericoronal**
  - Maxilla: Commonly near canine crown; preferred location for compound odontomas
  - Mandible: Most common in molar region; preferred location for complex odontomas
  - **Above IAN canal**
- High-density structures similar to or more dense than adjacent teeth
- Surrounded by cortical boundary with uniform **low-density rim within cortex**

TOP DIFFERENTIAL DIAGNOSES

- For compound odontoma = supernumerary teeth
  - Usually single well-formed tooth
- For complex odontoma = ossifying fibroma
  - Not as dense as odontoma

CLINICAL ISSUES

- Most common odontogenic tumor
- Often interferes with eruption of permanent teeth

DIAGNOSTIC CHECKLIST

- Consider: Multiple supernumerary teeth (cleidocranial dysplasia and Gardner syndrome)
- Check for uneven dilation of soft tissue capsule that would signal infection or dentigerous cyst formation if pericoronal

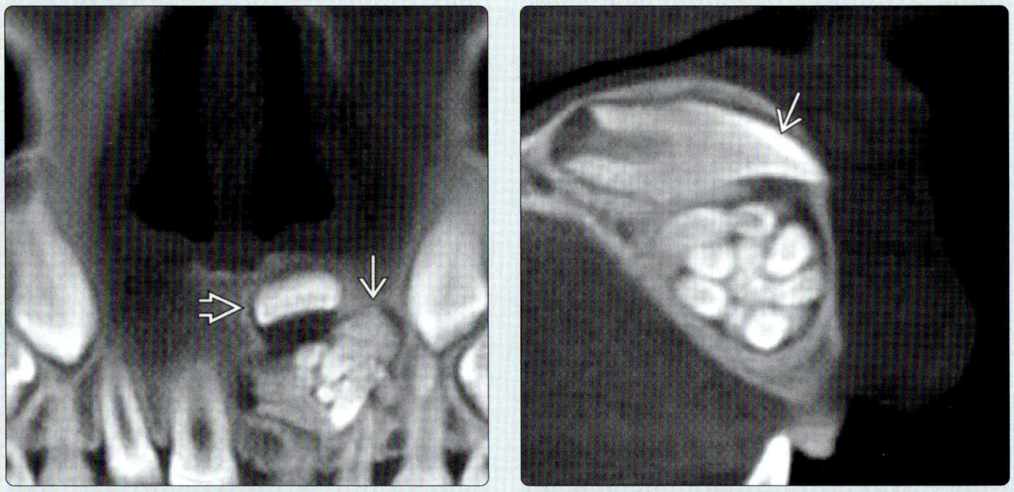

(Left) *CBCT panoramic reformat shows a compound odontoma ➡ impeding the eruption of the permanent maxillary left central incisor ➡. The permanent maxillary left lateral incisor is congenitally missing.* **(Right)** *CBCT cross section in the same patient shows the relationship of the odontoma to the impacted permanent maxillary left central incisor crown ➡. Note that the odontoma resembles a "bag of teeth."*

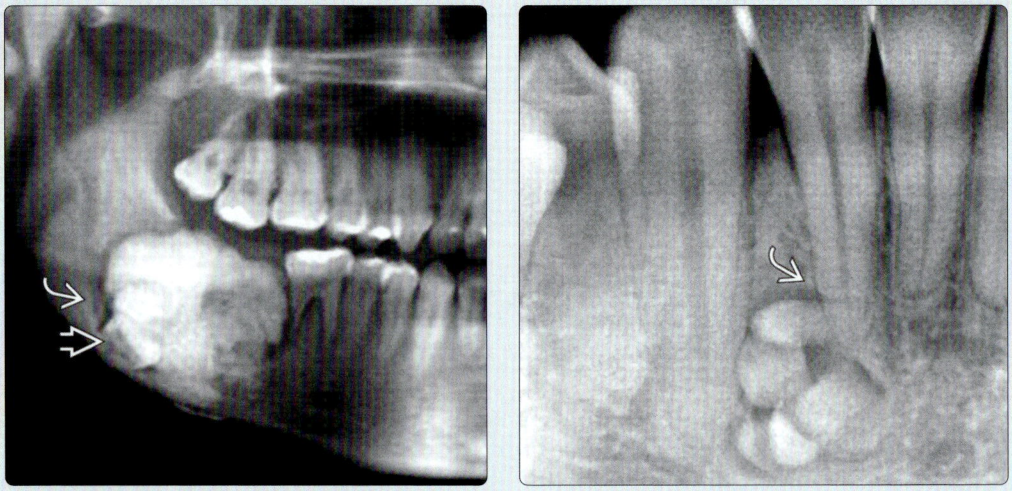

(Left) *Panoramic radiograph shows displacement of the mandibular right 2nd molar ➡ by a complex odontoma. The mandibular canal is displaced inferiorly ➡. Complex odontomas have a predilection for the posterior jaws. (Courtesy M. Noujeim, DDS.)* **(Right)** *Periapical radiograph shows a compound odontoma between the roots of the mandibular right lateral incisor and canine with slight mesial tipping of the root of the lateral incisor ➡. Compound odontomas have a predilection for the anterior jaws.*

TERMINOLOGY

Synonyms

- Odontome, compound composite odontoma, complex composite odontoma, odontogenic hamartoma, calcified mixed odontoma, cystic odontoma

Definitions

- Tumor that produces mature tooth structures: Enamel, dentin, cementum, pulp tissue
- Hamartoma of well-differentiated tooth structure
- 2 main types
    - **Compound**: Looks like **multiple small teeth**
    - **Complex**: Amorphous mineralized mass with **no resemblance to teeth**

IMAGING

General Features

- Best diagnostic clue
    - **Compound odontoma**
        - Small, tooth-like structures surrounded by **radiolucent (low-density) rim**
        - Multiple well-differentiated mini-teeth (**denticles**)
    - **Complex odontoma**
        - **Amorphous** mass of tooth-density material that may be similar to or exceed density of adjacent teeth
        - Surrounded by **low-density rim** and corticated periphery
        - If infected
            - Low-density capsule may be widened
            - Cortex may be thickened
            - Surrounding bone is sclerotic
- Location
    - **Tooth-bearing areas**: May be multiple &/or **pericoronal**
        - Maxilla
            - Most common anteriorly near canine crown
            - Preferred **location for compound odontomas**
        - Mandible
            - Most common in molar region
            - **Above** inferior alveolar nerve (**IAN**) **canal** (where tooth would normally develop)
            - Preferred **location for complex odontomas**
- Size
    - Varies dramatically: Small (mm) up to 6 cm or more in diameter
- Morphology
    - Compound
        - Varying number of small, **deformed teeth**
    - Complex
        - Amorphous, generally **homogeneously dense** material
        - Appears as clump of cotton
        - Difficult to make out denticles or separate components of tooth structure

Radiographic Findings

- Radiography
    - Surrounded by cortical boundary with uniform low-density rim within cortex
    - High-density structures similar to or more dense than adjacent teeth
    - **Dilated odontome** shares some features
        - Most extreme variant of dens invaginatus
        - Single calcified structure with central low-density area
        - Resembles **donut**
- Intraoral plain film
    - Differentiation of enamel, dentin, pulp, and periodontal ligament components can be made
    - Minute changes to adjacent teeth such as external resorption can be visualized
- Extraoral plain film
    - Panoramic
        - Mesiodistal extent of lesion (not faciolingual)
        - Relationship to adjacent teeth
        - Effect on eruption of adjacent teeth can be determined

CT Findings

- CBCT
    - Possible expansion of facial or lingual cortices of jaws
    - Will best show **relationship to incisive canal** (in anterior maxilla)
        - Can be located within or partially within canal
    - Will best show **relationship to IAN canal** (in mandible)
        - Pushes canal inferiorly

Imaging Recommendations

- Best imaging tool
    - **CBCT**
        - Shows relationship to adjacent structures in all dimensions
        - Can determine degree of impaction of tooth, if present, as well as faciolingual inclination of impacted tooth

DIFFERENTIAL DIAGNOSIS

Supernumerary Teeth (Hyperdontia)

- Usually **single, well-formed tooth**
- If multiple, they are of normal tooth shape and size and usually separate from one another
- Tooth can be of normal size or can be smaller (microdont)
- May be erupted into oral cavity or impacted

Ossifying Fibroma

- **Less dense** than complex odontoma
- Not usually associated with unerupted teeth
- Develops in young adults (juvenile variant has been described)
- Not self-limiting: Does not stop growing at end of odontogenesis

Periapical Osseous Dysplasia

- Late-stage periapical osseous dysplasia resembles complex odontoma
- Usually multiple
- Centered around **apices of teeth**
- Irregular sclerotic border and low-density rim
- Black middle-aged women or those of Asian descent more likely to develop

Ameloblastic Fibroodontoma

- Tooth structure is seen within larger, low-density lesion
- Calcifications do not make up majority of lesion, as in odontoma
- Not self-limiting: Does not stop growing at end of odontogenesis

Idiopathic Osteosclerosis

- Radiopacity with **no low-density rim**
- Can have ragged borders

Sclerosing Osteitis

- Odontogenic inflammation is causative factor so **located at apex**
- Associated with nonvital or inflamed tooth
- Widened periodontal ligament space between radiopacity and tooth but **no low-density rim**

Osteoma

- Usually less-dense radiopacity with **no low-density rim**
- Can have exophytic presentation with peduncle

PATHOLOGY

General Features

- Associated abnormalities
  - Odontomas have been reported in association with dentigerous cyst, adenomatoid odontogenic tumor, odontogenic keratocyst, and calcifying odontogenic cyst

Staging, Grading, & Classification

- Benign odontogenic tumor
- Mixed odontogenic epithelial and odontogenic mesenchymal tumor
- Hamartoma of dental tissues

Gross Pathologic & Surgical Features

- **Compound**
  - Separate tiny, tooth-like structures that may or may not be fused
- **Complex**
  - Clump of dentin-like material

CLINICAL ISSUES

Presentation

- Most common signs/symptoms
  - Lack of eruption of tooth
- Clinical profile
  - Most common odontogenic tumor
  - Prevalence exceeds all other odontogenic tumors combined
  - Often interferes with eruption of permanent teeth
  - May be associated with dentigerous cyst

Demographics

- Age
  - 2nd decade
  - Usually found when investigative radiography is done because tooth fails to erupt
- Gender
  - No sex predilection

Natural History & Prognosis

- Begins forming while normal dentition is forming
- Stops forming when normal tooth development ends
- Not locally invasive
- Some may erupt into oral cavity
- If excised, do not recur

Treatment

- Simple excision
- Consider proximity to adjacent structures when excising

DIAGNOSTIC CHECKLIST

Consider

- Multiple supernumerary teeth (cleidocranial dysplasia and Gardner syndrome)
- Ossifying fibroma

Image Interpretation Pearls

- Most common type of odontogenic tumor
- Prevalence exceeds all other odontogenic tumors combined (more likely to be odontoma than anything else in differential)

Reporting Tips

- Comment on effect on adjacent teeth
  - Displacement
  - Aplasia
  - Malformation
  - Impaction
- Check for uneven dilation of soft tissue capsule that would signal infection or dentigerous cyst formation if pericoronal
- Report on condition of surrounding bone and communication with crestal bone in cases of suspected infection

SELECTED REFERENCES

1. Dagrus K et al: Dentigerous cyst arising from a complex odontoma: an unusual presentation. BMJ Case Rep. 2016, 2016
2. Girish G et al: Compound composite odontoma. J Oral Maxillofac Pathol. 20(1):162, 2016
3. Jayachandran S et al: Dilated odontoma: A report of two cases from a radiological perspective. Contemp Clin Dent. 7(1):107-10, 2016
4. Santos LA et al: Complex odontoma: a case report with micro-computed tomography findings. Case Rep Dent. 2016:3584751, 2016
5. Sharma G et al: An erupted dilated odontoma: a rare presentation. Case Rep Dent. 2016:9750947, 2016
6. Verma S et al: Erupted complex odontoma of the posterior maxilla: A rarity. J Nat Sci Biol Med. 6(Suppl 1):S167-9, 2015
7. Chrcanovic BR et al: Two-stage surgical removal of large complex odontoma. Oral Maxillofac Surg. 14(4):247-52, 2010
8. Marques YM et al: Importance of cone beam computed tomography for diagnosis of calcifying cystic odontogenic tumour associated to odontoma. Report of a case. Med Oral Patol Oral Cir Bucal. 15(3):e490-3, 2010
9. Bhatavadekar NB et al: The use of digital volume tomography in imaging an unusually large composite odontoma in the mandible. Pediatr Dent. 31(5):438-41, 2009
10. Isler SC et al: Radiologic evaluation of an unusually sized complex odontoma involving the maxillary sinus by cone beam computed tomography. Quintessence Int. 40(7):533-5, 2009
11. Teruhisa U et al: A case of unerupted lower primary second molar associated with compound odontoma. Open Dent J. 3:173-6, 2009
12. Bordini J Jr et al: Multiple compound odontomas in the jaw: case report and analysis of the literature. J Oral Maxillofac Surg. 66(12):2617-20, 2008
13. Tam D et al: Compound odontoma causing airway obstruction of the newborn: a case report. J Laryngol Otol. 120(10):879-81, 2006
14. Litonjua LA et al: Erupted complex odontoma: a case report and literature review. Gen Dent. 52(3):248-51, 2004

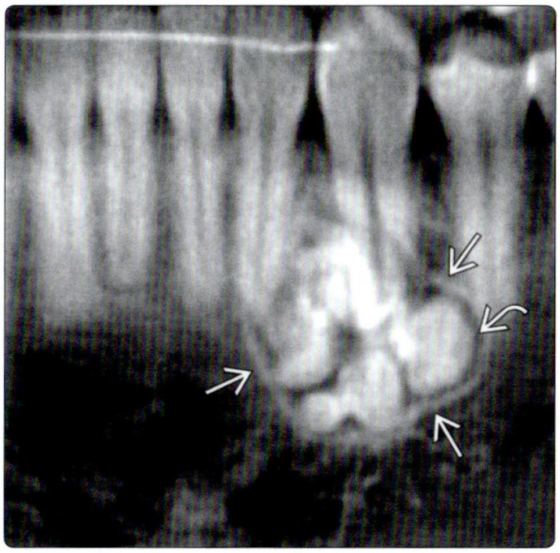

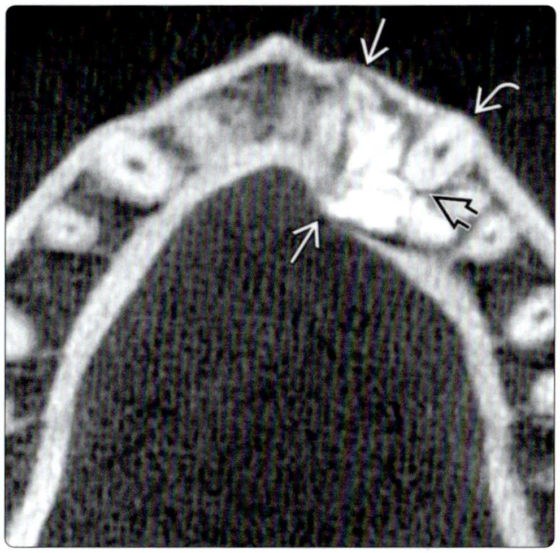

(Left) *CBCT panoramic reformat shows a compound odontoma at the root of the fully erupted permanent mandibular left canine. Note corticated border and low-density rim within.* **(Right)** *Axial CBCT in the same patient shows expansion and thinning of the lingual and facial cortices of the mandible in the area of the compound odontoma. A thin zone of radiolucency separates the permanent canine root from the odontoma.*

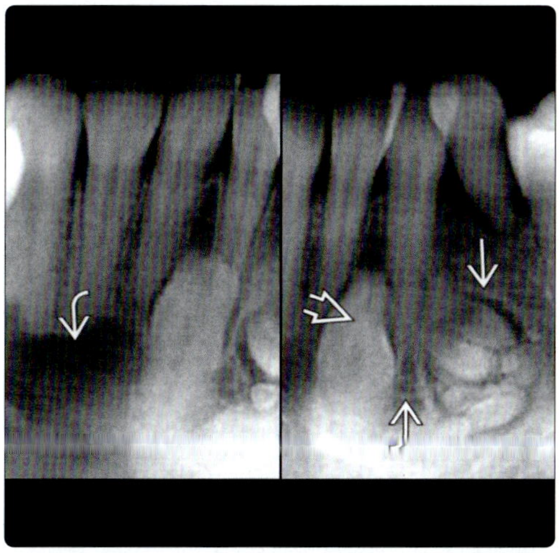

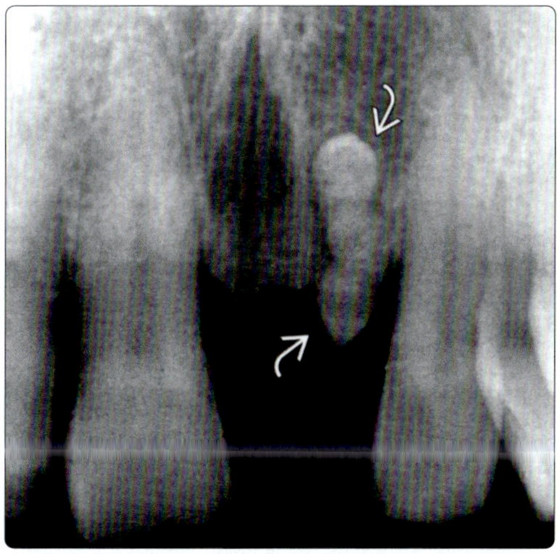

(Left) *Periapical radiographs of the left anterior mandible show an odontoma adjacent to the impacted mandibular left canine. The radiolucency associated with the canine proved to be an odontogenic keratocyst. Odontomas may often be found in association with other lesions. (Courtesy M. Pharoah, DDS.)* **(Right)** *Periapical radiograph shows agenesis of the permanent maxillary left central incisor. A partially erupted compound odontoma has formed in its place.*

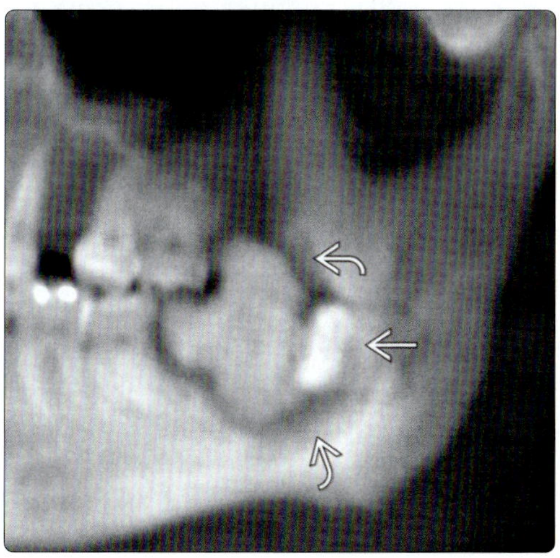

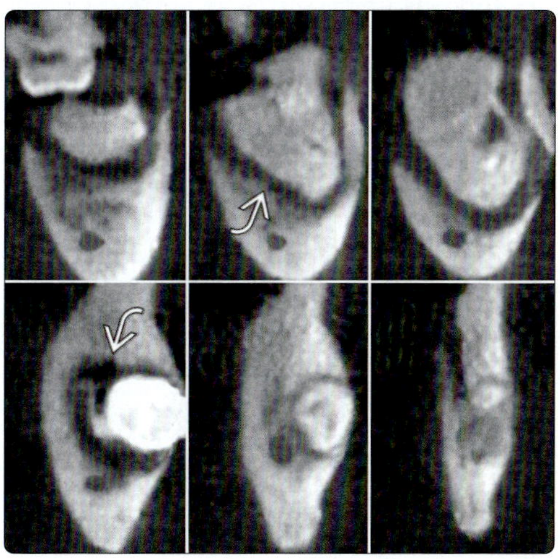

(Left) *CBCT panoramic reformat shows an infected, partially erupted complex odontoma pericoronal to the displaced mandibular left 3rd molar. Note widening of the low-density rim and sclerosis of the surrounding bone. The occlusal contact with the opposing molar may be the reason for the infection. (Courtesy M. Noujeim, DDS.)* **(Right)** *CBCT cross sections of infected complex odontoma in the same patient show ragged borders and sclerosis of surrounding bone. (Courtesy M. Noujeim, DDS.)*

Adenomatoid Odontogenic Tumor

KEY FACTS

TERMINOLOGY

- Adenomatoid odontogenic tumor (AOT)
- Definition: Odontogenic epithelial tumor, often containing calcifications
- Can be **central** or **peripheral**
- Can be **follicular** (pericoronal) or **extrafollicular** (with no associated tooth)
- Follicular type is more common in central lesions

IMAGING

- Well-corticated low-density lesion with small flecks of calcification; possibly related to impacted tooth
- Not necessarily attached to cemento-enamel junction (CEJ) of teeth
- Mostly in **anterior maxilla**
- Calcifications can vary from faint snowflake to small pebble appearance
- May have **peripheral band of radiolucency** void of any radiopaque flecks

TOP DIFFERENTIAL DIAGNOSES

- Calcifying odontogenic cyst
- Calcifying epithelial odontogenic tumor
- Ameloblastic fibro-odontoma
- Dentigerous cyst
- Odontogenic keratocyst

CLINICAL ISSUES

- Most common in **2nd decade** of life
- **Female patients** 2x as likely to develop AOT

DIAGNOSTIC CHECKLIST

- Check **relationship to CEJ to differentiate from dentigerous cyst**
- Look for faint calcifications when windowing and leveling
- Comment on position of impacted tooth and relationship with adjacent teeth

(Left) *Occlusal radiograph of the right anterior maxilla shows impaction of the lateral incisor due to an AOT. Note the faint calcifications → within the low-density body of the lesion. (Courtesy M. Noujeim, DDS.)* **(Right)** *Sagittal CBCT shows an AOT associated with a maxillary premolar. The corticated boundary of the lesion is attached to the midroot of the tooth →. Note calcifications are in the center of the lesion, and there is a peripheral zone of radiolucency often seen in AOT →. (Courtesy M. Noujeim, DDS.)*

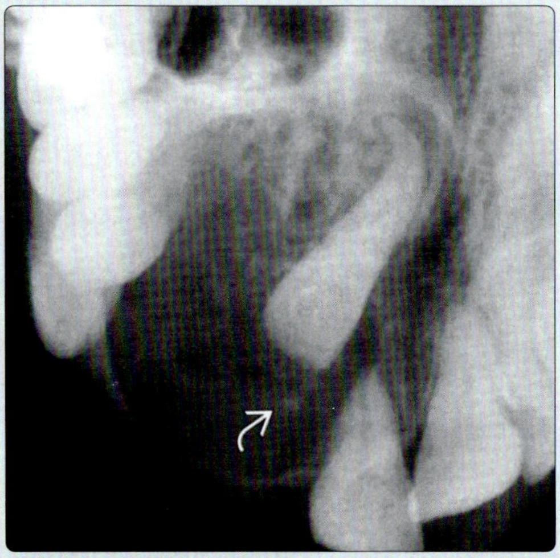

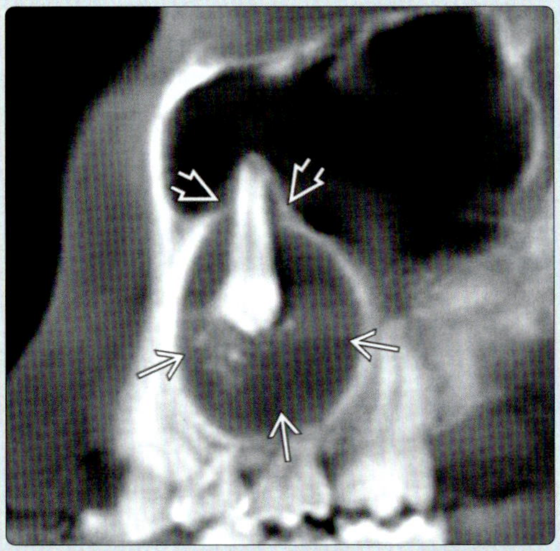

(Left) *Coronal CBCT shows an AOT surrounding the crown and the coronal 1/3 of the root of the maxillary left 2nd premolar with displacement into the maxillary sinus. Calcifications can be seen coronal to the tooth →. (Courtesy, M. Noujeim, DDS.)* **(Right)** *Periapical radiograph shows a completely radiolucent lesion of AOT between the roots of the permanent right maxillary lateral incisor (displaced) → and the primary canine →. The developing permanent canine is displaced →. (Courtesy M. Finklestein, DDS.)*

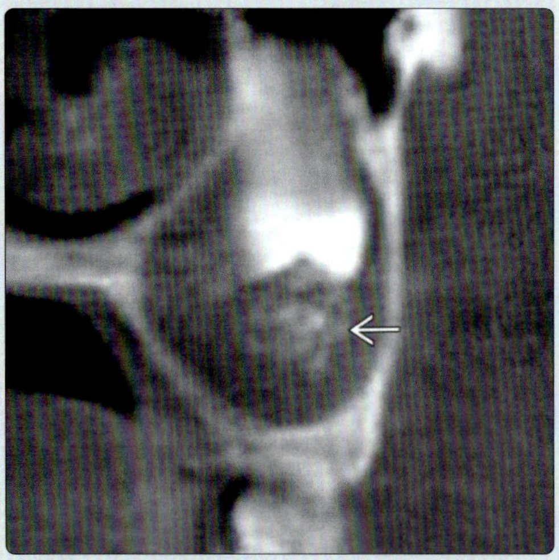

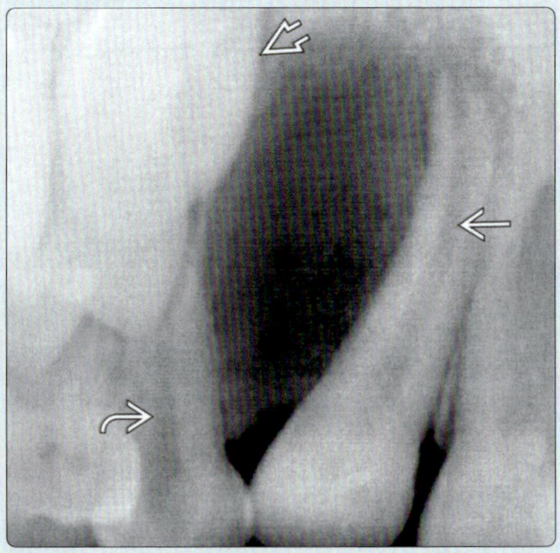

TERMINOLOGY

Abbreviations

- Adenomatoid odontogenic tumor (AOT)

Synonyms

- Adenoameloblastoma, ameloblastic adenomatoid tumor

Definitions

- Odontogenic epithelial tumor, often containing calcifications
- Can be **central** or **peripheral**
- Can be **follicular** (pericoronal) or **extrafollicular** (with no associated tooth)
- Follicular type is more common in central lesions

IMAGING

General Features

- Best diagnostic clue
  - Well-corticated low-density lesion with small flecks of calcification most often pericoronal to unerupted tooth
  - When pericoronal, does not necessarily attach near cemento-enamel junction (CEJ) of teeth
- Location
  - Mostly in **anterior maxilla**, canine area; rarely in mandible
  - 75% associated with unerupted permanent teeth
- Size
  - Seldom exceeds 3 cm in diameter
  - When large, can completely envelop tooth
- Morphology
  - Corticated boundary
  - Internal low density with varying degrees of calcified foci
  - 60% have internal calcifications
  - Calcifications can vary from **faint snowflake to small pebble appearance**
  - May have **peripheral band of radiolucency** void of any radiopaque flecks
- Related lesions
  - Cementoosseous reactive proliferation/dysplasia
  - Dentigerous cyst

Imaging Recommendations

- Best imaging tool
  - CBCT
    - Shows lesion in all dimensions
    - Shows position of impacted tooth, if present
    - Shows effect on surrounding structures

Radiographic Findings

- Intraoral plain film
  - Large corticated unilocular radiolucent lesion with internal calcifications
  - Can help show relationship of lesion to impacted tooth CEJ
  - Impaction &/or displacement of teeth
  - Minute root resorption can be detected, though rare
- Extraoral plain film
  - Shows mesiodistal extent of lesion
  - Shows involvement of teeth and extent of displacement

CT Findings

- CBCT
  - Faciolingual expansion can be appreciated
  - Exact localization of associated and adjacent teeth can be determined

DIFFERENTIAL DIAGNOSIS

Calcifying Odontogenic Cyst

- Difficult to differentiate from AOT
- Slightly older age group, especially maxillary lesions

Calcifying Epithelial Odontogenic Tumor

- More common in posterior mandible
- Older age group

Ameloblastic Fibro-Odontoma

- More common in posterior mandible

Dentigerous Cyst

- **Always pericoronal**: Lesion attaches near or **at CEJ**
- May look similar when AOT is devoid of calcifications

Odontogenic Keratocyst

- Can be confused with AOT when AOT is devoid of calcifications

PATHOLOGY

Staging, Grading, & Classification

- Benign odontogenic epithelial tumor

Gross Pathologic & Surgical Features

- Well encapsulated
- Easily separated from bone

Microscopic Features

- Tubular or duct-like structures surrounded by columnar or cuboidal epithelial cells are characteristic

CLINICAL ISSUES

Presentation

- Most common signs/symptoms
  - **Failure of tooth eruption**

Demographics

- Age
  - 5-50 years: Most common in **2nd decade** of life
- Gender
  - **Female patients** 2x as likely to develop AOT

Natural History & Prognosis

- Not locally invasive
- Stops developing when tooth development ceases
- Recurrence rate is 0.2%

Treatment

- Conservative surgical excision

SELECTED REFERENCES

1. Naidu A et al: Adenomatoid odontogenic tumor with peripheral cemento-osseous reactive proliferation: Report of 2 cases and review of the literature. Oral Surg Oral Med Oral Pathol Oral Radiol. 122(3):e86-93 2016

Ameloblastoma

KEY FACTS

TERMINOLOGY
- Definition: Benign but **locally aggressive** neoplasm originating from odontogenic epithelium
- Most common odontogenic tumor of clinical significance
- Solid/multicystic, unicystic, peripheral, and desmoplastic subtypes

IMAGING
- Well-defined, expansile, **multilocular** (80%) radiolucency in posterior mandible
- **Soap bubble pattern** of internal septa typical; not pathognomonic
- **Pericoronal relationship** to impacted and displaced molar tooth often in unicystic type
- Extensive expansion and thinning of cortices
- **Resorption** of adjacent teeth roots
- T1WI C+: Solid tumor components & cyst walls show strong enhancement
  - **Mural nodule enhances** in unicystic type

TOP DIFFERENTIAL DIAGNOSES
- Odontogenic myxoma
- Central giant cell granuloma
- Aneurysmal bone cyst
- Dentigerous cyst (DC)
- Odontogenic keratocyst (OKC)

CLINICAL ISSUES
- 3rd-5th decade; unicystic type at younger age
- Slow-growing, expansile, painless mass
- High recurrence rate
- Treatment requires resection with ≥ 1 cm margin of bone

DIAGNOSTIC CHECKLIST
- Larger dentigerous cyst & OKC most difficult to differentiate from unicystic ameloblastoma
  - Attachment at CEJ more likely indicates DC
  - Ameloblastomas more expansile in mandible than OKC
- **Follow-up for recurrence** is critical

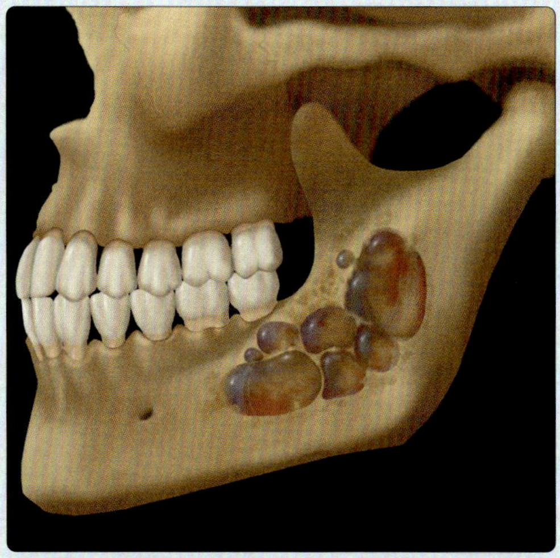
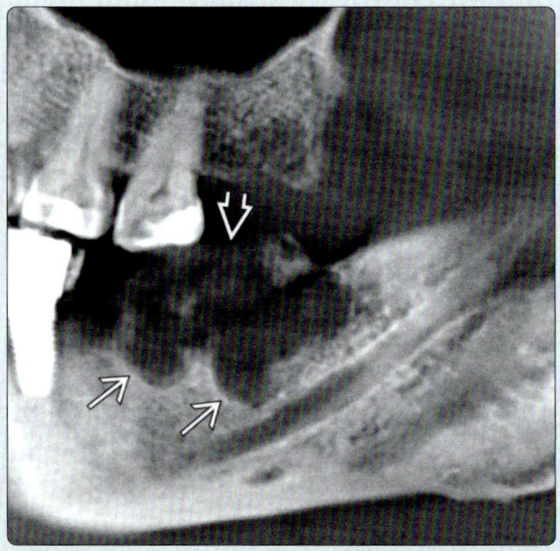

(Left) *Lateral graphic shows the multilocular and expansile nature of a mandibular ameloblastoma. The posterior mandible is the most common location for this tumor.* **(Right)** *Sagittal oblique CBCT of an ameloblastoma in a 49-year-old man shows a multilocular lesion with large, well-defined curves around the periphery ➡ separated by thick bony septa, giving a soap bubble appearance. It has caused expansion of the crest of the alveolar ridge ➡.*

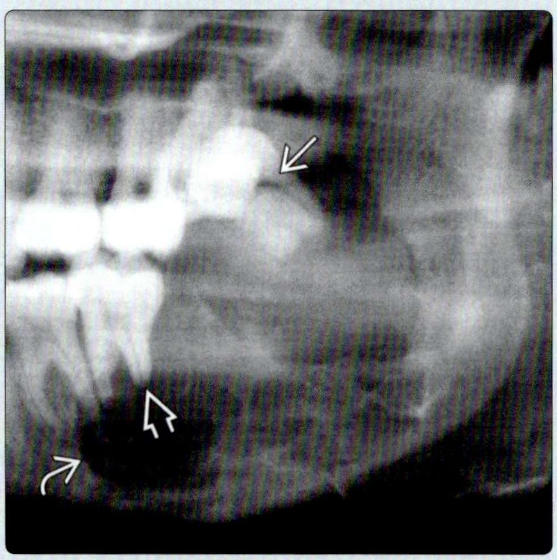
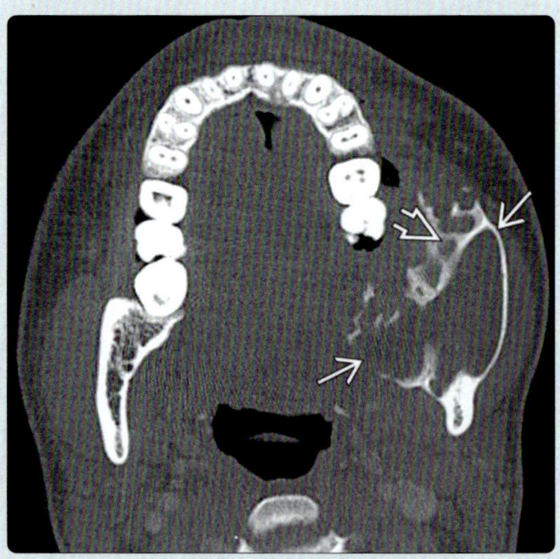

(Left) *Panoramic radiograph shows a large ameloblastoma in the left posterior mandible that is causing extreme displacement of the 3rd molar superiorly ➡ and displacement and root resorption of the 2nd molar ➡. The well-defined periphery ➡ and multilocular nature of the lesion are also appreciated.* **(Right)** *Axial bone CT of the same patient shows the extreme expansion of the buccal and lingual cortices ➡. The characteristic thick septa between the lesion loculations are also evident ➡.*

Ameloblastoma

TERMINOLOGY

Synonyms

- Adamantinoma (old term, now describes rare low-grade malignancy of long bones), adamantoblastoma

Definitions

- Locally aggressive, benign, odontogenic neoplasm of epithelial origin
- **Central** ameloblastoma: Develops within jaw bones, may be multi- or unilocular radiographically
  - **Solid/multicystic** ameloblastoma: Most common type
  - **Unicystic** ameloblastoma: Histologically presents as single cystic entity
    - Usually radiographically unilocular, but scalloping margins may give rise to multilocular appearance
- **Peripheral** ameloblastoma: Develops on gingiva or alveolar mucosa, not usually apparent radiographically
- **Desmoplastic** ameloblastoma: Subtype with distinct clinical, radiologic, and pathologic features

IMAGING

General Features

- Best diagnostic clue
  - Well-defined, expansile lesion with multilocular or **soap bubble** pattern in posterior mandible
- Location
  - Often associated with impacted tooth
  - **Mandible**:maxilla ratio = 5:1
  - Most common site: Mandibular 3rd molar, ramus regions
    - Desmoplastic type common in anterior/premolar area
  - In maxilla: May extend into maxillary sinus or nasal fossa
  - Peripheral type on alveolar mucosa or gingiva
- Size
  - > 2 cm at discovery in most cases
- Morphology
  - Unilocular pattern: Round, hydraulic, cyst-like lesion
  - Multilocular pattern (80%): Irregular or scalloped shape

Radiographic Findings

- Radiography
  - Periphery: **Well-defined**, corticated border
  - Internal structure: Reflects pathologic type
    - Unicystic subtype: Unilocular unless scalloped periphery gives multilocular appearance
      - **Radiolucent** with no internal septa
    - Solid/multicystic subtype: Most often multilocular radiographically
      - Bony **septa are thick and curved** forming round "soap bubble" loculations
      - But can have unilocular presentation
    - Desmoplastic subtype
      - Greater radiopaque component with sclerotic or granular bone, **may mimic fibroosseous lesion**
  - Local effects
    - Displacement and **resorption of tooth roots**, significant in large lesions
    - **Expansion of cortices**, can be extensive
    - Thinning and perforation of cortices
      - Loss of anterior border of ramus with unilocular, pericoronal lesion suggestive of unicystic ameloblastoma
    - Displacement of structures; nerve canal, floor of sinus, floor of nasal fossa

CT Findings

- CECT
  - Multicystic/solid lesions show strong enhancement of solid components
  - Unicystic lesions show **enhancement of wall and mural nodules**
  - Larger lesions with extraosseous extension show moderate soft tissue enhancement mixed with cystic (low-density) areas
    - Extraosseous extension is uncommon
- CBCT and bone CT
  - Low-attenuation osteolytic lesion
  - Uni- (20%) or **multilocular (80%)** with scalloped borders
  - **Soap bubble pattern** is typical; not pathognomonic
  - Extensive expansion and thinning of cortices
  - Resorption of adjacent teeth, often **"knife-edged"**
  - Desmoplastic subtype demonstrates internal granular calcification, honeycomb multilocularity

MR Findings

- T1WI
  - Solid tumor parts: Low to intermediate T1 signal intensity
  - Cystic parts: Low to intermediate T1 signal intensity
- T2WI
  - Solid and cystic components: High T2 signal intensity
- T1WI C+
  - Solid tumor components show strong enhancement
    - Thicker enhancing walls seen than in odontogenic cysts
    - Enhancement of **mural nodules** seen in unicystic ameloblastoma
  - Cystic areas show no enhancement

Imaging Recommendations

- Best imaging tool
  - Thin-section CECT with soft tissue and bone algorithm
- Protocol advice
  - CT best demonstrates internal morphology of septa and pattern of bone expansion
  - CECT delineates focal enhancing mural nodules
  - C+ MR best defines extraosseous components & association with critical neurovascular structures
  - Both CT & MR may be required to differentiate from other cystic lesions

DIFFERENTIAL DIAGNOSIS

Odontogenic Myxoma (Myxofibroma)

- Multilocular lesion in posterior maxilla or mandible
- **Finer and straighter** septations than ameloblastoma
- Less bony expansion than ameloblastoma
- Greater extension between roots **without resorption**

Central Giant Cell Granuloma

- Benign nonodontogenic reactive lesion with multilocular radiographic pattern
- More commonly presents **anterior to 1st molars**
- Periphery is less clearly corticated than ameloblastoma
- **Septa are wispy** and less well defined than ameloblastoma

Aneurysmal Bone Cyst

- Children > adults
- Bone CT: Greatly expansile, multilocular mass
- Septa are more granular and wispy, like central giant cell granuloma
- NECT or MR: **Fluid-fluid levels**

Dentigerous Cyst

- Unilocular cystic lesion surrounding **crown of impacted tooth**
- Lesion originating in follicle and attaching at cementoenamel junction
- CT/MR: No enhancing mural nodule
- Unicystic ameloblastoma may mimic dentigerous cyst

Odontogenic Keratocyst

- Uni- or multilocular cystic lesion often associated with unerupted tooth
- Fewer internal septa compared to multilocular/solid ameloblastoma
- Demonstrates **less bony expansion** in mandible with scalloping of cortices
- CT/MR: No enhancing mural nodule
- MR: More heterogeneous DWI signal intensities
- Unicystic & smaller solid ameloblastoma may mimic this tumor

PATHOLOGY

General Features

- Etiology
  - Benign tumor arising from odontogenic epithelium (rests of enamel organ or dental lamina)
  - Somatic mutations identified
    - Mitogen-activated protein kinase (MAPK) signaling pathway dysregulation: *BRAF* mutation
    - Hedgehog pathway: *SMO* mutation

Microscopic Features

- Proliferating sheets or islands of odontogenic epithelium in connective tissue stroma
  - Epithelial cells are ameloblast-like
    - Palisading, columnar cells with hyperchromatic nuclei polarized away from basement membrane
  - Small to macroscopic cysts form in epithelial islands
- Histologic types: Follicular, plexiform, acanthomatous, desmoplastic, basal cell, & granular cell
- Unicystic type: Ameloblastic epithelium in cyst lining
  - Epithelium may proliferate into cyst lumen (intraluminal type) or into cyst wall (mural type)

CLINICAL ISSUES

Presentation

- Most common signs/symptoms
  - Hard, painless facial or intraoral swelling

Demographics

- Age
  - Most commonly presents in patients 30-50 years old
  - Unicystic ameloblastoma often seen at younger age
- Gender
  - No significant gender predilection
- Epidemiology
  - 2nd most common odontogenic tumor but varies by population studied
  - Most common **clinically significant** odontogenic tumor
  - 1% of odontogenic lesions

Natural History & Prognosis

- Slow-growing, sometimes indolent, but aggressive benign neoplasm
- Tumor **recurrence is common**
  - Recurrence rate varies by treatment but is high (15%), even with adequate treatment
  - Unicystic tumor recurs less frequently
- Malignant transformation is rare (< 1%)
  - Ameloblastic carcinoma & malignant ameloblastoma may metastasize

Treatment

- Multilocular/solid lesions: **Complete surgical resection**
  - ≥ 1 cm margin past radiologic border advocated
  - Curettage no longer acceptable therapy (90% recurrence)
- Unicystic lesions without mural involvement may be treated more conservatively
- Chemotherapy & radiotherapy are contraindicated
- **Long-term follow-up** required
  - Late recurrence (> 5 years) is not uncommon

DIAGNOSTIC CHECKLIST

Consider

- Larger dentigerous cyst & pericoronal odontogenic keratocyst most difficult to differentiate from unicystic ameloblastoma

Image Interpretation Pearls

- Thick, curved septa within lesion creating **soap bubble** or honeycomb pattern
- Look for **mural nodule** in unicystic lesions to differentiate from odontogenic cyst

Reporting Tips

- Relationship to, or involvement of, inferior alveolar nerve canal in mandible
- Look for extension into adjacent spaces/structures

SELECTED REFERENCES

1. Almeida Rde A et al: Recurrence rate following treatment for primary multicystic ameloblastoma: systematic review and meta-analysis. Int J Oral Maxillofac Surg. 45(3):359-67, 2016
2. McClary AC et al: Ameloblastoma: a clinical review and trends in management. Eur Arch Otorhinolaryngol. 273(7):1649-61, 2016
3. Milman T et al: Ameloblastoma: 25 year experience at a single institution. Head Neck Pathol. 10(4):513-520, 2016
4. Luo J et al: Cone beam computed tomography signs of desmoplastic ameloblastoma: review of 7 cases. Oral Surg Oral Med Oral Pathol Oral Radiol. 118(4):e126-33, 2014

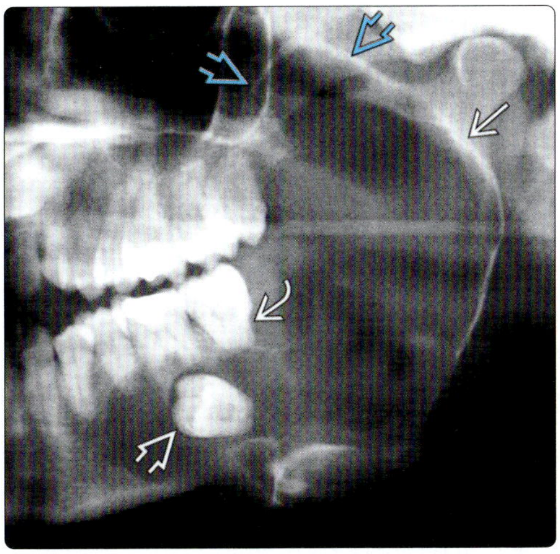

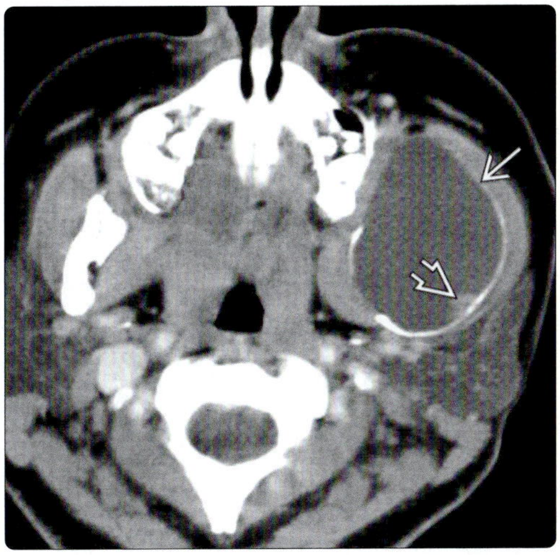

(Left) *Panoramic radiograph shows a large unicystic ameloblastoma in the left mandible with a well-defined, corticated periphery. Slight multilocular appearance is due to scalloping of margins. Note expansion into the coronoid process. Displaced 3rd molar and root resorption are also seen.* **(Right)** *Axial CECT in the same patient shows the expanded cortices. The internal low density is suggestive of a cystic lesion, but an enhancing mural nodule gives a clue to the correct diagnosis.*

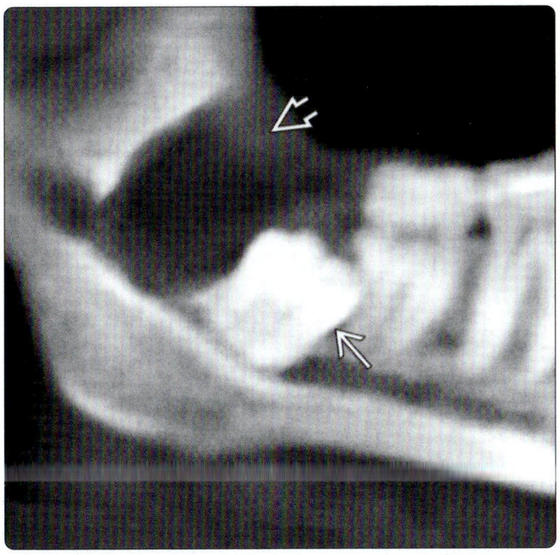

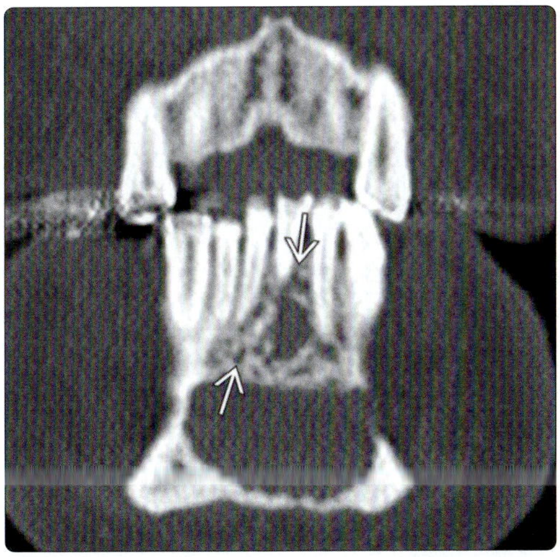

(Left) *Panoramic reformat CBCT shows a unicystic ameloblastoma in the right posterior mandible. Note the eccentric involvement of the impacted 3rd molar and the destruction of the anterior border of the ramus.* **(Right)** *Coronal CT in a 62-year-old man shows features characteristic of the desmoplastic-type ameloblastoma in the superior half of the lesion. Numerous small locules are interspersed with thick septa and coarse bone deposits. This type of ameloblastoma may mimic a fibroosseous lesion.*

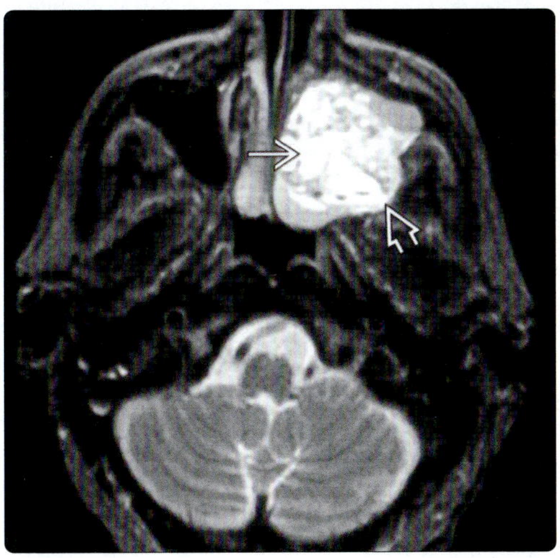

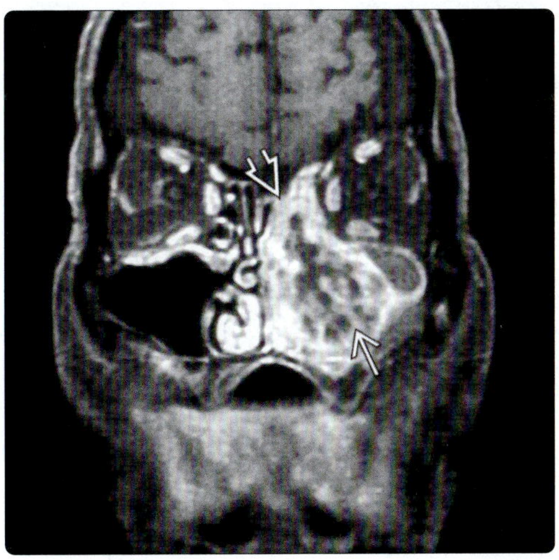

(Left) *Axial T2WI FS MR of a maxillary ameloblastoma shows both solid and cystic components in a multiloculated pattern. Note the typical bright T2 signal of the cystic components and the expansion of the posterior maxillary sinus walls.* **(Right)** *Coronal T1WI C+ FS MR in the same patient demonstrates the enhancement of the septations typically seen with ameloblastoma. The locally aggressive nature of this tumor is evident by its extension into the nasal cavity and ethmoid air cells.*

Ameloblastic Fibroma

KEY FACTS

TERMINOLOGY

- Synonyms: Soft odontoma, mixed odontogenic tumor, fibroadamantoblastoma, granular cell ameloblastic fibroma
- Definition: Benign odontogenic tumor containing ectomesenchyme resembling dental papilla and epithelial strands and nests resembling dental lamina and enamel organ

IMAGING

- Well-defined, corticated, often expansile **radiolucency without evidence of tooth structures** or calcifications within
- Associated with **crown of unerupted tooth** (pericoronal) in many cases
- Usually **posterior mandible of young patients**
- **Unilocular or multilocular** radiolucency
- CBCT best demonstrates expansion and loculations
- Large lesions may perforate buccal and lingual cortices

TOP DIFFERENTIAL DIAGNOSES

- Pericoronal: Hyperplastic follicular space, **dentigerous cyst**, unicystic ameloblastoma, odontogenic keratocyst (OKC)
- Multilocular: Ameloblastoma, central giant cell granuloma, OKC, odontogenic myxoma

CLINICAL ISSUES

- Slow growing but can reach large size
- Recurrence (~ 33%) higher with curettage, less with radical resection
- **Malignant transformation** reported at ~ 10%
- **Radiographic follow-up** recommended

DIAGNOSTIC CHECKLIST

- If pericoronal, look for hydraulic expansion to **rule out dentigerous cyst** (most common)
- If small, consider immature odontoma, ameloblastic fibroodontoma, and ameloblastic odontoma

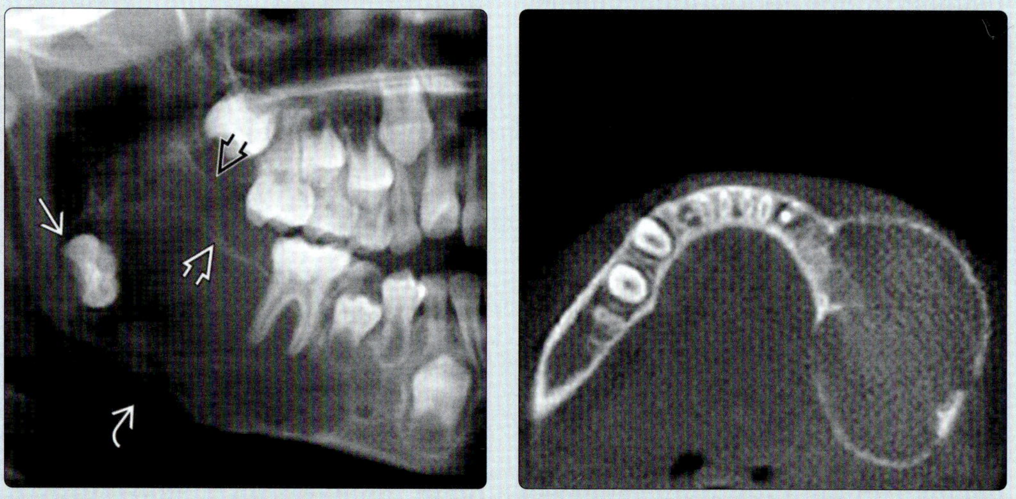

(Left) *Panoramic radiograph shows a large ameloblastic fibroma (AF) in the right posterior mandible. The lesion is pericoronal to the developing crown of the 2nd permanent molar, which has been displaced inferiorly and posteriorly by the lesion. Note expansion of the inferior border of the mandible and the anterior border of the ramus. A faint septum is evident. (Courtesy M. Noujeim, DDS.)* **(Right)** *Axial CBCT shows a large, expansile, unilocular AF in the left posterior mandible. (Courtesy M. Noujeim, DDS.)*

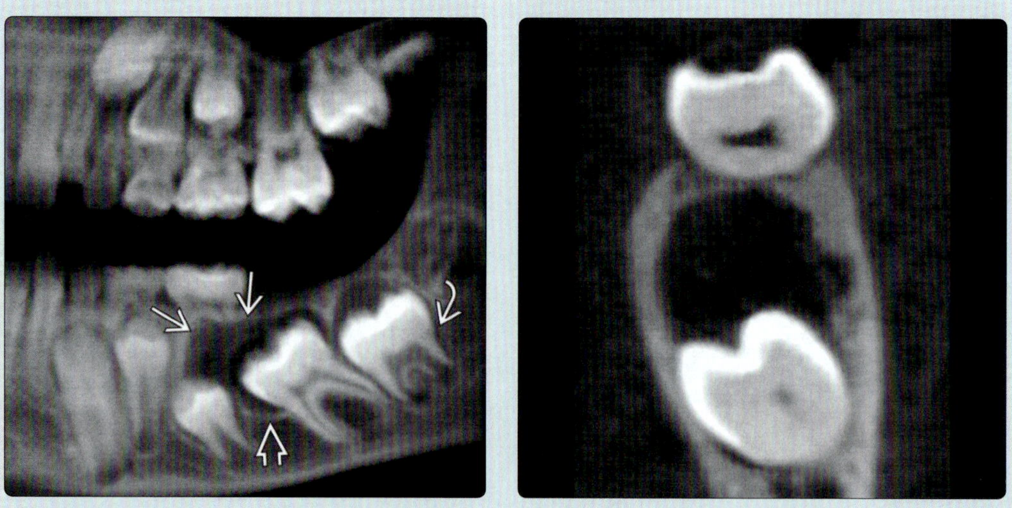

(Left) *Panoramic reformat CBCT shows an AF as an irregular pericoronal radiolucency associated with the unerupted left mandibular 1st permanent molar. This tooth and the developing 2nd premolar have been displaced. Note bulging at the attachment to the tooth compared to the adjacent normal follicular space. (Courtesy M. Noujeim, DDS.)* **(Right)** *Cross section CBCT in the same patient shows that the AF has not yet caused expansion. (Courtesy M. Noujeim, DDS.)*

TERMINOLOGY

Abbreviations

- Ameloblastic fibroma (AF)

Synonyms

- Soft odontoma
- Mixed odontogenic tumor
- Fibroadamantoblastoma
- Granular cell AF

Definitions

- Benign odontogenic tumor containing ectomesenchyme resembling dental papilla and epithelial strands and nests resembling dental lamina and enamel organ

IMAGING

General Features

- Best diagnostic clue
  - Well-defined, corticated, often expansile **radiolucency without calcifications**
    - Associated with **crown of unerupted tooth** (pericoronal) in many cases
    - Usually posterior mandible of young patients
- Location
  - **Mandible** > maxilla
    - **Posterior** > anterior
- Size
  - Small to very large (< 1 cm to 16 cm)
- Morphology
  - Well-defined **unilocular or multilocular** radiolucency
  - Typical neoplastic expansion: May form **acute angles with remaining cortex**

Imaging Recommendations

- Best imaging tool
  - CBCT will best show expansion
  - Panoramic and occlusal views
- Protocol advice
  - Bone window

Radiographic Findings

- Intraoral plain film
  - Well-defined radiolucency **without evidence of hard tissue structures**
    - Most often associated with **crown of impacted or unerupted tooth** (pericoronal)
    - **Corticated** border
- Extraoral plain film
  - Panoramic radiograph will demonstrate expansion in cephalad-caudal direction if present
    - Expansion and thinning of inferior cortex of mandible and external oblique ridge
    - Expansion into maxillary sinus or nasal cavity
  - Loculations may be present

CT Findings

- CBCT
  - Demonstrates buccal-lingual expansion
  - Loculations may be more evident
  - Large lesions may perforate buccal and lingual cortices

DIFFERENTIAL DIAGNOSIS

Hyperplastic Follicular Space

- Enlarged follicular space around crown of unerupted tooth
- Well-defined pericoronal radiolucency
- **Suspect pathology** if pericoronal space **> 3 mm**
- Look for morphology to follow outline of tooth crown

Dentigerous Cyst

- Accumulation of fluid between reduced enamel epithelium and crown of unerupted or impacted tooth
- Most common **pericoronal radiolucency**: Well defined, **unilocular**
- Follicular space takes on more **rounded** appearance
- **Hydraulic expansion**: Expanded cortex meets normal cortex at equal obtuse angles
- May not be able to differentiate if small

Unicystic (Mural) Ameloblastoma

- Ameloblastoma arising in wall of cyst (most commonly dentigerous cyst)
- Once infiltrates bone, behaves as ameloblastoma: May appear **multilocular**

Odontogenic Keratocyst

- Odontogenic neoplasm with thin para- or orthokeratinized epithelium
- **Does not expand** significantly in **mandible**
- Can be unilocular, multilocular, or pericoronal

Ameloblastoma

- Neoplasm of odontogenic epithelium
- **Multilocular** radiolucency
- Posterior mandible
- **Older** age group

Central Giant Cell Granuloma

- Reactive nonodontogenic lesion
- Usually **multilocular and expansile**
- Predilection for anterior mandible
- **Never pericoronal**

Odontogenic Myxoma

- Benign neoplasm of odontogenic ectomesenchyme
- **Multilocular with straight septa** making geometric shapes and letters

Immature Odontoma

- Hamartoma of odontogenic epithelium and ectomesenchyme
- Produces **radiopaque/high-density areas** consistent with tooth structure
- Unilocular
- May be **completely radiolucent prior to maturation**

Immature Ameloblastic Fibroodontoma

- Mixed odontogenic neoplasm
- Produces less calcified tooth structure than odontoma

Immature Ameloblastic Odontoma

- Mixed odontogenic neoplasm; more aggressive than odontoma and ameloblastic fibroodontoma (AFO)
- Very rare

PATHOLOGY

General Features

- Etiology
  - Unknown
- Genetics
  - Alteration of *TP53* gene in malignant transformations
- Associated abnormalities
  - Has been reported in **association with calcifying odontogenic cyst** (Gorlin cyst)
    - Strands of odontogenic epithelium are found in hypercellular connective tissue nodules located in cystic wall

Gross Pathologic & Surgical Features

- Encapsulated tumor mass

Microscopic Features

- Strands and nests of odontogenic epithelium in immature fibrous connective tissue stroma resembling dental papilla
  - Contains **no hard tissue** (tooth) structures
- Odontoma, AFO, and ameloblastic odontoma (AO), which contain tooth structure, may look similar prior to maturation when calcifications may not be radiographically evident
- Concept that AF represents immature form of odontoma, AFO, or AO is not supported by current data
  - Several residual and recurrent AFs have not demonstrated further maturation
  - AF is occasionally observed in older age group beyond period of odontogenesis
- Malignant transformation to **ameloblastic fibrosarcoma** occurs in mesenchymal component: Increased cellularity, mitosis, and anaplasia
  - Epithelial component disappears
  - Rarely metastasizes
- Malignant transformation to **ameloblastic carcinosarcoma** has been reported but is extremely rare
  - Epithelial component is retained and exhibits spectrum from normal palisading ameloblasts to frankly malignant cells showing pleomorphism and hyperchromatic nuclei
  - More likely to occur after multiple resections of AF
  - Metastasis to lungs and regional lymph nodes

CLINICAL ISSUES

Presentation

- Most common signs/symptoms
  - Hard swelling of jaws
    - Associated with multilocular lesions
  - Failure of eruption of involved tooth
- Other signs/symptoms
  - Occasionally pain &/or drainage
    - Symptomatic patients usually have multilocular lesions

Demographics

- Age
  - Childhood/adolescence
    - Mean: ~ 15 years
- Gender
  - Slight male predilection

Natural History & Prognosis

- Slow growing but can reach large size
- Recurrence (~ 33%) directly related to treatment modality
  - Recurrence higher with more conservative treatment
  - Longer period of nonrecurrence with more radical treatment
  - One study found recurrence rates of 41% and 69% at 5 and 10 years, respectively
- **Malignant transformation** reported at ~ 10%
  - Malignant transformation rate of 10% and 22% at 5 and 10 years, respectively
    - Malignant transformation less likely to occur in patients < 22 years
  - May recur multiple times and even cause death
  - Distant metastases rare

Treatment

- Curettage
- Enucleation
- Simple excision
- Radical resection for larger tumors
- Close **radiographic follow-up** recommended

DIAGNOSTIC CHECKLIST

Consider

- Odontoma, AFO, and AO if small
  - In early stages, these lesions may be completely radiolucent
- Ameloblastoma, central giant cell granuloma, and odontogenic keratocyst if multilocular

Image Interpretation Pearls

- If pericoronal, look for hydraulic expansion to rule out dentigerous cyst, which is most common pericoronal radiolucency

SELECTED REFERENCES

1. Bertoni F et al: Ameloblastic fibrosarcoma of the mandible evolving from a prior ameloblastic fibroma after two years: an unusual finding. Int J Surg Pathol. 24(7):656-9, 2016
2. Tozoglu S et al: Extensive ameloblastic fibroma of the mandibula in a female adult patient: a case report with a follow-up of 3 years. Eur J Dent. 10(1):139-43, 2016
3. Arora M et al: Ameloblastic fibroma with ghost cell differentiation and calcification: a unique case report. J Cancer Res Ther. 11(4):1033, 2015
4. de Vasconcellos SJ et al: Massive ameloblastic fibroma treated with surgical conservative treatment. J Craniofac Surg. 26(3):999-1000, 2015
5. Ealla KK et al: Ameloblastic fibroma of the maxilla with bilateral presentation: report of a rare case with review of the literature. Case Rep Pediatr. 2015:250713, 2015
6. Manzon S et al: Treatment of a recurrent ameloblastic fibroma. N Y State Dent J. 81(1):30-2, 2015
7. Melo Lde A et al: Ameloblastic fibroma: a rare case report with 7-year follow-up. Srp Arh Celok Lek. 143(3-4):190-4, 2015
8. de Castro JF et al: Ameloblastic fibroma: a rare case appearing as a mixed radiographic image. J Clin Exp Dent. 6(5):e583-7, 2014
9. Hu YY et al: Ameloblastic fibrosarcoma of the mandible: a case report and mini review. Exp Ther Med. 8(5):1463-1466, 2014
10. Buchner A et al: Ameloblastic fibroma: a stage in the development of a hamartomatous odontoma or a true neoplasm? Critical analysis of 162 previously reported cases plus 10 new cases. Oral Surg Oral Med Oral Pathol Oral Radiol. 116(5):598-606, 2013

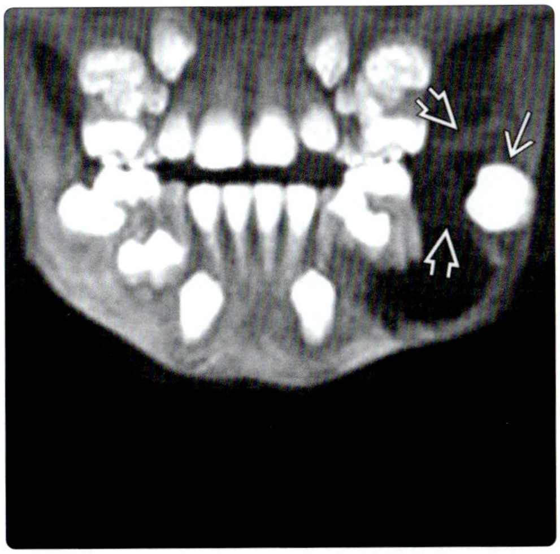

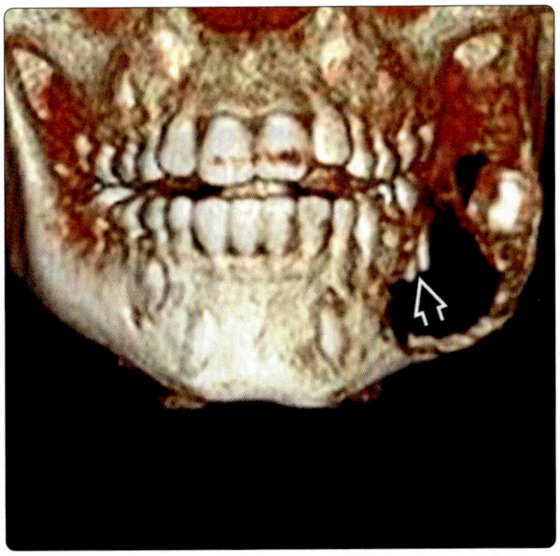

(Left) *Panoramic reformat CBCT shows a large AF in the left posterior mandible associated with the crown of the unerupted developing 2nd permanent molar. The lesion has expanded into the anterior border of the ramus, and septa are evident. (Courtesy M. Noujeim, DDS.)* **(Right)** *CBCT 3D reconstruction in the same patient shows the mandibular left 1st permanent molar roots visible within the AF. (Courtesy M. Noujeim, DDS.)*

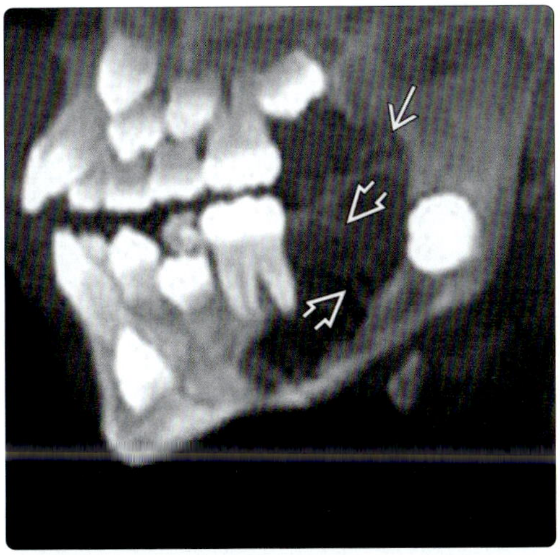

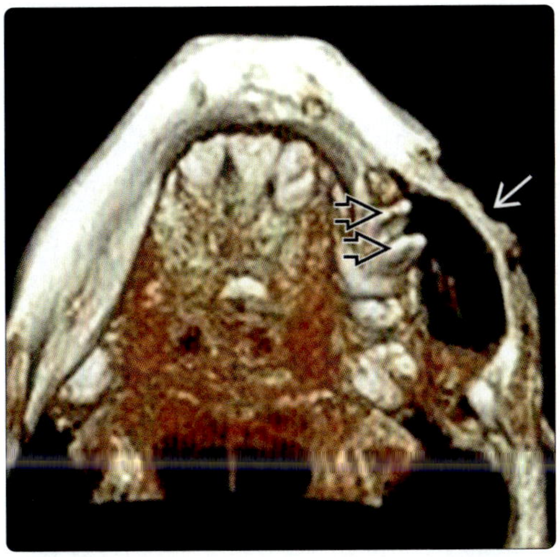

(Left) *Lateral CBCT in the same patient shows the lesion has extended into the coronoid process. Note fine septa within the lesion. (Courtesy M. Noujeim, DDS.)* **(Right)** *CBCT 3D reconstruction in the same patient shows the AF viewed from below. Note the buccal expansion and the mesial and distal roots of the 1st molar clearly visible within the lesion. The inferior border of the mandible has been spared. (Courtesy M. Noujeim, DDS.)*

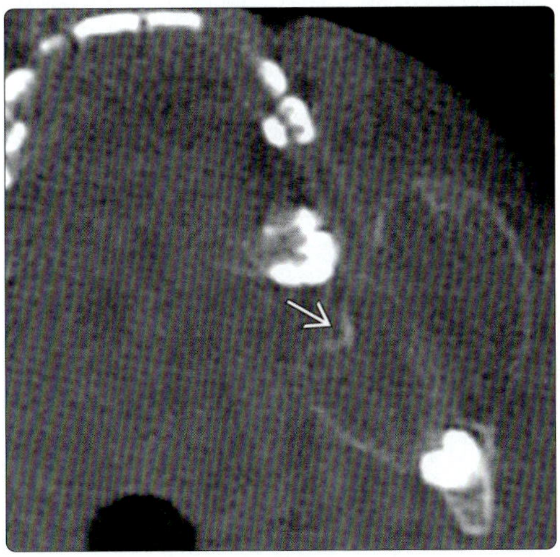

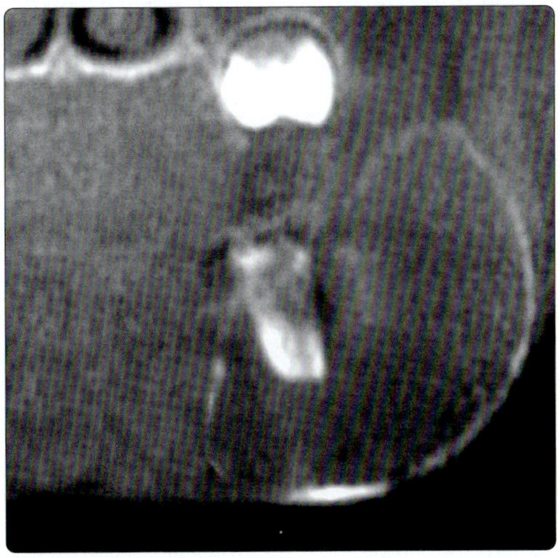

(Left) *Axial CBCT shows AF in the same patient. The cortex is expanded and thinned but not perforated. Note how the lesion curves back on itself to form an acute angle with the normal cortex. This is characteristic of a tumor rather than a cyst, which causes hydraulic expansion and produces more obtuse angles. (Courtesy M. Noujeim, DDS.)* **(Right)** *Coronal CBCT in the same patient shows the AF has expanded mainly in the buccal direction. (Courtesy M. Noujeim, DDS.)*

Ameloblastic Fibroodontoma

KEY FACTS

TERMINOLOGY

- Ameloblastic fibroodontoma (AFO)
- Definition: Tumor of mixed odontogenic epithelium and ectomesenchyme; similar to ameloblastic fibroma but with scattered collections of enamel and dentin

IMAGING

- Well-defined, sometimes corticated, lucent area with **specks of tooth-density material** within
- Calcifications may be **doughnut-shaped with rim of enamel density**
- Associated with **missing tooth** or unerupted tooth
- Most common in **posterior mandible** pericoronal to developing tooth
- May appear **as small as enlarged tooth follicles or few cm in diameter**
- Larger lesions have more calcified material
- CBCT will show **buccolingual expansion**

TOP DIFFERENTIAL DIAGNOSES

- Ameloblastic fibroma
- Odontoma
- Adenomatoid odontogenic tumor
- Calcifying odontogenic cyst
- Calcifying epithelial odontogenic tumor

PATHOLOGY

- Islands of odontogenic epithelium in loose primitive connective tissue resembling dental papilla

CLINICAL ISSUES

- Age: 2nd decade
- M = F
- Large lesions may present as painless bony swelling
- Treatment: Enucleation, recurrence rare
- Development of ameloblastic fibrosarcoma after curettage has been reported but is very rare

(Left) *3D reformation shows an impacted and displaced 2nd molar by an ameloblastic fibroodontoma (AFO). Note the small calcified tooth density material ➡ within the lesion.* **(Right)** *Axial CBCT in same patient shows that the AFO contains multiple small tooth density calcifications ➡. This slice is inferior to the impacted tooth. Note that the calcifications do not resemble teeth.*

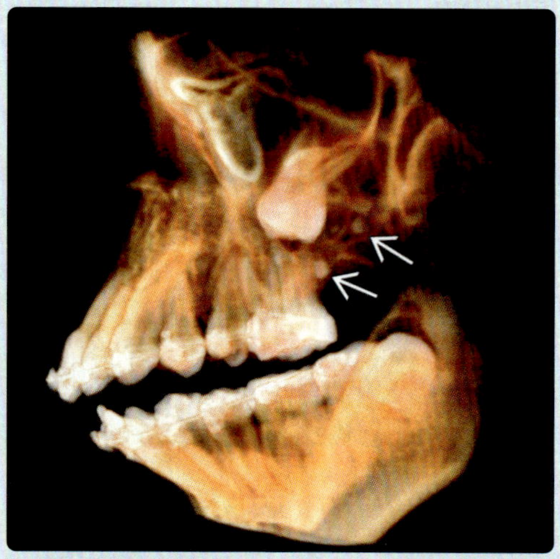

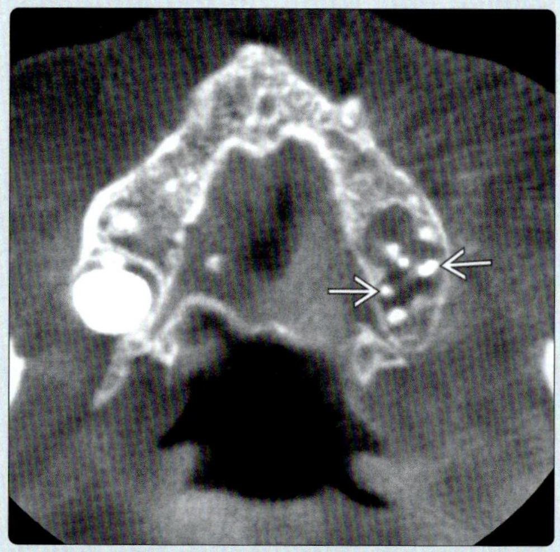

(Left) *Panoramic radiograph shows a large expansile AFO. Note the inferior displacement of the mandibular left 2nd molar ➡ and the doughnut-shaped calcifications ➡ signifying enamel and dentin deposition.* **(Right)** *Axial CBCT shows expansion of the facial cortex of the right anterior maxilla by an AFO. Tooth density material ➡ is seen within the low-density body of the lesion. (Courtesy M. Noujeim, DDS.)*

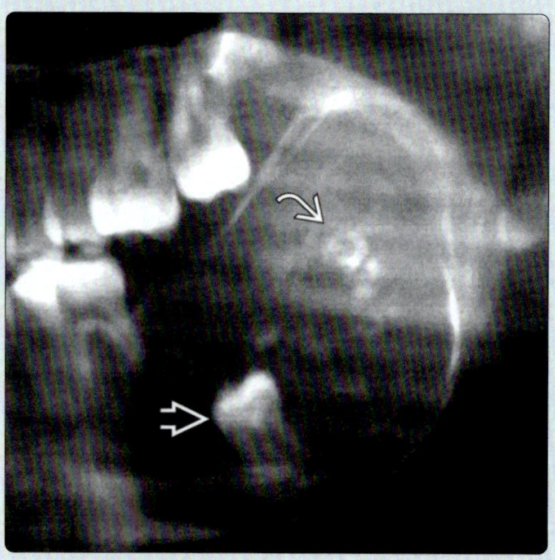

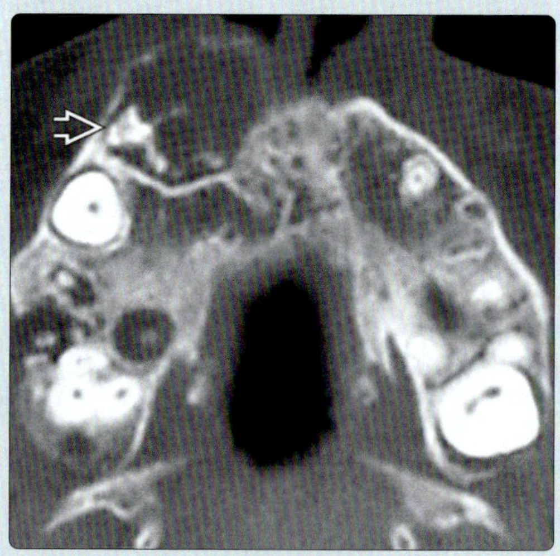

TERMINOLOGY

Abbreviations

- Ameloblastic fibroodontoma (AFO)

Definitions

- Tumor of mixed odontogenic epithelium and ectomesenchyme; similar to ameloblastic fibroma but with scattered collections of enamel and dentin

IMAGING

General Features

- Best diagnostic clue
  - Largely radiolucent area with **specks of tooth density material** within it associated with missing tooth or tooth that has not erupted
- Location
  - Most common in posterior mandible occlusal or **pericoronal** to developing tooth
- Size
  - May appear as small as enlarged tooth follicles or a few cm in diameter
- Morphology
  - Well defined
  - May or may not be corticated
  - Mixed density internal structure but **mostly radiolucent**
  - Larger lesions have more calcified material
  - Calcifications may be **doughnut-shaped** with rim of enamel density
  - Calcifications **do not resemble teeth**
  - Unilocular; rarely multilocular

Imaging Recommendations

- Best imaging tool
  - CBCT will show buccolingual expansion if present and relationship of related tooth to vital structures (inferior alveolar nerve canal or maxillary sinus)
  - Periapical or panoramic radiography may be 1st diagnostic imaging to determine cause of unerupted tooth

DIFFERENTIAL DIAGNOSIS

Ameloblastic Fibroma

- Entirely radiolucent
- Histology may show small foci of calcified material indicating AFO

Odontoma

- Larger amount of calcified material
- If odontoma is still developing, may look like AFO
- AFO calcified material never resembles teeth
- Odontoma is usually self limiting, stops growing after teeth development ends

Adenomatoid Odontogenic Tumor

- "Snow flake" or fine calcifications
- Mostly in anterior maxilla
- Mostly pericoronal

Calcifying Odontogenic Cyst

- Can be pericoronal
- Varied amounts of calcifications: If sparse, may resemble AFO
- Older mean age group

Calcifying Epithelial Odontogenic Tumor

- Occurs in older patients with prevalence in middle age
- Usually much larger

PATHOLOGY

Microscopic Features

- Small islands of odontogenic epithelium in loose primitive connective tissue that resembles dental papilla
- Calcified foci of enamel and dentin matrix formation in close relationship to epithelial structures

CLINICAL ISSUES

Presentation

- Most common signs/symptoms
  - Missing or unerupted tooth
  - Tooth may be displaced
  - Painless swelling of affected bone

Demographics

- Age
  - 2nd decade; Has been reported as young as 1 year old
  - Develops while teeth are developing
- Gender
  - No gender predilection

Treatment

- Enucleation
- Tumor separates easily from bony bed
- Recurrence is rare
- Development of ameloblastic fibrosarcoma after curettage has been reported but is very rare

DIAGNOSTIC CHECKLIST

Consider

- AFO is considered to be stage of development of odontoma and not separate entity by some investigators due to similarity in histopathology

SELECTED REFERENCES

1. Atarbashi Moghadam S et al: Peripheral developing odontoma or peripheral ameloblastic fibroodontoma: A rare challenging case. Case Rep Dent. 2016:9379017, 2016
2. Bhargava M et al: Ameloblastic fibrodentinoma: Report of a case in an infant. J Clin Diagn Res. 10(1):ZD06-7, 2016
3. Bhattacharyya I et al: Diagnostic discussion. Meloblastic fibro-odontoma. Todays FDA. 28(1):45-8, 2016
4. Ghandehari-Motlagh M et al: Ameloblastic fibro-odontoma in a 4-year-old boy. Iran J Pediatr. 26(2):e3124, 2016
5. De Riu G et al: Ameloblastic fibro-odontoma. Case report and review of the literature. J Craniomaxillofac Surg. 38(2):141-4, 2010
6. de Souza Tolentino E et al: Ameloblastic fibro-odontoma: a diagnostic challenge. Int J Dent. 2010, 2010
7. Phillips MD et al: Hybrid odontogenic tumor with features of ameloblastic fibro-odontoma, calcifying odontogenic cyst, and adenomatoid odontogenic tumor: a case report and review of the literature. J Oral Maxillofac Surg. 68(2):470-4, 2010
8. Cavalcante AS et al: Ameloblastic fibro-odontoma: a case report. Med Oral Patol Oral Cir Bucal. 14(12):e650-3, 2009
9. Neville BW et al: Oral and Maxillofacial Pathology. 3rd ed. St. Louis: Saunders Elsevier. 2009

Calcifying Epithelial Odontogenic Tumor

KEY FACTS

TERMINOLOGY

- Calcifying epithelial odontogenic tumor (CEOT)
- **Definition**: Odontogenic epithelial tumor that produces mineralized substance

IMAGING

- **CBCT**: Shows extent of lesion, displacement of structures, and buccolingual extent
- **Location**: Posterior mandible, less common in posterior maxilla
- Border may be well defined or ill defined
- Unilocular or multilocular
- Scattered high-density foci of calcification of varying size and density: Described as **driven snow**
- May be pericoronal to impacted tooth
  - Calcifications often cluster close to crown of tooth, impeding eruption
- Fine, sparse trabeculation may be present

TOP DIFFERENTIAL DIAGNOSES

- Adenomatoid odontogenic tumor (AOT)
- Ameloblastic fibroodontoma (AFO)
- Calcifying odontogenic cyst
- Dentigerous cyst

CLINICAL ISSUES

- Painless, slow-growing swelling of jaws
- Can occur at any age
- **Most common in 5th decade**
- M > F

DIAGNOSTIC CHECKLIST

- AOT most common in anterior maxilla
- AFO similar but in younger age group
- Early pericoronal lesions may be indistinguishable from pericoronal lesions that do not produce radiopacities: Most commonly dentigerous cyst

(Left) Axial bone CT shows a CEOT presenting as a large, expansile, mixed-density lesion in the posterior right maxilla of a 78-year-old man. There is a large focus of calcification noted in the lesion ➡ in addition to multiple small flecks of calcification. (Courtesy E. Bolideau, MD.) **(Right)** *Axial bone CT shows invasion of a CEOT into the right nasal cavity medially ➡ and the pterygopalatine fossa posteriorly ➡ with occupation of the right maxillary sinus. (Courtesy E. Bolideau, MD.)*

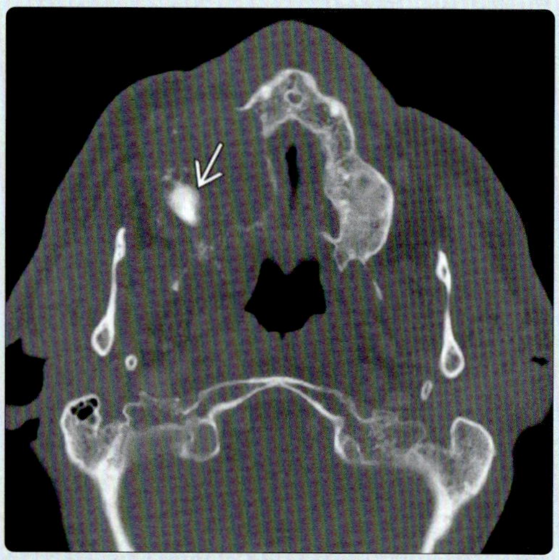

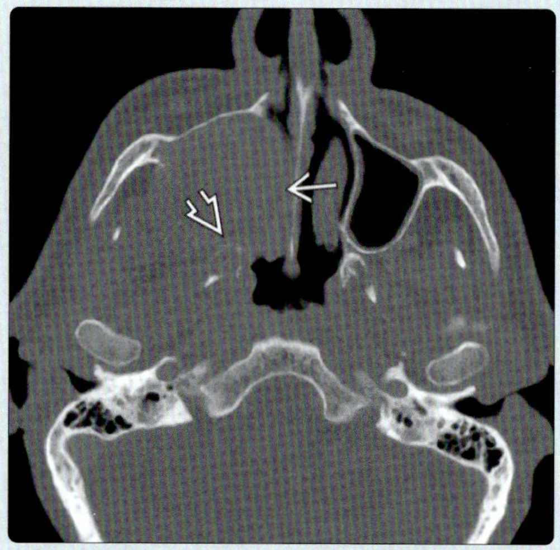

(Left) *Coronal CBCT shows a small CEOT at the apices of the right premolar. Faint calcifications ➡ are seen between the roots of the teeth. Note the thinning of the floor of the maxillary sinus ➡. (Courtesy E. Bolideau, MD.)* **(Right)** *Panoramic radiograph shows a pericoronal CEOT in the posterior right mandible. Note clustering of calcifications ➡ and driven snow appearance. Lesion showed malignant changes histologically and eventually led to the demise of the patient. (Courtesy K. Abramovitch, DDS.)*

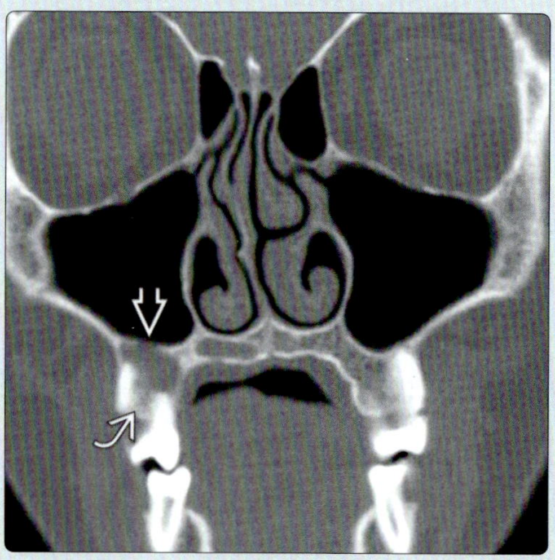

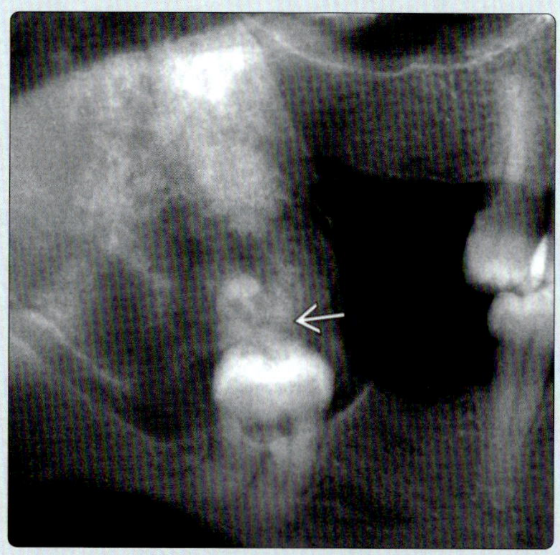

TERMINOLOGY

Abbreviations

- Calcifying epithelial odontogenic tumor (CEOT)

Synonyms

- Pindborg tumor

Definitions

- Odontogenic epithelial tumor that produces mineralized substance

IMAGING

General Features

- Best diagnostic clue
  - Unilocular or multilocular radiolucency with internal calcifications in posterior mandible
- Location
  - **Posterior mandible**, less common in posterior maxilla
  - May occur in anterior jaws but rare
  - May or may not be associated with impacted tooth
  - Extraosseous (peripheral) variety has been described
- Size
  - May be small radiolucency surrounding crown of unerupted tooth
  - May enlarge and extend into ramus of mandible or expand maxilla and into surrounding structures

Imaging Recommendations

- Best imaging tool
  - **CBCT**
    - Shows extent of lesion, displacement of structures, and buccolingual extent

CT Findings

- Border may be well defined or ill defined
- **Unilocular or multilocular**
- Scattered high-density foci of calcification of varying size and density: Described by some as having appearance of **driven snow**
- Calcifications may be clustered close to impacted tooth crown and impede eruption
- Fine, sparse trabeculation may be present
- Expansion of cortices of affected jaw
- Inferior displacement of inferior alveolar nerve canal if in posterior mandible

DIFFERENTIAL DIAGNOSIS

Adenomatoid Odontogenic Tumor

- **Anterior maxilla**
- Younger age group, 2nd decade
- More common in females

Ameloblastic Fibroodontoma

- Posterior mandible
- Tooth density calcifications
- **2nd decade of life**

Calcifying Odontogenic Cyst

- Anterior to 1st molar
- Peaks in 2nd decade, with mean age of 36 years

Dentigerous Cyst

- Most common pericoronal radiolucency
- Early pericoronal lesions of CEOT may be indistinguishable

PATHOLOGY

General Features

- Associated abnormalities
  - Single report of association of adenomatoid odontogenic tumor (AOT) component within CEOT
  - Single report of hybrid ameloblastoma/CEOT

Microscopic Features

- Islands, strands, or sheets of polyhedral epithelial cells in fibrous stroma
- Tumor islands enclose masses of amyloid-like material, giving cribriform appearance
- Calcifications develop within amyloid-like material in concentric rings **(Liesegang rings)**

CLINICAL ISSUES

Presentation

- Most common signs/symptoms
  - Painless, slow-growing swelling of jaws

Demographics

- Age
  - Can occur at any age, **most common in 5th decade**
- Gender
  - M > F

Natural History & Prognosis

- Malignant transformation due to loss of *TP53* (P53) transcriptional activity has been reported

Treatment

- Conservative local resection
- Lesions in posterior maxilla should be treated more aggressively as they can extend intracranially
- Recurrence is ~ 15%

DIAGNOSTIC CHECKLIST

Consider

- AOT may appear similar but most common in anterior maxilla
- Ameloblastic fibroodontoma can show same appearance but in younger age group

SELECTED REFERENCES

1. Caliaperoumal SK et al: Pindborg tumor. Contemp Clin Dent. 7(1):95-7, 2016
2. Mitra S et al: Pindborg tumor presenting as a nasal polyp: immunohistology and ultrastructural features of a rare case, with review of the literature. Int J Surg Pathol. 24(6):568-72, 2016
3. Rani V et al: Aggressive calcifying epithelial odontogenic tumor of the maxillary sinus with extraosseous oral mucosal involvement: a case report. Iran J Med Sci. 41(2):145-9, 2016
4. Rydin K et al: Clear cell variant of intraosseous calcifying epithelial odontogenic tumor: a case report and review of the literature. Oral Surg Oral Med Oral Pathol Oral Radiol. 122(4):e125-30, 2016
5. Demian N et al: Malignant transformation of calcifying epithelial odontogenic tumor is associated with the loss of p53 transcriptional activity: a case report with review of the literature. J Oral Maxillofac Surg. 68(8):1964-73, 2010

Cementoblastoma

KEY FACTS

TERMINOLOGY

- Synonyms
  - Benign cementoblastoma
  - True cementoblastoma
- Definition: Benign odontogenic neoplasm of cementoblasts and cementum

IMAGING

- Well-defined **radiopacity or mixed radiodensity** lesion **attached to** and **surrounding** root of **vital** tooth
  - May have amorphous or spoke-wheel pattern
  - Has **well-defined radiolucent rim**
  - **External root resorption** sometimes seen
  - Outline of root usually obscured
- Most commonly form on mandibular permanent **premolar or 1st molar**
  - **Mandible** > maxilla (4:1)
  - Rarely seen in primary dentition
- Large lesions may be expansile
- Usually no larger than 1-2 cm in diameter

TOP DIFFERENTIAL DIAGNOSES

- Periapical osseous (cemental) dysplasia
- Periapical sclerosing (condensing) osteitis
- Idiopathic osteosclerosis (enostosis)
- Hypercementosis

PATHOLOGY

- Closely resembles osteoblastoma microscopically

CLINICAL ISSUES

- Ranges from 12-65 years but predominantly seen in young adults; M > F
- **Pain** and swelling in some cases
- Associated **tooth is vital**
- Treatment: Excision and extraction of associated tooth or tumor amputation with endodontic treatment of associated tooth
- Recurrence as high as 37% has been reported

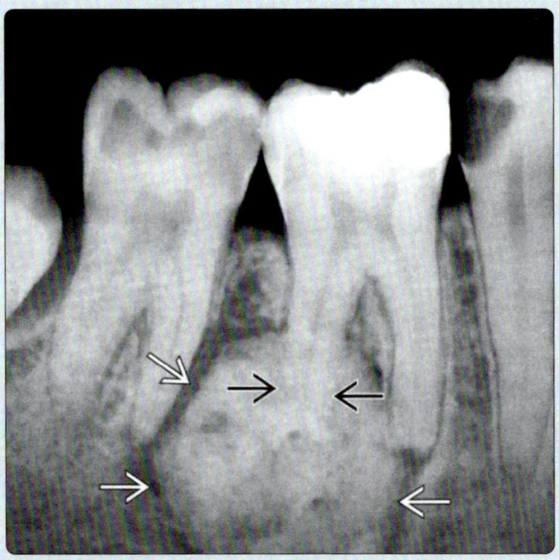

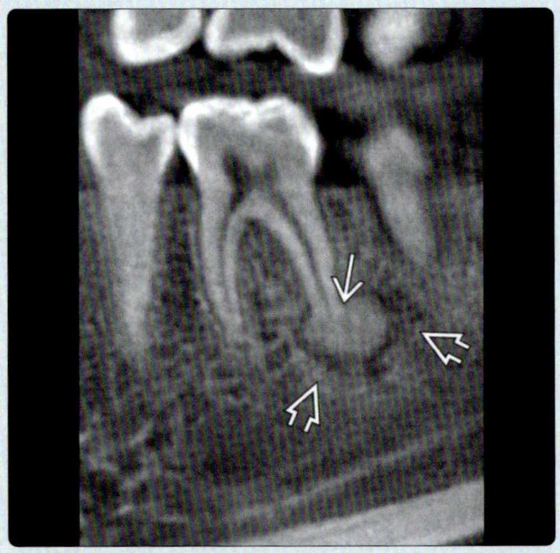

(Left) *Periapical radiograph shows classic appearance of a cementoblastoma attached to the distal root of the mandibular right 1st molar. Note the radiolucent periphery* ➡*. The lesion is directly attached to the distal root* ⇨*, and the apex is obscured.* **(Right)** *Sagittal reformatted CBCT exhibits a cementoblastoma on the distal root of the left mandibular 1st molar. There is root resorption and attachment to the root* ➡*. The hypodense border exhibits an unusual radiating pattern* ➡*.*

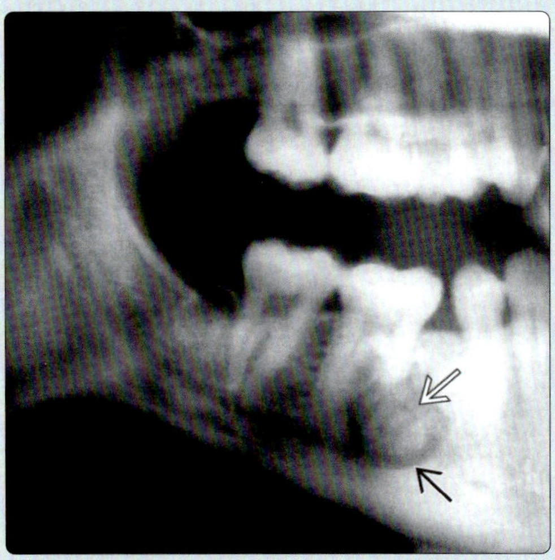

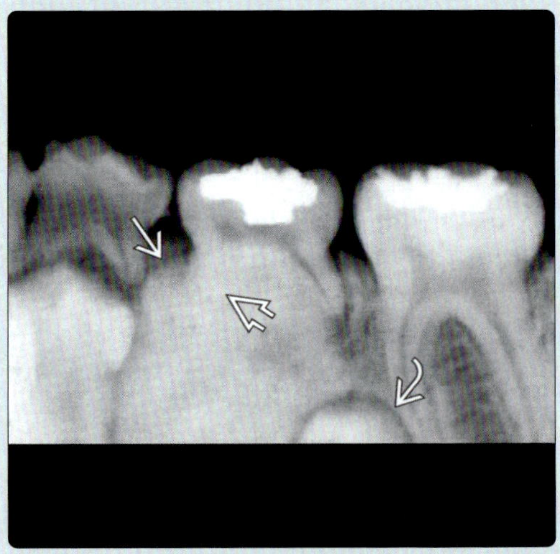

(Left) *Panoramic radiograph shows a cementoblastoma attached to the mesial root of the mandibular right 1st molar* ➡*. The 1st molar is most commonly affected by this lesion. Note the apex is not visible. The inferior alveolar nerve canal passes below the lesion* ⇨*.* **(Right)** *Periapical radiograph shows a rare cementoblastoma associated with a mandibular left primary 2nd molar. Note the fine radiolucent border* ➡ *and attachment to the mesial root* ➡*. The developing premolar is also displaced inferiorly and distally* ➡*.*

TERMINOLOGY

Synonyms

- Benign cementoblastoma
- True cementoblastoma

Definitions

- Benign odontogenic neoplasm of cementoblasts and cementum

IMAGING

General Features

- Best diagnostic clue
  - Bulbous mixed radiodensity lesion **attached to** and **surrounding** root of **vital tooth**
- Location
  - **Mandible** > maxilla (4:1)
  - Most common on permanent **premolar** or **1st molar**
  - Rare in primary dentition
- Size
  - Usually no larger than 1-2 cm in diameter

Imaging Recommendations

- Best imaging tool
  - Periapical or panoramic images
  - Occlusal and CBCT preferable modalities to exhibit expansion

Radiographic Findings

- Well-defined radiopacity or **mixed radiopaque-radiolucent mass**
  - May have amorphous or spoke-wheel pattern
- **Well-defined radiolucent rim** surrounding mass
- **External root resorption** may be seen
- Outline of **roots usually obscured**
- Large lesions may expand mandible; cortex remains intact

DIFFERENTIAL DIAGNOSIS

Periapical Osseous (Cemental) Dysplasia

- Well-defined periapical **radiopacity with radiolucent periphery or rim** (mature stage)
  - Occasionally radiolucent periphery is not discernible
  - Lesion **does not attach directly to root**
- Most commonly **mandibular anterior teeth, multiple**
- Affected **teeth are vital** and asymptomatic

Periapical Sclerosing (Condensing) Osteitis

- Thick, dense trabeculae at periphery of rarefying periapical inflammation; tooth is **nonvital**
- Apical **periodontal ligament (PDL) space is widened**
- Sclerotic bone **blends** with surrounding trabecular pattern
- **Does not have radiolucent rim or periphery**

Idiopathic Osteosclerosis (Enostosis)

- Well-defined radiopacity that does not blend with trabecular pattern
- Seen in all areas of jaws; most common in mandibular premolar-molar region
- When periapical, apical **PDL space is normal** width
- **Does not have radiolucent rim or periphery**

Hypercementosis

- Excessive cementum seen as irregular enlargement of tooth root
- Extra cementum is directly attached to tooth root **without separating radiolucency**
- Lamina dura and **PDL space are continuous** around enlargement

Osteoblastoma

- Rare in jaws; if seen, slight predilection for mandible
- **Pain** that is unrelieved by NSAIDs
- Well-defined or ill-defined radiolucency with **patchy areas of radiopacity**; usually > 2 cm

Osteoid Osteoma

- Very rare in jaws
- Nocturnal **pain relieved by NSAIDs**
- Mixed-density lesion with central nidus of radiolucency, surrounded by **zone of reactive sclerosis**; usually < 1 cm

PATHOLOGY

Microscopic Features

- Thick trabeculae of mineralized material with irregularly placed lacunae and prominent basophilic reversal lines
- Trabeculae lined by prominent cementoblasts
- Cellular fibroblastic tissue present between mineralized material
- Periphery is uncalcified matrix
- Multinucleated giant cells often present
- Closely resembles osteoblastoma

CLINICAL ISSUES

Presentation

- Most common signs/symptoms
  - **Pain** and swelling in some cases
  - Associated tooth is **vital**

Demographics

- Age
  - Ranges from 12-65 years but predominantly seen in young adults
- Gender
  - More common in males than females

Treatment

- Excision and extraction of associated tooth
- Tumor amputation with endodontic treatment of associated tooth
- Recurrence as high as 37% has been reported

SELECTED REFERENCES

1. Nuvvula S et al: Cementoblastoma relating to right mandibular second primary molar. Case Rep Dent. 2016:2319890, 2016
2. Huber AR et al: Cementoblastoma. Head Neck Pathol. 3(2):133-135, 2009
3. Neves FS et al: Benign cementoblastoma: case report and review of the literature. Minerva Stomatol. 58(1-2):55-9, 2009
4. Brannon RB et al: Cementoblastoma: an innocuous neoplasm? A clinicopathologic study of 44 cases and review of the literature with special emphasis on recurrence. Oral Surg Oral Med Oral Pathol Oral Radiol Endod. 93(3):311-20, 2002

KEY FACTS

TERMINOLOGY

- **Definition**: Benign tumor of odontogenic ectomesenchyme

IMAGING

- Mandible > maxilla; **premolar-molar** regions
- Unilocular or **multilocular radiolucency** with thin, straight internal septa
  - Septa may form **right angles** or geometric shapes
  - In larger lesions, septa may be coarse, curved ("soap bubble") and mimic ameloblastoma
- Borders may be well defined or ill defined; if well defined, often lobular or scalloped
- T2WI MR
  - ↑ signal: Establishes tumor extent

TOP DIFFERENTIAL DIAGNOSES

- Ameloblastoma
- Central giant cell granuloma
- Aneurysmal bone cyst
- Central hemangioma
- Osteosarcoma

CLINICAL ISSUES

- **Uncommon**; only 3-6% of odontogenic tumors
- Wide age range; average 25-30 years
- Slight female predilection
- May demonstrate rapid growth and expansion
- Infiltrates surrounding bone; does not metastasize
- Treatment: Curettage for small lesions
  - Extensive resection for large lesions
  - Complete removal difficult with **25% recurrence rate**: Follow-up required for at least 5 years

DIAGNOSTIC CHECKLIST

- Look for thin cortical margin to rule out osteosarcoma when pseudoperiosteal reaction present

(Left) *Cropped panoramic radiograph shows a large, loculated lesion that has displaced teeth ⇨. Straight septa at the expanded inferior cortex extend in a radiating pattern ➡ producing a pseudoperiosteal reaction. (Courtesy S. Kalathingal, DDS.)* **(Right)** *Axial bone CT in the same patient shows coarse, straight septa ➡ and radiating wisps of bone ➡ at the periphery of the lesion. The thin, corticated margin ➡ can be discerned and helps differentiate this lesion from an osteosarcoma. (Courtesy S. Kalathingal, DDS.)*

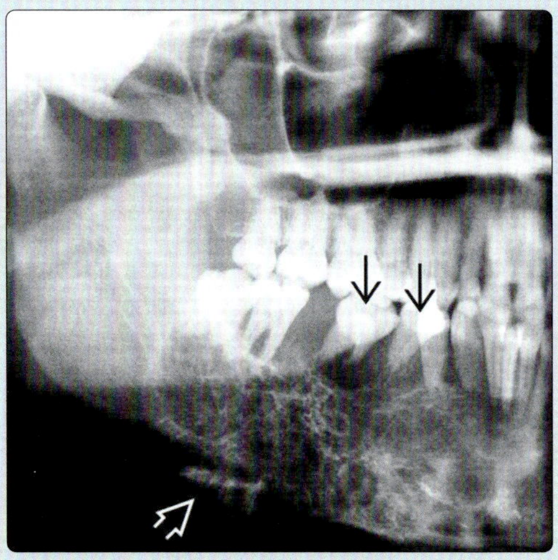

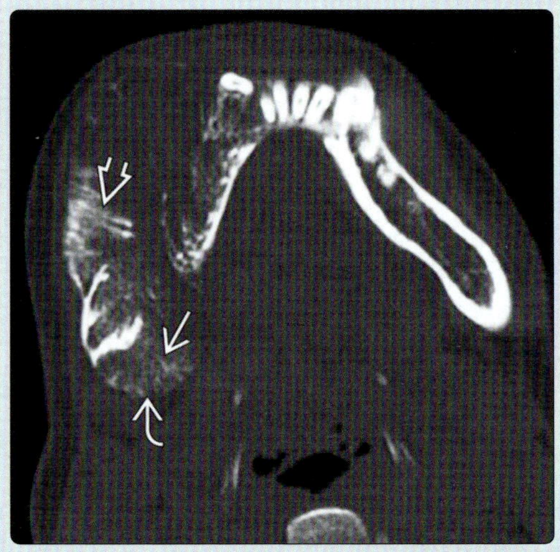

(Left) *Cropped panoramic CBCT reformat of a 30-year-old woman is shown. The multilocular appearance includes significant extent, external root resorption ➡, and tooth displacement ➡. Multiple thick internal trabeculae are present, some forming at approximately right angles ➡.* **(Right)** *Volume-rendered CBCT of the same patient reveals significant facial expansion ➡ and multiple thick internal trabeculae. In addition, external root resorption on the anterior teeth is visible.*

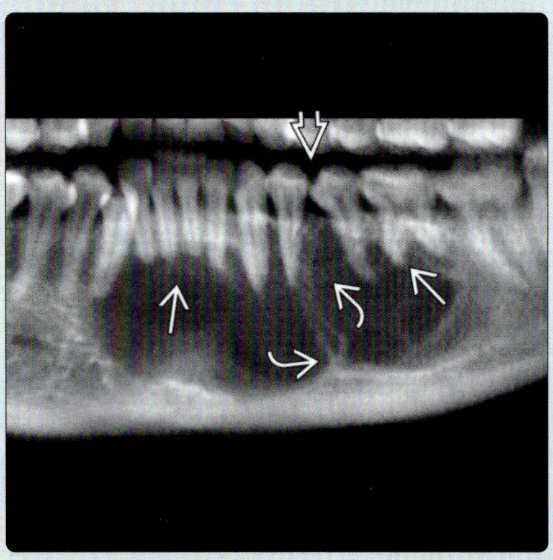

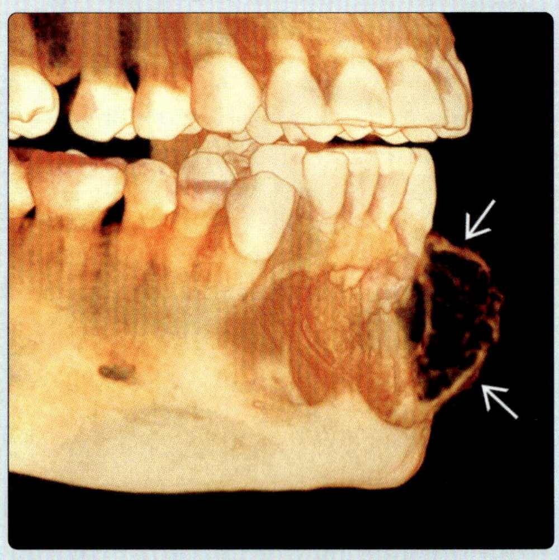

Odontogenic Myxoma

TERMINOLOGY

Synonyms

- Myxoma, myxofibroma, fibromyxoma

Definitions

- Benign tumor of odontogenic ectomesenchyme

IMAGING

General Features

- Best diagnostic clue
  - Multilocular radiolucency with thin, often straight, internal septa at right angles
- Location
  - Any area of jaws; mandible > maxilla (3:1)
  - Most common in premolar-molar regions
- Size
  - Variable, depending on when discovered

Imaging Recommendations

- Best imaging tool
  - CT or CBCT: Evaluation of extent & margins

Radiographic Findings

- Radiography
  - Small lesion may be unilocular and well defined
  - Larger lesion may be well defined or ill defined
    - Lobular or scalloped edges ± cortication
  - Internal septa often thin: May form right angles with each other or make geometric shapes
    - May be coarse and curved ("soap bubble") and mimic ameloblastoma
    - May extend at periphery in radiating pattern giving **pseudoperiosteal reaction**
  - If large, may displace teeth; tooth resorption rare

CT Findings

- CBCT or bone CT
  - Better determines extent of larger lesions
  - Thin cortical margin helps differentiate from osteosarcoma when pseudoperiosteal reactions are present

MR Findings

- T2WI
  - ↑ signal: Establishes tumor extent

DIFFERENTIAL DIAGNOSIS

Ameloblastoma

- Multilocular radiolucency, corticated border, and coarse, curved internal septa ("soap bubble")
- Most common in posterior mandible

Central Giant Cell Granuloma

- Multilocular radiolucency; well defined, noncorticated
- Wispy septa, some at right angles to periphery
- Anterior mandible most common; may cross midline

Aneurysmal Bone Cyst

- Multilocular radiolucency with well defined borders that are curved or "hydraulic"
- Internal septa wispy, ill defined; some at right angles to periphery
- Rapid expansion in posterior mandible typical

Central Hemangioma

- Multilocular radiolucency: Corticated or ill defined
- May see small compartments internally, similar to large marrow spaces surrounded by coarse trabeculae
- Slow enlargement of jaw, may or may not be painful
- May produce linear spicules ("sunray") at periphery

Osteosarcoma

- Spiculated periosteal reaction ("sunray"); **cortex not intact**

PATHOLOGY

Gross Pathologic & Surgical Features

- Not encapsulated
- Loose, **gelatinous consistency**; pathognomonic

Microscopic Features

- Resembles developing tooth mesenchyme (dental papilla)
- Stellate, spindle-shaped, or round cells in abundant loose myxoid stroma
- May see small islands of epithelium

CLINICAL ISSUES

Presentation

- Most common signs/symptoms
  - May expand bone
  - Variable growth pattern but can be rapid, painless

Demographics

- Age
  - Wide range; average: 25-30 years
- Gender
  - Slight female predilection
- Epidemiology
  - Uncommon; only 3-6% of odontogenic tumors

Natural History & Prognosis

- Infiltrates surrounding bone but does not metastasize
- May demonstrate rapid growth and expansion

Treatment

- Curettage for small lesions
- Extensive resection for large lesions
- Follow-up required for at least 5 years; complete removal difficult with **25% recurrence rate**

DIAGNOSTIC CHECKLIST

Image Interpretation Pearls

- Look for thin cortical margin to rule out osteosarcoma when pseudoperiosteal reaction present

SELECTED REFERENCES

1. Subramaniam SS et al: Odontogenic myxoma in the paediatric patient: a review of eight cases. Int J Oral Maxillofac Surg. 45(12):1614-1617, 2016
2. Kawase-Koga Y et al: Surgical management of odontogenic myxoma: a case report and review of the literature. BMC Res Notes. 7:214, 2014
3. Kumar N et al: Odontogenic myxoma. J Maxillofac Oral Surg. 13(2):222-6, 2014

Central Odontogenic Fibroma

KEY FACTS

TERMINOLOGY

- Synonyms: Simple odontogenic fibroma; odontogenic fibroma (WHO type); myxofibroma
- Definition: Tumor of odontogenic ectomesenchymal origin that may contain mature fibrous tissue (simple type) or is more cellular with possible calcifications (WHO type)

IMAGING

- Mandible: Premolar-molar region
- Maxilla: Anterior to 1st molar tooth
- Small lesions: Well-defined, **unilocular** radiolucency
- Large lesions: **Multilocular** radiolucency; septations can be fine and straight (differentiate from myxoma) or granular (differentiate from central giant cell granuloma)
- 12% have fine, unorganized, **radiopaque flecks**
- CBCT and bone CT findings
  - Expansion of bone cortices
  - Preservation of thin cortical boundary
  - Will detect any facial/lingual **root resorption**
  - Root divergence may be seen
  - May grow along length of bone with minimal expansion

TOP DIFFERENTIAL DIAGNOSES

- Periapical rarefying osteitis
- Lateral periodontal cyst
- Odontogenic keratocyst
- Odontogenic myxoma
- Central giant cell granuloma
- Central desmoplastic fibroma

CLINICAL ISSUES

- Bony expansion; loosening of teeth
- Often **depression on palate** adjacent to lesion
- Reported between 4-80 years with **mean age of 40 years**
- F:M = 2:1

(Left) *Periapical radiograph shows a well-defined radiolucency between the roots of the maxillary left 1st and 2nd premolar. Resorption of the root of 1st premolar is noted as well as slight lifting of the floor of the maxillary sinus. (Courtesy P. Sikorski, DDS.)* **(Right)** *Cropped panoramic radiograph shows a well-defined radiolucency between the roots of the maxillary left lateral incisor and canine. Note divergence of the roots, a common finding in COF. (Courtesy P. Sikorski, DDS.)*

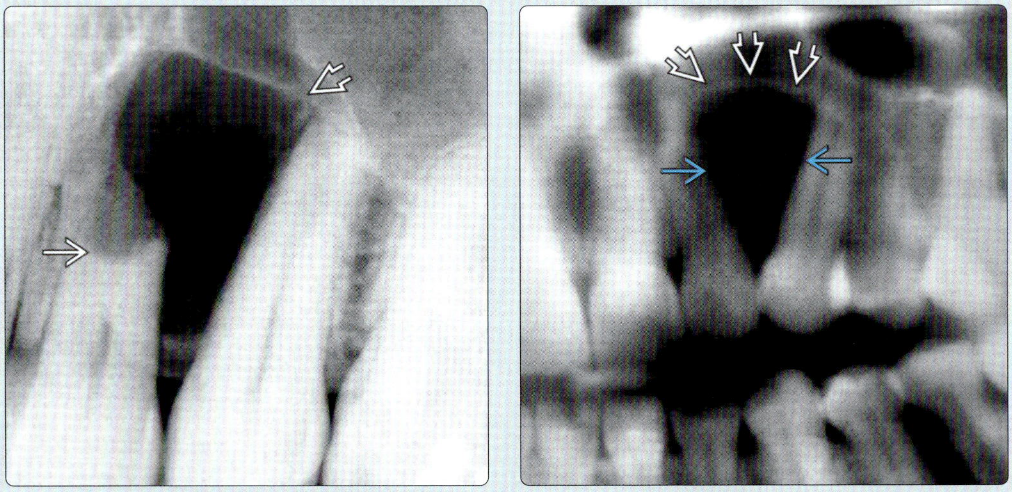

(Left) *Axial CBCT shows a COF in the anterior left maxilla exhibiting minimal expansion of the alveolar process with preservation and thinning of the lingual cortex. The lesion appears to be growing along the length of the bone. (Courtesy S. Gonzalez, DDS.)* **(Right)** *Sagittal CBCT in the same patient shows the COF resorbing the lingual aspect of the apical 1/3 of the maxillary canine. The lingual cortex of the alveolar process is barely visible. COFs may present clinically with a depression on the palate. (Courtesy S. Gonzalez, DDS.)*

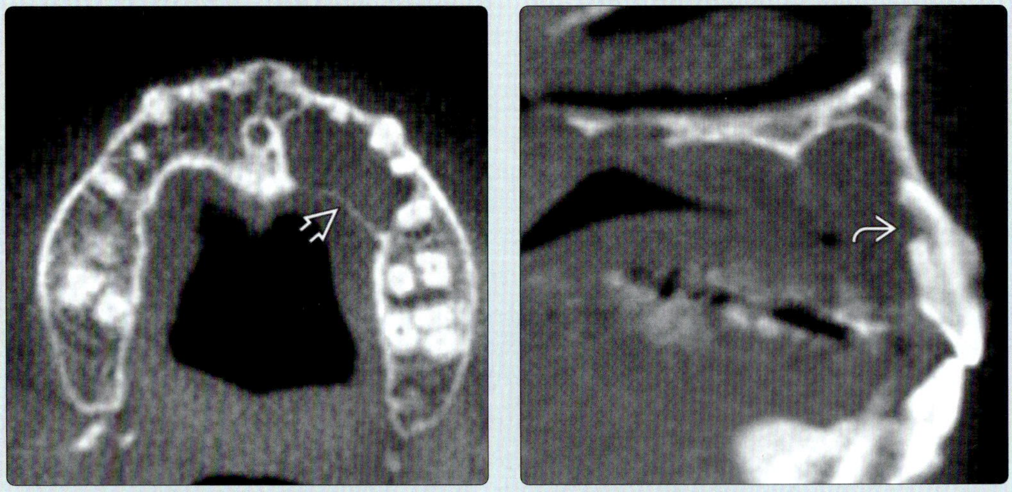

TERMINOLOGY

Abbreviations

- Central odontogenic fibroma (COF)

Synonyms

- Simple odontogenic fibroma; odontogenic fibroma (WHO type); myxofibroma

Definitions

- Tumor of odontogenic ectomesenchymal origin that may contain mature fibrous tissue (simple type) or is more cellular with possible calcifications (WHO type)

IMAGING

General Features

- Location
  - **Maxilla**: Anterior to 1st molar tooth
  - **Mandible**: Premolar-molar region

Radiographic Findings

- Radiography
  - **Small lesions**
    - Well defined
    - Unilocular
    - Completely radiolucent
  - **Large lesions**
    - Multilocular radiolucency
    - Septations can be fine and straight (differentiate from myxoma) or granular (differentiate from central giant cell granuloma)
    - 12% have fine, unorganized, radiopaque flecks (WHO type)

CT Findings

- CBCT
  - Expansion of cortices
  - **Preservation of thin cortical boundary**
  - **Root resorption** on facial or lingual surfaces of teeth can be detected
  - Root divergence may occur
  - May grow along length of bone with minimal expansion
  - Periosteal reaction can be seen in younger individuals

DIFFERENTIAL DIAGNOSIS

Periapical Rarefying Osteitis

- Apical radiolucency associated with pulpal pathology
- Tooth is **nonvital**
- Root resorption rare

Lateral Periodontal Cyst

- Unilocular, interradicular radiolucency
- Mandibular premolar areas most commonly
- Root resorption usually not seen

Odontogenic Keratocyst

- Loculations, if present, are usually large
- Tends to grow along length of bone, especially in mandible
- Root resorption rare

Odontogenic Myxoma (Myxofibroma)

- Fine, thin septations may be present in both myxomas and COFs
  - Septa tend to be straight or form geometric patterns
- Mandible > maxilla: Posterior > anterior

Central Giant Cell Granuloma

- Granular septations may be present in both
- Histopathology of COF may show **central giant cell granuloma (CGCG)-like component**

Central Desmoplastic Fibroma

- **More aggressive**
- May destroy cortices of bone
- May invade soft tissues
- Thick, straight, and angular septations

PATHOLOGY

General Features

- 2 types
  - **Simple**
    - Stellate fibroblasts arranged in **whorled patterns**
    - Collagen fibrils and substantial ground substance
  - **WHO type**
    - Cellular fibrous connective tissue with **collagen fibers arranged in interlacing bundles**
    - Odontogenic epithelium in **long strands or nests** is present and may make up bulk of lesion
    - **Calcifications** (dentinoid or cementoid material) may be present
- Examples of COF with giant cell granuloma-like components have been reported

CLINICAL ISSUES

Presentation

- Most common signs/symptoms
  - Bony expansion
  - Loosening of teeth
  - May see **depression on palate** adjacent to lesion
    - Occasional destruction of lingual cortex and exposure of tooth root

Demographics

- Age
  - Reported between 4-80 years with **mean age of 40 years**
- Gender
  - F:M = 2:1

Treatment

- Enucleation, **vigorous curettage**

SELECTED REFERENCES

1. Pippi R et al: The central odontogenic fibroma: How difficult can be making a preliminary diagnosis. J Clin Exp Dent. 8(2):e223-5, 2016
2. Santoro A et al: Central odontogenic fibroma of the mandible: A case report with diagnostic considerations. Ann Med Surg (Lond). 5:14-8, 2016
3. Anbiaee N et al: Central odontogenic fibroma (simple type) in a four-year-old boy: atypical cone-beam computed tomographic appearance with periosteal reaction. Imaging Sci Dent. 45(2):109-15, 2015
4. El Harti K et al: Central odontogenic fibroma of the maxilla. Indian J Dent. 6(4):217-20, 2015

Central Hemangioma

KEY FACTS

TERMINOLOGY

- Definition: Benign blood vessel proliferation (neoplasm) vs. mesenchymal cell proliferation (hamartoma)

IMAGING

- Uni- or multilocular; variable margins from ill defined to well defined with cortication
- Classic **sunray linear spicules** from surface of bone if cortical perforation present; often **honeycomb** (early) or **soap bubble** (late) internal trabecular appearance; others may be unilocular
- If mandibular canal involved, canal is widened with possible **serpentine shape**
- Possible **phleboliths** if lesion extends to soft tissue
- Adjacent **teeth often resorbed** or **displaced**
- Teeth developing adjacent to hemangioma may be **macrodonts** and **erupt earlier** than normal
- Mandible > maxilla; posterior body and within mandibular canal
- Imaging protocol
  - Panoramic radiography and CBCT initially, but CT bone/CECT best overall
  - Angiography to demonstrate vascularity and delineate lesion
  - High-resolution Doppler US for vascular flow

TOP DIFFERENTIAL DIAGNOSES

- Osteosarcoma
- Arteriovenous fistula
- Ameloblastoma
- Odontogenic myxoma
- Central giant cell granuloma
- Aneurysmal bone cyst

CLINICAL ISSUES

- Slow expansion; may throb ± bleeding around teeth
- Treatment: Embolization, en bloc resection with ligation of external carotid, or sclerosing techniques

(Left) *Axial CECT shows a highly expansile lytic lesion of the right mandibular ramus with thinned cortices ➔ and honeycomb internal trabecular pattern ➔. Bone CT/CBCT or panoramic radiograph would assess a possible increase in the mandibular canal width &/or serpentine morphology. (Courtesy M. Ayadi, MD.)* **(Right)** *Coronal CECT in same patient shows the thinned mandibular cortices ➔ due to expansion of the hemangioma. An air space ➔ within the buccal vestibule is also apparent.*

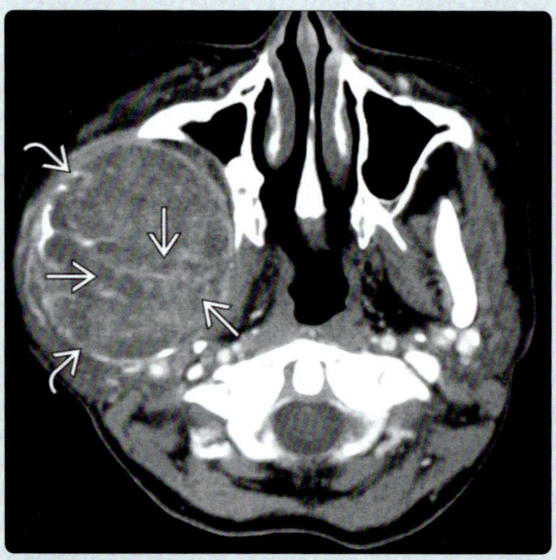

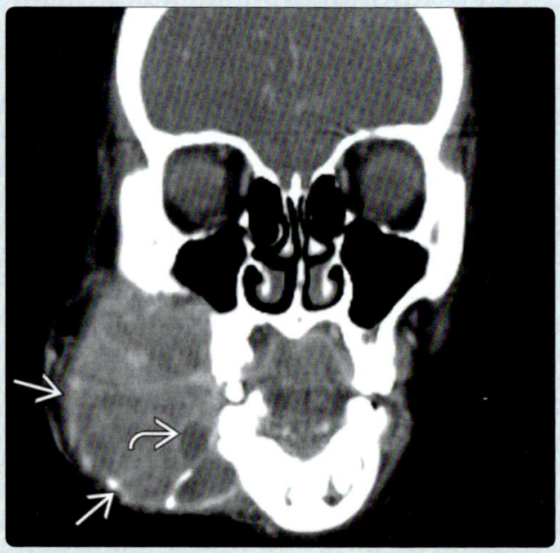

(Left) *Axial bone CT shows an intraosseous hemangioma with a soap bubble appearance. The expansile lesion ➔ arises from the malar eminence of the maxilla. Rapid blood loss may occur from inadvertent accidental or surgical trauma.* **(Right)** *Panoramic radiograph of the right mandibular ramus shows multiple phleboliths ➔ from a soft tissue hemangioma. Note the laminated vascular calcification morphology ➔.*

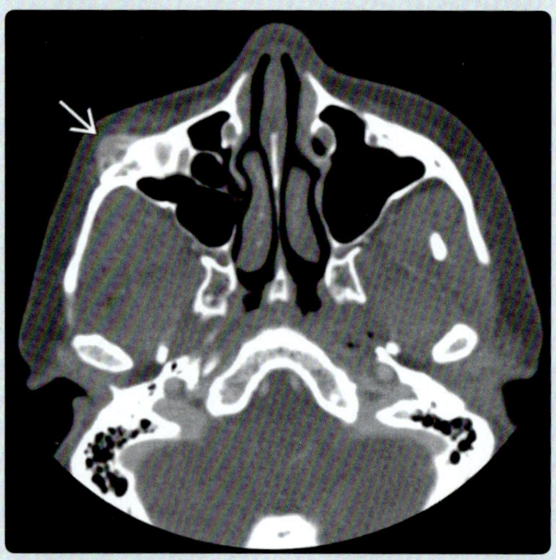

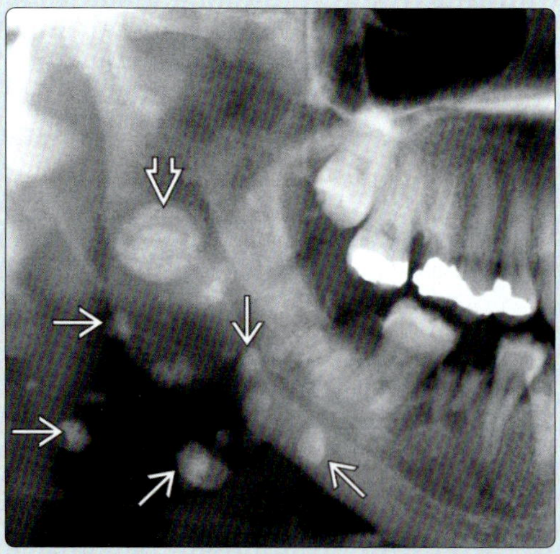

TERMINOLOGY

Definitions

- Benign blood vessel proliferation resembling neoplasm vs. hamartoma of mesenchymal cell proliferation

IMAGING

General Features

- Best diagnostic clue
  - Rare in jaws
  - **Uni- or multilocular radiolucency** with **honeycomb** or **soap bubble** trabecular appearance
  - Classic **sunray linear spicules** from surface of bone if cortical perforation present
  - When in mandibular canal, canal is widened and may have **serpentine** shape
- Location
  - Most common oral sites: Posterior mandibular body and within mandibular canal
- Morphology
  - Uni- or multilocular; variable margins from ill-defined to well-defined with cortication

Radiographic Findings

- Radiography
  - Often **honeycomb** (early) or **soap bubble** (late) trabecular appearance; others may be unilocular
  - Thinned, expanded cortices
  - Possible **sunray spicules** projecting at right angles from cortical surface
  - **Phleboliths** may be apparent if soft tissue extension
  - Adjacent **teeth often resorbed** or **displaced**
  - Teeth developing adjacent to hemangioma may be **macrodonts** and **erupt earlier** than normal

CT Findings

- Ill-defined lytic mass with moderate enhancement
- Sunray spicules and phleboliths common, especially with soft tissue extension

Ultrasonographic Findings

- Color Doppler
  - Ill-defined hypoechoic mass; pulsing on real-time US

Imaging Recommendations

- Protocol advice
  - Panoramic is most appropriate initially
  - CBCT, CECT, angiography, Doppler US

DIFFERENTIAL DIAGNOSIS

Osteosarcoma

- **Sunray appearance** is similar to hemangioma
- Sclerotic/osteolytic **destructive** lesion; ill-defined borders
- Symmetrically widened periodontal ligament space around a few teeth

Arteriovenous Fistula

- Radiographic appearance not specific
- Does not involve mandibular canal
- **Spontaneous hemorrhage** around teeth

Ameloblastoma

- Most common site is posterior mandible
- Uni- or multilocular, usually adjacent to impacted tooth
- Adjacent tooth **root resorption common**

Odontogenic Myxoma

- 3rd or 4th decade; mandible
- Lacy trabecular pattern resembles **tennis racquet**
- Dental root resorption rare

Central Giant Cell Granuloma

- Swelling may be only clinical sign; anterior mandible
- May be peripheral or central; mean age: 30 years
- Malposition and resorption of teeth are not unusual

Aneurysmal Bone Cyst

- 1st or 2nd decades; usually in posterior mandible
- Progressive jaw swelling with possible pain/tenderness
- Large mass with fluid-fluid levels on T2WI MR

PATHOLOGY

General Features

- Cavernous type: Deep soft tissue mass; **large vessels**
- Capillary type: Superficial strawberry appearance; **small vessels**

CLINICAL ISSUES

Presentation

- Most common signs/symptoms
  - Slowly expanding, bony hard swelling
  - May or may not be painful; may throb
  - Bleeding around loosened, migrating teeth with rebound mobility
  - **Aspiration**: arterial blood under pressure
- Other signs/symptoms
  - **Audible bruit** in highly expansile lesions

Natural History & Prognosis

- Female > male (2:1); most common in 2nd decade

Treatment

- Embolization, en bloc resection with ligation of external carotid, or sclerosing techniques

DIAGNOSTIC CHECKLIST

Image Interpretation Pearls

- Sunray appearance similar to osteosarcoma
- **Honeycomb** or **soap bubble** trabecular appearance

SELECTED REFERENCES

1. Jain S et al: Central hemangioma: A case report and review of literature. J Indian Soc Pedod Prev Dent. 34(1):87-91, 2016
2. Chetan BI et al: Diagnostic and surgical aspects of central hemangioma of mandible: a surgical approach for the reconstruction of mandible. J Int Oral Health. 7(1):56-8, 2015
3. Eliot CA et al: Intraosseous hemangioma of the anterior mandible. Head Neck Pathol. 4(2):123-5, 2010
4. Hansen T et al: Hemangioma of the mandible: case report with special emphasis on bone degradation. Oral Maxillofac Surg. 13(4):239-42, 2009
5. Oliveira AC et al: Central haemangioma of the mandible in a 7-year old child. Int J Paediatr Dent. 19(3):216-8, 2009
6. Nagpal A et al: Central haemangioma: variance in radiographic appearance. Dentomaxillofac Radiol. 34(2):120-5, 2005

Osteoid Osteoma

KEY FACTS

TERMINOLOGY

- Osteoid osteoma: Small, round, benign tumor of bone
  - 10-12% of all primary bone tumors

IMAGING

- Most common in long bones: Rare in jaws
  - Mandible > maxilla; posterior > anterior
- Central **radiolucent or mixed-density nidus** often with radiolucent rim surrounded by reactive sclerotic bone
- Radiolucent center **< 2 cm**
- Associated reactive **sclerotic bone may be extensive**
- May cause expansion of cortices
- T2WI MR: May show edema in adjacent soft tissues

TOP DIFFERENTIAL DIAGNOSES

- Osteoblastoma
- Cemento-ossifying fibroma
- Cementoblastoma
- Periapical cemental dysplasia

PATHOLOGY

- Central nidus contains osteoid ± trabeculae within vascularized fibrous connective tissue

CLINICAL ISSUES

- **Severe pain** worsening at night: Prostaglandins concentrated in nidus of lesion thought to play role
  - Relieved by **NSAIDs**
  - Pain reported less frequently in gnathic lesions than lesions in long bones
- Adjacent soft tissue may be tender
- 2nd and 3rd decades; range: 4-77 years
- M:F = 2:1
- Treatment: Excision preferred because of immediate relief of pain

DIAGNOSTIC CHECKLIST

- Some authors consider osteoid osteoma to be early stage in formation of osteoblastoma

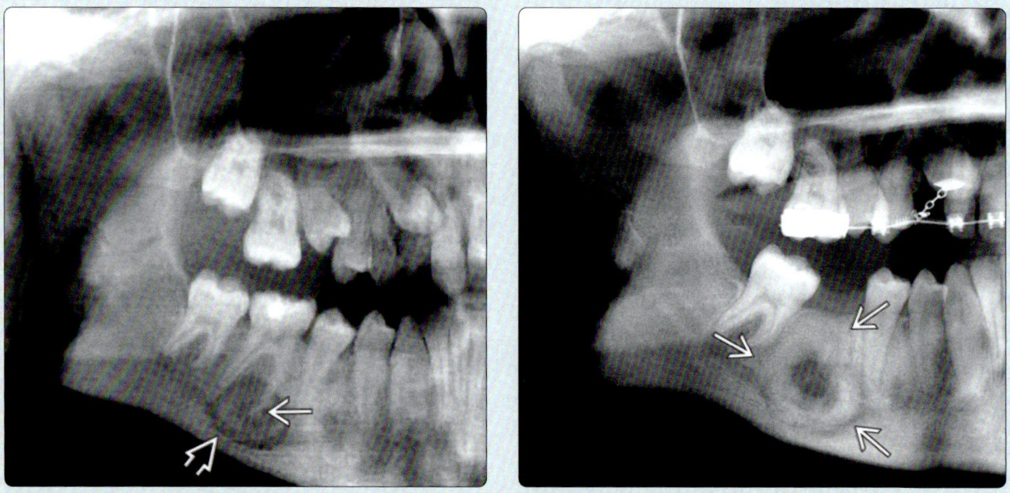

(Left) *Panoramic radiograph shows mixed radiopaque/radiolucent lesion at the apex of the mesial root of the mandibular right 1st molar. The working diagnosis for this lesion was cementoblastoma; however, the apex of the root ➡, normally not visible in cementoblastoma, is clearly seen. Note mild depression of the inferior alveolar canal ➡.* **(Right)** *Panoramic radiograph in the same patient 6 months postoperatively shows a central nidus of radiolucency and an extensive surrounding area of sclerotic bone ➡.*

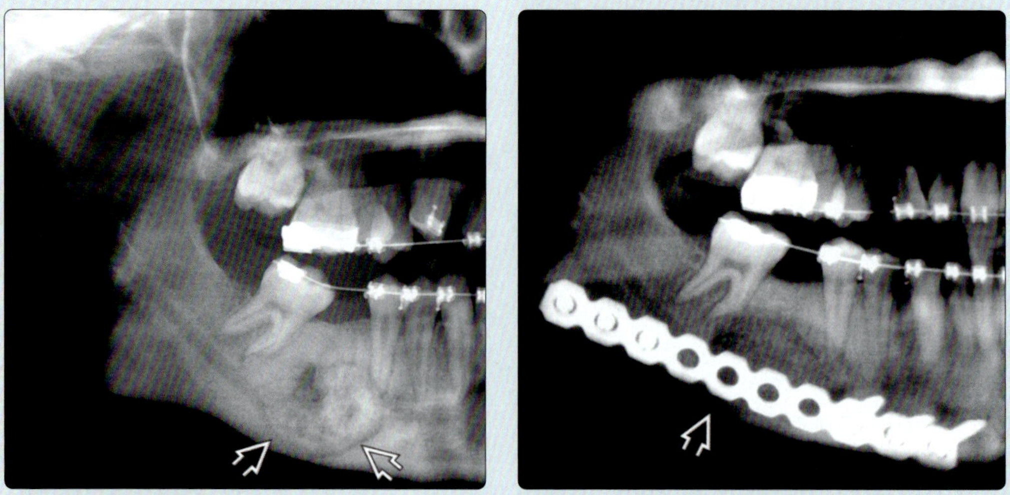

(Left) *Panoramic radiograph in the same patient 1 year postoperatively shows continued growth of the lesion and more severe depression of the inferior alveolar nerve ➡. The patient continued to complain of significant pain, and a 2nd opinion was sought. At the request of the radiologist, the histological slides were read by an oral pathologist. The diagnosis of osteoid osteoma was confirmed.* **(Right)** *Panoramic radiograph in the same patient following 2nd surgery shows loss of inferior cortex ➡ and healing lesion.*

Osteoid Osteoma

TERMINOLOGY

Definitions

- Small, round, benign tumor of bone
  - 10-12% of all primary bone tumors

IMAGING

General Features

- Best diagnostic clue
  - Central radiolucent or mixed-density nidus often with radiolucent rim and reactive sclerotic bone
- Location
  - Most common in long bones: Femur and tibia
  - Rare in jaws: Mandible > maxilla; posterior > anterior
    - Multifocal cases with multiple nidi reported
    - Classified according to location: Cortical, cancellous, or subperiosteal
    - Has been reported in condyle
- Size
  - Radiolucent center < 2 cm
  - Associated reactive sclerotic bone may be extensive
  - May cause expansion of cortices
- Morphology
  - Rounded lesion with well-defined borders

Radiographic Findings

- Intraoral and extraoral 2D imaging
  - Mixed-density lesion with central nidus of radiolucency or mixed density and surrounding sclerotic bone
  - If located near root apices, may appear similar to cementoblastoma initially

CT Findings

- CBCT and bone CT
  - Will demonstrate expansion, if present

MR Findings

- T2WI
  - May show edema in adjacent soft tissues

DIFFERENTIAL DIAGNOSIS

Osteoblastoma

- Thought by some authors to be same lesion as osteoid osteoma; others believe clinical and pathologic behavior differentiates
  - Less painful than osteoid osteoma and not relieved by nonsteroidal antiinflammatory agents
  - Considered to be more aggressive with greater growth potential

Cemento-Ossifying Fibroma

- Expands around epicenter, which is usually radiopaque
- Often has thin, radiolucent band at periphery representing fibrous capsule
- **Painless**

Cementoblastoma

- Benign tumor of cementum around apex of tooth
- **Root apex is resorbed or obscured** by lesion
- Center of lesion more sclerotic compared to osteoid osteoma

Periapical Cemental Dysplasia

- Usually **multifocal**; osteoid osteoma usually solitary
- Older age group: Middle-aged black women

Periapical Sclerosing Osteitis

- Reactive bone at apex of **nonvital tooth**
- Apical periodontal ligament space is widened

PATHOLOGY

Staging, Grading, & Classification

- Some authors do not consider osteoid osteoma to be true neoplasm but possibly of inflammatory origin or as result of unusual healing process

Gross Pathologic & Surgical Features

- Mixed soft and bony tissues
- Literature reports presence of distinguishable capsule at surgery

Microscopic Features

- Central nidus contains osteoid ± trabeculae within vascularized fibrous connective tissue
- Multinucleated giant cells rarely seen

CLINICAL ISSUES

Presentation

- Most common signs/symptoms
  - Severe pain worsening at night: Prostaglandins concentrated in nidus of lesion thought to play significant role
    - Relieved by NSAIDs
    - Pain reported less frequently in gnathic lesions than lesions in long bones
- Other signs/symptoms
  - Adjacent soft tissue may be tender

Demographics

- Age
  - 2nd and 3rd decades; range: 4-77 years
- Gender
  - M:F = 2:1

Treatment

- Excision: Spontaneous regression has been reported; however, excision preferred because of immediate relief of pain

DIAGNOSTIC CHECKLIST

Consider

- Some authors consider osteoid osteoma to be early stage in formation of osteoblastoma

SELECTED REFERENCES

1. Mortazavi H et al: Radiolucent rim as a possible diagnostic aid for differentiating jaw lesions. Imaging Sci Dent. 45(4):253-61, 2015
2. An SY et al: Unusual osteoid osteoma of the mandible: report of case and review of the literature. Oral Surg Oral Med Oral Pathol Oral Radiol. 116(2):e134-40, 2013
3. Jones AC et al: Osteoblastoma of the maxilla and mandible: a report of 24 cases, review of the literature, and discussion of its relationship to osteoid osteoma of the jaws. Oral Surg Oral Med Oral Pathol Oral Radiol Endod. 102(5):639-50, 2006

Osteoblastoma

KEY FACTS

TERMINOLOGY

- Definition: Benign tumor of bone arising from osteoblasts and accounting for ~ 1% of all bone tumors

IMAGING

- Most commonly in vertebral column
- Mandible > maxilla
  - Posterior > anterior; body of mandible most often
- Usually unilocular; rarely multilocular
- Radiodensity varies from radiolucent to mixed with abundant calcification
- Tooth roots may be displaced or resorbed
- If close to tooth root, may be confused with cementoblastoma or periapical pathology, especially if pain is present
  - Vitality testing and lack of etiology (caries/fracture) helps rule out pulpal pathology
- CBCT and bone CT: Will show expansion if present

TOP DIFFERENTIAL DIAGNOSES

- Osteoid osteoma
- Cementoblastoma
- Cemento-ossifying fibroma
- Osteosarcoma

PATHOLOGY

- Histologically identical to osteoid osteoma
- **Aggressive osteoblastoma**: Larger; rapid growth

CLINICAL ISSUES

- Swelling; pain or tenderness ~ 50%
- Complete excision ± chemotherapy if aggressive
- Recurrence low: 13%; aggressive osteoblastoma: 50%

DIAGNOSTIC CHECKLIST

- Some believe aggressive osteoblastoma represents low-grade osteosarcoma: Look for periosteal reactions

(Left) *Panoramic radiograph of an asymptomatic 17-year-old boy shows a mixed density lesion in the mandibular right 1st molar area. This osteoblastoma (OB) appears very similar to a cementoblastoma. The visible root apex ➡ differentiates. The mandibular canal is displaced ➡ inferiorly. (Courtesy K. Martonffy, MD.)* **(Right)** *Panoramic radiograph in a 13-year-old girl shows a poorly defined radiolucency ➡ below and between the mildly displaced roots of the mandibular left premolars. (Courtesy R. Urzúa, DDS.)*

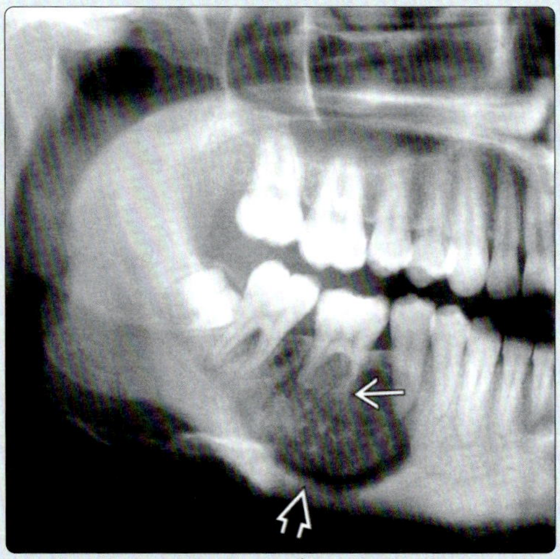

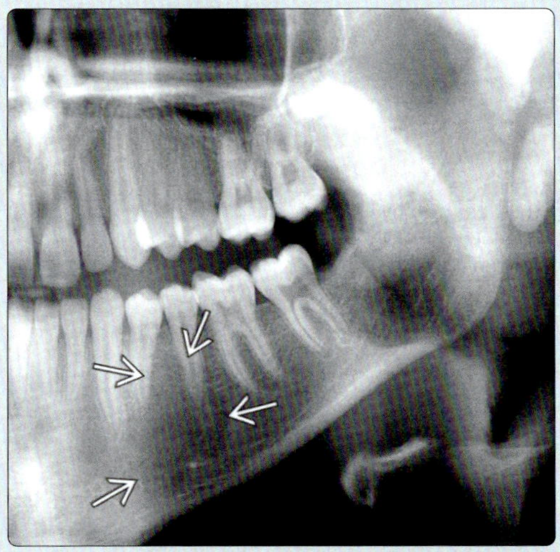

(Left) *Cross section CBCT in the same patient shows the contents of this OB appearing granular. Note extension into the lingual ➡ and buccal ➡ cortices and lack of expansion. (Courtesy R. Urzúa, DDS.)* **(Right)** *Axial CBCT in the same patient shows the cortical involvement and homogeneous granular appearance ➡. OBs in the jaws are most often found in the body of the mandible, and radiodensity varies from radiolucent to mixed with abundant calcifications. (Courtesy R. Urzúa, DDS.)*

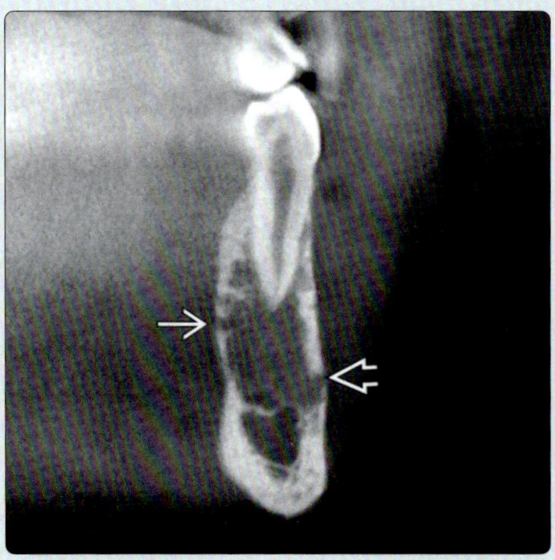

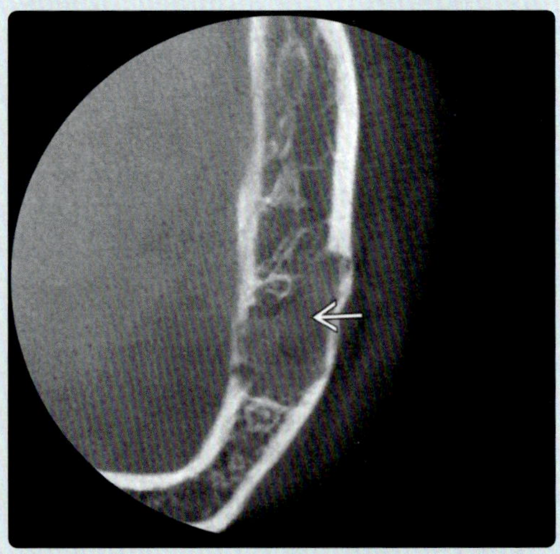

TERMINOLOGY

Synonyms

- Giant osteoid osteoma, giant osteogenic fibroma

Definitions

- Benign tumor of bone arising from osteoblasts and accounting for ~ 1% of all bone tumors

IMAGING

General Features

- Best diagnostic clue
  - Expansile, mixed radiopaque/radiolucent lesion in body of mandible
- Location
  - Most commonly in vertebral column, ribs, pelvis; craniofacial bones rarely
  - Mandible > maxilla; posterior > anterior
    - Body of mandible most commonly
    - TMJ cases reported
- Size
  - ≥ 1.5 cm at discovery; greater growth potential than osteoid osteoma
- Morphology
  - Well or ill defined; some may appear corticated or partly corticated
  - Usually unilocular; rarely multilocular
  - Radiodensity varies from radiolucent to mixed with abundant calcification

Radiographic Findings

- Intraoral and extraoral 2D imaging
  - Lesion of varying radiodensity
    - If close to tooth root, may be confused with cementoblastoma or periapical pathology, especially if pain is present
      - Vitality testing and lack of etiology (caries/fracture) helps rule out pulpal pathology
  - Tooth roots may be displaced or resorbed

CT Findings

- CBCT and bone CT
  - Expansion may be present
  - More aggressive: Spiculated (sunray) periosteal reactions may be present

DIFFERENTIAL DIAGNOSIS

Osteoid Osteoma

- Usually smaller than osteoblastoma; painful
- Radiolucent nidus with sclerotic periphery

Cementoblastoma

- Similar radiographic and histologic appearance to osteoblastoma but intimately related to tooth root
- Tooth **apex is lost in lesion**

Cemento-Ossifying Fibroma

- Peripheral zone of radiolucency with concentric growth pattern

Osteosarcoma

- Well-differentiated osteosarcoma histologically similar to osteoblastoma

PATHOLOGY

General Features

- Associated abnormalities
  - Osteoblastoma reported in association with simple bone cyst and aneurysmal bone cyst

Staging, Grading, & Classification

- **Aggressive (epithelioid) osteoblastoma** is subcategory
  - Larger, grows more rapidly, and tends to occur in older age group
  - May invade soft tissues

Microscopic Features

- Identical to osteoid osteoma
- Fibrous connective tissue stroma with spindle-shaped fibroblasts and vascular channels
- Osteoid and trabeculae rimmed with plump osteoblasts containing basophilic nuclei

CLINICAL ISSUES

Presentation

- Most common signs/symptoms
  - Swelling
  - Pain or tenderness ~ 50%
    - Differentiating from osteoid osteoma on presence/absence or degree of pain, not definitive
  - May be asymptomatic

Demographics

- Age
  - Range: 3-61 years; mean: Middle 3rd decade
- Gender
  - Males > females (2:1)

Natural History & Prognosis

- Prognosis is generally good
  - Spontaneous remission after biopsy reported
- **Sarcomatous change** reported in few cases

Treatment

- Complete excision
- Recurrence low: 13%; aggressive osteoblastoma: 50%
- Adjuvant chemotherapy recommended by some for lesions showing aggressive features because of difficulty differentiating from low-grade osteosarcoma
- Radiographic follow-up important

DIAGNOSTIC CHECKLIST

Consider

- Some believe aggressive osteoblastoma represents low-grade osteosarcoma: Look for periosteal reactions

SELECTED REFERENCES

1. Rana V et al: Epithelioid osteoblastoma of maxilla: A rare and aggressive variant of a benign neoplasm at an uncommon site. J Oral Maxillofac Pathol. 20(2):332, 2016
2. Mahajan A et al: Osteoblastoma in the retromolar region - Report of an unusual case and Review of literature. J Maxillofac Oral Surg. 12(3):338-40, 2013

Mandible-Maxilla Osteoma

KEY FACTS

TERMINOLOGY

- Definition: Benign bone-forming neoplasm producing either compact or cancellous bone

IMAGING

- Peripheral: Well-defined, bone density radiopacity arising from cortical plates
  - **Pedunculated or sessile** with broad base
- Central: Arising from endosteal surfaces of bone
  - **No radiolucent halo**; may cause expansion and displace teeth
- Mandible > maxilla: Posterior (especially ramus and condyle) > anterior
- CBCT and bone CT best show extent, size, location, and expansion if present

TOP DIFFERENTIAL DIAGNOSES

- Idiopathic osteosclerosis
- Sclerosing osteitis
- Buccal and lingual exostoses
- Mandibular tori

PATHOLOGY

- Associated with **Gardner syndrome** (GS) (familial adenomatous polyposis): Autosomal dominant
  - **Multiple osteomas precede presentation** of intestinal polyps, which have **100% potential for malignant change**

CLINICAL ISSUES

- Hard, bony swelling or expansion of jaws
- Can be painful especially if infected
- Age range: 13-69 years; mean: 40 years
- GS patients usually 20-40 years old
- Surgical excision for cosmetics and to restore function

DIAGNOSTIC CHECKLIST

- Consider GS if multiple lesions

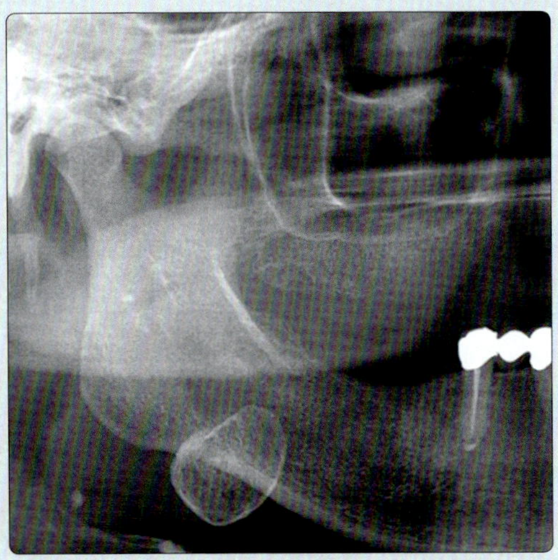

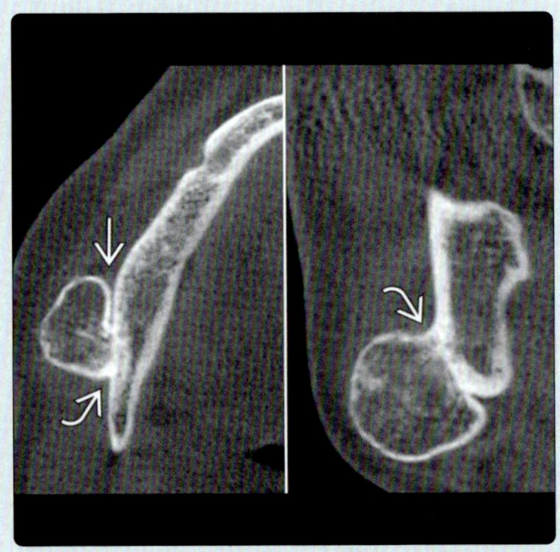

(Left) *Cropped panoramic radiograph shows a well-defined, corticated radiopacity centered over the inferior border of the right mandible just anterior to the angle. This osteoma was misdiagnosed 4 years earlier as a sialolith.* **(Right)** *Axial (left) and coronal (right) CBCT images of the same patient show the osteoma is not connected to the mandible anteriorly ➔ but has a pedunculated attachment to the mandibular cortex posteriorly ➔. The lesion was bony-hard and fixed, which differentiates from sialolith.*

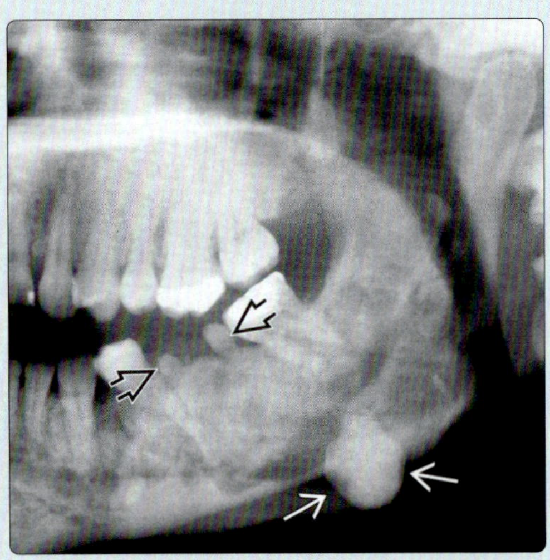

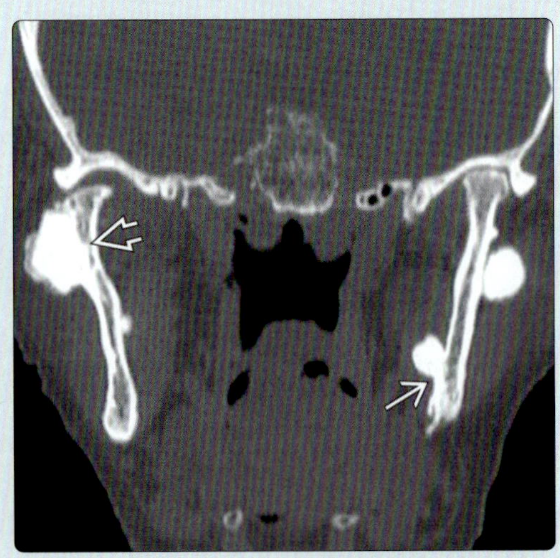

(Left) *Panoramic radiograph shows an osteoma ➔ at the inferior border of the left mandible in a patient with Gardner syndrome. Note small supernumerary teeth ➔ and increased density of mandible caused by central osteomas. (Courtesy B. Pass, DDS.)* **(Right)** *Coronal bone CT shows multiple exophytic peripheral osteomas in the ramus of the mandible in a patient with Gardner syndrome. The lesion on the lingual of the left ramus is pedunculated ➔, while the osteoma at the right condylar neck has a broad base ➔.*

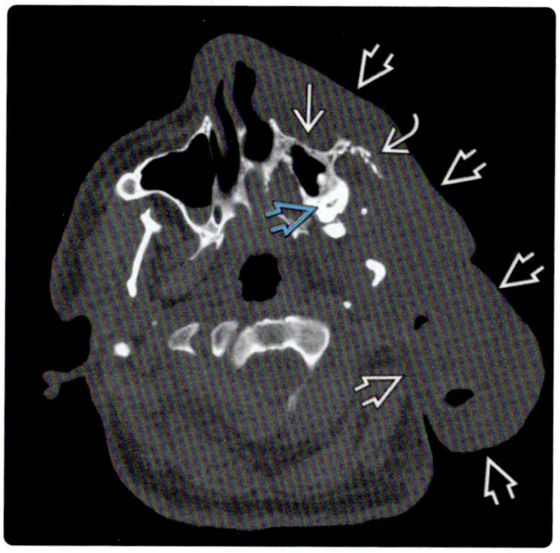

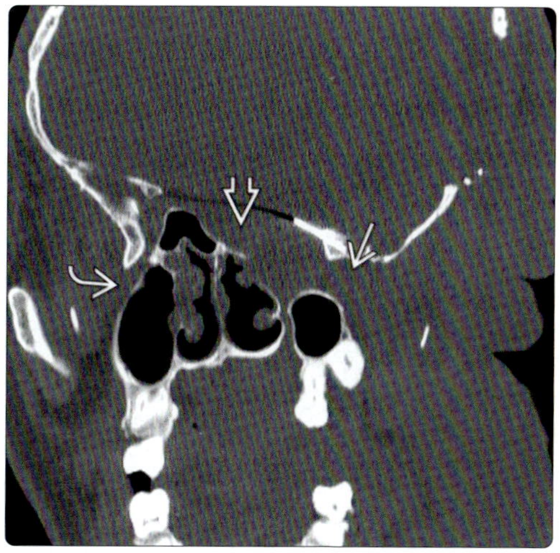

(Left) *Axial bone CT shows massive peripheral plexiform neurofibroma affecting the left maxilla in a 32-year-old man with NF1. There is remodeling of the anterior maxilla & patchy destruction of the zygomatic arch. Note displacement of molar tooth.* **(Right)** *Coronal oblique bone CT in the same patient shows extension of the neurofibroma through the pterygomaxillary fissure into the sphenoid sinuses. Note widening of the pterygomaxillary fissure compared to the normal contralateral side.*

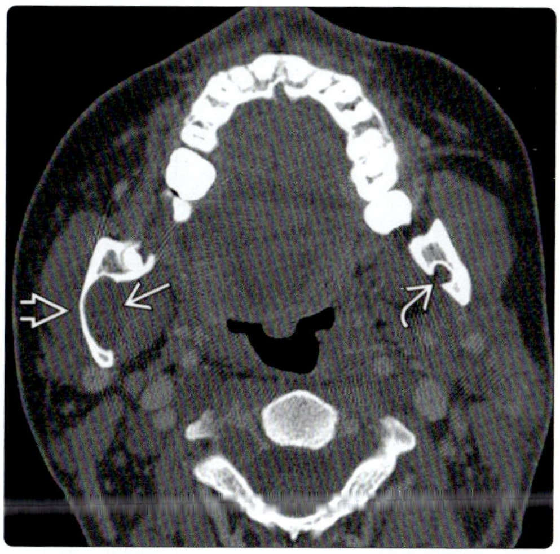

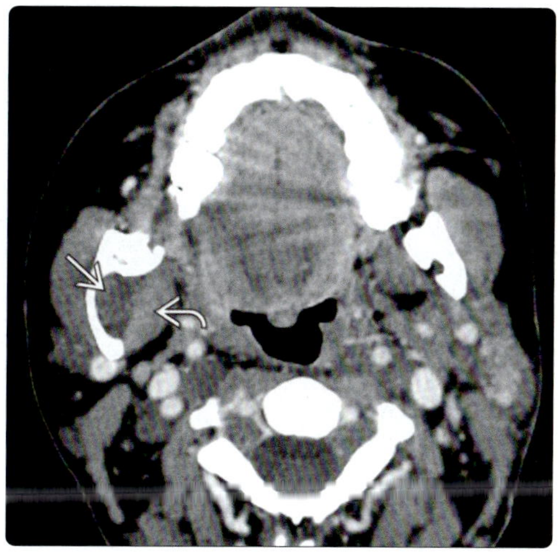

(Left) *Axial bone CT shows an expansile mass & bowing of the ramus typical of neurofibroma associated with the inferior alveolar nerve in a 31-year-old woman with NF1. Note enlargement of the mandibular foramen compared to the contralateral side. (Courtesy L. Ginsberg, MD.)* **(Right)** *Axial CECT in the same patient shows that the neurofibroma is hypodense compared to the adjacent medial pterygoid muscle. (Courtesy L. Ginsberg, MD.)*

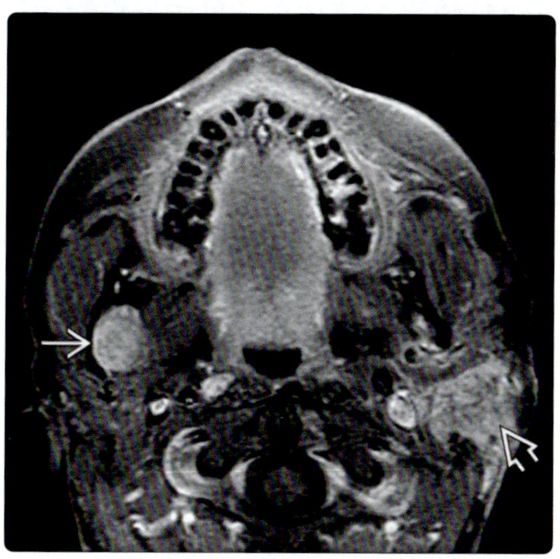

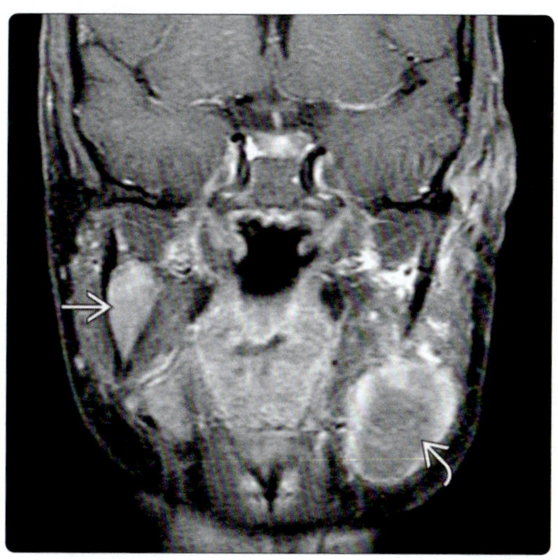

(Left) *Axial T1WI C+ FS MR in the same patient shows diffuse heterogeneous enhancement in the V3 lesion & an additional plexiform neurofibroma of the left parotid. (Courtesy L. Ginsberg, MD.)* **(Right)** *Coronal T1WI C+ FS MR in the same patient shows MPNST in the left submandibular region. Note heterogeneous enhancement of the MPNST & the V3 lesion. There is a 2-16% risk of malignant transformation of plexiform neurofibroma in patients with NF1. (Courtesy L. Ginsberg, MD.)*

Desmoplastic Fibroma

KEY FACTS

TERMINOLOGY

- Definition: Rare myofibroblastic tumor that accounts for < 1% of all bone neoplasms

IMAGING

- Multilocular radiolucency with **coarse straight septa**
- Mandible > > maxilla
  - Posterior > anterior; especially ramus
- Multilocular > > unilocular (3:1)
- Well defined > ill defined
- Root divergence or resorption
- **Expansion or cortical perforation** (29% of cases)
- Periosteal reactions may occasionally be seen: Sunray, mimicking osteogenic sarcoma
- CBCT/CT: Better demonstrates locularity and any cortical erosion or periosteal reactions
- MR for cases with cortical perforation
  - Determines extent of soft tissue involvement

TOP DIFFERENTIAL DIAGNOSES

- Aneurysmal bone cyst
- Odontogenic myxoma
- Ameloblastoma
- Central hemangioma
- Central odontogenic fibroma
- Simple (traumatic) bone cyst

CLINICAL ISSUES

- Painless expansile mass
- Limited opening/trismus, tooth displacement
- 1st-5th decades; 84% < 30 years; mean = 16 years
- Recommended treatment: Resection or wide excision
  - 70% recurrence with curettage

DIAGNOSTIC CHECKLIST

- Location below mandibular canal rules out odontogenic lesions

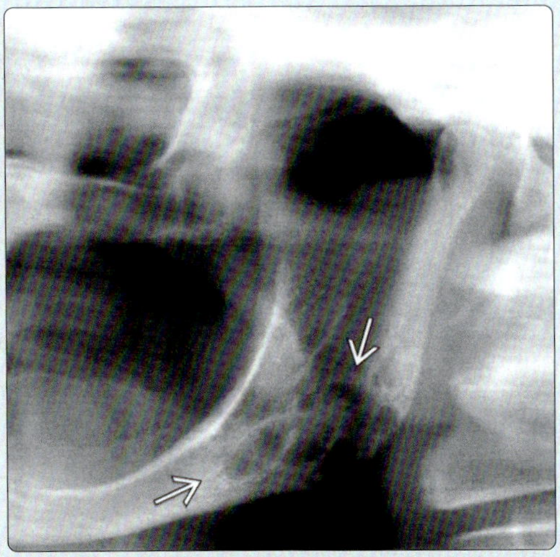
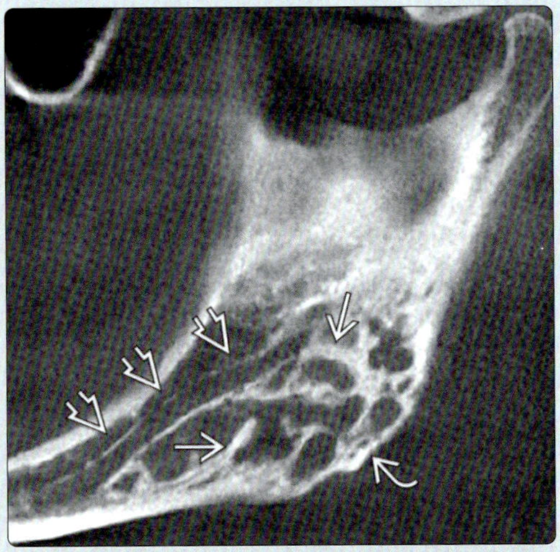

(Left) *Panoramic radiograph shows desmoplastic fibroma as a multilocular radiolucency ➡ in the left posterior mandible and angle. The relationship of the mandibular canal to the lesion is not clear. (Courtesy M. Noujeim, DDS.)* **(Right)** *Panoramic reformat CBCT in the same patient shows coarse septa ➡ and extension into inferior cortex ⇨, which remains intact. The mandibular canal ➡ is clearly visible and has been displaced superiorly. Location below the mandibular canal rules out odontogenic lesions. (Courtesy M. Noujeim, DDS.)*

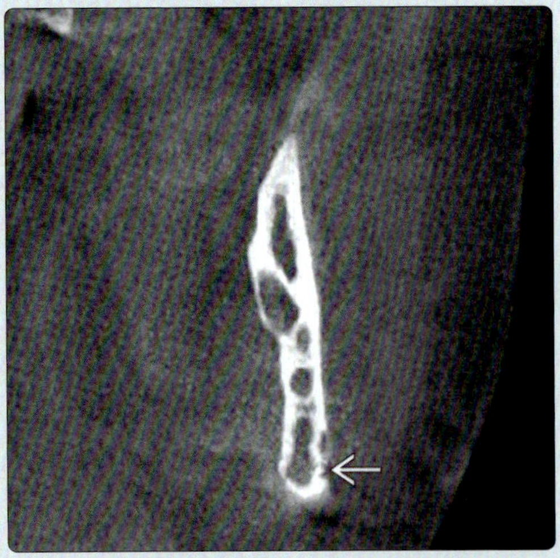
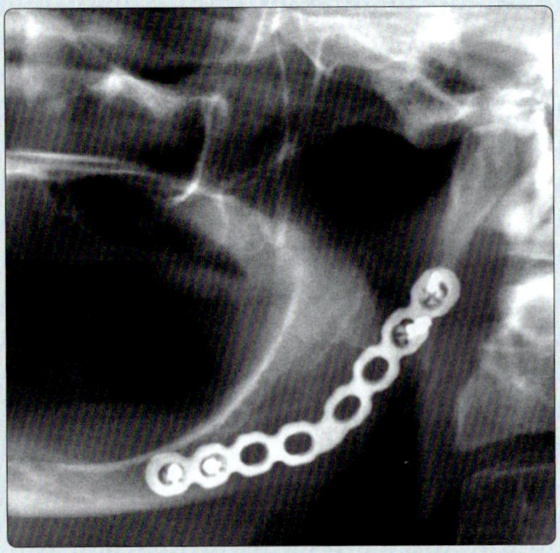

(Left) *Coronal CBCT in the same patient shows locularity of lesion and no expansion. The possibility of cortical erosion ➡ is noted at the buccal inferior margin. If soft tissue extension is suspected, MR is the imaging modality of choice. (Courtesy M. Noujeim, DDS.)* **(Right)** *Panoramic radiograph in the same patient, postoperatively, shows stabilizing surgical chain and healing bone. Resection or wide excision is recommended for these aggressive tumors to avoid the possibility of recurrence. (Courtesy M. Noujeim, DDS.)*

Desmoplastic Fibroma

TERMINOLOGY

Abbreviations

- Desmoplastic fibroma (DF)

Synonyms

- Aggressive fibromatosis is soft tissue counterpart

Definitions

- Rare myofibroblastic tumor that accounts for < 1% of all bone neoplasms

IMAGING

General Features

- Best diagnostic clue
  - Multilocular radiolucency with coarse straight septa
- Location
  - Jaws > femur > pelvic bones > radius > tibia
  - Mandible > > maxilla
    - Posterior > anterior; especially ramus
- Morphology
  - Multilocular > > unilocular (3:1)
    - Smaller lesions: Unilocular and may resemble simple bone cyst
    - Larger lesions: Multilocular with coarse straight septa
  - Well defined > ill defined

Radiographic Findings

- Intraoral and extraoral 2D imaging
  - Root divergence or resorption
  - **Expansion or cortical perforation** (29% of cases)
  - Periosteal reactions may occasionally be seen: Sunray, mimicking osteogenic sarcoma
  - Displacement of mandibular canal may be seen

CT Findings

- CBCT and bone CT
  - Better demonstrates locularity and any cortical erosion or periosteal reactions

Imaging Recommendations

- Best imaging tool
  - CBCT/CT to examine for cortical involvement and periosteal reactions
  - MR for cases with cortical perforation
    - Determines extent of soft tissue involvement

DIFFERENTIAL DIAGNOSIS

Aneurysmal Bone Cyst

- Multilocular radiolucency with **finer, wispy septa**
- Same age group; rapidly expanding

Odontogenic Myxoma (Myxofibroma)

- Multilocular radiolucency with **straight septa**
- Epicenter above mandibular canal

Ameloblastoma

- Multilocular radiolucency with curved or **"soap bubble" loculations**
- Epicenter above mandibular canal; older age group

Central Hemangioma

- Multilocular radiolucency; same age group

Central Odontogenic Fibroma

- Multilocular = unilocular; **root resorption**
- Older age group; F > M

Simple (Traumatic) Bone Cyst

- Unilocular radiolucency with **corticated border**
- May mimic small unilocular lesion of DF

Eosinophilic Granuloma

- Unilocular (punched-out) radiolucency without corticated border

PATHOLOGY

General Features

- Associated abnormalities
  - DF may appear as part of **Gardner syndrome**
  - Reported association with **tuberous sclerosis**

Microscopic Features

- Small elongated fibroblasts; abundant collagen fibers
- May appear **similar to well-differentiated fibrosarcoma**
- Biopsy center of lesion to avoid reactive bone → misdiagnosis of fibroosseous lesion or osteosarcoma

CLINICAL ISSUES

Presentation

- Most common signs/symptoms
  - Painless expansile mass
- Other signs/symptoms
  - Limited opening/trismus
  - Pain occasionally, especially if TMJ involved
  - Tooth mobility or displacement

Demographics

- Age
  - 1st-5th decades; 84% < 30 years; mean = 16 years
- Gender
  - M = F

Natural History & Prognosis

- Aggressive benign tumor; morbidity may be high
- Long-term follow-up to monitor for recurrence

Treatment

- Resection or wide excision
- Simple excision or enucleation: 20-40% recurrence
- Curettage: 70% recurrence
- Chemotherapy for cases not amenable to surgery

DIAGNOSTIC CHECKLIST

Image Interpretation Pearls

- Location below mandibular canal rules out odontogenic lesions

SELECTED REFERENCES

1. Khatib B et al: Desmoplastic fibroma of the mandible in young children-a case series. Int J Oral Maxillofac Surg. 46(2):173-180, 2017

Malignant Ameloblastoma and Ameloblastic Carcinoma

KEY FACTS

TERMINOLOGY

- **Ameloblastic carcinoma** exhibits histologic criteria of malignant neoplasm
- **Malignant ameloblastoma** is histologically similar to benign ameloblastoma but is metastatic clinically
  - Terms are sometimes used interchangeably due to similarities, but they are different entities

IMAGING

- Uni- or more commonly multilocular with **honeycomb/soap bubble** internal trabecular pattern; robust and **thick septa**
- Cortical destruction, extraosseous extension, extensive solid components
- Dental **root resorption** not uncommon, may **displace** teeth
- Lesion can **erode** through cortex with **extension** into surrounding oral mucosa
- May have **multiple, coarse internal calcifications**
- Imaging protocol
  - Panoramic radiograph, followed by CBCT or CECT
  - MR if simultaneous mixed solid and cystic

TOP DIFFERENTIAL DIAGNOSES

- Ameloblastoma
- Odontogenic keratocyst
- Odontogenic myxoma
- Central mucoepidermoid tumor
- Carcinoma ex dentigerous cyst
- Central giant cell granuloma

CLINICAL ISSUES

- Slow-growing expansile mass similar in appearance to benign ameloblastoma
- 3rd-5th decades
- Treatment: En bloc surgical resection
  - Initial treatment often inadequate as clinical, radiographic, and histologic appearance is similar to benign ameloblastoma

(Left) *Axial CBCT shows ameloblastic carcinoma in the maxillary right canine/premolar area. Note the buccal expansion → as well as perforation of the buccal cortex →. (Courtesy M. Ahmad, DDS.)* **(Right)** *Alveolar cross section reformatted CBCT in the same patient details expansion → and gross cortical perforation → of the buccal cortex and also advanced external dental root resorption → of the 1st premolar. (Courtesy M. Ahmad, DDS.)*

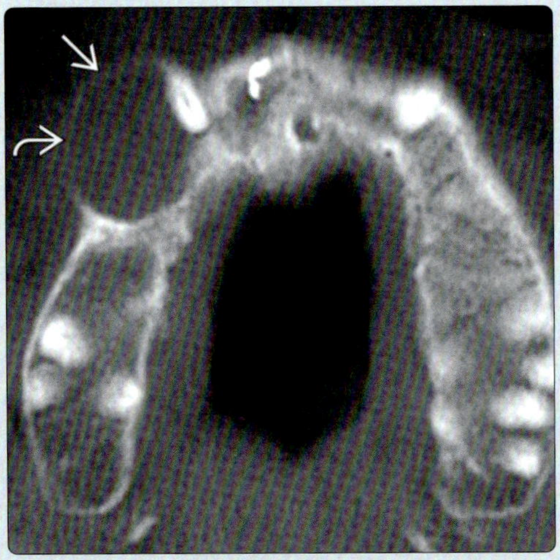

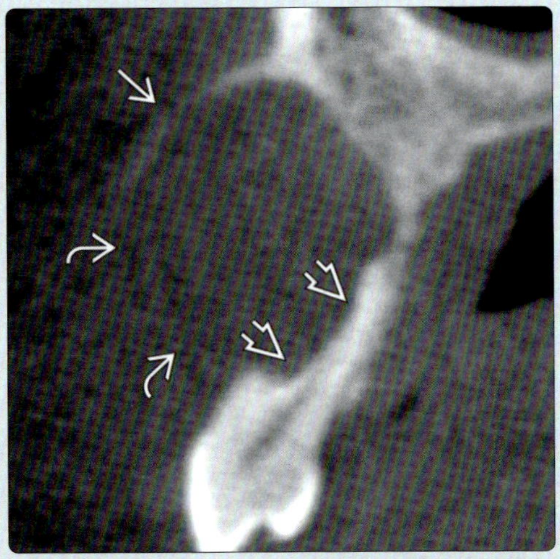

(Left) *Panoramic reformatted CBCT in the same patient depicts the dental root resorption → and well-defined radiolucent lesion →. (Courtesy M. Ahmad, DDS.)* **(Right)** *Axial CECT shows deformity of the left face → from previous resection of an ameloblastoma that has metastasized to the soft tissues of the neck and cervical vertebra. This is an example of malignant ameloblastoma looking histologically benign (as distinct from an ameloblastic carcinoma) but metastasizing to nodes or elsewhere.*

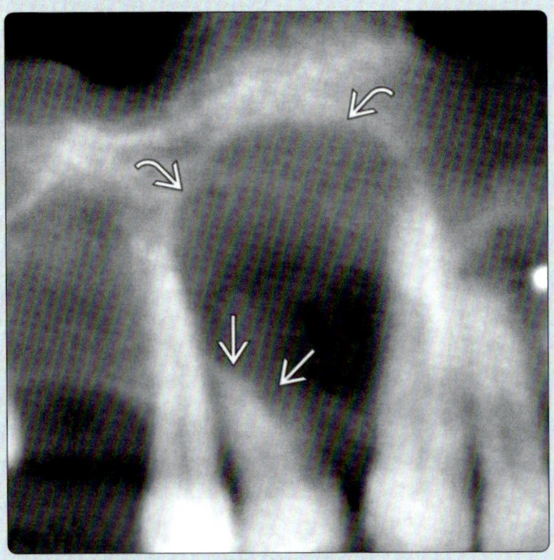

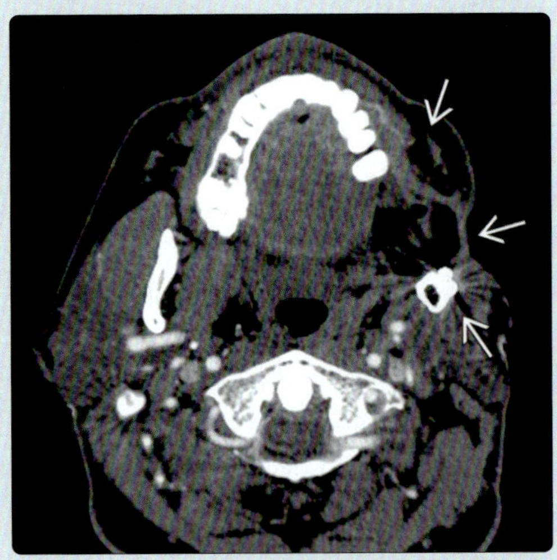

TERMINOLOGY

Definitions

- **Ameloblastic carcinoma** exhibits histologic criteria of malignant neoplasm
- **Malignant ameloblastoma** is histologically indistinguishable from ameloblastoma but is metastatic clinically
  - Terms are sometimes used interchangeably due to similarities between lesions, but they are indeed different entities

IMAGING

General Features

- Best diagnostic clue
  - Cortical destruction, extraosseous extension, extensive solid components
- Location
  - Mandible > maxilla; most often premolar/molar area
- Morphology
  - Well-defined border with cortication; crenations of scalloping borders
  - Malignant ameloblastoma may show malignant signs, such as loss of cortical integrity invading adjacent tissues
  - Uni- or more commonly multilocular with honeycomb/soap bubble internal trabecular pattern; **robust and thick septa**

Radiographic Findings

- Radiography
  - Radiographic features similar to benign ameloblastoma
    - Slow-growing expansile lesion
    - Adjacent **teeth** may be **displaced** or **resorbed**
    - Adjacent structures may be displaced

CT Findings

- Cystic areas of low attenuation with scattered isoattenuating regions
- Lesion can also **erode** through cortex with **extension** into surrounding oral mucosa
- May have multiple, coarse internal **calcifications**

MR Findings

- T1WI
  - Solid portions have intermediate signal intensity
  - Cystic components have homogeneous intermediate signal intensity
- T2WI
  - Solid portions have high signal intensity and enhance with gadolinium
  - Cystic components have homogeneous high signal intensity without enhancement with gadolinium
- Mural nodule or thickened wall can be detected

Imaging Recommendations

- Protocol advice
  - Panoramic radiograph followed by CBCT or CECT
  - MR imaging if simultaneous presence of mixed solid and cystic patterns

DIFFERENTIAL DIAGNOSIS

Ameloblastoma

- Well-defined, expansile, uni- or multilocular radiolucent lesion with honeycomb/soap bubble internal pattern; resorbs dental roots

Odontogenic Keratocyst

- Usually not expansile; dental root resorption rare

Odontogenic Myxoma (Myxofibroma)

- Straight, lacy septa making tennis racket-like internal pattern; moderate expansion

Central Mucoepidermoid Tumor

- Typically has benign radiographic features; longstanding expansion; F > M

Carcinoma Ex Dentigerous Cyst

- Arises from wall of dental follicular cyst
- Locally invasive

Central Giant Cell Granuloma

- Younger patient
- Anterior to permanent 2nd molar

PATHOLOGY

Microscopic Features

- Ameloblastic carcinoma: Abnormal mitoses and large hyperchromatic nuclei
- Malignant ameloblastoma: Proliferating sheets/islands of odontogenic epithelium typical of plexiform, follicular, and granular cell ameloblastoma variants

CLINICAL ISSUES

Presentation

- Most common signs/symptoms
  - Slow-growing asymptomatic expansile mass; similar appearance to benign ameloblastoma

Demographics

- 3rd-5th decades

Natural History & Prognosis

- Metastasis may not be apparent for months or years after initial treatment as benign ameloblastoma
- Most involved metastatic sites: Brain, lymph nodes, bone

Treatment

- En bloc surgical resection with 2- to 3-cm bony margins
- Initial treatment often inadequate as clinical, radiographic, and histologic appearance is similar to ameloblastoma
- Radiotherapy and chemotherapy of limited value except when not amenable to surgical resection

SELECTED REFERENCES

1. Yunaev M et al: A rare case of ameloblastic carcinoma. Ear Nose Throat J. 93(9):E34-6, 2014
2. Lai H et al: Benign metastasizing ameloblastoma or malignant ameloblastoma? J Craniofac Surg. 22(3):995-7, 2011
3. Matsuzaki H et al: Ameloblastic carcinoma: a case report with radiological features of computed tomography and magnetic resonance imaging and positron emission tomography. Oral Surg Oral Med Oral Pathol Oral Radiol Endod. 112(1):e40-7, 2011

Mandible-Maxilla Metastasis

KEY FACTS

TERMINOLOGY

- Definition: Spread of malignant disease from distant primary tumor

IMAGING

- Ramus, premolar-molar region of mandible most common
- Also mandibular angle, condyle, maxillary sinus, anterior palate
- Usually **poorly defined**, invasive margins
- Early disease: Patchy areas of bone destruction separated from each other by normal bone
- Late disease: Radiolucent areas coalesce, moth-eaten appearance
- Most malignancies cause bone destruction, but **breast** and **prostate** malignancies may cause **bone formation and sclerotic appearance**
- May cause symmetric widening of periodontal ligament space, loss of lamina dura, loss of crypt cortex
- **Spiculated periosteal reaction** occasionally seen, especially with prostate carcinoma

TOP DIFFERENTIAL DIAGNOSES

- Osteomyelitis
- Periapical inflammation
- Multiple myeloma

CLINICAL ISSUES

- Pain, swelling, **numbness, or paresthesia** of 3rd branch of trigeminal nerve, including **chin**
- 5th-7th decades most common
- Metastases to jaws rare and account for ~ 1% of oral malignancies
- Most common primary lesions from breast, lung, kidney, thyroid, prostate, colon, rectum, stomach, testis, bladder, cervix, and ovary
- Metastases to jaws associated with poor prognosis

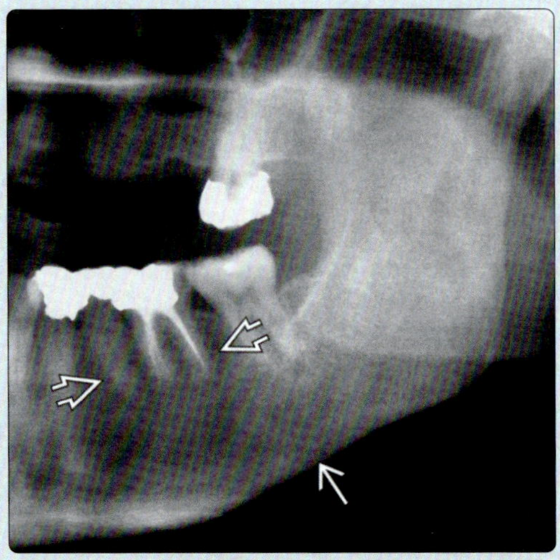
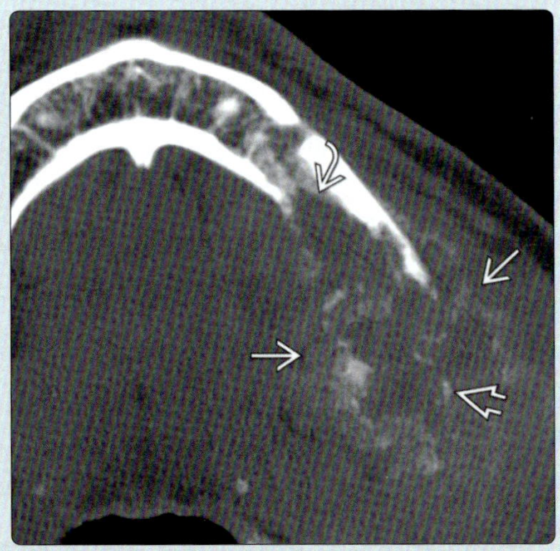

(Left) *Cropped panoramic radiograph shows breast metastases affecting the left mandible and ramus. Note the loss of inferior cortical border ➡, loss of lamina dura ➡, and loss of normal trabecular architecture.* **(Right)** *Axial bone CT shows colon metastases in the left mandible. There is frank bone destruction of the affected area with mandibular expansion ➡ and patchy residual trabecular bone ➡. Note the well-defined anterior margin ➡. Metastases to the jaws are indicative of a poor prognosis.*

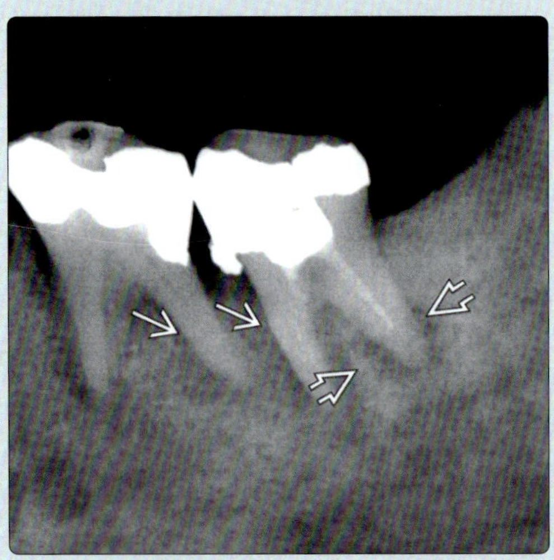
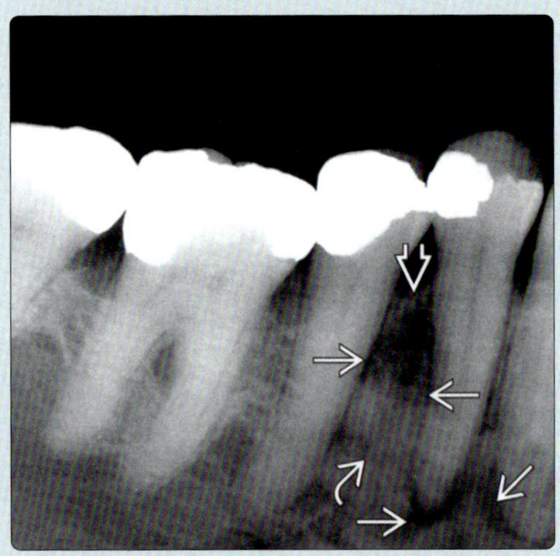

(Left) *Periapical radiograph shows breast metastases in the left mandible. The lamina dura are missing ➡, and there is symmetrical widening of the periodontal ligament spaces ➡. The bone pattern is sclerotic. This appearance mimics osteomyelitis.* **(Right)** *Periapical radiograph shows breast metastases in the right mandible. There is permeative destruction between the premolars near the alveolar crest ➡, sclerotic bone in the apical 1/2 ➡, and widening of the periodontal ligament spaces ➡.*

TERMINOLOGY

Synonyms

- Secondary malignancy

Definitions

- Spread of malignant disease from distant primary tumor

IMAGING

General Features

- Best diagnostic clue
  - Patchy or moth-eaten bone destruction with periodontal ligament space widening in patient with known primary carcinoma
- Location
  - Ramus, premolar-molar region of mandible most common; can be bilateral
  - Other sites: Mandibular angle, condyle, maxillary sinus, anterior palate
  - Occasionally at root apex or dental papilla of developing tooth and mimics periapical inflammation
- Morphology
  - Irregular shape, can be expansile

Imaging Recommendations

- Best imaging tool
  - CT or CBCT to determine extent and behavior of lesion

Radiographic Findings

- Usually **poorly defined**, invasive margins
- Early disease: Patchy areas of bone destruction separated from each other by normal bone
- Late disease: Radiolucent areas coalesce to form larger lesions
  - Generalized radiolucency, **moth-eaten appearance** or frank bony destruction
  - Pathologic fracture
- Most metastases cause bone destruction, but breast and prostate metastases may cause bone formation and sclerotic appearance
- **Spiculated periosteal reaction** occasionally seen, especially with prostate carcinoma
- May cause **symmetric widening of periodontal ligament space**, loss of lamina dura, loss of developing tooth crypt cortex

CT Findings

- May have associated soft tissue mass

DIFFERENTIAL DIAGNOSIS

Osteomyelitis

- Clinical signs and symptoms similar, but periosteal reaction in osteomyelitis is more often parallel to mandibular cortex

Periapical Inflammation

- Usually at root apex; metastases cause symmetric widening of entire periodontal ligament space

Multiple Myeloma

- Lesions well defined (punched out); metastases poorly defined and invasive

PATHOLOGY

General Features

- Etiology
  - Spread from primary tumor usually hematogenous

Microscopic Features

- Depend on origin of primary lesion

CLINICAL ISSUES

Presentation

- Most common signs/symptoms
  - Pain, swelling, numbness, or paresthesia of 3rd branch of trigeminal nerve, including chin
- Other signs/symptoms
  - Intraoral mass, tooth mobility, gingival irritation, halitosis
  - Occasionally pathological fracture or bleeding from tumor site
  - Extraction **socket may enlarge or not heal**

Demographics

- Age
  - 5th-7th decades most common
- Gender
  - Female predilection reported, likely because **breast carcinoma metastases most common** type
- Epidemiology
  - Metastases to jaws rare and account for ~ 1% of oral malignancies
  - Most common primary lesions from breast, lung, kidney, thyroid, prostate, colon, rectum, stomach, testis, bladder, cervix, and ovary

Natural History & Prognosis

- Metastases to jaws associated with **poor prognosis**

Treatment

- Radiotherapy, chemotherapy, surgery, or palliative Tx depending on type of primary lesion, extent of metastases, and symptoms

DIAGNOSTIC CHECKLIST

Consider

- Metastases may be discovered prior to primary tumor
- Consider medical history and suspect metastases if patient has known primary carcinoma

Image Interpretation Pearls

- Remember, metastases occasionally sclerotic
- Widespread areas of bone destruction suggest metastases

SELECTED REFERENCES

1. Torregrossa VR et al: Metastatic cervical carcinoma of the jaw presenting as periapical disease. Int Endod J. 49(2):203-11, 2016
2. Schneider KM et al: Large cell neuroendocrine carcinoma: topic review and a unique case of metastasis to the mandible. J Maxillofac Oral Surg. 14(Suppl 1):120-6, 2015
3. Hirshberg A et al: Metastatic tumors to the jaws and mouth. Head Neck Pathol. 8(4):463-74, 2014
4. Hirshberg A et al: Metastatic tumors to the jawbones: analysis of 390 cases. J Oral Pathol Med. 23(8):337-41, 1994

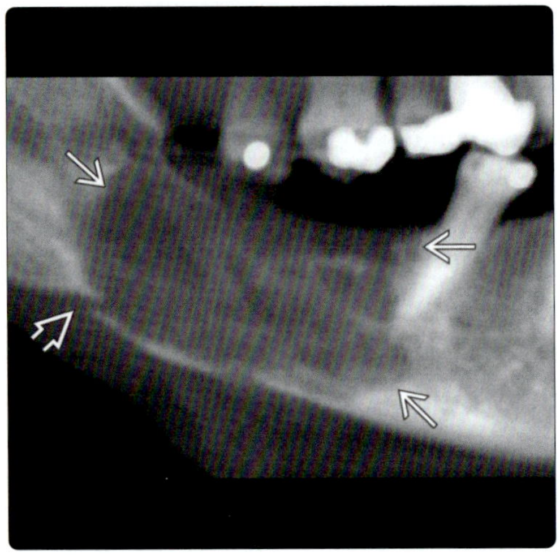
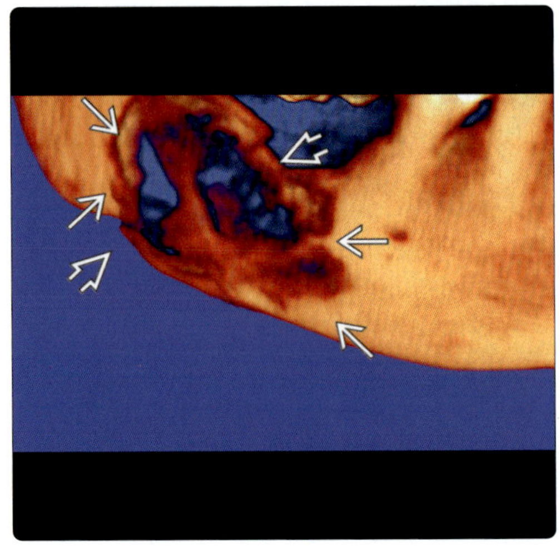

(Left) *Panoramic reformat CBCT shows breast metastases to the right mandible. The lesion is well defined* ➔ *and radiolucent with some residual internal trabeculae. There is a pathological fracture at the inferior border* ➔. **(Right)** *CBCT 3D reformation in the same patient shows the well-defined borders* ➔ *of the metastatic lesion and the pathological fracture* ➔ *at the inferior mandibular border and alveolar crest.*

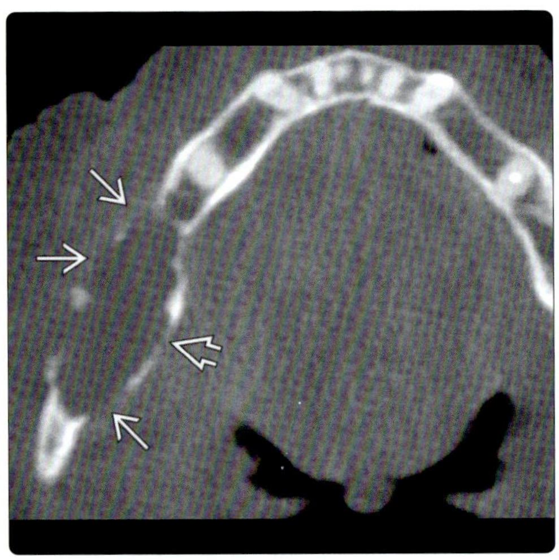
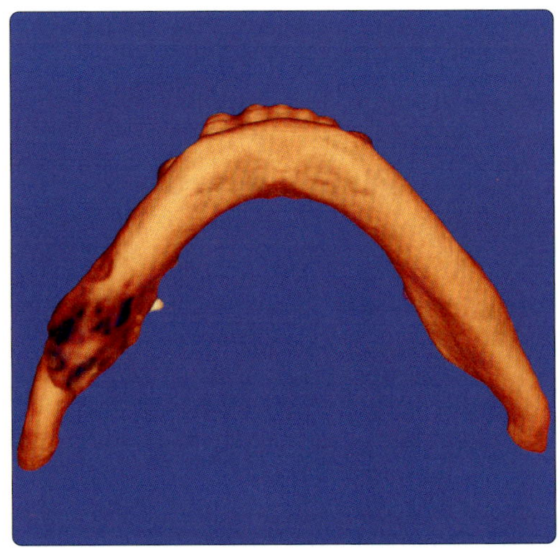

(Left) *Axial CBCT in the same patient shows destruction* ➔ *of the buccal and lingual mandibular cortices with lesion extension to the surrounding soft tissues. There is also cortical thinning and expansion* ➔. **(Right)** *CBCT 3D reformation in the same patient shows patchy destruction of the inferior mandibular cortex.*

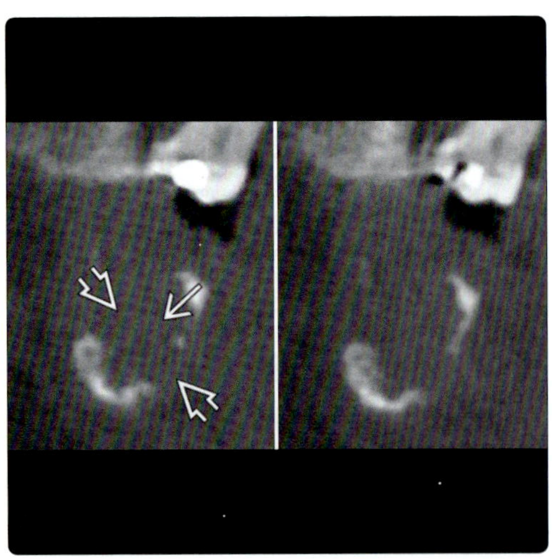
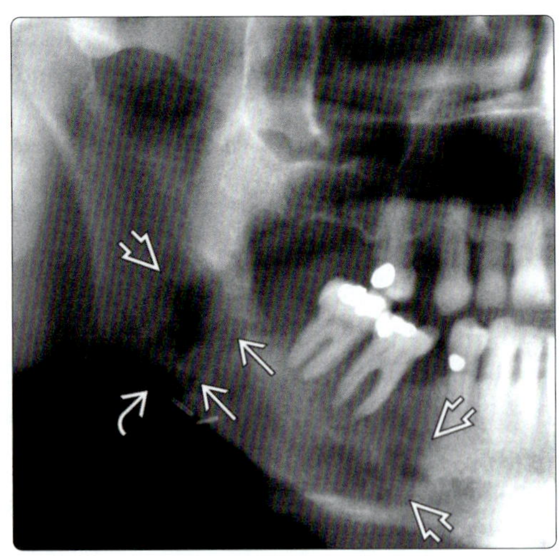

(Left) *Cross section CBCT in the same patient shows metastatic disease in the mandible resulting in loss of trabecular structure* ➔*and destruction of the mandibular cortices* ➔. **(Right)** *Panoramic radiograph shows metastatic disease (unknown primary tumor) in the right ramus and alveolar process of the mandible with a pathologic fracture* ➔. *Note the permeative borders* ➔, *thinning and destruction of the inferior cortex* ➔, *and widening of the periodontal ligament spaces of the molars.*

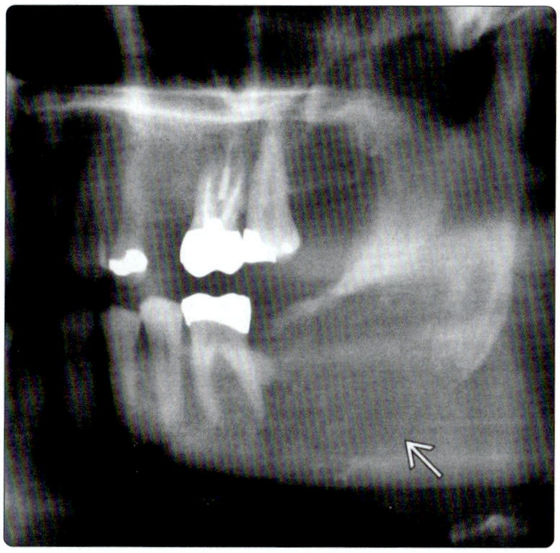

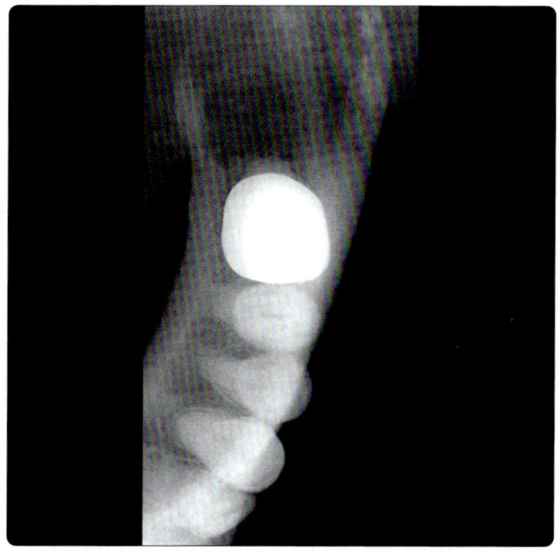

(Left) *Panoramic radiograph shows colon metastases in the left mandible. There is patchy destruction of the inferior mandibular cortex* ➔ *and destruction of the lamina dura of the involved mandibular teeth.* **(Right)** *Occlusal radiograph in the same patient shows patchy bone destruction posterior to the molar and lack of periosteal response.*

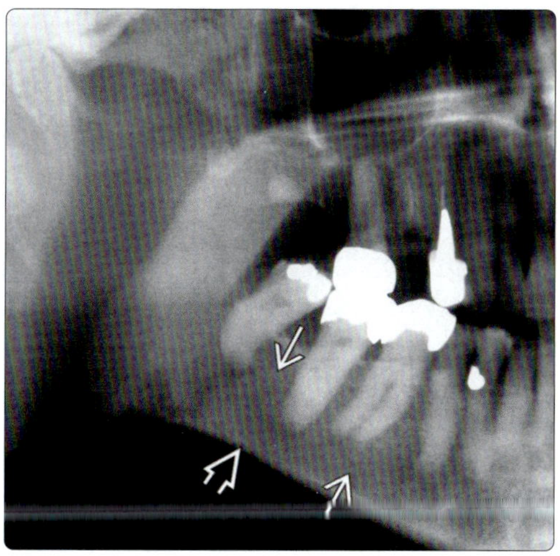

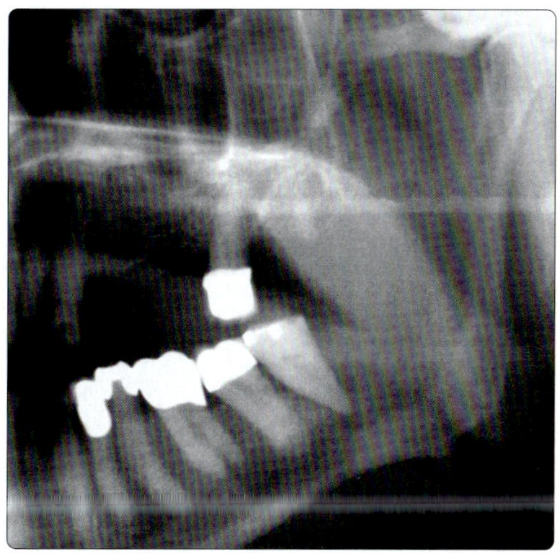

(Left) *Panoramic radiograph shows lung metastases in the right posterior mandible. The right ramus has been destroyed, the lamina dura of the posterior mandibular teeth are missing, and there is loss of normal trabecular architecture* ➔*. Note persistence of inferior cortex* ➔*.* **(Right)** *Panoramic radiograph in the same patient shows involvement of the left ramus, loss of lamina dura, and widening of the periodontal ligament spaces. The destruction of the rami is very symmetrical in this case.*

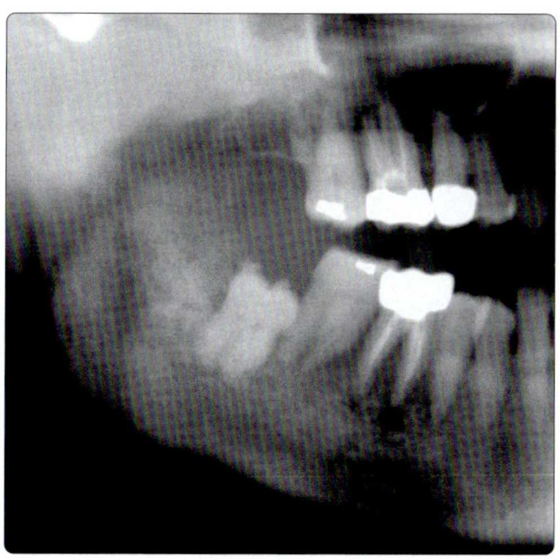

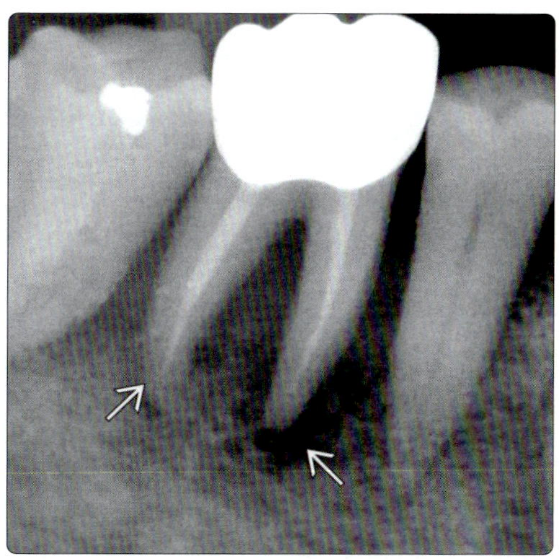

(Left) *Panoramic radiograph shows prostate metastases in the right mandible, including the ramus and coronoid process. There is increased bone density with ill-defined borders.* **(Right)** *Periapical radiograph in the same patient shows sclerotic metastases with patchy bone destruction at the molar tooth roots* ➔*. Note the symmetric widening of the periodontal ligament space of the 1st mandibular molar, which may have been mistaken for inflammatory disease and inappropriately endodontically treated.*

(Left) *Occlusal radiograph in the same patient shows patchy bone destruction, destruction of the normal buccal cortex* ➡*, and widening of the periodontal ligament spaces around the posterior teeth* ➡*.* **(Right)** *Periapical radiograph of the right mandibular cuspid area shows breast metastases to the mandible. The periodontal ligament spaces of the cuspid and incisors are widened* ➡*, and the lamina dura is missing. The trabecular bone pattern is otherwise unremarkable.*

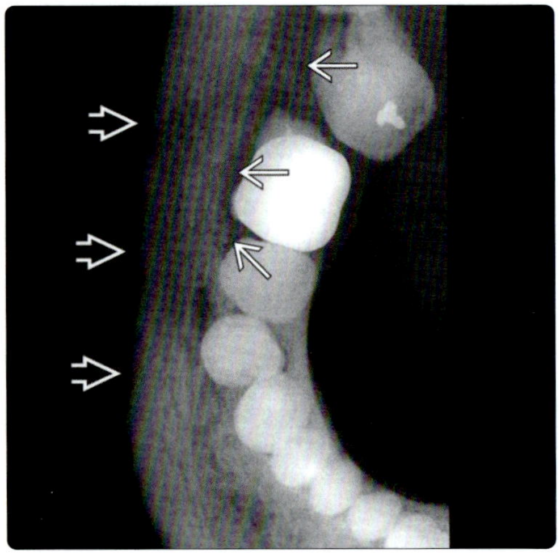

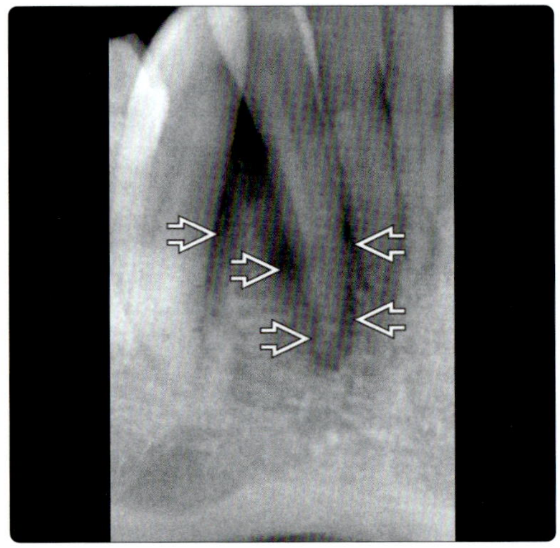

(Left) *Panoramic radiograph shows prostate metastases affecting the entire mandible. There is increased density of trabecular bone with no discernible borders. The lamina dura around the tooth roots are missing and the inferior cortex is no longer distinct.* **(Right)** *Occlusal radiograph in the same patient shows prostate metastases in the mandible. Note the bilateral finely spiculated periosteal reaction ("hair on end")* ➡ *frequently seen with prostate metastases.*

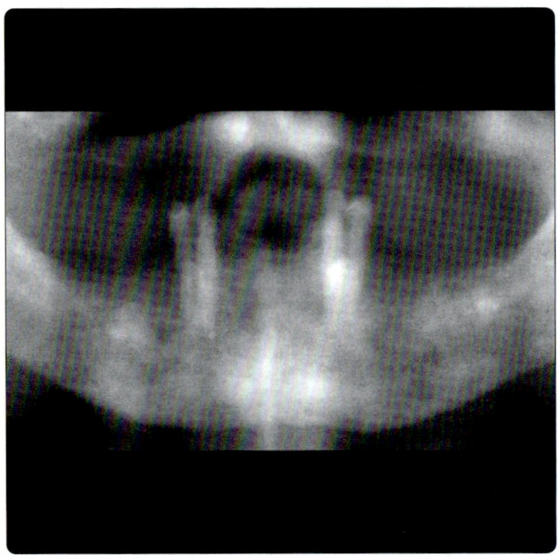

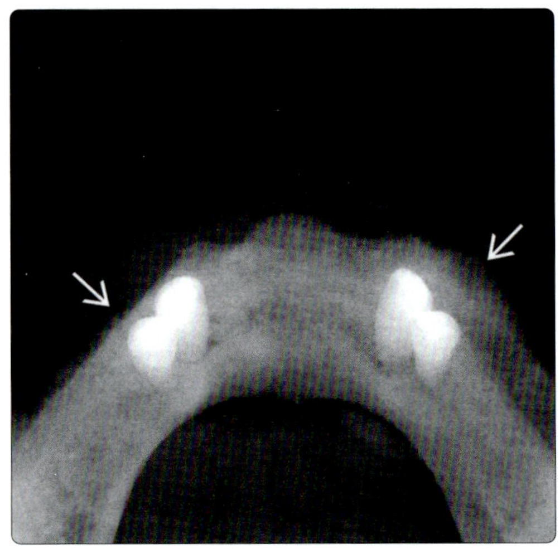

(Left) *Panoramic radiograph shows lung metastases in the right mandibular ramus and alveolus. The trabecular detail is lost, and the lamina dura around the tooth roots are not visible.* **(Right)** *Panoramic radiograph in the same patient shows similar changes in the left posterior mandible and symmetrical involvement of both sides of the mandible. The inferior cortex is unaffected.*

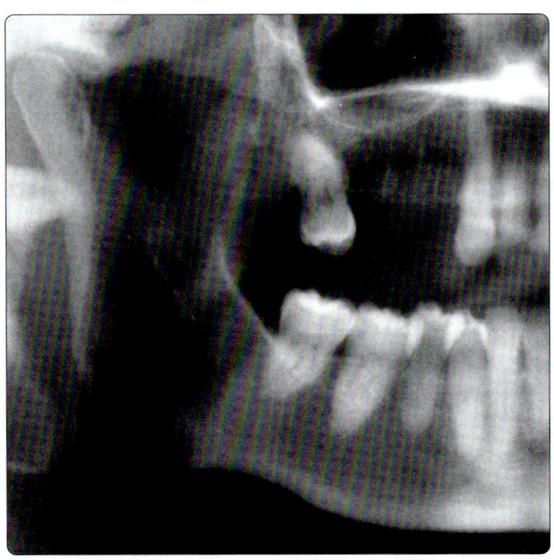

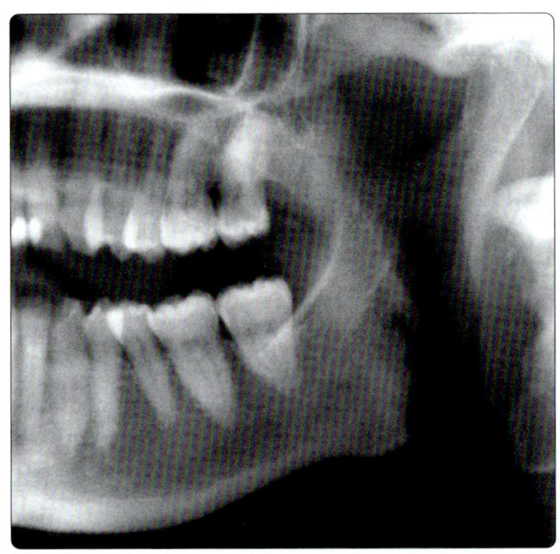

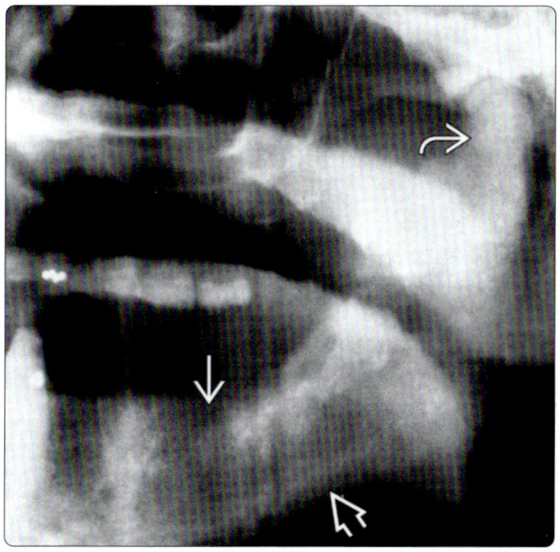

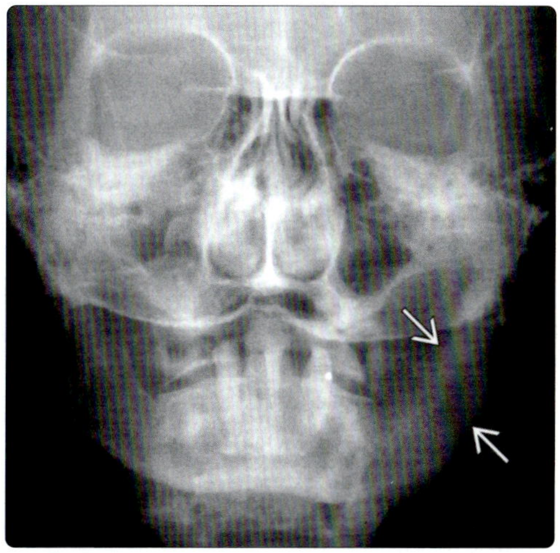

(Left) *Cropped panoramic radiograph shows prostate metastases presenting as a moth-eaten bone pattern in the left mandibular body* ➡ *with sclerotic metastases in the upper ramus and condyle* ➡*. The mandibular cortex is irregular due to a spiculated periosteal response* ➡*, resulting in bony enlargement. (Courtesy E. Lam, DMD.)* **(Right)** *PA radiograph of the skull in the same patient shows loss of normal cortical boundaries in the mandible* ➡ *and accompanying enlargement. (Courtesy E. Lam, DMD.)*

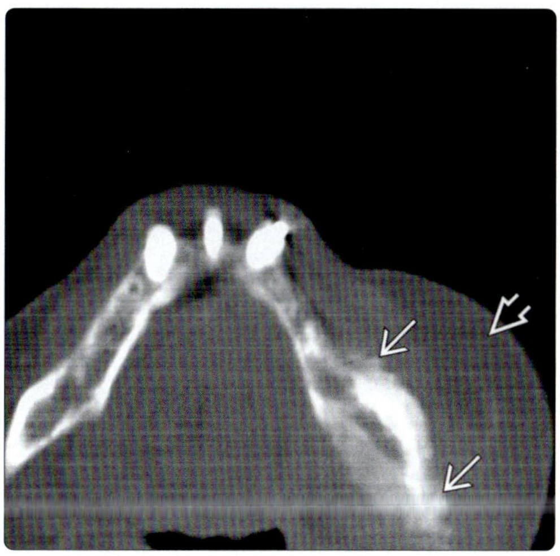

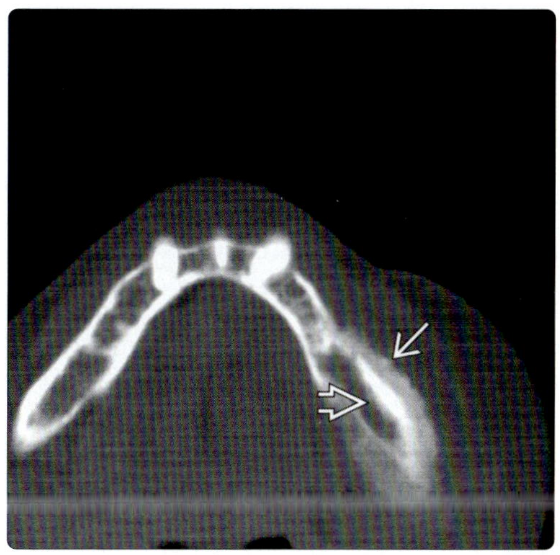

(Left) *Axial bone CT in the same patient shows an exuberant periosteal response, which is spiculated in some areas* ➡*. There is a prominent accompanying soft tissue mass* ➡*. (Courtesy E. Lam, DMD.)* **(Right)** *Axial bone CT in the same patient at a more inferior level shows the spiculated (beard-like) periosteal reaction* ➡ *and a very radiolucent body of the mandible* ➡ *due to bone destruction from the prostate metastases.*

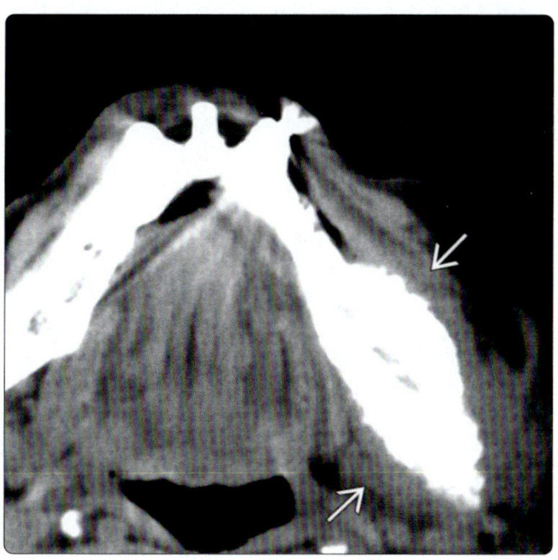

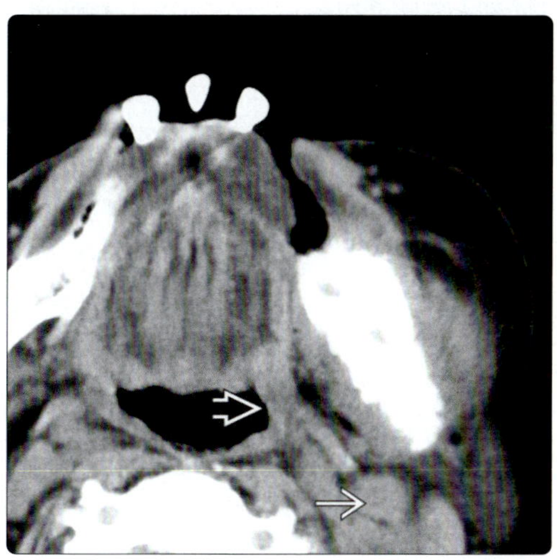

(Left) *Axial soft tissue window NECT in the same patient shows adjacent soft tissue* ➡ *involvement of the prostate metastases. (Courtesy E. Lam, DMD.)* **(Right)** *Axial soft tissue window NECT in the same patient at a lower level shows nodal enlargement* ➡ *and medial displacement of the pharyngeal constrictor muscle* ➡*. (Courtesy E. Lam, DMD.)*

Mandible-Maxilla Osteosarcoma

KEY FACTS

TERMINOLOGY

- Definition: Malignant bone tumor with ability to produce osteoid or immature bone

IMAGING

- Poorly defined **destructive** alveolar mass, ± tumor bone formation, with cortical erosion ± aggressive periosteal reaction
- Periosteal reaction may be **"hair on end"** or **"sunray spicules"** of new bone perpendicular to cortex
- **Symmetric widening of periodontal ligament space** of teeth in absence of dental disease
- Osteolytic: Entirely radiolucent, with nonspecific bone destruction
- Osteoblastic: Lesion is almost entirely radiopaque
- Mixture of osteolytic & osteoblastic
- Can resorb or displace tooth roots

TOP DIFFERENTIAL DIAGNOSES

- Osteomyelitis
- Metastasis
- Chondrosarcoma
- Fibrous dysplasia
- Ewing sarcoma

CLINICAL ISSUES

- Painless **swelling** in maxilla or mandible
- **Loose teeth** or nonhealing extraction site
- **Mean age: 35 years**, M:F = 2:1
- **Osteosarcoma less aggressive in jaws** than in long bones

DIAGNOSTIC CHECKLIST

- Consider infection or metastatic disease if no aggressive periosteal reaction
- Consider XRT-induced sarcoma if patient had radiation years prior

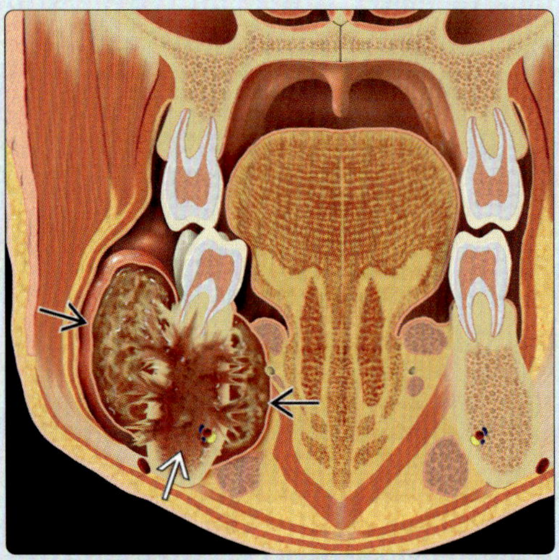

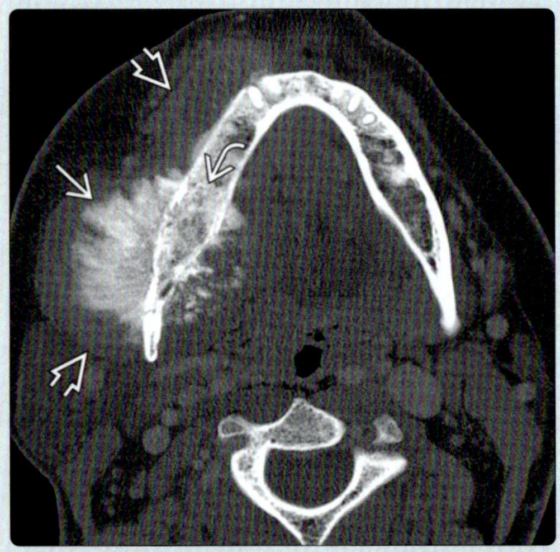

(Left) *Coronal graphic shows right mandible osteosarcoma. Note soft tissue mass perforating through cortex → & intramedullary tumor →.* **(Right)** *Axial bone CT shows a large, dense mass arising from the right mandible →. Mass has both an osteoid matrix & a periosteal reaction. This is the classic periosteal reaction associated with osteosarcomas where periosteum is lifted off perpendicular to bone. Marrow within involved portion of mandible is sclerotic →. Note the associated soft tissue mass →.*

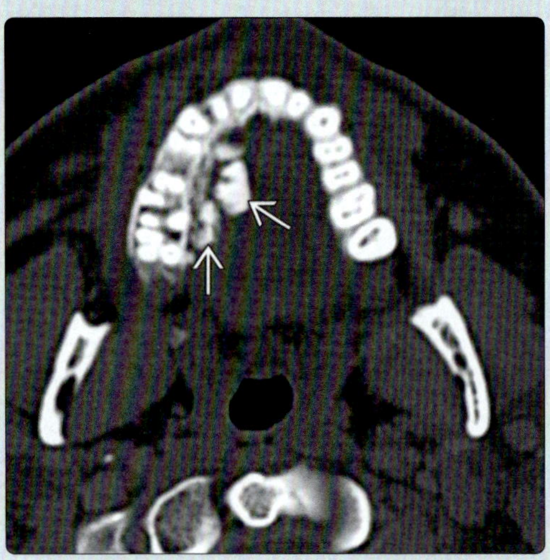

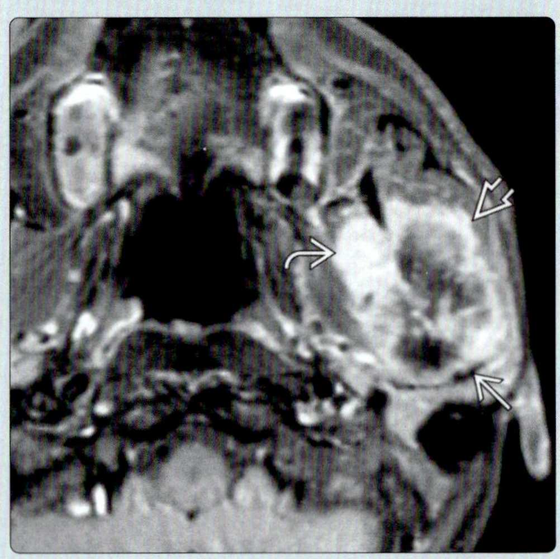

(Left) *Axial bone CT through the maxilla shows an exophytic mass with amorphous immature new bone → & cortical breakthrough. This is the parosteal form of osteosarcoma. Note the absence of significant associated nonossified soft tissue mass.* **(Right)** *Axial T1WI C+ FS MR shows heterogeneous enhancement of the soft tissue component of an osteosarcoma arising in the mandible. Note the tumor has infiltrated the parotid gland →, masseter →, & the pterygoid muscles →.*

TERMINOLOGY

Abbreviations

- Osteosarcoma (OS)

Synonyms

- Osteogenic sarcoma

Definitions

- Malignant bone tumor with ability to produce osteoid or immature bone

IMAGING

General Features

- Best diagnostic clue
  - Bone destruction with aggressive periosteal reaction ± tumor bone formation
- Location
  - Mandible > maxilla
    - Mandible: Angle, ramus, or body
    - Maxilla: Posterior alveolar ridge, maxillary sinus, posterior palate
  - Crosses midline
  - Often invades adjacent soft tissues & anatomic structures
- Size
  - Variable; usually < 10 cm
- Morphology
  - Destructive lesion with osteoid formation
  - Usually poorly defined border, but well-defined, noncorticated borders also seen

Radiographic Findings

- Radiography
  - Poorly defined alveolar mass, ± tumoral calcification, with cortical erosion ± aggressive periosteal reaction
    - Periosteal reaction may be **"hair on end"** or **"sunray spicules"** of new bone perpendicular to cortex
    - Tumor often destroys cortex & invades adjacent soft tissue, producing mass
  - Symmetric **widening of periodontal ligament space** of teeth in absence of dental disease
  - Radiographic variants
    - Osteolytic: Entirely radiolucent, with nonspecific bone destruction
    - Osteoblastic: Lesion is almost entirely radiopaque
    - Mixture of osteolytic & osteoblastic: Most common type
      - Mottled, granular ossification: Resembles fibrous dysplasia or ossifying fibroma
      - Other internal patterns: Cotton wool with distinct margin, patchy radiopacity, diffuse hazy opacification
      - Sunburst appearance: May see bone lamellae arising from focus, around central area of destruction
- Intraoral plain film
  - Symmetrical periodontal ligament space widening around teeth
  - Root resorption can occur but is uncommon
  - Tooth displacement can occur
- Extraoral plain film
  - Panoramic radiograph good to evaluate changes in mandibular canal
    - Irregular widening or narrowing of canal
    - Loss of canal cortical margins

CT Findings

- NECT
  - Soft tissue window may better show spiculated periosteal response & infiltration of adjacent soft tissues
- CECT
  - Moderate enhancement of solid components
- CBCT & bone CT
  - Expansile lesion with increased density, aggressive periosteal reaction, & bone erosion
  - Loss of anatomical cortices of maxillary sinus, nasal fossa, mandibular canal

MR Findings

- Heterogeneous signal intensity on T1 & T2
- Heterogeneous contrast enhancement

Nuclear Medicine Findings

- Bone scan
  - Increased tracer uptake

Imaging Recommendations

- Best imaging tool
  - CT best for demonstrating degree of bone involvement, osseous destruction, osteoid matrix
  - MR best for soft tissue & intramedullary extent, relationship of tumor to soft tissue anatomy

DIFFERENTIAL DIAGNOSIS

Osteomyelitis

- Bony destruction without osteoid formation; may see sequestrum formation
- Lytic bone destruction with exuberant periosteal reaction
  - Periosteal reaction is typically laminar (onion skin) rather than spicules perpendicular to cortex

Metastasis

- Consider metastasis if lesion primarily radiolucent
- Aggressive bony destructive changes
- No periosteal reaction or tumoral calcification
  - May have spiculated periosteal reaction in prostate or breast cancer metastasis

Chondrosarcoma

- Chondrosarcoma (CS) rarer in head & neck than OS
- Consider CS if some internal radiopacity present in tumor

Fibrous Dysplasia

- **Fibrous dysplasia narrows periodontal ligament space**; OS widens it
- Expansion more regular with fibrous dysplasia & no periosteal reaction

Ewing Sarcoma

- Irregular destructive lytic mass in mandible
- Does not produce osteoid matrix
- May have periosteal reaction: Sunburst or, less commonly, laminar

PATHOLOGY

General Features

- Etiology
  - Primary etiology unknown in most cases
    - Genetic mutation or viruses suggested
  - **May occur following radiation to face** (10% of cases)
    - Typically > 10 years after XRT
- Associated abnormalities
  - May be associated with Paget disease, fibrous dysplasia, giant cell tumor, osteochondroma, enchondroma, Ollier disease

Staging, Grading, & Classification

- Staging based on degree of differentiation, local vs. distant spread, & whether tumor has metastasized
- Grading (low, intermediate, high) based on degree of cellular atypia & histologic architecture
- Classification based on histology: Osteoblastic, chondroblastic, fibroblastic, telangiectatic, & juxtacortical types
- Classification based on location: Parosteal, periosteal, intracortical, medullary, extraskeletal
  - Parosteal type is less aggressive with less prominent bone invasion
  - Periosteal type very rare in jaws

Gross Pathologic & Surgical Features

- Heterogeneous mass with ossified & nonossified components
- Periosteal reaction: Spicules of new bone at lesion periphery

Microscopic Features

- Highly pleomorphic, spindle-shaped tumor cells producing different forms of osteoid

CLINICAL ISSUES

Presentation

- Most common signs/symptoms
  - Painless swelling in maxilla or mandible
- Other signs/symptoms
  - Presenting symptoms often nonspecific
  - Rapid **swelling**, submucosal mass
  - **Numbness** or altered sensation
  - **Loose teeth** or nonhealing extraction site
  - Erythema of overlying mucosa, ulceration
  - Nasal obstruction, epistaxis, exophthalmos
  - Trismus
- Clinical profile
  - 35-year-old man with painless rapidly enlarging jaw mass

Demographics

- Age
  - **Mean: 35 years old**
    - Wide age range: 4-84 years; peak in 4th decade
    - Occurs on average 10 years later than OS of long bones
- Gender
  - M:F = 2:1
    - Some studies found female predominance
- Epidemiology
  - OS is most common primary malignancy of bone = 1:100,000
    - Jaw lesions: < 10% of all osteosarcomas

Natural History & Prognosis

- **OS of jaws less aggressive** than OS of long bones
  - Jaw OS present in slightly older age group
  - Lower incidence of metastases than OS of other bones
  - Regional metastases in 10-15% of jaw cases
  - Distant metastases rare in absence of regional metastases
    - Distant metastases most common in lung, liver, & bone
- Prognosis depends on multiple factors
  - Pathologic type, size, location, presence of metastases
  - Poorer prognosis for maxillary lesions due to difficulty in obtaining adequate surgical margins
  - Prognosis better if no paresthesia, smaller tumor size, clear surgical margins, more differentiated histological grade of tumor, younger age
  - Radiographic appearance & histological type not related to survival
- **5-year survival: 40%**
  - Better survival in patient with less extensive disease
  - Mandibular lesions have better survival than maxillary
    - Maxillary sinus tumors have worst prognosis: Death from extension to skull

Treatment

- Complete resection with wide margins affords best chance of survival
- Radiation & chemotherapy usually used for controlling metastatic spread or for palliation

DIAGNOSTIC CHECKLIST

Consider

- Infection or metastatic disease if no aggressive periosteal reaction
- Consider XRT-induced sarcoma if patient had radiation years prior

Image Interpretation Pearls

- Presence of destructive, unicentric lesion with poorly-defined margins & predominantly lytic, sclerotic, or mixed bone pattern raises suspicion of OS
- Aggressive periosteal reaction suggests OS

SELECTED REFERENCES

1. Puranik SR et al: Parosteal osteosarcoma: report of a rare juxtacortical variant of osteosarcoma affecting the maxilla. J Oral Maxillofac Pathol. 18(3):432-6, 2014
2. Yildiz FR et al: Gnathic osteosarcomas, experience of four institutions from Turkey. Int J Clin Exp Pathol. 7(6):2800-8, 2014
3. van den Berg H et al: Osteosarcoma: a comparison of jaw versus nonjaw localizations and review of the literature. Sarcoma. 2013:316123, 2013
4. Kämmerer PW et al: Clinical, therapeutic and prognostic features of osteosarcoma of the jaws - experience of 36 cases. J Craniomaxillofac Surg. 40(6):541-8, 2012
5. Wang S et al: Osteosarcoma of the jaws: demographic and CT imaging features. Dentomaxillofac Radiol. 41(1):37-42, 2012

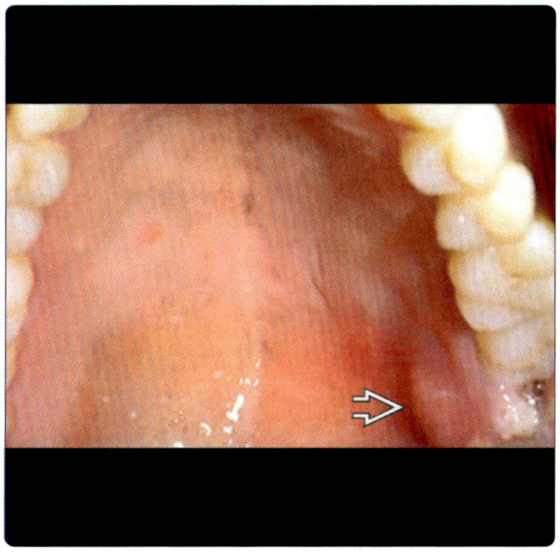

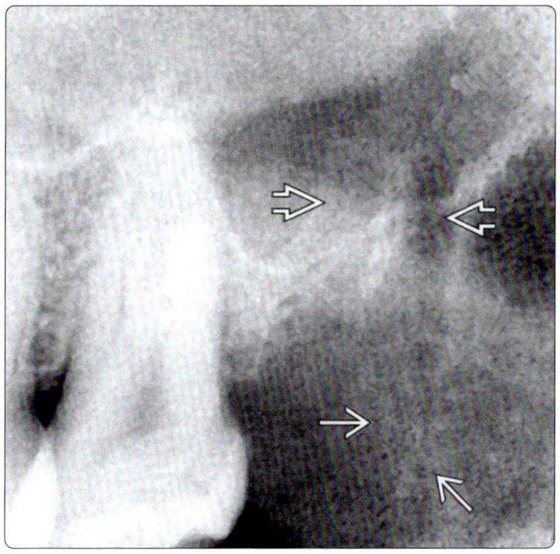

(Left) *Occlusal photograph of the maxilla shows a palatal swelling in the left 3rd molar area. The 3rd molar was removed, but the socket did not heal.* **(Right)** *Periapical radiograph of the same patient shows the maxillary left 3rd molar tooth socket & a soft tissue mass containing multiple foci of bone extending occlusally from the socket. Biopsy diagnosis was osteosarcoma.*

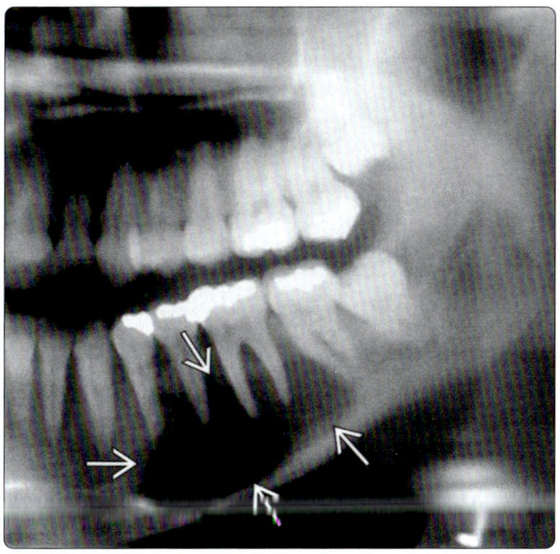

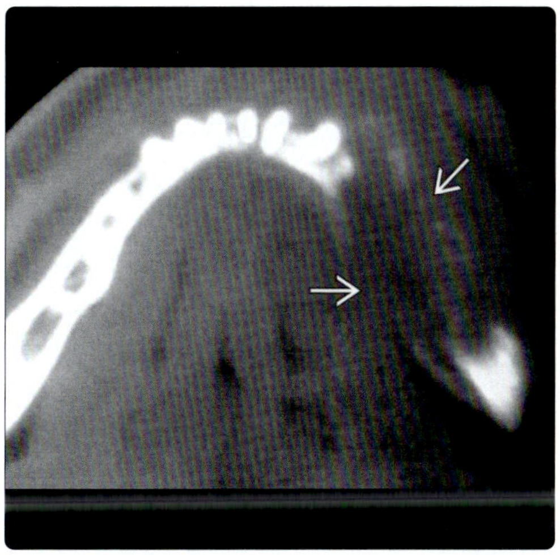

(Left) *Panoramic radiograph shows the lytic type of osteosarcoma in the left mandible. The lesion is well defined, & the internal aspect is radiolucent, resembling a large cyst. However, there is widening of the periodontal ligament spaces around the teeth, which suggests malignancy.* **(Right)** *Axial bone CT in the same patient shows destruction of the mandibular cortices. Compare the well-defined margins in the panoramic image with destructive margins seen in CT.*

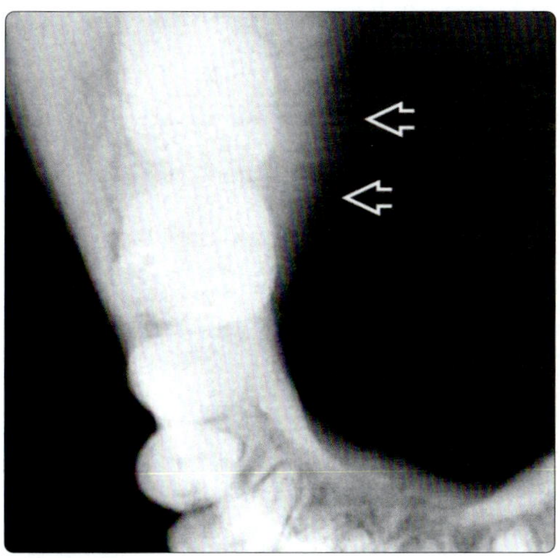

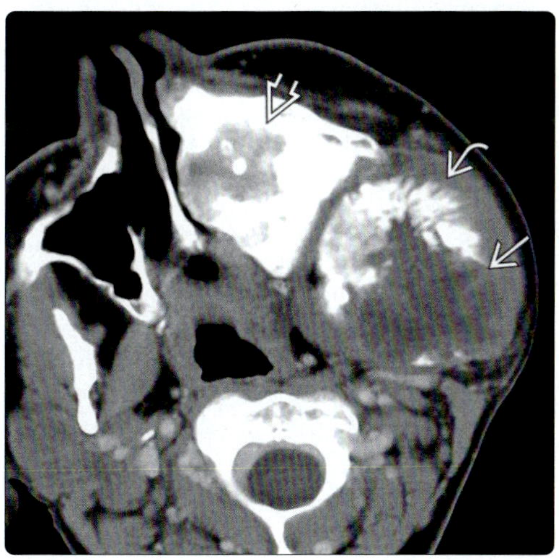

(Left) *Occlusal radiograph of the right mandible shows a finely spiculated periosteal reaction on the lingual aspect. This is a common feature of osteosarcoma but may also be seen in other malignancies.* **(Right)** *Axial CECT shows a new osteosarcoma in the mandible of a patient treated for fibrous dysplasia of the maxilla & mandible. Note the expansile destructive mass with classic periosteal reaction in contrast to the diffusely thickened bone in the maxilla, representing fibrous dysplasia.*

Mandible-Maxilla Chondrosarcoma

KEY FACTS

TERMINOLOGY

- Chondrosarcoma (CS): Malignant tumor arising from cartilage cells

IMAGING

- Irregularly shaped, permeative radiolucency with randomly scattered, patchy, radiopaque foci
- May be well defined and corticated or permeative
- If periosteal involvement, calcification perpendicular to bone surface: **Sunray or sunburst spicules**
- Appearance varies due to presence or absence of tumor calcification
- Internal calcifications may be cloud-like with **calcified whorls and arcs**
- Often **radiolucent center** in each radiopacity
- Maxilla = mandible but some reports maxilla > mandible
    - Maxilla: Anterior, nasal septum, paranasal sinuses
    - Mandible: Molar/ramus area, symphysis, condylar head and neck, coronoid process

TOP DIFFERENTIAL DIAGNOSES

- Osteosarcoma
    - Radiopacities do not have radiolucent centers
- Fibrous dysplasia
- Metastatic tumor

PATHOLOGY

- Histologic grade: Ranging from low to high (1, 2, 3)

CLINICAL ISSUES

- Painless, enlarging, firm mass
- Peak age is 3rd-6th decade

DIAGNOSTIC CHECKLIST

- Difficult to differentiate between benign and low-grade malignant chondrogenic tumors so **diagnosis often based on imaging findings**
- Permeative borders with infiltration of cortical or trabecular bone favors diagnosis of CS

(Left) *Periapical radiograph of the maxillary midline shows a chondrosarcoma that has caused characteristic malignant changes associated with the teeth. The periodontal ligament space is symmetrically widened around the incisor roots ➡. There is also destruction of the interdental bone between the left central and lateral incisor ⇨.* **(Right)** *Lateral radiograph of the anterior maxilla in the same patient shows irregular bony expansion ➡ without a corticated border and internal radiopacities of the lesion over the root of a maxillary incisor.*

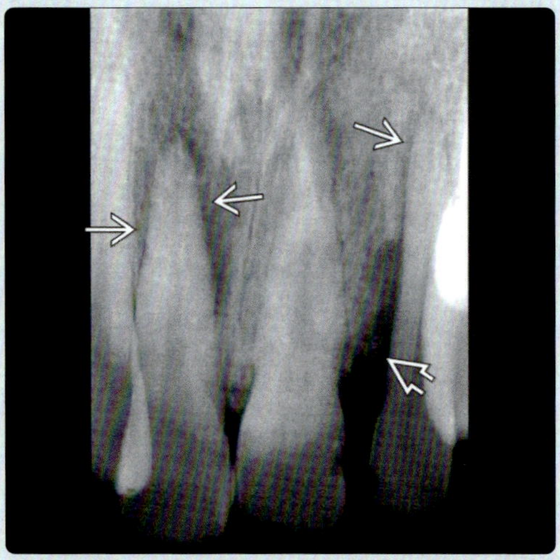

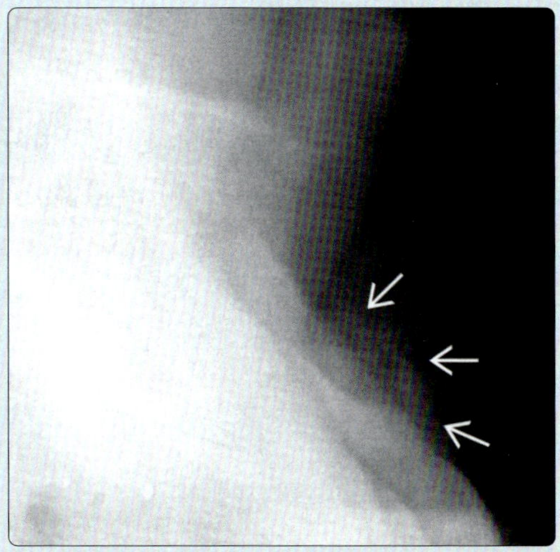

(Left) *Axial CBCT in a 48-year-old woman shows a chondrosarcoma presenting as a diffuse radiolucency in the anterior maxilla. The margins are poorly defined and the buccal cortex is lost ➡.* **(Right)** *Sagittal CBCT in the same patient shows loss of the floor of the nasal cavity with soft tissue extension ➡. The buccal cortex is lost ⇨ and the palatal cortex is thinned and irregular ↪. Buccal soft tissue swelling was reported clinically. The anterior maxilla is a common location for chondrosarcoma.*

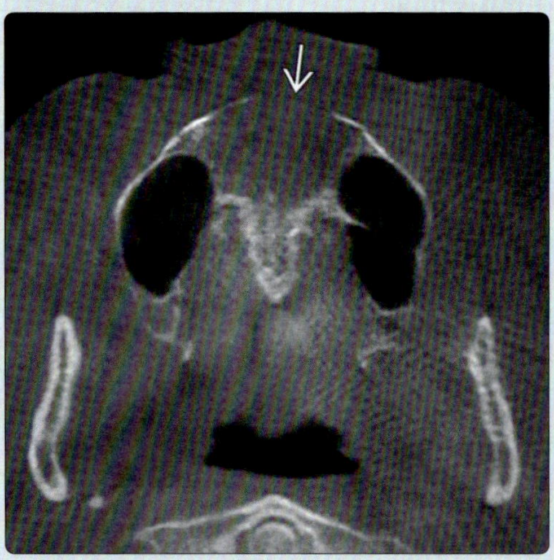

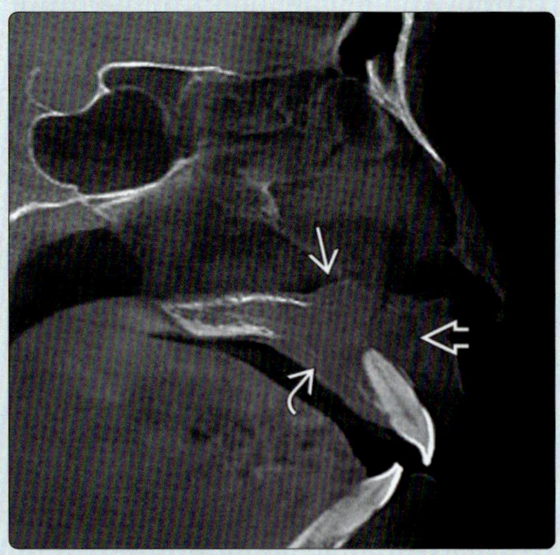

TERMINOLOGY

Abbreviations

- Chondrosarcoma (CS)

Synonyms

- Chondrogenic sarcoma

Definitions

- Malignant tumor arising from cartilage cells
- Can occur centrally in bone, on periphery of bone (parosteal CS), or in soft tissue
- Accounts for 11% of all primary malignant tumors, 2nd most common sarcoma after osteogenic sarcoma

IMAGING

General Features

- Best diagnostic clue
  - Irregularly shaped, permeative radiolucency with randomly scattered, patchy, radiopaque foci
- Location
  - More common in long bones, pelvis, and ribs
    - Only 1-2% occur in H&N region
  - Maxilla (Max) = mandible (Mand) but some reports Max > Mand
    - Max: Usually in anterior region, nasal septum, or paranasal sinuses
    - Mand: Molar/ramus area, symphysis, condylar head and neck, coronoid process
- Size
  - Variable, usually > 2 cm
- Morphology
  - Irregularly shaped borders
  - May be well defined and corticated or permeative
  - If periosteal involvement, calcification perpendicular to bone surface (sunray spicules)
  - May be lobulated

Radiographic Findings

- Radiography
  - Appearance varies due to presence or absence of tumor calcification
  - Some lesions entirely radiolucent, especially in mandible
    - Radiolucent area may have granular pattern
  - Internal calcifications may be **cloud-like with calcified whorls and arcs**
    - Often radiolucent center in each radiopacity
  - TMJ involvement: Enlarged condyle
    - Articular fossa may also enlarge if condylar lesion slow growing
- Intraoral plain film
  - Symmetrically **widened periodontal ligament** (PDL) space around involved teeth
  - Can displace teeth
  - Can resorb roots

CT Findings

- CBCT
  - CBCT and CT give better detail of cortical involvement
    - CT especially useful if trying to differentiate benign from low-grade malignant chondrogenic lesion
  - Mass with ill-defined borders and long zone of transition
  - May see new periosteal bone perpendicular to cortex: **Sunray** or **sunburst** periosteal reaction
  - Often cortical disruption
    - Slow-growing CS may expand rather than destroy cortices
  - May see endosteal scalloping
  - Soft tissue mass

MR Findings

- T1WI
  - **Low to intermediate** signal intensity relative to gray matter
    - Low-signal foci within tumor may suggest tumor calcifications
- T2WI
  - **High** T2 signal
  - Hypointense foci (calcifications) less conspicuous than on CT
- T1WI C+
  - Heterogeneously enhancing mass
    - Whorls of enhancing lines within tumor matrix often seen
    - Extent of enhancement depends on tumor grade
      - Greater enhancement in high-grade CS

Imaging Recommendations

- Best imaging tool
  - Bone CT or CBCT to characterize tumor matrix, cortical/periosteal involvement, & extent of tumor
  - MR to analyze bone marrow extension & involvement of adjacent soft tissue
- Protocol advice
  - When using CECT, view bone windows
    - Bone CT most likely to show characteristic calcifications
- CT or MR to determine nodal stage of H&N tumors

Nuclear Medicine Findings

- Bone scan
  - Increased uptake in central CS
  - Reveals metabolically active areas in peripheral CS
  - Whole-body scans
    - Identify metastases
    - No uptake: Rules out malignant transformation of osteochondroma

DIFFERENTIAL DIAGNOSIS

Osteosarcoma

- Primary malignancy of bone
- May not be able to distinguish from CS
- Radiopacities in osteosarcoma **do not have radiolucent centers**
- May have similar periosteal reactions

Fibrous Dysplasia

- Replacement of normal bone with fibrous tissue
- Granular bone pattern may resemble radiolucent CS
- Loss of lamina dura and **expansion**
- No soft tissue mass

- CS only in 1 bone; history and clinical findings different from polyostotic fibrous dysplasia
- Young females

Metastatic Tumor

- Bone CT: Destructive mass, often in mandible
- MR: Multiple enhancing, invasive lesions
- Usually known primary tumor

PATHOLOGY

General Features

- CS formed from cartilage in tissues not normally harboring cartilage or form in cartilage cap of exostosis or enchondroma
- Most cases sporadic (primary): 75% of cases
- Predisposing conditions (secondary)
  - Osteochondroma
  - Enchondroma
  - Ollier disease
  - Maffucci syndrome

Staging, Grading, & Classification

- Osseous vs. extraosseous
- Central (medullary) vs. peripheral (juxtacortical)
- Primary vs. secondary
- Histological subtype
  - Conventional
  - Clear cell
  - Dedifferentiated
  - Myxoid
  - Mesenchymal
- Histologic grade: Ranging from low to high (1, 2, 3)
  - Based on degree of cellularity, pleomorphism, mitoses, multinucleated cells, & necrosis

Gross Pathologic & Surgical Features

- Firm, bluish-white, pearly translucency with faceting or lobulation
- White or yellowish gritty speckling corresponding to calcified or ossified parts of tumor

Microscopic Features

- Hypercellular tumor composed of chondrocytes with hyperchromatic, pleomorphic nuclei, and prominent nucleoli
- Hyaline matrix may calcify in "**ringlets**"
- Intercellular matrix solid in hyaline type vs. mucinous/gelatinous matrix in myxoid or mixed types
- Histology may overlap with or be **confused with benign chondroid tumors**

CLINICAL ISSUES

Presentation

- Most common signs/symptoms
  - Painless, enlarging, firm mass
- Other signs/symptoms
  - Loose teeth
  - Altered sensation
  - Nasal obstruction
  - Epistaxis
  - Proptosis
  - Visual disturbances
  - Headache
  - If involves TMJ: Trismus or signs of TMJ dysfunction

Demographics

- Age
  - Most common in adults
    - Can occur at any age (mean: 47 years; range: 17 months to 75 years)
    - Mesenchymal CS occurs in younger age group (2nd to 3rd decade) and is more common in females
  - Peak age is 3rd-6th decade
  - Appears later and is less common than OS
- Gender
  - M = F
- Epidemiology
  - 2nd most common malignancy of bone (after osteosarcoma, excluding multiple myeloma)
  - CS: 15% of malignant bone tumors

Natural History & Prognosis

- Prognosis depends on adequacy of primary resection, tumor location & extent, and histological grade of neoplasm
  - Prognosis better than osteosarcoma
- High incidence of local recurrence
- Late recurrence can occur > 2 decades later
- Some tumors are slow growing
- Overall prognosis depends on tumor grade, size at presentation

Treatment

- Wide surgical excision since locally aggressive
- Role of radiation, chemotherapy, cryosurgery, and immunotherapy are controversial and evolving

DIAGNOSTIC CHECKLIST

Consider

- Difficult to differentiate between benign and low-grade malignant chondrogenic tumors, so **diagnosis often based on imaging findings**
  - Permeative borders with infiltration of cortical or trabecular bone favors diagnosis of CS
  - CS may have associated soft tissue extension
- Change in clinical symptoms in patient with known osteochondroma should raise suspicion of secondary CS

Image Interpretation Pearls

- Arc and whorl-like **radiopacities with radiolucent centers** favors CS

SELECTED REFERENCES

1. Chen Y et al: Myxoid chondrosarcoma of the mandible in a 22-year-old man: A case report. Mol Clin Oncol. 5(3):237-240, 2016
2. Coca-Pelaz A et al: Chondrosarcomas of the head and neck. Eur Arch Otorhinolaryngol. 271(10):2601-9, 2014
3. Pontes HA et al: Clinicopathological analysis of head and neck chondrosarcoma: three case reports and literature review. Int J Oral Maxillofac Surg. 41(2):203-10, 2012
4. Mohammadinezhad C: Chondrosarcoma of the jaw. J Craniofac Surg. 20(6):2097-100, 2009

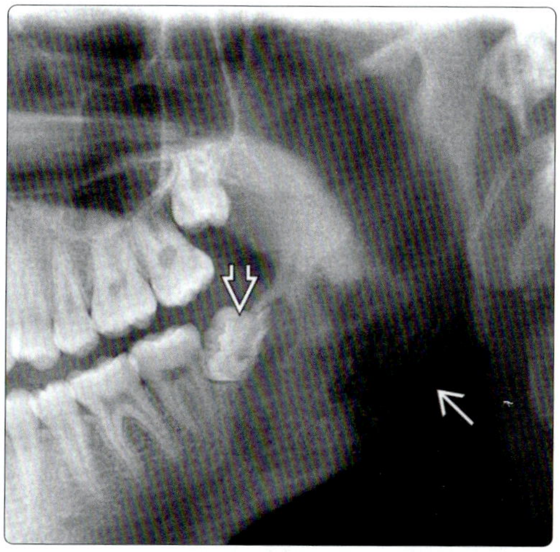
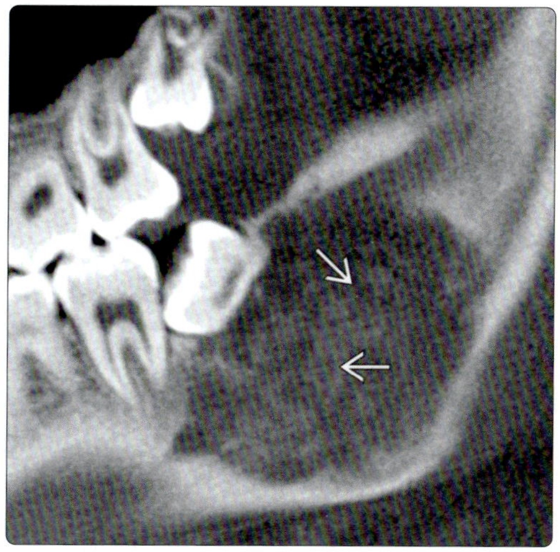

(Left) *Cropped panoramic radiograph of the left side shows a well-defined chondrosarcoma in the posterior mandible ➡. The lesion has displaced and rotated the developing 3rd molar ➡ mesially and occupies a large portion of the angle and ramus of the mandible.* **(Right)** *Panoramic reformat of a CBCT scan in the same patient shows arcs and whorls of calcification with radiolucent centers ➡. This characteristic helps to differentiate from osteosarcoma, which may appear similarly.*

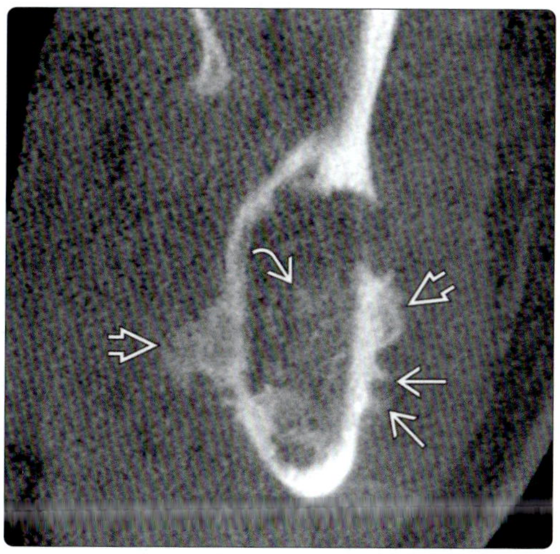
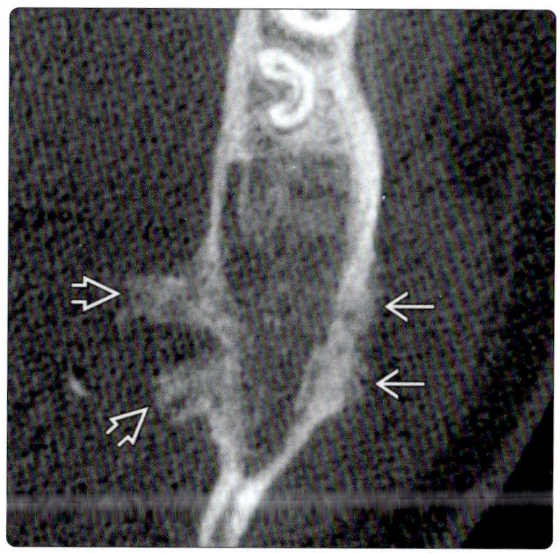

(Left) *Cross section CBCT in the same patient shows periosteal new bone perpendicular to the cortices (sunray spicules) ➡ and larger masses of periosteal new bone on the buccal and lingual surfaces ➡. There are faint internal calcifications of the tumor ➡.* **(Right)** *Axial CBCT in the same patient illustrates periosteal new bone formation perpendicular to the buccal ➡ and lingual ➡ cortices, more exuberant on the lingual aspect.*

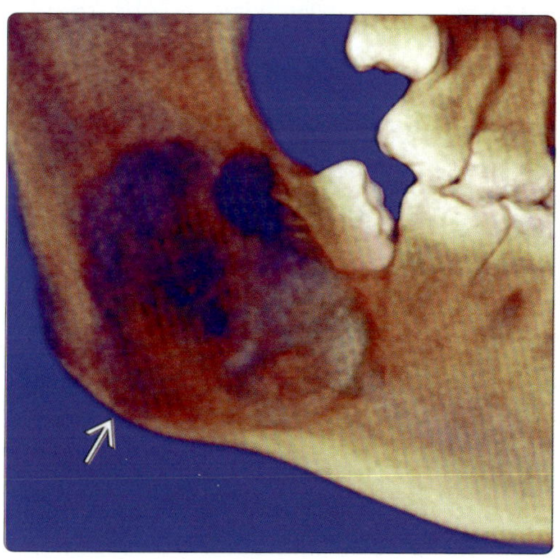
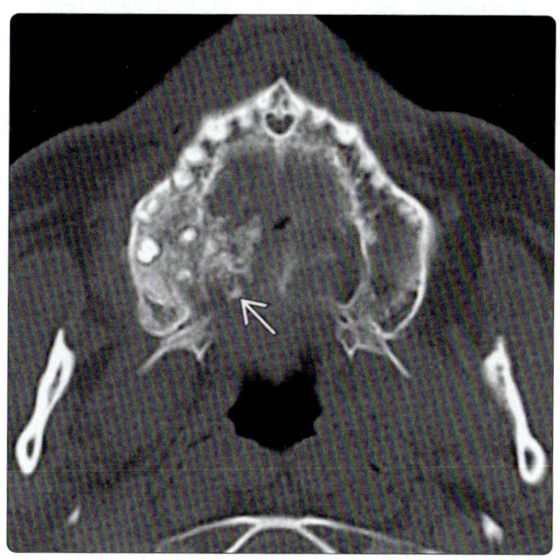

(Left) *Sagittal 3D reformation viewed from the lingual aspect in the same patient shows the degree of expansion at the inferior cortex ➡ and the lobulated nature of the lesion.* **(Right)** *Axial NECT shows a low-grade chondrosarcoma of the maxilla. There is a radiopaque mass ➡ arising from the alveolar portion of the right maxilla. This mass has irregular, almost shaggy margins, which favors a malignant lesion. The internal aspect has stippled mineralization.*

Primary Intraosseous Squamous Cell Carcinoma

KEY FACTS

TERMINOLOGY

- Primary intraosseous squamous cell carcinoma: Rare malignancy arising from odontogenic epithelium residues in bone
  - Does not include osseous spread from soft tissue carcinoma (gingiva, alveolar ridge, floor of mouth)

IMAGING

- **Mandible** > maxilla
- **Posterior** regions most common
  - In tooth-bearing parts of jaw
- **Usually ill-defined** borders but may be well defined **without cortication**
- **Radiolucent** with moth-eaten appearance
- Destroys anatomic cortices
- **Teeth "floating in space"** appearance; root resorption unusual
- Small lesions may resemble cyst
- Multilocular lesions reported

TOP DIFFERENTIAL DIAGNOSES

- Metastatic lesion
- Odontogenic cyst or tumor
- Central mucoepidermoid carcinoma

CLINICAL ISSUES

- **Early** cases **asymptomatic** so often diagnosed late
- **Swelling** and **pain**
- **Paresthesia** of lower lip or face, toothache, loose teeth, trismus, lymphadenopathy
- **4th-8th decade** (mean age: 45 years)
- M:F = 2:1
- Tx: Wide resection; high recurrence rate and metastasis

DIAGNOSTIC CHECKLIST

- **Can resemble benign odontogenic cysts or tumors** or have classical malignant appearance
- Malignant transformation of odontogenic cyst should be considered when cyst margins become diffuse and irregular

(Left) *Axial CBCT shows primary intraosseous squamous cell carcinoma (PIOSCC) with moth-eaten destruction of the buccal and lingual cortices ➡ and extension of bone destruction to the mesial root of the 1st molar ➡.* **(Right)** *Cross-section CBCT in the same patient shows patchy destruction of the buccal and lingual cortices ➡ and widening of the periodontal ligament space around the distal root of the 2nd molar ➡. The mandibular canal is evident ➡.*

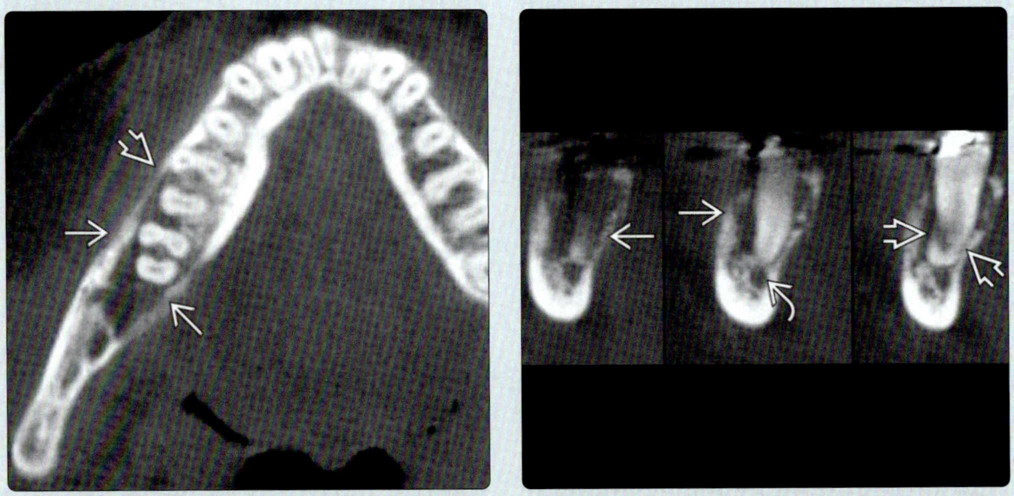

(Left) *Axial CBCT shows a nonkeratinizing PIOSCC presenting as an ill-defined, low-density lesion in the anterior maxilla. Note loss of buccal ➡ and palatal ➡ cortices with soft tissue extension palatally ➡. Differential includes chondrosarcoma.* **(Right)** *Axial bone CT shows PIOSCC in the left maxilla ➡. The borders are infiltrative and a large portion of the posterior alveolus is destroyed. There is a soft tissue mass ➡. This appearance suggests malignancy but not a definitive diagnosis of PIOSCC.*

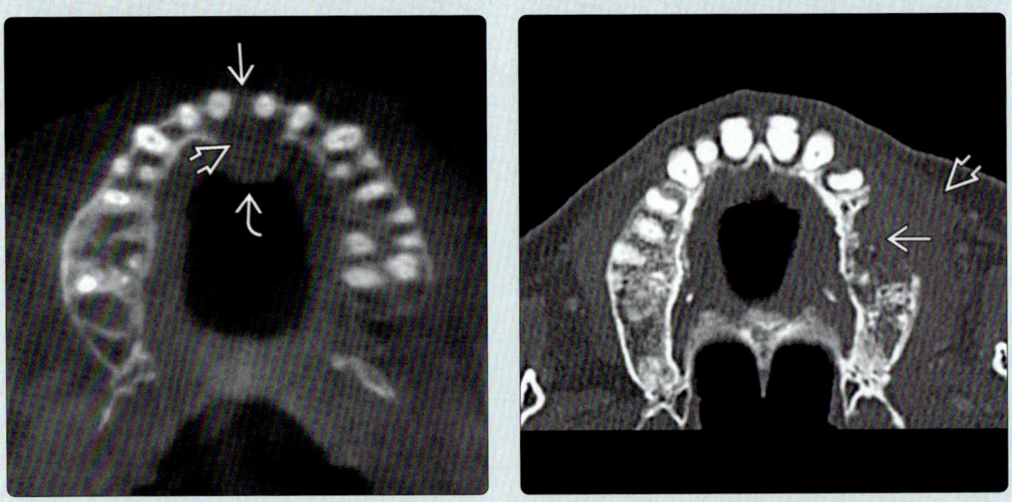

TERMINOLOGY

Abbreviations

- Primary intraosseous squamous cell carcinoma (PIOSCC)

Synonyms

- Central squamous cell carcinoma, primary intraosseous carcinoma, odontogenic squamous cell carcinoma, primary intraalveolar carcinoma, primary odontogenic carcinoma

Definitions

- Rare malignancy arising from odontogenic epithelium residues in bone
  - Arises **de novo** from intraosseous remnants of odontogenic epithelium: Rests of Malassez, remnants of dental lamina, or reduced enamel epithelium surrounding unerupted/impacted tooth
  - Covered by normal mucosa; no cystic component or other odontogenic tumor cells; absence of primary tumor elsewhere (not metastatic)
  - Does not include osseous spread from soft tissue carcinoma (gingiva, alveolar ridge, floor of mouth)

IMAGING

General Features

- Location
  - **Mandible** > maxilla
  - **Posterior** regions most common, in tooth-bearing parts of jaw
- Morphology
  - Irregular or round lesion ± soft tissue mass

Radiographic Findings

- Radiography
  - **Usually ill-defined** borders but may be well defined **without cortication**
    - Small lesions may resemble cyst
  - **Radiolucent** with moth-eaten appearance
    - May contain residual bone
    - Multilocular lesions reported

CT Findings

- Bone CT
  - Destroys anatomic cortices
  - **Teeth"floating in space"** appearance; root resorption unusual

MR Findings

- Signal intensity varies due to polymorphic features of lesions

Imaging Recommendations

- Best imaging tool
  - Bone CT or CBCT to view extent of lesion

DIFFERENTIAL DIAGNOSIS

Metastatic Lesion

- May be unable to differentiate PIOSCC and metastases until rule out primary tumor elsewhere

Odontogenic Cyst or Tumor

- PIOSCC may have well-defined borders and resemble benign cyst or tumor

Central Mucoepidermoid Carcinoma

- Indistinguishable from PIOSCC; need biopsy

PATHOLOGY

Microscopic Features

- Features of squamous cell carcinoma that may or may not be keratinizing
  - Degree of differentiation varies

CLINICAL ISSUES

Presentation

- Most common signs/symptoms
  - **Swelling** and **pain**
- Other signs/symptoms
  - **Paresthesia** of lower lip or face, toothache, loose teeth, trismus, lymphadenopathy

Demographics

- Age
  - **4th-8th decade** (mean: 45 years)
- Gender
  - M:F = 2:1
- Epidemiology
  - Alcohol, tobacco, or betel-quid abuse not usually present in PIOC cases
  - Most common risk factor: Reactive inflammatory stimulus ± predisposing genetic cofactor

Natural History & Prognosis

- **Early** cases **asymptomatic** so often diagnosed late
- Pathologic **fracture** secondary to large lesions
- Prognosis usually poor but better with adequate resection, early diagnosis, and for lesions arising in cysts
- Frequent regional lymph node metastasis, **high recurrence** rate
- 5-year survival: 30-40%

Treatment

- Wide resection
- Radiation and chemotherapy for lesions not completely removed at surgery

DIAGNOSTIC CHECKLIST

Consider

- **Can resemble benign odontogenic cysts or tumors** or have nonspecific malignant appearance
- Malignant transformation of odontogenic cyst should be considered when cyst margins become diffuse and irregular

SELECTED REFERENCES

1. Geetha P et al: Primary intraosseous carcinoma of the mandible: a clinicoradiographic view. J Cancer Res Ther. 11(3):651, 2015
2. Tamgadge S et al: Primary intraosseous squamous cell carcinoma arising from an odontogenic keratocyst: a case report and literature review. Ecancermedicalscience. 7:316, 2013

Central Mucoepidermoid Carcinoma

KEY FACTS

TERMINOLOGY

- Central mucoepidermoid carcinoma (CMC): Uncommon malignant epithelial tumor arising in bone, originating from odontogenic epithelium or from metaplasia of odontogenic cyst lining; most commonly dentigerous cyst

IMAGING

- Mandible > maxilla: Most common in **molar/premolar** regions, superior to mandibular canal
- Most often **resembles benign tumor or cyst**
  - Uni- or multilocular expansile radiolucency
  - May have **soap bubble** appearance, especially anterior mandible
- Regular or undulating/scalloped border
- Common appearance: Impacted **mandibular molar** with associated **cystic** lesion accompanied by **swelling** and **paresthesia**
- Less commonly has malignant characteristics: Infiltrative margins, soft tissue extension
  - More likely in longstanding cases

TOP DIFFERENTIAL DIAGNOSES

- Dentigerous cyst
- Ameloblastoma
- Glandular odontogenic cyst

CLINICAL ISSUES

- **Painless swelling**, often of long duration
- Most **4th-5th** decade; also reported in **teenagers and children**
- Locally invasive but sometimes metastasizes to regional lymph nodes

DIAGNOSTIC CHECKLIST

- Consider: CMC may be **indistinguishable** from **benign tumor or cyst**

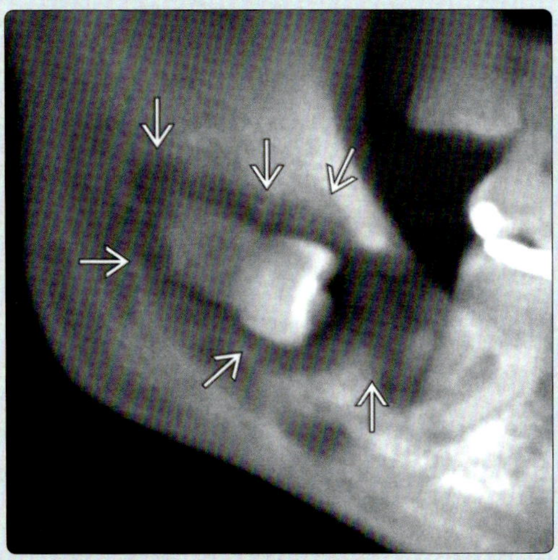
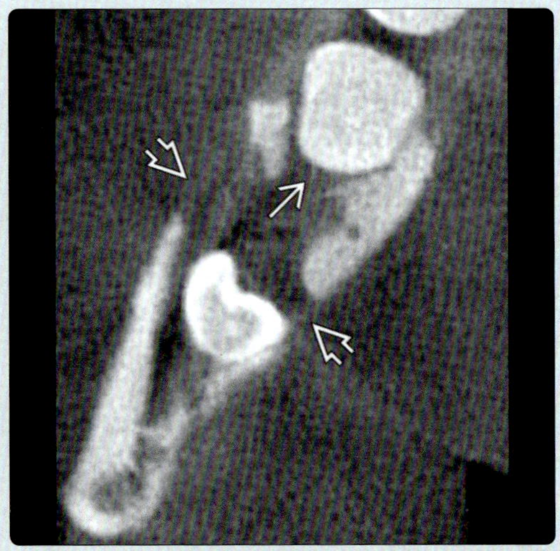

(Left) *Panoramic radiograph shows a CMC associated with an impacted right mandibular 3rd molar. The lesion is a well-defined, irregular radiolucency* ➡ *associated with the crown and extending around the root. This lesion is likely associated with a former dentigerous cyst or keratocyst and may be mistaken for osteomyelitis. (Courtesy M. Noujeim, DDS.)* **(Right)** *Axial CBCT in the same patient shows extension of the lesion to the periodontal ligament space of the 2nd molar* ➡*. Note cortical destruction* ➡*. (Courtesy M. Noujeim, DDS.)*

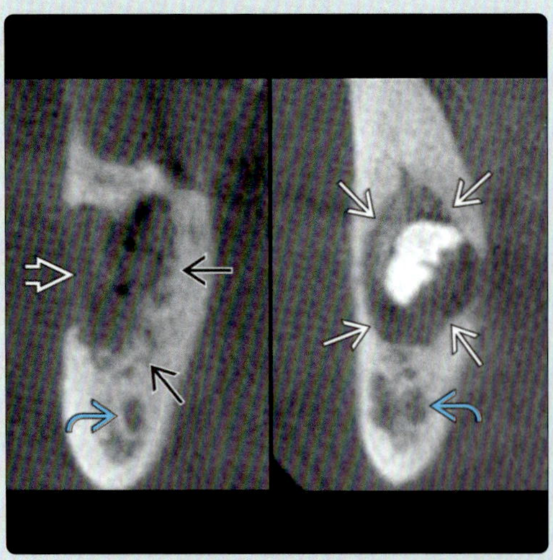
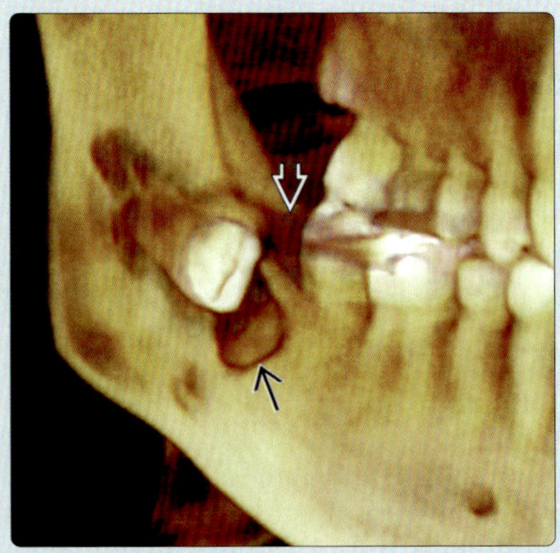

(Left) *Cross section CBCT in the same patient shows a well-defined lesion outline at the tooth crown* ➡ *with infiltrative margins further mesially at the lingual and inferior aspects* ➡*. The buccal cortex is destroyed* ➡*. Note uninvolved mandibular canal located inferiorly* ➡*. (Courtesy M. Noujeim, DDS.)* **(Right)** *Oblique 3D CBCT reformation in the same patient shows the well-defined, cyst-like mesial border of the lesion* ➡ *with irregular extension in the retromolar area* ➡*. (Courtesy M. Noujeim, DDS.)*

TERMINOLOGY

Abbreviations

- Central mucoepidermoid carcinoma (CMC)

Synonyms

- Mucoepidermoid carcinoma, central mucoepidermoid tumor

Definitions

- Uncommon malignant epithelial tumor arising in bone, originating from odontogenic epithelium or from **cyst lining**

IMAGING

General Features

- Best diagnostic clue
  - Impacted **mandibular molar** with associated **cystic** lesion accompanied by **swelling** and **paresthesia**
- Location
  - Mandible:maxilla = 2:1 (but 1:1 in children)
  - Most common in **molar/premolar** regions, superior to mandibular canal
  - Maxilla: Most common in molar-sinus-palatal area
- Size
  - Varies, often relatively large at diagnosis because patients may **wait months** before seeking treatment
- Morphology
  - Regular or undulating/scalloped border

Radiographic Findings

- Radiography
  - Most often **resembles benign tumor or cyst**
    - Well-defined, often corticated border
  - Uni- or multilocular expansile **radiolucency**
    - May have **soap bubble** appearance, especially anterior mandible
  - Ground-glass internal pattern reported
  - Mandibular canal may be **displaced**
  - Teeth usually unaffected, but root resorption and displacement reported
  - Less commonly has malignant characteristics: Infiltrative margins, soft tissue extension

CT Findings

- Irregular margins
- Cortical destruction and soft tissue extension more likely visible with CT
  - More likely in longstanding cases

Imaging Recommendations

- Best imaging tool
  - CBCT or CT to assess cortices and lesion extent

DIFFERENTIAL DIAGNOSIS

Dentigerous Cyst

- CMC may arise in cyst lining and have identical radiographic appearance
- No cortical erosion with dentigerous cyst
- No history of pain or paresthesia

Ameloblastoma

- Multilocular soap bubble appearance similar to CMC
- No cortical erosion
- No history of pain or paresthesia

Glandular Odontogenic Cyst

- Radiographic appearance can be identical to low-grade CMC
- Must rely on histologic findings to differentiate from CMC

PATHOLOGY

General Features

- Etiology
  - Mucous metaplasia of odontogenic cyst wall (50% of cases): Most commonly **dentigerous cyst**
  - Ectopic salivary gland tissue

Microscopic Features

- Multiple cystic structures lined with mucous or epidermoid cells in fibrous connective tissue stroma

CLINICAL ISSUES

Presentation

- Most common signs/symptoms
  - **Painless swelling**, often of long duration
  - Often **incidental** finding because asymptomatic
- Other signs/symptoms
  - Facial **asymmetry**, **pain**, **paresthesia**, dysphagia, trismus, edema, adenopathy, displaced or mobile teeth

Demographics

- Age
  - Most **4th-5th** decade; also reported in **teenagers and children**
- Gender
  - F:M = 2:1, although some reports 1:1

Natural History & Prognosis

- **Slow growing**: Patients may not seek treatment early
- Locally invasive but sometimes metastasizes to regional lymph nodes, ipsilateral clavicle, lung, or brain

Treatment

- Wide **resection**, otherwise recurrence common
- If metastases to regional lymph nodes or high-grade tumor: Radiation treatment

DIAGNOSTIC CHECKLIST

Consider

- CMC may be **indistinguishable** from **benign tumor or cyst**

Image Interpretation Pearls

- Tumor may not destroy cortices and may be well defined

SELECTED REFERENCES

1. Kechagias N et al: Central mucoepidermoid carcinoma of the anterior region of the mandible: report of an unusual case and review of the literature. Oral Maxillofac Surg. 19(3):309-13, 2015

Burkitt Lymphoma

KEY FACTS

TERMINOLOGY

- Definition: Undifferentiated malignant non-Hodgkin lymphoma

IMAGING

- Large **expansile osteolytic lesion** in mandible in young patient (endemic variant)
- Mandibular **poorly defined expansile mass** with mottled, permeative pattern of bone destruction
- **Erupted teeth and developing tooth buds in crypts displaced**, follicular spaces widened, periodontal ligament spaces widened
- **Teeth "floating in space,"** developing teeth erupting with little or no root formation
- Expansion may be balloon-like with associated soft tissue mass
  - Spiculated periosteal reaction may occur if periosteum involved

TOP DIFFERENTIAL DIAGNOSES

- Osteosarcoma
- Langerhans cell histiocytosis
- Metastatic disease
- Cherubism
- Osteomyelitis

CLINICAL ISSUES

- Tooth mobility, toothache, gingival enlargement, pain, paresthesia of inferior alveolar nerve or other sensory facial nerves
- Occurs predominantly in children
  - Adults have worse prognosis than children
- One of fastest growing malignancies in humans

DIAGNOSTIC CHECKLIST

- Consider other aggressive lesions in children: Osteosarcoma, Langerhans histiocytosis, metastatic disease

(Left) *Clinical photograph of young boy with Burkitt lymphoma shows marked right facial swelling of recent onset. (Courtesy C. Nortjé, BChD.)* **(Right)** *Panoramic radiograph in the same patient shows an ill-defined radiolucency in the right mandible ➡ with superior displacement of the developing 2nd permanent mandibular molar ⮫. There is a large radiolucency at the apex ⮫. The lamina dura and follicular cortices of the developing teeth are destroyed. (Courtesy C. Nortjé, BChD.)*

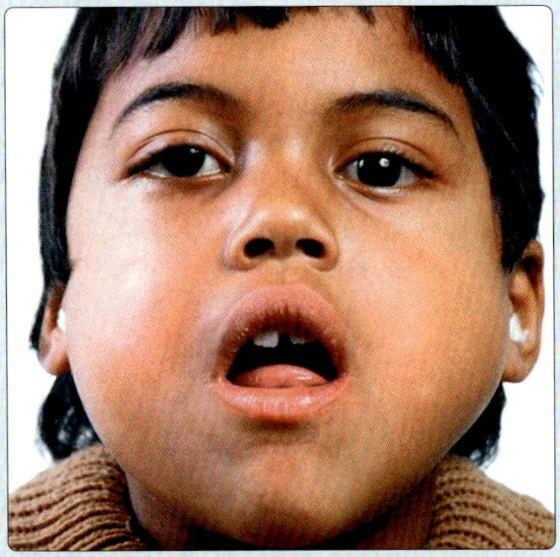

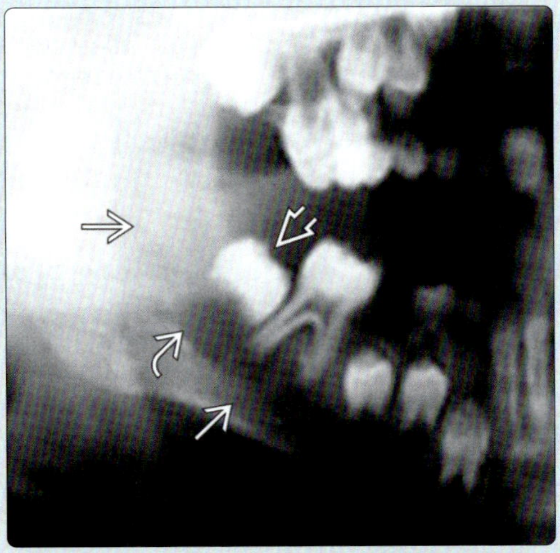

(Left) *Clinical photograph shows a Burkitt lymphoma patient with a rapidly growing left facial swelling and proptosis. (Courtesy C. Nortjé, BChD.)* **(Right)** *Axial NECT in the same patient shows infiltration of the Burkitt lymphoma tumor into the ethmoid and posterior orbital areas ➡. (Courtesy C. Nortjé, BChD.)*

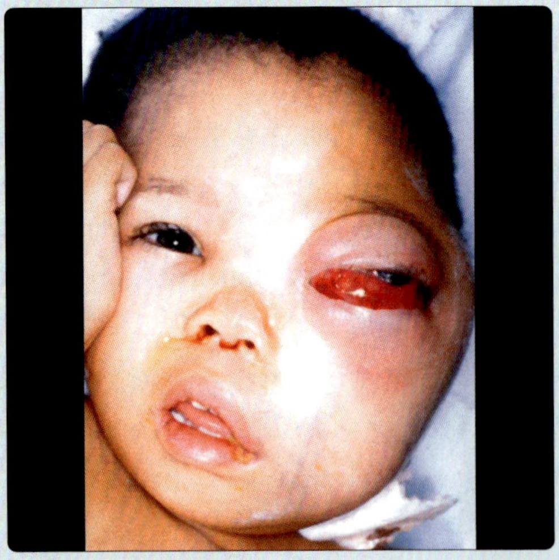

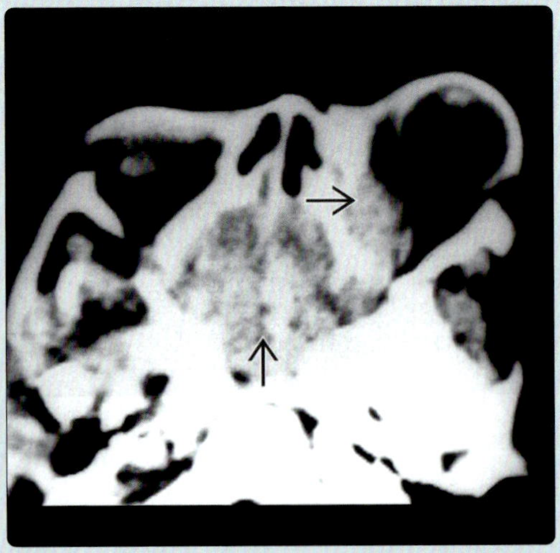

TERMINOLOGY

Synonyms

- Burkitt tumor, high-grade B-cell lymphoma, small noncleaved cell lymphoma, African jaw lymphoma, American Burkitt lymphoma

Definitions

- Burkitt lymphoma: Undifferentiated malignant non-Hodgkin lymphoma (NHL)
  - 3 distinct variants
    - Endemic (Africa & New Guinea, most common type)
    - Sporadic (throughout world)
    - Immunodeficiency-associated (primarily HIV)

IMAGING

General Features

- Best diagnostic clue
  - Large **expansile osteolytic lesion** in mandible in young patient (endemic variant)
- Location
  - Endemic variant: Involves **mandible** more commonly than maxilla, can affect both jaws
    - **Posterior regions** more common
    - If both jaws involved, disease usually ipsilateral
    - Can affect other bones such as pelvis, femur, tibia, humerus
  - Sporadic variant: Usually involves abdominal organs; jaws may not be affected
    - Most commonly involves distal ileum, cecum, or mesentery
    - Less commonly other abdominal organs, pelvic organs, & facial bones
    - May affect Waldeyer ring and lymph nodes
  - Immunodeficiency-associated: Usually involves abdominal organs and bone marrow
- Size
  - Tumors can reach large size because of **rapid growth**, resulting in significant facial deformity
- Morphology
  - Permeative bone marrow infiltration with associated **soft tissue mass**

Radiographic Findings

- Radiography
  - **Poorly defined expansile jaw mass** with mottled, permeative pattern of bone destruction
  - Expansion may be balloon-like with associated soft tissue mass
    - Spiculated periosteal reaction may occur if periosteum involved
  - **Erupted teeth and developing tooth buds in crypts displaced**, follicular spaces widened, periodontal ligament spaces widened
  - **Follicular cortices and lamina dura of teeth destroyed**, anatomical cortices thinned or destroyed
  - **Teeth "floating in space,"** developing teeth erupting with little or no root formation
  - Often multiple lesions; can be bilateral

CT Findings

- NECT
  - Destructive soft tissue mass, erodes adjacent bones and invades adjacent spaces
  - No tumor matrix or soft tissue calcification
- CECT
  - Mild to moderate enhancement of associated soft tissue mass

MR Findings

- T1WI
  - Diffuse infiltration with low signal intensity
- T2WI
  - Heterogeneous signal intensity: Hyper-, iso-, or hypointense
  - Fibrotic regions hypointense
- T1WI C+
  - Enhancement best defines soft tissue component and enlarged lymph nodes

Imaging Recommendations

- Best imaging tool
  - Panoramic or intraoral radiographs useful for evaluation of lamina dura and periodontal ligament spaces
  - Bone CT helpful to determine disease extent
  - MR best demonstrates marrow replacement and soft tissue component
- Protocol advice
  - Contrasted MR examination of face with fat saturation, including STIR

DIFFERENTIAL DIAGNOSIS

Osteosarcoma

- Osteolytic variant may grow rapidly and be indistinguishable from Burkitt lymphoma
- Both osteosarcoma and Burkitt lymphoma can have spiculated periosteal reaction

Langerhans Cell Histiocytosis

- Often other bones also involved, such as skull
- Lesions more well defined than in Burkitt lymphoma

Metastatic Disease

- Can have similar appearance
- Often multifocal disease

Cherubism

- **Bilateral** jaw expansion, but cortices intact
- Grows more slowly

Osteomyelitis

- Clinical history of slow jaw enlargement; Burkitt lymphoma grows rapidly
- Jaw expansion due to characteristic laminated periosteal reaction

PATHOLOGY

General Features

- Etiology
  - Etiology unclear; 2 main hypotheses

  - Proto-oncogene *C-MYC* translocation to region of vigorous gene transcription causes overproduction of c-myc product that may lead to B-cell proliferation
  - Immunosuppression caused by coexistent malaria or another infection; child is unable to mount appropriate response against B cells that are infected latently with EBV
    - Leads to excessive B-cell proliferations
- Associated abnormalities
  - Endemic variant strongly associated with EBV
  - EBV associated with 20% of sporadic and immunodeficiency variants
  - Immunodeficiency variant associated with HIV, congenital immunodeficiency diseases, or after organ transplantation
- Most primary lymphomas of bone are due to NHL
  - 6% are due to Hodgkin lymphoma

Staging, Grading, & Classification

- Ann Arbor staging classification
  - Stage I: Involvement of single lymph node region
  - Stage II: Involvement of ≥ 2 lymph node regions on same side of diaphragm
  - Stage III: Involvement of lymph node regions on both sides of diaphragm
  - Stage IV: Diffuse or disseminated involvement of ≥ 1 extralymphatic organ or tissues ± associated lymph node enlargement
- National Cancer Institute (NCI) system
  - A: Single solitary extraabdominal site
  - B: Multiple extraabdominal tumors
  - C: Intraabdominal tumor
  - D: Intraabdominal plus ≥ 1 extraabdominal site

Gross Pathologic & Surgical Features

- Gray-white, soft, fleshy, intraosseous component
- Extraosseous tissue with tan-white appearance; resembles lymphomatous lymph nodes

Microscopic Features

- B-cell neoplasm
  - Characterized by small, uniform, noncleaved cells
- Scattered macrophages with phagocytes cell debris

CLINICAL ISSUES

Presentation

- Most common signs/symptoms
  - Endemic variant: **Rapidly growing**, **painful jaw mass**
  - Other signs/symptoms
    - Tooth mobility or displacement, toothache, gingival enlargement, pain, paresthesia of inferior alveolar nerve or other sensory facial nerves
    - Rapidly growing, painless cervical lymph nodes or orbital mass
    - Extreme fatigue, weight loss, night sweats
  - Sporadic variant: Head & neck cases may have Waldeyer ring and nodal involvement
    - Airway compression, dysphagia, dyspnea, wheezing, airway obstruction
  - Immunodeficiency-associated: Abdominal mass
- Clinical profile
  - African child with rapidly enlarging, painful, firm mass at angle of jaw with associated cervical nodes

Demographics

- Age
  - Occurs predominantly in **children**
    - Endemic variant: Mean age 7 years
    - Sporadic variant: Children and young adults, mean age 11 years
    - Immunodeficiency-associated: Adults
- Gender
  - M:F = 3:1
- Epidemiology
  - Endemic variant is prevalent in central Africa (most common childhood malignancy in Africa)
    - Incidence: 3/100,000
  - Sporadic variant rare, with 100 new cases each year
    - Incidence: 0.16/100,000

Natural History & Prognosis

- Prior to aggressive therapy, children died quickly
- One of fastest growing malignancies in humans
- Diagnosis of Burkitt lymphoma usually made by bone marrow or node biopsy
- Prognosis is highly dependent on disease stage, extent, and patient age
  - Adults have worse prognosis than children
- Usually curable if treated aggressively with chemotherapy
  - Survival rate 60% with combination chemotherapy and CNS prophylaxis
  - Cure rate over 90% with limited disease
  - Cure rate 75% if disease spreads to marrow or CSF

Treatment

- Systemic chemotherapy is treatment of choice
  - Adjuvant radiotherapy may be added
  - CNS prophylaxis
    - Intrathecal methotrexate ± cytarabine & hydrocortisone

DIAGNOSTIC CHECKLIST

Consider

- Other aggressive lesions in children: Osteosarcoma, Langerhans histiocytosis, metastatic disease

Image Interpretation Pearls

- Cortex can be intact despite soft tissue extension
- Soft tissue portion often larger than intraosseous part

SELECTED REFERENCES

1. Derinkuyu BE et al: Imaging features of Burkitt lymphoma in pediatric patients. Diagn Interv Radiol. 22(1):95-100, 2016
2. Rebelo-Pontes HA et al: Burkitt's lymphoma of the jaws in the Amazon region of Brazil. Med Oral Patol Oral Cir Bucal. 19(1):e32-8, 2014
3. Kimura H et al: Epstein-Barr virus-associated lymphoid malignancies: the expanding spectrum of hematopoietic neoplasms. Nagoya J Med Sci. 75(3-4):169-79, 2013
4. Sasaki M et al: Bilateral numb chin syndrome leading to a diagnosis of Burkitt's cell acute lymphocytic leukemia: a case report and literature review. Oral Surg Oral Med Oral Pathol Oral Radiol Endod. 111(3):e11-6, 2011

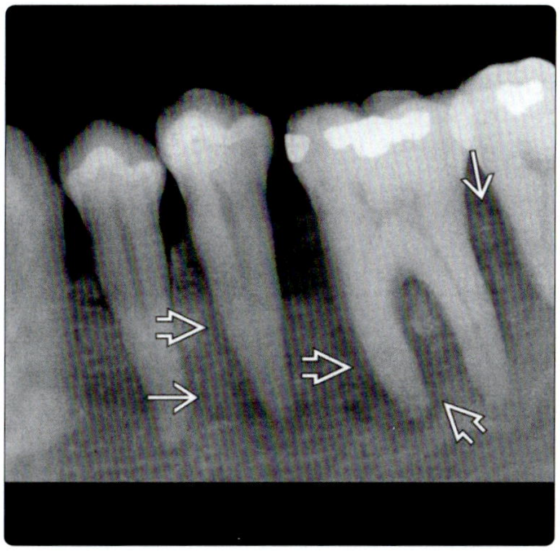

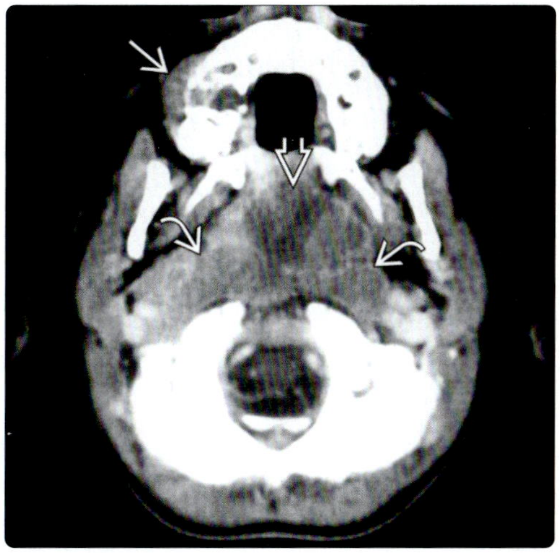

(Left) *Periapical radiograph shows Burkitt lymphoma affecting the left posterior mandible. The radiographic changes are not specific for Burkitt lymphoma but show malignant characteristics such as permeative bone destruction and symmetrically widened periodontal ligament spaces.* **(Right)** *Axial CECT of a patient with Burkitt lymphoma shows a maxillary lesion with an associated soft tissue mass. Note extensive adenoidal and retropharyngeal nodal involvement.*

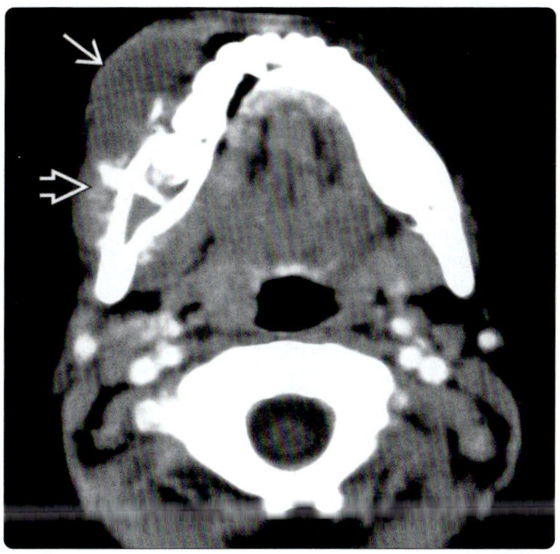

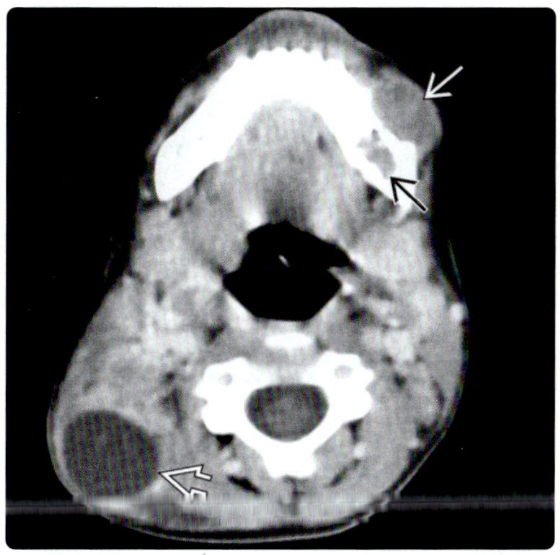

(Left) *Axial CECT shows a large mass arising from the right mandible with extension into the adjacent soft tissues. There is a spiculated periosteal response on the buccal aspect of the mandible. This appearance is also seen in osteosarcoma.* **(Right)** *Axial CECT shows an ill-defined lesion of Burkitt lymphoma in the left mandible with an associated soft tissue mass. A large necrotic posterior cervical node is also seen.*

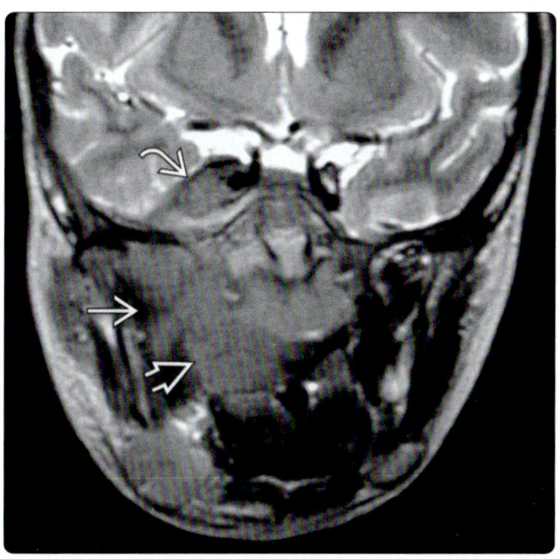

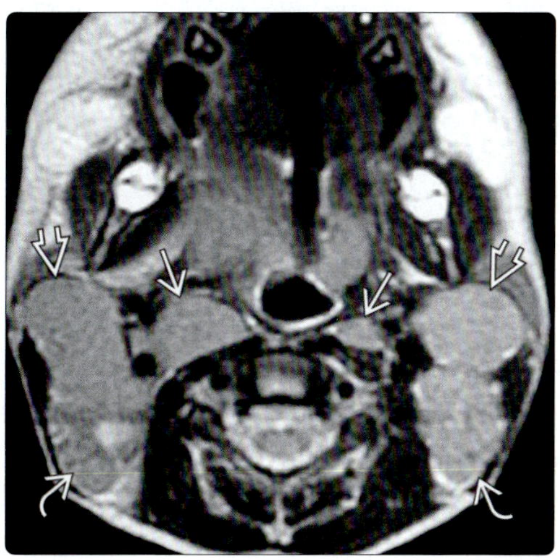

(Left) *Coronal T2WI MR shows transspatial Burkitt lymphoma involving the pharyngeal mucosal space, masticator space, and posterior right maxilla. There is also Meckel cave involvement.* **(Right)** *Axial T2WI MR shows nodal Burkitt lymphoma as a large, nonnecrotic retropharyngeal, deep cervical, and spinal accessory adenopathy.*

Non-Hodgkin Lymphoma of Pharyngeal Mucosal Space

KEY FACTS

TERMINOLOGY

- Non-Hodgkin lymphoma (NHL) of pharyngeal mucosal space (PMS)
- Multiple subtypes, usually B- or T-cell categories
- 3 subsites of Waldeyer lymphatic ring
    - Nasopharyngeal adenoids
    - Palatine tonsils
    - Lingual tonsil

IMAGING

- CECT: Minimally enhancing bulky mass filling PMS airway, often without deep extension
    - Associated NHL nodal disease present 50% of time
- T2WI MR: Varies in signal intensity (SI) depending on cellularity
- DWI MR: Restricted because of high cellularity

TOP DIFFERENTIAL DIAGNOSES

- Tonsillar lymphoid hyperplasia
- PMS benign mixed tumor
- Nasopharyngeal carcinoma
- Palatine tonsil squamous cell carcinoma (SCCa)
- Lingual tonsil SCCa
- Inflammatory pseudotumor/IgG4 disease
- PMS minor salivary gland malignancy

PATHOLOGY

- When in H&N, commonly involves Waldeyer ring

CLINICAL ISSUES

- Increased incidence in patients with AIDS, Sjögren syndrome, Hashimoto thyroiditis, IgG4 disease, some autoimmune conditions

DIAGNOSTIC CHECKLIST

- Consider NHL of PMS when imaging shows bulky mass of adenoids, tonsils, or base of tongue
- Note local or deep extension & associated adenopathy for staging & treatment planning

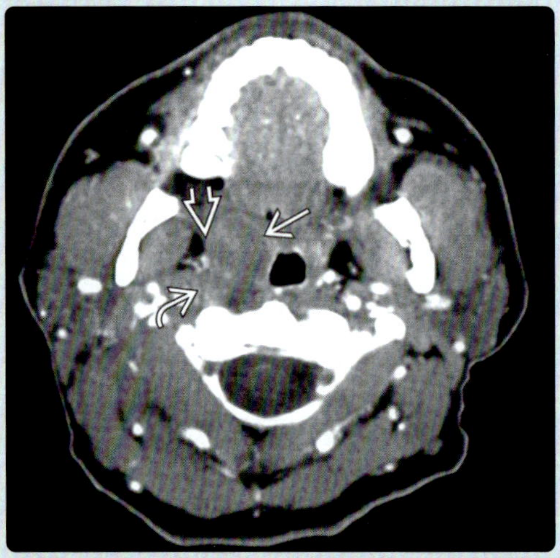
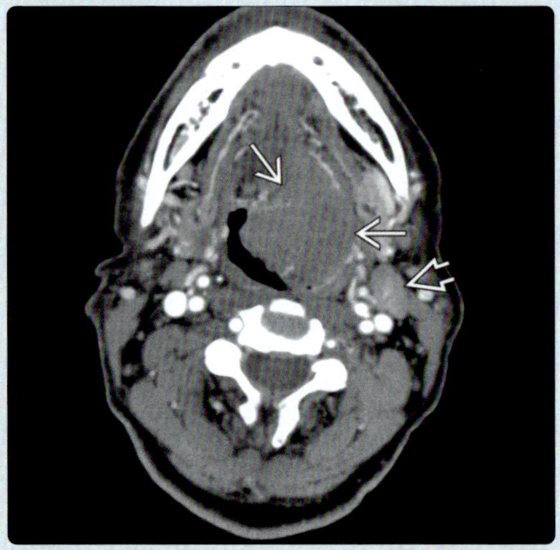

(Left) *CECT shows a large, low-density mass in right tonsil. Smooth interface between parapharyngeal fat implies no extension through lateral capsule, but note fullness in right prevertebral muscles, suggesting mass has invaded through posterior tonsillar capsule.* **(Right)** *Large, exophytic, minimally enhancing NHL arises in left lingual lymphoid tissue with near-complete airway obstruction. Note level IIA node with no central necrosis, a common finding in nodal lymphoma.*

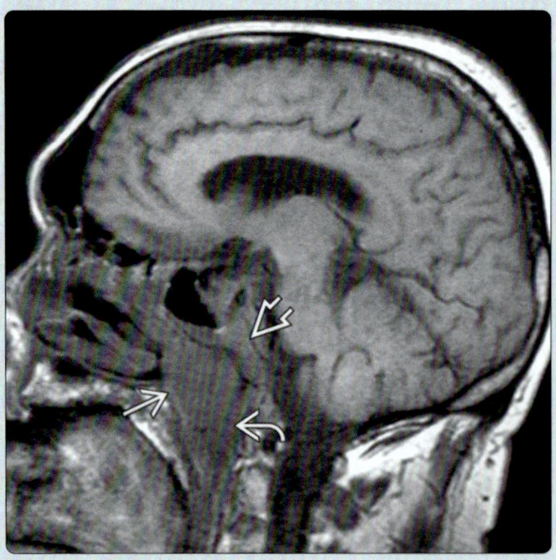
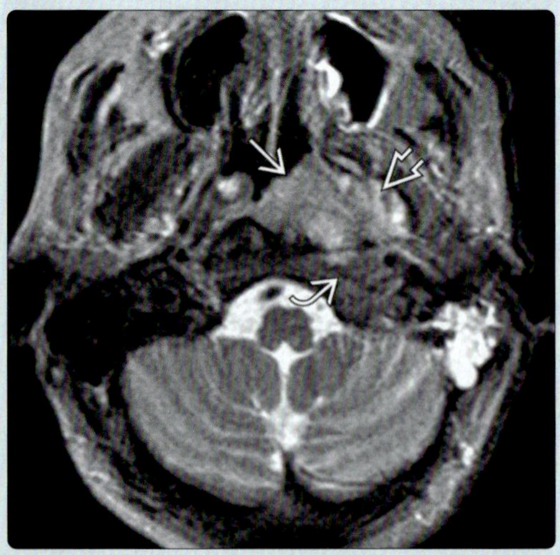

(Left) *Sagittal T1WI MR shows a bulky nasopharyngeal mass extending to oropharyngeal level. Abnormal signal intensity in clivus implies central skull base invasion.* **(Right)** *Axial T2WI FS MR in the same patient reveals mass is relatively low signal intensity with invasion of prevertebral muscles and parapharyngeal space. Note mastoid opacification from tumor invasion of eustachian tube orifice. Nasopharyngeal carcinoma could exactly mimic this imaging appearance.*

TERMINOLOGY

Abbreviations

- Non-Hodgkin lymphoma (NHL) of pharyngeal mucosal space (PMS)

Synonyms

- Multiple subtypes, usually B- or T-cell categories
  - B-cell types: Burkitt, diffuse large, follicular, immunoblastic large cell, mantle cell, chronic lymphocytic lymphoma, mucosa-associated lymphoid tissue (MALT)
  - T-cell types: Anaplastic large cell, precursor T-lymphoblastic, mycosis fungoides

Definitions

- 3 subsites of Waldeyer lymphatic ring: Adenoids, palatine tonsils, lingual tonsil

IMAGING

General Features

- Best diagnostic clue
  - Large PMS mass with associated cervical adenopathy > 50% of time
  - Imaging findings **may be identical to squamous cell carcinoma** (SCCa) of PMS
- Location
  - Most common sites of NHL of PMS
    - Palatine tonsil > nasopharyngeal adenoids > lingual tonsil
    - More than 1 site often involved
  - Nonnodal, extralymphatic NHL of sinus, orbit, parotid, larynx, or thyroid can rarely occur
- Size
  - Large, usually > 4 cm, at presentation
- Morphology
  - Poorly defined, diffusely infiltrative mass most common (mimics SCCa)
  - Unilateral, asymmetric, smooth mass in tonsil less common (mimics benign mixed tumor)

CT Findings

- CECT
  - Minimally enhancing bulky mass filling PMS airway
    - Often without deep extension into surrounding spaces
  - Associated NHL nodal disease present 50% of time
    - **Nodes** usually **large**, > 2 cm, & nonnecrotic
    - Nodes may be centrally necrotic in high-grade NHL
      - Especially AIDS-related NHL

MR Findings

- T1WI
  - Large PMS mass isointense to muscle
- T2WI
  - Varies in signal intensity (SI), depending on cellularity, but usually homogeneously intermediate SI
    - Highly cellular lesions generally less hyperintense on T2WI
  - Invasion into surrounding structures, including skull base, PPS, & prevertebral muscles, is common
- DWI
  - Restricted diffusion especially for FDG-avid lymphoma types
- T1WI C+
  - Enhancing palatine, lingual, or adenoidal tonsillar mass
  - No internal enhancing septa present, as compared with benign lymphoid hyperplasia or tonsillar infection

Nuclear Medicine Findings

- PET
  - NHL FDG avid
  - MALT-type lymphomas less FDG avid
  - PET/CT used to stage disease & for surveillance of posttreatment imaging
    - PET/CT limited sensitivity for lower grade NHL

Imaging Recommendations

- Best imaging tool
  - PET/CT best staging & surveillance modality
  - CECT recommended as part of PET/CT imaging
- Protocol advice
  - Imaging (CT or MR) should cover entire extracranial H&N from sellar floor above to clavicles below
    - Coverage should include PMS primary site as well as potential cervical adenopathy

DIFFERENTIAL DIAGNOSIS

Tonsillar Lymphoid Hyperplasia

- Patients < 20 years old (NHL usually > 40 years old)
- Symmetric enlargement of adenoidal & tonsillar tissue

Nasopharyngeal Carcinoma

- Poorly circumscribed nasopharyngeal PMS mass
  - Often mimics NHL on imaging alone
- Associated malignant, often necrotic, adenopathy

Palatine Tonsil Squamous Cell Carcinoma

- Invasive palatine tonsil mass
  - Often mimics NHL on imaging alone

Lingual Tonsil Squamous Cell Carcinoma

- Invasive lingual tonsil mass
  - Often mimics NHL on imaging alone

Pharyngeal Mucosal Space Minor Salivary Gland Malignancy

- May be indistinguishable from H&N SCCa
- Associated nodal metastases are rare

Pharyngeal Mucosal Space Benign Mixed Tumor

- Well-circumscribed, noninvasive PMS mass

Inflammatory Pseudotumor/IgG4 Disease

- Poorly defined autoimmune disease can present as PMS mass
- Spectrum that includes Sjögren syndrome, thyroiditis, autoimmune disease

PATHOLOGY

General Features

- Etiology
  - Primary malignancy of lymphatic system

- PMS NHL usually of B-cell origin
- Genetics
  - Cytogenetics of NHL complicated & related to subtype of lymphoma
- Associated abnormalities
  - Sjögren syndrome & Hashimoto thyroiditis associated with MALT, B-cell type, NHL
    - Currently being redefined as IgG4 disease
  - Posttransplant lymphoproliferative disorders associated with NHL from iatrogenic immunosuppression used for transplant patients
    - Spectrum of diseases from prominent lymphoid hyperplasia to malignant NHL

Staging, Grading, & Classification

- 2 prognostic groups: Indolent & aggressive
- NHL clinical staging (I-IV) Ann Arbor staging system
  - Stage I or IE
    - Single lymphatic site: Waldeyer lymphatic ring
    - IE: Single extralymphatic site + no nodal disease
  - Stage II or IIE
    - ≥ 2 nodal regions on same side of diaphragm
    - IIE: Single extralymphatic site & > 1 nodal region on same side of diaphragm
  - Stages III, IIIE, IIIS
    - ≥ 2 nodal regions on both sides of diaphragm
    - IIIE: Extralymphatic extension with adjacent lymph node involvement
    - IIIS: Splenic involvement
  - Stage IV: Diffuse or disseminated involvement of ≥ 1 extralymphatic organ(s) ± lymph node involvement

Gross Pathologic & Surgical Features

- Soft, bulky PMS lesion, may be submucosal or ulcerative

Microscopic Features

- Any of NHL patterns & cell types can be seen
- Most common histologic pattern is diffuse with immunoblastic or large cell (B cell) cytologic features & markers
  - Immunochemistry differentiates nasopharyngeal carcinoma (NPC) from NHL
    - Leukocyte common antigen (LCA) vs. cytokeratin
    - NHL, immunoblastic or large cell type: LCA(+), cytokeratin (-)
    - NPC, undifferentiated: LCA(-), cytokeratin (+)

CLINICAL ISSUES

Presentation

- Most common signs/symptoms
  - Presenting signs similar to SCCa
    - Nasopharyngeal adenoidal NHL: Nasal obstruction, serous otitis media
    - Palatine or lingual tonsil NHL: Sore throat, otalgia, tonsillar mass
  - Other signs/symptoms
    - B symptoms: Systemic complaints, such as fever, sweats, weight loss
    - Children with large PMS NHL may present with airway compromise
- Clinical profile
  - Most common presentation: Adult with PMS mass & neck mass
  - Increased incidence in patients with AIDS, Sjögren syndrome, Hashimoto thyroiditis, & other autoimmune conditions

Demographics

- Age
  - Adult more common than pediatric; > 50 years
- Gender
  - M:F = 1.5:1
- Epidemiology
  - NHL 5x as common as Hodgkin disease in H&N
  - 35% of extranodal NHL in H&N occurs in PMS
  - PMS is most common extranodal site in H&N
    - Palatine tonsil involved (50%)
    - Nasopharyngeal adenoids involved (35%)
    - Lingual tonsil involved (15%)
  - 50% of PMS NHL have malignant lymph nodes at presentation

Natural History & Prognosis

- Prognosis determined by both stage & aggressive vs. indolent types
  - High histopathologic grade & recurrent disseminated disease have poorest prognosis
  - AIDS-related NHL generally has poorer prognosis
- 2/3 of patients have remission after initial therapy
  - Of these, 2/3 are cured & have no further relapse
- 75% of those who relapse after achieving remission die of NHL

Treatment

- Based on clinical stage & aggressive vs. indolent subtypes at presentation
- Treatment regimens range from "watch & wait" for indolent types especially in elderly to combined chemoradiotherapy
- Complete remission & cure rates improved with development of combined chemotherapy options
- **Overall survival rate** for H&N PMS NHL is **60%**

DIAGNOSTIC CHECKLIST

Consider

- NHL of PMS when imaging shows bulky mass of adenoidal, tonsillar, or base of tongue (lingual tonsil)

Image Interpretation Pearls

- Local or deep extension important to recognize & map for staging & radiotherapy
- Associated cervical adenopathy common
  - Must scan entire neck

Reporting Tips

- Describe primary PMS lesion & adenopathy as both affect accurate staging

SELECTED REFERENCES

1. Heacock L et al: PET/MRI for the evaluation of patients with lymphoma: initial observations. AJR Am J Roentgenol. 204(4):842-8, 2015
2. Aiken AH et al: Imaging Hodgkin and non-Hodgkin lymphoma in the head and neck. Radiol Clin North Am. 46(2):363-78, ix-x, 2008

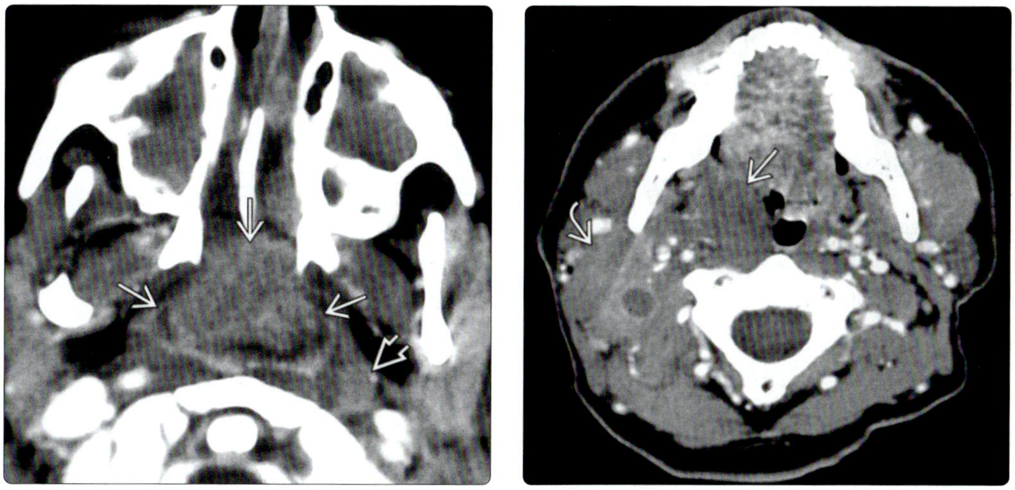

(Left) *Axial CECT in a child with AIDS shows heterogeneous enhancement in bulky adenoidal NHL ➔. Note the large left retropharyngeal lymph node ⇨ and near occlusion of nasopharyngeal airway. Benign secretions fill bilateral maxillary sinuses and nasal cavity.* **(Right)** *Axial CECT shows multifocal NHL with involvement in right tonsil ➔ and level II matted nodal mass ↪ with extranodal extension. Cervical adenopathy is present more than 50% of time with NHL of pharyngeal mucosal space (PMS).*

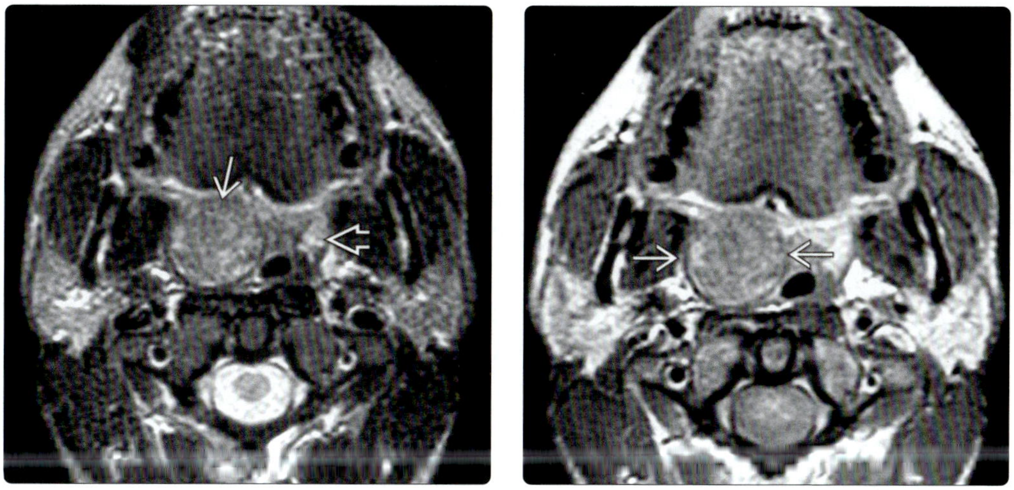

(Left) *Axial T2WI FS MR shows a well-circumscribed right tonsillar NHL ➔. Small left tonsil ⇨ is normal for adult as lymphoid tissue involutes with age. Squamous cell carcinoma of tonsil or benign mixed tumor could have identical appearance, and only biopsy would confirm NHL.* **(Right)** *Axial T1WI C+ MR in the same patient reveals homogeneous enhancement in tonsillar NHL ➔. Tonsillar infection should have a striated enhancement pattern; intratonsillar abscess would be centrally necrotic.*

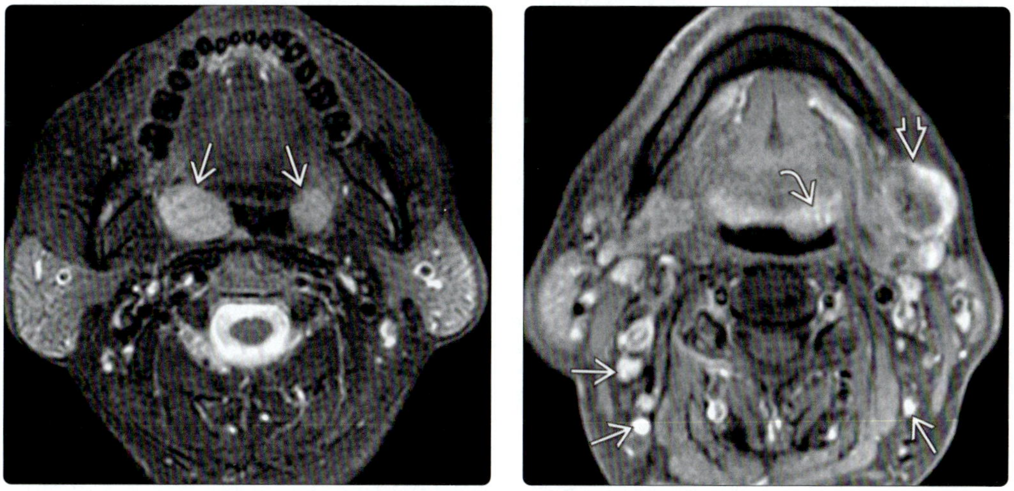

(Left) *Axial T2WI FS MR demonstrates multifocal NHL in both palatine tonsils ➔. Well-circumscribed appearance suggests that tumor remains within tonsillar capsules.* **(Right)** *Axial T1WI C+ FS MR in the same patient shows additional sites of NHL in left base of tongue lymphoid tissue ↪ and large necrotic left level IB node ⇨. Multiple small cervical nodes ➔ are present, and only a metabolic study, such as PET/CT, could determine involvement by NHL.*

Multiple Myeloma

KEY FACTS

TERMINOLOGY

- Synonyms: Plasmacytoma, plasma cell myeloma, myeloma
- Definition: Monoclonal malignant proliferation of plasma cells

IMAGING

- **Punched-out,** mostly well-defined, round radiolucencies without corticated border
- Most common locations: **Calvarium, mandible**, pelvis, sternum, clavicle, humerus, and femur
  - Mandible > maxilla; posterior > anterior
- Generalized rarefaction may be present
  - Lamina dura around tooth roots may be lost
  - Follicular cortical outline of developing teeth may be less distinct
- Skull lesions present in 45% of patients
- CT or CBCT for H&N lesions

TOP DIFFERENTIAL DIAGNOSES

- Metastasis
- Osteomyelitis
- Hyperparathyroidism
- Langerhans histiocytosis
- Simple (traumatic) bone cyst
- Primary intraosseous carcinoma

CLINICAL ISSUES

- Male > female; 50-80 years
- Persistent bone pain, usually lower back
- Paresthesia: Numb chin suggestive not pathognomic
- **Bence Jones protein** in urine → kidney failure
- **Pathologic fracture**

DIAGNOSTIC CHECKLIST

- When multiple lesions detected in mandible/maxilla, look for additional lesions in skull and spine

(Left) *Panoramic radiograph shows a large lytic lesion in the left posterior mandible and ramus in a patient with multiple myeloma. The lesion has destroyed the anterior border of the ramus → and coronoid process. Smaller punched-out radiolucencies → can still be seen. Smaller lesions may coalesce and become much larger.* **(Right)** *Axial NECT in the same patient shows a large lytic lesion in the right body of the mandible. Note destruction of the lingual cortex → and pathologic fracture →.*

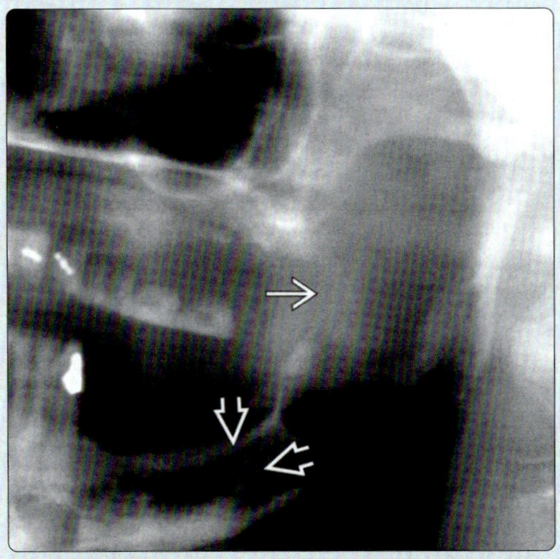

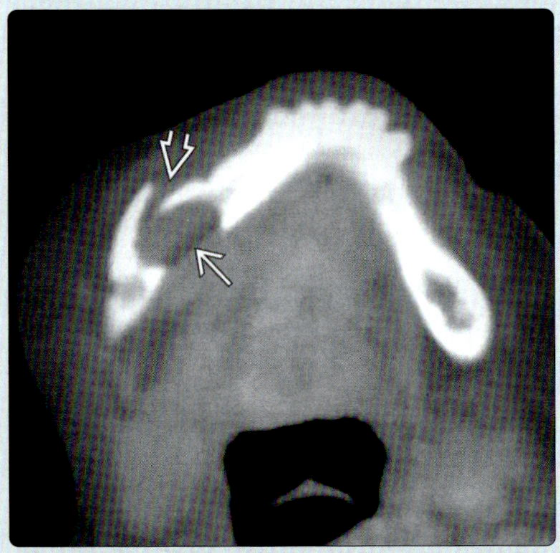

(Left) *Lateral cephalometric radiograph in the same patient shows numerous round or punched-out radiolucencies in the skull. Note that most of the lesions are well defined but not corticated, a classic feature of the lesions of multiple myeloma.* **(Right)** *AP radiographs in the same patient show numerous radiolucencies in the right humerus → and the left femur →. Note the pathologic fracture in the humerus →. The humerus and the femur are the most commonly involved long bones.*

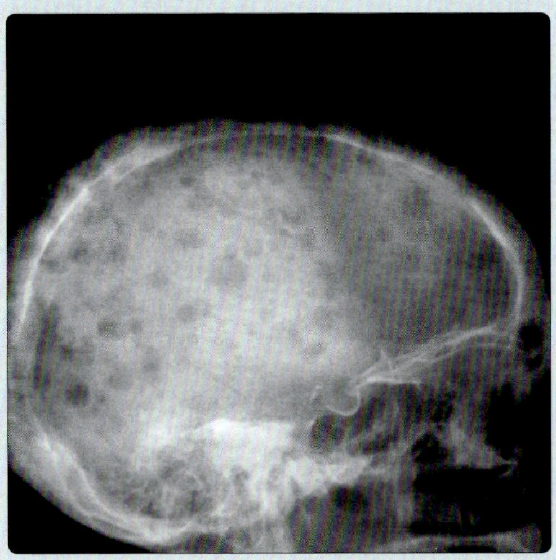

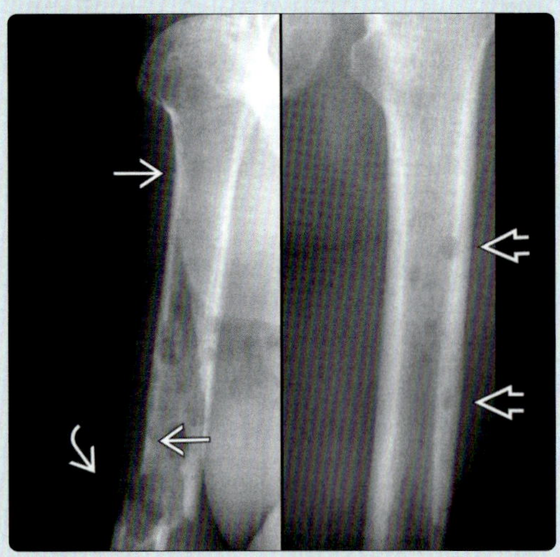

TERMINOLOGY

Abbreviations

- Multiple myeloma (MM)

Synonyms

- Plasmacytoma
- Plasma cell myeloma
- Myeloma

Definitions

- Monoclonal malignant proliferation of plasma cells
  - Solitary plasmacytoma is localized form
- MM is most common malignancy of bone in adults

IMAGING

General Features

- Best diagnostic clue
  - **Punched-out**, mostly well-defined, round radiolucencies without corticated border
- Location
  - Most common locations: **Calvarium, mandible**, pelvis, sternum, clavicle, humerus, and femur
  - In oral cavity
    - Mandible > maxilla
      - Posterior > anterior
- Size
  - Small: Usually < 1 cm at diagnosis; lesions may coalesce and become much larger
- Morphology
  - Multiple small, unilocular, round, or oval radiolucencies
    - Lesions that coalesce may appear multilocular
  - Occasionally lesions appear ill defined and infiltrative

Radiographic Findings

- Extraoral plain film
  - Panoramic imaging will show lesions in ramus and angle
  - Generalized rarefaction may be present
    - Lamina dura around tooth roots may be lost
    - Follicular cortical outline of developing teeth may be less distinct
  - Lateral cephalometric images will demonstrate skull lesions

CT Findings

- CBCT and bone CT
  - Best show extent of disease
  - Radiolucencies may be present in skull and cervical spine
    - Skull lesions present in 45% of patients

Imaging Recommendations

- Best imaging tool
  - CT or CBCT for H&N lesions
  - Screening for additional lesions in femur and humerus done with long-bone radiographs

DIFFERENTIAL DIAGNOSIS

Metastasis

- Radiolucent metastatic lesions **most difficult to differentiate from MM**
- Usually history of known primary; most commonly breast, lung, and prostate
  - Metastatic lesions to jaws as 1st sign of disease is rare

Osteomyelitis

- May present with moth-eaten radiolucent appearance
- Source of infection usually evident
- Often has associated surrounding areas of **sclerosis** representing reactive bone
- Periosteal reactions **parallel to cortex** may be present

Hyperparathyroidism

- Produces reduced density (radiolucency) throughout jaws that may also be seen in MM
- Females > males
- Increased serum calcium

Langerhans Histiocytosis

- Lesions of Langerhans histiocytosis are also described as punched out
- Langerhans histiocytosis in much younger age group
- Lesions in mandible may appear **scooped out** and any involved teeth may appear to be **floating**

Simple (Traumatic) Bone Cyst

- May appear similar to solitary mandibular lesion of MM
- More often corticated
- Lesions usually larger and **scallop between teeth**
- Seen in younger age group

Primary Intraosseous Carcinoma

- Usually solitary, ill-defined lesion
- May have associated soft tissue mass
- Rare in jaws

PATHOLOGY

General Features

- Etiology
  - Unknown
  - Solitary plasmacytoma may precede development of MM
    - ~ 70% convert to MM during average time span of 20 months
    - Mandibular plasmacytoma as 1st sign of MM reported in literature
- Genetics
  - Human leukocyte antigen studies suggest possible genetic predisposition

Staging, Grading, & Classification

- Plasma cells normally produce immunoglobulins; MM develops from single malignant plasma cell precursor
  - All subsequent cells have same genetic makeup, hence term **monoclonal**
- Monoclonal nature of cells demonstrated by antibodies directed against either lambda or kappa light chain of immunoglobulin
  - All cells in specimen take up only 1 type of antibody
  - In comparison, reactive infiltrate will mark for both
- **Monoclonal gammopathy**: Term used to describe overproduction of abnormal immunoglobulin

- Serum electrophoresis shows presence of myeloma protein (M protein) and is diagnostic
- 30-50% of patients have excess light chain immunoglobulins in urine: Known as **Bence Jones protein**

Gross Pathologic & Surgical Features

- Dark red, friable, soft tissue mass

Microscopic Features

- Diffuse monotonous sheets of plasmacytoid cells with varying degrees of differentiation
- Increased mitotic activity may be seen
- Biopsy specimen should show at least 10% of atypical plasma cells
- Amyloid may be present
  - Stains with Congo red show apple-green birefringence on polarized light

CLINICAL ISSUES

Presentation

- Most common signs/symptoms
  - Persistent bone pain, usually lower back
  - **Bence Jones protein** present in urine
    - Kidneys may eventually fail
- Other signs/symptoms
  - Paresthesia
    - **Numb chin**, not pathognomic for MM but sinister sign of malignancy
  - **Pathologic fracture**
  - Tooth mobility
  - Gingival hemorrhage/ulceration
  - Fever
  - Increased susceptibility to infections, especially of lungs and urinary tract
  - Fatigue
  - Temporal arteritis
  - 15% of patients show deposition of amyloid especially in tongue → macroglossia

Demographics

- Age
  - 50-80 years; mean: 60 years
- Gender
  - Male > female
- Epidemiology
  - MM accounts for 50% of all bone malignancies
    - 20-30% of these cases develop jaw lesions
    - Oral lesions rarely occur as 1st sign of disease
  - Blacks > whites
    - Most common hematologic disease in blacks living in USA

Natural History & Prognosis

- Prognosis is poor
  - Younger patients may live longer
- Prognosis only improved slightly over years
  - 5-year survival rate = 25%
- Serum levels of β_2 microglobulin and albumin may be helpful in determining prognosis
  - If β_2 microglobulin < 3.5 mg/L and albumin high, median survival = 5 years
  - Higher β_2 microglobulin level results in median survival of 2.5 years

Treatment

- Often multiagent chemotherapy
  - Alkylating agents, such as melphalan and cyclophosphamide with corticosteroid
  - Thalidomide has been used in some cases
- Bone marrow transplants for younger patients
- Radiation therapy for localized treatment of bone lesions
- Bisphosphonates: Pamidronate, clodronate, zoledronic acid (zoledronate)
  - Used to reduce morbidity and risk of pathologic fracture
  - Patients taking zoledronate at greatest risk for **medication-related osteonecrosis of jaws**; estimated incidence in MM patients is 6-8% and higher in patients taking combination pamidronate and zoledronate
    - Prior extraction is common predisposing factor

DIAGNOSTIC CHECKLIST

Image Interpretation Pearls

- When multiple lesions detected in mandible/maxilla, look for additional lesions in skull and spine

SELECTED REFERENCES

1. Choi WS et al: Medication-related osteonecrosis of the jaw: a preliminary retrospective study of 130 patients with multiple myeloma. Maxillofac Plast Reconstr Surg. 39(1):1, 2017
2. Kitagawa J et al: Efficacy and safety of denosumab in multiple myeloma. Rinsho Ketsueki. 57(5):592-6, 2016
3. Kucukkurt S et al: Solitary plasmacytoma of the mandible: report of two cases. BMJ Case Rep. 2016, 2016
4. Moura LB et al: Pathologic mandibular fracture as first sign of multiple myeloma. J Craniofac Surg. 27(2):e138-9, 2016
5. Yu WJ et al: [Osteonecrosis of the jaw associated with long time withdrawal of bisphosphonates in multiple myeloma: one case report.] Zhonghua Xue Ye Xue Za Zhi. 37(12):1089, 2016
6. Geng CJ et al: Ibandronate to treat skeletal-related events and bone pain in metastatic bone disease or multiple myeloma: a meta-analysis of randomised clinical trials. BMJ Open. 5(6):e007258, 2015
7. Goetze E et al: Osseous plasma cell neoplasm of the mandible for initial diagnosis of multiple myeloma: case report and literature review. J Maxillofac Oral Surg. 14(Suppl 1):469-74, 2015
8. Krstevska S et al: Osteonecrosis of the jaw after bisphosphonates treatment in patients with multiple myeloma. Med Arch. 69(6):367-70, 2015
9. Sun J et al: Bioinformatics analyses of differentially expressed genes associated with bisphosphonate-related osteonecrosis of the jaw in patients with multiple myeloma. Onco Targets Ther. 8:2681-8, 2015
10. Kamal M et al: Mandibular plasmacytoma of jaw - a case report. J Clin Diagn Res. 8(8):ZD20-1, 2014
11. Mohan RP et al: A multilocular radiolucency of mandible as the first evidence of multiple myeloma: A clinico-radiographic case report. Dent Res J (Isfahan). 11(2):272-5, 2014
12. Patel CG et al: Biomarkers of bone remodeling in multiple myeloma patients to tailor bisphosphonate therapy. Clin Cancer Res. 20(15):3955-61, 2014
13. Tejani N et al: Numb chin syndrome: a case series of a clinical syndrome associated with malignancy. J Med Imaging Radiat Oncol. 58(6):700-5, 2014
14. Troeltzsch M et al: Root resorption caused by jaw infiltration of multiple myeloma: report of a case and literature review. J Endod. 40(8):1260-4, 2014
15. George S et al: Plasma cell myeloma infiltrating the dental pulp: An interesting finding. J Oral Maxillofac Pathol. 17(3):417-9, 2013
16. Rodríguez-Caballero B et al: Mandibular solitary plasmocytoma of the jaw: A case report. Med Oral Patol Oral Cir Bucal. 16(5):e647-50, 2011
17. Elias HG et al: Multiple myeloma presenting as mandibular ill-defined radiolucent lesion with numb chin syndrome: a case report. J Oral Maxillofac Surg. 67(9):1991-6, 2009
18. Daneshbod Y et al: Jaw lesion as the first presentation of multiple myeloma diagnosed by fine needle aspiration. Acta Cytol. 52(2):268-70, 2008

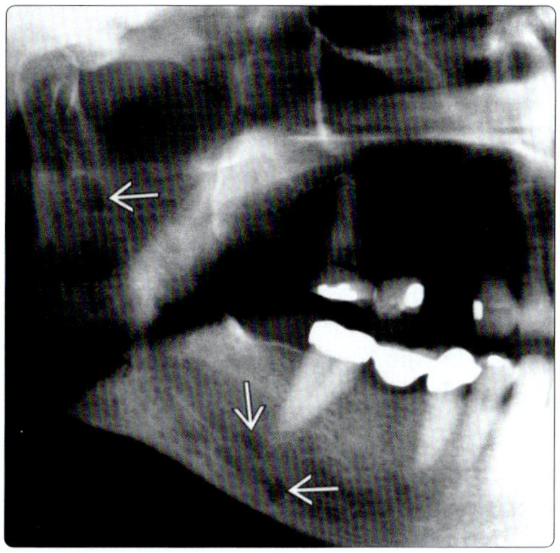

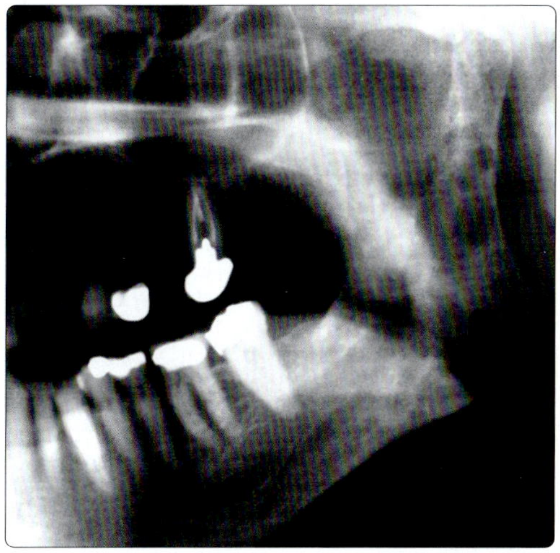

(Left) *Panoramic radiograph shows multiple well-defined, punched-out radiolucencies in the right mandibular body and ramus of an 80-year-old male patient with previously undiagnosed multiple myeloma.* **(Right)** *Panoramic radiograph in the same patient shows similar lesions in the left mandible. 20-30% of patients with multiple myeloma will develop jaw lesions, but it is rare that these are the 1st presentation of the disease.*

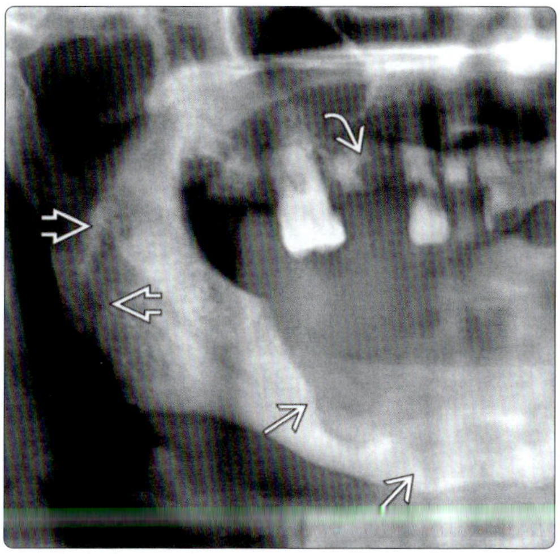

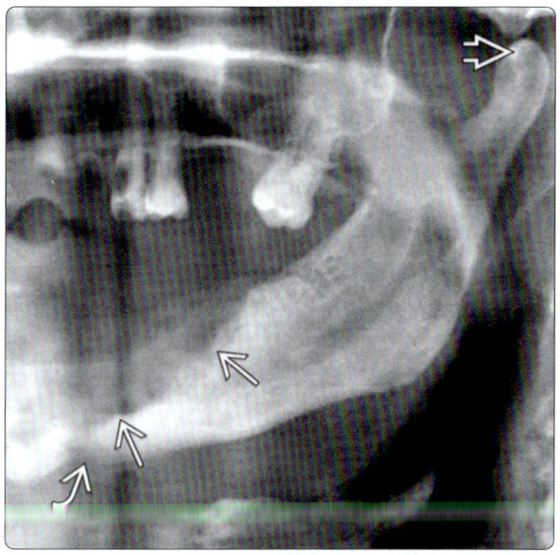

(Left) *Panoramic radiograph shows massive destruction of the anterior and body of the right mandible in a patient treated with bisphosphonates for multiple myeloma. Bisphosphonates are used to reduce morbidity of the disease and to aid in prevention of pathologic fractures. Note lytic lesions of multiple myeloma in the ramus and maxilla.* **(Right)** *Panoramic radiograph in the same patient shows similar destruction on the left side. Note pathologic fracture and small lesions in the condyle.*

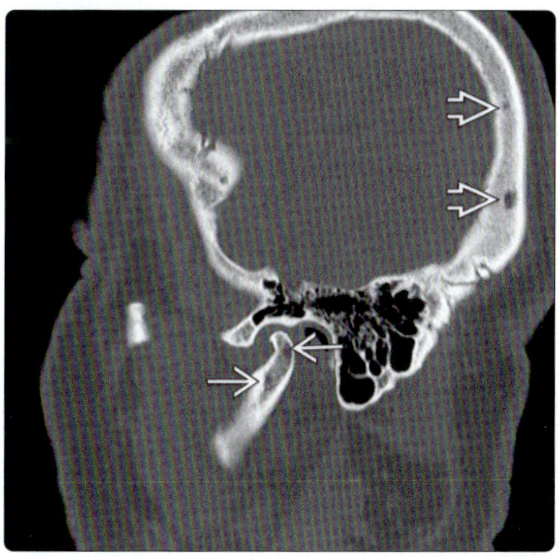

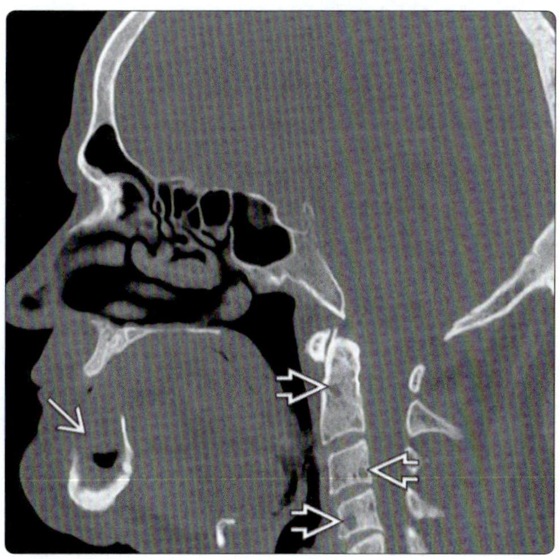

(Left) *Sagittal NECT through the left TMJ in the same patient shows small lesions of multiple myeloma in the head and neck of the condyle. Note also the well-defined lesions in the skull.* **(Right)** *Sagittal NECT in the same patient shows the large destructive lesion in the anterior mandible. Patients receiving IV zoledronic acid have the greatest risk for development of medication-related osteonecrosis of the jaws. Note numerous small round radiolucencies of multiple myeloma in the cervical spine.*

Ewing Sarcoma

KEY FACTS

TERMINOLOGY

- Abbreviations: Ewing sarcoma (ES)
- Synonyms: ES/primitive neuroectodermal tumor (ES/PNET); ES family of tumors (ESFT)

IMAGING

- Ill-defined, destructive radiolucency typical of malignancy
  - Bone destruction is not pathognomonic
- Mandible > maxilla (in one study, maxilla > mandible)
  - Mandible/maxilla > orbit > cranial bones > nasal cavity
  - Classic **onion peel** appearance rare in H&N
  - **Sun ray spicule** pattern occasionally
- Sinonasal ES rare: 20% of H&N
  - Maxillary sinus > ethmoid sinus > nasal cavity
  - Opacification of sinus with destruction of border
- CECT: Heterogeneously enhancing ± calcifications
- CBCT: Bone displacement/erosion/destruction
- T1WI isointense; T2WI/T1WI C+ hyperintense

TOP DIFFERENTIAL DIAGNOSES

- Osteosarcoma
- Rhabdomyosarcoma
- Olfactory neuroblastoma
- Mesenchymal chondrosarcoma
- Synovial sarcoma

CLINICAL ISSUES

- Swelling, pain, loosening of teeth, paresthesia, nasal obstruction, epistaxis
- Visual disturbance/loss; proptosis; eye swelling
- Usually 10-20 years; mean: 13; M > F
- H&N ES extremely rare
- 5-year survival: 54-69%
- Treatment: Surgery & radiation ± chemotherapy

DIAGNOSTIC CHECKLIST

- May not be possible to differentiate ES from other malignancies radiographically

(Left) *Panoramic reformat CBCT of an 8-year-old boy with a history of pain shows soft tissue density ➡ in the right maxillary sinus with loss of normal corticated boundary posteriorly ⇨. The oral surgeon noticed that follicle of 2nd molar ↪ went from 7 o'clock to 10 o'clock position in 2 weeks. (Courtesy M. Ahmad, DDS.)* **(Right)** *Axial CBCT in the same patient shows bowing of the wall ➡ of the maxillary sinus by Ewing sarcoma (ES). Unfortunately, the patient subsequently succumbed to the disease. (Courtesy M. Ahmad, DDS.)*

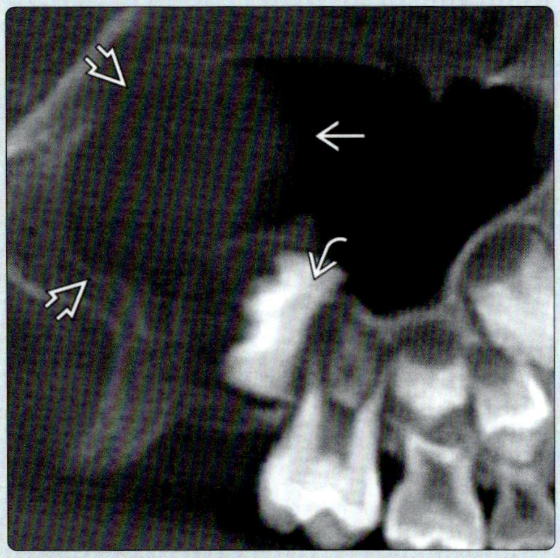

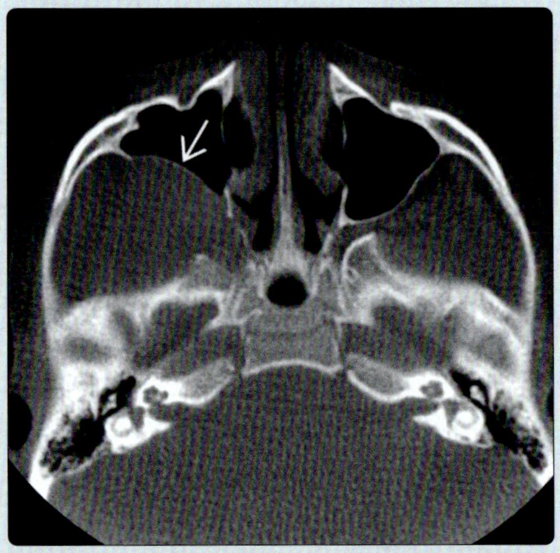

(Left) *Axial CECT bone window reveals ES of the mandibular ramus ➡ spreading into the masticator space ↪. The lesion is ill defined and has destroyed the mandibular ramus.* **(Right)** *Axial CECT soft tissue window in the same patient shows an invasive heterogeneous mass within the right masticator space ➡. The masticator space is a rare location for this malignant tumor.*

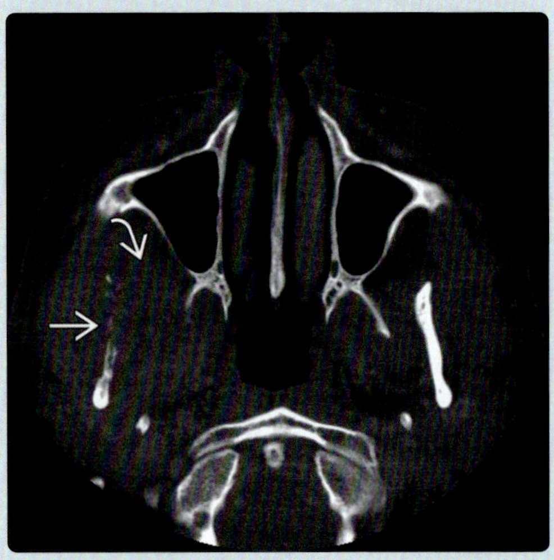

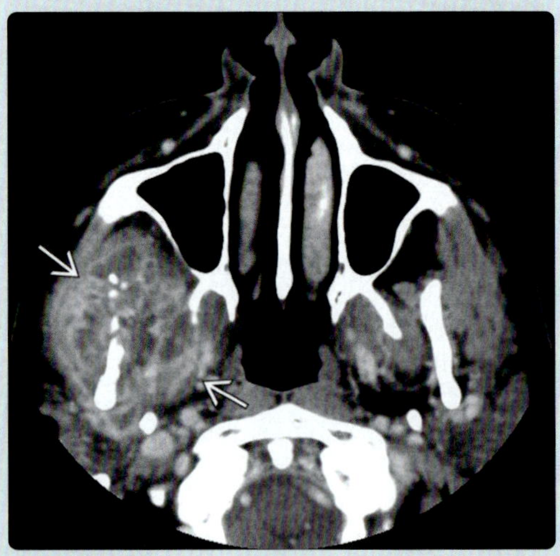

TERMINOLOGY

Abbreviations

- Ewing sarcoma (ES)

Synonyms

- ES/primitive neuroectodermal tumor (ES/PNET)
- ES family of tumors (ESFT)

Definitions

- Group of cancers including
  - Classic ES
  - PNET or primitive neuroepithelioma
  - Malignant small round cell tumor

IMAGING

General Features

- Best diagnostic clue
  - Bone destruction
    - Not pathognomonic
  - If sinus involvement: Opacification of sinus with destruction of border
    - Not pathognomonic
- Location
  - ES is rare, therefore preferential locations not well established
  - H&N ES = 3% of osseous ES (some reports range 1-9%)
    - Mandible > maxilla (in one study, maxilla > mandible)
      - Mandible/maxilla > orbit > cranial bones > nasal cavity
      - Studies too few and small for valid statistics
    - Sinonasal ES rare: 20% of H&N ES
      - Maxillary sinus > ethmoid sinus > nasal cavity
      - May involve more than 1 sinus and nasal cavity
      - Orbital extension reported with development of proptosis &/or diplopia
- Size
  - Varies, but often large on presentation if sinonasal
- Morphology
  - No distinct shape

Radiographic Findings

- Radiography
  - Ill-defined, destructive radiolucency typical of malignancy
  - Classic **onion skin** periosteal reaction rare in H&N
  - **Sun ray spicule** pattern occasionally

CT Findings

- CECT
  - Heterogeneously enhancing mass with soft tissue calcifications
  - Opacification of affected sinus
  - Bone displacement/erosion/destruction
- NECT or CBCT
  - Homogeneous mass causing displacement/erosion/destruction of osseous structures

MR Findings

- T1WI
  - Isointense
- T2WI
  - Hyperintense
- T1WI C+
  - Hyperintense
  - Inhomogeneous enhancement

Imaging Recommendations

- Best imaging tool
  - CT for bone involvement
  - MR for soft tissue involvement

DIFFERENTIAL DIAGNOSIS

Osteosarcoma

- Mandible more likely osteolytic
- Maxilla more likely osteogenic
- Widening of periodontal ligament space around involved teeth (Garrington sign)
- Both ES and osteosarcoma may have sun ray spicule appearance
- Need histopathology to differentiate from ES

Rhabdomyosarcoma

- Need histopathology to differentiate from ES
- ES may be positive for desmin, but diffusely positive for rhabdomyosarcoma
- ES is negative for myogenin and MyoD1, positive for rhabdomyosarcoma

Olfactory Neuroblastoma

- Need histopathology to differentiate from ES
- ES may have Homer Wright rosettes; olfactory neuroblastoma does not
- ES is 95% positive for CD99, olfactory neuroblastoma usually negative
- ES immunopositive for FLI-1, olfactory neuroblastoma negative for FLI-1

Mesenchymal Chondrosarcoma

- Young adults; extremely rare
- May have flocculent calcification
- Need histopathology to differentiate from ES

Synovial Sarcoma

- Rare in H&N
- Age: 15-35 years (median: 27 years)
- Up to 1/3 have punctate calcification, often at periphery but rarely more extensive
- Higher incidence of intratumoral hemorrhage
- Need histopathology to differentiate from ES

PATHOLOGY

General Features

- Etiology
  - Derived from pluripotential neuroectodermal cells
- Genetics
  - Translocation involving *EWSR1* at 22q12
    - Various translocations of chromosomes 11 and 22, t(11:22)(q24;q12)
  - Gene fusions, most commonly *EWS* to *ETS* family genes

Microscopic Features

- Small round cells; neuroendocrine type

- Positive for vimentin, CD99
- Positive focally for EMA

CLINICAL ISSUES

Presentation

- Most common signs/symptoms
  - Depends upon site and size
    - Swelling
    - Pain
    - In mandible
      - Loosening of teeth
      - Otitis media
      - Paresthesia
    - In sinonasal
      - Facial swelling
      - Nasal obstruction
      - Epistaxis
      - Visual disturbance/loss
      - Proptosis
      - Eye swelling
- Other signs/symptoms
  - In sinonasal
    - Rhinorrhea
    - Anosmia
    - Headache
    - Dizziness

Demographics

- Age
  - 8-44 years, most < 20
    - 26 cases total in world literature
    - Unusual over 30 years
- Gender
  - M > F (slight preponderance)
- Ethnicity
  - More common in USA Caucasians
- Epidemiology
  - Sinonasal ES extremely rare
  - ES 4-6% of all primary malignant tumors of bone
    - 2nd most common primary malignant tumor of bone in children 10-15 years
    - 1-9% of ES in H&N
  - ES 1 per million in USA population
    - Incidence between ages 10-19 years is 9-10 per million
    - More common in males
  - 1 case of extraskeletal metastasis to right ethmoid sinus from primary skeletal ES

Natural History & Prognosis

- 5-year survival: 54-69%
  - Depends on therapy and whether or not ES is localized
  - Survival directly related to tumor size and inversely to time of delay in seeking treatment
- 3-year event-free survival ~ 2x better for patients < 15 years than for patients > 15 years
- Sinonasal ES in patients <15 years may be 55%

Treatment

- Options, risks, complications
  - Surgery standard
    - Usually augmented by radiation &/or chemotherapy
  - Proton beam therapy has been suggested for sinonasal ES
    - Insufficient evidence to support or refute
  - Complications from radiation therapy
    - Osseous hypoplasia
    - Dental hypoplasia and malformation
      - Aplasia of some teeth
    - Xerostomia
    - Xerophthalmia
    - Cataracts
    - 2nd malignancy
  - Interval-compressed chemotherapy more effective without increase in toxicity
  - High percentage become resistant to chemotherapy
  - Vincristine, doxorubicin, and cyclophosphamide alternating with ifosfamide and etoposide

DIAGNOSTIC CHECKLIST

Consider

- May not be possible to differentiate ES from other malignancies radiographically
- Diagnosis requires histological, molecular, and genetic investigation

SELECTED REFERENCES

1. Leroy R et al: Proton Therapy in Children: A Systematic Review of Clinical Effectiveness in 15 Pediatric Cancers. Int J Radiat Oncol Biol Phys. 95(1):267-78, 2016
2. Qureshi SS et al: Local therapy in non-metastatic primary Ewing sarcoma of the mandible and maxilla in children. Int J Oral Maxillofac Surg. 45(8):938-44, 2016
3. Grevener K et al: Management and Outcome of Ewing Sarcoma of the Head and Neck. Pediatr Blood Cancer. ePub, 2015
4. Negru ME et al: Primary Ewing's sarcoma of the sinonasal tract, eroding the ethmoid and sphenoid sinus with intracranial extension: A rare case report. Mol Clin Oncol. 3(4):807-810, 2015
5. Ahmed AA et al: Therapy resistance mechanisms in Ewing's sarcoma family tumors. Cancer Chemother Pharmacol. 73(4):657-63, 2014
6. Li M et al: Primary Ewing's sarcoma of the ethmoid sinus with intracranial and orbital extension: case report and literature review. Am J Otolaryngol. 34(5):563-8, 2013
7. Yamaoka M et al: Multidisciplinary therapy including proton beam radiotherapy for a Ewing sarcoma family tumor of maxillary sinus in a 4-year-old girl. Head Neck. 35(12):E386-90, 2013
8. Rombi B et al: Proton radiotherapy for pediatric Ewing's sarcoma: initial clinical outcomes. Int J Radiat Oncol Biol Phys. 82(3):1142-8, 2012
9. Tanboon J et al: Primary intracranial Ewing sarcoma with an unusually aggressive course: a case report and review of the literature. Neuropathology. 32(3):293-300, 2012
10. Yeshvanth SK et al: Rare case of extraskeletal Ewings sarcoma of the sinonasal tract. J Cancer Res Ther. 8(1):142-4, 2012
11. Davido N et al: Case of Ewing's sarcoma misdiagnosed as a periapical lesion of maxillary incisor. J Endod. 37(2):259-64, 2011
12. Gradoni P et al: Clinical outcomes of rhabdomyosarcoma and Ewing's sarcoma of the head and neck in children. Auris Nasus Larynx. 38(4):480-6, 2011
13. Hayes SM et al: Solitary extra-skeletal sinonasal metastasis from a primary skeletal Ewing's sarcoma. J Laryngol Otol. 125(8):861-4, 2011

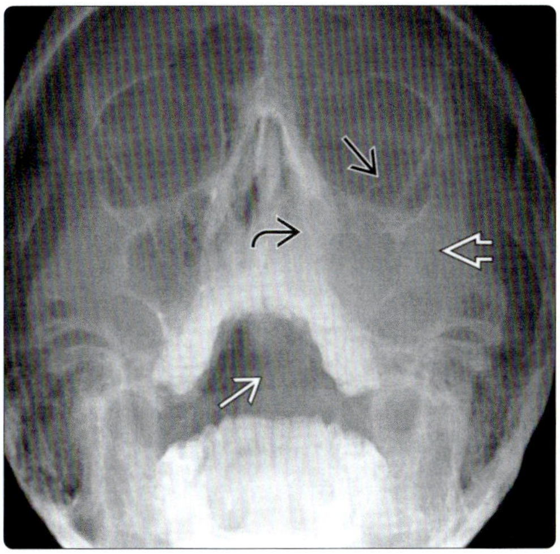

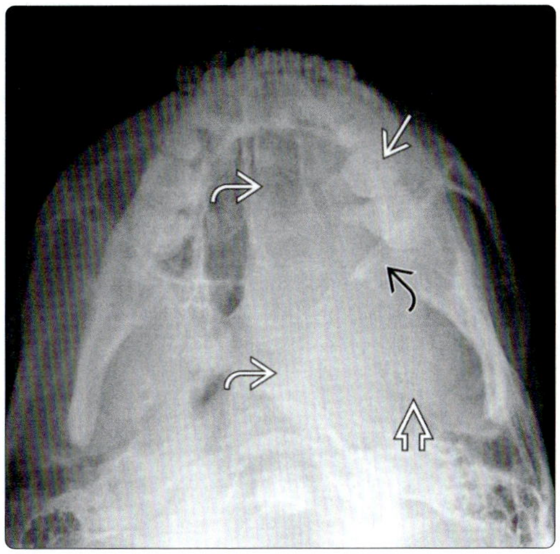

(Left) *Occipitomental radiograph shows a homogeneous radiopacity projecting over the left maxillary sinus extending inferiorly into the oropharynx . The medial wall of the left maxillary sinus is indistinct with lifting of the roof of the sinus . (Courtesy T. Moritani, MD.)* **(Right)** *Axial radiograph in the same patient shows the radiopacity projecting over left maxillary sinus , nasal & pharyngeal airway , and left skull base . Posterior wall of left maxillary sinus is indistinct. (Courtesy T. Moritani, MD.)*

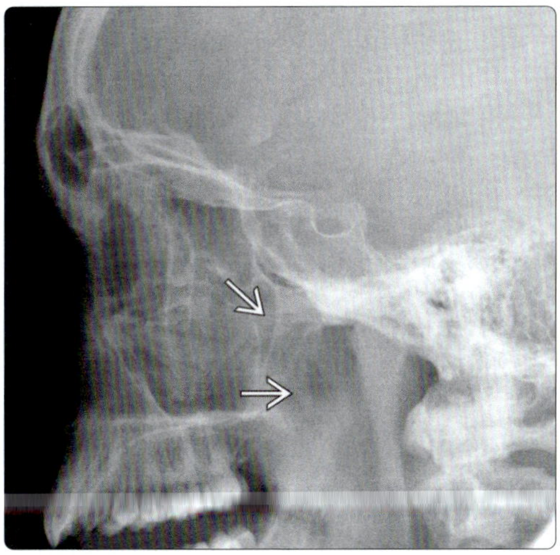

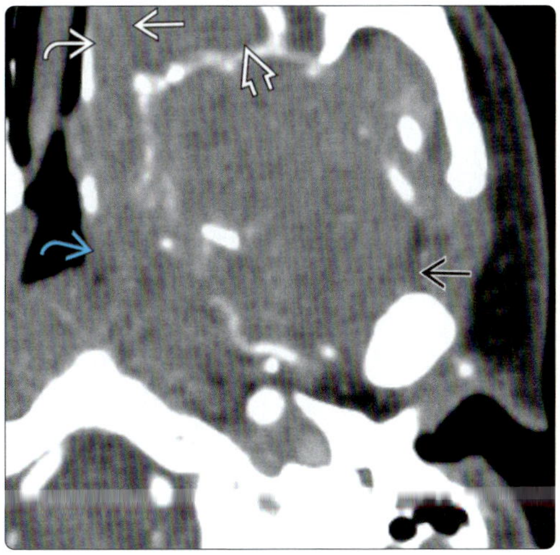

(Left) *Lateral skull radiograph in the same patient shows increased radiopacity of the nasopharyngeal area due to the mass . (Courtesy T. Moritani, MD.)* **(Right)** *Axial CECT soft tissue window shows a somewhat heterogeneous mass occupying the left maxillary sinus and nasal fossa , extending to the mandibular ramus and into the pharynx . There is disruption of the osseous borders of the left maxillary sinus . (Courtesy T. Moritani, MD.)*

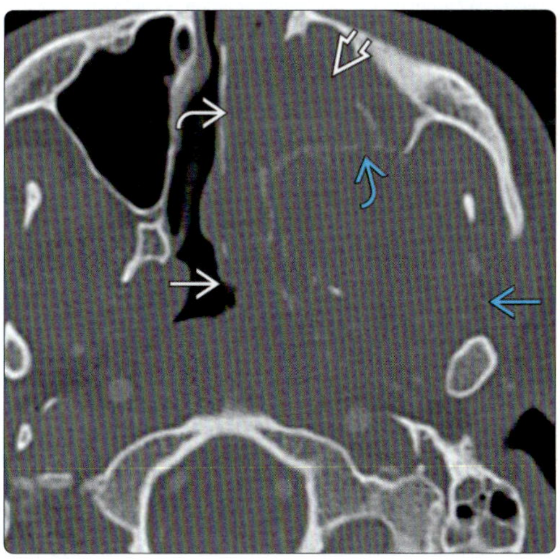

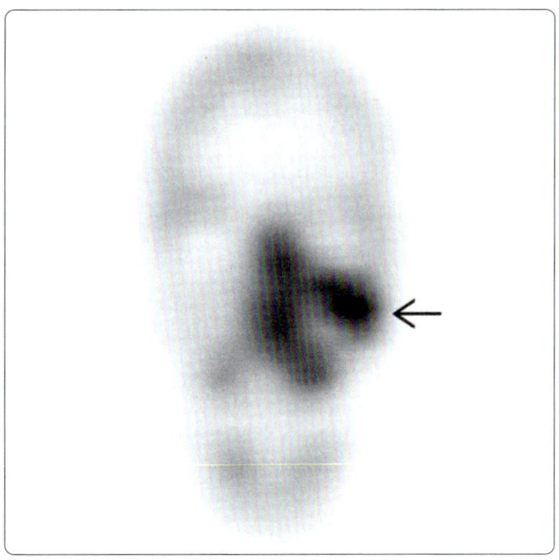

(Left) *Axial CECT bone window (same patient) shows a homogeneous mass occupying the left maxillary sinus and nasal fossa , extending to the mandibular ramus and into the pharynx . There is disruption of the osseous borders of the left maxillary sinus . (Courtesy T. Moritani, MD.)* **(Right)** *Tc-99m MDP image in the same patient shows active uptake in the left maxilla and nasal fossa, corresponding to location of mass seen on CT images. (Courtesy T. Moritani, MD.)*

Leukemia

KEY FACTS

TERMINOLOGY

- Synonyms: Acute lymphoblastic leukemia (ALL), acute nonlymphoblastic leukemia (ANL), chronic myelocytic leukemia (CML), chronic lymphocytic leukemia (CLL)
- Definition: Diverse spectrum of stem cell hematopoietic malignancies

IMAGING

- Acute: Lytic, blastic, or mixed lesion with ill-defined margins; **may simulate periodontal disease or periapical osteitis**
  - Hair on end pattern of new bone growth
  - Destruction of bone crypts of developing teeth
- Chronic: Osteolytic lesions < 3%
  - Foci of leukemic cells behaves like localized malignancy **(chloromas); may simulate periapical inflammatory lesions**
- Best imaging tool: Panoramic or intraoral radiographs, CBCT, bone CT, nuclear medicine
- Radiographically detectable lesions in 50-70% of children and < 10% of adults; radiologic signs more rare in chronic leukemia

TOP DIFFERENTIAL DIAGNOSES

- Neuroblastoma
- Lymphoma
- Metabolic disorders: Osteoporosis, osteopenia

CLINICAL ISSUES

- Presentation
  - Acute: Sudden onset of malaise, weakness, fever, bone pain, pallor, spontaneous bleeding
  - Chronic: Usually few or no symptoms

DIAGNOSTIC CHECKLIST

- **May simulate periodontal disease and periapical inflammatory lesions**
- **Radiographic signs may signal relapse**

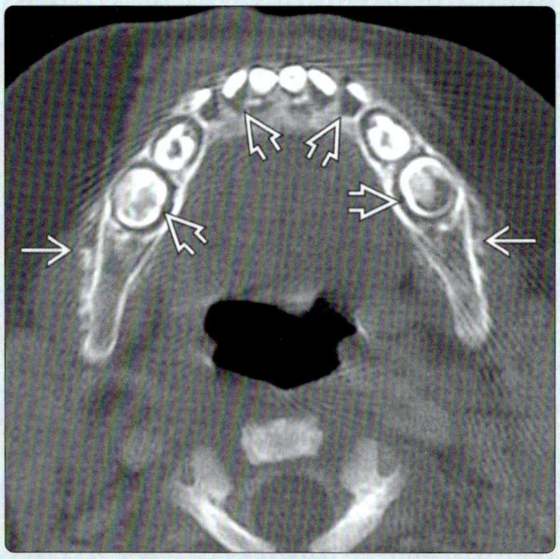
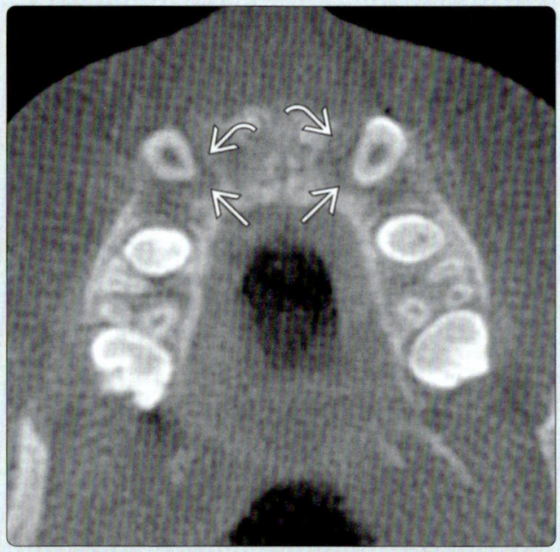

(Left) *Axial bone CT of the mandible of a young child shows loss of lamina dura and widened periodontal ligament spaces ➔. Diffuse osseous radiolucency is also evident with hair on end pattern of new bone formation ➔.* **(Right)** *Axial CBCT of an 11-year-old boy presenting for orthodontic treatment shows alveolar bone loss from leukemia ➔, which simulates periodontal disease not usually present in children. The lamina dura is not visualized, and the periodontal ligament space is widened ➔. (Courtesy M. Noujeim, DDS.)*

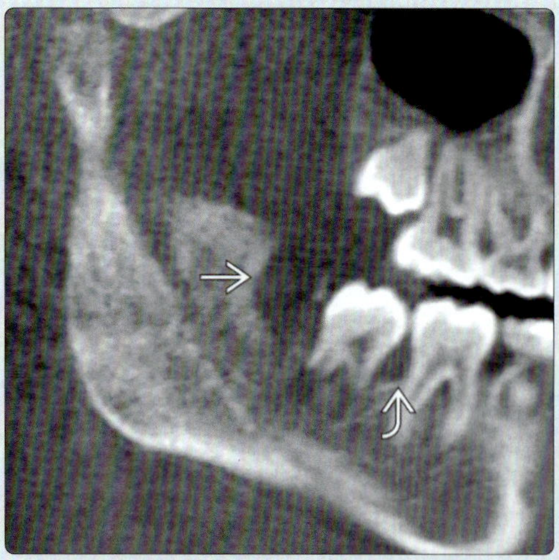
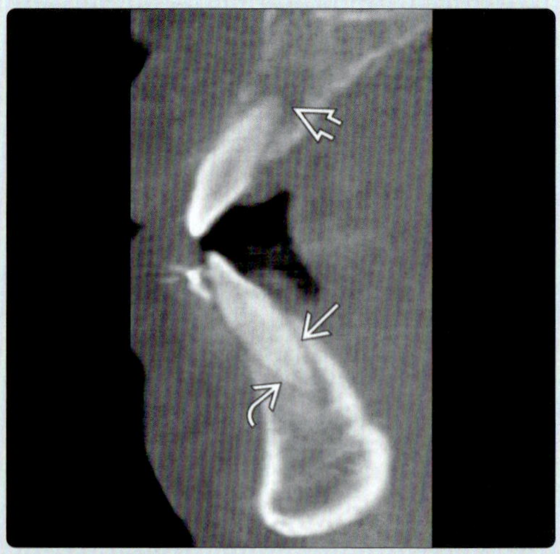

(Left) *Panoramic CBCT reformat of same patient shows minimally corticated tooth follicle displaced occlusally ➔. Crestal alveolar bone loss is also present ➔ simulating periodontal disease. (Courtesy M. Noujeim, DDS.)* **(Right)** *Cross section CBCT of same patient shows a widened periodontal ligament space ➔ and minimal lamina dura ➔. These findings are also found during active orthodontic treatment. Chloroma mimics a periapical inflammatory lesion at maxillary incisor apex ➔. (Courtesy M. Noujeim, DDS.)*

TERMINOLOGY

Synonyms

- Acute lymphoblastic leukemia (ALL), acute nonlymphoblastic leukemia (ANL), chronic myelocytic leukemia (CML), chronic lymphocytic leukemia (CLL)

Definitions

- Diverse spectrum of stem cell hematopoietic malignancies

IMAGING

General Features

- Best diagnostic clue
  - Radiographically detectable lesions in 50-70% of children and < 10% of adults; radiologic signs more rare in chronic leukemia
  - Acute: Lytic, blastic, or mixed lesion with ill-defined margins
    - **Effaced dental lamina dura with widened periodontal ligament spaces**
    - Premature loss of deciduous teeth
    - Destruction of bone crypts of developing teeth
  - Chronic: Osteolytic lesions < 3%
    - Foci of leukemic cells behaves like localized malignancy **(chloromas); may simulate periapical inflammatory lesions**

CT Findings

- Bone CT
  - Acute: Ill-defined margins with lytic, blastic, or mixed lesions; **may simulate periodontal disease**
    - Diffuse osteopenia; similar appearance to osteoporosis/osteopenia
    - Effacement of dental lamina dura and dental follicle cortices; widened periodontal ligament spaces
      - May simulate rarefying periapical osteitis and occlusal displacement of tooth follicles
    - **Hair on end** pattern of new bone growth
  - Chronic: < 3% have lytic lesions of bone, usually in femur and humerus

Imaging Recommendations

- Best imaging tool
  - Panoramic or intraoral radiographs, CBCT, bone CT, nuclear medicine

DIFFERENTIAL DIAGNOSIS

Neuroblastoma

- Primary cases: Very rare in jaws
- Metastatic cases: Jaw involvement primarily in mandibular molar area
  - May have rapid growth/swelling with moderate pain
  - One of most common childhood malignancies

Lymphoma

- Developing teeth may be displaced occlusally
- Difficult to distinguish from periapical rarefying osteitis
- Lesions spread along fat layers in soft tissue spaces and along bone surfaces

Metabolic Disorders

- Osteoporosis or osteopenia
  - Generalized osseous rarefaction and thin cortices

PATHOLOGY

General Features

- Genetics
  - Nonrandom chromosomal abnormalities are common
- Acute: Malignant blast cells displace normal marrow cells
  - Extend into peripheral blood circulation with spread to liver, spleen, lymph nodes, CNS, kidneys, and gonads
- Chronic: Massive appearance of mature lymphocytes in blood, bone marrow, and lymphoid organs

Staging, Grading, & Classification

- Based on clinical behavioral and histopathological criteria

CLINICAL ISSUES

Presentation

- Most common signs/symptoms
  - Acute: Sudden onset of malaise, weakness, fever, bone pain, pallor, spontaneous bleeding
    - Hepatomegaly, splenomegaly, lymphadenopathy
    - Oral symptoms commonly absent but variable (8-18% reported), e.g., petechiae, ulceration, and loose teeth; gingival enlargement most common in myelomonocytic type
  - Chronic: Usually few or no symptoms
- Other signs/symptoms
  - Rarely, pathologic mandibular fractures (0.47%)

Demographics

- Age
  - ALL (3-5 years), ANL (all ages), CML (> 10 years; median is 45 years), CLL (median is 60 years in 75% of cases)
- Gender
  - No gender predilection in ALL, ANL, or CML
  - M:F ratio: 2-3:1 in CLL

Treatment

- Chemotherapy ± bone marrow transplantation

DIAGNOSTIC CHECKLIST

Image Interpretation Pearls

- May simulate periodontal disease and periapical inflammatory lesions
- Radiographic signs may signal relapse

SELECTED REFERENCES

1. Guan G et al: Oral manifestations as an early clinical sign of acute myeloid leukaemia: a case report. Aust Dent J. 60(1):123-7, 2015
2. Zimmermann C et al: Dental treatment in patients with leukemia. J Oncol. 2015:571739, 2015
3. Padmini C et al: Oral and dental considerations in pediatric leukemic patient. ISRN Hematol. 2014:895721, 2014
4. Ali R et al: Acute lymphoblastic leukaemia: an unusual radiological presentation. Dentomaxillofac Radiol. 38(5):289-91, 2009
5. McKenna SJ: Leukemia. Oral Surg Oral Med Oral Pathol Oral Radiol Endod. 89(2):137-9, 2000

Mandible-Maxilla Central Giant Cell Granuloma

KEY FACTS

TERMINOLOGY

- Definition: Reactive intraosseous lesion of jaws

IMAGING

- General imaging findings
  - **Expansile lesion**, often poorly corticated periphery
  - Loculated with **granular, wispy septa**
  - **Mandible** > maxilla: **Anterior** to 1st molar
  - Root resorption
- Bone CT findings
  - Undulating, expansile margin
  - "Flow-around" of expanded border over original cortex
  - Septations at **right angle** to periphery
  - Variable granular bone deposits internally
- Best imaging tool: CECT

TOP DIFFERENTIAL DIAGNOSES

- Ameloblastoma
- Odontogenic myxoma
- Aneurysmal bone cyst
- Brown tumor of hyperparathyroidism
- Cherubism

PATHOLOGY

- Unknown etiology
  - Reactive granuloma vs. benign neoplasm
- Spectrum of behavior: Aggressive vs. nonaggressive
  - **Recurrence common with aggressive lesion**

CLINICAL ISSUES

- Presentation: **Swelling**, ± pain
- Age < 30 years, F > M
- Surgical excision treatment of choice: Calcitonin, intralesional steroids may be adjuncts

DIAGNOSTIC CHECKLIST

- Report cortical perforation
- Root resorption = sign of ↑ aggressiveness
- Test for hyperparathyroidism when CGCG diagnosed

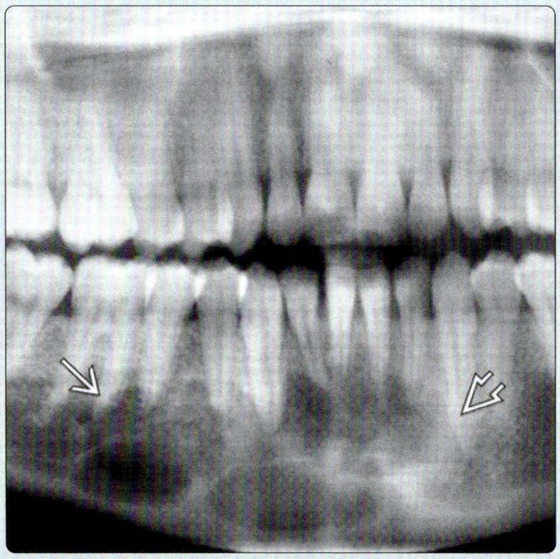

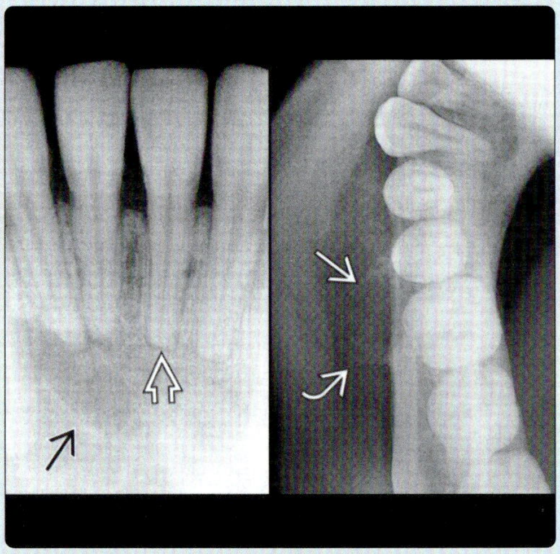

(Left) *Cropped panoramic radiograph shows a faintly corticated, multilocular lesion extending from the mandibular right 1st molar to the left canine. Note the inability to appreciate any expansion in this view.* **(Right)** *Periapical radiograph of the same patient shows faint septa and mild external root resorption. The occlusal radiograph, though subtle, shows prominent buccal expansion with wispy septa internally.*

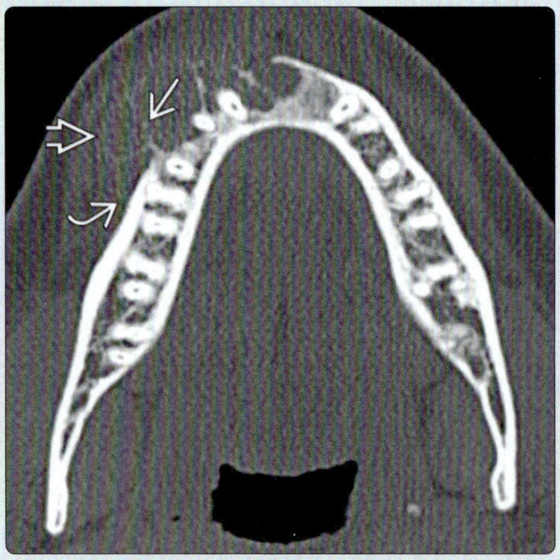

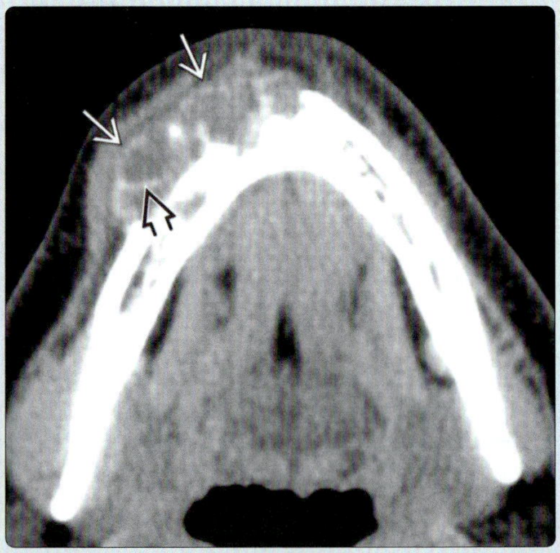

(Left) *Axial bone CT slice near the apices of the teeth of the same patient better demonstrates the granular, wispy septa within the lesion. Notice that the peripheral cortex is very faint and grainy. "Flow-around" of the expanded lesion border over the normal cortex is an aggressive feature.* **(Right)** *Axial NECT of the same patient shows the undulating, expansile, corticated periphery. Note the septa oriented at right angle to the outer corticated border, which is a characteristic feature of CGCG.*

TERMINOLOGY

Abbreviations

- Central giant cell granuloma (CGCG)

Synonyms

- Giant cell reparative granuloma

Definitions

- Reactive lesion of jaws with benign tumor-like behavior

IMAGING

General Features

- Best diagnostic clue
  - Multilocular lesion with **granular, wispy septa**
- Location
  - **Mandible** > maxilla
    - Most commonly **anterior** to 1st molar
    - May **extend across midline**
- Size
  - **Expansile**: May become large before detection

Imaging Recommendations

- Best imaging tool
  - CECT
- Protocol advice
  - Thin-section CECT
  - Bone CT shows extent and internal characteristics

Radiographic Findings

- Radiography
  - Unilocular or multilocular when large
  - Periphery well defined but **poorly corticated**
  - Undulating, expanded margins
  - **Wispy, faint septa** or **granular bone deposits**
  - **Root resorption** seen in ~ 1/3 of lesions
  - Tooth displacement common

CT Findings

- CECT
  - May see soft tissue involvement
  - Mild enhancement internally
- Bone CT/CBCT
  - Cortical expansion creates undulations
  - "Flow-around" of expanded border over original cortex
  - **Septa form at right angles** to outer boundaries
  - Varying amounts of granular bone internally, may form irregular septations

MR Findings

- T1/T2WI
  - Hypo- to isointense
- T1WI C+
  - Heterogeneous enhancement

DIFFERENTIAL DIAGNOSIS

Ameloblastoma

- Predominately 3rd-5th decade (**older than CGCG**)
- More likely to present posteriorly
- **Septations** tend to be **coarser than CGCG**
- Periphery more well corticated

Odontogenic Myxoma

- Older average age at presentation
- See **straighter and sharper septa**
- Generally less expansile than CGCG

Aneurysmal Bone Cyst

- Majority of lesions in posterior mandible
- Same radiographic characteristics as CGCG
- CT: Low density of large vascular spaces
- MR: **Fluid-fluid levels** on T2 sequence

Brown Tumor of Hyperparathyroidism

- Radiographic appearance often identical to CGCG
- Occurs in older patient than true CGCG
- Patients with diagnosis of CGCG histologically should be routinely tested for **hyperparathyroidism**

Cherubism

- Radiographic pattern may be identical to CGCG
- **Bilateral lesions** with epicenter posteriorly
- Autosomal dominant condition; young children

PATHOLOGY

General Features

- Etiology
  - Controversy over reactive lesion vs. benign neoplasm
    - Histopathology overlaps with giant cell tumor
- Associated abnormalities
  - Giant cell granulomas of jaws found in cherubism, Noonan syndrome, & neurofibromatosis type 1

Staging, Grading, & Classification

- 2 types considered: Aggressive vs. nonaggressive
- Aggressive: Rapid growth, root/cortical resorption
  - **↑ risk of recurrence**

Microscopic Features

- Stroma cellular to loose; spindle or ovoid fibroblasts
- Heterogeneous **clumps of multinucleated giant cells**
- Hemorrhage and osteoid; no necrosis

CLINICAL ISSUES

Presentation

- Most common signs/symptoms
  - Asymptomatic swelling; can have pain

Demographics

- Age
  - Wide range but majority < 30 years old; F:M = 2:1

Natural History & Prognosis

- High recurrence rate (11-20%)

Treatment

- Surgical excision: Treatment of choice
- Pharmacologic: Intralesional steroid injection, systemic calcitonin, α-interferon 2a, denosumab

SELECTED REFERENCES

1. Schreuder WH et al: Alternative pharmacologic therapy for aggressive central giant cell granuloma: denosumab. J Oral Maxillofac Surg. 72(7):1301-9, 2014

(Left) *Cropped panoramic radiograph in the maxillary right premolar and canine region shows that the periphery of this CGCG is not clearly corticated; however, a scalloped border extends into the maxillary sinus. Faint granular bone deposits, forming irregular, wispy septa, are seen internally.* **(Right)** *Occlusal radiograph of the same patient shows faint, wispy internal septa with 2 straight septa extending perpendicular to the periphery. The noncorticated periphery is also seen.*

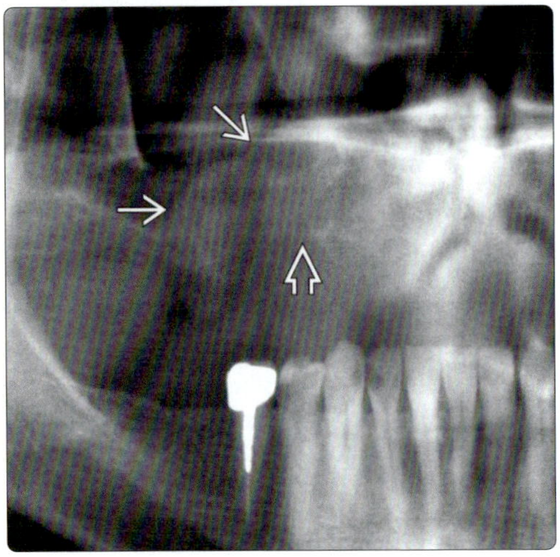

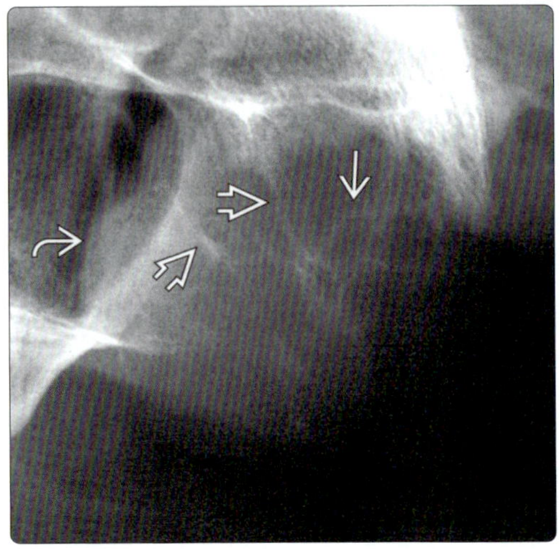

(Left) *Cropped panoramic radiograph of the left posterior mandible shows a CGCG that developed after extraction of a 3rd molar. The periphery is irregular but well defined. Faint, granular internal structure is seen. The molars are displaced anteriorly.* **(Right)** *Axial CECT, bone window, of the same patient shows prominent expansion of the mandible with undulating, expanded margins. Loculations are seen internally; however, the septa are not as coarse or defined as in an ameloblastoma.*

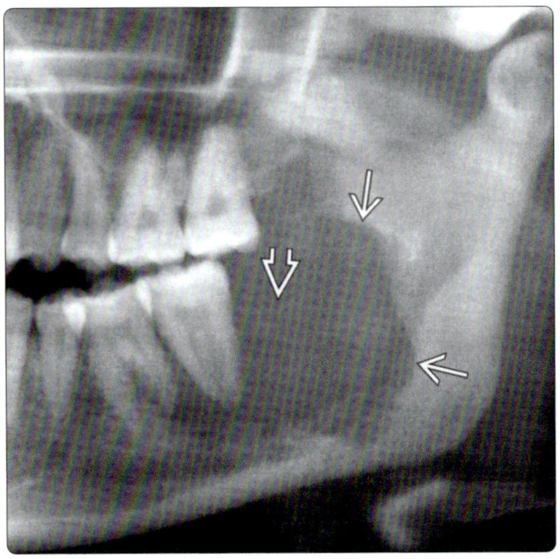

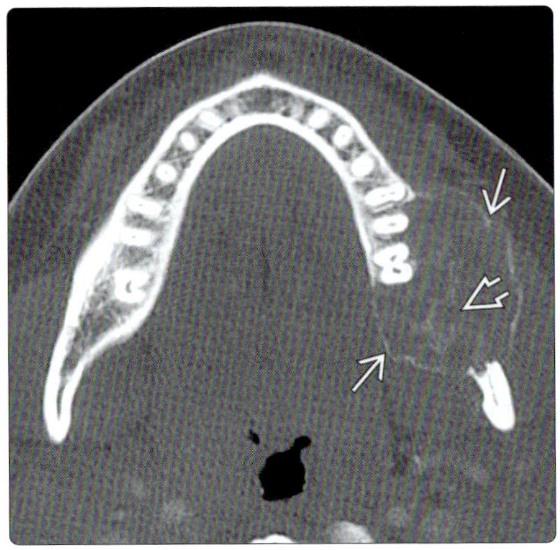

(Left) *Axial bone CT of a CGCG in the anterior mandible of a 15-year-old girl shows that the expanded cortices are faint and irregular.* **(Right)** *Axial bone CT of the same patient 4 months later, with no treatment, shows that the lesion has grown considerably and crossed the mandibular midline. Septa are extending at right angles from the lesion periphery. Irregular bone deposits are also seen internally. The buccal cortex is still faint and "flows-around" the normal cortex. (Courtesy C. Schatz, MD.)*

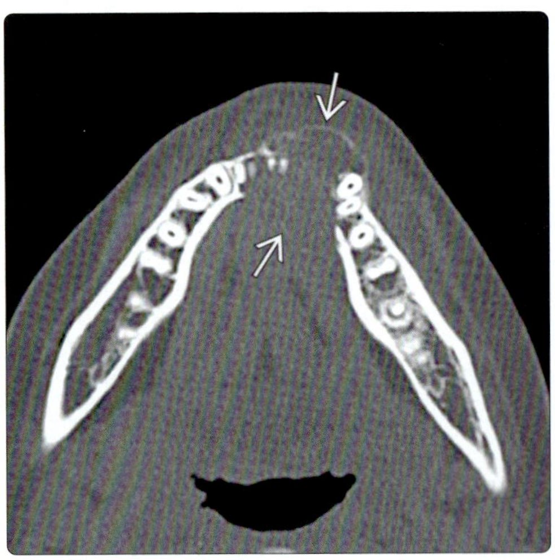

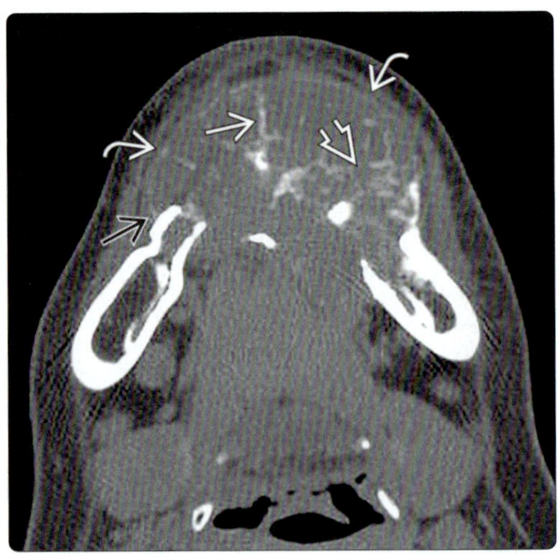

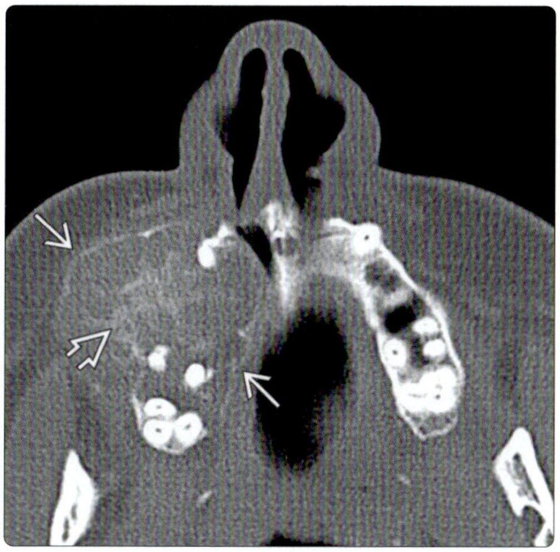

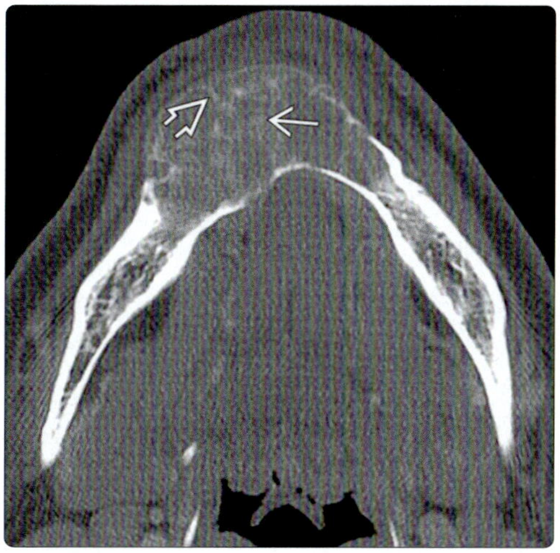

(Left) *Axial CECT, bone window, shows a very expansile CGCG in the right maxilla. The periphery is wispy and undulating, and there are granular bone formations internally.* **(Right)** *Axial bone CT shows a large CGCG extending across the mandibular midline. Multiple islands of granular bone are seen internally. One short septum is seen extending perpendicular from the buccal cortex.*

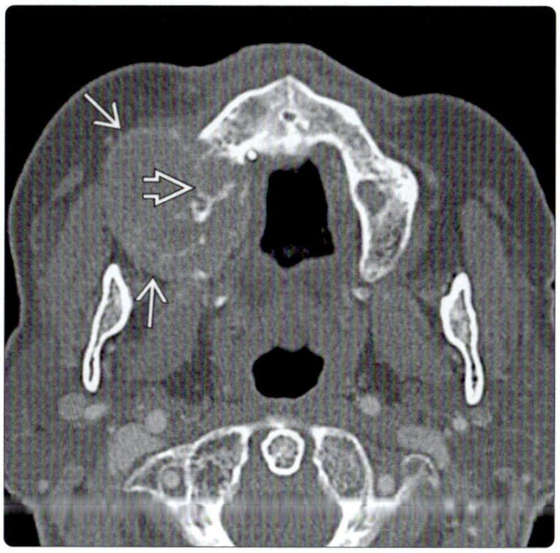

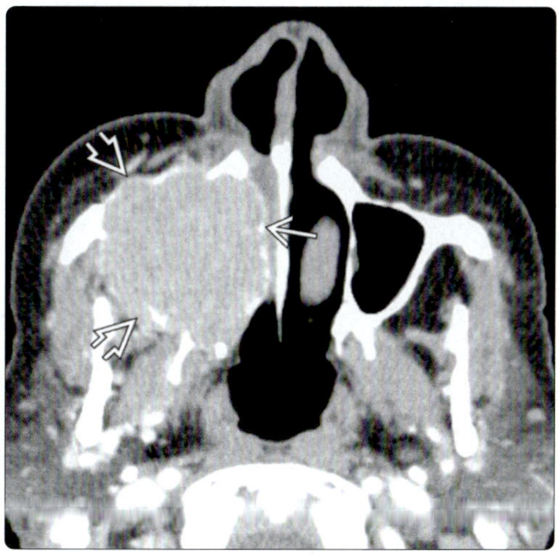

(Left) *Axial CECT, bone window, shows a large, expansile lesion in the right maxilla. The periphery is not well corticated but the surrounding fat planes are preserved. Some irregular internal septa are seen within the lesion.* **(Right)** *Axial CECT through the maxillary sinus of the same patient shows the lesion displacing the lateral wall of the nose. The anterior and posterolateral walls of the maxillary sinus are also resorbed and expanded. There is mild contrast enhancement of the lesion.*

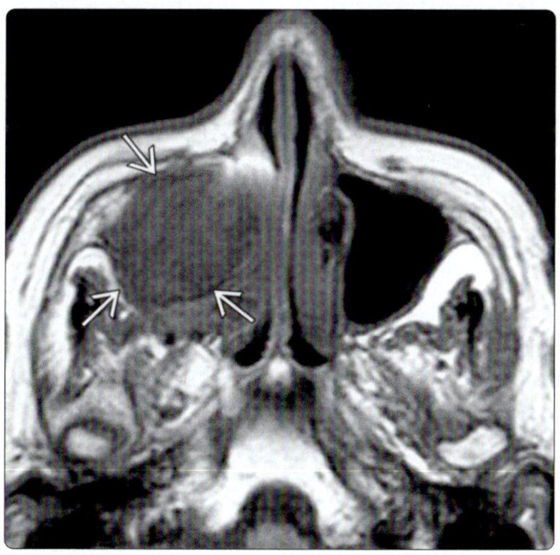

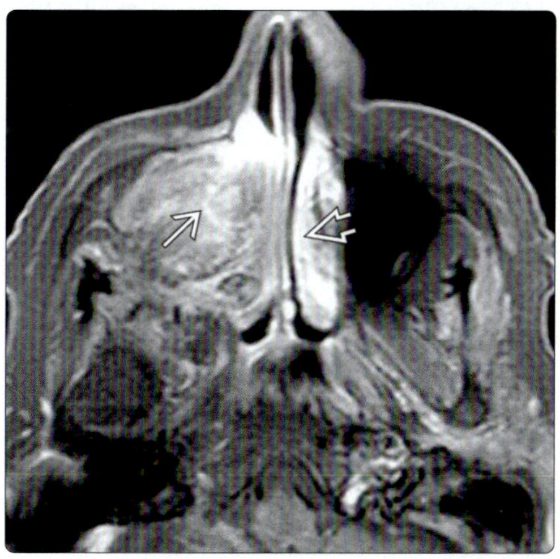

(Left) *Axial T1WI MR of the same patient shows that the lesion has a low to isointense internal signal. The periphery is well defined.* **(Right)** *Axial T1WI C+ FS MR of the same patient shows heterogeneous internal enhancement of the lesion, similar to the signal from the left inferior concha.*

Langerhans Histiocytosis

KEY FACTS

TERMINOLOGY

- Langerhans cell histiocytosis (LCH): Group of lesions affecting reticuloendothelial system and characterized by proliferation of **Langerhans cells**

IMAGING

- Well-defined or punched-out **radiolucency without corticated border**
- Bone lesions found in **skull**, femur, jaws, ribs, long bones, vertebrae, and pelvis
- **Mandible** > maxilla; posterior > anterior
- Bone may appear scooped out
- Teeth may appear to be floating
- Periosteal reaction parallel to cortex may be evident
- Skull lesions may be irregular (geographic skull)

TOP DIFFERENTIAL DIAGNOSES

- Localized aggressive periodontitis
- Squamous cell carcinoma
- Osteomyelitis
- Metastasis

PATHOLOGY

- Acute disseminated (Letterer-Siwe disease): Multiple organ involvement
- Chronic disseminated (Hand-Schüller-Christian): Triad of multiple bone lesions, diabetes insipidus, exophthalmos
- Chronic localized form (eosinophilic granuloma): Monostotic or polyostotic bone lesions without visceral involvement

CLINICAL ISSUES

- Mobility of teeth; intraoral mass/swelling; pain
- Overall prognosis related to age at onset and degree of organ dysfunction

DIAGNOSTIC CHECKLIST

- Lesions of multiple myeloma (MM) are also described as punched out, but MM occurs in much older age group

(Left) *Periapical radiograph shows a lesion of eosinophilic granuloma (EG) ➡, the localized form of Langerhans cell histiocytosis (LCH), appearing similar to localized aggressive periodontitis. Note total loss of alveolar crest and interproximal bone.* **(Right)** *Lateral oblique radiograph shows extensive bone loss in the posterior mandible ➡ in a patient with EG. Note the 1st molar ➡ appears to be floating. The radiolucencies at the apices ➡ of the 2nd molar are the follicles of the developing tooth roots.*

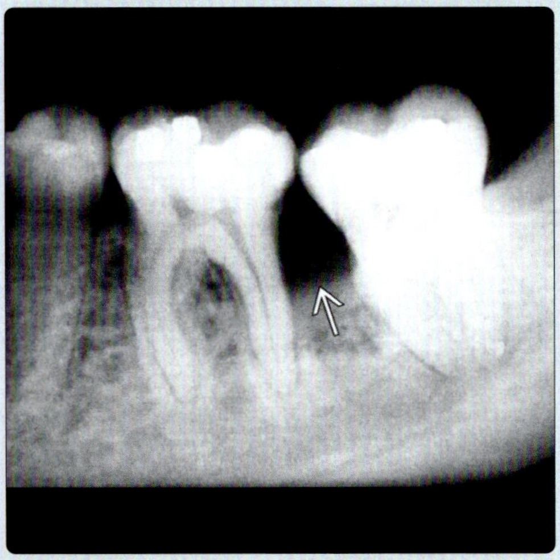

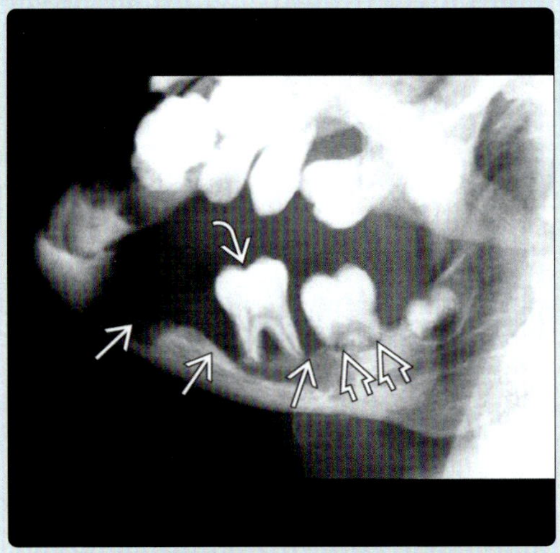

(Left) *Panoramic radiograph shows a fairly well-defined, radiolucent lesion ➡ of EG distal to the developing mandibular right 3rd molar. Note that the external oblique ridge ➡ is intact, which helps differentiate from pericoronitis or periodontal disease.* **(Right)** *Panoramic radiograph shows a large, irregular lytic lesion ➡ in the left posterior mandible. Note how the lesion curves back ➡ to meet the crest anteriorly, giving a somewhat scooped-out appearance typical of bone loss in EG.*

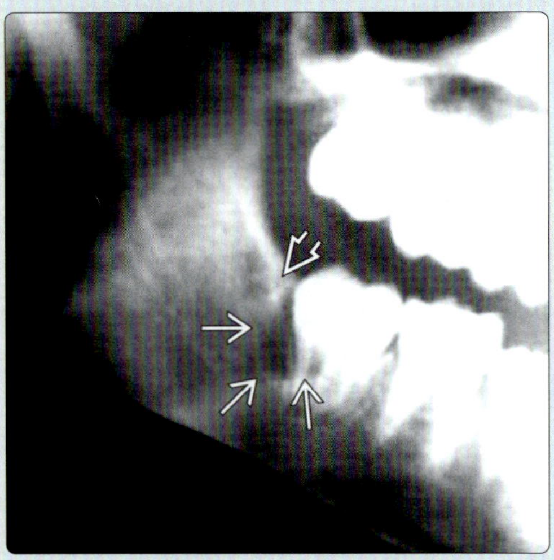

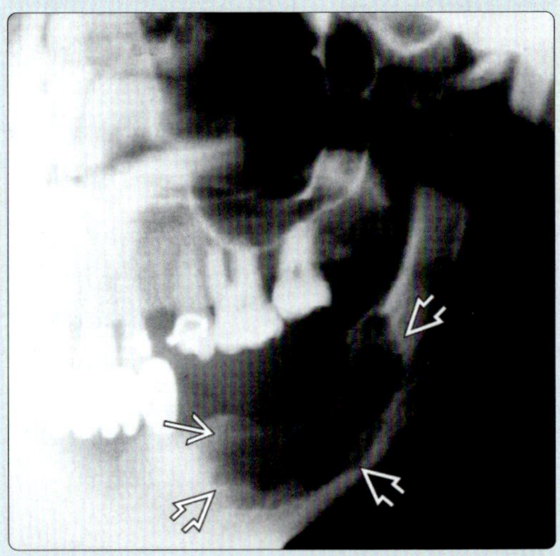

TERMINOLOGY

Abbreviations

- Langerhans cell histiocytosis (LCH)

Synonyms

- Histiocytosis X, idiopathic histiocytosis, Langerhans cell disease, Langerhans cell granulomatosis, Langerhans cell granuloma, eosinophilic granuloma (EG)

Definitions

- Group of lesions affecting reticuloendothelial system and characterized by proliferation of Langerhans cells

IMAGING

General Features

- Best diagnostic clue
  - Well-defined or punched-out **radiolucency without corticated border**
  - In alveolar process, teeth may appear to be floating in air
- Location
  - Bone lesions found in **skull**, femur, jaws, ribs, long bones, vertebrae, and pelvis
  - 50% of all bone lesions found in skull and facial bones
  - In oral cavity: Jaw lesions > oral soft tissues (2:1)
    - Jaws involved in 10-20% of all cases
    - **Mandible** > maxilla
      - Posterior > anterior; especially mandibular body and ramus
- Size
  - From small (punched-out) to large irregular lesions
- Morphology
  - Round or oval lesions at onset
  - As lesions progress, they may become irregular or coalesce

Radiographic Findings

- Intraoral and extraoral 2D imaging
  - Bone loss around root or whole tooth
  - May mimic periodontal disease; the following help differentiate
    - Periodontal disease begins at alveolar crest; **epicenter of LCH lesion usually midroot**
    - Bone may appear scooped out, unlike periodontal disease
  - Teeth may appear to be floating
  - Periosteal reaction parallel to cortex may be evident in panoramic images
- Cephalometric images
  - Will demonstrate skull lesions
    - Lesions may be punched out and relatively well defined
    - Lesions may have irregular shape and larger size, sometimes referred to as geographic skull

CT Findings

- Bone CT and CBCT
  - Will show extent of osteolytic lesions in maxilla and mandible
  - Depending on field of view, CBCT may demonstrate presence of skull lesions
  - Periosteal reactions are better detected

MR Findings

- T1WI
  - Isointense to muscle; moderately enhancing
- T2WI
  - Hyperintense

Nuclear Medicine Findings

- Lesions show avid uptake of Tc-99m: Useful for determining extent of disease

DIFFERENTIAL DIAGNOSIS

Localized Aggressive Periodontitis

- Aggressive form of periodontal disease affecting localized areas
  - 1st molars and incisors most commonly
  - Bone loss may form **arc pattern** in interproximal space
- Young patients, teenage years

Squamous Cell Carcinoma

- **Solitary** ill-defined radiolucency
  - Presence of multiple lesions rules out this diagnosis
- Destruction of bone around tooth roots may cause teeth to become mobile
- May have associated soft tissue mass
- Usually older age group

Osteomyelitis

- Ill-defined radiolucent or mixed lesions
- Often source of infection can be identified
- **Sequestra** are "hallmark"
- Periosteal reactions may be present

Metastasis

- Ill-defined radiolucency
- May grow within periodontal ligament space
- Usually history of known primary

Lymphoma

- Ill-defined radiolucency
- Preferential **growth in periodontal ligament space**
- May destroy developing tooth follicle
- Histologically, lymphoma may resemble EG if few eosinophils present

Leukemia

- Multifocal radiolucencies
- Widening of periodontal ligament space
- Fever, malaise

PATHOLOGY

Staging, Grading, & Classification

- Acute disseminated form (Letterer-Siwe disease): Multiple organ involvement
  - Hepatomegaly, splenomegaly, hemorrhage, anemia, lymphadenopathy, involvement of thymus and bone marrow, cutaneous lesions
  - Most likely represents malignant neoplastic process
  - 10% of all cases of LCH

- Chronic disseminated form (Hand-Schüller-Christian disease)
  - Triad: Multiple bone lesions, diabetes insipidus, exophthalmos
  - 20% of all cases of LCH
- Chronic localized form (eosinophilic granuloma): Monostotic or polyostotic bone lesions **without visceral involvement**
  - Polyostotic forms usually involve 2-4 bones
  - Eosinophilic granuloma accounts for **60-70 % of all cases of LCH**

Microscopic Features

- Aggregation of eosinophils interspersed with histiocyte-like cells
- Plasma cells, lymphocytes, and multinucleated giant cells sometimes seen
- Identification of Langerhans cells needed for diagnosis
  - Langerhans cells: Dendritic mononuclear cells found primarily in epidermis and bone marrow
    - Present antigens to T lymphocytes
    - Contain **Birbeck** granules in cytoplasm
      - Differentiates Langerhans cells from other mononuclear phagocytes
    - Immunohistochemistry: CD1a strongly positive; S100 positive

CLINICAL ISSUES

Presentation

- Most common signs/symptoms
  - Mobility of teeth
    - Sockets of lost teeth do not heal normally
  - Intraoral mass/swelling
  - Pain
- Other signs/symptoms
  - Gingivitis/bleeding
  - Ulcers
  - Impaired healing
  - Halitosis

Demographics

- Age
  - Acute disseminated: Infants < 3 years
  - Chronic disseminated: 1st decade
  - Localized (eosinophilic granuloma): Older children → adults
- Gender
  - M = F, although some report male preponderance for localized form (2:1)
- Epidemiology
  - 2-5 cases per 1 million
  - 50% < 15 years old

Natural History & Prognosis

- Overall prognosis related to age at onset and degree of organ dysfunction
- **Localized form: Good**
  - Spontaneous remission of eosinophilic granuloma following biopsy reported
  - Intralesional bone regeneration and malunion reported in adult following pathologic fracture without intervention
- **Chronic disseminated: Fair**
  - Progression to lethal dissemination may occur (10%)
- **Acute disseminated: Poor**
  - Invariably fatal in early infancy
  - Prognosis improves slightly after 2 years of age

Treatment

- Eosinophilic granuloma: Localized lesions of mandible/maxilla
  - Surgical curettage
  - Low-dosage radiation therapy ± chemotherapy for inaccessible lesions
    - Concern for malignancy induction with radiation therapy in younger patients
    - Radiation dose usually < 10 Gy
  - Recurrence from 1.6-25.0%
  - Recurrence may be less for surgery + radiation compared to surgery alone
  - Intralesion injection of corticosteroid reported successful in some lesions
- Chronic disseminated
  - Chemotherapy: Vinblastine sulphate, vincristine, etoposide ± corticosteroid (prednisone)
    - Prednisone thought to help decrease recurrence
- Acute disseminated: Multiple chemotherapeutic agents

DIAGNOSTIC CHECKLIST

Consider

- Although lesions of multiple myeloma (MM) are also described as punched out, MM occurs in much older age group

SELECTED REFERENCES

1. Azariah ED et al: "Histiocytosis X" - a rare case report. J Clin Diagn Res. 10(10):ZD19-ZD22, 2016
2. Gambirazi L et al: Diagnosis and intralesional corticotherapy in oral ulcers occurring as the sole manifestation of Langerhans cell histiocytosis. A Case Report. Open Dent J. 10:330-7, 2016
3. Plona GA et al: Spontaneous resolution of an eosinophilic granuloma of the mandible following open biopsy. Oral Surg Oral Med Oral Pathol Oral Radiol. 122(2):e60-3, 2016
4. Agarwal P et al: An unusual presentation of Langerhans cell histiocytosis. J Cytol. 31(4):227-9, 2014
5. Shi S et al: Multifocal Langerhans cell histiocytosis in an adult with a pathological fracture of the mandible and spontaneous malunion: A case report. Oncol Lett. 8(3):1075-1079, 2014
6. Cho YA et al: Hypothetical pathogenesis of eosinophilic infiltration in Langerhans cell histiocytosis of the jaw. Oral Surg Oral Med Oral Pathol Oral Radiol. 116(6):734-42, 2013
7. Lee BD et al: Eosinophilic granuloma in the anterior mandible mimicking radicular cyst. Imaging Sci Dent. 43(2):117-22, 2013
8. Lee SH et al: Intralesional infiltration of corticosteroids in the treatment of localized Langerhans cell histiocytosis of the mandible: report of two cases. Oral Surg Oral Med Oral Pathol Oral Radiol. 116(4):e255-60, 2013
9. Zajko J: Mandibular Langerhans cell histiocytosis in an adult. Bratisl Lek Listy. 114(8):488-90, 2013
10. Lajolo C et al: Langerhans's cell histiocytosis in old subjects: two rare case reports and review of the literature. Gerodontology. 29(2):e1207-14, 2012
11. Parihar A et al: Management of polyostotic eosinophilic granuloma. Dent Res J (Isfahan). 9(6):821-5, 2012
12. Zhao Y et al: [The expression of S-100 protein, CD1a, CD83 and Ki-67 in oral Langerhans cell histiocytosis.] Hua Xi Kou Qiang Yi Xue Za Zhi. 29(6):604-9, 2011

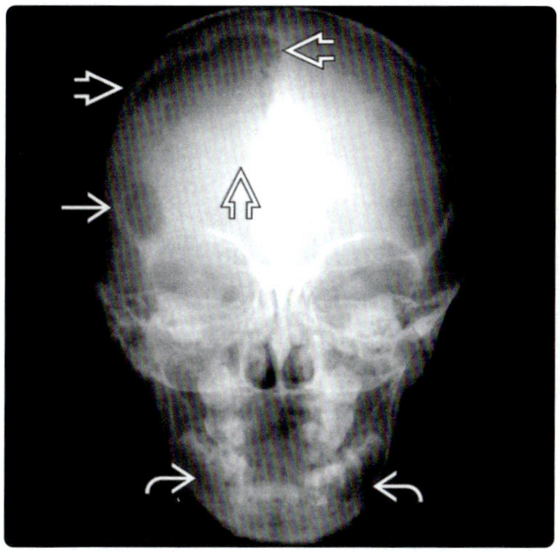

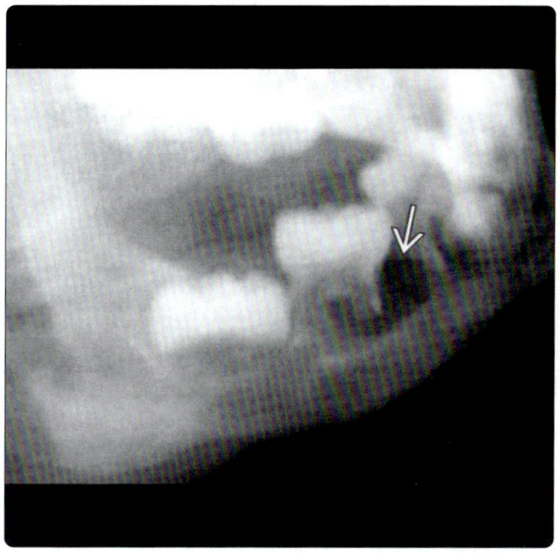

(Left) *PA radiograph shows 2 lesions of LCH in the frontal bone, a smaller, round, well-defined lesion* ➔ *and a larger irregular lesion* ⇨*. This appearance gave rise to the term geographic skull. Lesions are also present in the mandible* ↷*.* **(Right)** *Lateral oblique radiograph in the same patient shows round, scooped-out appearance* ➔ *of lesion around mesial root of developing 1st mandibular molar. The patient had the chronic disseminated form and presented clinically with exophthalmos.*

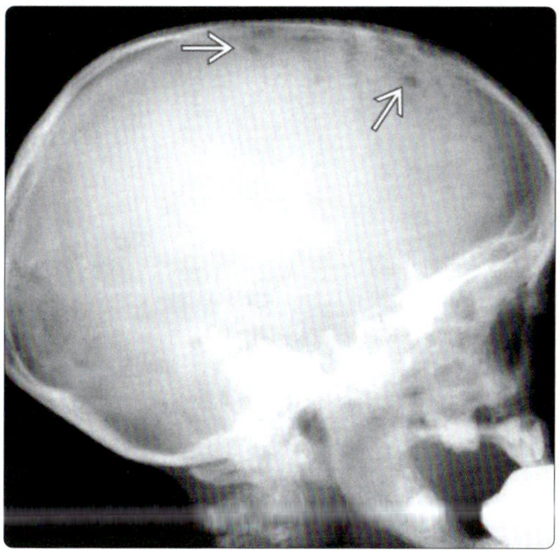

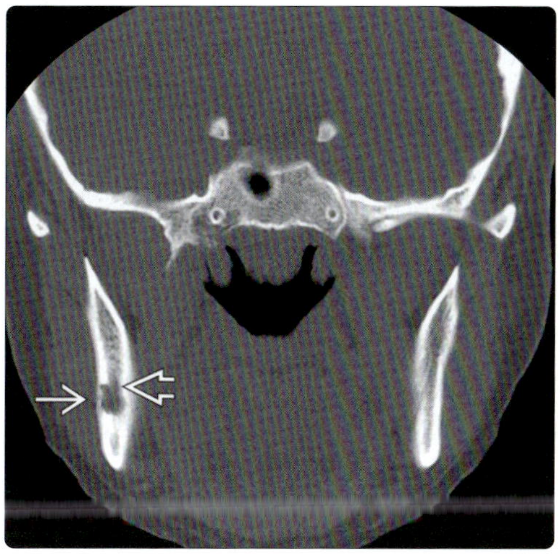

(Left) *Lateral cephalometric radiograph shows typical small, punched-out radiolucencies* ➔ *in the skull of a young patient with the chronic disseminated form of LCH.* **(Right)** *Coronal bone CT shows a small, well-defined lesion of eosinophilic granuloma in the right mandibular ramus of a 28-year-old woman. Note that the buccal cortex is thinned* ➔ *but not perforated. The lesion extends buccally around the mandibular canal* ⇨*, which lies superiorly.*

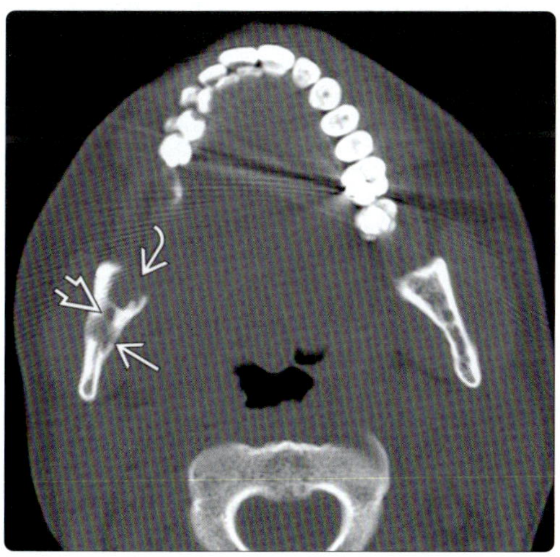

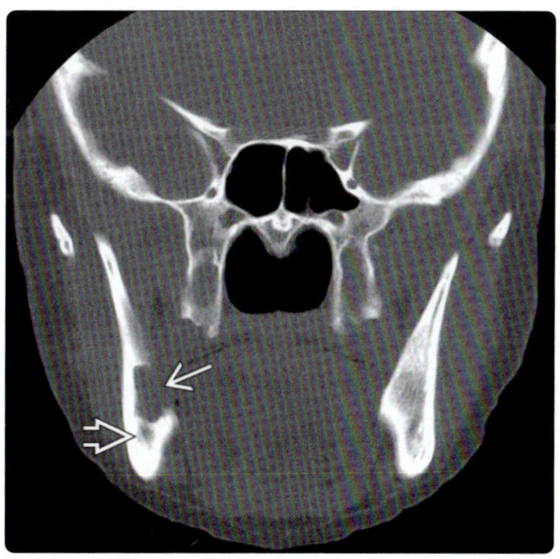

(Left) *Axial bone CT in the same patient shows the lesion in the ramus* ➔ *and a separate, more destructive, ill-defined lesion anteriorly* ↷*. The mandibular canal is evident between the lesions* ⇨*.* **(Right)** *Coronal bone CT in the same patient shows that the larger lytic lesion has caused destruction of the lingual cortex* ➔*. Note mandibular canal inferiorly* ⇨*. This was a case of monostotic eosinophilic granuloma with isolated lesions in the right ramus. Prognosis is good for these patients.*

PART II
SECTION 4

Temporomandibular Joint

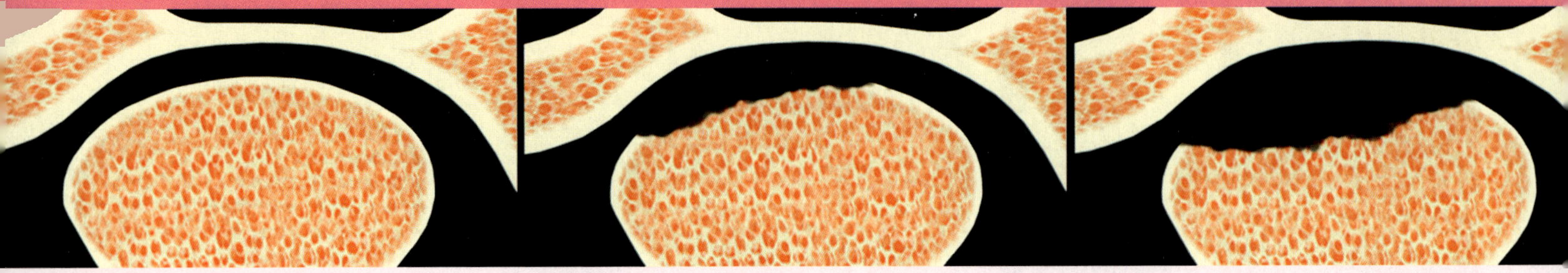

Congenital Disorders

Condylar Aplasia 540
Hemifacial Microsomia 542

Developmental Acquired Disorders

Condylar Hyperplasia 546
Coronoid Hyperplasia 552
Condylar Hypoplasia 556
Fibrous Ankylosis 560
Bony Ankylosis 562

Trauma

TMJ Fractures 564
TMJ Dislocation 570
Bifid Condyle 572
TMJ Osteochondritis Dissecans 576

Inflammation

TMJ Rheumatoid Arthritis 578
TMJ Juvenile Idiopathic Arthritis 584
TMJ Pigmented Villonodular Synovitis 590

Degenerative Disorders

Degenerative Joint Disease 592
TMJ Synovial Cyst 596
Progressive Condylar Resorption 598

Disc Derangement Disorders

Disc Displacement With Reduction 604
Disc Displacement Without Reduction 610
Adhesions 616

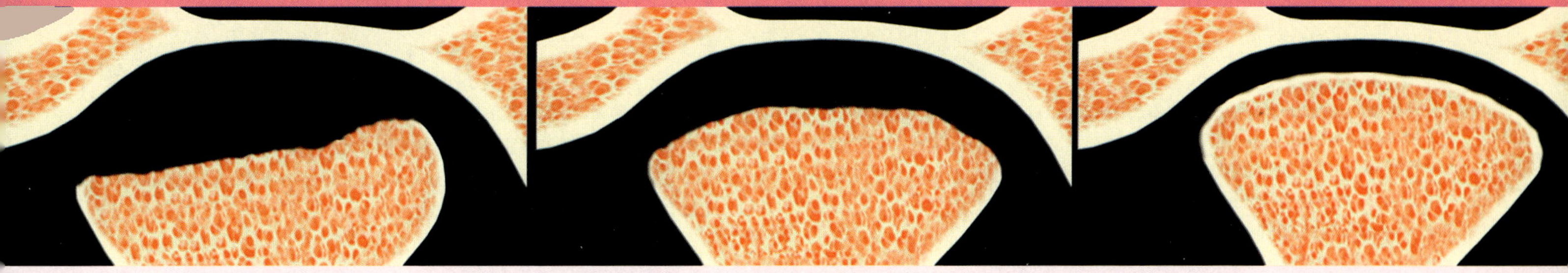

Neoplasm, Benign

TMJ Osteoma 618

TMJ Osteochondroma 620

Tumor-Like Lesions

TMJ Calcium Pyrophosphate Dihydrate Deposition Disease 626

TMJ Primary Synovial Chondromatosis 630

Neoplasm, Malignant

TMJ Osteosarcoma 634

TMJ Chondrosarcoma 636

TMJ Metastasis 640

Miscellaneous

TMJ Simple (Traumatic) Bone Cyst 642

Aneurysmal Bone Cyst 644

Condylar Aplasia

KEY FACTS

TERMINOLOGY

- Synonyms: Partial agnathia, hemignathia
- Definition: Anomaly of unknown origin that effects TMJ development, usually unilaterally

IMAGING

- Missing condyle
- Lack of development of glenoid fossa and articular eminence
- Facial soft tissue malformation
    - Ears, muscles, mouth
- Small ipsilateral ramus
    - Teeth developing in small ramus
- Body of mandible small
- CBCT or bone CT for size, shape, and quality of osseous anatomy
- Panoramic projection can provide overview assessment of mandible, TMJ, and maxilla

TOP DIFFERENTIAL DIAGNOSES

- Neonatal subcondylar fracture
- Juvenile idiopathic arthritis
- Progressive condylar resorption

PATHOLOGY

- May be feature of oculoauriculovertebral dysplasia, Goldenhar syndrome, 1st and 2nd branchial arch syndrome, type III hemifacial microsomia (HFM), Treacher Collins syndrome

CLINICAL ISSUES

- Preauricular tags or pits
- Facial asymmetry
- Reduction in ipsilateral facial volume
- Elevated occlusal plane
- Failure or reduced growth on involved side
- Asymmetry may be progressive

(Left) *Frontal CBCT 3D reformation of a 12-year-old boy with type III hemifacial microsomia shows a congenitally missing left condyle and superior portion of ramus. There is reduced lateral development of the left 1/2 of mandible, and the left orbit is enlarged. Mandibular osseous midline is shifted to small side, and the occlusal plane is elevated.* **(Right)** *Panoramic reformat CBCT shows absent condyle. The mandibular body has a short vertical dimension, and teeth are developing in the ramus.*

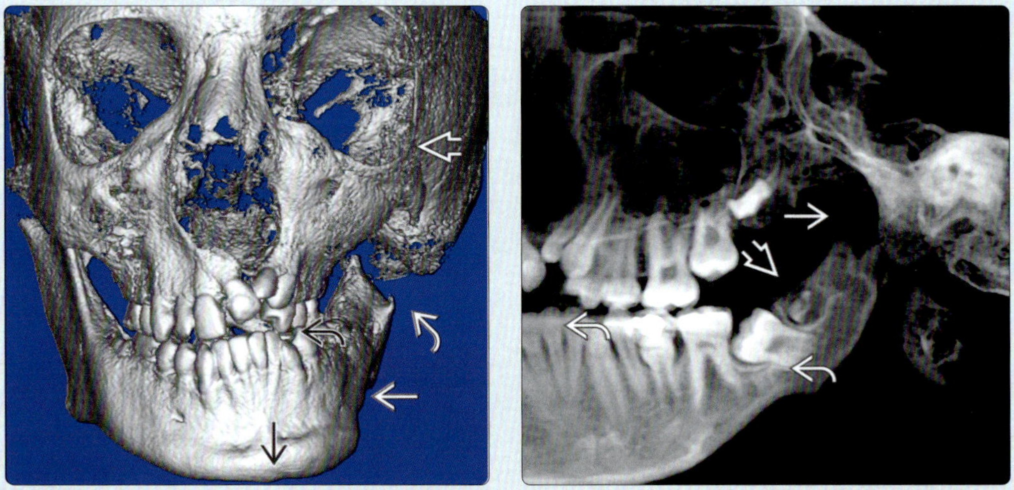

(Left) *Frontal CBCT 3D reformation of a 5-year-old girl with type III hemifacial microsomia shows reduced lateral development of the left 1/2 of the mandible. The left angle of the mandible is elevated when compared to the contralateral side. The mastoid process is inferiorly positioned.* **(Right)** *Panoramic reformat CBCT in the same patient shows missing left condyle and superior 1/2 of the left ramus. There is no development of the left glenoid fossa or articular eminence. Note dental crowding.*

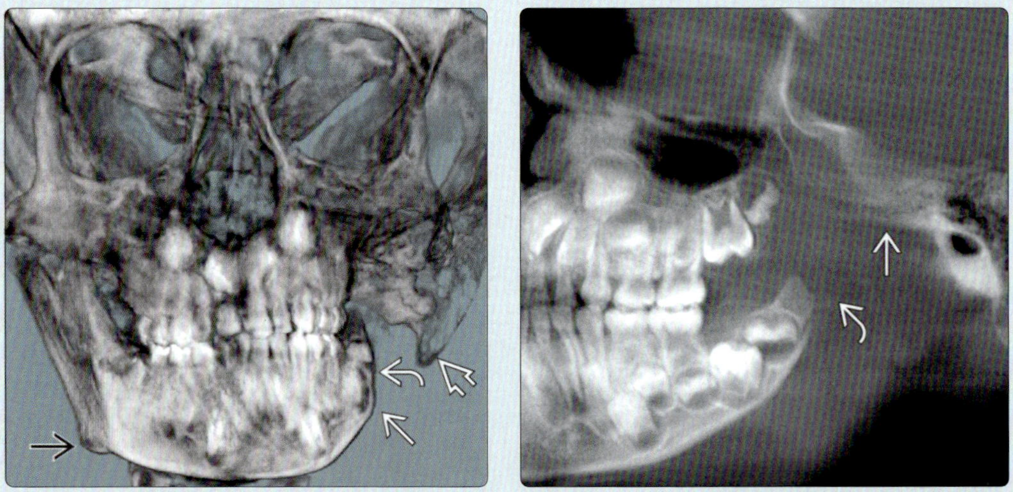

TERMINOLOGY

Synonyms

- Partial agnathia, hemignathia

Definitions

- Anomaly of unknown origin that effects TMJ development, usually unilaterally

IMAGING

General Features

- Best diagnostic clue
  - Missing condyle and associated lack of glenoid fossa development
  - Most often associated with ipsilateral facial malformations
- Location
  - Derivatives of 1st and 2nd branchial arches
    - Mandible
    - Muscles
    - Ear

CT Findings

- CBCT
  - Condyle absent
  - Lack of glenoid fossa and articular eminence development
  - Small ipsilateral ramus
    - Teeth developing in small ramus
  - Body of mandible is small
  - Defect rarely extends to bicuspid region
  - Hypoplasia of mastoid on affected side
  - Coronoid may be present or reduced in size

Imaging Recommendations

- Best imaging tool
  - CBCT or bone CT for size, shape, and quality of osseous anatomy
  - Panoramic projection can provide overview assessment of mandible, TMJ, and maxilla
- Protocol advice
  - Include jaws and cranial base

DIFFERENTIAL DIAGNOSIS

Neonatal Subcondylar Fracture

- Condyle (proximal segment) dislocates and heals in anterior, inferior, and medial position
- Anteroposterior dimensions of sigmoid (mandibular) notch narrows
- Sigmoid notch has V shape rather than typical U shape
- Short ascending ramus and body

Juvenile Idiopathic Arthritis

- Bilateral
- No facial soft tissue involvement
- Polyarticular systemic disease
- Serum indicators
- Pannus

Progressive Condylar Resorption

- Postpubertal onset in females
- Unilateral or bilateral
- Subtotal loss of condyle
- No facial soft tissue involvement

PATHOLOGY

General Features

- Etiology
  - Unknown etiology: Possibly hematoma in 1st and 2nd branchial arch regions or abnormal neural crest development and migration
- Associated abnormalities
  - May be feature of oculoauriculovertebral dysplasia, Goldenhar syndrome, 1st and 2nd branchial arch syndrome, type III hemifacial microsomia (HFM), Treacher Collins syndrome

CLINICAL ISSUES

Presentation

- Most common signs/symptoms
  - Congenitally missing condyle
- Other common signs/symptoms
  - Ears
    - Microtia
    - Preauricular tags or pits
    - Aural atresia
  - Face
    - Macrostomia
    - Facial asymmetry
    - Reduction in ipsilateral facial volume
  - Jaws and teeth
    - Elevated occlusal plane
    - Impaction of teeth on involved side

Natural History & Prognosis

- Failure or reduced growth on involved side
- Asymmetry may be progressive

Treatment

- Orthodontic and surgical management of jaws

DIAGNOSTIC CHECKLIST

Consider

- May be associated with syndrome

Image Interpretation Pearls

- Missing condyle and lack of development of glenoid fossa and articular eminence
- Facial soft tissue anomalies

SELECTED REFERENCES

1. Leoni C et al: Respiratory and gastrointestinal dysfunctions associated with auriculo-condylar syndrome and a homozygous PLCB4 loss-of-function mutation. Am J Med Genet A. 170(6):1471-8, 2016
2. Takano K et al: The association of external and middle ear anomaly and mandibular morphology in congenital microtia. Otol Neurotol. 37(7):889-94, 2016
3. Lin AE: The partnership of medical genetics and oral and maxillofacial surgery when evaluating craniofacial anomalies. J Oral Maxillofac Surg. 73(12 Suppl):S13-6, 2015
4. Shivhare P et al: Non-syndromic bilateral condylar aplasia: a rare case. Indian J Dent Res. 26(2):210-3, 2015

Hemifacial Microsomia

KEY FACTS

TERMINOLOGY

- Definition: Anomaly of unknown origin unilaterally affecting ear, face, mandible, teeth, and orbit
- Synonyms: Oculoauriculovertebral dysplasia, Goldenhar syndrome, 1st and 2nd branchial arch syndrome, lateral facial dysplasia, craniofacial microsomia

IMAGING

- Underdevelopment of mandibular condyle
    - Ranges from **small condyle to condylar aplasia**
    - Fossa development proportional to condylar development and function
- Decreased ipsilateral ramus and body development
- Small malar bone and zygomatic arch
- Hypoplasia of mastoid process
- Orbital dystopia: Orbit displaced laterally and inferiorly

TOP DIFFERENTIAL DIAGNOSES

- Fracture of condyle
- Condylar hypoplasia
- Degenerative disease of TMJ

CLINICAL ISSUES

- Preauricular tags or pits
- Facial asymmetry
    - **Chin deviated toward affected side**
- Reduced facial volume
- **Elevated occlusal plane** on involved side
- Impacted teeth on involved side

DIAGNOSTIC CHECKLIST

- Rule out subcondylar fracture dislocation at birth
- Mandibular asymmetry includes
    - Condyle, ramus, and mandibular body
    - Orbit, malar bone, ear, jaw muscles

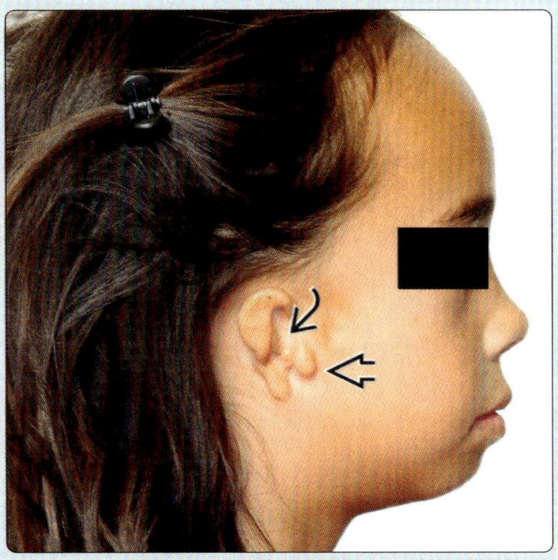
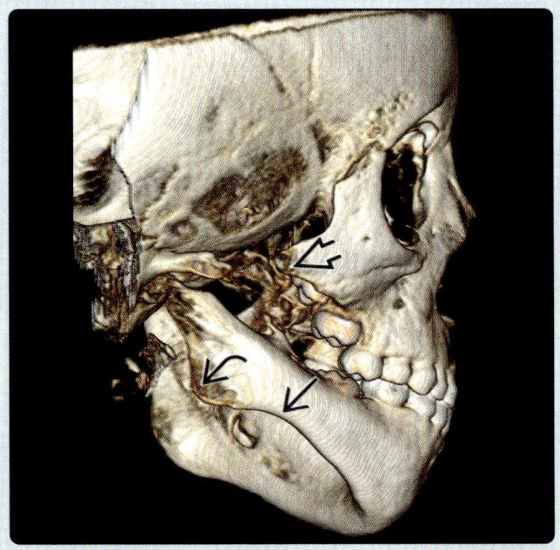

(Left) *Clinical photograph of a 7-year-old girl with hemifacial microsomia (HFM) shows characteristic ear changes: Microtia, aural atresia, and ear tags.* **(Right)** *3D CBCT reformation in the same patient shows a zygomatic arch defect, missing coronoid process, obtuse gonial angle, and prominent antegonial notch. The mandibular asymmetry is demonstrated by the different levels of the inferior mandibular borders of the right and left side.*

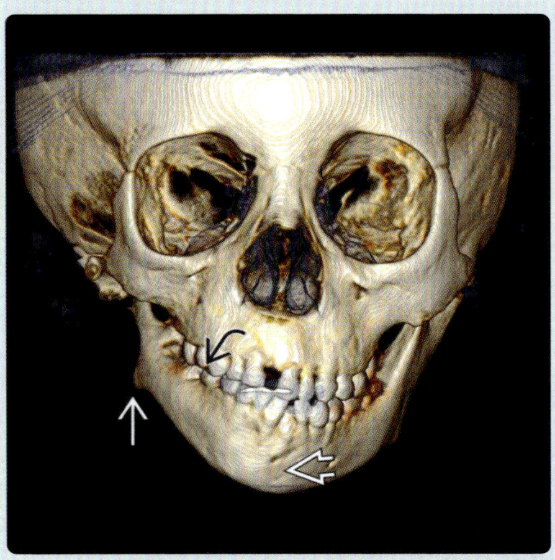
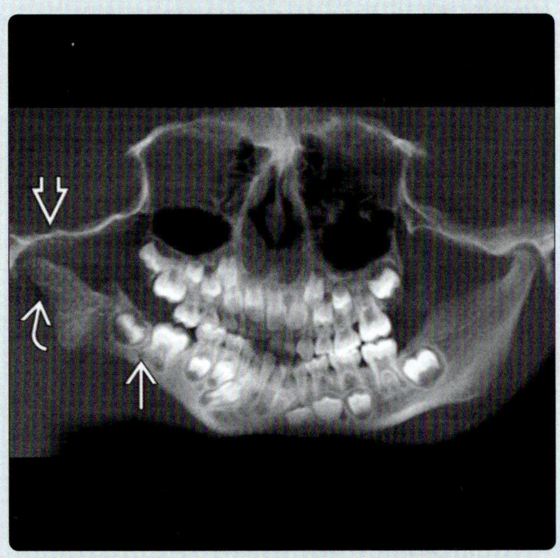

(Left) *AP CBCT 3D reformation in the same patient shows that the right occlusal plane is elevated with decreased lateral development of the right mandible and elevation of the right mandibular angle. Note shift of the mandibular midline to the right.* **(Right)** *Panoramic CBCT reformat in the same patient shows decreased vertical height of the mandibular body, short ramus, posterior inclination of the condylar process, and no articular eminence development. This is HFM type IIb.*

Hemifacial Microsomia

TERMINOLOGY

Abbreviations

- Hemifacial microsomia (HFM)

Synonyms

- Oculoauriculovertebral dysplasia, Goldenhar syndrome, 1st and 2nd branchial arch syndrome, lateral facial dysplasia, craniofacial microsomia (CFM)

Definitions

- Anomaly of unknown origin **unilaterally affecting ear, face, mandible, teeth, and orbit**

IMAGING

General Features

- Best diagnostic clue
  - Underdevelopment of mandibular condyle ranging from **small condyle to condylar aplasia** with reduced development of ipsilateral 1/2 of mandible
- Location
  - Derivatives of 1st and 2nd branchial arches: Jaws, muscles, ear
  - 5 major craniofacial manifestations of HFM
    - Ear: Most commonly involved soft tissue
    - Mandible: Most commonly involved skeletal structure
    - Orbit
    - Cranial nerves: Primarily CNVII
    - Facial soft tissue including masticatory muscles

CT Findings

- Small to absent condyle
- Fossa development proportional to condylar development and function
- Decreased ipsilateral ramus and body development
  - Ramus and mandibular body development proportional to condylar development
- **Occlusal plane elevated** on involved side
- Occasional cleft palate
- Small malar bone and zygomatic arch
- Hypoplasia of mastoid process
- Orbital dystopia: Orbit displaced laterally and inferiorly
- Middle and external ear defects

Imaging Recommendations

- Best imaging tool
  - CBCT, CT
  - Panoramic projection for overview of jaws

DIFFERENTIAL DIAGNOSIS

Fracture

- Condylar fracture in infancy: Proximal segment dislocates anteriorly, inferiorly, and medially and heals in this position
  - Sigmoid notch narrowed and shape changed
- Short ascending ramus and mandibular body

Condylar Hypoplasia

- Normal shape but small condyle
- Small ipsilateral 1/2 of mandible: Severity related to age of onset and severity of hypoplasia

Degenerative Disease

- Onset prior to puberty (unilateral): Small condyle and ipsilateral 1/2 of mandible

PATHOLOGY

General Features

- Etiology
  - Unknown: **Possibly hematoma** in 1st and 2nd branchial arch or abnormal neural crest development and migration

Staging, Grading, & Classification

- Type I: Mild hypoplasia of condyle, ramus, and body
- Type IIA: Small flat condyle, poorly developed or absent glenoid fossa, small abnormally shaped ramus, condyle normally positioned in fossa
- Type IIB: Same as IIA but condyle inferiorly, medially, and anteriorly positioned
- Type III: TMJ fails to form, small or absent ramus, small mandibular body

CLINICAL ISSUES

Presentation

- Most common signs/symptoms
  - Ears: Microtia, preauricular tags or pits, aural atresia
  - Face
    - Macrostomia
    - Facial asymmetry
      - **Chin deviated toward affected side**
      - Reduced facial volume
    - Jaws and teeth
      - Small condyle or condylar aplasia
      - Elevated occlusal plane
      - Impacted teeth on involved side

Natural History & Prognosis

- Failure or reduced growth on involved side results in asymmetry that may or may not be progressive

Treatment

- Orthodontics and surgery

DIAGNOSTIC CHECKLIST

Consider

- Subcondylar fracture dislocation at birth
- Condylar hypoplasia
- Prepubertal onset of degenerative joint disease

Image Interpretation Pearls

- Mandibular asymmetry (including condyle, ramus, and body), plus involvement of 1 or more of orbit, malar bone, ear, jaw muscles

SELECTED REFERENCES

1. Choi JW et al: Three-dimensional functional unit analysis of hemifacial microsomia mandible-a preliminary report. Maxillofac Plast Reconstr Surg. 37(1):28, 2015
2. Modica RF et al: Goldenhar syndrome associated with extensive arterial malformations. Case Rep Pediatr. 2015:954628, 2015

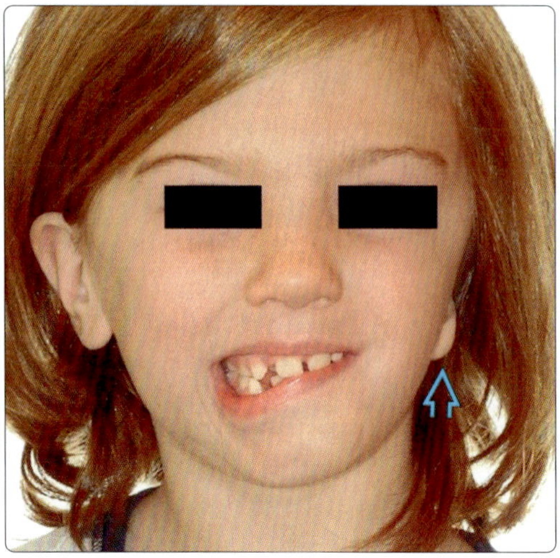

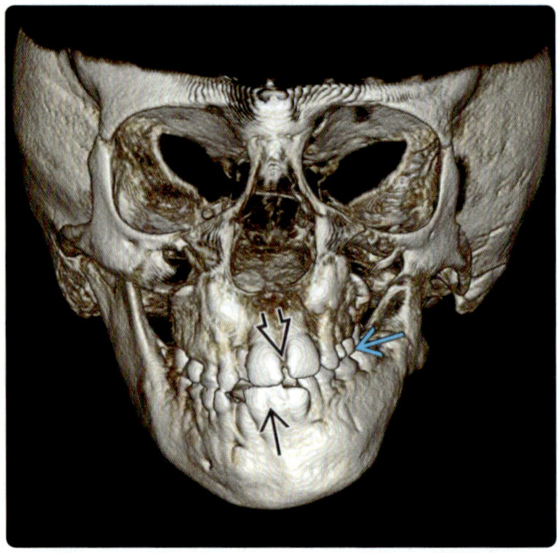

(Left) *Smile pose clinical photograph shows a 7-year-old girl with left side HFM and 7th nerve palsy of the left lower face. There is reduced soft tissue fullness of left side of face and deficient ear pinna.* **(Right)** *Volume-rendered CBCT of the same patient shows normal skeletal development of right side. The vertical and lateral dimensions of the left 1/2 of mandible are less than the right. The occlusal plane is elevated on the left side. The dental midline of the mandible is shifted to the right and the maxillary to the left.*

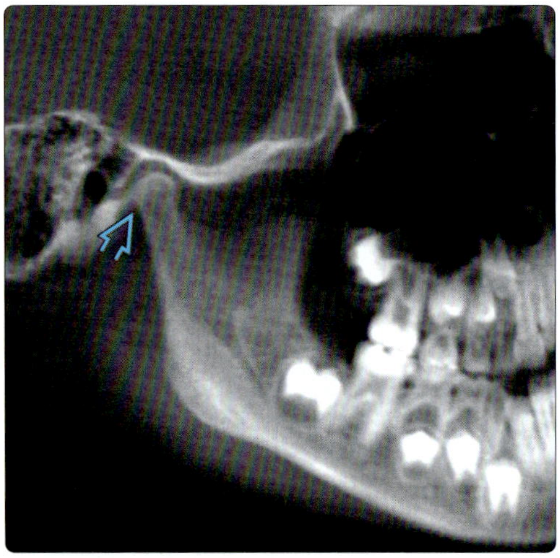

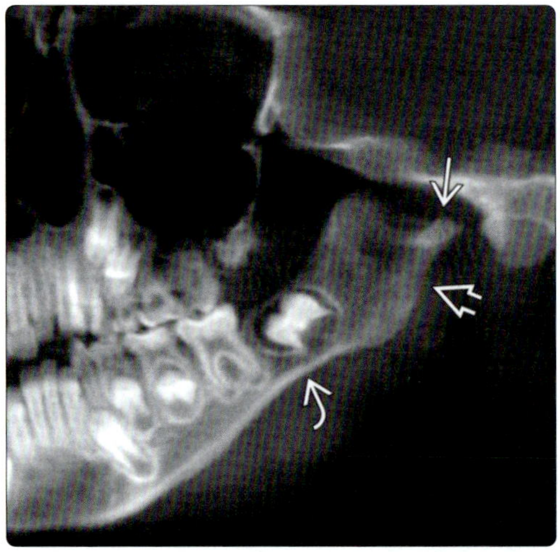

(Left) *CBCT reconstructed panoramic projection of the right side in the same patient shows normal development of the right condyle, mandible, and temporal bone.* **(Right)** *Panoramic reformat of the left side in the same patient shows the condylar process is small. The vertical dimensions of the left ramus and body of the mandible are less than the contralateral side.*

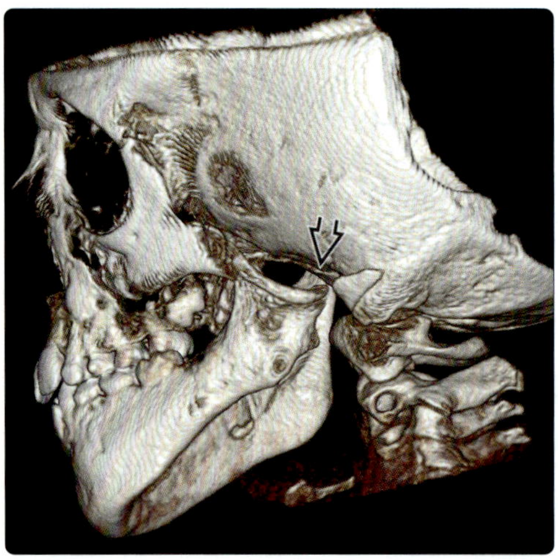

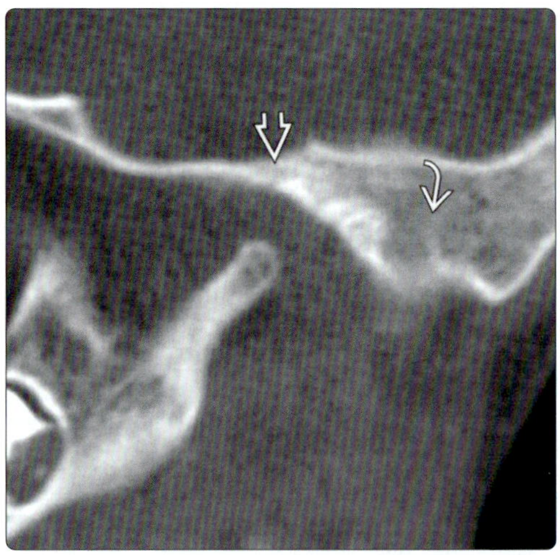

(Left) *Volume-rendered CBCT of the same patient shows a relatively small left side of mandible superimposed over the right side. There is a deficient zygomatic arch. The external auditory canal is absent.* **(Right)** *CBCT sagittal oblique reformat shows left TMJ and proximal 1/2 of mandible. Note the lack of eminence development. The mastoid process is small and there is an absence of external and internal ear structures.*

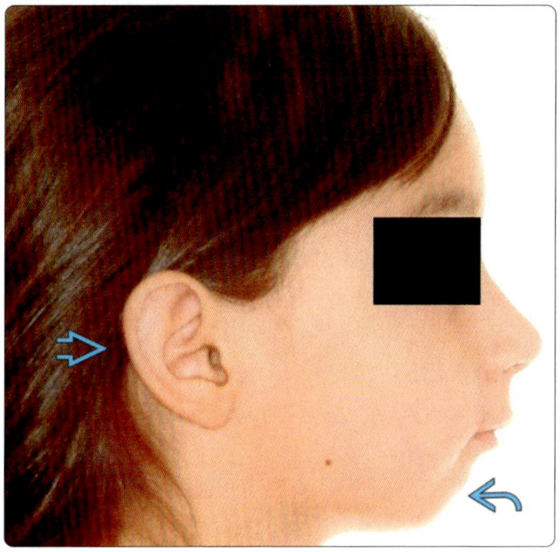

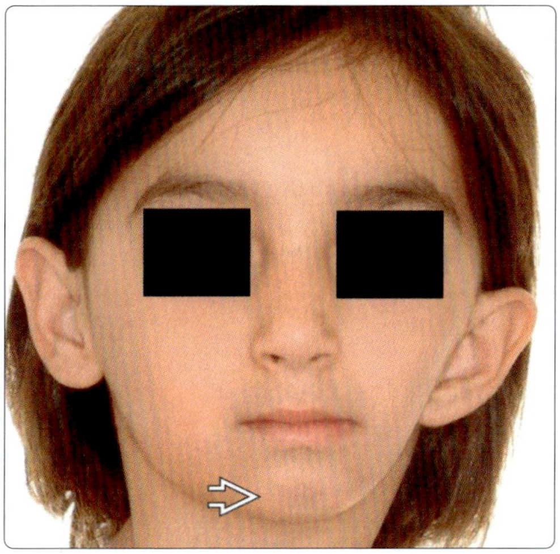

(Left) *Lateral photograph shows a 5-year-old girl with hemifacial microsomia. Note the recessive mandible but normal ear development on the right side. The mandible deviates to the short side and results in a reduction in anterior projection of the mandible.* **(Right)** *Frontal photograph of the same patient shows loss of facial volume on the affected left side, typical of HFM. Note deviation of the chin to the affected (left) side and the inferiorly positioned left ear.*

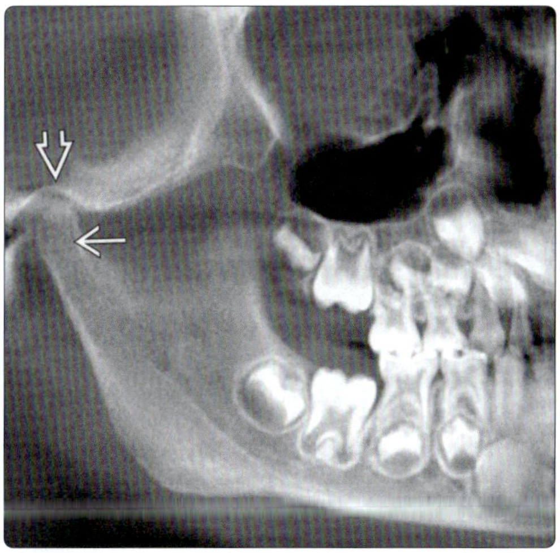

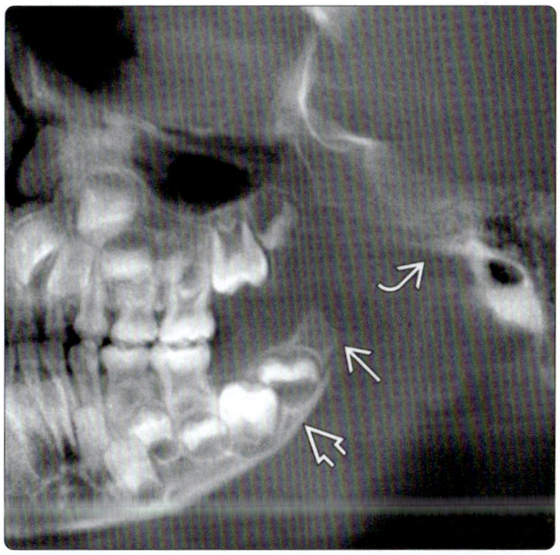

(Left) *Panoramic reformatted CBCT in the same patient shows normal development of the right mandible and right TMJ, including the condyle and glenoid fossa.* **(Right)** *Panoramic reformatted CBCT in the same patient shows lack of development of the left glenoid fossa, eminence, and condyle. Note the very short ramus and crowding of the mandibular posterior teeth. This is classified as HFM type III.*

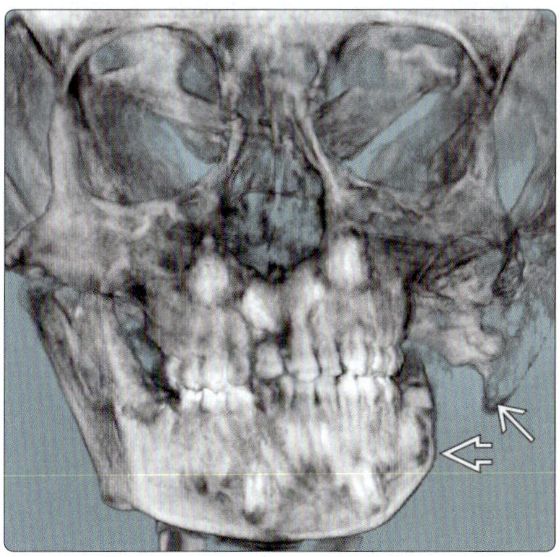

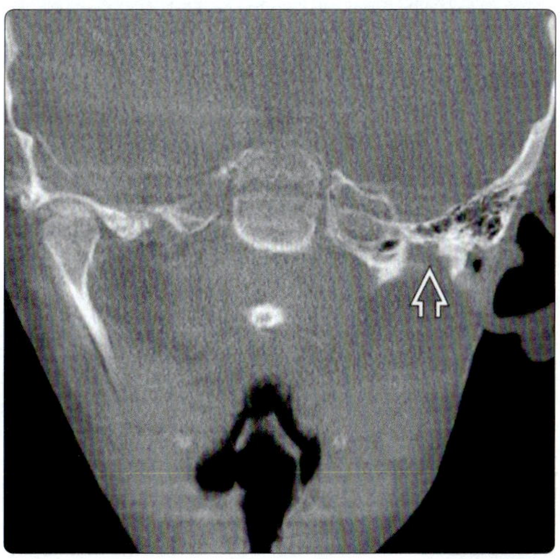

(Left) *Posteroanterior CBCT 3D reformat in the same patient shows deficient lateral development of mandible. The mastoid process is inferiorly positioned.* **(Right)** *Coronal CBCT in the same patient shows that the cranial base is inferiorly positioned on the left side. The cranial base typically exhibits compensatory downward growth when the condyle is small or absent.*

Condylar Hyperplasia

KEY FACTS

TERMINOLOGY

- Synonyms: **Hemimandibular hyperplasia**, **hemifacial hypertrophy**
- Definition: Unilateral overgrowth of mandibular condyle

IMAGING

- **Large condylar process with normal cortical borders and subchondral bone**
- Unilateral enlargement of ipsilateral condylar process, ascending ramus, and body of mandible
- Condylar process large compared to dimensions of ipsilateral fossa
- Posterior border of **ramus and lower border of mandible tend to be convex** rather than concave
- Condylar shape changes secondary to modeling by fossa constraints: Shape changes proportional to condylar size
- Osseous midline of mandible may shift to contralateral side

TOP DIFFERENTIAL DIAGNOSES

- Osteochondroma
- Condylar hypoplasia
  - Contralateral normal condyle can be confused for hypoplastic condyle

CLINICAL ISSUES

- Facial asymmetry
- No treatment in mild cases; condylar surface shave or high condylectomy in severe cases
- Continued growth up to 3rd decade

DIAGNOSTIC CHECKLIST

- Identify or rule out active condylar growth with bone scintigraphy (SPECT) scan
- **Imaging pearl**: Enlarged condyle and ipsilateral half of mandible

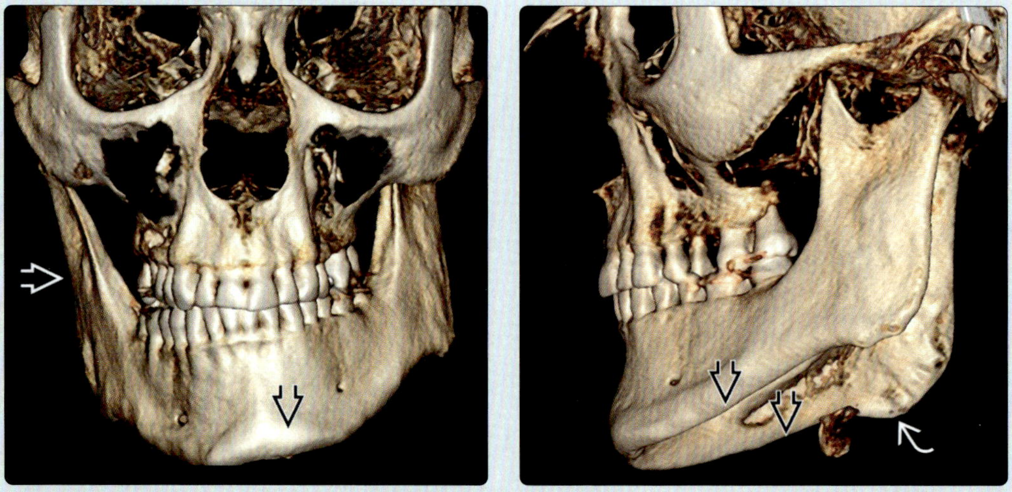

(Left) *Frontal CBCT volume-rendered image shows that the vertical heights of the right ascending ramus, mandibular body, and condylar process are larger than the left. The osseous midline of the mandible is shifted to the left.* **(Right)** *Lateral CBCT volume-rendered true lateral image in the same patient shows a proportionally large right side of the mandible. Note the different levels of the inferior mandibular borders.*

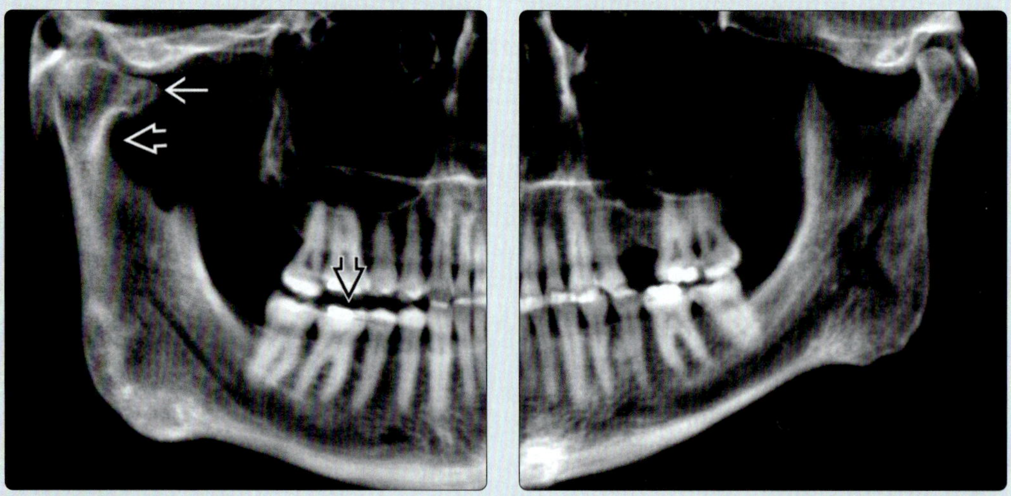

(Left) *Panoramic reformat CBCT shows enlargement of the right condyle compared to the ipsilateral glenoid fossa and contralateral condyle. The length and circumference of the right condylar neck are larger than the left. The right side occlusal plane is depressed due to the increased length of the right ramus, resulting in a right side posterior open bite.* **(Right)** *Panoramic reformatted CBCT in the same patient shows the left side of the mandible with anatomically normal size and shape.*

TERMINOLOGY

Abbreviations

- Condylar hyperplasia (CH)

Synonyms

- Hemimandibular hyperplasia
- Hemifacial hypertrophy

Definitions

- Slowly developing **unilateral overgrowth** of mandibular condyle
  - May also have elongation of condylar **neck**
  - Regional overgrowth of **ipsilateral half of mandible** proportional to condylar overgrowth

IMAGING

General Features

- Best diagnostic clue
  - Unilateral enlargement of mandibular condyle and regional enlargement of ipsilateral condylar process, ascending ramus, and mandibular body
- Location
  - Mandibular condyle, usually **unilateral**
- Size
  - **Varies** from mild to excessive enlargement of condyle and ipsilateral half of mandible
- Morphology
  - **Length and circumference** of condylar process relatively large compared to dimensions of ipsilateral fossa and contralateral condyle
  - Posterior border of ramus and inferior mandibular border often **convex** rather than usual concavity

CT Findings

- Large condylar process with **normal cortical borders and subchondral bone**
- Condylar **enlargement** greatest in **anteroposterior** and **vertical** dimensions
- Condylar **shape changes** secondary to modeling by fossa constraints
  - Shape changes generally proportional to condylar size
  - Conical, spherical, elongated, lobulated, or irregular outline
  - Condylar neck may be elongated, thickened, and bend laterally
- Fossa may remodel in response to functional demands
  - **Fossa** may be **enlarged**
- Increased vertical heights of condylar process, mandibular body, and ascending ramus
- Occlusal plane **depressed** on involved side
- Mandibular canal in same positional relationship to inferior mandibular cortex as contralateral side
- Posterior border of ramus and lower border of mandible convex
- Temporal fossa may be **elevated** on cranial base compared to contralateral side
- Osseous midline of mandible may **shift** to contralateral side
- Lateral development of involved half of mandible greater than opposite side
- Lower border of mandible on normal side **laterally** displaced
- **Lateral bowing** of involved ramus

MR Findings

- Normal bone marrow signal
- Condylar hyperplasia not related to disc position

Imaging Recommendations

- Best imaging tool
  - CBCT
    - Spatially accurate, ideal for serial comparisons of morphology
  - Panoramic projection for overview of mandibular asymmetry
    - Differentiates between hyperplasia and bony tumor
- Protocol advice
  - Skeletal imaging of temporomandibular joints, maxilla, mandible, and skull base

Nuclear Medicine Findings

- Bone scan
  - Increased uptake suggests active growth
    - Compare condyles side by side; > 55% uptake in affected side considered abnormal
  - May be calibrated to lumbar spine as uptake ratio

DIFFERENTIAL DIAGNOSIS

Osteochondroma, TMJ

- Well-defined osseous enlargement with cartilage cap
- **Well-localized growth** often extends from anterior or superior surfaces of condyle
- Does not cause regional enlargement of mandible

Condylar Hypoplasia, TMJ

- Mandibular asymmetry secondary to small condyle
- **Normal side** may be mistaken for hypoplastic condyle
  - Dimensions of normal condyle proportional to dimensions of ipsilateral fossa
  - Normal condyle has normal morphology

Acromegaly

- **Bilateral** condylar enlargement
- Enlarged sella turcica
- Bilateral posterior open bite

Osteoma

- Pedunculated or sessile osseous mass
- Extends from condyle or neck
- Smooth or lobulated margins
- Uniformly sclerotic or sclerotic margin and central trabecular bone

Hemimandibular Elongation

- Anteroposterior lengthening of mandible
- Negative overjet
- Osseous and dental midlines displaced to contralateral side

Odontogenic Lesions Extending Into Condyle

- Subchondral bone will have pattern characteristic of odontogenic pathosis

Fibrous Dysplasia

- Very rare; polyostotic form
- Subchondral bone will have bone pattern characteristic of fibrous dysplasia

PATHOLOGY

General Features

- Etiology
  - Overactive cartilage or persistent cartilage rests
  - Superior surface of condyle is growth site
  - Excessive condylar growth during skeletal development has regional effect on cranial base, maxilla, and remainder of ipsilateral half of mandible

Microscopic Features

- Thickening of cartilage layer and undifferentiated mesenchymal cells at growth site
- Cartilage islands in trabecular bone
  - Trabeculae may be thickened

CLINICAL ISSUES

Presentation

- Most common signs/symptoms
  - Progressive facial **asymmetry**
    - Chin **deviated** to unaffected side or unchanged
  - Variable growth rate
  - Changes in occlusion
    - Depression of occlusal plane on involved side ± open bite
    - Occasional contralateral side crossbite
- Other signs/symptoms
  - Altered mechanics of mandibular function may predispose to **dysfunction**
    - **Posterior displacement** of contralateral condyle
    - Internal derangement and associated degenerative joint disease in either joint
  - **Limited** condylar movement, deviated mandibular opening

Demographics

- Age
  - Onset varies: As early as 1st decade, but onset most often at **puberty**
    - Commonly presents between 10-25 years old
- Gender
  - M > F
- Epidemiology
  - CH most common postnatal growth abnormality of TMJ

Natural History & Prognosis

- Growth rate **variable**
- Continued growth up to 3rd decade
- Usually **self-limiting**

Treatment

- No treatment in mild cases
- Condylar surface shave or high condylectomy in severe cases
- Orthognathic surgery and **orthodontics after growth complete**

DIAGNOSTIC CHECKLIST

Consider

- Identify or rule out active condylar growth with bone scintigraphy (SPECT) scan
  - Superimpose serial image taken at 6-month to 1-year intervals

Image Interpretation Pearls

- Large condyle and enlargement of ipsilateral half of mandible
- Look for larger space between ascending ramus and maxilla compared to contralateral side in coronal views
- Posterior and inferior borders of mandible convex

SELECTED REFERENCES

1. Rodrigues DB et al: Condylar hyperplasia of the temporomandibular joint: types, treatment, and surgical implications. Oral Maxillofac Surg Clin North Am. 27(1):155-67, 2015
2. Wallender A et al: Neonatal coronoid hyperplasia: a report of a case and concepts to promote early diagnosis and treatment. J Oral Maxillofac Surg. 73(8):1615, 2015
3. Ferreira S et al: Unilateral condylar hyperplasia: a treatment strategy. J Craniofac Surg. 25(3):e256-8, 2014
4. Olate S et al: TMJ function after partial condylectomy in active mandibular condylar hyperplasia. Int J Clin Exp Med. 7(3):775-9, 2014
5. Singh V et al: Ortho-surgical management of condylar hyperplasia: Rare case reports. Natl J Maxillofac Surg. 5(1):54-9, 2014
6. Wen B et al: Clinical value of 99Tcm-MDP SPECT bone scintigraphy in the diagnosis of unilateral condylar hyperplasia. ScientificWorldJournal. 2014:256256, 2014
7. Wolford LM et al: A classification system for conditions causing condylar hyperplasia. J Oral Maxillofac Surg. 72(3):567-95, 2014
8. Xu M et al: Hemimandibular hyperplasia: classification and treatment algorithm revisited. J Craniofac Surg. 25(2):355-8, 2014
9. Karssemakers LH et al: Interobserver variation of single-photon emission computed tomography bone scans in patients evaluated for unilateral condylar hyperactivity. Oral Surg Oral Med Oral Pathol Oral Radiol. 115(3):399-405, 2013
10. Olate S et al: Facial asymmetry and condylar hyperplasia: considerations for diagnosis in 27 consecutives patients. Int J Clin Exp Med. 6(10):937-41, 2013
11. Olate S et al: Mandible condylar hyperplasia: a review of diagnosis and treatment protocol. Int J Clin Exp Med. 6(9):727-37, 2013
12. Stopa Z et al: Coronoid-condylar index in assessing of mandibular coronoid hyperplasia. Preliminary results. Adv Med Sci. 58(2):429-33, 2013
13. Verhoeven TJ et al: Unilateral condylar hyperplasia: a 3-dimensional quantification of asymmetry. PLoS One. 8(3):e59391, 2013
14. Walters M et al: Robust and regional 3D facial asymmetry assessment in hemimandibular hyperplasia and hemimandibular elongation anomalies. Int J Oral Maxillofac Surg. 42(1):36-42, 2013
15. Raijmakers PG et al: Female predominance and effect of gender on unilateral condylar hyperplasia: a review and meta-analysis. J Oral Maxillofac Surg. 70(1):e72-6, 2012
16. Mehrotra D et al: Condylar hyperplasia and facial asymmetry: report of five cases. J Maxillofac Oral Surg. 10(1):50-6, 2011
17. Villanueva-Alcojol L et al: Hyperplasia of the mandibular condyle: clinical, histopathologic, and treatment considerations in a series of 36 patients. J Oral Maxillofac Surg. 69(2):447-55, 2011
18. Shintaku WH et al: Imaging modalities to access bony tumors and hyperplasic reactions of the temporomandibular joint. J Oral Maxillofac Surg. 68(8):1911-21, 2010
19. Kawamoto HK et al: Differential diagnosis of the idiopathic laterally deviated mandible. Plast Reconstr Surg. 124(5):1599-609, 2009
20. Pirttiniemi P et al: Abnormal mandibular growth and the condylar cartilage. Eur J Orthod. 31(1):1-11, 2009
21. Saridin CP et al: Quantitative analysis of planar bone scintigraphy in patients with unilateral condylar hyperplasia. Oral Surg Oral Med Oral Pathol Oral Radiol Endod. 104(2):259-63, 2007
22. Sándor GK et al: Management of facial asymmetry. Oral Maxillofac Surg Clin North Am. 19(3):395-422, vi, 2007
23. Kajan ZD et al: Assessment of growth activity in the mandibular condyles by single-photon emission computed tomography (SPECT). Aust Orthod J. 22(2):127-30, 2006

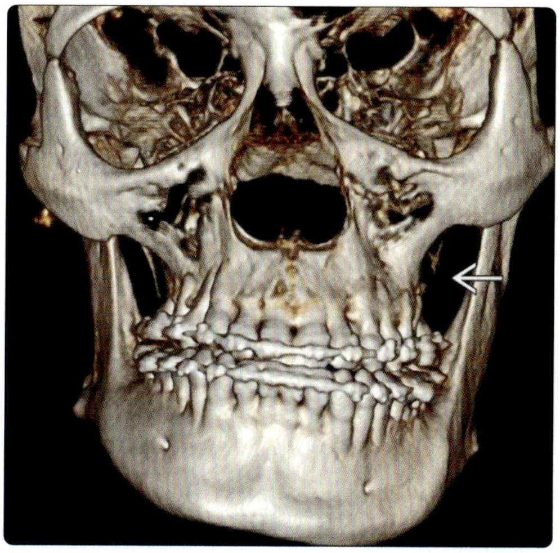

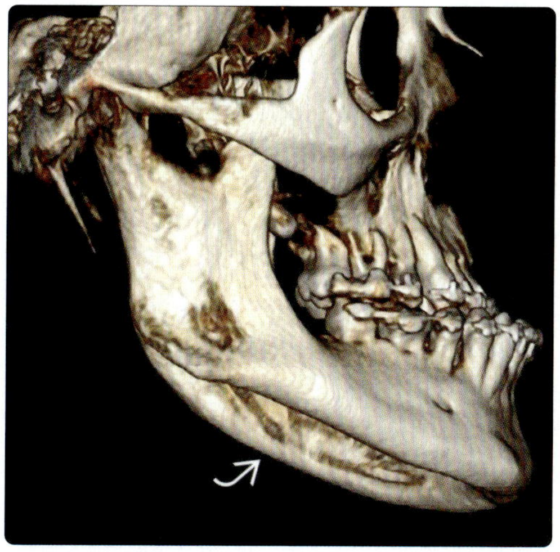

(Left) *AP CBCT 3D reformation shows a mandibular asymmetry with left side enlargement caused by condylar hyperplasia. The lateral development of the mandible is greater on the left side, demonstrated by the space between the ramus and maxilla. The occlusal plane is depressed on the left side.* **(Right)** *Lateral CBCT 3D reformation in the same patient demonstrates size and shape differences between the right and left halves of the mandible. The lower border of the affected side is convex.*

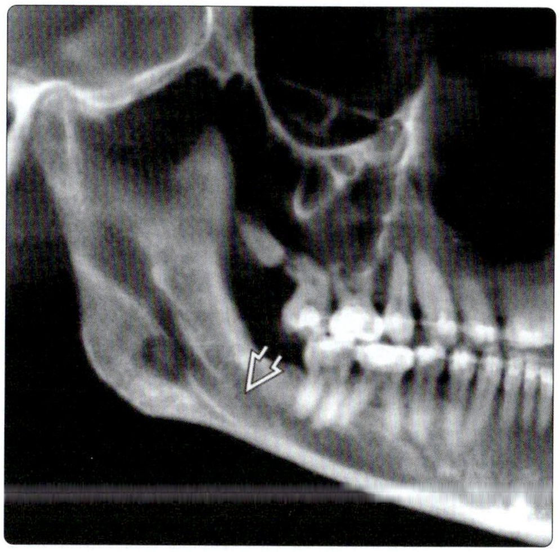

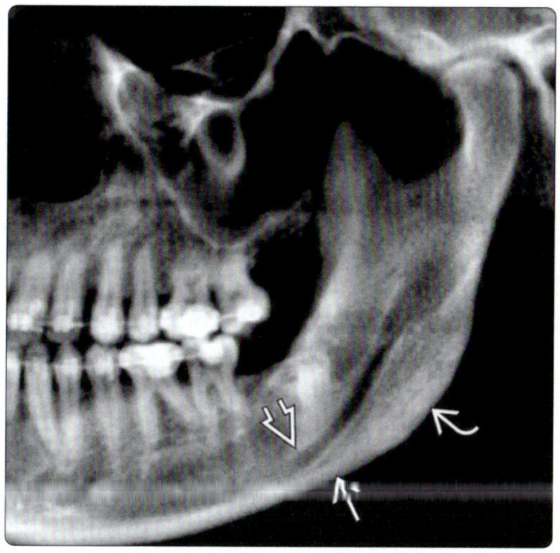

(Left) *Panoramic reformatted CBCT in the same patient shows normal size and shape of the right mandible. Note the position of the mandibular canal.* **(Right)** *Panoramic reformatted CBCT in the same patient shows that the vertical heights of the left condylar process, ascending ramus, and mandibular body are greater than the right. The inferior and posterior mandibular borders are convex. The mandibular canal maintains bilaterally symmetrical spatial relationships with the lower border of the mandible.*

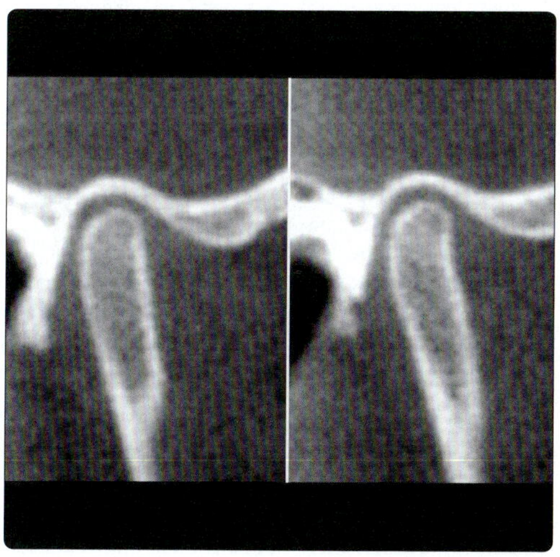

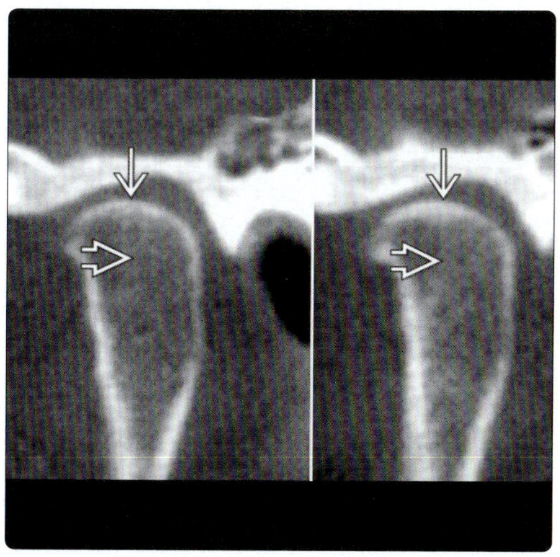

(Left) *Sagittal reformatted CBCT in the same patient shows that the right condyle has a normal size and shape. The proportional dimensions of the right condyle and fossa are also normal.* **(Right)** *Sagittal reformatted CBCT in the same patient shows that the left condyle is relatively large compared to the dimensions of the ipsilateral fossa and contralateral condyle. The condyle has a normal cortical outline and normal subchondral trabeculation.*

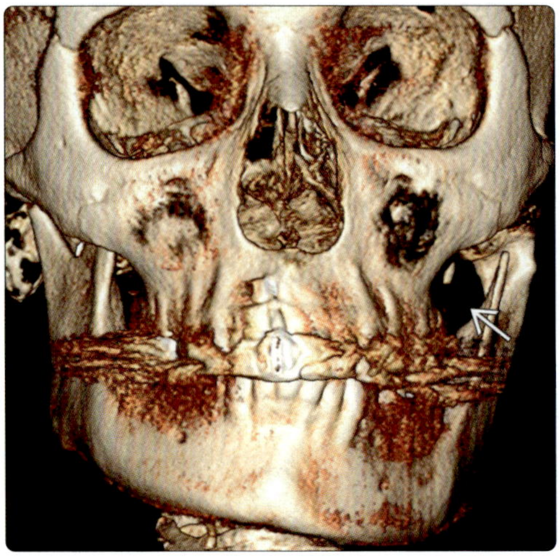
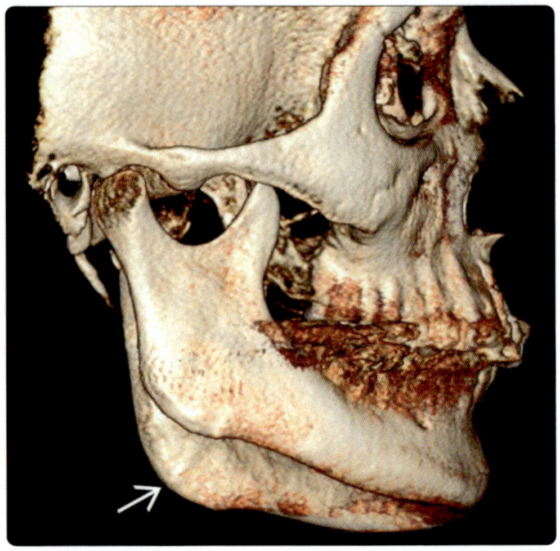

(Left) *PA CBCT 3D rendering shows greater lateral development of the left side of the mandible in a patient with left condylar hyperplasia. Note the increased space between the ramus and maxilla ➔.* **(Right)** *CBCT true lateral volume rendering in the same patient shows left mandibular enlargement ➔ and vertical discrepancy in lower border dimensions due to condylar hyperplasia on the left side.*

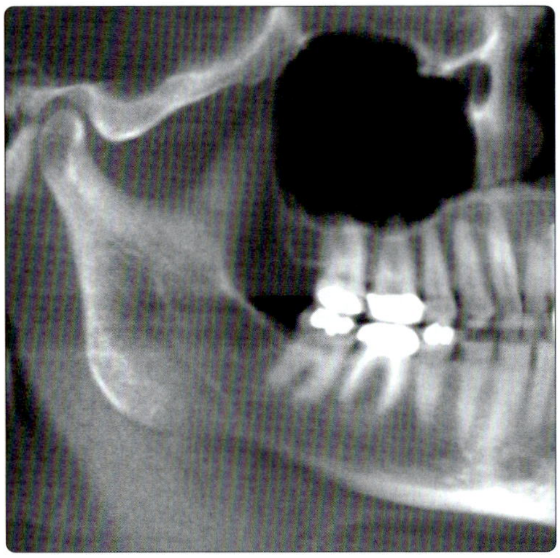
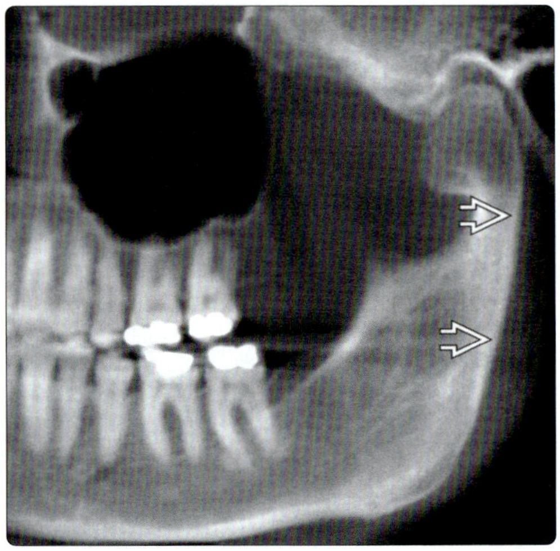

(Left) *Panoramic reformatted CBCT in the same patient shows normal size and shape of the right condylar process, ramus, and body of the mandible.* **(Right)** *Panoramic reformatted CBCT in the same patient shows the very large left condyle relative to the ipsilateral fossa and contralateral condyle. The condyle exhibits normal cortical outline and subchondral trabeculation. Note the convex shape ➔ of the neck of the condyle and posterior border of the ramus.*

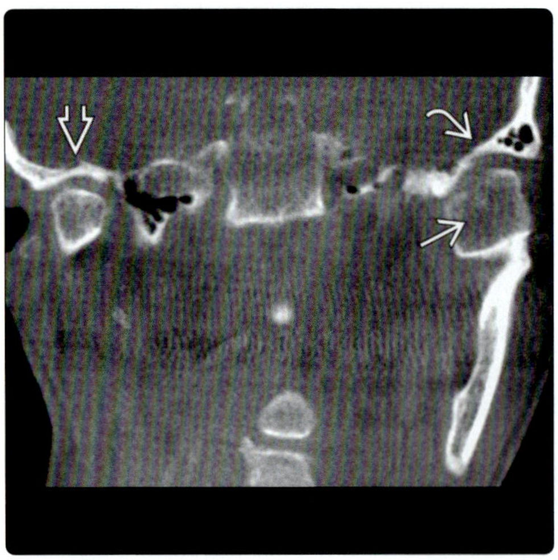
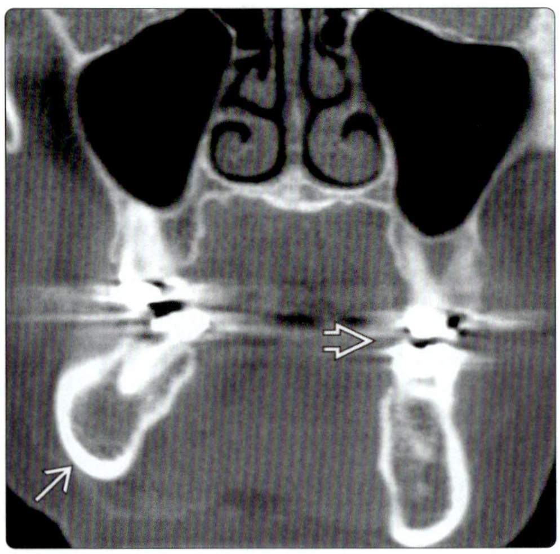

(Left) *Coronal CBCT in the same patient with the image plane through the TMJ shows elevation of the left glenoid fossa ➔ on the cranial base compared to the normal right side ➔. The condyle is enlarged in all planes, but the subchondral bone ➔ is normal.* **(Right)** *Coronal CBCT in the same patient shows lateral displacement of the right lower border of the mandible ➔. The occlusal plane ➔ is depressed on the long side.*

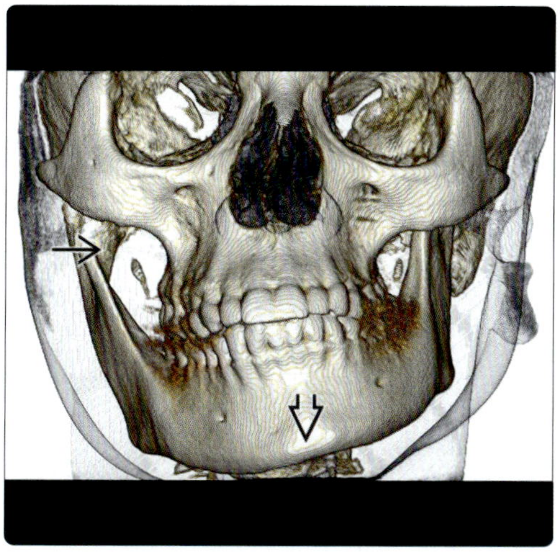

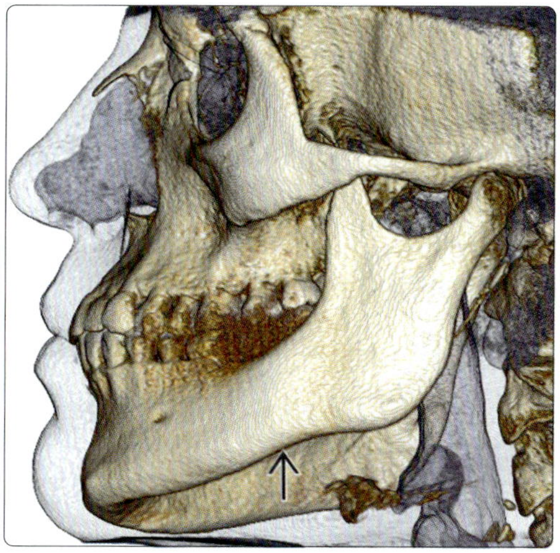

(Left) *AP CBCT 3D reformation shows increase in size of the right mandible due to right condylar hyperplasia. There is greater lateral development of the right mandible as evidenced by increase in maxilla to ramus width* ⇨ *compared to the contralateral side. Note the osseous mandibular midline shift to the left* ⇨. **(Right)** *CBCT true lateral volume in the same patient shows the difference in size between the normal left mandible* ⇨ *and the contralateral side.*

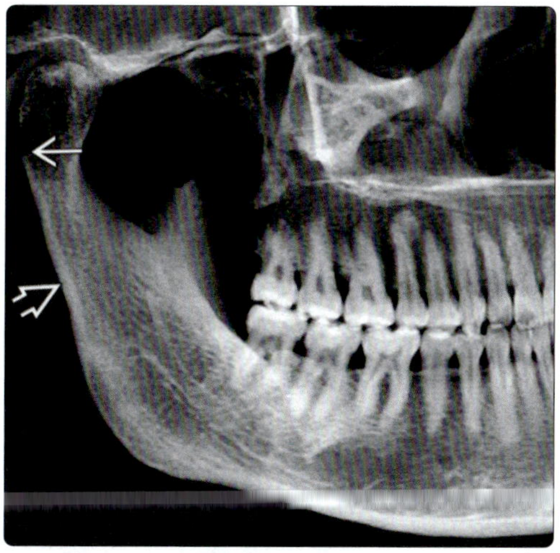

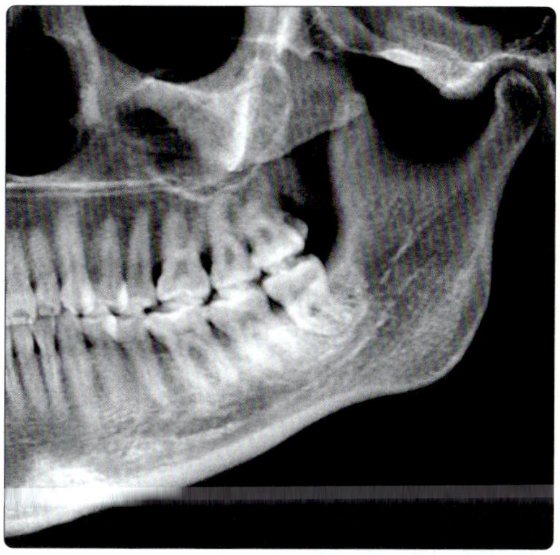

(Left) *Panoramic reformatted CBCT in the same patient shows the large right condyle relative to the ipsilateral fossa and contralateral condyle. The condyle exhibits normal cortical outline and subchondral trabeculation. Note the convex shape of the neck of the condyle* ➡ *and posterior border of the ramus* ➡ *compared to the contralateral side.* **(Right)** *Panoramic reformatted CBCT in the same patient shows normal size and shape of the left condylar process, ramus, and body of the mandible.*

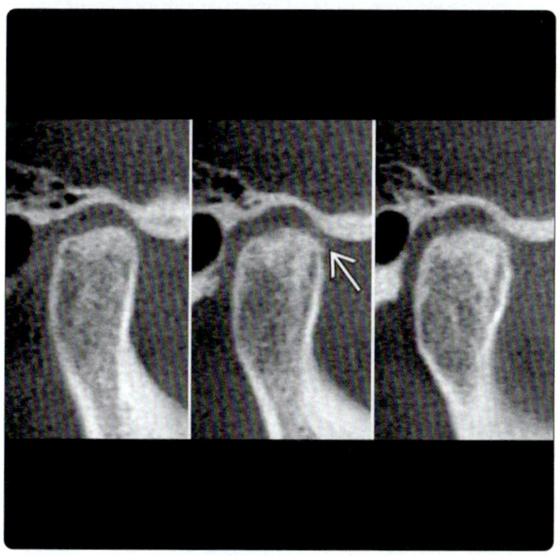

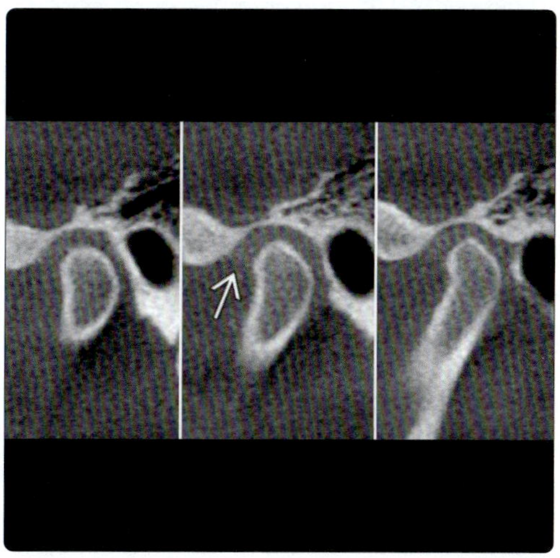

(Left) *Sagittal oblique CBCT images of the right TMJ in the same patient show a condyle that appears to be too large for the fossa. Note narrow anterior joint space* ➡. *The fossa and eminence are of similar size and morphology to the contralateral side. The condyle is corticated.* **(Right)** *Sagittal oblique CBCT images of the left TMJ in the same patient show a normal condyle, fossa, and eminence. The condyle is positioned centrally within the fossa, and the anterior joint space is within normal limits* ➡.

Coronoid Hyperplasia

KEY FACTS

TERMINOLOGY

- Definition: Uncommon unilateral or bilateral **elongation or enlargement** of coronoid process

IMAGING

- Tip extends **≥ 1 cm** above inferior rim of zygomatic arch
- Coronoid process impinges on medial surface of zygomatic arch, posterior zygomatic bone, or posterior maxilla during opening; restricts condylar translation
- Sagittal reformat: Coronoid process large but maintains normal shape or may **curve** anteriorly
- Initial detection may be in panoramic radiograph

TOP DIFFERENTIAL DIAGNOSES

- Osteochondroma
- Osteoma

PATHOLOGY

- Normal bone structure
- Associated with basal cell nevus syndrome and trismus-pseudocamptodactyly syndrome
- Acquired or developmental, but most cases are **idiopathic**
- May be related to increased temporalis muscle activity, trauma, or TMJ ankylosis

CLINICAL ISSUES

- **Progressive** decrease in range of opening
- Usually **painless**
- **Bilateral**:unilateral = 4.7:1.0
- If unilateral: Deviation to affected side on opening and facial asymmetry
- Mobile lump above zygomatic arch
- Onset often in **puberty**; age range: Birth-62 years
- M:F = 3.3:1.0 for bilateral presentation

DIAGNOSTIC CHECKLIST

- Use axial CBCT reformat in open position to see coronoid interference on opening

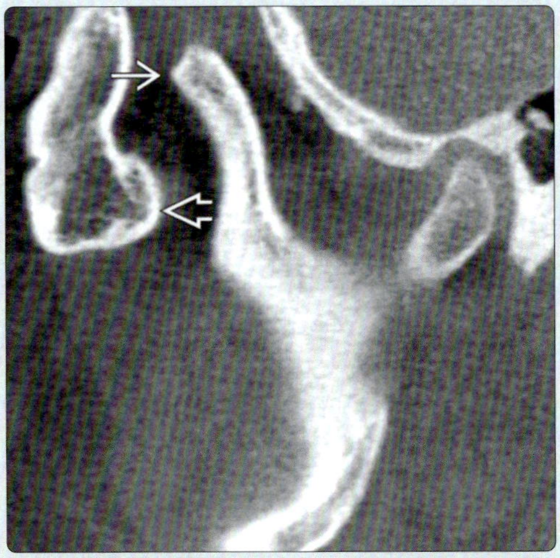
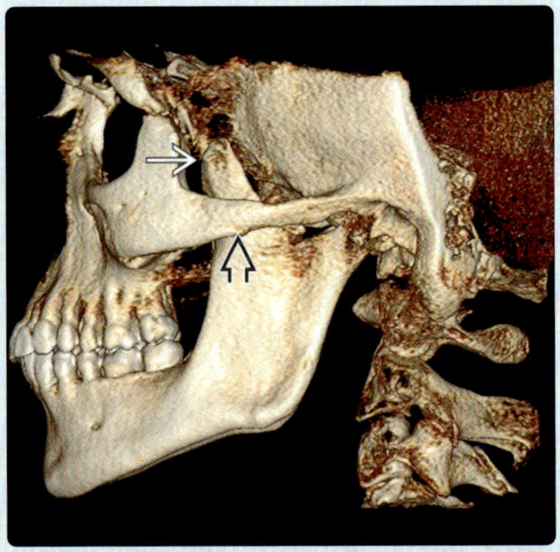

(Left) *Sagittal CBCT shows hyperplasia and elongation of the left coronoid process ➡. The coronoid process extends above the level of the zygomatic arch ➡ and is also thickened.* **(Right)** *Lateral 3D reformation in the same patient, in the closed position, shows the degree of elongation of the left coronoid process ➡. Note the length of the coronoid process projecting superior to the zygomatic arch ⇨.*

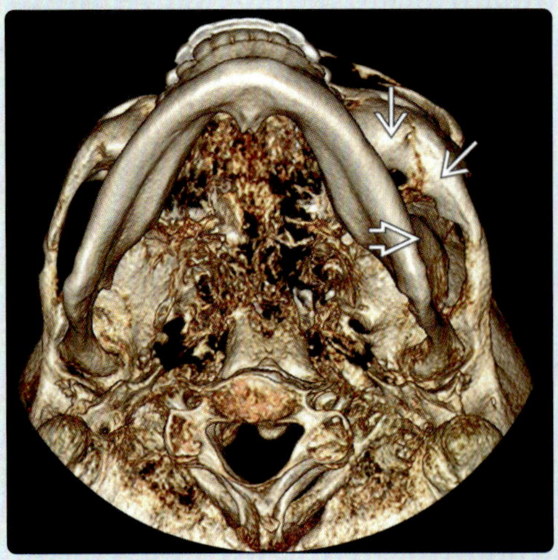
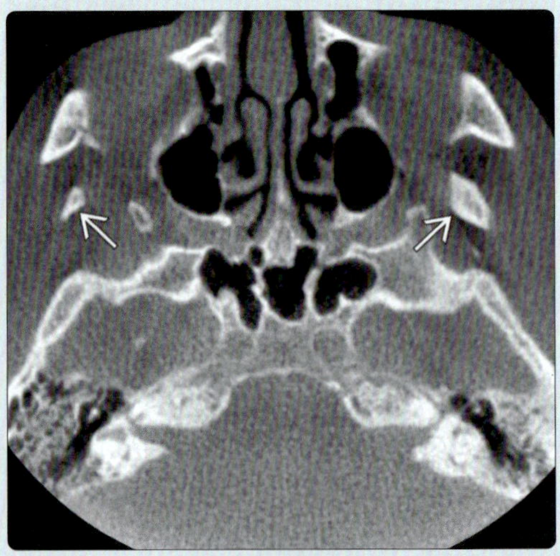

(Left) *Axial 3D reformation in the same patient shows enlargement of the medial aspect of the left zygoma ➡ compared to the right side. The elongated left coronoid process is visible ➡. Contact of the inner aspect of the zygomatic arch with the coronoid process may produce exostoses and a pseudoarthrosis.* **(Right)** *Axial CBCT at a level superior to the mandibular condyles shows the tips of bilaterally elongated coronoid processes ➡. The coronoid processes are not normally seen at this level.*

TERMINOLOGY

Synonyms

- Jacob disease: Coronoid process hyperplasia with pseudocartilaginous joint between coronoid process and zygoma

Definitions

- Uncommon unilateral or bilateral **elongation or enlargement** of coronoid process

IMAGING

General Features

- Best diagnostic clue
  - Elongated coronoid process, often seen in **panoramic** view

Radiographic Findings

- Radiography
  - Tip of coronoid process extends **≥ 1 cm** above inferior rim of zygomatic arch

CT Findings

- CBCT
  - Coronoid process impinges on medial surface of zygomatic arch, posterior zygomatic bone, or posterior maxilla during opening; restricts condylar translation
  - Axial reformat: **± exostosis** on inner aspect of zygomatic arch at contact point with coronoid process → pseudoarthrosis
  - Sagittal reformat: Coronoid process large but maintains normal shape or may **curve** anteriorly

Imaging Recommendations

- Best imaging tool
  - **Panoramic** radiograph for initial detection
  - CT or CBCT with 3D reformats to see morphology and extent of involvement
- Protocol advice
  - Axial and sagittal CT reformats in **open** position

DIFFERENTIAL DIAGNOSIS

Osteochondroma

- Tumor of bone and cartilage, has **irregular** shape

Osteoma

- Coronoid process has **irregular** shape

PATHOLOGY

General Features

- Etiology
  - Acquired or developmental but most cases **idiopathic**
    - Increased temporalis muscle activity, trauma, TMJ ankylosis, or masticatory parafunction (awake &/or sleep)
- Associated abnormalities
  - May be component of
    - Basal cell nevus syndrome
    - Trismus-pseudocamptodactyly syndrome

Microscopic Features

- Normal bone structure

CLINICAL ISSUES

Presentation

- Most common signs/symptoms
  - **Progressive** decrease in range of opening
    - May have apparent closed lock
  - Usually **painless**
- Other signs/symptoms
  - If unilateral: **Deviation** to affected side on opening, facial **asymmetry**
    - Affected malar bone may be more prominent
  - Mobile lump above superior zygomatic arch

Demographics

- Age
  - Onset often in **puberty**; age range: Birth-62 years
- Gender
  - M:F = 3.3:1 for bilateral presentation

Natural History & Prognosis

- 1 or both coronoid processes enlarge and impinge on medial aspect of zygomatic bone to restrict mouth opening
- **Bilateral**:unilateral = 4.7:1.0
  - Unilateral cases may show minor changes on contralateral side, suggesting spectrum of involvement
- Prognosis excellent with adequate treatment

Treatment

- Surgical removal of coronoid ± muscle myotomy/fasciotomy
- Postoperative physiotherapy important

DIAGNOSTIC CHECKLIST

Consider

- Some cases of limited mandibular movement due to normal coronoid process impinging on
  - **Tooth**, such as buccally positioned maxillary 2nd or 3rd molar
  - Enlarged and thickened maxillary **tuberosity**
- Superior repositioning of coronoid process secondary to loss of condylar length
  - Juvenile idiopathic arthritis (JIA), condylar fracture, progressive condylar resorption (PCR)
- Superior repositioning of coronoid process and coronoid process elongation
  - JIA, PCR, fracture, and coronoid enlargement secondary to muscle pull

Image Interpretation Pearls

- Use axial CBCT reformat in open position to see coronoid interference on opening

Reporting Tips

- Check contralateral side: May also be enlarged but to lesser extent

SELECTED REFERENCES

1. Torenek K et al: Clinical and radiological findings of a bilateral coronoid hyperplasia case. Eur J Dent. 9(1):149-52, 2015

(Left) *CBCT lateral 3D surface rendering of a patient with coronoid hyperplasia is shown. Note the coronoid process ⇨ extending above the superior border of the zygomatic arch.* **(Right)** *CBCT lateral 3D surface rendering (same patient) shows the mandible in the open position. There is limitation of opening noted, caused by the coronoid process and attached temporalis muscle not clearing the zygomatic bone ⇨.*

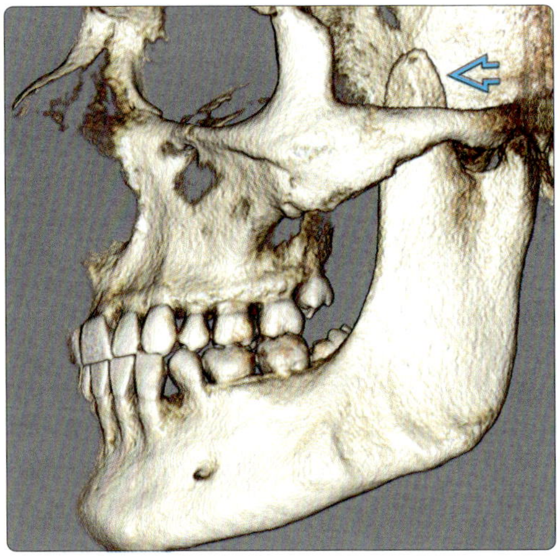

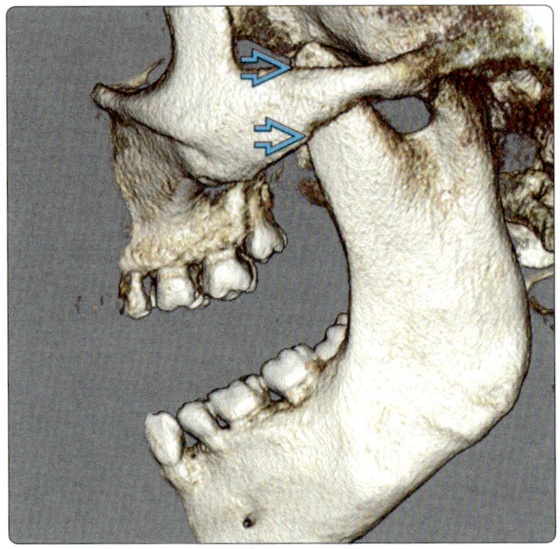

(Left) *Axial CBCT in the closed position in the same patient shows a thickened and elongated coronoid process ⇨ and bony apposition on the zygomatic arch ↷ opposing the large coronoid process.* **(Right)** *Axial CBCT in the open position in the same patient shows the proximity of the coronoid process to the zygomatic bone and the formation of a pseudocartilaginous joint ↷. There is no real bone-to-bone contact due to the presence of facial and temporalis muscle fibers on the coronoid process tip.*

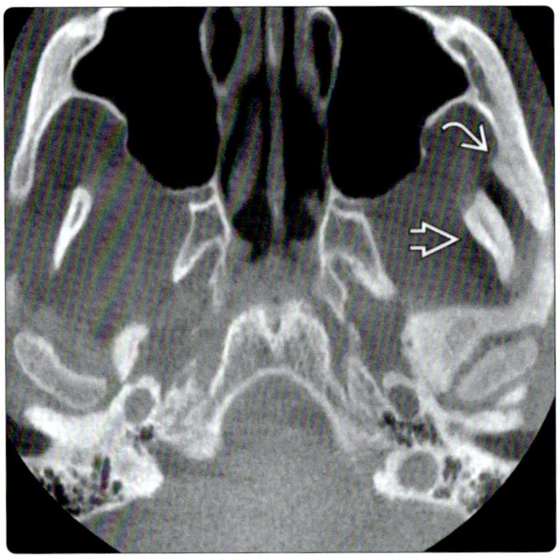

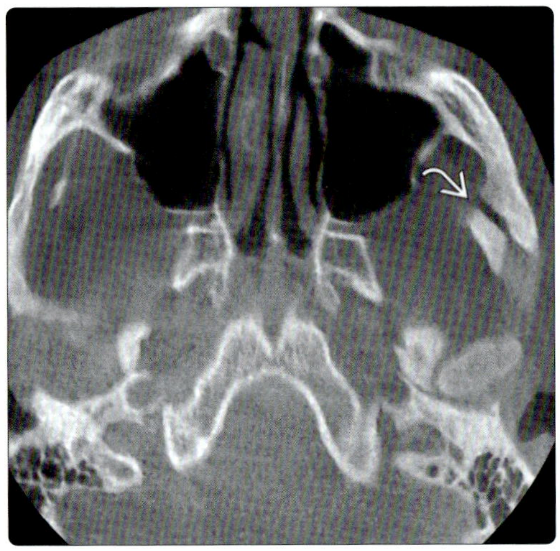

(Left) *Sagittal oblique CBCT in the closed position in the same patient shows the size of the coronoid hyperplasia in relation to the condyle. The condyle is seated in the fossa ⇨. The sigmoid notch is elevated ↷, creating the appearance of a short condyle.* **(Right)** *Sagittal oblique CBCT (same patient) shows the limited translation of the condyle ⇨ in the fossa due to the obstruction of the mandibular movement by the large coronoid abutting the zygoma ↷.*

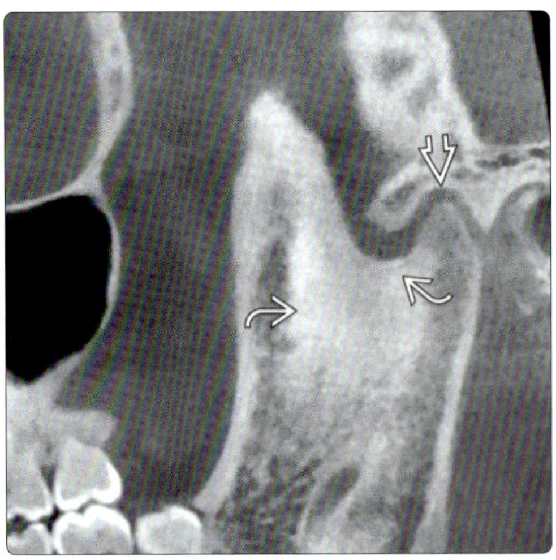

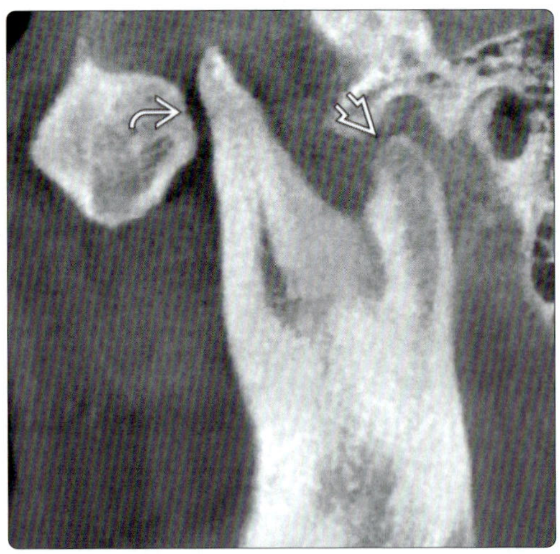

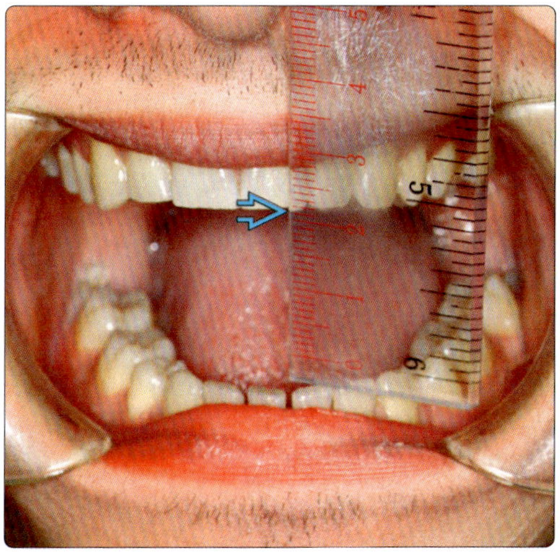

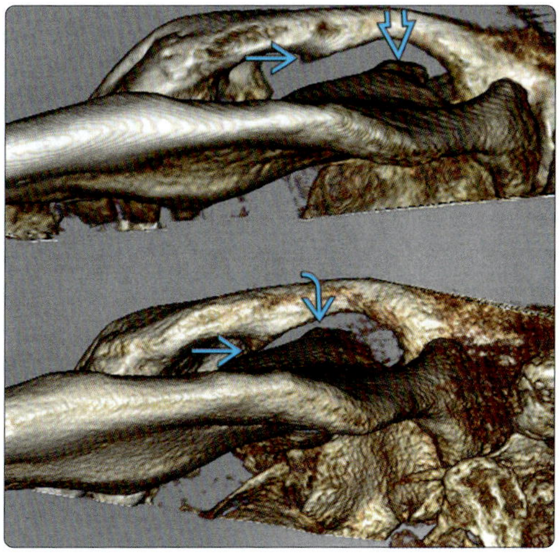

(Left) *Clinical photograph in the same patient shows limitation of opening (about 24 mm) due to the coronoid hyperplasia.* **(Right)** *CBCT inferior 3D surface rendering shows the position of the coronoid process in relation to the zygoma in the closed and open positions. Bony exostosis is noted on the medial surface of the zygoma.*

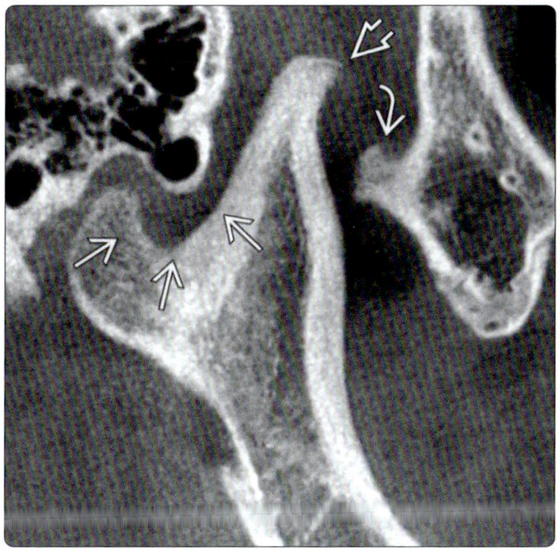

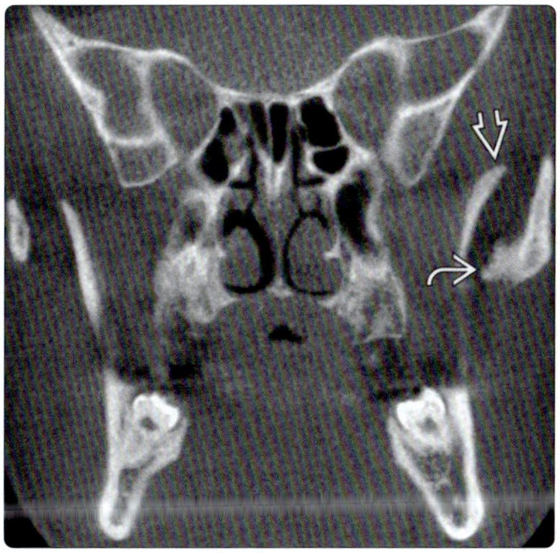

(Left) *Sagittal oblique CBCT in the closed position shows coronoid hyperplasia with an anterior hook formation. Upon opening, this hook engages an exostosis on the zygoma. The mandibular notch is shallow and the condyle, notch, and coronoid process resemble a "check mark" or "swoosh".* **(Right)** *Coronal CBCT in the same patient shows the lateral bowing of the left coronoid process forming a hook that, upon opening, engages with the exostosis on the zygoma.*

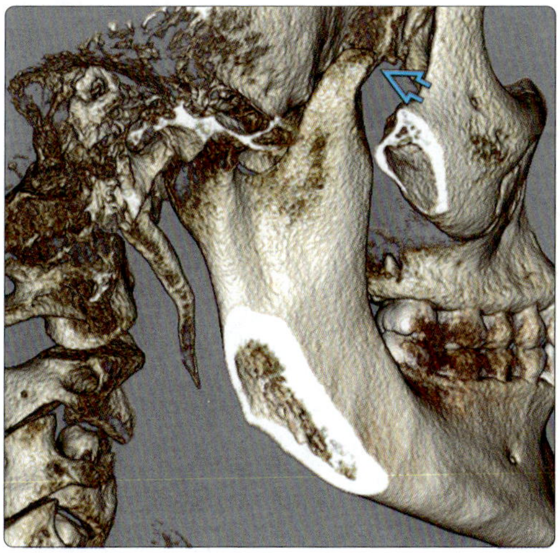

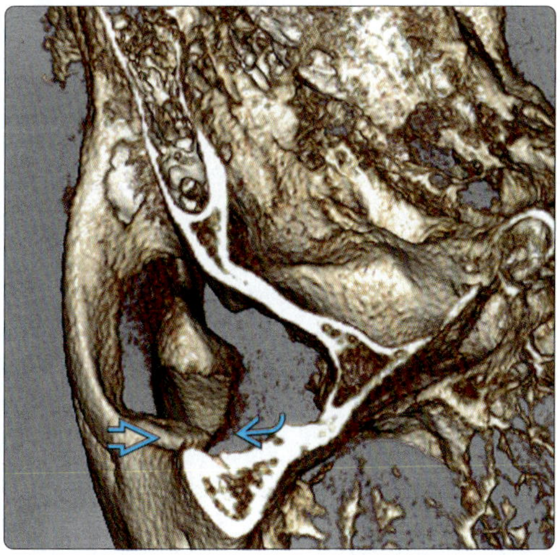

(Left) *CBCT lateral 3D surface rendering with sagittal clipping in the same patient shows the hook appearance of the coronoid process.* **(Right)** *CBCT inferior 3D surface rendering with axial clipping (same patient) shows the hook-shaped coronoid process engaging the exostosis on the zygoma upon opening.*

Condylar Hypoplasia

KEY FACTS

TERMINOLOGY

- Definition: Abnormally **small condyle** due to developmental abnormality
  - Development of ipsilateral half of mandible also affected; mandible also small on affected side

IMAGING

- Condyle small but morphology **normal**
- Affects **condyle** with underdevelopment of ipsilateral **ramus** and **mandibular body**
- **Unilateral** more common than bilateral
- Small condyle with normal shape and structure
- Condylar neck slender, may be shortened
- Mandibular fossa small
- Posterior ramus border and condylar neck may have **posterior inclination**
- Degree of hypoplasia ranges from mild condylar size alteration to severe condylar growth disturbance with marked facial asymmetry

TOP DIFFERENTIAL DIAGNOSES

- Normal variation
- Degenerative joint disease
- Juvenile arthritis

CLINICAL ISSUES

- Mandibular **asymmetry**, TMJ dysfunction
- Chin often **deviated** to affected side, mandible deviates to affected side on opening
- Usually component of mandibular growth deficiency
  - Degree of resulting asymmetry depends on **age** when condylar growth affected
  - Greater disturbance of condylar growth and ipsilateral facial development if it occurs **early**
- **Degenerative joint disease** often long-term sequela

DIAGNOSTIC CHECKLIST

- May be part of generalized hypoplasia (hemifacial microsomia) or syndrome

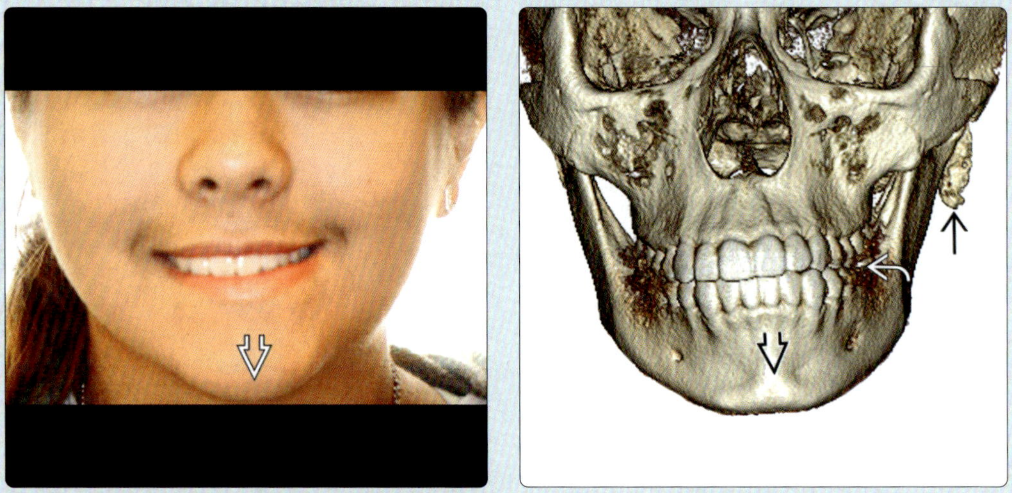

(Left) *Clinical photograph shows facial asymmetry and the chin to the left of the midline.* **(Right)** *Anteroposterior CBCT 3D reformation in the same patient shows asymmetry of the mandible due to left condylar hypoplasia. The mastoid process is visible on the left, indicating less lateral development of the left mandible. The dental midlines are coincident, but the mandibular osseous midline is shifted to the left. The occlusal plane is higher on the left, and there is a posterior crossbite.*

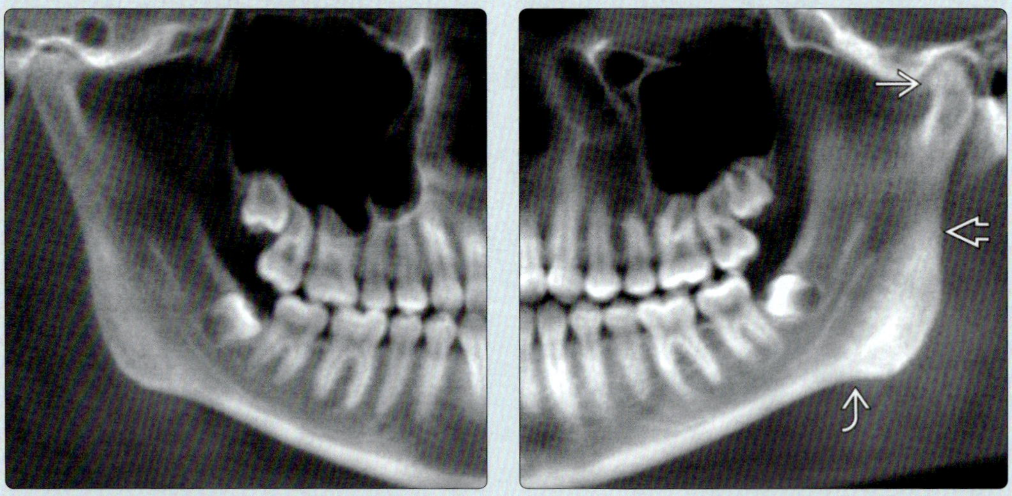

(Left) *Panoramic CBCT reformation in the same patient shows the normal right condyle and normal contour of the posterior ramus and angle of the mandible.* **(Right)** *Panoramic CBCT reformation in the same patient shows a small left condyle with otherwise normal morphology and signs of a small left mandible, including increased dorsal bend of the ramus and a deepened antegonial notch.*

TERMINOLOGY

Definitions

- Abnormally **small condyle** due to developmental abnormality
  - Development of ipsilateral half of mandible also affected; mandible also small on affected side
  - If additional structures of face affected: Hemifacial microsomia

IMAGING

General Features

- Best diagnostic clue
  - Condyle small but morphology **normal**
- Location
  - Affects **condyle** with underdevelopment of ipsilateral **ramus** and **mandibular body**
  - **Unilateral** more common than bilateral
- Size
  - Degree of hypoplasia ranges from mild condylar size alteration to severe condylar growth disturbance with marked facial asymmetry
- Morphology
  - Condyle has normal shape and bone pattern

CT Findings

- CBCT
  - Small condyle with normal shape and structure
  - Mandibular fossa small
  - Condylar neck slender, may be shortened or elongated
  - Coronoid process slender
  - **Ramus and mandibular body** on affected side small
  - **Deepened** antegonial notch

Imaging Recommendations

- Best imaging tool
  - CT or CBCT to view condyle and mandible in multiple planes
- Protocol advice
  - Panoramic reformat to assess mandibular asymmetry and dental crowding
  - Sagittal and coronal reformats of TMJs to assess condylar symmetry

DIFFERENTIAL DIAGNOSIS

Normal Variation

- Minor variability in condylar size is normal
- Not associated with mandibular asymmetry

Degenerative Joint Disease

- No mandibular hypoplasia unless occurs during growth
- Other joints may be involved

Juvenile Arthritis

- Condyle small but has abnormal shape due to destructive changes
- Other joints usually also involved

PATHOLOGY

General Features

- Etiology
  - Congenital or developmental abnormalities
    - Hemifacial microsomia, micrognathia, Treacher Collins syndrome, Pierre Robin sequence, Crouzon syndrome, auriculocondylar syndrome
    - Developmental abnormalities that manifest during growth usually unilateral
  - Acquired conditions
    - Trauma: Early injury or birth trauma
      - Affects mandibular growth center
    - Disc displacement in childhood may cause developmental disturbance in condylar growth
    - Tumor resection, radiation therapy

CLINICAL ISSUES

Presentation

- Most common signs/symptoms
  - Mandibular **asymmetry**, TMJ dysfunction
- Other signs/symptoms
  - Chin often **deviated** to affected side, mandible deviates to affected side on opening
  - Usually component of mandibular growth deficiency
  - May be associated with congenital defects of ear and zygomatic arch

Natural History & Prognosis

- Degree of resulting asymmetry depends on **age** when condylar growth affected
  - Greater disturbance of condylar growth and ipsilateral facial development if occurs early
- **Degenerative joint disease** often long-term sequela

Treatment

- Growing patients: Orthopedic treatment with functional appliances
- Older patients: Orthognathic surgery and orthodontics
- TMJ may have to be reconstructed

DIAGNOSTIC CHECKLIST

Consider

- May be part of generalized hypoplasia (hemifacial microsomia) or syndrome

Image Interpretation Pearls

- Condylar shape is **normal**, but condyle and ipsilateral mandible **small**

Reporting Tips

- Check for abnormalities of adjacent structures

SELECTED REFERENCES

1. Travieso R et al: A range of condylar hypoplasia exists in Treacher Collins syndrome. J Oral Maxillofac Surg. 71(2):393-7, 2013
2. Moze K et al: Cone beam computed tomography in the diagnosis of unilateral condylar hypoplasia: report of a case. West Indian Med J. 61(7):739-42, 2012
3. Papagrigorakis MJ et al: Auriculo-condylar syndrome. Angle Orthod. 82(3):556-64, 2012

(Left) *Volume-rendered CBCT in a 19-year-old woman with a left-side condylar hypoplasia shows that lateral development of the left mandible* ➔ *is less than the right. The mandibular angle* ➔ *and occlusal plane* ➔ *are elevated on the left side. The osseous midline of the mandible is shifted to the left* ➔*.* **(Right)** *Volume-rendered lateral view of the same patient shows elevation of the left angle of the mandible* ➔ *and a relatively prominent left antegonial notch* ➔*.*

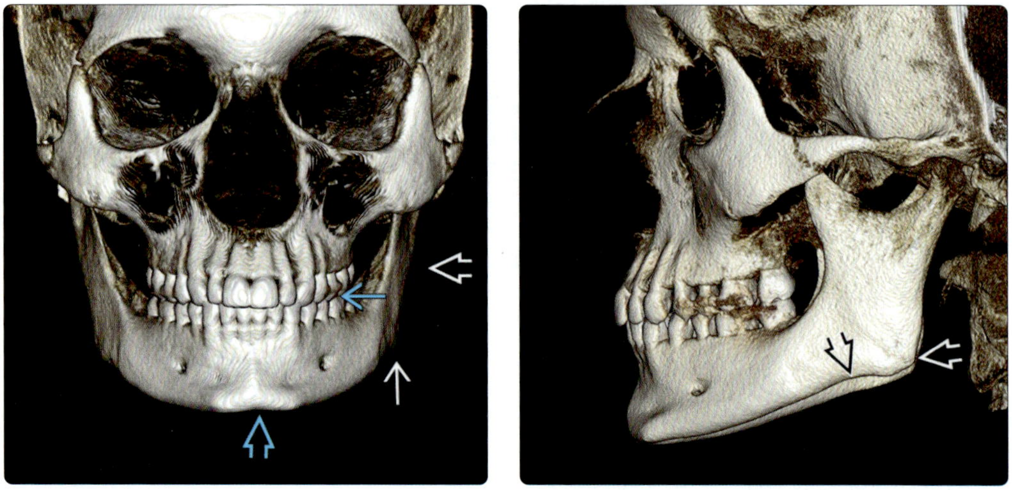

(Left) *CBCT panoramic reconstruction in the same patient shows normal size and shape of the right mandible.* **(Right)** *Panoramic reformat of the left mandible in the same patient shows the vertical dimensions of the body* ➔*, ascending ramus* ➔*, and condylar process* ➔ *of the mandible are shorter than the contralateral side.*

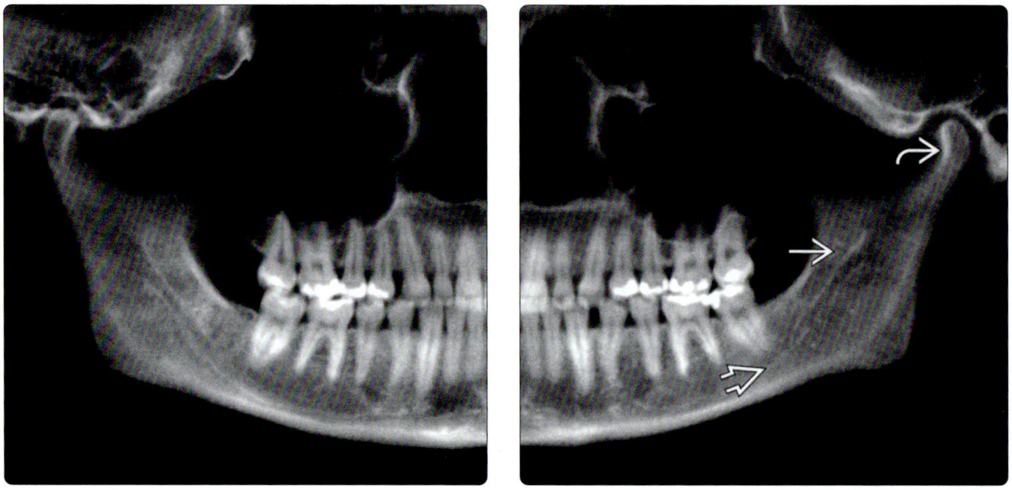

(Left) *CBCT sagittal oblique section of the same patient shows a right condyle with normal size and shape.* **(Right)** *CBCT sagittal oblique section of the same patient shows a small (hypoplastic) condyle with normal shape positioned posteriorly within the fossa. This posterior position may predispose to an anteriorly displaced disc. Disc displacement during somatic growth may be associated with condylar hypoplasia.*

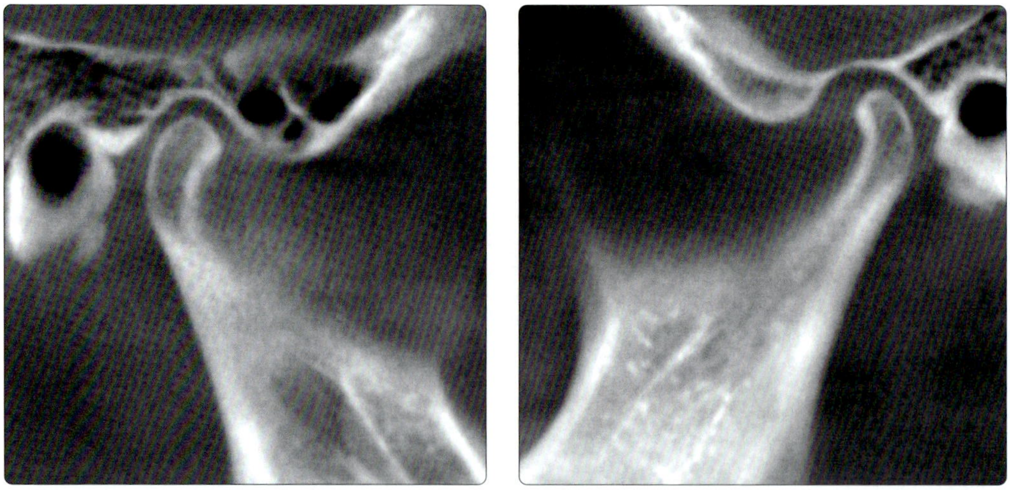

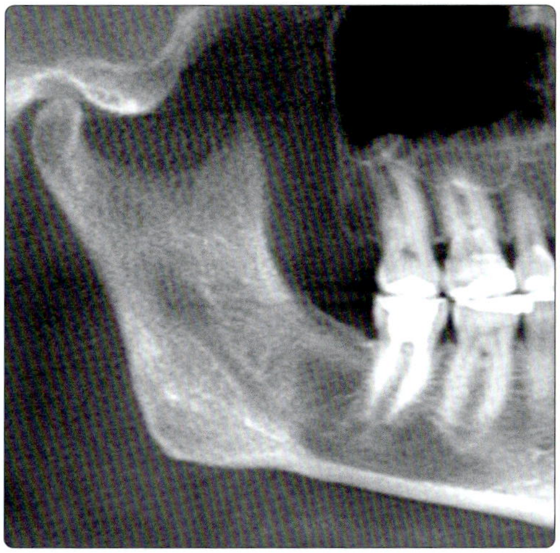
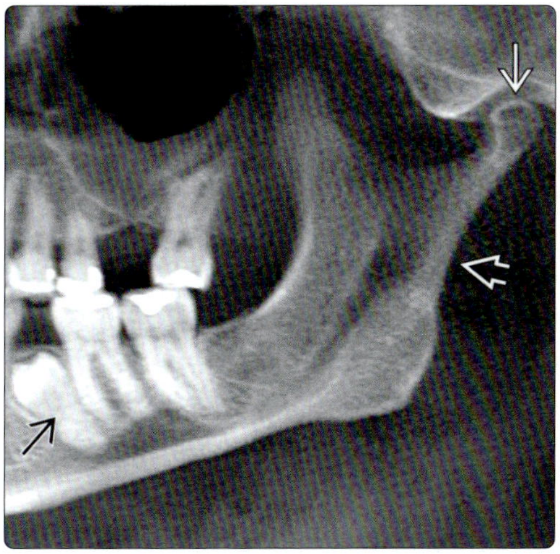

(Left) *Panoramic reformatted CBCT of a patient with left condylar hypoplasia shows the normal right side.* **(Right)** *Panoramic reformatted CBCT of the same patient shows a smaller condyle → on the left side, more pronounced dorsal bend → of the posterior ramus, and smaller mandibular height than on the contralateral side. The impacted mandibular bicuspid → is an incidental finding.*

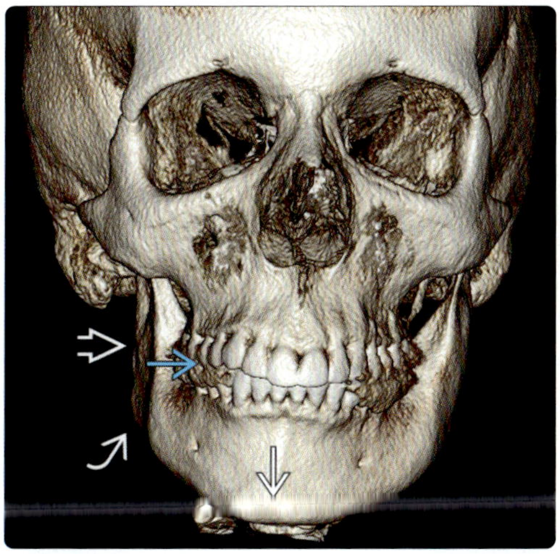
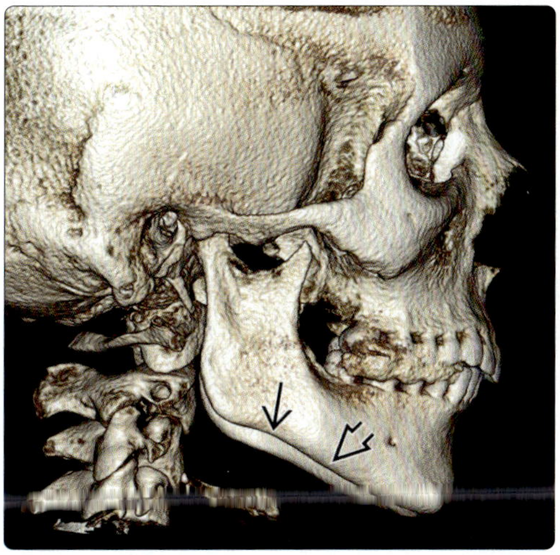

(Left) *Frontal volume-rendered CBCT shows a patient with right-side condylar hypoplasia. The osseous midline of the mandible is shifted to the right →. Lateral development of the right side of the mandible is decreased →. The right angle of the mandible → and the occlusal plane → are elevated.* **(Right)** *Lateral CBCT 3D rendering of the same patient shows elevation of the right side of the mandible →. The right antegonial notch → is more prominent than the left.*

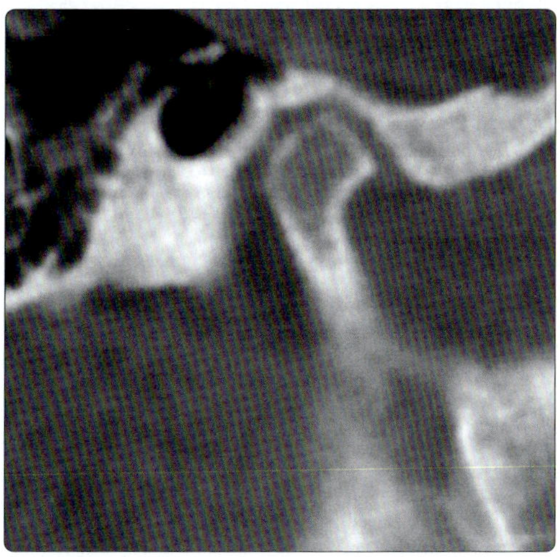
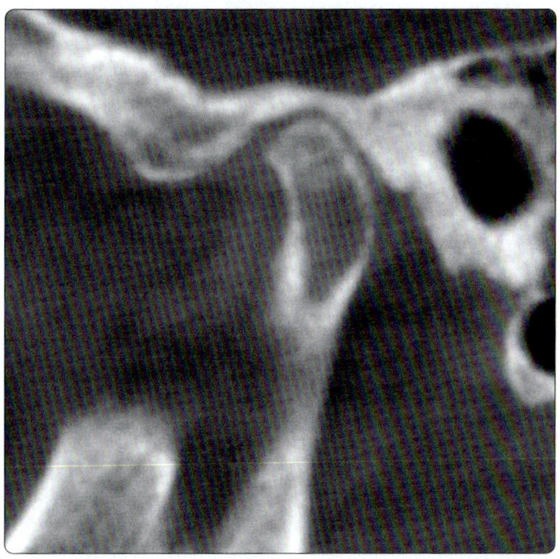

(Left) *CBCT parasagittal view of the right TMJ in the same patient shows a small condyle with a normal shape. Note thin superior joint space, which increases the probability of disc displacement. Disc displacement during somatic growth may be associated with condylar hypoplasia.* **(Right)** *Parasagittal CBCT of the left TMJ in the same patient shows that the left condyle has a normal size and shape.*

Fibrous Ankylosis

KEY FACTS

TERMINOLOGY

- Synonyms: Ankylosis, adhesions
- Definition: Unyielding restriction in condylar movement due to intraarticular fibrous tissue and not associated with pain

IMAGING

- Protocol advice
  - Open- and closed-mouth images
  - Images reconstructed parallel and perpendicular to mediolateral long axis of condyle
- CT or CBCT
  - Maintenance of joint space: Visible separation of condyle and fossa
  - No condylar translation
  - May have cortical irregularities
- MR
  - No joint effusion
  - No contrast enhancement

TOP DIFFERENTIAL DIAGNOSES

- Adhesions
- Bony ankylosis
- False ankylosis

PATHOLOGY

- Predisposing factors
  - Trauma (57-63%)
  - Inflammatory arthritides
  - Joint surgery
  - Infection

CLINICAL ISSUES

- Severely limited interincisor mouth opening
- Very limited condylar translation
- Treatment: Excision of fibrous and bony ankylotic mass
  - Achieve 35-mm opening and maintain with mobility exercises and physical therapy

(Left) *CBCT panoramic reformat in an 8-year-old girl shows a fibrous type of ankylosis secondary to trauma and a subcondylar fracture dislocation. A large osseous mass is attached to the temporal bone ➡ and mandible ⇨. A lucent zone ➡ is seen separating the masses, indicating maintenance of joint space.* **(Right)** *Sagittal oblique CBCT of the left TMJ of an adult woman shows a fibrous ankylosis secondary to a healed intracapsular infection. A thin, irregular joint space ➡ is noted between the condyle and fossa.*

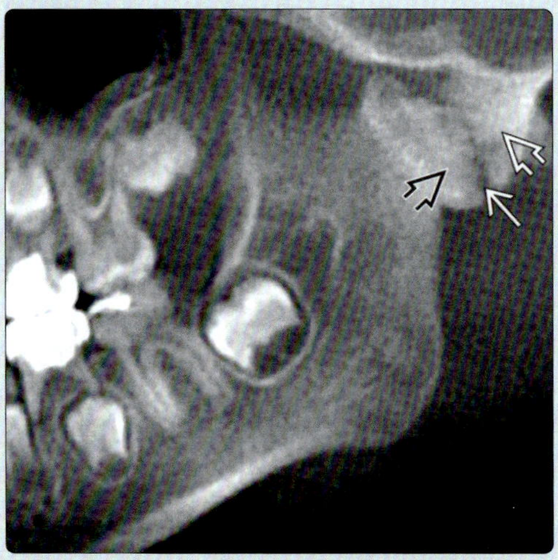

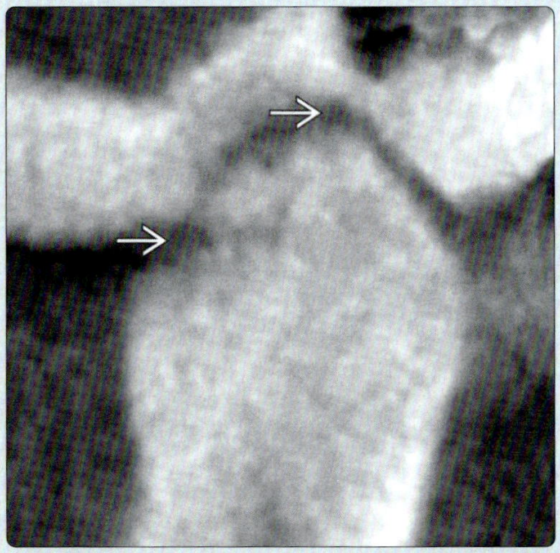

(Left) *CBCT 3D rendering in an adolescent patient shows abnormal, remodeled condyle ⇨ and fossa ⇨ representing ankylosis following a prior trauma. Note elongated abnormal hyperplastic coronoid process ⇨ extending above the superior border of the zygomatic arch.* **(Right)** *Sagittal oblique CBCT through the left ramus in the same patient shows maintenance of a thin band of radiolucency ⇨ between the temporal and mandibular components of the joint, indicating a fibrous rather than a bony union.*

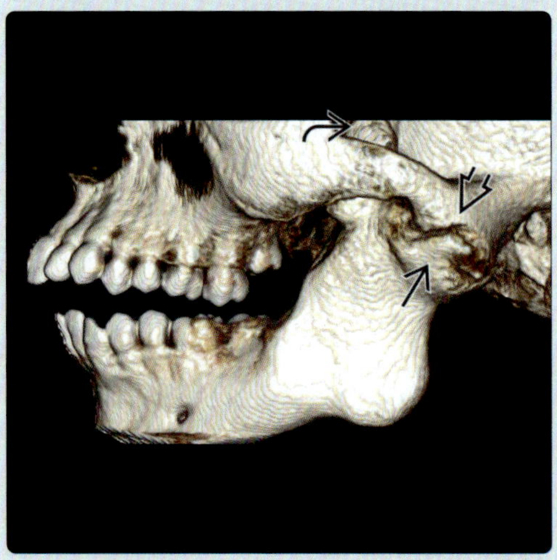

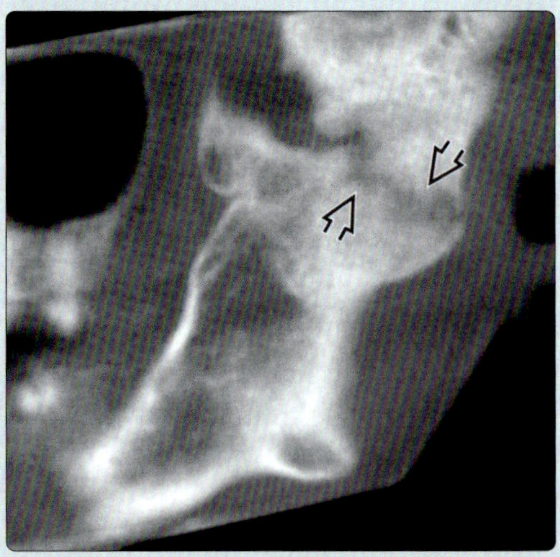

TERMINOLOGY

Synonyms

- Ankylosis, adhesions

Definitions

- Unyielding restriction in condylar movement due to intraarticular fibrous tissue and not associated with pain

IMAGING

General Features

- Best diagnostic clue
  - Lack of condylar translation
- Location
  - TMJ

CT Findings

- CBCT
  - Very limited or no condylar translation
  - Maintenance of joint space: Visible separation of condyle and fossa
  - May have cortical irregularities

MR Findings

- No joint effusion
- No contrast enhancement

Imaging Recommendations

- Best imaging tool
  - CT or CBCT
- Protocol advice
  - Open and closed mouth images
  - Images reconstructed parallel and perpendicular to mediolateral long axis of condyle
  - Panoramic reconstruction
    - Assessment of mandibular symmetry

DIFFERENTIAL DIAGNOSIS

Adhesions

- No disc motion
- Condylar translation, but limited

Bony Ankylosis

- Bone formation
- **Loss of joint space**

False Ankylosis

- Extracapsular causes of ankylosis include
  - Coronoid hyperplasia
  - Muscle abnormalities

PATHOLOGY

General Features

- Etiology
  - Predisposing events
    - Trauma (57-63%)
      - Extravasation of blood into joint
      - Disruption of fibrocartilage integrity
      - Ingrowth of fibrous connective tissue
      - ± ossification
      - Fusion of condyle to temporal bone
    - Inflammatory arthritides
      - Juvenile idiopathic arthritis
      - Rheumatoid arthritis
      - Ankylosing spondylitis
    - Joint surgery
    - Infection

Staging, Grading, & Classification

- Fibrous
  - Maintenance of joint space
  - Osseous surfaces may be irregular
- Fibroosseous
  - Bone formation
  - Maintenance of joint space
- Osseous
  - Bone formation
  - Loss of joint space

CLINICAL ISSUES

Presentation

- Most common signs/symptoms
  - Severely limited interincisor mouth opening
  - Very limited condylar translation
- Other signs/symptoms
  - No pain
  - No joint sounds
  - ± subcondylar fracture
  - Associated with **limited mandibular growth in children**
    - Short condylar process
    - Short ramus
    - Body of mandible with short vertical dimension
    - Elevation of ipsilateral occlusal plane
    - Obtuse gonial angle

Treatment

- Excision of fibrous and bony ankylotic mass
- Achieve passive intraoperative opening of 35 mm
  - Unilateral or bilateral coronoidectomy if 35-mm opening not achieved
- Replace native disc or line TMJ with temporalis myofascial flap
- Restore ramus length with distraction osteogenesis or costochondral graft and rigid fixation
- Early mobilization of jaw
- Aggressive physical therapy

DIAGNOSTIC CHECKLIST

Consider

- Rule out false ankylosis: Not related to joint

Image Interpretation Pearls

- Lack of condylar translation of intracapsular origin

SELECTED REFERENCES

1. Yan YB et al: A pilot trial on the molecular pathophysiology of traumatic temporomandibular joint bony ankylosis in a sheep model. Part II: The differential gene expression among fibrous ankylosis, bony ankylosis and condylar fracture. J Craniomaxillofac Surg. 42(2):e23-8, 2014
2. Yan YB et al: Current concepts in the pathogenesis of traumatic temporomandibular joint ankylosis. Head Face Med. 10:35, 2014

KEY FACTS

TERMINOLOGY

- Definition: Joint immobility characterized by formation of osseous or fibroosseous mass fused to skull

IMAGING

- Markedly **reduced or absent joint space** with irregular, enlarged joint margins with fibroosseous or bony bridging
- Bridge may fuse condyle to cranial base and obliterate joint space
- Can involve condyle, temporal bone, and zygomatic process
- Secondary degenerative joint disease common
- Associated changes
  - Elongation of coronoid process
  - **Deepened antegonial notch** on affected side due to muscle function during attempted opening
- Ankylosis in very young patients affects mandibular growth
  - Short ramus, prominent antegonial notching, steep mandibular plane: **Bird face**

TOP DIFFERENTIAL DIAGNOSES

- Osteochondroma
- Osteoma
- Fibrous ankylosis

CLINICAL ISSUES

- Most common signs: History of progressively restricted jaw opening or longstanding history of limited opening
- If unilateral ankylosis, usually have some opening due to flexing of mandible
- Limited or no protrusive or lateral movement, especially if bilateral ankylosis
- If ankylosis occurs in infancy, mandibular growth affected → **micrognathia**
- Prognosis varies: **May get recurrence** of ankylosis or limited mandibular movement
- Treatment: Surgical removal of osseous bridge, occasionally condylectomy or joint replacement

(Left) *Sagittal reformatted CBCT shows ankylosis of the left condyle. The condyle is sclerotic → and the joint space is absent → in the area of fusion. The temporal bone is sclerotic and irregular →. The glenoid fossa is flattened and the articular eminence is absent.* **(Right)** *Panoramic radiograph shows bony ankylosis of the left TMJ →. The joint space is not visible, and condylar morphology is poorly defined. The coronoid process → is elongated, and there is deepening of the antegonial notch →.*

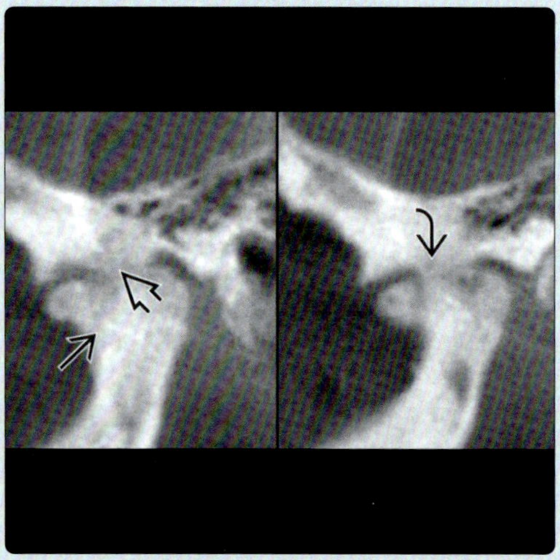

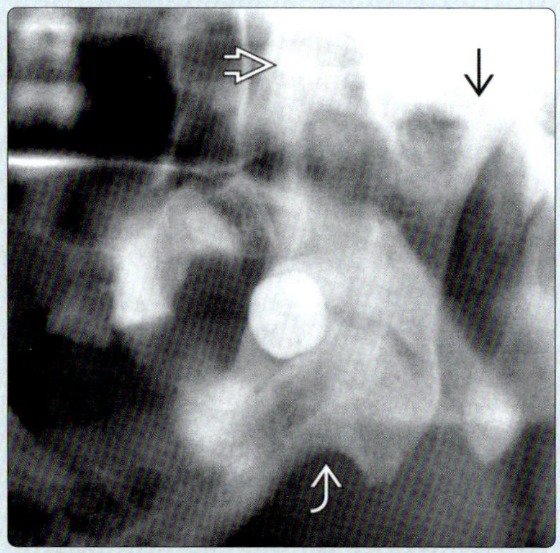

(Left) *Coronal NECT of the same patient shows gross enlargement of the right condyle, which is fused to the temporal bone by an osseous bridge → on the lateral aspect. The joint space is obliterated. The condylar neck and ramus → are thick.* **(Right)** *Axial NECT of the same patient shows sclerosis → and enlargement of the condyle in all dimensions with fusion → to the temporal bone and loss of joint space.*

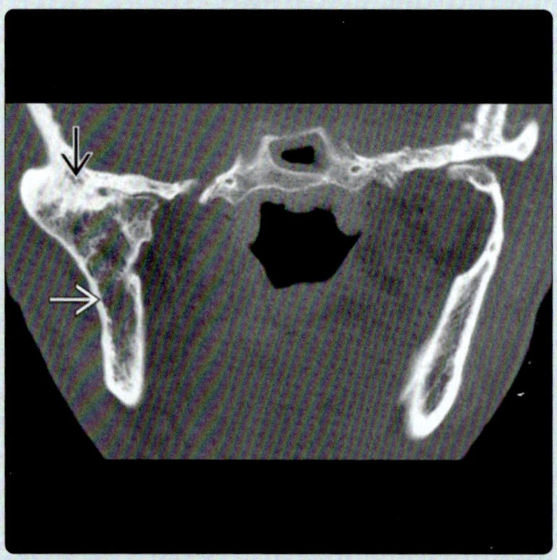

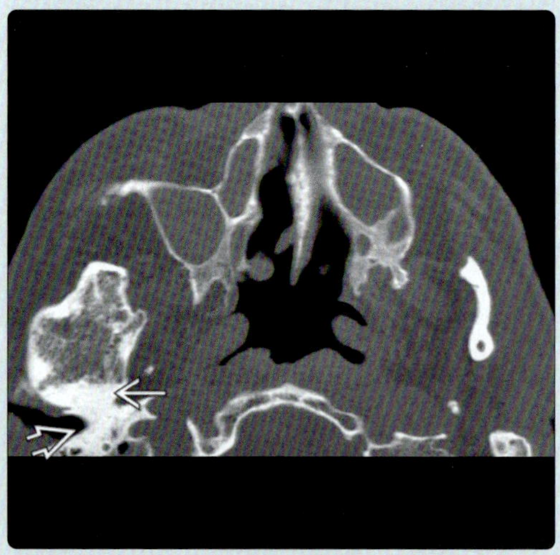

TERMINOLOGY

Definitions

- Joint immobility characterized by formation of osseous or fibroosseous mass fused to skull
  - Unilateral or bilateral

IMAGING

General Features

- Best diagnostic clue
  - Markedly reduced or absent joint space with irregular, enlarged joint margins with fibrous or bony bridging

CT Findings

- Joint space partly or completely obliterated by osseous bridge
  - Bridge may be **small bone segment** or **large bony mass** that extends medially and laterally beyond confines of capsule
    - Bridge may fuse condyle to cranial base and **obliterate joint space**
    - Ankylosis often develops lateral to condyle, especially if condyle medially displaced due to fracture
- Can involve condyle, temporal bone, and zygomatic process
- Flattening of glenoid fossa, which remodels to accommodate abnormal condyle
- Secondary degenerative joint disease common
- Associated changes
  - Elongation of coronoid process
  - **Deepened antegonial notch** on affected side due to muscle function during attempted opening
- Ankylosis in very young patients **affects mandibular growth**
  - Short ramus, prominent antegonial notching, steep mandibular plane: **Bird face**
  - Condyle and glenoid fossa more inferiorly positioned

Imaging Recommendations

- Best imaging tool
  - Bone CT or CBCT
- Protocol advice
  - Coronal images best

DIFFERENTIAL DIAGNOSIS

Osteochondroma

- No history of trauma, infection, or other joint diseases
- Osteochondroma can appear as large bony mass on condyle but **joint space still visible**

Osteoma

- May look similar if osteoma large and involves superior condylar surface; **joint space still visible**
- No history of trauma, infection, or other joint diseases

Fibrous Ankylosis

- Can simulate bony ankylosis due to hypomobility
- Joint components normal; **joint space narrowed but still visible**

PATHOLOGY

General Features

- Etiology
  - Trauma (most common)
  - Infection: Local or systemic
  - Systemic disease: Rheumatoid arthritis, psoriasis, ankylosing spondylitis
  - Most common cause of bilateral ankylosis is rheumatoid arthritis or bilateral condylar fractures
  - Ankylosis occurring in infancy often due to birth injury (condylar fracture)

Staging, Grading, & Classification

- Classification
  - **True**: Limited condylar movement due to mechanical problem in joint
    - Subclassified as bony, fibrous, or fibroosseous
    - Intra- or extracapsular
  - **False**: Limited condylar movement due to mechanical cause not related to joint components
    - Elongation of coronoid process or ankylosis of coronoid process to posterior maxilla
  - Congenital ankylosis reported: Etiology is condylar region malformation

CLINICAL ISSUES

Presentation

- Most common signs/symptoms
  - History of progressively restricted jaw opening or longstanding history of limited opening
- Other signs/symptoms
  - If unilateral ankylosis, usually have some opening due to flexing of mandible
  - Limited or no protrusive or lateral movement, especially if bilateral ankylosis
  - If ankylosis occurs in infancy, mandibular growth affected → **micrognathia**
    - Degree of mandibular growth retardation worse if ankylosis occurs at younger age
  - **Deviation** of mandible on opening

Natural History & Prognosis

- Trauma → intraarticular hematoma → fibrosis and excessive bone formation
- Prognosis varies: May get recurrence of ankylosis or limited mandibular movement after treatment

Treatment

- Surgical removal of osseous bridge, occasionally condylectomy or joint replacement
  - Early treatment preferred, especially in young patients
- Physiotherapy after surgical phase

SELECTED REFERENCES

1. Anyanechi CE: Temporomandibular joint ankylosis caused by condylar fractures: a retrospective analysis of cases at an urban teaching hospital in Nigeria. Int J Oral Maxillofac Surg. 44(8):1027-33, 2015
2. Vijay P et al: Unilateral ankylosis of temporomandibular joint (TMJ) with contralateral condylar aplasia and related orthopedic deformity - syndromic or nonsyndromic? J Clin Diagn Res. 9(1):ZD34-6, 2015

TMJ Fractures

KEY FACTS

TERMINOLOGY

- Usually occur at **condylar neck** and often accompanied by **dislocation** of condyle

IMAGING

- Best diagnostic clue
  - Condylar angle altered or condyle displaced from normal position
- Location
  - Condyle ("intracapsular") and condylar neck ("extracapsular")
- Irregular boundary or step defect of cortex at fx
- Fractured fragment often anterior-medially dislocated due to pull of lateral pterygoid muscle
- Occasionally disc disruption, capsular tear, retrodiscal tissue tear, hemarthrosis
- Best tool: **Panoramic** radiograph or CBCT or CT
- Overlap (telescoping) of fx borders can occur, seen on coronal

TOP DIFFERENTIAL DIAGNOSES

- Bifid condyle
- Condylar hypoplasia
- Hemifacial microsomia

PATHOLOGY

- Condyle fx often accompanied by fx of mandible or facial skeleton

CLINICAL ISSUES

- May be **asymptomatic**, especially in **young** patients
- **Unilateral**:bilateral = 3:1
- Fractured fragment may **ankylose** to ramus stump: **Bifid condyle** in coronal views
- If fx at **young age**: Mandibular **hypoplasia** on affected side with deviation of mandible

DIAGNOSTIC CHECKLIST

- Consider condylar fx in cases of chin/angle trauma

(Left) *CBCT panoramic reformat of a 17-year-old boy with a history of trauma to the right side of the mandible and resultant left-side TMJ pain shows normal right side mandibular anatomy. There is limited mandibular motion and deviation to the left on opening.* **(Right)** *Panoramic reformat of the left mandible in the same patient shows a dislocated condylar neck fracture. The proximal segment is displaced in the direction of pull of the lateral pterygoid muscle. Note the empty fossa.*

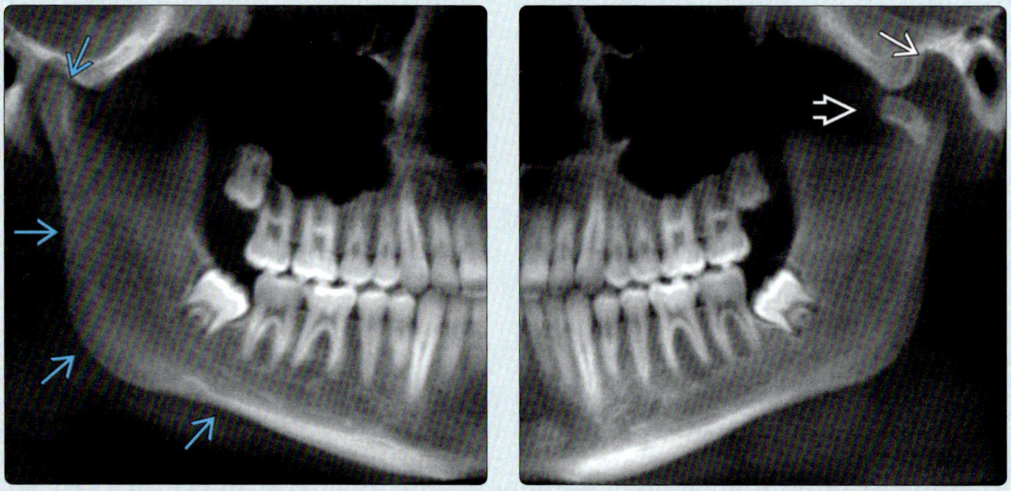

(Left) *Sagittal oblique CBCT in the same patient shows the left TMJ fracture. The proximal segment is displaced and opposes the apex of the articular eminence. Normal healing encourages function between the eminence and displaced proximal segment.* **(Right)** *Coronal oblique CBCT in the same patient shows the proximal segment located medially to the ramus. The main pull vector of the lateral pterygoid muscle is anteriorly and medially, therefore the proximal segment normally displaces in that direction.*

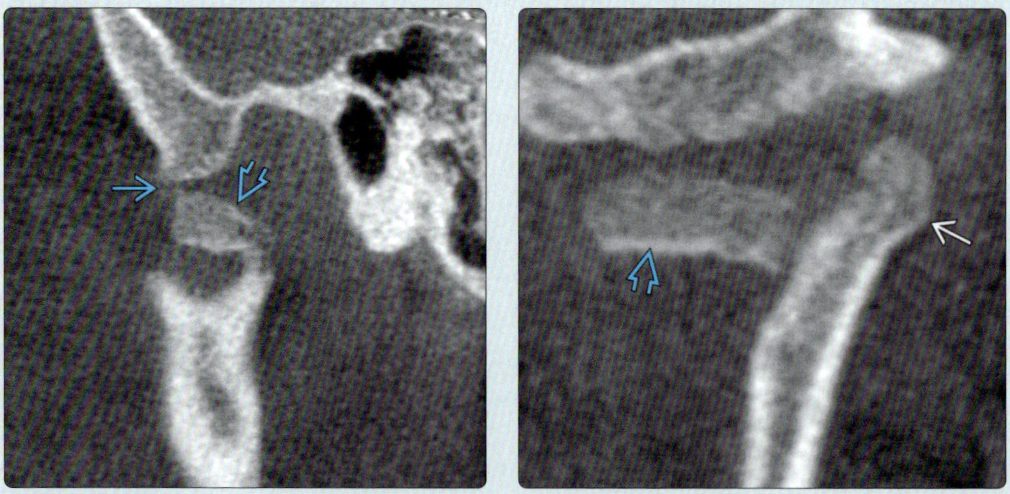

TERMINOLOGY

Definitions

- Usually occurs at **condylar neck** and often accompanied by **dislocation** of condyle

IMAGING

General Features

- Best diagnostic clue
  - Condylar angle altered or condyle displaced from normal position
- Location
  - Condyle ("intracapsular") and condylar neck ("extracapsular")
  - Rare: Fx of glenoid fossa roof or articular eminence, condylar displacement to external auditory meatus or middle cranial fossa

Radiographic Findings

- Radiography
  - Recent nondisplaced condylar neck fx: **Radiolucent line** limited to outline of condylar neck
    - Width of radiolucent line varies
      - Fragments aligned: Narrow line
      - Displacement: Wider line
      - Fragments overlap: Area of increased radiopacity instead of radiolucent line
  - Irregular boundary or step defect of cortex in fx area

CT Findings

- CBCT
  - Fx of condyle may be compressive or vertical type
  - Fractured fragment often anterior-medially dislocated due to pull of lateral pterygoid muscle

MR Findings

- Occasionally disc disruption, capsular tear, retrodiscal tissue tear, hemarthrosis

Imaging Recommendations

- Best imaging tool
  - **Panoramic** radiograph, CBCT, or CT
- Protocol advice
  - Use **3D** reformats to visualize position and displacement of fragments and to see comminution

DIFFERENTIAL DIAGNOSIS

Bifid Condyle

- Simulates condylar fx if deep notch or duplication of condyle
- May not be able to distinguish bifid condyle from old fx
- No history of trauma

Condylar Hypoplasia

- Condyle small but normal morphology

Hemifacial Microsomia

- May have temporal bone and zygoma involvement

PATHOLOGY

General Features

- Associated abnormalities
  - Condyle fx often accompanied by fx of mandible or facial skeleton

CLINICAL ISSUES

Presentation

- Most common signs/symptoms
  - May be **asymptomatic**, especially in **young** patients
  - **Swelling** over TMJ
  - **Limited range of motion** with deviation of chin to affected side on opening
  - Mandibular asymmetry; malocclusion; soft tissue contusion

Demographics

- Gender
  - M > F (3:1)
- Epidemiology
  - Condylar fxs often occur in conjunction with other mandibular fxs
  - **Unilateral**:bilateral TMJ fx = 3:1
  - Condylar and subcondylar fxs most common fxs of pediatric population

Natural History & Prognosis

- Fractured fragment may **ankylose** to ramus stump producing appearance of **bifid condyle** in coronal views
- Fractured fragment or ramus may **remodel** to produce "new" condyle or ramus
  - Mandibular fossa becomes flattened with loss of vertical height on affected side
- If fx at **young age**: Mandibular **hypoplasia** on affected side with deviation of mandible
  - Short condylar neck, flat glenoid fossa, irregular condylar angle
- **Degenerative** changes may occur with time; changes more severe if condyle displaced

Treatment

- **None** if normal mobility, otherwise surgical reduction
- Decision to treat based on patient age, coexistence of other fxs, unilateral or bilateral fx, displacement of fragment, dental occlusion

DIAGNOSTIC CHECKLIST

Consider

- Condylar fx in cases of chin trauma
- Rule out bilateral fx even if only symptomatic on 1 side
- May have additional fx(s) in mandibular body
  - Force of blow to mandibular body can cause fx of contralateral condyle

SELECTED REFERENCES

1. Nabil Y: Evaluation of the effect of different mandibular fractures on the temporomandibular joint using magnetic resonance imaging: five years of follow-up. Int J Oral Maxillofac Surg. 45(11):1495-1499, 2016
2. Cenzi R et al: Mandibular condyle fractures: evaluation of the Strasbourg Osteosynthesis Research Group classification. J Craniofac Surg. 20(1):24-8, 2009

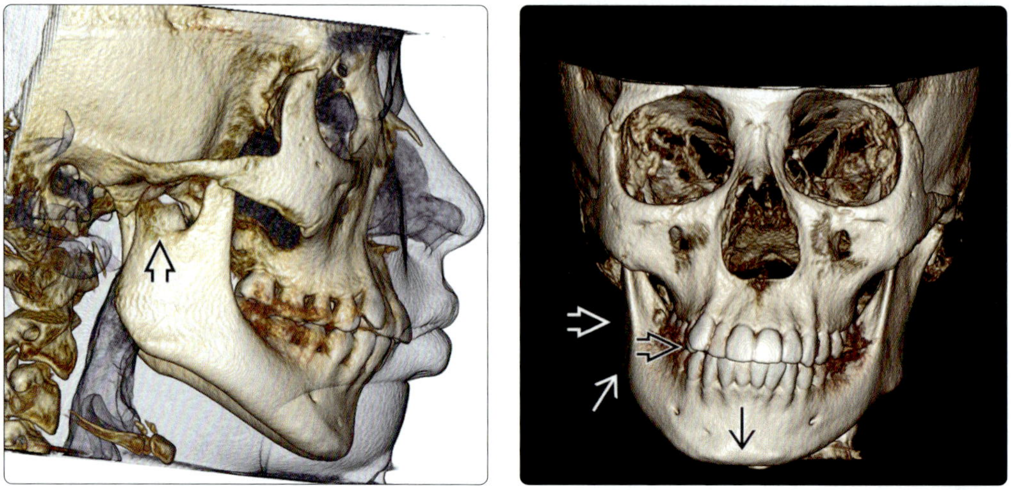

(Left) *CBCT volume rendering of a 15-year-old patient shows a perinatal condylar fracture dislocation. The proximal segment* → *is anteriorly displaced and has attached to the ramus.* **(Right)** *Volume-rendered frontal view of the same patient shows mandibular asymmetry. The right ascending ramus* → *is medially positioned, the right gonial angle* → *is superior, and the right side occlusal plane* → *is elevated. The osseous midline of the mandible* → *is shifted to the right.*

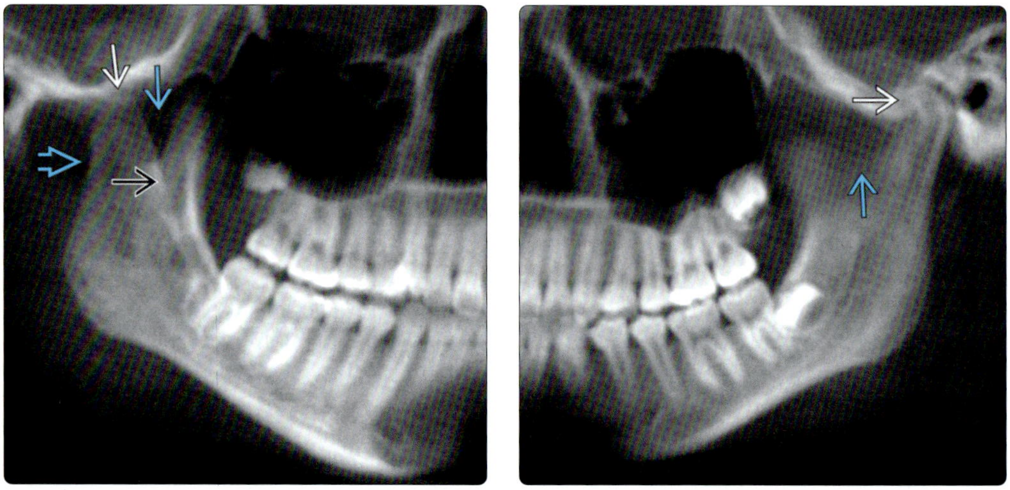

(Left) *CBCT panoramic reformat of right mandible in the same patient shows anterior positioning of the condylar process* →*. The condylar cortex* → *traverses the ramus. There is an acute angle* → *between the condylar and coronoid process. The posterior surface of the ramus and condylar process* → *has an anterior inclination.* **(Right)** *Panoramic reformat of the left mandible in the same patient shows no condylar dislocation* →*. The condylar cortex does not traverse the ramus and the sigmoid notch* → *is broad and smooth.*

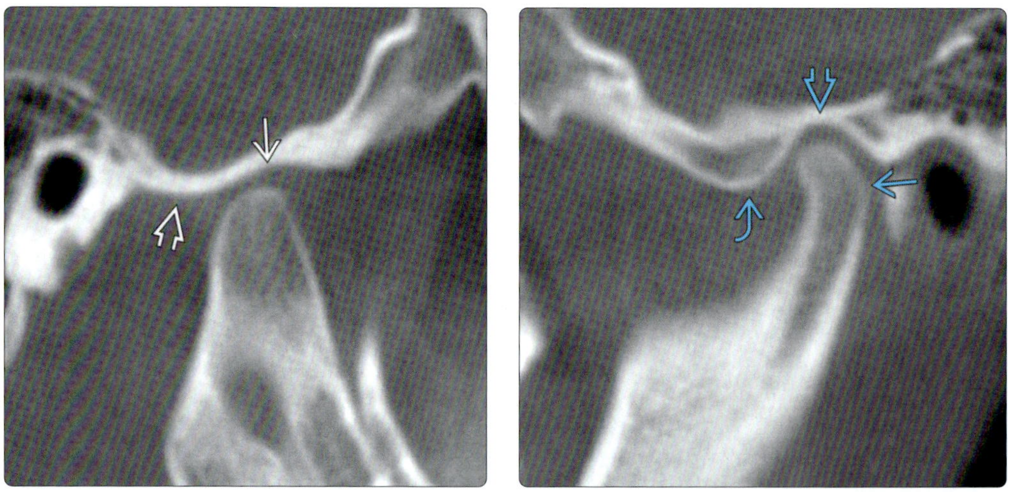

(Left) *Sagittal oblique CBCT of the right TMJ in the same patient shows an anteriorly positioned condylar process* → *on the cranial base and lack of eminence* → *development. Eminence development progresses from birth and is induced by normal condylar position and function. Lack of eminence development indicates early onset of injury.* **(Right)** *Sagittal oblique CBCT of the left TMJ in the same patient shows normal condylar* →*, fossa* →*, and eminence* → *development.*

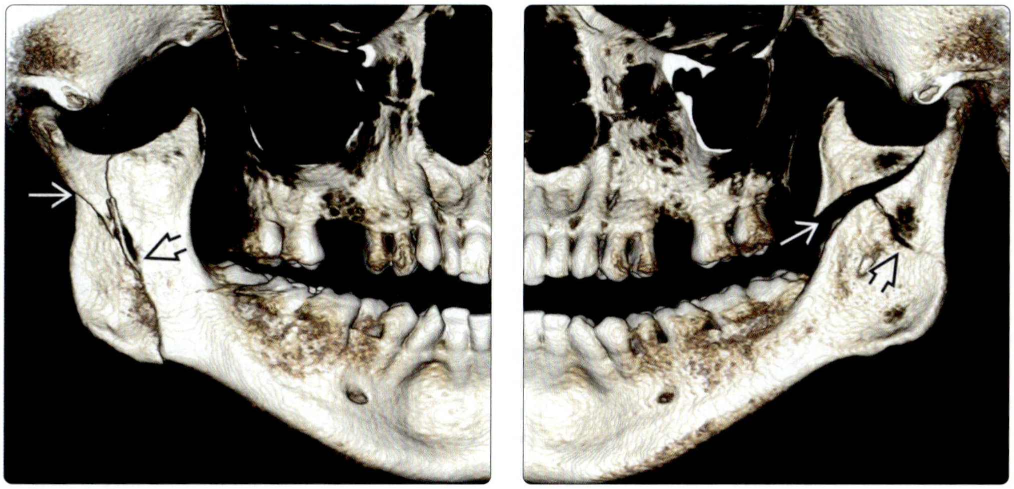

(Left) *CBCT volume-rendered panoramic reformat shows a complex mandibular fracture. There is a vertical right ramus fracture and a subcondylar fracture extending into the ramus.* **(Right)** *CBCT volume-rendered panoramic reformat of the left side in the same patient shows oblique ramus and coronoid fractures. It is not uncommon to see bilateral or multiple mandibular fractures.*

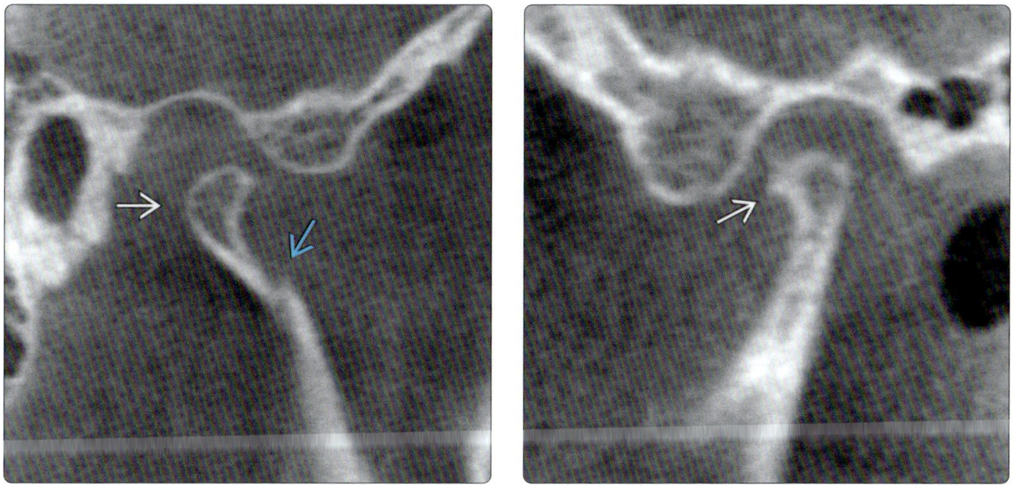

(Left) *Parasagittal CBCT in the same patient shows the anteroinferior positioning of the condyle within fossa. A subcondylar fracture and step deformity between the proximal and distal segments can be seen.* **(Right)** *Sagittal oblique CBCT of the left TMJ in the same patient shows that the condyle is small secondary to preexisting stable degenerative joint disease and is inferiorly positioned within its fossa.*

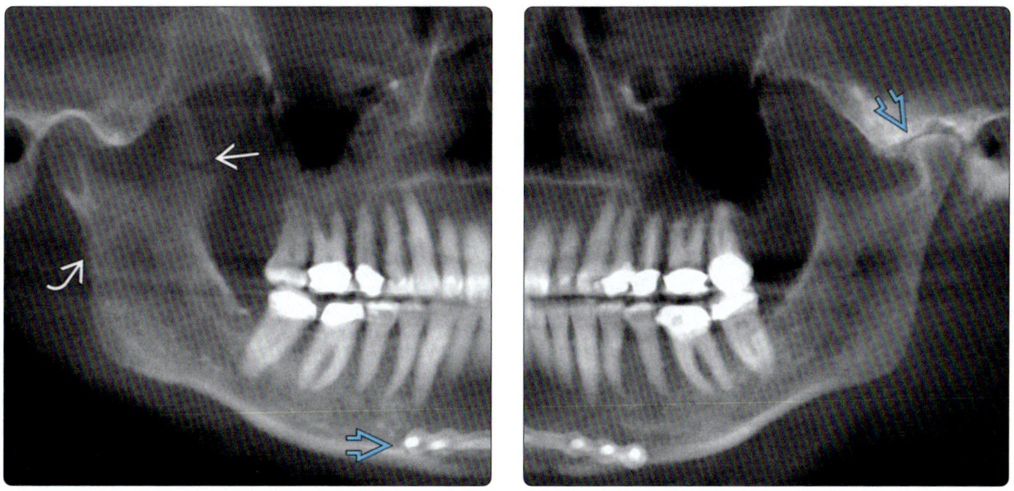

(Left) *CBCT right side panoramic reformat shows coronoid and subcondylar fractures following facial trauma. A fracture of the anterior mandible has been reduced surgically.* **(Right)** *CBCT left side panoramic reformat in the same patient shows absence of fracture in left TMJ. Degenerative changes, including sclerosis and congruent flattening of the eminence and condyle, are evident.*

(Left) *Sagittal oblique CBCT reformat shows a comminuted subcondylar fracture in the right TMJ. There is posterior displacement of the condyle within the fossa as evidenced by the increased anterior joint space. A coronoid process fracture is also seen.* **(Right)** *Coronal oblique CBCT in the same patient shows the comminuted subcondylar fracture. The inferior margin of the proximal segment has telescoped over the proximal segment, producing a step deformity. Callus formation is seen, indicating an active healing process.*

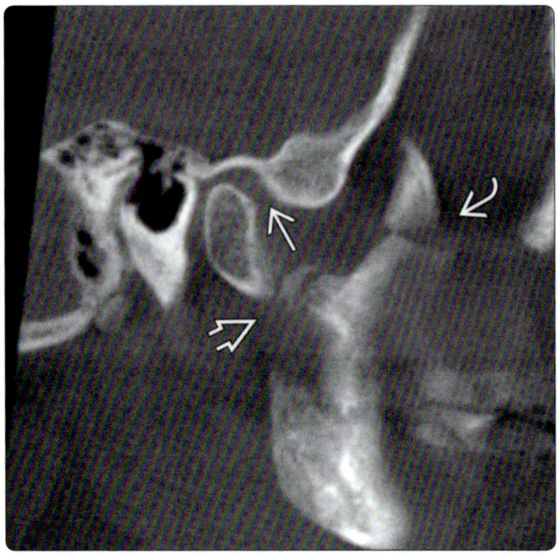

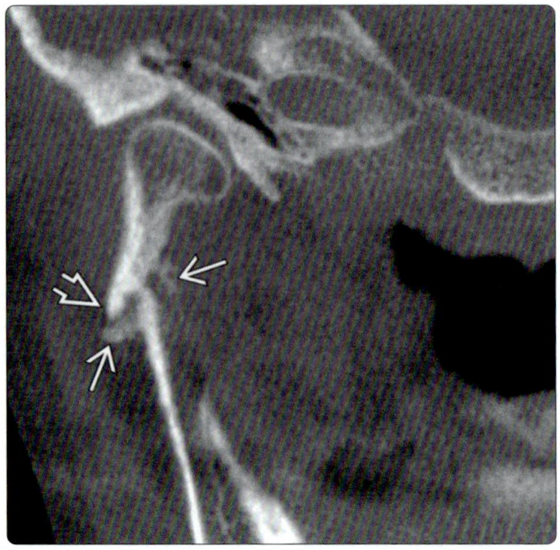

(Left) *CBCT panoramic reformat of an adult patient with a history of a posterosuperior vector of trauma to the right parasymphysis and a chief complaint of left TMJ pain shows a normal right condylar process and a normal condyle/fossa spatial relationship.* **(Right)** *CBCT panoramic reformat of the left mandible in the same patient shows no mandibular fractures. The left side condyle/fossa spatial relationships are not well visualized.*

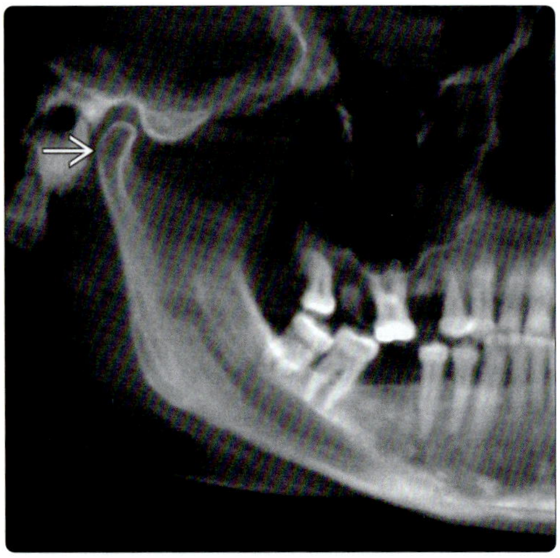

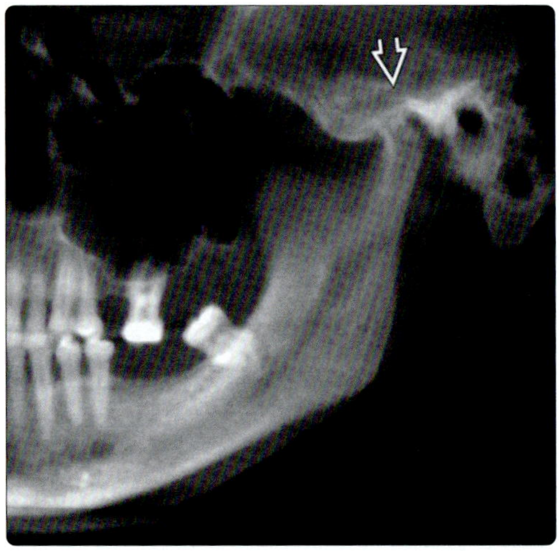

(Left) *Sagittal oblique CBCT of the left TMJ in the same patient shows a glenoid fossa fracture demonstrating several fragments of bone. Subchondral sclerosis along the anterosuperior surface of the left condyle and an erosion along its posterior surface are noted.* **(Right)** *Coronal oblique CBCT of the left TMJ in the same patient shows dehiscence in the roof of the glenoid fossa, suggestive of fracture.*

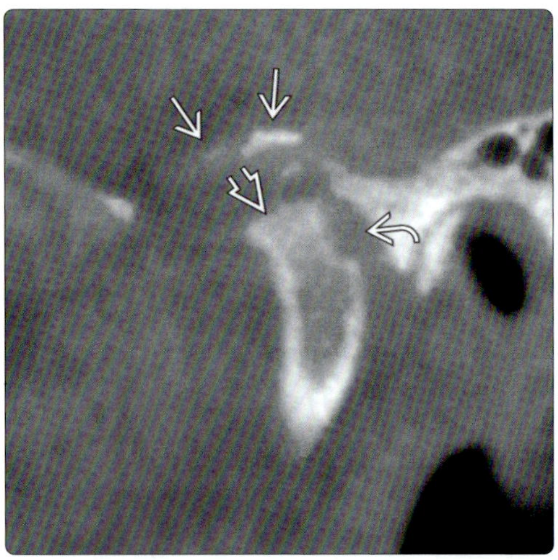

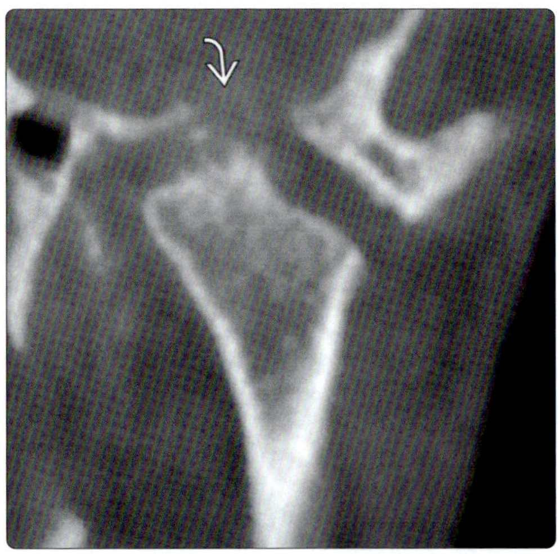

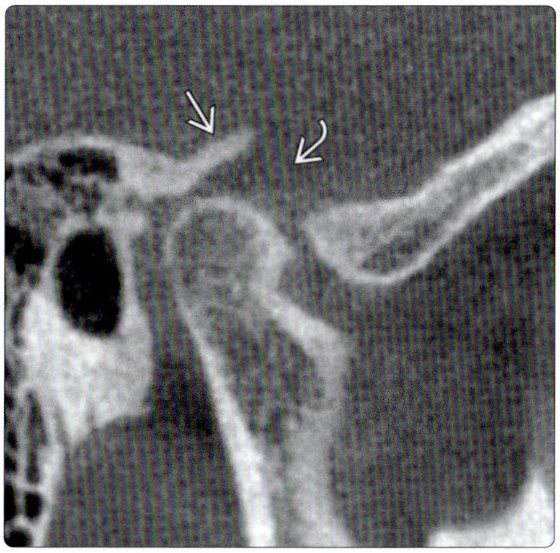

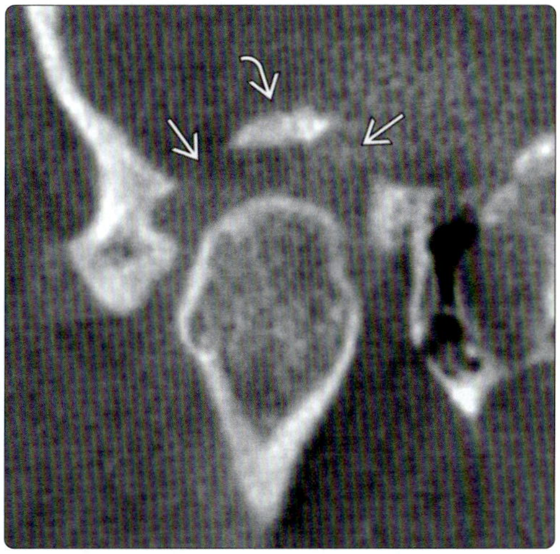

(Left) *Sagittal oblique CBCT of the right TMJ in a patient following left parasymphyseal trauma shows dehiscence ➡ in the roof of the glenoid fossa and elevation of the posterior margin of the fossa ➡ into the middle cranial fossa. The condyle is superiorly repositioned.* **(Right)** *Coronal oblique CBCT of the right TMJ in the same patient shows dehiscence ➡ of the roof of the glenoid fossa. An osseous segment ➡ is elevated into the middle cranial fossa. Note superior position of the condyle. Fossa fractures are rare. The left TMJ was normal.*

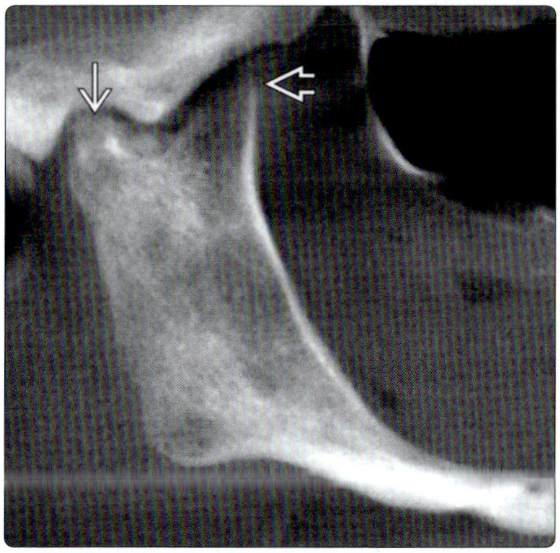

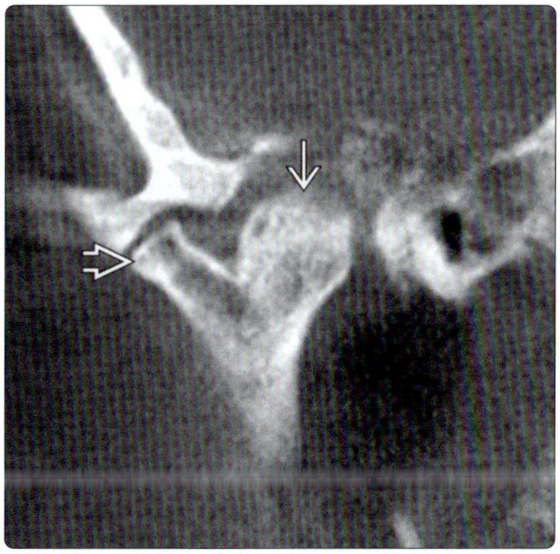

(Left) *CBCT panoramic reformat of the right mandible shows fracture of the condyle ➡. The condylar neck is absent, and the coronoid process appears relatively long ➡ due to the loss of condylar height.* **(Right)** *Coronal CBCT reformat of the same patient shows that the fractured condylar head ➡ has remodeled and attached to the medial aspect of the condylar neck and that the ramus stump on the lateral side has remodeled to form a "new" condylar head ➡. This has resulted in a bifid condyle with a medial and lateral lobe.*

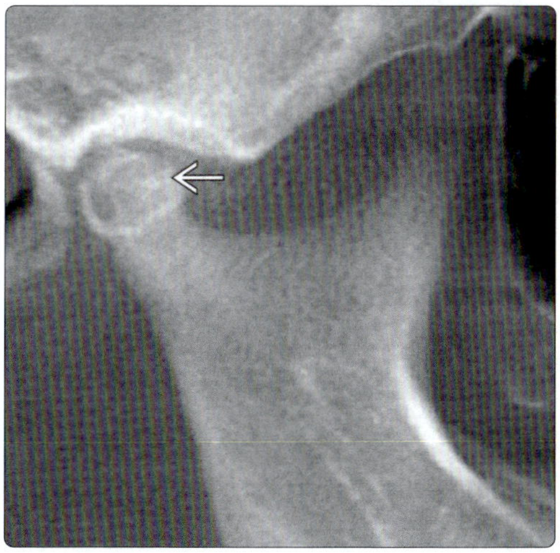

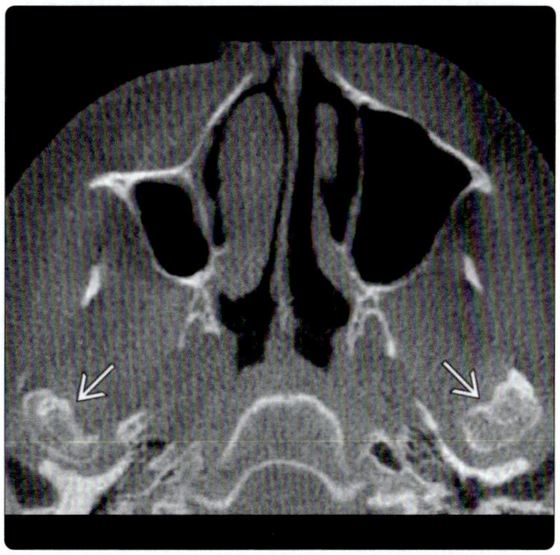

(Left) *CBCT panoramic reformat shows a crush fracture of the right condyle ➡. The glenoid fossa is normal.* **(Right)** *CBCT axial image in the same patient shows enlargement and abnormal morphology of both condyles ➡ as a result of bilateral crush fractures.*

TMJ Dislocation

KEY FACTS

TERMINOLOGY

- Definition: Condyle displaced out of glenoid fossa but remaining within joint capsule
- Synonyms: Subluxation, luxation

IMAGING

- Condyles lodged anteriorly and superiorly to articular eminence; **patient unable to close mouth**
- Best imaging tool: Bone CT or CBCT with 3D reformats to clearly demonstrate anatomic relationship of dislocated condyle

TOP DIFFERENTIAL DIAGNOSES

- TMJ hypermobility

PATHOLOGY

- Predisposing factors
  - **Prolonged mouth opening**, especially after dental procedures or general anesthetic
  - **Trauma**, abnormal chewing movements, abnormal TMJ ligaments, capsule laxity, masticatory muscle abnormalities
- Most common dislocation: **Bilateral anterior acute**
- **Superior** dislocation more common in **children** because condyle is small and round with underdeveloped medial and lateral poles

CLINICAL ISSUES

- Bilateral anterior dislocation: Patient unable to close after wide mouth opening (open lock)
- Open bite, deviated mandible, preauricular swelling
- Hollowness/depression anterior to tragus
- Pain, limited TMJ movement
- Treatment: Manual reduction

DIAGNOSTIC CHECKLIST

- Open TMJ views may suggest dislocation, but patient may still be able to close mouth (hypermobility)

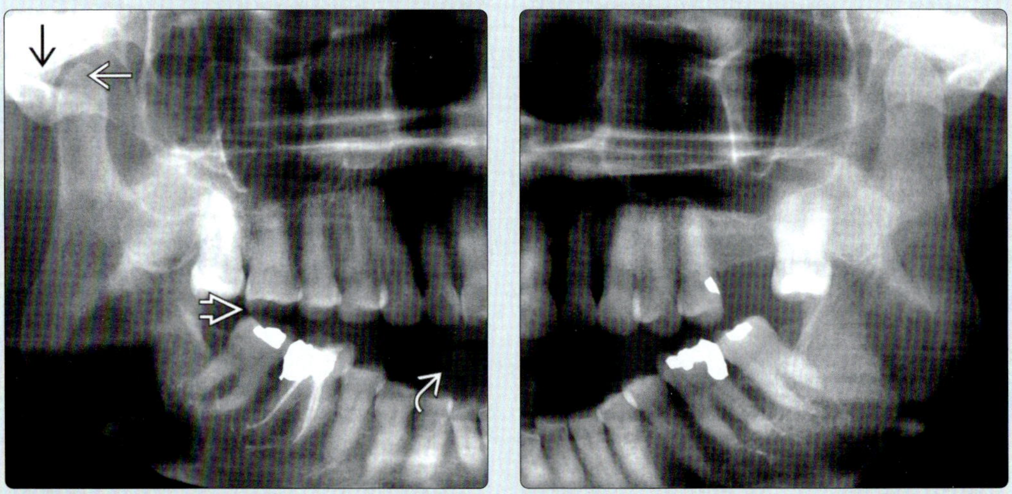

(Left) *Panoramic radiograph shows the right condyle positioned anteriorly and superiorly to the articular eminence in a case of bilateral anterior dislocation. There is a prominent anterior open bite, but the molars are in occlusion.* **(Right)** *Panoramic radiograph of the same patient shows similar changes on the left side. The open bite is due to the abnormal anterior condylar position, and the posterior tooth contacts are due to the associated superior condylar position.*

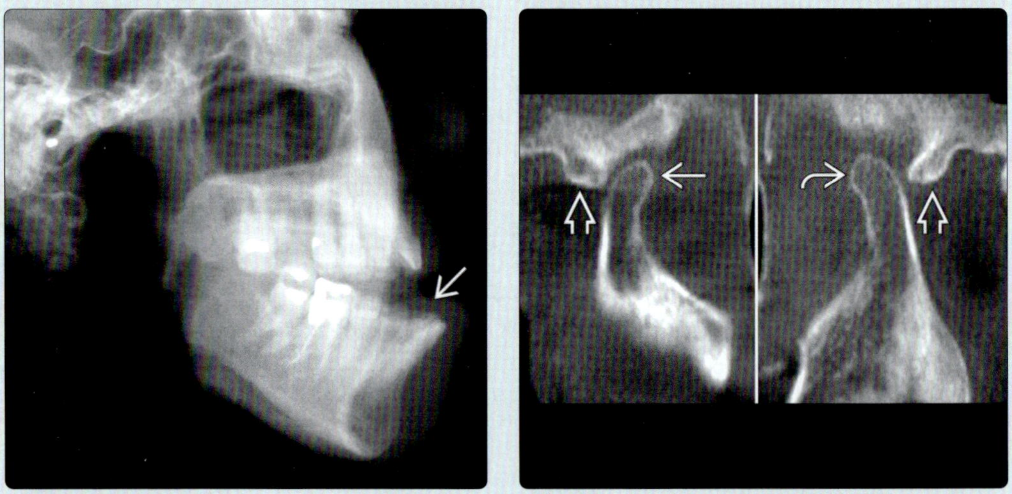

(Left) *Lateral radiograph of the same patient shows the prognathic mandibular position and anterior open bite due to the anterior-superior position of the mandibular condyles.* **(Right)** *Sagittal CBCT slices of the right and left condyles in the same patient show the condyles positioned anteriorly and superiorly to the articular eminentia. Note that the condyles exhibit normal cortication and morphology.*

TERMINOLOGY

Synonyms

- Luxation
- Subluxation = partial dislocation

Definitions

- Condyle displaced out of glenoid fossa but remaining within joint capsule

IMAGING

General Features

- Best diagnostic clue
  - Condyles lodged anteriorly and superiorly to articular eminence; patient unable to close mouth
- Location
  - Anterior dislocation most common, **often bilateral**

Radiographic Findings

- Radiography
  - Condyles positioned **anteriorly and superiorly to articular eminence**

CT Findings

- Bone CT and CBCT
  - Chronic dislocation: Articular eminence may be atrophic and glenoid fossa flattened

MR Findings

- Joint **effusion** and disc abnormalities common in chronic recurrent cases

Imaging Recommendations

- Best imaging tool
  - Panoramic radiograph good for initial evaluation
  - Bone CT or CBCT with 3D reformats to clearly demonstrate anatomic relationship of dislocated condyle

DIFFERENTIAL DIAGNOSIS

TMJ Hypermobility

- Wide range of motion on opening with condyle positioned anteriorly and superiorly to eminence
- **Patient able to close mouth**, and mouth does not remain in open locked position

PATHOLOGY

General Features

- Etiology
  - Predisposing factors: **Prolonged mouth opening**, especially after dental procedures or general anesthetic
    - Yawning, vomiting, extremes of masticatory effort, or laughing
  - **Trauma**, abnormal chewing movements, abnormal TMJ ligaments, capsule laxity, masticatory muscle abnormalities
  - More common in patients with general joint laxity &/or internal derangement
  - Systemic diseases resulting in hypermobility of TMJ, psychogenic or neurological disorders
  - Drugs causing extrapyramidal effects (e.g., antiemetics, phenothiazines)

Staging, Grading, & Classification

- Classification based on
  - **Number** of affected TMJs: Unilateral vs. bilateral
  - **Direction** of displacement: Anterior, posterior, medial, lateral, superior, combination
    - Anterior-medial often associated with mandibular fracture
    - Superior dislocation: Often due to trauma; condyle enters middle cranial fossa and may be associated with dural injury
  - **Duration** of dislocation: Acute, chronic, recurrent
- Most common dislocation: **Bilateral anterior acute**
- **Superior** dislocation more common in **children** because condyle is small and round with underdeveloped medial and lateral poles

CLINICAL ISSUES

Presentation

- Most common signs/symptoms
  - Bilateral anterior dislocation: Patient unable to close after wide mouth opening (open lock)
- Other signs/symptoms
  - Open bite, deviated mandible, preauricular swelling
  - Hollowness/depression anterior to tragus
  - Pain, limited TMJ movement

Natural History & Prognosis

- Prognosis improved with early treatment

Treatment

- Manual reduction
- May need intermaxillary fixation to prevent redislocation and help damaged ligaments heal
- Physiotherapy to prevent fibrosis
- Occasionally, surgery to create mechanical obstruction to limit extreme anterior translation of condyle or eminoplasty to prevent dislocation and locking anterior to eminence
- Superior dislocation: May need glenoid fossa reconstruction and craniotomy if dural injury

DIAGNOSTIC CHECKLIST

Consider

- Open TMJ views may suggest dislocation, but patient may still be able to close mouth (hypermobility)
  - History of trauma or prolonged wide mouth opening; patient unable to close mouth with true dislocation

Image Interpretation Pearls

- If superior dislocation, check integrity of glenoid fossa roof

Reporting Tips

- Check for morphological abnormalities of TMJ that predispose to recurrent dislocation

SELECTED REFERENCES

1. He Y et al: Treatment of traumatic dislocation of the mandibular condyle into the cranial fossa: development of a probable treatment algorithm. Int J Oral Maxillofac Surg. 44(7):864-70, 2015

Bifid Condyle

KEY FACTS

TERMINOLOGY

- Synonym: Bifid mandibular condyle
- Rare entity characterized by **partial division** of mandibular condyle

IMAGING

- Lobulated condyle in panoramic radiograph
- Unilateral or bilateral
- Varies from division of normal condyle to large irregular mass
- **Notch or depression** on superior condylar surface or **duplication** of condyle
- Orientation can be in **mediolateral or anteroposterior** plane
- Mediolateral case appears as **heart** shape in coronal images
- Anteroposterior case appears as **2 condyles**, one anterior to other, in sagittal reformat
- Bony **ankylosis** if trauma etiology

TOP DIFFERENTIAL DIAGNOSES

- Condylar fracture
- Normal anatomic variant

PATHOLOGY

- Congenital
- Developmental
- Acquired

CLINICAL ISSUES

- Usually **asymptomatic, incidental** finding
- **Pain, joint noises** most common if symptomatic
- Most patients diagnosed after 20 years old
- Treatment: None unless pain or functional impairment (condylectomy to restore function)

DIAGNOSTIC CHECKLIST

- Consider: Lack of trauma history not always reliable, especially if trauma occurred at young age

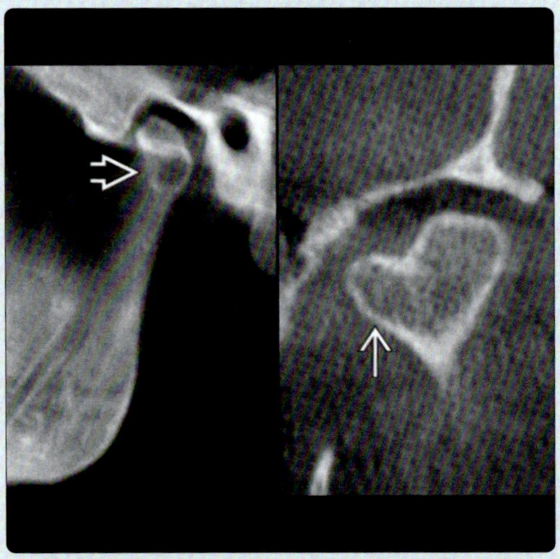

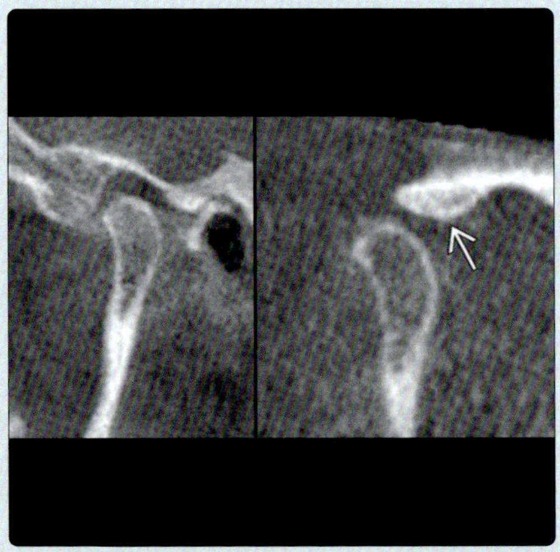

(Left) *CBCT panoramic reformat (L) shows unusual appearance of the left condyle. Coronal CBCT (R) shows heart-shaped bifid condyle. The outline of the smaller medial pole ➡ is seen inferior to the lateral pole in the panoramic reformat ➡.* **(Right)** *Sagittal CBCT of the same patient in closed position (L) shows the lateral pole of the bifid condyle seated in a relatively normal fossa. In open position (R), the condyle translates freely out of the fossa beyond the crest of the eminence ➡, indicating unrestricted range of motion.*

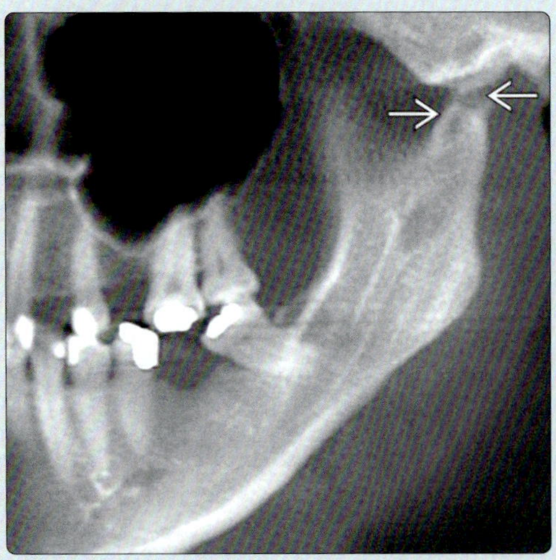

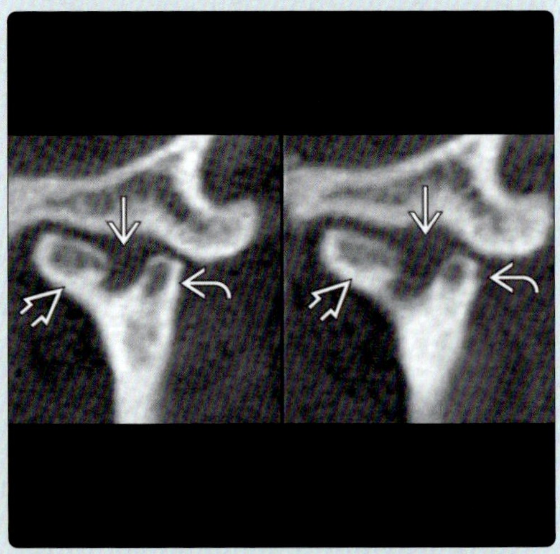

(Left) *Panoramic CBCT shows a bifid condyle on the left side. The condyle appears to have 2 separate lobes ➡ that are aligned in the vertical plane.* **(Right)** *Coronal CBCT in the same patient shows a deep depression in the center of the condyle ➡ with the appearance of a duplicate condyle on the medial ➡ and lateral ➡ aspects. The glenoid fossa has remodeled to accommodate the large articular surface.*

TERMINOLOGY

Synonyms

- Bifid mandibular condyle (BMC)

Definitions

- Rare entity characterized by **partial division** of mandibular condyle

IMAGING

General Features

- Best diagnostic clue
  - Lobulated condyle in panoramic radiograph
- Location
  - Unilateral:bilateral = 4:1
- Morphology
  - Condyle may be divided in medial-lateral or anterior-posterior plane
  - Variable appearance based on severity
    - Mild **notch**
    - Vertical **depression**
    - Broad cleft resulting in **duplication** of condyle

Radiographic Findings

- Radiography
  - Panoramic radiograph: Lobulated ± enlarged condyle

CT Findings

- Bone CT
  - **Depression or notch** on superior condylar surface or **duplication** of condyle: Cortex continuous
  - Orientation can be in **mediolateral or anteroposterior** plane
    - Mediolateral case appears as **heart** shape in coronal images
    - Anteroposterior case appears as **2 condyles**, one anterior to other, in sagittal reformat
  - Mandibular fossa may **remodel** to accommodate altered condylar morphology
  - Bony **ankylosis** if traumatic etiology

MR Findings

- Articular disc in normal position or displaced

Imaging Recommendations

- Best imaging tool
  - CBCT or CT
- Protocol advice
  - Coronal and sagittal reformats to determine orientation of bifid condyle
  - Sagittal CBCT or CT useful to differentiate duplicated head from coronoid process in anteroposterior BMC

DIFFERENTIAL DIAGNOSIS

Condylar Fracture

- Vertical fracture through condyle gives appearance of 2 condyles: Cortex discontinuous
- Healing of displaced segments may → appearance of BMC

Normal Anatomic Variant

- Mild depression on condylar articular surface simulates mild bifid condyle
- No clear definition to distinguish anatomic variant from bifid condyle

PATHOLOGY

General Features

- Etiology
  - Congenital
    - Genetic factors, endocrine disorders
  - Developmental
    - Obstructed blood supply during development, persistence of fibrovascular septa in developing condyle
  - Acquired
    - Teratogenic embryopathy, nutritional deficiency, infection, irradiation, trauma

CLINICAL ISSUES

Presentation

- Most common signs/symptoms
  - Usually **asymptomatic, incidental** finding
- Other signs/symptoms
  - **Pain, joint noises** most common if symptomatic
  - Swelling, limitation of motion
  - Deviation of mandible to affected side, facial asymmetry

Demographics

- Age
  - Most patients diagnosed after 20 years old
    - Reported 3-67 years old
- Gender
  - M = F

Natural History & Prognosis

- Many cases remain asymptomatic
- May develop TMJ dysfunction

Treatment

- None unless pain or functional impairment: Condylectomy to restore function

DIAGNOSTIC CHECKLIST

Consider

- Lack of trauma history not always reliable, especially if trauma occurred at young age

SELECTED REFERENCES

1. Haghnegahdar AA et al: Prevalence of bifid mandibular condyle in a selected population in South of iran. J Dent (Shiraz). 15(4):156-60, 2014
2. Cho BH et al: Nontraumatic bifid mandibular condyles in asymptomatic and symptomatic temporomandibular joint subjects. Imaging Sci Dent. 43(1):25-30, 2013
3. Miloglu O et al: The frequency of bifid mandibular condyle in a Turkish patient population. Dentomaxillofac Radiol. 39(1):42-6, 2010
4. Rehman TA et al: Bifid mandibular condyle with associated temporomandibular joint ankylosis: a computed tomography study of the patterns and morphological variations. Dentomaxillofac Radiol. 38(4):239-44, 2009

(Left) *Panoramic reformatted CBCT shows a right-side bifid condyle. There is a depression on the superior condylar surface, but the condyle is otherwise unremarkable. Note the increased superior joint space. The patient's teeth are biting together in occlusion.* **(Right)** *Panoramic reformatted CBCT of the same patient shows an apparently normal left condyle. Note that the superior joint space on this side is within normal limits compared to the contralateral side.*

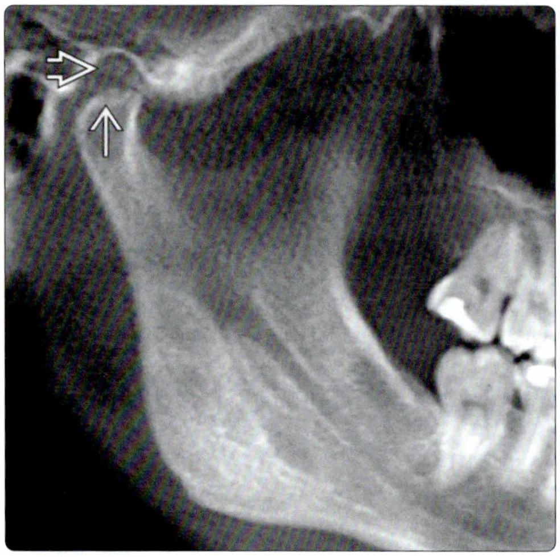

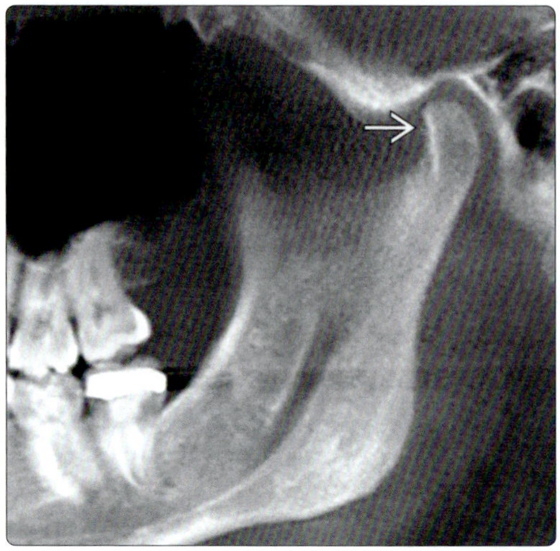

(Left) *Sagittal CBCT of the same patient shows a depression in the center of the right condyle. There is flattening of the articular eminence indicating remodeling and adaptation to the altered condylar shape.* **(Right)** *Sagittal CBCT of the same patient shows abnormal condylar shape on the left side that was not apparent in the panoramic reformat. There is a depression in the center of the condyle with apparent elongation of the anterior aspect.*

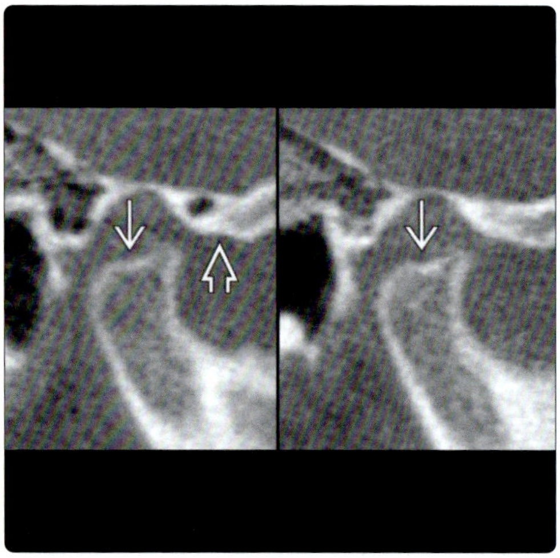

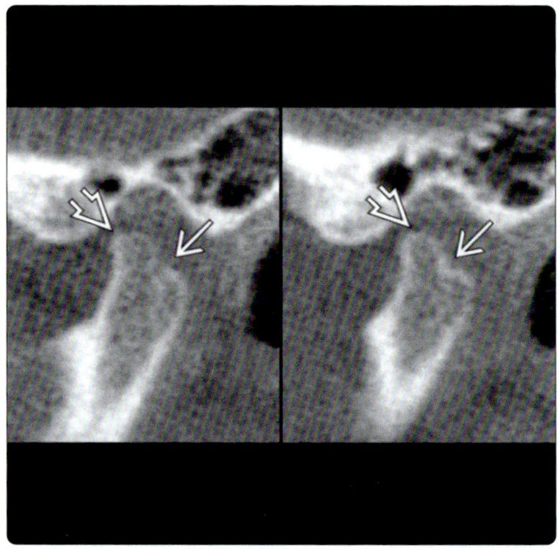

(Left) *Coronal CBCT of the same patient shows a shallow depression in the center of the right condyle, separating the head into medial and lateral lobes and giving it a characteristic heart shape. The condyle is otherwise evenly corticated.* **(Right)** *Coronal CBCT of the left condyle in the same patient shows a V-shaped depression on the lateral aspect of the condyle separating the head into a larger medial and smaller lateral lobe. This is an unusual case of bilateral bifid condyle.*

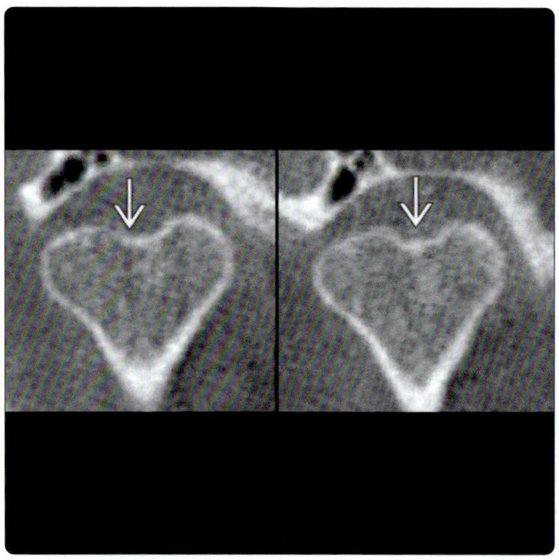

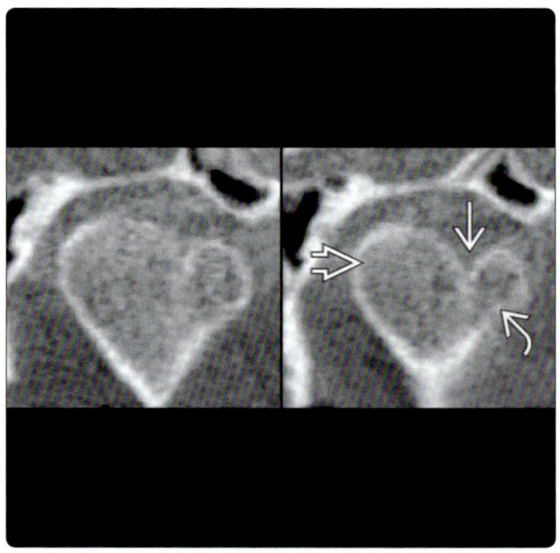

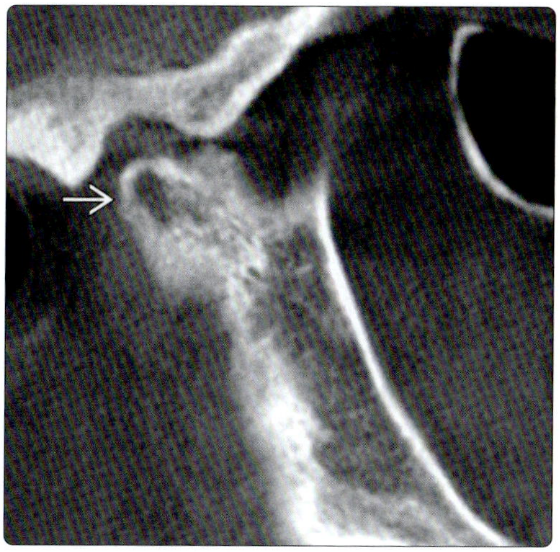

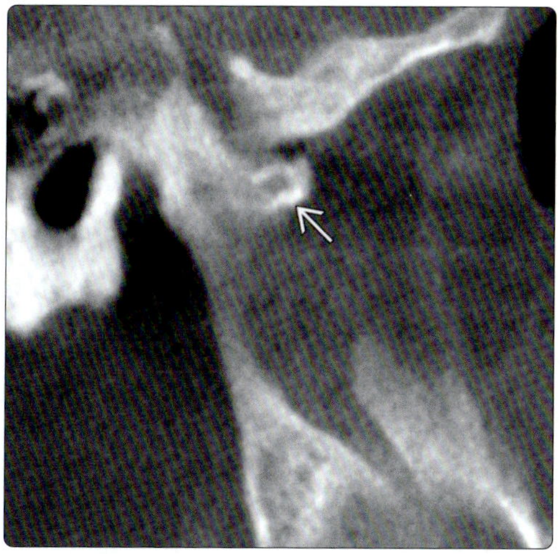

(Left) *Sagittal CBCT demonstrates a bifid condyle resulting from a right-sided condylar fracture. This image shows the lateral aspect of the condyle. The condylar neck is not visible, and the condyle is angled posteriorly.* **(Right)** *Sagittal CBCT in the same patient shows abnormal condylar shape and the appearance of an extra anterior lobe in this more medially located slice.*

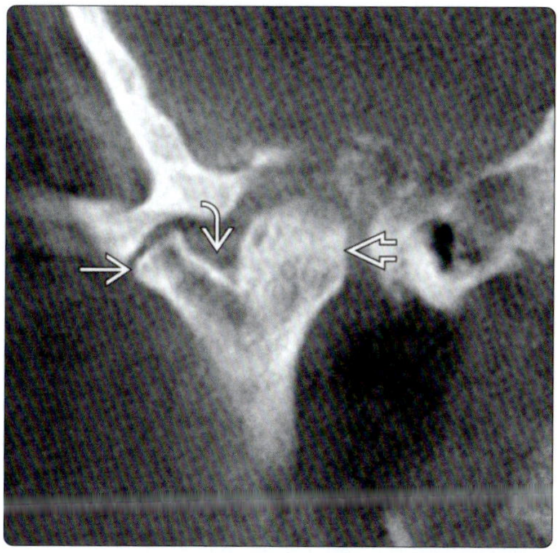

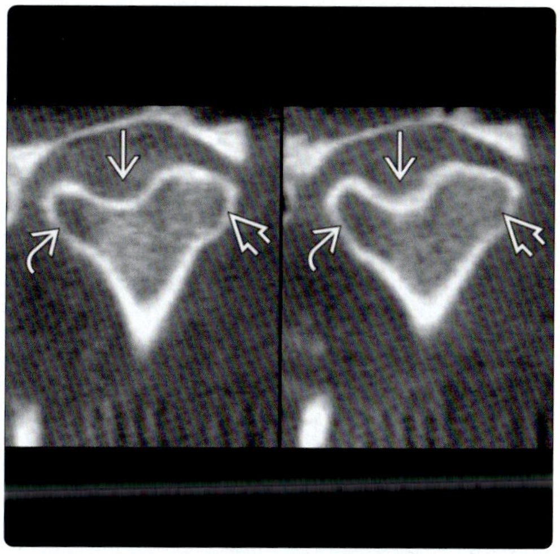

(Left) *Coronal CBCT in the same patient shows a smaller lateral condylar lobe and larger medial lobe with a V-shaped central depression. The medial lobe likely represents the original but remodeled condyle that reattached to the condylar neck after the fracture.* **(Right)** *Coronal CBCT shows a bifid condyle in the left TMJ with a moderately deep and broad central depression dividing the condyle into a larger lateral lobe and smaller medial lobe.*

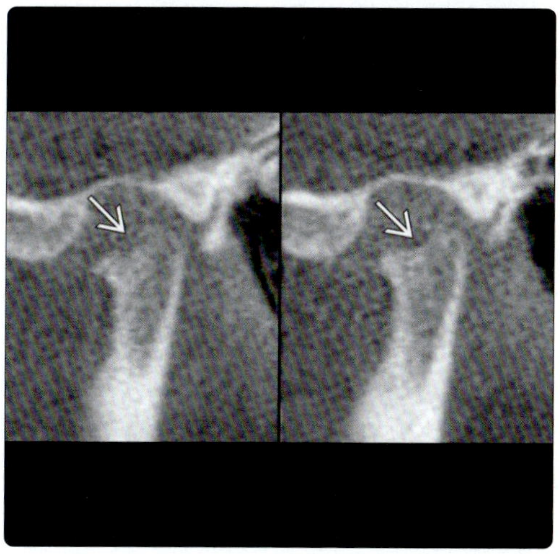

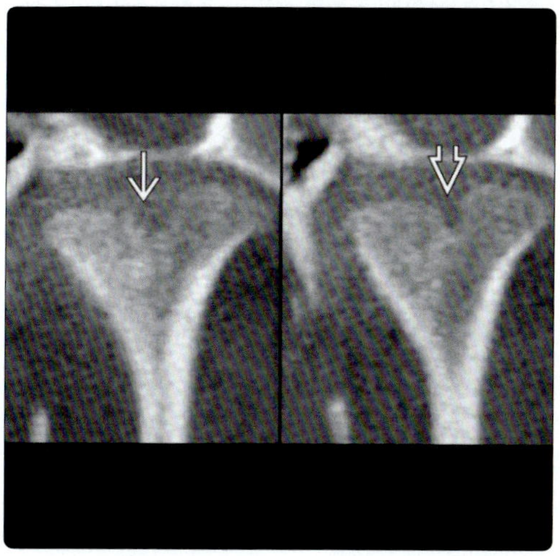

(Left) *Sagittal CBCT of a left bifid condyle shows a depression on the central aspect of the condyle. The glenoid fossa and articular eminence are normal.* **(Right)** *Coronal CBCT of the same patient shows the extent of the central depression, which is wider on the anterior aspect of the condyle than at the posterior aspect.*

TMJ Osteochondritis Dissecans

KEY FACTS

TERMINOLOGY

- Definition: Lesion of articular surface involving subchondral bone and surface fibrocartilage

IMAGING

- Best clue: Concave defect in anterosuperior surfaces of condyle ± osseous loose bodies in defect
- Location: Load-bearing surface of TMJ condyle
- CT findings occur late in process
- MR findings
  - **Early stage**: Subchondral stress reaction
  - Hypointensity T1, hyperintense on fluid-sensitive sequences; no fracture line
  - **Intermediate stage**: Fracture line forms, but articular surface intact
  - Focal T1 hypointensity may obscure fracture line
  - **Advanced stage**: Articular surface disrupted
  - Fluid from effusion surrounds fragment

TOP DIFFERENTIAL DIAGNOSES

- Degenerative joint disease (DJD)
- Synovial chondromatosis

CLINICAL ISSUES

- Pain
- Locking
- Limitation of jaw movement
- Stable lesions may return to full function
- Instability or loose bodies may result in persistent pain and mechanical symptoms
- Unstable lesions may lead to DJD
- Treatment
  - Palliative treatment preferred
  - Osteochondral loose body removed if interfering with function

(Left) *Sagittal oblique T2WI MR of the left TMJ shows stage I osteochondritis dissecans (OCD). There is an obvious fracture line ➔, but the articular surface ➔ is intact.* **(Right)** *Coronal oblique T2WI MR of the TMJ shows stage III OCD. There is an osteochondral fragment ➔ that has separated from the host bed ➔ but has not dislocated (in situ).*

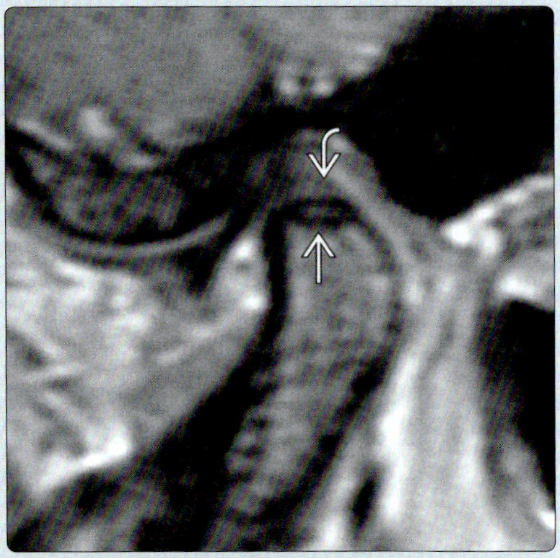

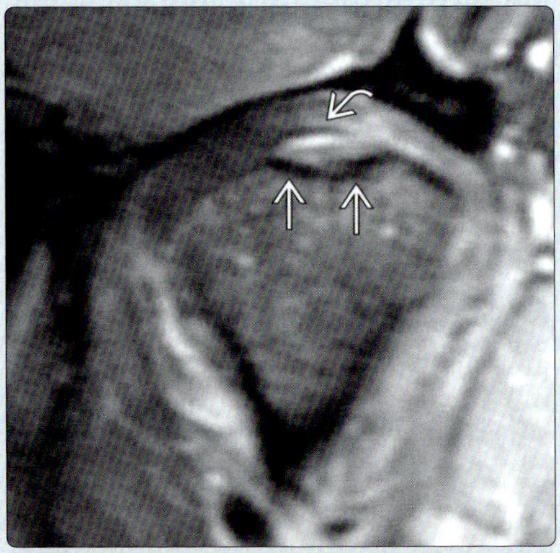

(Left) *Sagittal oblique CBCT of the right TMJ shows stage III OCD. There is an osteochondral fragment ➔ positioned superior to the host bed ➔. The subchondral bone inferior to the bed is sclerotic* ➔. **(Right)** *Coronal oblique CBCT of the same patient shows a stage III OCD involving the laterosuperior surfaces of the left condyle. This is a loaded articular surface. An in situ osteochondral fragment ➔ is positioned over the host bed* ➔.

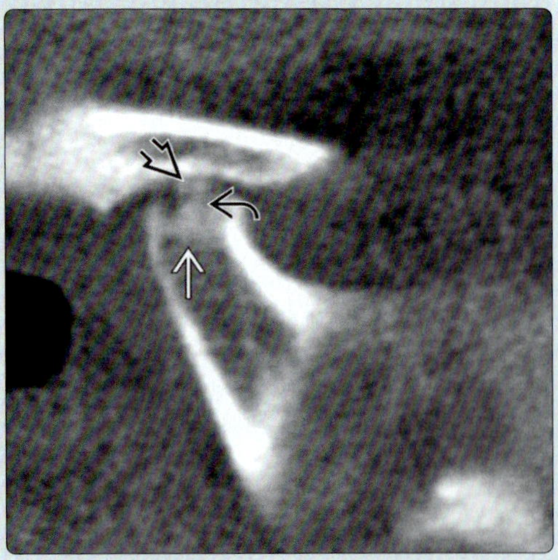

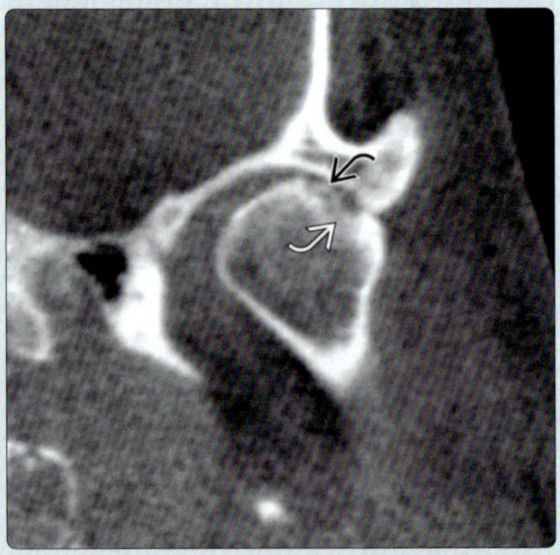

TERMINOLOGY

Abbreviations

- Osteochondritis dissecans (OCD)

Synonyms

- Osteochondral defects; osteochondritis

Definitions

- Lesion of articular surface involving subchondral bone and surface fibrocartilage

IMAGING

General Features

- Best diagnostic clue
  - Convex articular surface with concave defect, ± osseous body
- Location
  - Load-bearing surface of TMJ condyle
    - Anterosuperior surface
    - Unilateral

CT Findings

- CBCT
  - Concave defect in anterosuperior surfaces of condyle
    - Sclerotic margins
  - Osseous loose bodies in defect
  - CT findings occur late in process

MR Findings

- Early stage: Subchondral stress reaction
  - Hypointense on T1, hyperintense on fluid-sensitive sequences
  - No fracture line
  - Intact overlying fibrocartilage
- Intermediate stage: Fracture line forms, but articular surface intact
  - Focal T1 hypointensity may obscure fracture line
  - Focal hyperintensity on fluid-sensitive sequence
    - Central signal intensity variable: Low, high, or mixture of both
- Advanced stage: Articular surface disrupted
  - Fluid from effusion surrounds fragment

DIFFERENTIAL DIAGNOSIS

Degenerative Joint Disease

- Associated with **displaced disc**
- Defect begins at surface and enlarges into bone marrow
- Loose bodies not associated with defect

Synovial Chondromatosis

- Primary
  - Metaplasia of synovial lining into cartilaginous nodules that break free, creating loose bodies
- Secondary
  - Osteocartilaginous loose bodies associated with degenerative joint disease (DJD)

PATHOLOGY

General Features

- Etiology
  - Uncertain: Believed to be repetitive microtrauma or macrotrauma
    - Excessive bone strain leads to microfractures within subchondral bone
    - Subchondral trabecular microfracture coalesce into fracture line
    - May extend to overlying cartilage if injury pattern continues without protection
- Epidemiology
  - Rare in TMJ
  - Knee most common joint, followed in order by ankle, elbow, shoulder, and wrist

Staging, Grading, & Classification

- International Cartilage Repair Society: Classifies OCD at surgery
  - **Stage I**: Stable lesion in continuity with host bone, covered by intact cartilage
  - **Stage II**: Partial discontinuity, stable on probing
  - **Stage III**: Complete discontinuity of "dead in situ" lesion, but fragment not dislocated
  - **Stage IV**: Dislocated fragment

CLINICAL ISSUES

Presentation

- Most common signs/symptoms
  - Pain
- Other signs/symptoms
  - Locking
  - Swelling
  - Limitation of jaw movement

Natural History & Prognosis

- Stable lesions may return to full function
- Instability or loose bodies may result in persistent pain and mechanical symptoms
- Unstable lesions may lead to DJD

Treatment

- Palliative treatment preferred
- Osteochondral loose body removed if interfering with function

SELECTED REFERENCES

1. Misirlioglu M et al: Radiographic diagnosis of osteochondritis dissecans of the temporomandibular joint: two cases. Med Princ Pract. 23(6):580-3, 2014
2. Gomoll AH et al: The subchondral bone in articular cartilage repair: current problems in the surgical management. Knee Surg Sports Traumatol Arthrosc. 18(4):434-47, 2010
3. Madry H et al: The basic science of the subchondral bone. Knee Surg Sports Traumatol Arthrosc. 18(4):419-33, 2010
4. Madry H: The subchondral bone: a new frontier in articular cartilage repair. Knee Surg Sports Traumatol Arthrosc. 18(4):417-8, 2010
5. Orhan K et al: Temporomandibular joint osteochondritis dissecans: case report. Oral Surg Oral Med Oral Pathol Oral Radiol Endod. 102(4):e41-6, 2006
6. Campos PS et al: Osteochondritis dissecans of the temporomandibular joint. Dentomaxillofac Radiol. 34(3):193-7, 2005

KEY FACTS

TERMINOLOGY

- Rheumatoid arthritis (RA)
- Definition: Chronic inflammatory disease manifesting as synovial membrane inflammation in several joints; characterized by progressive bony erosions and cartilage destruction

IMAGING

- Erosion and flattening of anterior and posterior condylar surfaces, giving **sharpened pencil** appearance of condyle
- Anterior **open bite** due to anterior-superior positioning of condyles
- Narrowed joint space
- Generalized **osteopenia** of condyle and temporal component
- **Erosion** of articular eminence and anterior-superior medial surfaces of condyle
- Often **secondary degenerative joint disease (DJD)** with subchondral erosions; difficult to distinguish between RA and DJD

TOP DIFFERENTIAL DIAGNOSES

- Degenerative disease, TMJ
- Juvenile idiopathic arthritis, TMJ
- Psoriatic arthritis, TMJ

CLINICAL ISSUES

- More commonly affects small joints of hands (Bouchard nodes), wrists, knees, and feet
- TMJ: Preauricular **swelling**, pain, tenderness
- **Stiffness**, limited opening; crepitus
- Most frequent from 35-45 years old
- F:M = 2.5:1

DIAGNOSTIC CHECKLIST

- Erosive changes in RA usually more severe than DJD, but may see RA and DJD in same joint

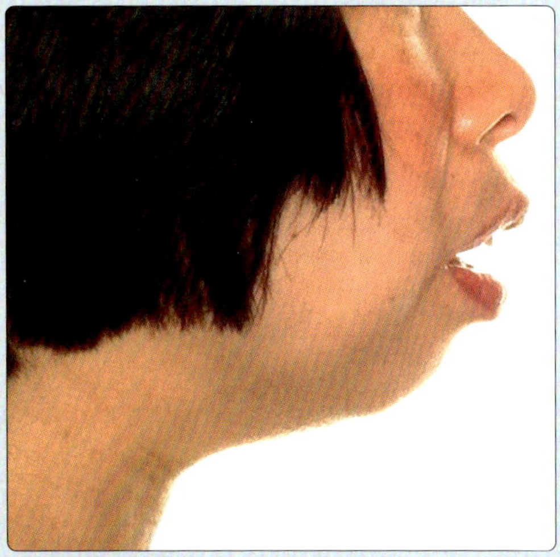

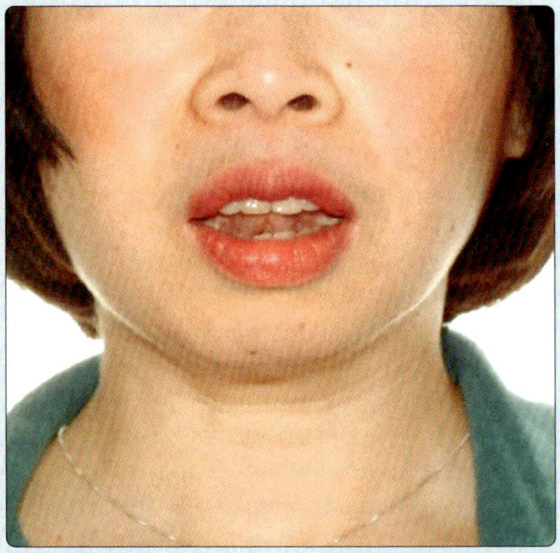

(Left) *Lateral photograph shows a 46-year-old patient with posterior teeth in occlusion. The chin is recessive. There is an anterior open bite and incompetent lip posture noted.* **(Right)** *Frontal photograph of the same patient shows an anterior open bite and a recessive mandible.*

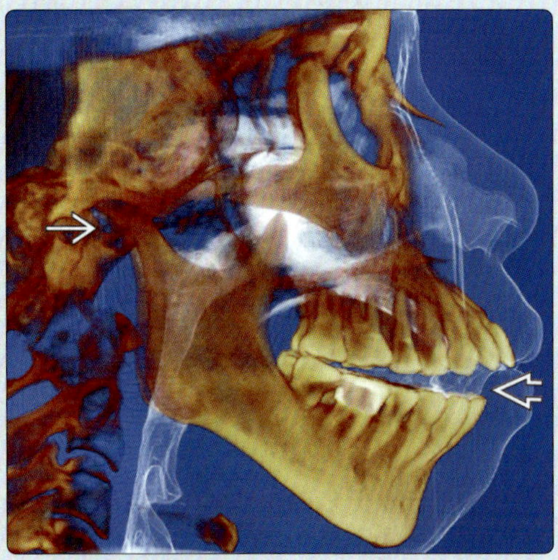

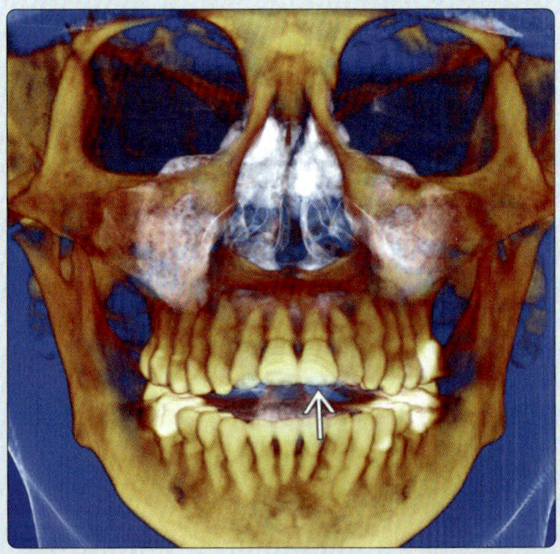

(Left) *CBCT volume-rendered image of the same patient shows a normal occlusal plane. Wear on the occlusal surface of posterior teeth is noted. The condylar process is short ➡. Normal size and shape of body and ramus of mandible indicates postsomatic growth condylar changes. The open bite ➡ indicates a clockwise rotation of mandible.* **(Right)** *CBCT volume-rendered frontal view of the same patient shows anterior open bite. Anterior tooth wear ➡ indicates an acquired open bite.*

TERMINOLOGY

Abbreviations

- Rheumatoid arthritis (RA)

Definitions

- Chronic **inflammatory** disease manifesting as synovial membrane inflammation in several joints; characterized by progressive bony erosions and cartilage destruction
- Villous synovitis leads to formation of synovial granulomatous tissue (pannus) that grows into fibrocartilage and bone, releasing enzymes that destroy articular surfaces and underlying bone

IMAGING

General Features

- Best diagnostic clue
    - Erosion and flattening of anterior and posterior condylar surfaces, giving **sharpened pencil** appearance of condyle
- Location
    - Condyle, glenoid fossa, articular eminence
    - Cervical spine, craniovertebral junction

Imaging Recommendations

- Best imaging tool
    - CT best for assessing bony abnormalities and MR best for condylar marrow abnormalities and joint effusion

Radiographic Findings

- Anterior **open bite** due to anterior-superior positioning of condyles
- Narrowed joint space

CT Findings

- Bone CT and CBCT
    - No radiographic changes in early phase of disease
    - Early changes may include generalized **osteopenia** of condyle and temporal component
    - **Erosion** of articular eminence and anterior-superior medial surfaces of condyle
        - Erosions can destroy entire condyle and articular eminence
        - Often **secondary degenerative joint disease (DJD)** with subchondral erosions; difficult to distinguish between RA and DJD
    - ± subchondral sclerosis
    - ± late fibrous or bony **ankylosis**
    - ± associated disc **displacement**

MR Findings

- T1WI
    - May see cortical erosions, decreased bone marrow density
    - Pannus (synovial granulomatous tissue) has intermediate signal intensity in T1 and T2
    - Disc displacement not associated with RA process but can occur
    - Pannus can displace temporal posterior attachment inferiorly and condylar posterior attachment posteriorly
- T2WI
    - ↑ signal intensity in both joint compartments representing joint fluid
    - ↑ signal intensity in condylar marrow due to edema, or ↓ signal intensity due to sclerosis

DIFFERENTIAL DIAGNOSIS

Degenerative Disease, TMJ

- Joint destruction in RA can lead to secondary DJD, so may see evidence of both diseases in joint
- **Subchondral sclerosis** and presence of osteophytes more often characteristic of DJD
- Osteopenia and severe erosions more characteristic of RA

Juvenile Idiopathic Arthritis

- Occurs in young patients
- Leads to marked mandibular hypoplasia
    - Steep mandibular plane
    - Obtuse gonial angle
- Fusion of spinous processes of cervical spine
- Narrowing of anterior-posterior dimension of vertebral bodies

Psoriatic Arthritis, TMJ

- Rule out by patient history
- Destructive changes less severe than RA

PATHOLOGY

General Features

- Etiology
    - Various theories
        - Infections: From *Mycoplasma* organisms, Epstein-Barr virus, parvovirus, rubella
        - Genetic: Shared epitope of HLA-DR4/DR1 cluster present in up to 90% of patients with RA
        - Immunologic
- Associated abnormalities
    - **Extraarticular** involvement of skin, heart, lungs, eyes
    - Rheumatoid factor (RF) not found in all patients, but increased levels of RF in combination with clinical signs of RA are more prognostic for severe disease

Staging, Grading, & Classification

- Classification (American College of Rheumatology)
    - Stage I (early RA)
        - No destructive changes seen in radiographic examination
        - May see osteopenia of joint components
    - Stage II (moderate progression)
        - Radiographic evidence of periarticular osteopenia ± slight subchondral bone ± cartilage destruction
        - May have limitation of movement but no joint deformity
        - Adjacent muscle atrophy
        - ± extraarticular soft tissue lesions (nodules, tenosynovitis)
    - Stage III (severe progression)
        - Radiographic evidence of cartilage and bone destruction with osteopenia
        - Joint deformity (e.g., subluxation, ulnar deviation, hyperextension) without fibrous or bony ankylosis
        - Extensive muscle atrophy
        - ± extraarticular soft tissue lesions

- Stage IV (terminal progression)
  - All stage III criteria with fibrous or bony ankylosis

Gross Pathologic & Surgical Features

- Inflammatory proliferation of synovium = pannus
  - Osteoclast-rich portion of synovial membrane destroys bone
- Enzymes secreted by synoviocytes and chondrocytes degrade cartilage

Microscopic Features

- Thickened synovium containing plasma cells, multinucleated giant cells, polymorphonuclear leukocytes and lymphocytes

CLINICAL ISSUES

Presentation

- Most common signs/symptoms
  - More commonly affects small joints of hands (Bouchard nodes), wrists, knees, and feet
  - TMJ: Preauricular **swelling**, pain, tenderness
  - **Bilateral** and **symmetrical** involvement
- Other signs/symptoms
  - **Stiffness** on opening or limited opening
    - Degree of limited opening correlates with duration and severity of disease
  - Crepitus
  - Tenderness in muscles of mastication
  - Receded chin; anterior open bite

Demographics

- Age
  - Most frequent from 35-45 years old
    - Occurs at any age, but incidence ↑ with age
- Gender
  - F:M = 2.5:1
- Epidemiology
  - 1-3% of population affected
    - TMJ involved in 4.7-84% of RA patients (mean = 50%)

Natural History & Prognosis

- Periods of remission and exacerbation of symptoms
- Main prognostic signs for patients with severe disease: Several swollen joints, high serum levels of acute phase reactants or IgM rheumatoid factor, early radiographic and functional abnormalities
- Radiographic progression varies and is **unpredictable**

Treatment

- Medical treatment
  - Corticosteroids
  - Disease-modifying agents slow disease progression
    - Tumor necrosis factor inhibitors, methotrexate (MTX), cyclosporine
      - Current smoking, female gender, longer symptom duration, and younger age predict worse response to MTX in patients with new-onset RA
    - Biological treatment, such as infliximab, for failure of initial MTX treatment
      - However, absence of convincing clinical difference at 24 months and substantially higher costs
  - Medications for pain relief, reduction, or antiinflammatory
- Physiotherapy
- Joint replacement surgery if severe joint destruction

DIAGNOSTIC CHECKLIST

Consider

- Erosive changes in RA usually more severe than DJD, but may see RA and DJD in same joint
- Evaluate craniovertebral junction
  - Chronic cases with marked destruction can lead to basilar impression due to cranial settling over C1 and C2 vertebra
  - Neurological conditions due to compression of brainstem possible
  - Possible compression of autonomic centers
    - Patient may experience labile blood pressures, arrhythmias, respiratory depression, or sudden death

SELECTED REFERENCES

1. Ahmed N et al: Deficient cytokine control modulates temporomandibular joint pain in rheumatoid arthritis. Eur J Oral Sci. 123(4):235-41, 2015
2. Ahmed N et al: Tumor necrosis factor mediates temporomandibular joint bone tissue resorption in rheumatoid arthritis. Acta Odontol Scand. 73(3):232-40, 2015
3. Ahola K et al: Impact of rheumatic diseases on oral health and quality of life. Oral Dis. 21(3):342-8, 2015
4. Hoyuela CP et al: Oro-facial evaluation of women with rheumatoid arthritis. J Oral Rehabil. 42(5):370-7, 2015
5. Malliari M et al: First diagnosis of rheumatoid arthritis in a patient with temporomandibular disorder: a case report. Int J Prosthodont. 28(2):124-6, 2015
6. Morales H et al: Imaging approach to temporomandibular joint disorders. Clin Neuroradiol. ePub, 2015
7. Sodhi A et al: Rheumatoid arthritis affecting temporomandibular joint. Contemp Clin Dent. 6(1):124-7, 2015
8. Ruparelia PB et al: Bilateral TMJ involvement in rheumatoid arthritis. Case Rep Dent. 2014:262430, 2014
9. Witulski S et al: Evaluation of the TMJ by means of clinical TMD examination and MRI diagnostics in patients with rheumatoid arthritis. Biomed Res Int. 2014:328560, 2014
10. Kretapirom K et al: MRI characteristics of rheumatoid arthritis in the temporomandibular joint. Dentomaxillofac Radiol. 42(4):31627230, 2013
11. Uchiyama Y et al: Temporomandibular joints in patients with rheumatoid arthritis using magnetic resonance imaging. Clin Rheumatol. 32(11):1613-8, 2013
12. Cunha CO et al: Bilateral asymptomatic fibrous-ankylosis of the temporomandibular joint associated with rheumatoid arthritis: a case report. Braz Dent J. 23(6):779-82, 2012
13. Bayar N et al: Temporomandibular joint involvement in rheumatoid arthritis: a radiological and clinical study. Cranio. 20(2):105-10, 2002
14. Treister N et al: Rheumatoid arthritis: a review and suggested dental care considerations. J Am Dent Assoc. 130(5):689-98, 1999
15. Gynther GW et al: Radiographic changes in the temporomandibular joint in patients with generalized osteoarthritis and rheumatoid arthritis. Oral Surg Oral Med Oral Pathol Oral Radiol Endod. 81(5):613-8, 1996
16. Larheim TA et al: Imaging temporomandibular joint abnormalities in patients with rheumatic disease. Comparison with surgical observations. Oral Surg Oral Med Oral Pathol. 73(4):494-501, 1992
17. Larheim TA et al: Rheumatic disease of the temporomandibular joint: MR imaging and tomographic manifestations. Radiology. 175(2):527-31, 1990
18. Tegelberg A: Temporomandibular joint involvement in rheumatoid arthritis. A clinical study. Swed Dent J Suppl. 49:1-133, 1987

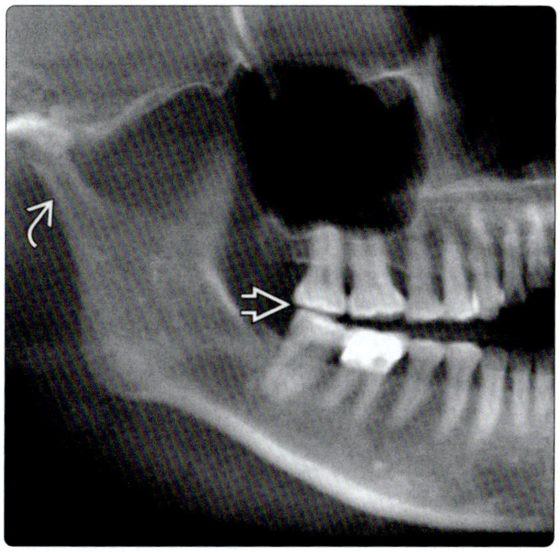

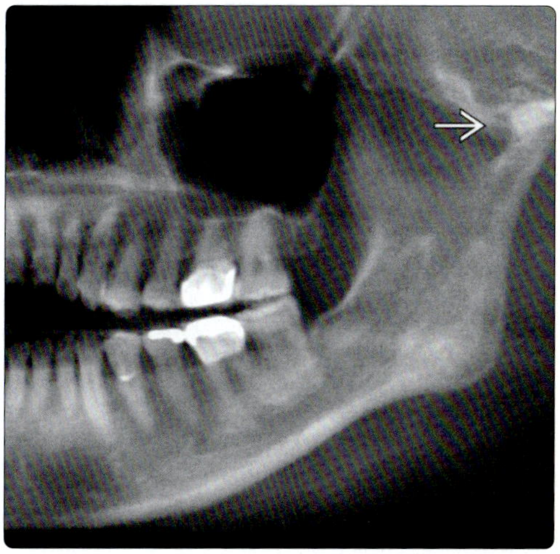

(Left) *Right side panoramic reformat of CBCT in same patient shows the condylar process is short and has a posterior inclination* →*. Tooth contact occurs between opposing 2nd molar teeth* →*.* **(Right)** *Left side panoramic reformat shows the left half of the mandible in the same patient. The left condylar process is short* → *and has a posterior inclination.*

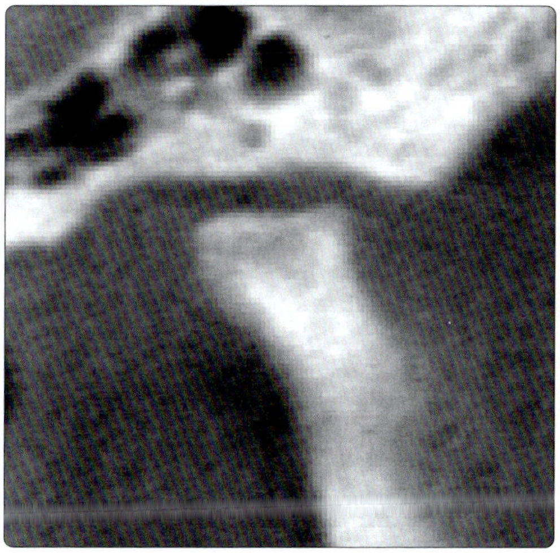

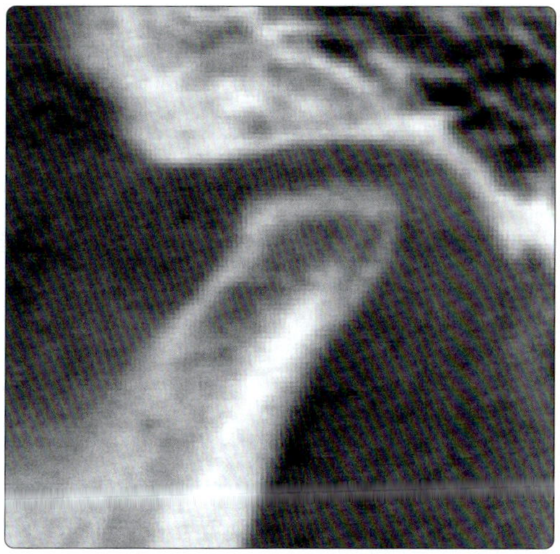

(Left) *Sagittal oblique CBCT section shows the right TMJ in the same patient. The condyle has lost vertical height and has a reduced volume. Sclerosis, flattening, and repaired erosions of the condyle and posterior slope of eminence are noted. The eminence slope is horizontal. The condyle is anteriorly repositioned within its fossa.* **(Right)** *Sagittal oblique CBCT section shows the left TMJ in the same patient.*

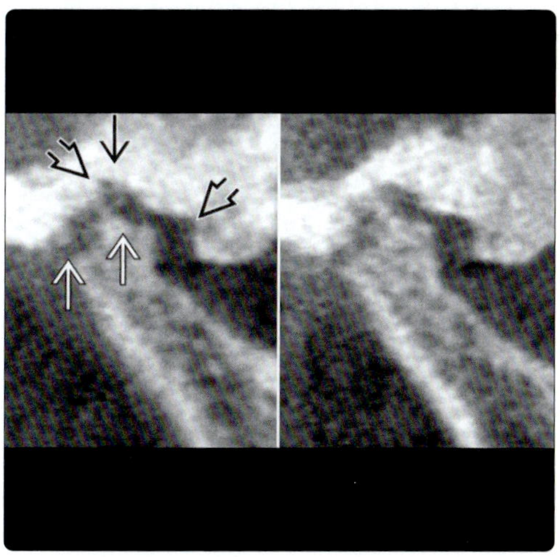

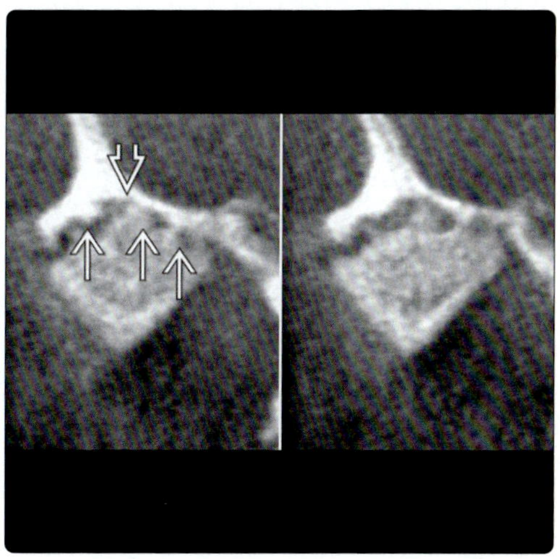

(Left) *Sagittal reformatted CBCT of RA in the right TMJ demonstrates sclerosis of the temporal bone* → *with large erosions* →*. The condyle is also irregularly eroded* →*.* **(Right)** *Coronal reformatted CBCT of the same patient shows a bony bridge* → *extending from the condyle to the temporal bone, suggesting bony ankylosis. Large erosions span the entire width of the condyle* →*. The temporal bone has adapted to accommodate the altered shape of the condyle.*

(Left) *Graphic depiction of a TMJ with RA shows the pannus formation in the joint spaces destroying the bone of the condyle and the eminence, and displacing the posterior attachments .* **(Right)** *T1 MR of TMJ in an RA patient shows erosions and flattening along the superior surface of the condyle and posterior slope of the eminence. Condylar process bone marrow with low signal is noted. Intermediate signal mass adjacent to condyle represents pannus . Note the inferior displacement of the temporal posterior attachment .*

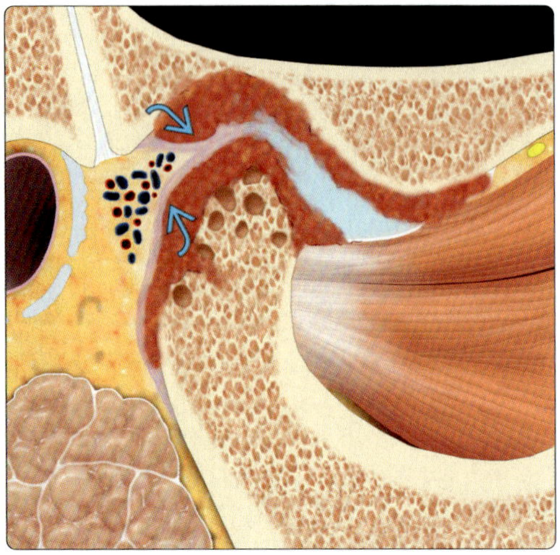

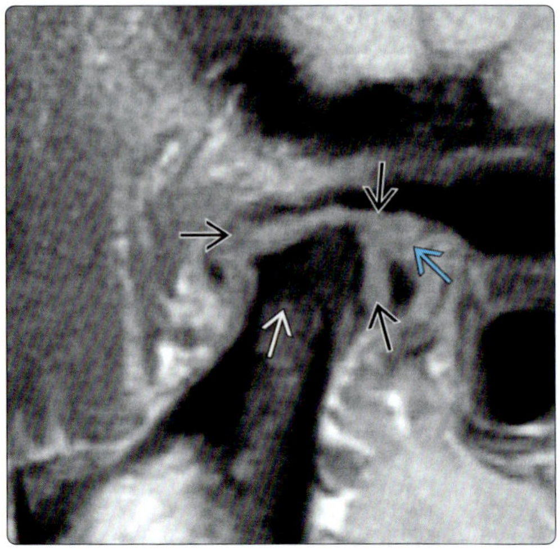

(Left) *Closed mouth T1 MR in an RA patient shows erosion on the superior surface of the condyle . An intermediate-signal mass, suggestive of a pannus, is seen expanding the joint compartments .* **(Right)** *T1 MR of TMJ in open-mouth position in the same patient shows the condyle is reduced in size along its posterior surface . An intermediate-signal mass, suggestive of a pannus , is noted expanding the volume of the joint compartments. The disc is not visible.*

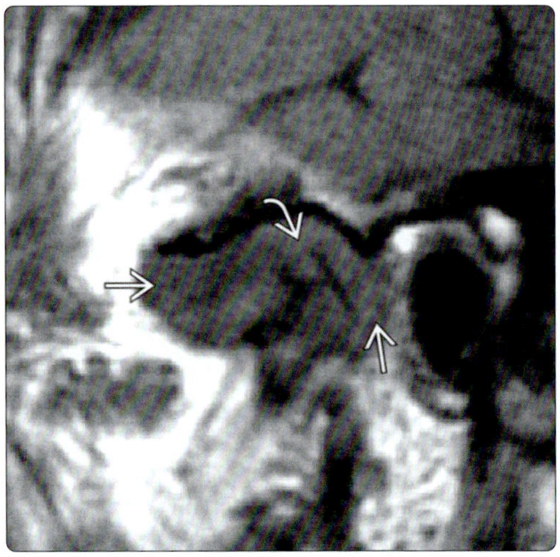

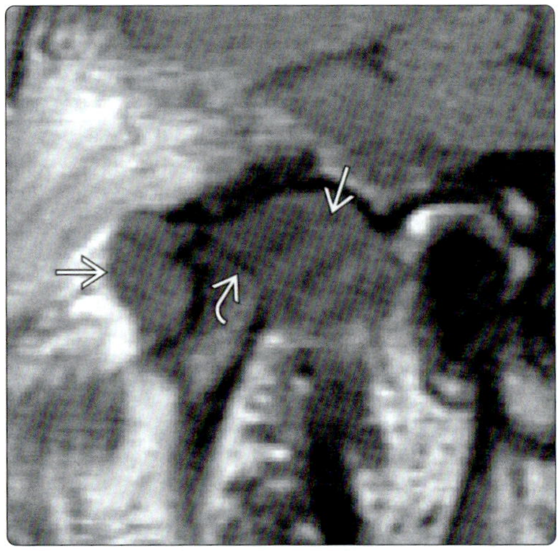

(Left) *Sagittal CT in an RA patient exhibits erosions along the posterior margin of the dens and widening of the anterior atlantodental interval (AADI) .* **(Right)** *Sagittal CT demonstrates marked erosive change of the dens . Erosion of the odontoid process frequently coincides with the development of anterior atlantoaxial subluxation. Widening of the AADI is also noted . There is narrowing of the posterior atlantodental interval , and the space for the cord is markedly narrowed.*

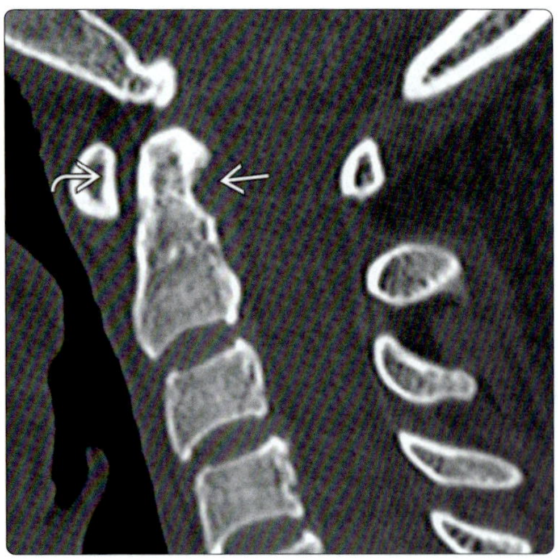

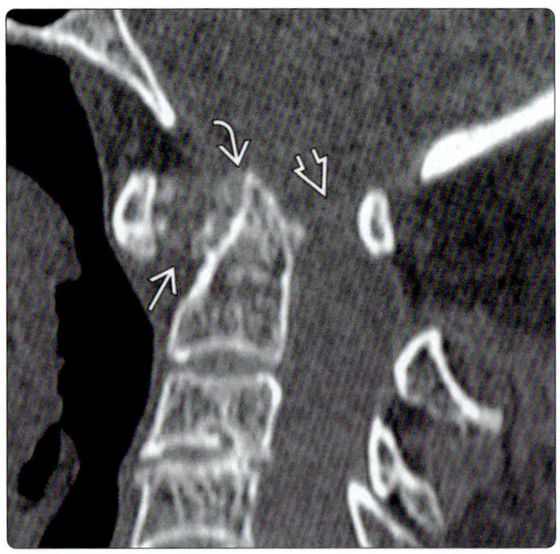

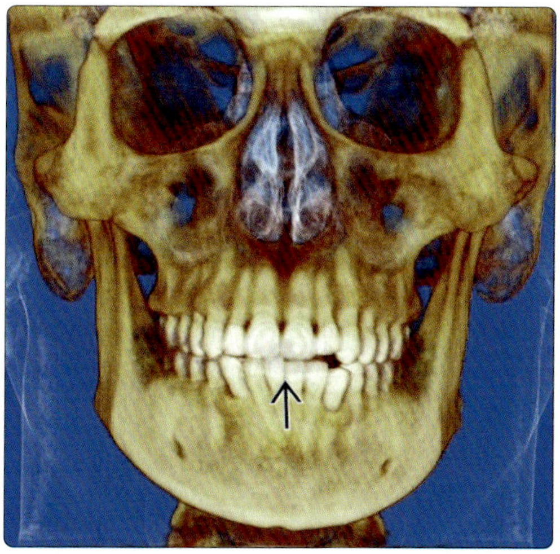

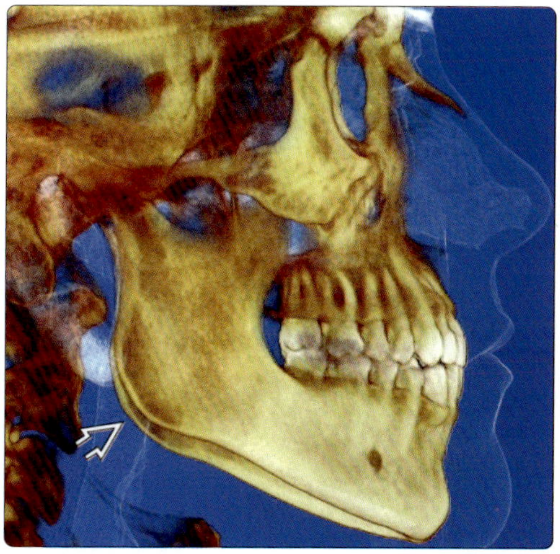

(Left) *Frontal view of a volume-rendered CBCT in a 34-year-old woman with RA is shown. Orthodontic therapy has reduced a large anterior open bite to a small left side anterior open bite. The mandibular dental midline → remains shifted to left.* **(Right)** *Volume-rendered CBCT lateral view of the same patient shows an asymmetrical mandible with a normally developing body and ramus. The gonial angle → and anterior projection of the mandible are normal.*

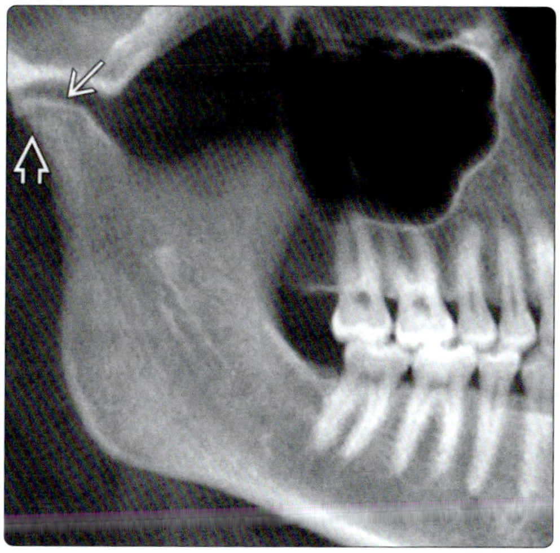

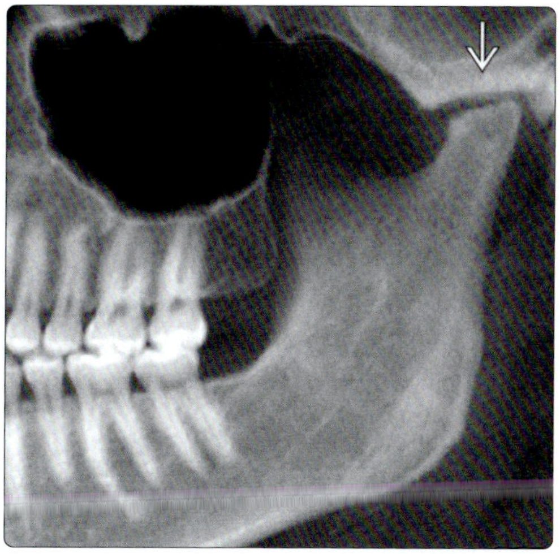

(Left) *Panoramic radiograph of the right side in the same patient with RA in the right TMJ shows the condyle has characteristic flattening → resulting in a pointed or sharpened pencil appearance of the posterior aspect →.* **(Right)** *Panoramic radiograph of the left side in the same patient shows similar changes in the left condyle with flattening and sclerosis of the left temporal component →.*

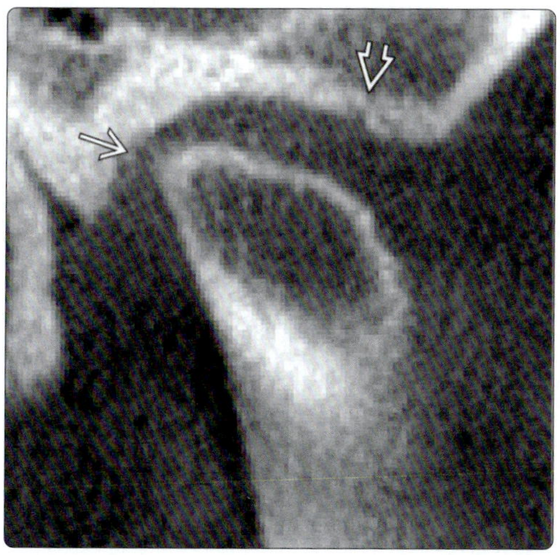

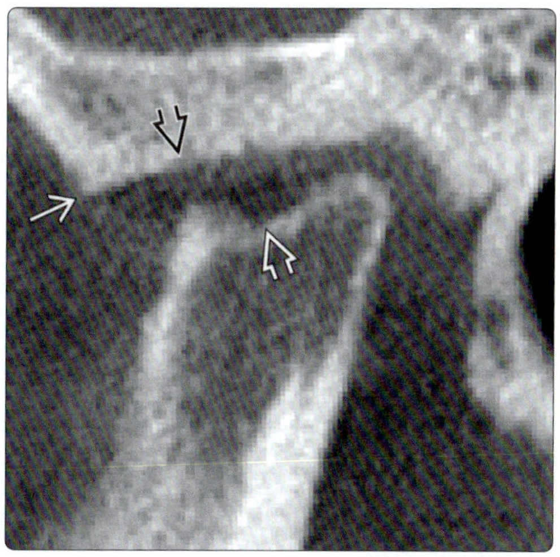

(Left) *Sagittal reformatted CBCT of RA in the right TMJ of the same patient shows the condyle is flattened with a sharpened pencil appearance → while the temporal component is flattened with sclerosis and erosions →.* **(Right)** *Sagittal reformatted CBCT of RA in the left TMJ of the same patient shows there is severe flattening and sclerosis of the temporal component →. The anterior-superior surface of the condyle is flattened with a large erosion in the center → of the condyle and smaller erosions in the glenoid fossa roof →.*

TMJ Juvenile Idiopathic Arthritis

KEY FACTS

TERMINOLOGY

- Juvenile idiopathic arthritis (JIA)
- Definition: Autoimmune musculoskeletal inflammatory disease in childhood

IMAGING

- Bone CT best demonstrates contours of TMJ
    - Flat, deformed, mandibular condyles & wide, flat condylar fossae
    - Condyle concavity or bifid
    - Bilateral disease more common than unilateral
    - May have secondary osteoarthritis with osteophytes
    - Condyle often repositions anterior and superiorly on flattened fossa
- MR may show joint space enhancement & early inflammation before joint destruction
    - TMJ discs thin, perforated, or absent
- In cervical spine, may see atlantoaxial subluxation, vertebral fusion and ↓ AP vertebral body dimension

TOP DIFFERENTIAL DIAGNOSES

- Condylar hypoplasia
- Degenerative disease

CLINICAL ISSUES

- JIA affects 1-22 per 1,000 children worldwide
- TMJ involved in 20-90% of children with JIA
    - More likely if systemic disease, young age at diagnosis, & long duration of activity
- F > M
- TMJ and masticatory muscle pain, decreased range of jaw motion, retrognathia, micrognathia
- **70% asymptomatic** when MR shows acute arthritis
- Treat with either local or systemic therapy (or combination of both)
    - Local: Occlusal devices, arthrocentesis, intraarticular injections
    - Systemic: NSAIDs, methotrexate, sulfasalazine

(Left) *Coronal bone CT in a 4-year-old girl with juvenile idiopathic arthritis (JIA) demonstrates irregular chronic erosion of right mandibular condyle ➡. Note also wide, flattened condylar fossa ➡.* **(Right)** *Coronal T1WI C+ FS MR in the same child with JIA reveals marked inflammatory enhancement involving the joint ➡ and marrow space of the right mandibular condyle ➡. The left TMJ ➡ shows no inflammatory change and no condylar deformity.*

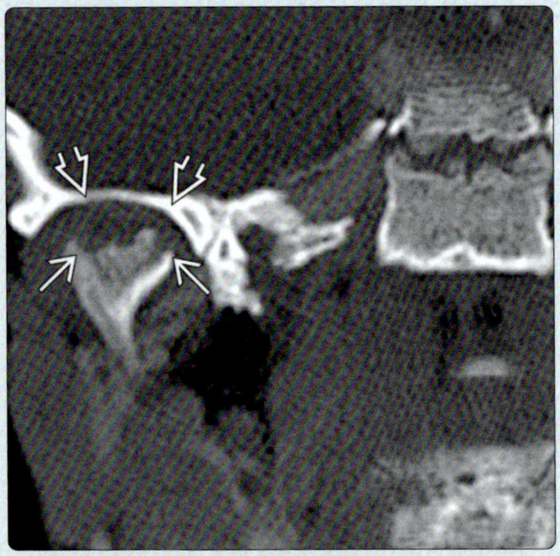

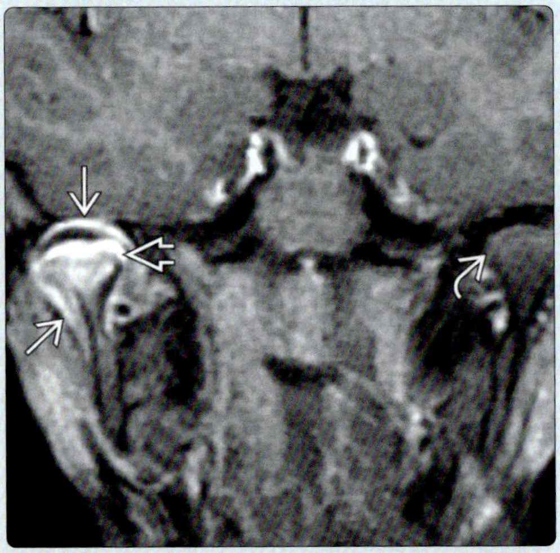

(Left) *Sagittal oblique T1WI C+ FS MR in a 21-year-old woman with longstanding JIA reveals a small mandibular condyle with irregular, low intensity sclerotic margins ➡ and a widened and flat fossa ➡. There is no inflammatory enhancement, but note the small anterior osteophyte ➡ from secondary osteoarthritis.* **(Right)** *Lateral radiograph in a 13-year-old girl with JIA demonstrates classic fusion of the posterior elements of C2-5 ➡ and decreased AP dimension of corresponding vertebral bodies ➡.*

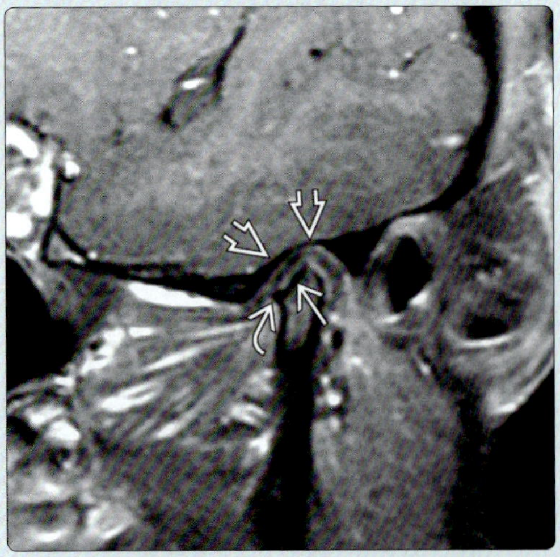

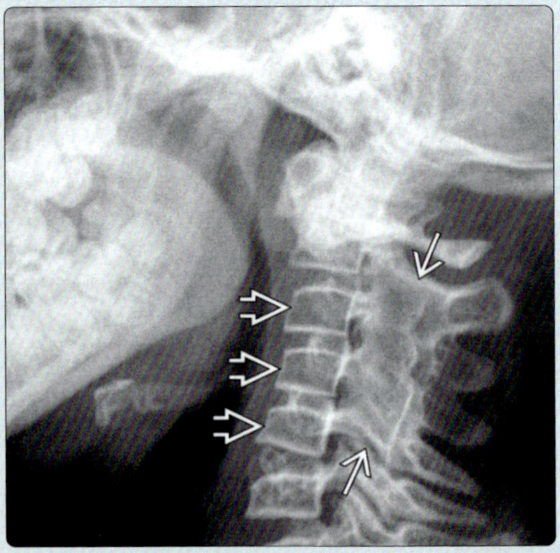

TERMINOLOGY

Abbreviations

- Juvenile idiopathic arthritis (JIA); temporomandibular joint (TMJ)

Synonyms

- Juvenile rheumatoid arthritis (JRA), juvenile chronic arthritis (JCA)
  - JIA is preferred term of International League of Associations for Rheumatology (ILAR)

Definitions

- **Autoimmune** musculoskeletal inflammatory disease of childhood

IMAGING

General Features

- Best diagnostic clue
  - Bilateral flat, deformed, mandibular condyles with wide glenoid fossae
- Location
  - Primarily large joints: Knees, wrists, ankles
    - Adult onset RA more common in small joints of hands and feet
  - In head and neck: TMJ, craniovertebral junction (CVJ), and cervical spine

CT Findings

- Bone CT
  - TMJ has flat, deformed, mandibular condyles and wide, flat glenoid fossae
    - **Condyle concavity** or bifid
    - Sclerotic margins when more advanced
  - Bilateral > unilateral
  - May have secondary osteoarthritis with joint space narrowing and osteophyte formation
  - Coronoid process often elongated and superiorly repositioned
  - Condyle may reposition anteriorly and superiorly on broad flat fossa
  - In cervical spine, may see **atlantoaxial subluxation**
    - Vertebral fusion and ↓ AP vertebral body dimension
  - Clockwise rotation of mandible may be associated with narrowing of airway dimensions

MR Findings

- T1WI
  - Mandibular condyles flat and deformed with wide, flat condylar fossae
    - Condyle concavity or bifid
- T2WI
  - Hyperintense joint effusion, bone marrow edema, &/or subchondral cysts less common
  - TMJ discs thin, perforated, or absent
- T1WI C+
  - **Joint space enhancement**
  - May see early inflammation before joint destruction
  - May be abnormal without symptoms
- **Dynamic imaging**: Decreased condyle translation
- **Cervical spine and CVJ**
  - Atlantoaxial subluxation
  - Cranial settling, basilar invagination
  - Fusions progress to ankylosis and decreased AP dimension of vertebral bodies
  - Growth disturbance

Imaging Recommendations

- Best imaging tool
  - MR with contrast

DIFFERENTIAL DIAGNOSIS

Condylar Hypoplasia

- Bilateral: Pierre Robin and Treacher Collins
- Unilateral: Hemifacial microsomia
- Classic condylar hypoplasia
  - Small condyle with normal shape
  - Ipsilateral 1/2 of mandible small
  - Often displaced disc

Degenerative Disease

- Articular disc displaced anterior in position
  - Perforated, fibrotic, or dysmorphic contours
- Loss of condylar volume
- ± osteophyte, subchondral bone cyst, congruent articulation
- Joint space narrowing

Synovitis/Capsulitis

- Enhancing synovium/capsule

Calcium Pyrophosphate Dihydrate Deposition Disease

- Metabolic disease with chondrocalcinosis
- Calcified, enhancing intracapsular mass

Progressive Condylar Resorption

- Postpubertal females
- Small condyle
- Often bilateral
- Retrognathia, mandibular asymmetry, and bite changes common
- Often displaced discs

Synovial Chondromatosis

- Chondrometaplasia of synovial membranes
- Cartilaginous nodules detach from synovium and calcify → intraarticular loose bodies

PATHOLOGY

General Features

- Genetics
  - Polymorphisms in *IL6* & *MIF* genes associated with susceptibility to JIA

Staging, Grading, & Classification

- **3 classification systems may be used**
  - (1) JRA criteria by American College of Rheumatology
  - (2) JCA criteria by European League Against Rheumatism
  - (3) International League of Associations for Rheumatology (ILAR)

- 6 subtypes based on clinical features during first 6 months of disease
  - Oligoarticular JIA (50-60%)
  - Polyarticular JIA rheumatoid factor positive and negative (30-35%)
  - Systemic JIA (10-20%)
  - Juvenile psoriatic arthritis (2-15%)
  - Enthesitis-related arthritis (1-7%)
  - Undifferentiated arthritis

Microscopic Features

- Infiltration by lymphocytes, plasma cells, macrophages, and dendritic cells associated with proliferation of fibroblasts and macrophage-like synoviocytes

CLINICAL ISSUES

Presentation

- Most common signs/symptoms
  - In children with MR findings of acute TMJ arthritis, **70% asymptomatic**
  - TMJ and masticatory muscle pain
  - Long term
    - Condyle and temporal bone deformity
      - Wide, flat fossa
      - Flat, deformed condyles
    - Abnormal disc morphology
      - Thin or perforation discs in normal position
      - Absent discs
    - Frequently degenerative joint disease and synovitis
- Other signs/symptoms
  - **Retrognathia** secondary to clockwise rotation of mandible
  - **Micrognathia** (33%) from secondary mandibular growth disturbance
  - Malocclusion 66%
  - Facial asymmetry
  - Chewing difficulties & decreased mouth opening (decreased maximal incisor opening) 36%

Demographics

- Epidemiology
  - Most common childhood autoimmune musculoskeletal inflammatory disease
    - 1-22 per 1,000 children worldwide
    - TMJ involved in 20-90% of children and ≤ 70% adults with longstanding JIA
    - TMJ involvement more likely if systemic disease, young age at diagnosis, and long duration of activity
  - F > M

Treatment

- Systemic therapy
  - NSAIDs, methotrexate, sulfasalazine
- Local therapy
  - Arthrocentesis
  - Occlusal devices and functional appliances
  - Intraarticular injections of steroids or sodium hyaluronate

SELECTED REFERENCES

1. Abramowicz S et al: Juvenile arthritis: current concepts in terminology, etiopathogenesis, diagnosis, and management. Int J Oral Maxillofac Surg. 45(7):801-12, 2016
2. Al-Shwaikh H et al: Radiologic features of temporomandibular joint osseous structures in children with juvenile idiopathic arthritis. Cone beam computed tomography study. Stomatologija. 18(2):51-60, 2016
3. Niibo P et al: Contemporary management of TMJ involvement in JIA patients and its orofacial consequences. EPMA J. 7:12, 2016
4. Resnick CM et al: Quantifying temporomandibular joint synovitis in children with juvenile idiopathic arthritis. Arthritis Care Res (Hoboken). ePub, 2016
5. Arvidsson LZ et al: Temporomandibular joint findings in adults with long-standing juvenile idiopathic arthritis: CT and MR imaging assessment. Radiology. 256(1):191-200, 2010
6. Fjeld M et al: Relationship between disease course in the temporomandibular joints and mandibular growth rotation in patients with juvenile idiopathic arthritis followed from childhood to adulthood. Pediatr Rheumatol Online J. 8:13, 2010
7. Parra DA et al: Use and accuracy of US guidance for image-guided injections of the temporomandibular joints in children with arthritis. Pediatr Radiol. 40(9):1498-504, 2010
8. Argyropoulou MI et al: Temporomandibular joint involvement in juvenile idiopathic arthritis: clinical predictors of magnetic resonance imaging signs. Eur Radiol. 19(3):693-700, 2009
9. Arvidsson LZ et al: Radiographic TMJ abnormalities in patients with juvenile idiopathic arthritis followed for 27 years. Oral Surg Oral Med Oral Pathol Oral Radiol Endod. 108(1):114-23, 2009
10. Farronato G et al: Craniofacial growth in children affected by juvenile idiopathic arthritis involving the temporomandibular joint: functional therapy management. J Clin Pediatr Dent. 33(4):351-7, 2009
11. Müller L et al: Early diagnosis of temporomandibular joint involvement in juvenile idiopathic arthritis: a pilot study comparing clinical examination and ultrasound to magnetic resonance imaging. Rheumatology (Oxford). 48(6):680-5, 2009
12. Ringold S et al: The temporomandibular joint in juvenile idiopathic arthritis: frequently used and frequently arthritic. Pediatr Rheumatol Online J. 7:11, 2009
13. Stoustrup P et al: Intra-articular vs. systemic administration of etanercept in antigen-induced arthritis in the temporomandibular joint. Part II: mandibular growth. Pediatr Rheumatol Online J. 7:6, 2009
14. Barr T et al: Juvenile idiopathic arthritis: a chronic pediatric musculoskeletal condition with significant orofacial manifestations. J Can Dent Assoc. 74(9):813-21, 2008
15. Pedersen TK et al: A prospective study of magnetic resonance and radiographic imaging in relation to symptoms and clinical findings of the temporomandibular joint in children with juvenile idiopathic arthritis. J Rheumatol. 35(8):1668-75, 2008
16. Ringold S et al: Intraarticular corticosteroid injections of the temporomandibular joint in juvenile idiopathic arthritis. J Rheumatol. 35(6):1157-64, 2008
17. Twilt M et al: Long-term followup of temporomandibular joint involvement in juvenile idiopathic arthritis. Arthritis Rheum. 59(4):546-52, 2008
18. Weiss PF et al: High prevalence of temporomandibular joint arthritis at disease onset in children with juvenile idiopathic arthritis, as detected by magnetic resonance imaging but not by ultrasound. Arthritis Rheum. 58(4):1189-96, 2008
19. Billiau AD et al: Temporomandibular joint arthritis in juvenile idiopathic arthritis: prevalence, clinical and radiological signs, and relation to dentofacial morphology. J Rheumatol. 34(9):1925-33, 2007
20. Twilt M et al: Incidence of temporomandibular involvement in juvenile idiopathic arthritis. Scand J Rheumatol. 36(3):184-8, 2007
21. Twilt M et al: Facioskeletal changes in children with juvenile idiopathic arthritis. Ann Rheum Dis. 65(6):823-5, 2006
22. Arabshahi B et al: Utility of corticosteroid injection for temporomandibular arthritis in children with juvenile idiopathic arthritis. Arthritis Rheum. 52(11):3563-9, 2005
23. Twilt M et al: Temporomandibular involvement in juvenile idiopathic arthritis. J Rheumatol. 31(7):1418-22, 2004
24. Martini G et al: Isolated temporomandibular synovitis as unique presentation of juvenile idiopathic arthritis. J Rheumatol. 28(7):1689-92, 2001
25. Sidiropoulou-Chatzigianni S et al: Dentoskeletal morphology in children with juvenile idiopathic arthritis compared with healthy children. J Orthod. 28(1):53-8, 2001
26. Walton AG et al: Oral health and juvenile idiopathic arthritis: a review. Rheumatology (Oxford). 39(5):550-5, 2000
27. Smith HJ et al: Rheumatic and nonrheumatic disease in the temporomandibular joint: gadolinium-enhanced MR imaging. Radiology. 185(1):229-34, 1992

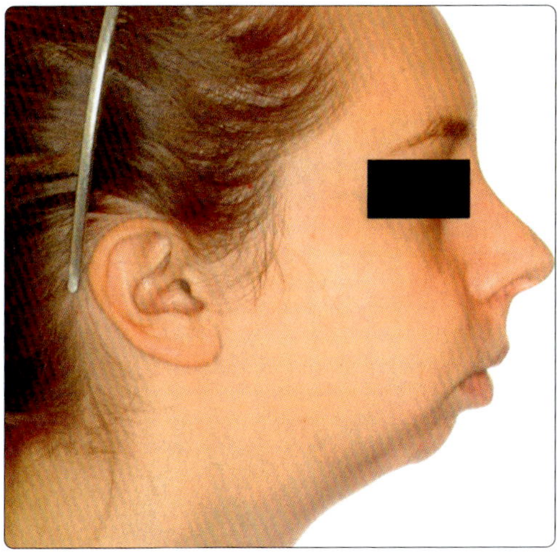

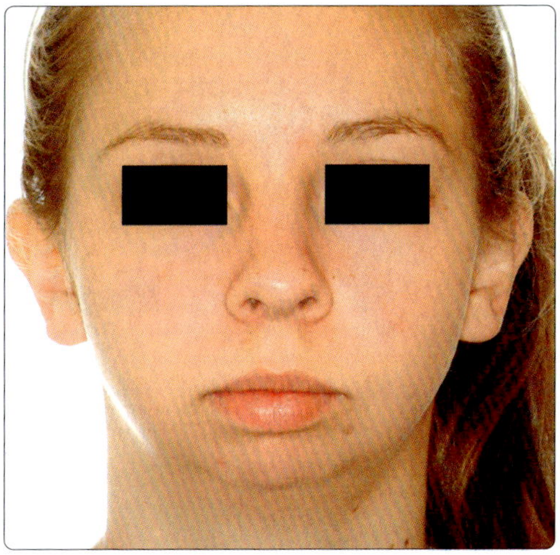

(Left) *Lateral face photograph shows a girl, age 17, with bilateral symmetrical JIA. The chin is recessive secondary to a clockwise rotation of the mandible and posteroinferior repositioning of the chin. The inferior 1/3 of the face has a short vertical dimension.* **(Right)** *Frontal face photograph of the same patient with JIA shows the mid and lower thirds of the face have a narrow mediolateral dimension. The lower 1/3 of the face has a short vertical dimension.*

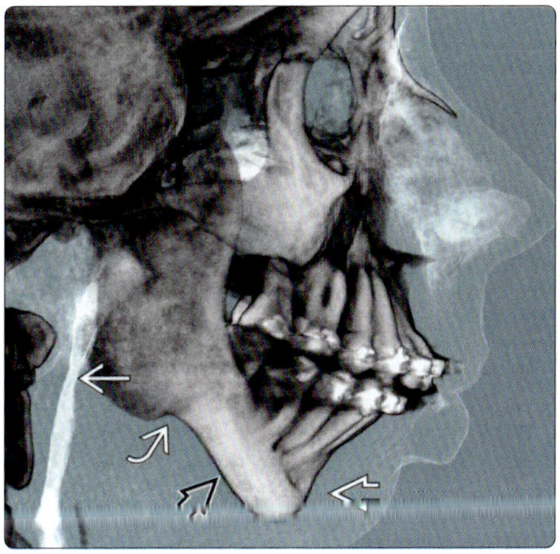

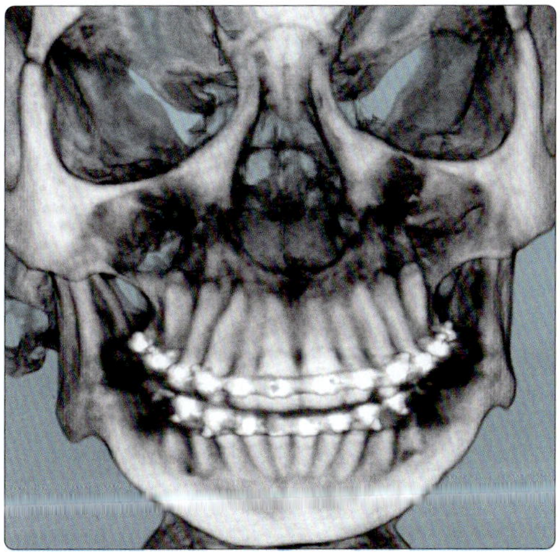

(Left) *Lateral CBCT 3D reformation of same patient shows the mandible is recessive ➡. The mandibular plane is steep ⇨ and there is a prominent antegonial notch ↪. The gonial angle is obtuse and there is airway narrowing ➡ secondary to posteroinferior repositioning of the chin and attached tongue muscles.* **(Right)** *Frontal CBCT 3D reformation of the same patient demonstrates the short rami and narrow coronal dimensions of mandible.*

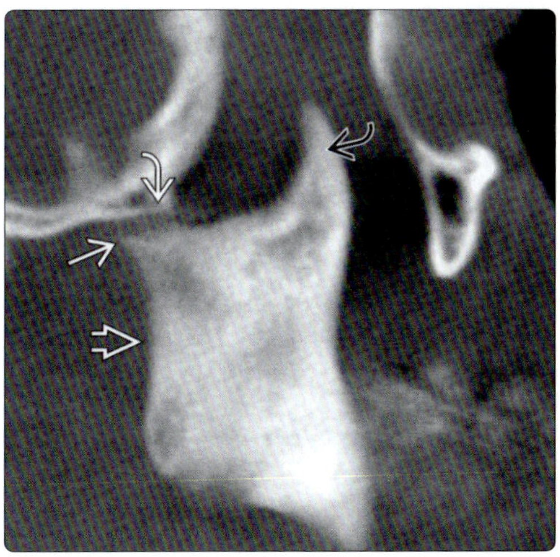

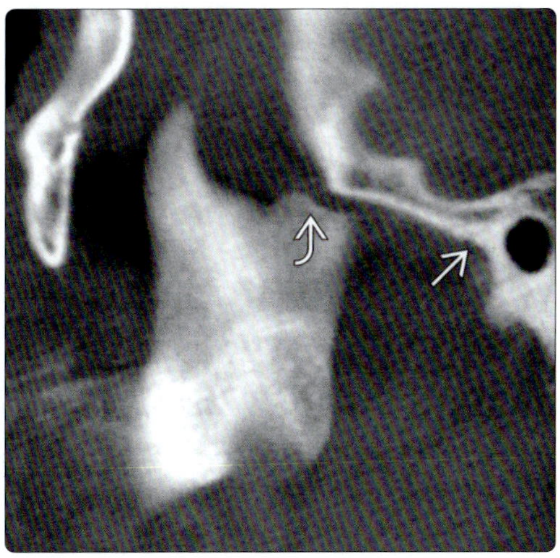

(Left) *Sagittal CBCT of the right side of the mandible in the same patient shows the condylar process is absent ➡. Note the flat and horizontal glenoid fossa/eminence ↪ and elongated coronoid process ↪. The posterior border of the ascending ramus is concave ⇨.* **(Right)** *Sagittal CBCT of the left side of the mandible in the same patient shows the short mandibular neck has a broad base ↪. The proximal end of the mandible is articulating anteriorly from the normal position in the glenoid fossa ➡.*

(Left) *Lateral face photograph shows a 12-year-old boy with JIA. Note the very recessive chin and short vertical dimension of lower 1/3 of the face.* **(Right)** *Lateral cephalometric projection of the same patient shows a steep mandibular plane, obtuse gonial angles, and short rami. The antegonial notches are prominent. There is posteroinferior repositioning of the chin and the condylar processes are very short.*

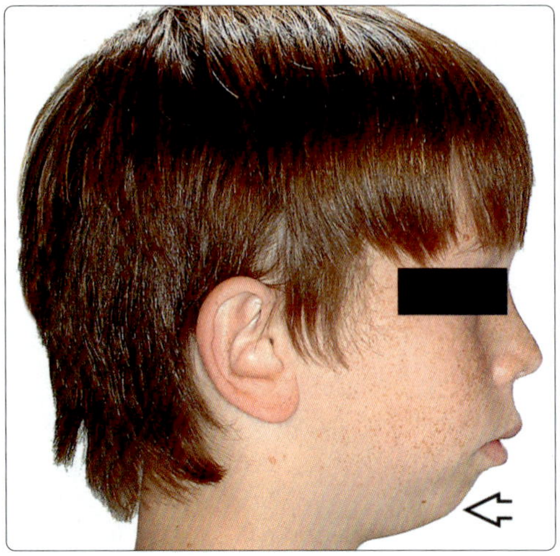

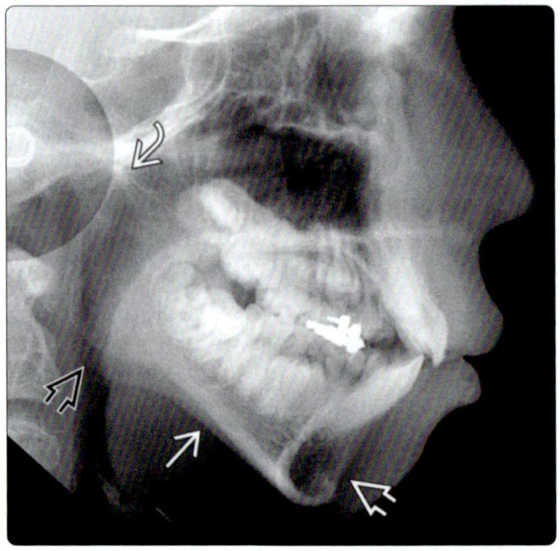

(Left) *Panoramic reformatted CBCT shows the right 1/2 of the mandible in a girl, age 15, with bilateral JIA. The coronoid process is elongated, and the condylar process is very short. The gonial angle is obtuse.* **(Right)** *Panoramic reformatted CBCT of the same patient shows a prominent antegonial notch. The ascending ramus is short and the posterior border is concave. The proximal end of the mandible has a broad base that articulates in the anterior region of the glenoid fossa.*

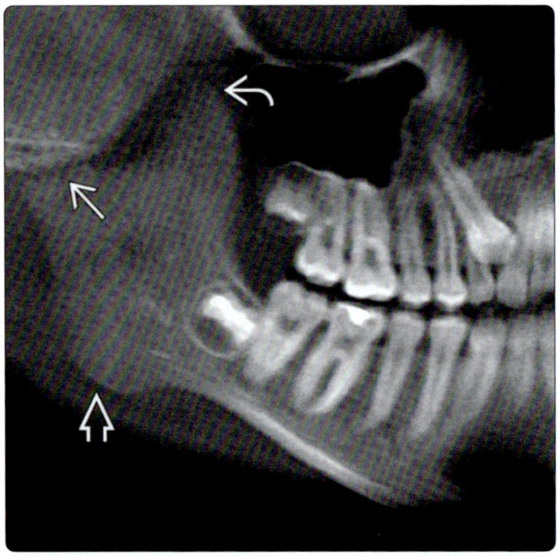

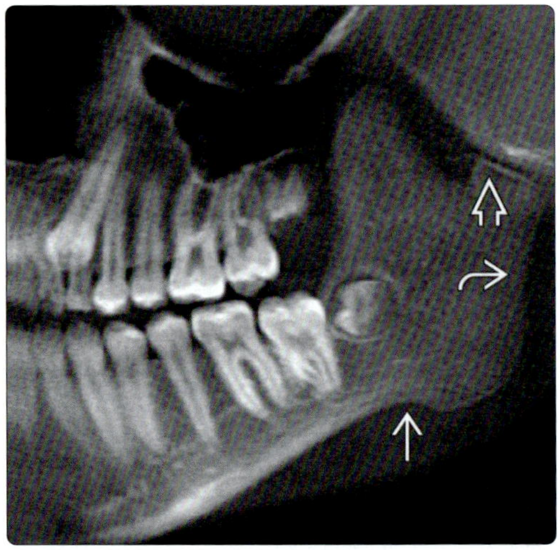

(Left) *Panoramic reformatted CBCT shows the right 1/2 of the mandible in a boy, age 15, with bilateral JIA. The condylar process is short and the posterior slope of the articular eminence is flat and horizontal. The antegonial notch is deep.* **(Right)** *Panoramic reformatted CBCT in the same patient shows a short mandibular ramus and the 3rd molar developing within the ramus. The mandibular plane is steep and there is prominent antegonial notching.*

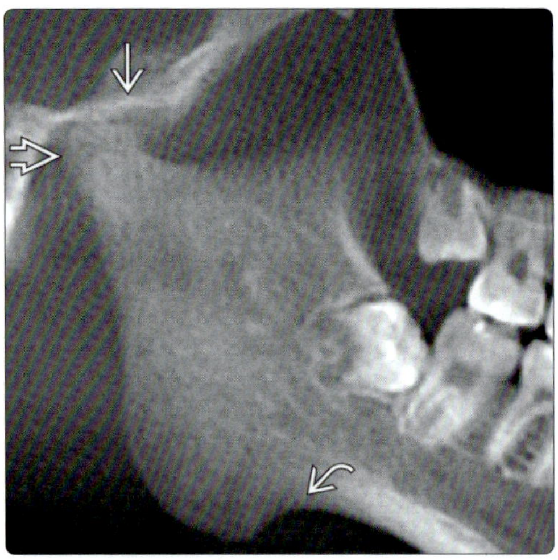

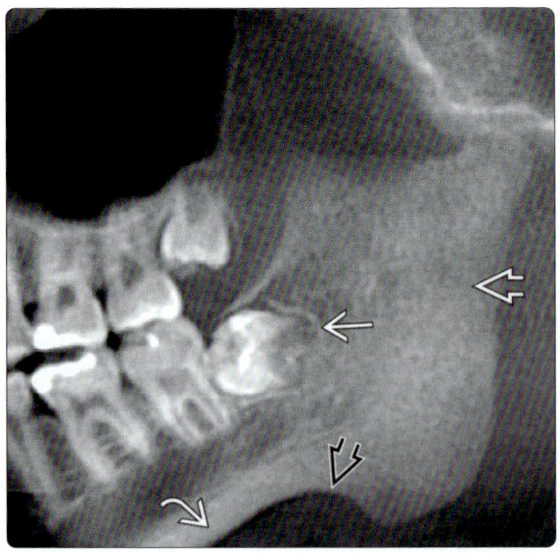

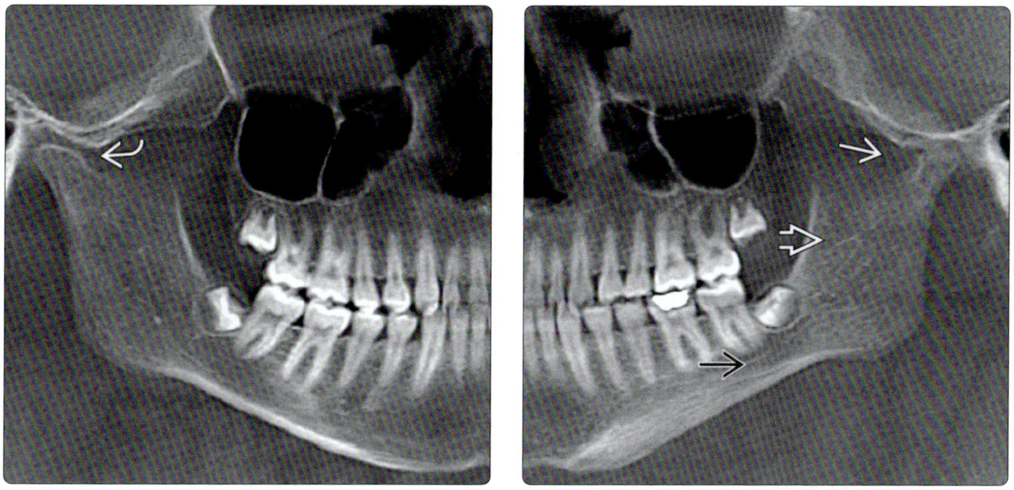

(Left) *Panoramic reformation of a CBCT shows JIA in right 1/2 of mandible. The condylar process is short and has a posterior inclination* ➡*. The ramus is relatively short. The teeth have a class II relationship and do not fully interdigitate.* **(Right)** *CBCT panoramic reformat of same patient showing the vertical dimensions of the left condylar process* ➡*, ascending ramus* ➡ *and body of mandible* ➡ *are short. The left antegonial notch is deep.*

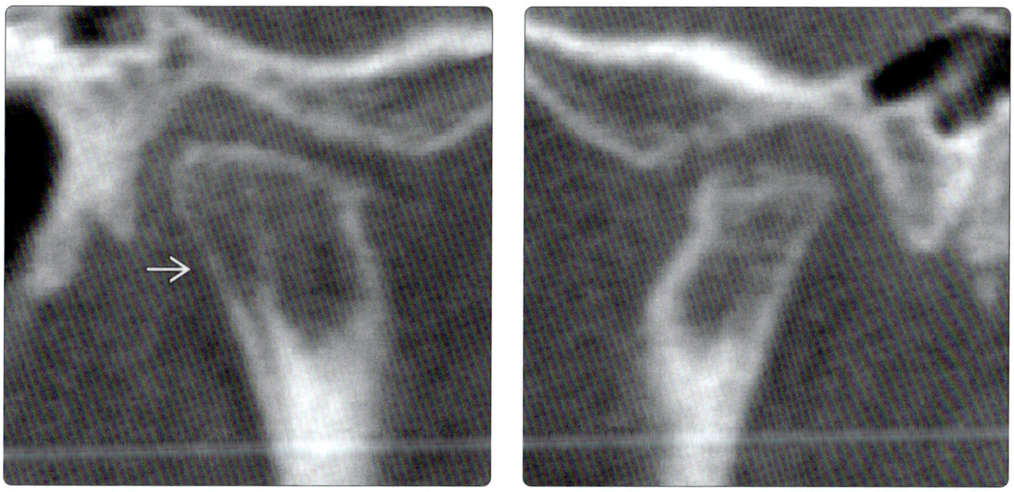

(Left) *CBCT sagittal oblique section on same patient shows a broad, shallow fossa. The condylar process has a short vertical dimension but large AP dimension. There is evidence of appositional type bone growth* ➡ *along the posterior surface of condyle.* **(Right)** *Sagittal oblique section shows left TMJ on same patient. Condylar process has a short vertical dimension and a posterior inclination. The condyle is anteriorly positioned within fossa.*

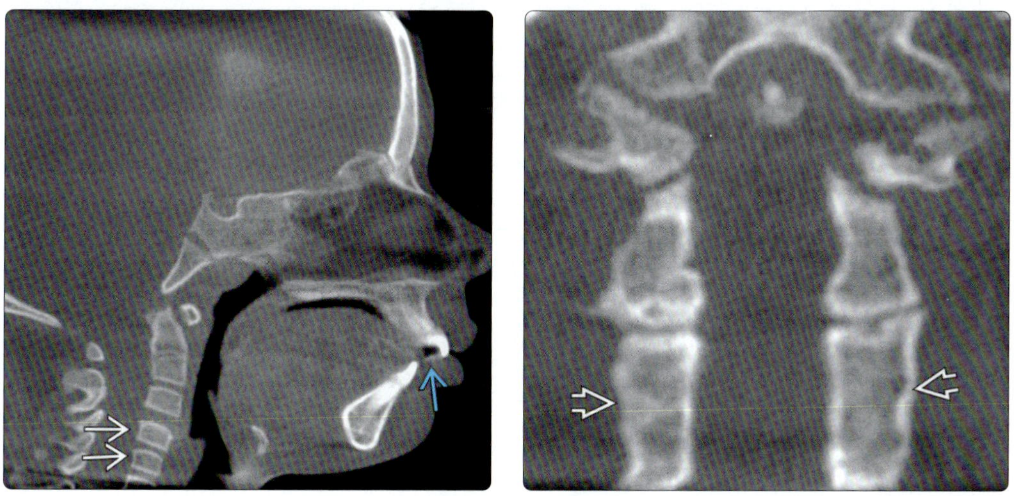

(Left) *CBCT midsagittal view of JIA patient shows a recessive mandible and associated small airway. There is a large anterior overjet* ➡*. The vertebral bodies have a short AP dimension* ➡*.* **(Right)** *CBCT coronal sections of same patient shows fusion of the facet joints of the lateral masses of the cervical vertebra* ➡*.*

TMJ Pigmented Villonodular Synovitis

KEY FACTS

TERMINOLOGY

- Pigmented villonodular synovitis **(PVNS)**
- Definition: Benign, locally aggressive tumefactive disease of synovium

IMAGING

- Best imaging tool: TMJ & skull base enhanced MR & thin-section bone CT
- CT: **Erosion** of mandibular **condyle** ± glenoid fossa
  - Lobulated, rounded lytic lesions
  - May extend to greater wing of sphenoid, temporal bone, intracranially
- T1 MR: **Hypointense**-to-isointense **mass** with peripheral rim of low signal
- T2 MR: **Hypointense** lobulated mass often with **peripheral rim of low signal**
  - Hypointensity due to hemosiderin deposition
- T1 C+ MR: Portions of mass show mild enhancement

TOP DIFFERENTIAL DIAGNOSES

- Giant cell tumor
- Chondrosarcoma
- Chondrocalcinosis disease
- Synovial chondromatosis

PATHOLOGY

- Etiology: Unknown
  - Monarticular hyperplastic inflammatory process involving TMJ

CLINICAL ISSUES

- Presenting symptoms: Preauricular pain, swelling, trismus
- Age: Between 20-50 years; gender: F:M = 3:1
- Treatment: Complete surgical resection

DIAGNOSTIC CHECKLIST

- Consider if lesion centered in TMJ or skull base

(Left) *Axial bone CT demonstrates widening of the right TMJ space ➔ and multiple rounded erosions of the adjacent skull base involving the internal aspect of the zygomatic arch ➔ and greater wing of the sphenoid up to the lateral margin of the foramen ovale ➔.* **(Right)** *Coronal T1WI MR shows a hypointense right TMJ mass ➔ with peripheral lower signal intensity. A hypointense contiguous middle cranial fossa extraaxial mass ➔ is evident with similar markedly low-signal peripheral rim.*

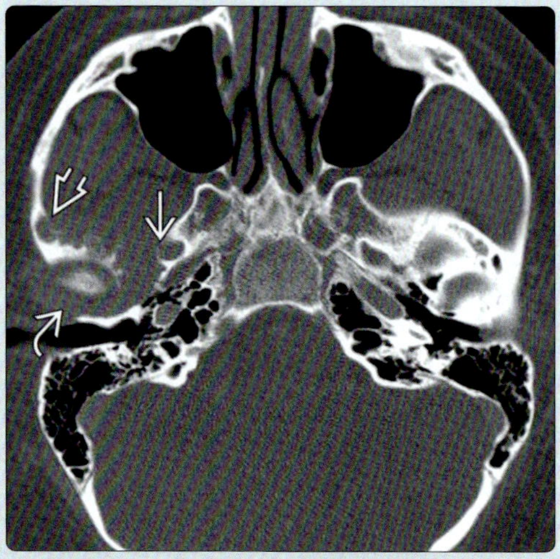

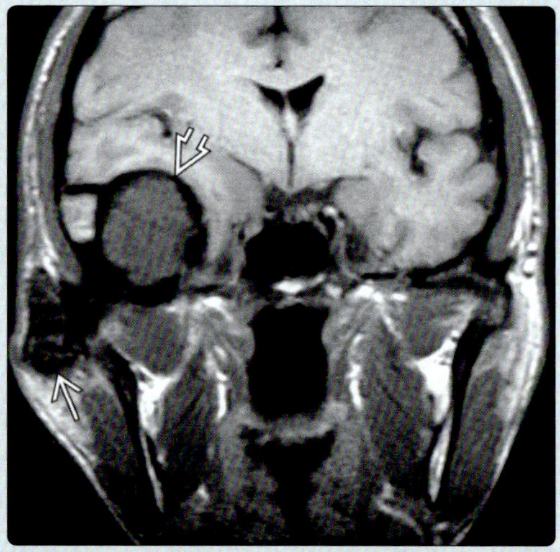

(Left) *Axial T2WI MR through the floor of the middle cranial fossa reveals a markedly low-signal mass ➔ above the area of the right TMJ. This mass represents the intracranial spread of pigmented villonodular synovitis from the TMJ.* **(Right)** *Axial T1WI C+ FS MR in the same patient reveals only mild enhancement of some of the solid portions of this pigmented villonodular synovitis mass ➔.*

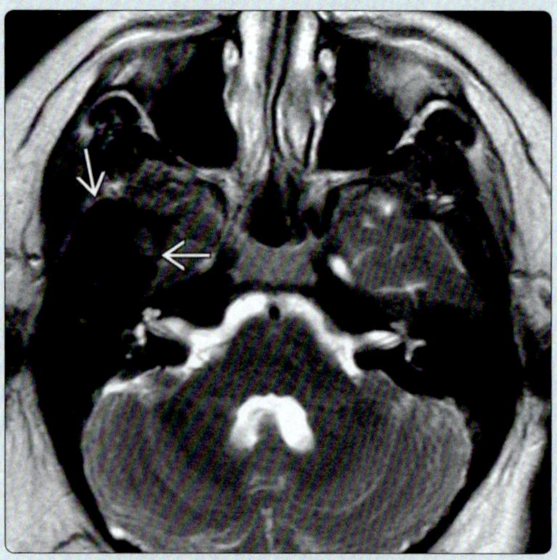

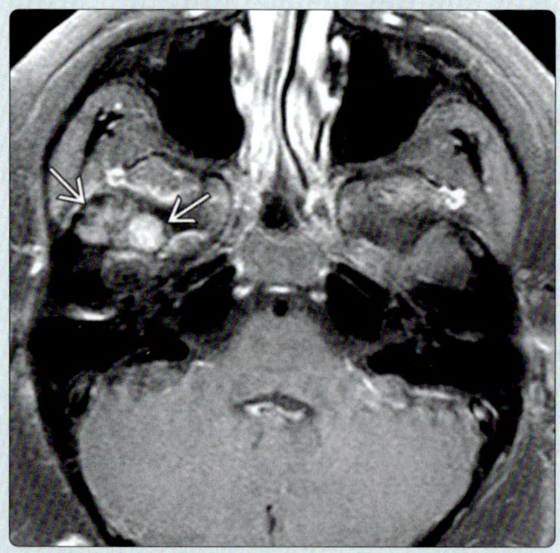

TMJ Pigmented Villonodular Synovitis

TERMINOLOGY

Abbreviations

- Pigmented villonodular synovitis **(PVNS)**

Definitions

- **Benign**, locally aggressive **tumefactive disease** of **synovium**

IMAGING

General Features

- Best diagnostic clue
  - **Monarticular hyperplastic, inflammatory process involving TMJ**
- Location
  - Rare in TMJ
    - More common in knee, hip, shoulder, ankle, wrist
    - Typically $\geq$ 1 cm at diagnosis

Imaging Recommendations

- Best imaging tool
  - T2WI & T1 C+ MR
  - TMJ & skull base enhanced MR & thin-section bone CT

CT Findings

- CBCT or bone CT
  - **Erosion** of mandibular condyle ± glenoid fossa
  - Lobulated, rounded lytic lesions
  - When large, erosive mass may extend to greater wing of sphenoid, temporal bone, & intracranially

MR Findings

- T1WI
  - Hypointense-to-isointense mass with **peripheral rim of low signal**
    - May have areas of ↑ T1 due to lipid in foamy macrophages
- T2WI
  - Hypointense lobulated mass often with peripheral rim of low signal
    - Hypointensity due to hemosiderin deposition
      - GRE MR will show characteristic hemosiderin bloom
  - Cystic areas of synovial fluid will be hyperintense
- T1WI C+
  - Mild enhancement of portions of mass common

DIFFERENTIAL DIAGNOSIS

Giant Cell Tumor

- In H&N, most commonly involves sphenoid & temporal bones
- Expansile mass with benign eggshell wall on bone CT
  - Multiple lytic lesions may have bubbly appearance
- May have hypointense rim on T1 & T2 MR
- Marked homogeneous or heterogeneous enhancement on CECT or T1 C+ MR

Chondrosarcoma

- Chondroid malignancy involving TMJ or petrooccipital fissure
- Calcification + bone destruction on CBCT or bone CT
- Hypointense on T1, hyperintense on T2 MR
- Heterogeneously enhancing on CECT or T1WI C+ MR

Chondrocalcinosis Disease

- Metabolic disease resulting in peri-/intraarticular chondrocalcinosis
- Diffusely calcified mass involving TMJ on CBCT or CT
  - Associated remodeling, erosion, or mass effect
- Hypointense T1, heterogeneously hypointense T2 MR
- Heterogeneously enhancing on T1WI C+ MR

Synovial Chondromatosis

- Synovial metaplasia with formation of hyaline cartilage foci
- Multiple calcified loose bodies in superior joint space
- CBCT or bone CT: Calcified nodules surrounding condyle
- MR: Multiple hypointense nodules in joint space T1

PATHOLOGY

General Features

- Etiology
  - Unknown: Thought to represent inflammatory or reactive synovial infiltrate

Gross Pathologic & Surgical Features

- Darkly pigmented, cystic-appearing mass

Microscopic Features

- Plump histiocytes with **giant cells** + **hemosiderin**
- Erosion into surrounding bone; no atypia or mitoses
- Lymphoplasmacytic infiltrate & chondroid metaplasia

CLINICAL ISSUES

Presentation

- Most common signs/symptoms
  - Preauricular pain, swelling, trismus

Demographics

- Age
  - Between 20-50 years; mean: 30 years
- Gender
  - F:M = 3:1

Natural History & Prognosis

- Low recurrence rate with complete resection

Treatment

- Complete surgical resection

DIAGNOSTIC CHECKLIST

Consider

- Whether lesion centered in TMJ or skull base
  - PVNS/TMJ vs. giant cell tumor/skull base
- Both giant cell tumor & chondrosarcoma tend to enhance more than PVNS

SELECTED REFERENCES

1. Baj A et al: Pigmented villonodular synovitis of temporomandibular joint: pathological aspects and surgical treatment. Minerva Stomatol. 64(4):213-8, 2015
2. Damodar D et al: Pigmented villonodular synovitis of the temporomandibular joint: case report and review of the literature. Head Neck. 37(12): E194-9, 2015

Degenerative Joint Disease

KEY FACTS

TERMINOLOGY

- Degenerative joint disease (DJD); osteoarthritis, osteoarthrosis (OA); arthrosis deformans (AD)
- Definition: Localized noninflammatory degenerative disorder of synovial joints characterized by destruction and repair of articular fibrocartilage and underlying subchondral bone

IMAGING

- Reduction in condylar size from superior surface ± evidence of sclerosis, flattening, **erosions, osteophytes and subchondral bone cyst**, joint space narrowing, disc displacement
- Location: Anterosuperior surface of condyle and opposing articular eminence
- Focal defect in articular soft tissues and subjacent bone enlarges to involve entire condyle
- Progressive vertical loss of condylar height

TOP DIFFERENTIAL DIAGNOSES

- Progressive condylar resorption
- Inflammatory (rheumatoid or juvenile idiopathic) arthritis
- Chondrocalcinosis

CLINICAL ISSUES

- Osseous signs of DJD are usually preceded by nonreducing anteriorly displaced disc
- Acute phase: Decrease in condylar size and motion
  - Joint pain and sounds, including crepitation
- Proliferative phase: Restores articular surface and may increase congruency and size of contact area
- End-stage DJD: Often accompanied by normal motion and pain-free function

DIAGNOSTIC CHECKLIST

- DJD may limit growth of ipsilateral half of mandible with **compensations in maxilla and cranial base**

(Left) *Sagittal oblique T1WI MR of TMJ in closed position shows loss of the low-signal rim with cavitation of the subchondral bone. The bone marrow produces a low T1 signal. A small segment of disc is anterior to condyle, and the remainder of disc is outside image plane. These changes indicate an active stage of degenerative joint disease (DJD) and associated bone marrow edema.* **(Right)** *Coronal oblique T1WI MR, same patient, shows superior cavitation in the condyle. There is anterior and medial displacement of the disc.*

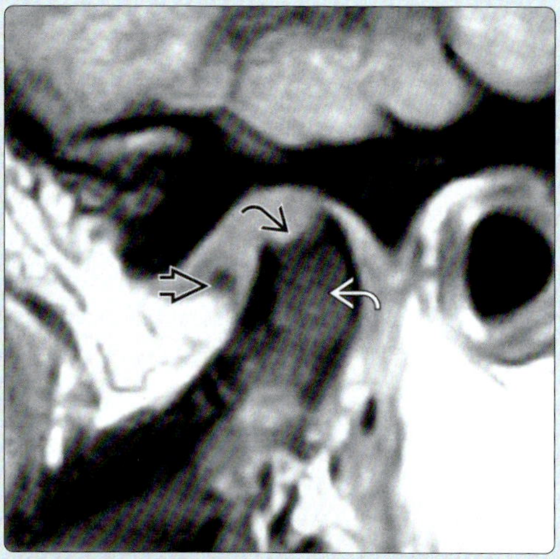

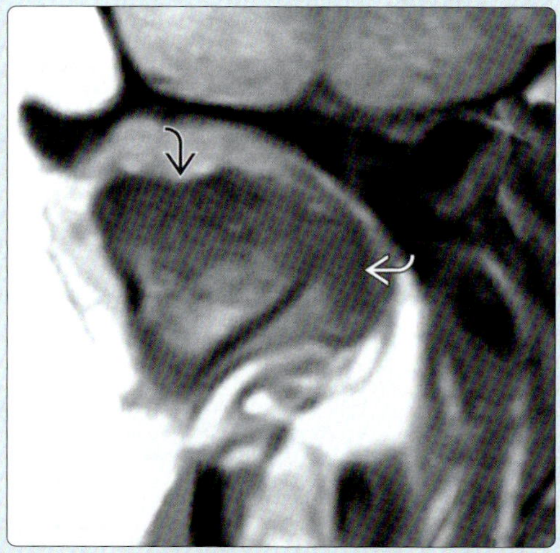

(Left) *Coronal oblique and sagittal oblique reformatted CBCTs show a condyle with loss of the superior cortex, cavitation of the subchondral bone, and a reduction in condylar volume. These changes indicate an active stage of DJD.* **(Right)** *Sagittal oblique T1WI FSE MR shows a small condyle with a thick, low-signal rim along its superior surface. The disc is anterior to the condyle in the closed position. This represents a stable end-stage DJD.*

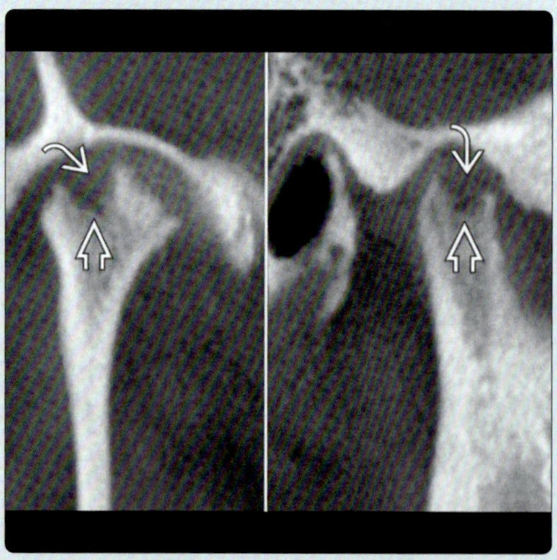

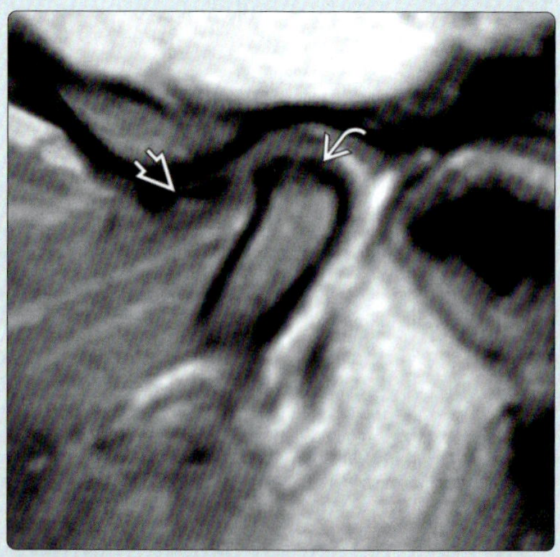

TERMINOLOGY

Synonyms

- Degenerative joint disease (DJD); osteoarthritis, osteoarthrosis (OA); arthrosis deformans (AD)

Definitions

- Localized, noninflammatory, degenerative disorder of synovial joints characterized by destruction and repair of articular fibrocartilage and underlying subchondral bone

IMAGING

General Features

- Best diagnostic clue
    - Reduction in condylar size from superior surface ± evidence of sclerosis, flattening, erosions, osteophytes and subchondral bone cyst, joint space narrowing, disc displacement
- Location
    - Anterosuperior surface of condyle and opposing articular eminence
- Size
    - Starts as focal defect in articular soft tissues and subjacent bone; may enlarge to involve entire condyle
- Morphology
    - Progressive vertical loss of condylar height

Imaging Recommendations

- Best imaging tool
    - CBCT or CT to determine size, shape, and quality of changes in osseous anatomy
    - MR for soft tissue and bone marrow
- Protocol advice
    - Axially corrected views to section perpendicular and parallel to mediolateral long axis of condyles

DIFFERENTIAL DIAGNOSIS

Inflammatory (Rheumatoid) Arthritis

- **Polyarticular** systemic disease
- Serum indicators
- Pannus formation

Progressive Condylar Resorption

- Degenerative process occurring in adolescent females

PATHOLOGY

General Features

- Functional loading of articular tissues beyond their adaptive capacity
    - Adaptive capacity may be reduced &/or functional loads may be too great
- Displacement of articular disc

Gross Pathologic & Surgical Features

- Soft tissue
    - Proteoglycan depletion, collagen fiber network disintegration, and fatty degeneration

CLINICAL ISSUES

Presentation

- Most common signs/symptoms
    - Joint pain and sounds including crepitation
    - Decrease in condylar motion
    - Jaw and neck muscle pain and dysfunction
    - Opening **deviation of mandible to affected side**
    - Change in occlusion: Contralateral posterior open bite

Demographics

- Age
    - Incidence is highest prior to age 40
        - Incidence peak for subgroup of females following puberty
    - Females are most susceptible between puberty and menopause
- Gender
    - Female > male = 8.5:1 for DJD

Natural History & Prognosis

- Soft tissue changes precede osseous changes
- Osseous signs of DJD are usually preceded by nonreducing anteriorly displaced disc
- DJD progresses until **equilibrium between form and function is achieved**
- Destructive (active) phase of DJD reduces condylar size
    - **Erosions**, concave articular surface
    - Formation of subchondral bone cysts
    - ± joint effusion
    - ± synovitis
    - Pain and limited opening during active phase
- Proliferative phase restores articular surface
    - **Sclerosis (eburnation)**, flattening, and osteophyte formation
    - May increase articular congruency and size of contact area
- End-stage DJD is often accompanied by normal motion and **pain-free** function

Treatment

- Conservative
    - Reduce joint loads during active phase
    - Manage joint inflammation with NSAIDs
    - Manage muscle hyperactivity and parafunction
- Surgical
    - Rarely indicated for joint pain and limited motion
    - Arthrocentesis; arthroscopy; disc repair or arthroplasty

DIAGNOSTIC CHECKLIST

Image Interpretation Pearls

- DJD may limit growth of ipsilateral half of mandible with **compensations in maxilla and cranial base**

SELECTED REFERENCES

1. Gunson MJ et al: Oral contraceptive pill use and abnormal menstrual cycles in women with severe condylar resorption: A case for low serum 17beta-estradiol as a major factor in progressive condylar resorption. Am J Orthod Dentofacial Orthop. 136(6):772-9, 2009
2. Sano T et al: Common abnormalities in temporomandibular joint imaging. Curr Probl Diagn Radiol. 33(1):16-24, 2004

(Left) *Closed-mouth sagittal oblique T1WI MR shows an early active stage of DJD. Loss of the superior surface of the condyle is evident as a low-signal rim, and the disc is anterior to the condyle. Note the mild loss of condylar volume and normal bone marrow signal.* **(Right)** *Sagittal oblique T1WI MR in the same patient in open-mouth position shows that the condyle translates to a point short of the summit of the eminence. The disc remains anterior to the condyle.*

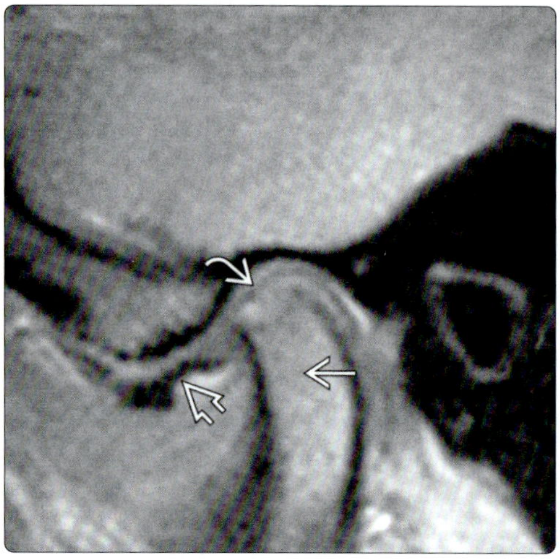

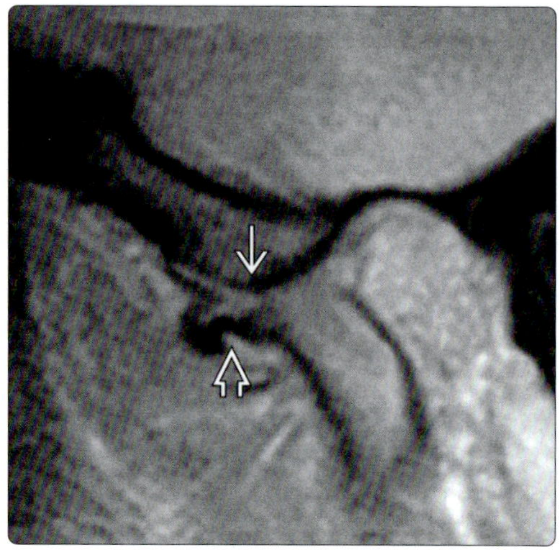

(Left) *Sagittal oblique T1WI MR of the opposite joint in the same patient, in closed-mouth position, shows a stable stage of DJD. Note that the condyle is small, and the low-signal rim has reformed following the erosive phase. The disc is anterior to the condyle.* **(Right)** *Sagittal oblique T1WI MR in the same patient in open-mouth position shows the condyle translated to a point short of the summit of eminence. The disc remains anterior to the condyle. This is a nonreducing displaced disc with limited motion.*

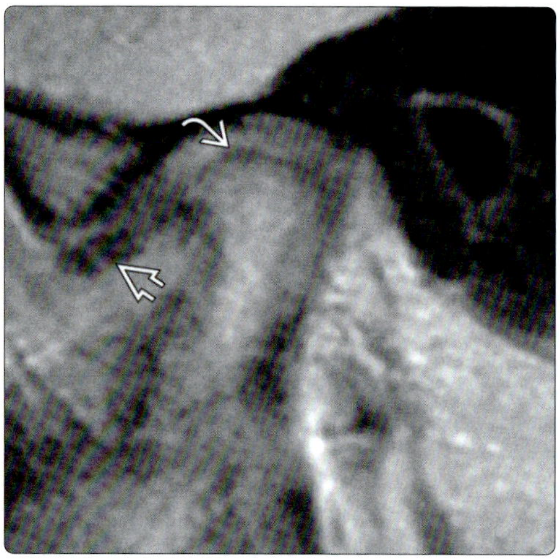

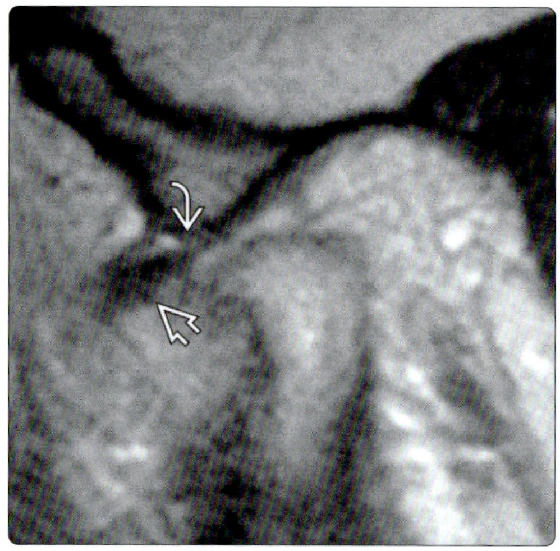

(Left) *Coronal oblique and sagittal oblique CBCT of a TMJ shows reparative phase of DJD. Note bone formation with congruent articulation between condyle and fossa, cortication of articular surface, and resultant large contact area. An osteophyte extends from the anterior surface of the condyle.* **(Right)** *Sagittal oblique CBCT shows end-stage DJD. The joint space is narrowed, and there is congruent articulation resulting in a large contact area. Note the subchondral bone cyst and osteophyte formation.*

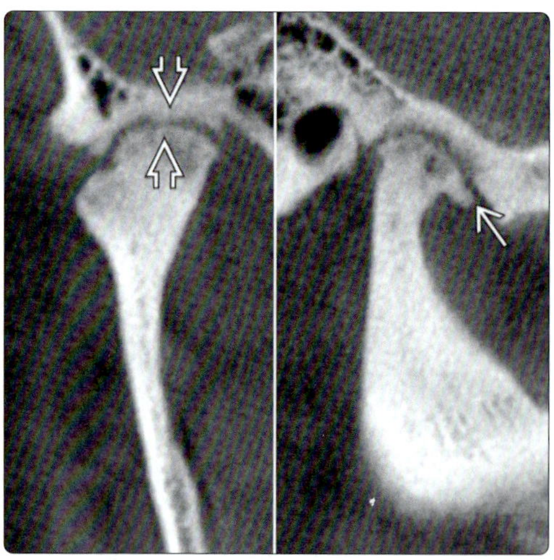

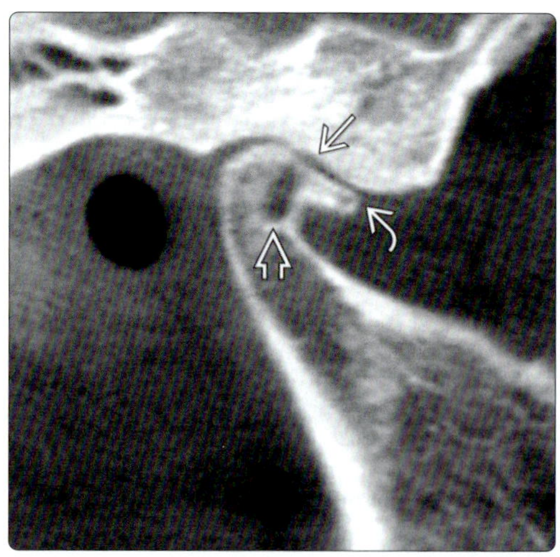

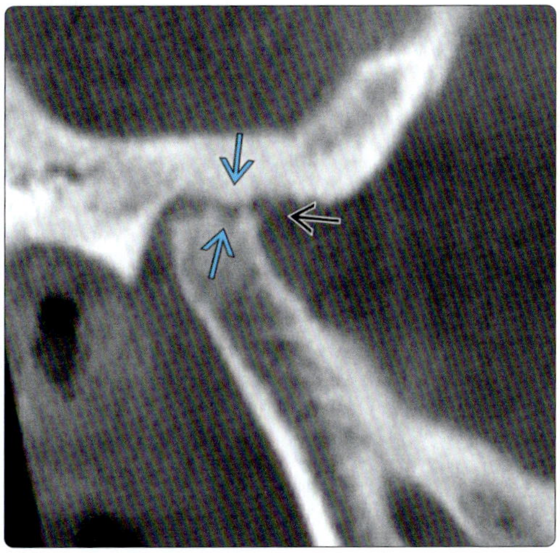

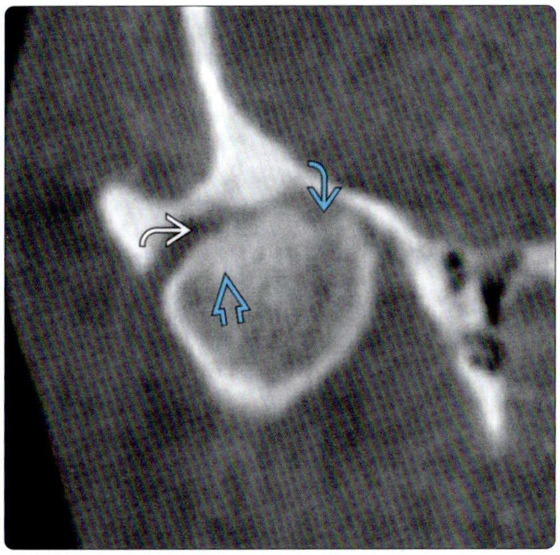

(Left) *CBCT sagittal oblique reformat of an adult woman shows an active stage of DJD. There is loss of condylar height from superior surface. Subchondral sclerosis, flattening, and erosions are seen along the superior surface of condyle and articular eminence. There is joint space narrowing.* **(Right)** *Coronal oblique section of right TMJ in the same patient shows erosions, subchondral sclerosis, and joint space narrowing.*

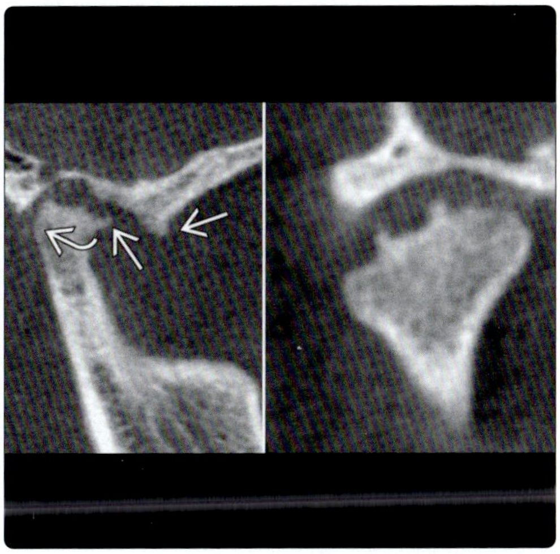

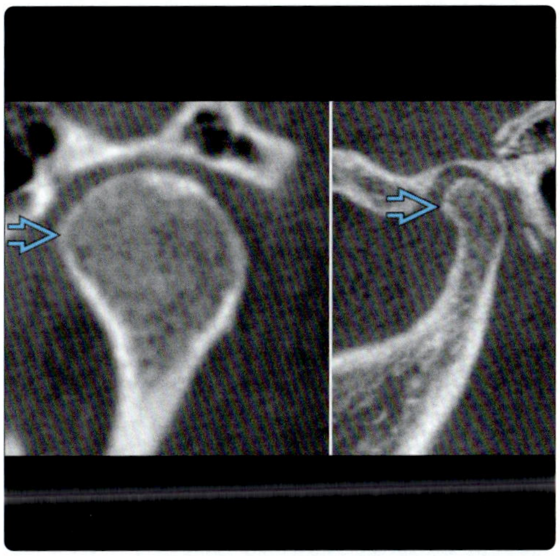

(Left) *CBCT sagittal oblique & coronal oblique images of right TMJ shows active DJD. Loss of vertical dimension from superior surface of condyle, erosions, flattening, & subchondral sclerosis are noted along superior surface of condyle and posterior slope of the articular eminence. Eminence and condylar osteophytes are seen. Note posterior height of contour near superior surface of condyle.* **(Right)** *Left TMJ in the same patient shows normal osseous components for comparison to normal contours and size.*

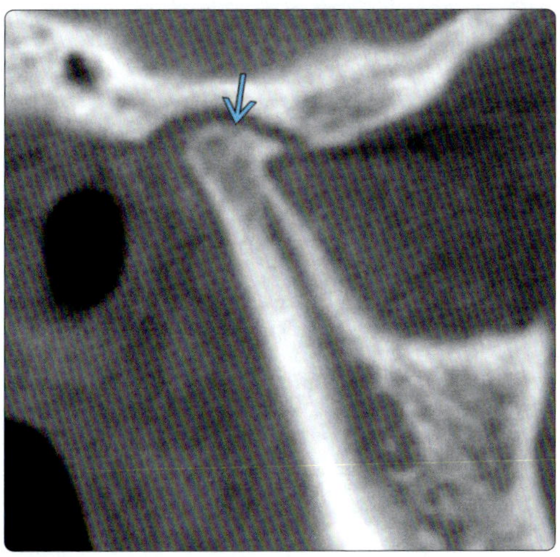

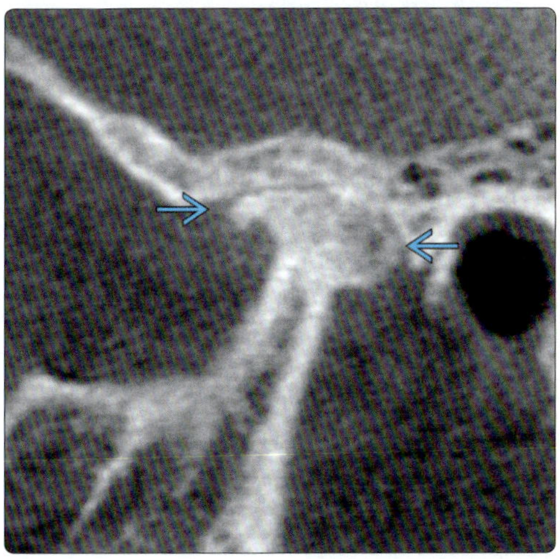

(Left) *CBCT sagittal oblique reformat of the right TMJ of an adult patient with radiographically stable DJD shows a condyle that has a short vertical dimension. Eminence and condylar flattening, sclerosis, and previous erosions are evident.* **(Right)** *Sagittal oblique reformat of CBCT shows proliferative DJD. The vertical dimension of condyle and eminence are short. The AP dimensions of condyle are increased. The opposing surfaces form a congruent articulation.*

TMJ Synovial Cyst

KEY FACTS

TERMINOLOGY

- Definition: Fluid-filled cysts, which have synovial membrane, caused by herniation of TMJ capsule into surrounding soft tissues

IMAGING

- Location: TMJ capsule → herniation
- Size: Usually < 1 cm at discovery
- CBCT
  - Normal
  - Possible soft tissue swelling
- T1WI MR
  - Hypointense to intermediate signal intensity
  - Hydraulic-shaped mass extending from joint capsule
- T2WI MR
  - Uniformly hyperintense cystic mass
  - May have stalk connecting cyst to joint

TOP DIFFERENTIAL DIAGNOSES

- Ganglion cyst
- Joint effusion
- Synovial chondromatosis
- Parotid mass

PATHOLOGY

- Etiology unknown
- Synovial cyst enlarges by **hydraulic pumping** of joint fluid
- 1-way flow of fluid from joint to cyst

CLINICAL ISSUES

- Pain and swelling in parotid region in 50% of cases
- Limitation of jaw motion
- Treatment: Open excision
  - Excision of stalk + small amount of capsule
- Recurrence rate is low

(Left) *Coronal T1WI MR of the left TMJ shows a homogeneous, intermediate signal, circular-shaped mass extending from the medial condylar pole region ⇨. The mass is well defined and has a hydraulic shape typical of cystic lesions.* **(Right)** *Sagittal T1WI MR of the left TMJ in the same patient shows a section medial to the left condyle. Note the superior ⇨ and inferior ➡ heads of the lateral pterygoid muscle. A homogeneous, hypointense, circular-shaped mass ↶ medial to the medial pole of the left condyle is visualized.*

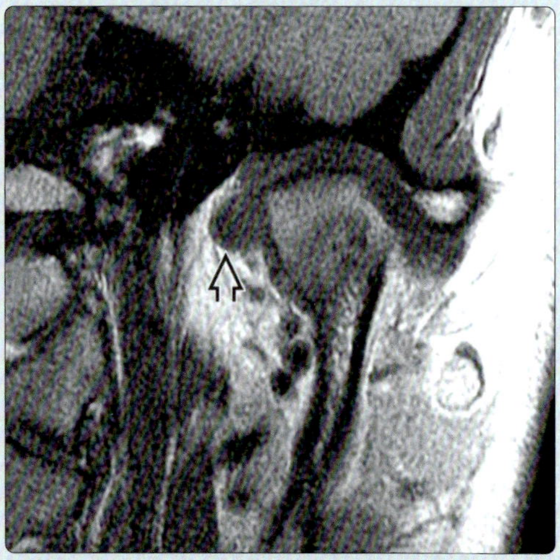

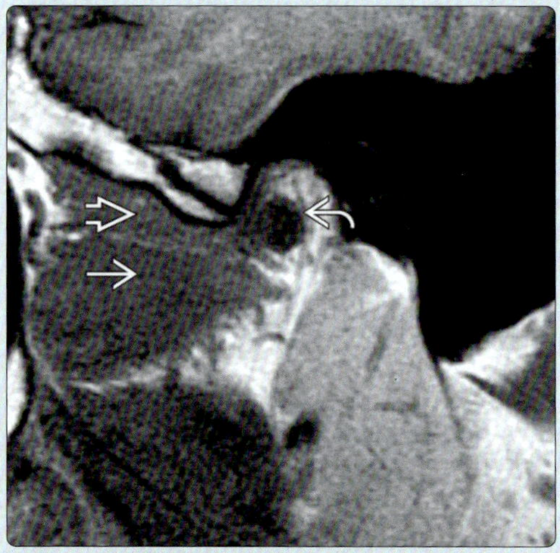

(Left) *Sagittal oblique T2WI MR of the left TMJ in the same patient shows a uniformly hyperintense, circular-shaped mass medial to the left condyle ↶, consistent with a synovial cyst.* **(Right)** *Open mouth sagittal oblique view shows an anteriorly displaced disc ➡. Note the teardrop-shaped hyperintense mass ⇨ posteroinferior to a condyle with a bottle neck-like extension ⇨ into the posterior recess of the superior joint compartment.*

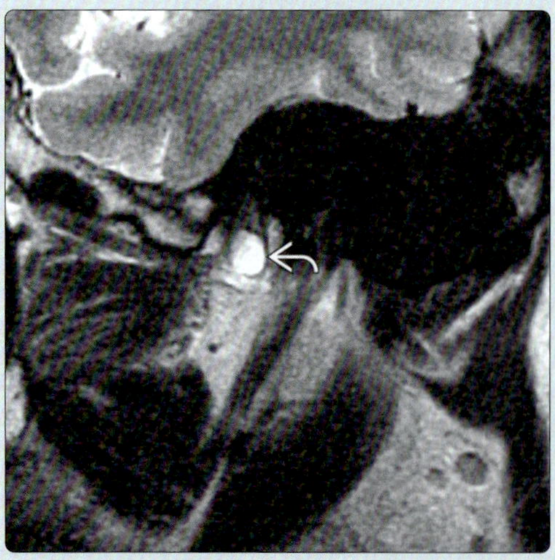

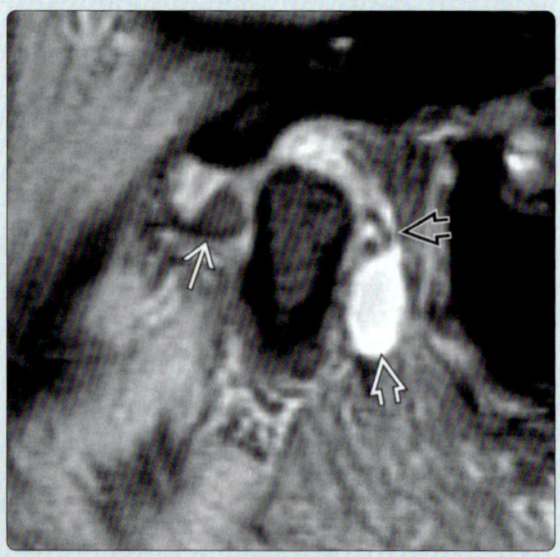

TERMINOLOGY

Definitions

- Fluid-filled cysts, which have synovial membrane, caused by herniation of TMJ capsule into surrounding soft tissues

IMAGING

General Features

- Location
  - TMJ capsule: Herniation may occur in different directions
    - Laterally anterior to tragus of ear
    - Posteriorly into external auditory meatus
    - Medially
- Size
  - Usually < 1 cm at discovery
  - Cyst may decrease in size with mouth opening
- Morphology
  - Hydraulic shape typical of cystic lesions

CT Findings

- CBCT
  - Normal
  - Possible soft tissue swelling

MR Findings

- T1WI
  - Hypointense to intermediate signal intensity
  - Hydraulic-shaped mass extending from joint capsule
- T2WI
  - Uniformly hyperintense cystic mass
  - May have stalk connecting cyst to joint

Imaging Recommendations

- Best imaging tool
  - MR
    - T1WI and T2WI
- Protocol advice
  - Parasagittal and paracoronal corrected to mediolateral long axis of condyle
  - Axial image

DIFFERENTIAL DIAGNOSIS

Ganglion Cyst

- Near joint
- Pseudocyst lined with fibrous connective tissue with myxoid degeneration
- No synovial cell lining
- Contains mucous extravasation
- Does not connect to joint cavity

Joint Effusion

- Fluid within joint cavity
- No capsular herniation
- Often associated with trauma or disc displacement

Synovial Chondromatosis

- May have expanded capsule
- Contains cartilaginous or osteocartilaginous loose bodies

Parotid Mass

- Mass in parotid gland and not at superior border
- Does not decrease in size with mouth opening

PATHOLOGY

General Features

- Etiology
  - Unknown
  - Capsular herniation into surrounding tissues occurs
    - Synovial cyst enlarges by **hydraulic pumping of joint fluid**
    - 1-way flow of fluid from joint to cyst
  - Theories leading to herniation
    - Increase in intraarticular pressure
      - **Blunt trauma**
      - TMJ dysfunction
    - Associated with inflammatory process
      - Rheumatoid arthritis
      - Synovitis
      - Osteoarthritis
    - Displacement of synovial tissues during embryogenesis

Microscopic Features

- Contains gelatinous fluid
- Lined by cuboidal to flattened cells consistent with synovial origin

CLINICAL ISSUES

Presentation

- Most common signs/symptoms
  - Pain and swelling in parotid region 50% of cases
- Other signs/symptoms
  - Limitation of jaw motion
  - Joint sounds
  - Chewing discomfort

Demographics

- Age
  - Average: 42 years; range: 22-65 years
- Gender
  - F:M = 7:2

Treatment

- Open excision
- Excision of stalk + small amount of capsule
- Repair capsule
- Recurrence rate is low

SELECTED REFERENCES

1. Levarek RE et al: Temporomandibular joint ganglion cyst: a unique case of complete resolution following subtotal excision. J Oral Maxillofac Surg. 74(9):1783-91, 2016
2. Partridge JC et al: Periarticular cysts of the temporomandibular joint are more frequently synovial than ganglion. J Oral Maxillofac Surg. 74(7):1396-402, 2016
3. LaBan MM et al: "Numb chin" syndrome: mental nerve mononeuropathy resulting from a synovial temporomandibular cyst. Am J Phys Med Rehabil. 94(7):e65, 2015
4. Steen MW et al: Ganglion and synovial cyst of the temporomandibular joint: a case report and literature review. Plast Reconstr Surg Glob Open. 3(9):e524, 2015
5. Spinzia A et al: Synovial cyst of the temporomandibular joint: a case report and literature review. Int J Oral Maxillofac Surg. 40(8): 874-7 2011

Progressive Condylar Resorption

KEY FACTS

TERMINOLOGY

- Synonyms: Juvenile degenerative joint disease, condylysis, idiopathic condylar resorption, osteoarthritis, degenerative joint disease, arthrosis deformans
- Definition: Localized noninflammatory degenerative disorder of TMJ characterized by lysis and repair of articular fibrocartilage and underlying subchondral bone following onset of puberty in females

IMAGING

- Best diagnostic clue: Unilateral (but often bilateral) resorption of superior portions of condyles
- Location: Anterosuperior surfaces of condyles and occasionally opposing articular eminentia
- CBCT or CT to determine size, shape, and quality of changes in osseous anatomy
- MR for evaluation of disc position and bone marrow
- Axially corrected views to section perpendicular and parallel to mediolateral long axis of condyles

TOP DIFFERENTIAL DIAGNOSES

- Juvenile idiopathic arthritis
- Degenerative joint disease

CLINICAL ISSUES

- TMJ and myofascial pain
- Joint sounds: Clicking and crepitation
- Nonreducing **anteriorly displaced disc**
- Destructive/active phase
    - **Cavitation defect** into subchondral bone
    - Reduction in condylar height
- Reparative phase
    - Condylar flattening and recortication
- Limited vertical growth of condylar process, ascending ramus, and body of mandible

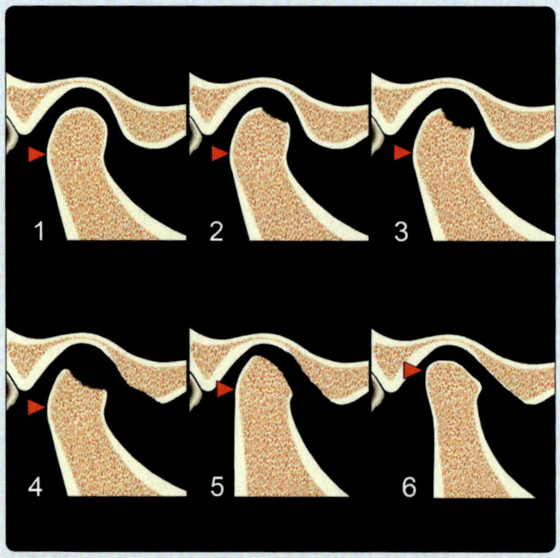

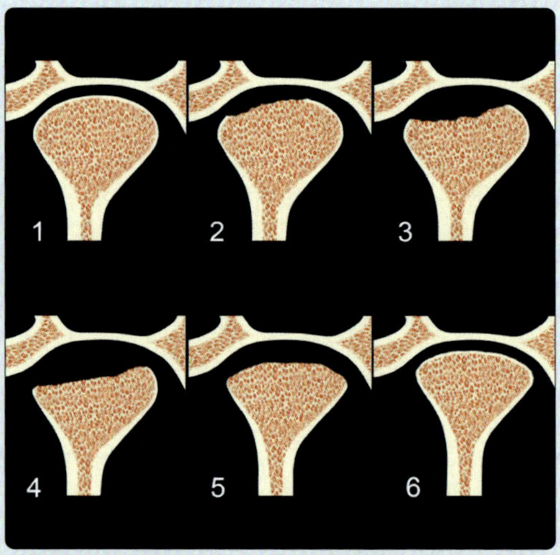

(Left) *Sagittal graphics show progression of progressive condylar resorption (PCR). Note position of posterior height of contour (red arrow) throughout series: (1) Normal condyle & fossa with normal spatial relationship, (2) early active phase with noncorticated erosion, (3) late active phase with condylar volume loss, (4) early repair with smoothing of defect, (5) incomplete repair with flattening of articular surfaces (congruence), (6) recortication & complete repair.* **(Right)** *Coronal graphics show same progression of PCR.*

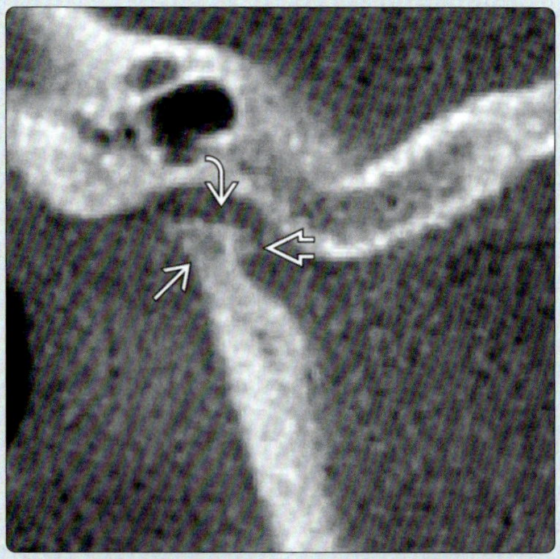

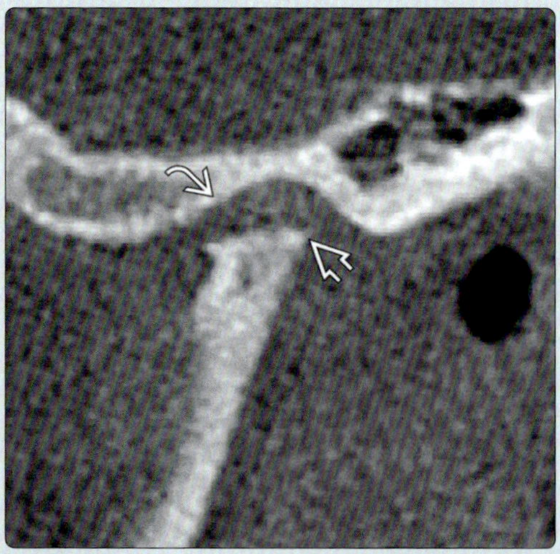

(Left) *Sagittal CBCT of the right TMJ shows a stable stage of PCR. Note the severe loss of condylar volume, a flat and corticated superior condylar surface, and a small osteophyte.* **(Right)** *Sagittal CBCT of the left TMJ in the same patient shows a small condyle. The posterior slope of the articular eminence is flat and forms a shallow incline. The posterior condylar height of contour is near the superior surface of the condyle.*

TERMINOLOGY

Synonyms

- Juvenile degenerative joint disease, condylysis, idiopathic condylar resorption, osteoarthritis, degenerative joint disease, arthrosis deformans

Definitions

- Localized noninflammatory degenerative disorder of TMJ that is characterized by lysis and repair of articular fibrocartilage and underlying subchondral bone following onset of puberty in females

IMAGING

General Features

- Best diagnostic clue
  - Unilateral (but often bilateral) resorption of superior portions of condyles
- Location
  - Anterosuperior surfaces of condyles and occasionally opposing articular eminentia
- Size
  - Initiates as focal defect with loss of articular soft tissue and subjacent bone
  - Lesion often enlarges, resulting in significant loss of condylar volume
- Morphology
  - Progressive vertical loss of condylar height and ramus height

Imaging Recommendations

- Best imaging tool
  - CBCT or CT to determine size, shape, and quality changes in osseous anatomy
  - MR for evaluation of disc position and bone marrow
- Protocol advice
  - Axially corrected views to section perpendicular and parallel to mediolateral long axis of condyles

DIFFERENTIAL DIAGNOSIS

Juvenile Idiopathic Arthritis

- Bilateral symmetrical destruction; may have cervical spine involvement

Degenerative Joint Disease

- Onset following skeletal maturity and normal serum levels of relaxin and β-estradiol

PATHOLOGY

General Features

- Etiology
  - Chemical transduction
    - Elevated or reduced serum levels of β-estradiol
    - Elevated serum levels of relaxin
  - Mechanotransduction
    - Functional loading of articular tissues beyond their adaptive capacity
    - Disc displacement alters loading, lubrication, and nutritional characteristics

Gross Pathologic & Surgical Features

- Soft tissues
  - Proteoglycan depletion
  - Collagen fiber network disintegration

CLINICAL ISSUES

Presentation

- Most common signs/symptoms
  - TMJ and myofascial pain
  - Joint sounds: Clicking and crepitation
  - Limited opening
- Other signs/symptoms
  - Change in occlusion
  - Skeletal asymmetry
  - Limited jaw development on ipsilateral side

Demographics

- Age
  - Closely follows onset of puberty and rare after age 20
- Gender
  - F:M = 9:1

Natural History & Prognosis

- Soft tissue changes precede osseous changes
  - Possible hypermobility/joint laxity
  - Nonreducing **anteriorly displaced disc**
  - Reduction in condylar mobility
- Destructive/active phase
  - **Cavitation defect** into subchondral bone
  - Reduction in condylar height
  - Active phase may be associated with limited condylar motion and pain
- Reparative/stable phase
  - Condylar flattening and recortication
  - Restoration of condylar motion and reduction in pain
- Limitation of growth on ipsilateral side
  - Limited vertical growth of condylar process, ascending ramus, and body of mandible
  - Compensations in maxilla and cranial base

Treatment

- Conservative
  - Reduce joint loads during active phase
  - Manage joint inflammation with NSAIDs
  - Manage muscle hyperactivity and parafunction

DIAGNOSTIC CHECKLIST

Consider

- CBCT scan for assessment of condylar size, shape, and quality
- MR useful for disc position evaluation

Image Interpretation Pearls

- Rapid loss of condylar volume

SELECTED REFERENCES

1. Hatcher DC: Progressive condylar resorption: pathologic processes and imaging considerations. Seminars in Orthodontics. 19(2): 96-105, 2013

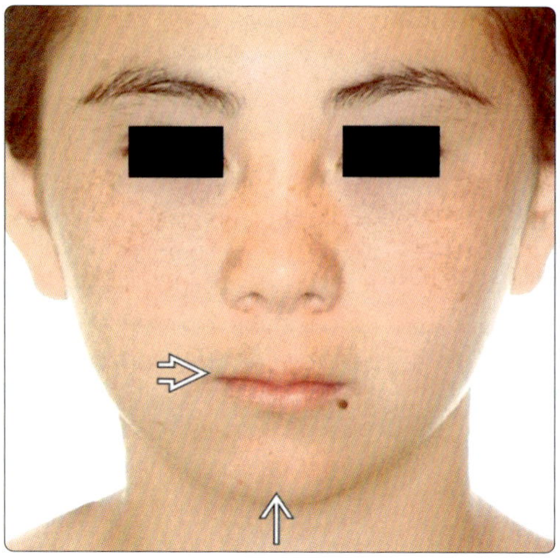

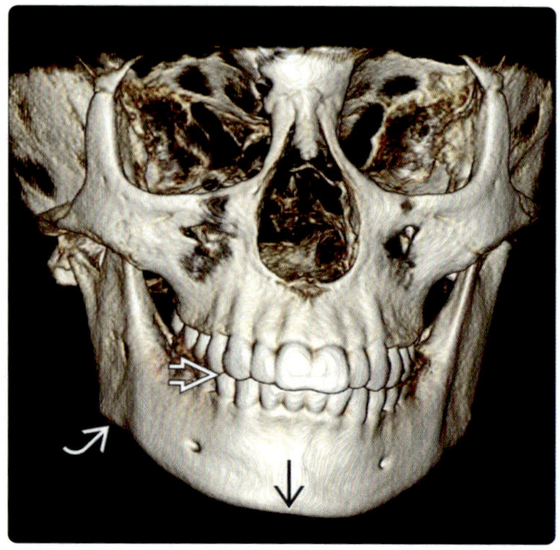

(Left) *Frontal facial photograph of a 13-year-old girl shows facial asymmetry associated with PCR of her right condyle. The soft tissue midline of the chin is displaced to the left. The right side lip commissure is elevated.* **(Right)** *Frontal CBCT of the same patient shows facial asymmetry. The osseous midline of the mandible is shifted to the right, and the right side occlusal plane is elevated. The right side mandibular angle is also elevated.*

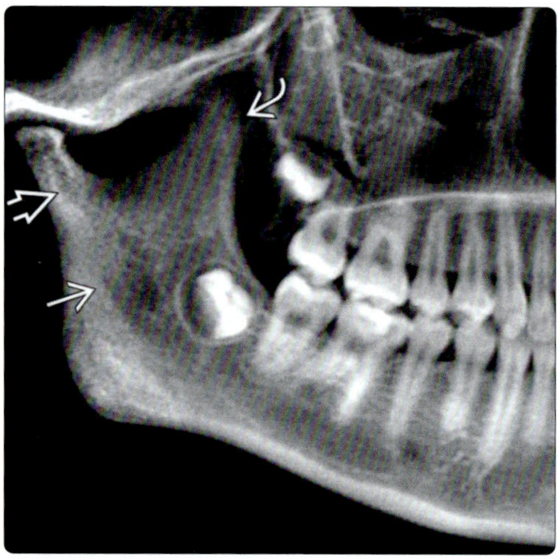

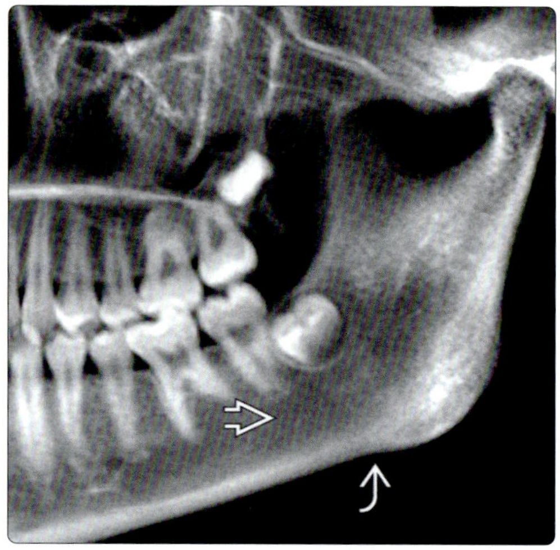

(Left) *Panoramic reformatted CBCT of the right side of the same patient shows reduced development. The right ramus is short compared to the contralateral side. The right coronoid process is elongated, and the right condylar process is short.* **(Right)** *Panoramic reformatted CBCT of the same patient shows normal development of the left side. The vertical height of the left body of the mandible is greater than the right, and the antegonial notch is shallow.*

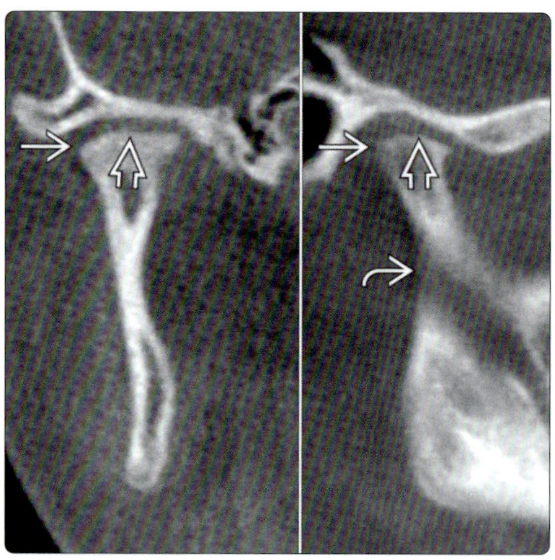

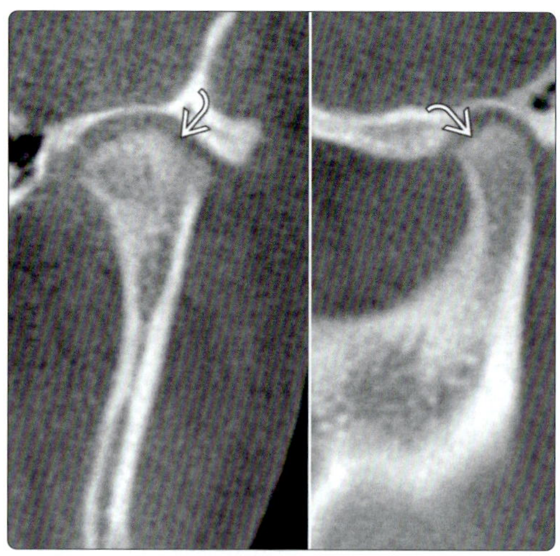

(Left) *Coronal oblique and parasagittal CBCT reconstructions of the right TMJ in the same patient show the TMJ at stable stage of PCR. The superior surface of the condyle is flat and corticated. Note the deep concavity in the posterior border of ramus and condylar heights of contour near the superior surface.* **(Right)** *CBCT of the left TMJ in the same patient shows normal development, but there is a small cortical defect along the superior surface of the condyle indicating early active PCR.*

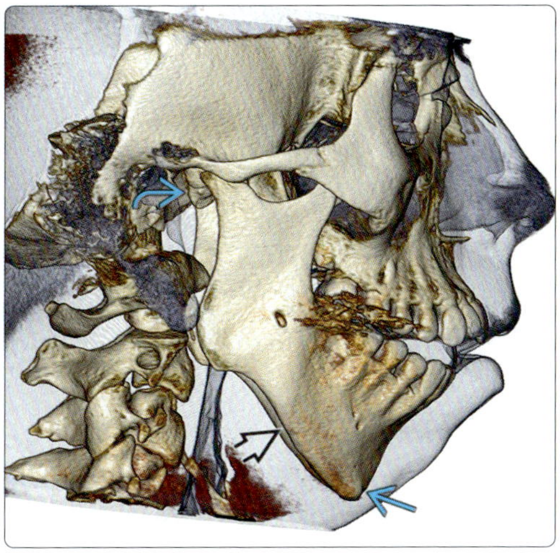

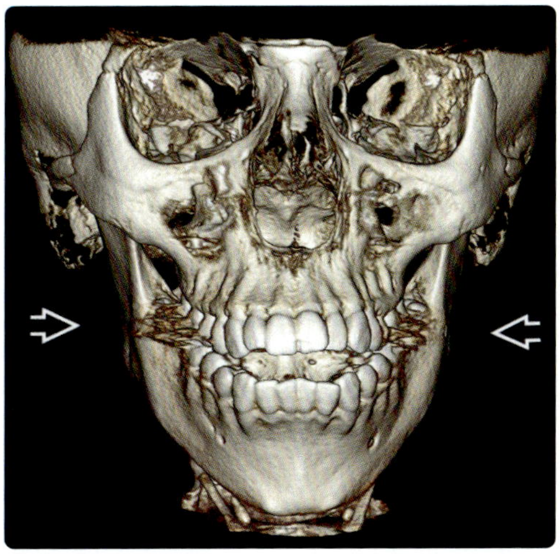

(Left) *Volume-rendered CBCT in a 16-year-old girl with advanced PCR is shown. The mandibular plane is steep, the gonial angles are obtuse, & there is posterior inclination of the condylar processes. There is a posteroinferior displacement of the chin. The vertical dimension of the anterior region of mandible is increased.* **(Right)** *Frontal view of same patient shows anterior open bite. The mediolateral dimensions of the maxilla and mandible alveolar processes are small. The lateral development of the mandible is reduced.*

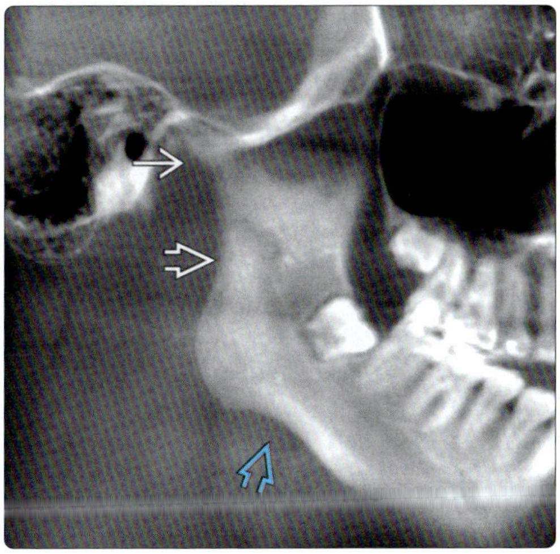

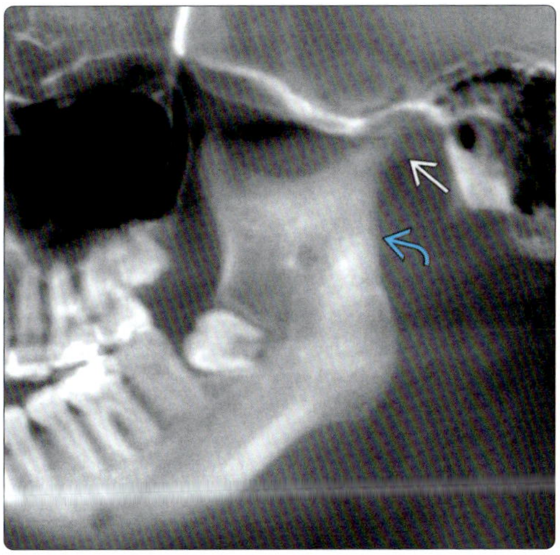

(Left) *CBCT panoramic reconstruction of the same patient shows a vertically short condylar process and ascending ramus. Prominent antegonial notch is also shown.* **(Right)** *Panoramic reconstruction of the left 1/2 of the mandible in the same patient shows posterior inclination of the left condylar process. The posterior border of the ascending ramus has an increase in the depth of the normally concave surface.*

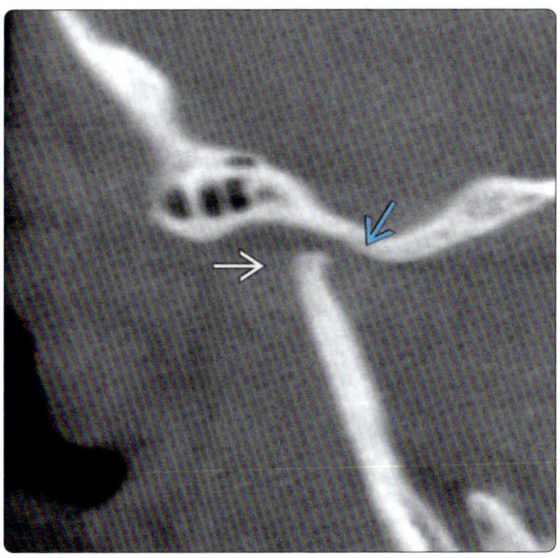

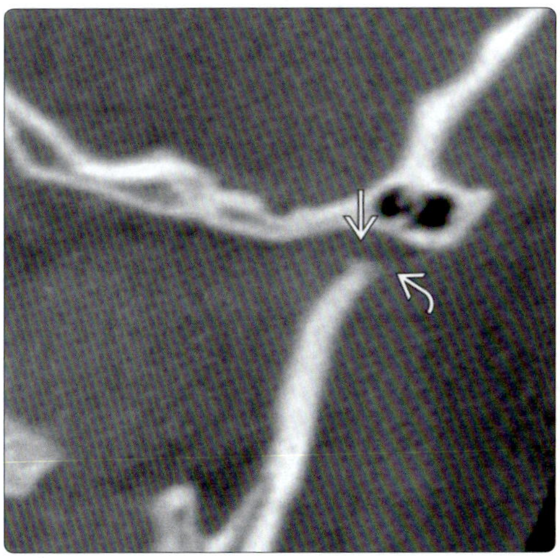

(Left) *Sagittal oblique CBCT section of the right TMJ in the same patient is shown. The condylar process is very small. The posterior slope of the articular eminence is flat and forms a shallow incline.* **(Right)** *Sagittal oblique section of the left TMJ in the same patient is shown. The posterior height of contour is near superior surface of the condyle, indicating an acquired shortening of the condyle through an erosive process. Small articular area may be associated with increased functional stress concentrations.*

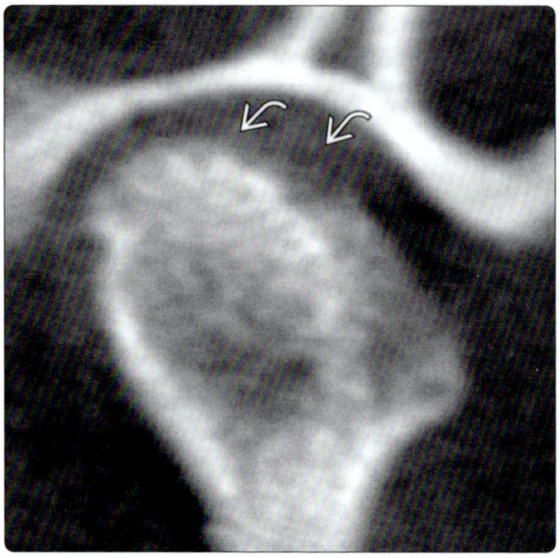
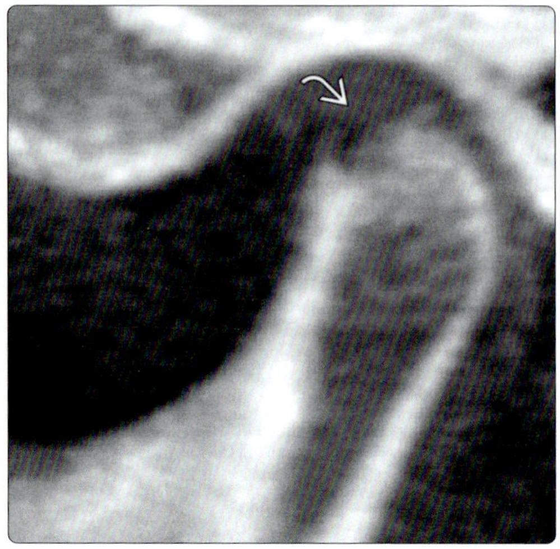

(Left) *Coronal oblique CBCT shows the left TMJ of a 12-year-old girl. This image demonstrates an early but active destructive phase of PCR. There is a superior surface defect characterized by a loss of cortex and minor loss of subchondral bone.* **(Right)** *Sagittal oblique CBCT in the same patient shows the left TMJ. The anterosuperior surface of the left condyle shows loss of cortex and some subchondral bone. Note that the bone loss corresponds to the functional loading regions.*

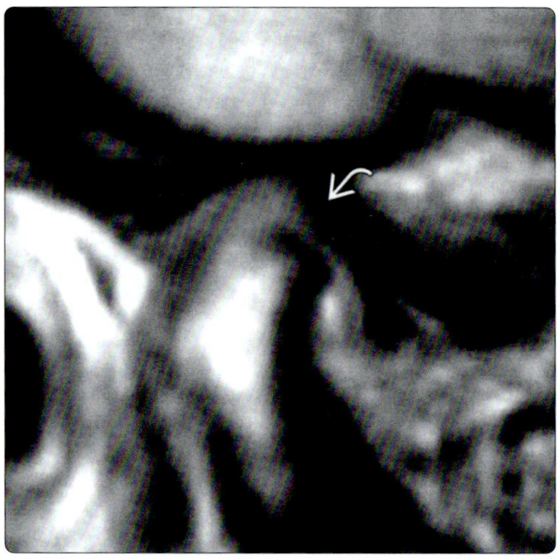
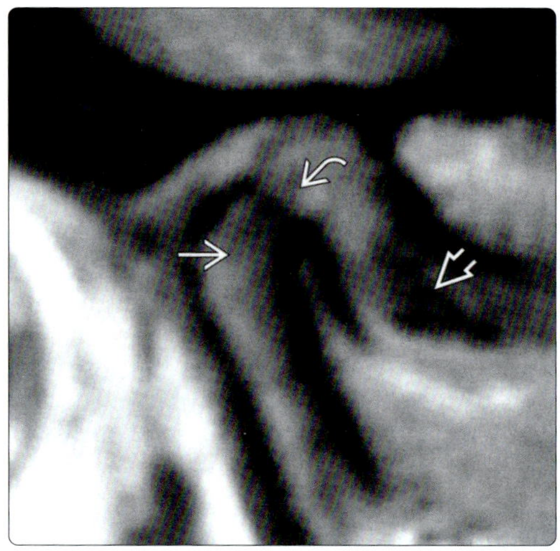

(Left) *Sagittal oblique T1WI MR of the right TMJ of a 15-year-old girl shows normal condylar size and shape. The disc is partially displaced in an anterior direction. Function is on the posterior band of the disc.* **(Right)** *Sagittal oblique T1WI MR in the same patient 11 months later shows right TMJ. There is a nonreducing, anteriorly displaced disc associated with early active PCR. Note the loss of low-signal rim and minor loss of condylar volume. Bone marrow has intermediate signal suggestive of edema.*

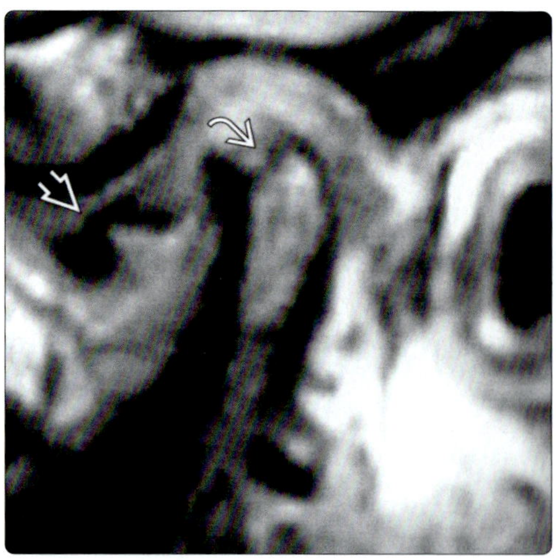
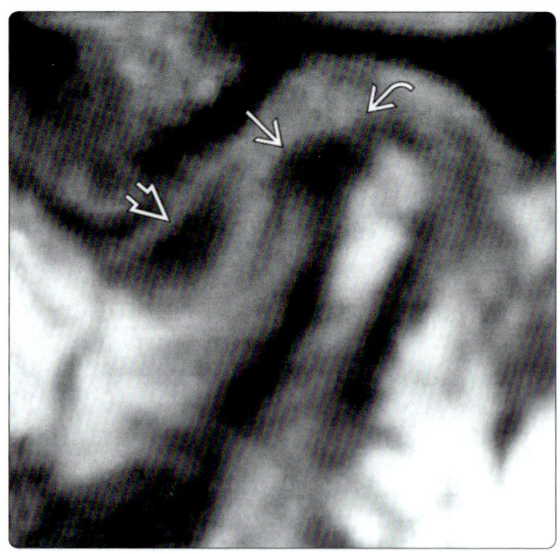

(Left) *Sagittal oblique T1WI MR in the same patient shows left TMJ at initial presentation. Note nonreducing, anteriorly displaced disc and cavitation defect on superior surface of condyle.* **(Right)** *Sagittal oblique T1WI MR in the same patient 11 months later shows left TMJ. The condyle has lost volume. The superior surface of the condyle has reformed a low-signal rim. Note low-signal beak extending from anterior surface of condyle. Disc morphology has changed since initial presentation.*

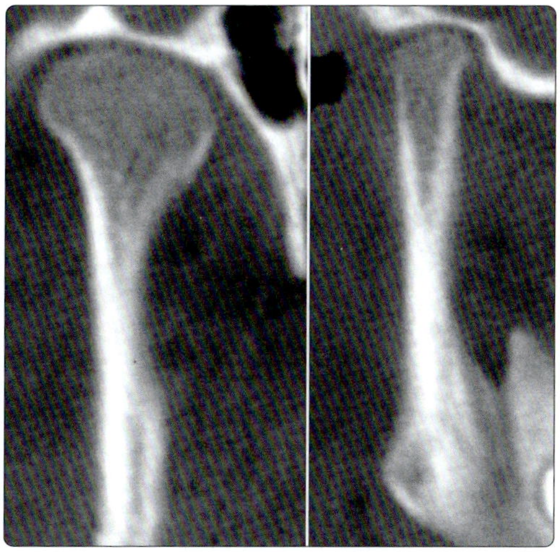

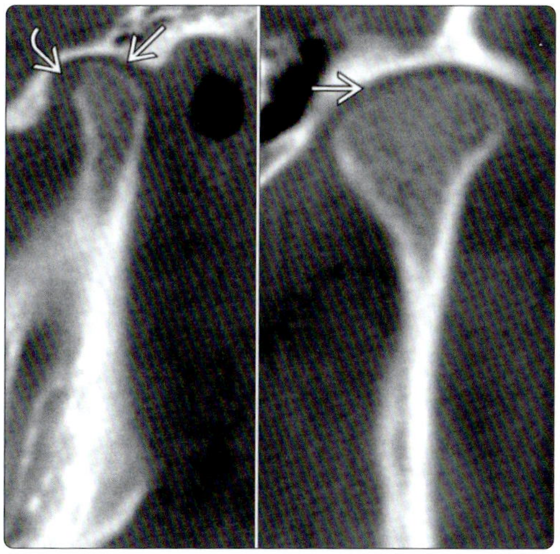

(Left) *Coronal oblique and sagittal oblique CBCT images show the right TMJ of a 12-year-old girl. The condyle has a normal size, shape, and quality. Narrowed joint space suggests soft tissue thinning &/or displaced disc.* **(Right)** *Coronal oblique and sagittal oblique CBCT images of the same patient show the left TMJ. There is a small cortical defect (erosion) with very minor loss of bone volume localized to the functional loading zone. This represents early active PCR. Note the thin superior joint space.*

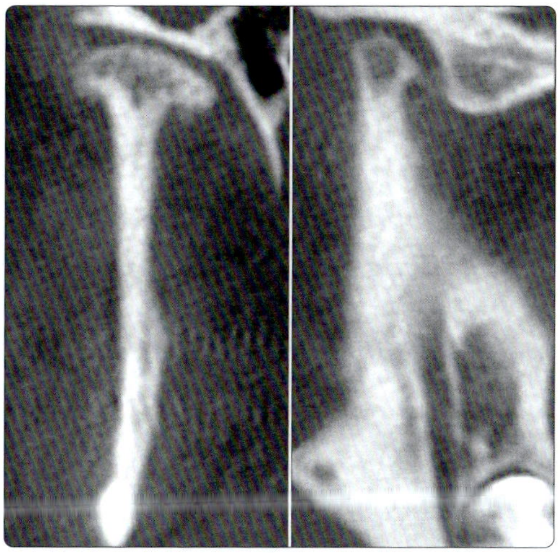

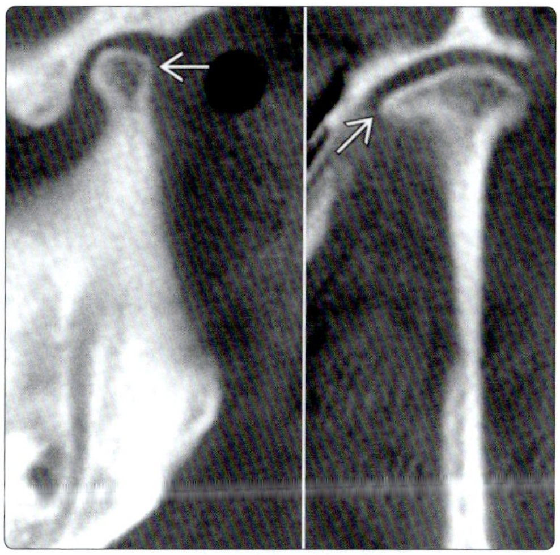

(Left) *Coronal oblique and sagittal oblique CBCT images of the same patient at age 15 show a stable stage of PCR in the right TMJ. Note the loss of condylar volume since initial scan. Superior surface of the condyle and posterior slope of articular eminence are flat and corticated.* **(Right)** *Coronal oblique and sagittal oblique CBCT images of the same patient at age 15 show a stable stage of PCR in the left TMJ. Note the heights of contour (poles) near the superior surface of the condyle and a short condylar process.*

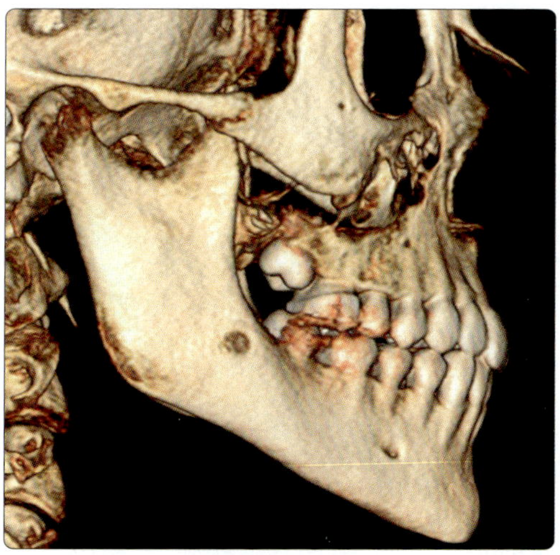

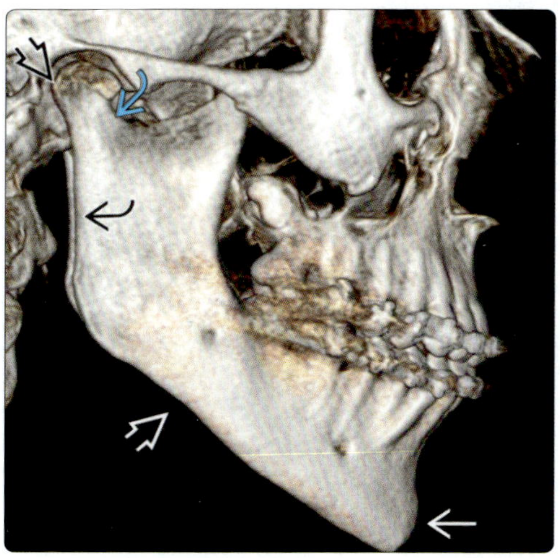

(Left) *Lateral CBCT 3D reformation shows the same patient at age 12. Note the normal size proportions between condylar process, ramus, and body of mandible as well as a normal anterior projection of the chin.* **(Right)** *Lateral CBCT 3D reformation shows the same patient at age 15. Note the short condylar process, concave posterior border of ramus, steep mandibular plane, recessive chin, and height of contour near the superior surface of the condyle.*

Disc Displacement With Reduction

KEY FACTS

TERMINOLOGY

- Definition: Disc displaced or misaligned with condyle in mandibular closed position improving to normal position with mouth opening

IMAGING

- Posterior band of disc located anterior to most superior aspect of condyle in closed mouth on oblique sagittal images
- Disc can displace in following directions
  - Anterior: Partial or complete
  - Anterior rotational: Medial and lateral
  - Sideways: Medial and lateral
  - Posterior: More likely subluxation of condyle
- CBCT: Disc is not seen
  - Thin superior joint space increases probability of displaced disc or thinning of soft tissues
- MR: Open- and closed-mouth T1-weighted images acquired **perpendicular** to mediolateral long axis of condyles
  - Closed-mouth T1-weighted images acquired **parallel** to mediolateral long axis of condyles

TOP DIFFERENTIAL DIAGNOSES

- Disc displacement without reduction
- Condylar subluxation
- Deviations of form and shape of articulating surfaces
- Loose bodies (e.g., synovial chondromatosis)
- Fibrous bands and adhesions in joint space
- Eminence click

CLINICAL ISSUES

- Clicking: Sharp, quick sound with jaw motion
  - Opening click
  - Closing click
- Female > > male
- Pain localized to TMJ region
- Muscle tenderness around TMJ
- May have increased range of anterior condylar translation

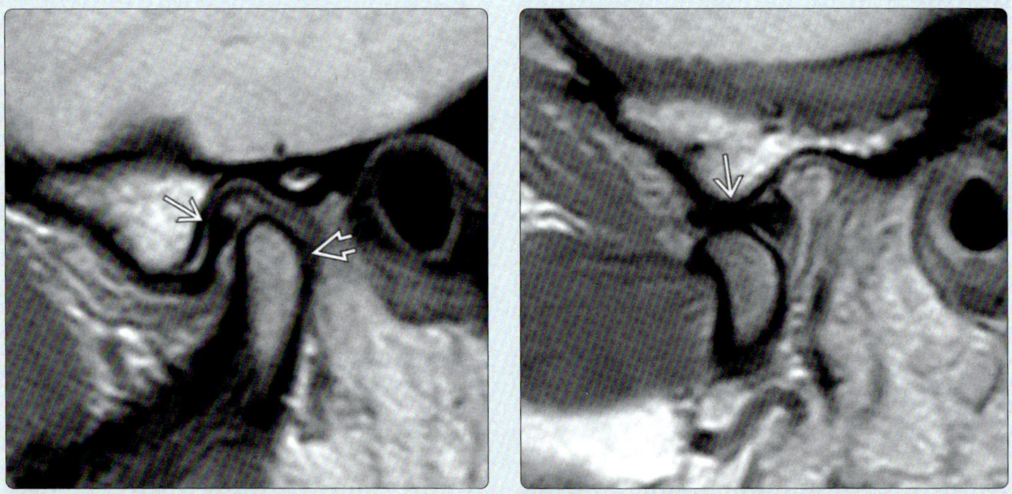

(Left) *Sagittal oblique PD MR shows anterior disc displacement with reduction. The most posterior aspect of the posterior band is in the 10 o'clock position ➡. The condyle is in a slightly posterior position to the center of the fossa ➡.* **(Right)** *Sagittal oblique PD MR in the open position in same patient shows that the intermediate zone of disc ➡ is interposed between the condyle and eminence indicating reduction of the disc upon opening. There is normal condylar translation.*

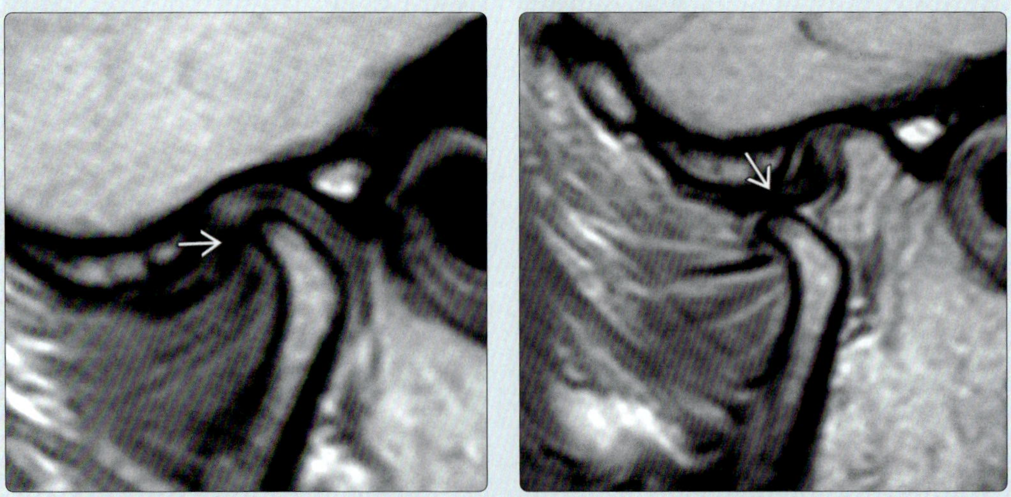

(Left) *Sagittal oblique PD MR shows the posterior band is in the 9-o'clock position on the condyle ➡. The disc has a biplanar shape and is anteriorly displaced.* **(Right)** *Open PD MR in same patient shows the intermediate zone of disc ➡ is interposed between the condyle and eminence. No disc translation is noted when compared to the closed view, suggestive of adhesion. Mild subnormal condylar translation is noted. Reduction of the disc occurs, but the disc is adhered (stuck) to the fossa.*

TERMINOLOGY

Abbreviations

- Disc displacement with reduction (DDwR)

Synonyms

- Reducing displaced disc, clicking jaw, disc displacement with recapture, reciprocal clicking

Definitions

- Disc displaced or misaligned with condyle in mandibular closed position reverting to normal position with mouth opening

IMAGING

General Features

- Best diagnostic clue
  - Posterior band of disc located anterior to most superior aspect of condyle in closed-mouth position on oblique sagittal MR
- Location
  - Disc can displace in following directions
    - Anterior: Partial or complete
    - Anterior-rotational: Medial or lateral
    - Sideways: Medial or lateral
    - Posterior: More likely subluxation of condyle
- Morphology
  - Disc usually with normal biconcave shape but may have deformed morphology
    - Displaced disc may have shortened anteroposterior dimensions
    - Posterior band may vertically thicken or thin
  - Disc displacement can be complete or partial
    - Partial: Displaced disc only partially recaptures on opening
      - Part of disc remains in displaced position and another part assumes normal condylar-disc position
      - Can occur in all forms of displacement
      - More common with medial and lateral displacement

CT Findings

- CBCT
  - Disc is not seen on CBCT
  - Thin superior or posterior joint spaces increase probability of displaced disc or thinning of soft tissues

Imaging Recommendations

- Best imaging tool
  - MR
    - Normal disc has low T1, T2 signal
    - Biconcave AP-sectional shape
      - Posterior band thickest and intermediate zone thinnest dimension
    - Disc degeneration: May see intermediate T1 signal
- Protocol advice
  - Bilateral surface coils
  - Open and closed PD or T1-weighted images acquired **perpendicular** to mediolateral long axis of condyles
  - PD or T1-weighted images acquired **parallel** to mediolateral long axis of condyles; closed position
  - Closed
    - Maximum tooth intercuspation
  - Open
    - Patient instructed to open jaw beyond opening click
    - Bite block (e.g., syringe wrapped with gauze) to stabilize jaw in open position

DIFFERENTIAL DIAGNOSIS

Disc Displacement Without Reduction

- 15% of joint clicking is disc displacement without reduction (DDwoR)
- Disc does not reduce to normal position in open-mouth position but is associated with clicking sound

Fibrous Bands and Adhesions (Stuck Disc)

- Disc adhered to eminence and does not translate relative to posterior slope of articular eminence
- Condyle translates along inferior surface of disc and can translate anterior to anterior band
- Irregular surfaces due to degenerative joint disease (DJD) provide frictional restrictions that can cause clicking sounds

Deviations of Form and Shape of Articulating Surfaces

- Irregular surfaces provide frictional restrictions that can cause clicking
- Sometimes indistinguishable from early stage disc displacement

Condylar Subluxation

- Condyle translates far anterior and superior to eminence and, rarely, to anterior band of disc
- Can be considered form of posterior displacement of disc
  - Condyle articulates against anterior capsule wall anterior to anterior band of disc
- Has been associated with clicking and catching or locking of jaw on opening (open lock)

Loose Bodies (e.g., Synovial Chondromatosis)

- Can produce joint sounds similar to clicks

Eminence Click

- Jolting or clunking sound that **occurs in same location on opening and closing paths**
- Skeletal incoordination between bony condyle, disc, and articular eminence
- History of jaw dislocation and subluxation
- Normal disc function and position
- No TMJ pain
- Deviations of jaw from midline are greater with eminence clicks than disc clicks

PATHOLOGY

General Features

- Etiology
  - Biomechanical
    - Trauma; direct and indirect
    - Parafunction
  - Biochemical
    - Estrogen and relaxin induction of matrix metalloproteinase and cytokines

Staging, Grading, & Classification

- Progression of disc displacement is associated with proteoglycan depletion from disc and stretching of disc attachments
- Rough correlation between condyle distance of opening click from fossa and distance of closing reciprocal click from fossa
  - Has important implications if anterior repositioning appliances are considered for treatment
- Early-opening recapture
  - Repositioning of disc related to condyle when condyle has moved along posterior 1/2 of slope to articular eminence
- Midopening recapture
  - Disc assumes normal relationship to condyle when condyle is at position between midpoint of slope and crest of articular eminence
- Late-opening recapture
  - Disc assumes normal relationship with condyle at or beyond apex of articular eminence

CLINICAL ISSUES

Presentation

- Most common signs/symptoms
  - Joint sounds/clicking
    - Usually reciprocal
    - Clicking: Sharp, quick sound with jaw motion
      - Opening click: Click timing can occur early, intermediate, or late in opening cycle
      - Closing click: Occurs just prior to tooth contact; not as loud as opening click and may not be detectable
    - Deflection in condylar path is associated with both opening and closing clicks
    - Sound thought to represent impact between condyle and temporal bone with soft tissues interposed
    - Some joints with DDwR do not click
    - Change in velocity of condylar movement associated with open and close clicks (6-36 milliseconds)
  - Pain localized to TMJ region
  - Muscle tenderness around TMJ
  - May have hypermobile condyle
- Other signs/symptoms
  - Prior to click, condyle slows its translation speed and distracts from eminence
    - Jaw deviates to involved side
  - At click, condyle accelerates its motion in anterosuperior direction
    - Jaw deviation corrects or overcorrects at time of click

Demographics

- Gender
  - Female > > male
- Epidemiology
  - Clicking sounds recognized in 14-44% of general population

Natural History & Prognosis

- 7% of patient population with benign clicking progress to symptomatic level
- Incidence of progression of reducing disc displacement to nonreducing disc displacement and DJD is unknown
- Up to 1/3 of asymptomatic patients may have displaced disc on MR
- 70% of symptomatic subjects have displaced disc (always correlate clinically)

Treatment

- Palliative treatment

Sonography

- Joint sound analysis currently being used to study diverse sounds emitted from TMJ in patients with facial pain and masticatory dysfunction
- Sound-power spectrum analysis can be used as screening modality to differentiate patients with TMJ internal derangement, separation of displacement vs. nondisplacement, and detection of degenerative arthritis with crepitus
- Determination of diagnostic specificity has not been established

DIAGNOSTIC CHECKLIST

Consider

- Confirm that posterior band of disc is displaced

Image Interpretation Pearls

- Actual configuration of disc probably more correctly assessed by examining its shape in open-mouth position
  - Disc reduces to normal anatomic relationship to condyle and eminence
- In open mouth, disc form can best be evaluated after reduction

Pitfalls

- MR appearance can be falsely normal if patient is not scanned in maximum intercuspation
- Volume averaging between top of condyle, disc, and glenoid fossa sometimes makes it difficult to evaluate posterior band of disc in closed position
- There may be maximal deformation of disc shape and configuration just before reduction of opening click
  - Can create overstaging of chronicity of internal derangement
- If patient is imaged in submaximal opening, DDwR can be mistaken for DDwoR

SELECTED REFERENCES

1. Bryndahl F et al: Cartilage changes link retrognathic mandibular growth to TMJ disc displacement in a rabbit model. Int J Oral Maxillofac Surg. 40(6):621-7, 2011
2. Balke Z et al: Prevalence of temporomandibular disorders: Samples taken from attendees of medical health-care centers in the Islamic Republic of Iran. J Orofac Pain. 24(4):361-6, 2010
3. Kalaykova S et al: Two-year natural course of anterior disc displacement with reduction. J Orofac Pain. 24(4):373-8, 2010
4. Zeng RZ et al: [Technical study of temporomandibular joint disc showing with 3T magnetic resonance imaging.] Hua Xi Kou Qiang Yi Xue Za Zhi. 28(6):619-22, 2010
5. Katzberg RW: Temporomandibular joint imaging. Radiology. 170(2):297-307, 1989
6. Miller TL et al: Temporomandibular joint clicking with nonreducing anterior displacement of the meniscus. Radiology. 154(1):121-4, 1985
7. Katzberg RW et al: Dislocation of jaws. Skeletal Radiol. 11(1):38-41, 1984

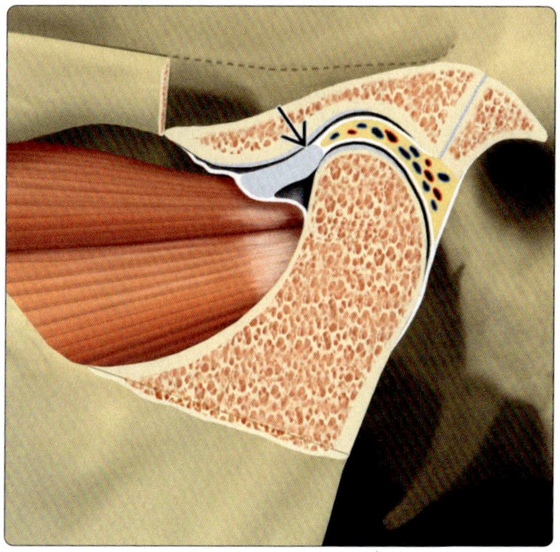

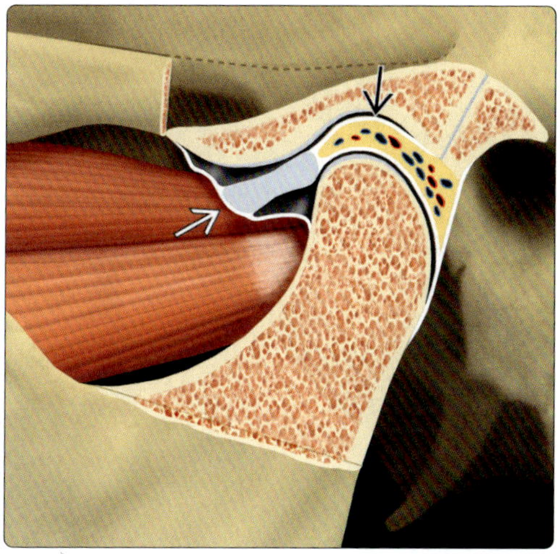

(Left) *Series of 8 graphics of the TMJ shows the position of the TMJ components with a pure anterior disc displacement with reduction during the opening and closing cycle. The condyle is seated in the fossa with a slightly more posterior and superior position due to the dislocation of the thick posterior band from its normal 12 o'clock position in relation to the condyle.* **(Right)** *The condyle starts to rotate, creating slightly more space in the superior aspect of the joint space, and the disc starts to become compressed anteriorly.*

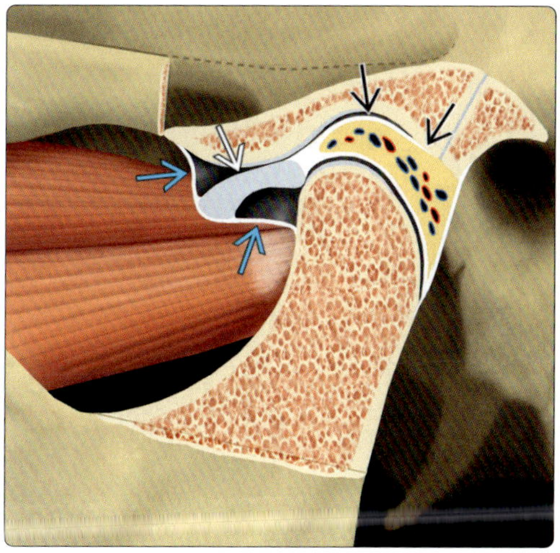

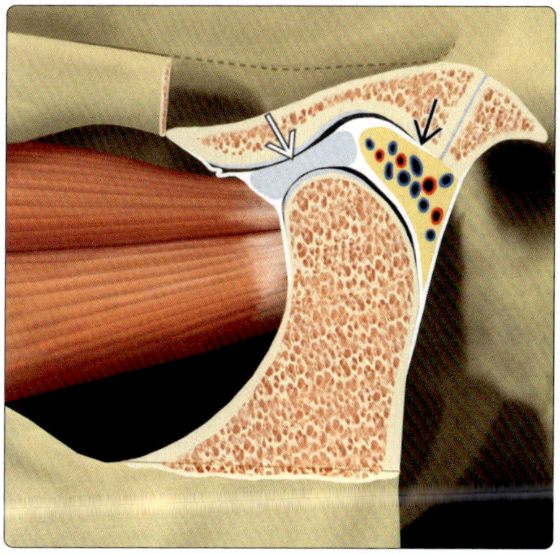

(Left) *Translation of the condyle starts and widening of the posterior and superior aspects of the joint space is seen. The disc is further compressed anteriorly and shows a deformation (folding) of its shape and stretching of the anterior capsule wall.* **(Right)** *The disc is recaptured by the condyle passing over the posterior band and engaging in the intermediate zone of the disc, resulting in a click. The retrodiscal tissues show dilation of the blood vessels that normally occurs with translation of the condyle.*

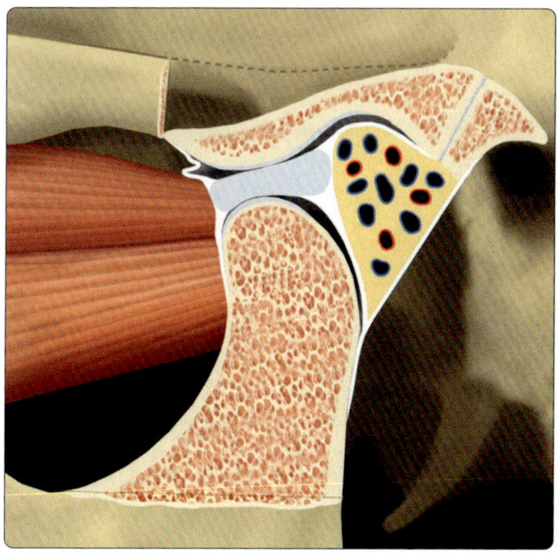

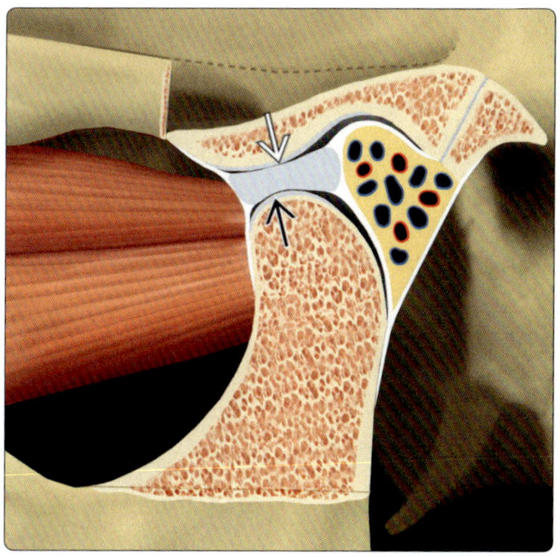

(Left) *The condyle continues translating forward to normal range of motion with the disc engaged.* **(Right)** *During the initial phases of closing, the disc and condyle maintain the reduced position, and the disc is relatively normal in shape (biconcave).*

(Left) *The condyle has not seated completely in the fossa, and the disc is still in the reduced position* ⇨. **(Right)** *At the terminal part of closing right before teeth contact, the condyle seats in the fossa and the disc becomes displaced again, resulting in the softer closing click. The posterior attachment is stretched and positioned at the 11 and 12 o'clock positions* ⇨ *of the condyle.*

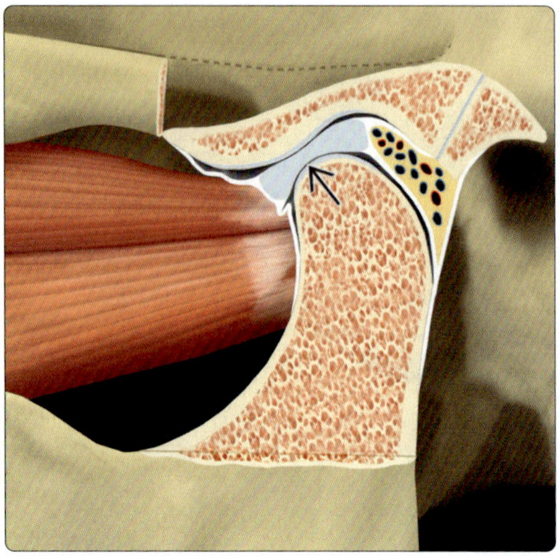

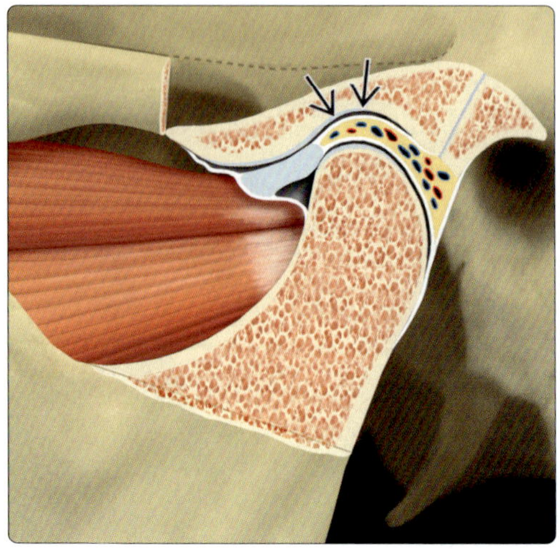

(Left) *Closed sagittal oblique PD MR shows a displaced disc in the anterior direction. The posterior band of the disc* ⇨ *is at the 10 o'clock position of the adjacent condyle. A more medial image showed a normal disc position; thus, this is a partially displaced disc.* **(Right)** *Sagittal oblique PD MR in the open position shows the intermediate zone* ➡ *between the condyle and the crest of the eminence. The diagnosis for this case is partial anterior displacement with reduction.*

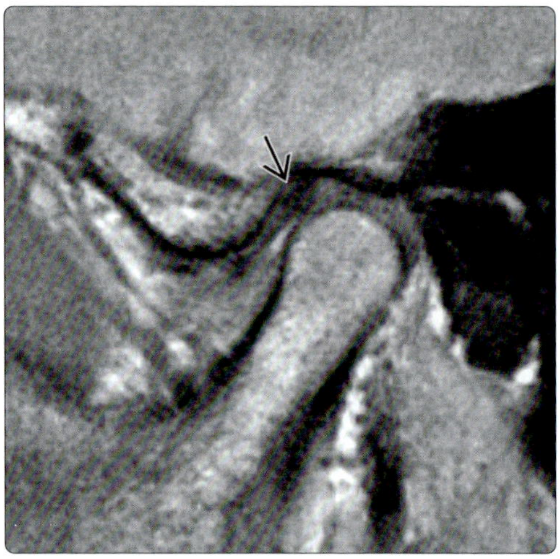

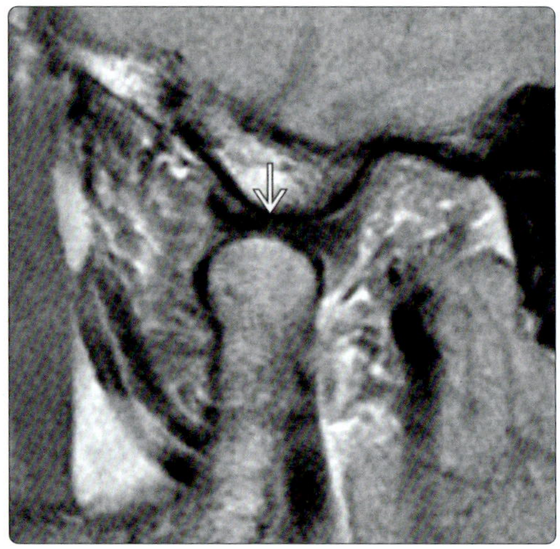

(Left) *Open oblique sagittal view from the central region of a TMJ shows a recaptured disc in this zone* ➡*. In the closed position (not shown), the disc was anteriorly displaced.* **(Right)** *Open oblique sagittal view in the same patient, medial to prior image, shows a partial recapture of disc. The posterior band* ➡ *of disc is interposed between the condyle and eminence. The diagnosis is anterior displacement with partial reduction.*

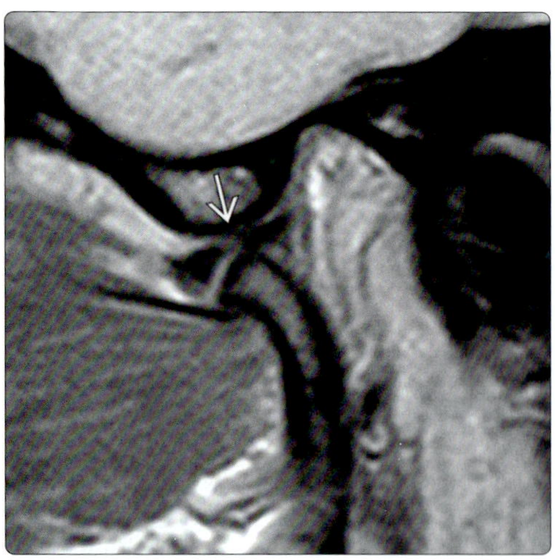

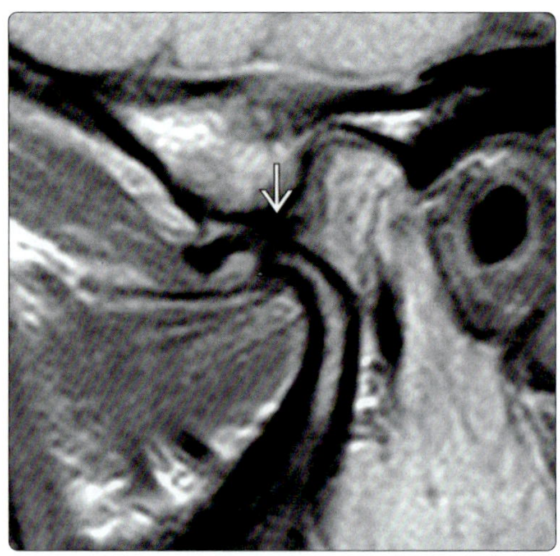

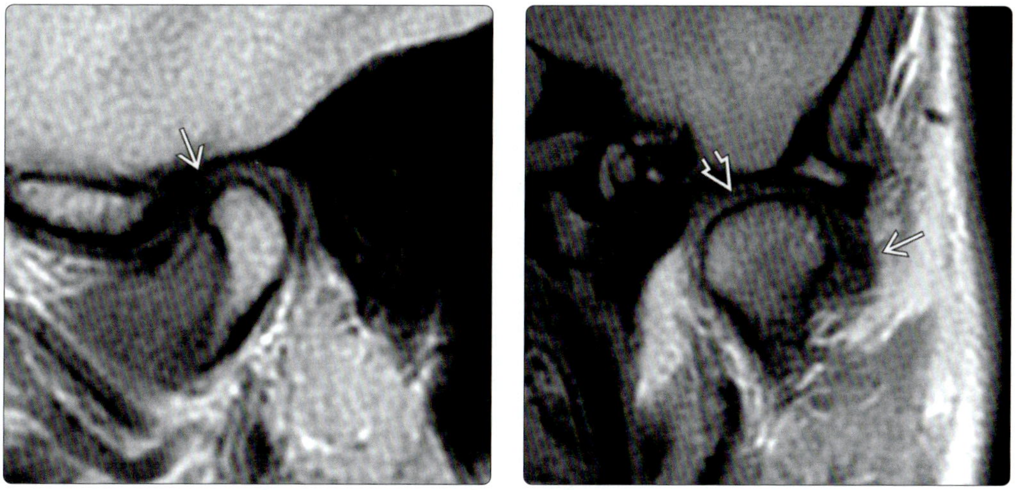

(Left) *Closed oblique sagittal MR from lateral region of a TMJ shows the posterior band is partially displaced opposite the 10 o'clock position of the condyle.* **(Right)** *Closed oblique coronal view in same patient shows a laterally directed sideways displacement of the disc. The disc is outside the plane of section in the medial region of the TMJ with elongation of the medial collateral attachment.*

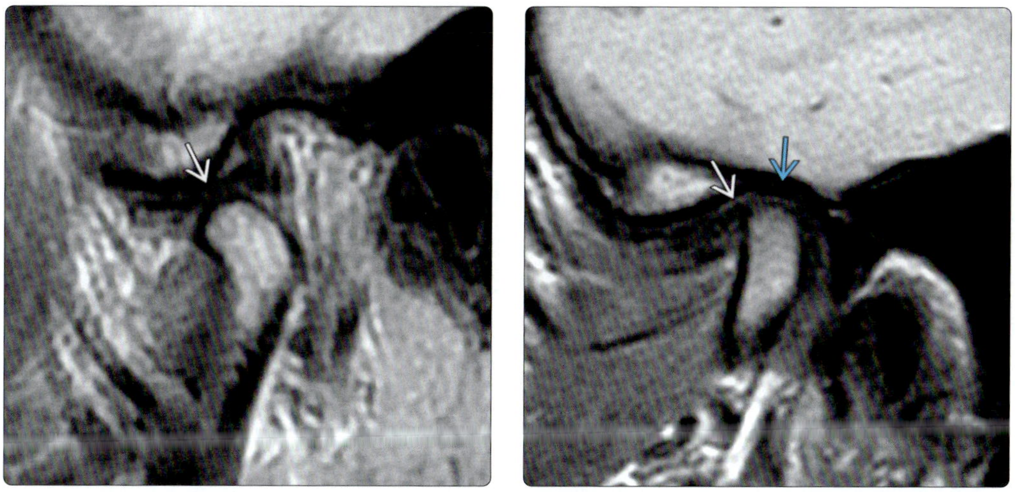

(Left) *Open oblique sagittal PD MR in the same patient shows the disc reducing so that the intermediate zone is interposed between the condyle and eminence. There is mildly subnormal condylar translation. The diagnosis is sideways lateral displacement with reduction.* **(Right)** *Closed sagittal oblique PD MR from medial region of a TMJ shows the posterior band of disc is flattened and positioned at the 10 to 11 o'clock position on the adjacent condyle. The thickened temporal posterior attachment is seen at the 12 o'clock position.*

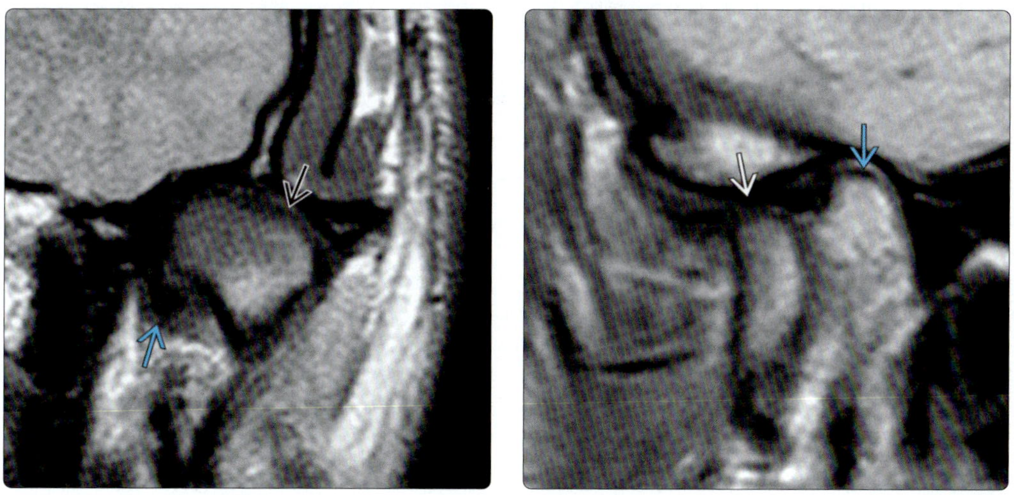

(Left) *Closed coronal oblique view in the same patient shows a sideways disc displacement in a medial direction. No disc is visualized in the lateral region of TMJ. There is elongation of the lateral collateral attachment.* **(Right)** *Open PD MR from the lateral region of the TMJ in same patient shows the intermediate zone of the disc is interposed between the condyle and eminence. The diagnosis is sideways medial displacement with reduction. Note the prominent temporal posterior attachment.*

Disc Displacement Without Reduction

KEY FACTS

TERMINOLOGY

- Disc displacement without reduction (DDwoR): Misaligned disc-condyle structural relationship that is maintained during all mandibular movement

IMAGING

- MR is best imaging tool
  - Normal disc has low T1, T2 signal
  - Disc degeneration produces intermediate T1 signal
- Open- and closed-mouth PD or T1-weighted images acquired **perpendicular** to mediolateral long axis of condyle
  - Open-mouth MR: Support occlusion at slightly submaximal opening with bite block
- Closed-mouth PD or T1-weighted images acquired **parallel** to mediolateral long axis of condyle
- Posterior band of disc not aligned with superior most point of condyle in closed and open positions
- Disc deforms after displacement
  - Biconcave: Shortstanding displacement
  - Biconvex and shortened AP dimensions: Longstanding anterior displacement

TOP DIFFERENTIAL DIAGNOSES

- Disc derangement with reduction
- Adhesions

CLINICAL ISSUES

- Female > male
- Acute displacement
  - History of click that suddenly stopped
  - Limited opening and jaw pain
  - Short window of time to potentially reduce displaced disc
- Chronic displacement
  - Restoration of jaw motion and reduction in pain
  - Palliative management
- DDwoR is risk factor for degenerative joint disease

(Left) *Sagittal oblique T2W MR in closed position shows that the condyle is posterior and inferior to the center of the fossa. The posterior band is anterior to the condyle. The posterior band is relatively large, and the intermediate zone is small. There is a fluid signal, primarily in the anterior recess of the superior joint compartment.* **(Right)** *MR of same patient in open position shows AP shortening and bowing of the disc that remains anterior to condyle. The fluid in superior compartment has shifted posteriorly with opening.*

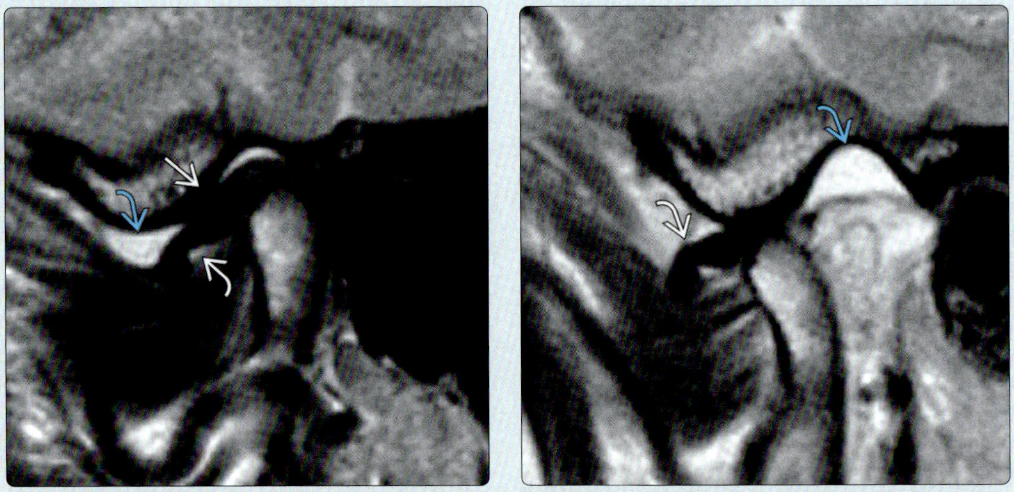

(Left) *Sagittal oblique T1W MR in closed position shows a large erosive defect and low signal intensity in superior surface of condyle. The disc has a biplanar shape and is anterior to condyle. The raphe between superior and inferior lateral pterygoid muscles appears of low signal intensity and should not be confused with the disc.* **(Right)** *Open sagittal oblique view for the same patient shows the disc remains anterior to condyle and demonstrates degeneration.*

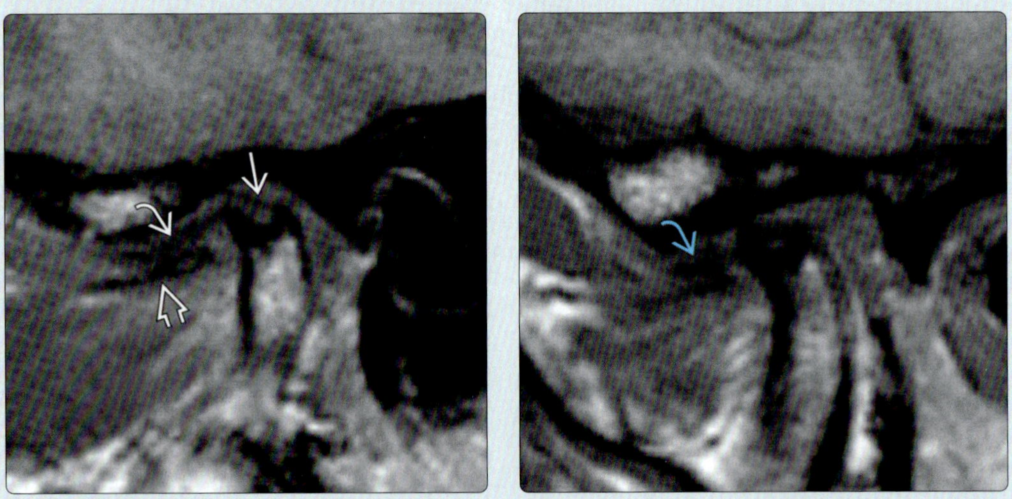

TERMINOLOGY

Abbreviations

- Disc displacement without reduction (DDwoR)

Synonyms

- Closed lock; nonreducing displaced disc (NRDD); disc displacement without recapture

Definitions

- Misaligned disc-condyle structural relationship that is maintained during all mandibular movement
  - Remains displaced despite jaw manipulation attempts by patient to normalize discal/condylar position

IMAGING

General Features

- Best diagnostic clue
  - Closed: Posterior band of disc not aligned with superior-most point of condyle
  - Open: Junction between anterior band and intermediate zone is not interposed between condyle and eminence
- Location
  - Disc can displace in following directions
    - Anterior (partial or complete), anterolateral and anteromedial rotation, or sideways (medial or lateral)
  - Anterior and anterolateral rotations are most common directions
  - Medial and lateral disc displacements may have lower tendency to reduce than pure anterior displacement
- Morphology
  - Disc deforms after displacement
    - Biconcave in acute displacement
    - Biconvex and shortened AP dimensions in longstanding anterior displacement

CT Findings

- CBCT
  - **Disc is not seen on CBCT**
  - Clues
    - Shifts in condylar position in relation to fossa may indicate disc displacement, especially posterior and mediolateral position of condyle
    - Axial view: Anterior concavity on condyle may indicate chronic disc displacement
    - Bony projections off superior aspect of condyle may indicate perforation of disc or posterior attachment
    - Appositional bone growth on surface of fossa may indicate chronic disc displacement (bone growing into space left by disc)
    - Disc displacement almost always precedes degenerative joint disease (DJD); if osseous changes are seen, disc is most likely displaced

MR Findings

- Normal disc has low signal intensity signal on T1, T2, and proton density (PD)
- Abnormal disc shape
  - In acute phase of displacement: Disc has normal thickness but may be folded (bowed) on opening
  - Normally thin intermediate zone of disc is nearly obliterated by progressive thickening of posterior band of disc, leaving only small groove on undersurface
  - This notch in this condition is useful landmark demarcating thickened posterior band from smaller anterior band
- Disc degeneration produces intermediate signal on T1
- Joint effusion produces high signal on T2 in upper, lower, or both joint compartments
  - Amount of effusion varies from subtle, thin line along articular surface to large significant collections
  - Thin, physiologic effusion can be seen in normal TMJs and may not be significant clinically
  - Large collections probably reflect inflammatory component of disease process
  - Marked joint effusion associated with painful joint
  - Effusion can provide arthrographic effect
    - Disc or posterior attachment perforation can be demonstrated by MR due to flow of joint effusion fluid from one compartment to other through perforation

Imaging Recommendations

- Best imaging tool
  - MR
- Protocol advice
  - Bilateral TMJ surface coils
  - 4 is number of excitations (NEX)
  - PD or T1- and T2-weighted images acquired **perpendicular** to mediolateral long axis of condyle **(axially corrected, sagittal oblique)**
    - Closed and open mouth
    - Support occlusion at slightly submaximal opening with bite block
  - PD or T1-weighted images acquired **parallel** to mediolateral long axis of condyle **(axially corrected, coronal oblique)**
    - Closed mouth

Pitfalls

- Retrodiscal tissues have high signal on T2 open mouth
  - Do not confuse with joint effusion
- Thickening of posterior attachment creates appearance of pseudodisc that does not appear displaced
- Thickening of fascia of inferior belly of lateral pterygoid muscle simulate disc tissue
- Appearance of flat, thin disc in superior position of condyle and in joint, representing capsular herniation with sideways displacement
  - Coronal oblique view important
  - Review entire series mediolaterally
- Stuck disc
  - Adhesions occurring in upper joint space manifested as movement of condyle underneath nonmovable disc, representing disc dysfunction with condylar translation
- MR is not sensitive to presence of perforations
  - Clues
    - If joint effusion is present, arthrographic effect of fluid moving from 1 compartment
    - Marked narrowing of joint space &/or bone-to-bone contact

DIFFERENTIAL DIAGNOSIS

Disc Derangement With Reduction

- On open-mouth view, junction between anterior band and intermediate zone is positioned between condyle and eminence

Adhesions

- Lack of anteroposterior disc motion
- Condyle translates along inferior surface of disc

PATHOLOGY

General Features

- Etiology
  - Biomechanical
    - Damage to disc attachments both posteriorly and laterally
      - Trauma, direct or indirect
      - Parafunction
  - Biochemical
    - Estrogen and relaxin induction of matrix metalloproteinase and cytokines
- Causes of pain
  - Squeezing force of condyle on well-innervated posterior disc attachments up against eminence
  - Trauma from disc impinging on inner aspect of anterior capsule
  - Inflammatory changes in disc and joint capsule secondary to disc displacement

Staging, Grading, & Classification

- RDC/TMD Validation Project scoring system classifies this as C
  - Further subclassified as
    - DDwoR **with** limited jaw opening
    - DDwoR **without** limited opening
- Often preceded by reducing displaced disc
- Progression of disc displacement is associated with proteoglycan depletion from disc, disc deformation, and stretching of disc attachments
- Considered intermediate progression of internal derangement
  - Most significant mechanical dysfunction of disc and condyle
- Perforations occur in cases of long history of chronic symptomatology
- Degenerative bony changes are almost always preceded by DDwoR

CLINICAL ISSUES

Presentation

- Most common signs/symptoms
  - Acute displacement
    - History of click that suddenly stopped
    - Limited opening ~ 25 mm interincisal
    - Multiple episodes of
      - Joint pain
      - Temporal headaches
      - Major mechanical symptoms (transient catching, locking, and sustained locks)
      - Restriction of motion
      - Difficulty of function (due to pain)
    - Jaw deviates to involved side on opening
- Other signs/symptoms
  - Chronic displacement
    - With time, jaw opening can increase and eventually become relatively normal again, even though disc is still displaced
    - Restoration of jaw motion with progressive increase in anterior translation
    - Reduction in pain to normal values
    - In closed lock
      - Deviation of jaw to affected side
      - Limited anterior condylar translation
    - Some have clicking due to multiple irregular surfaces that provide frictional restrictions such as in cases of
      - Adhesions
      - Advanced degenerative changes in condyle, disc, and fossa (crepitus also heard)
- Clinical profile
  - Clinical assessment and diagnosis (without imaging) of DDwoR with limited opening has high sensitivity and specificity
  - Clinical assessment and diagnosis (without imaging) of DDwoR without limited opening has low sensitivity and specificity

Demographics

- Gender
  - Female > male; bilateral involvement is greatest in female patients

Natural History & Prognosis

- DDwR is often precursor to DDwoR, but not always
- 7% of patient population with benign clicking progress to symptomatic level
- Clicking disappears
- Acute limitation of anterior condylar translation, resulting in restriction of mouth opening and deviation to affected side
- DDwoR is risk factor for DJD
- Incidence of progression of reducing displaced disc to nonreducing displaced disc and DJD is unknown

Treatment

- Acute displacement: Short window of time to reduce displaced disc
- Chronic displacement: Palliative management

SELECTED REFERENCES

1. Schiffman E et al: Diagnostic criteria for temporomandibular disorders (DC/TMD) for clinical and research applications: recommendations of the International RDC/TMD Consortium Network and Orofacial Pain Special Interest Group. J Oral Facial Pain Headache. 28(1):6-27, 2014
2. Palconet G et al: Correlating cone beam CT results with temporomandibular joint pain of osteoarthritic origin. Dentomaxillofac Radiol. 41(2):126-30, 2012
3. Look JO et al: Reliability and validity of Axis I of the Research Diagnostic Criteria for Temporomandibular Disorders (RDC/TMD) with proposed revisions. J Oral Rehabil. 37(10):744-59, 2010
4. Ahmad M et al: Research diagnostic criteria for temporomandibular disorders (RDC/TMD): development of image analysis criteria and examiner reliability for image analysis. Oral Surg Oral Med Oral Pathol Oral Radiol Endod. 107(6):844-60, 2009

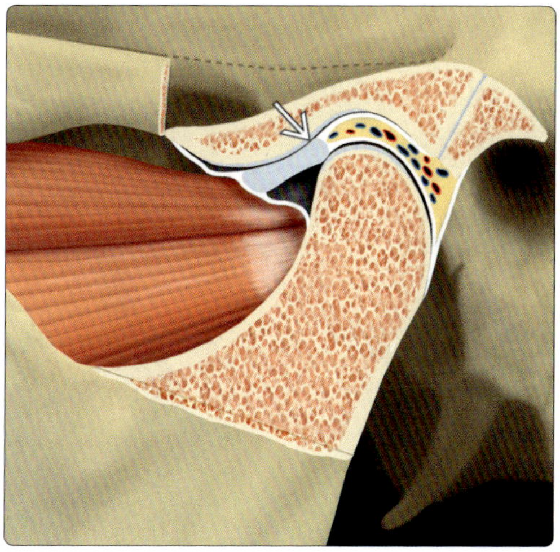

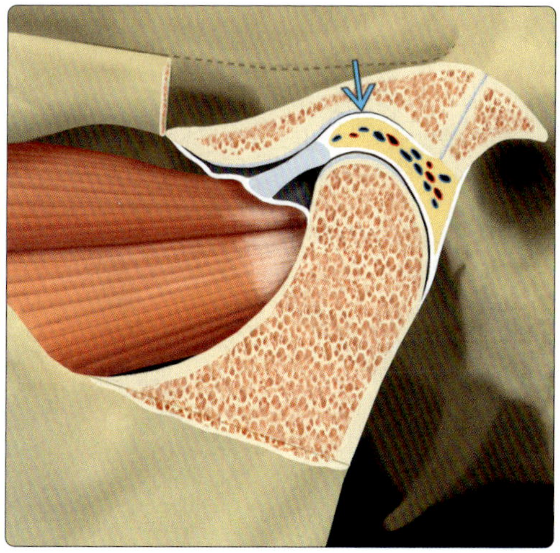

(Left) *Series of 8 graphics of the TMJ shows the position of the components of a TMJ with a pure anterior DDwoR during the opening and closing cycle. The condyle is seated in the fossa with a slightly more posterior and superior position due to the dislocation of the thick posterior band* → *from its normal 12-o'clock position in relation to the condyle.* **(Right)** *The condyle starts to rotate and translate, creating slightly more space in the superior aspect of the joint space* →*, and the disc starts to become compressed anteriorly.*

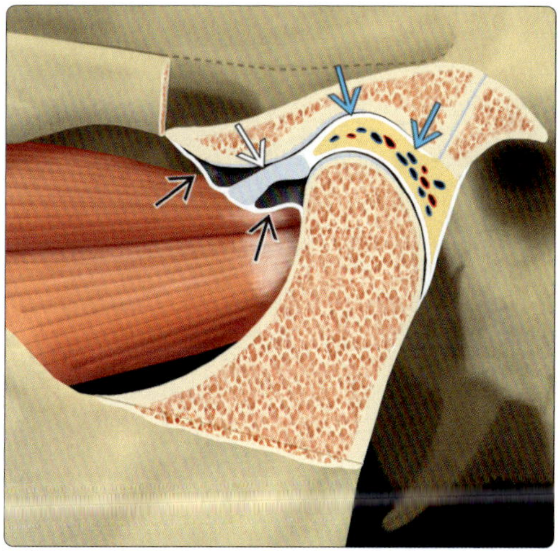

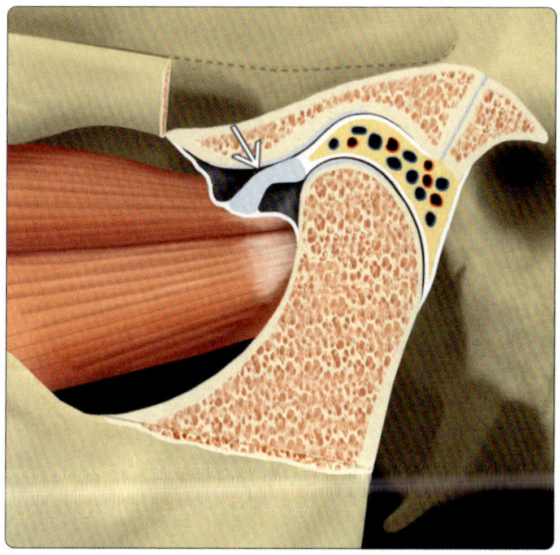

(Left) *Translation of the condyle continues, and widening of the posterior and superior aspects of the joint space* → *is seen. The disc is further compressed anteriorly and shows a deformation (folding)* → *of its shape and stretching of the anterior capsule wall* →*.* **(Right)** *The condyle continues to translate forward but does not pass over the posterior band of the disc to engage the intermediate zone. The disc continues to deform* →*.*

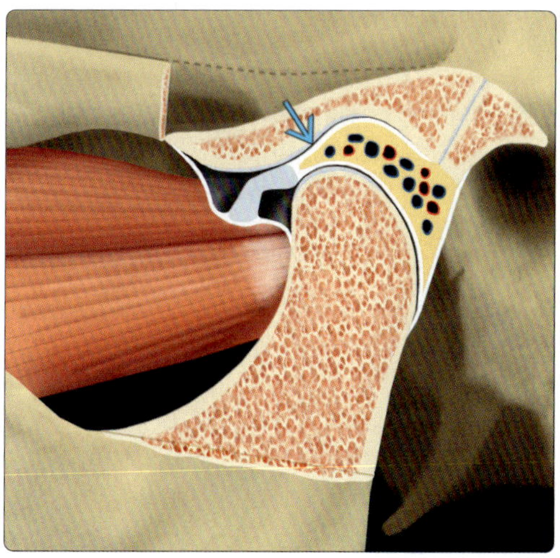

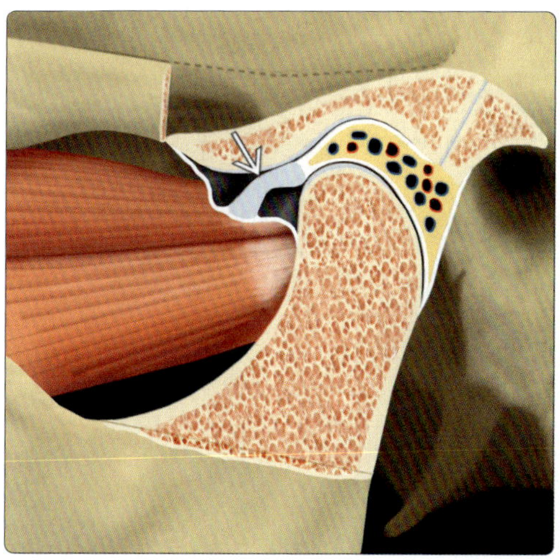

(Left) *At maximum opening, the condyle fails to recapture the disc. The posterior attachment is stretched* →*, and the disc remains anterior to the condyle. The range of motion of the condyle is initially mechanically limited (closed lock) but is regained with time as the tissue adapts.* **(Right)** *Initial closing phase starts to reposition the condyle in the fossa, and the disc deformation eases* →*. In chronic DDwoR, the disc may lose its structural integrity and atrophy, so this folding and unfolding may not be seen on MR.*

(Left) *The condyle has not seated completely in this image. The posterior attachment and anterior capsule walls remain stretched due to the displacement of the disc.* **(Right)** *Complete seating of the condyle is seen. The disc has not been recaptured in any of the phases of opening. With time and chronic irritation of the retrodiscal tissues through compression and stretching, breakdown of these tissues can occur (retrodiscitis, perforation, and fibrosis).*

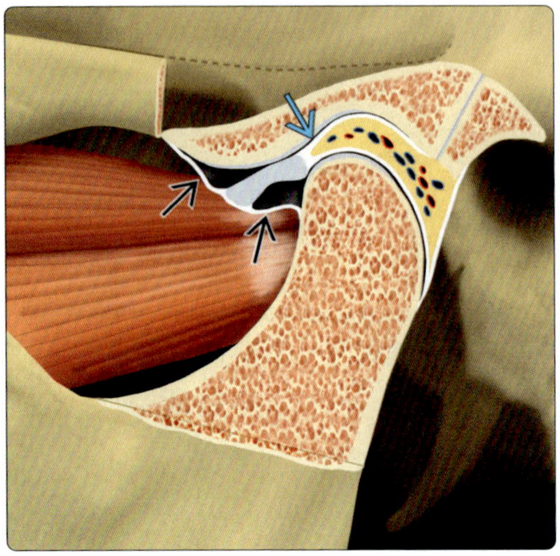

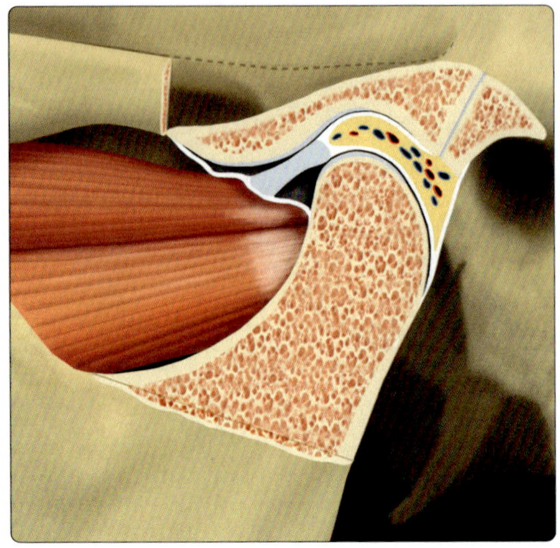

(Left) *PD MR shows a chronically anteriorly displaced disc that has lost its structural integrity and has atrophied. The condyle is superiorly positioned in the fossa with thinning of the posterior attachment soft tissues in the joint space.* **(Right)** *PD MR (same patient) in the open position shows the anterior position of the disc, the subnormal range of motion of the condyle, and the thinning of the soft tissue between the condyle and eminence, suggestive of possible posterior attachment perforation.*

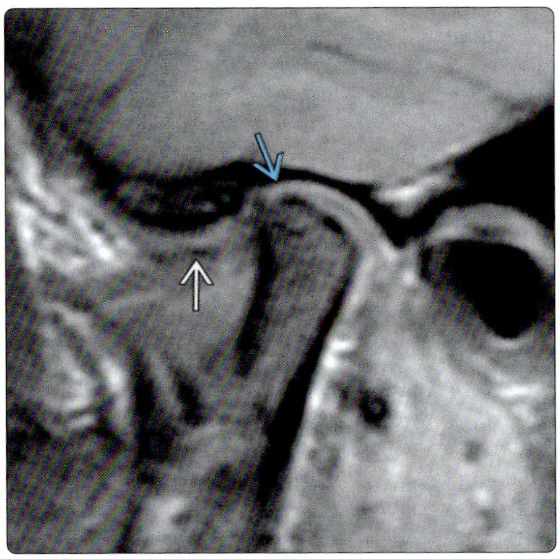

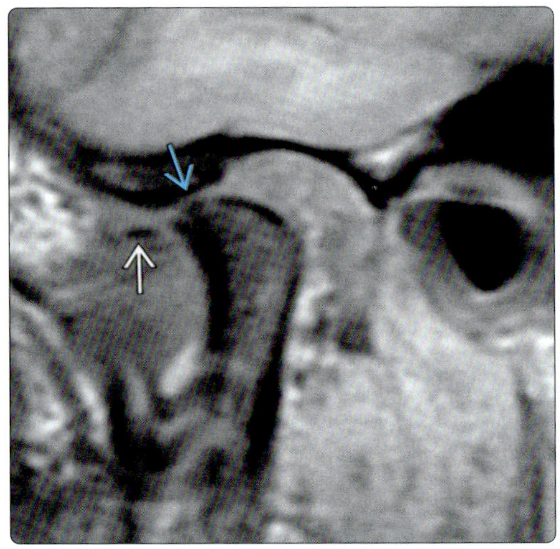

(Left) *Sagittal oblique PD MR in closed position shows a large posterior band of disc is anterior to condyle. The small condyle is superiorly positioned in fossa.* **(Right)** *Sagittal oblique PD MR of the same patient in the open-mouth position is shown. The condyle has normal translation, and the disc remains anterior to condyle. The disc folds into a biconvex shape. The posterior attachment is seen between the condyle and the eminence and should not be confused with the disc.*

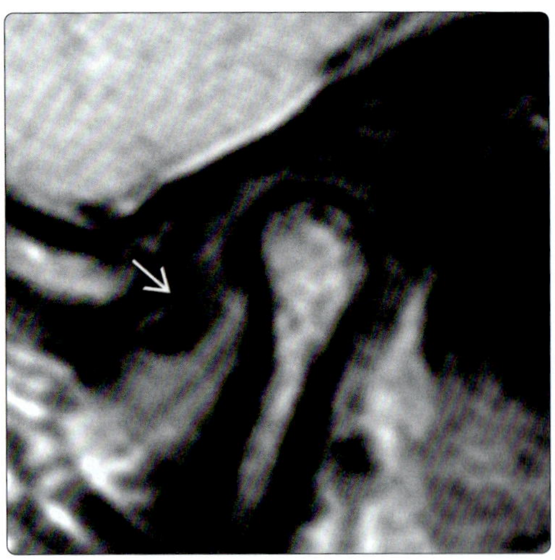

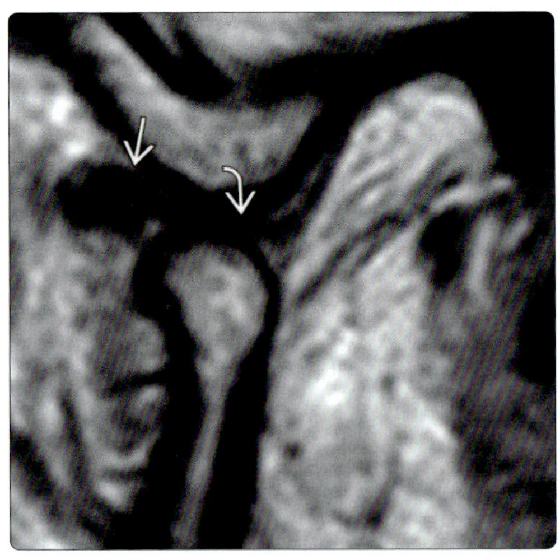

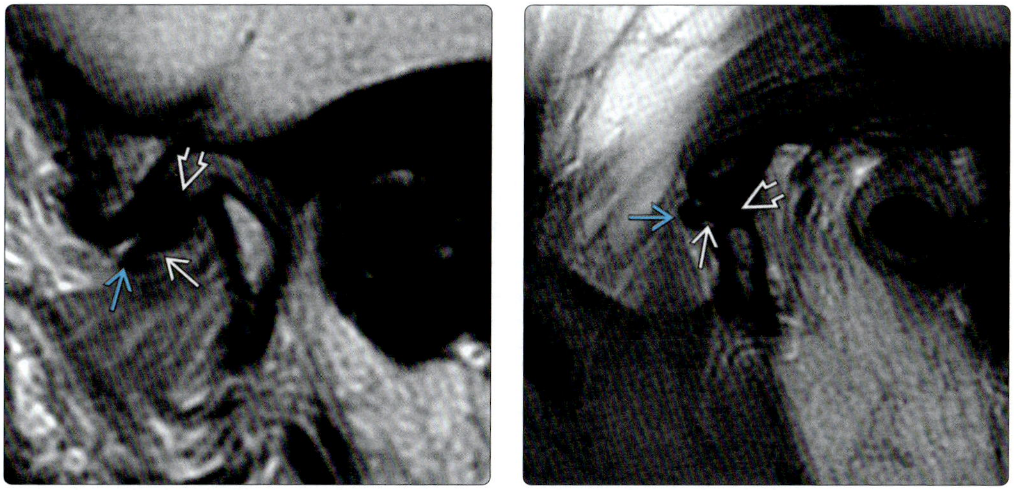

(Left) *PD MR of the mid section of a 29-year-old woman with DDwoR shows the thickening of the posterior band →, the smaller anterior band →, and the small notch where the intermediate zone would normally be →. The condyle is posteriorly positioned in fossa.* **(Right)** *PD MR of the same patient with open mouth shows the disc anterior to the condyle's lateral pole. The condyle does not re-engage the disc, and the posterior band →, anterior band →, and thin intermediate zone → remain anterior to the condyle.*

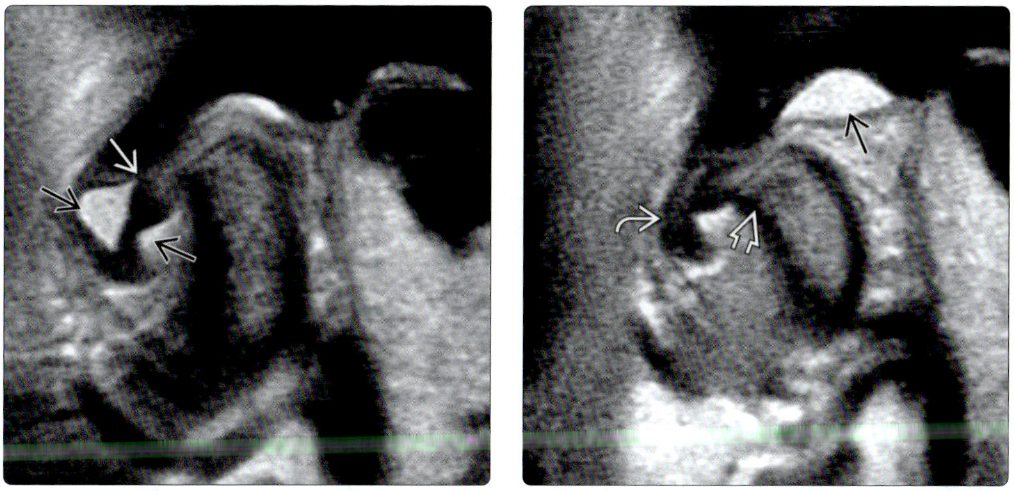

(Left) *Sagittal oblique T2WI MR in closed position shows the posterior band of the disc → is anterior to the condyle. There is reduction in the AP dimension of the disc and width of the intermediate zone. Fluid signal → is seen in the anterior recesses of both compartments.* **(Right)** *Sagittal oblique T2WI MR, same patient, in open position shows that disc → remains anterior to the condyle →. Note limited condylar translation & fluid signal in superior joint compartment →. This is relatively acute disc displacement with active DJD.*

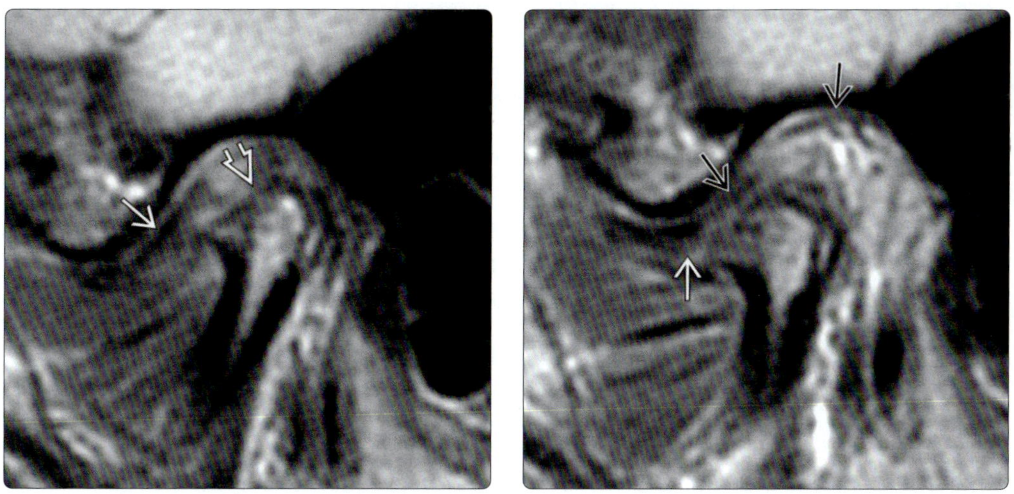

(Left) *Sagittal oblique PD MR of TMJ in closed position shows a small condyle → secondary to DJD. The posterior band of disc is anterior to condyle →.* **(Right)** *Sagittal oblique open view of same patient shows the condyle demonstrating subnormal motion. The posterior band of disc → remains anterior to the condyle. The superior lamina → of the posterior attachment is visible and should not be confused with the disc.*

KEY FACTS

TERMINOLOGY

- Definition: Connection of disc to fossa or eminence by fibrous connective tissue

IMAGING

- Best imaging tool: Arthrography
  - Visualize superior compartment using fluoroscope
- MR
- Adhesions most common in **superior joint compartment**
- **Lack of disc motion** relative to posterior slope of articular eminence
- Posterior band of disc may remain adhered to temporal bone in open position
- Maintenance of disc space and TMJ spatial relationships is seen

TOP DIFFERENTIAL DIAGNOSES

- Fibrous ankylosis
- False ankylosis

PATHOLOGY

- Various classifications, but most are based on type of adhesion &/or location of adhesions
  - Adhesion types: Filmy, band-like, and partition

CLINICAL ISSUES

- Trauma and displaced discs are predisposing factors
- May be **painful** at maximum opening
- Condyle translating along inferior surface of immobile disc may produce **joint sounds**
- Reduced condylar motion related to maturation of adhesions
- Treatment: Free adhesions with arthrocentesis or arthroscopy
  - Postsurgical management with jaw mobility exercises

DIAGNOSTIC CHECKLIST

- MR diagnosis based on lack of disc motion

(Left) *Sagittal oblique TMJ T1WI MR in closed position shows the posterior band ➡ of the disc in a normal position relative to the condyle.* **(Right)** *Sagittal oblique open-mouth TMJ T1WI MR of the same patient shows the posterior band of the disc ➡ remaining adhered to the most superior region of the glenoid fossa. The junction between the anterior band & the intermediate zone ➡ is interposed between the condyle & opposing eminence. There is no disc translation relative to the posterior slope of the eminence.*

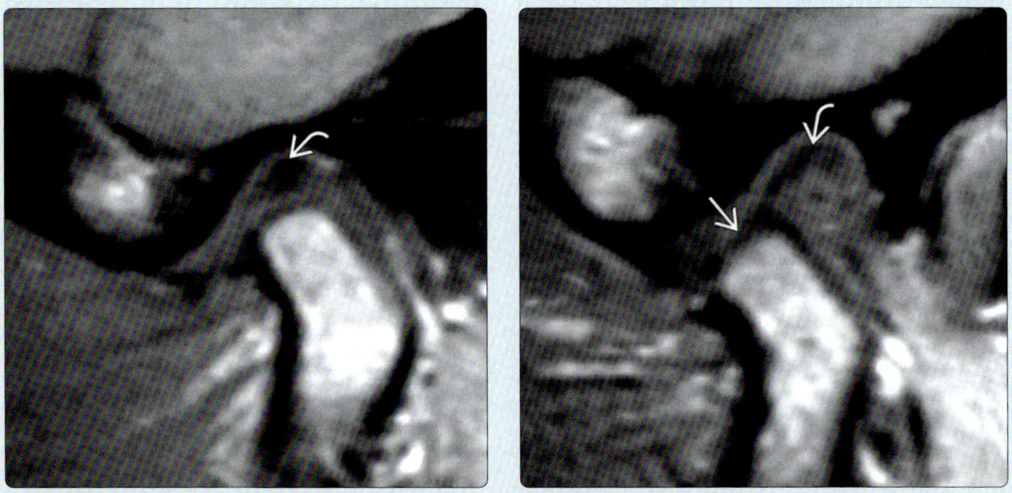

(Left) *Sagittal oblique T2WI MR of left TMJ in closed position shows posterior band ➡ and intermediate zone ➡ of the disc in a normal position relative to the condyle.* **(Right)** *Sagittal oblique T2WI MR of same patient in open-mouth position shows limited condylar translation. No disc translation is seen relative to posterior slope of eminence. Posterior band of disc ➡ is at most superior position of glenoid fossa. The junction between intermediate zone and anterior band ➡ is interposed between condyle and eminence.*

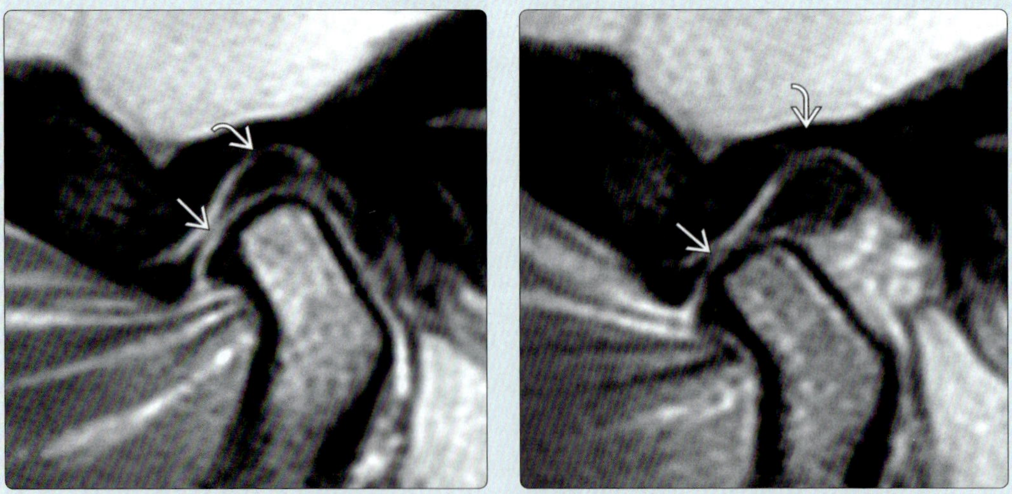

TERMINOLOGY

Synonyms

- Intraarticular adhesions (IA)

Definitions

- Connection of disc to fossa or eminence by fibrous connective tissue

IMAGING

General Features

- Best diagnostic clue
  - Lack of disc translation; maintenance of disc space
- Location
  - **Superior joint compartment**; anterior recess most common

MR Findings

- **Lack of disc motion** relative to posterior slope of articular eminence
- Posterior band of disc may remain adhered to temporal bone in open position

Imaging Recommendations

- Best imaging tool
  - Arthrography
    - Visualize superior compartment using fluoroscope
    - Irregularly shaped superior joint compartment
    - Hesitation of contrast to fill superior joint compartment
  - MR
  - MR arthrography
  - Arthroscope
- Protocol advice
  - Closed-mouth and maximum-opening images
  - Image sections corrected to perpendicular and parallel to mediolateral long axis of condyle

DIFFERENTIAL DIAGNOSIS

Fibrous Ankylosis

- No condylar translation
- Condyle adhered to temporal bone by fibrous connective tissue

False Ankylosis

- Normal joint spaces
- Limited condylar motion not related to joint components

PATHOLOGY

General Features

- Etiology
  - Hypothesis 1: Synovitis causes fibrin deposition, decrease in lubrication that leads to stiction effect (2 solid objects pressed against each other but not sliding), reduced disc mobility, and further increase in fibrin depositions and formation of fibrous adhesions
  - Hypothesis 2: Synovial membrane hematoma attracts fibroblasts and fibrocysts to area; healing process results in scar tissue formation on fibrous capsular wall
  - Hypothesis 3: Longstanding, nonreducing, anteriorly displaced disc, inflammation, and mechanical squeezing of synovium in anterior recess; vessel congestion and exudation from inflamed synovium accumulates and results in adhesions in anterior recess

Staging, Grading, & Classification

- Various classifications, but most based on type of adhesion &/or location of adhesions
  - Adhesion types: Filmy, band-like, and partition
  - Locations in superior joint compartment include 9-cell matrix: 3 cells extending from medial to lateral and 3 cells extending from anterior to posterior

CLINICAL ISSUES

Presentation

- Most common signs/symptoms
  - Restriction in disc and condylar translation
  - Associated with displaced disc
- Other signs/symptoms
  - May be **painful** at maximum opening
  - Condyle translating along inferior surface of immobile disc may produce **joint sounds**

Natural History & Prognosis

- Predisposing factors
  - Trauma
  - Displaced disc
- Severity of adhesions are proportional to patient age and severity of internal derangement
- Adhesion maturation increases with presence and duration of degenerative joint disease
- Reduced condylar motion related to maturation of adhesions

Treatment

- Free adhesions with arthrocentesis or arthroscopy
- Postsurgical management with jaw mobility exercises

DIAGNOSTIC CHECKLIST

Consider

- MR diagnosis based on lack of disc motion

Image Interpretation Pearls

- Adhesions generally localized to superior joint compartment

SELECTED REFERENCES

1. Juran CM et al: Engineered microporosity: enhancing the early regenerative potential of decellularized temporomandibular joint discs. Tissue Eng Part A. 21(3-4):829-39, 2015
2. Liu XM et al: Can puncture increase the risk of intra-articular adhesion in the temporomandibular joint? J Craniofac Surg. 25(1):e26-9, 2014
3. Shinohara Y et al: Inhibition of fibrous adhesion formation in the temporomandibular joint of tenascin-C knockout mice. Eur J Histochem. 58(4):2337, 2014
4. Shen P et al: Synovial tissue in internal derangement of temporomandibular joint. J Craniofac Surg. 24(3):748-52, 2013
5. Venetis G et al: The value of magnetic resonance arthrography of the temporomandibular joint in imaging disc adhesions and perforations. Dentomaxillofac Radiol. 40(2):84-90, 2011
6. Zhang S et al: Intra-articular adhesions of the temporomandibular joint: Relation between arthroscopic findings and clinical symptoms. BMC Musculoskelet Disord. 10:70, 2009

KEY FACTS

TERMINOLOGY

- Definition: Benign, **slow-growing**, bone-forming tumor characterized by proliferation of either compact or cancellous bone

IMAGING

- Best diagnostic clue: Well-defined bone-density lesion extending from condyle, neck of condyle, or upper ramus
- Jaw osteomas relatively uncommon
  - TMJ involvement **rare**
  - Additional sites: Mandibular notch below condylar neck, coronoid, glenoid fossa
- Homogeneous, well-defined, bone-based, **high-density** (radiopaque) mass
- Internal trabecular pattern is **normal**
- Morphology
  - Globular; may be pedunculated

TOP DIFFERENTIAL DIAGNOSES

- Osteochondroma, TMJ
- Condylar hyperplasia

CLINICAL ISSUES

- Usually **asymptomatic** and **incidental** finding on imaging
- Symptoms similar to **TMD**
  - Limitation of movement, occasional pain
- Facial **asymmetry** and swelling once enlarges
- Ipsilateral **open** bite if condyle involved
  - Deviation of mandible
- Age: 24-74 years old; most in 4th decade
- M = F for TMJ involvement
- Treatment: Excision or condylectomy

DIAGNOSTIC CHECKLIST

- Consider Gardner syndrome if multiple osteomas

(Left) *Coronal CBCT shows an ivory osteoma ➡ composed of dense bone arising from the lateral aspect of the left condylar neck. The lesion has a broad base and is smoothly rounded and symmetrical. (Courtesy M. Noujeim, DDS.)* **(Right)** *Axial CBCT of the same patient shows that the osteoma ➡ arises from the cortex and has not affected condylar cortical thickness or density. The lesion is symmetric, and the morphology of the condyle is otherwise normal. (Courtesy M. Noujeim, DDS.)*

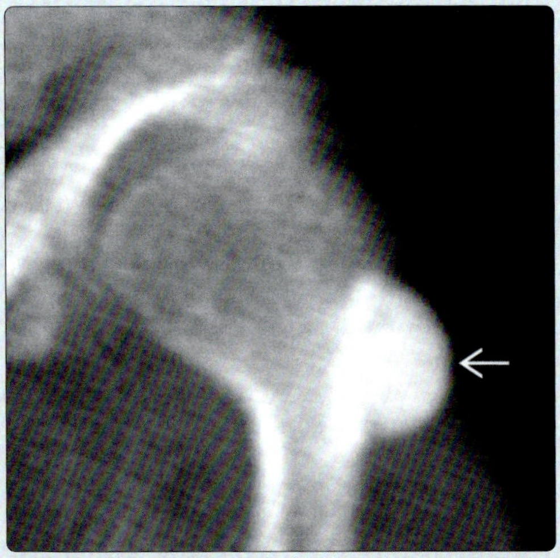

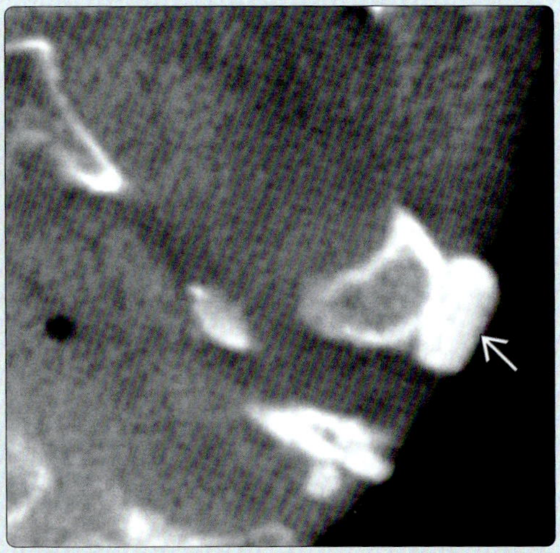

(Left) *Coronal CBCT shows a large osteoma ➡ arising from the left condyle and neck of the condyle. The osteoma is composed mostly of dense cortical bone, but the original cortex of the condylar neck is still visible ➡, helping to differentiate this osteoma from an osteochondroma.* **(Right)** *Axial CBCT in the same patient shows the large, somewhat lobulated appearance of the osteoma at the neck of the mandible, exhibiting a sessile attachment ➡ rather than pedunculated.*

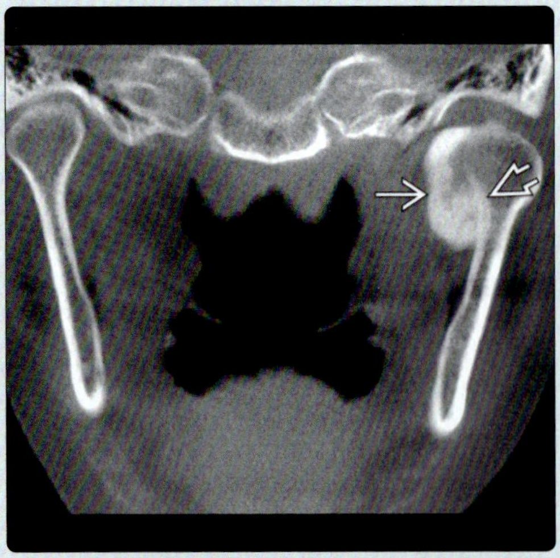

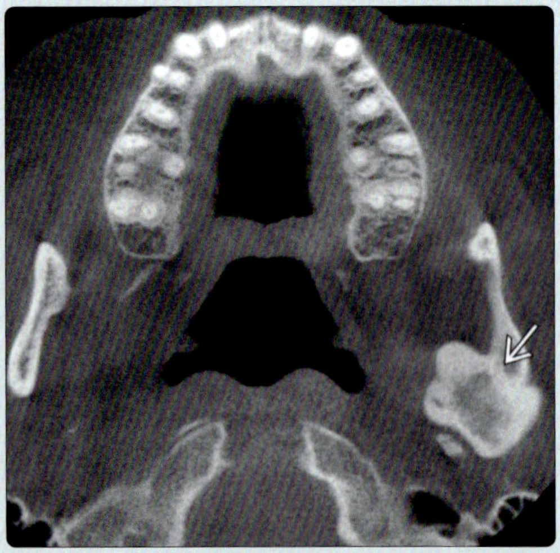

TERMINOLOGY

Definitions

- Benign, **slow-growing**, bone-forming tumor characterized by proliferation of either compact or cancellous bone

IMAGING

General Features

- Best diagnostic clue
  - Well-defined bone-density lesion extending from condyle, neck of condyle, or upper ramus
- Location
  - Almost exclusively found in craniofacial region
  - Paranasal sinuses most common site
  - Jaw osteomas relatively uncommon; TMJ involvement **rare**
    - Additional sites: Mandibular notch below neck of condyle, coronoid, glenoid fossa
- Size
  - Varies; some TMJ osteomas > 2 cm in diameter
- Morphology
  - Globular; grows from wide base or attached to cortex by pedicle

Radiographic Findings

- Well-defined bony radiopacity superimposed or extending from condyle or surrounding TMJ area
- ± peripheral cortex

CT Findings

- Bone CT
  - Homogeneous, well-defined, bone-based, **high-density** (radiopaque) mass
    - Internal trabecular pattern is **normal**

MR Findings

- T1WI
  - Low signal, but central yellow marrow may be high signal
- T2WI
  - Hypointense or follows marrow signal
  - May have hypointense cortical rim

Imaging Recommendations

- Best imaging tool
  - Bone CT or CBCT with sagittal and coronal reformats to illustrate relationship of lesion with TMJ components

DIFFERENTIAL DIAGNOSIS

Osteochondroma, TMJ

- Cartilage-capped lesion that undergoes endochondral ossification deep in tumor
  - Originates from cartilage areas of mandible: Articular surfaces of condyle, coronoid process
  - Osteoma originates from periosteal surfaces
- **Trabecular pattern** of condyle **continuous** with osteochondroma

Condylar Hyperplasia

- Condylar enlargement where condyle retains its original shape
  - Osteoma is pedunculated or lobulated

PATHOLOGY

General Features

- Etiology
  - Trauma
  - Congenital and hereditary endocrine disorders
  - Chronic inflammation or infection
- Associated abnormalities
  - **Gardner syndrome** (familial adenomatous polyposis)
    - Multiple osteomas of long bones, skull, and jaws
    - Premalignant colorectal polyposis
    - Multiple epidermoid or sebaceous cysts
    - Impacted permanent or supernumerary teeth

Staging, Grading, & Classification

- Compact (ivory) osteoma
  - Well-differentiated dense mature bone with scant marrow
- Cancellous osteoma
  - Lamellar trabeculae with abundant marrow

Microscopic Features

- Normal bone; may have normal cortical border
- Covered by periosteum; not encapsulated

CLINICAL ISSUES

Presentation

- Most common signs/symptoms
  - Usually **asymptomatic** and **incidental** finding on imaging
  - Symptoms similar to **TMJ dysfunction**: Limitation of movement and occasional pain
- Other signs/symptoms
  - Facial **asymmetry** and swelling once enlarges
  - Ipsilateral **open** bite if condyle involved
  - Deviation of mandible

Demographics

- Age
  - In TMJ: 24-74 years old; most in 4th decade
- Gender
  - M = F for TMJ involvement

Natural History & Prognosis

- Slow-growing, remains asymptomatic until large

Treatment

- Excision or condylectomy
- Orthodontic correction of any occlusal discrepancies
- No reported recurrence

DIAGNOSTIC CHECKLIST

Consider

- Gardner syndrome if multiple osteomas

SELECTED REFERENCES

1. Nojima K et al: Multidisciplinary treatment of peripheral osteoma arising from mandibular condyle in patient presenting with facial asymmetry. Bull Tokyo Dent Coll. 55(1):39-47, 2014
2. Almeida LE et al: Giant mandibular condyle osteoma. J Craniofac Surg. 22(3):1147-9, 2011

TMJ Osteochondroma

KEY FACTS

TERMINOLOGY

- Definition: Cartilage-capped exophytic lesion arising from bone
- Synonym: Osteocartilaginous exostosis

IMAGING

- Lesion cortex and internal aspect **continuous** with trabecular portion and cortex of originating bone
- **Coronoid** process and **condyle** most common sites in jaws
- Irregular, distorted, enlarged condyle; ipsilateral mandible normal size
- Border between lesion and underlying normal bone usually **indistinct**
- May appear as **pedunculated** mass of mixed density attached to condyle or coronoid process
- Often extends from anterior or anterior-medial surface of condyle at attachment of lateral pterygoid

TOP DIFFERENTIAL DIAGNOSES

- Condylar hyperplasia
- Degenerative joint disease
- Coronoid hyperplasia
- TMJ osteoma

CLINICAL ISSUES

- Painless, hard **swelling** over TMJ
- Facial **asymmetry** with vertical **elongation** of face on affected side; lateral open bite on affected side; crossbite on contralateral side
- Symptoms often mimic TMJ dysfunction: Hypomobility, TMJ clicking and locking
- Mean age for TMJ cases = 40 years; F > M (slight)

DIAGNOSTIC CHECKLIST

- Osteochondroma does not enlarge ipsilateral 1/2 of mandible as does condylar hyperplasia

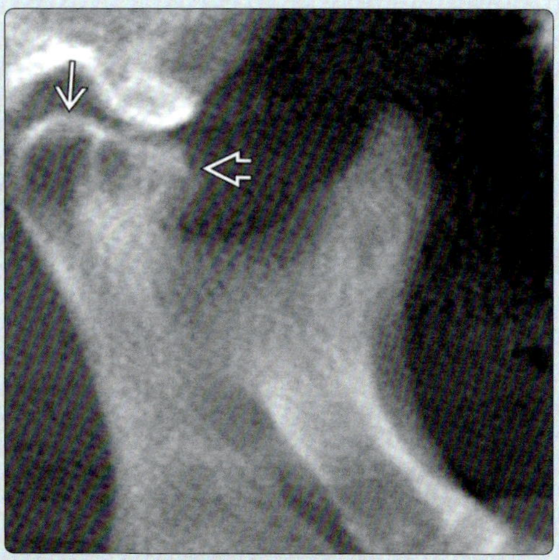

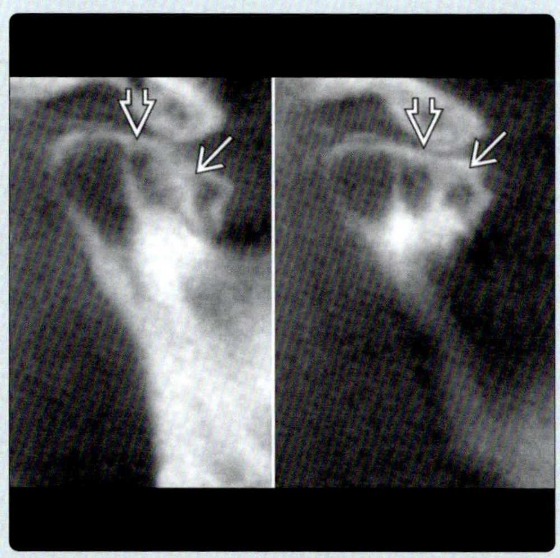

(Left) *Panoramic CBCT reformat shows an osteochondroma of the right condyle. The normal condylar outline is seen* ➡*, but a linear radiopacity, representing an osteochondroma* ➡*, extends anteriorly from the condyle. The lesion causes inferior displacement of the condyle because the lesion articulates with the articular eminence.* **(Right)** *Sagittal CBCT of the same patient shows the osteochondroma* ➡ *attached to the condyle by a narrow stalk* ➡*.*

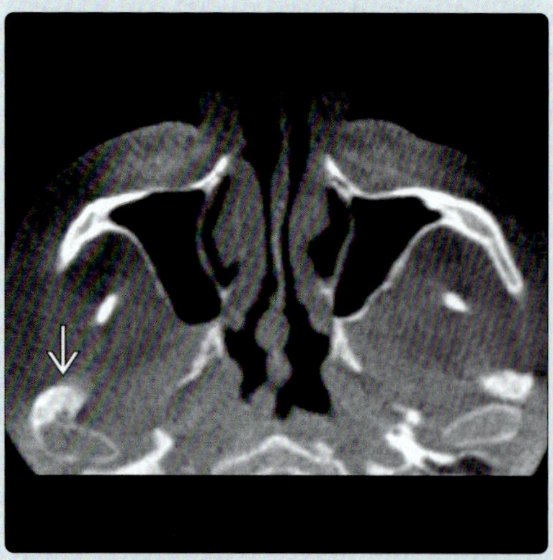

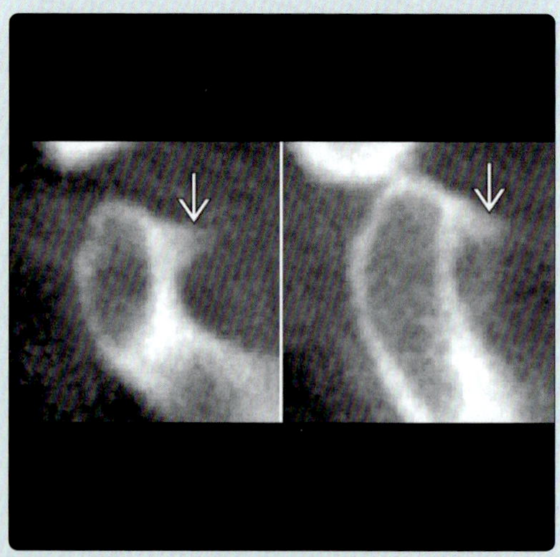

(Left) *Axial CBCT in the same patient shows continuity of the osteochondroma* ➡ *with the normal trabecular bone and cortex of the mandibular condyle. The lesion is oriented in the direction of the lateral pterygoid muscle fibers (medially and anteriorly).* **(Right)** *Sagittal CBCT images show a triangular-shaped osteochondroma* ➡ *extending from the anterior surface of the right condyle. This lesion could be mistaken for an osteophyte; however, there are no other signs of degenerative joint disease in the TMJ.*

TMJ Osteochondroma

TERMINOLOGY

Synonyms

- Osteocartilaginous exostosis

Definitions

- Cartilage-capped exophytic lesion arising from bone
  - Considered tumor by some and hamartoma by others

IMAGING

General Features

- Best diagnostic clue
  - Lesion cortex and internal aspect **continuous** with trabecular portion and cortex of originating bone
- Location
  - **Coronoid process** and **condyle** most common sites in jaws
    - Also reported in glenoid fossa, mandibular symphysis, zygoma, zygomatic arch, nasal septum, skull base
- Size
  - Varies from small exophytic lesion to very large mass distorting neighboring structures

Radiographic Findings

- Radiography
  - Irregular, distorted, enlarged condyle
    - Ipsilateral 1/2 of mandible **not** enlarged
  - Border between lesion and underlying normal bone usually **indistinct**
  - Condyle may resemble enlarged sclerotic mass
  - If originates from coronoid process, may see **mushroom-shaped** enlargement

CT Findings

- May appear as **pedunculated** mass of mixed density attached to condyle or coronoid process
- Often extends from anterior or anterior-medial surface of condyle at attachment of lateral pterygoid **muscle**
- Can **erode** adjacent structures

Imaging Recommendations

- Best imaging tool
  - CBCT or bone CT

DIFFERENTIAL DIAGNOSIS

Condylar Hyperplasia

- Enlarged condyle, but shape and proportions maintained
- Ipsilateral 1/2 of mandible also enlarged
- Normal cortical thickness and trabecular pattern

Degenerative Joint Disease

- Condylar osteophyte may resemble small osteochondroma; condyle will exhibit degenerative changes
- **Osteophyte adapts to space available**; osteochondroma usually displaces condyle

Coronoid Hyperplasia

- Enlarged coronoid process, but shape maintained
- Occasionally coronoid process curves anteriorly

TMJ Osteoma

- Dense cortical bone; sometimes trabecular bone

TMJ Chondrosarcoma

- Bone destruction with mottled densities
- Condyle may appear enlarged; may see condylar mass

PATHOLOGY

Microscopic Features

- Bony mass consisting of endochondral ossification in deepest part of cartilage with cartilaginous islands in subchondral bone, covered by cartilaginous cap

CLINICAL ISSUES

Presentation

- Most common signs/symptoms
  - Painless, hard **swelling** over TMJ
  - Facial **asymmetry** with vertical **elongation** of face on affected side
  - Lateral **open bite** on affected side, **crossbite** on contralateral side
- Other signs/symptoms
  - **Deviation** of mandible to unaffected side
  - May have pain
  - Symptoms often mimic TMJ dysfunction: Hypomobility, TMJ clicking and locking

Demographics

- Age
  - Mean age at diagnosis for TMJ cases = 40 years
- Gender
  - M:F = 1:1.5
- Epidemiology
  - Osteochondroma = 10-15% of all benign bone tumors, but rare in jaws

Natural History & Prognosis

- Most are **slow growing**

Treatment

- Surgical removal; recurrence rare

DIAGNOSTIC CHECKLIST

Consider

- Condylar hyperplasia more common

Image Interpretation Pearls

- Osteochondroma does not enlarge ipsilateral 1/2 of mandible
  - If mandibular enlargement, consider condylar hyperplasia

SELECTED REFERENCES

1. Venturin JS et al: Temporomandibular joint condylar abnormality: evaluation, treatment planning, and surgical approach. J Oral Maxillofac Surg. 68(5):1189-96, 2010
2. Etöz OA et al: Osteochondroma of the mandibular coronoid process: a rare cause of limited mouth opening. Br J Oral Maxillofac Surg. 47(5):409-11, 2009
3. González-Otero S et al: Osteochondroma of the mandibular condyle: Resection and reconstruction using vertical sliding osteotomy of the mandibular ramus. Med Oral Patol Oral Cir Bucal. 14(4):E194-7, 2009
4. Zhang J et al: Osteochondromas of the mandibular condyle: variance in radiographic appearance on panoramic radiographs. Dentomaxillofac Radiol. 37(3):154-60, 2008

(Left) *Sagittal CBCT shows a large osteochondroma of the right coronoid process* ➔*. The lesion has a bulbous, mushroom-shaped morphology and interferes with mandibular opening as it articulates with the zygomatic process of the maxilla* ⇨*. The differential diagnosis includes a hyperplastic coronoid process, but the morphology of the coronoid process would be normal with hyperplasia.* **(Right)** *Coronal CBCT of the same patient shows bulbous enlargement of the coronoid process osteochondroma* ➔*.*

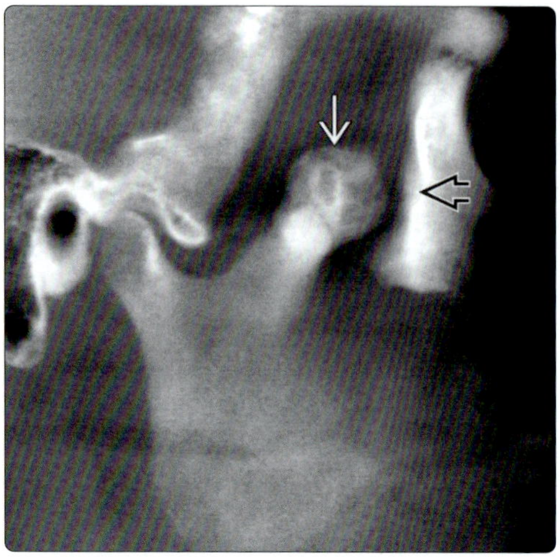

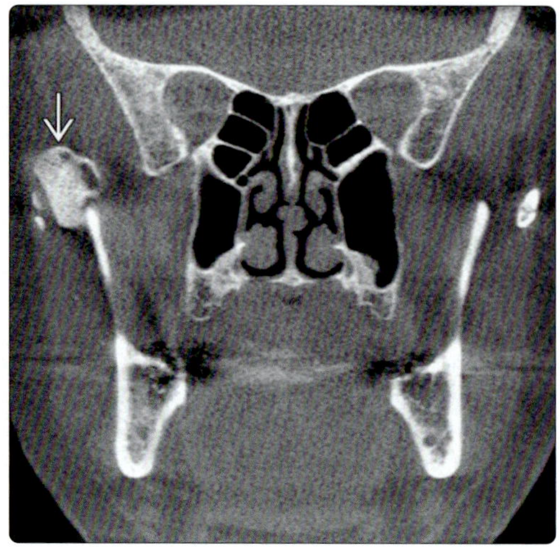

(Left) *Axial CBCT of the same patient shows the normal coronoid process on the left side* ➔ *compared to the coronoid process osteochondroma* ⇨ *on the contralateral side.* **(Right)** *Sagittal CBCT of the left condyle shows a large, bulbous osteochondroma* ➔ *extending from the anterior condylar surface. The internal aspect of the lesion is continuous with the normal trabecular bone of the condyle. The temporal bone has remodeled to accommodate the mass* ⇨*.*

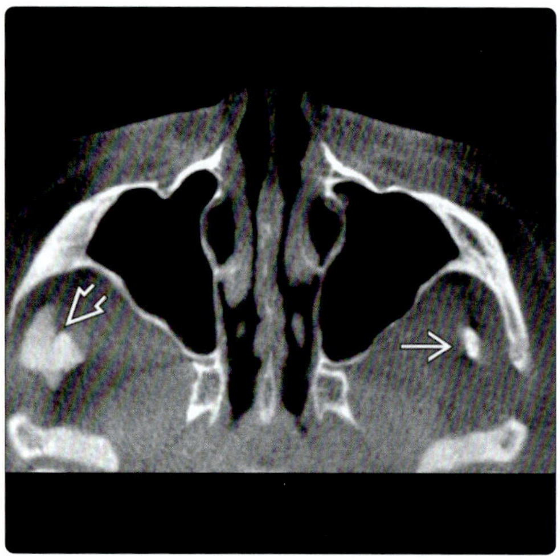

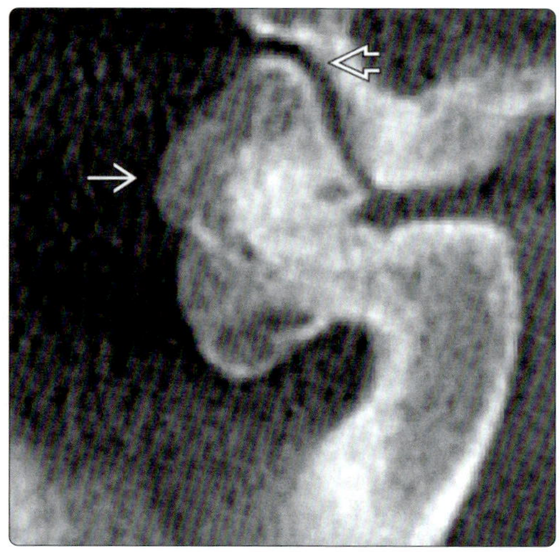

(Left) *Sagittal 3D reformation of the same patient shows the large condylar osteochondroma* ➔ *medial to the zygomatic arch and extending superiorly* ⇨ *above the arch.* **(Right)** *Coronal reformatted CBCT of the same patient shows the large, bulbous mass of the condylar osteochondroma. The internal aspect is composed of trabecular bone with a central, more sclerotic area* ⇨*. Note the thin cortication at the articulating surface* ➔*.*

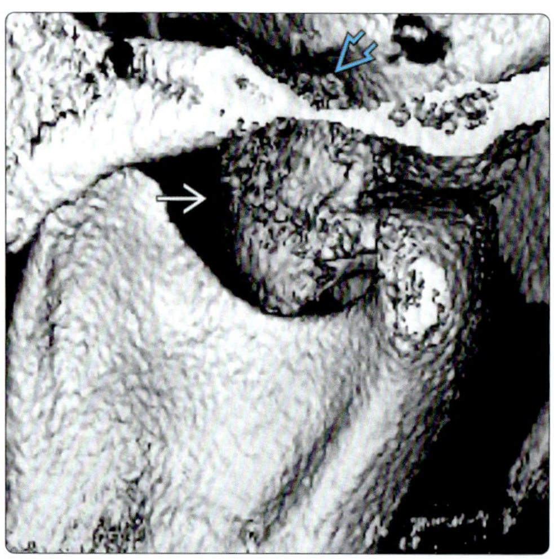

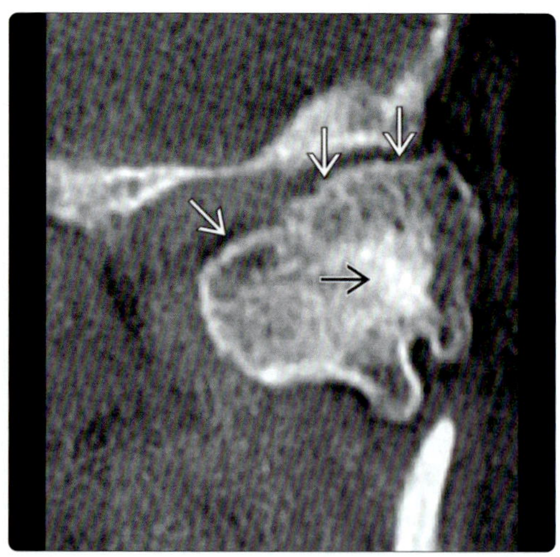

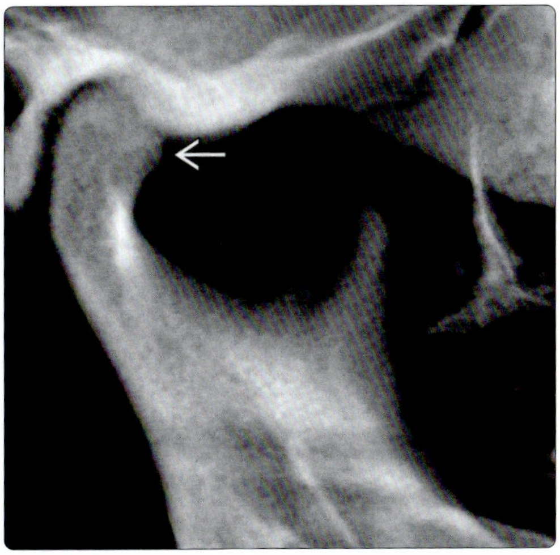

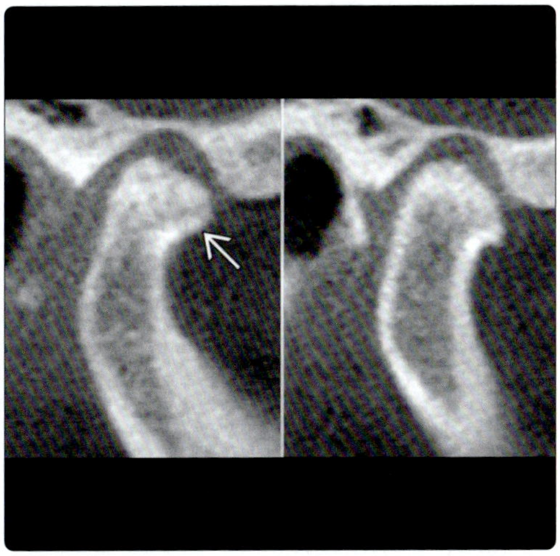

(Left) *Panoramic reformatted CBCT shows an osteochondroma of the right condyle that gives the appearance of an enlarged condyle. The ipsilateral body and ramus of the mandible are not enlarged, which helps to differentiate the lesion from condylar hyperplasia.* **(Right)** *Sagittal reformatted CBCT images of the same patient show that the osteochondroma has caused a slight bulbous shape to the condyle. The articular fossa is normal.*

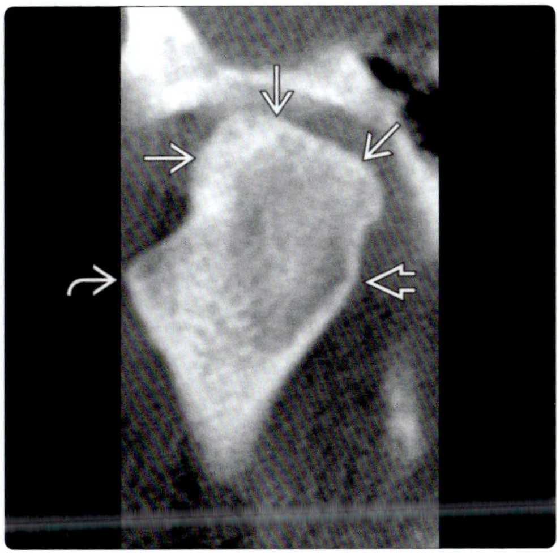

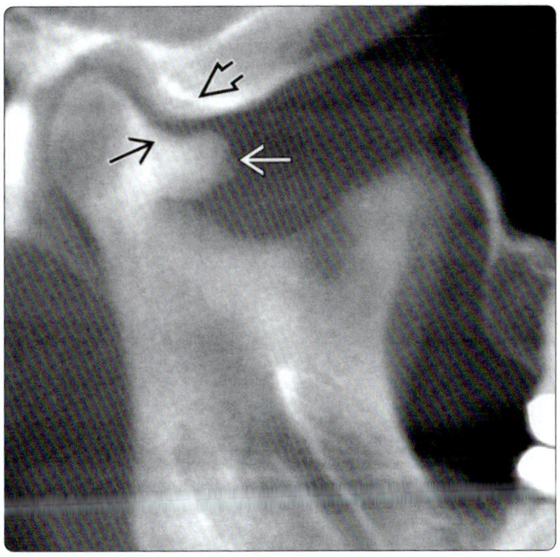

(Left) *Coronal reformatted CBCT of the same patient shows the osteochondroma extending from the superior condylar surface. The trabecular bone and cortex of the condyle are continuous with the internal aspect of the lesion. The normal medial and lateral condylar poles are visible.* **(Right)** *Panoramic reformatted CBCT shows an osteochondroma extending from the anterior surface of the right condyle. The superior lesion surface is curved to accommodate the articular eminence.*

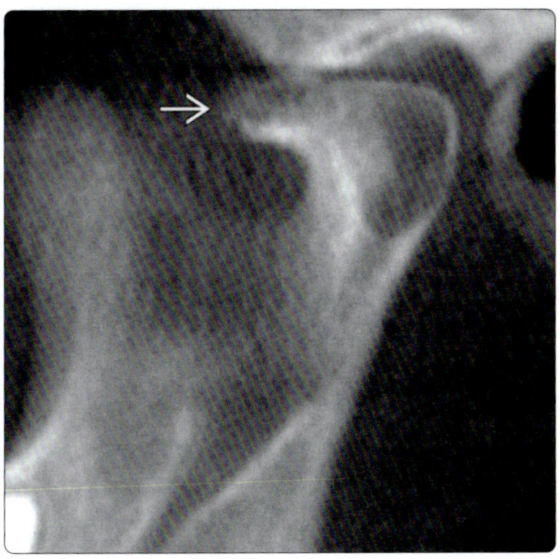

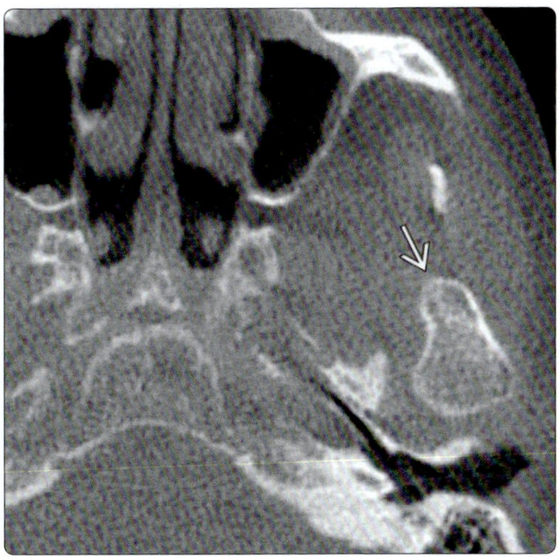

(Left) *Panoramic reformatted CBCT shows an osteochondroma extending from the anterior surface of the left condyle. The trabecular bone of the lesion is continuous and indistinguishable from the trabecular bone of the condyle. Note the inferior position of the condyle in fossa.* **(Right)** *Axial CBCT of the same patient shows the large osteochondroma extending from the anterior condylar surface. The cortex and trabecular bone of the lesion appear similar to the condyle.*

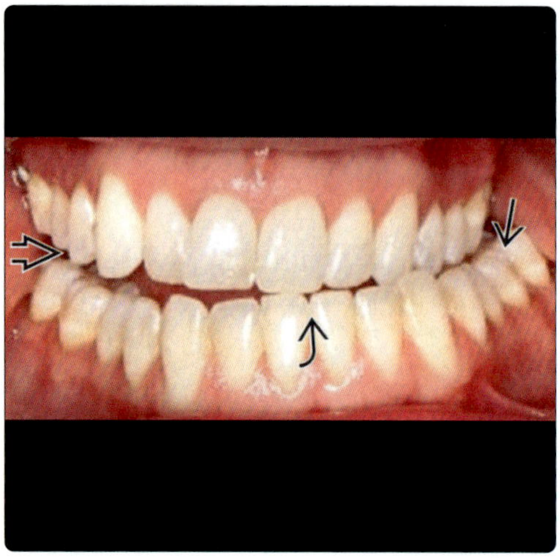

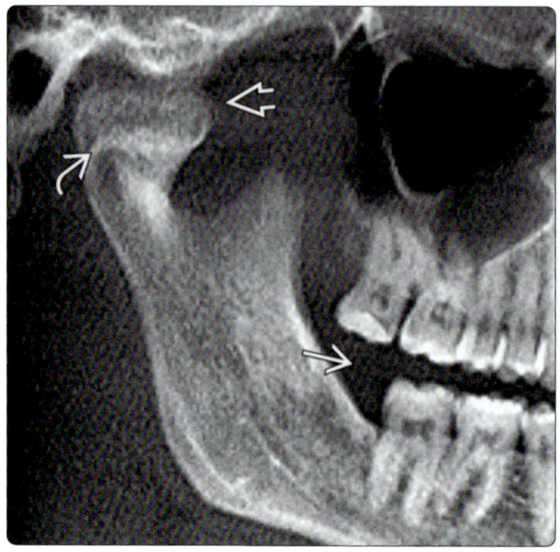

(Left) *Clinical photograph shows dentition in maximum intercuspation. There is an acquired right posterior open bite, left posterior crossbite, and shift of the mandibular dental midline to the left.* **(Right)** *CBCT panoramic reformation of the same patient shows an osteochondroma extending from the superior surface of the native condyle. The mass is displacing the mandible and altering the occlusion. (Courtesy D. Way, DDS.)*

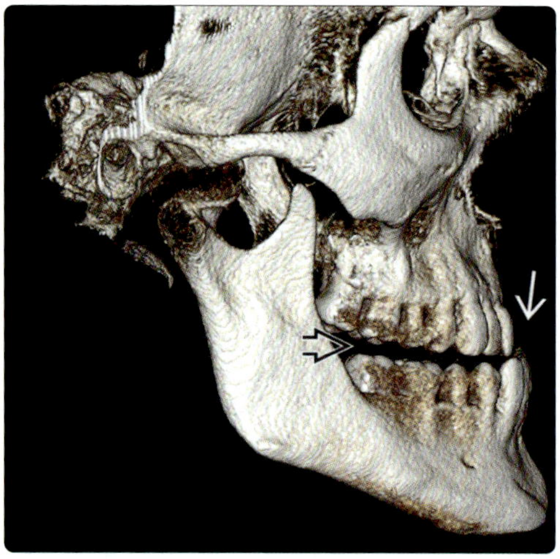

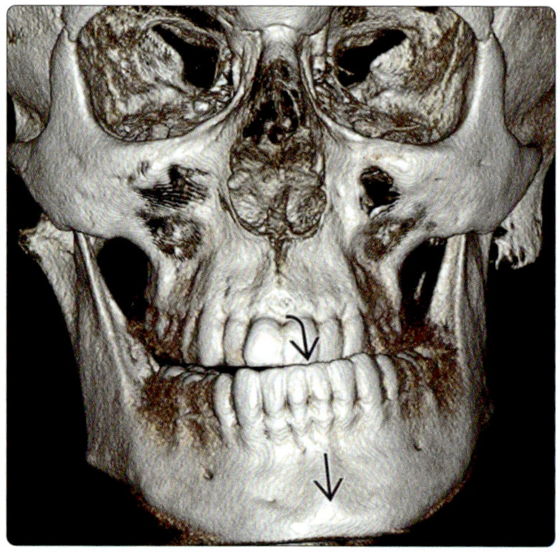

(Left) *CBCT surface rendering of the same patient shows the right posterior open bite and the negative anterior overjet.* **(Right)** *CBCT surface rendering of the same patient shows the mandibular displacement. The osseous and dental midlines of the mandible shift to the left.*

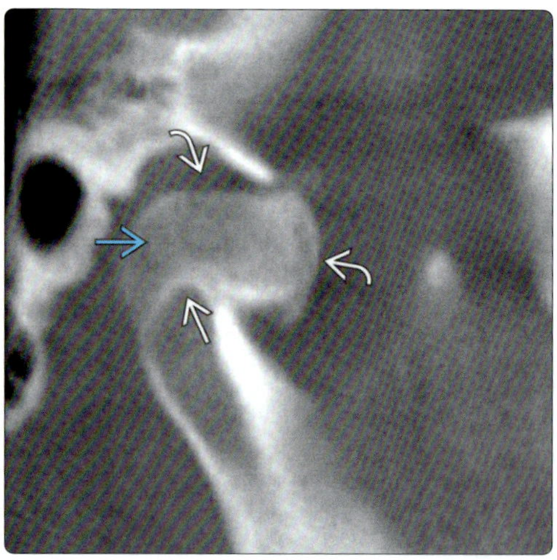

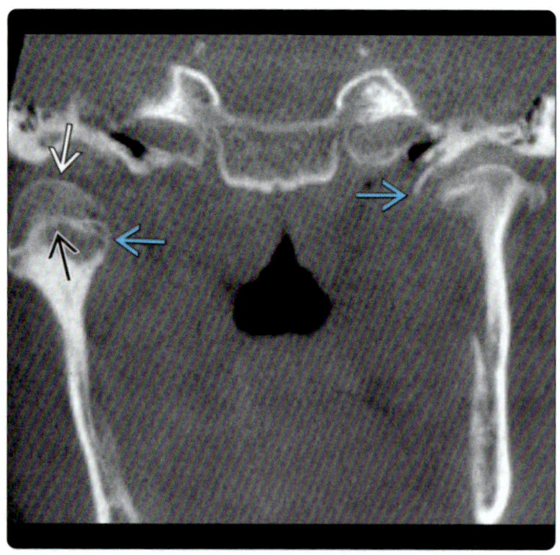

(Left) *CBCT sagittal oblique section of the same patient distinctly shows the intact native condyle. The margins of the osteochondroma are smooth and well defined. Medullary bone is observed internally.* **(Right)** *Coronal view of the same patient shows the mediolateral extent of the osteochondroma as it extends superiorly from the native condyle. Note the difference in axial levels between the 2 condyles due to the inferior displacement of the right condyle by the tumor.*

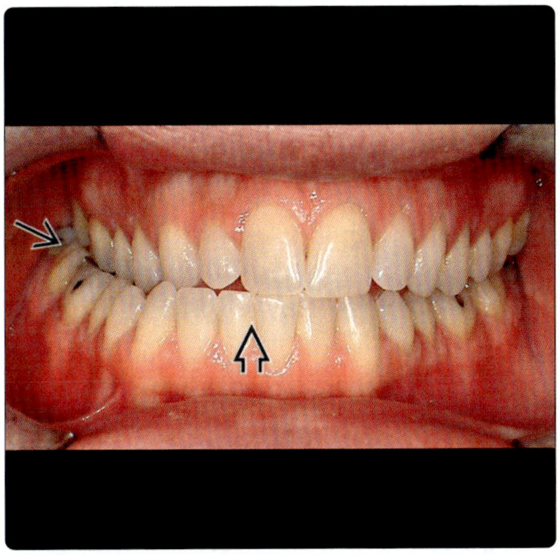

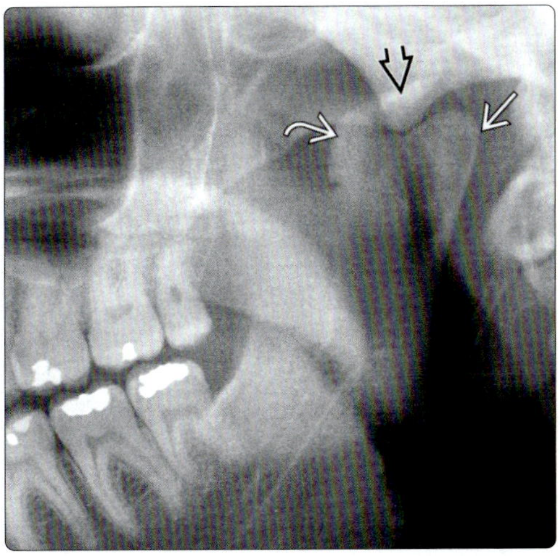

(Left) *Frontal photograph shows an acquired change in occlusion. The mandibular dental midline is shifted to the right, and there is a right posterior crossbite. (Courtesy J. Buchanan, DDS.)* **(Right)** *Panoramic projection of the same patient shows an osteochondroma extending from the anterior surface of the condyle, displacing the mandible to the contralateral side and articulating with the apex of the articular eminence.*

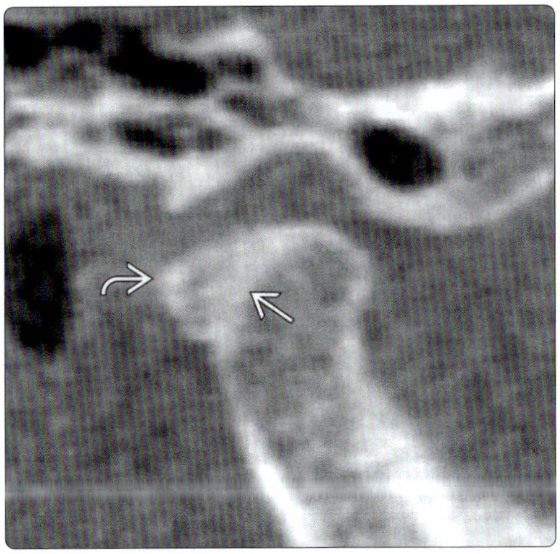

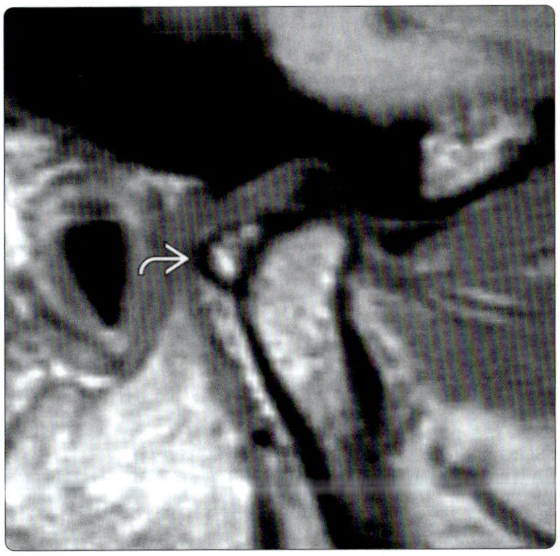

(Left) *Sagittal oblique CBCT of the right TMJ shows a lesion extending from the posterior surface of condyle. The condyle and right side of the mandible are displaced in an anteroinferior direction. The location of this lesion is more suggestive of an osteoma (coming from a periosteal surface and not the articular fibrocartilage surface).* **(Right)** *Sagittal oblique PD MR of the same patient shows the lesion extending from the native condyle. Note low signal rim around the lesion and internal bone marrow signal.*

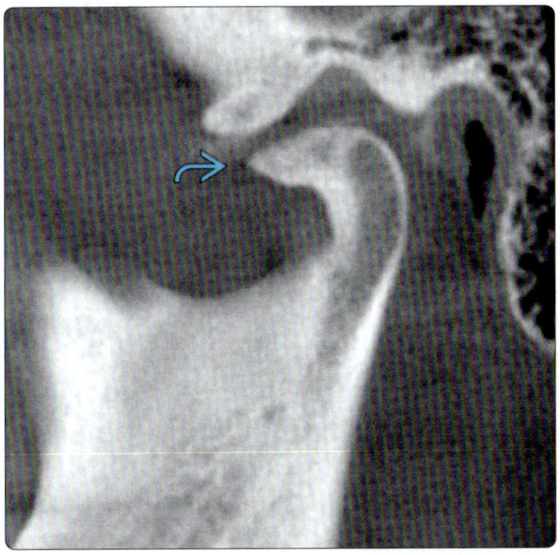

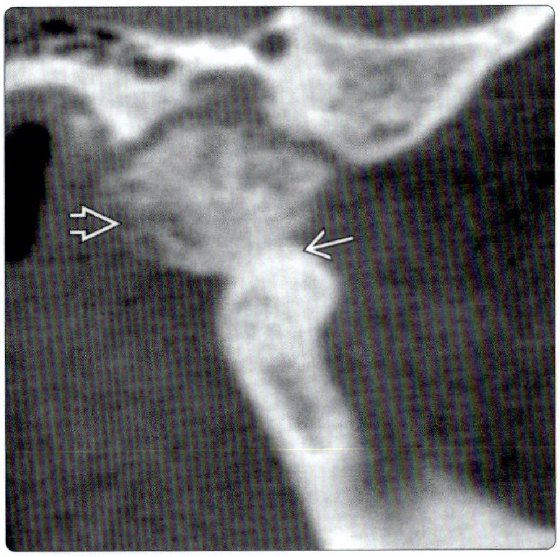

(Left) *CBCT sagittal oblique image shows an osteochondroma extending from the anterior surface of the condyle and articulating with the eminence apex. The condyle is inferiorly displaced from the fossa.* **(Right)** *CBCT sagittal oblique section of the right TMJ shows an osteochondroma extending from the posterosuperior surface of the condyle. The condyle and ipsilateral 1/2 of the mandible are anteroinferiorly displaced. (Courtesy C. Aichinger, DDS.)*

TMJ Calcium Pyrophosphate Dihydrate Deposition Disease

KEY FACTS

TERMINOLOGY

- Abbreviation: Calcium pyrophosphate dihydrate **(CPPD)**
- Synonyms: Pseudogout, chondrocalcinosis, tophaceous pseudogout
- Definition: **Metabolic disease** in which calcium pyrophosphate crystals deposited in synovial fluid result in calcification of articular cartilage, leading to acute arthritis in some patients

IMAGING

- Bone CT
  - **Fine, cloud-like** synovial calcifications with even distribution in joint space, often encircling condyle
  - Chunky, **diffusely calcified** mass
  - Associated remodeling, **erosion**, or **mass effect** on condyle and adjacent structures including skull base and external auditory canal
  - May **mimic malignancy (chondrosarcoma)** due to extensive bone destruction
- MR findings
  - T1: **Low**- to intermediate-signal lesion; capsule and joint space expansion
  - T2: **Hypointense**, somewhat heterogeneous mass
  - T1 C+: Heterogeneously enhancing TMJ lesion

TOP DIFFERENTIAL DIAGNOSES

- Synovial chondromatosis
- Chondrosarcoma
- Degenerative disease
- Chondroblastoma

CLINICAL ISSUES

- Preauricular pain, joint swelling from intermittent arthritic attacks
- Most common in middle age or elderly
- Treatment: Medications such as colchicine, steroids, NSAIDs, ASA; surgical removal of larger deposits and occasionally joint reconstruction

(Left) *Axial bone CT through the skull base reveals extensive calcific density surrounding the right mandibular condyle and condylar neck in a patient with CPPD deposition disease. Note the sparing of the joint space around the condyle.* **(Right)** *Sagittal bone CT reformation in the same patient better delineates the calcifications in relation to the TMJ. Note glenoid fossa demineralization and erosion resulting in a defect of the middle cranial fossa. The inferior joint space is compressed but spared.*

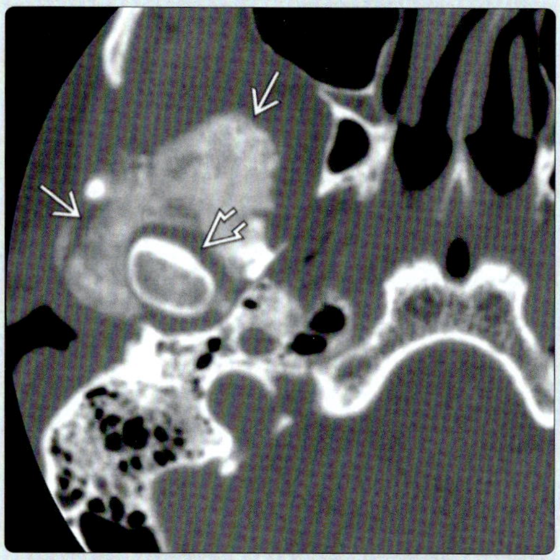

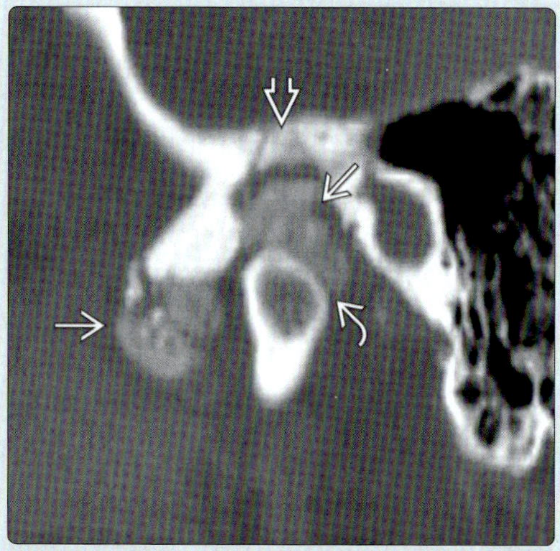

(Left) *Coronal bone CT in the same patient shows the calcifications laterally and medially to the condyle with sclerosis and erosion of the temporal component of the TMJ.* **(Right)** *Coronal bone CT in the same patient shows the calcifications located laterally to the condyle, which extend inferiorly to the condylar neck. There is extensive glenoid fossa erosion resulting in a large defect of the right middle cranial fossa.*

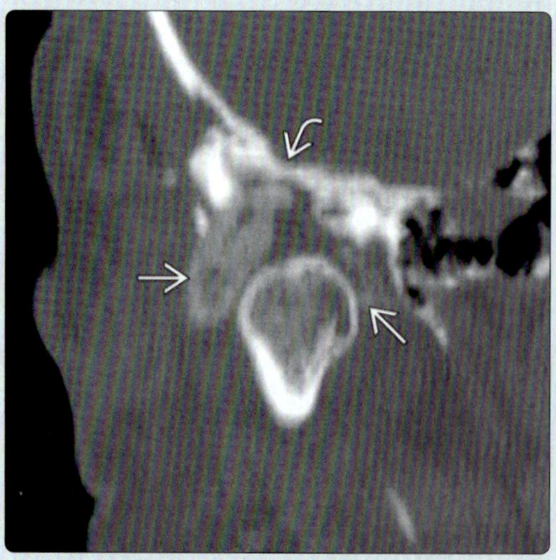

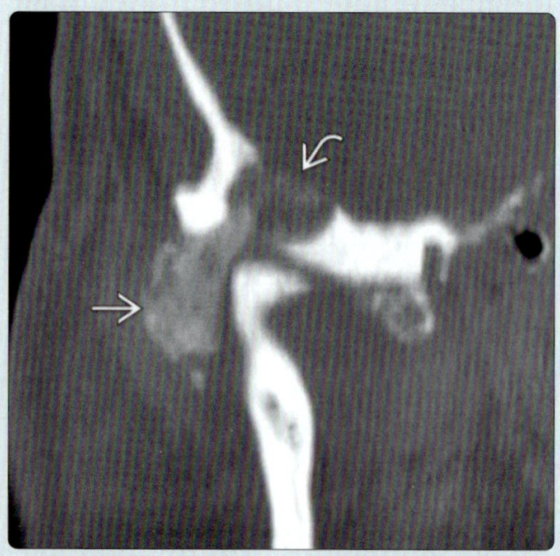

TERMINOLOGY

Abbreviations

- Calcium pyrophosphate dihydrate (CPPD)

Synonyms

- Pseudogout
- Chondrocalcinosis
- Tophaceous pseudogout

Definitions

- **Metabolic disease** in which calcium pyrophosphate crystals deposited in synovial fluid result in calcification of articular cartilage, leading to acute arthritis in some patients
  - **Tophaceous (tumoral) CPPD** deposition disease most prevalent in TMJ
  - Differs from gout, in which uric acid crystals are precipitated; therefore termed pseudogout

IMAGING

General Features

- Best diagnostic clue
  - Calcified TMJ **mass**
- Location
  - Predilection for joints with fibrocartilage: Knee, wrist, hip, shoulder, elbow
  - TMJ involvement **uncommon**
  - Intracapsular > extracapsular
    - May involve masticator space, parotid space, peri-TMJ skull base
    - **Unilateral** more common
- Size
  - Overall lesion typically 1 cm or larger
    - Calcifications fine and regular

CT Findings

- Bone CT and CBCT
  - Mild/early CPPD deposition disease
    - **Fine, cloud-like** synovial calcifications with even distribution in joint space, often encircling condyle
    - Linear calcification of articular cartilage
  - Late/severe CPPD deposition disease
    - Chunky, **diffusely calcified** mass
    - Calcified mass may have **ground-glass** appearance
    - Associated remodeling, **erosion**, or **mass effect** on condyle and adjacent structures
      - Bone density of condyle may be increased
    - May have associated demineralization/erosion of skull base, external auditory canal
      - May mimic **malignancy** due to extensive bone destruction
  - 50% have involvement of multiple joints: Knee, hand, wrist, shoulder, spine

MR Findings

- T1WI
  - **Low**- to intermediate-signal TMJ lesion
  - Calcified soft tissue mass in articular space
    - Expansion of joint capsule and joint space
    - ± joint effusion
  - Remodeling or erosion of mandibular condyle
- T2WI
  - **Hypointense**, somewhat heterogeneous periarticular mass
  - Soft tissue swelling and **edema** of surrounding muscles
- T1WI C+
  - Heterogeneously enhancing lesion

Imaging Recommendations

- Best imaging tool
  - Combination bone CT + TMJ MR
- Protocol advice
  - Thin-section bone CT-enhanced TMJ MR

DIFFERENTIAL DIAGNOSIS

Synovial Chondromatosis

- Synovial membrane metaplasia with formation of hyaline cartilage foci
- Multiple small, **calcified loose bodies** in superior joint space
  - Usually does not form contiguous solid mass
  - Loose bodies **larger** and more unevenly distributed than CPPD deposition disease
- Associated condylar osteoarthritis

Chondrosarcoma

- **Calcified** or partially calcified **TMJ mass**
- Tends to arise from or be intimately associated with condyle
- Condylar erosion, resorption
- T2 signal > CPPD deposition disease; more diffusely enhancing
- Often extends into masticator space, parotid space, skull base, temporal bone
- Solitary: Other joints often involved with CPPD deposition disease

Degenerative Disease

- Loose articular bodies ("joint mice") may simulate calcification of CPPD deposition disease
- Associated condylar osteoarthritis
- Joint mouse usually single and varies in size
  - CPPD deposition disease has finer calcifications and mass effect

Chondroblastoma

- Arises from epiphysis of distal femur, proximal tibia, proximal humerus
  - Rare in TMJ
- Lytic condylar expansion ± calcified mass
- May infiltrate through disc and capsule
- 3rd decade; male predilection

PATHOLOGY

General Features

- Etiology
  - Metabolic disturbance of phosphate metabolism
    - Elevated levels of inorganic phosphate in joint in combination with abnormal cartilage matrix serve as nucleation point for crystal formation
  - Various proposed etiologies
    - Hereditary: Often autosomal dominant or familial

- Sporadic (idiopathic)
- Associated with metabolic disease
  - Hyperparathyroidism
  - Hypothyroidism
  - Hypophosphatasia
  - Rheumatoid arthritis, other chronic arthritides
  - Hemochromatosis
  - Hypomagnesemia
  - Renal failure
- Associated with trauma or surgery

- Associated abnormalities
  - Often associated with disc **displacement**
  - Mass effect may occur due to crystal deposition in **adjacent** soft tissue structures

Staging, Grading, & Classification

- Classification
  - Pseudogout
    - **Acute** presentation of CPPD deposition disease
    - Crystals shed from cartilage surface, possibly precipitated by damage to cartilage, e.g., by trauma
  - Tophaceous pseudogout
    - **Massive** or **tumorous** calcium pyrophosphate crystal deposits
    - Often mistaken for benign or malignant cartilage lesion, such as **chondrosarcoma**

Gross Pathologic & Surgical Features

- Nodular, friable, gritty granulomatous tissue within joint space ± periarticular soft tissues
- Joint aspirate: Bloodstained, thick, and milky

Microscopic Features

- Calcium pyrophosphate **crystals** in synovial fluid is diagnostic
  - Crystals **birefringent** under polarized light
    - Gout = nonrefringent crystals of uric acid
- Metaplastic chondroid tissue
  - Pleomorphic hyperchromatic nuclei

CLINICAL ISSUES

Presentation

- Most common signs/symptoms
  - Preauricular pain
  - Joint swelling from intermittent arthritic attacks
  - Occasionally asymptomatic
- Other signs/symptoms
  - Crepitus in TMJ
  - Trismus
  - Malocclusion
  - Otalgia
  - Hearing loss
  - Tinnitus

Demographics

- Age
  - Most common in middle age or elderly
    - Increased prevalence with age
- Gender
  - Males > females
    - Some studies show female predominance

Natural History & Prognosis

- Acute attacks or chronic pain secondary to degenerative disease
  - Acute presentation mimics symptoms of **gout**
  - Chronic presentation mimics symptoms of **degenerative joint disease**

Treatment

- Basis of treatment
  - Prevention of crystal formation
  - Dissolution of crystals
  - Decreasing biologic consequences of crystal-cell interactions
- Acute: Medications such as colchicine, steroids, NSAIDs, ASA
- Large crystal deposits: Surgical debridement
- Occasionally, joint reconstruction

DIAGNOSTIC CHECKLIST

Consider

- Appearance may mimic malignancy: Chondrosarcoma

SELECTED REFERENCES

1. Laviv A et al: Pseudogout in the temporomandibular joint with imaging, arthroscopic, operative, and pathologic findings. Report of an unusual case. J Oral Maxillofac Surg. 73(6):1106-12, 2015
2. Abdelsayed RA et al: Tophaceous pseudogout of the temporomandibular joint: a series of 3 cases. Oral Surg Oral Med Oral Pathol Oral Radiol. 117(3):369-75, 2014
3. Lv H et al: A case of pseudogout of the temporomandibular joint with giant cell reparative granuloma of the temporal bone. Am J Otolaryngol. 34(6):762-5, 2013
4. Valentini V et al: Diagnosis and treatment of synovial chondromatosis of the TMJ: a clinical case. Ann Stomatol (Roma). 4(3-4):269-72, 2013
5. Magarelli N et al: Imaging of chondrocalcinosis: calcium pyrophosphate dihydrate (CPPD) crystal deposition disease – imaging of common sites of involvement. Clin Exp Rheumatol. 30(1):118-25, 2012
6. Matsumura Y et al: Synovial chondromatosis of the temporomandibular joint with calcium pyrophosphate dihydrate crystal deposition disease (pseudogout). Dentomaxillofac Radiol. 41(8):703-7, 2012
7. Srinivasan V et al: Calcium pyrophosphate deposition disease of the temporomandibular joint. J Neurol Surg Rep. 73(1):6-8, 2012
8. Zweifel D et al: Tophaceuos calcium pyrophosphate dihydrate deposition disease of the temporomandibular joint: the preferential site? J Oral Maxillofac Surg. 70(1):60-7, 2012
9. Meng J et al: A case of destructive calcium pyrophosphate dihydrate crystal deposition disease of the temporomandibular joint: a diagnostic challenge. Int J Oral Maxillofac Surg. 40(12):1431-7, 2011
10. Sklenicka S et al: Pseudogout of the temporomandibular joint: an uncommon cause of temporomandibular joint pain and swelling. Oral Surg Oral Med Oral Pathol Oral Radiol Endod. 111(6):709-14, 2011
11. Kamani T et al: Chondrocalcinosis of the temporomandibular joint: a rare but important diagnosis. Ear Nose Throat J. 88(9):E6-9, 2009
12. Naqvi AH et al: Calcium pyrophosphate dihydrate deposition disease (CPPD)/pseudogout of the temporomandibular joint - FNA findings and microanalysis. Cytojournal. 5:8, 2008
13. Reynolds JL et al: Tophaceous calcium pyrophosphate dihydrate deposition disease of the temporomandibular joint. J Rheumatol. 35(4):717-21, 2008
14. Marsot-Dupuch K et al: Massive calcium pyrophosphate dihydrate crystal deposition disease: a cause of pain of the temporomandibular joint. AJNR Am J Neuroradiol. 25(5):876-9, 2004
15. Greaves S et al: Bilateral temporomandibular joint pseudogout. Br Dent J. 192(1):25-7, 2002
16. Aoyama S et al: Differential diagnosis of calcium pyrophosphate dihydrate deposition of the temporomandibular joint. Br J Oral Maxillofac Surg. 38(5):550-3, 2000
17. Goudot P et al: A destructive calcium pyrophosphate dihydrate deposition disease of the temporomandibular joint. J Craniofac Surg. 10(5):385-8, 1999
18. Chuong R et al: Bilateral pseudogout of the temporomandibular joint: report of case and review of literature. J Oral Maxillofac Surg. 53(6):691-4, 1995
19. Ishida T et al: Tophaceous pseudogout (tumoral calcium pyrophosphate dihydrate crystal deposition disease). Hum Pathol. 26(6):587-93, 1995

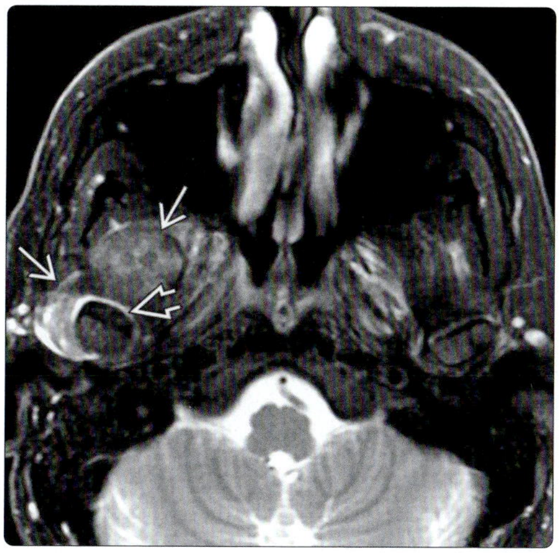

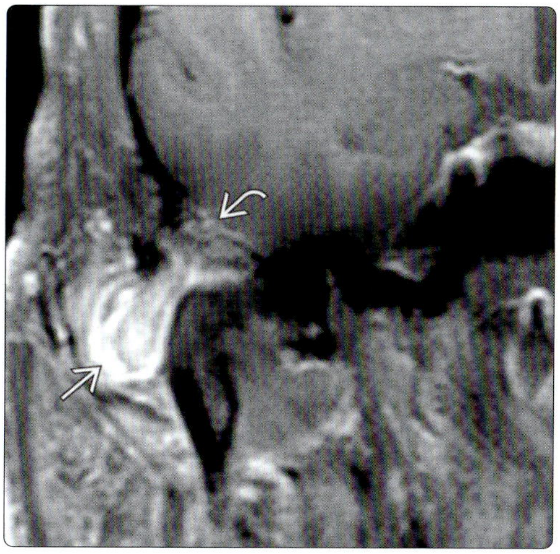

(Left) *Axial T2WI FS MR in a patient with CPPD deposition disease in the right TMJ shows a heterogeneous but predominantly low signal intensity lesion along the margins of the TMJ. Note the increased signal intensity from joint space fluid around the mandibular condyle.* **(Right)** *Coronal T1WI C+ FS MR in the same patient shows enhancement of the inferolateral mass. Note the glenoid fossa defect and mild dural enhancement but no intracranial extension.*

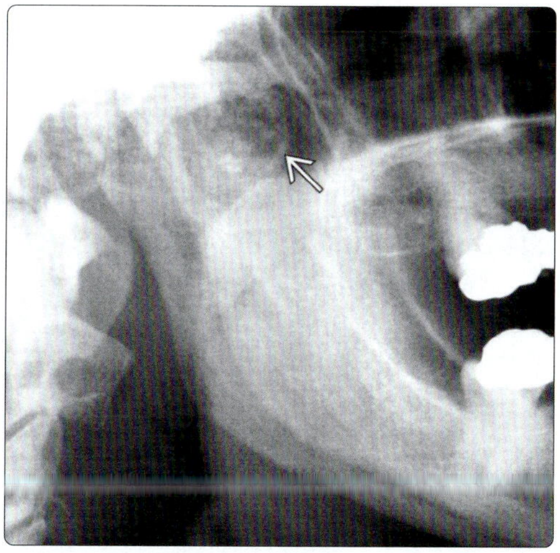

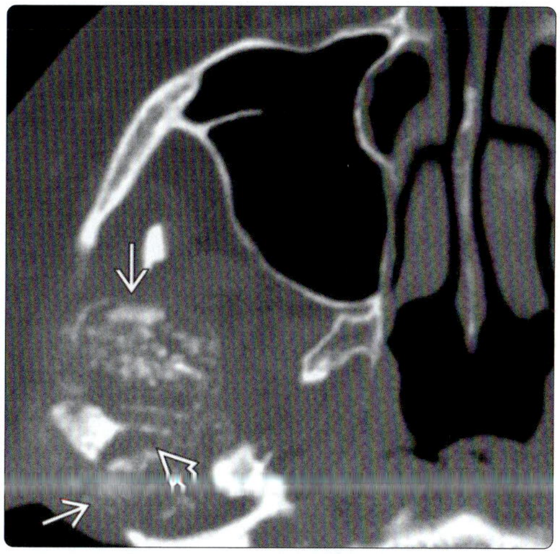

(Left) *Lateral radiograph of the mandible shows a large, diffusely calcified mass representing CPPD deposition disease associated with the TMJ. Due to superimposition of the 2 sides, it is not possible to distinguish whether the mass is on the right or left side.* **(Right)** *Axial bone CT in the same patient shows the extent of the well-defined mass located anteriorly and posteriorly to the right condyle. A large, radiolucent, erosive defect is visible at the medial aspect of the condyle.*

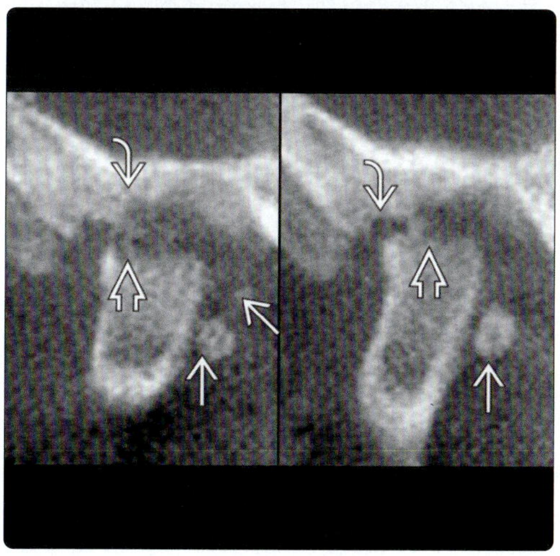

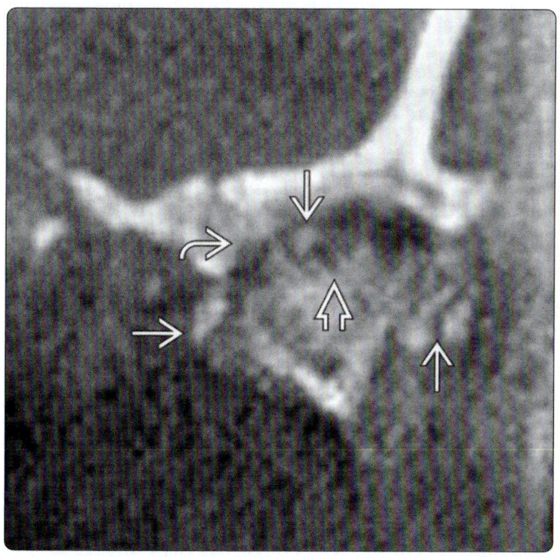

(Left) *Sagittal reformatted CBCT of CPPD deposition disease of the left TMJ shows large, radiopaque masses in the joint space and erosions of the condyle and glenoid fossa accompanied by sclerosis.* **(Right)** *Coronal reformatted CBCT in the same patient shows smaller calcified masses laterally, medially, and superiorly to the condyle. Note the extensive erosions of the condylar articulating surface and of the medial aspect of the glenoid fossa. This appearance simulates chondrosarcoma.*

TMJ Primary Synovial Chondromatosis

KEY FACTS

TERMINOLOGY

- Definition: Development of cartilaginous nodules within subsynovial connective tissue that subsequently detach, ossify, and form loose/free-floating bodies in joint space

IMAGING

- Most commonly in **superior** joint space of TMJ
- Multiple **calcified/ossified nodules** surrounding condyle
- Condylar articular surface **degenerative** changes (irregularity and sclerosis) commonly seen
- May see soft tissue **swelling** or mass with mixed-density solid portion representing metaplasia of synovial tissue
- MR: **Hypointense nodules** in superior joint space
  - Superior joint space **effusion ± expansion**
  - **Ring-like** signal: High-signal fluid surrounds collection of hypointense nodules

TOP DIFFERENTIAL DIAGNOSES

- Calcium pyrophosphate dihydrate deposition disease
- Osteochondritis dissecans
- Chondrosarcoma
- Degenerative disease, TMJ

CLINICAL ISSUES

- Preauricular pain, swelling
- Symptoms simulate **TMJ dysfunction**
- Adults (mean age: 4th decade)
- F:M = 4:1
- Recurrence rate low
- Malignant transformation reported but **rare**

DIAGNOSTIC CHECKLIST

- **CT for diagnosis**: May get false-negative diagnosis with 2D imaging
- Evaluate osseous components of TMJ to rule out presence of degenerative changes
  - Degenerative changes make diagnosis of secondary synovial chondromatosis more likely

(Left) *Axial bone CT of synovial chondromatosis shows multiple small, calcified nodules ➡ in the right temporomandibular joint (TMJ). The condyle is sclerotic and somewhat irregular ⇨ with anterior narrowing of the joint space due to degenerative change.* **(Right)** *Gross pathology specimens taken from the same patient vary in size from 2-10 mm, and the nodules have an irregular shape. The colors of the nodules range from milky white to almost translucent.*

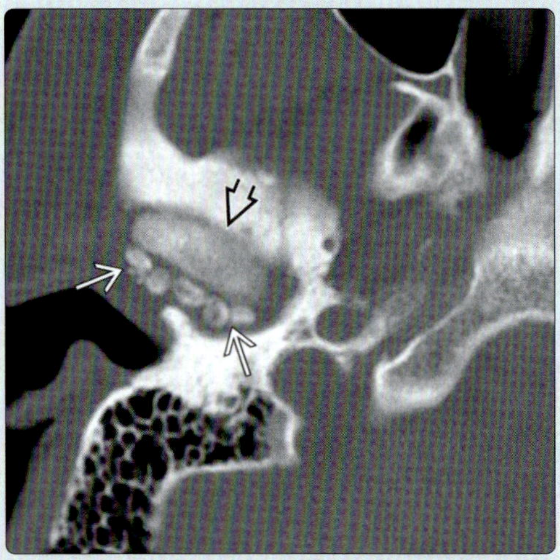

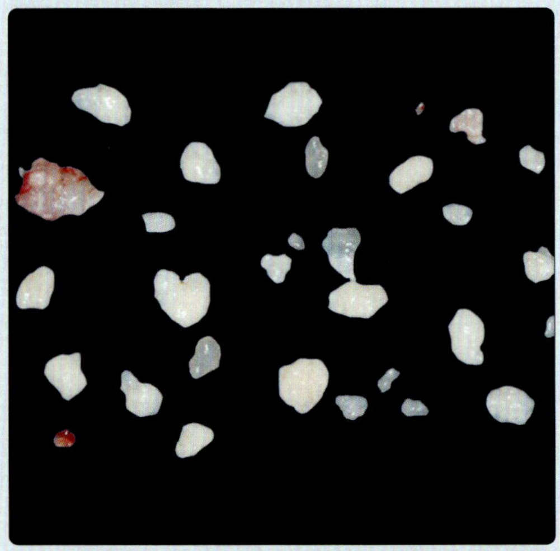

(Left) *Sagittal oblique T2 FS MR in the same patient shows distension of the right TMJ capsule with hyperintense fluid ➡ surrounding the low-signal, calcified loose bodies ⇨.* **(Right)** *Longitudinal oblique PD FSE MR in the same patient shows corticated, centrally isointense loose bodies ➡ in the superior joint space. Note the absence of cortical defects or marrow changes in the condyle ⇨, making the diagnosis of osteochondritis dissecans unlikely.*

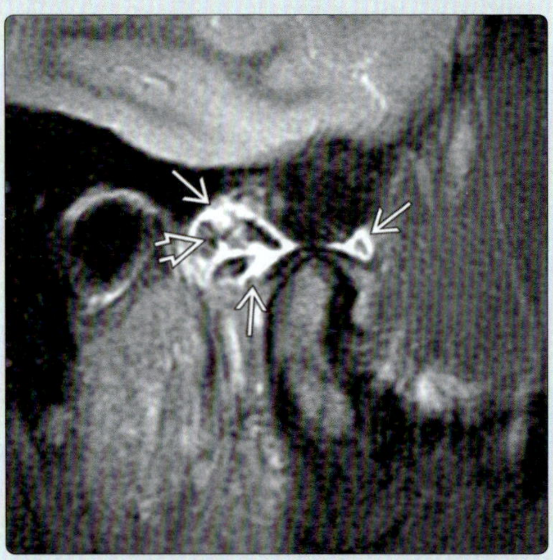

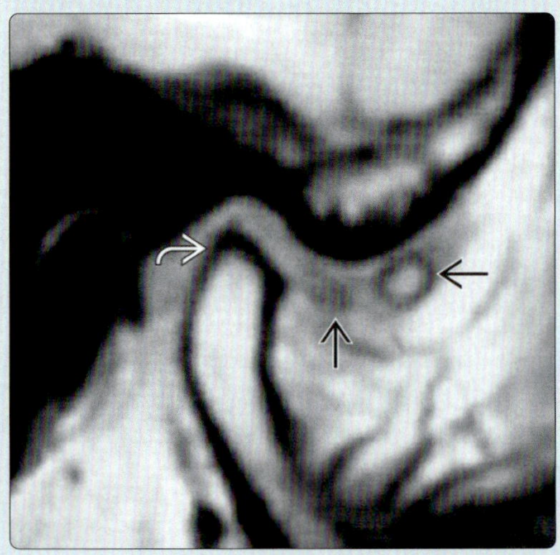

TERMINOLOGY

Synonyms

- Osteochondromatosis
- Synovial chondrometaplasia
- Synovial chondrosis

Definitions

- Development of cartilaginous nodules within subsynovial connective tissue that subsequently detach, ossify, and form loose/free-floating bodies in joint space
  - Nonneoplastic
  - Uncommon

IMAGING

General Features

- Best diagnostic clue
  - Multiple **ossified nodules** (loose bodies) in superior joint space
- Location
  - Usually affects larger diarthrodial joints
    - Knee, elbow, wrist, hip
  - If present in temporomandibular joint (TMJ), most commonly found in **superior** joint space
    - Reported predilection for right TMJ
  - Rarely extracapsular extension
    - Most common areas of spread include masticator space, parotid space, or middle cranial fossa
- Size
  - Calcifications **vary** from millimeters to centimeters

Imaging Recommendations

- Best imaging tool
  - TMJ MR ± bone CT
- Protocol advice
  - Use high-resolution CT or CBCT since loose bodies often < 1 mm in diameter and can otherwise be overlooked

CT Findings

- Bone CT
  - Multiple **calcified/ossified nodules** surrounding mandibular condyle
  - Condylar articular surface **degenerative** changes commonly seen
    - Irregularity and sclerosis
  - Widened joint space
  - May see soft tissue **swelling** or mass with mixed-density solid portion representing metaplasia of synovial tissue
  - **Intracranial** extension reported

MR Findings

- T1WI
  - MR helps define tissue planes between mass and surrounding soft tissue
    - Enables differentiation from parotid neoplasm
    - Helps exclude temporal lobe involvement in cases of intracranial extension
  - Multiple **hypointense nodules** in superior joint space
  - Synovial thickening
  - Separate from articular disc
- T2WI
  - Superior joint space **effusion ± expansion**
    - Mildly inhomogeneous bright signal may represent nonossified/calcified cartilage nodules
  - Occasionally will not see effusion, but may see heterogeneous signal intensity indicating soft tissue mass or cartilage nodules
  - **Ring-like** signal: High-signal fluid surrounds collection of hypointense nodules
- T1WI C+
  - Enhancing synovium

DIFFERENTIAL DIAGNOSIS

Calcium Pyrophosphate Dihydrate Deposition Disease

- Acute and chronic forms **rare** in TMJ
- Tophaceous pseudogout: Rare form of calcium pyrophosphate dihydrate deposition disease most frequent in TMJ
  - Calcified mass involving condyle or joint space
  - May mimic chondrosarcoma

Osteochondritis Dissecans

- Reactive joint condition that can cause **focal** calcifications but not accompanied by large calcifications as with synovial chondromatosis
- Results from transchondral **fracture**
  - Failure of healing and fragment displacement
- Condylar erosive defect with adjacent fragment

Chondrosarcoma

- Rarely arises directly from synovium
- **Destructive** and infiltrative with lytic condylar defects
- Associated intra- &/or extracapsular enhancing **mass**
  - May see small, focal calcifications within and around joint

Degenerative Disease, TMJ

- **Loose joint bodies** ("joint mice") a.k.a. secondary synovial chondromatosis
  - "Joint mice" usually **smaller** and **fewer** than seen in primary synovial chondromatosis

PATHOLOGY

General Features

- Etiology
  - Unknown

Staging, Grading, & Classification

- Primary
  - More **aggressive** course
  - Fibroblasts beneath synovial membrane undergo metaplasia and deposit chondromucin
  - Cartilage bodies enlarge and detach from synovial membrane
- Secondary
  - Associated with inflammatory joint disease, noninflammatory arthropathy, joint overuse, and microtrauma
  - Fragments of cartilaginous tissue become dislodged in synovial fluid and ossify over time

Gross Pathologic & Surgical Features

- Multiple hard, smooth-surfaced, gray-white nodules floating freely in joint space

Microscopic Features

- Synovial hyperplasia with round cellular cartilage islands within connective tissue ± loose bodies
- Synovial membrane **inflammation** with lymphocytes, macrophages, giant cells
- Cartilage metaplasia
- 3 histological phases (Milgram)
  - Stage 1 (early, active)
    - Intrasynovial involvement
    - Metaplasia only in synovial membrane
    - No loose bodies
      - Formation of cartilage islands confined to hyperemic and edematous subsynovial connective tissue
  - Stage 2 (intermediate, transitional)
    - Intrasynovial involvement
    - Loose bodies
    - Metaplasia in synovial membrane
  - Stage 3 (advanced)
    - Multiple loose bodies varying from 1 mm to > 10 mm
    - No sign of intrasynovial disease

CLINICAL ISSUES

Presentation

- Most common signs/symptoms
  - Preauricular pain, swelling
- Other signs/symptoms
  - Symptoms simulate **TMJ dysfunction**
    - Trismus
    - Crepitus
    - Malocclusion

Demographics

- Age
  - Adults
    - Mean: 4th decade
- Gender
  - F:M = 4:1

Natural History & Prognosis

- Recurrence rate low
- Malignant transformation reported but **rare**

Treatment

- Arthroscopy
  - Removal of joint loose bodies
- Synovectomy
- Condylectomy

DIAGNOSTIC CHECKLIST

Consider

- **CT for diagnosis**
  - 2D imaging often leads to false-negative diagnosis
- May not see loose bodies with MR but will see swelling and fluid in joint
- Evaluate osseous components of TMJ to rule out presence of degenerative changes
  - Degenerative changes make diagnosis of secondary synovial chondromatosis more likely

Image Interpretation Pearls

- Mixed-density solid portion and fluid in lesion help to distinguish from other entities

SELECTED REFERENCES

1. Liu X et al: Clinical and imaging findings of temporomandibular joint synovial chondromatosis: an analysis of 10 cases and literature review. J Oral Maxillofac Surg. 74(11):2159-2168, 2016
2. Chen MJ et al: Synovial chondromatosis of the tempromandibular joint: relationship between MRI information and potential aggressive behavior. J Craniomaxillofac Surg. 43(3):349-54, 2015
3. Ma X: [Diagnoses and treatment for synovial chondromatosis of temporomandibular joint.] Zhonghua Kou Qiang Yi Xue Za Zhi. 49(7):390-3, 2014
4. Peyrot H et al: Synovial chondromatosis of the temporomandibular joint: CT and MRI findings. Diagn Interv Imaging. 95(6):613-4, 2014
5. Sink J et al: Synovial chondromatosis of the temporomandibular joint: clinical, cytologic, histologic, radiologic, therapeutic aspects, and differential diagnosis of an uncommon lesion. Oral Surg Oral Med Oral Pathol Oral Radiol. 117(3):e269-74, 2014
6. Testaverde L et al: CT and MR findings in synovial chondromatosis of the temporo-mandibular joint: our experience and review of literature. Eur J Radiol. 78(3):414-8, 2011
7. Boffano P et al: Diagnosis and surgical management of synovial chondromatosis of the temporomandibular joint. J Craniofac Surg. 21(1):157-9, 2010
8. Guarda-Nardini L et al: Synovial chondromatosis of the temporomandibular joint: a case description with systematic literature review. Int J Oral Maxillofac Surg. 39(8):745-55, 2010
9. Meng J et al: Clinical and radiologic findings of synovial chondromatosis affecting the temporomandibular joint. Oral Surg Oral Med Oral Pathol Oral Radiol Endod. 109(3):441-8, 2010
10. Ida M et al: An investigation of magnetic resonance imaging features in 14 patients with synovial chondromatosis of the temporomandibular joint. Dentomaxillofac Radiol. 37(4):213-9, 2008
11. Balliu E et al: Synovial chondromatosis of the temporomandibular joint: CT and MRI findings. Dentomaxillofac Radiol. 36(1):55-8, 2007
12. Ardekian L et al: Synovial chondromatosis of the temporomandibular joint: report and analysis of eleven cases. J Oral Maxillofac Surg. 63(7):941-7, 2005
13. Wu CW et al: Primary synovial chondromatosis of the temporomandibular joint. J Otolaryngol. 33(2):114-9, 2004
14. Holmlund AB et al: Synovial chondromatosis of the temporomandibular joint: clinical, surgical and histological aspects. Int J Oral Maxillofac Surg. 32(2):143-7, 2003
15. von Lindern JJ et al: Synovial chondromatosis of the temporomandibular joint: clinical, diagnostic, and histomorphologic findings. Oral Surg Oral Med Oral Pathol Oral Radiol Endod. 94(1):31-8, 2002
16. Koyama J et al: Synovial chondromatosis in the temporomandibular joint complicated by displacement and calcification of the articular disk: report of two cases. AJNR Am J Neuroradiol. 22(6):1203-6, 2001
17. Milgram JW: The classification of loose bodies in human joints. Clin Orthop Relat Res. (124):282-91, 1977

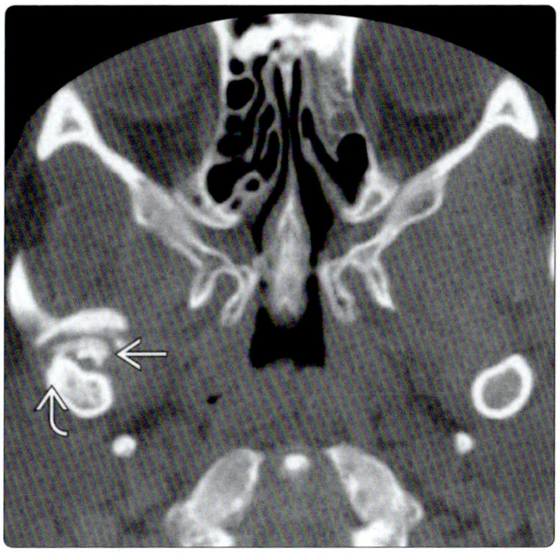

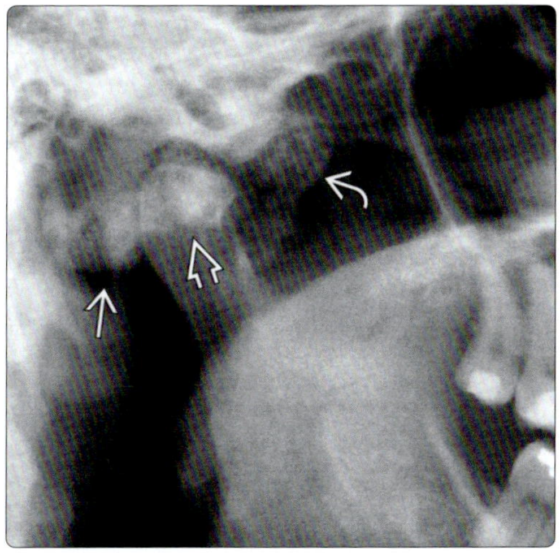

(Left) *Axial bone CT shows coarse calcifications located anteriorly to the condyle in the right TMJ. The condylar cortex is intact with lateral pole sclerosis due to degenerative changes.* **(Right)** *Panoramic projection of the right TMJ shows the condyle with a normal size and shape. A heterogeneous radiopacity is present anteriorly and posteriorly to the condyle. The large size of the mass will cause distension of the joint capsule.*

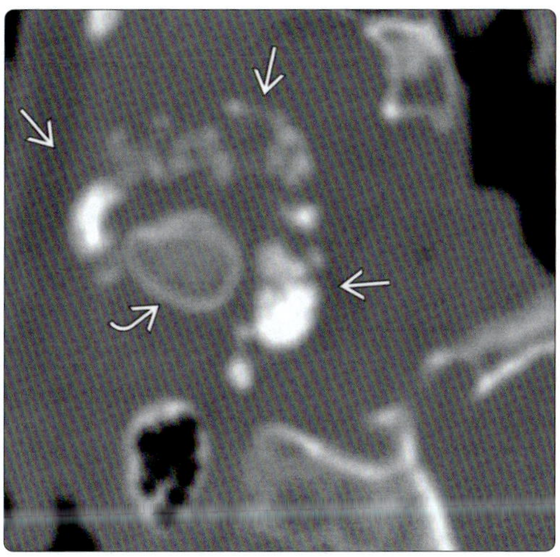

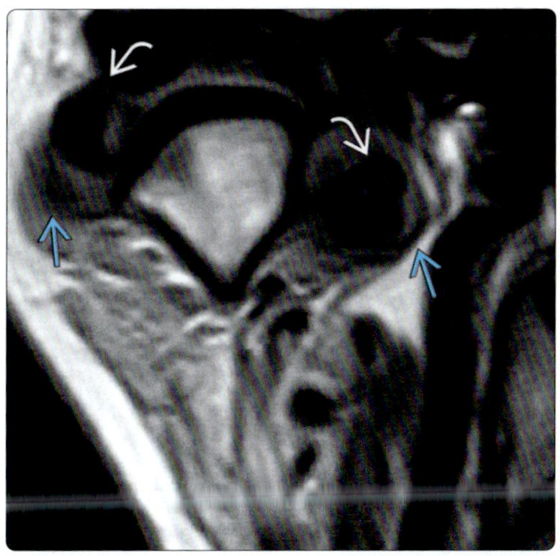

(Left) *Axial CT in the same patient shows multiple calcified/ossified loose bodies of various sizes distributed along the medial, lateral, and anterior aspects of the condyle. There is marked distension of the joint capsule.* **(Right)** *Coronal oblique T1 MR in the same patient shows low-signal ossified/calcified bodies within the confines of a distended capsule.*

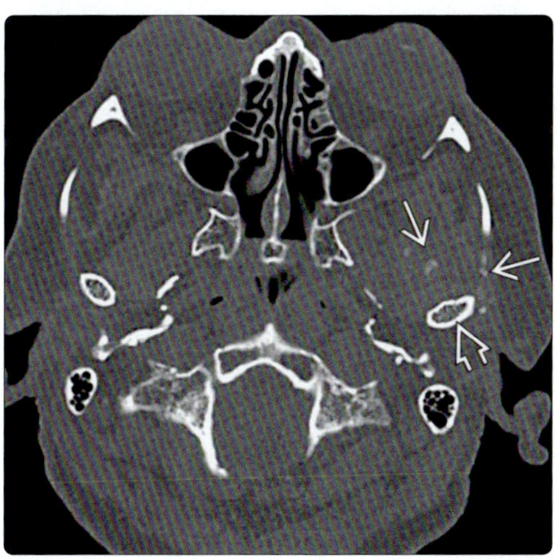

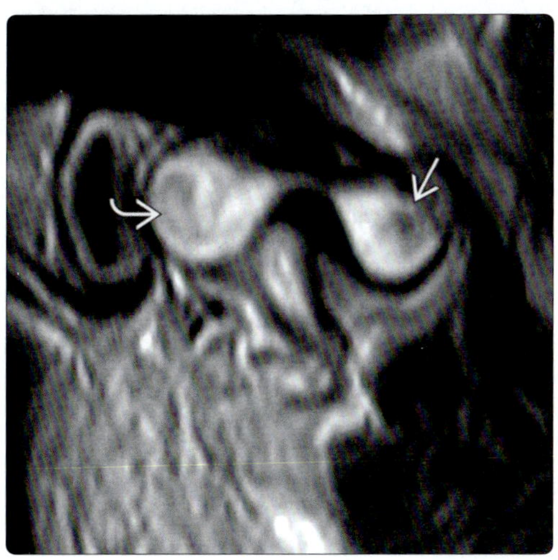

(Left) *Axial bone CT of a patient with synovial chondromatosis in the left TMJ shows a mass with multiple punctate calcifications located anteriorly and laterally to the condyle.* **(Right)** *Sagittal oblique T2 MR shows inhomogeneous signal consistent with cartilage nodules located posteriorly to the condyle and calcification/ossification located anteriorly to the condyle.*

TMJ Osteosarcoma

KEY FACTS

TERMINOLOGY

- Definition: Malignant bone tumor with ability to produce osteoid or immature bone

IMAGING

- Involvement of mandibular condyle **rare**
- Bone destruction with aggressive periosteal reaction ± tumor formation
  - Periosteal reaction: **"Hair on end"** or **sunburst spicules** of new bone perpendicular to cortex
- Often **invades** adjacent soft tissues and anatomic structures
- Can be **radiolucent, mixed, or sclerotic**
- **Poorly defined destructive** lesion of condyle with cortical erosion
- Mixture of radiolucent and sclerotic bone pattern most common type
- CT best for bone; MR best for soft tissue involvement
- Condyle may appear **enlarged** and composed of mottled bone pattern

TOP DIFFERENTIAL DIAGNOSES

- Metastatic disease
- Chondrosarcoma
- Aneurysmal bone cyst

CLINICAL ISSUES

- Similar to **arthrogenous TMD**: Decreased range of motion, restricted lateral movements, acquired occlusal changes, TMJ pain, headaches
- Preauricular swelling
- Mean age: 35 years; M > F
- Metastasizes later than osteosarcoma of other bones

DIAGNOSTIC CHECKLIST

- Consider metastatic disease if no aggressive periosteal reaction

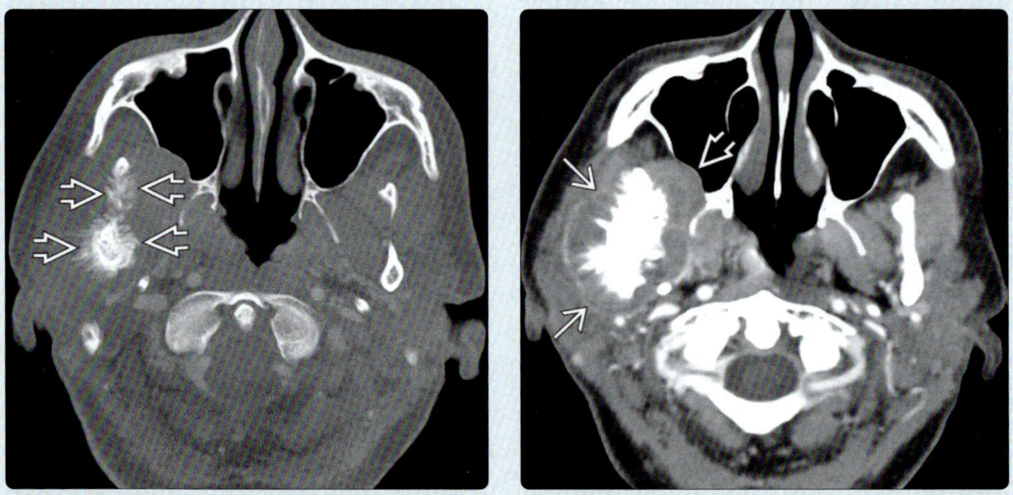

(Left) *Axial bone CT at the level of the sigmoid notch shows osteosarcoma involving the right mandibular ramus and condyle. The cortical margins are thickened and there is a spiculated periosteal reaction ➔ surrounding the affected bone. Note asymmetric swelling of the soft tissues of the right masticator space and overlying cheek.* **(Right)** *Axial CECT of the same patient shows the lesion displacing and likely invading the parotid gland posterolaterally ➔. The lesion extends to the right maxillary sinus ➔.*

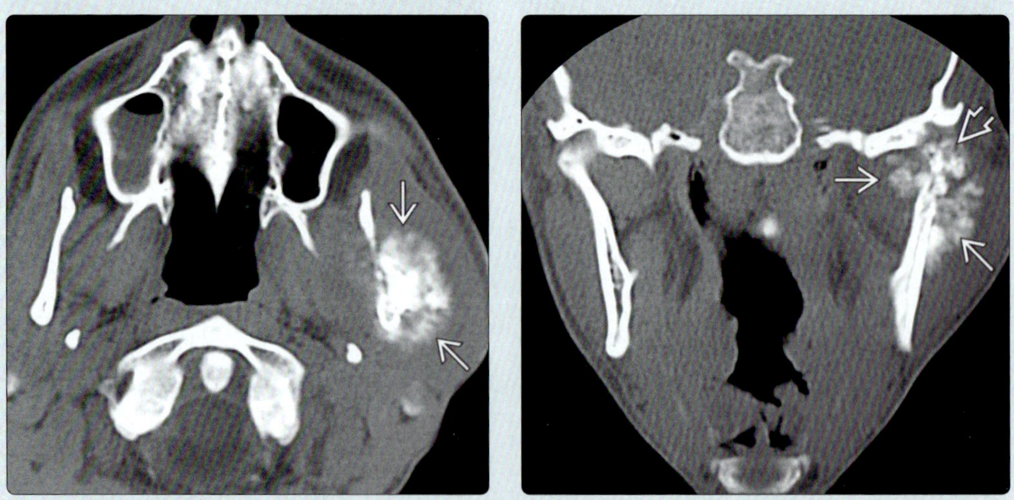

(Left) *Axial bone CT shows a large, aggressive osteosarcoma arising from the lateral surface of the superior aspect of the mandibular ramus. The lesion exhibits a sunburst periosteal reaction ➔ and formation of osteoid matrix.* **(Right)** *Coronal bone CT in the same patient shows the sunburst periosteal reaction involving the lateral and medial aspects of the ramus ➔ with patchy destruction and enlargement of the condyle ➔.*

TERMINOLOGY

Abbreviations

- Osteosarcoma (OS)

Definitions

- Malignant bone tumor with ability to produce osteoid or immature bone

IMAGING

General Features

- Best diagnostic clue
  - Bone destruction with aggressive periosteal reaction ± tumor formation
- Location
  - Mandible > maxilla
    - Body and angle of mandible most common maxillofacial sites; mandibular condyle **rare**
  - Often **invades** adjacent soft tissues and anatomic structures
- Morphology
  - Destructive lesion with osteoid formation

Radiographic Findings

- Can be **radiolucent, mixed, or sclerotic**
- **Poorly defined destructive** lesion of condyle with cortical erosion
- Occasional **periosteal** reaction: **"Hair on end"** or **sunburst spicules** of new bone perpendicular to cortex
  - May also be laminated

CT Findings

- CECT
  - Moderate enhancement of solid components
- CBCT and bone CT
  - Tumor often destroys cortex and invades adjacent soft tissue, producing **mass**
  - Condyle may appear **enlarged** and composed of mottled bone pattern

MR Findings

- Heterogeneous signal intensity on T1 and T2

Imaging Recommendations

- Best imaging tool
  - CT best for demonstrating degree of bone involvement, osseous destruction, osteoid matrix
  - MR best for soft tissue and intramedullary extent, relationship of tumor to soft tissue anatomy

DIFFERENTIAL DIAGNOSIS

Metastatic Disease to TMJ

- Appearance can be identical to OS
- Check patient history for primary tumor

Chondrosarcoma of TMJ

- Consider if some internal radiopacity present in tumor
- Chondrosarcoma radiopacities typically are shaped as arcs or whorls

Aneurysmal Bone Cyst of TMJ

- Expands rapidly, causes pain

PATHOLOGY

General Features

- Etiology
  - Jaw cases may occur after radiation to face

Staging, Grading, & Classification

- Several variants that differ in location, clinical behavior, and degree of cytologic atypia
- Conventional (classic) OS most frequent type

CLINICAL ISSUES

Presentation

- Most common signs/symptoms
  - Similar to arthrogenous TMD: Decreased range of motion, restricted lateral movements, acquired occlusal changes, TMJ pain, headaches
- Other signs/symptoms
  - Preauricular swelling

Demographics

- Age
  - Mean: 35 years
  - Occurs on average **10 years later than OS of long bones**
- Gender
  - M:F = 2:1
    - Some studies found female predominance
- Epidemiology
  - Only 5-6% of OSs occur in jaws; condylar involvement rare

Natural History & Prognosis

- OS of jaws **less aggressive** than OS of long bones
  - Metastasizes later than OS of other bones
  - Prognosis better if no paresthesia, smaller tumor size, clear surgical margins, more differentiated histological grade of tumor, younger age

Treatment

- Complete resection with wide margins
- Radiation and chemotherapy usually used for controlling metastatic spread or for palliation

DIAGNOSTIC CHECKLIST

Consider

- Metastatic disease if no aggressive periosteal reaction
- Consider XRT-induced sarcoma if patient had radiation years prior

Image Interpretation Pearls

- Aggressive periosteal reaction suggests OS

SELECTED REFERENCES

1. Uchiyama Y et al: MRI in a case of osteosarcoma in the temporomandibular joint. Dentomaxillofac Radiol. 43(2):20130280, 2014
2. Wang S et al: Osteosarcoma of the jaws: demographic and CT imaging features. Dentomaxillofac Radiol. 41(1):37-42, 2012
3. dos Santos DT et al: Osteosarcoma of the temporomandibular joint: report of 2 cases. Oral Surg Oral Med Oral Pathol Oral Radiol Endod. 94(5):641-7, 2002
4. Bennett JH et al: Osteosarcoma of the jaws: a 30-year retrospective review. Oral Surg Oral Med Oral Pathol Oral Radiol Endod. 90(3):323-32, 2000

TMJ Chondrosarcoma

KEY FACTS

TERMINOLOGY

- Chondrosarcoma (CS): Malignant tumor arising from cartilage cells

IMAGING

- Nonenhancing mass with flocculent calcifications around condyle and in joint space ± osseous **destruction**
- Internal calcifications may be **cloud-like** with calcified **whorls and arcs**
- Often erosion of articular fossa with involvement of infratemporal fossa, temporal bone, and middle cranial fossa
- **Widened** joint space
- Condyle may appear **enlarged** and lengthened
- Articular fossa may also enlarge if condylar lesion slow growing
- Bone CT or CBCT to show tumor extent, invasion of adjacent structures, and intralesional calcifications

TOP DIFFERENTIAL DIAGNOSES

- Synovial chondromatosis
- Calcium pyrophosphate dihydrate deposition disease
- Metastatic disease

CLINICAL ISSUES

- Preauricular **swelling**
- Mean: 50 years; range: 11-75 years
- F:M = 2:1
- Treatment: Wide surgical excision since locally aggressive

DIAGNOSTIC CHECKLIST

- Difficult to differentiate between benign and low-grade malignant chondrogenic tumors, so **diagnosis is often based on imaging findings**
- Permeative borders with infiltration of cortical or trabecular bone favors diagnosis of CS
- Arc and whorl-like radiopacities with **radiolucent centers** favor CS

(Left) *Cropped panoramic radiograph shows a chondrosarcoma (CS) of the left condyle. The lesion is radiolucent with well-defined borders and a lobulated appearance. The condyle is enlarged.* **(Right)** *Axial NECT of the same patient shows that the medial aspect of the CS in the left condyle is radiolucent. The lateral aspect has more internal radiopacity and has expanded laterally. Note the calcifications anterior and lateral to the condyle.*

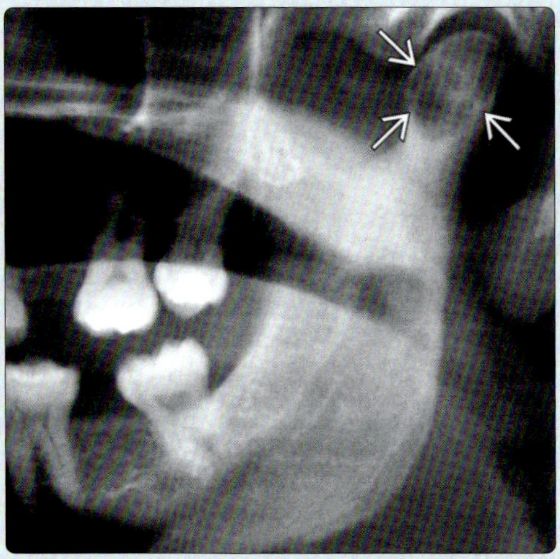

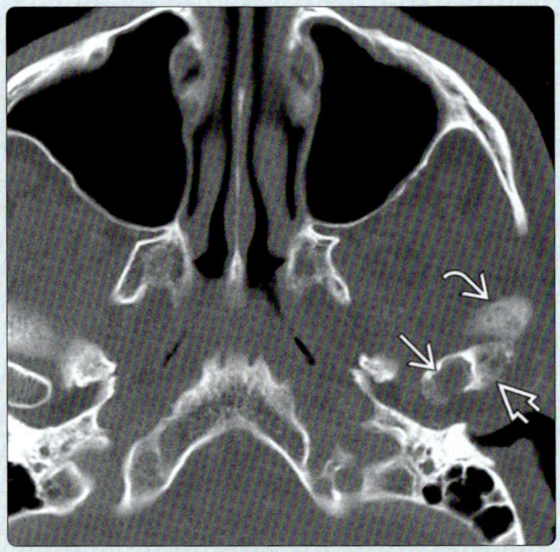

(Left) *Sagittal reformat NECT shows a CS of the left TMJ. Note the condylar deformity and flocculent whorl-like calcifications anterior and posterior to the condyle in the soft tissues surrounding the joint. The condyle is anteriorly displaced by the posterior mass.* **(Right)** *Axial NECT of the same patient shows an irregular sclerotic appearance of the condyle with multiple flocculent calcifications around the condyle.*

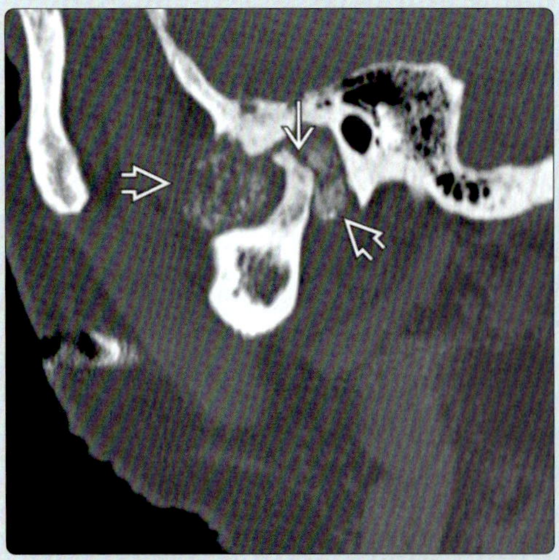

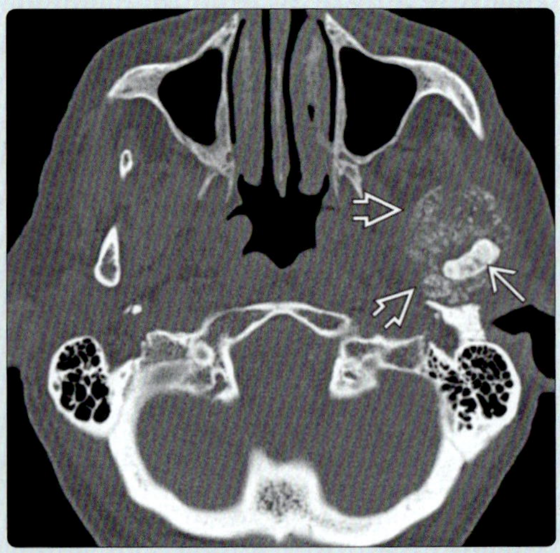

TERMINOLOGY

Abbreviations

- Chondrosarcoma (CS)

Synonyms

- Chondrogenic sarcoma

Definitions

- Malignant tumor arising from cartilage cells
- Can occur centrally in bone, on periphery of bone (parosteal CS), or in soft tissue

IMAGING

General Features

- Best diagnostic clue
  - **Ringlet** pattern of calcification in and around condyle ± **spiculated** periosteal reaction
- Location
  - More common in long bones, pelvis, and ribs
  - Only 1-2% occur in H&N region
  - Coronoid process more frequently affected than condyle
- Size
  - Variable, usually > 2 cm
- Morphology
  - Irregularly shaped borders
  - May be well defined and corticated or permeative
  - If periosteal involvement, calcification perpendicular to bone surface: **Sunray spicules**

Radiographic Findings

- Radiography
  - Appearance varies depending on degree of tumor calcification
  - Internal calcifications may be **cloud-like** with calcified **whorls and arcs**
    - Often **radiolucent center** in each radiopacity

CT Findings

- Bone CT
  - Nonenhancing mass with flocculent calcifications around condyle and in joint space **± osseous destruction**
  - Often, erosion of articular fossa with involvement of infratemporal fossa, temporal bone, and middle cranial fossa
  - **Widened** joint space
  - Condyle may appear **enlarged** and lengthened
    - Articular fossa may also enlarge if condylar lesion slow growing
  - Soft tissue **mass**

MR Findings

- T1WI
  - Low to intermediate signal intensity relative to gray matter
    - Low-signal foci within tumor may suggest tumor calcifications
- T2WI
  - High T2 signal
  - Hypointense foci (calcifications) less common than on CT
- T1WI C+
  - Heterogeneously enhancing mass
    - Whorls of enhancing lines within tumor matrix often seen

Imaging Recommendations

- Best imaging tool
  - Bone CT or CBCT to show tumor extent, invasion of adjacent structures, and intralesional calcifications
  - MR to analyze bone marrow extension and involvement of adjacent soft tissue
- Protocol advice
  - Sagittal, coronal, and axial reformats of TMJ and surrounding structures

Nuclear Medicine Findings

- Bone scan
  - Increased uptake in central CS
  - Reveals metabolically active areas in peripheral CS
  - Whole-body scans
    - Identify **metastases**
    - No uptake: Rules out malignant transformation of osteochondroma

DIFFERENTIAL DIAGNOSIS

Synovial Chondromatosis

- Radiographic and histological findings can mimic CS
- Differentiation based on clinical and radiographic behavior
  - CS shows destructive behavior and invasion

Calcium Pyrophosphate Dihydrate Deposition Disease

- Crystals in articular and periarticular structures
- Calcified material in joint space and degenerative joint disease of TMJ
- Acute attacks, pain, preauricular swelling, trismus, mandibular deviation

Metastatic Disease

- Radiolucent destruction of condyle in patient with primary malignancy
- TMJ involvement usually associated with mandibular or skeletal metastases
- Metastases can be radiopaque and mimic CS
  - Breast
  - Prostate

Osteosarcoma

- **Rare** in TMJ
- Typically destructive
- Varied radiographic appearance: Radiolucent, mixed, radiopaque
- May have **sunray** or spiculated periosteal reaction

PATHOLOGY

General Features

- Associated abnormalities
  - Maffucci syndrome: Short stature, underdeveloped muscles, and multiple enchondromas; CSs may develop
- CS formed from cartilage in tissues not normally harboring cartilage or form in cartilage cap of exostosis or enchondroma

- Forerunner may be vestigial rests of multipotential differentiation of mesenchymal cells

Staging, Grading, & Classification

- Classification
  - Primary CS arising from undifferentiated perichondrial cells
  - Secondary CS arising from metamorphosed cells either in enchondroma or osteochondroma
  - Mesenchymal CS arising from primitive mesenchymal cells (rare)
- Alternate classification
  - Clear cell
  - Dedifferentiated
  - Myxoid
  - Mesenchymal
- Evans classification
  - Grading based on relative degrees of cellularity, atypia, and pleomorphism
  - Grade I (low grade): Chondroid matrix with scattered clusters of chondrocytes with near-normal nuclei and no mitotic figures
  - Grade II: Higher degree of cellularity with less chondroid matrix, increased mitotic figures, multinucleation, and hyperchromatic vesicular nuclei
  - Grade III (high grade): Irregularly shaped chondrocytes in myxoid matrix with increased nuclear pleomorphism

Gross Pathologic & Surgical Features

- Firm, bluish-white, pearly translucency with faceting or lobulation
- White or yellowish gritty speckling corresponding to calcified or ossified parts of tumor

Microscopic Features

- Hypercellular tumor composed of chondrocytes with hyperchromatic, pleomorphic nuclei and prominent nucleoli
- Hyaline matrix may calcify in ringlets
- Intercellular matrix solid in hyaline type compared to mucinous/gelatinous matrix in myxoid or mixed types
- Histology may overlap with or be **confused with benign chondroid tumors**

CLINICAL ISSUES

Presentation

- Most common signs/symptoms
  - Preauricular **swelling**
- Other signs/symptoms
  - Mandibular deviation
  - Occlusal changes
  - Preauricular pain
  - Pain on mastication
  - May have hearing loss
  - Limitation of motion

Demographics

- Age
  - Mean: 50 years
    - Range: 11-75 years
- Gender
  - F:M = 2:1
- Epidemiology
  - CS more common than osteosarcoma in condyle but still very rare

Natural History & Prognosis

- Local recurrence in TMJ independent of tumor grading
  - Prognosis factors
    - Inadequate surgical therapy
    - Tumor location and extent
      - 5-year survival = 90% for grade I CS
      - 5-year survival = 50% for grades II and III CS
- Metastatic rate low
  - Metastases to lungs and vertebrae
- Death often due to local recurrence and invasion of cranial base
- Distant metastases can occur > 2 decades later
  - Prognostic indicators are size, location, grade, and surgical resectability of tumor

Treatment

- Wide surgical excision since locally aggressive
- ± radiation therapy &/or chemotherapy
- Occasionally immunotherapy, cryosurgery

DIAGNOSTIC CHECKLIST

Consider

- Difficult to differentiate between benign and low-grade malignant chondrogenic tumors, so **diagnosis is often based on imaging findings**
  - Permeative borders with infiltration of cortical or trabecular bone favors diagnosis of CS

Image Interpretation Pearls

- Arc and whorl-like radiopacities with **radiolucent centers** favors CS

SELECTED REFERENCES

1. Giorgione C et al: Temporo-mandibular joint chondrosarcoma: case report and review of the literature. Acta Otorhinolaryngol Ital. 35(3):208-11, 2015
2. Kumar Reddy DS et al: Central chondrosarcoma of a pediatric mandibular condyle: a case report and review. Ann Maxillofac Surg. 4(1):85-9, 2014
3. Rath R et al: Dedifferentiated chondrosarcoma of temporomandibular joint: atypical features of a rare case. J Clin Diagn Res. 8(9):ZD09-11, 2014
4. Goutzanis L et al: Chondrosarcoma of the mandibular condyle in a patient with Werner syndrome: a case report. J Craniomaxillofac Surg. 41(7):e170-4, 2013
5. Ramos-Murguialday M et al: Chondrosarcoma of the mandible involving angle, ramus, and condyle. J Craniofac Surg. 23(4):1216-9, 2012
6. González-Pérez LM et al: Temporomandibular joint chondrosarcoma: case report. J Craniomaxillofac Surg. 39(1):79-83, 2011
7. Xu B et al: Secondary chondrosarcoma in the mandibular condyle. Dentomaxillofac Radiol. 40(5):320-3, 2011
8. Garzino-Demo P et al: Chondrosarcoma of the temporomandibular joint: a case report and review of the literature. J Oral Maxillofac Surg. 68(8):2005-11, 2010
9. Gallego L et al: Chondrosarcoma of the temporomandibular joint. A case report and review of the literature. Med Oral Patol Oral Cir Bucal. 14(1):E39-43, 2009
10. Oliveira RC et al: Chondrosarcoma of the temporomandibular joint: a case report in a child. J Orofac Pain. 23(3):275-81, 2009
11. Warner BF et al: Temporomandibular joint neoplasms and pseudotumors. Adv Anat Pathol. 7(6):365-81, 2000
12. Sesenna E et al: Chondrosarcoma of the temporomandibular joint: a case report and review of the literature. J Oral Maxillofac Surg. 55(11):1348-52, 1997

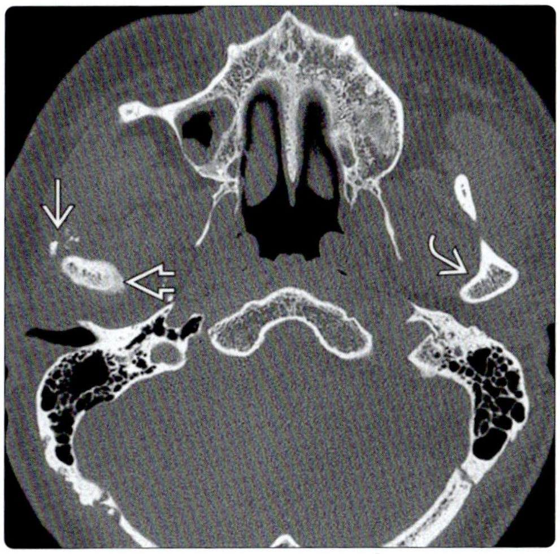

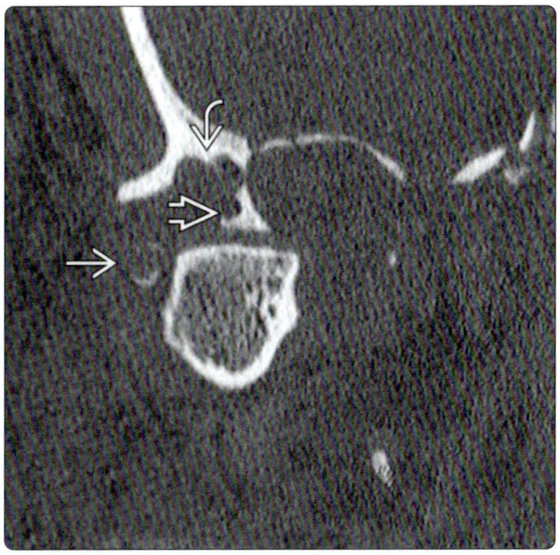

(Left) *Axial NECT shows CS of the right condyle. Radiopacities are visible lateral to the condyle, but a soft tissue mass is not present. The medial aspect of the condyle is sclerotic. Note the difference in condylar appearance from the normal left condyle.* **(Right)** *Coronal reformat NECT of the same patient shows a ring-like calcification with a radiolucent center in soft tissue. There is destruction of the glenoid fossa and greater sphenoid wing. The condyle is enlarged.*

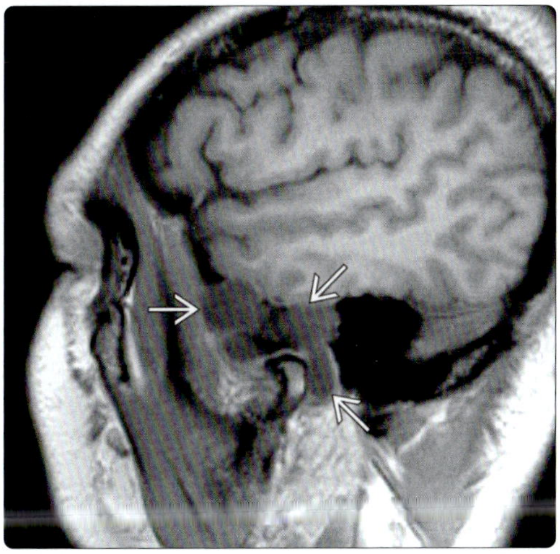

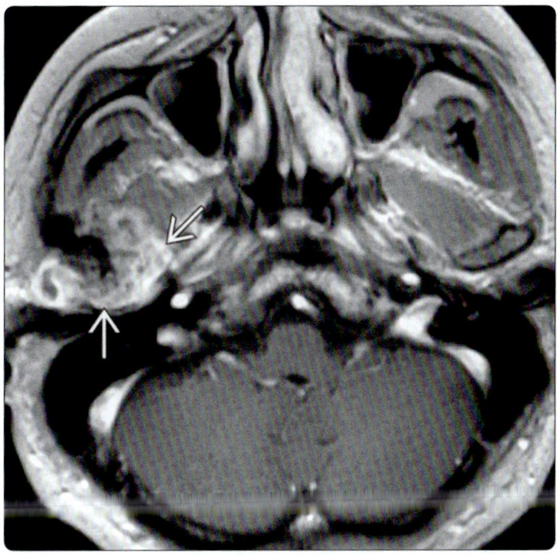

(Left) *Sagittal T1WI MR of the same patient shows a lobulated mass around the condyle involving the glenoid fossa and greater sphenoid wing.* **(Right)** *Axial T1WI C+ FS MR of the same patient shows extensive solid enhancement of the lesion surrounding the condyle, indicating the lesion is not inflammatory.*

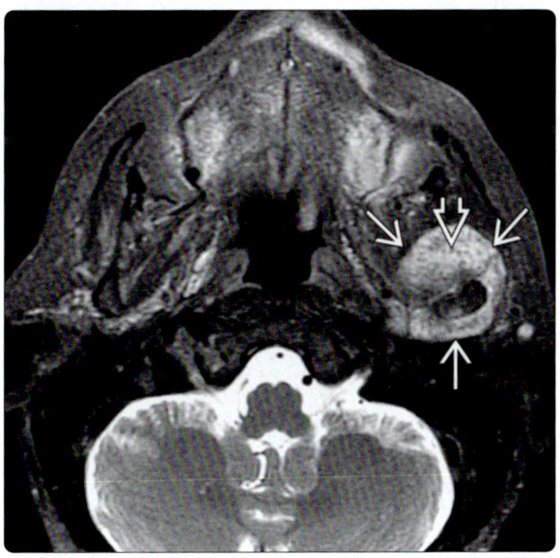

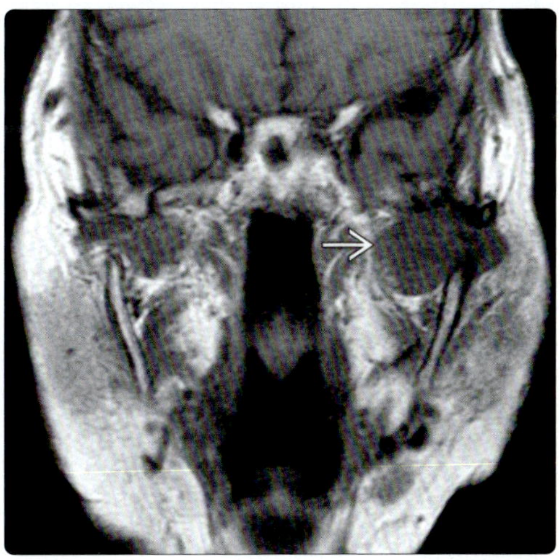

(Left) *Axial T2WI FS MR of CS of the left TMJ shows that the soft tissue component surrounding the condyle is heterogeneous but with overall high T2 signal intensity that is typical of chondroid tumors. The stippled low-intensity foci are from multiple tumoral calcifications.* **(Right)** *Coronal T1WI C+ FS MR of the same patient shows intense enhancement of the joint mass, indicating that this is a solid neoplasm and not due to a fluid-distended joint.*

TMJ Metastasis

KEY FACTS

IMAGING

- Radiolucent **destruction** of mandibular condyle in patient with **history of distant primary malignancy**
- Breast, prostate, and lung metastases may cause bone formation resulting in **mixed or sclerotic** radiographic appearance
- Metastasis to TMJ **rare**, but incidence may be underreported
- Usually **unilateral**, but bilateral TMJ involvement reported
- Solitary metastasis to TMJ rare
  - TMJ involvement usually associated with mandibular or generalized skeletal metastases
- Usually **poorly defined, invasive** margins
- May see destruction of **neighboring** anatomic structures, including skull base
- May have associated soft tissue mass
- MR: May see increased signal or enhancing mass in mandibular condyle

TOP DIFFERENTIAL DIAGNOSES

- Osteosarcoma
- Chondrosarcoma
- Multiple myeloma
- Osteomyelitis

PATHOLOGY

- Most common primary malignancies metastasizing to TMJ are breast, lung, and prostate

CLINICAL ISSUES

- Symptoms mimic **TMJ dysfunction**
- Most patients > 40 years; highest incidence: 6th decade
- Prognosis generally **poor**; most patients die within 1 year after diagnosis

DIAGNOSTIC CHECKLIST

- Consider metastatic disease in patient with symptoms of TMJ dysfunction if **history of primary malignancy**

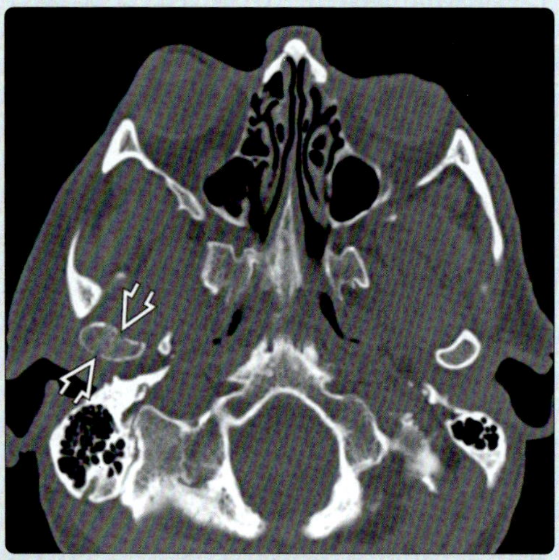
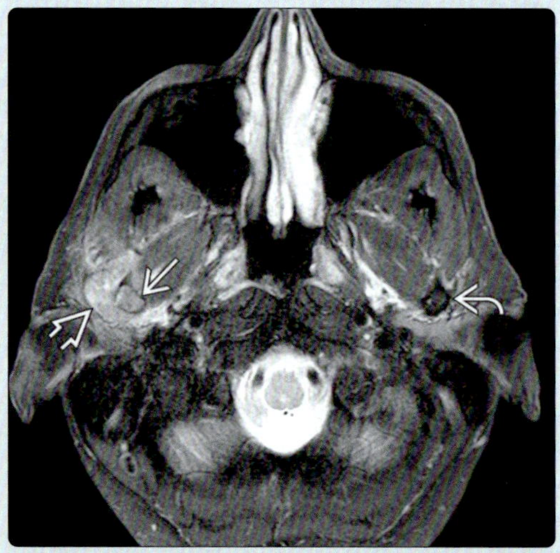

(Left) *Axial bone CT shows metastatic hepatocellular carcinoma involving the right mandibular condyle. There is cortical thinning and interruption of cortices on the anterior and posterior surfaces of the condyle.* **(Right)** *Axial T2WI FS MR in the same patient shows pathologically increased signal within the right mandibular condyle. Compare to normal left condyle. There is a soft tissue mass adjacent to the right condyle.*

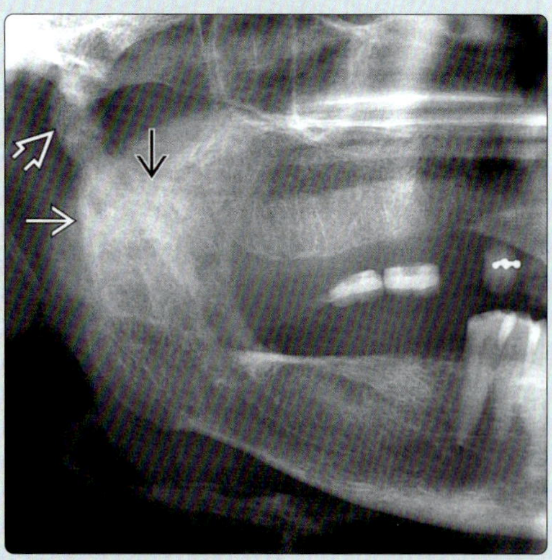
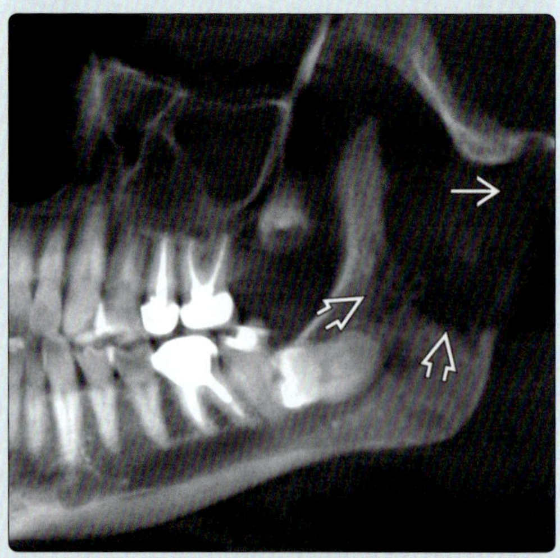

(Left) *Panoramic radiograph shows breast metastases to the mandible. The upper right ramus is sclerotic with loss of cortical boundaries and irregularity of the posterior border. The condyle is sclerotic with patchy areas of destruction. This case demonstrates both blastic and lytic bone metastases.* **(Right)** *Panoramic CBCT reformat in a 45-year-old woman with metastatic breast carcinoma shows destruction of the left ramus with complete loss of the left condyle. Note the infiltrative, ill-defined margins.*

TERMINOLOGY

Synonyms

- Secondary malignancy

Definitions

- Spread of malignant disease from distant primary tumor

IMAGING

General Features

- Best diagnostic clue
  - Radiolucent **destruction** of mandibular condyle in patient with **history of malignancy**
- Location
  - Posterior region of mandible most common
  - Metastasis to TMJ **rare**, but incidence may be underreported
    - Usually **unilateral**, but bilateral TMJ involvement reported
    - Solitary metastasis to TMJ rare: TMJ involvement usually associated with mandibular or generalized skeletal metastases
- Morphology
  - Irregular shape; can be expansile

Radiographic Findings

- Usually **poorly defined, invasive** margins
- **Destruction** of mandibular condyle
- Most metastases cause bone destruction, but breast, prostate, and lung metastases may cause bone formation and **mixed or sclerotic** radiographic appearance

CT Findings

- May have associated soft tissue mass
- May see destruction of **neighboring** anatomic structures, including skull base
- CT may show TMJ involvement not seen in panoramic radiography

MR Findings

- May see increased signal or enhancing mass in mandibular condyle

Imaging Recommendations

- Best imaging tool
  - CT or CBCT for initial investigation

DIFFERENTIAL DIAGNOSIS

Osteosarcoma

- Destructive changes to condyle similar to metastases, but osteosarcoma often has spiculated periosteal response

Chondrosarcoma

- Most common primary malignancy of condyle

Multiple Myeloma

- Lesions well defined; usually see additional lesions in mandible or other bones

Osteomyelitis

- Clinical signs and symptoms similar, but periosteal reaction in osteomyelitis more often parallel to cortex

PATHOLOGY

General Features

- Most common primary malignancies metastasizing to TMJ are breast, lung, prostate, kidneys, and thyroid
- Spread from primary tumor usually **hematogeneous**
- Metastases to TMJ rare because of paucity of red marrow in condyle and because condyle has separate blood supply from circular penetrating branches of maxillary artery and superficial temporal artery

CLINICAL ISSUES

Presentation

- Most common signs/symptoms
  - Symptoms mimic **TMJ dysfunction**: Pain, **trismus**, malocclusion, mandibular deviation, limited lateral movement, crepitation, clicking
- Other signs/symptoms
  - Preauricular **swelling**, mandibular paresthesia, pathological fracture
  - Symptoms due to tumor extension to neighboring structures: Hearing loss, decreased visual acuity, tinnitus, facial asymmetry

Demographics

- Age
  - Most > 40 years; highest incidence: 6th decade
  - Mean age: 54 years
- Epidemiology
  - 1-8% of tumors metastasize to maxillofacial area

Natural History & Prognosis

- Prognosis generally **poor**; most patients die within 1 year after diagnosis
  - Often other distant metastases at presentation

Treatment

- Surgery if disease controlled and there is only solitary metastasis to TMJ
- Radiation therapy ± chemotherapy; palliation for advanced cases

DIAGNOSTIC CHECKLIST

Consider

- Consider metastatic disease in patient with symptoms of TMJ dysfunction if **history of primary malignancy**
- Some cases of jaw metastases are 1st indication of occult malignancy or 1st evidence of primary tumor dissemination

SELECTED REFERENCES

1. Della Chiesa A et al: Metastatic breast cancer in the mandibular condyle mimicking temporomandibular joint (TMJ) disease. J Surg Case Rep. 2014(1), 2014
2. Kolokythas A et al: Metastatic pancreatic adenocarcinoma to the mandibular condyle: a rare clinical presentation. J Oral Maxillofac Surg. 72(1):83-8, 2014
3. Qiu YT et al: Metastatic spread to the mandibular condyle as initial clinical presentation: radiographic diagnosis and surgical experience. J Oral Maxillofac Surg. 71(4):809-20, 2013
4. Kruse AL et al: Temporomandibular disorders associated with metastases to the temporomandibular joint: a review of the literature and 3 additional cases. Oral Surg Oral Med Oral Pathol Oral Radiol Endod. 110(2):e21-8, 2010

TMJ Simple (Traumatic) Bone Cyst

KEY FACTS

TERMINOLOGY

- Definition: Solitary, empty, or partially empty bony cavity
- "Cyst" designation misnomer; lacks epithelial lining

IMAGING

- **Single corticated radiolucent** area in mandibular body, ramus, or condyle
- Well defined, thinly corticated in condyle
- Most nonexpansile but **occasional expansion**
- Occasionally **multilocular**
- Reported in condyle, condylar neck, and coronoid process
  - Can extend to condyle from ramus or be isolated to condyle
  - Condylar lesions often found in medial or lateral pole

TOP DIFFERENTIAL DIAGNOSES

- TMJ degenerative disease: Large **subchondral bone cyst** can simulate simple bone cyst
- Giant cell granuloma
- Langerhans histiocytosis
- Aneurysmal bone cyst

PATHOLOGY

- Empty/partially empty bone cavity with straw-colored fluid or old necrosis
- Unknown etiology: May be growth disturbance

CLINICAL ISSUES

- Incidental finding on imaging
  - 50% of condylar cases are tender or painful
- Condylar lesions often seen in patients who are 7-25 years old but only occasionally in older patients
- Gender: M = F for condylar lesions
- Slowly expanding growth; most are **incidental** findings
- Treatment = curettage, but some cases **heal spontaneously**; conservative radiographic follow-up may be indicated in young patients
- Recurrence uncommon

(Left) *Sagittal oblique (L) & coronal oblique (R) CBCT images of the right condyle show a simple bone cyst (SBC) appearing as a small well-corticated radiolucency ➡. This lesion appears similar to an Ely cyst, but morphology of the condyle ➡, fossa, & eminence ➡ are relatively normal.* **(Right)** *Sagittal oblique (L) and coronal oblique (R) CBCT images show an SBC presenting as a large radiolucency in the left condyle. The cortex is thinned but intact, and there is evidence of endosteal scalloping ➡.*

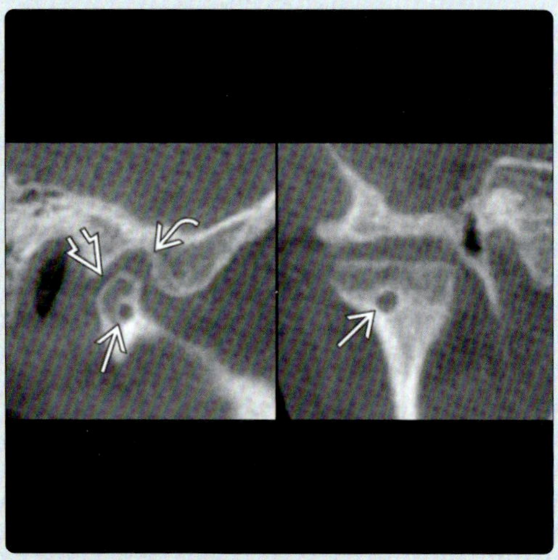

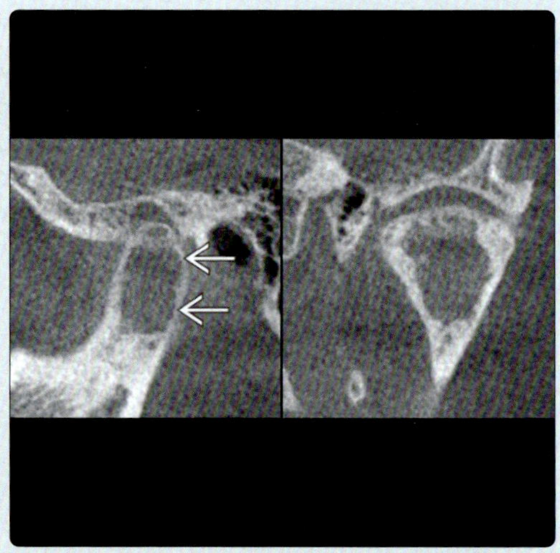

(Left) *Axial bone CT shows an SBC in the right condyle. There is a well-defined, mildly expansile radiolucent lesion ➡ in the right mandibular condyle. The condylar cortex is thinned but intact. The cyst walls are mildly scalloped, but there are no internal septations.* **(Right)** *Coronal bone CT of the same patient shows the lesion extending into and expanding the condylar neck and ramus ➡ with mild scalloping of the endosteal surface.*

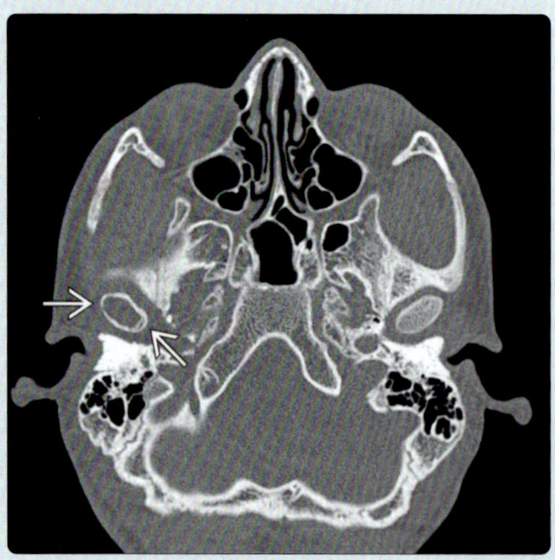

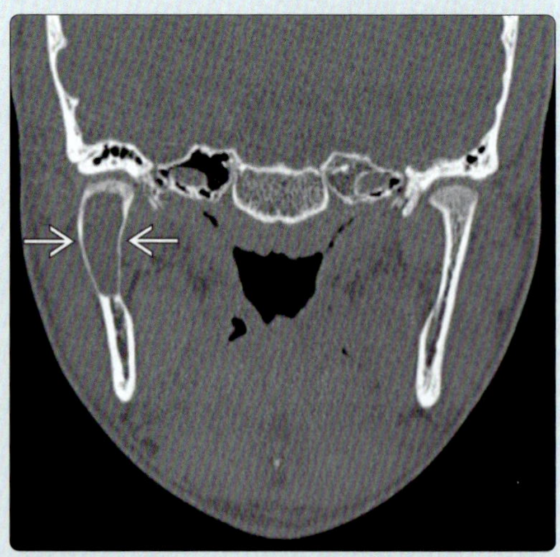

TERMINOLOGY

Abbreviations

- Simple bone cyst (SBC)

Synonyms

- Solitary bone cyst, traumatic bone cyst, hemorrhagic bone cyst, idiopathic bone cavity, extravasation cyst, unicameral bone cyst

Definitions

- Solitary, empty, or partially empty bony cavity
    - "Cyst" designation misnomer; lacks epithelial lining

IMAGING

General Features

- Best diagnostic clue
    - **Single corticated radiolucent** area in mandibular body, ramus, or condyle
- Location
    - Anywhere in mandible; most common in posterior molar regions, ramus
    - **Condylar** and maxillary lesions **rare**
        - Reported in condyle, condylar neck, and coronoid process
            - Can extend to condyle from ramus or be isolated to condyle
        - Condylar lesions often found in medial or lateral pole
- Size
    - Depends on when lesion discovered; typically 1 cm or larger
        - Condylar lesions may be **smaller**
- Morphology
    - Well defined; corticated
    - Most nonexpansile but **occasional expansion**

CT Findings

- CECT
    - Mildly enhancing at periphery
- CBCT and bone CT
    - Solitary thinly corticated radiolucency in condyle
        - Occasionally multilocular
    - Typically **nonexpansile**; if present, mild
        - Bone margins uniform but may display **endosteal scalloping**

MR Findings

- T2WI
    - Homogeneous hyperintensity without fluid-fluid levels
- T1WI C+
    - Mildly enhancing

DIFFERENTIAL DIAGNOSIS

TMJ Degenerative Disease

- Large **subchondral bone cyst** can simulate SBC
- Degenerative joint disease (DJD) rare in children; would see other radiographic signs of DJD in TMJ

Giant Cell Granuloma

- Large lesions usually have septations (multilocular)
- Tends to be expansile

Langerhans Histiocytosis

- Usually sharply defined punched-out areas but occasionally poorly defined
- Condylar involvement rare
- M:F = 2.7:1 for condylar lesions
- Age: 6-50 years

Aneurysmal Bone Cyst

- Ballooning of cortex, multilocular radiolucency
- TMJ lesions often associated with pain and trismus
- **Fluid-fluid levels** on T2 MR

PATHOLOGY

General Features

- Etiology
    - Unknown: May be growth disturbance, calcification abnormality, abnormal mesenchymal differentiation, or degeneration of another lesion, such as central giant cell granuloma
    - Previously thought to occur from medullary infarct following trauma

Gross Pathologic & Surgical Features

- Empty/partially empty bone cavity with straw-colored fluid or old necrosis

Microscopic Features

- Cystic cavity with connective tissue membrane; **no epithelial lining**

CLINICAL ISSUES

Presentation

- Most common signs/symptoms
    - Incidental finding on imaging
- Other signs/symptoms
    - Pain, swelling if associated with trauma
        - 50% of condylar cases are tender or painful

Demographics

- Age
    - Condylar lesions often seen in patients 7-25 years old but only occasionally in older patients

Natural History & Prognosis

- Slowly expanding growth; most are incidental findings
- Recurrence uncommon

Treatment

- Some cases heal spontaneously: Conservative radiographic follow-up may be indicated in young patients
- Curettage: Induction of bleeding in cavity to promote healing

SELECTED REFERENCES

1. Kim KA et al: Recurrent simple bone cyst of the mandibular condyle: a case report. Imaging Sci Dent. 43(1):49-53, 2013
2. Saia G et al: Intraoral endoscopic enucleation of a solitary bone cyst of the mandibular condyle. Int J Oral Maxillofac Surg. 41(3):317-20, 2012
3. Magliocca KR et al: Traumatic bone cyst of the condylar region: report of 2 cases. J Oral Maxillofac Surg. 65(6):1247-50, 2007
4. Hudson JW et al: Condylar lesion. J Oral Maxillofac Surg. 61(7):824-6, 2003
5. Minowa K et al: Evaluation of static bone cavities with CT and MRI. Dentomaxillofac Radiol. 32(1):2-7, 2003

Aneurysmal Bone Cyst

KEY FACTS

TERMINOLOGY

- Definition: Reactive lesion of bone that contains many large blood-filled spaces separated by connective tissue septa and containing **giant cells**
- Devoid of epithelial lining, therefore **not true cyst**
- Hydraulic-appearing outer margins ("ballooning" of cortex) gave rise to term "aneurysmal"

IMAGING

- Very expansile: **Well-defined hydraulic margins**
- Septate (multilocular) lesion containing fluid
  - Septa orient at **right angles to outer cortex**
- Subacute blood = hyperintense on T2WI MR
- Fluid-fluid levels best visualized on T2WI MR

TOP DIFFERENTIAL DIAGNOSES

- Central giant cell granuloma
  - May not be as large as aneurysmal bone cyst

PATHOLOGY

- Large blood-filled spaces separated by fibrous septa

CLINICAL ISSUES

- 80% are < 20 years of age
- Slight female predominance
- Firm nonpulsatile swelling
- ~ 50% with pain
- Crepitus with firm palpation
- Treatment: Excision, enucleation, block resection, curettage, embolization if vascular and grafting
  - High recurrence with curettage

DIAGNOSTIC CHECKLIST

- Expanding multilocular lesion with hydraulic margin
- Adapts to space available **without significant displacement** of mandible

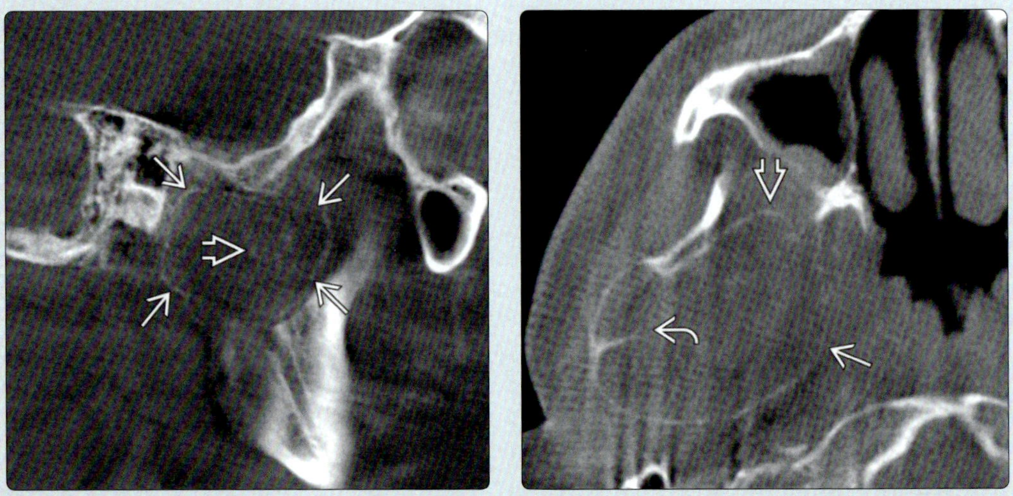

(Left) *Sagittal CBCT of a 22-year-old man shows a very expansile lesion of aneurysmal bone cyst (ABC) in the right condylar process. Note the thin well-defined surrounding cortex ➡ and wispy internal bony septa ⇨. The mandible was not inferiorly displaced. (Courtesy D. Levin, DDS.)* **(Right)** *Axial CBCT in the same patient shows hydraulic or ballooning-type expansion medially ➡ and anteriorly ⇨. Note that the trabecula is oriented perpendicular to the outer cortex ⇨, which is characteristic of this lesion. (Courtesy D. Levin, DDS.)*

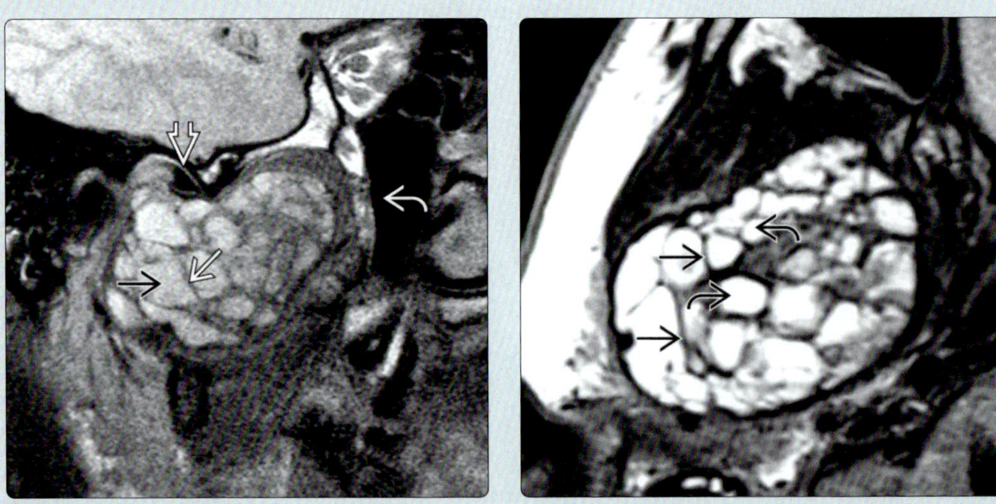

(Left) *Sagittal T1WI MR of the same patient shows a large expansile lesion in the condyle. The displaced soft tissues anterior to the lesion encroach upon the posterior region of the maxillary sinus ⇨. The disc is visualized superior to the ABC ⇨, and multiple locules ➡ separated by thin septa ⇨ are noted within the lesion. (Courtesy D. Levin, DDS.)* **(Right)** *Axial T2WI MR of the same patient shows the fluid signal partitioned into locules ⇨ by low-signal septa ➡. No fluid-fluid levels are noted. (Courtesy D. Levin, DDS.)*

TERMINOLOGY

Abbreviations

- Aneurysmal bone cyst (ABC)

Synonyms

- Benign central giant cell tumor, central giant cell lesion

Definitions

- Reactive lesion of bone that contains many large blood-filled spaces separated by connective tissue septa and containing giant cells
- Devoid of epithelial lining; therefore, **not true cyst**
- Hydraulic-appearing outer margins ("ballooning" of cortex) gave rise to term "aneurysmal"

IMAGING

General Features

- Best diagnostic clue
  - Very expansile lesion with well-defined hydraulic margins
  - Septate lesion containing fluid
- Location
  - Incidence in cranial and maxillofacial area ~ 5% of bone lesions
  - Mandible:maxilla = 3:1
  - Molar/ramus area most common
  - **Rare in condyle** and coronoid process
- Size
  - Can be quite large relative to all other TMJ lesions
- Morphology
  - Oval or fusiform

CT Findings

- NECT
  - Loculations
  - Soft-tissue window may show low density vascular space
- CECT
  - Septal uptake and multiple fluid levels
- CBCT
  - Fine trabeculae that may orient at **right angles (perpendicular) to outer cortex**
  - Delicate outer cortex
    - Hydraulic form

MR Findings

- T2WI
  - Subacute blood = hyperintense
  - Fluid-fluid levels

DIFFERENTIAL DIAGNOSIS

Central Giant Cell Granuloma

- Expansile multilocular lucent lesion generally **anterior to 1st mandibular molars**
- Septa form at right angles to outer cortex and may look identical to ABC
- May not be as large as ABC

PATHOLOGY

General Features

- Etiology
  - Nonneoplastic
  - Reactive process to trauma, preexisting lesion, or altered hemodynamic state
  - Considered by some to be variant of central giant cell granuloma
  - May be associated with other lesions such as fibrous dysplasia, osteosarcoma, central giant cell granuloma, simple bone cyst, nonossifying fibroma, central hemangioma, & osteoblastoma

Gross Pathologic & Surgical Features

- Large blood-filled spaces separated by fibrous septa
- Septa composed of connective tissue containing osteoid deposits, spicules of woven bone, deposits of hemosiderin, and extravasated erythrocytes
- Contains varying numbers of **multinucleated giant cells**

CLINICAL ISSUES

Presentation

- Most common signs/symptoms
  - Firm **nonpulsatile** swelling
- Other signs/symptoms
  - ~ 50% with pain
  - No bruit
  - Crepitus with firm palpation

Demographics

- Age
  - 80% are < 20 years of age
- Gender
  - Slight female predominance

Natural History & Prognosis

- High recurrence (up to 80%) with curettage

Treatment

- Excision, enucleation, block resection, curettage, embolization if vascular, and grafting

DIAGNOSTIC CHECKLIST

Image Interpretation Pearls

- Expanding multilocular lesion with hydraulic margin
- Adapts to space available without significant displacement of mandible

SELECTED REFERENCES

1. Ettl T et al: Recurrent aneurysmal bone cyst of the mandibular condyle with soft tissue extension. Int J Oral Maxillofac Surg. 38(6):699-703, 2009
2. Park W et al: Intraosseous lesion in mandibular condyle mimicking temporomandibular disorders: report of 3 cases. J Orofac Pain. 22(1):65-70, 2008
3. Smolka W et al: Aneurysmal bone cyst of the tuberculum articulare of the temporomandibular joint: a case report. Quintessence Int. 39(8):679-83, 2008
4. Warner BF et al: Temporomandibular joint neoplasms and pseudotumors. Adv Anat Pathol. 7(6):365-81, 2000
5. Svensson B et al: Benign osteoblastoma associated with an aneurysmal bone cyst of the mandibular ramus and condyle. Oral Surg Oral Med Oral Pathol. 76(4):433-6, 1993

(Left) *Clinical photograph shows an 8-year-old girl with a rapidly enlarging, nonpainful right facial swelling ⇗ resulting from a giant cell lesion containing focal areas of ABC.* **(Right)** *Volume-rendered CBCT of the same patient shows facial swelling ⇨.*

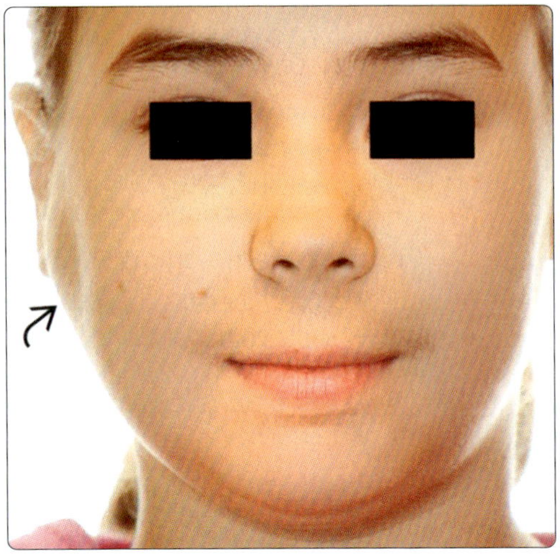

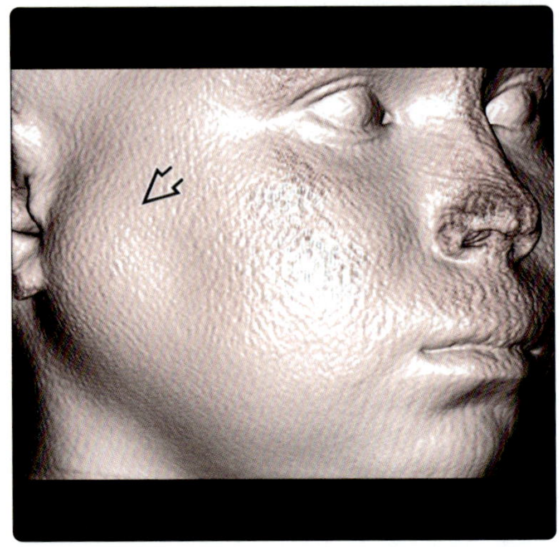

(Left) *CBCT sagittal oblique view of right TMJ shows an expansile lytic lesion with its epicenter within the condyle. The lesion margins are relatively well defined and mostly corticated ➡. The condyle is not displaced.* **(Right)** *Coronal CBCT section of the right TMJ in the same patient shows medial and lateral expansion. The lateral surface of the lesion shows thin cortex ➡ exhibiting hydraulic-type expansion.*

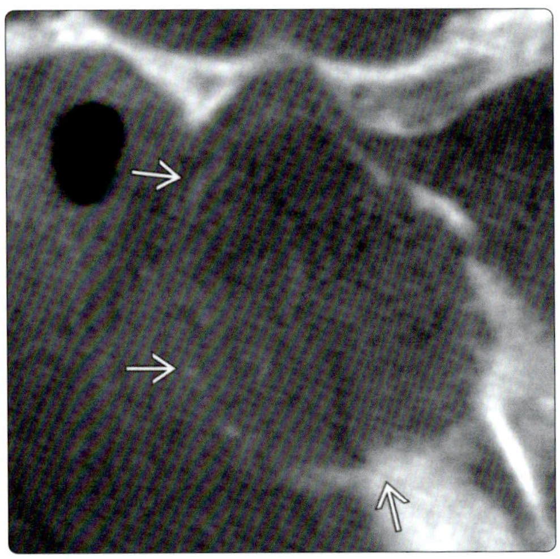

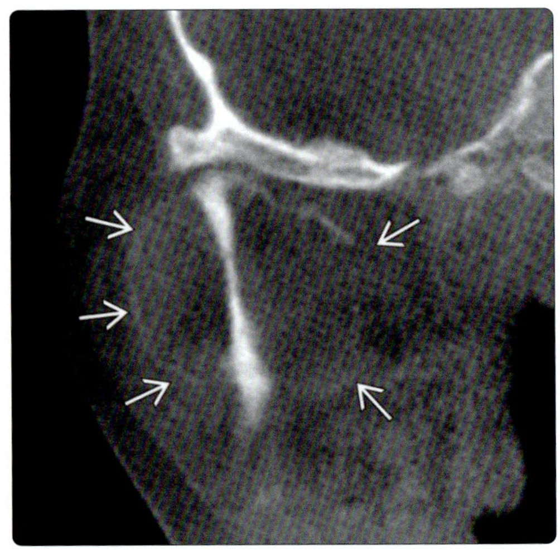

(Left) *CBCT panoramic reconstruction of the right side for the same patient shows the enlarged proximal end of mandible with hydraulic-like corticated expansion ➡. The teeth are in maximum interdigitation, indicating no displacement of condyle/mandible.* **(Right)** *CBCT panoramic reconstruction of the left 1/2 of the mandible for same patient shows occlusion and condyle/fossa spatial relationships are maintained.*

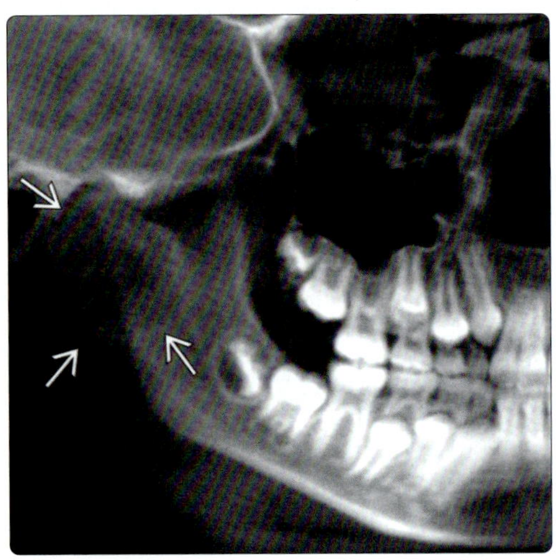

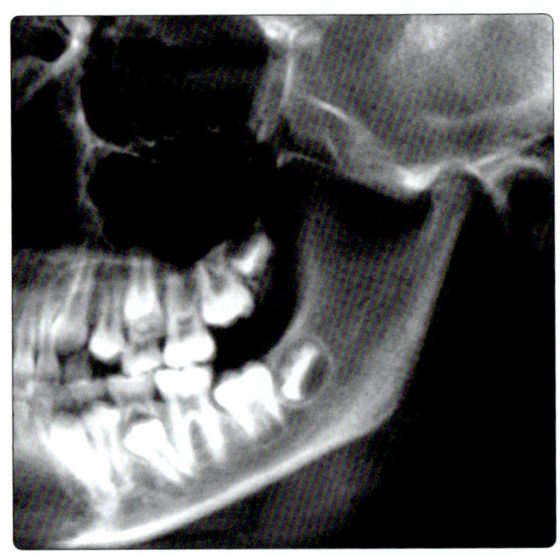

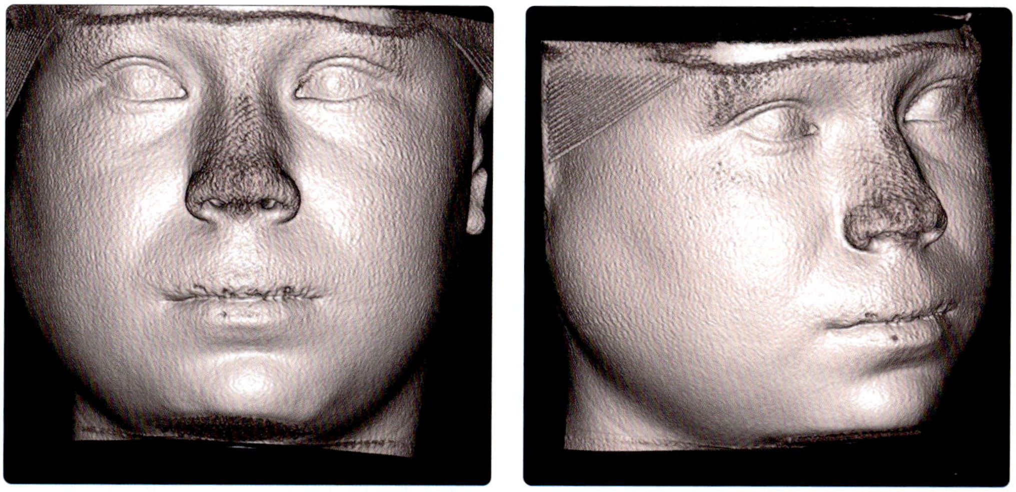

(Left) *Volume-rendered CBCT shows the same patient at age 11. Patient has been under treatment with doxycycline. There is an increase in the enlarged right side of the face since age 8.* **(Right)** *Oblique volume-rendered CBCT shows a diffuse area of facial swelling.*

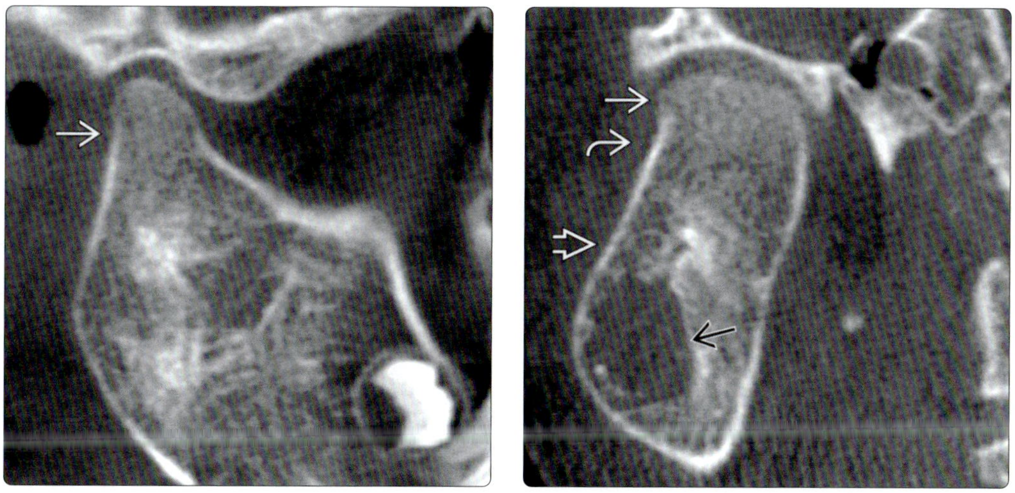

(Left) *CBCT sagittal oblique view of the right condylar process and ramus shows overall circumferential enlargement of condylar process* ➡ *and ascending ramus without significant change in vertical dimensions. The enlarged region has mostly filled with bone since the age of 8.* **(Right)** *Coronal oblique CBCT of the same patient shows mediolateral enlargement of the condyle* ➡*, neck* ➡*, and ramus* ➡*. There is a central low-attenuation region without bone fill, representing a persistent area of activity* ➡*.*

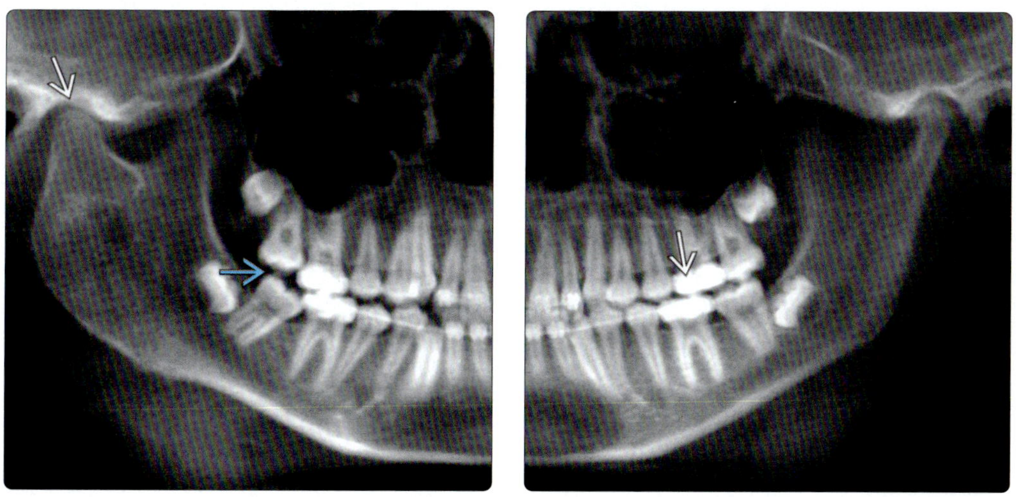

(Left) *CBCT panoramic reconstruction of the right 1/2 of mandible for the same patient shows a significant change in size and shape of the mandible without displacement of condyle* ➡ *or change in occlusion* ➡*.* **(Right)** *Panoramic reconstruction of the left 1/2 of the mandible shows a normal class I occlusion* ➡ *and mandibular growth.*

PART II
SECTION 5
Maxillary Sinus and Nasal Cavity

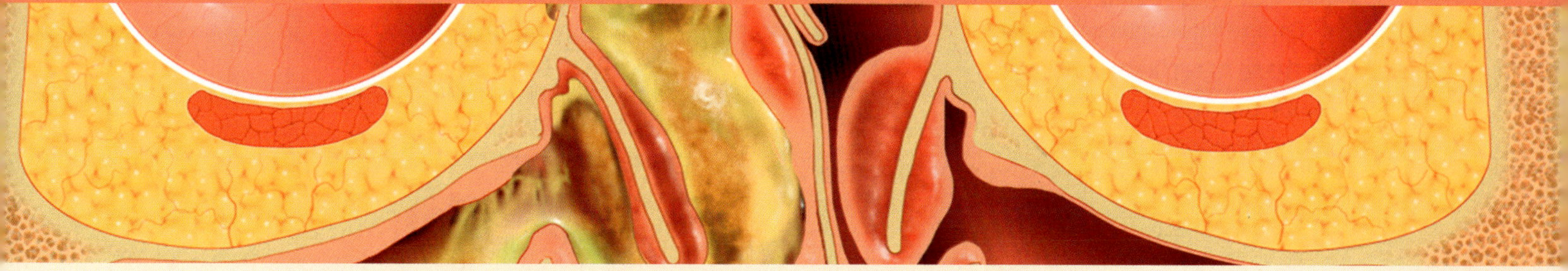

Normal Variants

Deviated Nasal Septum 650
Concha Bullosa 652
Accessory Ostia 656

Developmental

Hypoplasia/Aplasia 658

Inflammation

Mucus Retention Pseudocyst 662
Sinonasal Mucocele 664
Sinonasal Granulomatosis With Polyangiitis (Wegener Granulomatosis) 668
Sinonasal Polyposis 672
Acute Rhinosinusitis 676
Chronic Rhinosinusitis 680
Odontogenic Sinusitis 684
Allergic Fungal Sinusitis 686
Invasive Fungal Sinusitis 688
Mycetoma 692
Invasive Pseudotumor 694

Neoplasm, Benign

Sinonasal Inverted Papilloma 696
Sinonasal Osteoma 700

Neoplasm, Malignant

Sinonasal Squamous Cell Carcinoma 704
Sinonasal Adenoid Cystic Carcinoma 706
Nasopharyngeal Carcinoma 708
Sinonasal Malignant Melanoma 712

Fibroosseous Lesions

Sinonasal Fibrous Dysplasia 714
Sinonasal Ossifying Fibroma 718

Deviated Nasal Septum

KEY FACTS

IMAGING

- Marked deviation from midline position of nasal septum, creating **nasal fossae of unequal size**
- Best tool: CBCT or bone CT without contrast
  - Coronal reconstructions are best

TOP DIFFERENTIAL DIAGNOSES

- **Septal tubercle**
  - Normal localized enlargement of septum
  - May be mistaken for deviation of septum on panoramic radiograph
- **Fracture of septum**
  - Fracture segments may be displaced laterally
- **Intranasal neoplasm**
  - Deviation or destruction of septum by mass
- **Marfan syndrome**
  - High palatal arch; long narrow face
- **Septal spur**
  - Septum straight but has lateral projection

PATHOLOGY

- Etiology: **Developmental** (congenital) or **trauma**
- Classification
  - Vertical superior or inferior
  - Horizontal anterior or posterior
  - S-shaped vertically or horizontally
  - Combination of any of those above
  - Septal spur

CLINICAL ISSUES

- Difficulty breathing/nasal congestion
- Rhinosinusitis
- May complicate nasotracheal intubation for oral surgery

DIAGNOSTIC CHECKLIST

- Reporting tips: **State if mild, moderate, or severe** and orientation of spur if present
  - State degree of reduction of nasal airway on side of deviation

(Left) *Coronal CBCT shows deviation of the nasal septum to the left, severely reducing the nasal fossa airway on the left compared to the right.* **(Right)** *Axial CBCT shows deviation of the nasal septum to the left. The airway is deceased in size in this region, compared to the right, but is still patent.*

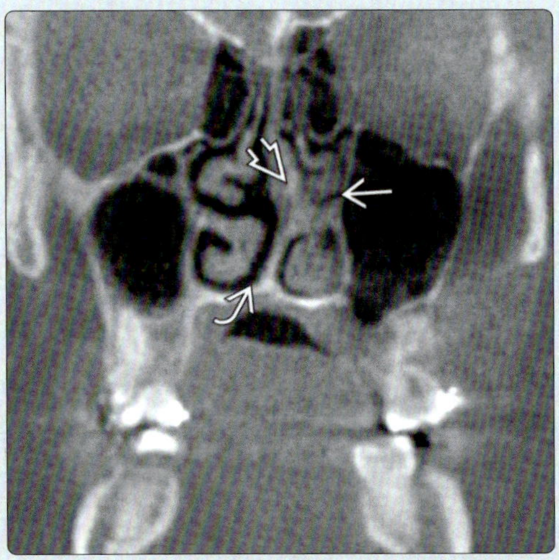

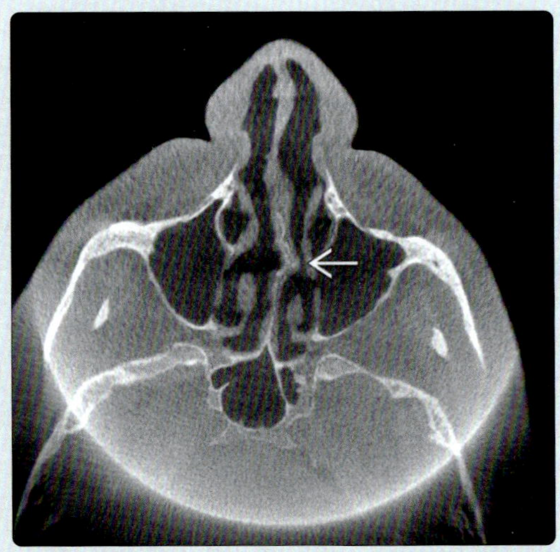

(Left) *Coronal CBCT shows a mild inferior septal deviation convex to the right. The inferior concha is large, and thus this part of the airway is restricted.* **(Right)** *Coronal bone CT demonstrates a large, broad-based, bony nasal septal spur extending toward the left middle meatus. Note obstruction of air space.*

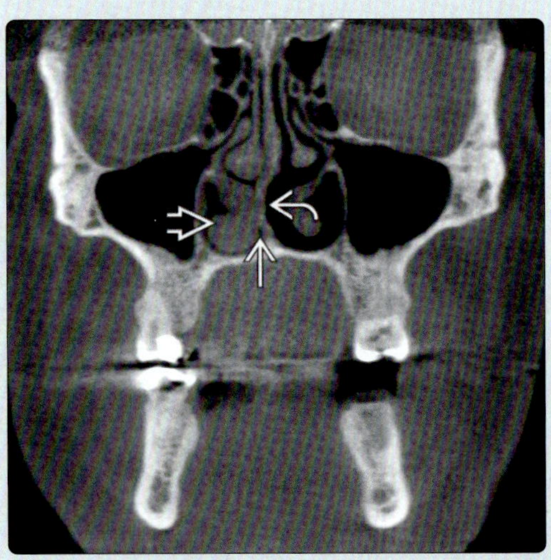

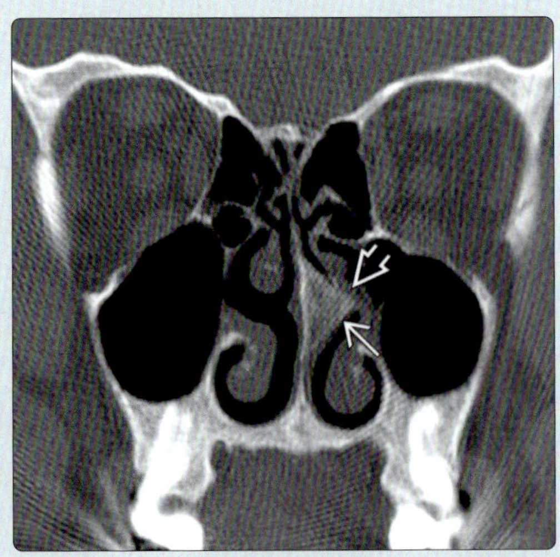

TERMINOLOGY

Abbreviations

- Deviated nasal septum (DNS)

Definitions

- Displacement of septum laterally that may be sufficient to cause rhinosinusitis or difficulty breathing through affected nasal fossa

IMAGING

General Features

- Best diagnostic clue
  - Marked lateral displacement (deviation) of midline septum
- Location
  - Midline/paramidline between left and right nasal fossa
- Morphology
  - Septum deviates to one side, making nasal fossae of unequal size
  - Middle and inferior conchae larger on concave side

Imaging Recommendations

- Best imaging tool
  - CT or CBCT
- Protocol advice
  - Bone algorithm CT or CBCT without contrast enhancement
  - Coronal and axial reconstructions are best

CT Findings

- Bone CT
  - Marked deviation from midline position of nasal septum
  - May see blockage of maxillary sinus ostium

DIFFERENTIAL DIAGNOSIS

Septal Tubercle

- Synonyms
  - Septal tumescence
  - Septal swell body
  - Septal turbinate
  - Kiesselbach body
  - Septal cavernous body
  - Septal erectile tissue
- Normal localized enlargement of septum may be mistaken for deviation of septum, especially on pantomograph, when both sides of tubercle are not visible

Fracture of Septum

- Fracture segments may be displaced laterally

Intranasal Neoplasm

- Deviation or destruction of septum by adjacent mass

Marfan Syndrome

- High palatal arch
- Long narrow face
- Malocclusion (dental crowding)

PATHOLOGY

General Features

- Etiology
  - Development (congenital)
  - Trauma
- Associated abnormalities
  - Rhinosinusitis
  - Difficulty breathing/nasal congestion
  - Marfan syndrome
  - Cleft palate

Staging, Grading, & Classification

- Classification
  - Minimal: Not included
  - Vertical: Superior or inferior
  - Horizontal: Anterior or posterior
  - S-shaped: Vertically or horizontally
  - Combination of any of those above
  - Septal spur

CLINICAL ISSUES

Presentation

- Most common signs/symptoms
  - May be silent if mild
  - Difficulty breathing; may lead to mouth breathing
- Other signs/symptoms
  - Rhinosinusitis
  - Nosebleed
  - Noisy breathing when asleep
- May complicate nasotracheal intubation for oral surgery

Demographics

- Age
  - At birth if developmental
  - Any age if posttraumatic
- Ethnicity
  - More common in individuals of European descent than African descent

Treatment

- Decongestants to manage symptoms
- Surgery

DIAGNOSTIC CHECKLIST

Consider

- **Septal tubercle**
  - Natural minor asymmetry of nasal fossae

Reporting Tips

- State mild, moderate, or severe depending on presentation
- State orientation of spur if present
- State degree of reduction of nasal airway on side of deviation

SELECTED REFERENCES

1. Sedaghat AR et al: Radiographic evaluation of nasal septal deviation from computed tomography correlates poorly with physical exam findings. Int Forum Allergy Rhinol. 5(3):258-62, 2015

Concha Bullosa

KEY FACTS

TERMINOLOGY

- Synonyms
  - **Concha pneumatization**
  - **Turbinate pneumatization**
- Definitions
  - Extension of sinus into concha
  - Pneumatization of 50% or more of vertical height of middle concha
  - Invagination of epithelium into inferior concha during development

IMAGING

- Location: Middle > superior > inferior concha, may be bilateral
- Size: Over 50% of vertical height of middle concha
- Extension of adjacent sinus into concha or invagination of inferior concha
- Best imaging tool: Coronal CBCT or bone CT
  - **Internal radiolucency of bulbous portion of concha**

CLINICAL ISSUES

- **Asymptomatic** but may have
  - Sinusitis
  - Blockage of nasal fossa
  - Blockage of sinus drainage
  - Headache if concha bullosa contacts other mucosal areas
- Developmental variant
- Nonprogressive
- **No treatment** if asymptomatic
- May complicate endoscopy or nasal intubation

DIAGNOSTIC CHECKLIST

- **Consider**: Increased spiral of normal middle concha
- Image interpretation pearls
  - Check patency of nasal fossa airway
  - Check sinuses for mucosal thickening indicating possible blockage
- Reporting tip: **Note possible loss of airway patency**

(Left) *Coronal CBCT reconstruction shows pneumatization of both the right and left middle conchae. There is slight deviation of the nasal septum to the left.* **(Right)** *Sagittal CBCT reconstruction through right middle concha in the same patient shows connection of right larger concha bullosa air cell to the other ethmoid air cells. It can be seen as an outpouching of the ethmoid air cells.*

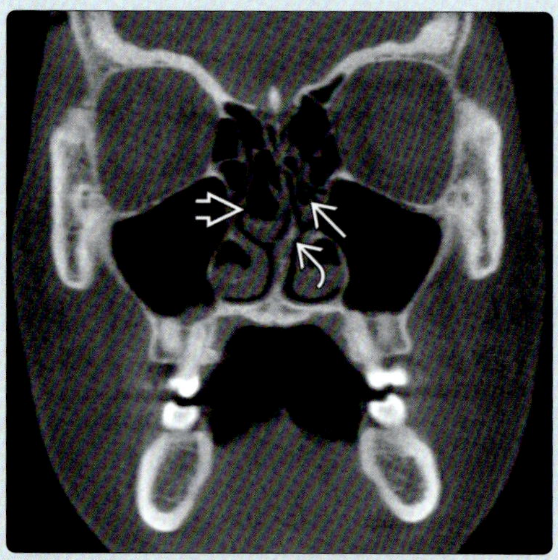

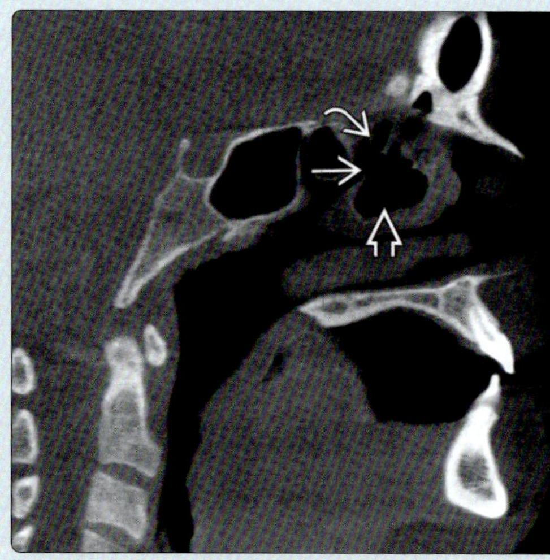

(Left) *Axial CBCT in the same patient shows concha bullosa of the right middle concha. The smaller left concha bullosa is not seen at this slice level. The airway is markedly decreased at this level of the apparent greatest enlargement of the air cell, even though the nasal septum is deviated to the left.* **(Right)** *Coronal CBCT shows unilateral middle concha bullosa on the left.*

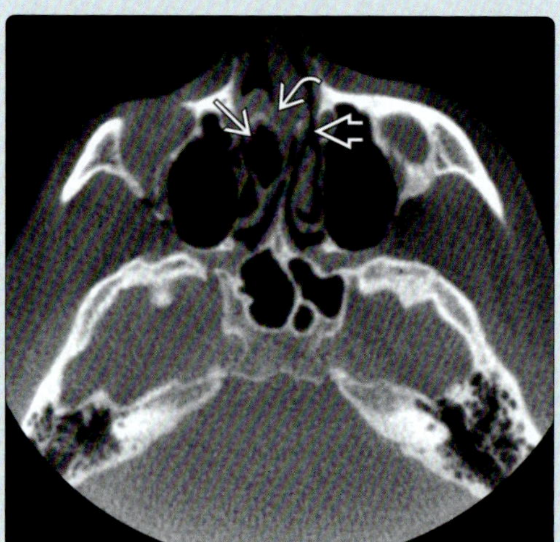

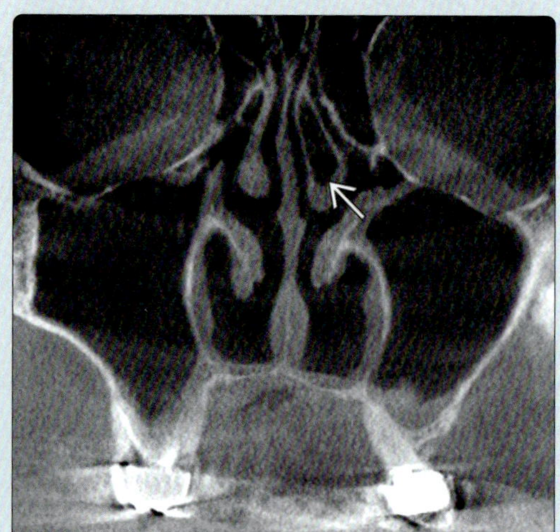

TERMINOLOGY

Synonyms

- Concha pneumatization
- Turbinate pneumatization

Definitions

- Extension of sinus into concha
- Invagination into double lamella of inferior concha during development
- Pneumatization of 50% or more of vertical height of middle concha

IMAGING

General Features

- Best diagnostic clue
  - Pneumatization of bulbous portion of concha
- Location
  - Middle > superior > inferior concha, may be bilateral
- Size
  - Over 50% of vertical height of middle concha, variable in other conchae
- Morphology
  - Possible enlargement of concha
  - Extension of ethmoid air cell into middle or superior concha
  - Extension of maxillary sinus into inferior concha or invagination from surface

CT Findings

- Bone CT
  - Internal radiolucency of bulbous portion of affected concha on coronal CT

Imaging Recommendations

- Best imaging tool
  - Coronal CT, bone algorithm, or coronal CBCT

CLINICAL ISSUES

Presentation

- Most common signs/symptoms
  - Asymptomatic
- Other signs/symptoms
  - May have sinusitis
  - Blockage of nasal fossa
  - Blockage of sinus drainage
  - Headache if concha bullosa contacts other mucosal areas
- Clinical profile
  - May complicate endoscopy or nasal intubation

Natural History & Prognosis

- Developmental variant
- Nonprogressive

Treatment

- None if asymptomatic

DIAGNOSTIC CHECKLIST

Consider

- Increased spiral of normal concha

Image Interpretation Pearls

- Check patency of nasal fossa airway
- Check sinuses for mucosal thickening indicating possible blockage

Reporting Tips

- Make note of possible loss of airway patency

SELECTED REFERENCES

1. Loftus PA et al: Anatomic variants of the paranasal sinuses in patients with recurrent acute rhinosinusitis. Int Forum Allergy Rhinol. 6(3):328-33, 2016
2. Min HJ et al: The potential significance of concha bullosa during nasotracheal intubation. J Craniofac Surg. 27(2):e153-4, 2016
3. Rusu MC et al: The pterygopalatine recess of the superior nasal meatus. Surg Radiol Anat. 38(8):979-82, 2016
4. Shin JM et al: Analysis of sinonasal anatomical variations associated with maxillary sinus fungal balls. Auris Nasus Larynx. 43(5): 524-8, 2016
5. Tomblinson CM et al: The impact of middle turbinate concha bullosa on the severity of inferior turbinate hypertrophy in patients with a deviated nasal septum. AJNR Am J Neuroradiol. 43(5):524-8, 2016
6. Bandyopadhyay R et al: Osteomeatal complex: a study of its anatomical variation among patients attending north bengal medical college and hospital. Indian J Otolaryngol Head Neck Surg. 67(3):281-6, 2015
7. Cantone E et al: Concha bullosa related headache disability. Eur Rev Med Pharmacol Sci. 19(13):2327-30, 2015
8. Demir UL et al: Anatomical correlation between existence of concha bullosa and maxillary sinus volume. Surg Radiol Anat. 37(9):1093-8, 2015
9. Göçmen G et al: Effect of septal deviation, concha bullosa and Haller's cell on maxillary sinus's inferior pneumatization; a retrospective study. Open Dent J. 9:282-6, 2015
10. Khojastepour L et al: Anatomical variations of ostiomeatal complex in CBCT of patients seeking rhinoplasty. J Dent (Shiraz). 16(1):42-8, 2015
11. Lee JH et al: Underestimation of rhinogenic causes in patients presenting to the emergency department with acute headache. Acta Neurol Taiwan. 24(2):37-42, 2015
12. Măru N et al: Variant anatomy of nasal turbinates: supreme, superior and middle conchae bullosae, paradoxical superior and inferior turbinates, and middle accessory turbinate. Rom J Morphol Embryol. 56(3):1223-6, 2015
13. Tiwari R et al: Study of anatomical variations on CT in chronic sinusitis. Indian J Otolaryngol Head Neck Surg. 67(1):18-20, 2015
14. Worrall DM et al: Concha bullosa: a shield against allergens? ORL J Otorhinolaryngol Relat Spec. 77(5):281-6, 2015
15. Javadrashid R et al: Concha bullosa, nasal septal deviation and paranasal sinusitis; a computed tomographic evaluation. B-ENT. 10(4):291-8, 2014
16. San T et al: Bilateral superior concha bullosa: a rare case overlooked. Kulak Burun Bogaz Ihtis Derg. 24(5):292-4, 2014
17. San T et al: Bilateral triple concha bullosa: a very rare anatomical variation of intranasal turbinates. Case Rep Otolaryngol. 2014:851508, 2014
18. Jain R et al: Comparison of anatomical abnormalities in patients with limited and diffuse chronic rhinosinusitis. Int Forum Allergy Rhinol. 3(6):493-6, 2013
19. Ozturan O et al: Pneumo-concha dilatans: middle concha growing in anterior and lateral directions. J Craniofac Surg. 24(4):e444-6, 2013
20. Ozturan O et al: 'Conchae bullosis': a rare case with bilateral triple turbinate pneumatisations. J Laryngol Otol. 127(1):73-5, 2013
21. Pittore B et al: Concha bullosa of the inferior turbinate: an unusual cause of nasal obstruction. Acta Otorhinolaryngol Ital. 31(1):47-9, 2011
22. Homsioglou E et al: Pneumatized superior turbinate as a cause of headache. Head Face Med. 3:3, 2007
23. Kiroglu AF et al: Isolated turbinitis and pneumatization of the concha inferior in a child. Am J Otolaryngol. 28(1):67-8, 2007
24. Hatipoğlu HG et al: Concha bullosa types: their relationship with sinusitis, ostiomeatal and frontal recess disease. Diagn Interv Radiol. 11(3):145-9, 2005
25. Alper F et al: A massive superior concha bullosa: case report and literature review. Rhinology. 42(1):38-40, 2004
26. Stallman JS et al: The incidence of concha bullosa and its relationship to nasal septal deviation and paranasal sinus disease. AJNR Am J Neuroradiol. 25(9):1613-8, 2004
27. Yanagisawa E et al: An unusual lateral ostium of a concha bullosa of the middle turbinate. Ear Nose Throat J. 82(3):159-60, 2003
28. Maru YK et al: Concha bullosa: Frequency and appearances on sinonasal CT. Indian J Otolaryngol Head Neck Surg. 52(1):40-4, 1999
29. Clerico DM: Pneumatized superior turbinate as a cause of referred migraine headache. Laryngoscope. 106(7):874-9, 1996

(Left) *Coronal CBCT reconstruction shows concha bullosa* ➡ *of the left inferior concha extending from the left maxillary sinus with no separating osseous border* ➡. *There is soft tissue thickening in the concha bullosa* ⇨. **(Right)** *Coronal CBCT reconstruction with bilateral superior conchae bullosa* ➡ *in a 53-year-old man is shown. (Courtesy F. Badr, BDS.)*

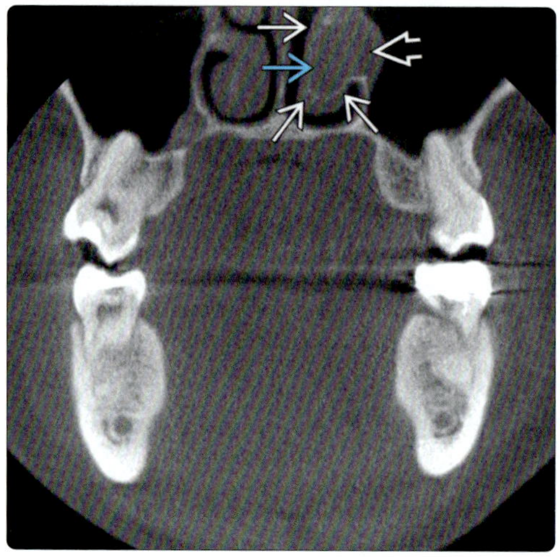

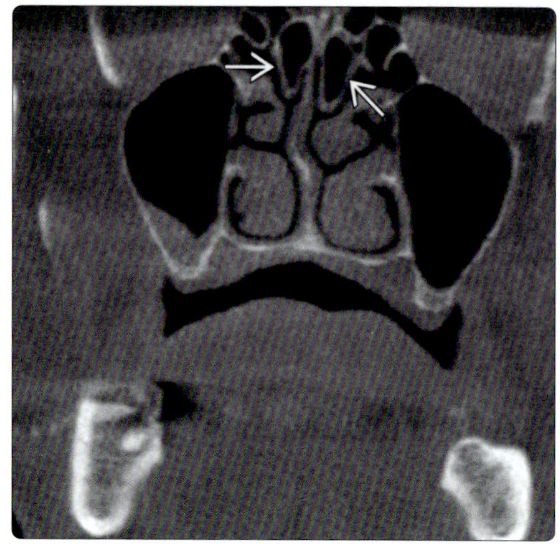

(Left) *Coronal CBCT reconstruction shows bilateral superior conchae bullosa* ➡ *in a 67-year-old man. (Courtesy W. Mohammed, BDS.)* **(Right)** *Coronal CBCT reconstruction shows bilateral superior conchae bullosa* ➡ *in a 53-year-old woman. (Courtesy F. Baabdullah, BDS.)*

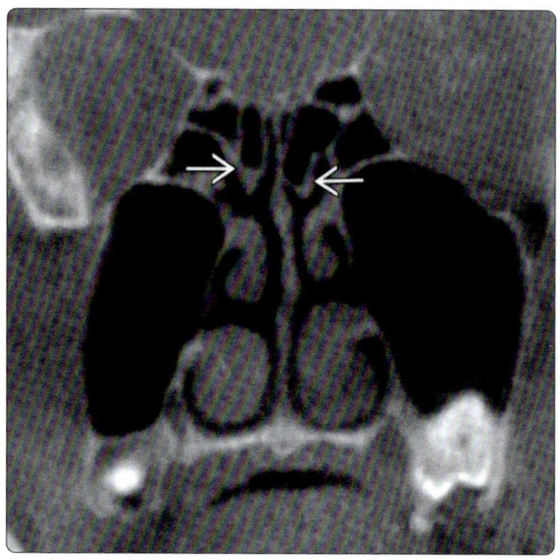

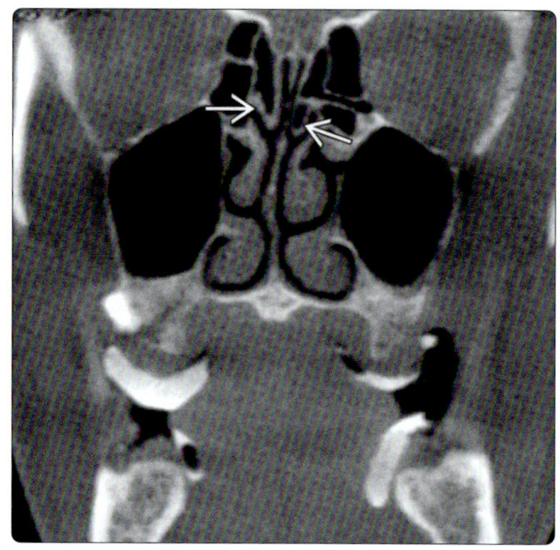

(Left) *Coronal CBCT reconstruction of a 77-year-old woman shows bilateral conchae bullosa* ➡ *within the lamellar portion of the conchae.* **(Right)** *Axial CBCT reconstruction of the same patient shows bilateral middle conchae bullosa* ➡.

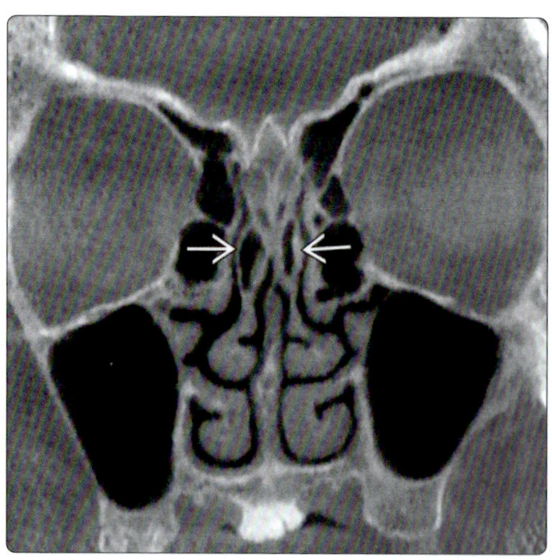

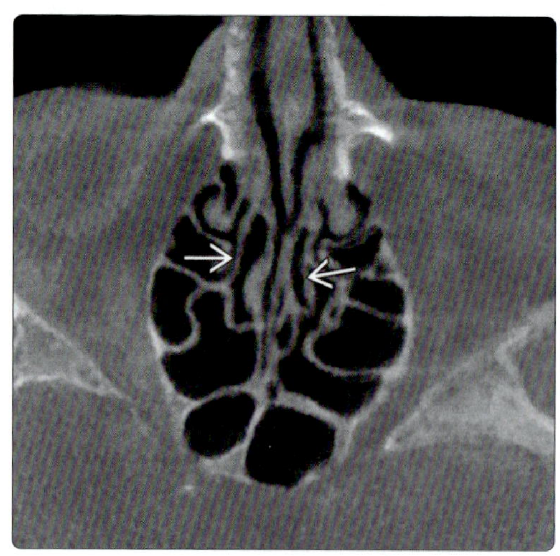

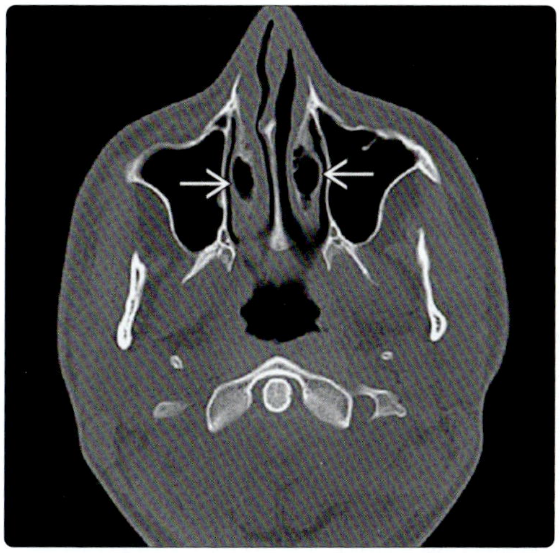

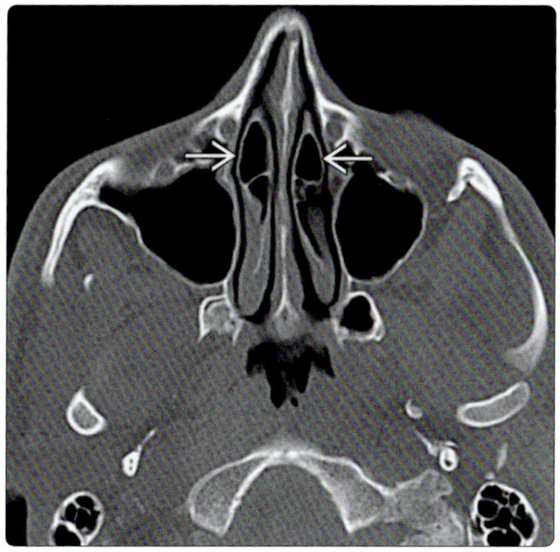

(Left) *Axial CBCT reconstruction in a 23-year-old man with bilateral inferior conchae bullosa → is shown. (Courtesy O. Ozturan, MD; A. Yenigun, MD; N. Degirmenci, MD; and F. Yilmaz, MD.)* **(Right)** *Axial CBCT reconstruction a 23-year-old man with bilateral middle conchae bullosa → is shown. (Courtesy O. Ozturan, MD; A. Yenigun, MD; N. Degirmenci, MD; and F. Yilmaz, MD.)*

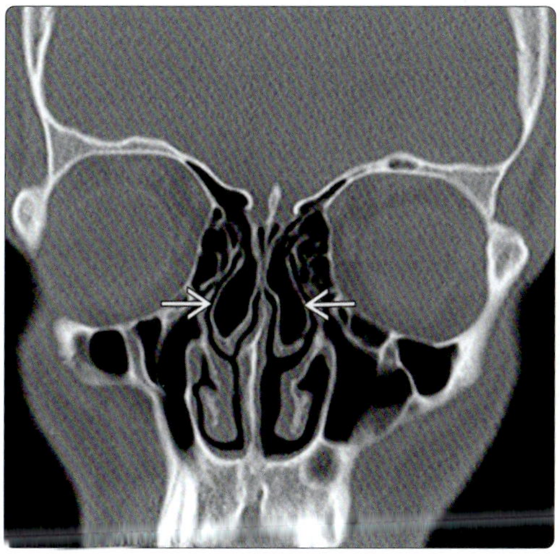

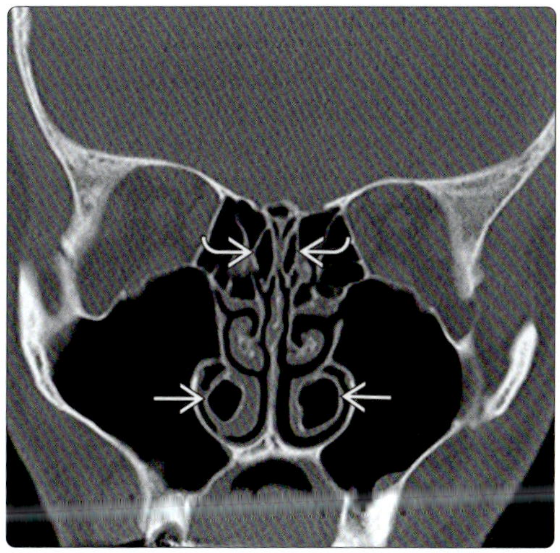

(Left) *Coronal CBCT reconstruction in a 23-year-old man with bilateral middle conchae bullosa → is shown. (Courtesy O. Ozturan, MD; A. Yenigun, MD; N. Degirmenci, MD; and F. Yilmaz, MD.)* **(Right)** *Coronal CBCT reconstruction in a 23-year-old man with bilateral superior → and inferior conchae bullosa → is shown. (Courtesy O. Ozturan, MD; A. Yenigun, MD; N. Degirmenci, MD; and F. Yilmaz, MD.)*

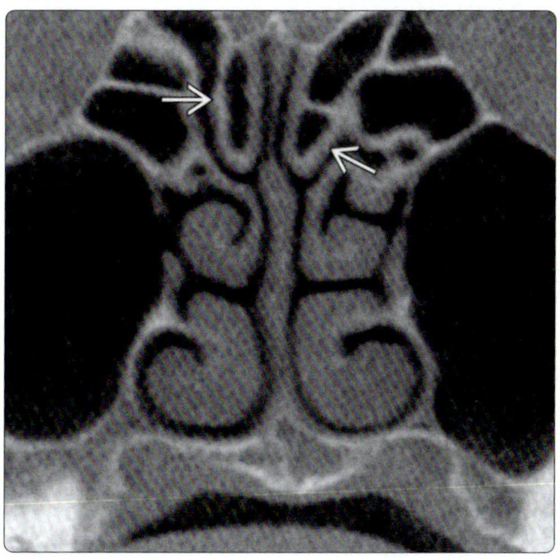

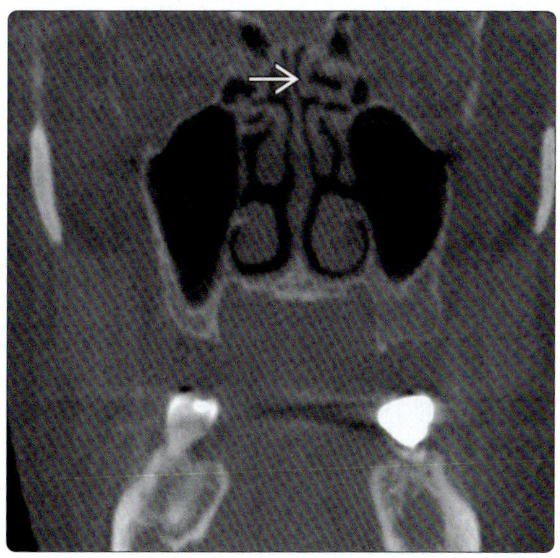

(Left) *Coronal CBCT reconstruction shows bilateral superior conchae bullosa →.* **(Right)** *Coronal CBCT reconstruction shows concha bullosa of the left superior concha → in a 45-year-old man. (Courtesy P. Wong, DMD.)*

Accessory Ostia

KEY FACTS

TERMINOLOGY

- Synonym: Ostia maxillare accessoria
- Definition: Additional openings between sinus and nasal fossa

IMAGING

- Best clue: **Discontinuity in medial wall of maxillary sinus** other than primary ostium
- Location
  - Medial wall of maxillary sinus
  - Infundibulum or region of anterior or posterior nasal fontanelles
  - Anterior fontanelle: Inferior and anterior to uncinate process
  - Posterior fontanelle: Between posterior end of uncinate process and palatine bone
- Size: Most < 10 mm in largest diameter
- Shape: Oval to variable
- Best imaging tool: Bone CT or CBCT
  - Axial and coronal sections

TOP DIFFERENTIAL DIAGNOSES

- Surgical defect
- Bone window but still closed/covered by mucous membrane
- Destruction of wall by malignant lesion

PATHOLOGY

- May have mucus ring as mucus enters accessory ostium and exits primary ostium

CLINICAL ISSUES

- Incidence of 18-30% in general population
- Asymptomatic, usually incidental finding
- Chronic maxillary sinusitis may be associated

DIAGNOSTIC CHECKLIST

- Consider: Thin wall that is lost by volume averaging
- Check ostium is seen on **both coronal and axial views**

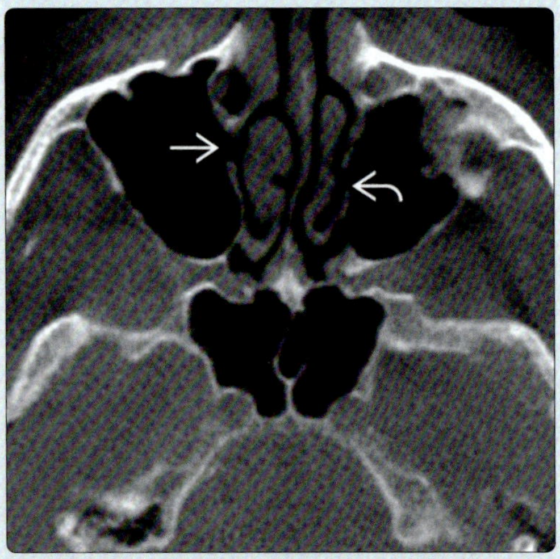
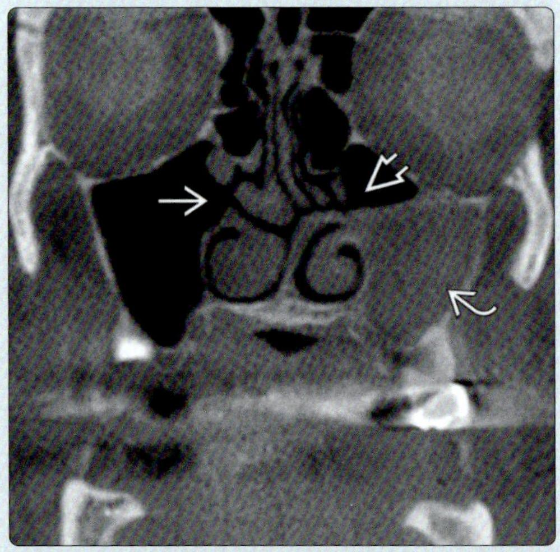

(Left) *Axial CBCT shows an accessory ostium on the right → and the left →, both inferior to their respective uncinate processes. The primary ostia are at a different level and not visible in this slice.* **(Right)** *Coronal CBCT in the same patient shows accessory ostia on the right → and left →. The primary ostia are not visible in this slice. Note opacification → of the majority of the left maxillary sinus.*

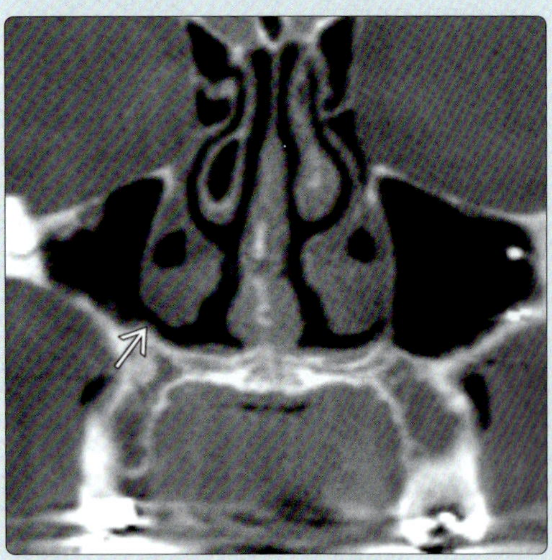
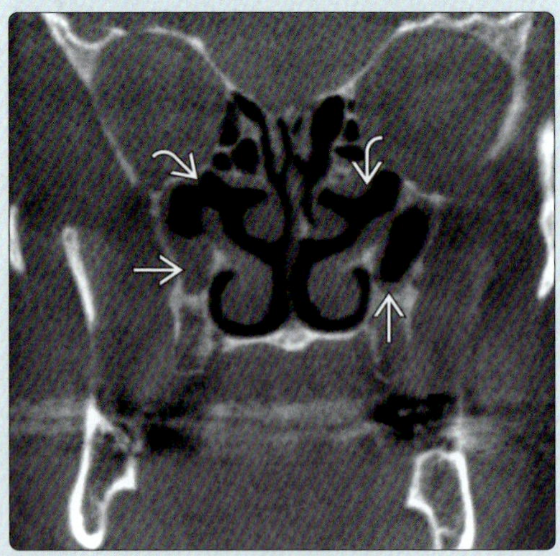

(Left) *Coronal CBCT reconstruction shows an anterior accessory ostium →. (Courtesy M. Tahmasbi, DDS.)* **(Right)** *Coronal CBCT shows accessory ostia → on the left and right, posterior to the primary ostia. The appearance is consistent with surgical intervention due to chronic sinusitis. There is soft tissue thickening → from chronic sinusitis seen in both maxillary sinuses.*

Accessory Ostia

TERMINOLOGY

Synonyms

- Ostia maxillare accessoria
- Accessory sinus ostia
- Accessory maxillary ostia
- Accessory openings
- Supplementary ostia
- 2 holes syndrome

Definitions

- Additional openings between sinus and nasal fossa

IMAGING

General Features

- Best diagnostic clue
  - **Discontinuity in medial wall of maxillary sinus** other than primary ostium
- Location
  - Medial wall of maxillary sinus
    - Infundibulum or region of anterior or posterior nasal fontanelles
      - Anterior fontanelle: Inferior and anterior to uncinate process
      - Posterior fontanelle: Between posterior end of uncinate process and palatine bone
- Size
  - Usually < 10 mm in largest diameter
- Morphology
  - Oval to variable

Imaging Recommendations

- Best imaging tool
  - CBCT or bone CT
    - If developmental
      - Discontinuity in wall between nasal fossa and maxillary sinus on coronal and axial reconstructions
      - Other anatomical architecture (conchae turbinates, uncinate process) is normal
    - If postsurgical
      - Ostium is usually larger
      - Other anatomical architecture (conchae turbinates, uncinate process) totally or partially missing or altered in morphology
- Protocol advice
  - Both **axial and coronal** sections
    - NECT bone window
    - CBCT

DIFFERENTIAL DIAGNOSIS

Surgical Defect

- History of chronic sinusitis
- Opening usually larger

Destruction of Wall by Malignant Lesion

- Look for soft tissue density adjacent to opening

PATHOLOGY

General Features

- Associated abnormalities
  - May have maxillary sinusitis
  - May have mucus ring as mucus enters accessory ostium and exits primary ostium
  - May have adjacent mass of malignant neoplasm

Staging, Grading, & Classification

- Anterior accessory ostia and posterior accessory ostia

CLINICAL ISSUES

Presentation

- Incidence of 18-30% in general population
- Most common signs/symptoms
  - Asymptomatic, usually incidental finding
  - Chronic maxillary sinusitis may be associated
- Other signs/symptoms
  - May have circulating mucus ring exiting primary ostium and reentering accessory ostium

Natural History & Prognosis

- May cause no problems
- May be cause or result of maxillary sinusitis
- May cause recirculation of mucus cleared via primary ostium

Treatment

- If recirculation of mucus, removal of bone between ostia to create 1 ostium

DIAGNOSTIC CHECKLIST

Consider

- Thin wall that is lost by volume averaging
- Osseous discontinuity but still mucous membrane over defect (i.e., normal fontanelle)

Image Interpretation Pearls

- Check that ostium is seen on **both coronal and axial views**

SELECTED REFERENCES

1. Magomedov MM et al: [The role of accessory ostia of the maxillary sinuses in pathogenesis of acute and chronic maxillary sinusitis.] Vestn Otorinolaringol. 80(5):98-100, 2015
2. Berjis N et al: Some anatomical variation of paranasal sinuses using sinus endoscopic approach on "cadaver" in Isfahan, Iran. Adv Biomed Res. 3:51, 2014
3. Jain R et al: Comparison of anatomical abnormalities in patients with limited and diffuse chronic rhinosinusitis. Int Forum Allergy Rhinol. 3(6):493-6, 2013
4. Na Y et al: The quantitative effect of an accessory ostium on ventilation of the maxillary sinus. Respir Physiol Neurobiol. 181(1):62-73, 2012
5. Zhu JH et al: Effect of accessory ostia on maxillary sinus ventilation: a computational fluid dynamics (CFD) study. Respir Physiol Neurobiol. 183(2):91-9, 2012
6. Mladina R et al: The two holes syndrome. Am J Rhinol Allergy. 23(6):602-4, 2009
7. Genc S et al: Development of maxillary accessory ostium following sinusitis in rabbits. Rhinology. 46(2):121-4, 2008
8. Gutman M et al: Iatrogenic maxillary sinus recirculation and beyond. Ear Nose Throat J. 82(1):61-3, 2003
9. Chung SK et al: Computed tomogram findings of mucous recirculation between the natural and accessory ostia of the maxillary sinus. Am J Rhinol. 16(5):265-8, 2002
10. Kumar H et al: Accessory maxillary ostia; topography and clinical application. J Anat Soc India. 50(1):3-5, 2001

Hypoplasia/Aplasia

KEY FACTS

TERMINOLOGY

- Abbreviations: Frontal sinus hypoplasia/aplasia (FSH/FSA); maxillary sinus hypoplasia/aplasia (MSH/MSA)
- Definition: Underdevelopment or lack of development of paranasal sinus(es) &/or nasal fossa(e) (NF)

IMAGING

- Frequency
  - Frontal > ethmoid > sphenoid > maxillary
  - MSH more common; MSA rare
- Smaller or absent air space of lumen of sinus due to ↓ distance between nonsclerotic osseous borders
  - **Mucosal thickening often associated, but osseous cavity is smaller**
- Normal maxillary sinus (MS) volume: 15 mL
  - Height: ~ 33 mm; width: 23-25 mm; AP length: 34 mm

TOP DIFFERENTIAL DIAGNOSES

- Chronic rhinosinusitis
- Fibrous dysplasia
- Odontogenic cysts

PATHOLOGY

- Type 1: Mild to moderate MSH; normally developed uncinate process; well-defined infundibulum; variable soft tissue thickening
- Type 2: Marked MSH; hypoplastic uncinate process; ill-defined or absent infundibulum; complete opacification of sinus by soft tissue
- Type 3: Profound MSH or MSA; absent or markedly hypoplastic uncinate process

CLINICAL ISSUES

- Often incidental finding
- Nasal obstruction; postnasal drainage; headache
- No treatment indicated in most isolated cases

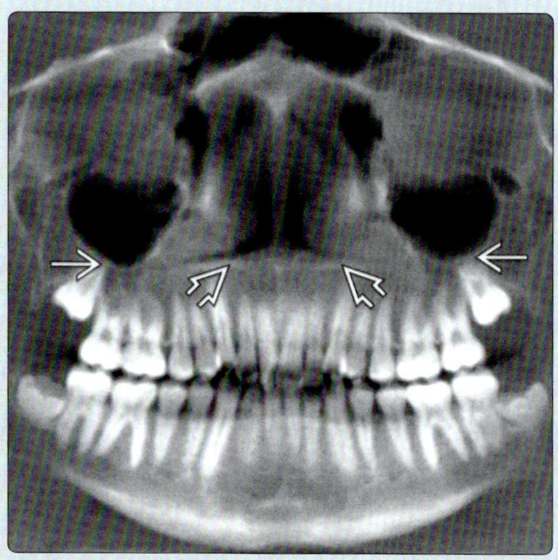
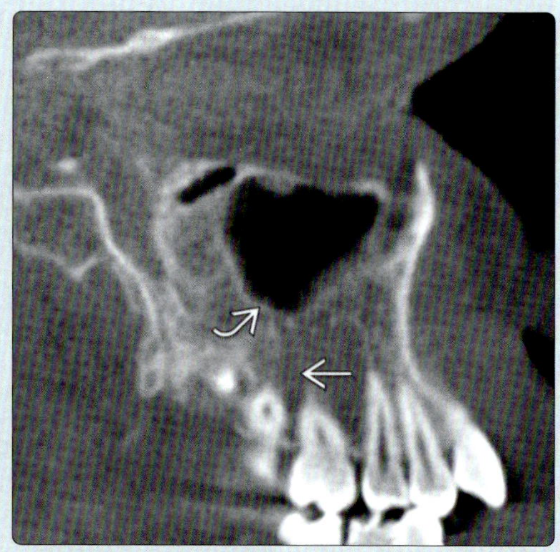

(Left) *Panoramic reformat CBCT shows bilateral hypoplasia of the maxillary sinuses (MS). Note the level of the floor of the MS ➡ is above the level of the floor of the nose ➡, which is a classic sign of maxillary sinus hypoplasia (MSH). This is type 1 MSH.* **(Right)** *Sagittal CBCT in the same patient shows the hypoplastic MS floor ➡ well above the apices of the teeth ➡. There is no evidence of any space-occupying lesion causing displacement of the MS floor that would account for the reduction in sinus size.*

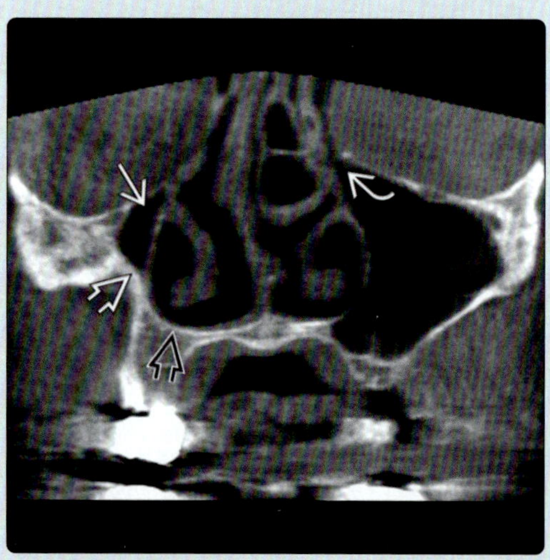
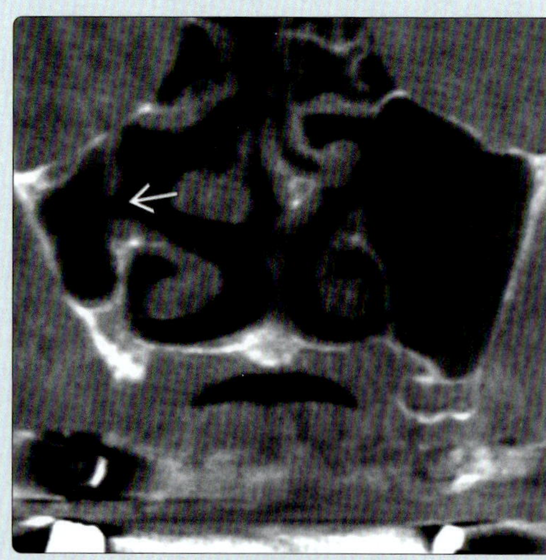

(Left) *Coronal CBCT shows the marked difference in size between the right hypoplastic MS ➡ and the left normal sinus. The floor ➡ of the right sinus is superior to the floor of the nasal fossa ➡, and the sinus does not extend laterally past the midline of the orbit. Note normal patent ostiomeatal unit ➡ on the left, which is absent on the right. This is type 2 MSH.* **(Right)** *Coronal CBCT in the same patient shows a posterior accessory ostia ➡ on the right, which provides a drainage pathway to the small hypoplastic sinus.*

TERMINOLOGY

Abbreviations

- Frontal sinus hypoplasia/aplasia (FSH/FSA)
- Maxillary sinus hypoplasia/aplasia (MSH/MSA)

Synonyms

- Hypogenesis/agenesis of specific sinuses &/or nasal fossae (NF)

Definitions

- Underdevelopment or lack of development of frontal sinus(es) (FS), ethmoid air cells [sinus(es)], sphenoid sinus(es), or maxillary sinus(es) (MS), &/or NF

IMAGING

General Features

- Best diagnostic clue
  - Smaller or absent air space of sinus lumen due to decreased distance between nonsclerotic osseous borders
    - Mucosal thickening often associated, but osseous cavity is smaller
- Location
  - May involve 1 or multiple sinuses and NF
  - Frequency
    - Frontal > ethmoid > sphenoid > maxillary
    - MSH more common; MSA rare
    - FSH variable, FSA not rare
- Size
  - Decreased size or absence of involved sinus
    - Normal MS volume: 15 mL
      - Height: ~ 33 mm
      - Width: 23-25 mm
      - AP length: 34 mm
    - Normal FS volume most variable of all sinuses
  - MS present at birth and fully developed around age 3
  - Ethmoid sinuses present at birth and fully developed around age 3
  - Sphenoid sinuses present around age 3 and fully developed around age 12
  - FS present around age 3 and fully developed around age 12
- Morphology
  - MSH: Morphology is normal but smaller
  - MSA: Complete absence

Radiographic Findings

- Radiography
  - Failure of MS to descend below level of nasal floor
  - Lack of pneumatization of alveolar process around apices of posterior maxillary teeth
  - Other sinuses smaller than normal

CT Findings

- CBCT and bone CT
  - Small or absent MS
    - If small, mucosal thickening in sinus
  - Small or absent uncinate process and infundibulum
  - Small or absent NF is rare
  - 4 of 5 of the following for MS in coronal plane
    - Failure of floor of sinus to descend below level of nasal floor
    - Smaller and oval-shaped sinus
    - Larger and oval-shaped orbit
    - Medial position of sinus border is lateral to medial border of orbit
    - Lateral position of sinus border is medial to middle of orbit at level of infundibulum
  - Small or absent FS
    - Failure of sinus to project over orbit
  - Small or absent SS
    - Failure or minimal aeration of body of sphenoid bone

Imaging Recommendations

- Best imaging tool
  - CBCT or bone CT
- Protocol advice
  - Include all paranasal sinuses and NF

DIFFERENTIAL DIAGNOSIS

Chronic Rhinosinusitis

- Sclerotic wall of sinus reduces lumen

Odontogenic Cysts/Neoplasms

- Border of sinus directionally displaced by encroaching lesion
  - Border "bulges" into lumen of sinus

Fibrous Dysplasia

- Encroaches upon ≥ 1 paranasal sinus
  - Border is displaced but remains intact
- Trabecular bone pattern is altered

Silent Sinus Syndrome

- Maxillary ostium is obstructed
  - Rather than hypodevelopmental, sinus becomes progressively smaller
  - Blockage thought to produce negative pressure
  - Hypoglobus
  - Inward retraction of medial and superior walls

Gaucher Disease

- Enlargement of marrow spaces results in enlargement of bone
  - Enlarged bone encroaches on sinuses
  - Bone may have frothy pattern due to many larger marrow spaces

PATHOLOGY

General Features

- Etiology
  - MSH/MSA is developmental
  - Smaller sinus also results from trauma, irradiation, surgery, neoplasm, systemic illness
  - Silent sinus syndrome may cause 2° acquired smaller sinus through progressive decrease in sinus volume
    - Probably due to ostium obstruction and resultant negative pressure
    - Often associated with hypoglobus and enophthalmos
- Genetics
  - Most MSH or MSA is not inherited

- May be associated with various genetically inherited syndromes
- Associated abnormalities
  - Absence or hypoplasia of other paranasal sinuses
    - MS least common
  - Many developmental abnormalities, including:
    - Mandibulofacial dysostosis (Treacher-Collins syndrome)
    - Craniofacial dysostosis (Crouzon disease)
    - Cleidocranial dysplasia
    - Acrocephalosyndactyly (Apert syndrome)
    - Thalassemia
    - Sickle cell anemia
    - Cretinism
    - Cleft palate
    - Hemifacial microsomia (Goldenhar syndrome)
    - Osteopetrosis (Albers Schönberg disease)
    - Pyknodysostosis
    - Trisomy 21 (Down syndrome)
    - Maxillomandibular dysplasia (Binder syndrome)
    - Progressive diaphyseal dysplasia (Camurati-Engelmann disease)
    - Generalized cortical hyperostosis (van Buchem disease)
    - Osteodystrophy (Melnick-Needles syndrome)
    - Craniometaphyseal dysplasia
    - Craniodiaphyseal dysplasia
    - Elfin face syndrome (Williams-Beuren syndrome)
    - Tricho-dento-osseous dysplasia
    - Homozygous delta F508 mutations in cystic fibrosis

Staging, Grading, & Classification

- Type 1
  - Mild to moderate sinus hypoplasia
  - Normally developed uncinate process
  - Well-defined infundibulum
  - Variable amount of sinus soft tissue thickening
- Type 2
  - Marked sinus hypoplasia
  - Hypoplastic uncinate process
  - Ill-defined or absent infundibulum
  - Complete opacification of sinus by soft tissue
- Type 3
  - Profound sinus hypoplasia or aplasia
    - Sinus is shallow cleft in lateral wall of NF
  - Absent or markedly hypoplastic uncinate process

Gross Pathologic & Surgical Features

- Small or absent MS and uncinate process

CLINICAL ISSUES

Presentation

- Most common signs/symptoms
  - Often incidental finding
  - Complaint of nasal obstruction
  - Postnasal drainage
  - Headache
- Other signs/symptoms
  - Facial asymmetry
  - Hypoglobus
  - Enophthalmia
  - Mucosal thickening/sinusitis
- Clinical profile
  - May be part of larger disorder

Demographics

- Age
  - Best assessed after 18 years

Natural History & Prognosis

- Occurs during time of sinus development

Treatment

- No treatment may be indicated in most isolated cases
- Depends upon associated abnormalities

DIAGNOSTIC CHECKLIST

Consider

- Chronic sclerosing rhinosinusitis
- Ethmomaxillary sinus
- Associated syndrome or systemic abnormality

Image Interpretation Pearls

- Note location of inferior border of MS relative to level of nasal floor
- Note size and shape (smaller and oval) of sinus
- Note size and shape (larger and oval) of ipsilateral orbit
- Note if medial position of sinus border is lateral to medial border of orbit
- Note if lateral position of sinus border is medial to middle of orbit at level of infundibulum
- Check morphology/presence of infundibulum and uncinate process
- Note if maxillary ostium is patent
- Check other paranasal sinuses for hypoplasia/aplasia

Reporting Tips

- Report absence of uncinate process, as this alters functional endoscopic sinus surgery approaches

SELECTED REFERENCES

1. Martínez-Capoccioni G et al: Silent sinus syndrome an acquired condition and the essential role of otorhinolaryngologist consultation: a retrospective study. Eur Arch Otorhinolaryngol. 273(10):3183-8, 2016
2. Angulo-Pérez G et al: [Prevalence, location and tomographic severity of chronic rhinosinusitis in adult patients with common variable immunodeficiency.] Rev Alerg Mex. 62(1):15-21, 2015
3. Demir UL et al: Anatomical correlation between existence of concha bullosa and maxillary sinus volume. Surg Radiol Anat. 37(9):1093-8, 2015
4. Göçmen G et al: Effect of septal deviation, concha bullosa and Haller's cell on maxillary sinus's inferior pneumatization; a retrospective study. Open Dent J. 9:282-6, 2015
5. Selcuk OT et al: Do altitude and climate affect paranasal sinus volume? J Craniomaxillofac Surg. 43(7):1059-64, 2015
6. Chrcanovic BR et al: Maxillary sinus aplasia. Oral Maxillofac Surg. 14(3):187-91, 2010
7. Güven DG et al: Combined aplasia of sphenoid, frontal, and maxillary sinuses accompanied by ethmoid sinus hypoplasia. J Craniofac Surg. 21(5):1431-3, 2010
8. Whyte MP et al: Dysosteosclerosis presents as an "osteoclast-poor" form of osteopetrosis: comprehensive investigation of a 3-year-old girl and literature review. J Bone Miner Res. 25(11):2527-39, 2010
9. Nagasao T et al: A rare case of congenital unilateral hypoplasia of the nose. J Plast Reconstr Aesthet Surg. 62(9):e305-8, 2009
10. Song SY et al: Volume and distances of the maxillary sinus in craniofacial deformities with midfacial hypoplasia. Otolaryngol Head Neck Surg. 141(5):614-20, 2009

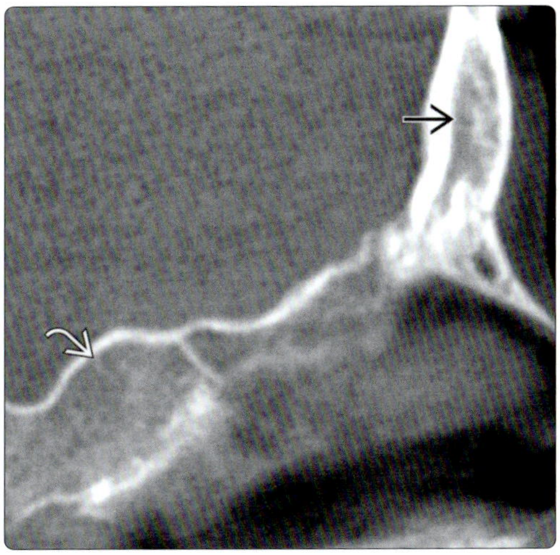

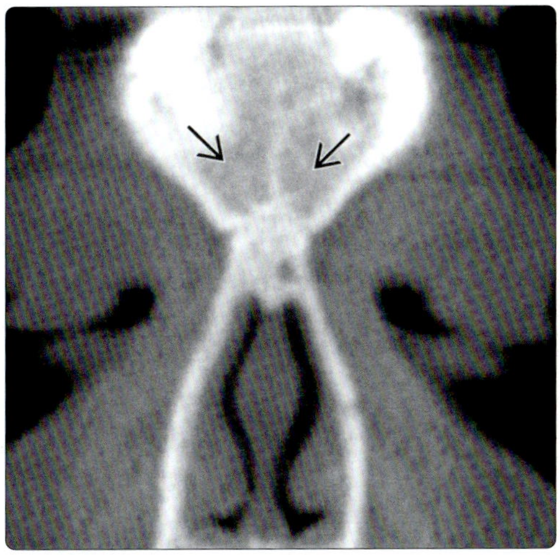

(Left) *Sagittal CBCT reconstruction shows aplasia of the sphenoid ➡ and frontal ⇨ sinuses in a patient who also has maxillary sinus hypoplasia.* **(Right)** *Coronal CBCT reconstruction in the same patient shows no evidence of frontal sinuses bilaterally, consistent with aplasia of the frontal sinuses ⇨. The frontal sinuses exhibit hypoplasia/aplasia more commonly than any of the other paranasal sinuses.*

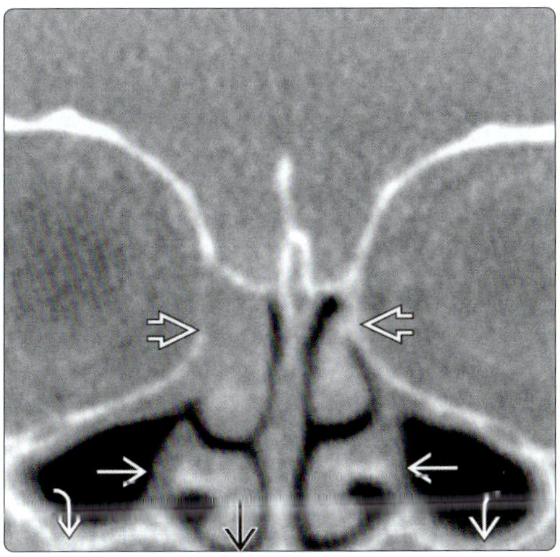

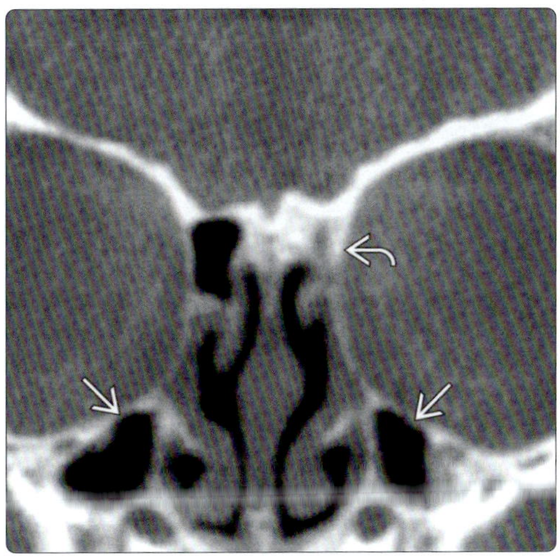

(Left) *Coronal CBCT of a limited volume shows the floor of the hypoplastic MS ➡ at the bottom of the image. The floor of the MS is above the level of the floor of the nasal fossae ⇨ (not shown). There is mucosal thickening ➡ in both sinuses. There is no evidence of the ethmoid sinuses ➡.* **(Right)** *Coronal CBCT shows bilateral hypoplastic MS ➡ and unilateral aplasia of the left ethmoid sinus ➡.*

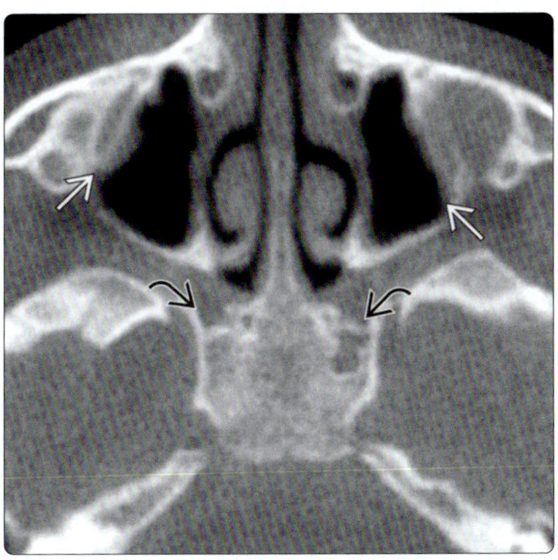

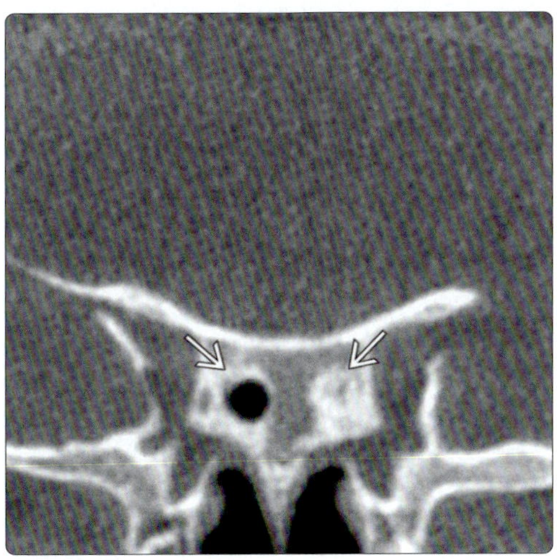

(Left) *Axial CBCT reconstruction of the previous patient shows hypoplastic maxillary sinuses ➡ and only rudimentary sphenoid sinuses consistent with extreme hypoplasia of both sphenoid sinuses ⇨.* **(Right)** *Coronal CBCT reconstruction of the same patient shows 2 extremely hypoplastic sphenoid sinuses ➡. It is less common to see hypoplasia/aplasia in the sphenoid sinuses than in the ethmoid or frontal sinuses.*

Mucus Retention Pseudocyst

KEY FACTS

TERMINOLOGY

- Synonyms: Mucus retention phenomenon, mucus retention pseudocyst
- Definition: Accumulation of mucus within soft tissue lining in paranasal sinus due to obstruction of gland within lining
- Not surrounded by epithelium, hence **"pseudocyst"**

IMAGING

- Common incidental finding
- **Dome-shaped mass** in sinus without change in sinus wall
- **No corticated border** around lesion
- Maxillary sinus floor or wall most common
  - Sphenoid sinus floor or wall next most common
- Varies from very small up to occupying most of sinus lumen
- Usually no accompanying soft tissue thickening
- **Border of sinus intact** and not displaced
- T1WI: Intermediate to low signal
- T2WI: Bright signal
- May be multiple

TOP DIFFERENTIAL DIAGNOSES

- Sinusitis
- Radicular cyst encroaching on sinus
  - Elevation of sinus floor at apex of **nonvital tooth**
- Dentigerous cyst encroaching on sinus
  - Associated with crown of **impacted tooth**
- Periostitis
- Mucositis, localized
- Malignant neoplasm in sinus
  - Border of sinus destroyed

CLINICAL ISSUES

- Slight male preponderance
- Occurs in all ages and populations
- Usually asymptomatic
- No treatment required: Self-limiting due to rupture

DIAGNOSTIC CHECKLIST

- Check that adjacent **sinus border is intact**

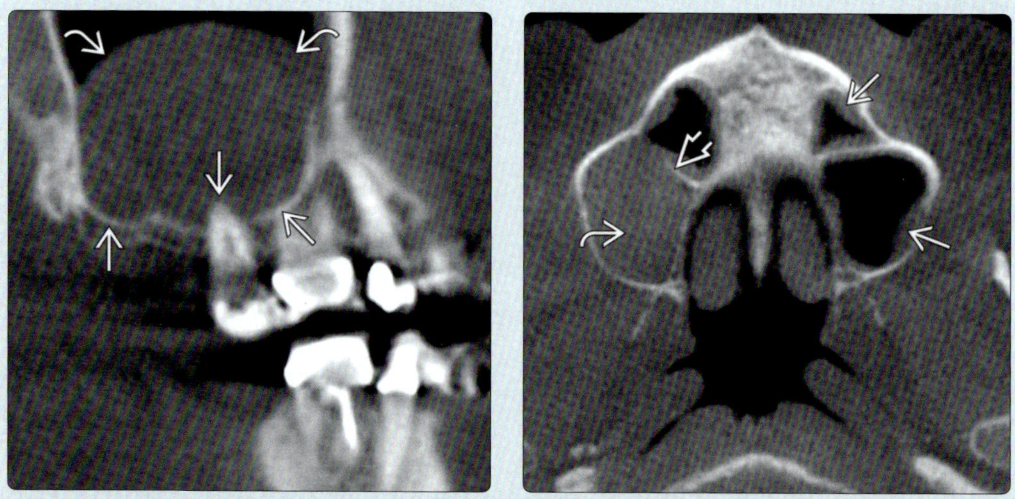

(Left) *Sagittal CBCT reconstruction shows a large, dome-shaped, noncorticated soft tissue density (relative to air) mass consistent with a mucus retention pseudocyst in the maxillary sinus. The adjacent border of the sinus is intact.* **(Right)** *Axial CBCT reconstruction shows a mucus retention pseudocyst occupying all of a loculus of the right maxillary sinus at this level. It is important not to confuse a sinus septum with a corticated margin. Note mild mucosal thickening in the locules of the left maxillary sinus .*

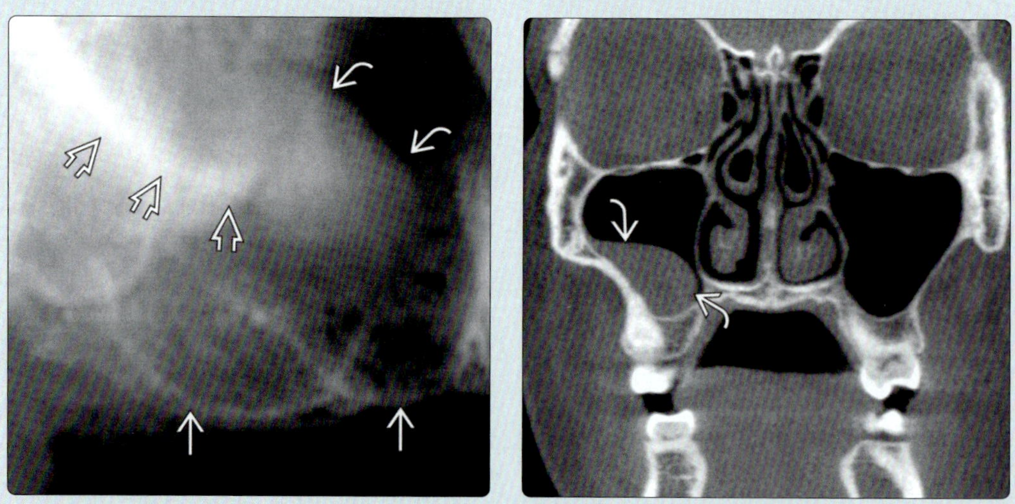

(Left) *Periapical radiograph of the right posterior edentulous maxilla shows a dome-shaped radiopaque (relative to air) mass in the maxillary sinus. The adjacent border of the sinus is intact. Note superimposition of the zygomatic process .* **(Right)** *A coronal CBCT reconstruction shows a dome-shaped mucus retention pseudocyst in the right maxillary sinus. The mass is noncorticated, and the sinus borders are intact. (Courtesy V. Allareddy, BDS.)*

TERMINOLOGY

Synonyms

- Mucus retention cyst, mucus retention phenomenon

Definitions

- Accumulation of mucus within soft tissue lining in paranasal sinus due to obstruction of gland within lining
- Elevation of floor of sinus by accumulation of mucus
- Not surrounded by epithelium, hence **"pseudocyst"**

IMAGING

General Features

- Best diagnostic clue
  - **Dome-shaped** mass in sinus **without cortication** or change in sinus wall
- Location
  - Maxillary sinus floor or wall most common
  - Sphenoid sinus floor > ethmoid > frontal
- Size
  - May be very small or occupy most of sinus
- Morphology
  - Dome-shaped; may be multiple

Imaging Recommendations

- Best imaging tool
  - Periapical or panoramic radiograph for maxillary sinus lesion
  - CBCT or bone CT if large or in other paranasal sinuses
    - CT evaluation if any doubt that sinus borders are intact
- Protocol advice
  - None; usually incidental finding

MR Findings

- T1WI
  - Intermediate to low signal
- T2WI
  - Bright signal

Imaging Features

- **Dome-shaped** radiopaque mass arising from floor/wall of sinus
- Usually no accompanying soft tissue thickening
- **No corticated border** around lesion
- Border of sinus intact and not displaced

DIFFERENTIAL DIAGNOSIS

Sinusitis

- More generalized soft tissue thickening
- Prolific polypoid mucosal thickening may appear in part as mucus retention pseudocyst

Radicular Cyst Encroaching on Sinus

- **Corticated border/radiopaque halo** around mass
- Associated with root(s) of carious tooth or recent extraction site
- See loss of lamina dura at apex of associated tooth

Dentigerous Cyst Encroaching on Sinus

- **Corticated border** around mass
- Associated with crown of impacted tooth
- Tooth displaced into sinus

Mucositis, Localized

- Localized soft tissue thickening
- **Sessile**, not dome-shaped

Antrochoanal Polyps

- Located on roof of sinus as well

Malignant Neoplasm in Sinus

- Border of sinus destroyed

Mucocele

- Entire sinus is radiopaque
- Associated with blocked ostium
- Sinus border displaced

PATHOLOGY

General Features

- Etiology
  - Unknown

Gross Pathologic & Surgical Features

- Fluid-filled swelling of soft tissue of sinus

CLINICAL ISSUES

Presentation

- Most common signs/symptoms
  - Usually asymptomatic
- Other signs/symptoms
  - Vague feeling of nasal/antral stuffiness or fullness
  - Vague pain

Demographics

- Age
  - Any age
- Gender
  - Slight male preponderance

Natural History & Prognosis

- Usually self-limiting due to rupture

Treatment

- Usually no treatment required

DIAGNOSTIC CHECKLIST

Consider

- Adjacent sinus border is intact

Image Interpretation Pearls

- **No corticated border** around mass

Reporting Tips

- Usually of no clinical significance
- Check patency of ostiomeatal unit if large

SELECTED REFERENCES

1. Giotakis EI et al: Cysts of the maxillary sinus: a literature review. Int Forum Allergy Rhinol. 3(9):766-71, 2013

Sinonasal Mucocele

KEY FACTS

IMAGING

- Opacified, **expanded** sinus with **smooth remodeling** of walls
  - May occur in septated sinuses & pneumatized anatomic variant air cells
  - **Frontal (60-65%)** > **ethmoid (25%)** > maxillary (5-10%) > sphenoid (2-5%)
- CT: Thin-section CT with coronal & sagittal reformat helpful for surgical planning & delineation of adjacent normal anatomy
  - Low-density or soft tissue density opacification of sinus with expansion
  - Bony sinus walls remodeled
  - No central enhancement; ± minimal peripheral enhancement
- MR: Enhanced MR recommended for detection of intracranial involvement & identifying obstructing neoplasm as underlying cause
  - High water content of mucous interior yields ↓ T1 signal, ↑ T2 signal

TOP DIFFERENTIAL DIAGNOSES

- Allergic fungal sinusitis
- Sinonasal polyposis
- Sinonasal solitary polyps

PATHOLOGY

- Results from obstruction of primary ostium of affected sinus

CLINICAL ISSUES

- Most common expansile lesion of paranasal sinuses
- Slowly progressive symptoms that vary depending upon lesion location without signs of acute infection
  - > 90% have ophthalmic symptoms & signs
- Surgical cure is goal & expected result when mucocele is present

(Left) *Coronal graphic shows a large, left anterior ethmoid mucocele extending into the left frontal sinus. The affected sinuses are expanded without evidence of aggressive bone destruction.* **(Right)** *Coronal bone CT shows the typical features of a right ethmoid mucocele. The sinus is opacified, and there is remodeling of the surrounding bony walls with erosion of the lamina papyracea ➡. Note the mass effect upon the orbit with lateralization of the globe ➡.*

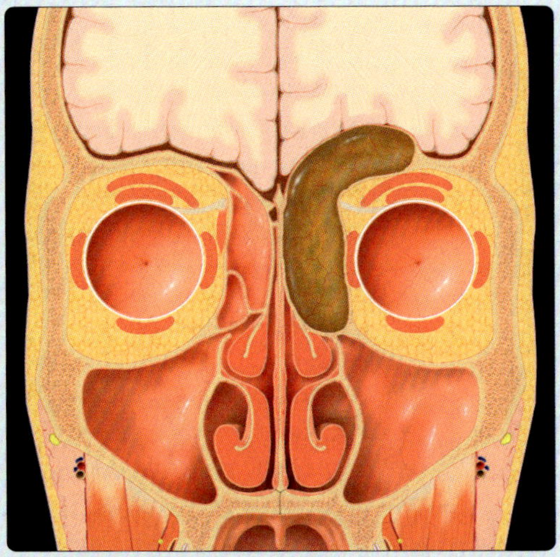

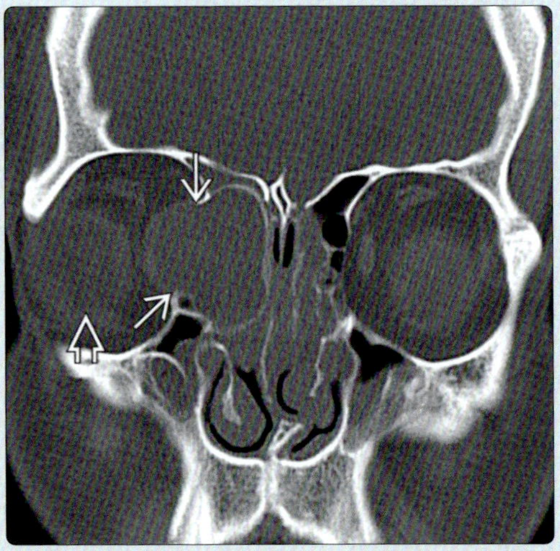

(Left) *Coronal CECT bone window of a 51-year-old woman shows an adenoid cystic carcinoma ➡ obstructing the left maxillary ostium, resulting in a mucocele in the left maxillary sinus ➡. (Courtesy A. Mancuso, MD and J. Bennett, MD.)* **(Right)** *Coronal CECT soft tissue window in the same patient better demonstrates the enhancement of the tumor ➡ obstructing the left maxillary ostium compared to the nonenhancing mucocele in the left maxillary sinus ➡. (Courtesy A. Mancuso, MD and J. Bennett, MD.)*

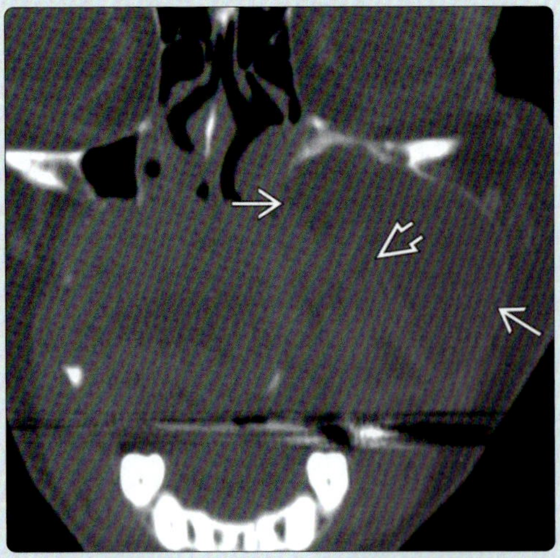

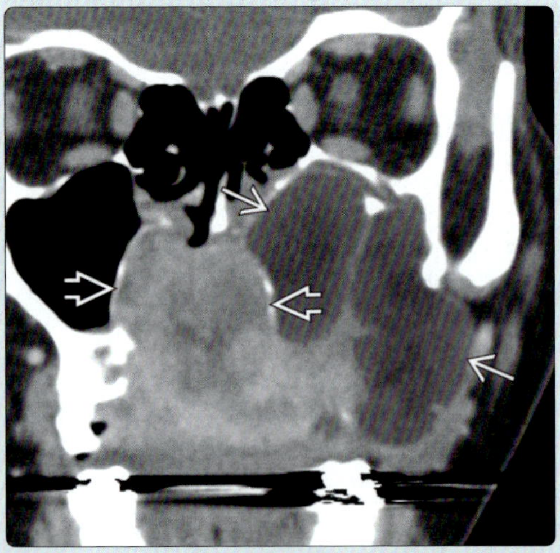

TERMINOLOGY

Definitions

- Opacified, mucus-containing, expanded sinus lined by respiratory epithelium & resulting from chronic major ostial obstruction
  - From Latin "muco" = mucus + Greek "kele" = tumor or "mucous tumor"
- If infected, called pyomucocele or pyocele

IMAGING

General Features

- Best diagnostic clue
  - Opacified, expanded sinus with smooth remodeling of walls
- Location
  - > 90% in frontal & ethmoid sinuses
    - **Frontal (60-65%)** > ethmoid (25%) > maxillary (5-10%) > sphenoid (2-5%)
  - May occur in septated sinuses & pneumatized anatomic variant air cells
  - Ethmoid mucoceles have greatest potential for intraorbital extension
  - Sphenoid mucoceles have greatest potential for intracranial extension
- Size
  - Usually involves whole sinus
  - Sinus may expand
- Morphology
  - Frontal mucocele: Expands anteriorly into skin of forehead or posteriorly into anterior cranial fossa
  - Ethmoid mucocele: Thins & remodels lamina papyracea (lateral ethmoid air cell wall), bowing it into orbit
  - Maxillary mucocele: Expands into ipsilateral nasal cavity, usually in area of secondary ostium of maxillary sinus or into premaxillary soft tissues
  - Sphenoid sinus mucocele: Expands anterolaterally into posterior ethmoids & orbital apex

Radiographic Findings

- Radiography
  - Frontal & maxillary sinus mucocele can be suggested from 2D imaging findings
    - "Clouding" of expanded sinus with loss of normal mucoperiosteal line of sinus wall
  - Ethmoid & sphenoid mucocele may be missed

CT Findings

- CECT
  - No central enhancement; ± minimal peripheral enhancement
    - Thick peripheral enhancement raises suspicion of superinfection (mucopyocele)
- Bone CT
  - Low-density or soft tissue density opacification of sinus with **expansion**
    - High-density areas related to desiccation of secretions or fungal colonization
  - Bony sinus walls remodeled
    - May be thinned, focally absent, or normal thickness

MR Findings

- T1WI
  - High water content of mucous interior yields ↓ T1 signal
    - When protein content high, ↑ T1 signal
- T2WI
  - High water content of mucous interior yields ↑ T2 signal
    - When areas of inspissated mucus exist, may be very low signal
- T1WI C+
  - No central enhancement; ± minimal peripheral enhancement
    - Thickened peripheral mucosa suggests infected mucocele (mucopyocele)
    - If associated nodule of enhancement seen, consider tumor obstruction of sinus with secondary mucocele
- MRS
  - N-acetyl compounds (N-acetylglucosamine, N-acetylgalactosamine) may cause peak at 2.0 ppm, mimicking brain N-acetylaspartate

Imaging Recommendations

- Best imaging tool
  - Small mucocele may require only unenhanced coronal bone CT
  - Larger mucocele with significant regional compression may benefit from enhanced MR with bone-only CT in axial and coronal planes
- Protocol advice
  - Thin-section CT with coronal & sagittal reformat helpful for surgical planning and delineation of adjacent normal anatomy
  - Enhanced MR recommended for detection of intracranial involvement & identifying obstructing neoplasm as cause of mucocele

DIFFERENTIAL DIAGNOSIS

Allergic Fungal Sinusitis

- Typically expansile, especially if seen with polyps
- Involves multiple sinuses
- High central density on CT; mixed MR signal

Sinonasal Polyposis

- Involves multiple sinuses **and** nasal cavity
- May have multiple small mucoceles associated

Sinonasal Solitary Polyps

- "Dumbbell" cystic mass that fills maxillary antrum, herniates through sinus ostium into adjacent nasal cavity

Slow-Growing Benign or Malignant Tumor

- May mimic mucocele when seen on bone/unenhanced CT
- Central, nodular enhancement on CT/MR differentiates from mucocele

PATHOLOGY

General Features

- Etiology
  - Results from **obstruction of primary ostium** of affected sinus

    - Obstruction from inflammation, trauma, functional endoscopic sinus surgery, or any space-occupying sinonasal mass
    - Secretion of mucus into obstructed sinus creates mucocele
    - Sinus expansion from pressure necrosis with slow erosion of inner surface of bony sinus wall matched by new bone formation on outer periosteal surface
- Associated abnormalities
    - Obstructing mass at ostium may cause secondary mucocele

Staging, Grading, & Classification

- 2 types
    - Internal: Herniation of cyst into submucosal tissue adjacent to sinus bony wall
    - External: Herniation of cyst through bony wall with extension into subcutaneous tissue or intracranial cavity

Gross Pathologic & Surgical Features

- Mucocele lumen filled with thick mucoid or gelatinous secretions

Microscopic Features

- Histologically indistinguishable from polyps & retention cysts
- Flattened, pseudostratified, ciliated columnar epithelium = mucus-secreting respiratory epithelium
    - Squamous metaplasia can be seen in longstanding cases
- Retained mucous secretions are sterile
    - Purulent exudate present in cases of mucopyocele
- Reactive bone formation or bony remodeling of adjacent sinus walls may be present

CLINICAL ISSUES

Presentation

- Most common signs/symptoms
    - > 90% have ophthalmic signs & symptoms
    - Principal presenting symptoms depend on site of involvement
        - Frontal mucocele: Forehead bossing, proptosis, diplopia, and mass in superomedial orbit or headache, retro-orbital pain, facial pressure, visual disturbance from intracranial extension
        - Ethmoid mucocele: Proptosis, blurred vision ± visual loss, periorbital swelling
        - Maxillary mucocele: Nasal obstruction from medial projection with cheek pressure, rhinorrhea
        - Sphenoid mucocele: Visual loss, oculomotor palsy, headache
- Other signs/symptoms
    - Epiphora, decreased color vision, hypoglobus (downward displaced eye)
    - Amaurosis uncommon complication in 5%
    - If pain present, consider mucopyocele
- Clinical profile
    - Slowly progressive symptoms that vary depending upon lesion location without signs of acute infection
    - Diagnosis requires correlation between clinical, radiographic, and pathologic findings, as diagnosis on histopathology alone can be difficult

Demographics

- Age
    - Most common in adults
        - Occurs in all age groups
    - In children, look for obstructing mass or underlying disorder (cystic fibrosis, immotile cilia syndrome)
- Epidemiology
    - Most common expansile lesion of paranasal sinuses
    - Although rare, sphenoid mucocele has highest complication rate due to proximity of vital structures

Natural History & Prognosis

- Gradual, clinically silent enlargement over months to years
- Cranial neuropathy (CNII-VI) may not recover following surgery if chronic at time of presentation
- Complications in untreated cases
    - Include superimposed infection (mucopyocele), meningitis ± brain abscess

Treatment

- Surgical cure is goal & expected result when mucocele is present
    - Endoscopic sinus surgery
        - Reserved for uncomplicated maxillary or ethmoid mucocele
    - Most frontal mucoceles treated with osteoplastic flap ± obliteration
    - Transfacial surgical approaches
        - Reserved for deeper posterior ethmoid or sphenoid mucocele
    - Transcranial surgical approach
        - Reserved for mucoceles with intracranial extension or causing compression of bone structures with optic pathway neurological symptoms

DIAGNOSTIC CHECKLIST

Consider

- Extensive peripheral enhancement may suggest **mucopyocele**
- If central enhancement present, consider neoplasm

Image Interpretation Pearls

- Look for thin peripheral rim of expanded bone
- No central enhancement on postcontrast CT or MR

SELECTED REFERENCES

1. DeParis SW et al: Paranasal sinus mucocele as a late complication of dacryocystorhinostomy. Ophthal Plast Reconstr Surg. ePub, 2015
2. Huang KL et al: An isolated intracranial mucocoele herniated from the frontal sinus. B-ENT. 11(3):245-7, 2015
3. Sari K et al: Concha bullosa mucopyocele: a Case Report. Acta Medica (Hradec Kralove). 58(4):147-9, 2015
4. Simões JC et al: Visual loss: a rare complication of maxillary sinus mucocele. Braz J Otorhinolaryngol. 81(4):451-3, 2015
5. Topdag M et al: Paranasal sinus mucoceles: our clinical experiments. Int J Clin Exp Med. 8(10):18518-22, 2015
6. Lee JT et al: Intracranial mucocele formation in the context of longstanding chronic rhinosinusitis: A clinicopathologic series and literature review. Allergy Rhinol (Providence). 4(3):e166-75, 2013
7. Verillaud B et al: Mucocele after transnasal endoscopic repair of traumatic anterior skull base fistula in children. Int J Pediatr Otorhinolaryngol. 75(9):1137-42, 2011
8. Lee TJ et al: Extensive paranasal sinus mucoceles: a 15-year review of 82 cases. Am J Otolaryngol. 30(4):234-8, 2009

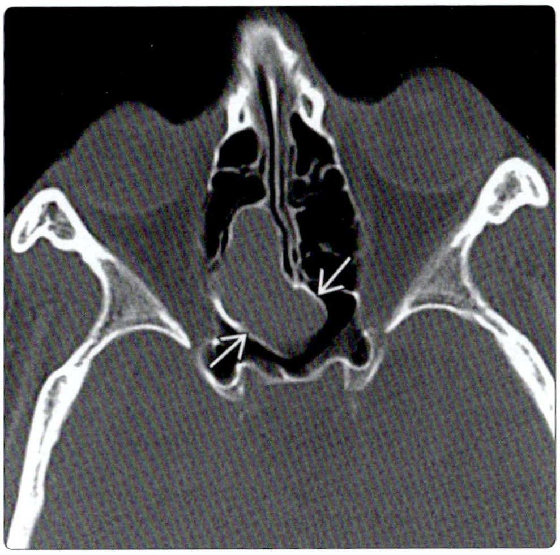

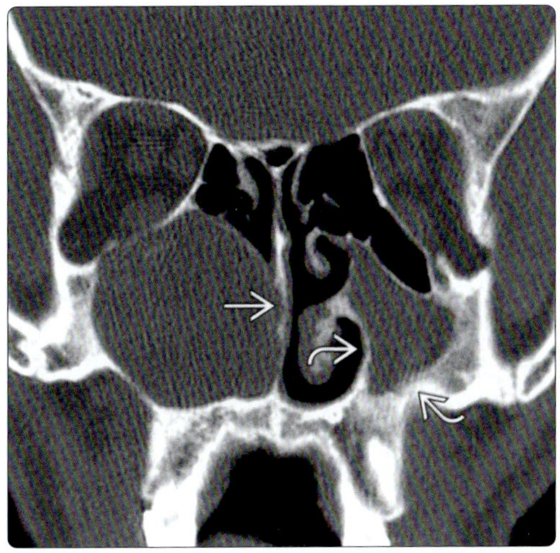

(Left) *Axial bone CT demonstrates a posterior ethmoid mucocele that extends into the sphenoid sinuses rather than into the orbit. The bone surrounding the lesion is thinned and remodeled.* **(Right)** *Coronal bone CT shows a large mucocele arising within the right maxillary sinus, an unusual location for a mucocele. The lesion occludes the nasal airway. Note the changes of chronic sinusitis of the left maxillary sinus with decreased volume and thickening of the walls.*

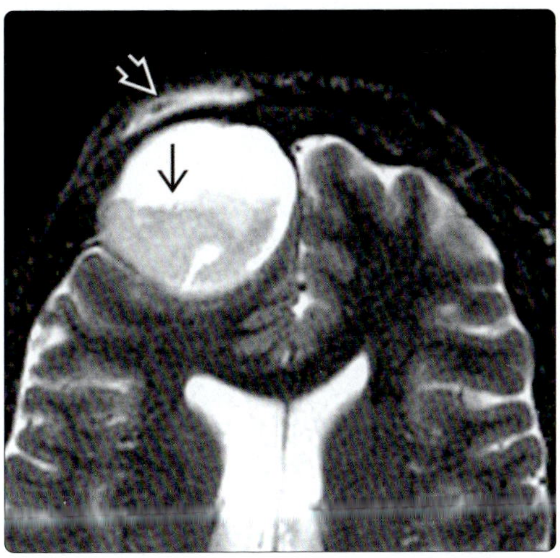

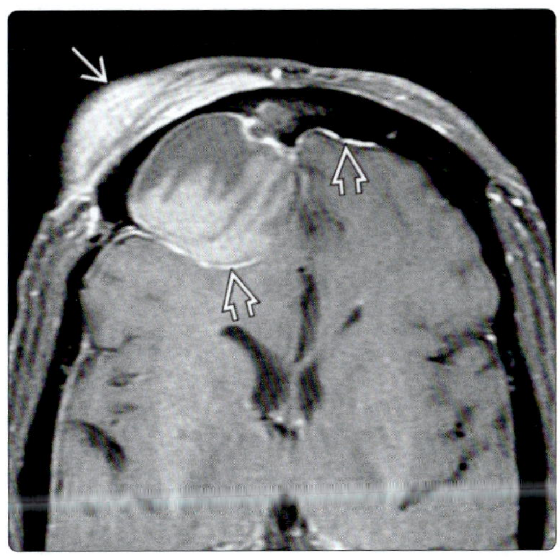

(Left) *Axial T2WI FS MR shows a large right frontal mucocele containing a fluid-fluid level with material of varying signal intensities. This mucocele extended into the superficial soft tissues, causing swelling and edema.* **(Right)** *Axial T1WI C+ FS MR in the same patient shows superficial soft tissue swelling and enhancement over the ruptured mucocele. There is also enhancement of the dura in the anterior fossa consistent with early meningeal inflammation.*

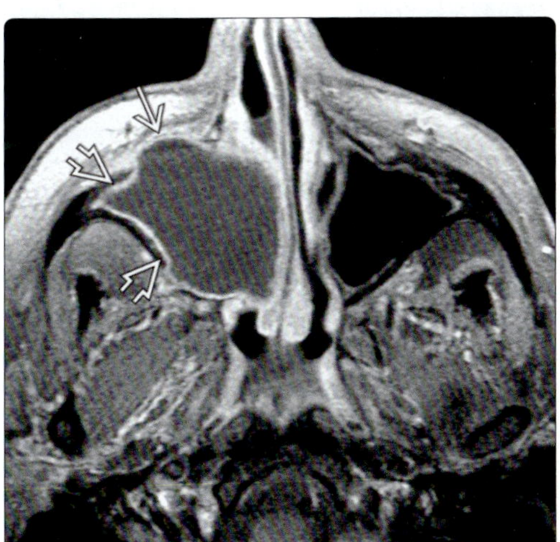

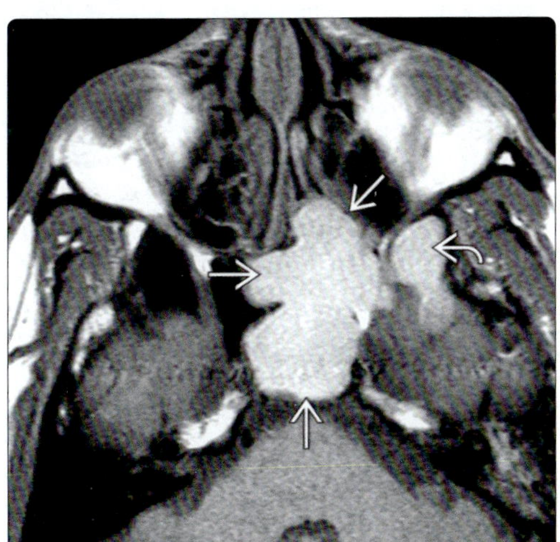

(Left) *Axial T1WI C+ FS MR shows a mucocele of the right maxillary sinus with erosion of the anterior wall and extension into the nasal cavity. There is peripheral mucosal enhancement but no central enhancement. This helps distinguish a mucocele from a neoplasm.* **(Right)** *Axial T1WI MR demonstrates a large mucocele of the left sphenoid sinus. The lesion is homogeneously hyperintense, likely related to highly proteinaceous contents. Note the involvement of the lateral recess.*

Sinonasal Granulomatosis With Polyangiitis (Wegener Granulomatosis)

KEY FACTS

TERMINOLOGY

- Abbreviation: Granulomatosis with polyangiitis (GPA)
- Definition: Idiopathic **necrotizing granulomatous vasculitis** that preferentially involves upper & lower respiratory tracts, kidneys, skin, & joints

IMAGING

- Nodular soft tissue in nose with **septal & nonseptal bone destruction**
  - **Orbital invasion** most common extrasinonasal H&N site
- Coronal bone CT is best tool for initial evaluation

TOP DIFFERENTIAL DIAGNOSES

- Sinonasal sarcoidosis
- Sinonasal non-Hodgkin lymphoma
- Nasal cocaine necrosis
- Chronic rhinosinusitis
- Invasive fungal sinusitis

CLINICAL ISSUES

- H&N involvement in 73-99% of GPA patients
  - Rhinologic symptoms in > 80%
- Symptoms mimic chronic rhinosinusitis (CRS)
  - Nasal obstruction & epistaxis
  - Diagnosis often delayed because symptoms mistaken for CRS
- Typically 4th & 5th decade & M > F
- Generally indolent but may transition to fulminating disease

DIAGNOSTIC CHECKLIST

- Consult with clinician for history of other organ system involvement (GPA vs. sarcoidosis) or cocaine abuse
- Can be **impossible to differentiate from sinonasal sarcoidosis or lymphoma** on imaging

(Left) *Coronal bone CT shows the classic features of sinonasal involvement by granulomatosis with polyangiitis (GPA). Nodular soft tissue ➔ is seen in the nasal cavity with an associated septal perforation ➔.* **(Right)** *Coronal bone CT shows extensive thickening & sclerosis of the maxillary sinus walls ➔, consistent with a chronic inflammatory process. Soft tissue lines the nasal cavity, & the inferior turbinates ➔ have been destroyed by the granulomatous disease.*

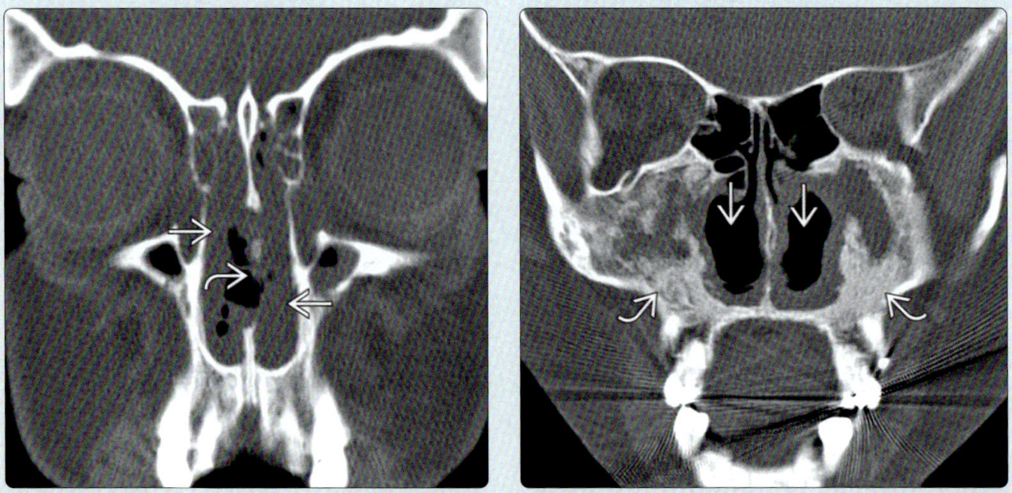

(Left) *Coronal bone CT in a case with severe sinonasal GPA shows extensive soft tissue thickening in the maxillary & ethmoid sinuses & nasal cavity. The nasal septum ➔, inferior & middle turbinates, & multiple ethmoid septations ➔ are destroyed.* **(Right)** *Axial STIR MR shows hyperintense soft tissue filling the maxillary & sphenoid sinuses. There is complete destruction of the nasal septum ➔. Thickening of the sinus walls is difficult to appreciate on the MR.*

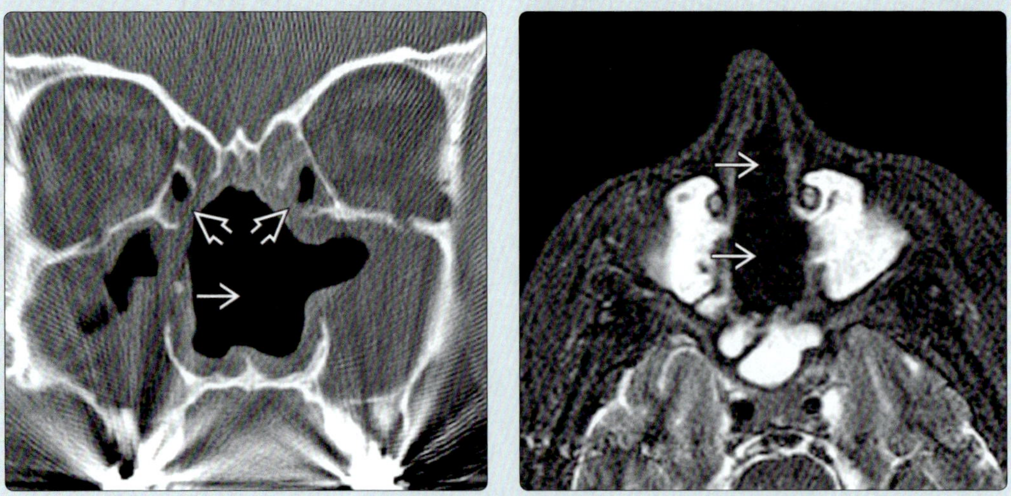

TERMINOLOGY

Abbreviations

- Granulomatosis with polyangiitis (GPA)

Definitions

- Idiopathic **necrotizing granulomatous vasculitis** that preferentially involves upper & lower respiratory tracts, kidneys, skin, & joints
- One of antineutrophil cytoplasmic antibody (ANCA)-related vasculitides

IMAGING

General Features

- Best diagnostic clue
  - Nodular soft tissue in nose with septal & nonseptal bone destruction
- Location
  - Nasal cavity (septum > turbinates) > sinuses (maxillary > ethmoid > frontal > sphenoid)
  - Other H&N sites
    - Orbital invasion most common extrasinonasal site
    - Nasopharynx, subglottic larynx, oral cavity, temporal bone, & salivary glands
- Morphology
  - Ulcerative ± nodular disease
  - No pathognomonic imaging features

CT Findings

- NECT
  - Nodular soft tissue masses centered in nasal cavity with associated chronic paranasal sinus inflammatory changes
  - Periantral soft tissue infiltration
  - Orbital extension often 1st extrasinonasal site of invasion
    - Less commonly involves infratemporal fossa, nasopharynx, skull base
- CECT
  - Inflamed nodular masses & mucosa enhance
- Bone CT
  - Nasal **septal perforation** common
  - Punctate foci of bone demineralization
    - Along pathways of perforating arteries indicative of vasculitis
  - Turbinates & lateral nasal wall **destruction** (uncinate process & medial wall maxillary sinus)
    - Starts in septum & conchae, spreads bilaterally to maxillary sinuses & then remaining sinuses
  - Hard palate not usually involved, but may extend through hard palate leading to sinonasal-oral fistula
  - Chronic obstruction & inflammation of adjacent sinuses may result in mucosal thickening & osteogenesis
    - Areas of less dense bone, but area ahead of spread is corticated

MR Findings

- T1WI
  - Low- to intermediate-signal nodular masses
- T2WI
  - ↓ signal nodular masses (compared to inflamed mucosa = ↑ T2 signal)
  - ↑ signal edema of soft tissues during acute exacerbations with extension into adjacent soft tissues
- T1WI C+
  - Homogeneous enhancement
  - Meningeal thickening with enhancement < 5% (late finding in those with skull base invasion)

Imaging Recommendations

- Best imaging tool
  - Bone-only coronal sinus CT or CBCT is best tool for initial evaluation
    - Axial MDCT with reformats also very helpful for identifying bone erosion
- Protocol advice
  - If orbital, deep facial, skull base, or meningeal involvement suspected from CT or clinical symptoms → enhanced, fat-saturated MR

DIFFERENTIAL DIAGNOSIS

Sinonasal Sarcoidosis

- Systemic granulomatous disease
  - Sinonasal involvement less common than GPA
  - More common in blacks
- Usually no airway mass
- Adenopathy
- May be indistinguishable from GPA on imaging

Nasal Cocaine Necrosis

- Septal perforation with nasal inflammatory changes
- May be less nodular than GPA

Chronic Rhinosinusitis

- Symptoms of GPA mimic chronic sinusitis
- Bone thickening & sclerosis **not** destruction
- No systemic disease

Invasive Fungal Sinusitis

- Rapidly progressive sinonasal destructive process in immunocompromised patient
- Sinus > nasal cavity site of origin; destroys any adjacent bone

Sinonasal Non-Hodgkin Lymphoma

- Midline soft tissue mass with septal & nonseptal bone destruction or remodeling
  - NK-/T-cell type lymphoma (a.k.a. lethal midline granuloma)
- May exactly mimic GPA on imaging
  - Has more lymphocytes in biopsy than GPA

PATHOLOGY

General Features

- Etiology
  - Autoimmune disease in which ANCA target proteinase 3, which is primarily expressed in B lymphocytes
    - ANCA targets proteinase-3 on neutrophils → cascade that ↑ adhesion of neutrophils to endothelium → release of lytic enzymes → necrotizing granulomas & vasculitis
- Associated abnormalities
  - Secondary sinus bacterial infections common

- Other organ system involvement
  - **Lungs (95%)**, **kidneys (85%)**, joints (65%)
  - Intracranial abnormalities include **meningeal enhancement** & brain infarcts
- 2 forms: Limited & severe
  - **Limited**: If produces no **immediate** threat to life or vital organs
    - May be locally destructive & progress to other organs
  - **Severe**: Does produce such threat

Gross Pathologic & Surgical Features

- Initially: Diffuse mucosal ulcerations with crusting
- Advanced: Septal perforation → saddle nose deformity

Microscopic Features

- Noncaseating, necrotizing, multinucleated, & giant cell granulomas
- Acute ± chronic inflammatory cell infiltrate
- Fibrinoid necrosis of small to medium-sized vessels
- Sinonasal GPA may mimic IgG4-related disease (IgG4-RD) when ↑ IgG4(+) cells found
  - ~ 19% in sinonasal & orbital/periorbital GPA
  - Inflammatory background rich in plasma cells, fibrosis, & obliterated blood vessels

CLINICAL ISSUES

Presentation

- Most common signs/symptoms
  - Nasal obstruction & epistaxis
    - Symptoms mimic chronic rhinosinusitis
- Other signs/symptoms
  - Pain, anosmia, purulent rhinorrhea
  - Septal ulcerations & perforation can lead to **saddle nose** deformity
  - Hoarseness (larynx), stridor (trachea), hearing loss & ear pain (temporal bone)
  - Constitutional symptoms: Fatigue, night sweats, weight loss
- Clinical profile
  - Classic clinical triad
    - Necrotizing granulomas of upper & lower respiratory tracts
    - Necrotizing vasculitis of both arteries & veins
    - Glomerulonephritis
  - Orbital GPA
    - May extend into sinuses
    - May have pseudotumor & proptosis
    - May mimic Ig4-related disease
  - Diagnosis made by biopsy of affected area (nose, sinus, lung, kidney)
    - Multiple biopsies may be inconclusive
      - Nasal biopsies positive in ~ 40%
  - Laboratory findings
    - ↑ **c-ANCA** (85-98% specificity for GPA)
      - c-ANCA titers followed for response to therapy
    - ↑ erythrocyte sedimentation rate
    - ↑ serum creatinine signals presence of renal GPA

Demographics

- Age
  - Typically 40-60 years
- Gender
  - M > F [except laryngeal form (M < F)]
    - At younger age may be F > M
    - Some studies show no sex predilection
- Epidemiology
  - Uncommon: Prevalence in USA ~ 3:100,000, 2,300 annually
    - More common in 4th & 5th decades
  - H&N involvement in 73-99%
  - Rhinologic symptoms in > 80%
  - 10-45% effect CNS

Natural History & Prognosis

- 3-year lag in diagnosis common because initially mistaken for chronic sinusitis
  - Better prognosis if diagnosed at younger age
- Generally indolent disease
  - Limited disease, localized to nose or orbit
    - Appropriate treatment → good to excellent prognosis
  - May transition to fulminating disease resulting in total nasal destruction (autorhinectomy) &/or death
    - Untreated, aggressive disease can be fatal 2° to renal failure or sepsis
- Long-term remissions have been achieved
  - Length of remission difficult to predict
  - Spontaneous remissions have been reported

Treatment

- Medical treatments include immunosuppressive agents, cyclophosphamide, & rituximab
  - Fulminant disease treated with high-dose prednisone followed by cyclophosphamide
  - **Limited form**: Usually responds well to less toxic regimens of methotrexate & glucocorticoids
  - **Severe form**: Usually requires aggressive treatment with glucocorticoids & cyclophosphamides
- Surgery reserved for selected head & neck manifestations, such as saddle nose deformity & subglottic stenosis
  - Surgical manipulation may exacerbate neoosteogenesis in sinonasal cavities

DIAGNOSTIC CHECKLIST

Consider

- GPA should be considered when **destructive process** centered **in nasal cavity**, particularly when septal perforation is present
- Consult with clinician for history of other organ system involvement (GPA vs. sarcoidosis) or cocaine abuse

Image Interpretation Pearls

- Can be **impossible to differentiate from sinonasal sarcoidosis or lymphoma** on imaging

SELECTED REFERENCES

1. Pakalniskis MG et al: The many faces of granulomatosis with polyangiitis: a review of the head and neck imaging manifestations. AJR Am J Roentgenol. 205(6):W619-29, 2015

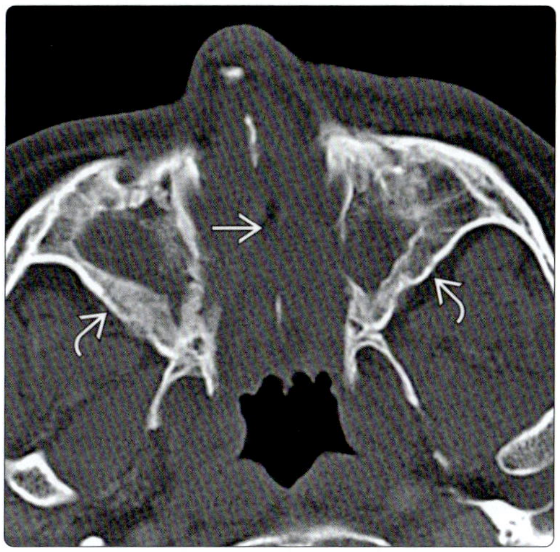

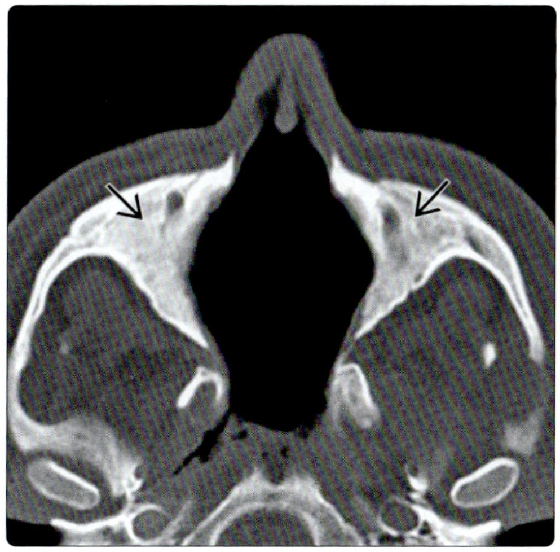

(Left) *Axial bone CT shows extensive nodular soft tissue filling the nasal cavity with opacification of the maxillary sinuses. A septal perforation is present, & there is thickening & sclerosis of the sinus walls, all findings consistent with GPA.* **(Right)** *Axial bone CT in an advanced case of GPA shows destruction of the bony anatomy of the nasal cavity including the septum. The maxillary sinuses are obliterated by thickened bone.*

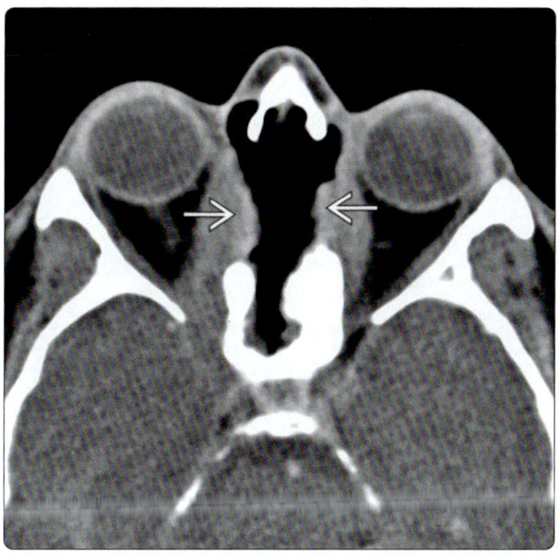

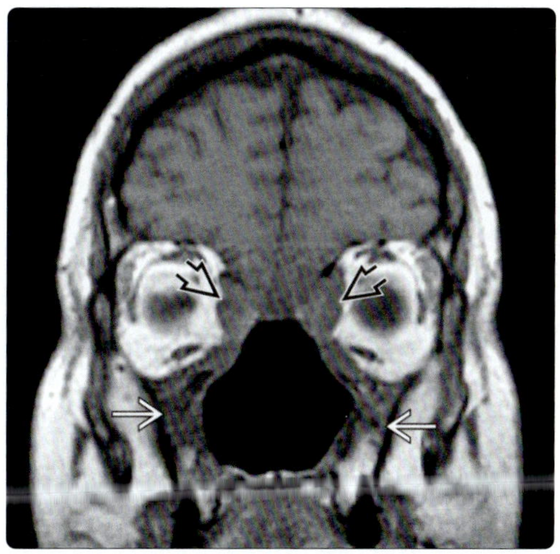

(Left) *Axial NECT shows destruction of the superior nasal septum, ethmoid septations, & the lamina papyracea bilaterally. In this case, there is bilateral orbital involvement by the granulomatous disease.* **(Right)** *Coronal T1WI MR in the same patient again shows the loss of normal nasal anatomy & thickening of the maxillary walls. The fat planes between the abnormal soft tissue & the medial rectus & superior oblique muscles are obscured.*

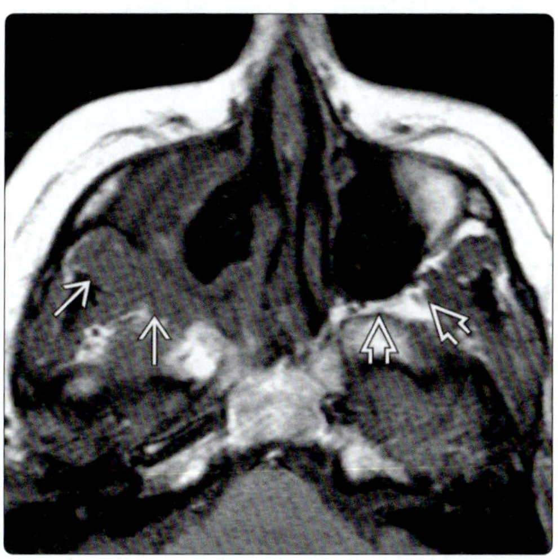

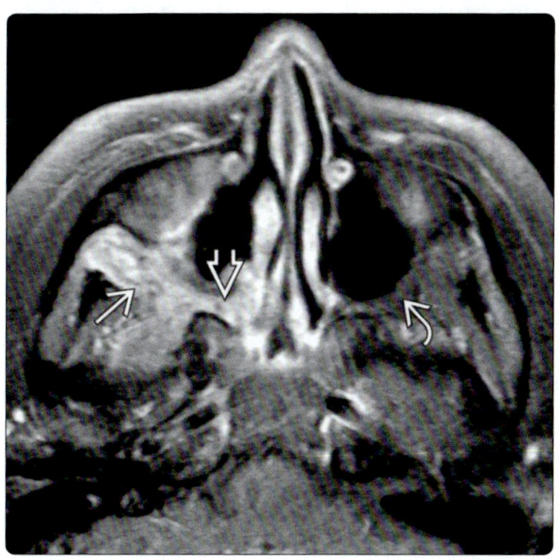

(Left) *Axial T1WI MR shows unilateral involvement of the right maxillary sinus with GPA. There is extension beyond the sinus lumen into the masticator space. Note the replacement of the normal retroantral fat signal compared to the normal left side.* **(Right)** *Axial T1WI FS MR in the same patient shows enhancement of the abnormal retroantral soft tissue & the pterygopalatine fossa. Note the normal suppression of fat on the left.*

Sinonasal Polyposis

KEY FACTS

TERMINOLOGY

- Definition: Nonneoplastic, inflammatory swelling of sinonasal mucosa that buckles to form polyps

IMAGING

- Involves nasal cavity & paranasal sinuses (vs. retention pseudocysts mainly within sinuses)
  - Predominantly along lateral nasal wall & roof of nasal cavity
  - Anterior > posterior
  - Primarily mucoid or soft tissue density
  - Remodeling of sinonasal bones common in severe cases
- MR imaging with gadolinium helpful for differentiating sinonasal polyposis (SNP) from neoplasm & to assess extrasinus extent

TOP DIFFERENTIAL DIAGNOSES

- Mucus retention pseudocyst
- Allergic fungal sinusitis
- Solitary polyp
- Sinonasal granulomatosis with polyangiitis (Wegener granulomatosis)

PATHOLOGY

- Formal pathogenesis of SNP has not been clarified
  - Chronic inflammation is major factor
  - Associated with allergy, asthma, primary ciliary dyskinesia, aspirin sensitivity, & cystic fibrosis

CLINICAL ISSUES

- Although not life threatening, persistent SNP unresponsive to therapy can be chronic, debilitating disease
- Medical therapy = treatment of choice
  - Topical & oral corticosteroids to reduce rhinitis symptoms, ↓ polyp size, & reduce recurrence
- Surgery reserved for symptomatic relief & correction of cosmetic deformities, orbital and intracranial involvement

(Left) *Coronal bone CT shows the classic appearance of sinonasal polyposis with multiple lobular soft tissue masses involving the nasal cavity → and paranasal sinuses →. In this case, the involvement is diffuse and bilateral without expansion.* **(Right)** *Coronal T1WI MR shows multiple intermediate signal intensity polyps → filling the nasal cavity, maxillary, and ethmoid sinuses. Trapped secretions with high protein content → (T1 shortening) are also noted.*

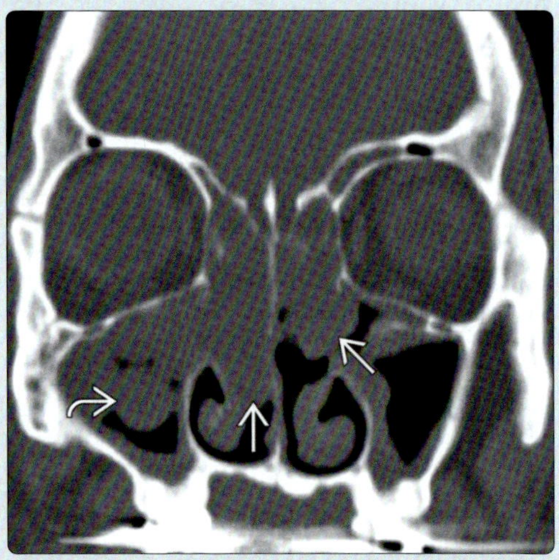

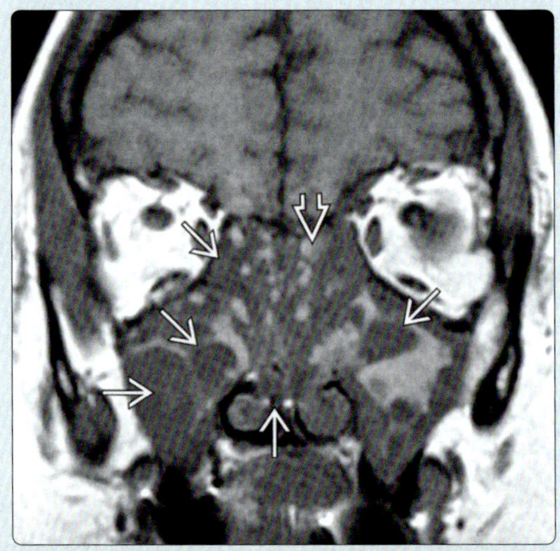

(Left) *Axial CBCT shows multiple polypoid masses → in the left maxillary sinus and thickening of the sinus mucosa. The right sinus is normal →. There is no evidence of polyps in the nasal fossae → (although the fossae were not completely imaged).* **(Right)** *Sagittal CBCT in the same patient shows polypoid thickening of the left maxillary sinus →. There is no apical pathosis associated with the teeth to suggest an odontogenic relationship to the polyposis.*

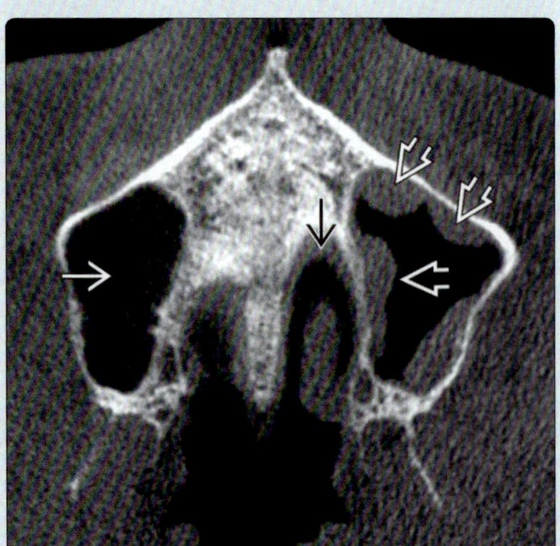

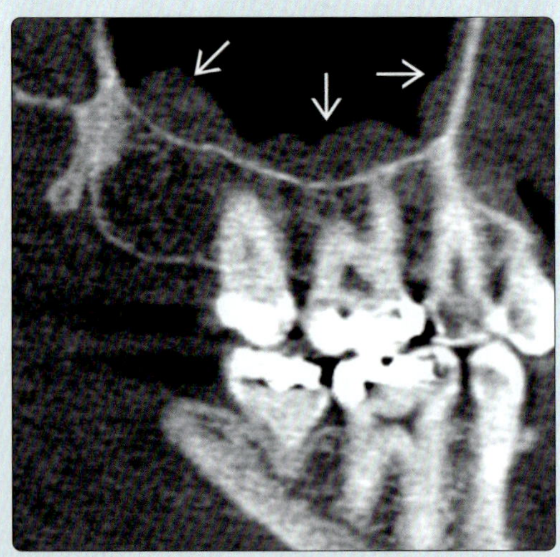

TERMINOLOGY

Abbreviations

- Sinonasal polyposis (SNP)

Synonyms

- Polyposis nasi, hypertrophic polypoid rhinosinusitis, polypoid sinusitis

Definitions

- Nonneoplastic, inflammatory swelling of sinonasal mucosa that buckles to form polyps

IMAGING

General Features

- Best diagnostic clue
  - Polypoid masses involving nasal cavity & paranasal sinuses mixed with chronic inflammatory secretions
- Location
  - Predominantly along lateral nasal wall (near middle meatus) & roof of nasal cavity & ethmoids
  - Anterior sinonasal cavities > posterior
  - Involves nasal cavity & paranasal sinuses (vs. retention pseudocysts mainly within sinuses)
  - Usually **multiple & bilateral**; may be unilateral
- Size
  - Variable; up to several centimeters
- Morphology
  - Polypoid, lobular

CT Findings

- NECT
  - Primarily mucoid or soft tissue density
    - May be hyperdense with ↑ protein, ↓ water content, or colonization with fungal elements
- CECT
  - Mucosal enhancement at periphery of polyps
    - **No central enhancement** as in neoplasms
- Bone CT & CBCT
  - Multiple, polypoid, soft tissue masses within nasal cavity and paranasal sinuses
  - **Remodeling** of sinonasal **bones** common in severe cases
    - May have areas of **bone erosion**
  - Other findings
    - Ethmoid sinus remodeling with trabecular loss and convex lateral walls bulging into orbits
    - **Air-fluid levels** may signal superinfection or merely **trapped fluid**

MR Findings

- T1WI
  - Fresh mucus (high water content) is hypointense
  - Bizarre mixture of layered signals seen in sinuses & nose
    - Results from polyps mixed with various ages of mucus
- T2WI
  - Fresh mucus is hyperintense
  - Chronic, inspissated mucus can appear **low signal** (mimics air)
- T1WI C+
  - Thin mucosal enhancement between polypoid soft tissue lesions without central enhancement

Imaging Recommendations

- Best imaging tool
  - Bone CT or CBCT in coronal plane is adequate for most cases
- Protocol advice
  - If orbital or intracranial extension is suspected based on dehiscent bone on CT, enhanced MR imaging done to assess extrasinus extent
  - MR imaging with gadolinium helpful for differentiating SNP from neoplasm in difficult cases

DIFFERENTIAL DIAGNOSIS

Mucus Retention Pseudocyst

- Clinically asymptomatic or sinusitis history
- Lesions usually occur within sinuses with relative sparing of nasal cavity
- Maxillary sinus mucus retention pseudocyst (MRPC) appears as smooth **dome-shaped** soft tissue density frequently arising from sinus floor
- Difficult to distinguish from polyps based on density/signal intensity alone
  - Fluid density/signal on CT/MR; no central enhancement

Allergic Fungal Sinusitis

- Atopic patient with multiple unilateral or pansinus involvement
- May mimic SNP; frequently seen in association with polyps
- CT shows high-density central material with low-density rim in expanded sinuses
- MR may show low signal on both T1 & T2 images

Sinonasal Solitary Polyps

- Unilateral, solitary lesion
- Extends from antrum through widened infundibulum into nasal cavity

Sinonasal Granulomatosis With Polyangiitis (Wegener Granulomatosis)

- Multisystem granulomatous disease involving lung and kidney
- Nodular soft tissue most often involving septum, inferior turbinates, and lateral nasal wall
- Bony destruction (septal perforation) rather than remodeling

Sinonasal Sarcoidosis

- Multisystem granulomatous disease
- Nodular soft tissue most often involving septum and turbinates

PATHOLOGY

General Features

- Etiology
  - Inflammatory swelling of unstable respiratory mucosa
  - Formal pathogenesis of SNP has not been clarified; chronic persistent inflammation is major factor
    - Principal hypothesis: Allergy & inflammation cause unstable mucosa with epithelial cell proliferation and morphologic changes
    - Others factors implicated

- Cytokines (IL-5, granulocyte-macrophage colony stimulating factor, tumor necrosis factor)
- Mechanical forces in areas of contact between opposing mucosal membranes
- Role of bacterial biofilms current area of investigation

- Genetics
  - No causative chromosomal aberrations identified
  - ↑ in cystic fibrosis patients (autosomal recessive)
- Associated abnormalities
  - Associated with chronic rhinosinusitis (CRS), allergy, asthma, primary ciliary dyskinesia, aspirin sensitivity, & cystic fibrosis
  - Polyposis & allergic fungal sinusitis (AFS) are **frequently** seen in association (~ 66% of cases)

Gross Pathologic & Surgical Features

- Pinkish, fleshy, pedunculated polypoid sinonasal masses with glistening mucoid surface

Microscopic Features

- Intact surface respiratory epithelium
- Underlying stroma is edematous with inflammatory cellular infiltrate & variable vascularity, glands, & goblet cells
- Seromucinous glands usually absent
- Eosinophil-dominated inflammation with component of neutrophils & mast cells
- May show squamous, cartilaginous, or osseous metaplasia ± surface ulceration & granuloma formation
  - Superinfecting bacteria include *Pseudomonas aeruginosa*, *Bacteroides fragilis*, *Staphylococcus aureus*

CLINICAL ISSUES

Presentation

- Most common signs/symptoms
  - Progressive nasal stuffiness & obstruction
  - Sensation of secretions that cannot be expelled
- Other signs/symptoms
  - Rhinorrhea, facial pain, headaches, & anosmia
  - Cosmetic deformity, hypertelorism in cases of "polypoid mucocele"
- Clinical profile
  - Allergic patient with progressive nasal stuffiness
  - Polyps identified with nasal endoscopy

Demographics

- Age
  - Most common in adults > 20 years old
  - Rare in children < 5 years old
- Epidemiology
  - Frequency of polyps
    - 1-2% of normal population
    - 5% of extrinsic asthma patients
    - 13% of intrinsic bronchial asthma patients
    - 16% of "dental" sinusitis patients
    - 20% of cystic fibrosis patients
    - > 50% of aspirin-intolerant patients

Natural History & Prognosis

- Often waxing & waning; chronic, relentless disease
- Left unattended, may become highly deforming in central facial region
- Although not life threatening, persistent SNP unresponsive to therapy can be chronic, debilitating disease

Treatment

- Medical therapy = treatment of choice
  - Topical & oral corticosteroids to reduce rhinitis symptoms, ↓ polyp size, & reduce recurrence
  - Antibiotics when superinfected
- Surgery reserved for symptomatic relief & correction of cosmetic deformities, orbital and intracranial involvement
  - Endoscopic polypectomy, functional endoscopic sinus surgery (FESS), or sphenoethmoidectomy
  - Usually only temporary relief

DIAGNOSTIC CHECKLIST

Consider

- If density of expansile polyps is increased ± signal heterogeneous on MR, AFS in setting of polyposis is likely

Image Interpretation Pearls

- Polyps occur in sinuses **and** nasal cavity
  - Mucous retention pseudocysts typically located in sinuses only
- Individual polyps cannot be differentiated from mucous retention cysts based on density or signal characteristics alone
- Do not be alarmed if areas of **bone erosion** are present in addition to remodeling
  - If predominant pattern is aggressive-appearing bone destruction, must rule out malignancy or granulomatous disease

SELECTED REFERENCES

1. Cahill KN et al: Impaired E prostanoid2 expression and resistance to prostaglandin E2 in nasal polyp fibroblasts from subjects with aspirin-exacerbated respiratory disease. Am J Respir Cell Mol Biol. 54(1):34-40, 2016
2. Stutzki M et al: Indications of cone beam CT in head and neck imaging. Acta Otolaryngol. 135(12):1337-43, 2015
3. Balikci HH et al: Antrochoanal polyposis: analysis of 34 cases. Eur Arch Otorhinolaryngol. 270(5):1651-4, 2013
4. Blomqvist EH et al: A randomized prospective study comparing medical and medical-surgical treatment of nasal polyposis by CT. Acta Otolaryngol. 129(5):545-9, 2009
5. Pearlman AN et al: Relationships between severity of chronic rhinosinusitis and nasal polyposis, asthma, and atopy. Am J Rhinol Allergy. 23(2):145-8, 2009
6. Bonfils P et al: Evaluation of combined medical and surgical treatment in nasal polyposis - III. Correlation between symptoms and CT scores before and after surgery for nasal polyposis. Acta Otolaryngol. 128(3):318-23, 2008
7. Can IH et al: The expression of MMP-2, MMP-7, MMP-9, and TIMP-1 in chronic rhinosinusitis and nasal polyposis. Otolaryngol Head Neck Surg. 139(2):211-5, 2008
8. Corradini C et al: Hyperproliferation in nasal polyposis tissues is not associated with somatic genomic instability. J Otolaryngol Head Neck Surg. 37(4):510-4, 2008
9. Kahveci OK et al: The role of MMP-9 and TIMP-1 in nasal polyp formation. Swiss Med Wkly. 138(45-46):684-8, 2008
10. Mladina R et al: Biofilm in nasal polyps. Rhinology. 46(4):302-7, 2008
11. Mortuaire G et al: Lund-Mackay score is predictive of bleeding in ethmoidectomy for nasal polyposis. Rhinology. 46(4):285-8, 2008
12. Konstantinidis I et al: Olfactory dysfunction in nasal polyposis: correlation with computed tomography findings. ORL J Otorhinolaryngol Relat Spec. 69(4):226-32, 2007
13. Gosepath J et al: Current concepts in therapy of chronic rhinosinusitis and nasal polyposis. ORL J Otorhinolaryngol Relat Spec. 67(3):125-36, 2005

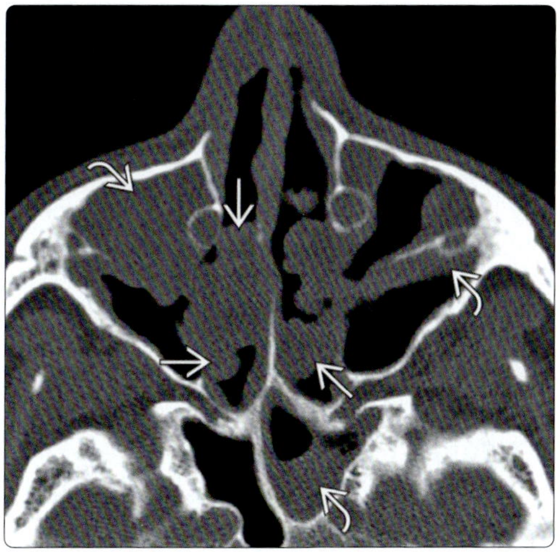

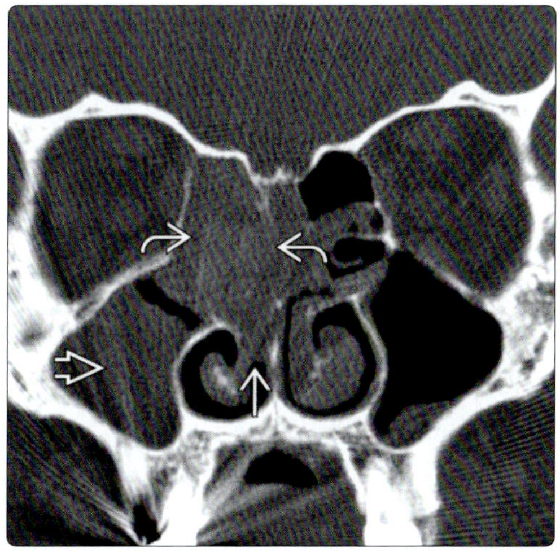

(Left) *Axial bone CT shows the typical features of sinonasal polyposis with multiple polypoid soft tissue lesions involving the nasal cavity. Mucosal thickening is seen in the maxillary and left sphenoid sinuses.* **(Right)** *Coronal bone CT shows increased density, expansile soft tissue in the right ethmoid sinuses with extension of polypoid soft tissue into the nasal cavity. Trapped secretions are noted in the right maxillary sinus.*

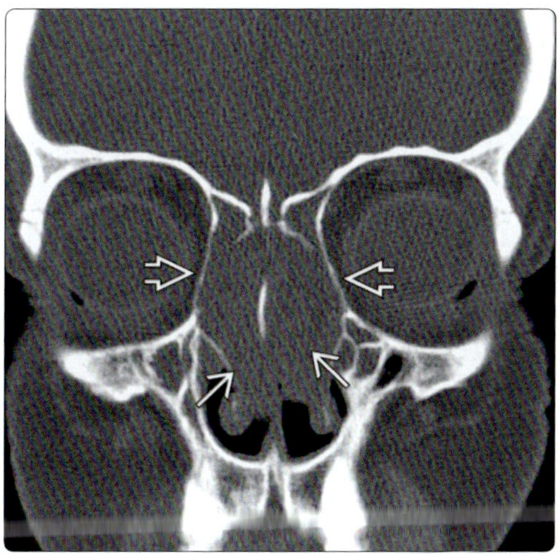

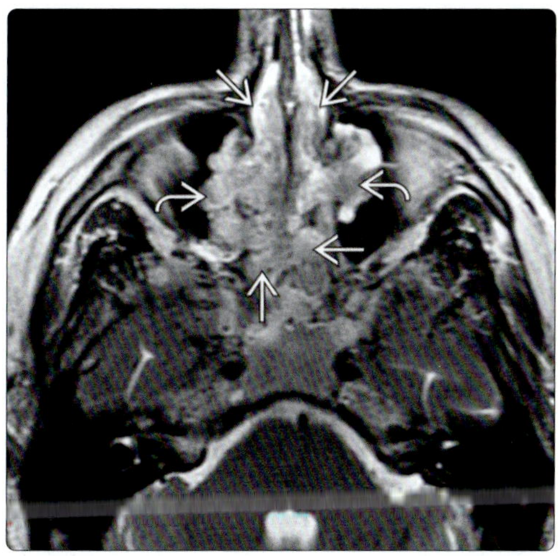

(Left) *Coronal CECT in a patient with polyposis shows polyps involving the nasal cavity bilaterally. Polypoid material also opacifies the ethmoid air cells. The expansion with lateral remodeling of the lamina papyracea helps to differentiate polyps from mucosal thickening.* **(Right)** *Axial T2WI MR in a severe case of polyposis shows multiple hyperintense polyps filling the nasal cavity and involving the medial portions of the maxillary sinuses.*

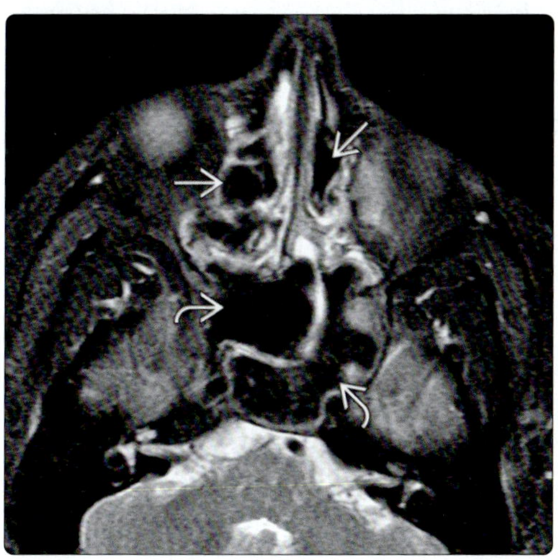

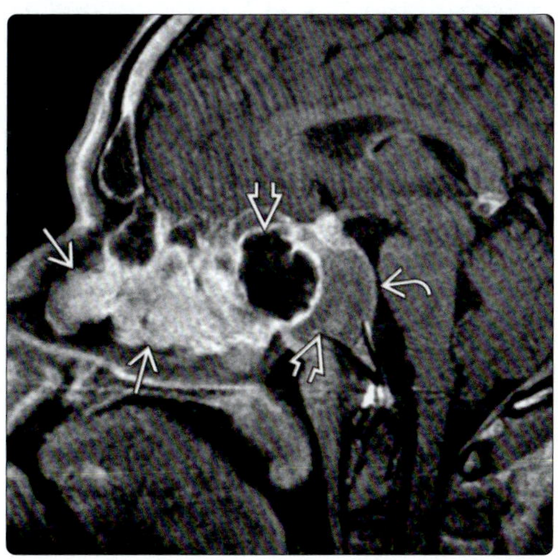

(Left) *Axial T2WI FS MR demonstrates hypointense polyps filling and expanding the ethmoid and sphenoid sinuses. On this sequence, the polyps mimic the hypointense signal of air-filled sinuses.* **(Right)** *Sagittal T1WI C+ MR in the same patient shows enhancement in multiple nasal cavity polyps. The sphenoid polyps show mixed signal intensity. Note the marked thinning of the clival cortex.*

Acute Rhinosinusitis

KEY FACTS

TERMINOLOGY

- Abbreviation: Acute rhinosinusitis (ARS)
- Definition: Acute inflammation of sinonasal mucosa lasting ≤ 4 weeks

IMAGING

- ARS is clinical diagnosis
- Most common in ethmoid & maxillary sinuses
- CT: Confirms diagnosis; evaluates patients not responding to medical therapy; delineates anatomic variants
  - Axial ≤ 1-mm slice thickness with coronal & sagittal reconstructions
  - Best sign: Air-fluid level ± bubbly or strandy-appearing secretions within sinus with mucosal thickening
- MR: Useful to evaluate for orbital or intracranial complications, fungal disease, neoplasm

TOP DIFFERENTIAL DIAGNOSES

- Pseudo-fluid level
- Posttraumatic blood level
- Postobstructive secretions

PATHOLOGY

- Most cases follow viral upper respiratory infection
- May be caused by vasomotor dysfunction; associated with allergy, odontogenic disease, or barotrauma
- Predisposing systemic disorders: Allergies, immunoglobulin deficiency, immotile cilia syndrome, cystic fibrosis

CLINICAL ISSUES

- Nasal congestion & purulent discharge, facial pain/pressure, headache, olfactory dysfunction, fever, cough
- Affects nearly 31 million in USA annually

DIAGNOSTIC CHECKLIST

- Fluid levels are most specific indicator in absence of recent nasal lavage or presence of nasogastric tube
- Normal nasal mucosal cycle may be impossible to distinguish from ARS mucosal thickening on MR

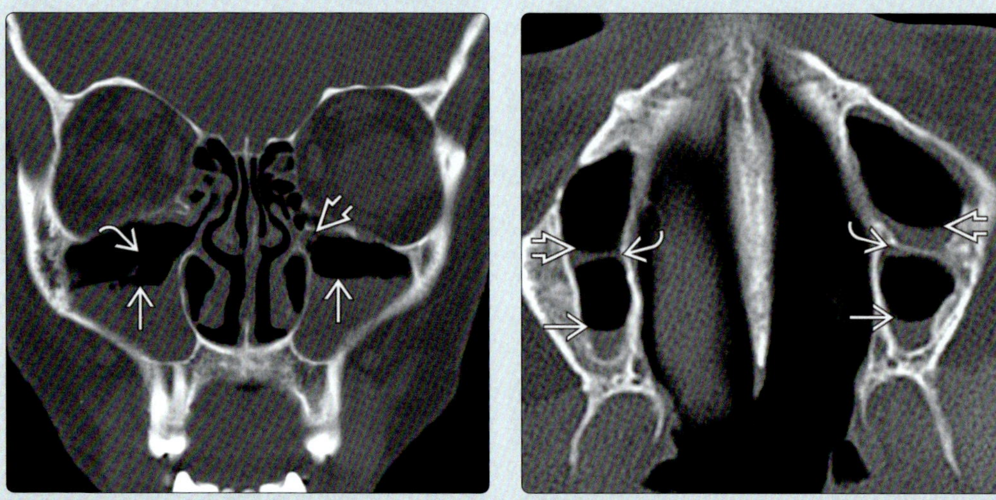

(Left) *Coronal bone CT in a patient with symptoms of acute rhinosinusitis shows bilateral maxillary sinus air-fluid levels → with bubbly appearing secretions on the right →. Note mucosal thickening occluding the left infundibulum →.* **(Right)** *Axial bone CT shows fluid levels → on posterior walls of maxillary sinuses (evident when the patient's head is supine in MDCT). Secondary fluid levels → are present due to septa → within the sinus acting as shelves to hold fluid.*

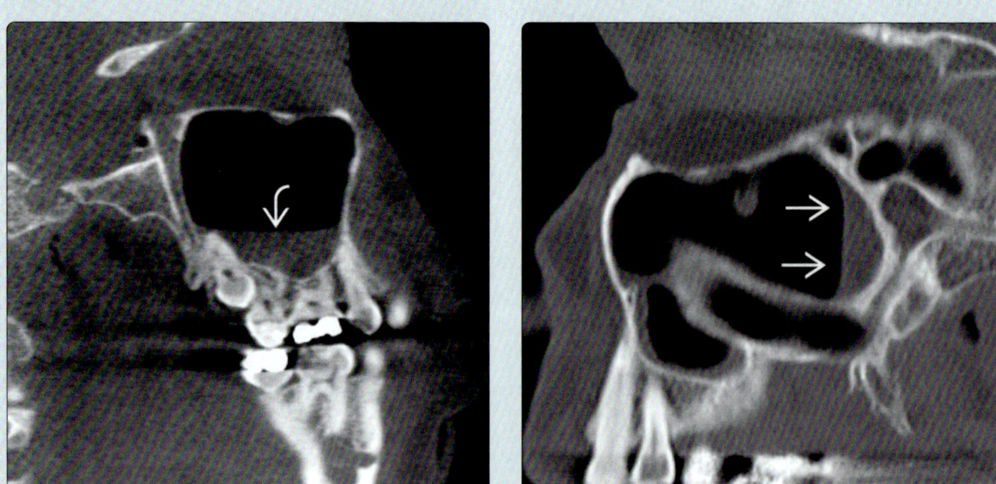

(Left) *Sagittal CBCT shows a fluid level → in the inferior part of the maxillary sinus. The floor of the sinus is the most dependent part of the sinus in the majority of CBCTs in comparison to traditional MDCTs.* **(Right)** *Sagittal bone CT shows a fluid level → on the posterior wall of the maxillary sinus. Patient was scanned with the head supine, and thus the posterior walls of the sinuses were the most dependent during the scan in comparison to the previous CBCT.*

TERMINOLOGY

Abbreviations

- Acute rhinosinusitis (ARS)

Synonyms

- Acute bacterial rhinosinusitis (ABRS)

Definitions

- Acute inflammatory process of sinonasal mucosa lasting ≤ 4 weeks

IMAGING

General Features

- Best diagnostic clue
  - **Air-fluid level** ± bubbly or strandy-appearing secretions within sinus with mucosal thickening
- Location
  - Most common in ethmoid & maxillary sinuses
  - Allergic sinusitis tends to be generalized
    - ABRS affects sinuses asymmetrically
- Size
  - Normal sinus lumen size
    - No expansion (mucocele) or reduced volume (chronic rhinosinusitis)

Radiographic Findings

- Radiography
  - Mucosal thickening or **opacification of sinus**
  - Air-fluid level in maxillary sinus
    - Can be difficult to identify in other sinuses

CT Findings

- CECT
  - Enhancement of inflamed mucosa
  - Central secretions do not enhance
- NECT and bone CT
  - **Air-fluid level**, bubbly or strandy-appearing secretions
    - Air-fluid level is parallel to floor; follows gravity
      - If patient scanned supine, air-fluid level will be parallel to coronal plane
      - If patient is scanned upright, air-fluid level will be parallel to axial plane
  - Mucosal thickening
  - Inflammatory tissue **obstructing drainage pathways** of ostiomeatal complex (OMC)

MR Findings

- T1WI
  - Mucosal thickening isointense to other soft tissue
  - Fluid signal layering within sinus
  - ↑ signal with elevated protein content
  - Air, cortical bone appear as signal voids
- T2WI
  - ↑ signal fluid & edematous mucosa
  - Secretions ↓ in signal with ↑ protein content/inspissation
- T1WI C+
  - Enhancement of inflamed peripheral mucosa
  - Central secretions do not enhance

Imaging Recommendations

- Best imaging tool
  - ARS is clinical diagnosis
  - Radiographs inaccurate in assessing extent of inflammation
    - Particularly in ethmoid, frontal, & sphenoid sinuses
  - CT: Confirms diagnosis
    - Evaluates patients not responding to medical therapy
    - Delineates anatomic variants
  - MR: Useful to evaluate for orbital or intracranial complications, fungal disease, neoplasm
- Protocol advice
  - Bone CT
    - Axial ≤ 1-mm slice thickness with coronal, sagittal reconstructions to evaluate OMC and frontal recess, respectively
    - Axial plane useful for evaluating sphenoid & posterior ethmoid regions, posterior wall of frontal sinus
  - MR
    - 4-mm slice thickness T1, T2, STIR sequences; axial & coronal planes
    - Use fat suppression post contrast

DIFFERENTIAL DIAGNOSIS

Pseudo-Fluid Level

- Flaccid mucus retention pseudocyst (MRP) mimics air-fluid level
- Fluid level not persistent through entire sinus; rounded edge usually found

Posttraumatic Blood Level

- Clinical history of recent facial injury
- Increased attenuation of layering fluid (blood)
- Associated sinus wall fractures
- Can be seen if injury to posterior superior alveolar canal during sinus lift surgery occurs

Postobstructive Secretions

- Lesion obstructs sinus drainage pathway, trapping fluid
- MR differentiates tumor from obstructed secretions

PATHOLOGY

General Features

- Etiology
  - Most cases of ARS follow viral upper respiratory infection (URI)
    - URI → mucosal swelling → sinus outflow obstruction → infection
    - Symptoms > 10 days or worsening after 5-7 days suggest bacterial superinfection
  - May be caused by vasomotor dysfunction or associated with allergy or barotrauma
  - Other important cause: **Odontogenic sinusitis** (communication of dental inflammation with lumen of sinus by effacing floor of maxillary sinus)
- Genetics
  - Cystic fibrosis (autosomal recessive disorder) predisposes to rhinosinusitis
- Associated abnormalities
  - Structural abnormalities may narrow drainage pathways

 - Anatomic variants of septum, uncinate process, middle turbinate, frontal recess, ethmoid sinuses
 - Benign or malignant neoplasms
 - Predisposing systemic disorders: Allergies, immunoglobulin deficiency, immotile cilia syndrome, cystic fibrosis

Staging, Grading, & Classification

- Can be classified according to etiology: Viral, bacterial, vasomotor

Gross Pathologic & Surgical Features

- Edematous, erythematous mucosa with ostial obstruction, purulent secretions

Microscopic Features

- Tissue-invasive bacteria
- Luminal exudate of neutrophils, eosinophils

CLINICAL ISSUES

Presentation

- Most common signs/symptoms
 - Symptoms: Nasal congestion & purulent discharge, facial pain/pressure, headache, olfactory dysfunction, fever, cough
 - Often worst in morning; improves in upright position/**worsens when bending over**
 - Signs: Facial swelling & erythema, nasal turbinate edema, nasal crusting, purulent nasal cavity/pharynx
- Other signs/symptoms
 - Maxillary: Infraorbital, cheek, upper teeth, or gum pain
 - Ethmoid: Lacrimal, periorbital, or temporal region tenderness
 - Frontal: Headache localized to forehead, supraorbital region
 - Sphenoid: Pain radiates to occiput ± skull vertex; infection near cavernous sinus may cause CNII-IV, V1, V2, or VI dysfunction
- Clinical profile
 - Pediatric or adult patient with nasal discharge & obstruction frequently following viral URI; lasting ≤ 4 weeks
 - Laboratory results
 - Nasal cultures nonspecific, often contaminated with *Staphylococcus aureus*
 - Endoscopic paranasal sinus aspiration more specific

Demographics

- Age
 - Typically follows viral URI in children
- Epidemiology
 - Sinonasal inflammatory disease is ubiquitous
 - 90% of patients with common cold have viral or bacterial rhinosinusitis
 - Rhinosinusitis affects nearly 31 million patients annually in USA
 - > 1 billion physician office visits due to viral & bacterial rhinosinusitis annually in USA

Natural History & Prognosis

- Usually self-limited if viral
- ABRS course may be shortened by medical therapy, surgical drainage
- If untreated, **ABRS complications** ensue
 - Orbital cellulitis, subperiosteal abscess, meningitis, subdural empyema, brain abscess, venous sinus thrombosis

Treatment

- Medical therapy
 - Saline nasal sprays & irrigants, mucolytics
 - Decongestants, antihistamines, antibiotics (amoxicillin)
 - Topical steroids
- Surgical therapy
 - More often performed for chronic RS
 - Drainage procedures performed in acute disease (frontal and sphenoid) to prevent development of complications

DIAGNOSTIC CHECKLIST

Consider

- Bone CT to confirm diagnosis if in doubt & to determine extent
 - Use ≤ 1-mm axial slices with coronal and sagittal reformations
- CT limitations
 - Cannot differentiate viral from bacterial disease
 - High incidence of sinus mucosal abnormalities in asymptomatic patients

Image Interpretation Pearls

- Fluid levels are most specific indicator in absence of recent nasal lavage or presence of nasogastric tube
- Normal nasal mucosal cycle may be impossible to distinguish from ARS mucosal thickening on MR
- Look for signs of invasive fungal sinusitis if immunocompromised patient

SELECTED REFERENCES

1. Dass K et al: Diagnosis and management of rhinosinusitis: highlights from the 2015 practice parameter. Curr Allergy Asthma Rep. 16(4):29, 2016
2. Loftus PA et al: Anatomic variants of the paranasal sinuses in patients with recurrent acute rhinosinusitis. Int Forum Allergy Rhinol. 6(3):328-33, 2016
3. Orlandi RR et al: International consensus statement on allergy and rhinology: rhinosinusitis. Int Forum Allergy Rhinol. 6 Suppl 1:S22-S209, 2016
4. Costa ML et al: Medical therapy vs surgery for recurrent acute rhinosinusitis. Int Forum Allergy Rhinol. 5(8):667-73, 2015
5. Dankbaar JW et al: Imaging findings of the orbital and intracranial complications of acute bacterial rhinosinusitis. Insights Imaging. 6(5):509-18, 2015
6. Joshi VM et al: Imaging in sinonasal inflammatory disease. Neuroimaging Clin N Am. 25(4):549-68, 2015
7. Lee JH et al: Underestimation of rhinogenic causes in patients presenting to the emergency department with acute headache. Acta Neurol Taiwan. 24(2):37-42, 2015
8. Namin AW et al: Facial paresis secondary to an aggressive acute bacterial rhinosinusitis. JAMA Otolaryngol Head Neck Surg. 141(9):856-7, 2015
9. Rosenfeld RM et al: Clinical practice guideline (update): adult sinusitis. Otolaryngol Head Neck Surg. 152(2 Suppl):S1-S39, 2015
10. Stutzki M et al: Indications of cone beam CT in head and neck imaging. Acta Otolaryngol. 135(12):1337-43, 2015
11. Javadrashid R et al: Concha bullosa, nasal septal deviation and paranasal sinusitis; a computed tomographic evaluation. B-ENT. 10(4):291-8, 2014
12. Bayonne E et al: Intracranial complications of rhinosinusitis. A review, typical imaging data and algorithm of management. Rhinology. 47(1):59-65, 2009
13. Madani G et al: Sinonasal inflammatory disease. Semin Ultrasound CT MR. 30(1):17-24, 2009

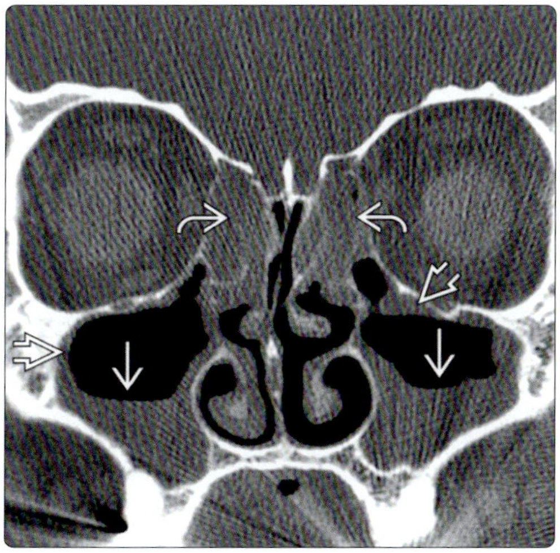

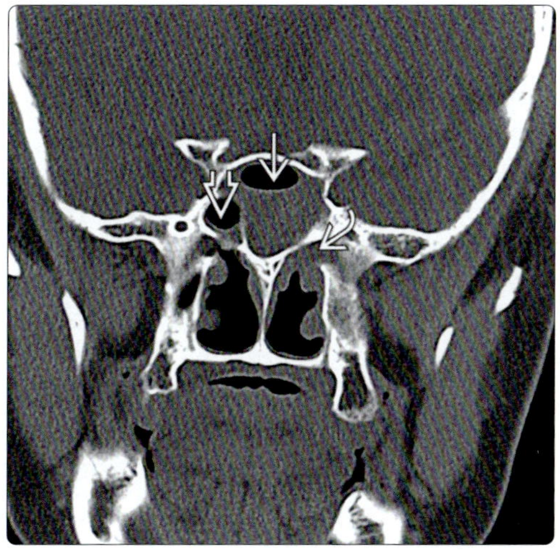

(Left) *Coronal bone CT shows findings consistent with acute bilateral maxillary sinusitis. Air-fluid levels and mucosal thickening are seen. Additional mucosal thickening is seen throughout the ethmoid sinuses.* **(Right)** *Coronal bone CT in a patient with acute sphenoiditis demonstrates large left and smaller right sphenoid sinus air-fluid levels. Mucosal thickening in the sphenoethmoid recess and posterior nasal cavity is likely contributing to the sphenoid disease.*

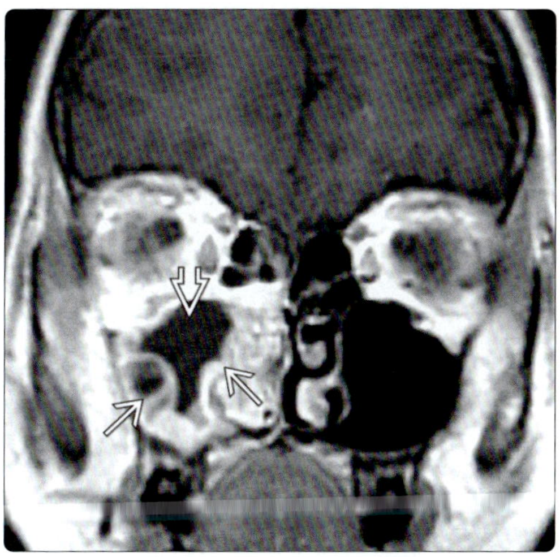

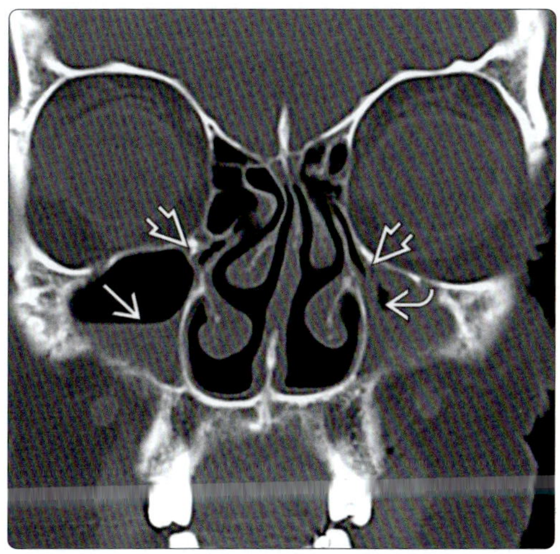

(Left) *Coronal T1WI C+ MR shows the typical features of maxillary sinusitis. There is lobular mucosal thickening at the periphery of the right maxillary sinus that enhances avidly. Trapped fluid is noted centrally within the sinus.* **(Right)** *Coronal bone CT in a patient with bilateral maxillary sinusitis shows an air-fluid level on the right and mucosal thickening on the left. The maxillary ostia are occluded bilaterally.*

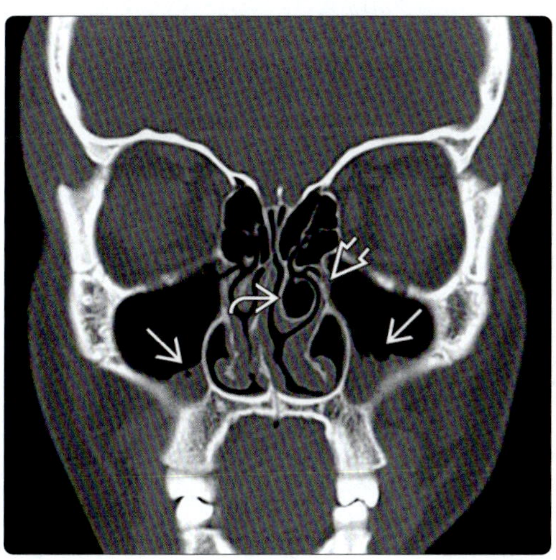

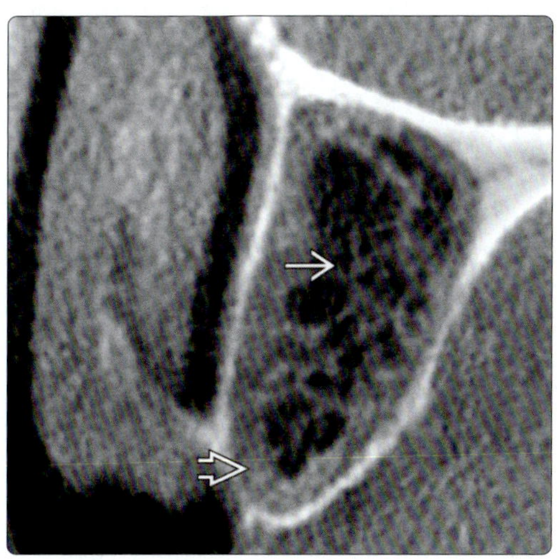

(Left) *Coronal bone CT in a patient with symptoms of acute sinusitis shows bilateral maxillary air-fluid levels. The left infundibulum is occluded by mucosal thickening. Incidental note is made of a left concha bullosa. This anatomic variant slightly narrows the left middle meatus.* **(Right)** *Coronal CBCT shows mucosal thickening and a bubbly or strandy appearance in the left maxillary sinus consistent with acute maxillary sinusitis.*

Chronic Rhinosinusitis

KEY FACTS

TERMINOLOGY

- Chronic rhinosinusitis (CRS)
- Definition: Group of disorders characterized by inflammation of nose & sinuses ≥ **12 consecutive weeks** of duration

IMAGING

- Bone CT is modality of choice
  - Mucosal thickening or soft tissue opacification with thickening & **sclerosis of bony walls**
  - Involved sinus normal or ↓ volume

TOP DIFFERENTIAL DIAGNOSES

- Fungal mycetoma
- Allergic fungal sinusitis
- Sinonasal polyposis
- Wegener granulomatosis
- Sarcoidosis

PATHOLOGY

- Causes of CRS are numerous, disparate, & frequently overlapping; many factors play role in etiology

CLINICAL ISSUES

- Often associated conditions, such as allergy, underlying anatomic variations
- Often present with nasal obstruction, nasal discharge, hyposmia, anosmia
- **Pharmacologic therapy**: Antibiotics, antifungals, decongestants, antihistamines, topical steroids (allergic cases)

DIAGNOSTIC CHECKLIST

- Coronal sinus CT is study of choice for evaluating changes in bone & identifying anatomic variants that may predispose to recurrent disease
- There is lack of correlation between symptomatology & imaging findings

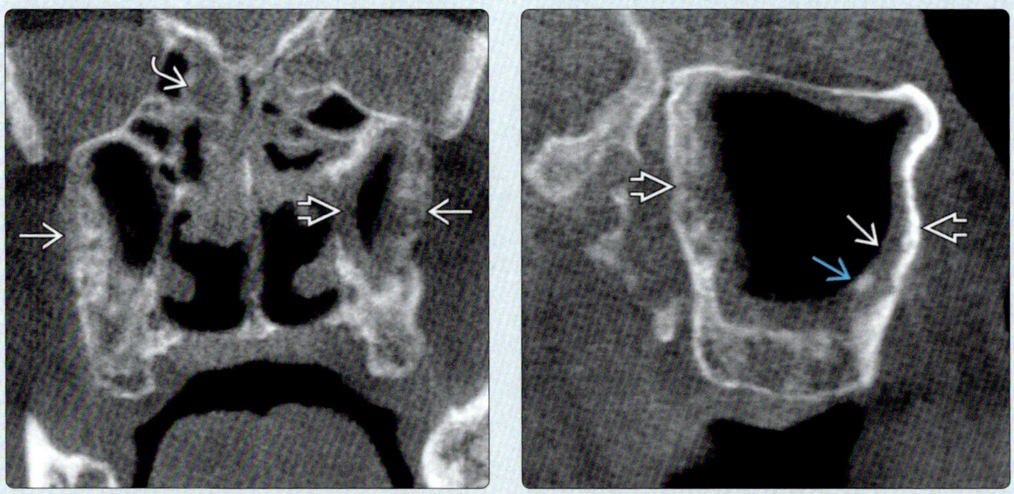

(Left) *Coronal CBCT shows findings of chronic bilateral maxillary sinusitis. There is mucosal thickening in the maxillary ➔ and ethmoid ↪ sinuses. Note thickening and sclerosis of the lateral maxillary sinus walls ⇨.* **(Right)** *Sagittal CBCT in the same patient shows thickening of the osseous borders ⇨ and mucosa ➔ consistent with chronic sinusitis. An antrolith is noted in the mucosal thickening ➔.*

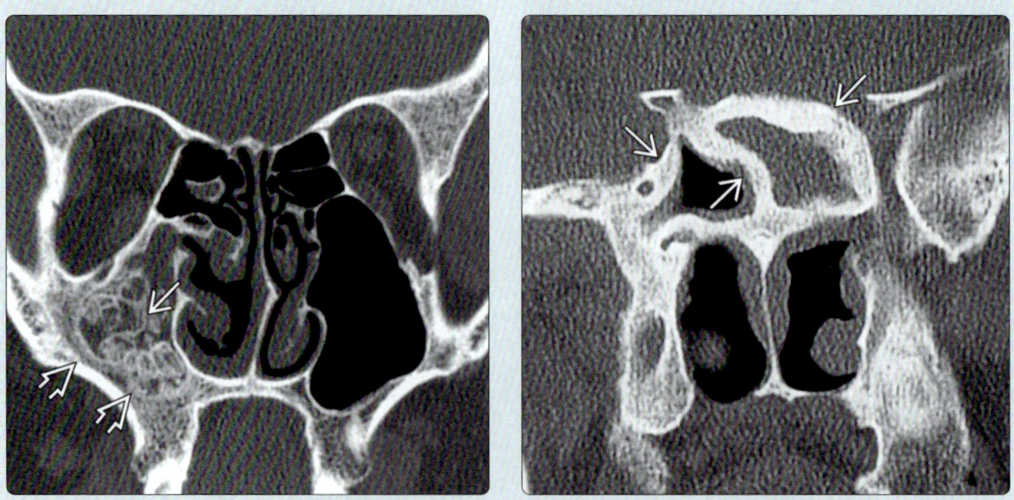

(Left) *Coronal bone CT in a patient with longstanding right maxillary inflammation shows prominent calcifications ➔ within the inspissated right maxillary sinus secretions. Osteitis of the walls of the sinus is also present ⇨. This appearance is similar to fibrous dysplasia; however, lack of expansion and mucosal thickening favor chronic rhinosinusitis (CRS).* **(Right)** *Coronal bone CT shows mucosal thickening in the right sphenoid sinus and opacification of the left sphenoid sinus with chronic osteitis of both sinus walls ➔.*

TERMINOLOGY

Abbreviations

- Chronic rhinosinusitis (CRS)

Synonyms

- Rhinosinusitis (RS)

Definitions

- CRS: Group of disorders characterized by inflammation of nose & sinuses ≥ **12 consecutive weeks** of duration

IMAGING

General Features

- Best diagnostic clue
  - Mucosal thickening or soft tissue opacification with thickening & sclerosis of bony walls
- Location
  - Ethmoid sinus > maxillary sinus > frontal & sphenoid sinuses
- Size
  - Involved sinus normal or ↓ volume
    - No sinus expansion
- Morphology
  - Normal morphology or concavity of walls (↓ sinus volume)

Radiographic Findings

- Radiography
  - Peripheral soft tissue thickening or opacification of sinus
  - Sclerotic, thickened sinus walls
  - Helpful for confirming diagnosis in symptomatic patients with equivocal physical exam findings
  - Low sensitivity & specificity

CT Findings

- CECT
  - Enhancement of inflamed mucosa may be seen
  - Contrast administration **not** necessary
- CBCT and bone CT
  - Mucosal thickening or opacification of sinus without expansion of sinus
  - Variable density of secretions
    - Isodense to hyperdense depending on protein, water, and fungal content
  - Occasionally, **calcifications may be present**
  - Bony walls of sinus thickened & **sclerotic**

MR Findings

- T1WI
  - Thickened mucosa isointense to other soft tissue
  - Variable signal of retained secretions depending on variable water & protein content
    - ↑ protein:water ratio → ↑ T1 signal
  - Bone thickening & sclerosis difficult to see with MR
- T2WI
  - Mucosa typically hyperintense
  - Retained secretions range from hyperintense (↑ water content) to hypointense (↓ water, desiccated)
  - Thickened sinus walls evident on T2 MR
- T1WI C+
  - Mucosal enhancement typical
  - Contrast administration not necessary

Imaging Recommendations

- Best imaging tool
  - Thin-section axial bone CT with coronal reformatted images
  - CT detects luminal sinus disease beyond what is seen endoscopically
- Protocol advice
  - 1.00- to 1.25-mm thick axial CT in bone algorithm with coronal ± sagittal reformatted images

DIFFERENTIAL DIAGNOSIS

Fungal Sinusitis, Mycetoma

- Sinus opacified
- Calcifications common
- Often seen in clinical setting of CRS
  - Bony changes may mimic CRS

Allergic Fungal Sinusitis

- Form of CRS in patients with asthma, allergy
- Involved sinuses opacified and expanded with central high-attenuation material

Sinonasal Polyposis

- Multiple variable-density polypoid soft tissue masses in nasal cavity & sinuses
- Expansion, remodeling of bony walls may be present

Sinonasal Wegener Granulomatosis

- Nodular soft tissue thickening ± bone erosion
- Tends to affect nasal cavity > sinuses
  - Involves septum and turbinates

Sinonasal Sarcoidosis

- Nodular soft tissue thickening ± bone erosion
- Sinonasal involvement less common than in Wegener
- Predilection for nasal cavity with septal and turbinate involvement similar to Wegener

Fibrous Dysplasia

- Sclerotic bone of CRS may mimic bone in fibrous dysplasia
- Sinus may be encroached upon, but "increased radiopacity" of sinus is bone, not swollen soft tissue
- **Expansile** unlike CRS

Acute Rhinosinusitis

- Clinical course of shorter duration often following viral upper respiratory tract infection
- Air-fluid levels & bubbly secretions in addition to mucosal thickening
- No bone changes

PATHOLOGY

General Features

- Etiology
  - Unified understanding is still being sought
  - Causes of CRS are numerous, disparate, & frequently overlapping
    - Inflammation plays greater role than infection

- Biofilms (antibiotic-resistant bacterial colonies) decrease antibiotic efficacy and release inflammatory mediators
- Many factors & processes play role in etiology of CRS
  - Systemic host factors: Allergic, immunodeficiency, genetic/congenital alterations, mucociliary dysfunction, endocrine, neuromechanism
  - Local host factors: Anatomic variants, neoplasms, acquired mucociliary dysfunction
  - Environmental: Microorganisms, noxious chemicals, medications, trauma, surgery
- Genetics
  - Sporadic disease in most cases
  - Genetics play role when underlying systemic disorder present
    - Cystic fibrosis, primary ciliary dysmotility, immunodeficiency in this category
- Associated abnormalities
  - Asthma, allergy (> 50% of CRS patients)
  - Dental disease (maxillary)
  - Sinonasal polyposis

Staging, Grading, & Classification

- CRS: 5 clinical categories
  - Acute, subacute, chronic, recurrent acute, acute exacerbation of CRS
- CRS may be bacterial, allergic, or fungal in nature
  - **Bacterial CRS**
    - Bacteria may initiate CRS, cause disease persistence, or exacerbate noninfectious inflammation
    - Common organisms: *Staphylococcus aureus*, coagulase-negative *Staphylococcus*, anaerobic & gram-negative bacteria
  - **Allergic CRS**
    - Cytokines & allergic mediators → nasal allergic inflammation → mucosal swelling → obstruction of ostia
  - **Allergic fungal sinusitis**
    - Inflammatory response to presence of noninvasive fungal elements

Gross Pathologic & Surgical Features

- Mucosal swelling, purulent discharge, polypoid changes, erythema

Microscopic Features

- Mixed inflammatory infiltrate of lymphocytes, plasma cells, eosinophils, interleukin-8, and interferon-γ
- Changes in adjacent bone similar to osteomyelitis

CLINICAL ISSUES

Presentation

- Most common signs/symptoms
  - Often present with nasal obstruction, nasal discharge, hyposmia, anosmia
- Other signs/symptoms
  - Facial pain & pressure, headache
- CRS definition: Sinonasal infection/inflammation ≥ **12 weeks of duration**
- Nasal endoscopy & CT performed to quantify mucosal disease and target culturing

Demographics

- Age
  - All ages affected
- Epidemiology
  - CRS results in 18-22 million office visits in USA annually
  - Prevalence of CRS difficult to determine due to heterogeneity of disease & diagnostic imprecision

Natural History & Prognosis

- Persistent, recurrent sinusitis often refractory to medical therapy
- Often associated conditions, such as allergy, underlying anatomic variations
  - Patients with mucosal eosinophilia have poorer outcomes
- Nasal endoscopy best objective indicator of early recurrent disease

Treatment

- **Pharmacologic therapy**: Antibiotics, antifungals, decongestants, antihistamines, topical steroids (allergic cases)
- Treatment of comorbid conditions (inhalant sensitivities, polyps, infections, immune deficiencies) critical for treatment success of CRS
- Surgery reserved for cases recalcitrant to medical therapy
  - **Functional endoscopic sinus surgery** (FESS) current surgical treatment of choice
  - External approaches/sinus obliteration (frontal) reserved for cases of FESS failure or when FESS cannot be performed due to anatomic considerations

DIAGNOSTIC CHECKLIST

Consider

- Coronal sinus CT imaging study of choice in CRS
  - Evaluates changes in bone & identifying anatomic variants that may predispose to recurrent disease

Image Interpretation Pearls

- Mucosal thickening or opacification in nonexpanded sinus with associated bone thickening/sclerosis most consistent with CRS
- CT yields little information about etiology of mucosal changes
- Note: There is lack of correlation between symptomatology & imaging findings

SELECTED REFERENCES

1. Novis SJ et al: A diagnostic dilemma: chronic sinusitis diagnosed by non-otolaryngologists. Int Forum Allergy Rhinol. 6(5):486-90, 2016
2. Orlandi RR et al: International consensus statement on allergy and rhinology: rhinosinusitis. Int Forum Allergy Rhinol. 6 Suppl 1:S22-S209, 2016
3. Angulo-Pérez G et al: [Prevalence, location and tomographic severity of chronic rhinosinusitis in adult patients with common variable immunodeficiency.] Rev Alerg Mex. 62(1):15-21, 2015
4. Bothur S et al: Asymptomatic chronic rhinosinusitis and osteitis in patients treated with multiple zygomatic implants: a long-term radiographic follow-up. Int J Oral Maxillofac Implants. 30(1):161-8, 2015
5. Hamilos DL: Pediatric chronic rhinosinusitis. Am J Rhinol Allergy. 29(6):414-20, 2015
6. Joshi VM et al: Imaging in sinonasal inflammatory disease. Neuroimaging Clin N Am. 25(4):549-68, 2015

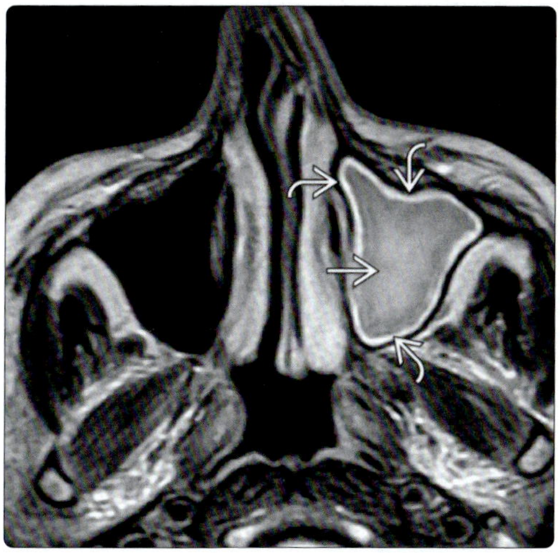

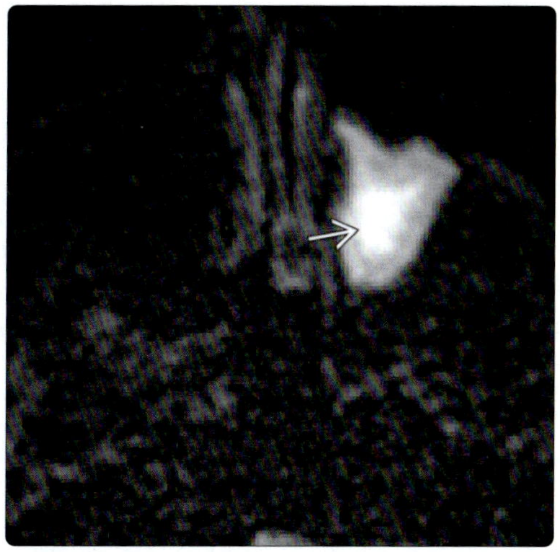

(Left) *Axial T2WI MR in a patient with CRS shows opacification of the left maxillary sinus. The central secretions are somewhat hypointense due to low water and high protein content* ➔. *Hyperintense inflamed mucosa is noted at the periphery* ↪. **(Right)** *Axial DWI MR in the same patient shows increased signal throughout the left maxillary sinus secretions, suggesting restricted diffusion. The restricted diffusion is greatest centrally* ➔.

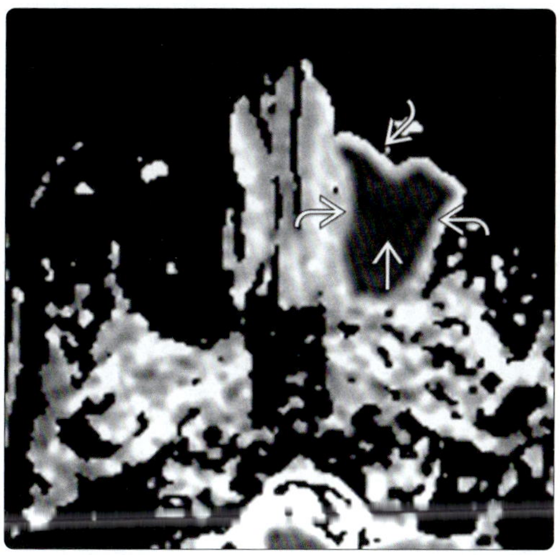

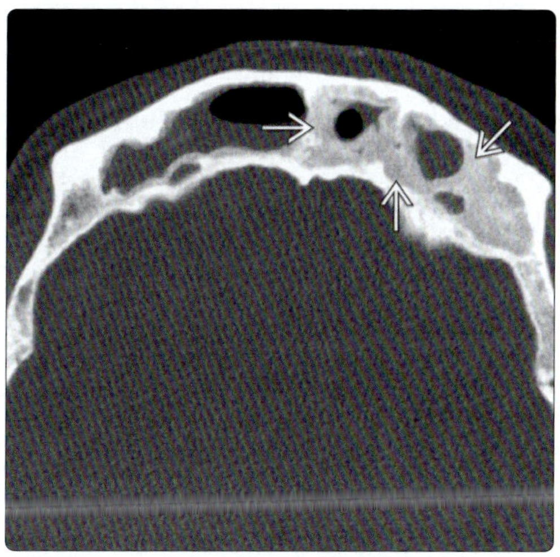

(Left) *Axial ADC in the same patient confirms that restricted diffusion was the cause of the high signal on the DWI. Diminished signal on the ADC is noted in the secretions* ➔ *with high signal in the peripheral mucosa* ↪. **(Right)** *Axial bone CT in a patient with chronic frontal sinusitis shows mucosal thickening in both frontal sinuses. There is marked thickening of the sinus walls, particularly on the left* ➔. *The changes on the left mimic fibrous dysplasia, but the area lacks expansion.*

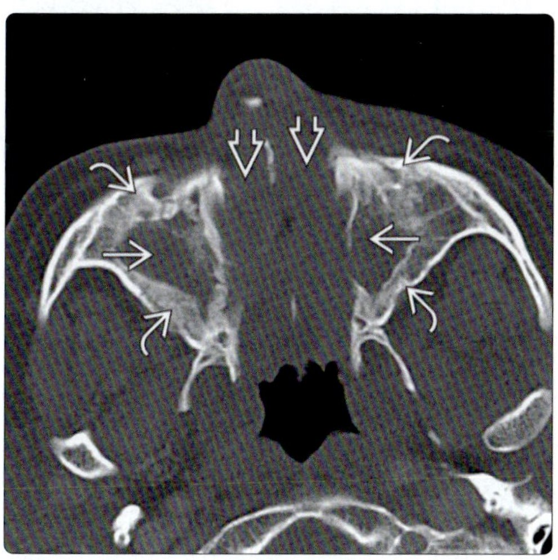

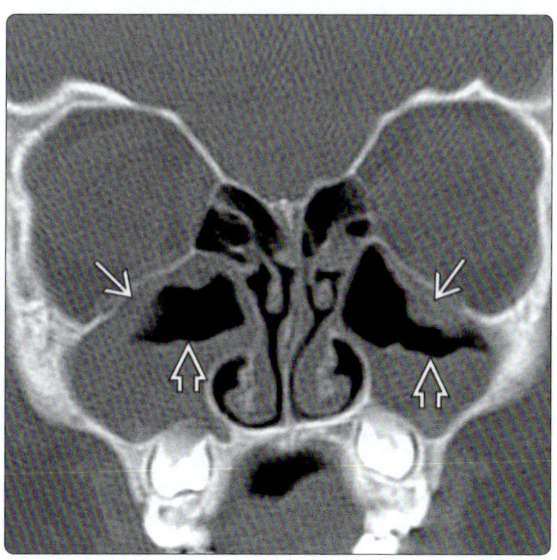

(Left) *Axial bone CT in a Wegener granulomatosis patient shows typical changes of CRS involving maxillary sinuses. Soft tissue opacifies the sinuses* ➔ *& nasal cavity* ⇨. *There is prominent osteitis involving the sinus walls* ↪. **(Right)** *Coronal bone CT in a child with cystic fibrosis shows lobular mucosal thickening in both maxillary sinuses* ➔. *Fluid levels are present* ⇨, *suggesting acute infection superimposed on chronic inflammation. Osteitis has not yet developed in this young patient.*

Odontogenic Sinusitis

KEY FACTS

TERMINOLOGY

- Definition: Inflammation of maxillary sinus(es) due to **extension of odontogenic inflammatory disease** or entry into sinus during dental treatment

IMAGING

- Best tool: Periapical or **panoramic** radiographs
- Nonenhanced bone window CT or CBCT
  - Air-fluid interface better visualized
- Soft tissue thickening in maxillary sinus
  - Located near **badly carious tooth with rarefying osteitis** or tooth with **advanced periodontal bone loss**
- Discontinuity of sinus floor if oroantral fistula (OAF)
- Tooth, tooth fragment, or foreign body in sinus
- Periosteal new bone on sinus border near tooth
  - **Radiopaque halo**/periphery to periapical pathology
- Lack of sinus floor disruption radiographically does not rule out microscopic communication of odontogenic infection

TOP DIFFERENTIAL DIAGNOSES

- Multiple mucus retention pseudocysts
- Allergic fungal sinusitis
- Sinusitis or OAF of nonodontogenic origin

CLINICAL ISSUES

- **Pain**: Remove dental cause via **extraction** or **endodontic treatment**
- Any foreign material in sinus must be removed
- **Antibiotics** for anaerobic as well as aerobic bacteria
- If ostium blocked, open or create secondary ostium
- Closure of oroantral fistula

DIAGNOSTIC CHECKLIST

- Odontogenic lesions (inflammatory or neoplastic) will displace floor of maxillary sinus superiorly
- Identify causative tooth
- Check if border of sinus is intact
- Check patency of ostiomeatal complex

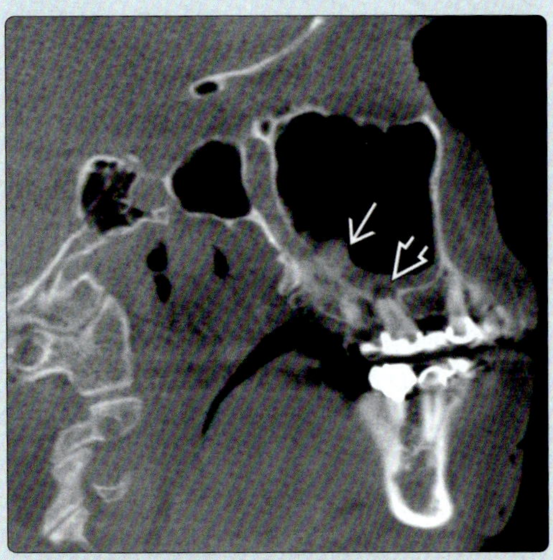
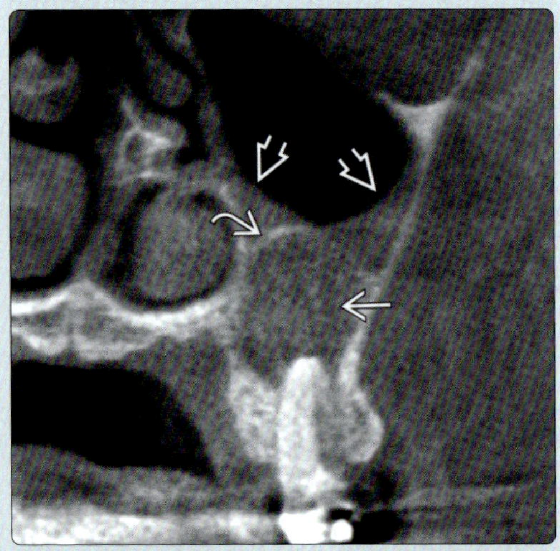

(Left) *Sagittal CBCT shows rarefying osteitis (abscess, cyst, &/or granuloma) at the apex of the maxillary left permanent 1st molar with a periosteal reaction ➔ and extension of the inflammatory response ➔ to the left maxillary sinus.* **(Right)** *Coronal CBCT shows left maxillary sinusitis ➔ caused by a large radicular cyst ➔. Note elevation of the sinus floor and well-corticated margin ➔. The radiopaque halo signifies pathology originating from outside the sinus rather than from within.*

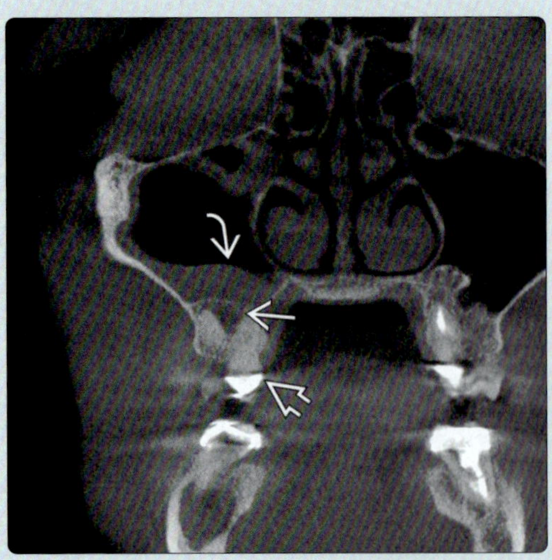
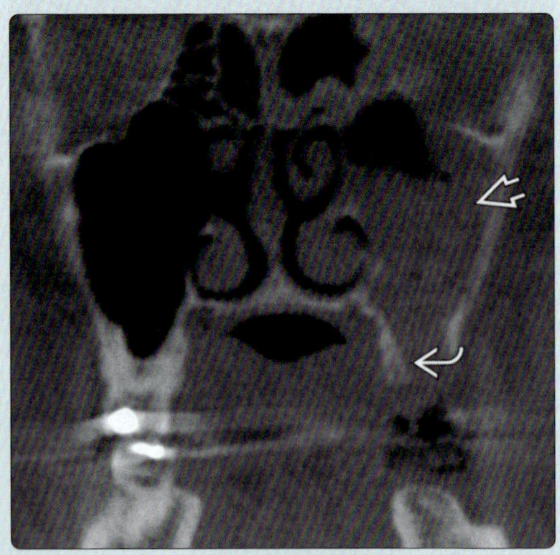

(Left) *There is a periapical inflammatory lesion (rarefying osteitis) ➔ at the apices of the maxillary right first molar ➔ resulting in inflammation (sinusitis) ➔ of the maxillary right sinus. (Courtesy P. Wong DMD.)* **(Right)** *Coronal cone-beam CT shows an oroantral fistula ➔ involving the left maxillary sinus. Almost all of the sinus is filled with thickened inflamed mucous membrane ➔ consistent with odontogenic sinusitis.*

TERMINOLOGY

Synonyms

- Sinusitis of odontogenic origin

Definitions

- Inflammation of maxillary sinus(es) due to extension of **odontogenic inflammatory disease** or entry into sinus during dental treatment [oroantral fistula (OAF)]

IMAGING

General Features

- Best diagnostic clue
  - Soft tissue enlargement in maxillary sinus
  - Badly carious or periodontally involved tooth near sinus
  - Periapical radiolucent lesion near sinus
- Location
  - Floor of maxillary sinus near badly carious or periodontally involved molar or premolar with rarefying osteitis in close proximity
- Size
  - Variable
- Morphology
  - Irregular soft tissue thickening in maxillary sinus
  - Possible loss of air space in sinus
  - Discontinuity of sinus floor if OAF present

Periapical/Occlusal Radiographic or Pantomographic Findings

- Any 1 or combination of following
  - Badly carious tooth with periapical radiolucent lesion near sinus
  - Advanced periodontal bone loss/periostitis extending to periapical area of tooth
  - Periosteal new bone on sinus border near tooth
  - Soft tissue thickening in sinus
  - Disruption of border of sinus (OAF)
  - Tooth, tooth fragment, or foreign body in sinus

CT Findings

- May better visualize
  - Air-fluid interface
  - Disruption of floor of sinus
    - Lack of sinus floor disruption radiographically does not rule out microscopic communication of odontogenic infection
  - Tooth, tooth fragment, or foreign body in sinus

Imaging Recommendations

- Best imaging tool
  - Periapical and **panoramic** radiographs, noncontrast CT or CBCT
- Protocol advice
  - Bone window

DIFFERENTIAL DIAGNOSIS

Multiple Mucus Retention Pseudocysts

- **Dome-shaped** soft tissue density **without cortication**, usually on floor of sinus
- Spontaneously regress

Allergic Fungal Sinusitis

- **Heterogeneous** mass (soft tissue) in sinus

Sinusitis of Nonodontogenic Origin

- Due to allergies or infection not dentally related
- Oroantral fistula of nonodontogenic origin

PATHOLOGY

General Features

- Depends on cause
  - Badly carious tooth with pathology at apex
  - Oroantral fistula with or without following objects in sinus
    - Tooth, fragment of tooth, or dental foreign body

Staging, Grading, & Classification

- Localized inflammation of mucous membrane of sinus without acute pain
- Generalized inflammation of mucous membrane of sinus without acute pain
- Generalized inflammation of mucous membrane of sinus with acute pain

CLINICAL ISSUES

Presentation

- Most common signs/symptoms
  - Pain (less than nonodontogenic sinusitis initially)
- Other signs/symptoms
  - Cacosmia
  - Mucopurulent discharge from sinus ostium &/or oroantral fistula

Natural History & Prognosis

- Prognosis good if dental cause removed &/or OAF repaired
- Rarely may spread to ethmoid air cells

Treatment

- Dental cause must be removed via extraction or endodontic treatment
- Any foreign material in sinus must be removed
- Antibiotics for anaerobic as well as aerobic bacteria
  - If ostium blocked, open or create secondary ostium
- Closure of oroantral fistula

DIAGNOSTIC CHECKLIST

Consider

- Fungal organisms

Image Interpretation Pearls

- Usually unilateral

Reporting Tips

- Identify causative tooth
- Check if floor of sinus is intact
- Check patency of ostiomeatal complex

SELECTED REFERENCES

1. Akhlaghi F et al: Etiologies and treatments of odontogenic maxillary sinusitis: a systematic review. Iran Red Crescent Med J. 17(12):e25536, 2015

Allergic Fungal Sinusitis

KEY FACTS

TERMINOLOGY

- Severe form of chronic rhinosinusitis (CRS) with polyposis
- Allergic response to fungi characterized by eosinophilic mucin with noninvasive fungal hyphae

IMAGING

- Opacification and expansion of multiple sinuses with inspissated material
- Centrally hyperdense and peripherally hypodense on CT
- Expansion of sinus with bony remodeling and erosion
- Hypointense on T2 MR; may mimic air

TOP DIFFERENTIAL DIAGNOSES

- Sinonasal polyposis
- Eosinophilic mucin rhinosinusitis
- Sinus fungal mycetoma
- Sinonasal solitary polyp
- Sinonasal mucocele
- Sinonasal non-Hodgkin lymphoma

PATHOLOGY

- **Type 1**, IgE-mediated hypersensitivity
- Immune response to fungal antigens
- Viscous, eosinophilic mucin with fungal hyphae
- **Absence** of tissue invasion

CLINICAL ISSUES

- Symptoms: Nasal obstruction, rhinorrhea
- Immunocompetent patient with longstanding CRS
- Serum eosinophilia, elevated IgE
- Cutaneous sensitivity to fungal antigens
- Topical steroids 1st-line medical therapy
- Surgical debridement + perioperative systemic steroids
- Topical and systemic antifungal agents controversial

DIAGNOSTIC CHECKLIST

- Consider allergic fungal sinusitis in polyposis patients with increased density and expansion involving multiple sinuses

(Left) *Coronal graphic shows classic features of allergic fungal sinusitis (AFS), including opacification and expansion of multiple paranasal sinuses and the nasal cavity. Centrally inspissated material is present, surrounded by peripheral edematous mucosa.* **(Right)** *Axial NECT shows unilateral involvement of AFS. The involved sinuses are expanded, with centrally dense inspissated material and a peripheral rim of low attenuation. Sinus involvement with AFS may be unilateral or bilateral.*

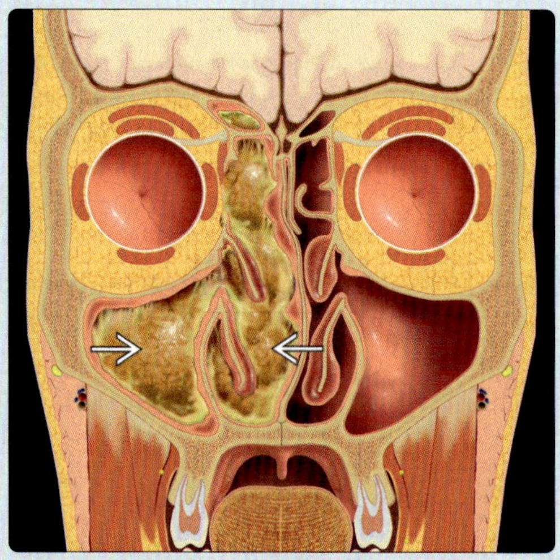

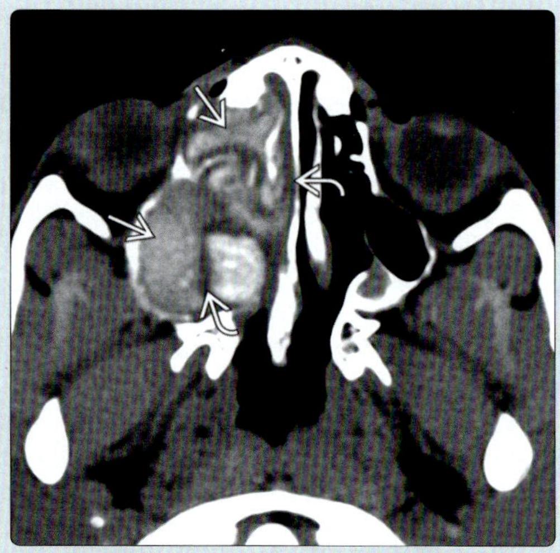

(Left) *Axial T2WI MR in a patient with bilateral AFS shows diffuse, hypointense signal within the involved ethmoid air cells. There is mild sinus expansion with lateral bowing of the lamina papyracea. Note that the very low signal mimics normal sinus aeration.* **(Right)** *Axial T1WI C+ MR in the same patient confirms that the ethmoid sinuses are not aerated but are in fact completely opacified. The surrounding mucosa shows peripheral linear enhancement.*

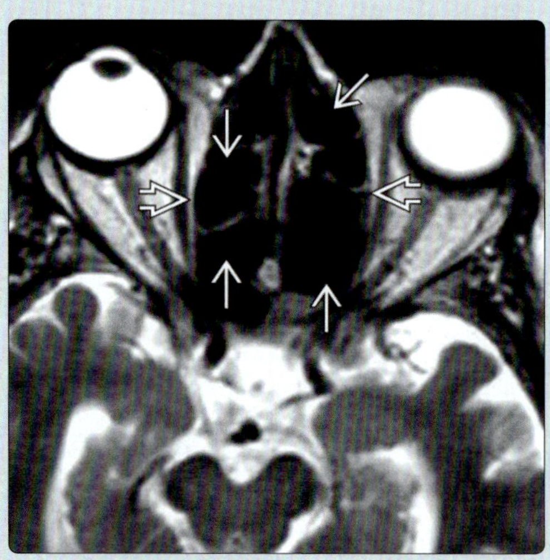

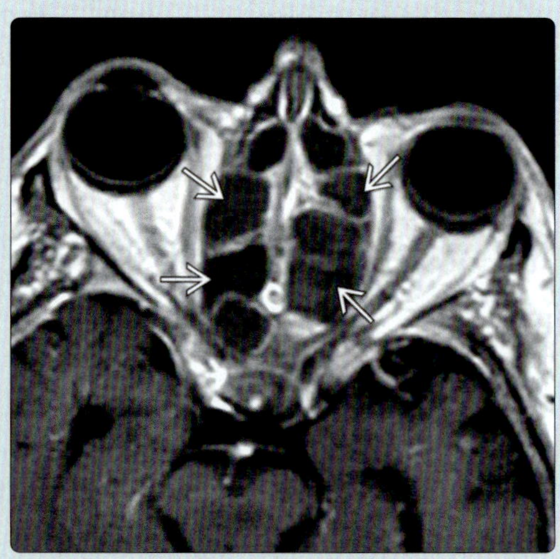

Allergic Fungal Sinusitis

TERMINOLOGY

Abbreviations

- Allergic fungal sinusitis (AFS) or rhinosinusitis (AFRS)

Definitions

- Severe form of chronic rhinosinusitis (CRS) with polyposis
  - Allergic response to fungi in susceptible individuals
- Characterized by production of eosinophilic mucin containing **noninvasive fungal hyphae**

IMAGING

General Features

- Best diagnostic clue
  - **Opacification** and **expansion** of multiple sinuses with inspissated material
  - Centrally **hyperdense** and peripherally **hypodense** on CT
  - Hypointense on T2 MR; may **mimic air**
- Location
  - Involves **multiple sinuses**
  - Unilateral or bilateral (50/50); R > L

CT Findings

- NECT
  - Hyperdense material **centrally** within opacified sinuses
  - Hypodense **rim of mucosa**
  - **Expansion** of sinus with bony remodeling and erosion

MR Findings

- T1WI
  - Signal **variable** (water, protein, and fungal content)
- T2WI
  - **Hypointense** signal **centrally** due to dense fungal concretions and heavy metals; may mimic air
- T1WI C+
  - Peripheral inflamed mucosa enhances

DIFFERENTIAL DIAGNOSIS

Sinonasal Polyposis

- Common form of CRS with polyposis
- Absence of specific antigenic or atopic etiology

Eosinophilic Mucin Rhinosinusitis

- Similar to AFS but without identifiable hyphae
- Systemic immune dysregulation; more often bilateral

Sinus Fungal Mycetoma

- Noninvasive fungal colonization without hyperimmunity
- Isolated, especially maxillary; hyperdense with fine calcifications

Sinonasal Solitary Polyp

- Low-density mass with rim enhancement
- Classic antrochoanal polyp (ACP)

Sinonasal Mucocele

- Isolated postobstructive lesion
- Chronic expansile features with bony remodeling

Sinonasal Non-Hodgkin Lymphoma

- Sinonasal mass with bone destruction or remodeling

PATHOLOGY

General Features

- Etiology
  - **Type 1**, IgE-mediated hypersensitivity
    - Immune response to **fungal antigens**

Gross Pathologic & Surgical Features

- Viscous brown or greenish black mucus with peanut butter/cottage cheese consistency

Microscopic Features

- Viscous, eosinophilic mucin with fungal hyphae
- Organisms: *Aspergillus*, *Curvularia*, *Bipolaris*, *Pseudallescheria*, and *Fusarium*
- **Absence** of tissue invasion

CLINICAL ISSUES

Presentation

- Most common signs/symptoms
  - Nasal obstruction, rhinorrhea
- Clinical profile
  - **Immunocompetent** patient with longstanding CRS
  - Polyposis history
  - Serum eosinophilia, elevated IgE
  - Cutaneous sensitivity to fungal antigens

Demographics

- Age
  - Primarily young adults (mean: ~ 30 years)
- Gender
  - Male predominance
- Epidemiology
  - Asthma history in 40%
  - Higher incidence in patients of African descent
  - Predilection for warm, humid climates

Natural History & Prognosis

- Slow, indolent course in face of CRS and allergy

Treatment

- Topical steroids 1st-line medical therapy
- Surgical debridement + perioperative systemic steroids
- Topical and systemic antifungal agents may be beneficial
  - Controversial effectiveness and risks

DIAGNOSTIC CHECKLIST

Consider

- AFS in polyposis patient with increased density and expansion involving multiple sinuses

Image Interpretation Pearls

- Hypointense on T2WI; may **mimic air**

SELECTED REFERENCES

1. Hull BP et al: Refractory chronic rhinosinusitis with nasal polyposis. Otolaryngol Clin North Am. 50(1):61-81, 2017
2. Rick EM et al: Allergic fungal airway disease. J Investig Allergol Clin Immunol. 26(6):344-354, 2016
3. Uri N et al: Allergic fungal sinusitis and eosinophilic mucin rhinosinusitis: diagnostic criteria. J Laryngol Otol. 127(9):867-71, 2013

KEY FACTS

TERMINOLOGY

- Acute invasive fungal rhinosinusitis (AIFRS): Rapidly progressive fungal sinus infection in immunocompromised patients that involves bone and adjacent soft tissues via vascular spread

IMAGING

- AIFRS is most common in maxillary and ethmoid sinuses followed by sphenoid sinus
- CT: Sinus opacification with **focal bone erosion**, adjacent soft tissue infiltration
- MR: Superior for evaluating intraorbital and intracranial extension

TOP DIFFERENTIAL DIAGNOSES

- Acute rhinosinusitis with complication
- Sinonasal Wegener granulomatosis
- Sinonasal squamous cell carcinoma
- Sinonasal non-Hodgkin lymphoma

PATHOLOGY

- Present classification based upon International Society for Human and Animal Mycology Group, February 2008
  - **Acute invasive** (fulminant) FRS
  - **Granulomatous invasive** FRS (GIFRS)
  - **Chronic invasive** FRS (CIFRS)

CLINICAL ISSUES

- AIFRS: Acute-onset fever, painless nasal septal ulcer, sinusitis
  - Can be rapidly progressive and fatal in days to weeks
  - Orbital and intracranial involvement are most dreaded complications
- GIFRS: Enlarging cheek, orbit, or sinonasal mass
- CIFRS: Sinus pain, nasal discharge, epistaxis, fever, polyposis

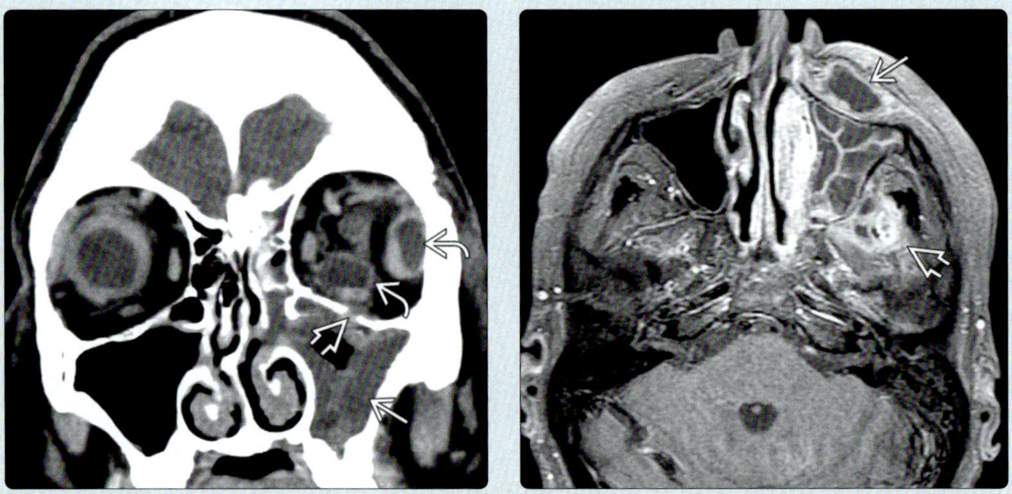

(Left) *Coronal NECT in a diabetic patient with mucormycosis infection shows extensive disease in the left maxillary sinus → with intraorbital extension of infection through a defect → in the infraorbital canal. Low-attenuation abscesses are seen involving the lateral and inferior rectus muscles →.* **(Right)** *Axial T1WI C+ FS MR in the same patient shows additional extension of the invasive fungal infection in the premaxillary soft tissues → and masticator space →.*

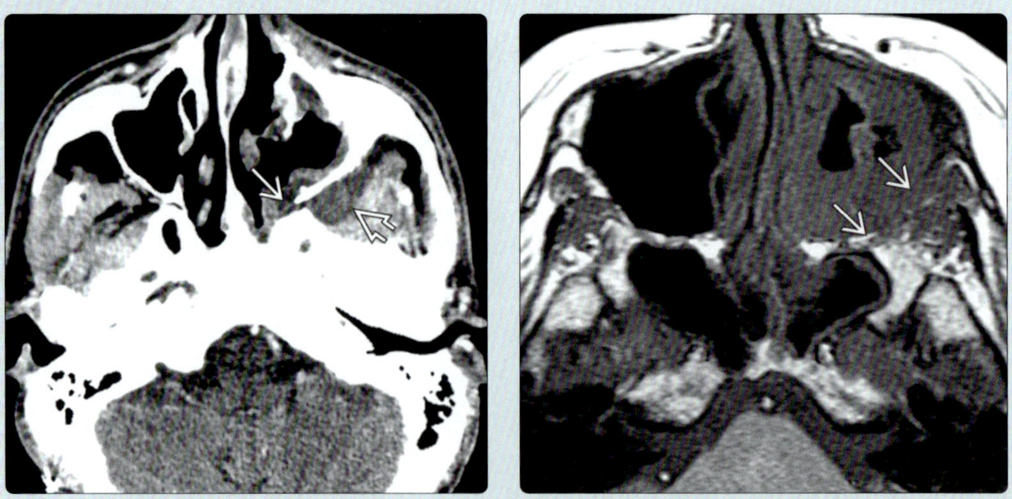

(Left) *Axial CECT in a patient with mucormycosis shows circumferential soft tissue in the left maxillary sinus. Destruction of the posterior wall of the sinus → is noted medially, and there is infiltration of the retroantral fat → consistent with fungal spread beyond the sinus.* **(Right)** *Axial T1WI MR shows extensive fungal involvement of the left maxillary sinus. The posterior sinus wall is eroded →, with extension of infection into the left retromaxillary fat pad.*

TERMINOLOGY

Abbreviations

- Invasive fungal sinusitis (IFS)

Synonyms

- Acute invasive fungal rhinosinusitis (AIFRS): Acute necrotizing FRS
- Granulomatous invasive fungal rhinosinusitis (GIFRS): Primary paranasal granuloma, indolent fungal sinusitis

Definitions

- AIFRS: Rapidly progressive fungal sinus infection in immunocompromised patients that crosses mucosa to involve blood vessels, bone, soft tissues, orbit, intracranial cavities
- GIFRS: Rarely seen in USA; indolent but profuse fungal growth with noncaseating granulomas
- Chronic invasive fungal rhinosinusitis (CIFRS): Dense hyphal accumulation resembling mycetoma (from which it may arise); associated with orbital apex syndrome, diabetes mellitus (DM), corticosteroid therapy

IMAGING

General Features

- Best diagnostic clue
  - Sinus opacification with **focal bone erosion**, adjacent soft tissue infiltration
- Location
  - AIFRS: Most common in maxillary and ethmoid sinuses followed by sphenoid sinus
    - Spread from sinuses can extend in any direction
  - CIFRS: Most common in ethmoid and sphenoid sinuses
- Morphology
  - Ill-defined or mass-like soft tissue lesion

CT Findings

- NECT
  - Complete or partial soft tissue opacification of affected sinus; mucosal thickening
  - Hyperattenuation of secretions suggests fungal infection; more typical of chronic than acute
  - Focal areas of sinus wall erosion
    - **Bone erosion** may be **subtle** as fungi extend along vessels
  - Infiltration of adjacent fat and soft tissues
    - Maxillary sinus: **Perimaxillary fat infiltration** (anterior, premaxillary, or retroantral fat)
    - Can be present without bone destruction via perivascular channels
    - May be due to edema from vascular congestion, tissue infiltration by fungal elements
- CECT
  - Periantral soft tissues, adjacent musculature may enhance
- CTA
  - May show arterial or venous narrowing/occlusion
    - Pseudoaneurysm formation
  - CTV: Better for confirming cavernous sinus thrombosis

MR Findings

- T1WI
  - Variable signal of material within involved sinus
    - Depends on protein/water content, presence of fungal elements
  - Diminished signal, similar to soft tissue, within periantral fat
- T2WI
  - Variable signal of sinus secretions
    - Fungal elements may cause hypointense T2 signal
  - High-signal edema in involved soft tissues may be seen with fat suppression
- T1WI C+
  - Enhancement of involved soft tissues
  - Leptomeningeal enhancement
- MRA
  - Vascular involvement (narrowing, dissection, thrombosis)

Angiographic Findings

- Vascular involvement (narrowing, dissection, thrombosis, pseudoaneurysm formation)

Imaging Recommendations

- Best imaging tool
  - CECT with soft tissue and bone windows to evaluate bone erosion, soft tissue infiltration
  - MR superior for evaluating intraorbital and intracranial extension
- Protocol advice
  - Axial helical CECT ≤ 1-mm slice thickness reconstructed in bone and soft tissue algorithm, coronal reconstructions
  - T1 C+ FS MR recommended to map disease spread beyond sinuses

DIFFERENTIAL DIAGNOSIS

Complicated Rhinosinusitis

- Patient may not be immunocompromised
- Bone erosion less likely
- Homogeneous air-fluid level, peripheral mucosal thickening in sinus
- Complications of subperiosteal postseptal abscess, cavernous sinus thrombosis, meningitis, and cerebral abscess appear similar to AIFRS

Granulomatosis With Polyangiitis

- Usually involves nasal cavity (septum and turbinates)
- Less mass-like soft tissue, prominent bone erosion
- Orbit and skull base involvement possible

Sinonasal Squamous Cell Carcinoma

- Typically immunocompetent patient
- Maxillary antrum most common site
- Solid mass with bone destruction

Sinonasal Non-Hodgkin Lymphoma

- Solid, homogeneous mass in nasal cavity
- ↓ T2 signal due to ↑ nuclear:cytoplasmic ratio could mimic fungus

PATHOLOGY

General Features

- Etiology
  - AIFRS: Vascular and soft tissue invasion by fungi in patients with variety of predisposing conditions
    - **Neutropenia**/neutrophil dysfunction
    - Uncontrolled **DM**
    - Hematologic malignancy, aplastic anemia
    - Hemochromatosis
    - Chronic **immunosuppressive therapy**, post transplantation/chemotherapy
  - Spread from sinuses via vascular invasion

Staging, Grading, & Classification

- Current classification based on International Society for Human and Animal Mycology Group, February 2008
  - Based on histopathologic finding of mucosal invasion
    - **Acute invasive** (fulminant) FRS, **granulomatous invasive** FRS, **chronic invasive** FRS

Gross Pathologic & Surgical Features

- AIFRS: Necrotic involved tissue, discoloration 2° to presence of fungus

Microscopic Features

- AIFRS
  - Hyphal invasion of mucosa, submucosa, and blood vessels
  - Prominent tissue infarction, neutrophilic infiltrates
- GIFRS
  - Noncaseating granulomatous response with considerable fibrosis and scant hyphae
  - Vasculitis, vascular proliferation, perivascular fibrosis
  - *Aspergillus flavus* most common
- CIFRS
  - Dense accumulation of hyphae with occasional vascular invasion
  - Sparse inflammatory reaction
  - > 50% *Aspergillus fumigatus*

CLINICAL ISSUES

Presentation

- Most common signs/symptoms
  - AIFRS: Acute-onset fever, painless nasal septal ulcer, sinusitis, and progression to headache/orbital symptoms
  - GIFRS: Enlarging cheek, orbit, or sinonasal mass
  - CIFRS: Sinus pain, nasal discharge, epistaxis, fever, polyposis
- Clinical profile
  - AIFRS: Rapidly progressive (< 4 weeks) invasive fungal infection in immunocompromised patient
    - Spreads from sinuses via vascular invasion
  - GIFRS: Immunocompetent host with > 12-week course of enlarging cheek, orbit, or sinonasal mass
  - CIFRS: Slowly destructive process (> 12 weeks) seen in patients with AIDS, DM, or on corticosteroids
    - Can be seen in immunocompetent patients
    - Symptoms may take months/years to develop; may persist and recur

Demographics

- Age
  - Typically in adults
- Epidemiology
  - Diabetic or immunocompromised patients with predisposing conditions
  - GIFRS: Seen primarily in Sudan, India, Pakistan, and Saudi Arabia

Natural History & Prognosis

- AIFRS: Can be rapidly progressive and fatal in days to weeks without appropriate surgical-medical therapy
  - Mortality (50-80%)
  - Fair prognosis if limited to sinus and immediately adjacent tissues
  - Orbital and intracranial involvement are most dreaded complications
  - AIFRS of sphenoid sinus can lead to cavernous sinus thrombosis, carotid occlusion, mycotic aneurysm formation, cranial nerve dysfunction, cerebral infarction

Treatment

- Radical debridement until histopathologically normal tissue reached
- Antifungal therapy with amphotericin B (*Mucor* species not sensitive to "azole" antifungals)
- Treat underlying condition responsible for immunocompromised state
  - Reversal of these conditions may ↓ mortality to 18%

DIAGNOSTIC CHECKLIST

Consider

- AIFRS in diabetic/immunocompromised patients with maxillary disease; "dirty" periantral fat, even if no bone erosion present

Image Interpretation Pearls

- Do not confuse normal variability in volume of periantral fat or normal musculature with fat infiltration
- Evaluate orbit, intracranial cavities for involvement (leptomeningeal enhancement)
- Closely examine cavernous sinus, internal carotid artery in sphenoid AIFRS

SELECTED REFERENCES

1. Goldfarb JM et al: Update on nonmalignant lesions of the inferior turbinate. Curr Opin Otolaryngol Head Neck Surg. 25(1):69-72, 2017
2. D'Anza B et al: Chronic invasive fungal sinusitis: characterization and shift in management of a rare disease. Int Forum Allergy Rhinol. 6(12):1294-1300, 2016
3. Humphrey JM et al: Invasive aspergillus sinusitis in human immunodeficiency virus infection: case report and review of the literature. Open Forum Infect Dis. 3(3):ofw135, 2016
4. Kim YK et al: Extrasinonasal infiltrative process associated with a sinonasal fungus ball: does it mean invasive fungal sinusitis? Diagn Interv Radiol. 22(4):347-53, 2016
5. Richter AL et al: Chronic invasive fungal sinusitis causing a pathologic Le Fort I fracture in an immunocompetent patient. Ear Nose Throat J. 95(9):E1-3, 2016
6. Smith A et al: Invasive fungal sinusitis in the pediatric population: Systematic review with quantitative synthesis of the literature. Int J Pediatr Otorhinolaryngol. 90:231-235, 2016
7. Chakrabarti A et al: Fungal rhinosinusitis: a categorization and definitional schema addressing current controversies. Laryngoscope. 119(9):1809-18, 2009

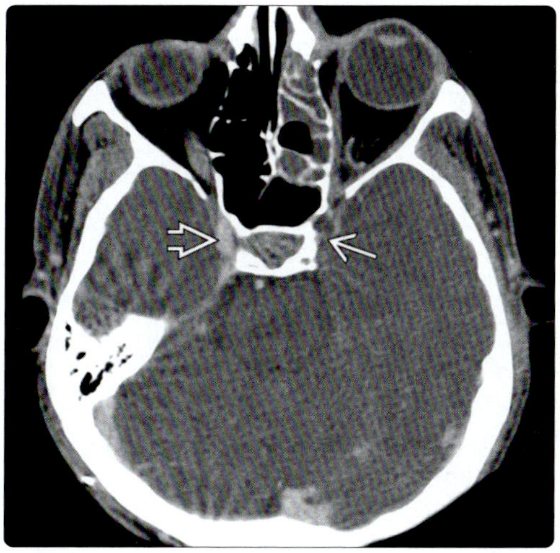
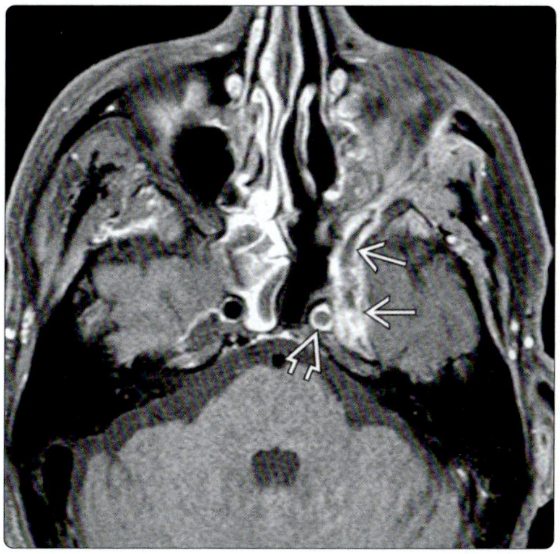

(Left) *Axial CECT in a patient with invasive mucormycosis involving the left maxillary and ethmoid sinuses reveals thrombosis of the left cavernous sinus and cavernous internal carotid artery (ICA). Note the normal enhancement within the right ICA.* **(Right)** *Axial T1WI C+ FS MR in the same patient shows extensive left cavernous sinus involvement. The intracranial ICA is occluded, and the vessel is engulfed by the invasive fungal disease in the left cavernous sinus.*

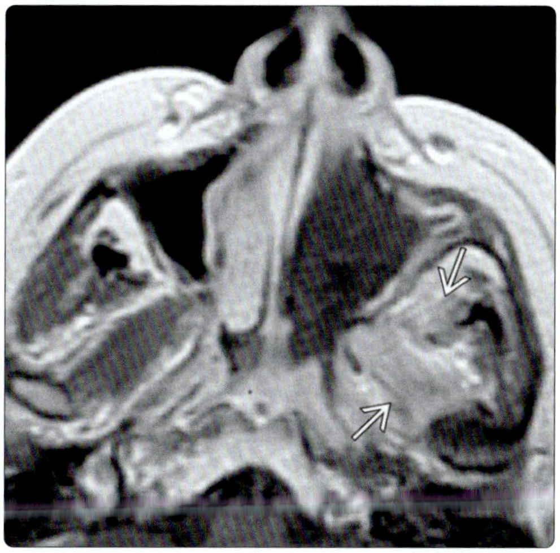
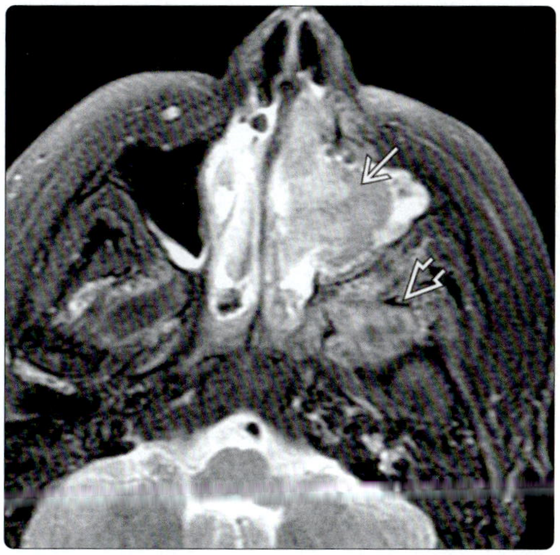

(Left) *Axial T1WI C+ MR shows a typical case of maxillary fungal sinusitis that has spread from the maxillary antrum to surrounding soft tissues. Spread into the masticator space is noted with enhancement of the muscles of mastication.* **(Right)** *Axial T2WI FS MR in the same patient shows hypointense signal characteristic of fungal material within the antrum. Hyperintense signal is noted within the involved masticator space musculature.*

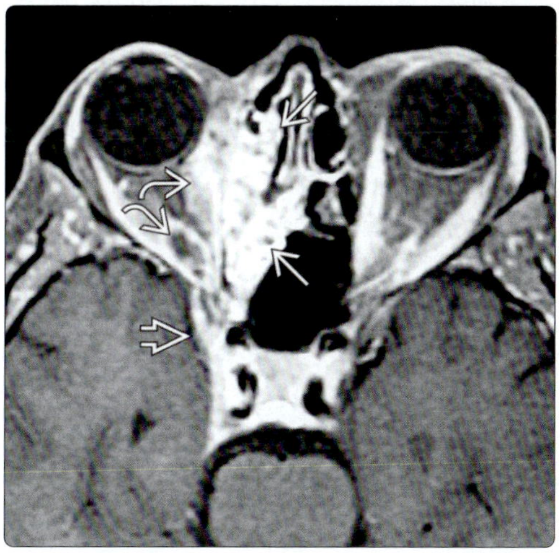
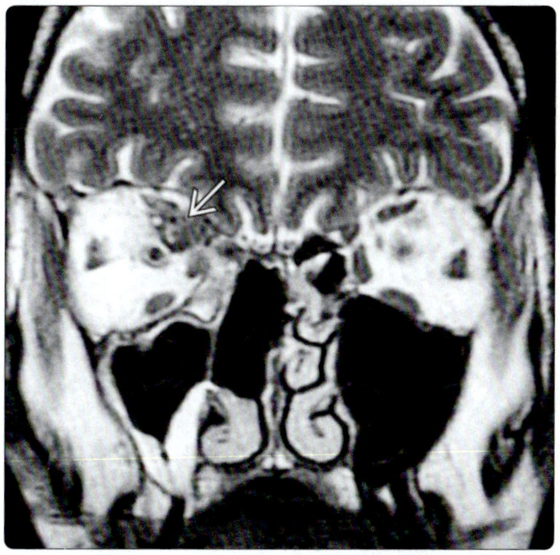

(Left) *Axial T1WI C+ FS MR in an immunosuppressed transplant patient shows invasive fungal sinusitis involving the right ethmoid air cells. There is extension of infection into the right orbit around the rectus muscles and at the orbital apex. Intracranial extension via the superior orbital fissure is noted.* **(Right)** *Coronal T2WI MR in the same patient shows hypointense signal, characteristic of fungal disease, in the superomedial aspect of the involved orbit.*

Mycetoma

KEY FACTS

TERMINOLOGY

- Synonyms: Fungus ball, aspergilloma
- Definition: Chronic, **noninvasive form** of fungal sinus infection in which material within sinonasal cavity is colonized by fungus

IMAGING

- Paranasal sinus containing **high-density material** with fine, round to linear matrix **calcifications**
- Usually affects **single sinus**
  - Maxillary > sphenoid > > frontal > ethmoid
- **Hypointense** T2: Macromolecular protein binding

TOP DIFFERENTIAL DIAGNOSES

- Chronic rhinosinusitis
- Allergic fungal sinusitis
- Mucocele
- Invasive fungal sinusitis

PATHOLOGY

- Deficient mucociliary clearance mechanism → inadequate clearance of fungal organisms → fungus germinates and replicates → incites inflammatory response

CLINICAL ISSUES

- Asymptomatic or mild sensation of pressure overlying sinuses
  - Indolent course for up to several years
- Commonly older females; may occur in all ages
- **Immunocompetent**, nonatopic, healthy patient

DIAGNOSTIC CHECKLIST

- Do not mistake low T2 signal for air
  - Correlate T2 appearance with other sequences ± CT
- Be sure to look for any signs of invasive disease

(Left) *Coronal bone CT shows the classic features of a mycetoma within the right maxillary sinus. The sinus is opacified but not expanded. Mixed-density material consistent with fungal elements and calcium deposits* ➡ *are present in the sinus.* **(Right)** *Axial T2WI MR is slightly degraded by motion but shows a classic fungus ball* ➡ *in the left maxillary sinus. The mycetoma is hypointense compared to inflamed mucosa* ➡ *at the periphery. Thickening of the bony sinus walls is also noted.*

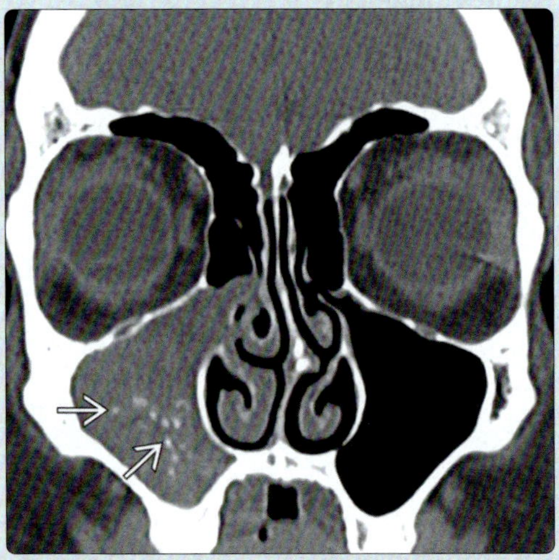

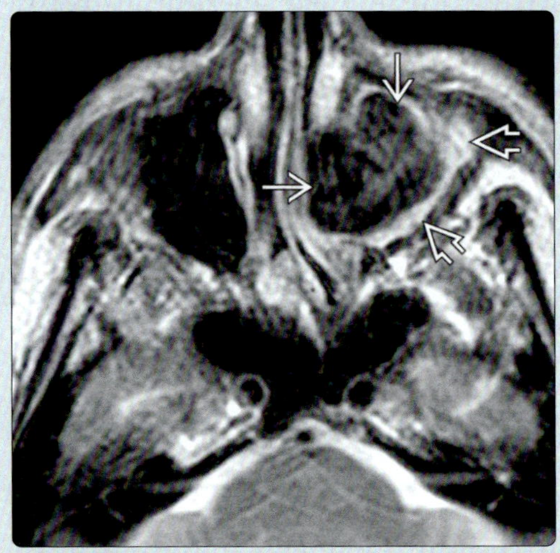

(Left) *Coronal CECT in a patient with a sphenoid sinus mycetoma demonstrates multiple foci of calcification* ➡ *within the fungus ball. The sinus is opacified, and there is no expansion.* **(Right)** *Sagittal T1WI C+ MR in the same patient shows a somewhat lamellated appearance of the material within the mycetoma* ➡*. The signal varies within the mycetoma from hypointense to hyperintense from anterior to posterior. Enhancement of inflamed mucosa* ➡ *is seen anteriorly.*

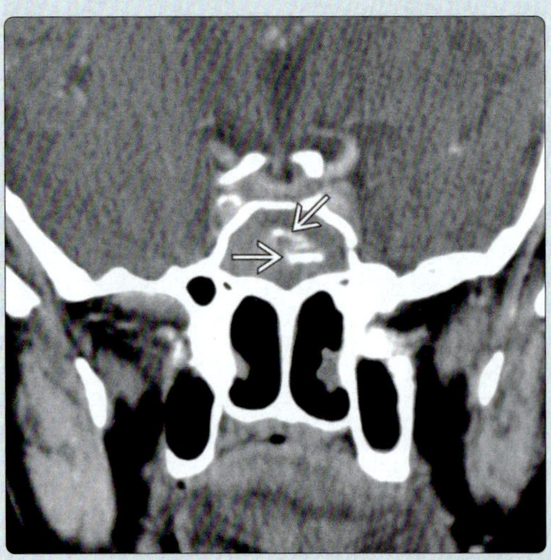

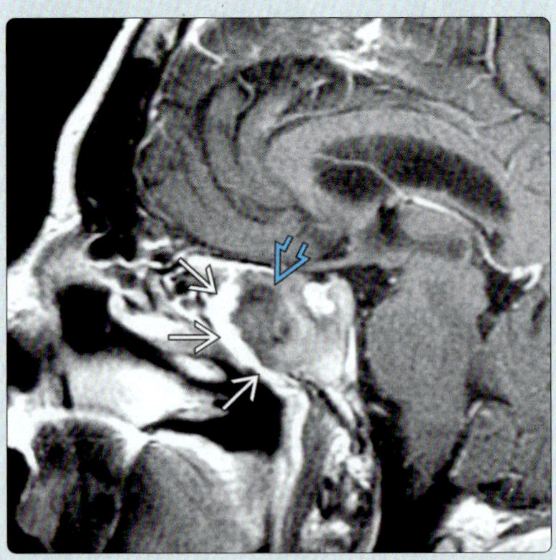

TERMINOLOGY

Synonyms

- Fungus ball, aspergilloma

Definitions

- Chronic, noninvasive form of fungal sinus infection in which material within sinonasal cavity is colonized by fungus

IMAGING

General Features

- Best diagnostic clue
  - Single paranasal sinus containing high-density material with fine, round to linear matrix calcifications (Ca++)
- Location
  - Usually affects single sinus
  - Maxillary > sphenoid > > frontal > ethmoid sinuses
- Size
  - Sinus typically normal, nonexpanded
- Morphology
  - May conform to sinus shape or be ovoid (ball-shaped) within sinus lumen

CT Findings

- CECT
  - Thickened, inflamed mucosa at periphery of sinus may enhance
- Bone CT
  - Opacification or focal mass within sinus lumen
  - Central areas of **high density ± calcification**
  - Thick, sclerotic bony sinus walls from chronic inflammation

MR Findings

- T1WI
  - Variable signal material in affected sinus
    - Usually ↓ **T1 signal** due to absence of free water in thick, solid, mycetomatous mass
- T2WI
  - **Hypointense** mass from macromolecular protein binding may be mistaken for air
- T1WI C+
  - Inflamed peripheral mucosa may enhance

Imaging Recommendations

- Best imaging tool
  - NECT features diagnostic in typical cases; better for detecting Ca++

DIFFERENTIAL DIAGNOSIS

Chronic Rhinosinusitis

- Less likely to appear mass-like
- Ca++ less likely

Allergic Fungal Sinusitis

- Atopic patient with multiple unilateral or pansinus involvement
- High-density (CT)/low T1/T2 (MR) material within expanded sinuses

Sinonasal Mucocele

- Sinus opacified and expanded
- Frontal and ethmoid > > > maxillary and sphenoid

Invasive Fungal Sinusitis

- Immunocompromised patient
- Bone destruction and soft tissue invasion

Sinonasal Inverted Papilloma

- Mass in nasal cavity centered at middle meatus
- Convoluted, cerebriform architecture

PATHOLOGY

General Features

- Etiology
  - Deficient mucociliary clearance mechanism → inadequate clearance of fungal organisms → fungus germinates & replicates → incites inflammatory response
  - Saprophytic fungal growth within paranasal sinus

Gross Pathologic & Surgical Features

- Thick, cheesy, semisolid lesion

Microscopic Features

- Tightly packed fungal hyphae with no allergic mucin (compared to allergic fungal sinusitis)
- No tissue (mucosal, blood vessel, bone) invasion compared to acute invasive fungal sinusitis

CLINICAL ISSUES

Presentation

- Most common signs/symptoms
  - Asymptomatic or mild sensation of pressure overlying sinuses
- Clinical profile
  - Immunocompetent, nonatopic, otherwise healthy patient with no or minimal symptoms

Demographics

- Age
  - Most common in older patients but may occur in all ages
- Gender
  - Female predilection
- Epidemiology
  - Mycetoma and allergic fungal sinusitis are most common forms of fungal sinusitis

Natural History & Prognosis

- Indolent course for up to several years

Treatment

- Surgical excision is treatment of choice and is curative

SELECTED REFERENCES

1. Robey AB et al: The changing face of paranasal sinus fungus balls. Ann Otol Rhinol Laryngol. 118(7):500-5, 2009
2. Daudia A et al: Advances in management of paranasal sinus aspergillosis. J Laryngol Otol. 122(4):331-5, 2008
3. Palacios E et al: Sinonasal mycetoma. Ear Nose Throat J. 87(11):606-8, 2008
4. Grosjean P et al: Fungus balls of the paranasal sinuses: a review. Eur Arch Otorhinolaryngol. 264(5):461-70, 2007
5. Som PM et al: Hypointense paranasal sinus foci: differential diagnosis with MR imaging and relation to CT findings. Radiology. 176(3):777-81, 1990

Invasive Pseudotumor

KEY FACTS

TERMINOLOGY

- Invasive pseudotumor (IPT): Benign tumor of unknown origin
    - Encompassing term for group of nonspecific inflammatory expansile lesions
- May represent 2 distinct groups of lesions
    - Histopathologically inflammatory and reparative lesions
    - Neoplasms that are histopathologically and clinically benign, aggressive, or malignant
- Many now considered part of IgG4-related disease (IgG4-RD)

IMAGING

- Most often **diagnosis of exclusion**
- < 5% in H&N
    - Orbit most common H&N site
    - Less common in larynx, paranasal sinuses, soft tissues of neck, esophagus, and skull base
- Homogeneous soft tissue mass
- Usually appears benign
- May show peripheral infiltration of surrounding tissues
- In paranasal sinus, mass may fill sinus
- Can fill sinus and **displace** or **erode** sinus walls

TOP DIFFERENTIAL DIAGNOSES

- Chronic rhinosinusitis
- Wegener granulomatosis
- Eosinophilic angiocentric fibrosis
- Sarcoidosis
- Squamous cell carcinoma

CLINICAL ISSUES

- In orbit: Pain, diplopia, proptosis, ↓ extraocular muscle mobility
- Fever, anorexia, malaise, somnolence in < 30%
- Orbital IPT fairly responsive to steroids
- 17-52% recurrence rate
- Resection may be necessary

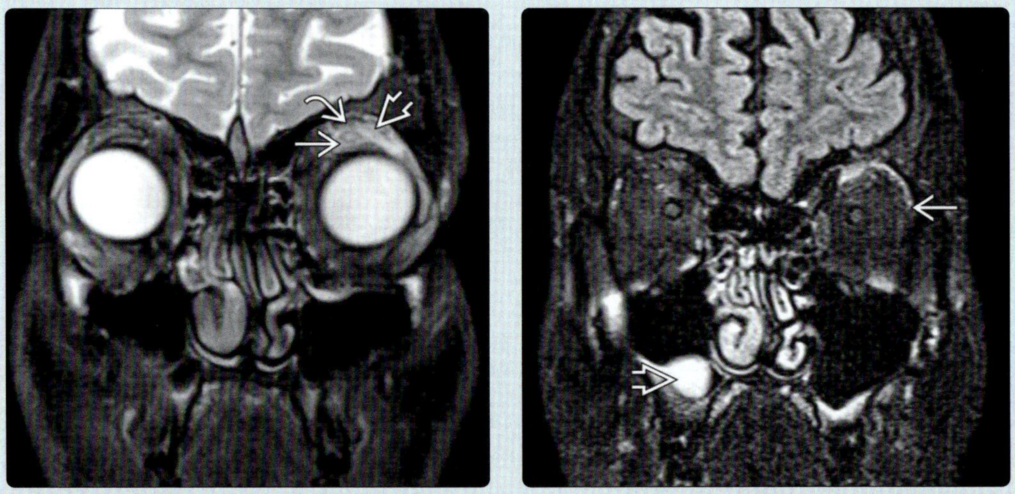

(Left) *Coronal T2WI MR shows a bright signal ➡ in the region of superior rectus ➡ and levator palpebrae superioris ➡, muscles consistent with inflammation of a pseudotumor.* **(Right)** *Coronal FLAIR MR in the same patient shows a bright signal superior to the globe, around superior rectus and levator palpebrae superioris muscles, extending laterally to the lateral rectus muscle ➡, consistent with inflammation of a pseudotumor. A mucus retention pseudocyst ➡ is in the right maxillary sinus.*

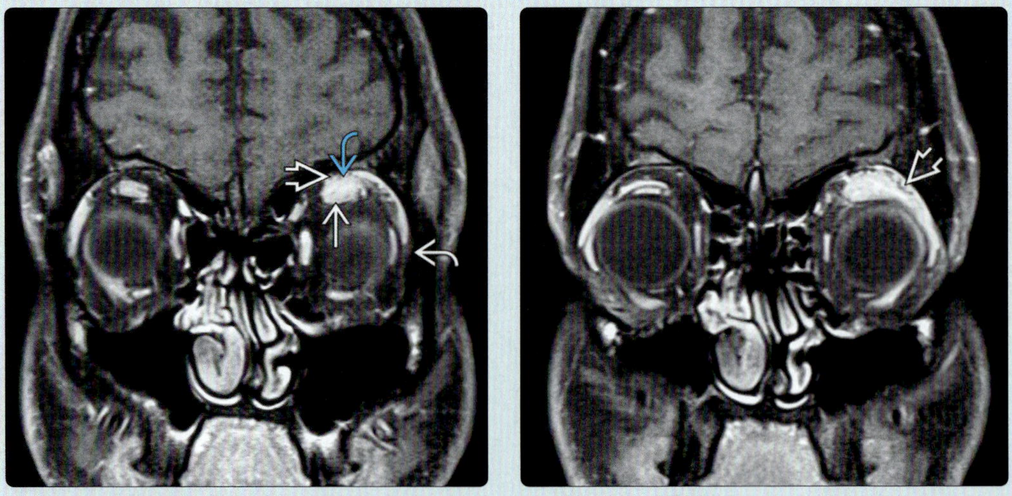

(Left) *Coronal T1WI C+ FS MR in the same patient shows a bright signal ➡ superior to the globe, around and between superior rectus ➡ and levator palpebrae superioris ➡ muscles, and extending laterally to the lateral rectus muscle ➡, consistent with inflammation of a pseudotumor.* **(Right)** *Coronal T1WI C+ FS MR in the same patient shows the bright signal ➡ of the pseudotumor superior and lateral to the globe.*

TERMINOLOGY

Abbreviations

- Invasive pseudotumor (IPT)

Synonyms

- Inflammatory myofibroblastic tumor; inflammatory pseudotumor; plasma cell granuloma; pseudosarcomatous myofibroblastic proliferation; spindle cell pseudotumor; mast cell granuloma; xanthogranuloma, IgG4-related disease (IgG4-RD)

Definitions

- Many now considered part of IgG4-RD
    - Considered immune-mediated condition, part of group of disorders with common clinical, pathologic, and serologic characteristics

IMAGING

General Features

- Best diagnostic clue
    - Most often **diagnosis of exclusion**
- Location
    - Most common in lungs
    - Of extrapulmonary sites
        - < 5% in H&N
            - Orbit most common; less common in larynx, paranasal sinuses, soft tissues of neck, esophagus, and skull base
            - Rare in nasopharynx; also seen in gingiva & periodontal tissues, tonsils
- Size
    - May be quite large on presentation
    - Can fill sinus and **displace** or **erode** walls
    - May **extend** to other air spaces and sinuses
- Morphology
    - Benign-appearing mass

CT Findings

- NECT
    - Homogeneous soft tissue mass
        - Usually appears benign
        - May show peripheral infiltration of surrounding tissues
        - In orbit, may displace globe
        - In either orbit or sinus
            - Displacement or erosion of bony walls

MR Findings

- T1WI
    - Hypo- or isointense to brain
- T2WI
    - Hypo- or isointense to brain

DIFFERENTIAL DIAGNOSIS

Chronic Rhinosinusitis

- Mucosal thickening and sclerosis of bony walls

Wegener Granulomatosis

- Lobular soft tissue lesions on nasal septum and conchae; may have septal perforation

Eosinophilic Angiocentric Fibrosis

- Rare fibrotic disease of idiopathic origin of sinonasal tract and upper airway; M:F = 1:1.3
- CT shows opacification of nasal cavity and sinuses ± bone erosion

Sarcoidosis

- Septum and conchae common sites
- Usually superficial nodular appearance

Squamous Cell Carcinoma

- Poorly defined bone destruction
- M > F; 95% > 40 years

PATHOLOGY

General Features

- Etiology
    - Unknown
        - IgG4-RD has features of autoimmune and allergic disorder

Microscopic Features

- Lymphoplasmacytic tissue infiltration predominantly IgG4(+) plasma cells and CD4(+) T lymphocytes
- Fibrosis with characteristic storiform pattern
- Obliterative phlebitis
- ↑ IgG4 serum levels
- Modest tissue eosinophilia

CLINICAL ISSUES

Presentation

- Most common signs/symptoms
    - Local swelling and pain
- Other signs/symptoms
    - In orbit: Pain, diplopia, proptosis, ↓ extraocular muscle mobility
    - Fever, anorexia, malaise, somnolence in < 30%

Natural History & Prognosis

- Pathogenesis of IgG4-RD poorly understood
- ↑ myofibroblastic/fibroblastic phenotype → ↑ local aggression and recurrence rate

Treatment

- Orbital IPT fairly responsive to steroids
    - 17-52% recurrence rate
- Resection may be necessary

DIAGNOSTIC CHECKLIST

Consider

- May not be possible to differentiate IPT from other lesions radiologically; image-guided biopsy may be indicated

SELECTED REFERENCES

1. Chen BN: IgG4-related disease presenting with destructive sinonasal lesion mimicking malignancy. Eur Arch Otorhinolaryngol. 273(11):4027-4029, 2016
2. Desai SV et al: Sinonasal and ventral skull base inflammatory pseudotumor: a systematic review. Laryngoscope. 125(4):813-21, 2015
3. Yokoi H et al: An inflammatory pseudotumor arising from pterygopalatine fossa with invasion to the maxillary sinus and orbital cavity. Case Rep Otolaryngol. 2015:950823, 2015

Sinonasal Inverted Papilloma

KEY FACTS

IMAGING

- Typical location: Along lateral nasal wall **centered at middle meatus** ± extension into antrum
- CT findings
  - 40% show entrapped bone
  - Focal hyperostosis of adjacent bone may indicate point of tumor attachment
- MR findings
  - T2: Predominantly hyperintense to skeletal muscle
  - T2 & T1 C+ FS: Curvilinear striations or **convoluted, cerebriform pattern** is distinctive
  - If portion of tumor appears invasive or necrosis present → consider synchronous squamous cell carcinoma (SCCa)
  - Multiplanar imaging optimal for tumor mapping & differentiating tumor from obstructed secretions
- PET cannot be reliably used to distinguish benign inverted papilloma & SCCa

TOP DIFFERENTIAL DIAGNOSES

- Solitary sinonasal (antrochoanal) polyp
- Sinonasal squamous cell carcinoma
- Sinonasal polyposis

PATHOLOGY

- Hyperplastic squamous epithelium replaces seromucinous ducts & glands in stroma with endophytic growth pattern
- **10%** either degenerate into or **coexist with SCCa**
  - SCCa may be either synchronous (7%) or metachronous (4%)

CLINICAL ISSUES

- Typically 30-60 years
- M > F = 4-5:1
- Strong potential for local recurrence if incompletely resected

(Left) *Coronal graphic shows an inverted papilloma (IP)* ➡ *originating near the middle meatus & extending into the left maxillary sinus. Blocked secretions are noted in the ethmoid* ➡ *& maxillary* ➡ *sinuses.* **(Right)** *Axial bone CT shows a mass in the right nasal cavity* ➡ *along the lateral wall near the middle meatus. The maxillary sinus is opacified, but it is difficult to differentiate obstructed secretions from papilloma on the CT. MR in such a case would be helpful to delineate the margins of the mass.*

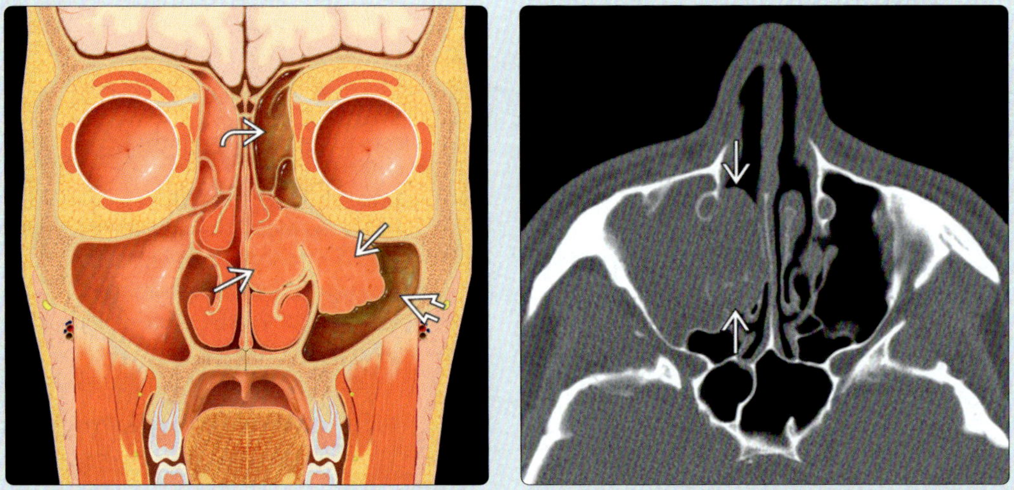

(Left) *Coronal T2WI FS MR shows characteristic features of an IP that involves the right maxillary sinus & nasal cavity. The lesion has a convoluted, cerebriform architecture. Note the inferior displacement of the inferior turbinate* ➡*.* **(Right)** *Axial T1WI C+ FS MR shows classic features of IP. The lesion is centered at the middle meatus with nasal cavity* ➡ *& antral* ➡ *components. This lesion, like the one in the previous image, shows characteristic architecture.*

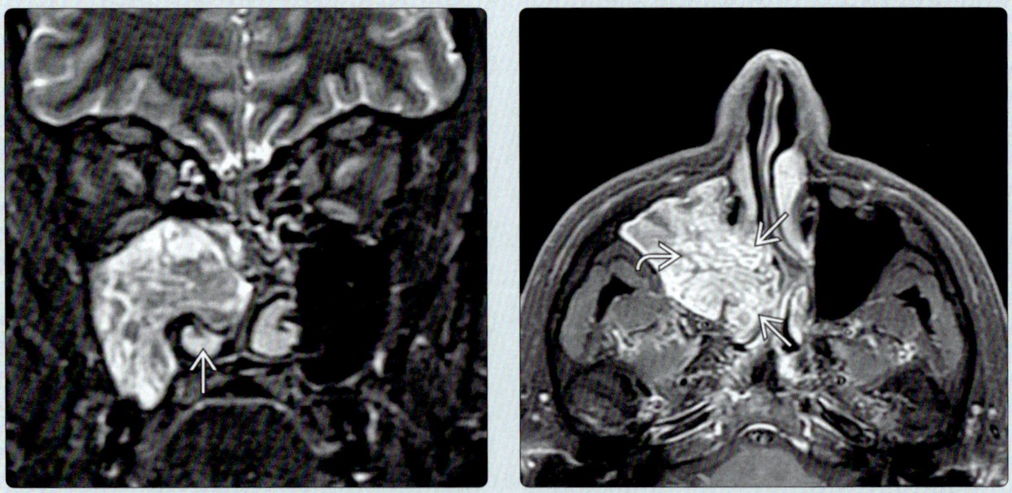

TERMINOLOGY

Abbreviations

- Inverted papilloma (IP)

Synonyms

- Endophytic papilloma, Schneiderian papilloma, squamous cell papilloma, transitional cell papilloma, cylindrical epithelioma

Definitions

- Benign, locally aggressive, epithelial tumor of nasal mucosa with histology showing epithelium proliferating into underlying stroma

IMAGING

General Features

- Best diagnostic clue
  - Mass along lateral nasal wall **centered at middle meatus** ± extension into antrum with local bone remodeling & obstructive sinus disease
- Location
  - Most commonly originates along lateral nasal wall near middle meatus
  - Spreads into adjacent sinuses
    - Maxillary (69%), ethmoid (50-90%), sphenoid (10-20%), frontal (10-15%), orbit & CNS (~ 30%)
  - Uncommonly originates in maxillary antrum, sphenoid, frontal, or ethmoid sinuses
- Size
  - Small IP: < 3 cm centered in middle meatal region of lateral wall of nose
  - Large IP: > 3-cm mass that remodels nasal cavity, invades or obstructs ipsilateral sinuses
- Morphology
  - Architecture described as convoluted, cerebriform pattern

CT Findings

- NECT
  - Soft tissue mass along lateral nasal wall at middle meatus ± extension into maxillary sinus
    - 40% show entrapped bone
    - 10% show tumorous calcification
    - Focal hyperostosis of adjacent bone (plaque or cone-shaped) may indicate point of tumor attachment
  - Unilateral obstruction yields ostiomeatal unit pattern of inflammatory sinus disease
    - Frontal, anterior ethmoid, & maxillary sinuses opacified
  - Small IP may show no bone changes, making identification of tumor difficult
  - Larger IP shows bone remodeling & mass effect in middle meatal region
    - If bony destruction present, consider synchronous squamous cell carcinoma (SCCa)
  - Focal underlying sclerosis suggests origin site
- CECT
  - IP enhances, whereas obstructed sinus secretions do not
    - Variable enhancement pattern from diffuse to heterogeneous
    - **Convoluted, cerebriform appearance** evident with contrast

MR Findings

- T1WI
  - Isointense to slightly hyperintense to soft tissue & muscle
- T2WI
  - Heterogeneous, predominantly hyperintense to skeletal muscle
    - Curvilinear striations or **convoluted, cerebriform pattern** is distinctive
      - □ Alternating bright layers (less cellular edematous stroma) & darker layers (highly cellular metaplastic epithelium)
  - Areas of necrosis & postobstructive secretions brighter on T2
- T1WI C+
  - Enhancement may have convoluted, cerebriform appearance
  - If portion of tumor appears invasive or necrosis present, consider synchronous SCCa

Imaging Recommendations

- Best imaging tool
  - Tumor usually 1st detected on sinus CT performed for evaluation of sinusitis symptoms
  - When mass found on CT, MR completed for preoperative tumor mapping
- Protocol advice
  - Multiplanar MR optimal for tumor mapping & differentiating tumor from obstructed secretions
  - T1 & T2 C+ FS sequences best show internal architecture

Nuclear Medicine Findings

- PET/CT
  - High FDG uptake with SUV max ≥ 3.0 typical in IP with higher SUV in associated SCCa
    - PET cannot be reliably used to distinguish benign IP & SCCa

DIFFERENTIAL DIAGNOSIS

Sinonasal Solitary Polyps

- Antrochoanal polyp: Dumbbell-shaped lesion involving maxillary antrum & ipsilateral nasal cavity
- Peripheral, **not central**, enhancing lesion with mucus or fluid density (CT) or intensity (MR)

Sinonasal SCCa

- In most cases, destroys rather than remodels bones
- Typically originates within maxillary antrum > nasal cavity

Sinonasal Polyposis

- Polypoid lesions in nasal cavity & paranasal sinuses
- Bone remodeling & sinus expansion

Juvenile Angiofibroma

- Adolescent males with nose bleeds
- Mass centered on margin of sphenopalatine foramen in posterior nasal cavity
- Intense enhancement of this highly vascular mass is typical

Esthesioneuroblastoma

- Typically centered in superior nasal cavity near cribriform plate
- Intense enhancement; more likely to invade orbit/anterior skull base

PATHOLOGY

General Features

- Etiology
  - Maturation of sinonasal mucosa into ciliated columnar epithelium & mucous glands gives rise to papillomas
  - Most commonly originates along lateral nasal wall
    - Local extension to maxillary & ethmoid sinuses
    - Rare in frontal & sphenoid sinuses
  - Neither etiology nor factors responsible for malignant transformation are fully elucidated
    - Viral origin has been postulated (e.g., HPV)
    - Epigenetic events contribute to underlying pathogenesis (promoter hypermethylation of *CDKN2B* gene)
    - Outdoor & industrial occupations may be potential risk factors
    - Does not result from allergy, noxious agents, or chronic infection
- Associated abnormalities
  - **10%** either degenerate into or **coexist with SCCa**
    - SCCa may be either synchronous (7%) or metachronous (4%)

Staging, Grading, & Classification

- 3 schneiderian papilloma types arise from nasal mucosa
  - IP (62%) (range = 47-78%)
  - Fungiform papilloma (32%) (range = 6-50%)
    - Occurs on nasal septum in young males & is rarely imaged prior to surgical treatment
  - Oncocytic papilloma (6%) (range = 2-26%)
- Not widely accepted, clinically relevant staging system

Gross Pathologic & Surgical Features

- Endoscopic or surgical observations
  - Bulky, opaque, polypoid mucosal mass with red-gray color characteristic of lobulated tumor surface

Microscopic Features

- Hyperplastic squamous epithelium replacing seromucinous ducts & glands in underlying stroma
  - Endophytic growth pattern
- Respiratory epithelium & calciform cells, abundant cytoplasm, eccentric nucleus
- Stroma lax or fibrous, inflammatory cells in epithelium
- May see hypergranulosis, hyperkeratosis, or parakeratosis
- Surrounding nasal mucosa often shows squamous metaplasia
- Mitoses rare, occur in basal & parabasal layers

CLINICAL ISSUES

Presentation

- Most common signs/symptoms
  - Similar to recurrent sinusitis with nasal obstruction & discharge
- Other signs/symptoms
  - Epistaxis, rhinorrhea, anosmia, headache, pain
- Clinical profile
  - Adult **male** patient with symptoms similar to chronic rhinosinusitis

Demographics

- Age
  - Typically 30-60 years
- Gender
  - M > F = 4-5:1
- Epidemiology
  - 0.4-4.0% of all sinonasal tumors
  - Involves at least 1 paranasal sinus in 82%
  - Typically unifocal
    - Multifocal in 4%
  - Bilateral in up to 13% due to transseptal extension

Natural History & Prognosis

- Benign but locally aggressive tumor
  - Grows centrifugally
  - Strong potential for local recurrence if incompletely resected &/or HPV(+)
    - 20% require repeat surgery
- History of repeated nasal polyposis & polypectomy

Treatment

- Type of surgery depends on location & size of lesion as well as involvement of critical structures
  - Surgical resection using variety of methods
    - Endoscopic resection is effective for most smaller tumors
    - Midfacial degloving & sublabial approaches for larger lesions
    - Medial maxillectomy through lateral rhinotomy + wide en bloc excision in more extensive IP

DIAGNOSTIC CHECKLIST

Consider

- T1 C+ FS MR used to search for convoluted, cerebriform appearance
- MR used to evaluate for extension beyond sinonasal cavities & differentiate tumor from secretions

Image Interpretation Pearls

- Identify invasion of deeper areas (ethmoid sinuses, pterygopalatine fossa, orbit) at imaging as this may alter surgical approach
- Areas of necrosis or frank bony destruction should raise suspicion for coexistent SCCa
- Look for additional masses as 4% are multifocal
- Associated cervical lymphadenopathy rare → consider other malignant lesions

SELECTED REFERENCES

1. Chawla A et al: Imaging features of sinonasal inverted papilloma: a pictorial review. Curr Probl Diagn Radiol. 45(5):347-53, 2016
2. Jalilvand S et al: The prevalence of human papillomavirus infection in Iranian patients with sinonasal inverted papilloma. J Chin Med Assoc. 79(3):137-40, 2016
3. Cannady SB et al: New staging system for sinonasal inverted papilloma in the endoscopic era. Laryngoscope. 117(7):1283-7, 2007

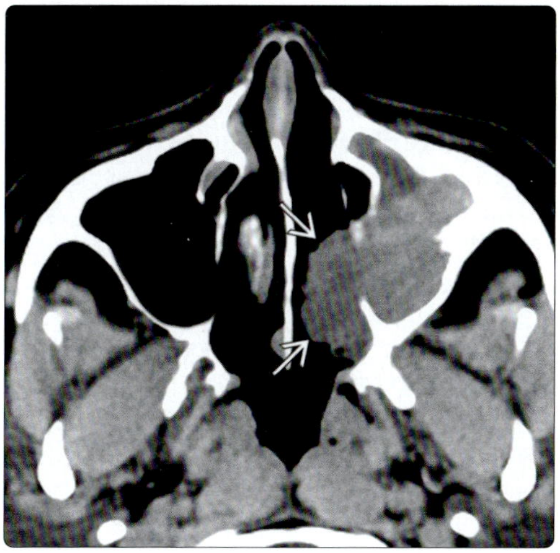
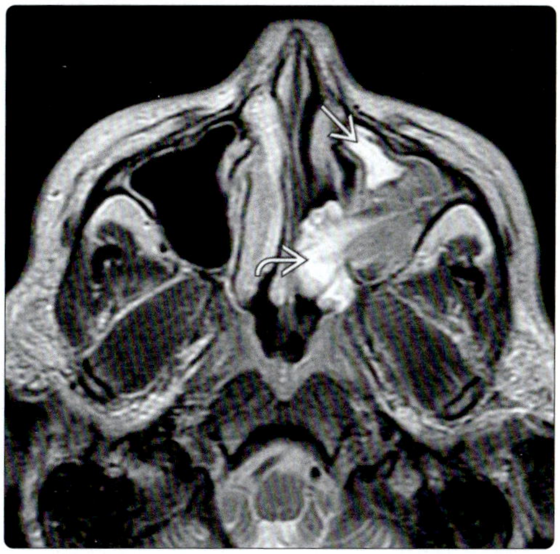

(Left) *Axial NECT shows a slightly lobular soft tissue mass within the left nasal cavity ➡ with extension into the left maxillary sinus. The location is typical of a papilloma. It is difficult to differentiate the mass from obstructed secretions.* **(Right)** *Axial T2WI MR in the same patient shows that the mass occupies most of the maxillary antrum & is hypointense compared to secretions ➡ trapped anteromedially. The nasal component of this papilloma ➡ is hyperintense.*

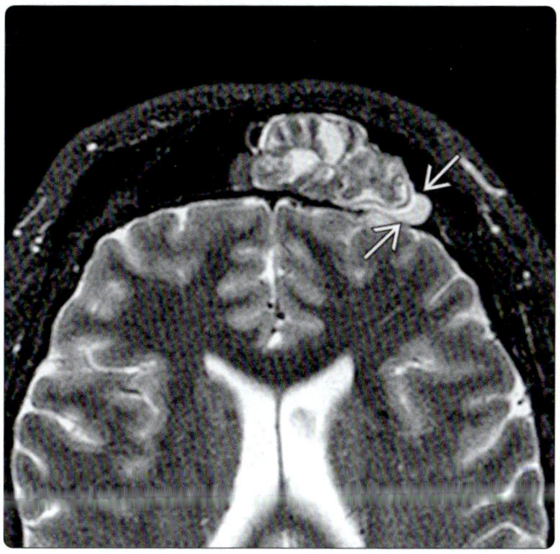
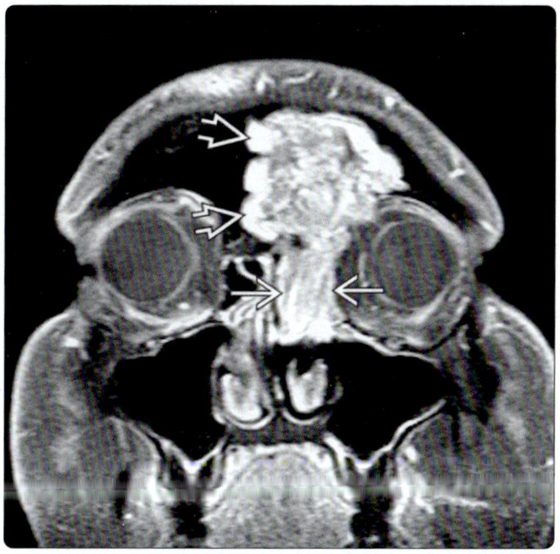

(Left) *Axial STIR MR shows the classic architecture of IP. The lesion shows a convoluted, cerebriform appearance. Trapped secretions laterally ➡ are hyperintense compared to the mass. The frontal sinus is an unusual location for this lesion.* **(Right)** *Coronal T2WI FS MR in the same patient shows that the papilloma involves the ethmoid sinuses ➡ in addition to the frontal sinus. Trapped secretions ➡ along the margin of frontal tumor component are proteinaceous with T1 shortening.*

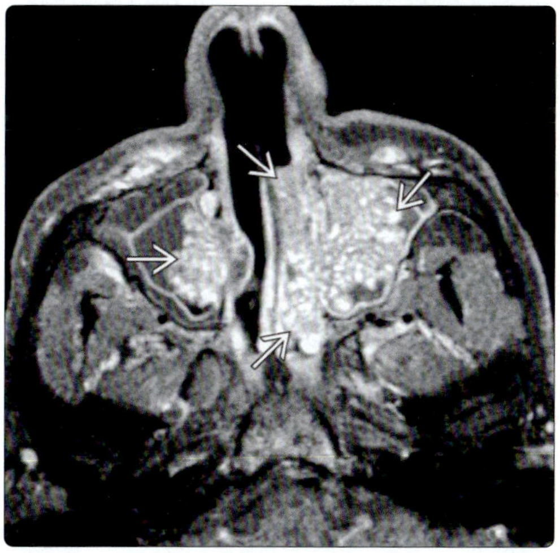
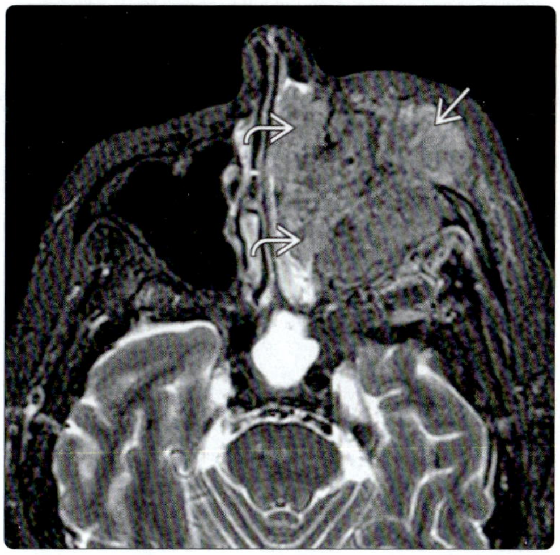

(Left) *Axial T1WI C+ MR shows an unusual case of bilateral IP ➡ due to transseptal extension involving the maxillary sinuses. The larger lesion on the left nearly fills the nasal cavity. Both lesions demonstrate the convoluted appearance typical of these lesions.* **(Right)** *Axial STIR MR demonstrates a squamous cell carcinoma arising within an IP. The carcinoma has destroyed the anterior maxillary wall ➡, & the papilloma extends into the left nasal cavity ➡.*

KEY FACTS

IMAGING

- Mostly in craniofacial bones and mandible
- **Frontal sinus** > ethmoid sinus > maxillary sinus > sphenoid sinus
- Usually 0.5-10 cm, but larger ones occur
- Varies from sessile dome-shaped or bumpy surface to pedunculated (mushroom-shaped)
- Mass with radiopacity of bone
- Cortical osteoma predominantly homogeneously radiopaque; more radiolucent at place of attachment to bone of origin
- Cancellous osteoma radiopaque with radiolucent areas intermixed, like cancellous bone
- Intracranial complications (mucocele, abscess) better evaluated with contrast

TOP DIFFERENTIAL DIAGNOSES

- Sinonasal fibrous dysplasia
- Sinonasal ossifying fibroma
- Sinonasal osteosarcoma
- Osteoblastoma
- Antrolith

CLINICAL ISSUES

- Most common neoplasm of paranasal sinuses
- Prevalence 0.014% to 3% radiographically, but many are silent
- Average age: 37; M:F = 3:2 to 3.1:1
- Continues to grow if not treated
- If small, may have no symptoms
- Frontal sinus osteoma associated with headaches
- No malignant potential, but may impinge on important structures
- Treatment: May follow if small, otherwise resection if occupying > 50% of sinus

DIAGNOSTIC CHECKLIST

- Consider **Gardner syndrome** if multiple

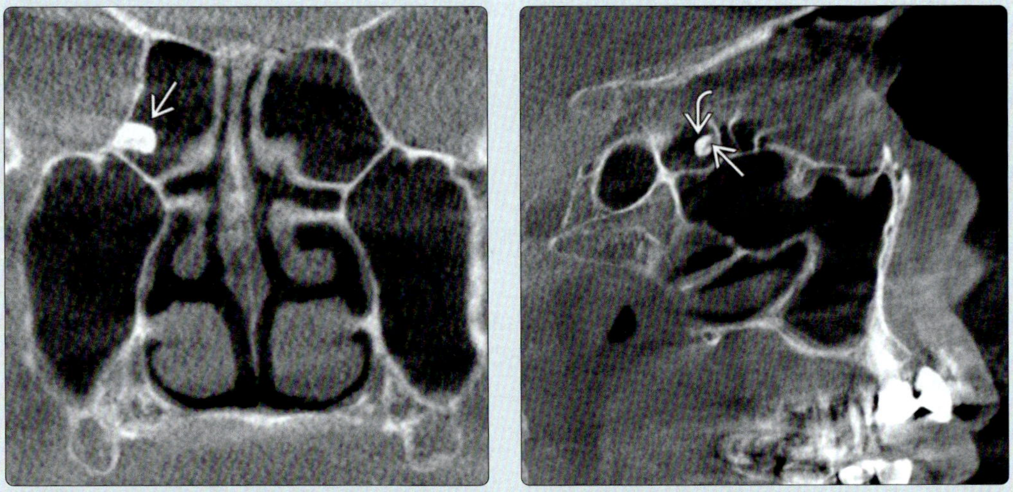

(Left) *Coronal CBCT shows a small cortical osteoma ➔ on the lateral wall of a large right ethmoid air cell. There is a more radiolucent cancellous core with a cortical bone outer layer. The air cell itself has no evidence of associated sinusitis.* **(Right)** *Sagittal CBCT shows a cortical osteoma in an ethmoid air cell. The bulk of the osteoma is cortical bone ➔. The core ➔, where the osteoma arises from the wall, looks like cancellous bone. There is no evidence of sinusitis in the air cell.*

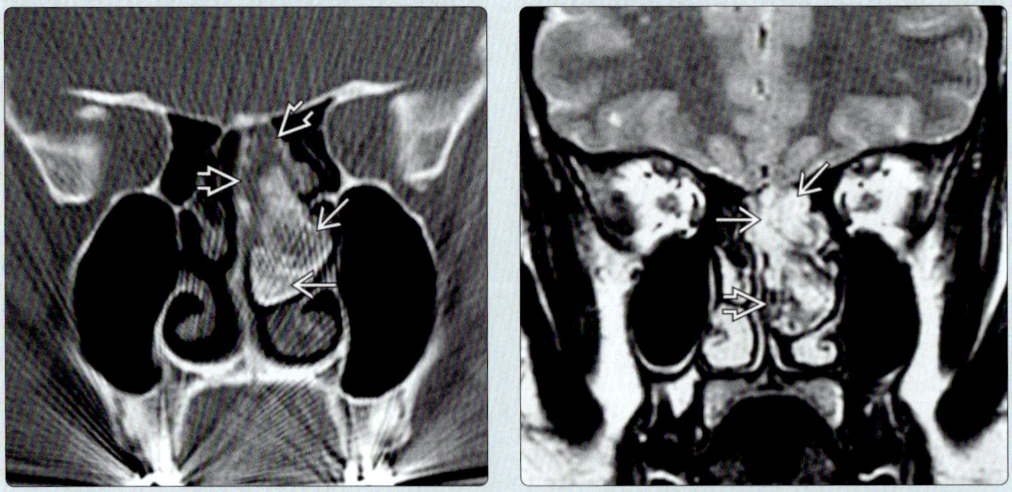

(Left) *Coronal bone CT shows a mixed calcified ➔ and soft tissue density ➔ mass involving the left ethmoid sinus and nasal cavity. Using imaging alone, it would be difficult to distinguish this osteoma from other fibroosseous lesions.* **(Right)** *Coronal T2WI MR in the same patient shows high signal in the more fibrous component of the lesion ➔ superiorly and low signal intensity in the ossified portions ➔ inferiorly.*

TERMINOLOGY

Definitions

- **Benign neoplasm of bone** in paranasal sinus or nasal fossa

Associated Syndromes

- Gardner syndrome (GS) (a.k.a. Fitzgerald-Gardner syndrome)

IMAGING

General Features

- Location
  - Mostly in craniofacial bones and mandible
  - **Frontal sinus** > ethmoid sinus > maxillary sinus > sphenoid sinus
- Size
  - Usually 0.5-10 cm, but larger ones occur
    - Since **growth is continuous**, could become extremely large in size if not treated
- Morphology
  - Varies from sessile dome-shaped or bumpy surface to pedunculated (mushroom-shaped)

Radiographic Findings

- Radiography
  - Mass with radiopacity of bone in paranasal sinus or nasal fossa
  - Surface smooth and possibly lobulated
  - Sessile or pedunculated
  - May have associated **sinusitis** or **mucocele**

CT Findings

- Bone CT
  - **Cancellous osteoma** radiopaque with radiolucent areas intermixed, like cancellous bone
  - **Cortical osteoma** predominantly homogeneously radiopaque, more radiolucent at place of attachment to bone of origin

MR Findings

- T1WI: ↓ signal all sequences; can be confused with air
- T2WI: Hypointense or follows marrow signal
- T1WI C+: No appreciable enhancement (except fibrous area)

Imaging Recommendations

- Best imaging tool
  - Thin-slice bone **CT without contrast or CBCT**
- Protocol advice
  - When larger osteoma involves dural surface, MR may be warranted before surgery
    - Enhanced MR best for assessing adjacent orbital & intracranial structures

DIFFERENTIAL DIAGNOSIS

Sinonasal Fibrous Dysplasia

- Expansile lesion of bone typically with ground-glass matrix

Sinonasal Ossifying Fibroma

- Thick, mature bony wall → immature woven bone centrally
- Most of center of lesion is more radiolucent on CT

Sinonasal Osteosarcoma

- Bone-forming, malignant neoplasm of bone
- Periosteal elevation; permeative margins present
- Soft tissue component often present

Osteoblastoma

- Benign, but can have more aggressive imaging features (surrounding bone edema & periosteal reaction)

Antrolith

- Deposition of $CaCO_3$, $Ca_3(PO_4)_2$, $Mg_3(PO_4)_2$, or $MgCO_3$ salts on nidus such as inspissated mucus
- Benign but can cause inflammatory change

PATHOLOGY

General Features

- Genetics
  - Usually **not familial**
  - If multiple osteomas, possible GS
- Associated abnormalities
  - GS: **Multiple osteomas**, intestinal polyps, soft tissue neoplasms, supernumerary teeth, odontomas

Staging, Grading, & Classification

- Cortical (ivory) osteoma
- Cancellous or mature osteoma
- Mixed cortical/cancellous osteoma

CLINICAL ISSUES

Presentation

- Most common signs/symptoms
  - If small, may have no symptoms
  - Frontal sinus osteoma associated with headaches: Constant or intermittent, minimal or severe
- Other signs/symptoms
  - Diplopia &/or proptosis, facial deformity, sinusitis symptoms, dizziness, acute or chronic rhinosinusitis, nasal discharge/obstruction, dacryocystitis, epistaxis

Demographics

- Age
  - 12-70 years; median = 37
- Gender
  - M:F = 3:2 to 3.1:1

Treatment

- Resection if occupies > 50% of sinus

DIAGNOSTIC CHECKLIST

Consider

- **Gardner syndrome** if multiple

Reporting Tips

- Relative size of osteoma to sinus (i.e., > or < 50%)

SELECTED REFERENCES

1. Lee JH et al: Underestimation of rhinogenic causes in patients presenting to the emergency department with acute headache. Acta Neurol Taiwan. 24(2):37-42, 2015
2. Almasi M et al: Sinolith in the ethmoid sinus: report of two cases and review of the literature. Eur Arch Otorhinolaryngol. 267(10):1649-52, 2010

(Left) *Coronal bone CT shows a very large, mixed density osteoma involving the right maxillary sinus, ethmoid sinuses, and nasal cavity. There is thinning of the orbital floor. The nasal turbinates on the right are not visible. The lesion outline follows but does not expand the anatomical boundaries.* **(Right)** *Axial bone CT shows a dense osteoma of the left ethmoid labyrinth. The lesion extended into the extraconal space of the left orbit and caused proptosis in this patient.*

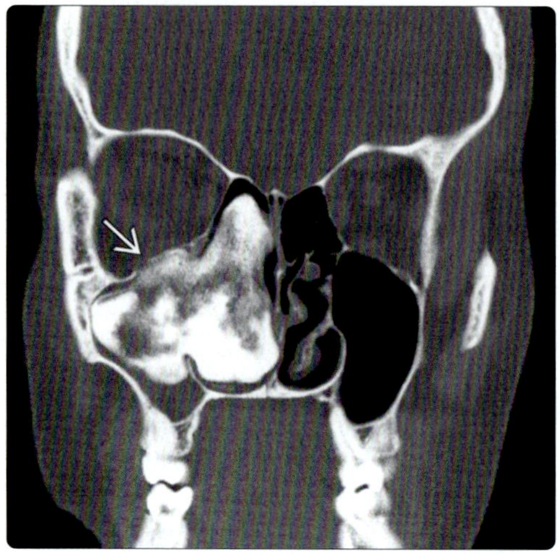

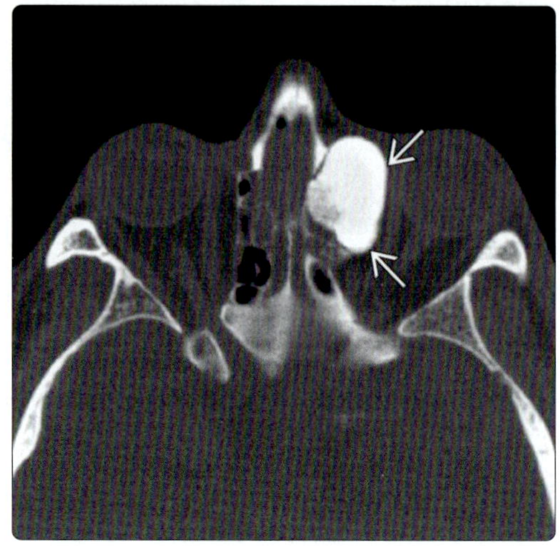

(Left) *Coronal CT reconstruction shows a large, lobulated ivory osteoma extending from the left ethmoid labyrinth into the medial aspect of the orbit and to the superior aspect of the left maxillary sinus. Proptosis was present clinically.* **(Right)** *Sagittal CT reconstruction shows a large, lobulated ivory osteoma involving the posterior aspect of the right maxillary sinus. The mass extended superiorly into the posterior aspect of the orbit and caused proptosis in this patient.*

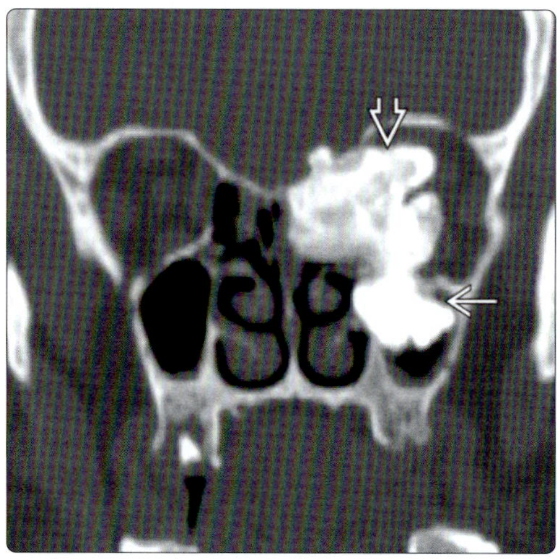

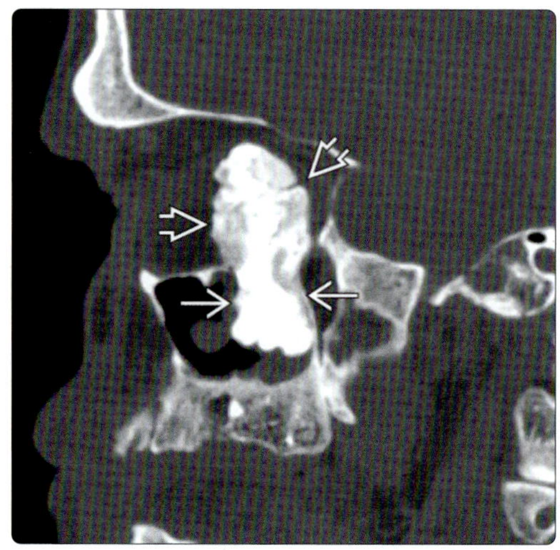

(Left) *Axial NECT of a patient with Gardner syndrome shows a small, pedunculated cortical osteoma in the right maxillary sinus. The sinus shows no evidence of sinusitis. There is a large osteoma associated with each mandibular ramus.* **(Right)** *Sagittal NECT in the same patient shows multiple osteomas in the maxilla and mandible. Note unerupted teeth typically seen in Gardner syndrome.*

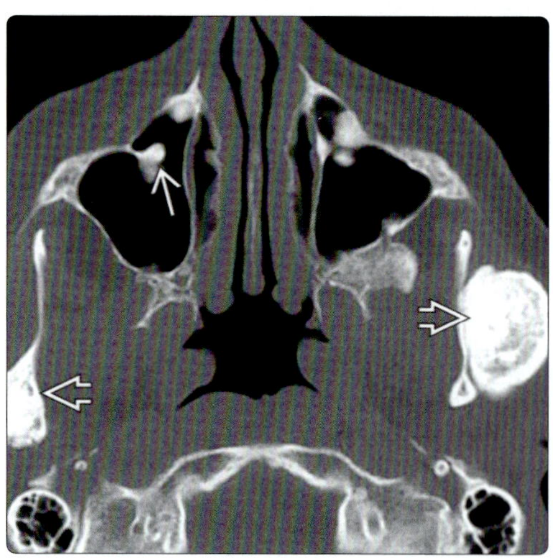

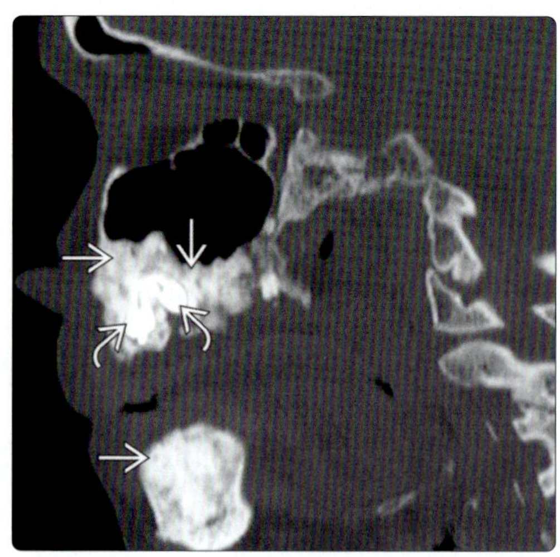

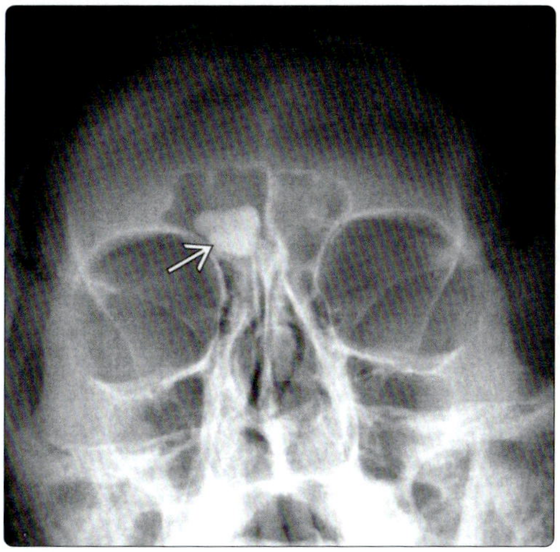

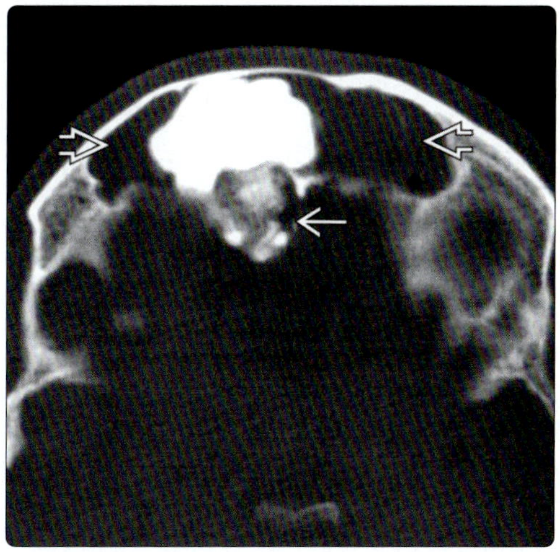

(Left) *Anteroposterior radiograph shows the classic appearance of an ivory osteoma in the inferomedial aspect of the right frontal sinus ➡. The sinus is otherwise well aerated.* **(Right)** *Axial bone CT demonstrates a dense ivory osteoma of the right frontal sinus crossing the midline to the left and extending intracranially ➡. Trapped secretions are seen in both frontal sinuses ➡. Osteomas are seen more frequently in the frontal sinus than any other paranasal sinus.*

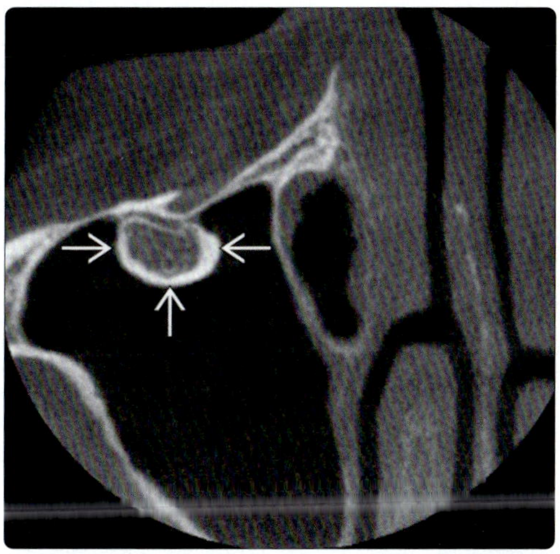

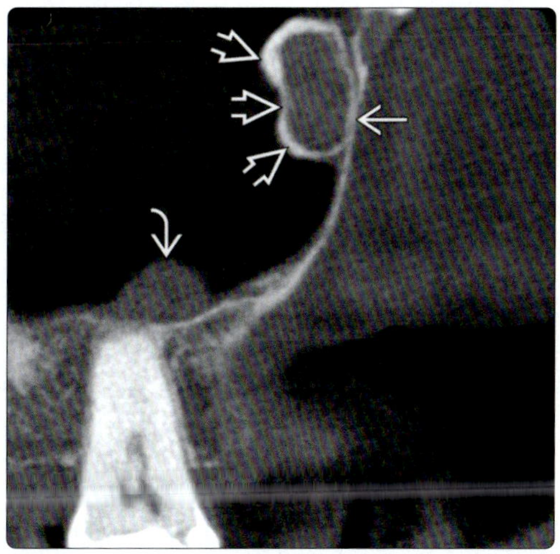

(Left) *Axial CBCT shows a cancellous osteoma ➡ arising from the anterior wall of the right maxillary sinus. The lesion has a thick, smooth cortical boundary with a core comprised of cancellous bone.* **(Right)** *Sagittal CBCT in the same patient shows the sessile nature of the osteoma attachment to the anterior maxillary sinus wall ➡. Note the irregular thickness and contour of the cortical margin ➡. A mucous retention pseudocyst arises from the sinus floor ➡. The pseudocyst lacks a cortex and has a homogeneous internal density.*

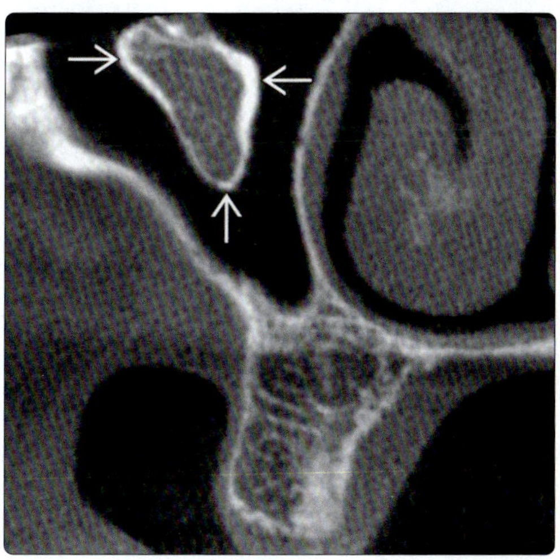

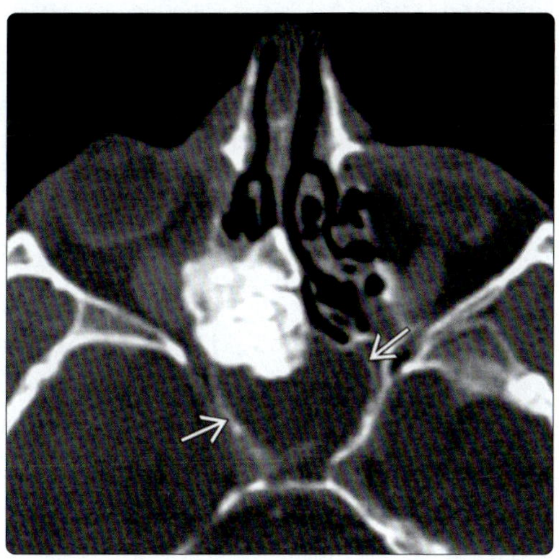

(Left) *Coronal CBCT reformat in the same patient shows the irregular shape of the cancellous osteoma ➡. There is no evidence of sinusitis because the osteoma is located inferior to the sinus ostium and does not interfere with sinus drainage.* **(Right)** *Axial bone CT reveals a large ivory osteoma originating from the right sphenoethmoid recess. The sphenoid sinus ostium is occluded with secondary development of a right sphenoid mucocele ➡.*

Sinonasal Squamous Cell Carcinoma

KEY FACTS

TERMINOLOGY

- Definition: Malignant epithelial neoplasm originating in respiratory mucosa of nasal fossae and paranasal sinuses

IMAGING

- Location: Maxillary and ethmoid sinuses and nasal fossa: > 93%; frontal: < 7%; sphenoid rare
- Sinus neoplasms often large when discovered
- Mass displacing or eroding osseous structures
- CECT: Focal or moderate enhancement
- Inversion recovery FSE: Hypointense with trapped sinus secretions
  - Hyperintense to muscle; isointense with cortex
- T2WI MR distinguishes from edematous mucosa

TOP DIFFERENTIAL DIAGNOSES

- Non-Hodgkin lymphoma
- Inverted papilloma

PATHOLOGY

- 80-90% of all nasal neoplasms
- Evidence that tobacco use is risk factor
- Inverted papilloma has 5% conversion rate to sinonasal squamous cell carcinoma

CLINICAL ISSUES

- Often insidious onset
- Nasal obstruction, facial pain, rhinorrhea, epistaxis
- Predominantly males
- Sinonasal squamous cell carcinoma is rare
- Overall prognosis poor: 5-year survival rate is 30-50%
  - Prognosis in nasal cavity better than in sinuses due to earlier diagnosis
- Moderate tendency to invade nerves (22%)
- Surgery + radiotherapy in advanced stages

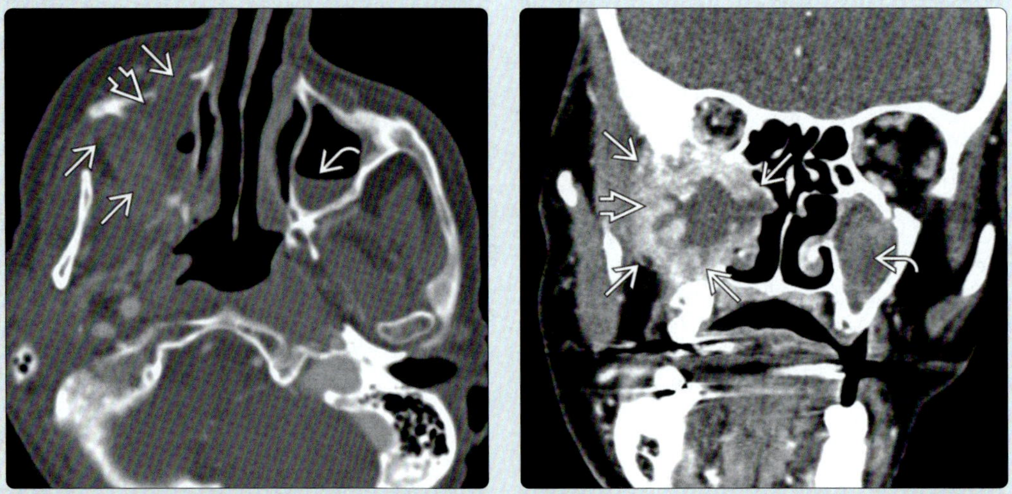

(Left) *Axial CECT (bone window) shows almost complete radiopacification ➡ of the right maxillary sinus by squamous cell carcinoma (SCCa). There is destruction of the walls of the sinus ➡ and an air-fluid interface in the left sinus ➡.* **(Right)** *Coronal CECT shows a SCCa in the right maxillary sinus exhibiting peripheral enhancement ➡. The lesion has displaced and destroyed most of the borders ➡ of the sinus. The radiopacity in the left sinus represents fluid ➡ in the most dependent part of the sinus.*

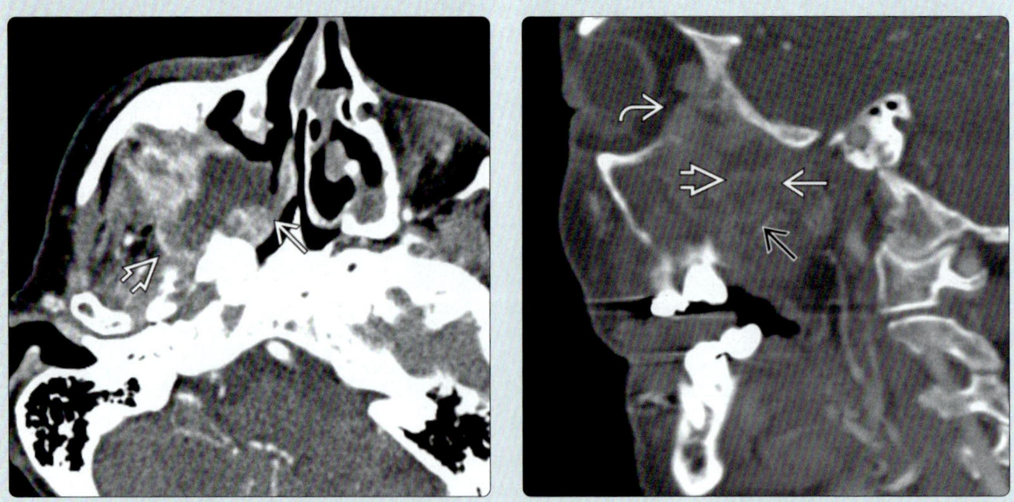

(Left) *Axial CECT shows displacement ➡ and destruction ➡ of the walls of the right maxillary sinus by a SCCa.* **(Right)** *Sagittal CECT (bone window) of the right maxillary sinus shows complete radiopacification ➡ with displacement ⇨ and destruction ➡ of the walls of the sinus by SCCa with invasion of the orbit ➡.*

TERMINOLOGY

Abbreviations

- Sinonasal squamous cell carcinoma (SNSCCa)

Definitions

- Malignant epithelial neoplasm originating in respiratory mucosa of nasal fossae and paranasal sinuses
- Basaloid squamous cell carcinoma is more aggressive subset

IMAGING

General Features

- Location
  - Nasal fossa: 50%; paranasal sinuses: 50% (predominantly maxillary)
    - Maxillary and ethmoid sinuses and nasal fossa: > 93%; frontal: < 7%; sphenoid rare
- Size
  - Varies: Sinus neoplasms often large when discovered
- Morphology
  - Mass displacing or eroding neighboring osseous structures

CT Findings

- CECT
  - Mass in nasal fossa or sinus
  - Focal or moderate enhancement
  - Bone erosion
- CBCT and bone CT
  - Mass in nasal fossa or sinus
  - Bone erosion

MR Findings

- Inversion recovery FSE
  - Hypointense with trapped sinus secretions
  - Hyperintense to muscle
  - Isointense with cortex

Imaging Recommendations

- Best imaging tool
  - CT and MR
- Protocol advice
  - Thin-slice CT to delineate bony erosion
  - T2WI to distinguish tumor from edematous mucosa and retained secretions
  - Fat-saturated MR if orbit involved to distinguish tumor from orbital fat

DIFFERENTIAL DIAGNOSIS

Non-Hodgkin Lymphoma

- Usually in nasal cavity with nasal septal destruction
- CT: Homogeneous and may be more hyperdense than other soft tissue
- MR: Homogeneous signal and enhancement; decreased T2 signal

Inverted Papilloma

- CT: Polypoid mass near middle meatus with extension into sinus

Invasive Fungal Sinusitis

- Maxillary or ethmoid sinus→ nasal cavity

Esthesioneuroblastoma

- Dumbbell-shaped mass centered at cribriform plate

PATHOLOGY

General Features

- Etiology
  - Occupational exposure to leather dust, wood dust, nickel, arsenic, formaldehyde have been suggested
  - Smoking increases risk 2-3x
  - Inverted papilloma has 5% conversion rate to SNSCCa (2-29% SNSCCa arise from inverted papilloma)

Prevalence

- 80-90% of all nasal neoplasms

CLINICAL ISSUES

Presentation

- Most common signs/symptoms
  - Often insidious onset
  - Nasal obstruction, facial pain, rhinorrhea, epistaxis

Demographics

- Age
  - Range: 9-86 years; mean: 50-60 years, most common 6th and 7th decades
- Gender
  - 2:1 M:F
- Epidemiology
  - Rare but more common than other sinonasal malignancies

Natural History & Prognosis

- Overall prognosis poor; 5-year survival rate reported as 30-77%
  - Nasal fossa > maxillary sinus > ethmoid sinus
- Regional lymph node involvement low at presentation (~ 10-20%)
- ~ 10% had distant mets at follow-up, almost all associated with locoregional recurrence
- Local recurrence is main cause of death
- Moderate tendency to invade nerves (22%)
- 5-year survival: ~ 18-69% (reports vary), inversely with increasing T#

Treatment

- Surgery, followed by radiotherapy in advanced stages
- Definitive radiotherapy itself may be as good as surgery and postoperative radiotherapy

DIAGNOSTIC CHECKLIST

Consider

- Lymphoma

SELECTED REFERENCES

1. Lewis JS Jr: Sinonasal squamous cell carcinoma: a review with emphasis on emerging histologic subtypes and the role of human papillomavirus. Head Neck Pathol. 10(1):60-7, 2016

Sinonasal Adenoid Cystic Carcinoma

KEY FACTS

TERMINOLOGY

- Malignant salivary type of sinonasal adenocarcinoma

IMAGING

- Location: **Maxillary sinus** > nasal cavity
- Low grade: Solidly enhancing, well-defined soft tissue mass
- High grade: Poorly defined, heterogeneous + bone destruction ± perineural tumor spread (PNTS)
- Multiplanar, **gadolinium-enhanced MR with fat suppression** recommended
  - Improves detection of PNTS

TOP DIFFERENTIAL DIAGNOSES

- Sinonasal squamous cell carcinoma
- Sinonasal adenocarcinoma (intestinal type)
- Esthesioneuroblastoma
- Sinonasal undifferentiated carcinoma

PATHOLOGY

- 3 histologic types
  - Cribriform (52%): Best survival
  - Tubular (20%)
  - Solid (29%): Worst outcome; ↑ tendency for PNTS
- Most patients present with **T4 disease (65%)**

CLINICAL ISSUES

- Sinonasal adenoid cystic carcinoma (ACCa) accounts for 10-25% of H&N ACCa
- Symptoms mimic sinusitis
  - **Facial pain ± numbness** (V2) → PNTS
- More common in Caucasians
- Overall 5-year survival: 50-86%
  - **Late recurrences**: > 15 years post initial therapy

DIAGNOSTIC CHECKLIST

- Be sure to **assess for skull base invasion and PNTS**

(Left) *Axial NECT shows a large, somewhat heterogeneous soft tissue mass centered in the sphenoid sinuses. There is extension laterally into the right infratemporal fossa ➡ and posteriorly into the clivus ↪. Typical of sinonasal adenoid cystic carcinoma (ACCa), this patient presented at an advanced T stage.* **(Right)** *Axial T1WI C+ MR in the same patient demonstrates diffuse, but heterogeneous enhancement throughout the mass. There is extensive clival invasion ➡. The lesion extends into nasal cavity ↪.*

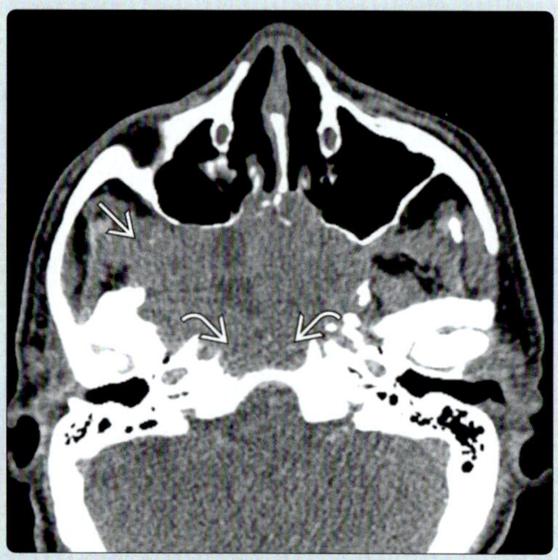

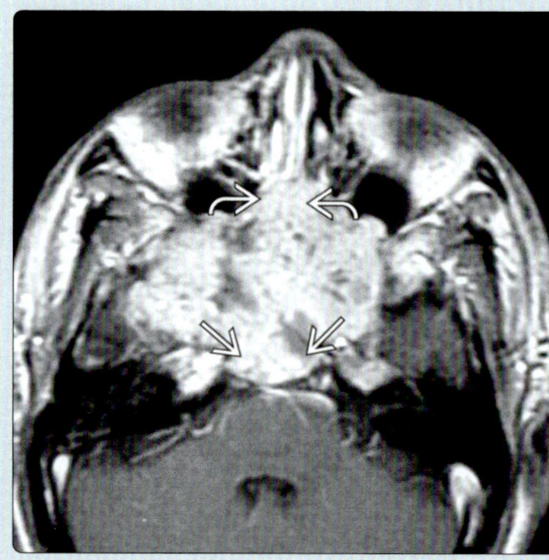

(Left) *Coronal bone CT shows opacification of the right maxillary sinus by a large, expansile ACCa. The medial maxillary wall is eroded and the mass extends into the nasal cavity. Note leftward deviation of the nasal septum ↪.* **(Right)** *Axial T2WI MR in the same patient shows slightly heterogeneous high signal throughout the mass. Slight extension into the premaxillary soft tissues is noted ➡. The relatively well-defined appearance of the ACCa may suggest a lower grade histology.*

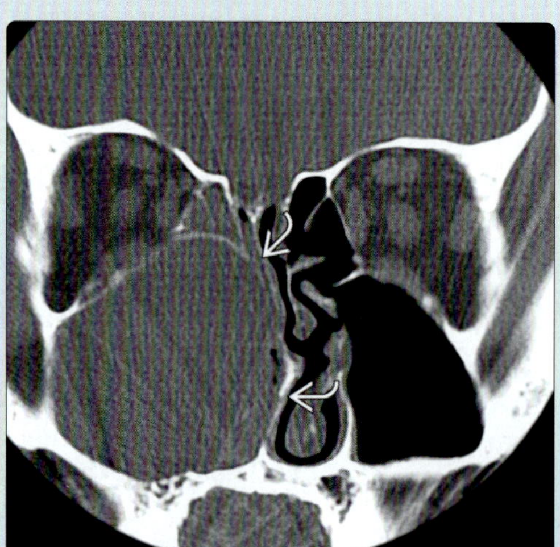

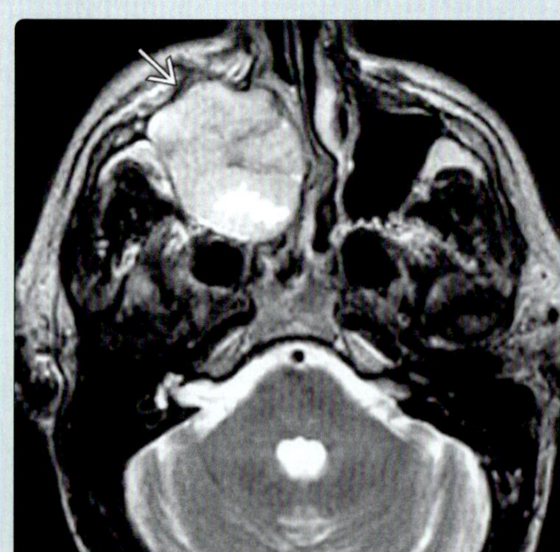

TERMINOLOGY

Abbreviations

- Adenoid cystic carcinoma (ACCa)

Definitions

- Malignant salivary type of sinonasal adenocarcinoma

IMAGING

General Features

- Best diagnostic clue
  - **Ill-defined maxillary sinus or nasal cavity mass** with perineural tumor spread (PNTS)
- Location
  - **47% maxillary, 30% nasal cavity**, 11% ethmoid, 5% sphenoid, 2% frontal
- Size
  - Tumors frequently **large at presentation** (> 4 cm)
- Morphology
  - Well circumscribed (low grade) to poorly defined (higher grade)

Imaging Recommendations

- Best imaging tool
  - Multiplanar, gadolinium-enhanced MR
- Protocol advice
  - **Fat suppression** on postcontrast sequences improves detection of PNTS

CT Findings

- CECT
  - **Low grade: Solidly enhancing**, well-defined soft tissue mass
  - Larger, **higher grade** lesions more poorly defined and **heterogeneously enhancing**
- Bone CT
  - Low-grade lesions may remodel bone
  - Higher grade: Infiltration and marked bone destruction

MR Findings

- T1WI
  - **Low to intermediate signal** (similar to muscle)
- T2WI
  - **Heterogeneous, intermediate signal** (> muscle); higher grade lesions → **lower T2 signal**
- T1WI C+ FS
  - Diffuse enhancement with more heterogeneity in higher grade, larger lesions
  - Enhancement and enlargement of adjacent nerves (especially V2) is indicative of PNTS

DIFFERENTIAL DIAGNOSIS

Sinonasal Squamous Cell Carcinoma

- Most common in maxillary sinus
- Aggressive bone destruction
- Imaging features can be identical to ACCa

Sinonasal Adenocarcinoma (Intestinal Type)

- Propensity for ethmoid site of origin
- Less likely to show PNTS

Esthesioneuroblastoma

- Originates in superior nasal cavity

Sinonasal Undifferentiated Carcinoma

- Aggressive with more rapid growth than ACCa

Hard Palate Minor Salivary Gland Malignancy

- Lesion extending into rather than from maxillary sinus

PATHOLOGY

General Features

- Associated abnormalities
  - Propensity for PNTS and bone invasion

Staging, Grading, & Classification

- 3 histologic types
  - Cribriform (52%): Best survival
  - Tubular-trabecular (20%)
  - Solid (29%): Worst outcome, higher rate of PNTS
- Staged using TNM classification
  - Most patients present with T4 disease (65%)

CLINICAL ISSUES

Presentation

- Most common signs/symptoms
  - **Nasal obstruction, facial pain, epistaxis**
- Other signs/symptoms
  - Nasal drainage, V2 numbness, oral and facial swelling, anopsia, anosmia, epiphora, oral ulcers

Demographics

- Age
  - Early teens to 80s (mean: 51 years)
- Ethnicity
  - More common in Caucasians
- Epidemiology
  - Sinonasal ACCa accounts for 10-25% of H&N ACCa, 1% of H&N malignancies, **1.3-11.5% of sinonasal malignancies**

Natural History & Prognosis

- Patients tend to present with advanced-stage disease due to delay in diagnosis as symptoms mimic sinusitis
- Overall 5-year survival: 50-86%
  - Nasal cavity primaries have best survival and sphenoid has worst
  - Recurrence rate unrelated to age or histopathological type
  - Recurrence rate greater if bony involvement
- **Late recurrences** not uncommon even > 15 years post initial therapy
- **Sinonasal ACCa ↓ distant mets than other ACCa**
  - Local recurrence 52%, distant mets 40%, regional lymph nodes 19%

Treatment

- **Surgical resection** + postoperative radiation therapy

SELECTED REFERENCES

1. Tabrizi R et al: Association between clinical features, treatment, and recurrence rate of adenoid cystic carcinoma of the palate: a 10-year retrospective study. Br J Oral Maxillofac Surg. 54(6):648-51, 2016

Nasopharyngeal Carcinoma

KEY FACTS

TERMINOLOGY

- Nasopharyngeal carcinoma (NPC)
- Mucosal tumor of lateral pharyngeal recess (fossa of Rosenmüller), strongly associated with EBV infection

IMAGING

- MR best demonstrates parapharyngeal fat, skull base infiltration, and intracranial tumor
- Nodal disease in 90% at presentation: Retropharyngeal, levels II and V most common
- Metastatic nodes often large ± necrosis
- NPC is markedly FDG avid

TOP DIFFERENTIAL DIAGNOSES

- Adenoidal benign lymphoid hyperplasia
- Nasopharyngeal non-Hodgkin lymphoma
- Nasopharyngeal minor salivary gland malignancy
- Pituitary macroadenoma

PATHOLOGY

- **25%: Keratinizing NPC** (previously type I)
- **75%: Nonkeratinizing NPC** (NK NPC)
  - Strongly associated with EBV
  - **15% differentiated** (previously type II)
  - **60% undifferentiated** (previously type III)
- Rare: Basaloid squamous cell carcinoma

CLINICAL ISSUES

- Peak incidence: 40-60 years
- Pediatric NPC rare; most often undifferentiated NK
- Clinical presentations
  - Bloody nasal discharge or epistaxis
  - 50-70% present with mass from metastatic nodes
  - Serous otitis from eustachian tube obstruction
- NK NPC has 5-year survival ~ 75%
- Keratinizing NPC has 5-year survival 20-40%

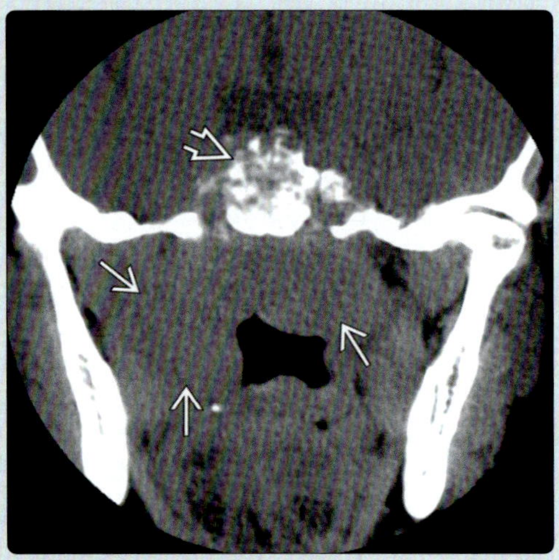
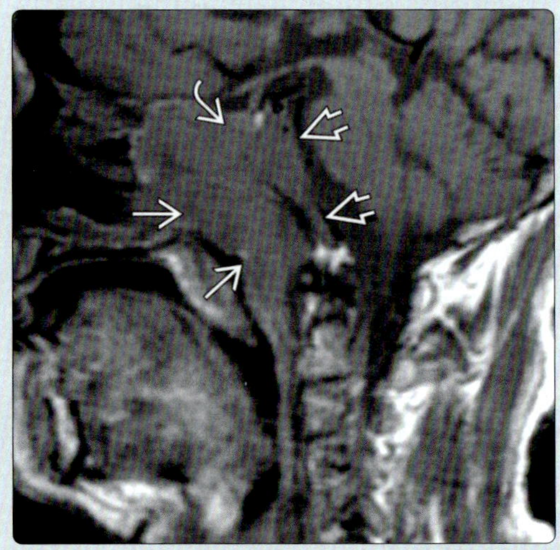

(Left) *Coronal NECT of paranasal sinuses, performed in a 62-year-old Asian man for evaluation of nasal stuffiness and epistaxis, demonstrates an asymmetric bulky mass of nasopharynx ➔ with heterogeneous, mottled texture of clivus ➔.* **(Right)** *Sagittal T1WI MR in the same patient reveals a large soft tissue mass in the nasopharynx ➔ extending superiorly to the sphenoid bone and sella ➔. There is replacement of normally hyperintense fatty marrow of the clivus ➔ without clival expansion.*

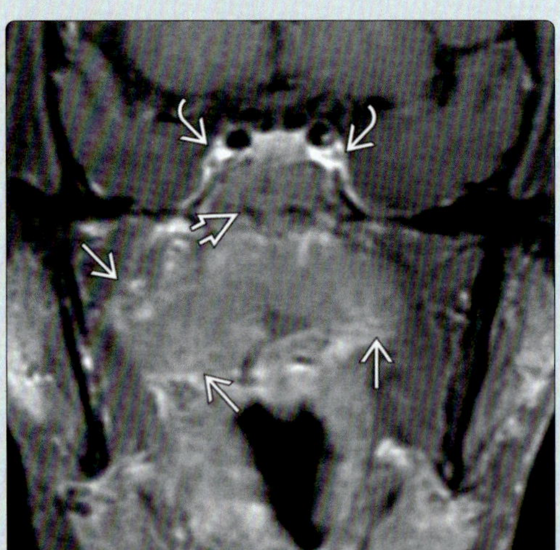
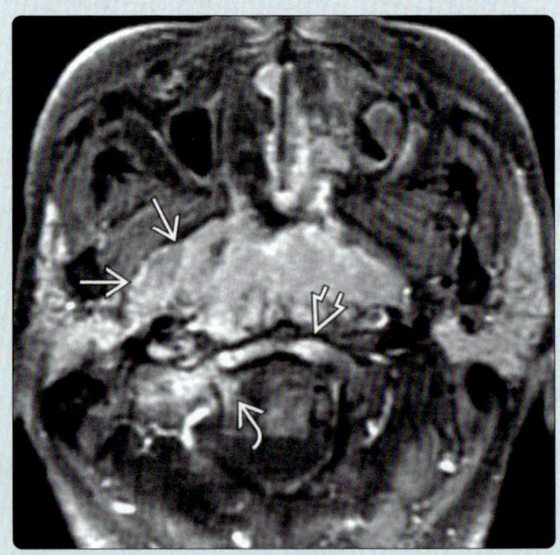

(Left) *Coronal T1WI C+ FS MR reveals moderate enhancement of a bulky mass ➔ filling the nasopharynx with an indistinct right lateral margin. Enhancing tumor extends cranially to infiltrate the sphenoid bone ➔. There is no abnormality of cavernous sinuses ➔.* **(Right)** *Axial T1WI C+ FS MR shows infiltration of parapharyngeal fat ➔. There is abnormal enhancement of basisphenoid ➔ consistent with marrow infiltration. More significantly, however, there is abnormal right hypoglossal nerve enhancement ➔. This is a T4 tumor.*

TERMINOLOGY

Abbreviations

- Nasopharyngeal carcinoma (NPC)

Definitions

- Primary mucosal malignancy arising in nasopharynx, most strongly associated with EBV infection

IMAGING

General Features

- Best diagnostic clue
  - Lateral pharyngeal recess mass with deep extension and cervical adenopathy
- Location
  - Arises in lateral pharyngeal recess, a.k.a. fossa of Rosenmüller
- Morphology
  - Poorly marginated mucosal mass with deep extension and invasion
  - Nodal disease in 90% at presentation

CT Findings

- CECT
  - Mildly enhancing **off-midline nasopharyngeal mass**
  - Metastatic nodes often large, ± necrosis
  - Retropharyngeal nodes often subtle on imaging, as they appear isodense to muscle
- Bone CT
  - May show destruction of clival cortex or pterygoid plates

MR Findings

- T1WI
  - **Asymmetric** mass, hypo- to isointense to muscle
  - Sensitive for infiltration of parapharyngeal fat and marrow involvement
- T2WI
  - Moderate hyperintensity of NPC compared with muscle
- T1WI C+ FS
  - Best illustrates infiltration of deep face, intracranial, and cavernous sinus disease
    - Coronal images aid in this evaluation
  - Mild homogeneous tumor enhancement

Nuclear Medicine Findings

- PET/CT
  - Markedly **FDG-avid** tumor, nodes, and metastases
  - If small primary, can miss with thick slices due to brain FDG uptake

Imaging Recommendations

- Best imaging tool
  - MR is recommended by American Joint Committee on Cancer (AJCC) for staging
    - Most sensitive for skull base and intracranial tumor spread
    - More sensitive than clinical exam/US/CT for detection of retropharyngeal nodes
    - CECT is alternative choice
  - PET/CT often obtained if N2/3 disease at staging or recurrent tumor
- Protocol advice
  - T1 MR best shows infiltration of skull base with loss of fat signal
  - Postcontrast axial and coronal images best demonstrate intracranial spread

DIFFERENTIAL DIAGNOSIS

Adenoidal Benign Lymphoid Hyperplasia

- Large adenoids seen in children, teens, and HIV patients
- Symmetric enlargement without infiltration of adjacent tissues

Nasopharyngeal Non-Hodgkin Lymphoma

- Midline symmetric mass, ± deep infiltration to prevertebral muscles
- In clivus, tends to expand rather than infiltrate

Nasopharyngeal Minor Salivary Gland Malignancy

- Uncommon primary tumor, nodal metastases uncommon
- May be small primary with extensive infiltration

Pituitary Macroadenoma

- Large sella mass extending through sphenoid to nasopharynx
- Expansion of sella is key imaging finding

Pharyngeal Mucosal Space Sarcoma

- Rare; more common differential in children
- Submucosal, aggressive mass

PATHOLOGY

General Features

- Etiology
  - **Nonkeratinizing (NK)** strongly associated with **prior EBV infection**
    - EBV DNA found in tumor cells and in premalignant (dysplastic, in situ) lesions
  - Other proposed factors
    - Carcinogens (nitrosamines) in food eaten as child
    - Genetic predisposition
      - Increased risk in 1st-degree relatives
      - HLA-A2 + HLA-Bsin2 → increased risk for NPC
    - Prior radiation (XRT)
    - Tobacco and alcohol most associated with basaloid squamous cell carcinoma (BSCCa) and keratinizing NPC

Staging, Grading, & Classification

- **AJCC Classification, 2010**
  - TNM staging; NPC has **unique nodal staging**

Gross Pathologic & Surgical Features

- Pathological types classified by World Health Organization
- **Keratinizing NPC** (previously type I)
  - Poorly, moderately, or well differentiated
- **NK NPC**
  - PCR for EBV positive 75-100%
    - Differentiated (previously type II)
    - Undifferentiated (previously type III)
- **BSCCa**
  - Typically EBV and HPV negative

AJCC Nasopharynx Staging (2010)

Tumor or Metastatic Stage (T or M)	Nodal Stage (N)
T1: Confined to nasopharynx or extension to oropharynx or nasal cavity	**N1**: ≥ 1 unilateral metastasis ≤ 6 cm &/or unilateral/bilateral retropharyngeal nodes ≤ 6 cm
T2: Extension to parapharyngeal fat	**N2**: Bilateral nodal metastases ≤ 6 cm
T3: Clivus or paranasal sinus invasion	**N3a**: Nodal metastases > 6 cm
T4: Intracranial spread, cranial nerve, orbit, hypopharynx, masticator space	**N3b**: Nodal metastasis to supraclavicular fossa
M0: No distant metastasis	
M1: Distant metastasis	

Note: This nodal staging is unique to nasopharyngeal carcinoma. Adapted from 7th edition AJCC Staging Forms.

CLINICAL ISSUES

Presentation

- Most common signs/symptoms
  - Conductive hearing loss secondary to middle ear obstruction
    - Obstruction or infiltration of eustachian tube
  - Bloody nasal discharge or epistaxis
  - 50-70% present with mass from metastatic nodes
- Other signs/symptoms
  - Uncommonly presents with cranial neuropathies

Demographics

- Age
  - Peak incidence: 40-60 years
  - Pediatric NPC rare; most often undifferentiated NK
- Gender
  - M:F = 2.5:1
- Ethnicity
  - NK NPC endemic in southern China
    - 800 cases per 1 million
    - Most of rest of world < 10 per 1 million
  - ↓ risk in 2nd- and 3rd-generation American-born Chinese
  - In children in USA, ↑ risk in African Americans
- Epidemiology
  - Worldwide, most common NP adult malignancy
    - Most common cancer in Asian men
  - NK NPC 75% > keratinizing NPC 25% > BSCCa rare

Natural History & Prognosis

- Keratinizing NPC: Poorest prognosis; 5-year survival 20-40%
- NK NPC: Radiosensitive, better prognosis; 5-year survival ~ 75%
- BSCCa: Generally poor
- Most NPC presents as **stage III** (T3 &/or N2), **stage IVA** (T4), or **stage IVB** (N3)
- ≥ 90% have nodal metastases at presentation, often bilateral
  - Retropharyngeal nodes primary site
  - Level II and V nodes next most common
- 5% have distant metastases at presentation, poorer prognosis
- ≤ 30% recur with distant metastases
  - Bone: Sclerotic or lytic lesions
  - Chest and liver also common sites

Treatment

- Generally radiosensitive, especially NK NPC
  - T1: XRT alone
  - T2-T4: XRT + chemotherapy
  - M1: Chemotherapy; XRT only if good response
- Neck dissection for residual disease post treatment

DIAGNOSTIC CHECKLIST

Consider

- Carefully evaluate nasopharynx whenever middle ear obstruction in adult
- Lymphoma is main differential with NP mass ± adenopathy
  - More often midline and expands clivus

Image Interpretation Pearls

- T1 MR sensitive for parapharyngeal space and bone marrow invasion
- T1 C+ key for intracranial, perineural, and cavernous sinus invasion

Reporting Tips

- Certain key tumor findings should be sought
  - Parapharyngeal fat infiltration (T2)
  - Skull base invasion (T3)
  - Intracranial or cranial nerve involvement (T4)
- Nodal disease is common; nodes often large
  - Retropharyngeal, levels II and V nodes most often
  - Supraclavicular nodes = N3b
    - Important, therefore, to describe any low neck nodes (IV or VB) as potentially supraclavicular

SELECTED REFERENCES

1. King AD et al: Detection of nasopharyngeal carcinoma by MR imaging: diagnostic accuracy of MRI compared with endoscopy and endoscopic biopsy based on long-term follow-up. AJNR Am J Neuroradiol. 36(12):2380-5, 2015
2. Lan M et al: Prognostic value of cervical nodal necrosis in nasopharyngeal carcinoma: analysis of 1800 patients with positive cervical nodal metastasis at MR imaging. Radiology. 276(2):536-44, 2015
3. Lee AW et al: Management of nasopharyngeal carcinoma: current practice and future perspective. J Clin Oncol. 33(29):3356-64, 2015
4. Zhang GY et al: Prognostic value of grading masticator space involvement in nasopharyngeal carcinoma according to MR imaging findings. Radiology. 273(1):136-43, 2014
5. Chan AT: Current treatment of nasopharyngeal carcinoma. Eur J Cancer. 47 Suppl 3:S302-3, 2011

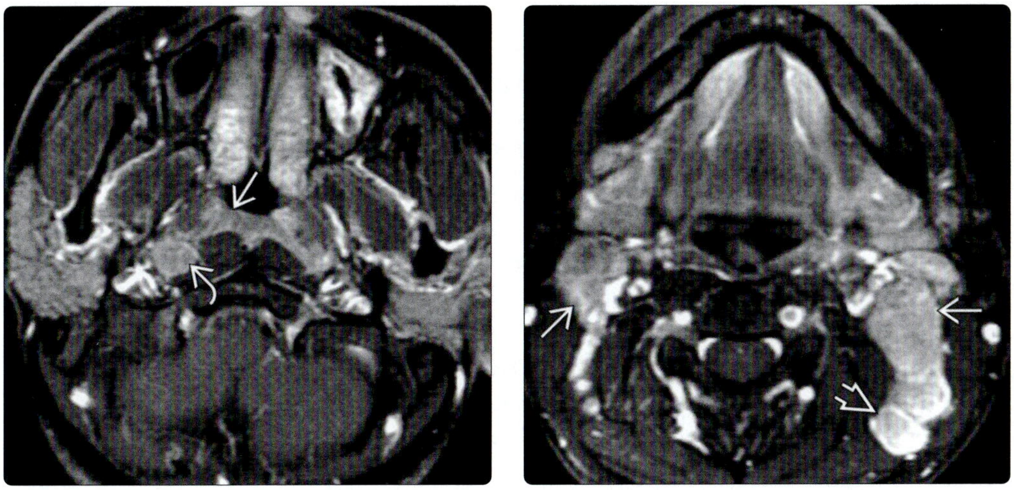

(Left) *Axial T1WI C+ FS MR in a 26-year-old Asian man presenting with neck masses demonstrates subtly asymmetric soft tissue fullness of nasopharynx mucosa ➡, though without infiltration of the prevertebral muscles. Enlarged right retropharyngeal node is evident ➡.* **(Right)** *Axial T1WI C+ FS MR in the same patient demonstrates bilateral enlarged level II ➡ and left level V ➡ nodes, which proved to be undifferentiated nonkeratinizing carcinoma, positive for EBV. This is staged as T1N2, stage III disease.*

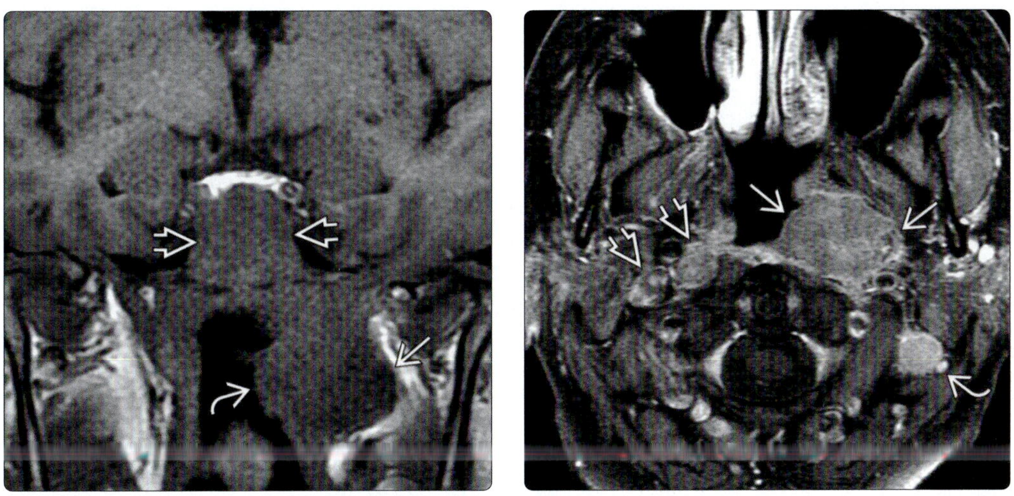

(Left) *Coronal T1 MR shows an infiltrative T1 hypointense mass in the superior lateral nasopharynx ➡, extending into the clivus ➡ and the left parapharyngeal space ➡. Endoscopic biopsy showed nonkeratinizing nasopharyngeal carcinoma (NPC).* **(Right)** *Axial T1 C+ FS in same patient shows NPC in left lateral nasopharyngeal recess extending in the parapharyngeal space ➡. Contralateral retropharyngeal ➡ and ipsilateral level IIB ➡ nodal metastases are well seen. This is staged as T3N2 or stage III.*

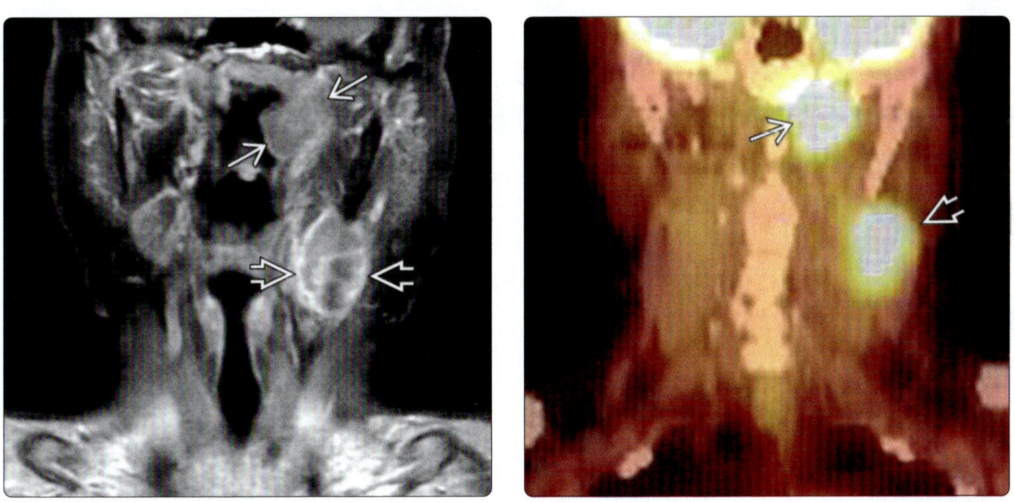

(Left) *Coronal T1WI C+ FS MR in a 65-year-old woman with newly diagnosed NPC demonstrates an ulcerated enhancing mass in the left nasopharynx ➡ associated with necrotic ipsilateral level II nodes ➡. Contralateral nodes were also found. Biopsy showed poorly differentiated keratinizing carcinoma.* **(Right)** *Coronal fused PET/CT shows intense FDG uptake in a left NPC ➡ and in level II node ➡. No distant metastases were found. This NPC was staged as T2N2M0, stage III disease.*

Sinonasal Malignant Melanoma

KEY FACTS

TERMINOLOGY

- Sinonasal melanoma (SNM)
- Definition: Neural crest cell malignancy arising from melanocytes in sinonasal and nasopharyngeal mucosa

IMAGING

- Location: Lateral wall of **nasal fossa, nasal septum, and maxillary sinus most common**
- Size: < 0.3 cm to large, filling nasal fossa &/or sinuses
- Morphology: Polypoid or sessile
- Bone CT or CBCT: Bone destruction ± remodeling
- Best imaging tool: Multiplanar MR
- **Melanotic** melanoma: **T1WI ↑ signal, T2WI ↓ signal**
- **Amelanotic** melanoma: **T1WI intermediate signal, T2WI variable signal**
- Avidly enhancing

TOP DIFFERENTIAL DIAGNOSES

- Sinonasal squamous cell carcinoma
- Sinonasal non-Hodgkin lymphoma
- Esthesioneuroblastoma
- Juvenile angiofibroma

PATHOLOGY

- SNM does not usually spread to regional lymph nodes 1st, therefore **no sentinel nodes**

CLINICAL ISSUES

- Nasal obstruction and epistaxis
- AJCC stage III or IV disease usual at presentation
- Range: 20-80 years; **mean: 65**
- 6-17% 5-year survival rate

DIAGNOSTIC CHECKLIST

- Check for involvement of orbit or skull base
- On CBCT, be suspicious of any soft tissue density that expands or destroys the bony architecture of the sinonasal complex

(Left) *Coronal graphic shows a darkly pigmented (highly melanotic) mass centered in the nasal cavity. Invasion of the skull base ➡, orbit ↶, and lateral nasal wall is seen, but the septum is deviated rather than invaded. Trapped secretions ⇨ are noted in the left maxillary sinus.* **(Right)** *Coronal bone CT in a patient with left nasal obstruction and epistaxis shows a mass in the left nasal cavity with erosion of the left middle turbinate ➡ and portions of the lateral nasal wall ↶. Opacification is noted in left maxillary sinus and ethmoid air cells.*

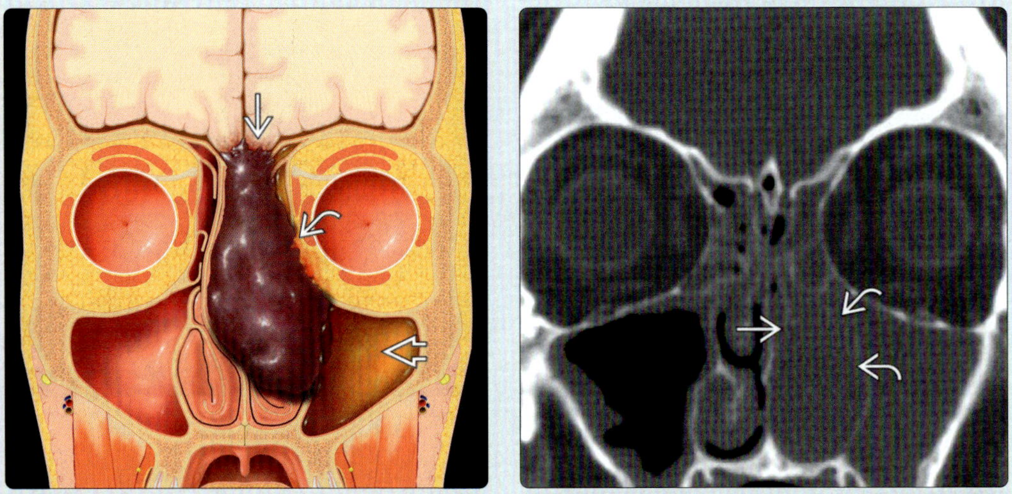

(Left) *Axial T1WI MR demonstrates a mass in the left nasal cavity with maxillary sinus extension. The lesion is heterogeneous with areas of T1 shortening ➡ and intermediate signal ↶. T1 shortening on unenhanced images may indicate the presence of melanin.* **(Right)** *Axial T2WI FS MR shows a lobular melanoma ➡ within the left nasal cavity. It is somewhat hypointense and is readily distinguishable from the hyperintense obstructed secretions ↶ in the left maxillary sinus.*

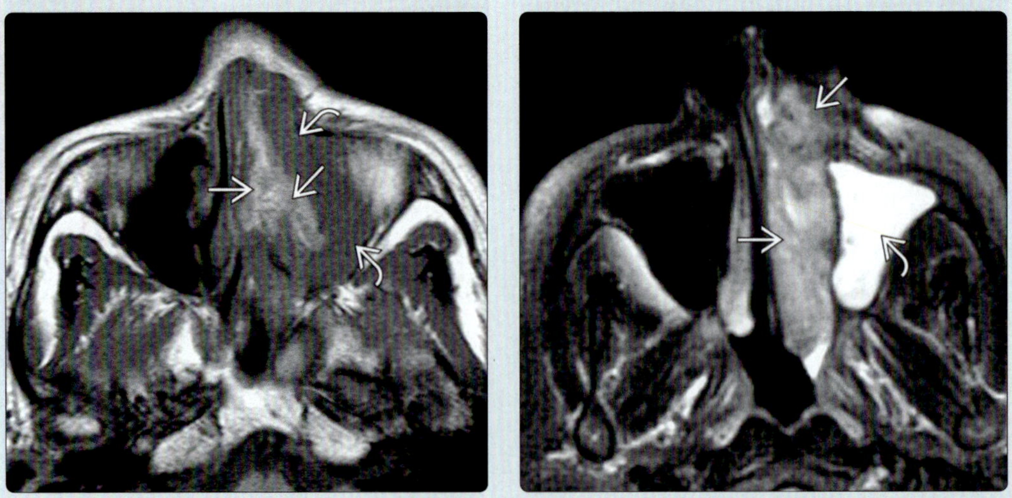

TERMINOLOGY

Abbreviations

- Sinonasal melanoma (SNM), mucosal melanoma (MM)

Definitions

- Neural crest cell malignancy arising from melanocytes in sinonasal and nasopharyngeal mucosa

IMAGING

General Features

- Best diagnostic clue
  - ↑ T1 MR signal in nasal cavity
- Location
  - Lateral wall of **nasal fossa, nasal septum, and maxillary sinus** most common
  - Ethmoid sinus
- Size
  - < 0.3 cm to large, filling nasal fossa &/or sinus
- Morphology
  - Polypoid or sessile

CT Findings

- CECT
  - Diffuse enhancement
- NECT bone window or CBCT
  - Lobular soft tissue mass in nasal fossa
  - Bone destruction ± remodeling

MR Findings

- T1WI
  - **Melanotic** melanoma: **↑ signal** due to melanin, free radicals, metal ions, hemorrhage
  - **Amelanotic** melanoma: Intermediate (soft tissue) signal
- T2WI
  - **Melanotic melanoma: ↓ signal**
  - **Amelanotic** melanoma: Variable signal
- T2* GRE
  - Hemorrhagic areas may show blooming
- T1WI C+
  - Avidly enhancing
    - Difficult to appreciate if ↑ precontrast T1 signal

Imaging Recommendations

- Best imaging tool
  - **Multiplanar MR**
  - Precontrast T1 sequence to look for T1 shortening
  - Full-body PET/CT has been recommended as follow-up

DIFFERENTIAL DIAGNOSIS

Sinonasal Squamous Cell Carcinoma

- Antrum > nasal fossa
- Aggressive bone destruction; heterogeneous with variable enhancement

Sinonasal Non-Hodgkin Lymphoma

- Nasal fossa mass with bone destruction ± remodeling
- Homogeneous; ↓ T2 signal; ↑ density on NECT

Esthesioneuroblastoma

- Mass near cribriform plate with bone destruction
- ± intratumoral Ca++ or cyst formation at brain tumor interface

Juvenile Angiofibroma

- Young male
- Posterior nasal fossa near sphenopalatine foramen

PATHOLOGY

General Features

- Etiology
  - Suggested association with **occupational exposure to formalin** and other chemicals but not confirmed
- Genetics
  - Varies in different populations
  - Mutations &/or increased number of *KIT* gene and increased expression of KIT protein

Staging, Grading, & Classification

- **AJCC classification**
  - AJCC 2002 better prognosticator than AJCC 2009

Gross Pathologic & Surgical Features

- SNM does not usually spread to regional lymph nodes 1st; therefore, **no sentinel nodes**

Microscopic Features

- ≥ 10 mitoses/HPF → poor prognosis
- Most MM can be diagnosed with H&E stain

CLINICAL ISSUES

Presentation

- Most common signs/symptoms
  - **Unilateral nasal obstruction and epistaxis, progressive**
  - Stage III or IV disease most common at presentation
- Other signs/symptoms
  - Sometimes melanorrhea
  - Epiphora, facial pain, swelling
  - Possible visual disturbances

Demographics

- Age
  - Range: 20-80 years; **mean: 65 years**
- Epidemiology
  - Rare but incidence appear to be increasing
  - < 7% of sinonasal tract neoplasms

Natural History & Prognosis

- 50% with **local control develop distant mets**
- 6-40% 5-year survival rate

Treatment

- **Surgery** ± **radiation therapy**

DIAGNOSTIC CHECKLIST

Reporting Tips

- Check for involvement of orbit or skull base

SELECTED REFERENCES

1. Lazarev S et al: Mucosal Melanoma of the Head and Neck: A Systematic Review of the Literature. Int J Radiat Oncol Biol Phys. 90(5):1108-1118, 2014

Sinonasal Fibrous Dysplasia

KEY FACTS

TERMINOLOGY

- Abbreviation: Fibrous dysplasia (FD)
- Monostotic FD (MFD): Involves only 1 bone
- Polyostotic FD (PFD): Involves 2 or more bones
- Craniofacial FD (CFD): PFD in craniofacial regions
- Jaffe-Lichtenstein syndrome: MFD with cutaneous pigmentation
- McCune-Albright syndrome: PFD with cutaneous pigmentation and endocrinopathies

IMAGING

- Altered bone pattern often with **ground-glass** density within intact, thinned, and expanded cortex
- **Lesion blends** into surrounding bone
- MFD = 80% of FD; 20% occur in facial region
- Maxilla > mandible; commonly **unilateral**
- Possible encroachment on paranasal sinuses, nasal fossae, orbits, foramina, and canals

TOP DIFFERENTIAL DIAGNOSES

- Osteoma
- Ossifying fibroma
- Juvenile ossifying fibroma

CLINICAL ISSUES

- Usually asymptomatic expansion of associated bone
- Monostotic type likely to stop growth at puberty
- Craniofacial type may continue to grow after puberty
- M < F, especially polyostotic forms
- Malignant transformation → sarcoma < 1%
- Usually no treatment during somatic growth due to marked growth potential

DIAGNOSTIC CHECKLIST

- Lesion must be **within outer cortex**

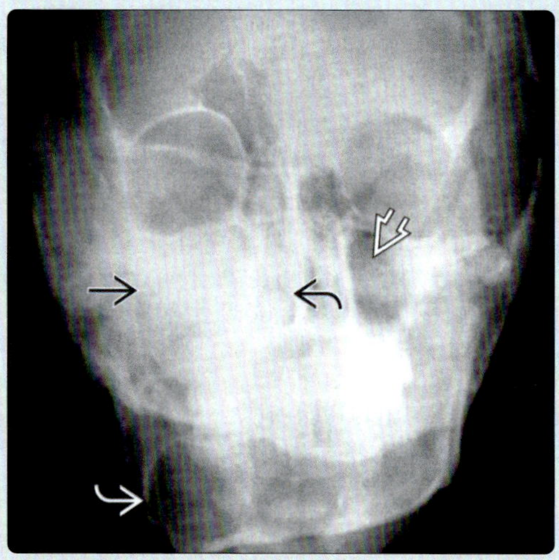
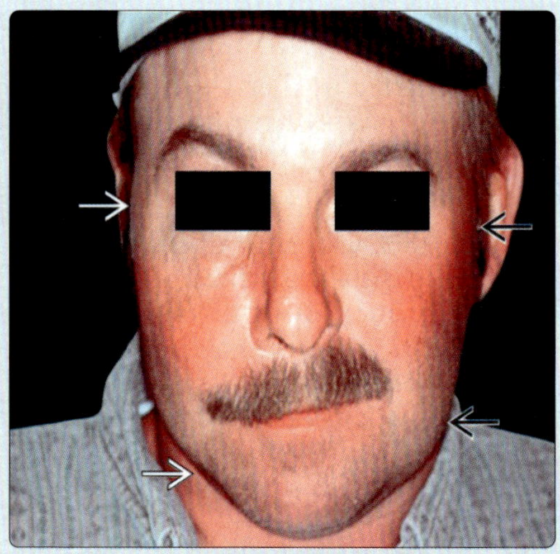

(Left) *Posteroanterior radiograph of the skull shows the osseous growth of polyostotic fibrous dysplasia (PFD) encroaching on the right maxillary sinus and nasal fossa. There is loss of the radiolucent lumen of the sinus compared to the contralateral side. Note a radiolucent lesion of FD in the right mandible.* **(Right)** *Clinical photograph of the same patient with PFD shows that the right maxilla and mandible have enlarged in a vertical direction compared to the normal left side.*

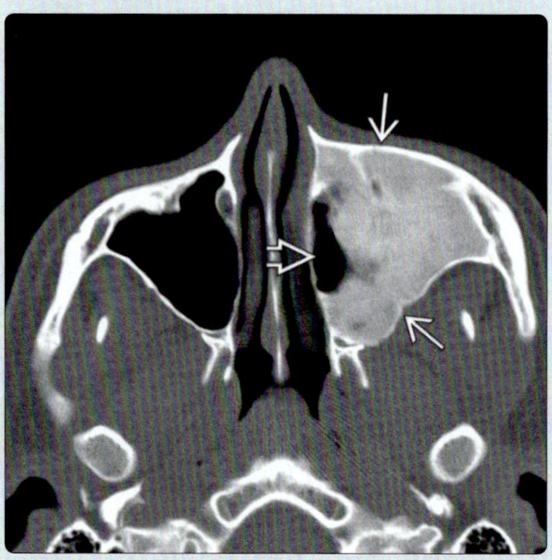
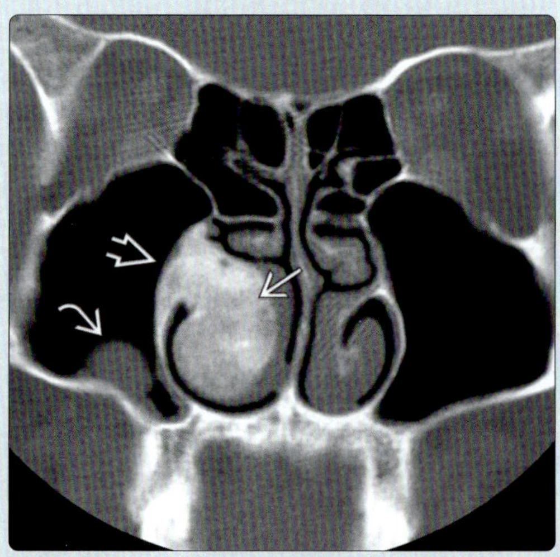

(Left) *Axial bone CT shows classic FD exhibiting expansion of the left maxillary sinus walls and a ground-glass appearance. Note the diminished volume of the left maxillary sinus. FD in the maxillofacial area is more likely to be monostotic, and the maxilla is affected more than the mandible.* **(Right)** *Coronal bone CT shows FD affecting the right inferior turbinate and lateral wall of the nasal fossa, reducing the volume of the right maxillary sinus. The mucus retention pseudocyst is an incidental finding.*

TERMINOLOGY

Abbreviations

- Fibrous dysplasia (FD)

Definitions

- Monostotic FD (MFD): Involves only 1 bone
- Polyostotic FD (PFD): Involves 2 or more bones
- Craniofacial FD (CFD): PFD in craniofacial regions
- Jaffe-Lichtenstein syndrome: MFD with cutaneous pigmentation
- McCune-Albright syndrome (MAS): PFD with associated cutaneous pigmentation and endocrinopathies, such as precocious sexual development

IMAGING

General Features

- Best diagnostic clue
  - Altered bone pattern, often with **ground-glass density** within intact, but thinned and expanded, cortex of involved bone(s)
  - **Lesion blends** into surrounding bone
- Location
  - In various bones of face or cranium
    - Subclinical lesions may confound frequency of bones involved
    - Maxilla > mandible > frontal bone > ethmoid and sphenoid bones > temporal bone
      - 2 cases of MFD reported in turbinate bone only
      - Usually **unilateral** in oral and maxillofacial region
  - MFD = 80% of FD; 10-20% of MFD occur in facial region (may be underreported)
  - PFD next most common; 50-100% of PFD occur in facial region
  - MAS least common
  - NIH study of 106 subjects with CFD found 92% sinonasal involvement
- Size
  - Varies from small and localized to involving most or all of several bones
- Morphology
  - Overgrowth of bone, independent of function
    - **Asymmetry** if overgrowth unilateral
  - Possible encroachment on paranasal sinuses, nasal fossae, orbits, foramina, and canals

Radiographic Findings

- Radiography
  - Abnormal bone pattern with areas of lesser and greater radiopacity
    - **Ground-glass** (extraoral radiographs) or orange peel (peau d'orange) appearance on intraoral radiographs
    - Radiolucent, mixed radiolucent and radiopaque, or completely radiopaque
    - Usually **radiopaque in maxilla**
  - Maintenance of cortex of involved bones, albeit probably thinned
  - Altered morphology and overgrowth of bone
  - Encroachment on surrounding structures such as sinuses, nasal fossae, orbits, canals, and foramina
  - May have associated simple bone cysts that present as well-defined radiolucent areas

CT Findings

- NECT or CBCT
  - Intact/expanded cortex of bones
  - Altered morphology of bones

MR Findings

- T1WI
  - Variable intensity based upon fibrous:mineralized tissue ratio
  - Not pathognomonic
- T2WI
  - Homogeneous, intermediate to hypointense
    - Ground-glass = ↓ signal; fibrous tissue = intermediate to ↑ signal
- T1WI C+ FS
  - May be useful to show associated aneurysmal bone cysts in CFD

Imaging Recommendations

- Best imaging tool
  - Periapical or panoramic radiograph to see internal structure and extent of lesion
  - NECT (bone window) or CBCT to evaluate effect on surrounding structures
- Protocol advice
  - Noncontrast CT or CBCT

DIFFERENTIAL DIAGNOSIS

Osteoma

- Usually **more radiopaque** than FD
- Median age: ~ 35 years

Ossifying Fibroma

- Tends to be separated from bone, unlike FD, which tends to blend with bone
- Often has **radiolucent periphery** consistent with capsule
- Unlike FD, expands around **center**
- Mutation in *GNAS1* absent

Juvenile Ossifying Fibroma

- Separated from bone
- More rapidly growing in young individuals

Paget Disease

- Patients generally over 40 years old
- Does not usually encroach on paranasal sinuses

Cherubism

- Usually **bilateral** and diagnosed before 6 years of age
- Usually starts in mandible
- May be in all 4 quadrants of dental arches
  - Maxillary lesions may enlarge into maxillary sinuses
- Radiolucent (multilocular) initially; as child matures, lesions **become more granular**

Osteomyelitis

- Enlargement of bone due to subperiosteal new bone outside cortex
- May see breaks in cortex under new bone

Osteosarcoma

- Pattern of bone may be similar
- May have Garrington sign of **widened periodontal ligament space**
- Periosteal reaction of Codman triangles or sunray spicules
- Could arise from FD but low malignant transformation likelihood (< 1%)

PATHOLOGY

General Features

- Etiology
  - Somatic mutation of *GNAS1* gene on 20q13
    - *GNAS1* encodes for Gsα subunit of Gs protein that stimulates adenylyl cyclase enzyme and overproduction of 3',5'-cyclic adenosine monophosphate
    - ↑ cAMP may cause downregulation of osteoblastic transcription factor Runx2 → abnormal osteoblastic differentiation and osteoclast recruitment and activation → ↑ interleukin 6 → ↑ bone resorption
    - Causes ↑ proliferation of osteogenesis associated cells
- Genetics
  - Usually not familial
- Associated abnormalities
  - Café au lait spots with MAS
  - **Endocrinopathies** with MAS
  - Simple bone cysts
  - Aneurysmal bone cysts (CFD)

Staging, Grading, & Classification

- Subclinical
  - Incidental finding on radiographs
- Clinical monostotic
  - Change in morphology in 1 bone is visible clinically or has caused symptoms such as pain
- Clinical polyostotic
  - Change in morphology in multiple bones is visible clinically as altered contours
  - Symptoms such as pain or blindness due to constriction of neural foramina

Gross Pathologic & Surgical Features

- Tan-white to yellow, soft, rubbery, gritty, or firm tissue

Microscopic Features

- Normal bone replaced by irregular whorled distribution of spindle-shaped fibroblast-like cells
- May have so-called **Chinese or Hebrew character** or **alphabet soup** pattern of woven bone trabeculae

CLINICAL ISSUES

Presentation

- Most common signs/symptoms
  - Enlargement/expansion of associated bone
  - Usually **asymptomatic** but pain and blindness possible
- Other signs/symptoms
  - Teeth displaced
  - Possible mucocele in paranasal sinuses
  - Nasal airway compromised → recurrent rhinosinusitis, hypo/anosmia
  - Trigeminal neuralgia

Demographics

- Age
  - Usually in first 2 decades of life
  - In younger patients, mean age = 13 years; tends to be progressive
  - In older patients, mean age = 25 years; tends not to be progressive
- Gender
  - More common in **females**, especially polyostotic forms

Natural History & Prognosis

- Most lesions stop growing at end of somatic growth
  - Monostotic type likely to stop growth at puberty
  - Craniofacial type may continue to grow after puberty
- Simple bone cyst or aneurysmal bone cyst may develop in association
- Spontaneous malignant transformation → sarcoma < 1%

Treatment

- Usually none during somatic growth due to marked growth potential
- Surgical recontouring to improve function or esthetics
- Resection and reconstruction if vital structures are impinged upon
- **Radiation therapy contraindicated** due to risk of sarcomatous change

DIAGNOSTIC CHECKLIST

Image Interpretation Pearls

- Lesion must be within outer cortex

SELECTED REFERENCES

1. Kim KS: Headache attributed to fibrous dysplasia of the ethmoid bone mimicking menstrual migraine without aura. J Craniofac Surg. 27(4):e417-9, 2016
2. Min HJ et al: Headache induced by fibrous dysplasia of the sphenoid sinus: a case report. Headache. 56(8):1348-51, 2016
3. Ciniglio Appiani M et al: Ossifying fibromas of the paranasal sinuses: diagnosis and management. Acta Otorhinolaryngol Ital. 35(5):355-61, 2015
4. DeKlotz TR et al: Sinonasal disease in polyostotic fibrous dysplasia and McCune-Albright syndrome. Laryngoscope. 123(4):823-8, 2013
5. Park HJ et al: Fibrous dysplasia of the inferior turbinate. Int J Clin Exp Pathol. 6(3):531-5, 2013
6. Karligkiotis A et al: Monostotic fibrous dysplasia of the inferior turbinate. Otolaryngol Head Neck Surg. 146(6):1035-6, 2012
7. Schreiber A et al: Fibrous dysplasia of the sinonasal tract and adjacent skull base. Curr Opin Otolaryngol Head Neck Surg. 20(1):45-52, 2012
8. Lee YH et al: Decortication of fibrous dysplasia of the maxillary sinus. J Craniofac Surg. 22(1):139-41, 2011
9. Char DH et al: Fibrous dysplasia. Orbit. 29(4):216-8, 2010
10. Shekhar MG et al: Juvenile aggressive ossifying fibroma of the maxilla. J Indian Soc Pedod Prev Dent. 27(3):170-4, 2009
11. Mansilla-Lory J et al: Leontiasis ossea: a paleopathologic case report. J Clin Rheumatol. 13(5):269-72, 2007
12. Eller R et al: Common fibro-osseous lesions of the paranasal sinuses. Otolaryngol Clin North Am. 39(3):585-600, x, 2006
13. Akintoye SO et al: Analyses of variable panoramic radiographic characteristics of maxillo-mandibular fibrous dysplasia in McCune-Albright syndrome. Oral Dis. 10(1):36-43, 2004
14. Crawford LB: An unusual case of fibrous dysplasia of the maxillary sinus. Am J Orthod Dentofacial Orthop. 124(6):721-4, 2003

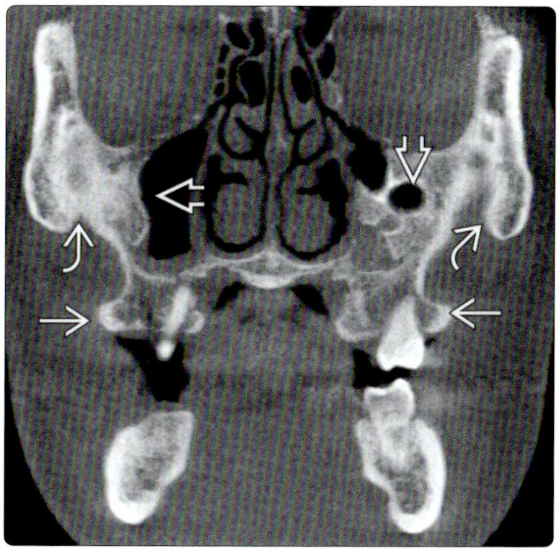

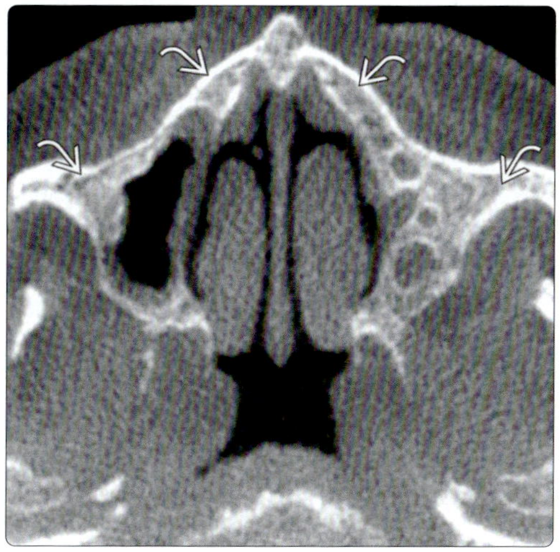

(Left) *Coronal CBCT shows the altered bone pattern of craniofacial FD (CFD) encroaching upon the maxillary sinuses , reducing the volume bilaterally. The alveolar processes of the maxilla are altered in morphology, showing buccal exostoses that are unrelated to the CFD.* **(Right)** *Axial CBCT in the same patient shows the altered bone pattern of CFD throughout the maxilla and zygomatic bones. The bone cortices have remained intact and there are no signs of cortical expansion in this slice.*

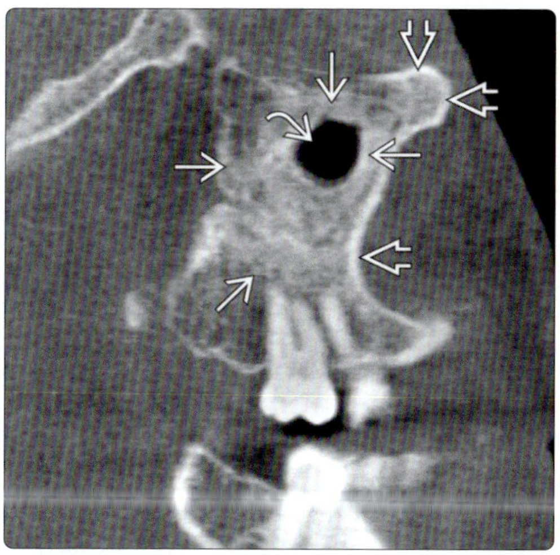

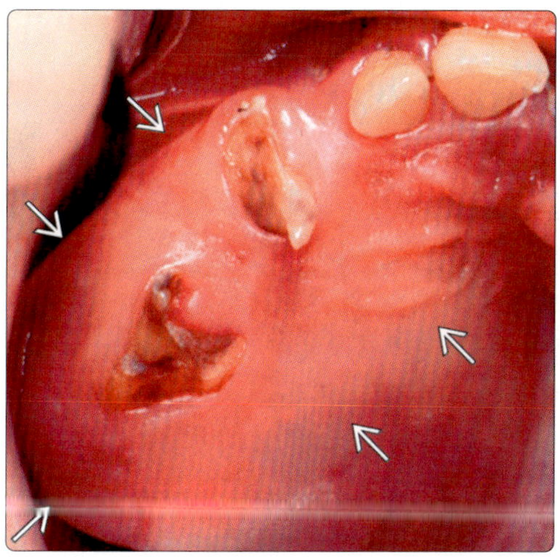

(Left) *Sagittal reformat CBCT in the same patient shows the coarse bone pattern of CFD with encroachment of the left maxillary sinus, which is markedly decreased in volume . Note the normal cortical bone thickness and density .* **(Right)** *Intraoral clinical photograph shows unilateral enlargement of the alveolar process due to FD. The enlargement extends to the palatal midline. Note the normal overlying mucosa. The carious teeth are not causally related.*

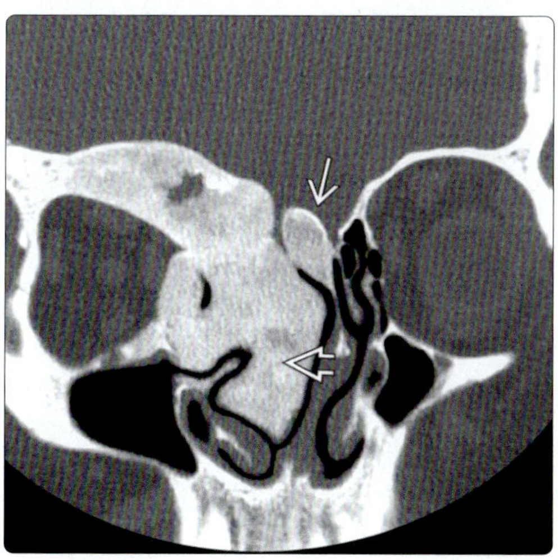

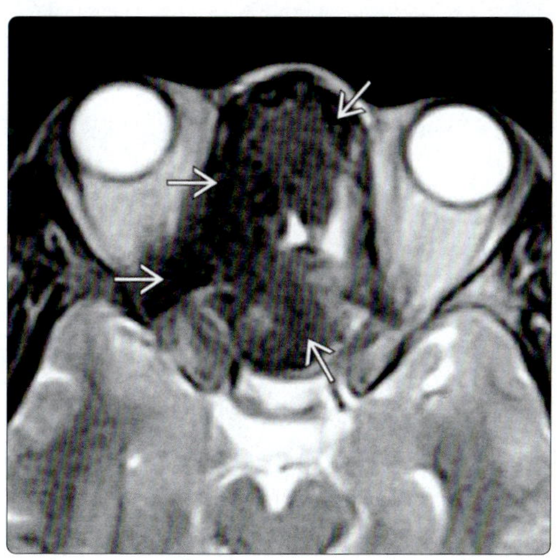

(Left) *Coronal bone CT shows PFD affecting the orbit, crista galli , ethmoids, and middle turbinate on the right. Note the typical ground-glass appearance. The nasal septum is deviated to the left.* **(Right)** *Axial T2WI MR in the same patient shows marked hypointense signal in the involved bones . The lesion is homogeneous, consistent with the ground-glass appearance on CT. If more fibrous tissue were present, foci of higher, long TR signal would be expected.*

Sinonasal Ossifying Fibroma

KEY FACTS

TERMINOLOGY

- Ossifying fibroma (OF): Benign, fibroosseous neoplasm composed of mixture of fibrous tissue & mature bone

IMAGING

- Most common craniofacial site is mandible (75%)
- 10-20% of craniofacial OFs arise from maxilla
- Imaging appearance depends on age (↑ ossified portions with age)
    - Classic appearance: Thick, bony peripheral rim surrounding fibrous center
- CT: **Expansile mass** with **soft tissue density** (fibrous) **central** area surrounded by **ossified rim**
    - May be indistinguishable from fibrous dysplasia & osteoma
- MR: Intermediate to low T1 signal throughout tumor
    - T2: Mixed low-signal (ossified) & high-signal (fibrous) areas
    - Inhomogeneous enhancement of fibrous components

TOP DIFFERENTIAL DIAGNOSES

- Sinonasal fibrous dysplasia
- Sinonasal osteoma

PATHOLOGY

- May originate from mesenchyme of periodontal ligament: Varying amounts of cemental tissue

CLINICAL ISSUES

- Generally asymptomatic & found incidentally
- 20-40 year olds most common
- M:F = 1:5
- Slow growing but may be locally aggressive
    - May obstruct sinus drainage, cause cosmetic deformity & ocular dysfunction
- Mimics other fibroosseous lesions: **Diagnosis not made on basis of imaging alone**

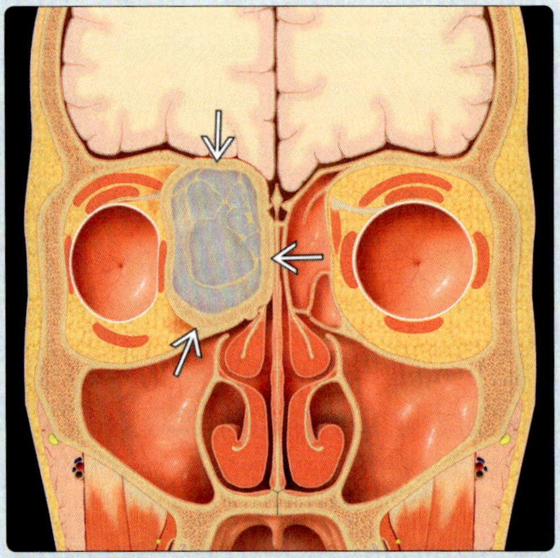
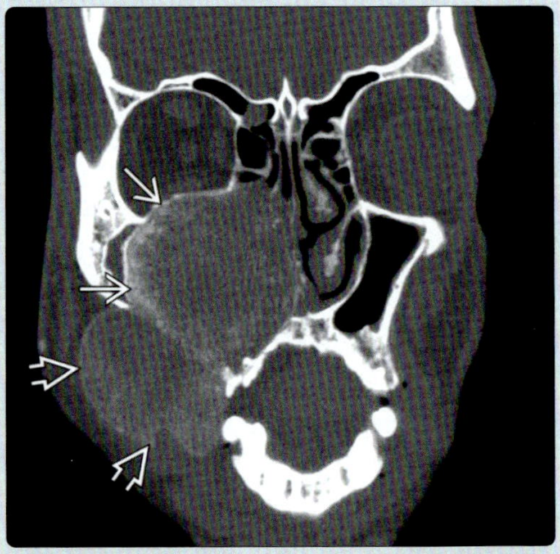

(Left) *Coronal graphic shows an ossifying fibroma (OF) of the ethmoid region with dense osseous material peripherally → and a fibrous center. The margins are well defined. There is mass effect on the orbital contents.* **(Right)** *Coronal bone CT demonstrates a very large, bilobed, OF with a large maxillary antral portion and smaller component extending into the buccal space ⇒. Peripheral ossification → of the maxillary component is noted.*

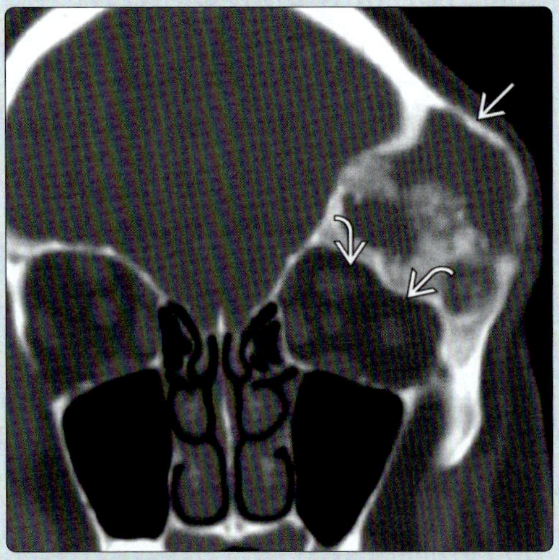
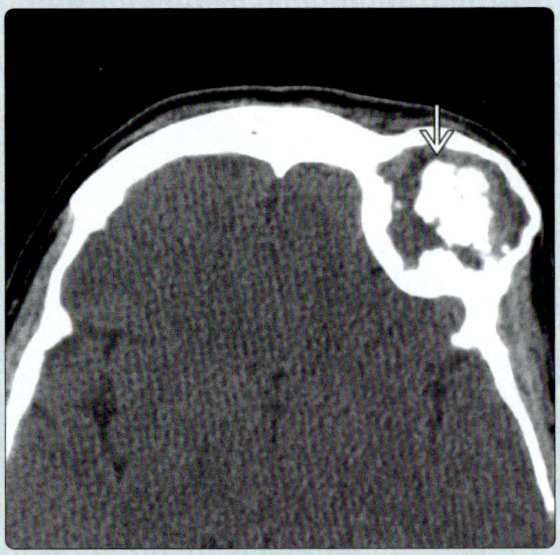

(Left) *Coronal bone CT shows a large OF of the orbital plate of the frontal bone with mixed ossified and fibrous density. It is expansile, and the patient presented with cosmetic deformity from forehead swelling → and proptosis from orbital mass effect ⇒.* **(Right)** *Axial NECT in the same patient shows that the dominant focus of ossification in this case is central → with surrounding soft tissue density rather than the classic pattern with peripheral ossification.*

Sinonasal Ossifying Fibroma

TERMINOLOGY

Abbreviations

- Ossifying fibroma (OF)

Synonyms

- Cementoossifying fibroma, cementifying fibroma, psammomatoid ossifying fibroma, juvenile-aggressive ossifying fibroma, juvenile trabecular ossifying fibroma, juvenile psammomatoid ossifying fibroma

Definitions

- **Benign, fibroosseous neoplasm** composed of mixture of fibrous tissue & mature bone

IMAGING

General Features

- Best diagnostic clue
  - **Well-demarcated, expansile mass** with soft tissue density (fibrous) central area surrounded by ossified rim
- Location
  - 10-20% of craniofacial OFs arise from maxilla
    - Most common craniofacial site is mandible (75%)
  - Characteristically **monostotic**
- Size
  - 0.5-15 cm
- Morphology
  - Well circumscribed, expansile

CT Findings

- NECT
  - Well-circumscribed, expansile mass with mixed soft tissue & bone density
  - Most often unilobular
- CECT
  - Fibrous areas may show subtle to more avid enhancement
- Bone CT or CBCT
  - Imaging appearance depends on age of OF (↑ **ossified portions with age**)
  - Classic appearance
    - **Thick, bony peripheral rim** surrounding low-attenuation fibrous center
  - Other appearance
    - Radiopaque center with **radiolucent (fibrous) rim** surrounded by thin cortex
    - Scattered foci of soft tissue density among ossified areas
    - Thin, eggshell appearance of peripheral bone
  - CT appearance may be indistinguishable from fibrous dysplasia & osteoma
  - May resorb maxillary tooth roots

MR Findings

- T1WI
  - **Intermediate to low signal** throughout tumor
    - Fibrous areas have intermediate signal (classically central)
    - Ossified areas hypointense (classically peripheral)
- T2WI
  - **Mixed low- & high-signal** areas
    - Fibrous areas hyperintense (usually lesion center)
    - Ossified areas hypointense (usually lesion periphery)
  - **Obstructed secretions** behind lesion & associated mucocele **hyperintense**
  - Fluid-fluid levels in portions of these tumors have been reported
- T1WI C+
  - Inhomogeneous enhancement of fibrous portions of tumor matrix
  - Enhancement of outer shell & septa may be seen

Imaging Recommendations

- Best imaging tool
  - Fibroosseous lesions of craniofacial area best studied with **bone algorithm CT**
- Protocol advice
  - **Thin-slice bone CT** in axial plane with coronal ± sagittal reformatted images
  - Enhanced T1 fat-saturated MR provides complete presurgical roadmap of surrounding soft tissues at risk

Nuclear Medicine Findings

- Increased Tc-99m MDP uptake

DIFFERENTIAL DIAGNOSIS

Sinonasal Fibrous Dysplasia

- **Poorly defined expansion** of maxillofacial bones
- Classic ground-glass appearance
- Mixed pattern of less active ground-glass areas and more active fibrous areas
- May be monostotic (70%) or polyostotic (30%)
- Encompasses rather than resorbs healthy tooth roots
- Blends into surrounding normal bone

Cementoosseous Dysplasia

- **Absence of concentric bony expansion**
- Usually no tooth root resorption
- Most often **multiple lesions**

Sinonasal Osteoma

- Mass comprised of mostly solid lamellar bone
- **Frontal sinus** common location
- No radiolucent rim

Sinonasal Osteosarcoma

- **Destructive, aggressive** lesion of craniofacial bones
- Tumor "new bone" in mass matrix
- "Sunburst" periosteal reaction
- Most common in adolescent males or as long-term complication of XRT

Cementoblastoma

- Benign tumor of cementum in young males
- Dense mass attached to resorbed tooth root
- **Not located in frontal, ethmoid, sphenoid sinuses**

PATHOLOGY

General Features

- Etiology
  - May originate from mesenchyme of periodontal ligament: Varying amounts of cemental tissue

- Presumed to originate from mesenchymal blast cells, but not all arise in dental area
- Densely cellular, well-defined fibrous tumor with ossification progressing from periphery toward center
  - Early stage: Primarily fibrous
  - Late stage: Fills in with mature bone
- Associated abnormalities
  - Large lesions may result in cosmetic **deformity**, ocular dysfunction
  - May **obstruct sinus drainage** pathways and lead to mucocele formation
  - Intracranial extension complicated by tension pneumocephalus has been reported
  - Associated simple bone cyst has been reported
  - May be associated with neurofibromatosis, Sturge-Weber syndrome, encephalocraniocutaneous lipomatosis, oculocerebrocutaneous (Delleman) syndrome

Staging, Grading, & Classification

- Subtypes described
  - (Adult) ossifying fibroma
  - Juvenile ossifying fibroma
    - Juvenile psammomatoid ossifying fibroma
    - Juvenile trabecular ossifying fibroma

Gross Pathologic & Surgical Features

- Gritty, gray to white, hard lesion

Microscopic Features

- Islands of osteoid rimmed by osteoblasts forming lamellar bone ± cementum-like tissue
- Central OF contains immature (woven) bone while periphery has more mature (lamellar) bone
- Fibrous stroma shows parallel & whorl arrangement of collagen & fibroblasts
  - May be densely cellular with hemorrhage, inflammation, & giant cells
- OF may be histologically indistinguishable from active form of fibrous dysplasia

CLINICAL ISSUES

Presentation

- Most common signs/symptoms
  - Generally **asymptomatic** & found incidentally
  - Size at presentation often larger than OFs in other locations, as OFs in sinus more difficult to detect
- Other signs/symptoms
  - Chronic sinusitis symptoms: Rhinorrhea, pain, cheek swelling, nasal obstruction
  - Displaced or partially resorbed teeth
  - Exophthalmos, diplopia, visual acuity loss due to orbital mass effect
- Clinical profile
  - **20- to 40-year-old woman** with mixed soft tissue-ossified sinus lesion incidentally detected on CT performed for other reasons
  - Appearance mimics other fibroosseous lesions, & **diagnosis not made on basis of imaging alone**
    - Based on combination of clinical, radiological, & pathological criteria

Demographics

- Age
  - 20-40 years most common
  - Wide range reported: 1st-9th decade
- Gender
  - M:F = 1:5
- Epidemiology
  - **10-20%** of craniofacial OFs arise in **maxilla**
  - < 0.5% risk of malignant degeneration

Natural History & Prognosis

- Slow growing but may be locally aggressive
  - OF of paranasal sinuses more aggressive than OF of mandible
  - Juvenile variant (active ossifying fibroma) may have aggressive, locally destructive behavior
- Prognosis excellent after complete resection
- High rate of recurrence if incompletely resected

Treatment

- Complete surgical excision is treatment of choice as permitted by OF location
- Lesions with benign behavior that do not produce deformity may be treated with curettage and ostectomy
  - Recurrence rates higher with this approach
  - Long-term follow-up (> 10 years) recommended

DIAGNOSTIC CHECKLIST

Consider

- May not have classic appearance of bony rim with fibrous center
  - Densities may be patchy & randomly distributed

Image Interpretation Pearls

- MR appearance of OF highly variable & lesion may appear more aggressive
  - Careful correlation with CT important
- May be **indistinguishable from fibrous dysplasia** in imaging
  - Refer to more generically as fibroosseous lesion
  - If polyostotic process, fibrous dysplasia more likely

Reporting Tips

- Be sure to describe position in relation to sinus drainage pathways
- Be sure to describe mass effect upon adjacent structures, such as orbit, neural foramina, & intracranial cavity

SELECTED REFERENCES

1. Zhang R et al: Incidental Detection of Ossifying Fibroma of the Frontal Sinus on 99mTc-MDP Bone Scan. Clin Nucl Med. 41(1):e51-2, 2016
2. Ciniglio Appiani M et al: Ossifying fibromas of the paranasal sinuses: diagnosis and management. Acta Otorhinolaryngol Ital. 35(5):355-61, 2015
3. Gantala R et al: Psammomatoid Juvenile Ossifying Fibroma Involving Upper Jaw: A Rare Case Report. J Clin Diagn Res. 9(7):ZD17-9, 2015
4. Mahomed F et al: Ossifying Fibroma in a Patient With Oculocerebrocutaneous (Delleman) Syndrome. J Oral Maxillofac Surg. 73(7):1314-9, 2015
5. Misra SR et al: Giant central ossifying fibroma of the maxilla presenting with a pus discharging intra-oral sinus. J Clin Diagn Res. 9(1):ZD08-11, 2015
6. Pinto WB et al: Ossifying fibroma of the maxilla and tuberous sclerosis complex. Neurology. 84(15):1611-2, 2015
7. Shaik M et al: Juvenile ossifying fibroma of the maxilla: a case report. J Maxillofac Oral Surg. 14(Suppl 1):69-72, 2015

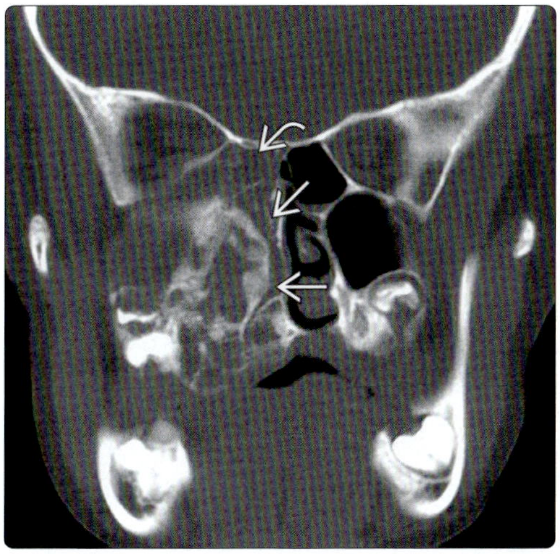

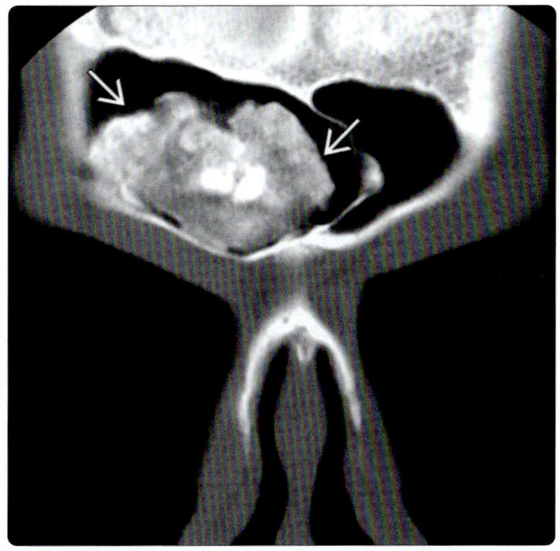

(Left) *Coronal bone CT shows a large maxillary ossifying fibroma that nearly fills the entire right maxillary antrum. The right nasal airway is obstructed* ➔*, and there are postobstructive secretions in the right ethmoid sinuses* ↪*.* **(Right)** *Coronal bone CT shows an atypical appearance of an OF. This frontal sinus lesion* ➔ *demonstrates diffuse, slightly heterogeneous ossification with little fibrous component, mimicking the appearance of an osteoma.*

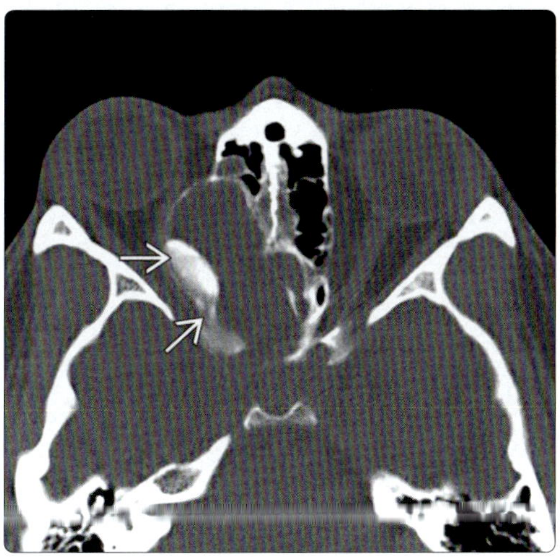

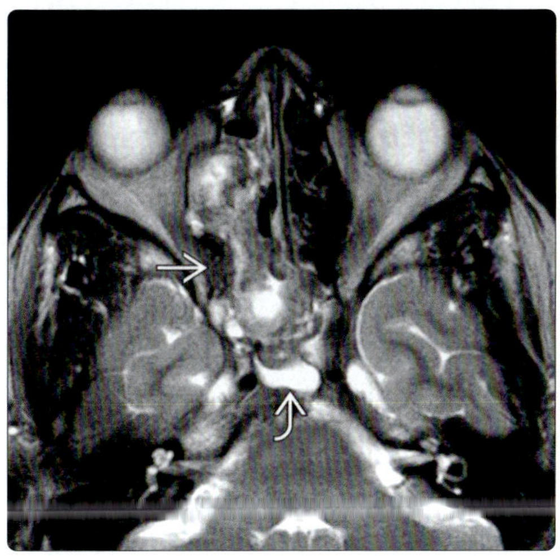

(Left) *Axial bone CT demonstrates an expansile, predominantly soft tissue density mass within the posterior ethmoid region. A focus of peripheral ossification* ➔ *along the lateral margin suggests that this is a fibroosseous lesion, in this case an OF.* **(Right)** *Axial T2WI MR in the same patient shows hypointense signal in the ossified portion* ➔ *of the lesion. Note the hyperintense obstructed secretions* ↪ *in the sphenoid sinus posterior to the lesion.*

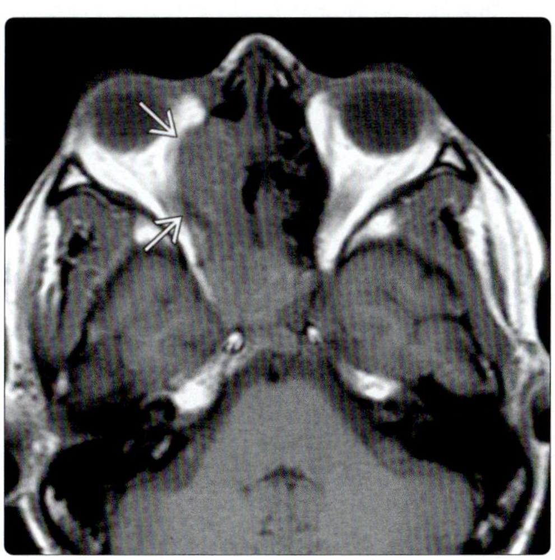

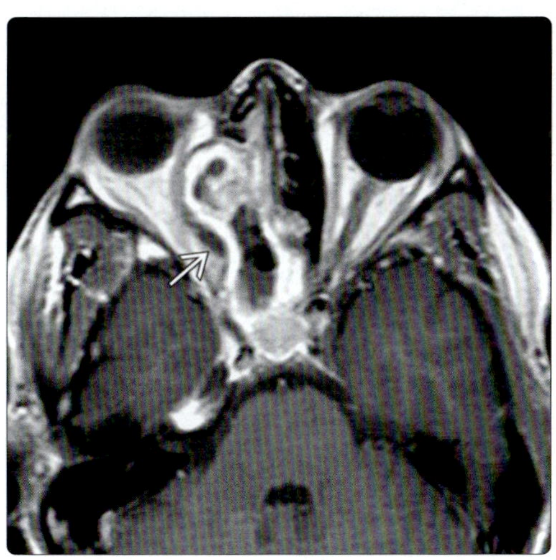

(Left) *Axial T1WI MR in the same patient shows signal intensity similar to that of muscle within the majority of the OF. The margins are well defined. Note the mass effect upon the right orbital contents* ➔*, causing diplopia in this patient.* **(Right)** *Axial T1WI C+ MR in the same patient reveals heterogeneous enhancement throughout the lesion. The fibrous portions of OF typically enhance, and there is little or no enhancement in the ossified* ➔ *portions.*

PART II
SECTION 6
Masticator Space

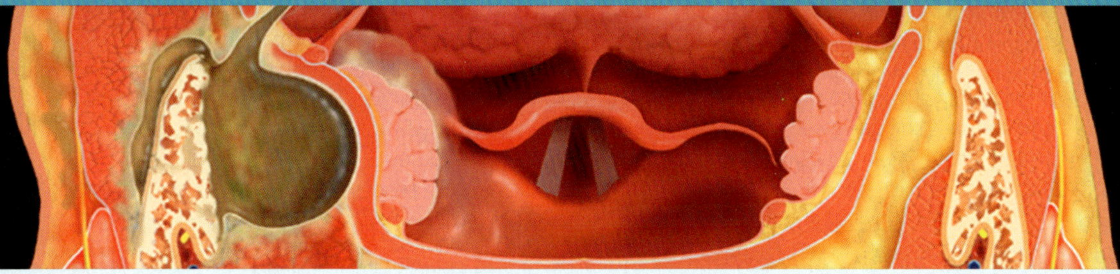

Infection

Masticator Space Abscess 724

Degenerative

Masticator Muscle Atrophy 728

Neoplasm, Benign

Masticator Space CNV3 Schwannoma 732

Neoplasm, Malignant

Masticator Space Chondrosarcoma 734
Masticator Space Sarcoma 738
Masticator Space CNV3 Perineural Tumor 742

Miscellaneous/Idiopathic

Benign Masticator Muscle Hypertrophy 746

Masticator Space Abscess

KEY FACTS

TERMINOLOGY

- Masticator space (MS) abscess: Abscess within MS from molar tooth infection or following dental procedure

IMAGING

- Bone CT: Posterior body of mandible-ramus osteomyelitis ± 2nd or 3rd molar tooth infection
- CECT: Focal fluid density within muscles of mastication with thick, enhancing rim = MS abscess
  - Adjacent muscles swollen, enhancing without associated fluid = myositis
- In setting of acutely infected patient with trismus, limited jaw movement, CECT viewed in soft tissue & bone algorithm is best imaging approach

TOP DIFFERENTIAL DIAGNOSES

- Masticator muscle hypertrophy
- Masticator muscle atrophy
- Cellulitis-phlegmon of MS
- Mandibular osteoradionecrosis
- Sarcoma of MS
- TMJ degenerative disease

CLINICAL ISSUES

- Principal symptom: Trismus
- Initial presentation may be confused clinically with TMJ dysfunction (i.e., TMJ pain and trismus)
- Early MS abscess treated with aggressive intravenous (IV) antibiotics
- Late abscess treatment: Surgical drainage + IV antibiotics

DIAGNOSTIC CHECKLIST

- Questions for radiologist to answer in MS abscess
  - Is mandibular osteomyelitis present
  - Is masticator space only space with abscess
  - Is suprazygomatic masticator space involved

(Left) *Axial graphic depicts a masticator space abscess ➔ arising from the infected posterior mandibular molar tooth ➔. Notice the sinus tract ➔ leading from the tooth to the abscess.* **(Right)** *Axial CECT in a 31 year old presenting with facial swelling, pain, and trismus demonstrates a right medial masticator space abscess containing gas ➔. There is inflammatory change in the lateral masticator space with edema and enlargement of the masseter muscle ➔.*

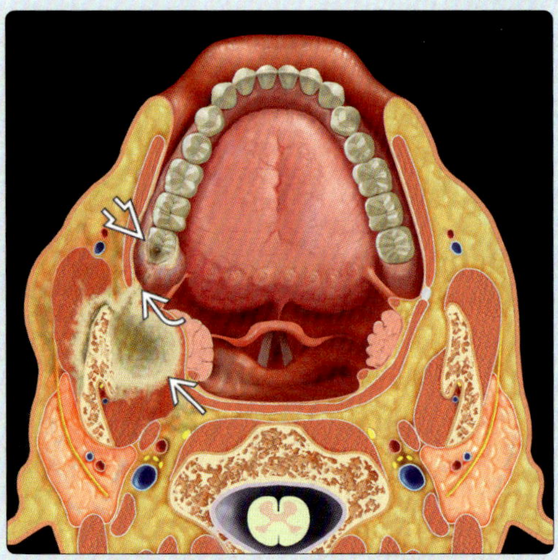

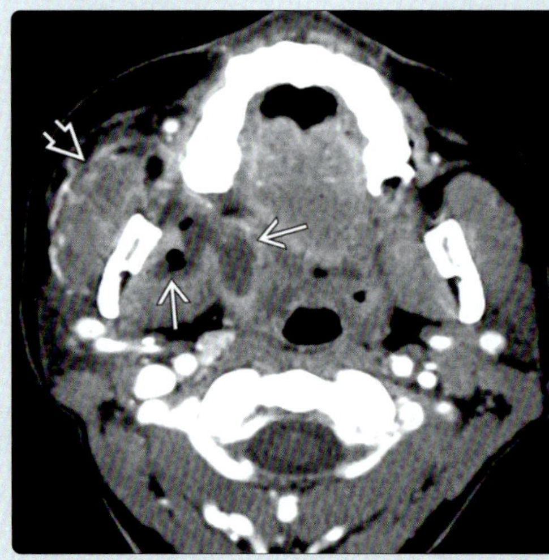

(Left) *Axial CECT in the same patient shows further inferior extent of the medial masticator space abscess ➔ as well as the lateral masticator space abscess ➔. Dental caries involving a molar tooth is the origin of this patient's infection.* **(Right)** *Axial CECT in the same patient reveals inferior extension of the abscess into the right submandibular space ➔. Reactive level II lymphadenopathy is present ➔.*

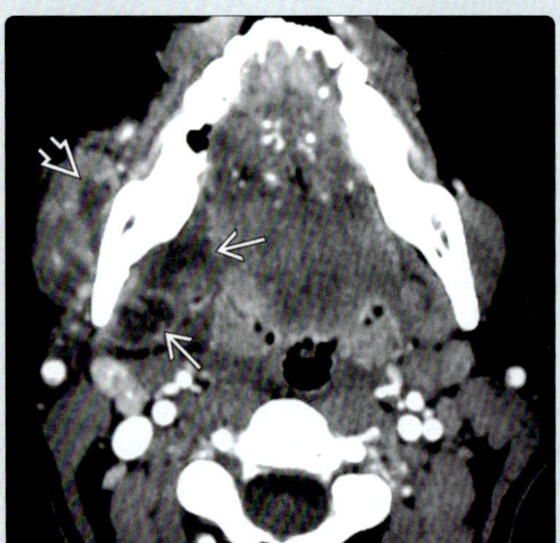

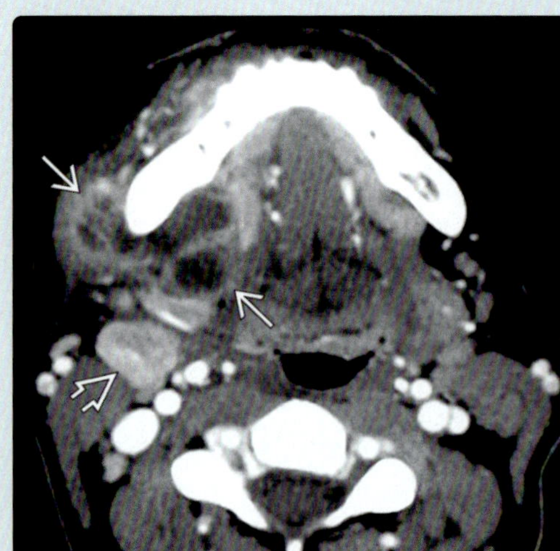

TERMINOLOGY

Abbreviations

- Masticator space (MS) abscess

Definitions

- Abscess within MS from molar tooth (odontogenic) infection or following dental procedure

IMAGING

General Features

- Best diagnostic clue
  - CECT: Fluid with enhancing wall within MS ± posterior mandibular osteomyelitis
- Location
  - Lower MS adjacent to posterior body & ramus of mandible
- Size
  - Early abscess: Often small (1 cm) fluid collection adjacent to mandible
  - Late, severe MS abscess: May be many centimeters, filling entire MS & beyond
- Morphology
  - Ovoid to round
  - If breaks into adjacent deep facial spaces, may be lobulated & irregular

CT Findings

- CECT
  - MS mass lesion with compression of parapharyngeal space from anterolateral to posteromedial
  - Focal fluid density within muscles of mastication with thick, enhancing rim = **MS abscess**
    - Adjacent muscles are swollen, enhancing without associated fluid = **myositis**
    - Adjacent fatty planes are "dirty" = **cellulitis**
  - **Linear markings** in subcutaneous fat & thickening of skin when associated help differentiate infection from malignant tumor
- CBCT & bone CT
  - Posterior body of mandible-ramus osteomyelitis ± 2nd or 3rd molar tooth infection
    - **Mandibular osteomyelitis**: Cortical destruction ± periosteal reaction; **sequestra** are hallmark
    - **Molar tooth infection**: Empty socket or lucency around molar tooth root ± sinus tract leading from tooth through perforation in cortex into adjacent soft tissue
- CTA
  - If abscess extends to parapharyngeal or retropharyngeal spaces, proximal internal carotid artery (ICA) may show spasm

MR Findings

- T1WI
  - Low-signal perimandibular area
- T2WI
  - Focal, high-signal foci represent MS abscess
- T1WI C+
  - Focal, low-signal area surrounded by enhancing wall defines MS abscess
  - Sinus tract from mandible may be visible
- MRA
  - If MS abscess has spread to involve either parapharyngeal or retropharyngeal spaces, ICA spasm may be seen

Nuclear Medicine Findings

- Bone scan
  - Can be used to follow mandibular osteomyelitis response to antibiotic therapy

Intraoral or Panoramic Findings

- Often nonvital carious tooth with associated apical rarefaction ± sequestra & periosteal reaction

Imaging Recommendations

- Best imaging tool
  - **CECT** preferred imaging modality in suspected infection
    - MR less sensitive to dental infection & osteomyelitis
- Protocol advice
  - In setting of acutely infected patient with trismus, limited jaw movement, CECT viewed in soft tissue & bone algorithm is best imaging approach
    - Rapid scan time important for sick patient
    - Shows extent of soft tissue abscess cavity
    - Identifies offending tooth & extent of osteomyelitis if not obscured by dental amalgam or other metal artifact

DIFFERENTIAL DIAGNOSIS

Masticator Muscle Hypertrophy

- Clinical: Asymmetric chewing, TMJ dysfunction, or nocturnal grinding
- Imaging: Masticator muscles show unilateral enlargement
  - No focal, rim-enhancing fluid or other cellulitis, myositis, or fasciitis

Masticator Muscle Atrophy

- Clinical: CNV, mandibular branch injured
- Imaging: Muscle of mastication atrophy with normal side appearing enlarged

Cellulitis-Phlegmon of Masticator Space

- Clinical: Painful, swollen MS; same as with MS abscess
- Imaging: Swollen MS with cellulitis, myositis ± fasciitis **without** focal rim-enhancing fluid

Mandibular Osteoradionecrosis

- Clinical: History of H&N radiation therapy in last year
- Imaging: Permeative-destructive focal area of mandible bone
  - Soft tissue swelling may be associated
  - Rarely fluid with enhancing wall
    - When seen, may require needle aspiration to exclude infection

Sarcoma of Masticator Space

- Clinical: Rock-hard cheek mass ± CNV symptoms
- Imaging: Infiltrating MS mass with significant enhancement & minimal adjacent skin or soft tissue changes
  - Lacks cellulitis, myositis, or fasciitis that might suggest infection

TMJ Degenerative Disease

- Clinical: TMJ pain, trismus, or other symptoms of TMJ dysfunction
- Imaging: Degenerative findings in TMJ
  - No MS abscess seen

PATHOLOGY

General Features

- Etiology
  - Dental infection (molar) or dental treatment results in osteomyelitis of posterior body of mandible with cortical dehiscence rupturing pus into MS
- Anatomic considerations
  - Superficial layer, deep cervical fascia circumscribes MS tissues
  - MS contains muscles of mastication, posterior body, ramus & condyle of mandible, & V3 as it passes into mandibular foramen
  - 2nd & 3rd molar abut anterior surface of MS
  - Temporal fossa is actually suprazygomatic MS
  - Infratemporal fossa is nasopharyngeal MS + retromaxillary fat pad (high posterior buccal space)

Gross Pathologic & Surgical Features

- Irregular cystic lesion filled with green-white thick fluid (pus) surrounded by thick wall made up of fibrous connective tissue
- Surrounding tissues are edematous

CLINICAL ISSUES

Presentation

- Most common signs/symptoms
  - Principal symptom: **Trismus**
  - Other signs/symptoms
    - Fever, high white blood cell count
    - Tender, swollen cheek
    - History of **poor dentition**, 2nd or **3rd molar extraction**, or root canal therapy common
    - Physical exam: Tenderness & limited mouth opening makes examination difficult
    - CECT becomes critical part of physical exam when patient cannot open mouth
- Other signs/symptoms
  - Initial presentation may clinically mimic **TMJ dysfunction** (i.e., TMJ pain and trismus)

Demographics

- Age
  - Younger patients more likely to have periosteal reactions; periosteum loosely attached
  - Older patients more likely to be medically compromised → increased susceptibility to osteomyelitis
- Epidemiology
  - Common cause of MS lesion
  - In countries where antibiotics & dental care readily available, MS involvement rare
  - When dental care & antibiotics unavailable, MS abscess from dental decay is common affliction

Natural History & Prognosis

- Previous oral antibiotic treatment has inadequately treated simmering MS infection
- After termination of oral antibiotic, clinical recrudescence occurs
- Adequate drainage of pus loculi leads to rapid cure

Treatment

- Removal of involved molar(s) 1st line of treatment
- Aggressive intravenous antibiotics for early abscess
- Surgical drainage combined with intravenous antibiotics needed in most cases
- Mandibular osteomyelitis may require subperiosteal drain, removal of sequestra, & prolonged intravenous antibiotics

DIAGNOSTIC CHECKLIST

Consider

- Questions for radiologist to answer in MS abscess
  - Is mandibular osteomyelitis present
    - If so, requires more extensive surgical intervention & protracted antibiotic therapy
  - Is masticator space only space with abscess
    - Surgeon needs 1 drain in each affected space or break through adjacent fascia
  - Is suprazygomatic masticator space involved
    - Infection tends to spread upward because superficial layer, deep cervical fascia is firmly attached to inferior margin of mandible below

Image Interpretation Pearls

- Differentiate cellulitis in MS from abscess
- If subtle fluid seen, consider delayed CECT
  - Multidetector CT may finish data acquisition before contrast reaches abscess wall
  - If so, existing abscess may be missed

SELECTED REFERENCES

1. Sakamoto H et al: A case of brain abscess extended from deep fascial space infection. Oral Surg Oral Med Oral Pathol Oral Radiol Endod. 108(3):e21-5, 2009
2. Hasegawa T et al: Two cases of masticator space abscess initially diagnosed as temporomandibular joint disorder. Kobe J Med Sci. 54(3):E163-8, 2008
3. Schuknecht B et al: Masticator space abscess derived from odontogenic infection: imaging manifestation and pathways of extension depicted by CT and MR in 30 patients. Eur Radiol. 18(9):1972-9, 2008
4. Jones KC et al: Chronic submasseteric abscess: anatomic, radiologic, and pathologic features. AJNR Am J Neuroradiol. 24(6):1159-63, 2003
5. Bratton TA et al: Management of complex multi-space odontogenic infections. J Tenn Dent Assoc. 82(3):39-47, 2002
6. Plaza Mayor G et al: Is conservative treatment of deep neck space infections appropriate? Head Neck. 23(2):126-33, 2001
7. Yuan WH et al: Image evaluation of suprazygomatic masticator space lesions. Kaohsiung J Med Sci. 17(3):139-49, 2001
8. Sivarajasingam V et al: Ultrasound-guided needle aspiration of lateral masticator space abscess. Oral Surg Oral Med Oral Pathol Oral Radiol Endod. 88(5):616-9, 1999
9. Yonetsu K et al: Deep facial infections of odontogenic origin: CT assessment of pathways of space involvement. AJNR Am J Neuroradiol. 19(1):123-8, 1998
10. Ginsberg LE: Inflammatory and infectious lesions of the neck. Semin Ultrasound CT MR. 18(3):205-19, 1997
11. Kim HJ et al: Odontogenic versus nonodontogenic deep neck space infections: CT manifestations. J Comput Assist Tomogr. 21(2):202-8, 1997
12. Chong VF et al: Pictorial review: radiology of the masticator space. Clin Radiol. 51(7):457-65, 1996

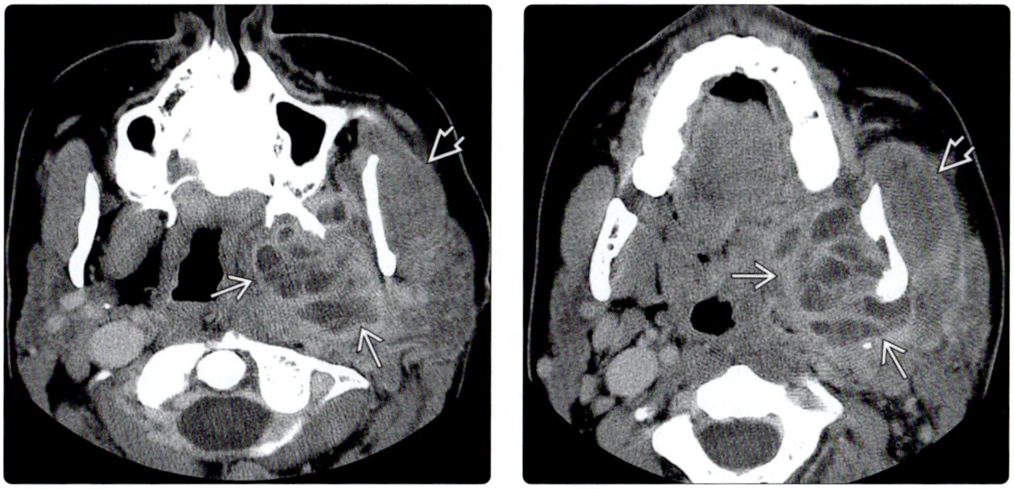

(Left) *Axial CECT demonstrates a large, multiloculated medial MS abscess involving the pterygoid musculature ➡. Note edema and swelling in the masseter muscle in the lateral masticator space ➡. The patient is a 21 year old who underwent a left molar tooth extraction 9 months previously. Since then, she has complained of trismus and otalgia misdiagnosed as TMJ syndrome.* **(Right)** *Axial CECT in the same patient shows further inferior extent of medial MS abscess ➡ and masseter edema ➡.*

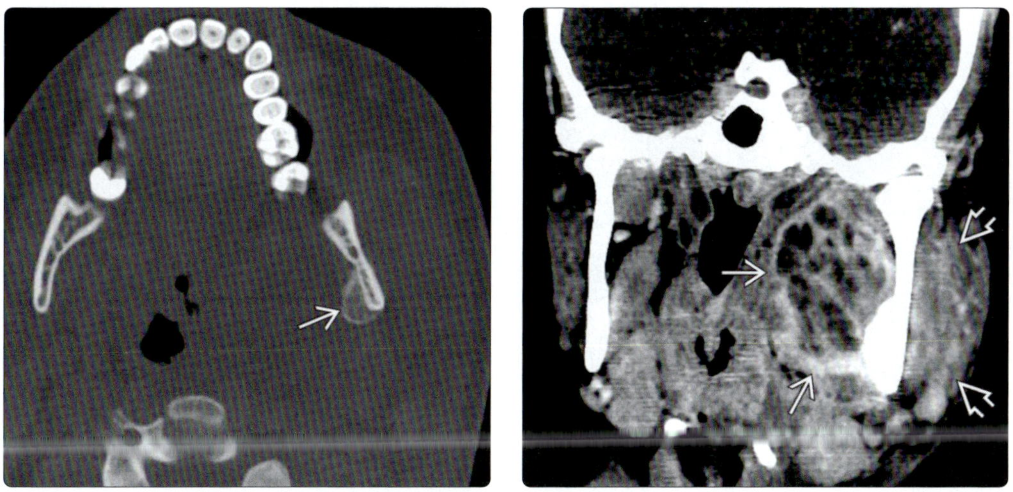

(Left) *Axial bone CT in the same patient reveals periosteal new bone formation indicative of mandibular osteomyelitis ➡.* **(Right)** *Coronal CECT in the same patient demonstrates medial masticator space multiloculated abscess ➡ and lateral masticator space masseter muscle edema and enlargement ➡.*

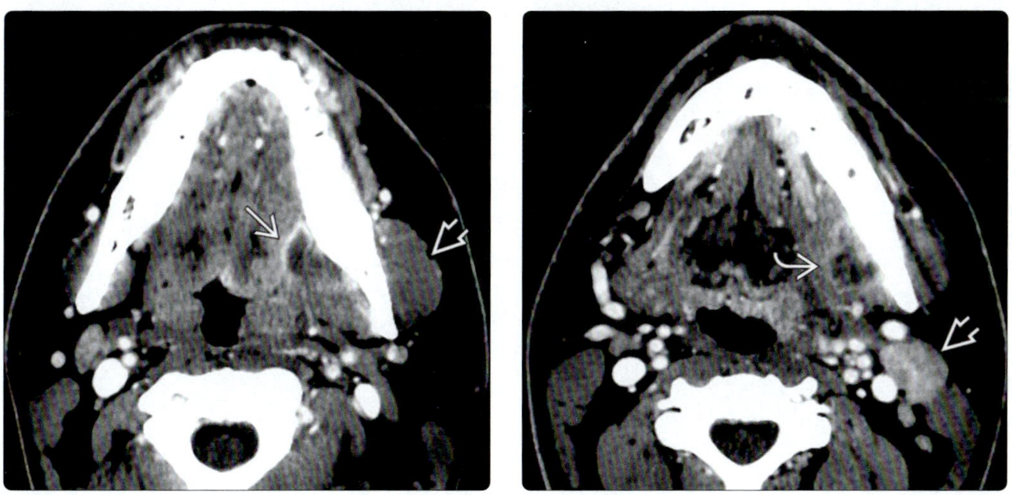

(Left) *Axial CECT demonstrates left medial masticator space abscess involving the inferior aspect of the medial pterygoid muscle ➡ with masseter muscle myositis ➡. Patient is a 22 year old with an infected molar tooth not responding to antibiotic treatment, presenting with pain, swelling, and trismus.* **(Right)** *Axial CECT in the same patient reveals inferior spread of abscess into the left submandibular space ➡. Level II reactive lymphadenopathy is also seen ➡.*

Masticator Muscle Atrophy

KEY FACTS

TERMINOLOGY

- Alteration in appearance of muscle groups from loss of innervation by mandibular nerve
    - Mandibular nerve = 3rd division (CNV3) of trigeminal nerve (CNV); only division with motor function
- Denervation pattern identified
    - **Acute** (< 1 month): Muscles slightly enlarged with edema; enhancement seen
    - **Subacute** (1-12 months): Fatty replacement & atrophy begin
    - **Chronic** (12-20 months): Fatty atrophic muscles with significant volume loss

IMAGING

- Acute: Increased T2 signal intensity with edema of muscles & abnormal contrast enhancement
- Subacute: T2 prolongation & abnormal contrast enhancement with early fatty replacement
- Chronic: Fatty infiltration of muscles with volume loss of muscles of mastication
- Location: **Masticator space** (muscles of mastication), nasopharynx (tensor veli palatini), & floor of mouth (anterior belly digastric & mylohyoid)

PATHOLOGY

- Malignant or benign tumors involving CNV3
- Surgical trauma 2nd most frequent cause

CLINICAL ISSUES

- May present as difficulty chewing or facial asymmetry

DIAGNOSTIC CHECKLIST

- 1st: Determine that CNV3 denervation is present by analyzing muscles involved
- 2nd: Determine cause of CNV3 denervation
- Review history for episodes of trauma or surgery
- If none, malignant tumor must be excluded
    - Search for CNV3 perineural tumor

(Left) *Axial T2WI FS MR demonstrates increased signal in the pterygoid muscles → & deep portion of the temporalis muscle →. Mastoid opacification → indicates eustachian tube obstruction due to tensor veli palatini dysfunction. This patient had meningioma in Meckel cave (not shown).* **(Right)** *Coronal T1WI C+ FS MR in the same patient shows mild pterygoid muscle enhancement → as well as small size of left torus tubarius →, consistent with subacute denervation atrophy of CNV3.*

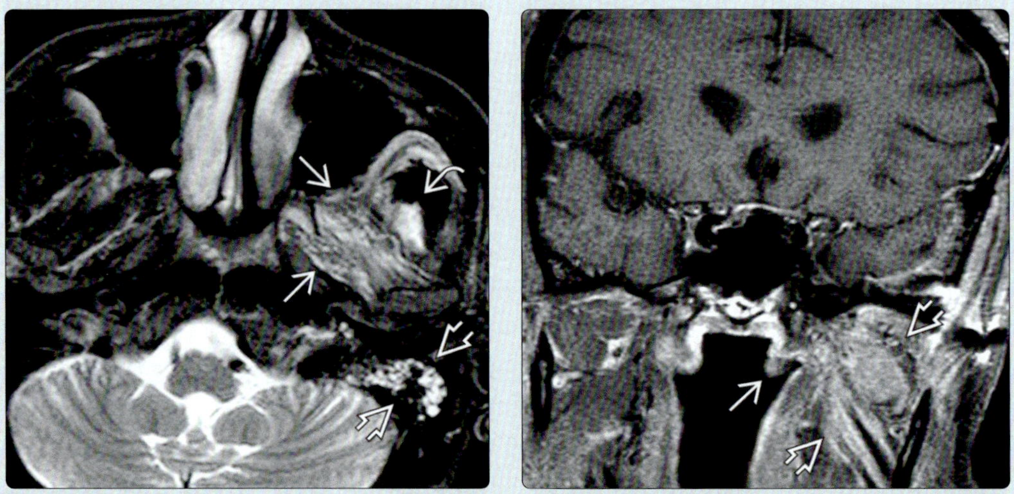

(Left) *Coronal T1WI MR reveals chronic fatty atrophy of the left temporalis → & masseter → muscles, indicating CNV3 injury. Left mylohyoid muscle is also small with fatty infiltration compared to the normal right muscle →.* **(Right)** *Axial T1WI MR in the same patient demonstrates the normal right mylohyoid muscle → & platysma muscle →. Their absence on the left indicates that both CNV3 (mylohyoid) & CNVII (platysma) are chronically injured.*

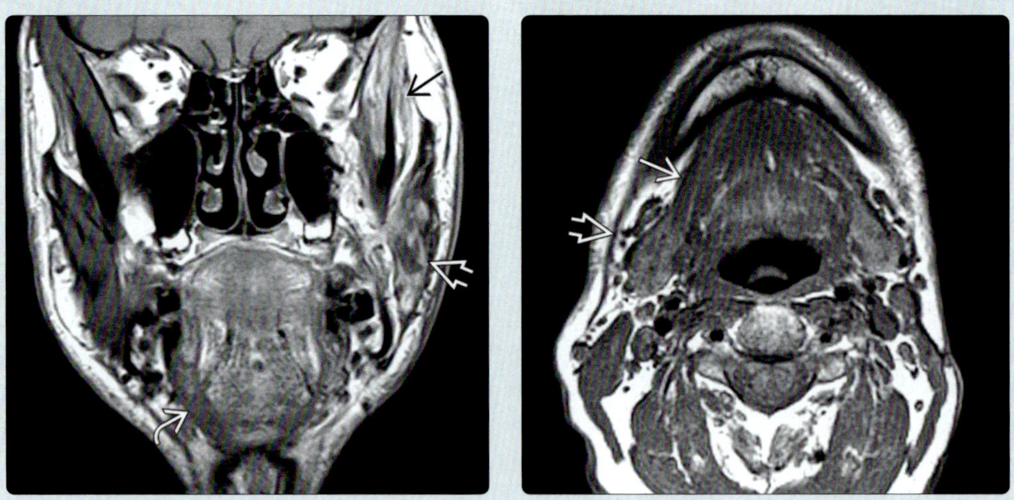

Masticator Muscle Atrophy

TERMINOLOGY

Synonyms

- Denervation atrophy

Definitions

- Alteration in appearance of muscle groups from loss of innervation by mandibular nerve
  - Mandibular nerve = 3rd division (CNV3) of trigeminal nerve (CNV); only division with motor function
- **CNV3 motor innervation**
  - Muscles of mastication
    - Medial & lateral pterygoid, masseter, & temporalis muscles
  - Tensor muscles
    - Tensor veli palatini & tensor tympani muscles
  - Floor of mouth muscles
    - Mylohyoid & anterior belly digastric muscles
- Denervation pattern identified
  - **Acute** (< 1 month): Muscles slightly enlarged with edema; enhancement seen
  - **Subacute** (1-12 months): Fatty replacement & atrophy begin
  - **Chronic** (12-20 months): Fatty atrophic muscles with significant volume loss

IMAGING

General Features

- Best diagnostic clue
  - Acute: Increased T2 signal intensity with edema of muscles & abnormal contrast enhancement
  - Subacute: T2 prolongation & abnormal contrast enhancement with early fatty replacement
  - Chronic: Fatty infiltration of muscles with volume loss of muscles of mastication
- Location
  - Most frequently unilateral process
  - **Masticator space** (muscles of mastication), nasopharynx (tensor veli palatini), & floor of mouth (anterior belly digastric & mylohyoid)
- Size
  - Acute: Muscles slightly enlarged
  - Subacute: Muscles may be normal size
  - Chronic: Muscles atrophic
- Morphology
  - Initially muscle edema, later fatty replacement & atrophy

CT Findings

- CECT
  - Acute & subacute V3 denervation atrophy
    - Altered density & enhancement may be difficult to identify
  - Chronic V3 denervation atrophy
    - Fatty atrophic change readily evident

MR Findings

- T1WI
  - Acute: Reduced muscle signal intensity from edema
  - Subacute: Increased signal intensity starts with fatty replacement
  - Chronic: Increased signal intensity with fatty atrophy
- T2WI
  - Acute: Increased T2 signal intensity of muscles (edema)
  - Subacute: Increased T2 signal intensity (early fat)
  - Chronic: Volume loss & fatty infiltration
- T1WI C+
  - **Acute**: Muscle **enhancement**
  - Subacute: Muscle enhancement more subtle
  - Chronic: No contrast enhancement

Imaging Recommendations

- Best imaging tool
  - MR best characterizes changes of muscles
    - Most sensitive to altered contrast enhancement
  - CT readily identifies chronic fatty atrophic changes
    - Relatively insensitive to earlier changes
- Protocol advice
  - Fat saturation/STIR makes ↑ T2 signal more evident
  - Contrast distinguishes acute & subacute from chronic

DIFFERENTIAL DIAGNOSIS

Masticator Muscle Hypertrophy

- Clinical: TMJ dysfunction or bruxism (nocturnal teeth grinding)
- CT/MR: Normal side appears too small compared to hypertrophic muscles
  - Masseter most frequently enlarged of masticator muscles
  - Mylohyoid, anterior belly digastric not affected
  - Normal muscle signal intensity & no abnormal contrast enhancement

Masticator Space Perineural Tumor, V3

- Clinical: Usually from squamous cell carcinoma of chin skin, mandibular alveolar ridge, deep palatine tonsil
- CT/MR: Thickened, enhancing CNV3
  - If nerve injury present, perineural tumor & V3 motor atrophy may coexist

Masticator Space Abscess

- Clinical: Presents with pain, fever, & elevated WBC
- CT/MR: Will not involve all muscle groups
  - Look particularly at temporalis, mylohyoid, & digastric muscles
  - Look for dental source of infection

Masticator Space Chondrosarcoma

- Clinical: History of new or treated deep facial malignancy
- CT/MR: Will not involve all muscle groups

PATHOLOGY

General Features

- Etiology
  - Malignant or benign tumors involving mandibular division CNV
  - Surgical trauma 2nd most frequent cause
  - Hemifacial atrophy can rarely occur from unilateral bulbar poliomyelitis infection
- Associated abnormalities
  - Other cranial nerves may also be affected

    - CNVII, X, XI, ± XII (depending on size/location of offending lesion)
- 2 denervation patterns recognized
  - Injury to CNV3 **proximal to** masticator nerve ramification (occurs just after CNV3 emerges from foramen ovale)
    - All muscles innervated by CNV3 undergo stages of atrophy
      - Medial & lateral pterygoid, masseter, temporalis
      - Tensor veli palatini & tensor tympani
      - Mylohyoid & anterior belly digastric
  - **Distal to** mandibular-masticator nerve bifurcation
    - Mylohyoid & anterior belly digastric muscles alone undergo stages of atrophy
    - Muscles of mastication spared
  - May be helpful in identifying site of injury
    - If only mylohyoid & anterior belly of digastric muscle involved, lesion is between skull base & mandibular foramen
    - If all CNV3-innervated muscles involved, lesion is between root exit zone of lateral pons & foramen ovale

Gross Pathologic & Surgical Features

- Loss of muscle bulk & tone with fatty change

Microscopic Features

- Denervated muscle shows relatively increased tissue water
- Atrophy of muscle fibers develops in subacute to chronic phases with fatty infiltration
- Denervated, atrophic muscle shows greater concentration of capillaries for muscle volume

CLINICAL ISSUES

Presentation

- Most common signs/symptoms
  - Difficulty chewing
  - In chronic atrophy, facial asymmetry from masseter muscle volume loss visible
  - Denervation difficult to detect clinically
    - Paralysis, loss of tone & reflexes, fasciculations
  - STIR MR signal intensity changes precede electromyography changes
- Other signs/symptoms
  - Serous otitis media from eustachian tube dysfunction with tensor veli palatini denervation

Demographics

- Age
  - Adults due to prevalence of H&N tumors & surgery
- Epidemiology
  - CNV most frequent of cranial nerves to show motor denervation

Natural History & Prognosis

- With peripheral neuropathies, acute & subacute changes may resolve spontaneously or with nerve grafting
  - Not so with cranial neuropathies
  - Cranial nerve grafting does not significantly reverse V3 atrophy
- Acute denervation signal intensity & contrast enhancement pattern expected to progress to chronic pattern with time

Treatment

- No effective treatment

DIAGNOSTIC CHECKLIST

Consider

- If CNV3 atrophy discovered without known cause, search for causal lesion must be completed

Image Interpretation Pearls

- First determine that V3 denervation is present by analyzing muscles involved
  - Look at all muscles innervated by CNV3
    - Muscles of mastication
    - Mylohyoid, anterior belly digastric muscles
    - Tensor veli palatini dysfunction → small torus tubarius & ipsilateral middle ear/mastoid fluid
    - Tensor tympani dysfunction not apparent by imaging
- Next, determine cause of CNV3 denervation
  - Review history for obvious episodes of trauma or surgery
    - If none, malignant tumor must be excluded
      - Check for perineural CNV3 malignancy
      - Check for masticator space malignancy
      - Follow course of CNV from lateral pons to mandibular foramen
- Finally, look for MR evidence of other cranial nerve dysfunction (especially CNVII, X-XII)

SELECTED REFERENCES

1. Wilson MH et al: Focal atrophy of the masticatory muscles caused by pure trigeminal motor neuropathy: case report. Br J Oral Maxillofac Surg. 54(1):e13-4, 2016
2. Chiba M et al: Unilateral atrophy of the masticatory muscles and mandibular ramus due to pure trigeminal motor neuropathy: a case report. Oral Surg Oral Med Oral Pathol Oral Radiol. 113(6):e30-4, 2012
3. Chong V: Imaging the cranial nerves in cancer. Cancer Imaging. 4 Spec No A:S1-5, 2004
4. Ho TL et al: Subacute mandibular and hypoglossal nerve denervation causing oedema of the masticator space and tongue. Neuroradiology. 45(4):262-6, 2003
5. Ariji Y et al: Denervation atrophy of the masticatory muscles in a patient with nasopharyngeal cancer: MR examinations before and after radiotherapy. Dentomaxillofac Radiol. 31(3): 204-8, 2002
6. Fischbein NJ et al: MR imaging in two cases of subacute denervation change in the muscles of facial expression. AJNR Am J Neuroradiol. 22(5):880-4, 2001
7. Antoniades K et al: Hemifacial atrophy secondary to poliomyelitis. Int J Oral Maxillofac Surg. 26(3):215-6, 1997
8. Russo CP et al: MR appearance of trigeminal and hypoglossal motor denervation. AJNR Am J Neuroradiol. 18(7):1375-83, 1997
9. Petersilge CA et al: Denervation hypertrophy of muscle: MR features. J Comput Assist Tomogr. 19(4): 596-600, 1995
10. West GA et al: Magnetic resonance imaging signal changes in denervated muscles after peripheral nerve injury. Neurosurgery. 35(6): 1077-85; discussion 1085-6, 1994
11. Fleckenstein JL et al: Denervated human skeletal muscle: MR imaging evaluation. Radiology. 187(1):213-8, 1993
12. Uetani M et al: Denervated skeletal muscle: MR imaging. Work in progress. Radiology. 189(2): 511-5, 1993
13. Schellhas KP: MR imaging of muscles of mastication. AJR Am J Roentgenol. 153(4):847-55, 1989
14. Polak JF et al: Magnetic resonance imaging of skeletal muscle. Prolongation of T1 and T2 subsequent to denervation. Invest Radiol. 23(5): 365-9, 1988
15. Shabas D et al: Magnetic resonance imaging examination of denervated muscle. Comput Radiol. 11(1): 9-13, 1987
16. Harnsberger HR et al: Major motor atrophic patterns in the face and neck: CT evaluation. Radiology. 155(3):665-70, 1985

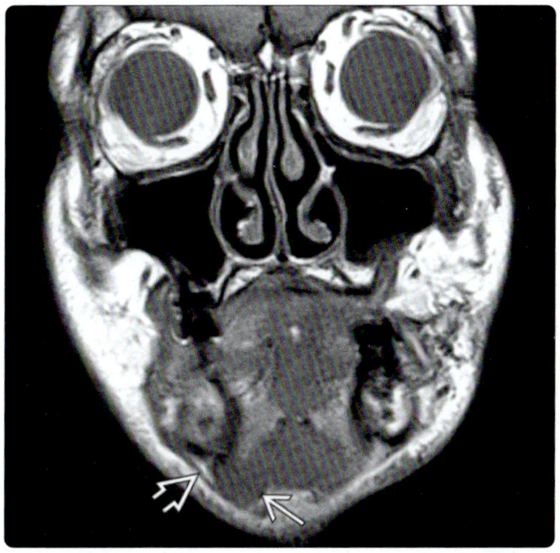

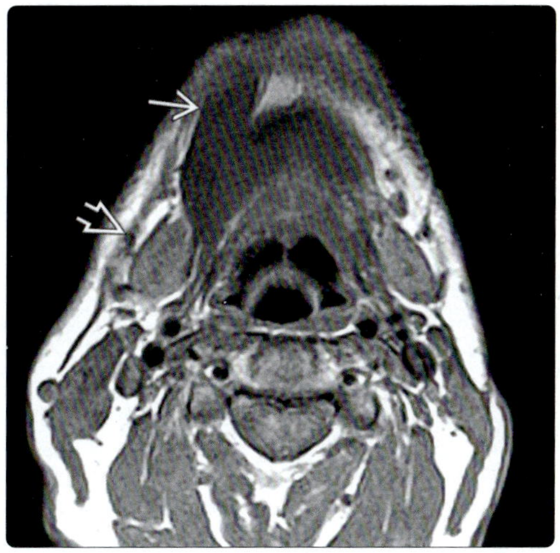

(Left) *Coronal T1WI MR reveals normal right anterior belly of digastric muscle ➡ & platysma muscle ➡. The left-sided mylohyoid & platysma are unseen as a result of chronic CNV3 & CNVII injury, respectively.* **(Right)** *Axial T1WI MR in the same patient shows a normal right anterior belly of digastric muscle ➡ & normal platysma muscle ➡. Both muscles on the left have undergone fatty atrophy & are not visible. Skull base malignant tumor was found affecting the foramen ovale & geniculate fossa.*

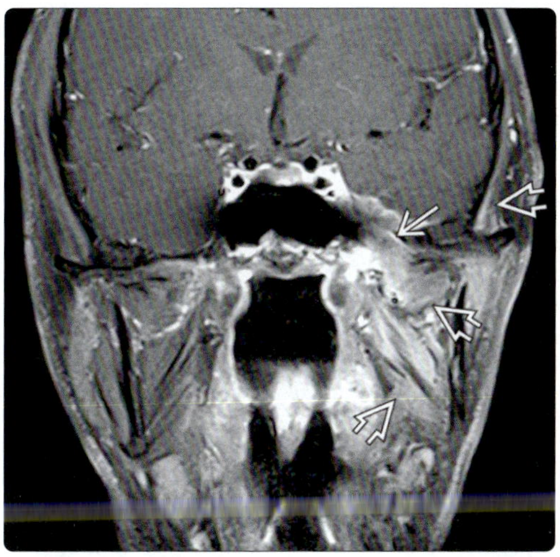

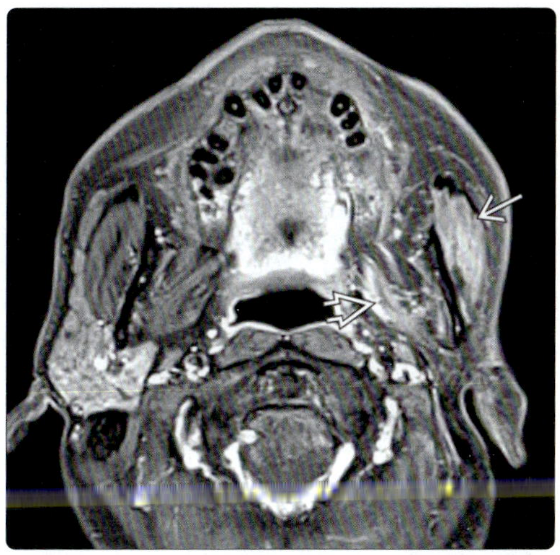

(Left) *Coronal T1WI C+ FS MR reveals adenoid cystic carcinoma spreading intracranially through the foramen ovale ➡. Subacute masticator muscle denervation ➡ causes muscle enhancement.* **(Right)** *Axial T1WI C+ FS MR in the same patient demonstrates the masseter ➡ & lateral pterygoid ➡ muscle enhancement typical of subacute denervation. The muscles are beginning to lose volume, indicating that they are in the late subacute phase of denervation.*

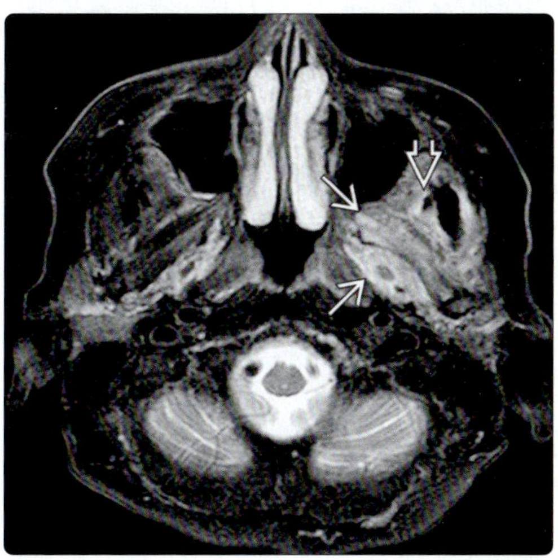

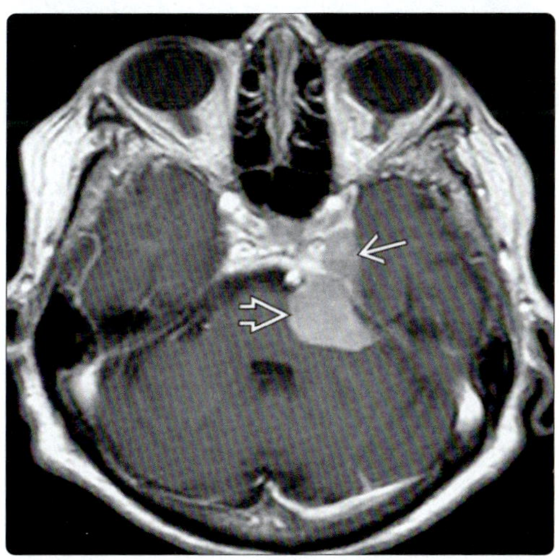

(Left) *Axial T2WI FS MR demonstrates T2 hyperintensity & swelling in the pterygoid ➡ & temporalis ➡ muscles, indicating acute to subacute denervation atrophy.* **(Right)** *Axial T1WI C+ MR in the same patient shows cavernous sinus ➡ & prepontine cistern ➡ meningioma, which is the cause of the denervation changes.*

Masticator Space CNV3 Schwannoma

KEY FACTS

TERMINOLOGY

- Abbreviations: Masticator space (MS), mandibular branch of trigeminal nerve (CNV3)
- Definition: Encapsulated tumor of Schwann cell origin, which displaces rather than infiltrates fascicles of CNV3 in MS

IMAGING

- CBCT & bone CT findings
  - Smooth enlargement of bony foramen involved
  - Foramen ovale most commonly enlarged by CNV3 schwannoma
  - Mandibular foramen, inferior alveolar nerve canal, or mental foramen enlargement occurs when rarer distal CNV3 schwannoma present
- Enhanced MR findings
  - Homogeneous or heterogeneous enhancement
  - Intramural cysts are characteristic of schwannoma
  - Masticator muscle atrophy possible

TOP DIFFERENTIAL DIAGNOSES

- CNV3 neurofibroma
- Perineural tumor CNV3 in MS
- CNV3 malignant nerve sheath tumor
- MS sarcoma
- Hemangioma

CLINICAL ISSUES

- Most common asymptomatic mass in deep facial soft tissues; even large lesions may be asymptomatic

DIAGNOSTIC CHECKLIST

- Determine whether patient has neurofibromatosis type 2
- MS mass without history of H&N squamous cell carcinoma or sepsis (MS abscess) should suggest MS sarcoma
- Smaller, low-grade sarcoma may mimic V3 schwannoma if centered on V3
- Well-circumscribed, fusiform, or ovoid mass following course of V3 suggests V3 schwannoma diagnosis

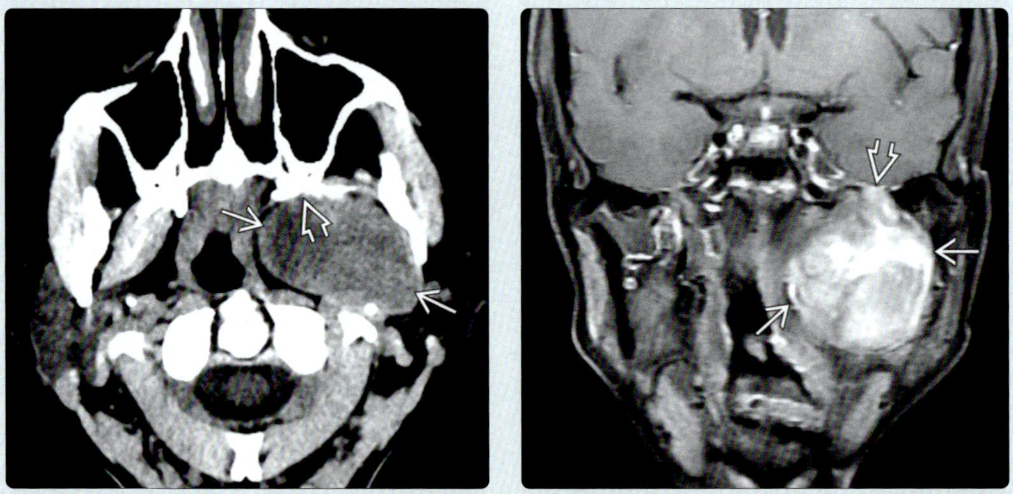

(Left) *Axial NECT in a patient with CNV3 schwannoma shows a circumscribed, heterogeneous solid mass in the left masticator space ➡ with remodeling of the pterygoid plates ➡ suggesting a slow-growing lesion.* **(Right)** *Coronal T1-enhanced fat-saturated MR in the same patient shows a heterogeneously enhancing masticator space schwannoma ➡ minimally projecting intracranially through an enlarged foramen ovale ➡.*

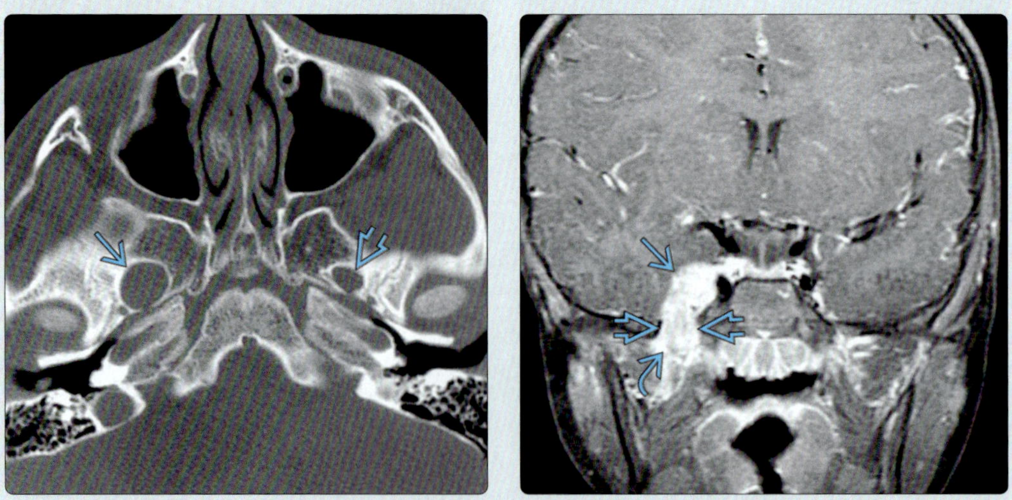

(Left) *Axial bone CT in a patient with known neurofibromatosis type 2 reveals a large right foramen ovale ➡. Note the normal left foramen ovale ➡. This foraminal enlargement with preservation of its cortical margin is characteristic of benign nerve sheath tumors.* **(Right)** *Coronal T1-enhanced fat-saturated MR in the same patient shows a tubular, enhancing CNV3 schwannoma coursing from the parasellar region ➡ through the enlarged foramen ovale ➡ and into the nasopharyngeal masticator space ➡.*

Masticator Space CNV3 Schwannoma

TERMINOLOGY

Abbreviations

- Masticator space (MS), mandibular branch of trigeminal nerve (CNV3)

Synonyms

- Neuroma, neurilemmoma, neurinoma

Definitions

- Encapsulated tumor of Schwann cell, which displaces rather than infiltrates fascicles of CNV3 in MS

IMAGING

General Features

- Best diagnostic clue
  - Sharply & smoothly marginated soft tissue mass along course of CNV3 branch of CN5
- Location
  - From Meckel cave to MS along CNV3
  - Rarely affects CNV3 branches (inferior alveolar or mental nerves)
- Size
  - Variable, from < 1 cm to 3-4 cm in diameter
- Morphology
  - Ovoid to fusiform/tubular

Radiographic Findings

- Radiography
  - Enlargement of inferior alveolar nerve canal or mental foramen on 2D imaging, panoramic, or periapical films

CT Findings

- CECT
  - Lesion enhances mildly to moderately
  - Homogeneous or heterogeneous enhancement
- CBCT & bone CT
  - **Smooth enlargement** of involved bony foramen
    - **Foramen ovale** most commonly enlarged
    - Mandibular foramen, inferior alveolar nerve canal, or mental foramen may show enlargement when rarer distal V3 schwannoma present

MR Findings

- T1WI
  - Iso- or hypointense to muscles of mastication
  - Hyperintense areas if hemorrhage present
  - Masticator muscle atrophy (↑ signal fat + ↓ volume)
- T2WI
  - Variable, iso- to hyperintense
    - More cellular tumors, isointense to muscle
  - Myxoid or cystic changes: ↑ signal intensity
  - Foci of hypointensity common in larger tumors
- T1WI C+
  - Homogeneous or heterogeneous enhancement
    - **Intramural cysts** somewhat characteristic
  - Sometimes rim enhances; appear mostly cystic

Imaging Recommendations

- Best imaging tool
  - T1WI C+ MR with fat sat in axial & coronal plane

DIFFERENTIAL DIAGNOSIS

CNV3 Neurofibroma

- Neurofibromatosis type 1 (NF1); rarely isolated

Perineural Tumor CNV3 in Masticator Space

- Known squamous cell carcinoma from chin skin, mandibular alveolar ridge, oral tongue, oropharynx

CNV3 Malignant Nerve Sheath Tumor

- Invasive mass centered on CNV3 within MS

Masticator Space Sarcoma

- More aggressive bony changes in adjacent mandible, zygomatic arch

Hemangioma

- Enlarged mandibular canal appears **serpiginous**

PATHOLOGY

General Features

- Etiology
  - Unknown in sporadic cases
- Genetics
  - Associated with NF2
    - Mutation on chromosome 22
    - Bilateral acoustic & peripheral schwannomas

Microscopic Features

- Proliferating Schwann cells in collagenous matrix with fibrous capsule
- 2 Antoni tissue types (may coexist in single lesion)
  - Antoni A type: Compact, hypercellular
  - Antoni B type: Looser architecture; cystic changes
- Cystic degeneration (intramural cysts) common

CLINICAL ISSUES

Presentation

- Most common signs/symptoms
  - Most common asymptomatic mass in deep facial soft tissues; even large lesions may be asymptomatic
  - Other signs/symptoms
    - Atypical facial pain, ↓ chin sensation

Demographics

- Age
  - Predominantly 3rd-4th decades
  - Younger in patients with NF2
- Epidemiology
  - Peripheral CNV3 schwannomas: 5% of all trigeminal schwannomas

Natural History & Prognosis

- Gradually enlarging MS mass

Treatment

- Surgical resection
- Gamma knife

SELECTED REFERENCES

1. Younes M et al: [Inferior alveolar nerve malignant schwannoma.] Rev Stomatol Chir Maxillofac. 113(6):465-7, 2012

Masticator Space Chondrosarcoma

KEY FACTS

TERMINOLOGY

- Masticator space chondrosarcoma (CS-MS)

IMAGING

- Soft tissue mass in MS adjacent to mandible with variable calcification pattern
- In mandible, molar region and ramus most frequent
- May extend down from skull base or temporomandibular joint (TMJ)
- CT shows characteristic calcifications, but MR better delineates extent of tumor
- Bone CT findings
  - Radiolucent lesion ± areas of calcification
  - **Rings and crescents of calcification**: Low-grade tumors
  - Amorphous or no calcification: High-grade tumors
  - Periosteal reaction usually mild, if present
- MR findings
  - Greater T1 C+ enhancement in high-grade CS
  - T1 C+ heterogeneous, predominantly peripheral enhancement
  - Invasion of bone best delineated on C-T1
  - High signal typical on T2

TOP DIFFERENTIAL DIAGNOSES

- MS infection
- TMJ synovial chondromatosis
- Mandibular osteosarcoma

CLINICAL ISSUES

- Expanding painless preauricular mass

DIAGNOSTIC CHECKLIST

- Unless characteristic calcifications seen, variable appearance of CS makes precise diagnosis difficult
- Infection far more common than sarcoma in MS
- If no calcifications, consider infection 1st
- MS masses should be followed to resolution to ensure that they are not sarcomas

(Left) *Axial T1WI MR shows an intermediate-signal mass ➡ distending the masticator space and causing anterior bowing of the posterior wall of the left maxillary sinus ➡. A large focal calcification is seen as low signal intensity ➡ on all sequences.* **(Right)** *Axial T2WI MR in the same patient shows the mass ➡ with characteristic pronounced T2 hyperintensity of chondroid tumors.*

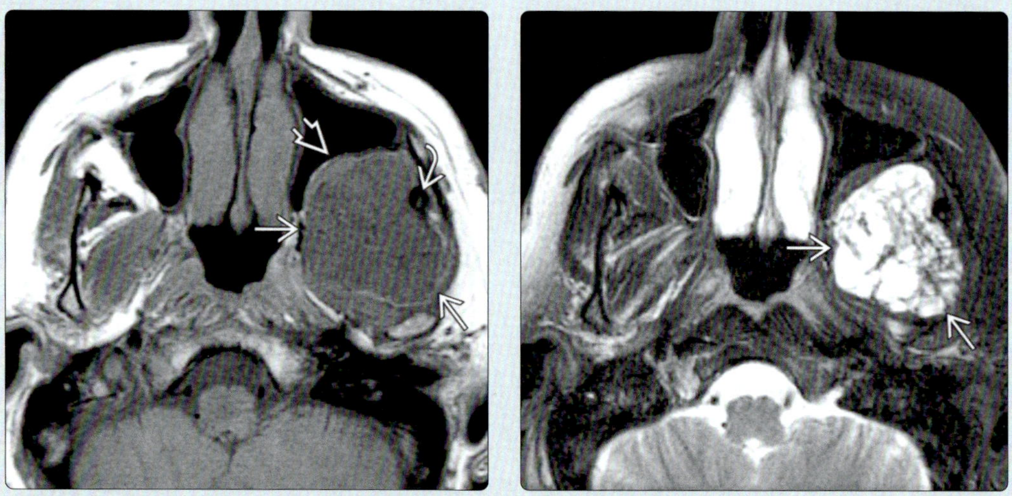

(Left) *Axial T1WI C+ MR in the same patient shows the tumor ➡ is generally heterogeneous with intense enhancement with gadolinium.* **(Right)** *Axial CECT presented with bone window in the same patient shows a large mass with intrinsic calcifications ➡, which are "fluffy," with rings and arcs. These are typical of chondroid calcifications. Chondrosarcomas with visible chondroid calcifications usually indicate a low-grade tumor is present.*

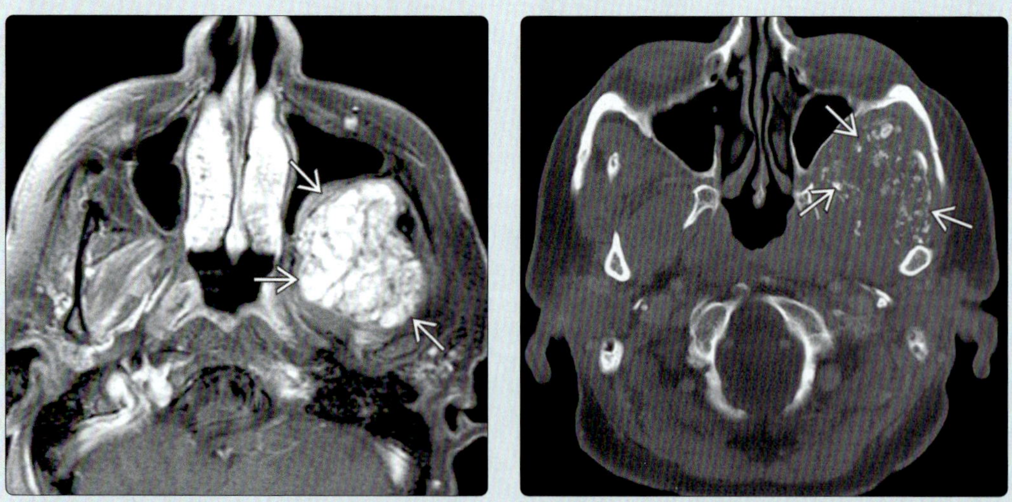

TERMINOLOGY

Abbreviations

- Masticator space chondrosarcoma (CS-MS)

Definitions

- Malignant tumor of cartilage that originates in masticator space

IMAGING

General Features

- Best diagnostic clue
  - Soft tissue mass in MS adjacent to mandible with variable calcification pattern
- Location
  - Adjacent to (inseparable from) bone of origin
  - In mandible, molar region and ramus most frequent
  - May extend down from skull base or temporomandibular joint (TMJ)
- Size
  - At presentation, most > 3 cm
- Morphology
  - Round with lobular margin

Radiographic Findings

- Radiography
  - Widened periodontal ligament spaces, better visualized on panoramic and periapical radiographs

CT Findings

- CECT
  - Heterogeneous, predominantly peripheral enhancement
  - Mass with ill-defined borders and long zone of transition
- Bone CT
  - Shows radiolucent lesion ± areas of **calcification**
    - Presence and degree of calcification depends on tumor grade
    - **Rings and crescents** of calcium most characteristic of **low-grade tumors**
    - **Amorphous calcification** or no calcification seen in **high-grade tumors**
  - Erosion of bone of origin and surrounding bones (e.g., skull base)
  - Widening of joint (when arising from TMJ)
  - Periosteal reaction usually mild, if present

MR Findings

- T1WI
  - Homogeneous intermediate signal
  - Cartilage matrix or calcification make signal heterogeneous
  - Invasion of bone best delineated on unenhanced images
    - Replacement of marrow fat
- T2WI
  - **High signal** typical
  - Homogeneous or heterogeneous, depending on degree and type of calcification
  - Marrow, soft tissue edema may be seen
- T1WI C+
  - Enhancement may be focal (often peripheral) or diffuse
  - Extent of enhancement depends on tumor grade
    - Greater enhancement in high-grade CS

Imaging Recommendations

- Best imaging tool
  - CT shows characteristic calcifications, but MR better delineates extent of tumor
- Protocol advice
  - When using CECT, view bone windows
    - Bone CT most likely to show characteristic calcifications

DIFFERENTIAL DIAGNOSIS

Masticator Space Infection

- Most frequent cause of MS mass
- Usually of dental origin
- Noncalcifying CS-MS may mimic MS infection on imaging

Temporomandibular Joint Synovial Chondromatosis

- Calcified loose bodies in soft tissues around TMJ
- Grains of rice appearance
- Abnormalities usually confined to expanded synovial cavity but can erode skull base

Mandibular Osteosarcoma

- Most frequent MS sarcoma of bone
- Cumulus cloud pattern of new bone formation
- Sunburst pattern of periosteal reaction
- Osteosarcoma has poorer prognosis than CS-MS

Mandibular Metastasis

- Calcification seen in lung, prostate, breast, colon metastases
- Amorphous calcification of mucinous metastases may be confused with chondroid calcification
- Sites of metastasis include jaw, skull base, soft tissues

PATHOLOGY

General Features

- Etiology
  - CS-MS mostly sporadic (75%)
  - May be associated with other conditions or cases of benign chondroid tumors
    - Osteochondroma
    - Enchondroma
    - Ollier disease
    - Maffucci syndrome
    - Paget disease
    - Fibrous dysplasia
    - Synovial chondromatosis
    - Radiation exposure
    - Thorotrast exposure
- CS-MS may or may not occur at cartilaginous joints (TMJ)
  - TMJ CS represents tumoral differentiation of pluripotent mesenchymal cells

Staging, Grading, & Classification

- Osseous vs. extraosseous
- Central (medullary) vs. peripheral (juxtacortical)
- Primary vs. secondary (secondary associated with enchondroma or osteochondroma)
- Histological subtype

- Conventional
- Myxoid
- Clear cell
- Mesenchymal
- Dedifferentiated
- Histologic grade (degree if differentiation)
  - Grade I (well differentiated): Calcification and bone formation frequent
  - Grade II (moderately differentiated): Matrix more myxoid than chondroid
  - Grade III (poorly differentiated): No matrix, high mitotic rate (rare)

Gross Pathologic & Surgical Features

- Firm, nodular mass
- Tan-white to opalescent blue-gray
- Gross hemorrhage in high-grade tumors

Microscopic Features

- Matrix of lobular hyaline cartilage
- Multinucleated lacunes with variable nucleoli
- May be difficult to distinguish from chondroblastic osteosarcoma
- Low-grade neoplasms hard to distinguish from enchondroma

CLINICAL ISSUES

Presentation

- Most common signs/symptoms
  - Expanding painless preauricular mass
    - Rate of enlargement depends on tumor grade
    - May be mistaken for parotid mass
  - Other signs/symptoms
    - Headache
    - Loose or displaced teeth
    - CNV (V3) dysfunction
    - CSa arising from TMJ often painful

Demographics

- Age
  - Any, but 30-45 years most common
- Epidemiology
  - 2nd most common malignancy of bone (after osteosarcoma, excluding multiple myeloma)
  - CS: 15% of malignant bone tumors
  - 5-10% of CSa occur in head and neck
    - Larynx, jaws, facial bones, skull base, TMJ affected
    - Orbit more common location in children

Natural History & Prognosis

- Local recurrence problematic (50%)
  - Late recurrence (10-20 years) possible
- Metastases unusual (7%)
- 5-year overall survival: 68% (90% grade I; 50% combined grade II and III)
- Overall prognosis depends on tumor grade, size at presentation
- May dedifferentiate into osteosarcoma, malignant fibrous histiocytoma, or fibrosarcoma

Treatment

- Wide local excision
- Role of radiation, chemotherapy, cryosurgery, and immunotherapy are controversial and evolving

DIAGNOSTIC CHECKLIST

Consider

- Infection far more common than sarcoma in MS
  - If no calcifications, consider infection 1st
- If MS mass without clinical suggestion of infection, consider tumor as possibility
  - 1st consider perineural tumor on V3 from squamous cell carcinoma (SCCa) of chin skin, mandibular alveolar ridge, retromolar trigone
  - If no evidence for SCCa invasion of MS, then consider primary MS sarcoma

Image Interpretation Pearls

- MS masses should be followed to resolution to ensure that they are not sarcomas
- Unless characteristic calcifications seen, variable appearance of CS makes precise diagnosis difficult
  - Suggestion of tumor is critical; exact pathology can be determined at surgery

SELECTED REFERENCES

1. Coca-Pelaz A et al: Chondrosarcomas of the head and neck. Eur Arch Otorhinolaryngol. 271(10):2601-9, 2014
2. Pontes HA et al: Clinicopathological analysis of head and neck chondrosarcoma: three case reports and literature review. Int J Oral Maxillofac Surg. 41(2):203-10, 2012
3. Oliveira RC et al: Chondrosarcoma of the temporomandibular joint: a case report in a child. J Orofac Pain. 23(3):275-81, 2009
4. Acar GO et al: Chondrosarcoma of the mandible extending to the infratemporal fossa: report of two cases. Oral Maxillofac Surg. 12(3):173-6, 2008
5. Sammartino G et al: Chondrosarcoma of the jaw: a closer look at its management. J Oral Maxillofac Surg. 66(11):2349-55, 2008
6. Angiero F et al: Mesenchymal chondrosarcoma of the left coronoid process: report of a unique case with clinical, histopathologic, and immunohistochemical findings, and a review of the literature. Quintessence Int. 38(4):349-55, 2007
7. Saini R et al: Chondrosarcoma of the mandible: a case report. J Can Dent Assoc. 73(2):175-8, 2007
8. Van Damme PA et al: Juxtacortical chondrosarcoma of the mandible: report of a unique case and review of the literature. Int J Oral Maxillofac Surg. 34(1):94-8, 2005
9. Atanasov DT et al: Sarcomas of the mandible. Literature review and case reports. Folia Med (Plovdiv). 46(2):31-5, 2004
10. Bernasconi G et al: Parosteal chondrosarcoma, a very rare condition of the mandibular condyle. Clin Imaging. 28(1):64-8, 2004
11. Antonio SM et al: Mesenchymal chondrosarcoma presenting as an external auditory canal mass. Otol Neurotol. 24(2):344-5, 2003
12. Gorsky M et al: Craniofacial osseous and chondromatous sarcomas in British Columbia--a review of 34 cases. Oral Oncol. 36(1):27-31, 2000
13. Koch BB et al: National cancer database report on chondrosarcoma of the head and neck. Head Neck. 22(4):408-25, 2000
14. Saito K et al: Chondrosarcoma of the jaw and facial bones. Cancer. 76(9):1550-8, 1995
15. Takahashi K et al: Mesenchymal chondrosarcoma of the jaw--report of a case and review of 41 cases in the literature. Head Neck. 15(5):459-64, 1993
16. Wanebo HJ et al: Head and neck sarcoma: report of the Head and Neck Sarcoma Registry. Society of Head and Neck Surgeons Committee on Research. Head Neck. 14(1):1-7, 1992

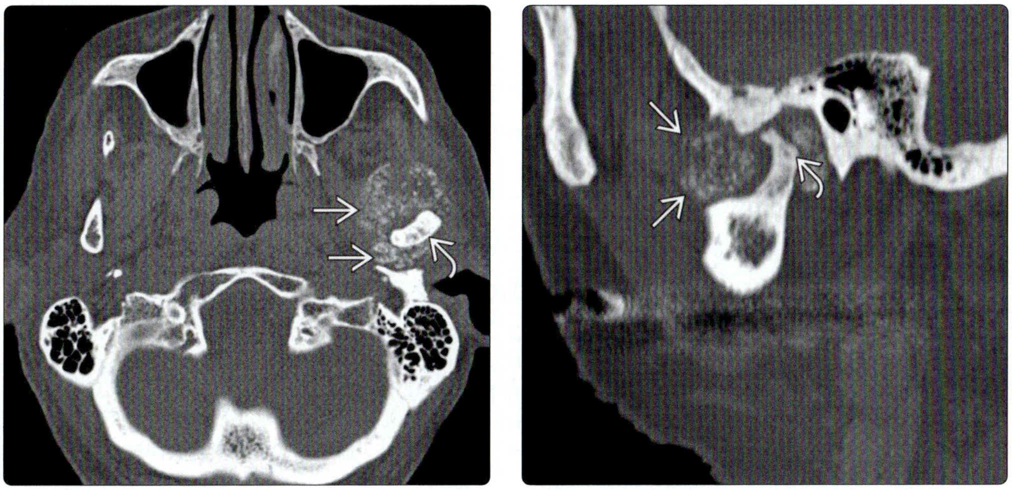

(Left) *Typical case of chondrosarcoma involving the TMJ with multiple calcific foci is shown. Axial bone CT through the left TMJ reveals irregular sclerotic appearance of mandibular condyle* ➡ *and multiple small, focal calcifications* ➡ *within and around the joint.* **(Right)** *Sagittal reformat in the same patient shows condylar deformity* ➡ *and also suggests that some of the calcifications* ➡ *reside within a soft tissue component outside the joint.*

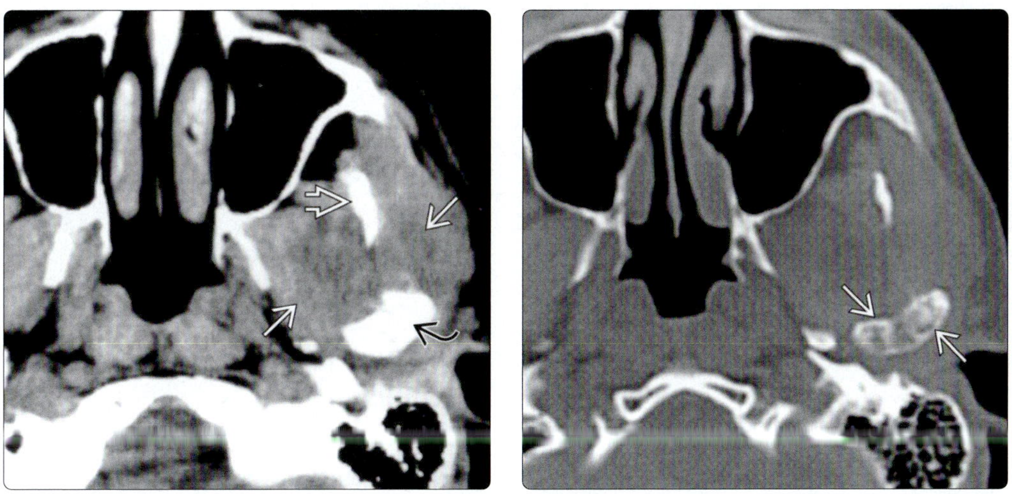

(Left) *Axial CECT with soft tissue window, in a variant case of masticator space chondrosarcoma without calcifications, shows a low-density mass* ➡ *surrounding the ramus of the mandible, extending around the coronoid process* ➡ *and condyle* ⇨*.* **(Right)** *Axial bone CT shows expansion of the condyle and neck of the mandible containing chondroid calcifications* ➡*. The absence of the characteristic calcifications of chondrosarcoma in the soft tissue component makes the diagnosis difficult in this case.*

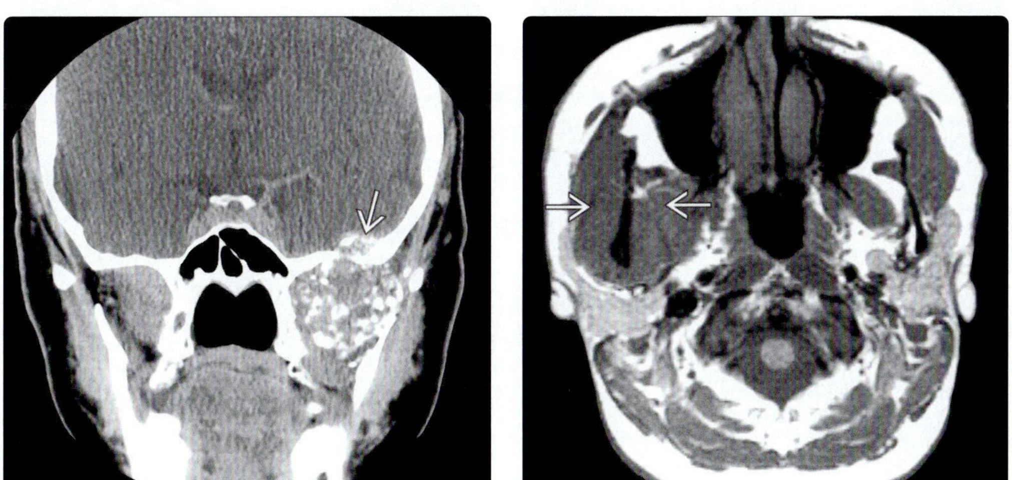

(Left) *Coronal CECT reveals a calcified masticator space mass extending through the skull base* ➡*. Calcification pattern is characteristic of well-differentiated chondrosarcoma.* **(Right)** *Axial T1WI MR shows an intermediate-signal mass* ➡ *surrounding the right mandibular ramus. This masticator space chondrosarcoma imaging appearance is nonspecific.*

Masticator Space Sarcoma

KEY FACTS

TERMINOLOGY

- Sarcoma, masticator space (Sa-MS): Malignant tumor of soft tissue origin (fat, muscle, nerve, joint, blood vessel, or deep skin tissues) in MS of suprahyoid neck

IMAGING

- Aggressive, poorly marginated MS mass with bone destruction and invasion of adjacent fascial planes/spaces
- Thin-section bone CT combined with T1 C+ MR
- Bone CT: Allows assessment of sarcoma matrix ± bone destructive changes
- MR: Evaluation of soft tissues, possible mandibular invasion
  - Perineural tumor spread along CNV3

TOP DIFFERENTIAL DIAGNOSES

- MS venous malformation
- MS abscess
- Mandibular osteomyelitis
- Invasive squamous cell carcinoma (SCCa)
  - Palatine tonsil SCCa
  - Retromolar trigone SCCa
- Perineural tumor of CNV3 in MS

CLINICAL ISSUES

- Enlarging soft tissue mass over mandible with increasing pain
- Mean age: 35 years old
- Sarcoma location, in addition to pathology and TNM stage, is important when planning treatment

DIAGNOSTIC CHECKLIST

- In absence of known systemic malignancy, head and neck malignancy, or septic symptoms (MS abscess), MS mass should suggest diagnosis of sarcoma
- **Symptoms of numbness along distribution of V3, masticator muscle paralysis, or increasing mandibular pain should alert clinician to possibility of Sa-MS**

(Left) *Axial CECT shows a large, heterogeneous, centrally necrotic mass with scattered coarse calcifications in the masticator space. The lesion surrounds the mandible and engulfs the medial and lateral pterygoid muscles, the temporalis, and the masseter muscle.* **(Right)** *Axial T1WI MR in the same patient shows the mass to be slightly hyperintense relative to the normal sternocleidomastoid muscle. Loss of marrow fat within the mandible suggests tumor infiltration.*

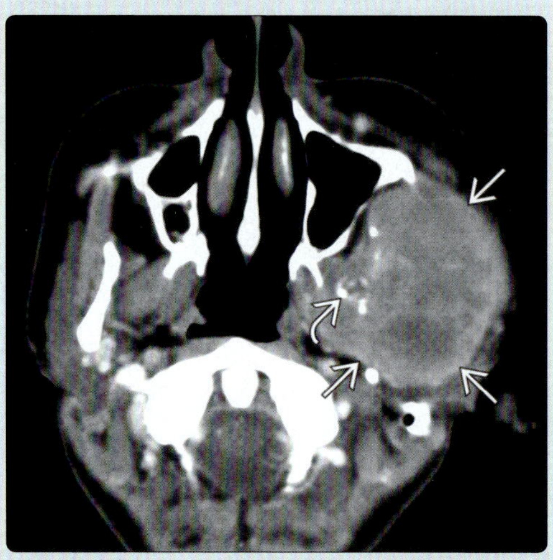

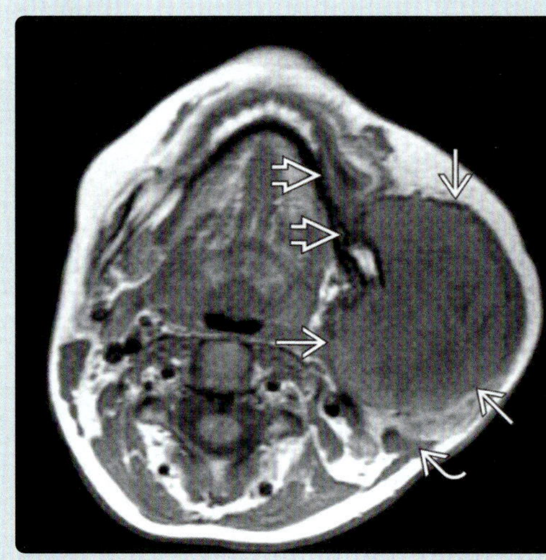

(Left) *Axial T2WI MR in the same patient shows the mass is diffusely increased in signal.* **(Right)** *Coronal T1WI C+ FS MR in the same patient shows heterogeneous enhancement of the mass. The mass abuts the skull base. This patient had a history of prior irradiation, putting the patient at risk for radiation-induced sarcomas. In this case, the lesion was an unusual tumor: An undifferentiated pleomorphic sarcoma.*

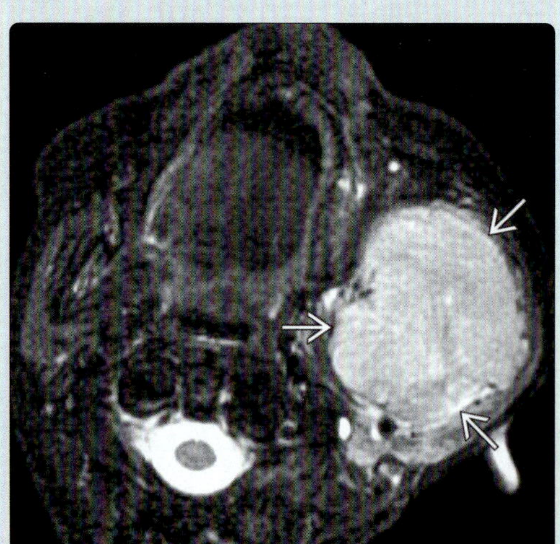

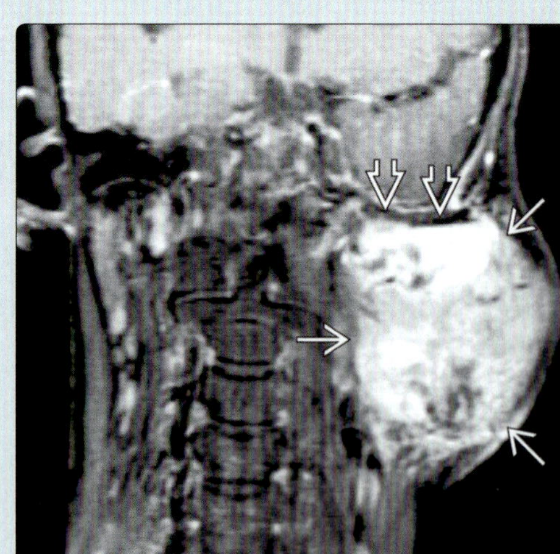

TERMINOLOGY

Synonyms

- Sarcoma, masticator space (Sa-MS)
- Sarcoma, other: Rhabdomyosarcoma, leiomyosarcoma, Ewing sarcoma, synovial sarcoma, liposarcoma, fibrosarcoma

Definitions

- Sa-MS: Malignant tumor of soft tissue origin (fat, muscle, nerve, joint, blood vessel, or deep skin tissues) in masticator space (MS) of suprahyoid neck

IMAGING

General Features

- Best diagnostic clue
  - Aggressive, poorly marginated MS mass with bone destruction and invasion of adjacent fascial planes/spaces
- Location
  - MS; frequently extends outside of MS
- Size
  - Often **large** (> 4 cm) despite superficial MS location
- Morphology
  - Poorly marginated ± multilobulated

CT Findings

- CECT
  - Variable enhancement pattern
    - Typically heterogeneous
- Bone CT
  - **Invasive MS mass** with mandibular, zygomatic arch, or pterygoid plate **destruction**
  - **Bone production** or **calcification** can be present in any sarcoma
    - Most commonly seen in osteosarcoma, chondrosarcoma, synovial sarcoma, and Ewing sarcoma
- CBCT
  - Same as bone CT with less soft tissue definition
  - Sometimes only clue to presence is effect on surrounding bone (e.g., periosteal reaction)

MR Findings

- T1WI
  - Iso- to hyperintense to normal muscle, often heterogeneous
  - Mandible involvement shows replacement of normal marrow signal
- T2WI
  - Heterogeneously hyperintense to muscle
- STIR
  - Heterogeneously hyperintense to muscle
- T1WI C+
  - Heterogeneous enhancement is typical

Nuclear Medicine Findings

- Bone scan
  - Tc-99m bone scans can assist with evaluation
- PET
  - F18 FDG avid
  - Role in directing biopsy, predicting tumor grade, and assessing treatment response under investigation

Imaging Recommendations

- Best imaging tool
  - Thin-section bone CT combined with T1 C+ MR
    - MR for evaluation of soft tissues, possible mandibular invasion, and evaluation for **perineural tumor spread along CNV3**
    - Bone CT allows assessment of sarcoma matrix ± bone destructive changes

DIFFERENTIAL DIAGNOSIS

Masticator Space Venous Malformation

- Multiloculated mass with possible "flow voids" and calcified phleboliths

Masticator Space Abscess

- Rim-enhancing MS fluid collection ± mandibular osteomyelitis

Mandibular Osteomyelitis

- Bony destruction without osteoid formation
- May see sequestrum formation
- May see linear periosteal reaction

Invasive Squamous Cell Carcinoma

- Palatine tonsil squamous cell carcinoma (SCCa)
  - Palatine tonsil mass invades subjacent MS
- Retromolar trigone SCCa
  - Retromolar triangle mass invades MS

Perineural Tumor of CNV3 in Masticator Space

- Chin skin SCCa or SCCa primary of oral cavity or oropharynx
- Malignancy spreads along CNV3 into MS

Mandible Metastasis

- Aggressive bony destructive changes
- Without periosteal reaction or tumoral calcification

PATHOLOGY

General Features

- Etiology
  - **Ionizing radiation** (XRT) (most commonly from XRT to treat other tumors)
    - Accounts for < 5% of sarcomas
    - 10 years is average time between XRT and sarcoma diagnosis
  - Family history
    - Gardner syndrome: Risk of desmoid tumors (low-grade fibrosarcoma) in abdomen
    - Li-Fraumeni syndrome: Increased risk of developing soft tissue sarcomas and bone sarcomas
    - Retinoblastoma (inherited form): Increased risk of developing bone or soft tissue sarcomas
  - Nodal injury
    - Lymphangiosarcomas rarely found following surgical nodal dissection or in XRT fields
- Genetics
  - DNA mutations common in soft tissue sarcoma

Staging, Grading, & Classification

- Histologic grading system
  - G1: Microscopically normal tissue (slow growing)
  - G2: Microscopically similar to normal tissue (somewhat faster growing)
  - G3: Microscopically only slightly similar to normal tissue (faster growing)
  - G4: Microscopically abnormal (fastest growing)
- T staging system
  - T1: Tumor < 5 cm
  - T2: Tumor > 5 cm
    - a: Superficial tumor
    - b: Deep tumor
- AJCC anatomic stages/prognostic groups
  - Stage IA: G1-2, T1 (a or b), N0, M0
  - Stage IB: G1-2, T2a, N0, M0
  - Stage IIA: G1-2, T2b, N0, M0
  - Stage IIB: G3-4, T1 (a or b), N0, M0
  - Stage IIC: G3-4, T2a, N0, M0
  - Stage III: G3-4, T2b, N0, M0
  - Stage IVA: Any G, any T, N1, M0
  - Stage IVB: Any G, any T, any N, M1

Gross Pathologic & Surgical Features

- Pathologic findings depend on sarcoma type
- Heterogeneous mass with ossified (yellow-white, firm) and nonossified components (soft, tan, with foci of hemorrhage ± necrosis)
- Periosteal reaction: Lamellae of new bone at lesion periphery

Microscopic Features

- Low-grade lesions
  - Few mitotic figures, little if any cellular atypia, and relatively noninfiltrative growth pattern
- High-grade lesions
  - Marked cellular atypia, hyperchromatism, nuclear pleomorphism, and infiltrative growth pattern

CLINICAL ISSUES

Presentation

- Most common signs/symptoms
  - Enlarging soft tissue mass over mandible with increasing pain
  - Other signs/symptoms
    - Cranial nerve deficits (numbness, masticator muscle paralysis) common if skull base involved

Demographics

- Age
  - Mean age: 35 years old
- Gender
  - M:F = 2:1
- Epidemiology
  - ~ 8,000 new cases in USA per year

Natural History & Prognosis

- Stage I: 5-year survival: 99%; recurrence: 20%
- Stage II: 5-year survival: 80%; recurrence: 35%
- Stage III: 5-year survival: 50%; recurrence: 65%
- Stage IVB: 5-year survival: 10%

Treatment

- Sarcoma location, in addition to pathology and TNM stage, is important when planning treatment
  - Multimodality treatment usually recommended
- Stage I: Surgically removed; XRT may be added if inadequate margins
  - XRT may be utilized primarily if tumor unresectable (i.e., encasing critical structures)
- Stage II: Surgical excision with 2-cm normal margin is goal
  - Pre- or postoperative XRT common; chemotherapy less commonly given
- Stage III: Surgery and XRT commonly used with chemotherapy to reduce recurrences
- Stage IV: Surgery and XRT with metastatic surgical excision
- Experimental treatments, such as interleukin-2 immunotherapy, are being researched
- Possible role for adjuvant chemotherapy in unusual cases
- Radiofrequency ablation has been used in recurrent rhabdomyosarcoma

DIAGNOSTIC CHECKLIST

Consider

- In absence of known systemic malignancy, head and neck malignancy, or septic symptoms (MS abscess), MS mass should suggest diagnosis of sarcoma
- Mandibular destruction ± perineural tumor spread along CNV3 toward skull base both suggest sarcoma diagnosis from imaging perspective

Image Interpretation Pearls

- CT or MR of MS mass suspected of being malignant
  - Carefully evaluate inferior alveolar canal, mandibular foramen, foramen ovale, and remainder of CNV3 course for perineural tumor spread

SELECTED REFERENCES

1. van den Berg H et al: Incidence and grading of cranio-facial osteosarcomas. Int J Oral Maxillofac Surg. 43(1):7-12, 2014
2. Abdel Razek AA et al: Role of diffusion-weighted MRI in differentiation of masticator space malignancy from infection. Dentomaxillofac Radiol. 42(4):20120183, 2013
3. Wang S et al: Osteosarcoma of the jaws: demographic and CT imaging features. Dentomaxillofac Radiol. 41(1):37-42, 2012
4. Abrigo JM et al: MRI of radiation-induced tumors of the head and neck in post-radiation nasopharyngeal carcinoma. Eur Radiol. 19(5):1197-205, 2009
5. Niedzielska I et al: Low-grade myofibroblastic sarcoma of the mandible: a case report. J Med Case Reports. 3:8458, 2009
6. Makimoto Y et al: Imaging findings of radiation-induced sarcoma of the head and neck. Br J Radiol. 80(958):790-7, 2007
7. Nashida Y et al: Radiofrequency ablation used for the treatment of frequently recurrent rhabdomyosarcoma in the masticator space in a 10-year-old girl. J Pediatr Hematol Oncol. 29(9):640-2, 2007
8. Shuman AG et al: Successful multimodal treatment of a carcinosarcoma of the masticator space. J Otolaryngol. 36(3):E28-30, 2007
9. Zaytoun G et al: Atypical lipomatous tumors of the face: a controversial issue. Eur Arch Otorhinolaryngol. 263(12):1065-9, 2006
10. Atanasov DT et al: Sarcomas of the mandible. Literature review and case reports. Folia Med (Plovdiv). 46(2):31-5, 2004
11. Carlson ER et al: Sarcoma of mandible. J Oral Maxillofac Surg. 62(1):81-7, 2004
12. Hain SF et al: Can FDG PET be used to successfully direct preoperative biopsy of soft tissue tumours? Nucl Med Commun. 24(11):1139-43, 2003
13. Pandey M et al: Soft tissue sarcoma of the head and neck region in adults. Int J Oral Maxillofac Surg. 32(1):43-8, 2003
14. Potter BO et al: Sarcomas of the head and neck. Surg Oncol Clin N Am. 12(2):379-417, 2003

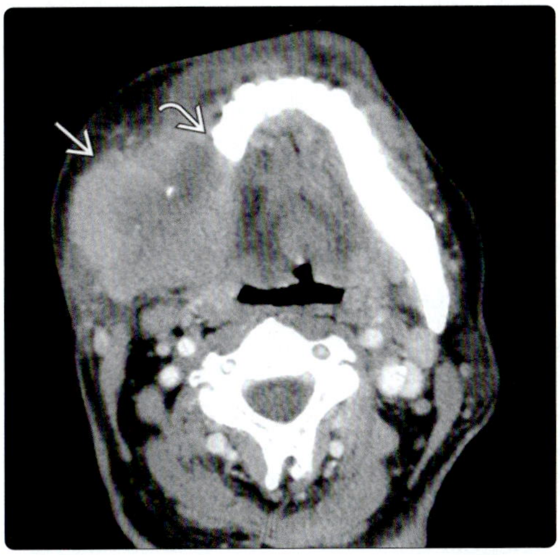

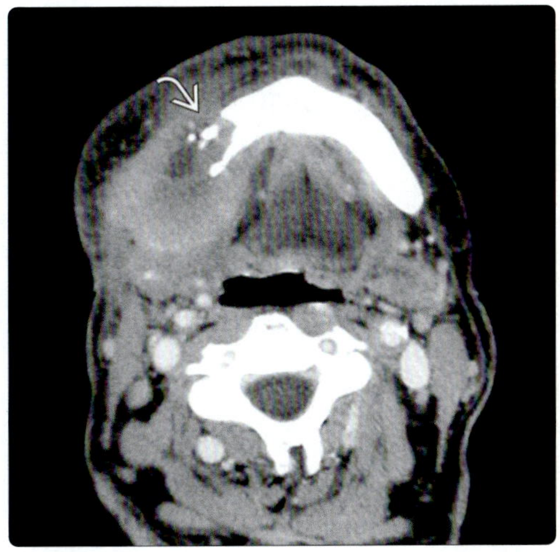

(Left) *Axial CECT shows a masticator space and mandible malignant fibrous histiocytoma. The lesion is seen as a solid, mildly enhancing right masticator space mass ➡ with mandibular destruction ➡, including both the ramus and body. The masticator space is known as a deep facial location where sarcoma arises.* **(Right)** *Axial CECT in the same patient demonstrates the right masticator space mass with extensive mandibular destruction ➡. Note the facial asymmetry on the affected side.*

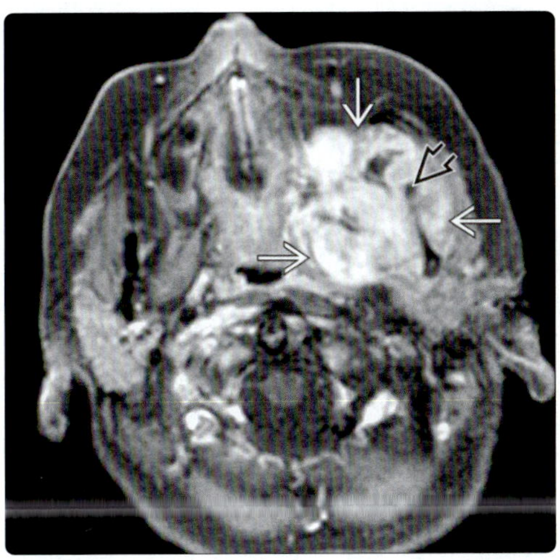

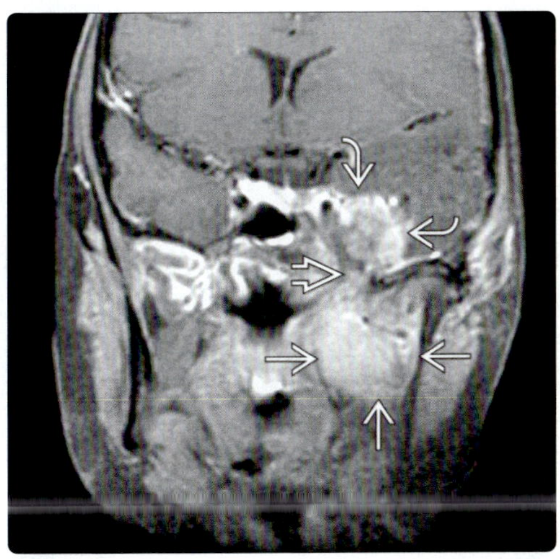

(Left) *Axial T1WI C+ FS MR shows a high-grade leiomyosarcoma of the masticator space. The tumor is a heterogeneously enhancing mass ➡ involving the mandible ➡. It is not possible to differentiate most masticator space sarcoma types with imaging unless osteo- or chondrosarcoma matrix is present.* **(Right)** *Coronal T1WI C+ FS MR in the same patient shows an enhancing mass ➡ with intracranial spread through the foramen ovale ➡, which allows the tumor to involve the cavernous sinus ➡.*

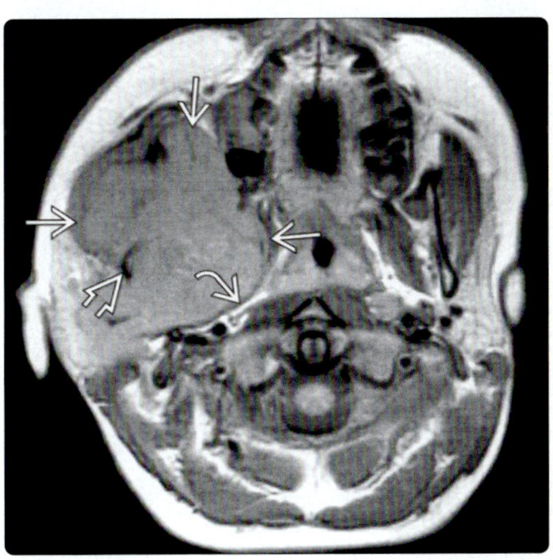

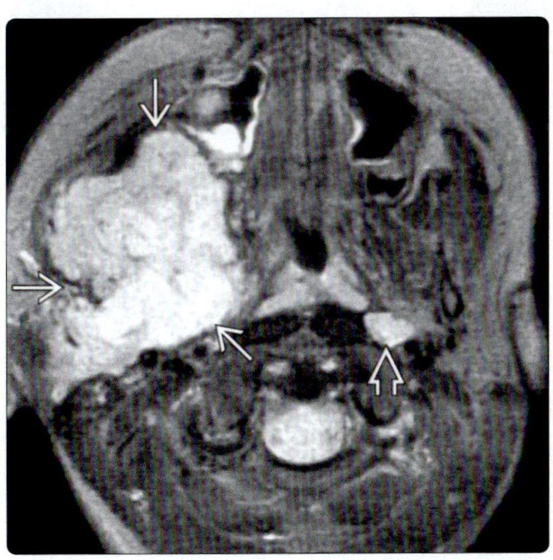

(Left) *Axial T1WI MR shows a Ewing sarcoma arising in the masticator space. Notice the very large mass is hyperintense to muscle on T1WI ➡. The mandibular ramus is destroyed and only a small fragment is visible in this image ➡. The parapharyngeal fat stripe ➡ is displaced medially.* **(Right)** *Axial T2WI FS MR in the same patient shows the tumor is markedly hyperintense but heterogeneous on T2WI ➡. A prominent left retropharyngeal node ➡ is incidentally noted.*

Diagnoses: Masticator Space

KEY FACTS

TERMINOLOGY

- Perineural tumor (PNT), masticator space (MS), mandibular branch of trigeminal nerve (CNV3)
- CNV3 PNT: Extension of malignancy along CNV3 from MS though foramen ovale into Meckel cave

IMAGING

- PNT spread can occur along all or segments of CNV3 from mental foramen to lateral pons root entry zone
  - Nerve enlarged; may reach 1 cm in diameter
  - CNV3 may be normal in size in early PNT
- CBCT & bone CT findings
  - **Enlarged** mandibular **inferior alveolar canal**, **mandibular foramen**, **foramen ovale**
- MR findings
  - Coronal T1 C+ best shows CNV3 abnormal extracranial, foramen ovale, & intracranial-enhancing PNT
  - Fat saturation increases conspicuity of PNT
  - Coronal T1 C- MR **without** fat saturation useful for obliteration of fat pads below foramen ovale

TOP DIFFERENTIAL DIAGNOSES

- Normal pterygoid venous plexus asymmetry
- Normal vasa nervosa CNV3
- CNV3 schwannoma
- CNV3 neurofibroma
- Skull base meningioma

DIAGNOSTIC CHECKLIST

- Primary malignancy sites of origin that may yield CNV3 PNT spread
  - Skin of chin & jaw [squamous cell carcinoma (SCCa) or melanoma]
  - Alveolar ridge (gingival), retromolar trigone, deep tonsillar SCCa, nasopharyngeal SCCa
  - MS malignancy (sarcoma, non-Hodgkin lymphoma)
  - Parotid carcinoma

(Left) *Coronal graphic depicts a classic example of malignant masticator space tumor ➡ with perineural V3 spread ➡ through the foramen ovale ⇨ into the intracranial compartment.* **(Right)** *This patient presented with a history of treated buccal space adenoid cystic carcinoma. New chin numbness creates concern for perineural CNV3 recurrence. Coronal T1WI C+ MR reveals perineural tumor (PNT) involving CNV3 in the nasopharyngeal masticator space ➡ passing through the foramen ovale ➡ & beginning to invade Meckel cave ➡.*

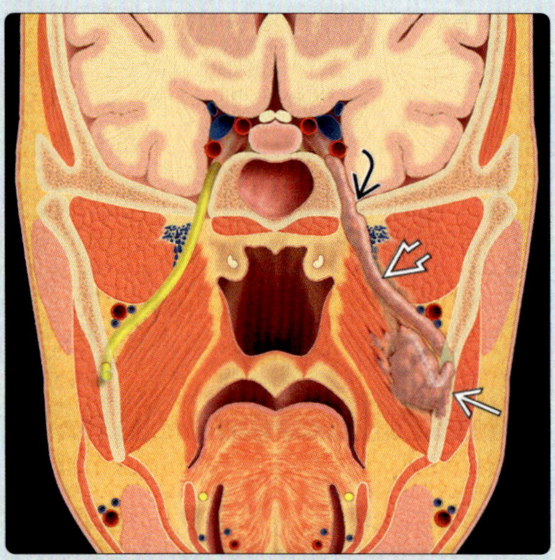

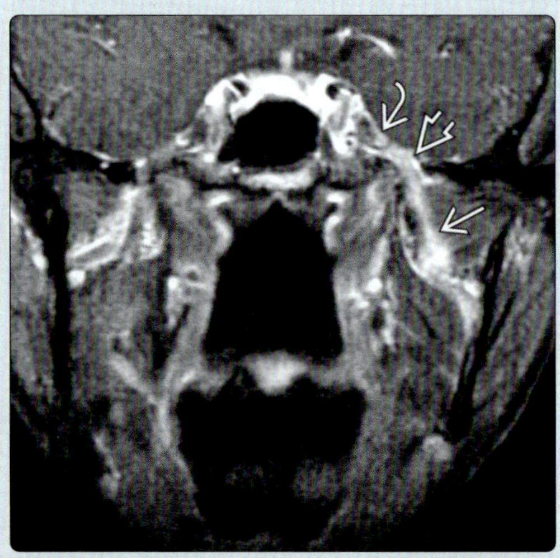

(Left) *Axial T1WI C+ FS MR in the same patient demonstrates the PNT at the mandibular foramen ➡. Notice the minimal enhancement in the contralateral mandibular foramen ➡. Clearly, if the radiologist does not look for this specific finding, the observation of PNT will not be made.* **(Right)** *Axial T1WI C+ FS MR in the same patient shows enhancing PNT ➡ surrounding the CNV3 ➡ on its way to the foramen ovale.*

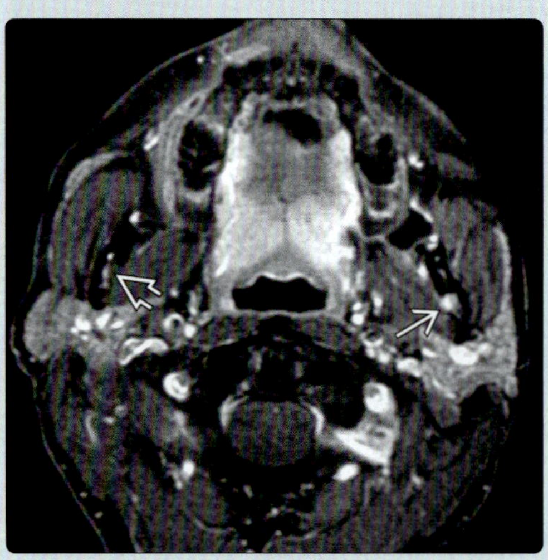

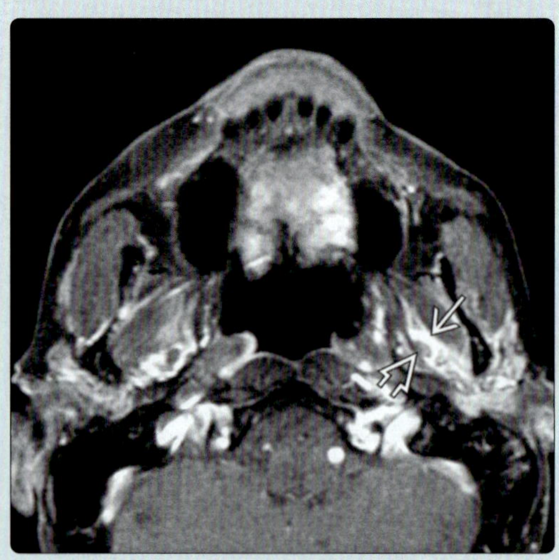

TERMINOLOGY

Abbreviations

- Perineural tumor (PNT), masticator space (MS), mandibular branch of trigeminal nerve (CNV3)

Synonyms

- PNT spread, PNT invasion

Definitions

- CNV3 PNT: Extension of malignancy along CNV3 from MS though foramen ovale into Meckel cave (MC)
- CNV3: 3rd division of trigeminal nerve (CNV)
- MC: Small cistern for CNV
  - Trigeminal ganglion on anterior aspect of MC
- Trigeminal ganglion (gasserian ganglion, semilunar ganglion): Major ganglion for CNV in MC

IMAGING

General Features

- Best diagnostic clue
  - T1 C+ MR shows **enlarged, enhancing V3**
- Location
  - PNT spread can occur along all or segments of CNV3 from mental foramen to root entry zone of CNV on lateral pons
    - **Inferior alveolar nerve**: In inferior alveolar canal from mental foramen to mandibular foramen
    - **Mandibular branch, CNV3**: Spans distance from mandibular foramen to foramen ovale in MS
    - **Foramen ovale**: Skull base foramen through which CNV3 passes
    - **MC**: Contains trigeminal ganglion; inferior, medial, & posterior to cavernous sinus
    - **Preganglionic segment CNV**: Spans distance from MC to root entry zone on lateral pons
- Size
  - Nerve usually enlarged; may reach 1 cm in diameter
  - Nerve may be normal in size early in PNT process
- Morphology
  - Linear, along expected course of V3

CT Findings

- CECT
  - CNV3 enhancement & enlargement
  - Abnormal enhancement, convexity to cavernous sinus & MC
- CBCT & bone CT
  - **Enlarged inferior alveolar canal in mandible**
  - Widened mandibular foramen
  - Foramen ovale enlargement

MR Findings

- T1WI
  - Infiltration of MS muscle & fat surrounding CNV3
  - Tissue within mandibular foramen; intermediate signal replacing marrow fat of mandibular ramus
  - Obliteration of fat pad below foramen ovale
  - Enlargement of CNV3
  - Fatty infiltration of muscles of mastication (chronic CNV3 atrophy)
- T2WI
  - Enlargement of MC with loss of normal fluid signal
  - Increased signal of edematous nerve is difficult & unreliable sign
- T1WI C+
  - Enlarged, enhancing extracranial CNV3
    - Inferior alveolar canal of mandible (inferior alveolar nerve)
    - Mandibular foramen to foramen ovale (mandibular nerve)
  - Enhancement of nerve in foramen ovale
    - Normal nerve: Low signal
    - Beware vasa nervosa (veins accompanying nerve)
    - Beware of normal pterygoid venous plexus enhancement
  - Enlargement, enhancement of MC
  - Enhancing MS muscles (acute-subacute V3 denervation)

Nuclear Medicine Findings

- PET
  - Uptake along V3 often difficult to differentiate from brain & primary tumor
  - Combined PET/CT useful; not as good as MR

Imaging Recommendations

- Best imaging tool
  - CECT insensitive for PNT; MR recommended
  - MR very sensitive but not specific for CNV3 PNT
    - Normal nerves asymmetrically enhance in 5% of patients
- Protocol advice
  - Coronal T1 C+ best shows CNV3 abnormal extracranial, foramen ovale, & intracranial-enhancing PNT
    - Fat saturation increases conspicuity of PNT
  - Coronal T1 C- MR **without** fat saturation useful for obliteration of fat pads below foramen ovale

DIFFERENTIAL DIAGNOSIS

Pterygoid Venous Plexus Asymmetry

- Normal venous plexus in & around pterygoid muscles in MS
- May extend to foramen ovale but does not enter
- Asymmetry common

CNV3 Schwannoma in MS

- Benign neoplasm of CNV3 nerve sheath
- Intermediate T1, heterogeneously bright T2
- Heterogeneous enhancement with intramural cysts possible
- When crossing foramen ovale, dumbbell-shaped on coronal images
- May arise anywhere along course of CNV

CNV3 Neurofibroma

- Uncommon site for neurofibroma
- When crossing foramen ovale, dumbbell-shaped on coronal images
- Uniform enhancement
- May follow branches of CNV3

Normal Skull Base Marrow Around Foramen Ovale

- Marrow fat in skull base around foramen ovale has inherent high T1 signal
- High T1 signal alongside foramen ovale
- Dark cortical bone separates marrow from nerve within foramen
- Fat-saturated T1 clarifies fat vs. enhancement

Skull Base Meningioma

- Benign neoplasm of brain coverings
- Isodense to brain on T1 & T2 images
- Uniform, brisk enhancement
- May extend into foramen ovale & beyond

Vasa Nervosa CNV3

- Normal small veins accompanying CNV3 through foramen ovale
- Vague peripheral enhancement on T1 C+ MR
- Nerve itself remains dark on T1 C+ MR

Normal Fat Pad, CNV3

- Fat pads normally seen at exit points of cranial nerves
- High inherent T1 signal surrounding nerve
- Does not extend into foramen ovale
- Fat-saturated T1 C+ MR clarifies fat vs. enhancement

PATHOLOGY

General Features

- Etiology
  - "Path of least resistance" for tumors predisposed to PNT spread
  - Tumor expression of nerve growth factor or neural cell adhesion molecules may correlate with propensity to PNT spread
- Tumor may spread outside nerve sheath or may involve support tissues within sheath (endoneurium, perineurium, epineurium)
- **Any malignant tumor may undergo PNT spread**

Gross Pathologic & Surgical Features

- Enlargement of nerve complex
- Encasement replacement of CNV3

Microscopic Features

- Perineural spread = gross pathologic or radiographic diagnosis of tumor along nerve
- Perineural invasion = microscopic finding of tumor within nerve bundles

CLINICAL ISSUES

Presentation

- Most common signs/symptoms
  - Often asymptomatic (40%)
  - Paresthesias of lower face
  - Jaw pain or numbness
  - Masticator muscle denervation atrophy

Demographics

- Age
  - 50-80 years (for common primary tumors)
- Gender
  - M > F, because squamous cell carcinoma (SCCa), which is frequently involved in CNV3 PNT spread, is more common in men
- Epidemiology
  - Tumors with greatest propensity for perineural spread
    - **Adenoid cystic carcinoma**
    - **Squamous cell carcinoma**, pharynx or skin
    - Desmoplastic melanoma, skin
    - Non-Hodgkin lymphoma (NHL)
    - Mucoepidermoid carcinoma

Natural History & Prognosis

- PNT spread strongly affects patient prognosis
- PNT is **very poor prognostic sign**
  - ↑ local recurrence
  - ↑ distant metastases
  - ↑ meningeal carcinomatosis
  - ↓ survival
- Cranial nerve defects unlikely to resolve with therapy

Treatment

- Radiotherapy ± surgery & chemotherapy

DIAGNOSTIC CHECKLIST

Consider

- Primary malignancy sites of origin that may yield CNV3 PNT spread
  - Skin of chin & jaw (SCCa or melanoma)
  - Alveolar ridge (gingival), retromolar trigone, deep tonsillar SCCa, nasopharyngeal SCCa
  - MS malignancy (sarcoma, NHL)
  - Parotid malignancy
    - May spread from CNVII along **auriculotemporal nerve** to CNV3

Image Interpretation Pearls

- If suspect PNT spread along CNV3, inspect CNV from mental foramen of mandible to root entry zone of lateral pons
  - Look for asymmetric CNV3 enlargement & enhancement
  - Use T1 C+ axial & coronal **fat-saturated** MR to increase lesion conspicuity
- Do not confuse normal pterygoid venous plexus with PNT spread
  - Look for CNV3 nerve enhancement to distinguish
- Beware of "**skip lesions**"
  - Interval of normal nerve between noncontiguous areas of PNT

SELECTED REFERENCES

1. Badger D et al: Imaging of perineural spread in head and neck cancer. Radiol Clin North Am. 55(1):139-149, 2017
2. Bourque PR et al: Combined isolated trigeminal and facial neuropathies from perineural invasion by squamous cell carcinoma: a case series and review of the literature. J Clin Neurosci. 35:5-12, 2017
3. Dulamea AO et al: Perineural spreading along the trigeminal nerve in a squamous cell carcinoma of the tongue. Acta Neurol Belg. 115(4):699-701, 2015
4. Warden KF et al: Perineural spread of cancer along the three trigeminal divisions. J Neuroophthalmol. 29(4):300-7, 2009
5. Ojiri H: Perineural spread in head and neck malignancies. Radiat Med. 24(1):1-8, 2006

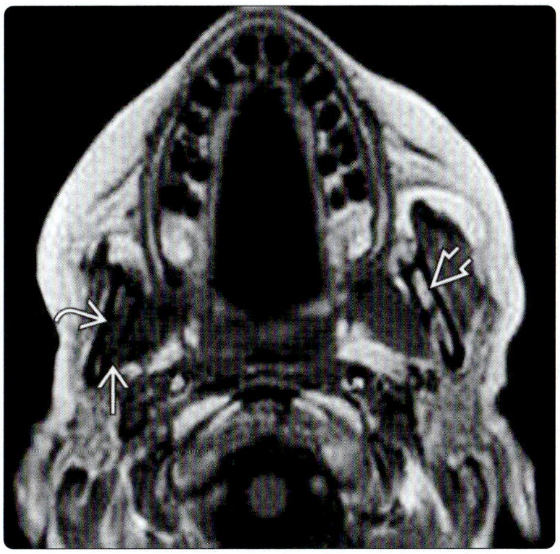

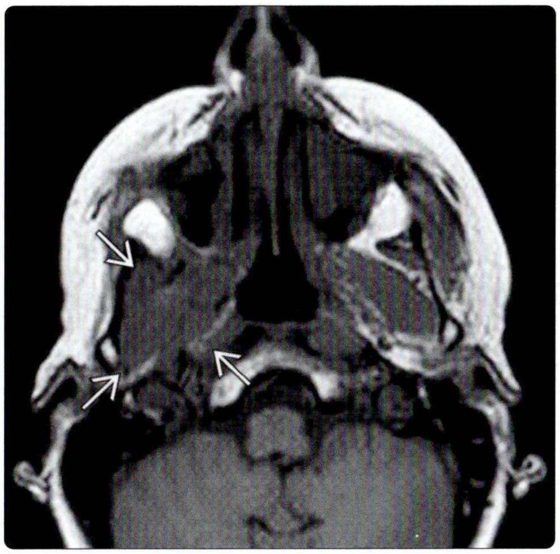

(Left) *Axial T1WI MR in a patient presenting with a history of previously treated nasopharyngeal squamous cell carcinoma shows replacement of the normal marrow fat in the right mandibular ramus & abnormal soft tissue at the level of mandibular foramen related to PNT spread along CNV3. Note normal high-signal marrow fat in the left mandibular ramus .* **(Right)** *Axial T1WI MR in the same patient shows CNV3 PNT spread with obliteration of normal fat planes in masticator space .*

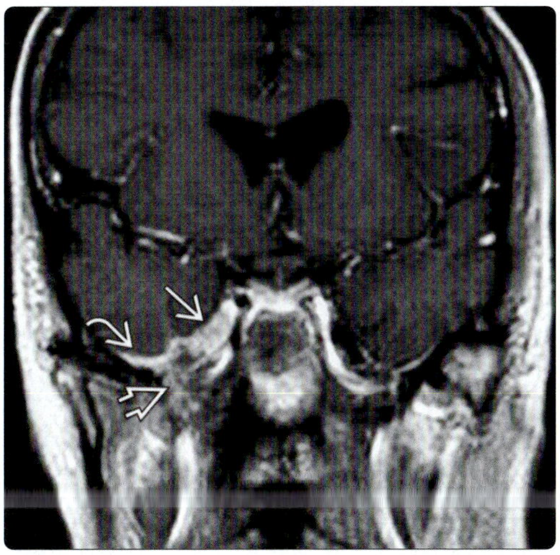

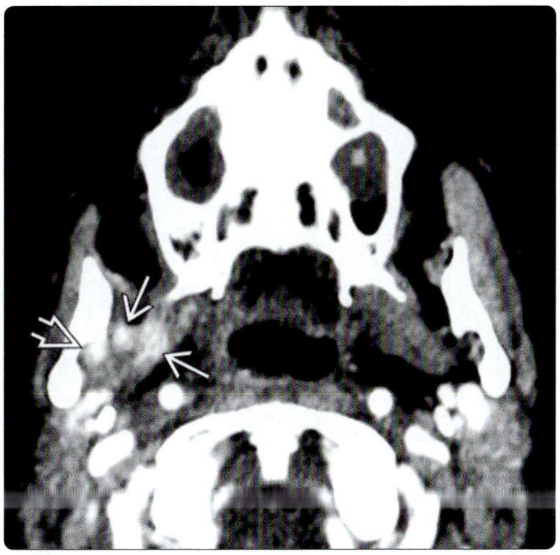

(Left) *Coronal T1WI C+ MR in the same patient demonstrates PNT extending along CNV3 through the foramen ovale & into the Meckel cave . There is also spread of tumor laterally along the dura of the middle cranial fossa.* **(Right)** *Axial CECT in the same patient shows enhancing tumor in the right mandibular foramen as well as areas of abnormal enhancement along the mandibular branch of V3 in the masticator space .*

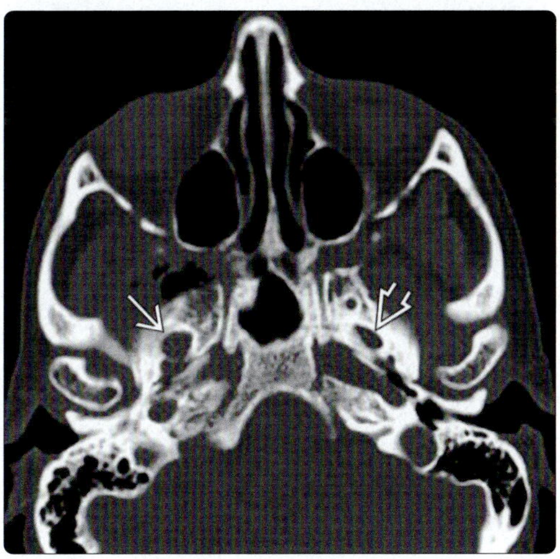

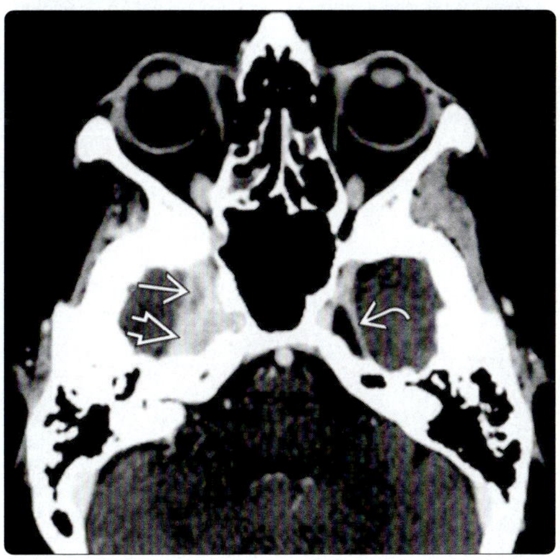

(Left) *Axial bone CT reveals an enlarged right foramen ovale compared to the normal left foramen ovale . CNV3 PNT is responsible for the foramen enlargement.* **(Right)** *Axial CECT in the same patient shows that the perineural CNV3 tumor has extended through foramen ovale into the Meckel cave & the middle cranial fossa . Note the normal CSF density Meckel cave on the left .*

Benign Masticator Muscle Hypertrophy

KEY FACTS

TERMINOLOGY

- Definition: Benign enlargement of muscles of mastication (temporalis, masseter, medial & lateral pterygoids)

IMAGING

- Smooth, diffuse enlargement of masticator muscles
  - Masseter muscle most obviously affected
  - Masticator muscles enhance normally
- 50% bilateral, usually asymmetric
- Flaring & irregularity of mandibular angle
- CT: Enlarged, normal-density masticator muscles
  - Cortical thickening of mandible & zygomatic arch
- MR: Enlarged, normal-intensity masticator muscles

TOP DIFFERENTIAL DIAGNOSES

- Masticator space pseudolesion
- Masticator space abscess
- Masticator space sarcoma
- Masticator space squamous cell carcinoma

PATHOLOGY

- Etiology: **Bruxism** (nocturnal teeth grinding), habitual gum chewing, TMJ dysfunction

CLINICAL ISSUES

- Nontender lateral facial mass that enlarges with jaw clenching; masseter muscle most obvious clinically
- M > F
- Slowly progressive masticator muscle enlargement
- Treat with surgery only for cosmetic reasons
- Treat TMJ dysfunction or parafunctional habit, if present

DIAGNOSTIC CHECKLIST

- Enlarged muscle(s) should be isodense (CT) or isointense (MR) to normal skeletal muscle

(Left) *Axial CECT demonstrates incidental asymmetric enlargement of the right masseter* ➔ *& medial pterygoid* ↩ *muscles. Enhancement & density of these muscles are equal to the opposite side.* **(Right)** *Frontal 3D CBCT of a patient with a history of bruxism shows irregularity & flaring of the mandibular angles bilaterally* ➔. *The irregular outline simulates the appearance of exostoses in the areas of attachment of the masseter muscles & is a remodeling response to the muscular hyperactivity.*

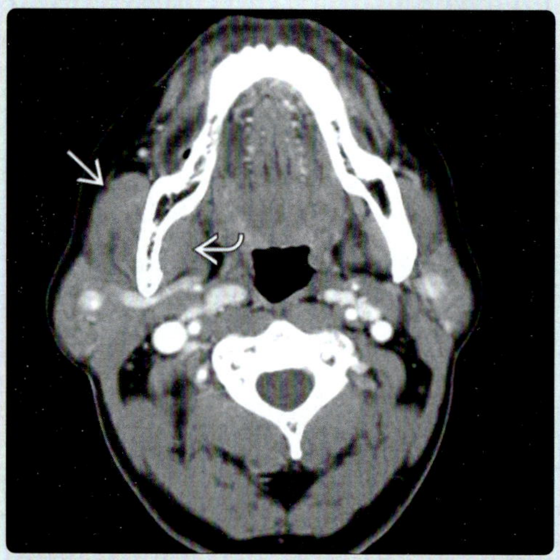

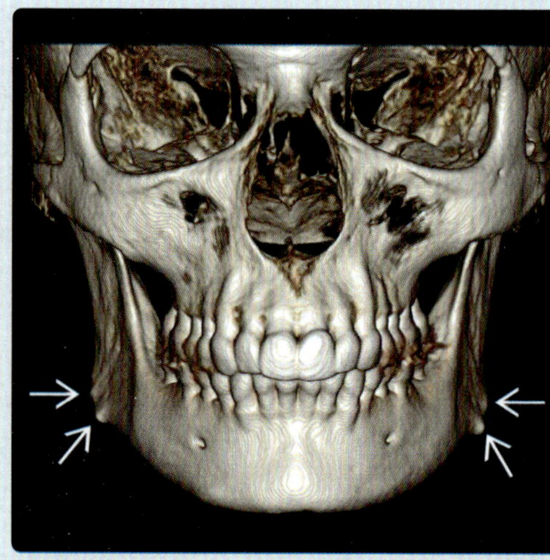

(Left) *Clinical photograph demonstrates the clinical appearance of a patient with unilateral benign masticator muscle hypertrophy. Note the broad, smooth cheek bulge secondary to the enlarged masseter muscle* ➔ *at its insertion into the angle of the mandible.* **(Right)** *Axial T2 MR in a typical case of unilateral benign masticator muscle hypertrophy shows that the right masseter* ➔ *& medial pterygoid* ↩ *muscles are enlarged but have identical signal intensity compared to those on the left.*

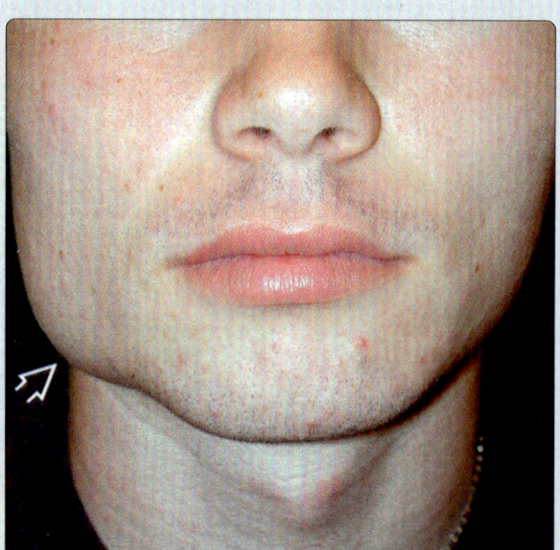

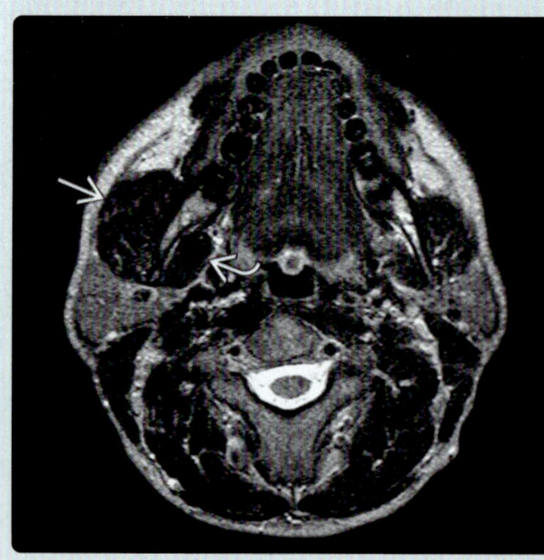

Benign Masticator Muscle Hypertrophy

TERMINOLOGY

Abbreviations

- Benign masticator muscle hypertrophy (BMMH)

Synonyms

- Benign masseteric hypertrophy

Definitions

- Benign enlargement of muscles of mastication (temporalis, masseter, medial & lateral pterygoids)

IMAGING

General Features

- Best diagnostic clue
  - Smooth, diffuse enlargement of masticator muscles
- Location
  - Masticator space (MS); masseter muscle most obviously affected
  - 50% bilateral, usually asymmetric

Radiographic Findings

- Radiography
  - Flaring of mandibular angle with exostosis at masseteric insertion

CT Findings

- NECT
  - Enlarged, normal-density masticator muscles
- CECT
  - Enlarged masticator muscles enhance normally
- CBCT & bone CT
  - Cortical thickening of mandible & zygomatic arch
  - Irregularity in outline of cortex at mandibular angle

MR Findings

- T1WI
  - Enlarged, normal-intensity masticator muscles
  - Decreased marrow signal in areas of cortical thickening (mandible, zygomatic arch)
- T2WI
  - Enlarged, normal-intensity masticator muscles
- T1WI C+
  - Enlarged masticator muscles enhance normally

Ultrasonographic Findings

- Enlarged masseter muscle with normal echogenicity

Nuclear Medicine Findings

- May have intense FDG uptake on PET

Other Modality Findings

- Sialography: Parotid duct displaced by large masseter

Imaging Recommendations

- Best imaging tool
  - CECT or T1 C+ MR excellent in evaluating MS lesions
- Protocol advice
  - Bone & soft tissue algorithms on CECT data

DIFFERENTIAL DIAGNOSIS

Masticator Space Pseudolesion

- Contralateral small masticator muscles make normal MS appear hypertrophic

Masticator Space Abscess

- Rim-enhancing fluid in MS ± mandibular osteomyelitis

Masticator Space Sarcoma

- Primary malignancy of MS

Masticator Space Squamous Cell Carcinoma, Direct Invasion or Perineural Tumor (V3)

- Enters MS directly (retromolar trigone, faucial tonsil)
- Enters MS via perineural V3 from chin skin squamous cell carcinoma or squamous cell carcinoma (mandibular alveolar ridge)

PATHOLOGY

General Features

- Etiology
  - **Bruxism** (nocturnal teeth grinding), gum chewing, TMJ dysfunction
  - Anabolic steroids ± unilateral chewing

Microscopic Features

- Normal skeletal muscle
- Process may involve hyperplasia (↑ number of fibers) rather than true hypertrophy

CLINICAL ISSUES

Presentation

- Most common signs/symptoms
  - Nontender lateral facial mass that enlarges with jaw clenching

Demographics

- Age
  - BMMH usually begins in adolescence
- Gender
  - M:F = 2:1

Natural History & Prognosis

- Slowly progressive masticator muscle enlargement

Treatment

- Surgery only for cosmetic reasons
- Botulinum toxin A injection
- Treat TMJ dysfunction of parafunctional habit, if present

DIAGNOSTIC CHECKLIST

Image Interpretation Pearls

- Enlarged muscle(s) should be isodense (CT) or isointense (MR) to normal skeletal muscle

SELECTED REFERENCES

1. Graziano P et al: Bilateral hypertrophy of masseteric and temporalis muscles, our fifteen patients and review of literature. Eur Rev Med Pharmacol Sci. 20(1):7-11, 2016
2. Fyfe EC et al: Magnetic resonance imaging in the diagnosis of asymmetrical bilateral masseteric hypertrophy. Dentomaxillofac Radiol. 28(1):52-4, 1999

PART II
SECTION 7
Parotid Space

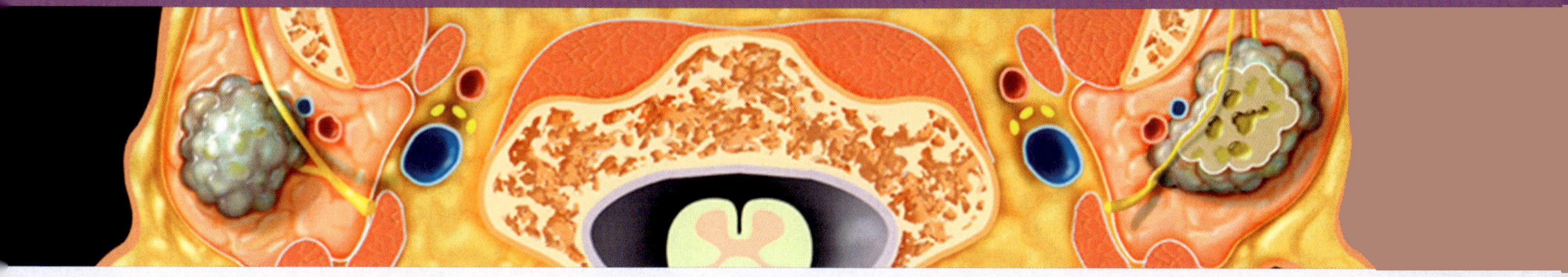

Inflammation

Benign Lymphoepithelial Lesions: HIV 750
Parotid Sialadenitis 754

Neoplasm, Benign

Parotid Benign Mixed Tumor 756
Warthin Tumor 760
Parotid Schwannoma 764

Neoplasm, Malignant

Parotid Malignant Mixed Tumor 766
Parotid Mucoepidermoid Carcinoma 768
Parotid Adenoid Cystic Carcinoma 772
Parotid Non-Hodgkin Lymphoma 774
Metastatic Disease of Parotid Nodes 778

Autoimmune

Sjögren Syndrome 782

Miscellaneous/Idiopathic

Parotid Sialoliths 784

Benign Lymphoepithelial Lesions: HIV

KEY FACTS

TERMINOLOGY

- 3-tiered classification
  - Persistent generalized parotid lymphadenopathy: **Solid** lesions
  - Benign lymphoepithelial lesions (BLEL): **Mixed** solid & cystic lesions
  - Benign lymphoepithelial cysts: **Cystic** lesions

IMAGING

- Enhanced CT or MR: Multiple bilateral, well-circumscribed cystic & solid masses within enlarged parotid glands
- Look for other CECT findings associated with HIV
  - **Reactive cervical adenopathy**
  - Adenoid, palatine, & lingual **tonsillar hypertrophy**

TOP DIFFERENTIAL DIAGNOSES

- 1st branchial cleft cyst
- Parotid Sjögren syndrome
- Non-Hodgkin lymphoma in parotid nodes
- Metastatic disease to parotid nodes

CLINICAL ISSUES

- Bilateral painless enlargement of both parotid glands
- BLEL may precede HIV seroconversion
- Historically, **5%** of HIV-positive patients develop BLEL

DIAGNOSTIC CHECKLIST

- Nonnecrotic cervical adenopathy with tonsillar hypertrophy can be important clue to BLEL diagnosis with CECT
- When BLE cysts present as unilateral cystic intraparotid mass, may be mistaken for 1st branchial cleft cyst
- When BLEL presents as unilateral solid intraparotid mass, may be mistaken for parotid tumor

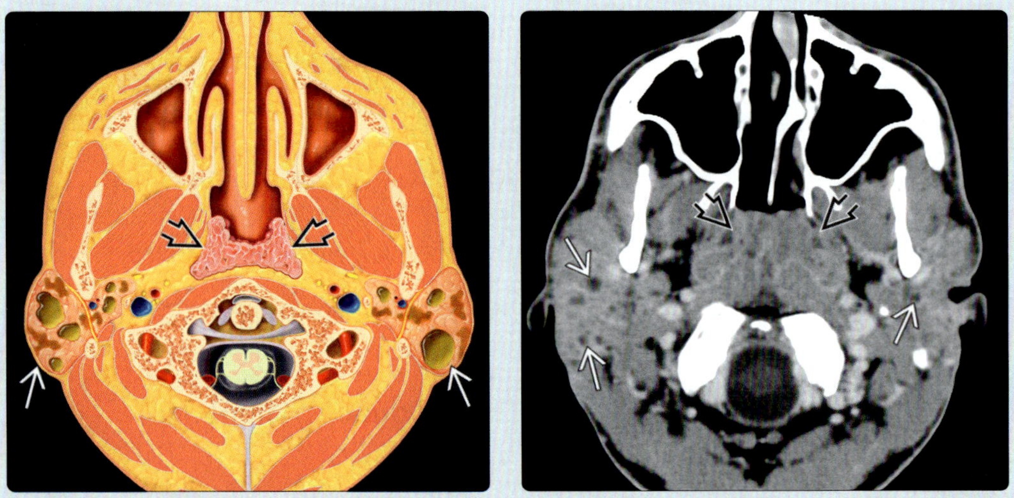

(Left) *Axial graphic shows classic findings of benign lymphoepithelial lesions (BLEL) as bilateral intraparotid cysts mixed with bilateral, solid lymphoid aggregates ➡. Note associated adenoid hypertrophy ⇨.* **(Right)** *Axial CECT shows microcysts ➡ scattered throughout both parotid glands in an HIV-positive patient, findings most consistent with benign lymphoepithelial (BLE) cysts. Note associated adenoid hypertrophy ⇨.*

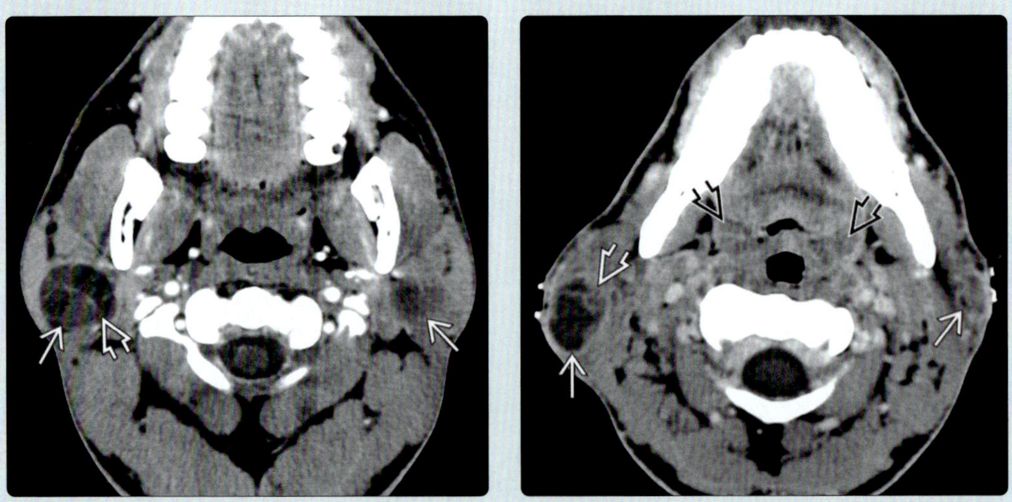

(Left) *Axial CECT in an HIV-positive patient shows loculated cystic masses ➡ in both parotid glands. Septations can sometimes be seen within BLE cysts ⇨.* **(Right)** *Axial CECT in an HIV-positive patient shows bilateral cystic masses ➡ with mural nodularity ⇨ in both parotid glands. BLEL can have both cystic & solid components. Note the associated tonsillar hypertrophy ⇨.*

TERMINOLOGY

Abbreviations

- Benign lymphoepithelial lesions (BLEL): HIV

Synonyms

- AIDS-related parotid cysts (ARPC)
  - Patient need only be HIV positive to manifest BLEL
    - May not have full-blown AIDS with BLEL
    - Avoid ARPC synonym

Definitions

- Multifocal mixed **cystic** & **solid** intraparotid masses found in HIV-infected patients
- 3-tiered classification
  - Persistent generalized parotid gland lymphadenopathy: Solid lesions
  - BLEL: Mixed solid & cystic lesions
  - Benign lymphoepithelial cysts: Cystic lesions

IMAGING

General Features

- Best diagnostic clue
  - Multiple cystic & solid masses enlarging both parotid glands associated with **tonsillar hyperplasia** & **reactive cervical adenopathy**
- Location
  - Intraglandular
  - **Bilateral** parotid space
  - Rarely seen in submandibular or sublingual salivary glands
    - Only parotid has intrinsic lymphoid tissue
- Size
  - Variable: Typically several mm, up to 3.5 cm
- Morphology
  - Cysts are well circumscribed, rounded
  - Solid lymphoid aggregates may be poorly defined
  - Bilateral parotid enlargement
  - Often innumerable small masses

CT Findings

- NECT
  - Multiple bilateral, well-circumscribed cystic & solid masses within enlarged parotid glands
- CECT
  - Thin rim enhancement of cystic lesions with heterogeneous enhancement of solid lesions
  - Other CECT findings associated with HIV
    - Reactive cervical adenopathy
    - Adenoid, palatine, & lingual tonsillar hypertrophy

MR Findings

- T1WI
  - Low signal intensity cystic lesions
  - Heterogeneous, variable signal in solid lesions
    - Normal parotid fat provides good inherent contrast
- T2WI
  - Hyperintense, bilateral, well-circumscribed, round to ovoid intraparotid lesions
  - Hyperintense, bilateral cervical lymphadenopathy
  - Waldeyer lymphatic ring enlargement with high signal
- STIR
  - Improves lesion conspicuity
- T1WI C+
  - Thin rim enhancement in cystic lesions with variable heterogeneous enhancement of solid lesions
  - Solid lesions may be less conspicuous on enhanced than unenhanced images because of surrounding fat

Ultrasonographic Findings

- Spectrum of sonographic findings ranging from simple cysts to mixed masses with predominantly solid components
  - Cystic lesions not purely anechoic but contain internal network of thin septa supplied by vessel pedicles
    - 40% have mural nodules
  - Solid lesions may resemble parotid neoplasms

Imaging Recommendations

- Best imaging tool
  - Either CECT or MR from skull base to clavicles will show signature findings of bilateral parotid masses, tonsillar hyperplasia, & cervical adenopathy

DIFFERENTIAL DIAGNOSIS

1st Branchial Cleft Cyst

- Clinical: Recurrent unilateral inflammatory parotid mass
- Imaging: Unilateral oval cystic intraparotid mass

Parotid Sjögren Syndrome

- Clinical: Older women with Sicca syndrome (dry eyes, dry mouth, dry skin) & connective tissue disorder (rheumatoid arthritis); antinuclear antibodies
- Imaging: May be identical to BLE cysts

Parotid Sarcoidosis

- Clinical: Intraparotid sarcoid is very rare
- Imaging: Cervical & mediastinal lymph nodes
  - May be identical to BLEL

Warthin Tumor

- Clinical: Solitary or multifocal parotid masses
- Imaging
  - Solid or mixed cystic-solid parotid masses with nodular walls
  - 20% are multifocal but never innumerable
  - Lacks associated tonsillar hyperplasia & cervical adenopathy

Non-Hodgkin Lymphoma in Parotid Nodes

- Clinical: Chronic systemic non-Hodgkin lymphoma (NHL) usually already apparent
- Imaging: Bilateral solid masses in parotid
  - May be identical to persistent parotid gland lymphadenopathy
- Primary parotid NHL rare
  - Unilateral, multifocal, solid intraparotid masses

Metastatic Disease to Parotid Nodes

- Clinical: Primary malignancy & other metastatic deposits already apparent
- Imaging: Unilateral multifocal solid parotid masses

PATHOLOGY

General Features

- Etiology
  - Hypothesis 1: Periductal lymphoid aggregates cause ductal radicular obstruction, periductal atrophy, & distal cyst formation
  - Hypothesis 2: Cyst formation occurs in included glandular epithelium within intraparotid nodes
    - So-called **cystification**
  - Does not arise directly from intraparotid lymph nodes
- Associated abnormalities
  - Cervical lymphadenopathy & nasopharyngeal lymphofollicular hyperplasia
- Cystic spaces lined by squamous epithelium accompanied by abundant lymphoid stroma
- Rare transformation to B-cell lymphoma reported

Gross Pathologic & Surgical Features

- Diffusely enlarged parotid glands with multiple well-delineated nodules with rubbery consistency & smooth, tan-white, fleshy appearance

Microscopic Features

- Thin, smooth-walled cysts measuring few mm to 3-4 cm
- Aspiration of cyst fluid reveals foamy macrophages, lymphoid & epithelial cells, & multinucleated giant cells
  - Intense immunoexpression of S100 & p24 (HIV-1) protein in multinucleated giant cells

CLINICAL ISSUES

Presentation

- Most common signs/symptoms
  - Bilateral painless parotid gland enlargement
- Other signs/symptoms
  - Cervical lymphadenopathy
  - Tonsillar swelling
- Clinical profile
  - Bilateral parotid masses in HIV-positive patient
    - Initially seen in HIV-positive patients prior to AIDS onset
      - BLEL may precede HIV seroconversion
      - BLEL not considered precursor to AIDS

Demographics

- Age
  - Any age infected with HIV
- Epidemiology
  - Historically, **5%** of HIV-positive patients develop BLEL
  - BLEL seen less frequently since institution of combination antiviral therapy

Natural History & Prognosis

- Left untreated, may grow into chronic, mumps-like state with significant bilateral parotid enlargement
- Rarely may transform into B-cell lymphoma
- Patient prognosis dependent on other HIV- & AIDS-related diseases, not on BLEL

Treatment

- Combination antiretroviral therapy for HIV will completely or partially treat BLEL of parotid glands
- Radiotherapy yields mixed, nonlasting regression
- BLE cysts: Intralesional doxycycline or alcohol sclerotherapy if painful or if not antiviral candidate
- Surgical excision not recommended in AIDS patients

DIAGNOSTIC CHECKLIST

Consider

- Consider using T2 FS MR to make lesions more conspicuous
- Image from skull base to clavicles to fully evaluate extent of parotid involvement & adenopathy

Image Interpretation Pearls

- Bilateral cystic & solid masses within enlarged parotids in HIV-positive patient should be considered BLEL until proven otherwise
- Nonnecrotic cervical adenopathy with tonsillar hypertrophy can be important clue to BLEL diagnosis with CECT
- When BLE cysts present as unilateral cystic intraparotid mass, may be mistaken for 1st branchial cleft cyst
- When BLEL presents as unilateral solid intraparotid mass, may be mistaken for parotid tumor

Reporting Tips

- BLE may be 1st sign of HIV infection; recommend HIV testing in characteristic cases

SELECTED REFERENCES

1. Berg EE et al: Office-based sclerotherapy for benign parotid lymphoepithelial cysts in the HIV-positive patient. Laryngoscope. 119(5):868-70, 2009
2. Gupta N et al: Multinucleated giant cells in HIV-associated benign lymphoepithelial cyst-like lesions of the parotid gland on FNAC. Diagn Cytopathol. 37(3):203-4, 2009
3. Kothari KS et al: Cystic lymphoepithelial lesion of the parotid as an early indicator of HIV infection. J Postgrad Med. 55(2):135-6, 2009
4. Meyer E et al: Alcohol sclerotherapy of human immunodeficiency virus related parotid lymphoepithelial cysts. J Laryngol Otol. 123(4):422-5, 2009
5. Wu L et al: Lymphoepithelial cyst of the parotid gland: its possible histopathogenesis based on clinicopathologic analysis of 64 cases. Hum Pathol. 40(5):683-92, 2009
6. Dave SP et al: The benign lymphoepithelial cyst and a classification system for lymphocytic parotid gland enlargement in the pediatric HIV population. Laryngoscope. 117(1):106-13, 2007
7. Marsot-Dupuch K et al: Head and neck lesions in the immunocompromised host. Eur Radiol. 14 Suppl 3:E155-67, 2004
8. Tripathi AK et al: HIV disease presenting as parotid lymphoepithelial cysts: a presumptive diagnosis of diffuse infiltrative lymphocytic syndrome (DILS). J Assoc Physicians India. 52:921-3, 2004
9. Hamilton BE et al: Earring lesions of the parotid tail. AJNR Am J Neuroradiol. 24(9):1757-64, 2003
10. Plaza G et al: Bilateral parotid cysts as presentation of Sjogren's syndrome. J Laryngol Otol. 117(2):151-2, 2003
11. Brudnicki AR et al: HIV-associated (non-thymic) intrathoracic lymphoepithelial cyst in a child. Pediatr Radiol. 31(8): 603-5, 2001
12. Mandel L: Ultrasound findings in HIV-positive patients with parotid gland swellings. J Oral Maxillofac Surg. 59(3): 283-6, 2001
13. Mandel L et al: HIV-associated parotid lymphoepithelial cysts. J Am Dent Assoc. 130(4): 528-32, 1999
14. Uccini S et al: The benign cystic lymphoepithelial lesion of the parotid gland is a viral reservoir in HIV type 1-infected patients. AIDS Res Hum Retroviruses. 15(15): 1339-44, 1999
15. Chetty R: HIV-associated lymphoepithelial cysts and lesions: morphological and immunohistochemical study of the lymphoid cells. Histopathology. 33(3): 222-9, 1998
16. Craven DE et al: Response of lymphoepithelial parotid cysts to antiretroviral treatment in HIV-infected adults. Ann Intern Med. 128(6): 455-9, 1998
17. Kooper DP et al: Management of benign lymphoepithelial lesions of the parotid gland in human immunodeficiency virus-positive patients. Eur Arch Otorhinolaryngol. 255(8): 427-9, 1998
18. Lustig LR et al: Doxycycline sclerosis of benign lymphoepithelial cysts in patients infected with HIV. Laryngoscope. 108(8 Pt 1): 1199-205, 1998

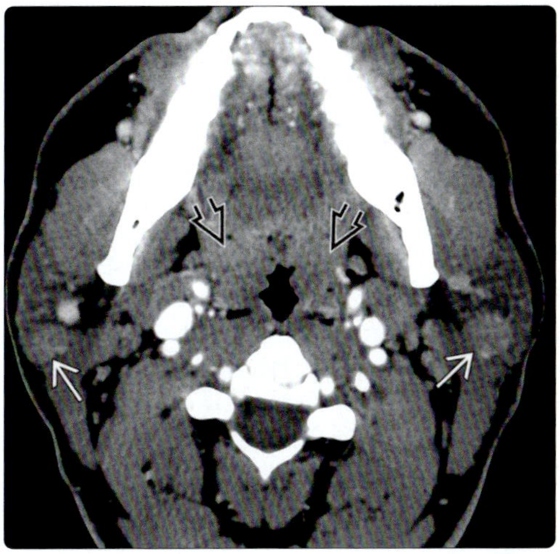
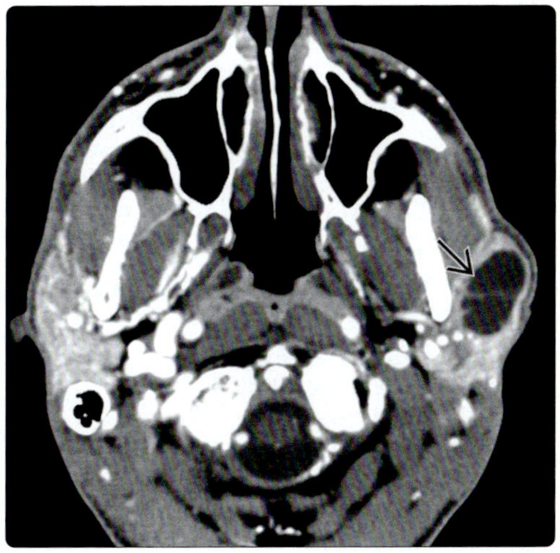

(Left) *Axial CECT shows bilateral, well-defined, enhancing, solid masses ➡ in both parotid glands. Although metastases & lymphoma may have a similar appearance, the presence of tonsillar hypertrophy ⇨ should suggest the diagnosis of BLEL or persistent parotid gland lymphadenopathy from HIV.* **(Right)** *Axial CECT shows a solitary septate mass ⇨ in the left parotid gland. BLEL are generally multiple but can present as a solitary mass.*

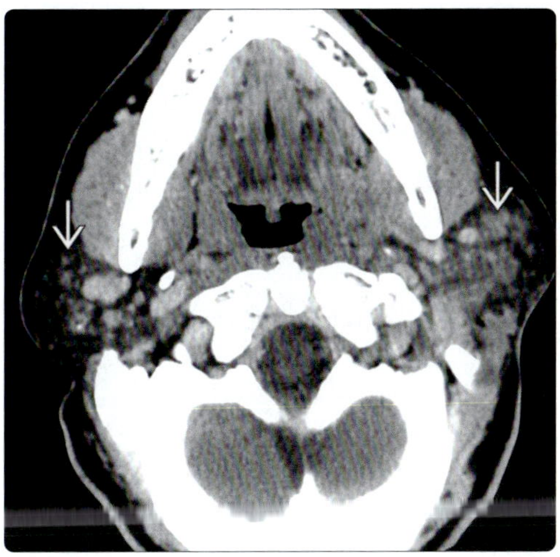
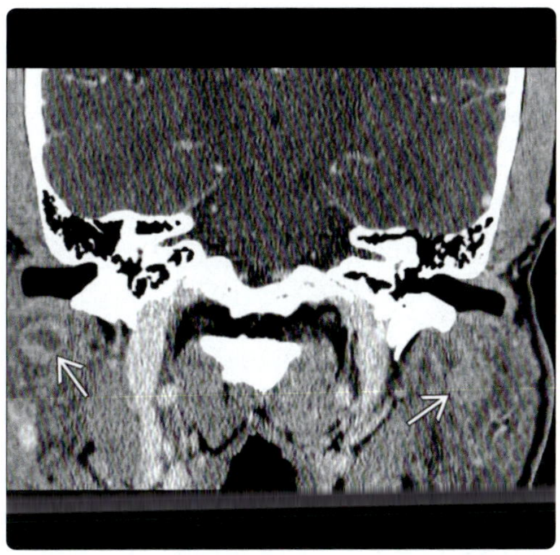

(Left) *Axial CECT shows innumerable small, enhancing nodules ➡ scattered throughout both parotid glands, characteristic of persistent generalized parotid gland lymphadenopathy. The nodules represent enlarged lymph nodes.* **(Right)** *Coronal reformatted CECT in a patient with HIV shows bilateral parotid lesions ➡ with both cystic & solid components, consistent with BLEL of HIV.*

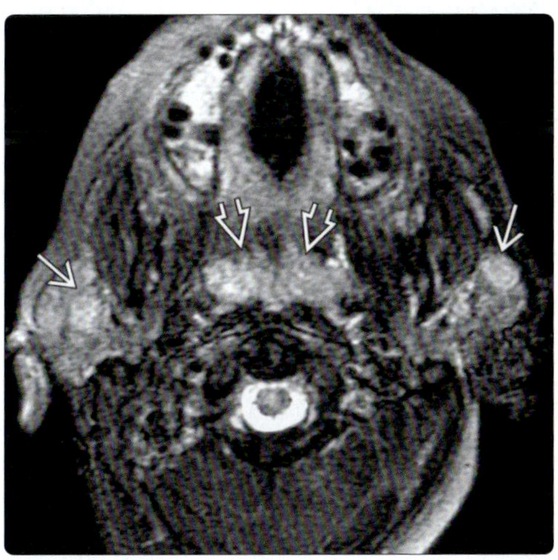
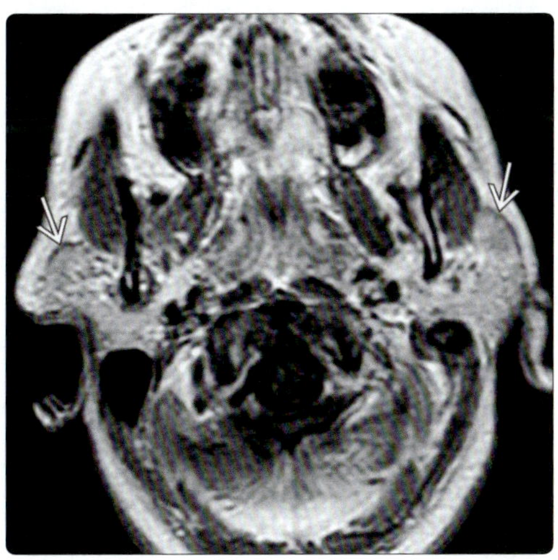

(Left) *Axial T2 FS MR shows bilateral parotid masses ➡ with high T2 signal. Both solid & cystic BLEL will have high T2 signal. Note the enlarged adenoids ⇨.* **(Right)** *Axial T1 C+ MR shows bilateral parotid masses ➡ with rim enhancement. Solid BLEL may be harder to recognize on contrast-enhanced images because the enhancement blends into the background fat of the parotid gland.*

Parotid Sialadenitis

KEY FACTS

TERMINOLOGY

- Definition: Inflammation or infection of parotid gland
  - Bacterial, viral or obstruction-induced by sialolith

IMAGING

- Sialography or MR sialography for ductal involvement
- CT or ultrasound for parenchymal involvement
- Conventional sialography
  - Dilated ducts **"reverse ductal architecture"** with intermittent ductal dilation/stricture **"sausage link"** (sialodochitis)
- CT
  - Acute: Diffuse radiodense lesion in enlarged parotid (bacterial/viral)
  - Chronic: Heterogeneous atrophied glands
  - Enlarged ducts with possible visualized sialolithiasis
  - Sialectasia and ductal changes are variable
  - **Abscess** cavities: Low density with **enhancing rim**
  - **May mimic mass lesion** or malignant neoplasm
- MR
  - Diffuse high signal with sporadic higher intensity foci (abscesses)
  - Diffuse enhancement of enlarged or atrophied gland

TOP DIFFERENTIAL DIAGNOSES

- **Sjögren syndrome**
- HIV-related benign lymphoepithelial cysts
- Malignant tumor

DIAGNOSTIC CHECKLIST

- Glandular swelling/enlargement in acute parotitis
- Parenchymal atrophy in chronic parotid sialolithiasis
- Possible **sialoliths** indicative of obstructive etiology
- Look for "reverse ductal architecture" and abnormal morphology of ductal system
- Look for globular and destructive sialectasia in more advanced cases
- **Rule out neoplasia**

*(**Left**) Conventional sialography of parotid sialadenitis shows minor ductal enlargement (reverse architecture) ➔ with minimal visualization of terminal ducts ➔ and acini. A radiolucent sialolith ➔ is present in the distal portion of the Stensen duct. (**Right**) Coronal reconstructed CECT of acute viral parotitis in a 7 year old shows hyperenhancement and enlargement of the right parotid gland ➔. The left parotid is normal ➔. There is no abscess formation, lymphadenopathy, or visible calculus.*

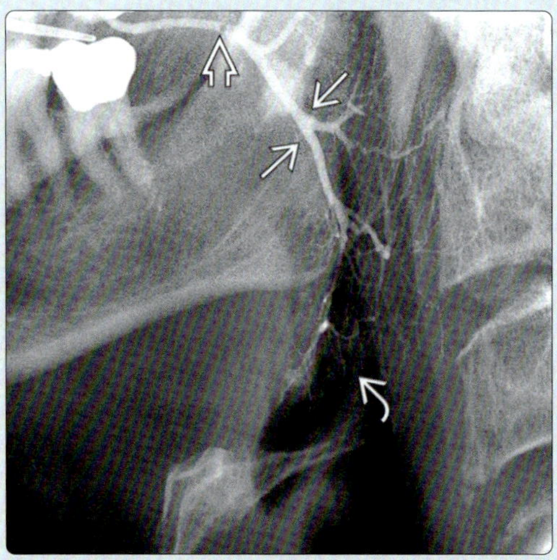

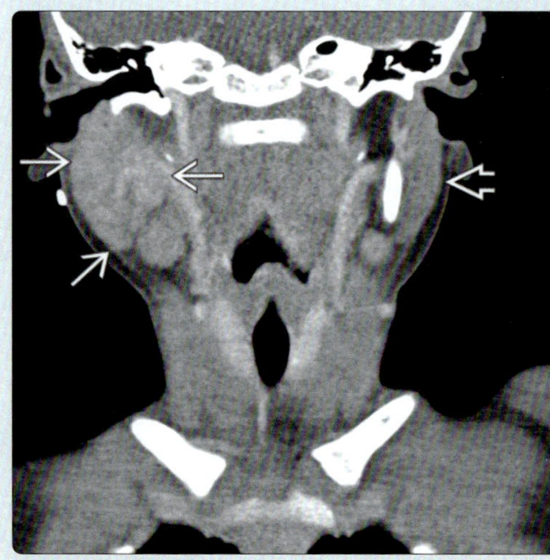

*(**Left**) Axial MR STIR of obstructive acute sialadenitis shows diffuse higher signal in left parotid gland compared to right ➔. Ductal obstruction ➔ and extraglandular main duct enlargement ➔ visualized. Obstruction from small stone or ductal stenosis is the cause of this parotitis. (**Right**) Axial CECT shows chronic parotitis. Both parotids are atrophied and slightly heterogeneous in density. On left side, there is intraglandular duct dilation ➔ and marked dilation of the Stensen duct ➔. No calculi are seen.*

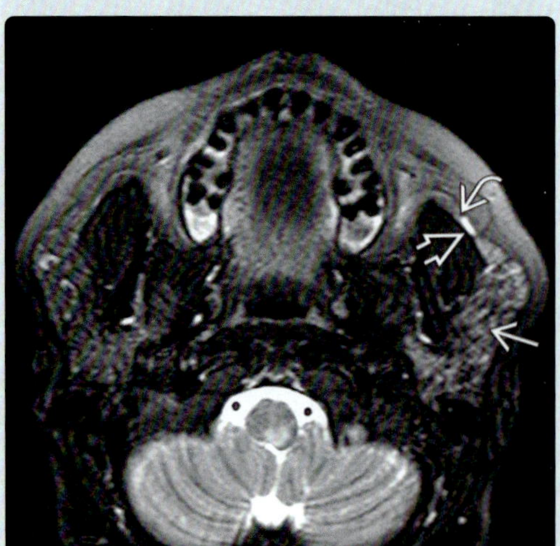

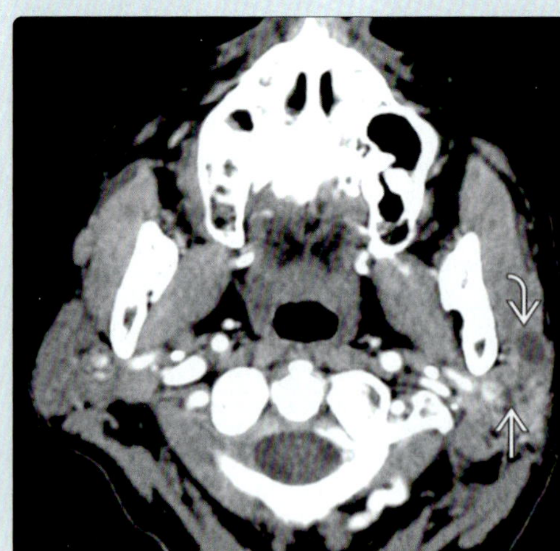

TERMINOLOGY

Synonyms

- Parotitis

Definitions

- Inflammation or infection of parotid gland
  - Bacterial: Acute suppurative (usually localized)
  - Viral: Acute viral parotid sialadenitis (epidemic parotitis)
  - Obstruction-induced by sialolith: Secondary sialadenitis
  - Unknown etiology: Juvenile recurrent parotitis

IMAGING

General Features

- Best diagnostic clue
  - Enlarged parotids in acute; atrophied parenchyma in chronic
- Location
  - Parotid space
  - Acute usually unilateral; chronic usually bilateral

Radiographic Findings

- Conventional or CBCT sialography
  - **"Reverse ductal architecture"**: Ducts are larger proximally, rather than smaller, due to dilation
  - Intermittent dilation/stricture **"sausage link"** (sialodochitis)
  - Extravasated/**extraacinar accumulations of contrast** agent (globular and destructive sialectasia)
  - Indicated for ductal inflammation and sialoliths (especially minimally calcified ones)
  - Contraindicated for mass lesions and acute infection

CT Findings

- NECT
  - Hyperdense parotid with irregular margins (bacterial/viral)
  - **Sialoliths** usually visualized
- CECT
  - Acute
    - Diffuse radiodense lesion in enlarged parotid (bacterial/viral)
    - Sialoliths usually visualized but small enhancing vessels may mimic appearance
    - Sialectasia and ductal changes are variable
    - Abscess cavities: Low density with enhancing rim
    - May mimic mass lesion or malignant neoplasm
    - Enlarged intrinsic lymph nodes difficult to differentiate from primary neoplasia
    - Enlarged deep lobe may create mass effect on lateral wall of parapharyngeal space
  - Chronic
    - Heterogeneous, atrophied glands
    - Enlarged ducts with possible visualized sialolithiasis

MR Findings

- T1WI
  - Diffuse high signal with sporadic higher intensity foci (abscesses)
- T2WI FS
  - MR sialography
- T1WI C+
  - Diffuse enhancement of enlarged parotid
  - **Rim-enhancing** low-signal fluid collections (abscesses)

Ultrasonographic Findings

- Enlarged hypoechoic heterogeneous parotid
- Sialoliths and abscess cavities may be detected

Imaging Recommendations

- Best imaging tool
  - Conventional sialography or MR for ductal involvement
    - MR sialography advantageous in acute infection
  - CT or ultrasound for parenchymal involvement
  - US initially in children to minimize radiation risk

DIFFERENTIAL DIAGNOSIS

Sjögren Syndrome

- Punctate sialectasia with multiple intraparotid cystic and solid masses
- May have secondary sialodochitis/sialadenitis

HIV-Related Benign Lymphoepithelial Cysts

- Multiple intraparotid cystic and solid masses mimicking Sjögren syndrome
- Tonsillar hyperplasia and cervical reactive adenopathy

Malignant Tumor

- Intraparotid cystic and solid masses with **invasive margins**

CLINICAL ISSUES

Presentation

- Most common signs/symptoms
  - Preauricular swelling
  - Pain ± suppuration (bacterial infection)
  - Decreased salivary flow

Demographics

- Acute bacterial: Neonates and elderly debilitated
- Acute viral: < 15 years
- Obstructive sialadenitis: Adults

Treatment

- Sialogogues (sugarless gum or sour candy); ↑ liquid intake
- Antibiotic therapy
- Ductal dilation or surgical sialolithectomy
- Surgical removal of entire gland

DIAGNOSTIC CHECKLIST

Consider

- Sjögren syndrome, neoplasia, and multicystic HIV disease

Image Interpretation Pearls

- Look for enlarged ducts and sialoliths
- Look for **"reverse architecture"** and abnormal duct morphology
- Parenchymal atrophy in chronic parotid sialolithiasis
- **Rule out neoplasia**

SELECTED REFERENCES

1. Prasad RS: Parotid gland imaging. Otolaryngol Clin North Am. 49(2):285-312, 2016

Parotid Benign Mixed Tumor

KEY FACTS

TERMINOLOGY

- Synonym: Pleomorphic adenoma

IMAGING

- Contrast-enhanced CT or MR adequate to answer most imaging questions
  - MR best if specific signs (↑ T2 signal, ↑ ADC) present
- CT findings
  - Smoothly marginated, homogeneously enhancing, ovoid mass
  - **Pear-shaped** when in deep lobe & extending through stylomandibular notch
  - Dystrophic calcification may be present
- MR findings
  - ↑ T1 signal in hemorrhagic lesions
  - **Very high T2** signal **specific for benign mixed tumor (BMT)**
  - ADC values higher than other parotid tumors

TOP DIFFERENTIAL DIAGNOSES

- Warthin tumor
- Metastatic nodes in parotid
- Parotid adenoid cystic carcinoma
- Mucoepidermoid carcinoma
- Parotid non-Hodgkin lymphoma

CLINICAL ISSUES

- Facial nerve paralysis is rare: Suggests malignancy
- Multifocal primary BMT rare (< 1%)
- Rapid enlargement concerning for malignant degeneration (carcinoma ex pleomorphic adenoma)

DIAGNOSTIC CHECKLIST

- Infiltrative margins, multicentricity, or hypointense T2 signal suggests malignancy
- Relationship of BMT to CNVII critical for surgical planning

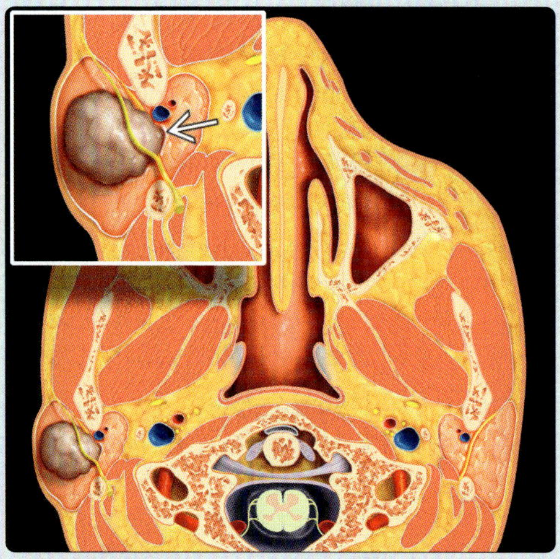

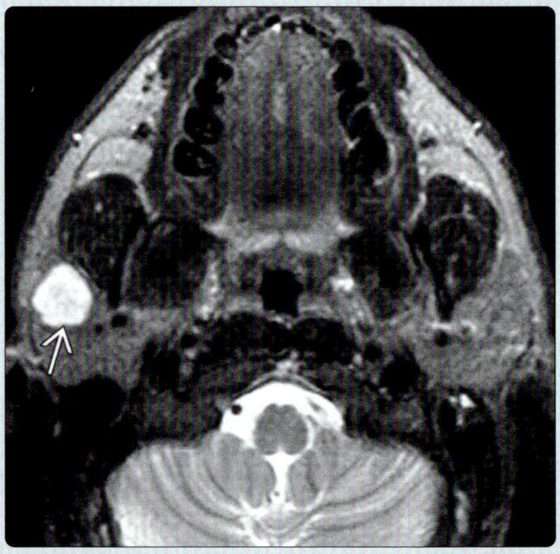

(Left) *Axial graphic depicts a small predominantly superficial lobe benign mixed tumor (BMT). Notice on insert that the tongue of the tumor has insinuated itself between 2 facial nerve branches to involve the deep lobe →.* **(Right)** *Axial T2WI FS MR reveals a sharply circumscribed, high-signal BMT → in the superficial lobe of the parotid gland. This tumor at the very least abuts, if not crosses, the plane of the intraparotid facial nerve.*

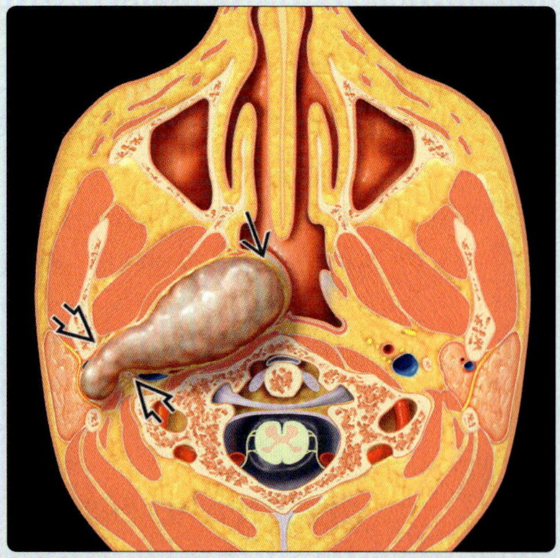

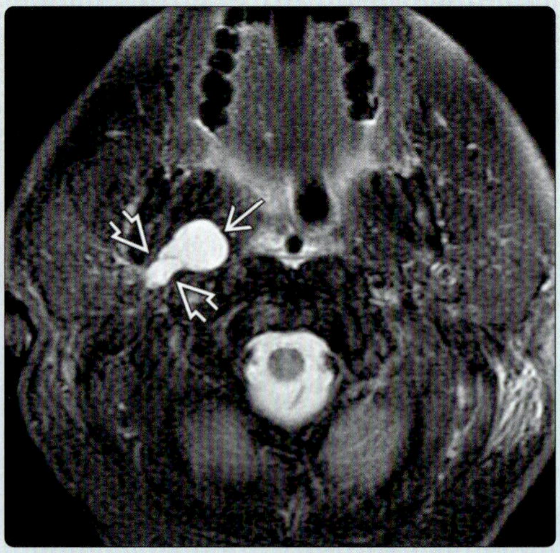

(Left) *Axial graphic reveals a pear-shaped BMT of the deep lobe of the parotid gland. Despite the size of this tumor, the parapharyngeal fat can still be seen → as it is pushed superomedially. Note the widened stylomandibular notch/canal →.* **(Right)** *Axial T2WI FS MR shows a pear-shaped mass → in the parapharyngeal space. The neck of the pear is the portion of the tumor extending through the stylomandibular notch →. Note the extremely high T2 signal (higher than CSF), which further suggests BMT.*

TERMINOLOGY

Synonyms

- Papillary cystadenoma lymphomatosum, adenolymphoma, lymphomatous adenoma

Definitions

- Benign tumor with characteristic histopathologic appearance: Papillary structures, mature lymphocytic infiltrate, & cystic changes

IMAGING

General Features

- Best diagnostic clue
  - Sharply marginated parotid tail mass with heterogeneous parenchyma
- Location
  - Intraparotid > > periparotid > upper cervical nodes
  - Most common mass to arise in parotid tail superficial to angle of mandible
  - **20% multifocal**
    - Multiple lesions in 1 gland or bilateral lesions
    - May be synchronous or metachronous
- Size
  - Typically 2- to 4-cm diameter
  - Neglected lesions > 10-cm diameter
- Morphology
  - Round to ovoid, well-circumscribed encapsulated mass or masses
  - **Parenchymal heterogeneity** is **characteristic**

CT Findings

- CECT
  - Solitary small, ovoid, smoothly marginated masses in posterior aspect of superficial lobe of parotid
  - No calcification
  - Cystic component in 30% with thin, uniform walls & CT density of 10-20 HU
    - Large cystic component, septa, or multiple adjacent cystic lesions
      - May be difficult to differentiate from 1st branchial cleft cyst, infected lymph node, or other cystic mass
    - **Mural nodule** more suggestive of Warthin tumor
  - Minimal enhancement of solid components
  - Dynamic CT behavior
    - Rapid enhancement with rapid washout

MR Findings

- T1WI
  - Low signal in both solid & cystic components
  - Cystic areas may show high signal secondary to proteinaceous debris ± hemorrhage
- T2WI
  - Intermediate to high T2 signal in solid component
  - High T2 signal in cystic foci
- STIR
  - Lesions more conspicuous, especially cystic component
- DWI
  - ADC values lower than benign mixed tumor (BMT) but similar to carcinoma
- T1WI C+
  - Minimal contrast enhancement of solid components
  - Dynamic contrast imaging: Rapid enhancement with rapid washout
    - Similar to some carcinomas

Ultrasonographic Findings

- Well-defined anechoic mass or masses with multiple anechoic areas at lower pole of superficial parotid
- Heterogeneous echotexture in septate or complicated intralesional cystic components

Nuclear Medicine Findings

- PET
  - Increased uptake of FDG
    - Benign parotid tumors (Warthin, oncocytoma) often incidentally seen on PET
- Technetium-99m
  - Increased uptake within mitochondrial-rich oncocytes of Warthin tumors
  - Delayed washout following sialogogue administration

Imaging Recommendations

- Best imaging tool
  - Contrast-enhanced CT or MR provides adequate presurgical information

DIFFERENTIAL DIAGNOSIS

Benign Lymphoepithelial Lesions: HIV

- When unilateral & singular, may strongly mimic Warthin tumor
- Tonsillar hyperplasia & cervical adenopathy help differentiate

Parotid Benign Mixed Tumor

- Well-circumscribed, homogeneous, intraparotid mass when small
- Larger lesions may be heterogeneous & mimic Warthin

Malignant Parotid Tumor

- Parotid adenoid cystic carcinoma
  - Low-grade tumor may be well demarcated & mimic Warthin tumor
  - High-grade tumor invasive appearance is distinctive
  - Perineural tumor spread common
- Parotid mucoepidermoid carcinoma
  - Low-grade tumor may be well demarcated & mimic Warthin tumor
  - High-grade tumor invasive appearance is distinctive
  - Adjacent malignant nodes common

Parotid Metastatic Nodal Disease

- Primary malignancy on or around skin of ear
- Single or multiple parotid masses with invasive margins
- Central necrosis may mimic cystic change of Warthin tumor

Parotid Non-Hodgkin Lymphoma

- Multiple solid, uniformly enhancing, intraparotid lesions
- Cervical adenopathy may help differentiate from Warthin tumor

PATHOLOGY

General Features

- Etiology
  - **Smoking-induced**, benign tumor arising from salivary-lymphoid tissue in intraparotid & periparotid nodes
  - Theorized heterotopic salivary gland parenchyma present in preexisting intra- or periparotid lymph nodes
  - Reported association with **Epstein-Barr virus**
    - Patients with multifocal or bilateral lesions
- Associated abnormalities
  - Increased incidence in patients with autoimmune disorders
- Embryology
  - Parotid gland undergoes "**late encapsulation**," incorporating lymphoid tissue/nodes within superficial layer of deep cervical fascia
    - Warthin tumor arises within this lymphoid tissue

Gross Pathologic & Surgical Features

- Encapsulated, soft, ovoid mass with smooth, lobulated surface
- Tan tissue with cystic spaces that contain tenacious, mucoid, brown fluid or thin, yellow fluid with cholesterol crystals
  - Papillary projections can be seen within cystic areas

Microscopic Features

- Epithelial & lymphoid components dominate histopathologic picture
- Papillary projections are lined with double epithelial layer
  - Inner luminal layer: Tall columnar cells with nuclei oriented toward lumen
  - Outer basal layer: Cuboidal or polygonal cells with vesicular nuclei
- Inner lymphoid component of papillary projection is composed of mature lymphoid aggregates with germinal centers

CLINICAL ISSUES

Presentation

- Most common signs/symptoms
  - Angle of mandible (tail of parotid) mass
  - Painless
  - Multiple masses ~ 20%
- Other signs/symptoms
  - Facial nerve weakness very rare; suggests malignancy
- Clinical profile
  - **90%** of patients with Warthin tumor **smoke**
  - Increased incidence with radiation exposure

Demographics

- Age
  - Mean age at presentation: 60 years
- Gender
  - Earlier reports have M:F = 3:1
  - More recent reports show more equal gender incidence (likely related to smoking patterns)
- Epidemiology
  - **2nd** most frequent benign parotid tumor (after BMT)
  - 10% of all salivary gland epithelial tumors
  - 12% of benign parotid gland tumors
  - 20% multifocal: May be unilateral or bilateral, synchronous or metachronous
  - **5-10%** arise in **extraparotid** locations (periparotid & upper neck lymph nodes)

Natural History & Prognosis

- Slowly growing, benign tumor
- Malignant transformation (carcinoma or lymphoma) reported in < 1%
- "Recurrent" Warthin tumor may be from inadequate resection or metachronous 2nd lesion

Treatment

- Biopsy (or excision) needed for confirmation of benign nature
- Resection of mass within collar of normal parotid tissue without injury to intraparotid facial nerve is treatment goal

DIAGNOSTIC CHECKLIST

Consider

- Consider CECT to help identify cystic areas within Warthin tumor to help differentiate from small BMT
- Enhanced T1 with fat saturation to determine intra- vs. periparotid tumor location & to define plane of facial nerve

Image Interpretation Pearls

- Be sure to carefully examine for multiplicity & bilaterality
- Well-circumscribed heterogeneous multiple or bilateral parotid masses in asymptomatic smoker should be considered Warthin tumor

SELECTED REFERENCES

1. Berger MH et al: Case of parotid mucoepidermoid carcinoma: expanding the spectrum of von Hippel-Lindau-related neoplasms. Head Neck. 39(3):E51-E54, 2017
2. Kulkarni M et al: Incidental Warthin tumor on pertechnetate scintigraphy. Clin Nucl Med. 41(9):728-9, 2016
3. Luers JC et al: The incidence of Warthin tumours and pleomorphic adenomas in the parotid gland over a 25-year period. Clin Otolaryngol. 41(6):793-797, 2016
4. Sagiv D et al: Warthin tumor within the superficial lobe of the parotid gland: a suggested criterion for diagnosis. Eur Arch Otorhinolaryngol. ePub, 2016
5. Yu C et al: Mucoepidermoid carcinoma arising in Warthin's tumor of the parotid gland: clinicopathological characteristics and immunophenotypes. Sci Rep. 6:30149, 2016
6. Habermann CR et al: Diffusion-weighted echo-planar MR imaging of primary parotid gland tumors: is a prediction of different histologic subtypes possible? AJNR Am J Neuroradiol. 30(3):591-6, 2009
7. Ethunandan M et al: Factors influencing the occurrence of multicentric and 'recurrent' Warthin's tumour: a cross sectional study. Int J Oral Maxillofac Surg. 37(9):831-4, 2008
8. Yerli H et al: Dynamic multislice computed tomography findings for parotid gland tumors. J Comput Assist Tomogr. 31(2):309-16, 2007
9. Hamilton BE et al: Earring lesions of the parotid tail. AJNR Am J Neuroradiol. 24(9):1757-64, 2003
10. Marioni G et al: Facial nerve paralysis secondary to Warthin's tumour of the parotid gland. J Laryngol Otol. 117(6):511-3, 2003
11. Zeebregts CJ et al: Synchronous tumours of the unilateral parotid gland: rare or undetected? J Craniomaxillofac Surg. 31(1):62-6, 2003
12. Laane CJ et al: Role of Epstein-Barr virus and cytomegalovirus in the etiology of benign parotid tumors. Head Neck. 24(5):443-50, 2002
13. Lewis PD et al: Mitochondrial DNA mutations in the parotid gland of cigarette smokers and non-smokers. Mutat Res. 518(1):47-54, 2002
14. Maiorano E et al: Warthin's tumour: a study of 78 cases with emphasis on bilaterality, multifocality and association with other malignancies. Oral Oncol. 38(1):35-40, 2002
15. Sungur N et al: Clinicopathological evaluation of parotid gland tumors: a retrospective study. J Craniofac Surg. 13(1):26-30, 2002

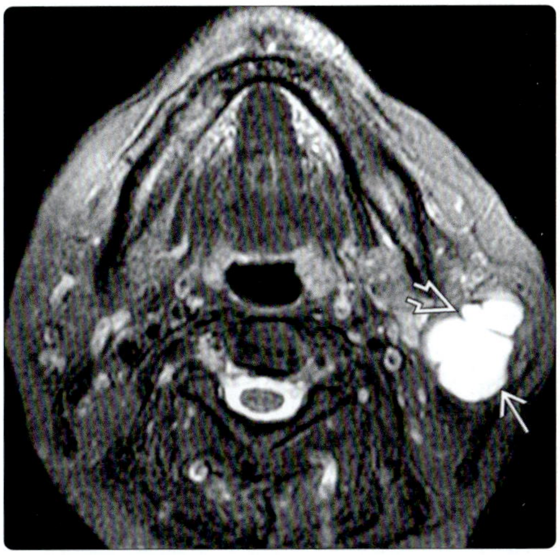

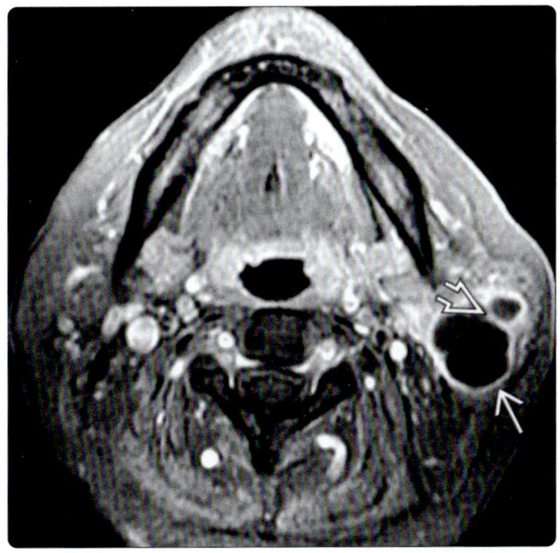

(Left) *Axial T2WI FS MR shows a high-intensity mass ➡ with septations ➡ in the superficial lobe of the parotid gland. Cystic Warthin tumors can be confused with simple cysts.* **(Right)** *Axial T1WI C+ FS MR in the same patient reveals a septated ➡ low-intensity mass ➡ with an enhancing rim. This enhancement can help to distinguish Warthin tumors from simple cysts but may be mistaken for a parotid abscess. Note the lack of surrounding fat stranding, which argues against abscess.*

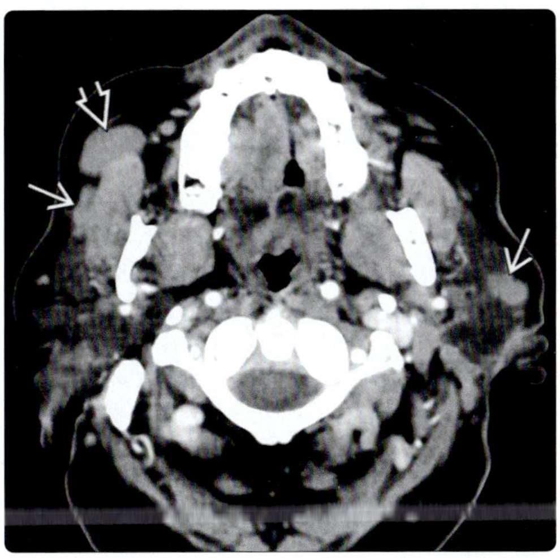

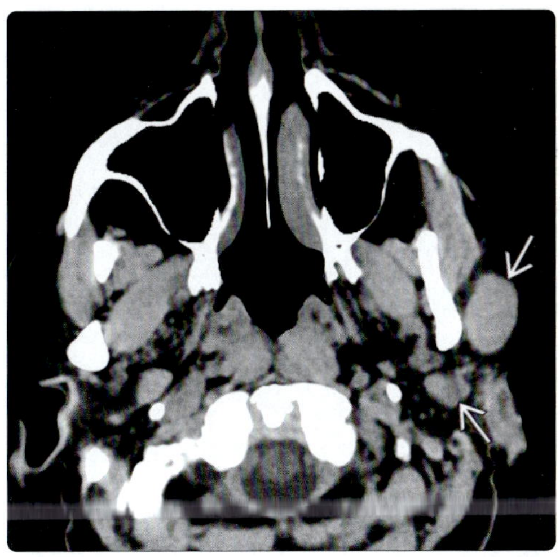

(Left) *Axial CECT shows multiple bilateral, ovoid, poorly enhancing Warthin tumors ➡ within the parotid glands. Note, in particular, the tumor involving the right accessory parotid lobe ➡.* **(Right)** *Axial NECT shows multiple well-defined, ovoid Warthin tumors ➡ of varying size within the left parotid gland. 20% of patients with Warthin tumors have multifocal disease, which may be multiple lesions in a single gland or bilateral lesions.*

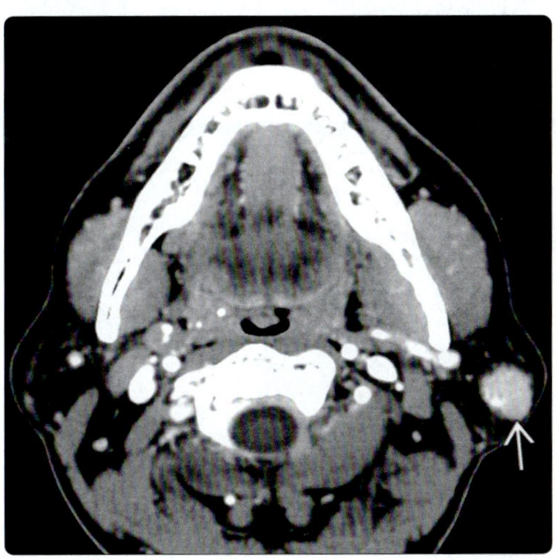

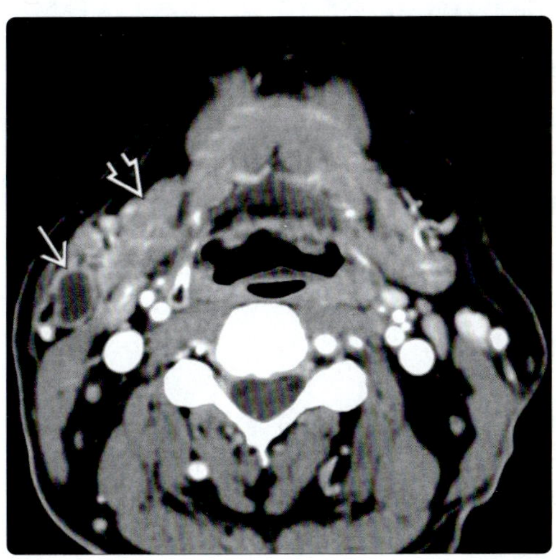

(Left) *Axial CECT shows a round, uniformly enhancing mass ➡ in the superficial lobe of the parotid gland. Smaller Warthin tumors may enhance homogeneously, but larger tumors are generally heterogeneous.* **(Right)** *Axial CECT shows a cystic mass ➡ lateral to the submandibular gland ➡ near the parotid tail. Although most Warthin tumors arise within the parotid gland, some are found in periparotid lymph nodes.*

Parotid Schwannoma

KEY FACTS

TERMINOLOGY

- Benign neoplasm of Schwann cells surrounding intraparotid facial nerve branches

IMAGING

- Heterogeneously enhancing tumor with intramural cystic areas when large
  - Cystic areas may be small, multifocal, or large
- May extend toward or into stylomastoid foramen
- Similar appearance to schwannomas in other anatomic locations

TOP DIFFERENTIAL DIAGNOSES

- Parotid benign mixed tumor
- Warthin tumor
- Parotid metastatic nodal disease
- Parotid mucoepidermoid carcinoma

PATHOLOGY

- Type A: Exophytic off CNVII branch; no CNVII resection required
- Type B: Intrinsic to facial nerve branch; branch resection required
- Type C: Intrinsic to facial nerve trunk; resection and reconstruction required
- Type D: Encases main trunk and branches; resection and reconstruction required

CLINICAL ISSUES

- Presents like any parotid mass; difficult to differentiate clinically or radiographically
  - Facial nerve palsy uncommon
- Associated with neurofibromatosis type 2
- Treatment controversial; tumor easily dissected from CNVII, but palsy may result nonetheless
- Stereotactic radiosurgery may be used if CNVII intact

(Left) *Axial T1WI C+ FS MR shows a rounded mass ➡ in the anterior aspect of the superficial parotid lobe. There are areas of heterogeneous enhancement with scattered cystic regions. Note the parotitis ⇨ that results from ductal obstruction by the schwannoma.* **(Right)** *Axial T2WI FS MR shows a round mass ➡ with heterogeneous high signal in the anterior aspect of the superficial parotid lobe. This lesion appearance would be difficult to distinguish from the far more common benign mixed tumor.*

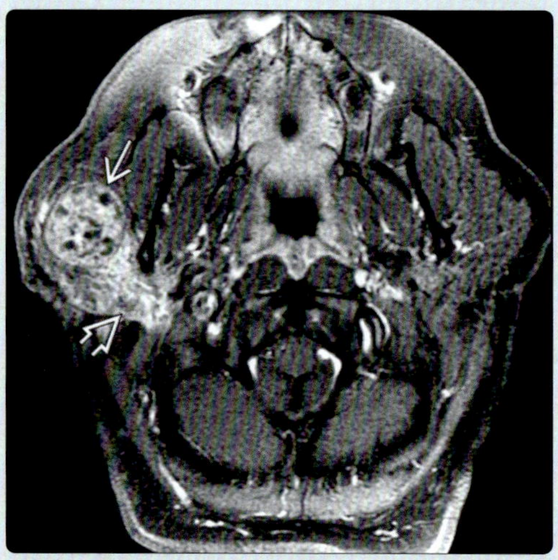

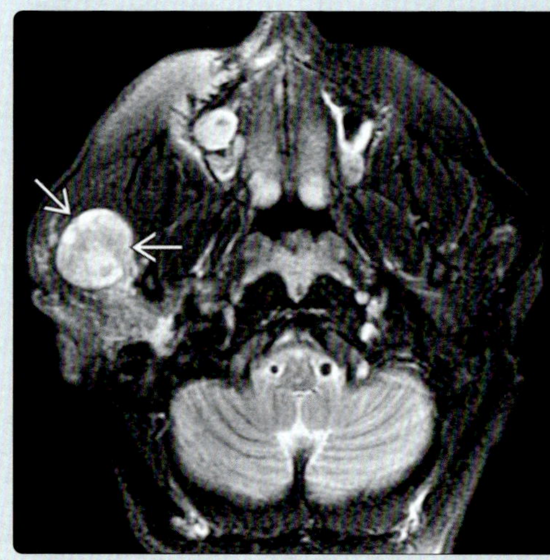

(Left) *Axial CECT in a patient with neurofibromatosis type 2 shows a round subcentimeter mass ➡ in the anterior aspect of the superficial parotid lobe. This schwannoma has heterogeneous enhancement but no cystic areas because of its small size.* **(Right)** *Coronal bone CT shows smooth expansion of the vertical segment of the facial canal ➡. The facial nerve schwannoma extends from the parotid gland ⇨ up through the stylomastoid foramen.*

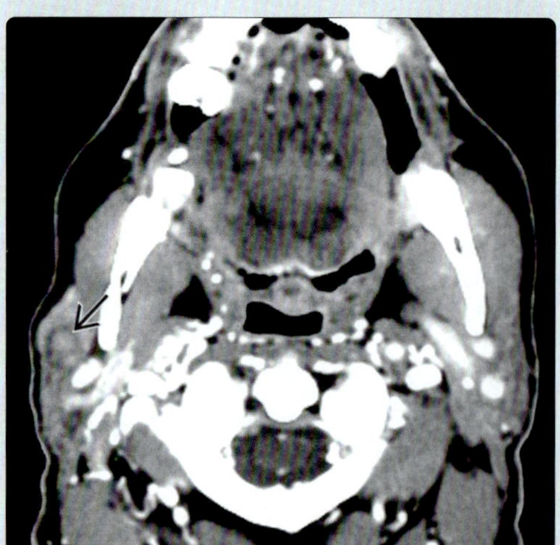

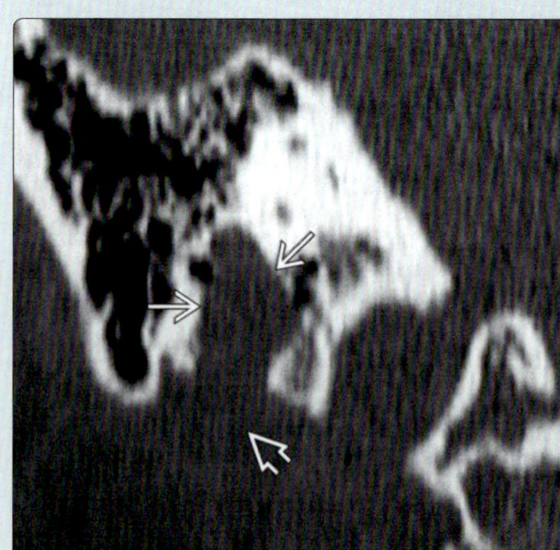

TERMINOLOGY

Synonyms

- Facial neuroma, intraparotid neurilemmoma

Definitions

- Benign neoplasm of Schwann cells surrounding facial nerve branches within parotid gland

IMAGING

General Features

- Best diagnostic clue
  - Heterogeneously enhancing + **intramural cysts**
    - Cystic areas may be small, multifocal, or large
- Location
  - Along CNVII plane within parotid
  - May extend toward or into stylomastoid foramen

Imaging Recommendations

- Best imaging tool
  - T1WI C+ FS MR best demonstrates cystic areas

CT Findings

- CECT
  - Well-defined intraparotid round or oval mass
  - Intramural cysts within larger (> 2 cm) lesions
  - Enlarged stylomastoid foramen in proximal lesions

MR Findings

- T1WI
  - Tumor isointense to muscle, well defined
- T2WI
  - Slightly hyperintense to brain, muscle
  - Larger lesions with high-intensity cysts
- T1WI C+ FS
  - Enhancing and cystic regions + peripheral enhancement

DIFFERENTIAL DIAGNOSIS

Parotid Benign Mixed Tumor

- Similar appearance on CT and MR
- Parotid schwannoma usually mistaken for this tumor

Warthin Tumor

- Cystic areas seen in both lesions

Parotid Metastatic Nodal Disease

- Often multiple

Parotid Mucoepidermoid Carcinoma

- Low-grade form well defined

PATHOLOGY

General Features

- Etiology
  - Arises from differentiated neoplastic Schwann cells wrapping around CNVII

Staging, Grading, & Classification

- Type A: Exophytic off CNVII branch; no CNVII resection required
- Type B: Intrinsic to CNVII branch; branch resection required
- Type C: Intrinsic to CNVII trunk; resection and reconstruction required
- Type D: Encases main CNVII trunk and branches; resection and reconstruction required

Gross Pathologic & Surgical Features

- Smooth, rubbery, yellow, encapsulated fusiform mass

Microscopic Features

- Same as schwannomas in other anatomic locations

CLINICAL ISSUES

Presentation

- Most common signs/symptoms
  - Slowly enlarging cheek mass
    - Often symptomatic for > 10 years
- Other signs/symptoms
  - Presents like any parotid mass; difficult to differentiate clinically or radiographically
    - Rarely diagnosed preoperatively
  - Facial nerve palsy not common but sometimes seen
  - Associated with neurofibromatosis type 2

Demographics

- Age
  - Can affect any age group

Natural History & Prognosis

- Slow, continuous enlargement
- Eventually causes mass effect or cosmetic issues

Treatment

- Controversial: Tumor is easily dissected from nerve, but facial nerve palsy may result nonetheless
  - Types C and D lesions at greater risk of postoperative facial nerve palsy
  - Choice of treatment depends on function of facial nerve and location of tumor
- Stereotactic radiosurgery may be used if CNVII intact

DIAGNOSTIC CHECKLIST

Consider

- Which branch of facial nerve involved
  - Main trunk most common
- Relationship of mass to stylomastoid foramen
  - Extent into mastoid segment of bony facial nerve canal

Image Interpretation Pearls

- Difficult to make radiographic diagnosis
  - Tissue sampling required but excisional biopsy risky
  - Image-guided biopsy (CT or US) very useful
    - Core needle biopsy required (fine-needle aspiration inadequate)

SELECTED REFERENCES

1. Damar M et al: Facial nerve schwannoma of parotid gland: difficulties in diagnosis and management. Case Rep Otolaryngol. 2016:3939685, 2016
2. Guraya SS et al: Peripheral nerve sheath tumors arising in salivary glands: A clinicopathologic study. Ann Diagn Pathol. 23:38-42, 2016
3. Zhang GZ et al: Clinical retrospective analysis of 9 cases of intraparotid facial nerve schwannoma. J Oral Maxillofac Surg. 74(8):1695-705, 2016
4. Jaiswal A et al: Intraparotid facial nerve schwannoma: A case report. World J Clin Cases. 3(3):322-6, 2015

Parotid Malignant Mixed Tumor

KEY FACTS

TERMINOLOGY

- Malignant mixed tumor (MMT)
- Synonym: Carcinoma ex pleomorphic adenoma
- 2 types of MMT
  - Carcinoma ex pleomorphic adenoma (far more common)
  - Carcinosarcoma (very rare)

IMAGING

- Early MMT: Encapsulated mass with gross appearance of benign mixed tumor (BMT)
- Late MMT: Extensive aggressive parotid mass with erosion of surrounding structures
  - Has characteristics of malignant cell type
  - Residual BMT usually still visible
- MR best for extent of lesion, invasion, & characterizing different tumor regions
  - Unenhanced T1 sequences very useful because of inherent contrast from parotid gland fat
  - Native BMT has high T2 signal, but most carcinomas have lower T2 signal
  - Native BMT has high diffusibility, but carcinomas have low diffusibility

CLINICAL ISSUES

- Rapid enlargement of longstanding parotid mass is most suggestive history
- Other signs
  - Facial nerve weakness & pain
- Early MMT may be incidentally discovered on histologic examination of pleomorphic adenoma
- Prior radiation may increase risk
- 5-10% of BMT degrade into MMT
  - All BMT should be surgically removed before they transform into MMT

DIAGNOSTIC CHECKLIST

- Sudden enlargement of longstanding parotid mass is suggestive history

(Left) *Axial T1WI C+ FS MR shows an aggressive mass ➡ at the stylomandibular tunnel with direct invasion of the mastoid bone ➡. This appearance is consistent with any aggressive parotid tumor, but histology revealed a myoepithelial carcinoma arising within a BMT.* **(Right)** *Axial CECT reveals a heterogeneously enhancing, irregularly calcified mass ➡ centered in the region of the parotid tail. Although BMT may calcify, these calcifications are from a chondrosarcoma that arose in a BMT.*

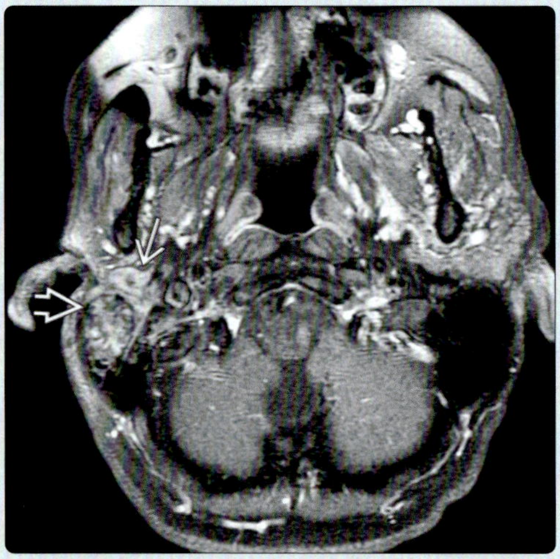

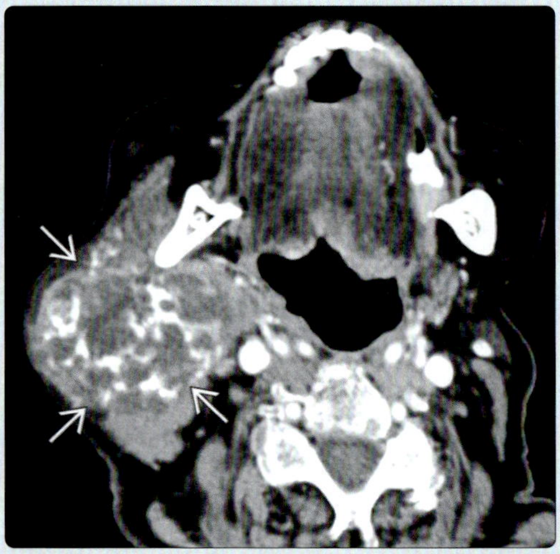

(Left) *Axial CECT demonstrates an ill-defined, invasive mass ➡ in the accessory lobe of the parotid, where the patient had sudden enlargement of a longstanding mass. This is salivary ductal carcinoma, the most common malignancy to arise from a BMT.* **(Right)** *Axial T1WI C+ FS MR shows an aggressive, heterogeneously enhancing mass ➡ replacing the parotid gland. Histologically, this malignancy showed areas of carcinoma and sarcoma, as well as residual BMT, which confirmed the diagnosis of "true" MMT.*

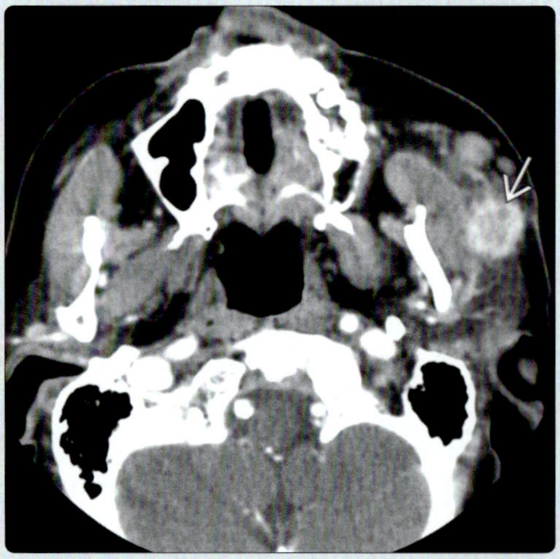

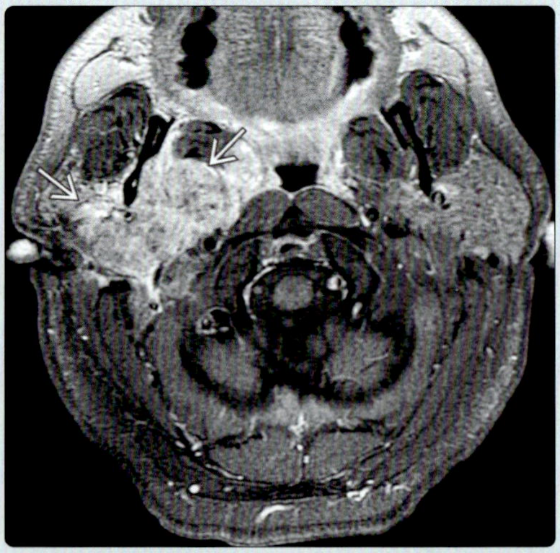

TERMINOLOGY

Abbreviations

- Malignant mixed tumor (MMT)

Synonyms

- **Carcinoma ex pleomorphic adenoma**

Definitions

- Malignant tumor arising within parotid benign mixed tumor (BMT)
- 2 types of MMT
  - **Carcinoma ex pleomorphic adenoma**
    - Common MMT type
    - Consists of single malignant cell type
  - **Carcinosarcoma** ("true" MMT)
    - Consists of multiple malignant cell types
    - Very rare (< 70 in literature)

IMAGING

General Features

- Best diagnostic clue
  - Early MMT: Not distinguishable from surrounding BMT
  - Late MMT: Aggressive parotid mass with extensive invasion of surrounding tissues
    - Tumor has characteristics of malignant cell type
    - Residual BMT may still be visible

MR Findings

- T2WI
  - Native BMT has high T2 signal, often heterogeneous
  - Some carcinomas (mucoepidermoid, salivary ductal) have low T2 signal
- DWI
  - Native BMT has high diffusivity (↓ DWI signal)
  - Carcinomas have low diffusivity (↑ DWI signal)

Imaging Recommendations

- Best imaging tool
  - MR best for extent of lesion, invasion, & characterizing different tumor regions
- Protocol advice
  - Unenhanced T1 sequences very useful because of inherent contrast from parotid gland fat

DIFFERENTIAL DIAGNOSIS

Parotid Benign Mixed Tumor

- Sharp margins
- MR: T2 mostly hypertense; T1 C+ heterogeneous

Warthin Tumor

- Typically at tail of parotid
- May be multiple, solid, or cystic
- MR: T2 bright if cystic or solid

Parotid Mucoepidermoid Carcinoma

- Well-defined or infiltrative PS mass
- MR: Lower T2 signal than adenoid cystic carcinoma; nodes common

Parotid Adenoid Cystic Carcinoma

- Well-defined or infiltrative PS mass
- MR: Higher T2 signal than parotid mucoepidermoid carcinoma; perineural tumor

PATHOLOGY

General Features

- Carcinoma ex pleomorphic adenoma: Malignant degeneration of 1 cell line in BMT
  - Most often salivary ductal carcinoma
  - Residual BMT needed to definitively diagnose carcinoma ex pleomorphic adenoma
- Parotid carcinosarcoma: Etiology controversial
  - Likely represents malignancy from pluripotent cell that differentiates in multiple directions while maintaining malignant potential
  - May represent collision tumor of multiple carcinomas ex pleomorphic adenoma
  - Carcinoma component of "true MMT" usually salivary gland carcinoma
    - Sarcoma component usually chondrosarcoma
    - Glandular & spindle cell components common

CLINICAL ISSUES

Presentation

- Most common signs/symptoms
  - Rapid enlargement of longstanding parotid mass
- Other signs/symptoms
  - Facial nerve weakness & pain
  - Early MMT may be incidentally discovered on histologic evaluation of pleomorphic adenoma

Demographics

- Prior radiation may increase risk
- 5-10% of BMT degrade into MMT
  - All BMTs should be surgically removed before they degrade

Natural History & Prognosis

- Carcinoma ex pleomorphic adenoma: Prognosis depends on histologic type, grade, & stage
- Carcinosarcoma: Aggressive tumor with poor prognosis
  - Mean survival: 3.6 years even with treatment

Treatment

- Trimodality therapy (surgery, chemotherapy, radiation)

DIAGNOSTIC CHECKLIST

Image Interpretation Pearls

- Sudden enlargement of longstanding parotid mass is suggestive history
- Look for CNVII & CNV perineural spread

SELECTED REFERENCES

1. Phan HN et al: Primary carcinosarcoma of the parotid gland mimicking as parotid abscess with deep neck infection. J Craniofac Surg. ePub, 2017
2. Enokida T et al: Combined salivary duct carcinoma and squamous cell carcinoma suspected of carcinoma ex pleomorphic adenoma. Pathol Int. 66(8):460-5, 2016
3. Feng D et al: Carcinosarcoma of parotid gland (malignant mixed tumor). Ann Maxillofac Surg. 5(2):240-3, 2015

Parotid Mucoepidermoid Carcinoma

KEY FACTS

TERMINOLOGY

- Parotid mucoepidermoid carcinoma (MECa): Malignant epithelial salivary gland neoplasm composed of mixture of both epidermoid & mucus-secreting cells arising from ductal epithelium

IMAGING

- Imaging appearance based on histologic grade
  - **Low-grade MECa**: Well-circumscribed, heterogeneous parotid space (PS) mass
  - **High-grade MECa**: Invasive, ill-defined PS mass with associated malignant nodes
- If lesion high grade, infiltrative, or near stylomastoid foramen, **perineural spread** on **CNVII** may occur
- High-grade MECa often has **nodal metastases**
- MR findings
  - Areas of **low T2 signal** are characteristic but not pathognomonic
  - T1 C+ shows heterogeneous tumor enhancement
  - Enhanced images may "hide" lesion
  - MR useful for extent of lesion & facial nerve **perineural spread**

TOP DIFFERENTIAL DIAGNOSES

- Parotid benign mixed tumor (BMT)
- Warthin tumor
- Parotid adenoid cystic carcinoma
- Parotid non-Hodgkin lymphoma

CLINICAL ISSUES

- MECa is most common primary parotid malignancy
- Recurrence & survival rates depend heavily on histologic grade
- Late local recurrence (after 5 years) possible

DIAGNOSTIC CHECKLIST

- Low-grade MECa may exactly mimic BMT
- In all parotid masses, check for **CNVII perineural spread**

(Left) *Axial CECT reveals a well-defined mass ➡ in the superficial lobe of the parotid gland. It has a thick rind of peripheral enhancement and is centrally cystic. This is a characteristic imaging appearance for a low-grade mucoepidermoid carcinoma (MECa).* **(Right)** *Axial CECT shows a mass in the parotid gland with ill-defined lateral borders ➡ and well-defined medial borders ➡. The tumor enhances uniformly. Although nonspecific, this is the expected appearance of an intermediate-grade MECa.*

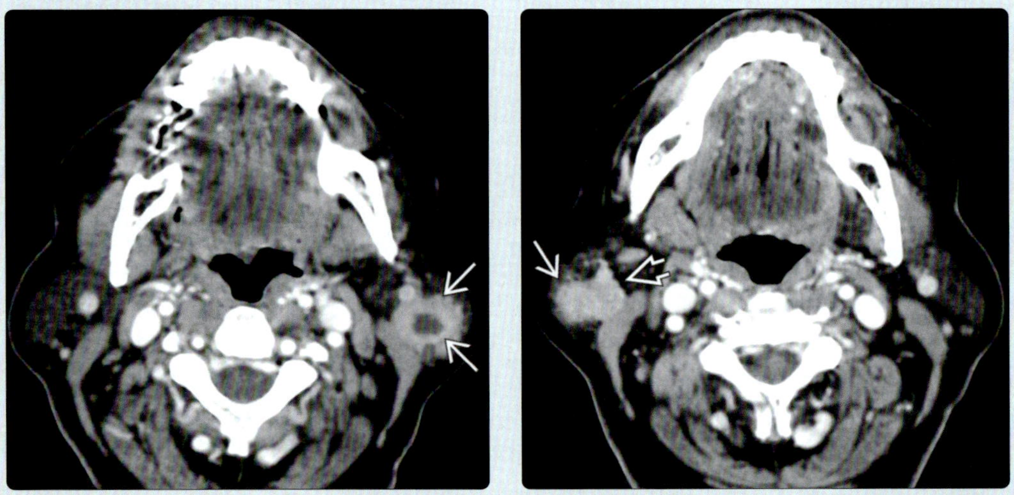

(Left) *Axial CECT shows a large, heterogeneous mass with cystic areas ➡, heterogeneous enhancement, and ill-defined borders ➡. The masseter muscle is invaded ➡. This is a characteristic appearance of a high-grade MECa.* **(Right)** *Axial T2WI FS MR shows an irregular mass in the parotid with mixed T2 signal. Laterally, there are high-signal cystic areas ➡, but medially, there is a low-signal region ➡. Low T2 signal within the solid components of the tumor is characteristic of MECa.*

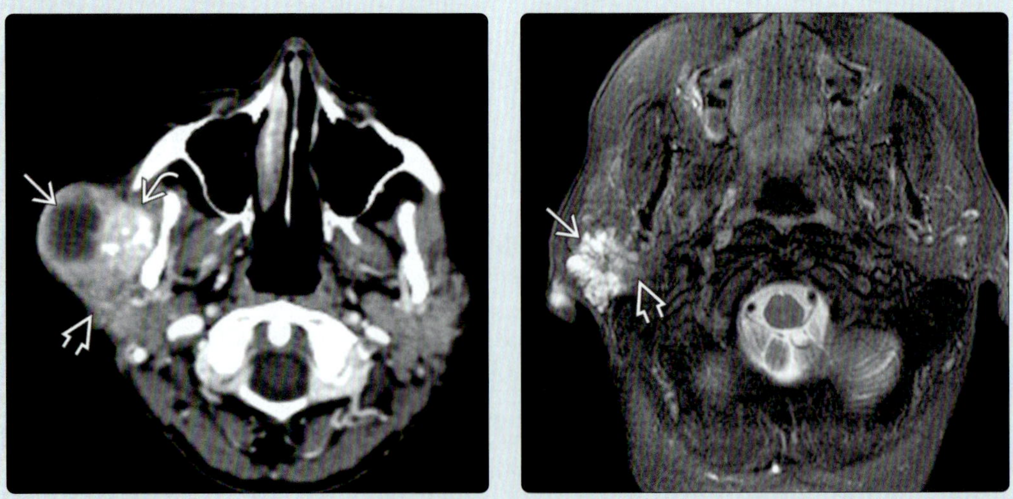

TERMINOLOGY

Abbreviations

- Mucoepidermoid carcinoma (MECa)

Definitions

- Malignant epithelial salivary gland neoplasm composed of variable mixture of both epidermoid & mucus-secreting cells arising from ductal epithelium

IMAGING

General Features

- Best diagnostic clue
  - Imaging appearance based on histologic grade
  - Low-grade MECa: Well-circumscribed, heterogeneous parotid space (PS) mass
  - High-grade MECa: **Invasive**, ill-defined PS mass with associated **malignant nodes**
- Location
  - Superficial lobe > > deep lobe parotid
- Size
  - Usually 1-4 cm at presentation
- Morphology
  - Low grade: Ovoid, well circumscribed
    - Cystic areas may be single & large or small & multifocal
  - High grade: Amorphous, infiltrating mass
- **Malignant adenopathy** often present
  - 1st-order nodes = jugulodigastric nodes (level II)
  - Intrinsic parotid nodes & parotid tail nodes also involved

CT Findings

- CECT
  - Low-grade MECa
    - Enhancing heterogeneous mass with well-defined margins
    - Mucus cystic deposits create cystic areas
  - High-grade MECa
    - Enhancing invasive mass with ill-defined margins
    - Intraparotid & cervical metastatic nodes

MR Findings

- T1WI
  - Low-grade MECa: Heterogeneous, well-defined mass with predominantly low signal
  - High-grade MECa: Solid, infiltrative mass with intermediate signal
- T2WI
  - Low-grade MECa: Heterogeneous signal
    - Areas of low signal are characteristic but not pathognomonic
    - Cystic areas have high signal
  - High-grade MECa: Intermediate signal infiltrating mass
- DWI
  - ADC value lower than benign mixed tumor (BMT) but similar to Warthin tumor
    - Not reliable enough to avoid biopsy
- T1WI C+
  - Heterogeneous enhancement
    - Cystic areas have no enhancement
  - If lesion high grade, infiltrative, or near stylomastoid foramen, perineural spread on CNVII may occur

Nuclear Medicine Findings

- No pertechnetate uptake (unlike Warthin tumor)

Imaging Recommendations

- Best imaging tool
  - MR useful for extent of lesion & perineural spread
  - No radiographic modality provides definitive diagnosis
- Protocol advice
  - T1 unenhanced images best delineate MECa because high-signal fat of normal parotid tissue provides natural contrast
  - Enhanced images may "hide" lesion even if fat saturation used
  - Long-term (at least 10 years) imaging follow-up recommended because of late recurrences

DIFFERENTIAL DIAGNOSIS

Parotid Benign Mixed Tumor

- Most common parotid mass
- Small BMT: Well demarcated, solid, homogeneous, ovoid
- Large BMT: Heterogeneous, lobulated
- Low-grade MECa may be confused with BMT

Warthin Tumor

- Multicentric (20%)
- CECT: 30% with cystic components
- T1WI C+ MR: Heterogeneous enhancement, well circumscribed
- Cystic areas of low-grade MECa appear similar to cystic areas of Warthin tumor

Parotid Adenoid Cystic Carcinoma

- 2nd most common parotid malignancy
- Homogeneous; may be well defined or poorly defined (depending on grade)
- Prone to perineural spread

Parotid Non-Hodgkin Lymphoma

- Primary parotid lymphoma: Invasive parenchymal tumor indistinguishable from high-grade MECa or adenoid cystic carcinoma (ACCa)
- Primary nodal lymphoma: Multiple bilateral intraparotid masses

Parotid Metastatic Nodes

- Primary lesion usually on or around skin of ear (squamous cell carcinoma, melanoma)
- Multiple intraparotid masses, often with central necrosis

Parotid Ductal Carcinoma

- Salivary ductal carcinoma similar to high-grade MECa on CT & MR
- Low T2 signal, infiltrative mass characteristic of both histologies
- Cannot differentiate preoperatively

PATHOLOGY

General Features

- Etiology

- Exposure risk: Radiation
  - Latency: 7-32 years

Staging, Grading, & Classification

- TNM staging
  - T1: Tumor ≤ 2 cm without extraparenchymal extension
  - T2: Tumor 2-4 cm without extraparenchymal extension
  - T3: Tumor 4-6 cm with extraparenchymal extension
  - T4: Tumor > 6 cm or invades adjacent structures
    - Mandible, skull base, deep spaces of suprahyoid neck
- Histologic grading (low vs. intermediate vs. high) correlates best with prognosis

Gross Pathologic & Surgical Features

- Gray, tan-yellow, or pink

Microscopic Features

- Mixture of epidermoid & mucus-secreting cells with some cells intermediate between these
- Cellular atypia & pleomorphism
- Arises in glandular ductal epithelium

CLINICAL ISSUES

Presentation

- Most common signs/symptoms
  - Palpable parotid mass, usually rock hard
  - Other signs/symptoms
    - Facial pain, otalgia
    - Facial nerve paralysis
    - Other cranial nerve involvement (V3)
  - Clinical presentation depends on tumor grade
    - Low grade: Painless, mobile, slowly enlarging
    - High grade: Painful, immobile, rapidly enlarging

Demographics

- Age
  - Usually 35-65 years
  - May be seen in pediatric population
- Epidemiology
  - **MECa** is **most common** primary parotid malignancy
  - MECa: 10% of all salivary gland tumors
  - MECa: 30% of all salivary gland malignancies
  - Majority (60%) occur in parotid
    - Also other salivary glands, any mucosal surface (especially larynx), or within bone (mandible)

Natural History & Prognosis

- Recurrence & survival rates depend heavily on histologic grade
  - Low grade: 6% local recurrence; 90% 10-year survival rate
  - Intermediate grade: 20% local recurrence; 80% 10-year survival rate
  - High grade: 78% local recurrence; 27% 10-year survival rate
  - Distant mets common in high grade; uncommon in low/intermediate
- Poor prognostic signs
  - Male gender
  - Age > 40 years
  - Fixed tumor, invasion of surrounding structures
  - Higher TNM stage or histologic grade
  - Cellular markers (p53, Ki-67)
- Late local recurrence (after 5 years) possible

Treatment

- Low-grade MECa
  - Wide local excision with preservation of facial nerve
  - Superficial parotidectomy if possible
  - Total parotidectomy may be necessary if tumor involves deep lobe
  - Postoperative radiotherapy
- High-grade MECa
  - Wide local excision; extended total parotidectomy
  - Facial nerve sacrifice often necessary
  - Neck dissection routine
  - Postoperative radiotherapy with large port

DIAGNOSTIC CHECKLIST

Consider

- In all parotid masses, check for **perineural spread** along **CNVII**
  - Replaced fat in stylomastoid foramen
  - Enhancement of vertical (mastoid) segment of CNVII
  - Extension along V3 (foramen ovale) if deep lobe parotid or **auriculotemporal nerve** involved
- Check for invasion of surrounding structures: Mandible, skull base, deep fascial spaces

Image Interpretation Pearls

- Low-grade MECa may exactly mimic BMT
- High-grade MECa has nonspecific invasive appearance
  - Remember to look for nodal metastases
  - Also check stylomastoid foramen & mastoid segment CNVII for perineural tumor spread
- General evaluation of PS masses
  - 1st decide whether lesion is **intraparotid** (BMT, Warthin, MECa, ACCa) or **extraparotid** (skin or different suprahyoid space)
  - If intraparotid, distinguish superficial vs. deep lobe
    - Divided by facial nerve plane, just lateral to retromandibular vein
  - Sharpness of margins helps distinguish benign from malignant lesions
    - Caveat: Benign tumors can incite sialadenitis, & low-grade malignancy may have sharp margins

SELECTED REFERENCES

1. Mao MH et al: Surgery combined with postoperative 125 I seed brachytherapy for the treatment of mucoepidermoid carcinoma of the parotid gland in pediatric patients. Pediatr Blood Cancer. 64(1):57-63, 2017
2. Ata-Ali J et al: [Mucoepidermoid carcinoma of the parotid gland.] An Pediatr (Barc). ePub, 2016
3. Berger MH et al: Case of parotid mucoepidermoid carcinoma: Expanding the spectrum of von Hippel-Lindau-related neoplasms. Head Neck. ePub, 2016
4. Bidari-Zerehpoosh F et al: Sclerosing mucoepidermoid carcinoma of the parotid gland. Iran J Otorhinolaryngol. 28(87):281-5, 2016
5. Gherghina FL et al: Parotid sclerosing mucoepidermoid carcinoma: a case report and immunohistochemical study. Rom J Morphol Embryol. 57(3):1107-1116, 2016
6. Lewis AG et al: Diagnosis and management of malignant salivary gland tumors of the parotid gland. Otolaryngol Clin North Am. 49(2):343-80, 2016
7. Yu C et al: Mucoepidermoid carcinoma arising in Warthin's tumor of the parotid gland: Clinicopathological characteristics and immunophenotypes. Sci Rep. 6:30149, 2016

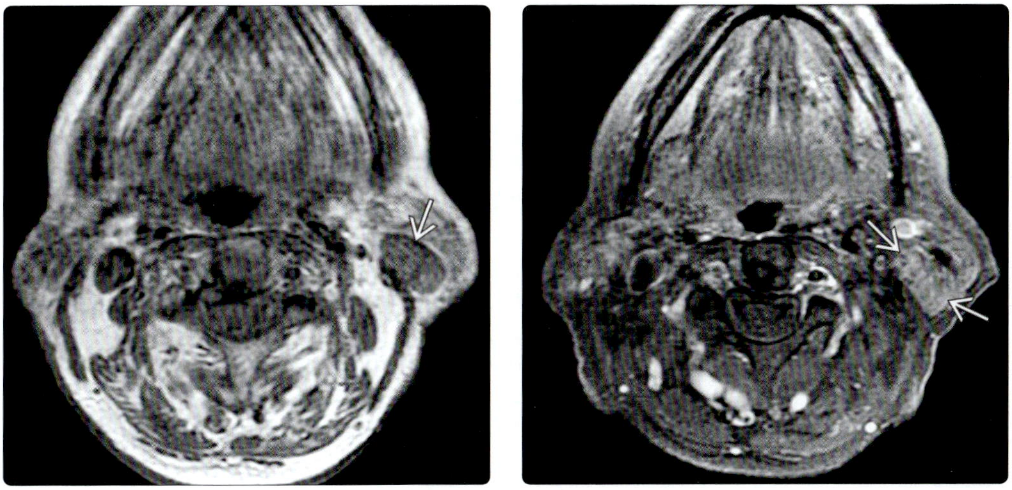

(Left) *Axial T1WI MR shows an ovoid well-defined mass ➡ of intermediate signal in the parotid tail. Note this low-grade MECa is easily distinguished from the surrounding gland on this unenhanced image.* **(Right)** *Axial T1WI C+ FS MR in the same patient shows a well-defined ovoid MECa ➡ that is almost indistinguishable from the surrounding parotid gland. The administration of contrast can sometimes obscure parotid masses if the enhancement matches the inherent fat signal in the gland.*

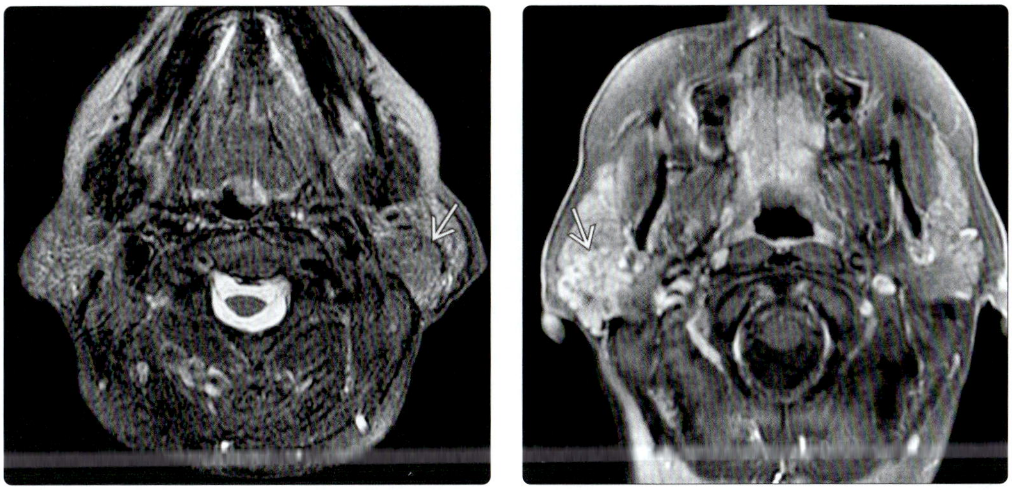

(Left) *Axial T2WI FS MR in the same patient demonstrates a low-signal well-defined ovoid mass ➡ in the parotid gland. Low T2 signal is unusual and is most frequently a sign of MECa.* **(Right)** *Axial T1WI C+ FS MR shows a lobular, well-defined mass ➡ in the parotid gland with numerous smaller cystic spaces. The cystic areas in MECa can be either 1 large cyst or multiple smaller cysts.*

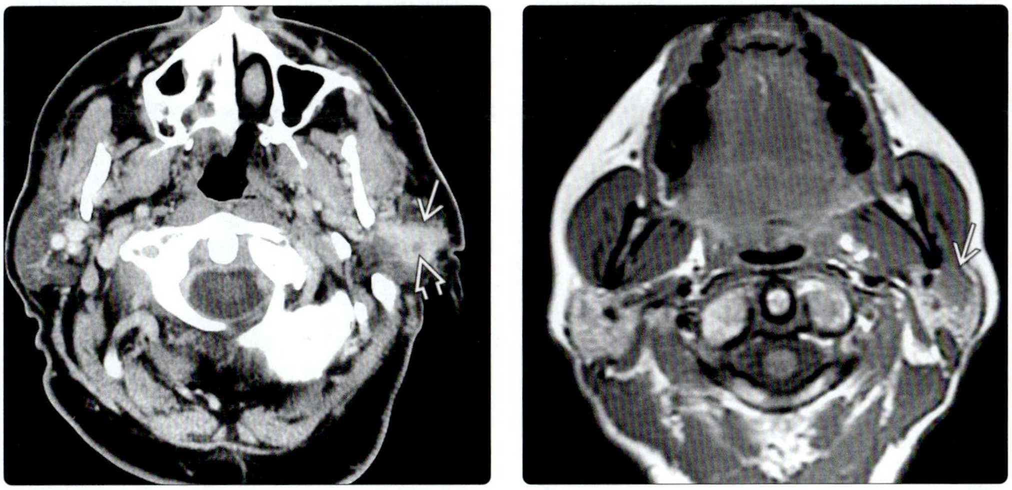

(Left) *Axial CECT reveals an ill-defined enhancing mass ➡ in the left parotid gland with a small central cystic area ➡. This is a characteristic imaging appearance for intermediate-grade MECa.* **(Right)** *Axial T1WI MR shows a well-defined intermediate-signal mass ➡ in the superficial lobe of the parotid gland. There are no features that specifically distinguish this mass as a low-grade MECa, which is why biopsy is needed in almost all parotid masses.*

Parotid Adenoid Cystic Carcinoma

KEY FACTS

TERMINOLOGY

- Malignant salivary gland neoplasm arising in peripheral parotid ducts; adenoid cystic carcinoma (ACCa) is **2nd most frequent** 1° parotid malignancy

IMAGING

- **Low-grade ACCa**: Well-circumscribed, homogeneously enhancing parotid mass
- **Higher grade ACCa**: Infiltrative, homogeneously enhancing parotid mass
- MR findings
    - Moderate T2 signal intensity
    - High-grade ACCa: Lower in signal intensity
    - Look for **perineural tumor** CNVII or CNV3
- Imaging findings often nonspecific for other parotid space (PS) tumors

TOP DIFFERENTIAL DIAGNOSES

- PS benign mixed tumor
- Warthin tumor
- PS mucoepidermoid carcinoma
- Intraparotid metastatic nodal disease

PATHOLOGY

- Tumor grading based on dominant histologic pattern
    - Tubular = grade 1, cribriform = grade 2, solid = grade 3

CLINICAL ISSUES

- Greatest propensity of all H&N tumors to spread via perineural pathway
- **Late local recurrence**, up to 20 years after diagnosis
- Favorable short-term, but poor long-term, prognosis
- Metastatic spread to lungs & bones > than lymph nodes
- 33% present with pain & CNVII paralysis
- Postoperative radiotherapy for all but lowest grade

DIAGNOSTIC CHECKLIST

- Look carefully for **perineural tumor** with any parotid neoplasm but particularly ACCa

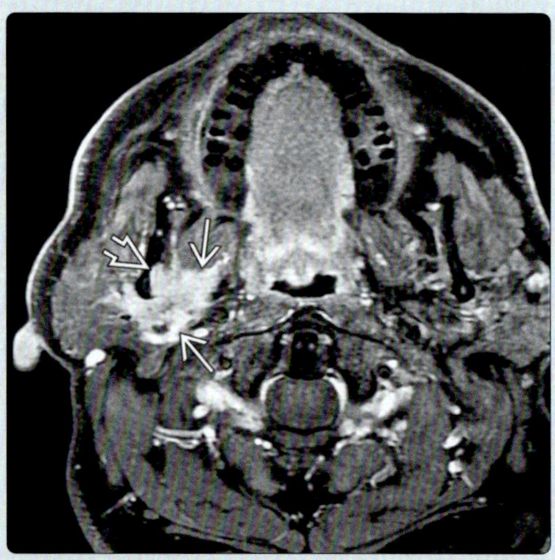
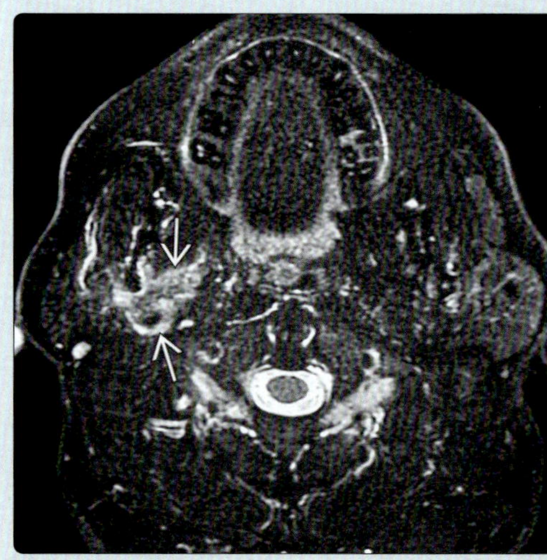

(Left) *Axial T1WI C+ FS MR shows an infiltrative uniformly enhancing mass ➡ replacing the deep lobe of the parotid gland. Tumor extends into the mandibular foramen ⇨ along the inferior alveolar nerve. The perineural spread provides a clue that this is adenoid cystic carcinoma (ACCa) but is not a specific finding.* **(Right)** *Axial T2WI FS MR shows an ill-defined intermediate-signal mass ➡ in the deep lobe of the parotid gland. Unlike mucoepidermoid carcinoma, this ACCa lacks cystic areas and low T2 signal.*

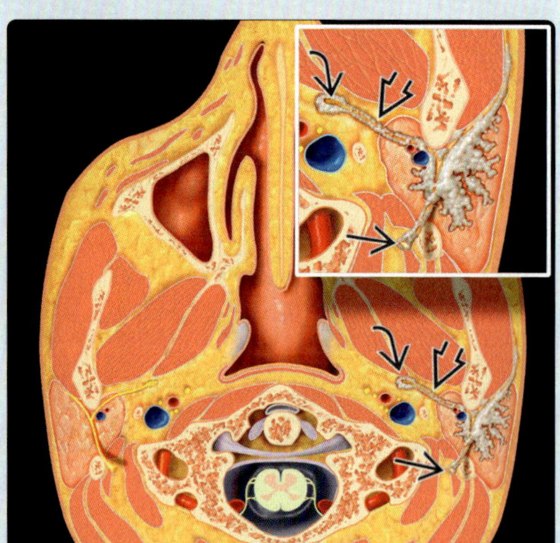
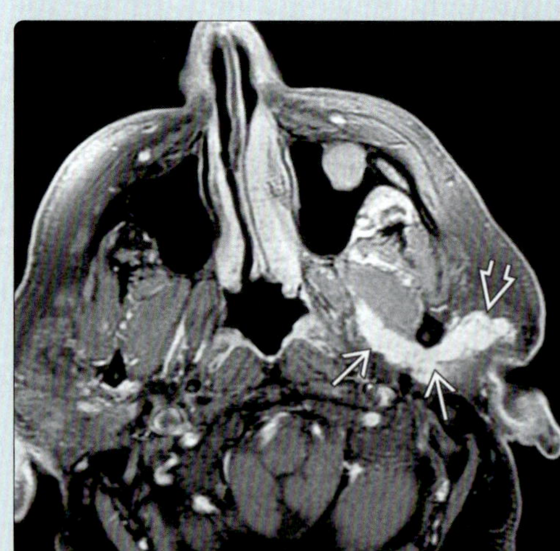

(Left) *Axial graphic depicts high-grade parotid ACCa spreading in a perineural fashion along the proximal facial nerve toward the stylomastoid foramen ➡ and via the auriculotemporal nerve ➡ to the mandibular branch (CNV3) of the trigeminal nerve ↪.* **(Right)** *Axial T1WI C+ FS MR shows marked thickening and enhancement of the auriculotemporal nerve ➡ from perineural spread of ACCa that originated in the superficial lobe of the parotid gland ⇨.*

TERMINOLOGY

Abbreviations

- Adenoid cystic carcinoma (ACCa)

Synonyms

- Previously called cylindroma

Definitions

- Malignant salivary gland neoplasm arising in peripheral parotid ducts
- **2nd most frequent** primary parotid malignancy (after mucoepidermoid carcinoma)

IMAGING

General Features

- Best diagnostic clue
  - **Low-grade ACCa**: Well-circumscribed, homogeneously enhancing parotid mass
  - **Higher grade ACCa**: Infiltrative, homogeneously enhancing parotid mass
- Location
  - May involve superficial or deep lobe

CT Findings

- CECT
  - Homogeneously enhancing parotid space (PS) mass with well-defined (low-grade) or ill-defined (high-grade) margins

MR Findings

- T1WI
  - Low to intermediate signal intensity PS mass
- T2WI
  - Moderate signal intensity PS mass
  - High-grade tumors usually lower in signal intensity
- T1WI C+
  - Homogeneously enhancing PS mass
  - **Perineural tumor** spread on **mastoid CNVII**

DIFFERENTIAL DIAGNOSIS

Parotid Space Benign Mixed Tumor

- Well-defined, homogeneous ovoid PS mass indistinguishable from low-grade ACCa

Warthin Tumor

- Well-defined PS mass, more heterogeneously enhancing than ACCa

Parotid Space Mucoepidermoid Carcinoma

- Well-defined or infiltrative PS mass; depends on grade
- More likely cystic or with lower T2 signal than ACCa

Intraparotid Metastatic Nodal Disease

- Primary lesion on skin of ear, forehead, or external auditory canal
- Often central necrosis; may be multiple nodes

PATHOLOGY

Staging, Grading, & Classification

- Tumor grading based on dominant histologic pattern
  - Tubular = grade 1, cribriform = grade 2, solid = grade 3

Gross Pathologic & Surgical Features

- Pink-tan with mottled surface; rarely necrotic
- Infiltrative margins; no capsule

Microscopic Features

- 3 distinct histological patterns
  - Cribriform, tubular, & solid
  - Tumor may have 1, 2, or 3 of these

CLINICAL ISSUES

Presentation

- Most common signs/symptoms
  - Painful, hard parotid mass; present months to years
  - 33% present with pain & CNVII paralysis

Demographics

- Age
  - Peak: 5th to 7th decades; rare < 20 years
- Epidemiology
  - 7-18% parotid tumors
  - Greatest propensity of all H&N tumors to spread via perineural pathway

Natural History & Prognosis

- **Late local recurrence**
  - Up to 20 years after diagnosis
- Favorable short-term, but poor long-term, prognosis
- Metastatic spread to lungs & bones more frequent than lymph nodes
- Predictors of distant metastasis: Tumor > 3 cm, solid pattern, local recurrence, node disease

Treatment

- Surgical plan is wide resection with negative margins
- Postoperative radiotherapy for all but lowest grade

DIAGNOSTIC CHECKLIST

Consider

- Look carefully for **perineural tumor** with any parotid neoplasm but particularly ACCa
  - CNVII & CNV
  - **Auriculotemporal nerve** runs behind mandible
    - Alternate course for intracranial spread via CNV3
- Ill-defined margins suggest higher grade lesion

Image Interpretation Pearls

- Imaging findings often nonspecific & similar to other parotid tumors
- Imaging is for extent of mass, perineural tumor, & adenopathy

SELECTED REFERENCES

1. INTERNATIONAL HEAD AND NECK SCIENTIFIC GROUP.: Cervical lymph node metastasis in adenoid cystic carcinoma of the major salivary glands. J Laryngol Otol. 131(2):96-105, 2017
2. Lee A et al: Patterns of care and survival of adjuvant radiation for major salivary adenoid cystic carcinoma. Laryngoscope. ePub, 2017
3. Das S et al: Adenoid cystic carcinoma of accessory parotid gland: a case report. J Oral Maxillofac Surg. 74(5):1097.e1-5, 2016
4. Lewis AG et al: Diagnosis and management of malignant salivary gland tumors of the parotid gland. Otolaryngol Clin North Am. 49(2):343-80, 2016

Parotid Non-Hodgkin Lymphoma

KEY FACTS

TERMINOLOGY

- 3 forms of parotid involvement with non-Hodgkin lymphoma (NHL)
- **Nodal NHL**
  - **Primary nodal NHL**
  - **Systemic NHL** involving parotid nodes
- **Primary parenchymal NHL**, often MALT (mucosa-associated lymphoid tissue) lymphoma

IMAGING

- Nodal NHL: Multiple well-defined homogeneous parotid masses
- Primary parotid NHL: Infiltrative or solid/cystic mass
- Periparotid & upper cervical lymphadenopathy often
- Ultrasound shows hypoechoic intraparotid mass(es)
- Color Doppler shows hypervascular mass(es)
- PET/CT typically markedly FDG avid
- MALT-type lymphoma variable; often less FDG avid

TOP DIFFERENTIAL DIAGNOSES

- Benign lymphoepithelial lesions: HIV
- Parotid Sjögren syndrome
- Warthin tumor
- Parotid nodal metastatic disease

CLINICAL ISSUES

- Overall 5-year survival: 72%
- Systemic NHL involves parotid in 1-8%
- Primary parotid NHL ~ 2-5% of parotid malignancies
- Chemotherapy & radiation remain mainstay of treatment

DIAGNOSTIC CHECKLIST

- Beware: Isodense NHL may be "invisible" on CECT
- Parotid lesions best seen on T1 or T2 FS/STIR
- Heterogeneous parotids with new parotid mass
  - Suspect NHL complicating Sjögren disease
  - **Sjögren may not be previously diagnosed**

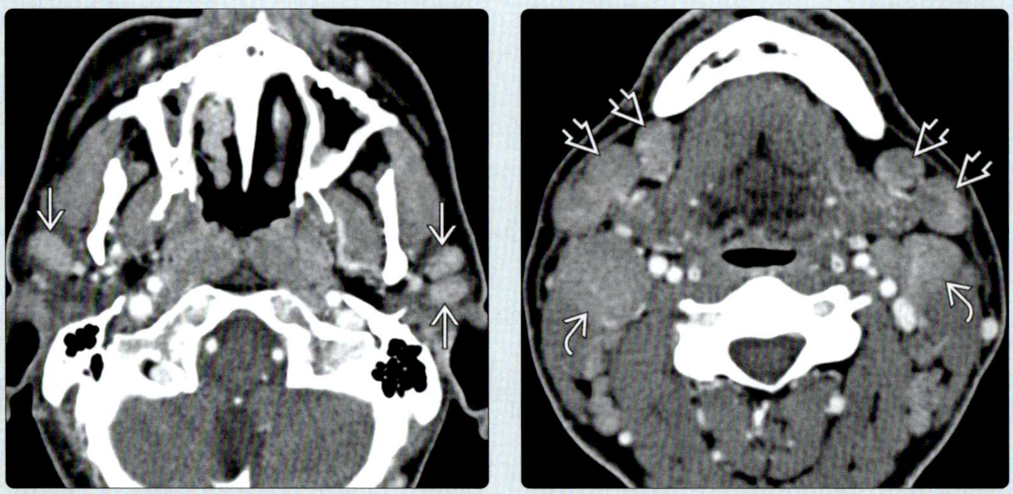

(Left) *Axial CECT shows multiple bilateral, well-defined, homogeneously enhancing masses ➡. Nodules ≥ 1 cm in parotid gland deserve further evaluation as they may represent multiple Warthin tumors, multiple metastatic nodes, or multiple lymphoma nodes. Remaining neck should be evaluated for lymphadenopathy as 1st step.* **(Right)** *Axial CECT in the same patient shows extensive lymphadenopathy in the upper neck, including levels I ⇨ and II ↪. This case shows parotid node involvement with systemic lymphoma.*

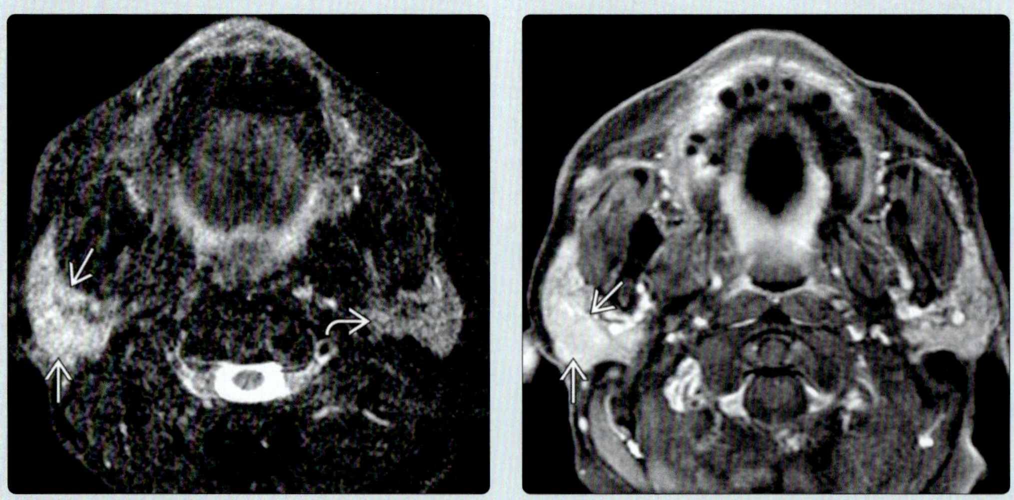

(Left) *Axial T2WI FS MR in a patient presenting with fullness of right cheek demonstrates subtle enlargement and diffuse hyperintensity of right parotid gland ➡ as compared to left side ↪. Prior CECT study had no reported abnormality or calculi.* **(Right)** *Axial T1 C+ FS MR in the same patient reveals diffuse enhancement of right parotid with more conspicuous ill-defined, but homogeneous, lesion ➡ in superficial lobe. Fine-needle aspiration revealed MALT-type (mucosa-associated lymphoid tissue) primary parotid lymphoma.*

TERMINOLOGY

Abbreviations

- Non-Hodgkin lymphoma (NHL)
- Mucosa-associated lymphoid tissue (MALT) lymphoma

Definitions

- 3 forms of parotid involvement with NHL
  - Nodal NHL
    - **Primary nodal NHL**
    - **Systemic NHL** involving parotid nodes
  - **Primary parenchymal lymphoma**
    - Most often MALT-type NHL

IMAGING

General Features

- Best diagnostic clue
  - Nodal NHL: Multiple homogeneous, well-defined parotid masses & upper cervical adenopathy
  - Parenchymal NHL: Infiltrative parotid mass
- Location
  - Parotid gland ± ipsilateral neck nodes
- Size
  - Nodal masses: 1-3 centimeters
  - Primary lymphoma may involve most of gland
- Morphology
  - Most often: Multiple round or ovoid, well-circumscribed masses
    - Unilateral with primary or systemic NHL
    - Bilateral with systemic NHL
  - Primary parotid lymphoma: Diffusely infiltrating process
    - Occasionally bilateral parotid masses
    - May be solid & cystic mass

CT Findings

- CECT
  - Nodal NHL: Multiple well-defined intraparotid masses
    - Mild to moderate homogeneous enhancement
    - Necrosis, calcification, & hemorrhage rare
  - Primary parenchymal NHL: Invasive mass or solid/cystic mass
  - Periparotid & upper cervical lymphadenopathy often present

MR Findings

- T1WI
  - Homogeneous intermediate signal nodules or infiltrative mass, seen in hypointense parotid
- T2WI FS
  - Fat sat or STIR makes parotid lesions more conspicuous
  - Homogeneous intermediate to low signal intensity nodules or solid/cystic mass
- T1WI C+
  - Mild to moderate homogeneous enhancement

Ultrasonographic Findings

- Grayscale ultrasound
  - Solitary or multiple uniform **hypoechoic** intraparotid masses
- Color Doppler
  - **Hypervascular** compared to adjacent parotid parenchyma

Nuclear Medicine Findings

- PET/CT
  - **Nodal NHL typically markedly FDG avid**
    - Multifocal nodular uptake in parotid ± neck nodes
    - Benign parotid lesions may also be FDG avid
  - **MALT-type lymphoma variable, often less FDG avid**
    - Role of PET controversial
- Ga-67 scintigraphy
  - Foci of ↑ activity within normal parotid uptake
  - Improved visualization with SPECT
  - Sialadenitis after chemotherapy or radiation therapy may have identical appearance
- Tc-99m pertechnetate
  - Cold lesion(s) within normal uptake of parotid

Other Modality Findings

- MR sialography or conventional sialography
  - Smooth displacement of ducts around ovoid masses
  - Normal arborization pattern without dilation of parotid ductal system
    - Unless in setting of Sjögren syndrome

Imaging Recommendations

- Best imaging tool
  - CECT to identify intraparotid lesions & allow evaluation of cervical lymphadenopathy for staging
    - Beware: Isodense lesions may be "invisible"
  - Intraparotid lesions more conspicuous on T1 or with T2 FS or STIR
- Protocol advice
  - Be sure to image from skull base to clavicles to aid in staging
  - PET/CT typically performed for complete staging

DIFFERENTIAL DIAGNOSIS

Benign Lymphoepithelial Lesions: HIV

- Mixed cystic & solid intraparotid lesions enlarge both parotid glands
- If AIDS patient has NHL, imaging may be complex

Parotid Sjögren Syndrome

- Older woman with connective tissue disease, dry eyes, dry mouth
- Bilateral enlarged parotid glands, small or large cysts ± lymphoid aggregates
- Chronic: Atrophied, heterogeneous glands ± calcifications
- Sjögren syndrome has 40x > incidence than NHL

Warthin Tumor

- Painless parotid mass in older male smoker
- Solid, cystic, or mixed
- 20% multiple, may be bilateral
- Lacks periparotid & cervical lymphadenopathy

Parotid Nodal Metastatic Disease

- Multiple unilateral or bilateral masses with invasive margins, often central necrosis
- Often other nodal metastases: Levels II & V
- Periparotid skin & scalp primaries most frequent

PATHOLOGY

General Features

- Etiology
  - Unknown; possibly multifactorial
    - Environmental, genetic, viral, prior radiation
  - Increased incidence with autoimmune disorders
    - **Sjögren syndrome** most commonly
    - Rheumatoid arthritis, systemic lupus
  - Increased incidence with **immunosuppression**

Staging, Grading, & Classification

- **Modified Ann Arbor staging system** is for clinical staging, treatment, & prognosis of NHL
  - Stage I: Single node region or lymphoid structure (e.g., spleen) or single extralymphatic site (IE)
  - Stage II: ≥ 2 node regions on same side of diaphragm (II) or contiguous extranodal organ/site + regional nodes ± other nodes on same side of diaphragm (IIE)
  - Stage III: Node regions on both sides of diaphragm (III), spleen (IIIS), extranodal (IIIE), both (IIISE)
  - Stage IV: Disseminated disease: ≥ 1 extranodal organ or tissue, ± nodes or isolated extralymphatic disease with distant nodes
- **World Health Organization** is NHL histological classification (2008)
  - Based on immunophenotype & morphology
  - B-cell (≤ 85%), T-cell, & putative NK-cell neoplasms

Gross Pathologic & Surgical Features

- Well-circumscribed, encapsulated, soft fleshy masses

Microscopic Features

- Sheets of homogeneous lymphoid cells arranged in diffuse or follicular pattern
  - Subdivided into small-cleaved & large-cell variants
- Primary parotid lymphoma
  - Most often MALT-type NHL
  - Unilateral diffuse invasion of ductal & acinar tissue

CLINICAL ISSUES

Presentation

- Most common signs/symptoms
  - Slowly enlarging painless parotid mass ± cervical lymphadenopathy
- Other signs/symptoms
  - Fever, weight loss, & night sweats are referred to as systemic "B" symptoms; "A" (absence of symptoms) & "B" are used to clarify stage (e.g., stage II-B)
- Clinical profile
  - Middle-aged men with painless cheek mass

Demographics

- Age
  - Mean age at presentation: 55 years
- Gender
  - M:F = 1.5:1
- Ethnicity
  - Whites > > blacks, Hispanic, or Asian
  - Rare T-cell lymphomas more common in young black male patients
- Epidemiology
  - Primary parotid NHL uncommon; 2-5% of parotid malignancies
  - Systemic NHL involves parotid in 1-8%

Natural History & Prognosis

- Depends on histology, morphology, & stage
- **Overall 5-year survival**: **72%**
  - High-grade disease: Rapidly progressive, aggressive
  - Low-grade lesions: Indolent, minimal treatment, & slow progression over years
    - Best prognosis: Small-cleaved cell & follicular forms
- Generally good prognosis with primary parotid NHL
  - Usually diagnosed early: Stage I or II
  - Radiation ± chemotherapy

Treatment

- Tumor debulking of parotid mass may be performed for cosmetic purposes
- Chemotherapy & radiation remain mainstay of treatment

DIAGNOSTIC CHECKLIST

Consider

- CECT from skull base to clavicles for intraparotid lesions & fully evaluate extent of cervical disease
- Beware: Isodense NHL may be "invisible" on CECT
- T2 MR, fat sat, or STIR make intraparotid lesions more conspicuous

Image Interpretation Pearls

- Carefully evaluate contralateral parotid, other salivary & lacrimal glands, & extent of cervical nodes
- PET/CT typically performed as work-up for systemic lymphoma
- In patient with new parotid mass, background heterogeneous parotids suggest NHL + Sjögren
  - **Sjögren may not be previously diagnosed**

SELECTED REFERENCES

1. Aydın S et al: Extranodal marginal zone lymphoma of the parotid gland. J Maxillofac Oral Surg. 15(Suppl 2):346-50, 2016
2. Dey B et al: A rare cytological diagnosis of primary non-Hodgkin lymphoma of the parotid gland. J Cytol. 33(2):108-10, 2016
3. Zhu L et al: Dynamic contrast-enhanced MR in the diagnosis of lympho-associated benign and malignant lesions in the parotid gland. Dentomaxillofac Radiol. 45(4):20150343, 2016
4. Bennett JA et al: Epstein-barr virus-associated extranodal marginal zone lymphoma of mucosa-associated lymphoid tissue (MALT Lymphoma) arising in the parotid gland of a child with ataxia telangiectasia. J Pediatr Hematol Oncol. 37(2):e114-7, 2015
5. Ciccia F et al: Interleukin (IL)-22 receptor 1 is over-expressed in primary Sjogren's syndrome and Sjögren-associated non-Hodgkin lymphomas and is regulated by IL-18. Clin Exp Immunol. 181(2):219-29, 2015
6. Nishishinya MB et al: Identification of lymphoma predictors in patients with primary Sjögren's syndrome: a systematic literature review and meta-analysis. Rheumatol Int. 35(1):17-26, 2015
7. Picard A et al: Extranodal lymphoma of the head and neck: a 67-case series. Eur Ann Otorhinolaryngol Head Neck Dis. 132(2):71-5, 2015
8. Shum JW et al: Parotid lymphoma: a review of clinical presentation and management. Oral Surg Oral Med Oral Pathol Oral Radiol. 118(1):e1-5, 2014
9. Smith J et al: Parotid gland follicular lymphoma lacking both cytoplasmic and surface light chains: a rare case. Int J Clin Exp Pathol. 7(10):7100-4, 2014
10. Risselada AP et al: Clinical features distinguishing lymphoma development in primary Sjögren's Syndrome–a retrospective cohort study. Semin Arthritis Rheum. 43(2):171-7, 2013
11. Zhu L et al: Non-Hodgkin lymphoma involving the parotid gland: CT and MR imaging findings. Dentomaxillofac Radiol. 42(9):20130046, 2013

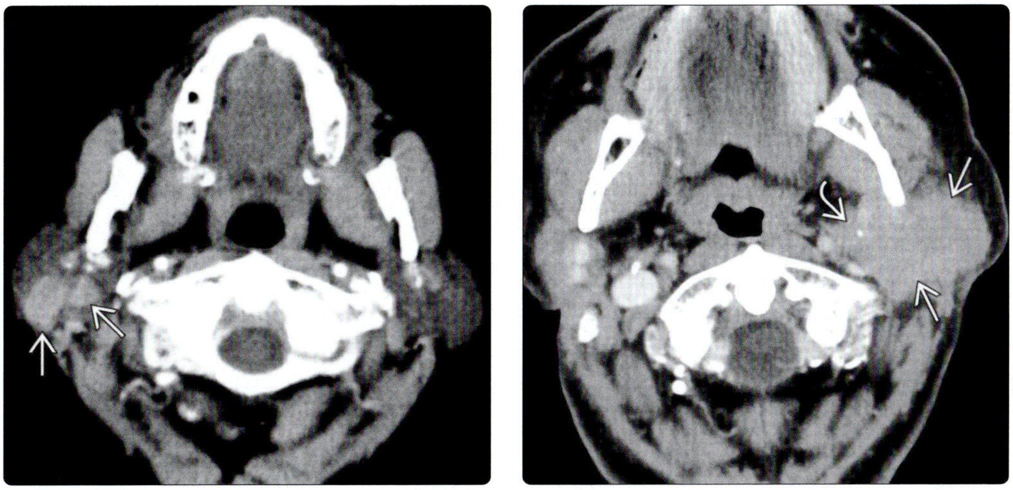

(Left) *Axial CECT shows multiple unilateral intraparotid masses* ➡ *with well-defined borders and uniform enhancement on right side. No evidence of disease was found elsewhere, so this patient was diagnosed with primary parotid nodal NHL.* **(Right)** *Axial CECT demonstrates primary MALT lymphoma of the parotid. The infiltrative mass involves the superficial* ➡ *and deep* ➡ *lobes, mimicking aggressive primary salivary gland malignancy. Lymphocytic lymphomas may have better defined margins.*

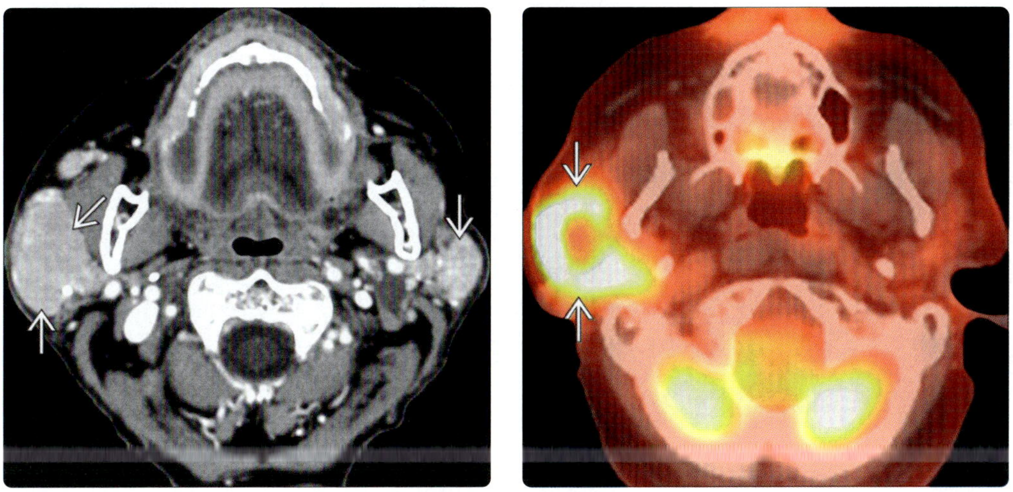

(Left) *Axial CECT shows bilateral, homogeneous enhancing parotid fullness* ➡ *found to be bilateral primary lymphoma in a patient with longstanding Sjögren syndrome. Patients with Sjögren syndrome have 40x increased risk of parotid lymphoma, and this is typical of MALT type.* **(Right)** *Corresponding axial fused PET/CT shows marked FDG uptake* ➡ *that is typically found with lymphoma. Interestingly, for such a homogeneous lesion on CT, the lesion has little central uptake suggesting necrosis.*

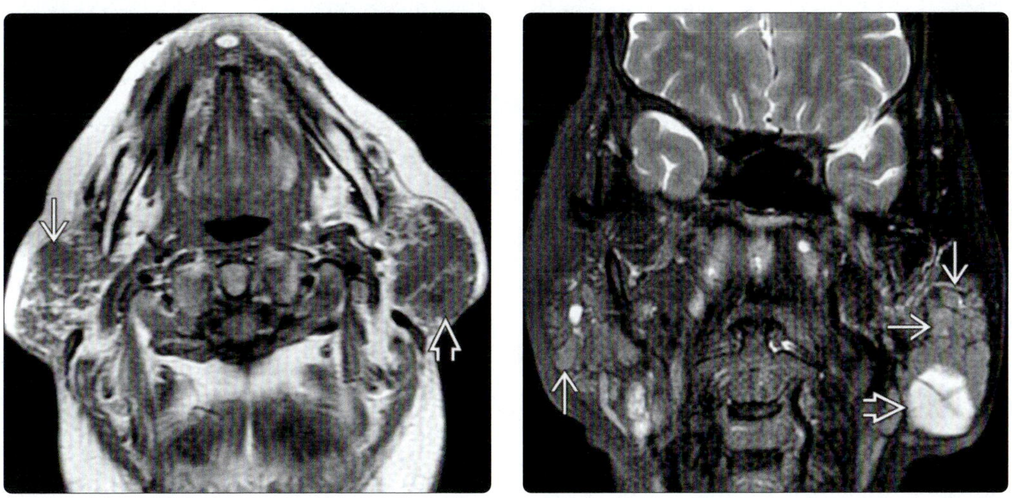

(Left) *Axial T1WI MR demonstrates markedly the heterogeneous appearance of enlarged parotid glands. Patient reported 10-year history of Sjögren disease and now palpable left parotid mass* ➡. *Clinician felt additional mass on right* ➡. **(Right)** *Coronal T2WI FS MR in the same patient reveals multiple intermediate-signal masses bilaterally* ➡ *and a solid and cystic lesion on left side* ➡. *Aspiration of this and right parotid revealed MALT lymphoma in both. Patient was treated with radiation therapy.*

Metastatic Disease of Parotid Nodes

KEY FACTS

TERMINOLOGY

- Definition: Lymphangitic or hematogenous tumor spread to intraglandular parotid lymph nodes
- Parotid & periparotid nodes = 1st-order nodal station for skin squamous cell carcinoma (SCCa) & melanoma from scalp, auricle, & face

IMAGING

- Nodes usually well defined, but infiltrative if extranodal spread
- Nodes may be homogeneous or heterogeneous with central necrosis
- PET/CT most sensitive for identification of small nodes
- MR most sensitive for extranodal spread & perineural tumor spread on CNVII

TOP DIFFERENTIAL DIAGNOSES

- Benign lymphoepithelial lesions: HIV
- Sjögren syndrome, parotid
- Warthin tumor
- Parotid non-Hodgkin lymphoma

PATHOLOGY

- Skin of face, external ear, & scalp accounts for 75% of primary tumors
- Systemic metastases to parotid nodes rare

CLINICAL ISSUES

- Prognosis depends on presence of extracapsular spread (8% vs. 79% local recurrence)
- Metastatic SCCa involving parotid gland & neck nodes is aggressive form of SCCa with tendency for infiltrative growth pattern & multiple recurrences

DIAGNOSTIC CHECKLIST

- If asked to image parotid nodal metastases from skin cancer, also scan cervical nodes to clavicle

(Left) *Axial CECT shows multiple enhancing masses ➡ of varying size within the left parotid gland. This patient has squamous cell carcinoma of the face, and these nodes represent 1st-order lymphatic drainage.* **(Right)** *Axial T1WI C+ FS MR shows an ill-defined mass ➡ replacing the left parotid gland. The primary tumor, postauricular squamous cell carcinoma, is partially visible ➡. The ill-defined margins of the intraparotid metastasis indicate extracapsular spread.*

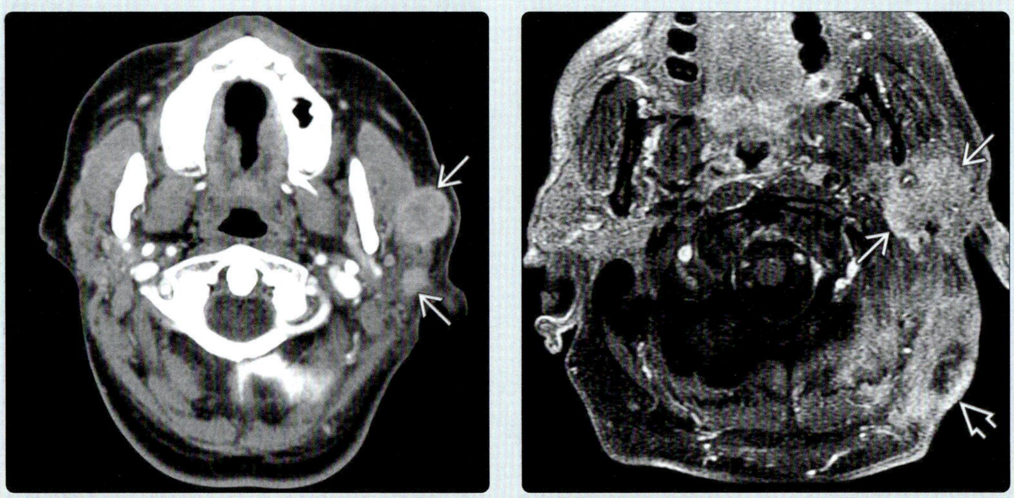

(Left) *Axial T1WI MR reveals numerous small masses ➡ in the left parotid gland. These regional metastases are clearly visible on unenhanced images because of the contrast with the surrounding fat.* **(Right)** *Axial T2WI FS MR in the same patient shows numerous masses ➡ in the left parotid gland with mildly increased T2 signal. Metastases may be more conspicuous on STIR images than on T2 images. These are regional metastases from a lymphoepithelial carcinoma of the base of tongue.*

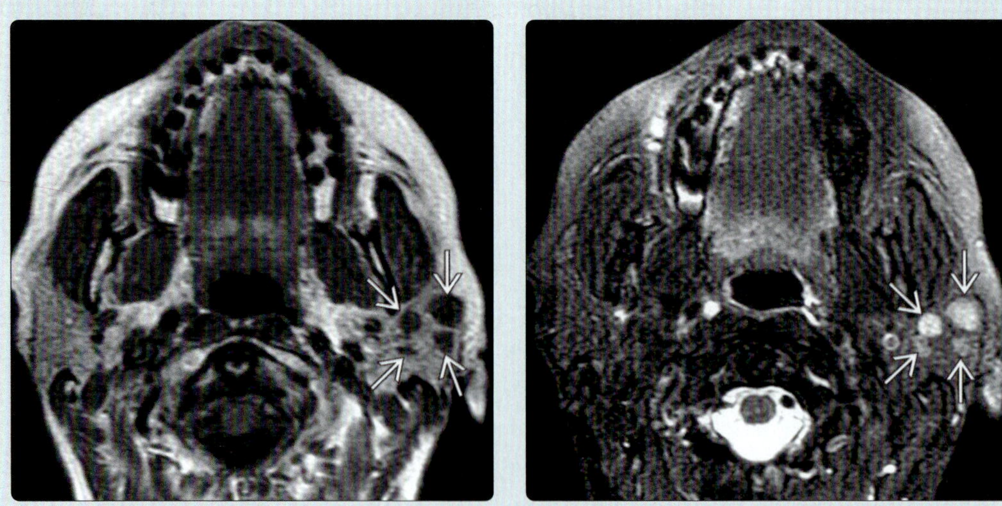

Metastatic Disease of Parotid Nodes

TERMINOLOGY

Definitions

- Lymphangitic or hematogenous tumor spread to intraparotid lymph nodes
- Parotid & periparotid nodes = **1st-order nodal station** for skin squamous cell carcinoma (SCCa) & melanoma from **scalp**, **auricle**, **& face**

IMAGING

General Features

- Best diagnostic clue
  - Multiple parotid masses in setting of known head & neck malignancy
  - 1 or more focal masses in superficial or deep lobe of parotid gland
    - Often with associated preauricular ± cervical nodal masses
- Location
  - Intraparotid ± periparotid
- Size
  - 5 mm to 4 cm, usually 1-3 cm
- Morphology
  - Ovoid or round
  - Usually well defined, but infiltrative if extranodal spread

CT Findings

- CECT
  - 1 or more intraparotid masses with sharp margins (early) or invasive margins (late, extranodal spread)
    - If extranodal, check for perineural tumor on CNVII
    - See if fat in stylomastoid foramen replaced with tumor
  - Nodes may be homogeneous or heterogeneous with central necrosis
  - Preauricular ± cervical nodal metastases may also be present
  - Periauricular or scalp skin thickening (primary skin malignancy)

MR Findings

- T1WI
  - Single or multiple intermediate signal masses
- T2WI
  - Uniform high signal or heterogeneous signal (necrosis)
- T1WI C+
  - Enhancing solid or cystic (central nodal necrosis) intraparotid nodal masses
  - If extranodal spread, may appear invasive

Nuclear Medicine Findings

- PET
  - If used in staging of primary tumor, may show intraparotid activity

Imaging Recommendations

- Best imaging tool
  - PET/CT most sensitive for identification of small nodes
  - MR most sensitive for extranodal spread & perineural tumor spread on CNVII
- Protocol advice
  - Image primary site, parotid, & remainder of neck nodal chains to clavicles
- MR imaging is best tool to evaluate uncertain parotid masses
  - Deep tissue spread & perineural tumor are better defined by MR
  - T1 nonfat-suppressed, unenhanced images often best delineate mass (inherent contrast between mass & fatty gland)
- All patients with invasive skin SCCa or melanoma on skin of face, scalp, & auricle should undergo staging PET/CT for intraparotid nodes ± nodes in cervical neck
  - MR obtained if PET/CT is positive

DIFFERENTIAL DIAGNOSIS

Benign Lymphoepithelial Lesions: HIV

- HIV or AIDS patient
- Multiple small, bilateral parotid cystic & solid lesions

Sjögren Syndrome, Parotid

- Autoimmune disease affecting salivary tissue
- Enlarged salivary glands
- Cystic dilation of intraglandular ducts + lymphoid aggregates

Warthin Tumor

- Male smokers with painless cheek mass
- Often cystic on CT or MR
- 20% multifocal

Parotid Non-Hodgkin Lymphoma

- Patient usually has systemic non-Hodgkin lymphoma (NHL)
- Bilateral, multiple intraparotid nodes
- Very difficult to distinguish from metastases if no known primary

Recurrent Parotid Benign Mixed Tumor

- History of benign mixed tumor (BMT) surgical removal
- Multifocal masses; cluster of grapes appearance

PATHOLOGY

General Features

- Etiology
  - Lymphangitic or hematogenous spread of tumor
  - Skin of face, external ear, & scalp accounts for 75% of primary tumors
  - Systemic metastases to parotid nodes rare
- Parotid has intraglandular lymph nodes (unlike submandibular & sublingual glands)
- Normal parotid: ~ 20 intraglandular nodes
- Embryology/anatomy
  - Parotid undergoes late encapsulation, incorporating nodes within its parenchyma
  - Parotid is "**forgotten nodal station**"

Gross Pathologic & Surgical Features

- Nodes may remain encapsulated or undergo extracapsular spread
- SCCa node: Tan-yellow nodules within parotid
- Melanoma node: Black, brown, or white rubbery mass

Microscopic Features

- Most common skin carcinomas
  - Squamous cell (60%)
  - Melanoma (15%)
- Systemic metastases: Lung, breast primaries most common
- SCCa: Lymph node is partially or entirely replaced by epithelial-lined structure ± central cystic change
  - Epithelium lining of cystic spaces is composed of hypercellular & pleomorphic cell population, with loss of polarity & ↑ mitotic activity
- Melanoma: Diffuse proliferation of epithelioid ± spindle cells with abundant eosinophilic cytoplasm & prominent nucleoli
  - Immunochemistry: S100 protein & HMB-45 present

CLINICAL ISSUES

Presentation

- Most common signs/symptoms
  - External ear, scalp, upper face skin cancer with enlarging parotid mass
  - CNVII dysfunction
  - Facial pain
  - Nonhealing sore (skin SCCa or melanoma) on skin of face, scalp, or auricle-external auditory canal associated with cheek mass

Demographics

- Age
  - 7th decade most frequent
- Gender
  - M:F = 2:1
- Epidemiology
  - Occurs in 1-3% of patients with H&N SCCa
  - Metastases = 4% of all salivary neoplasms
  - Intraparotid nodes more common in geographic regions of ↑ sun exposure

Natural History & Prognosis

- Prognosis depends heavily on presence of extracapsular spread (8% vs. 79% local recurrence)
- 5-year parotid control = 78%, but overall survival = 54%
- Metastatic SCCa involving parotid gland & neck nodes is aggressive form of SCCa with tendency for infiltrative growth pattern & multiple recurrences
- Some primary subsites (e.g., external ear) have worse prognosis
- Melanoma: Poor prognosis; rare long-term survivors

Treatment

- Parotidectomy, neck dissection + radiation therapy
- SCCa: Parotidectomy & neck dissection dictated by imaging & physical exam
  - Postoperative radiotherapy
- Melanoma: Parotidectomy & neck dissection dictated by lymphatic mapping & sentinel node identification
  - Adjuvant radiotherapy ± chemotherapy depends on context

DIAGNOSTIC CHECKLIST

Consider

- If asked to image parotid nodal metastases from skin cancer, also scan cervical nodes to clavicle
- If SCCa or melanoma found in parotid nodes, check external ear & scalp for primary
- Skin cancer may be hidden above hairline at time of presentation of parotid node

Image Interpretation Pearls

- Multifocal unilateral disease is most suggestive of 1st-order nodal disease from adjacent skin sites
- Presence of bilateral nodes suggests systemic disease or hematogenous metastatic spread

Reporting Tips

- Differential diagnosis for multifocal unilateral parotid masses with cervical adenopathy: Regional metastases, local NHL
- Differential diagnosis for multifocal unilateral parotid masses without cervical adenopathy: Warthin tumor, recurrent BMT, regional metastases
- Differential diagnosis for multifocal bilateral parotid masses: Systemic metastases, systemic NHL, Warthin tumors, benign lymphoepithelial lesions: HIV, Sjögren syndrome

SELECTED REFERENCES

1. Guzzo M et al: Major and minor salivary gland tumors. Crit Rev Oncol Hematol. 74(2):134-48, 2010
2. Turner SJ et al: Metastatic cutaneous squamous cell carcinoma of the external ear: a high-risk cutaneous subsite. J Laryngol Otol. 124(1):26-31, 2010
3. Dong XR et al: Parotid gland metastasis of nasopharyngeal carcinoma: case report and review of the literature. J Int Med Res. 37(6):1994-9, 2009
4. Ch'ng S et al: Parotid and cervical nodal status predict prognosis for patients with head and neck metastatic cutaneous squamous cell carcinoma. J Surg Oncol. 98(2):101-5, 2008
5. Hinerman RW et al: Cutaneous squamous cell carcinoma metastatic to parotid-area lymph nodes. Laryngoscope. 118(11):1989-96, 2008
6. Veness MJ et al: Cutaneous head and neck squamous cell carcinoma metastatic to parotid and cervical lymph nodes. Head Neck. 29(7):621-31, 2007
7. Ch'ng S et al: Parotid metastasis--an independent prognostic factor for head and neck cutaneous squamous cell carcinoma. J Plast Reconstr Aesthet Surg. 59(12):1288-93, 2006
8. Bron LP et al: Primary and metastatic cancer of the parotid: comparison of clinical behavior in 232 cases. Laryngoscope. 113(6):1070-5, 2003
9. Cole MD et al: Evaluation of nodal patterns for melanoma of the ear. Plast Reconstr Surg. 112(1):50-6, 2003
10. O'Brien CJ et al: Significance of clinical stage, extent of surgery, and pathologic findings in metastatic cutaneous squamous carcinoma of the parotid gland. Head Neck. 24(5):417-22, 2002
11. delCharco JO et al: Carcinoma of the skin metastatic to the parotid area lymph nodes. Head Neck. 20(5):369-73, 1998

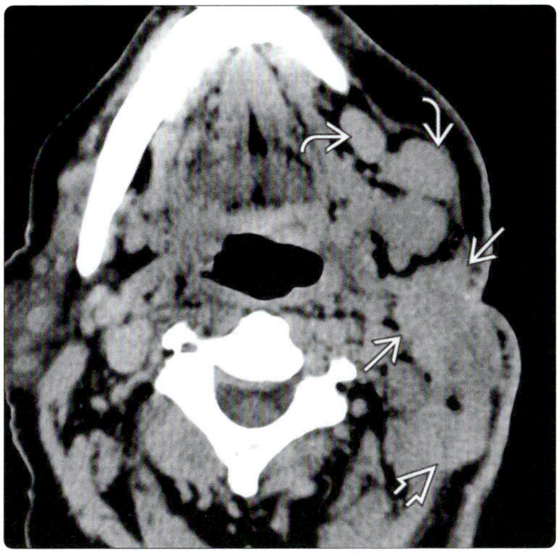

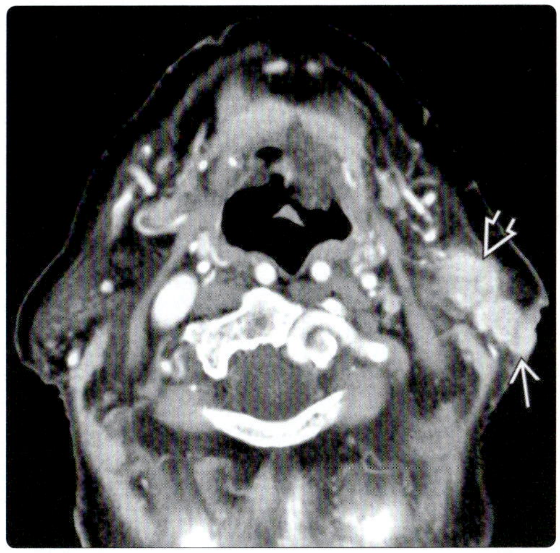

(Left) *Axial CECT shows a confluent mass ➡ replacing the tail of the left parotid. Extensive level I ➡ and level II ➡ metastases are also seen. This patient had squamous cell carcinoma of the lateral scalp.* **(Right)** *Axial CECT demonstrates aggressive primary skin squamous cell carcinoma ➡ spreading into deep subcutaneous soft tissues. Note that the 1st-order parotid tail lymph node ➡ is affected.*

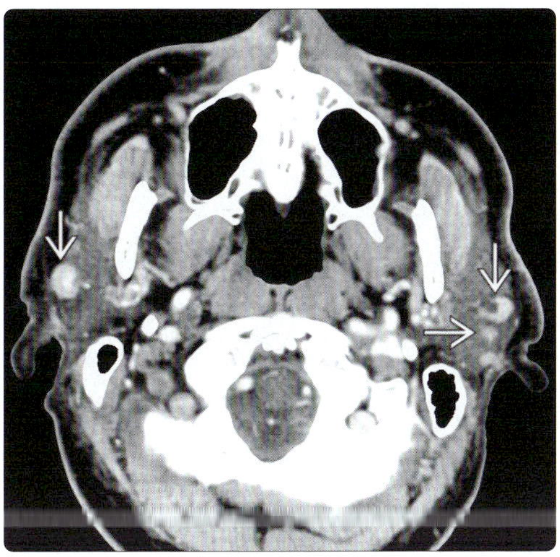

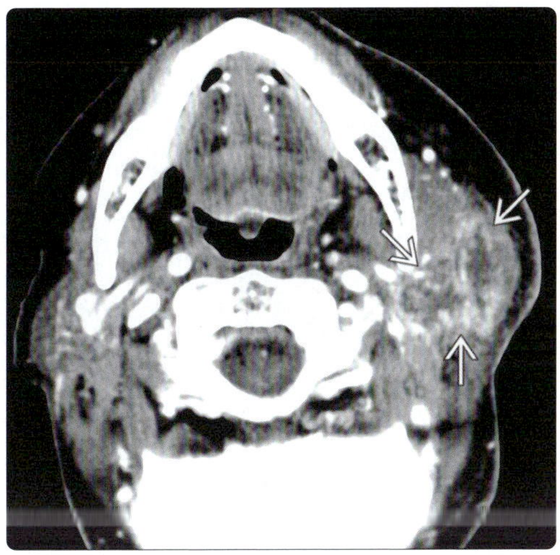

(Left) *Axial CECT reveals bilateral enhancing parotid masses ➡. These represent systemic metastatic disease from chronic lymphocytic leukemia. They were accompanied by extensive cervical adenopathy (not shown).* **(Right)** *Axial CECT shows an ill-defined, heterogeneously enhancing mass ➡ in the left parotid gland. The central necrosis and ill-defined margins are indicative of extracapsular spread. These are regional metastases from an angiosarcoma of the scalp*

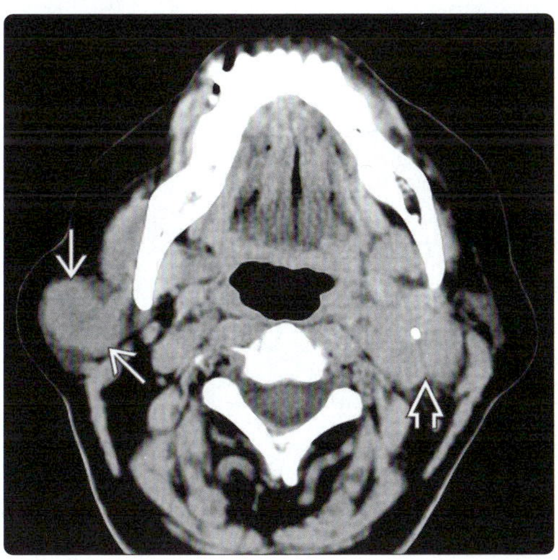

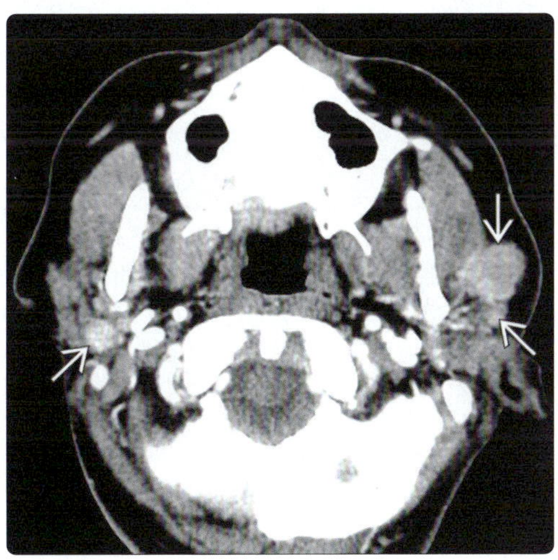

(Left) *Axial NECT shows a large, well-defined mass ➡ in the right parotid gland representing hematogenous metastasis from lung cancer. A large regional metastasis ➡ is also seen in contralateral level II, but no ascending cervical adenopathy was present on the right.* **(Right)** *Axial CECT demonstrates numerous bilateral, well-defined, uniformly enhancing parotid masses ➡ in a patient with known breast cancer. These masses represent hematogenous metastases.*

Sjögren Syndrome

KEY FACTS

TERMINOLOGY

- Synonyms: Sicca syndrome, myoepithelial sialadenitis
- Definition: Systemic autoimmune disease characterized by **lacrimal and salivary dysfunction**; secondary Sjögren syndrome (SS) associated with rheumatic disease

IMAGING

- Classification stages based on radiographic features of conventional or MR sialography (Rubin & Holt)
  - 1: Punctate sialectasia/↑ signal, smooth oval ≤ 1 mm
  - 2: Globular sialectasia/↑ signal, somewhat smooth oval 1-2 mm
  - 3: Cavitary sialectasia/↑ signal, somewhat smooth oval > 2 mm
  - 4: Destructive sialectasia/↑ signal, irregular > 2 mm
- Bilateral enlargement and possible punctate calcifications in major salivary glands
- Multiple cystic or solid intraglandular masses: Miliary pattern
- **Investigate rapid gland enlargement**, discrete swelling, or lymphadenopathy for lymphoma

TOP DIFFERENTIAL DIAGNOSES

- **Benign lymphoepithelial lesions**
- Warthin tumor
- Sarcoidosis
- Non-Hodgkin lymphoma, parotid nodes

CLINICAL ISSUES

- **Xerostomia and xerophthalmia (sicca syndrome)**
- Average onset 4th and 5th decades, but any age group
- 9:1 female predilection
- 2nd most common autoimmune rheumatoid disease (USA)
- **19x ↑ risk for non-Hodgkin lymphoma** in late stages of SS, especially parotid
- Treatment: Symptomatic management of dry eyes and mouth, therapeutic management of systemic rheumatic disease, **fluoride for caries prevention**

(Left) *Conventional sialography (lateral view) shows multiple punctate sialectasia with the cherry blossom or branchless fruit tree appearance indicative of Sjögren syndrome (SS) ➡ in right parotid gland. Note the "sausage-link" intermittent ductal dilation and stricture appearance of chronic infection (sialodochitis) ➡ in Stensen duct.* **(Right)** *Axial T2WI FS MR shows multiple tiny cysts ➡ scattered throughout the entire parotid parenchyma bilaterally. This is termed a miliary pattern of multicystic change.*

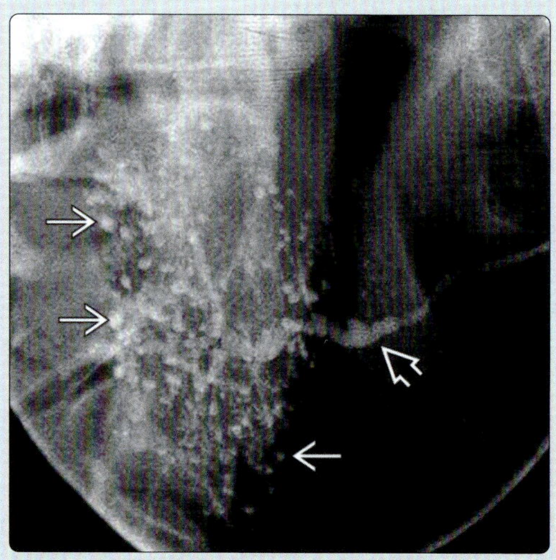

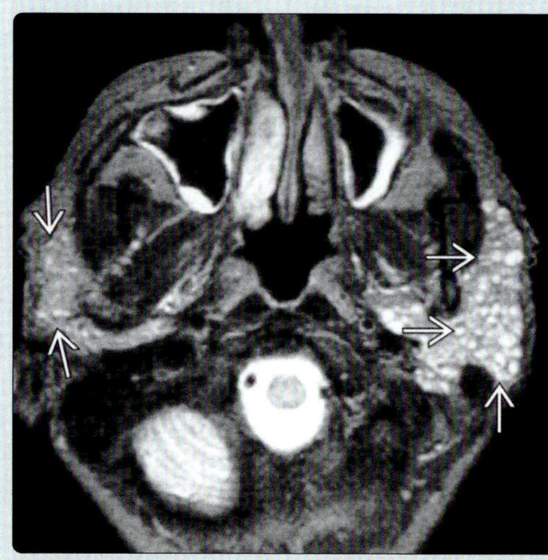

(Left) *Axial CECT shows features of SS involving the submandibular glands bilaterally. A mottled, heterogeneous pattern of density is visualized within the submandibular glands ➡ with slight enlargement of the gland on the right.* **(Right)** *Axial CECT reveals markedly heterogeneous, abnormal-appearing parotid glands with solid tissue ➡ interspersed with more cystic-appearing areas ➡. Subtle foci of calcification are also seen ➡.*

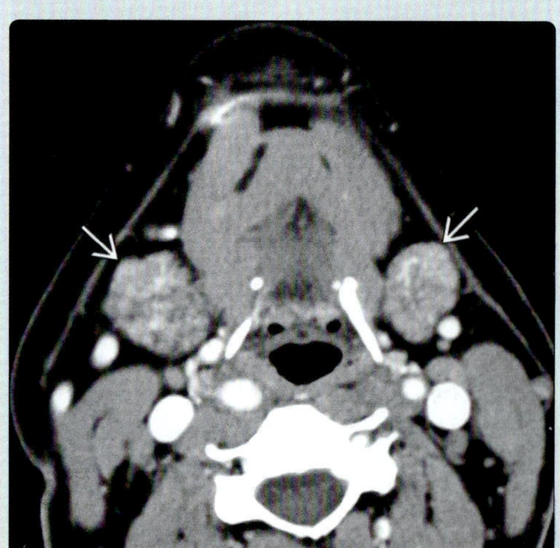

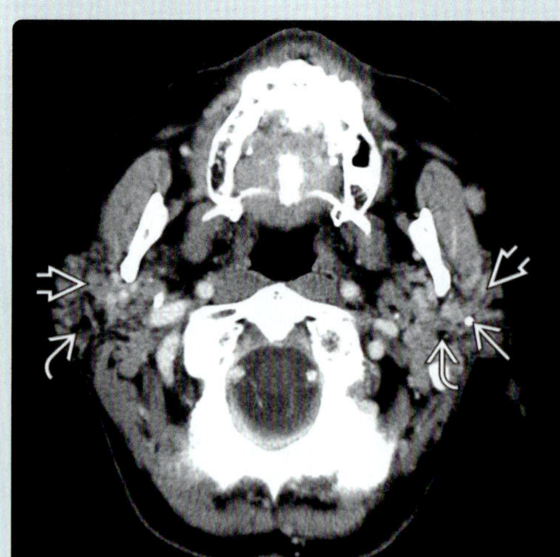

TERMINOLOGY

Abbreviations

- Sjögren syndrome (SS)

Synonyms

- Sicca syndrome
- Myoepithelial sialadenitis

Definitions

- Systemic autoimmune disease characterized by lacrimal and salivary gland dysfunction
- Secondary SS associated with another rheumatic disease (e.g., rheumatoid arthritis, systemic lupus erythematosus)

IMAGING

General Features

- Best diagnostic clue
  - Classification based on radiographic features of conventional or MR sialography (Rubin and Holt)
    - Stage 1: Punctate sialectasia/high signal, smooth oval ≤ 1 mm (sometimes termed **cherry blossom** or branchless fruit tree appearance)
    - Stage 2: Globular sialectasia/high signal, somewhat smooth oval 1-2 mm
    - Stage 3: Cavitary sialectasia/high signal, somewhat smooth oval > 2 mm
    - Stage 4: Destructive sialectasia/high signal, irregular > 2 mm
- Location
  - Lacrimal and major salivary glands bilaterally
- Morphology
  - Parotid heterogeneity/abnormal diffuse fat tissue deposition highly sensitive for SS on CT/MR/US

Radiographic Findings

- Multiple punctate sialectasia on sialography

CT Findings

- Bilateral enlargement of major salivary glands
- Possible punctate calcifications in major salivary glands
- Multiple cystic or solid intraglandular masses: Miliary pattern

MR Findings

- Multiple cystic or solid intraglandular masses on both T1WI/T2WI: Miliary pattern

Imaging Recommendations

- Investigate rapid gland enlargement, discrete swelling, or lymphadenopathy for lymphoma

DIFFERENTIAL DIAGNOSIS

Benign Lymphoepithelial Lesions

- Multiple cystic and solid intraglandular masses may exactly mimic SS
- HIV(+)
- Tonsillar hyperplasia with reactive cervical adenopathy

Warthin Tumor

- Inhomogeneous solid masses usually single but not always; unilateral or bilateral

Sarcoidosis

- Cystic and solid intraglandular masses with nonreactive cervical adenopathy

Non-Hodgkin Lymphoma, Parotid Nodes

- Part of systemic disease with unilateral or bilateral nodules

PATHOLOGY

General Features

- Periductal lymphocytic aggregates invade and destroy salivary acinar parenchyma

Staging, Grading, & Classification

- Histopathologic grading of minor **salivary gland lip biopsies** based on aggregation foci of lymphocytes, histiocytes, and plasma cells (1 focus = 50 aggregates per 4 mm of tissue)
- Revised classification criteria for SS requires presence of signs, symptoms, and laboratory findings

CLINICAL ISSUES

Presentation

- Most common signs/symptoms
  - Bilateral enlargement of major salivary glands
  - **Xerostomia and xerophthalmia (sicca syndrome)**
- Other signs/symptoms
  - Rampant dental caries secondary to xerostomia
  - Candidiasis
  - Dysgeusia
  - Dysphagia
  - Burning mouth
  - Peripheral neuropathies
- Diagnosis not straightforward; subjective and vague symptoms

Demographics

- Age
  - Average onset 4th and 5th decades but can occur in any age group
- Gender
  - 9:1 female predilection
- 2nd most common autoimmune rheumatic disease (USA)

Natural History & Prognosis

- **19x ↑ risk for non-Hodgkin lymphoma** in late stages of SS, especially parotid

Treatment

- Symptomatic management of dry eyes and mouth with artificial lubricants
- Therapeutic management of systemic rheumatic disease
- **Fluoride treatment for caries prevention**

SELECTED REFERENCES

1. Gomes Pde S et al: Diagnostic approaches to Sjögren's syndrome: a literature review and own clinical experience. J Oral Maxillofac Res. 3(1):e3, 2012
2. Sun Z et al: Diagnostic accuracy of parotid CT for identifying Sjögren's syndrome. Eur J Radiol. 81(10):2702-9, 2012
3. Bayetto K et al: Sjögren's syndrome: a review of aetiology, pathogenesis, diagnosis and management. Aust Dent J. 55 Suppl 1:39-47, 2010

Parotid Sialoliths

KEY FACTS

TERMINOLOGY

- Synonyms: Sialolithiasis, salivary stone, mucus plug, salivary calculus of parotid
- Definition: Calcified obstruction of parotid salivary duct

IMAGING

- Morphology: Somewhat smooth oval/round; may have concentric laminations
- Typically single or multiple **small radiopacities**; average diameter: 6.4 mm (range: 1-31 mm)
- **80% of parotid sialoliths are radiolucent** as they are not significantly calcified (mucus plugs)
- **83% in Stensen duct and 17% intraparenchymal**
- Duct proximal to obstruction may demonstrate intermittent dilation/stricture
- Imaging protocol
  - Conventional 2D imaging for screening
  - Conventional sialography presents best image of ductal system but is invasive
  - Conventional **sialography can visualize radiolucent sialoliths** as well as assess status of sialodochitis
  - CT, MR, or US if sialolith not visualized on 2D imaging and if conventional sialography not available or contraindicated

TOP DIFFERENTIAL DIAGNOSES

- Palatine tonsillolith
- Dystrophic calcification of lymph nodes
- Phlebolith/vascular malformation

PATHOLOGY

- May result in salivary stasis
- May result in sialodochitis/sialadenitis

CLINICAL ISSUES

- **Often multiple** and associated with sialadenitis
- Fullness/**discomfort at meal time**; may be asymptomatic
- Preauricular swelling
- Facilitate discharge with **sialogogues**

(Left) *Cropped panoramic radiograph shows multiple sialoliths of varying size in the right parotid ➡. The differential includes palatine tonsilloliths and a calcified lymph node; the latter usually has a more irregular or cauliflower-like morphology. Multiple sialoliths are somewhat common.* **(Right)** *Cropped axial CBCT shows sialolith in the parenchyma of the posterior lobe of the right parotid ➡. Approximately 17% of parotid sialoliths are located intraparenchymally.*

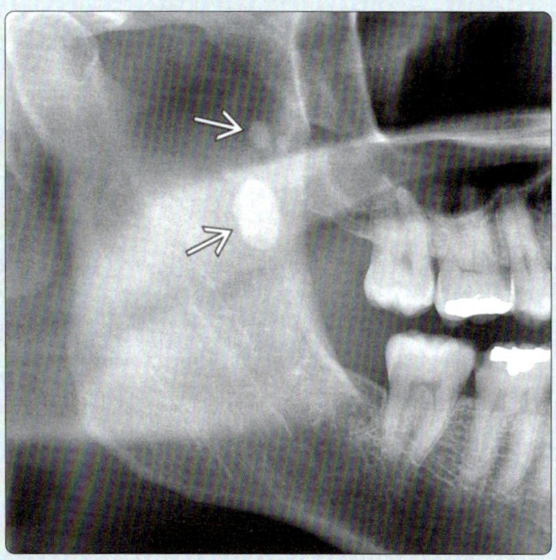

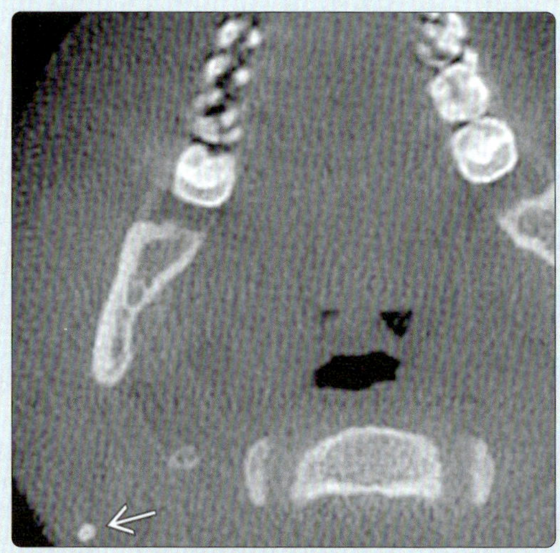

(Left) *Embossed conventional sialogram shows a minimally calcified sialolith (mucus plug) in Stensen duct presenting as a filling void ➡. Intermittent ductal dilation and stricture proximal to obstructions indicate sialodochitis.* **(Right)** *CECT in the axial plane shows typical acute parotitis with intense contrast enhancement ➡ associated with a sialolith (ductal calculus) ➡ in the distal segment of Stensen duct. There is also stranding of the overlying platysma ➡ and subcutaneous fat in keeping with this acute inflammatory process.*

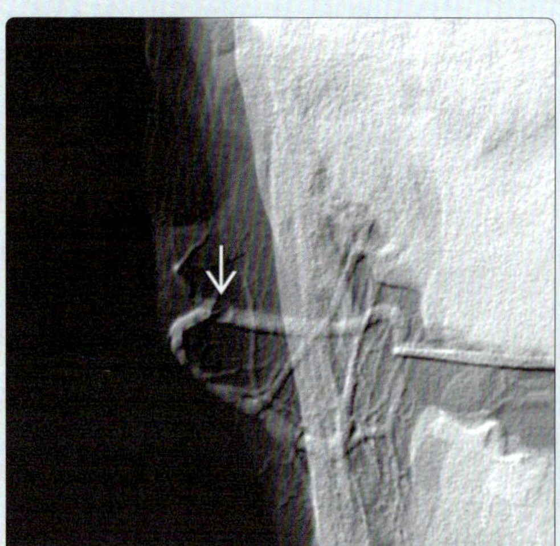

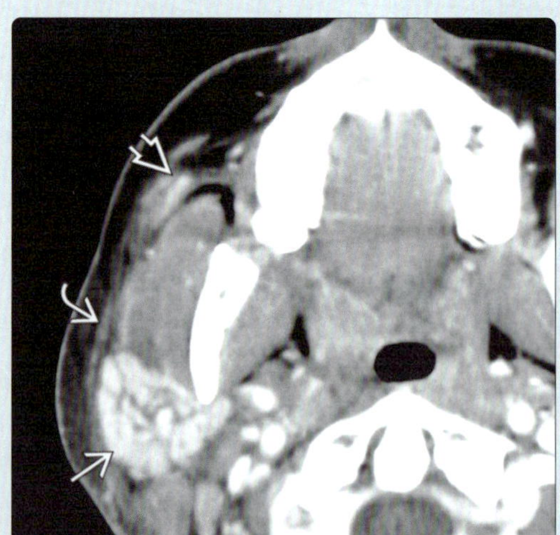

Parotid Sialoliths

TERMINOLOGY

Synonyms

- Sialolithiasis, salivary stone, mucus plug, salivary calculus of parotid

Definitions

- Calcified obstruction of parotid salivary duct

IMAGING

General Features

- Best diagnostic clue
    - Typically single or multiple **small radiopacities**; average diameter: 6.4 mm (range: 1-31 mm)
    - 80% are radiolucent as they are not significantly calcified (mucus plugs)
    - Duct proximal to obstruction may demonstrate intermittent dilation/stricture (sialodochitis)
- Location
    - **83% in Stensen duct and 17% intraparenchymal**
    - Sialoliths are more common in submandibular gland than in parotid due to serous nature of parotid saliva
- Morphology
    - Somewhat smooth oval/round; concentric laminations

Radiographic Findings

- Radiography
    - Radiopaque or radiolucent **ductal filling void** on conventional sialography
    - Intermittent dilation and stricture of duct from secondary ductal infection on conventional sialography
- Extraoral plain film
    - Oval radiopacity, sometimes laminated
    - May be visualized on panoramic radiograph or anteroposterior 2D imaging projected parallel to lateral aspect of mandibular ramus with cheek puffed out

CT Findings

- CECT
    - Density along path of Stensen duct if sialolith is significantly calcified; minimally calcified not visualized
- CBCT
    - Sialography with CBCT may help visualize ductal structures and obstruction

MR Findings

- T2WI
    - **Low-signal void** in parotid duct or at hilum
    - Difficult to visualize if poor salivary flow is present

Ultrasonographic Findings

- Ductile, highly mineralized sialoliths > 1.5 mm imaged with 99% accuracy
- Typical post acoustic shadow

Imaging Recommendations

- Best imaging tool
    - Conventional 2D imaging for screening
    - Conventional sialography presents best image of ductal system but is invasive
        - Conventional sialography can visualize radiolucent sialoliths as well as assess status of sialodochitis
    - CT, MR, or US if not visualized on 2D imaging and if conventional sialography not available or contraindicated

DIFFERENTIAL DIAGNOSIS

Palatine Tonsillolith

- Appears similar to parotid sialolith on panoramic radiographs
    - Superimposed over mandibular ramus on panoramic radiograph
    - Usually multiple and **irregularly shaped**
- Medial to mandibular ramus in tonsillar fossa on CT/CBCT/MR

Dystrophic Calcification of Lymph Nodes

- Typical multilobular or **cauliflower** appearance
- More inferior than parotid sialoliths; typical linear "chains"

Phlebolith/Vascular Malformation

- **Concentric**, **laminated**, oval radiopacities in soft tissue

PATHOLOGY

Gross Pathologic & Surgical Features

- May result in salivary stasis
- May result in sialodochitis/sialadenitis

CLINICAL ISSUES

Presentation

- Most common signs/symptoms
    - Fullness/**discomfort at meal time**; may be asymptomatic
    - Preauricular swelling
    - Progressive discomfort and possible sialadenitis

Natural History & Prognosis

- Good prognosis with treatment

Treatment

- Facilitate discharge with **sialogogues**
- Surgical removal of sialolith if in favorable location; sialendoscopy
- Lithotripsy with US guidance; risk of parenchymal damage/fibrosis
- Surgical removal of entire gland as last resort

DIAGNOSTIC CHECKLIST

Image Interpretation Pearls

- **Often multiple** and associated with sialadenitis
- Ductal dilation is typically present
- Only 20% of parotid sialoliths are radiopaque

SELECTED REFERENCES

1. Sigismund PE et al: Nearly 3,000 salivary stones: some clinical and epidemiologic aspects. Laryngoscope. 125(8):1879-82, 2015
2. Capaccio P et al: Modern management of obstructive salivary diseases. Acta Otorhinolaryngol Ital. 27(4):161-72, 2007
3. Konstantinidis I et al: Bilateral multiple sialolithiasis of the parotid gland in a patient with Sjögren's syndrome. Acta Otorhinolaryngol Ital. 27(1):41-4, 2007
4. Andretta M et al: Current opinions in sialolithiasis diagnosis and treatment. Acta Otorhinolaryngol Ital. 25(3):145-9, 2005
5. Rabinov K et al: Calculi and inflammation. In Radiology of Salivary Glands. Boston: G.K. Hall. 153-69, 1985

PART II
SECTION 8
Cervical Spine

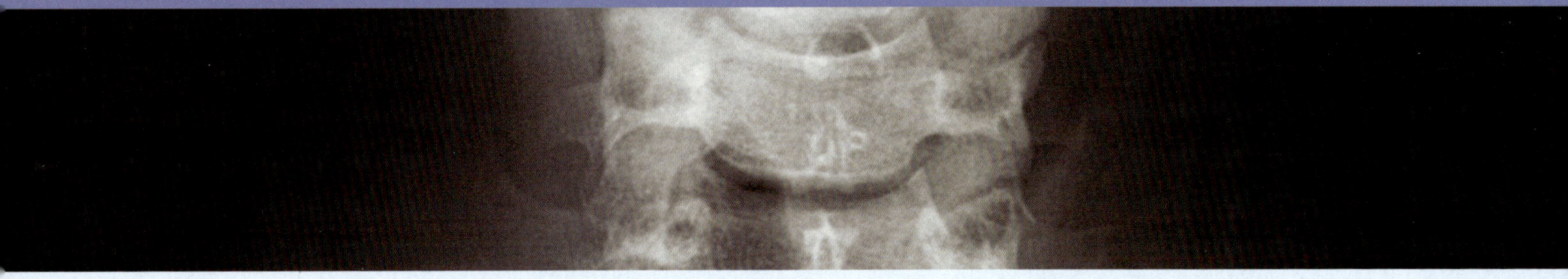

Developmental Alterations

C2-C3 Fusion 788
C1 Assimilation 790
Ponticulus Posticus 792
Ossiculum Terminale 794
Split Atlas 796
Os Odontoideum 798
Os Avis (Fused to Clivus) 802
Odontoid Hypoplasia/Aplasia 804
Failure of Formation 806
Failure of Segmentation 810

Degenerative Disorders

Degenerative Joint Disorders of Craniovertebral Junction 814
Ossification of Posterior Longitudinal Ligament 818
Diffuse Idiopathic Skeletal Hyperostosis 822
Cervical Facet Arthropathy 826

Tumor and Tumor-Like Lesions

Hemangioma, Cervical Spine 830
Lytic and Blastic Metastases 834

Fibroosseous

Fibrous Dysplasia, Cervical Spine 838

Miscellaneous

Tumoral Calcinosis 840

C2-C3 Fusion

KEY FACTS

TERMINOLOGY

- Congenital C2-C3 vertebral segmentation failure

IMAGING

- Rudimentary C2-C3 intervertebral disc space with narrow "waist"
  - C2-C3 disc space smaller than normal disc spaces in remainder of cervical spine
  - ± facet fusion
- Chiari 1 malformation may be present
- Spinal cord compression, syringomyelia unusual

TOP DIFFERENTIAL DIAGNOSES

- Juvenile inflammatory arthritis
- Surgical fusion
- Chronic sequelae of discitis

PATHOLOGY

- Congenital cervical fusion
  - Secondary to failure of normal cervical somite segmentation (3rd → 8th weeks)
- C2-C3 fusion [type II Klippel-Feil spectrum (KFS)] → autosomal dominant with variable penetrance

CLINICAL ISSUES

- Usually asymptomatic
  - Identified incidentally during spinal imaging for other reasons
- Predisposition to accelerated degenerative changes below fused level

DIAGNOSTIC CHECKLIST

- C2-C3 segmentation failure is usually incidental finding discovered while imaging for other reasons
- Less often it is associated with multiple vertebral segmentation anomalies (KFS)

(Left) *Sagittal T1WI MR of the craniovertebral junction demonstrates the characteristic rudimentary C2-C3 disc space ➡ with normal vertebral body marrow and intervertebral disc signal. The fused C2 and C3 spinous processes ➡ are relatively inapparent on MR.* **(Right)** *Sagittal bone CT of the craniovertebral junction depicts incomplete vertebral segmentation at C2-C3 ➡, with characteristic rudimentary intervertebral disc space (narrow "waist") and fusion of the spinous processes ➡.*

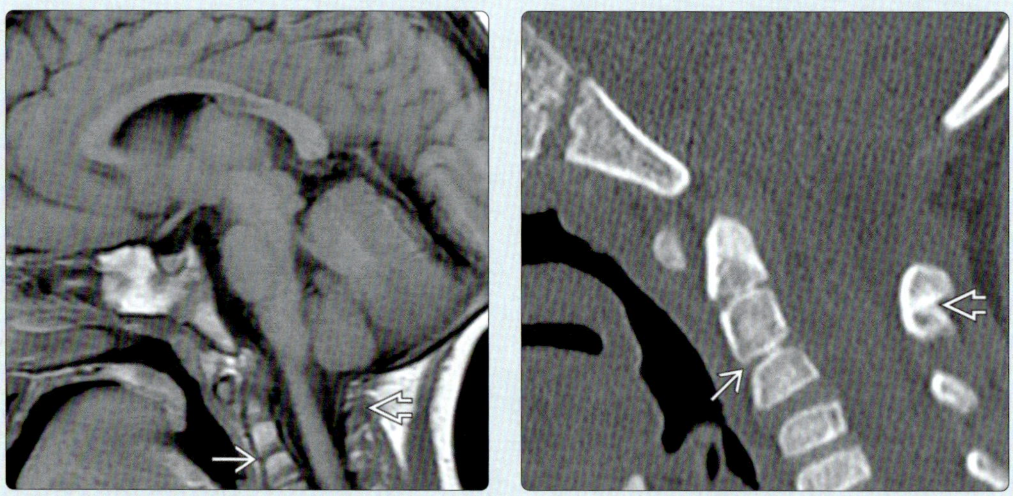

(Left) *Coronal bone CT of the craniovertebral junction confirms asymmetric, incomplete C2-C3 segmentation ➡ that results in mild upper cervical curvature convex to the right. The atlantooccipital and atlantoaxial articulations are normal.* **(Right)** *Coronal bone CT obtained through the posterior elements reveals bilateral fusion of the C2 and C3 lateral masses ➡ as well as unilateral (right) C4-C5 facet fusion ➡.*

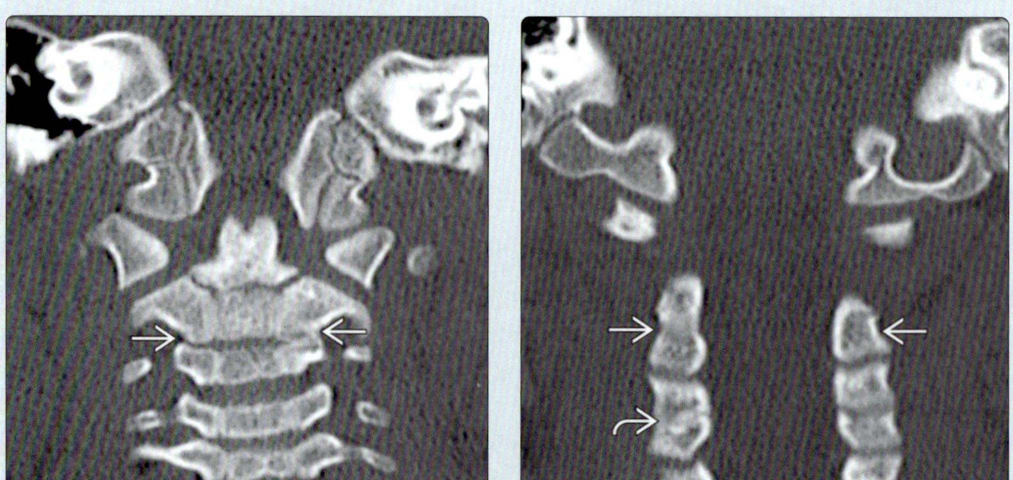

TERMINOLOGY

Definitions

- Congenital segmentation failure at C2-C3
  - Some consider congenital C2-C3 fusion within the mild Klippel-Feil spectrum (KFS)
  - May be isolated or found in conjunction with multiple congenital anomalies (more severe KFS)

IMAGING

General Features

- Best diagnostic clue
  - Narrow C2-C3 disc space ± fused facets
- Location
  - C2 and C3 vertebra
- Size
  - C2-C3 intervertebral disc space smaller than normal disc spaces in remainder of cervical spine
- Morphology
  - Rudimentary C2-C3 disc space with narrow "waist"
  - ± facet fusion

CT Findings

- Bone CT
  - Rudimentary C2-C3 intervertebral disc space with narrow "waist"
  - ± C2-C3 facet fusion
  - ± additional upper CVJ osseous anomalies

MR Findings

- T1WI
  - Rudimentary C2-C3 disc space with narrow "waist" ± C2-C3 facet fusion
    - Spinal cord and canal diameter usually normal
  - Normal marrow signal in C2 and C3 vertebral bodies, posterior elements
- T2WI
  - Same as T1WI
  - Cord compression, syringomyelia unusual
  - ± Chiari 1 malformation

Imaging Recommendations

- Best imaging tool
  - Multiplanar MR and bone CT both demonstrate osseous findings well
  - MR superior for demonstrating posterior fossa, spinal cord abnormalities

DIFFERENTIAL DIAGNOSIS

Juvenile Idiopathic Arthritis

- May be difficult to distinguish from congenital vertebral segmentation failure
- Clinical scenario very helpful
  - Identifying other affected joints and appropriate history helps make diagnosis

Surgical Fusion

- No disc space "waist," facets infrequently ankylosed
- Often surgical plate or removed hardware screw holes visible
- Surgical history key to making diagnosis

Chronic Sequelae of Discitis

- Irregular endplate margins, no "waist," ± kyphosis
- Confirm history of prior spinal infection

PATHOLOGY

General Features

- Etiology
  - Congenital cervical fusion secondary to failure of normal segmentation of cervical somites (3rd → 8th weeks)
  - No universally accepted etiology; embryonic insult postulated between 4th → 8th weeks
  - Putative environmental causative factors include teratogens, maternal alcoholism
- Genetics
  - C2-C3 fusion (type II KFS) → autosomal dominant with variable penetrance

Gross Pathologic & Surgical Features

- Surgical observations correlate to imaging findings

Microscopic Features

- Histologically normal bone, intervertebral disc

CLINICAL ISSUES

Presentation

- Most common signs/symptoms
  - Usually asymptomatic; identified incidentally during imaging for other reasons
- Other signs/symptoms
  - Cervical motion limitation most likely clinical finding in symptomatic patients

Natural History & Prognosis

- Predisposed to accelerated degenerative changes below fused level

Treatment

- None necessary

DIAGNOSTIC CHECKLIST

Consider

- C2-C3 segmentation failure is usually incidental finding discovered while imaging for other reasons
- Less often it is associated with multiple vertebral segmentation anomalies (KFS)

SELECTED REFERENCES

1. Goel A: C2-3 fusion, C3-4 cord compression and C1-2 posterior facetal instability: an evaluation of treatment strategy based on four surgically treated cases. Asian Spine J. 10(3):430-5, 2016
2. Naikmasur VG et al: Type III Klippel-Feil syndrome: case report and review of associated craniofacial anomalies. Odontology. 99(2):197-202, 2011
3. Menezes AH: Craniocervical developmental anatomy and its implications. Childs Nerv Syst. 24(10):1109-22, 2008
4. Samartzis D et al: 2008 Young Investigator Award: The role of congenitally fused cervical segments upon the space available for the cord and associated symptoms in Klippel-Feil patients. Spine (Phila Pa 1976). 33(13):1442-50, 2008
5. Samartzis DD et al: Classification of congenitally fused cervical patterns in Klippel-Feil patients: epidemiology and role in the development of cervical spine-related symptoms. Spine (Phila Pa 1976). 31(21):E798-804, 2006

C1 Assimilation

KEY FACTS

TERMINOLOGY

- Synonyms: Atlantooccipital assimilation, atlantal assimilation, "occipitalization"

IMAGING

- Partial or complete atlas assimilation into occipital bone
  - ± C1 ring hypoplasia → canal stenosis
  - ± posterior C2 arch hypertrophy → canal stenosis
- ± posterior fossa, spinal cord anomalies

TOP DIFFERENTIAL DIAGNOSES

- Juvenile idiopathic arthritis
- Craniovertebral junction surgical fusion

PATHOLOGY

- Inappropriate *PAX1* repression (humans) probably contributory, not sole mechanism
- Associated anomalies include
  - Atlantoaxial instability (up to 60%)
  - C2/3 segmentation failure
  - Klippel-Feil syndrome
  - Basilar invagination
  - Chiari 1 malformation

CLINICAL ISSUES

- May remain asymptomatic throughout life
- Symptomatic patients report neck pain, stiffness, myelopathy
  - Neurological deficits usually begin in 3rd-4th decade, worsen with age

DIAGNOSTIC CHECKLIST

- Clinical symptoms related to presence of atlantoaxial instability, cervical stenosis, and severity of associated anomalies

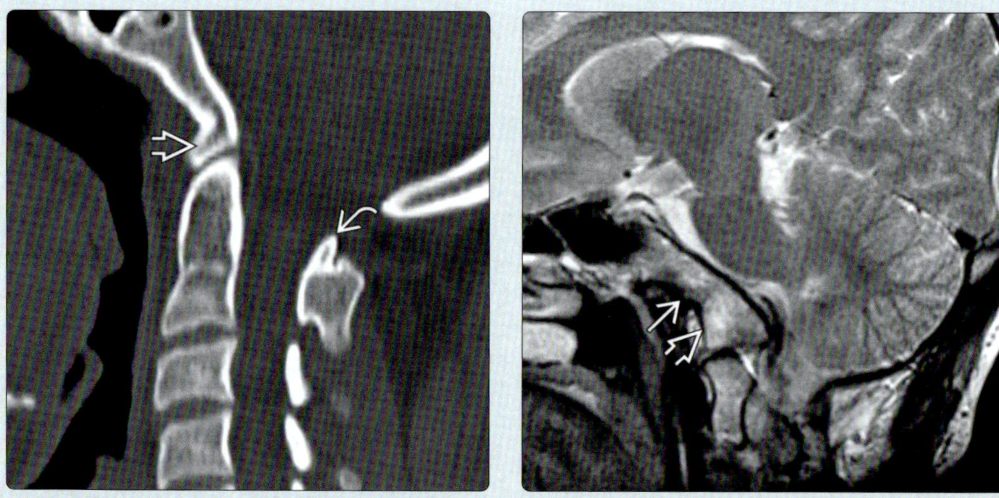

(Left) *Sagittal bone CT shows assimilation of the anterior C1 ring* ➡ *with the clivus (zone 1 assimilation) as well as aberrant fusion of the posterior C1 ring* ↶ *with the C2 spinous process.* **(Right)** *Sagittal T2WI MR shows segmentation failure of the occipital condyles* ➡ *and C1 lateral masses* ➡ *(zone 2 assimilation).*

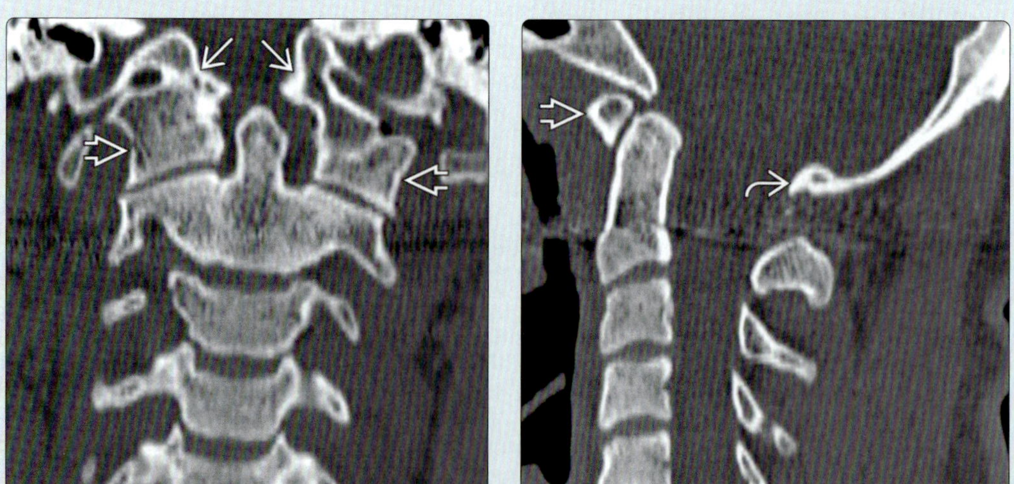

(Left) *Coronal bone CT confirms segmentation failure of the occipital condyles* ➡ *and C1 lateral masses* ➡ *(zone 2 assimilation). Formation of the proatlas is asymmetric, producing a mild head tilt to the right.* **(Right)** *Sagittal bone CT obtained in the midline shows normal alignment of clivus and odontoid tip. The anterior C1 ring* ➡ *is in normal position, but the posterior C1 ring* ↶ *is fused to the foramen magnum opisthion (zone 3 assimilation).*

TERMINOLOGY

Synonyms

- Atlantooccipital assimilation, atlantal assimilation, "occipitalization"

Definitions

- Nonresegmentation of proatlas sclerotome → failure of C1 to correctly segment from occipital bone

IMAGING

General Features

- Best diagnostic clue
  - Atlas fusion to occipital bone
- Location
  - Craniovertebral junction (CVJ)
- Morphology
  - Ranges from partial → complete atlas assimilation
  - May be unilateral or bilateral

CT Findings

- Bone CT
  - Atlas fusion to occipital bone
  - C1 ring ± hypoplastic → canal stenosis
  - ± posterior C2 arch hypertrophy → canal stenosis

MR Findings

- T1WI
  - Osseous findings same as bone CT
  - ± posterior fossa, spinal cord anomalies
- T2WI
  - Same as T1WI

Imaging Recommendations

- Best imaging tool
  - Bone CT with multiplanar reformats

DIFFERENTIAL DIAGNOSIS

Juvenile Idiopathic Arthritis

- Cervical spine subluxation, ankylosis
- Cranial settling, basilar invagination common
- Clinical history helpful

Craniovertebral Junction Surgical Fusion

- Current or previous surgical hardware presence usually visible
- Clinical history helpful

PATHOLOGY

General Features

- Etiology
  - Inappropriate *PAX1* repression (humans) probably contributory, not sole mechanism
  - Inactivation of *HOXD3* gene expression (mice) → anterior homeotic transformation at CVJ
    - C1 vertebra takes on occipital identity (assimilation), head–neck transitional zone moves caudally to C1–C2
    - *HOX* gene contribution in humans unclear
- Associated abnormalities
  - Atlantoaxial instability
  - C2/3 segmentation failure
  - Klippel-Feil syndrome
  - Basilar invagination
  - Chiari 1 malformation

Staging, Grading, & Classification

- 3 atlantooccipital assimilation zones
  - Zone 1: Anterior C1 arch (20%)
  - Zone 2: C1 lateral masses (17%)
  - Zone 3: Posterior C1 arch (13%)
  - Multiple zones involved in > 50% of patients

Gross Pathologic & Surgical Features

- Up to 60% of patients with C1 assimilation also have C1-C2 instability
  - Atlantal assimilation transfers 1st mobile segment (and motion stresses) to C1–C2 junction
  - Atlantoaxial instability incidence ↑ if C2/3 fusion also present

CLINICAL ISSUES

Presentation

- Most common signs/symptoms
  - Asymptomatic
- Other signs/symptoms
  - Neck pain, stiffness
  - Myelopathy (especially if C1-C2 instability)

Demographics

- Epidemiology
  - Prevalence 0.08% to 2.80% in general population

Natural History & Prognosis

- May remain asymptomatic throughout life
- Neurological deficits (when present) usually begin in 3rd-4th decade, worsen with age

Treatment

- Asymptomatic: Observation
- Symptomatic: Surgical stabilization, treatment of associated malformations

DIAGNOSTIC CHECKLIST

Consider

- Clinical symptoms related to presence of cervical stenosis, atlantoaxial instability, severity of associated anomalies

SELECTED REFERENCES

1. Pang D et al: Embryology and bony malformations of the craniovertebral junction. Childs Nerv Syst. 27(4):523-64, 2011
2. Tubbs RS et al: Morphometry of the outlet of the foramen magnum in crania with atlantooccipital fusion. J Neurosurg Spine. 15(1):55-9, 2011
3. Ahmed R et al: Fusions at the craniovertebral junction. Childs Nerv Syst. 24(10):1209-24, 2008
4. Menezes AH: Craniocervical developmental anatomy and its implications. Childs Nerv Syst. 24(10):1109-22, 2008
5. Gholve PA et al: Occipitalization of the atlas in children. Morphologic classification, associations, and clinical relevance. J Bone Joint Surg Am. 89(3):571-8, 2007

Ponticulus Posticus

KEY FACTS

TERMINOLOGY

- Latin: Little posterior bridge
- Synonyms: Arcuate foramen, sagittal foramen, canalis vertebralis, retroarticular canal, retroarticular/retrocondylar vertebral artery ring, upper retroarticular foramen, and atlantal posterior foramen

IMAGING

- Osseous roof along superior C1 arch covers C1 vertebral artery foramen
  - Vertebral artery passes through osseous tunnel
- May be partial or complete
- Unilateral or bilateral

TOP DIFFERENTIAL DIAGNOSES

- Broad C1 posterior arch

PATHOLOGY

- Postulated to arise from ossification of lateral segment of posterior atlantooccipital ligament or joint capsule
- Morphologically normal bone

CLINICAL ISSUES

- Most common: Asymptomatic
- Other symptoms
  - Vertebrobasilar ischemia or infarction
  - Vertigo
  - Headache
  - Neck pain

DIAGNOSTIC CHECKLIST

- Vertebral arteries predisposed to surgical injury during lateral mass screw placement
- Multiplanar bone CT with 3D reformats best demonstrate ponticulus posticus
- Presence of elongated styloid processes have been noted in cases with ponticulus posticus
  - Clinical significance of this association is unknown

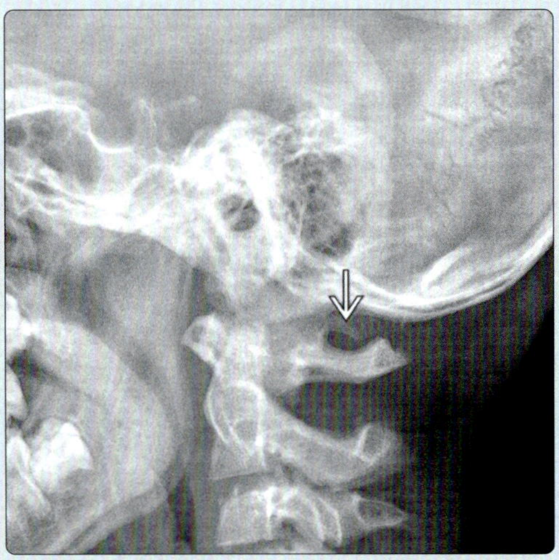
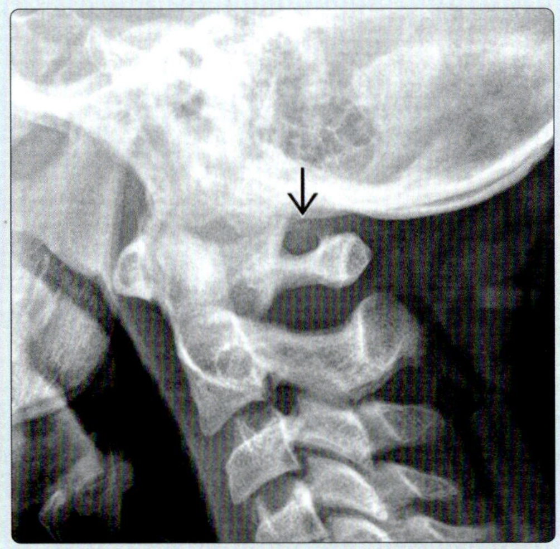

(Left) *Lateral radiograph of the upper cervical spine demonstrates a partial osseous roof ➡ over the C1 vertebral artery foramen, characteristic of ponticulus posticus (incomplete variant).* **(Right)** *Lateral radiography of the upper cervical spine reveals a complete osseous roof ⇨ over the C1 vertebral artery foramen, typical of classic ponticulus posticus (complete variant).*

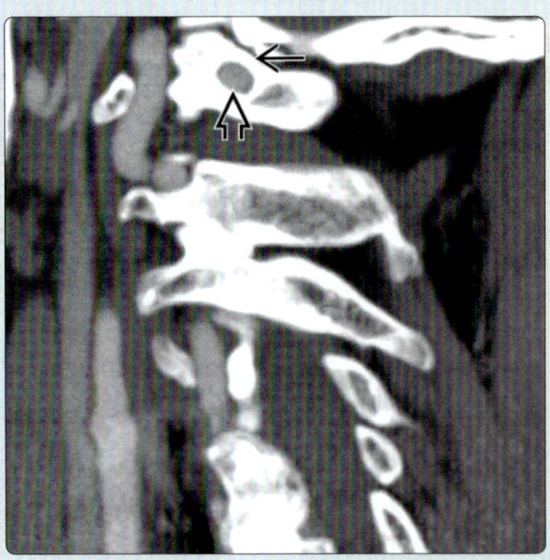
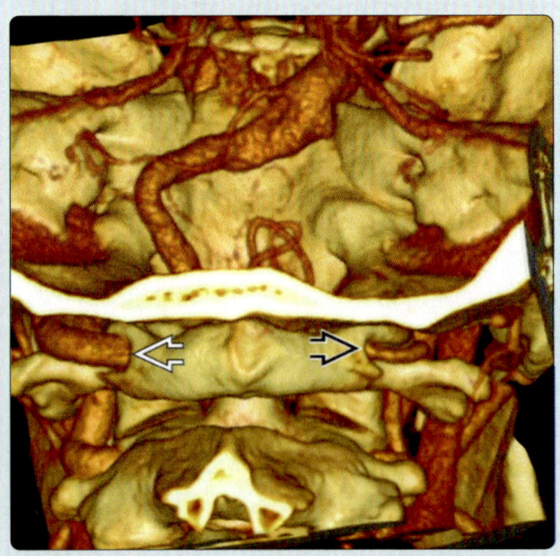

(Left) *Sagittal CTA depicts a complete C1 arch, with a robust osseous covering (complete ponticulus posticus) ⇨ over the vertebral artery ⇨, along the superior aspect of the C1 arch.* **(Right)** *Anteroposterior view of a CTA 3D reformat shows a dominant left vertebral artery ➡ and smaller (nondominant) right vertebral artery ⇨. Both are covered by a complete osseous bridge along the superior aspect of the C1 arch.*

TERMINOLOGY

Synonyms

- Arcuate foramen, sagittal foramen, canalis vertebralis, retroarticular canal, retroarticular/retrocondylar vertebral artery ring, upper retroarticular foramen, and atlantal posterior foramen

Definitions

- Osseous arch connecting retroglenoid tubercle with posterior C1 arch
- Latin: Little posterior bridge

IMAGING

General Features

- Best diagnostic clue
  - Osseous "bridge" along superior C1 arch covers vertebral artery
- Location
  - C1 arch vertebral foramen
  - Unilateral or bilateral
- Morphology
  - May be partial or complete

Radiographic Findings

- Radiography
  - Partial or complete osseous roof over C1 vertebral artery foramen

CT Findings

- Bone CT
  - Complete or incomplete osseous "bridge" covers C1 vertebral foramen
- CTA
  - Vertebral artery passes through osseous tunnel formed by ponticulus posticus

MR Findings

- Partial or complete osseous roof over C1 vertebral artery foramen
- MRA
  - Contains ipsilateral vertebral artery

Imaging Recommendations

- Best imaging tool
  - Multiplanar bone CT with 3D reformats

DIFFERENTIAL DIAGNOSIS

Broad C1 Posterior Arch

- Mistaking ponticulus posticus for broad posterior C1 arch → vertebral artery injury during C1 lateral mass screw placement

PATHOLOGY

General Features

- Etiology
  - Postulated to arise from ossification of lateral segment of posterior atlantooccipital ligament or joint capsule
- Associated abnormalities
  - None

Staging, Grading, & Classification

- Full: Complete osseous ring
- Incomplete: Portions of osseous ring absent
- Calcified: Linear or amorphous calcification

Gross Pathologic & Surgical Features

- Morphologically normal bone
- May mimic posterior C1 arch

CLINICAL ISSUES

Presentation

- Most common signs/symptoms
  - Asymptomatic
- Other signs/symptoms
  - Vertebrobasilar ischemia or infarction
  - Vertigo
  - Headache
  - Neck pain
  - Shoulder/arm pain

Demographics

- Age
  - No association
- Gender
  - F > M
- Epidemiology
  - 3-38%

DIAGNOSTIC CHECKLIST

Consider

- Vertebral arteries predisposed to surgical injury during lateral mass screw placement
- Multiplanar bone CT with 3D reformats best demonstrate ponticulus posticus

SELECTED REFERENCES

1. Zhang XL et al: The feasibility of inserting a C1 pedicle screw in patients with ponticulus posticus: a retrospective analysis of eleven patients. Eur Spine J. ePub, 2016
2. Chen CH et al: Prevalence of ponticuli posticus among patients referred for dental examinations by cone-beam CT. Spine J. 15(6):1270-6, 2015
3. Huang DG et al: Ponticulus posticus. Spine J. 15(11):e17-9, 2015
4. Krishnan P et al: Ponticulus posticus: an anatomical curiosity with clinical implications. Neurol India. 63(5):805-6, 2015
5. Sekerci AE et al: Is there a relationship between the presence of ponticulus posticus and elongated styloid process? Clin Imaging. 39(2):220-4, 2015
6. Sekerci AE et al: Prevalence and morphologic characteristics of ponticulus posticus: analysis using cone-beam computed tomography. J Chiropr Med. 14(3):153-61, 2015
7. Bayrakdar IS et al: Cone beam computed tomography imaging of ponticulus posticus: prevalence, characteristics, and a review of the literature. Oral Surg Oral Med Oral Pathol Oral Radiol. 118(6):e210-9, 2014
8. Geist JR et al: A cone beam CT investigation of ponticulus posticus and lateralis in children and adolescents. Dentomaxillofac Radiol. 43(5):20130451, 2014
9. Greiner HM et al: Rotational vertebral artery occlusion in a child with multiple strokes: a case-based update. Childs Nerv Syst. 26(12):1669-74, 2010
10. Koutsouraki E et al: Kimmerle's anomaly as a possible causative factor of chronic tension-type headaches and neurosensory hearing loss: case report and literature review. Int J Neurosci. 120(3):236-9, 2010
11. Cushing KE et al: Tethering of the vertebral artery in the congenital arcuate foramen of the atlas vertebra: a possible cause of vertebral artery dissection in children. Dev Med Child Neurol. 43(7):491-6, 2001
12. Wight S et al: Incidence of ponticulus posterior of the atlas in migraine and cervicogenic headache. J Manipulative Physiol Ther. 22(1):15-20, 1999

Ossiculum Terminale

KEY FACTS

TERMINOLOGY

- Synonym: Ossiculum terminale persistens
- Persistence of unfused odontoid tip ossification center into adulthood

IMAGING

- Separate ossicle with intact cortical margin positioned above normal-sized odontoid process in adolescent or adult
  - May be dystopic or orthotopic
- Soft tissue pannus suggests atlantoaxial instability
- Myelomalacia, brainstem compression in rare cases

TOP DIFFERENTIAL DIAGNOSES

- Os odontoideum
- Type I or II odontoid fracture
- Normal unfused odontoid tip synchondrosis
- Degenerative remodeling of odontoid process

PATHOLOGY

- Terminal ossicle normally appears by age 3 years, fuses with odontoid body by age 12 years
- Terminal ossicle located above transverse ligament
  - Atlantoaxial instability less common than with os odontoideum
  - Unstable ossiculum terminale usually dystopic

CLINICAL ISSUES

- Usually asymptomatic
- Uncommonly, neck pain or myelopathy related to CVJ instability

DIAGNOSTIC CHECKLIST

- Consider ossiculum terminale in patients > 12 years with persistent terminal ossicle at odontoid tip
- Evaluate for atlantoaxial instability if dystopic ossicle, excessive soft tissue pannus, or trisomy 21 patient

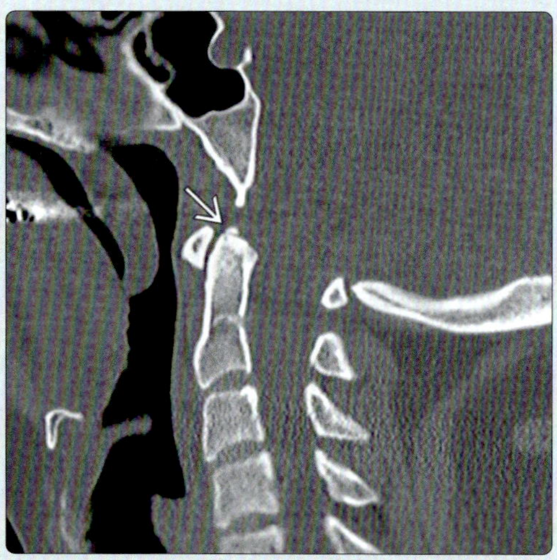

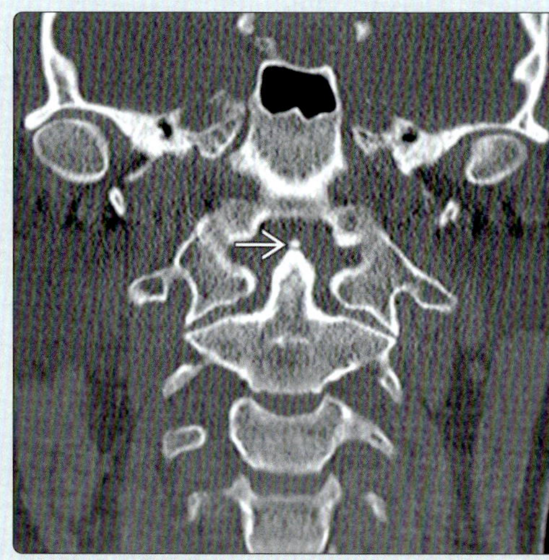

(Left) *Sagittal bone CT demonstrates a small ossiculum terminale ➡ located adjacent to the odontoid tip. The ossicle is in orthotopic position, and craniovertebral junction alignment is normal.* **(Right)** *Coronal bone CT confirms orthotopic placement of a small orthotopic ossiculum terminale ➡. Note that there is minimal flattening of the odontoid tip adjacent to the ossicle, supporting classification as a persistent terminal odontoid ossicle.*

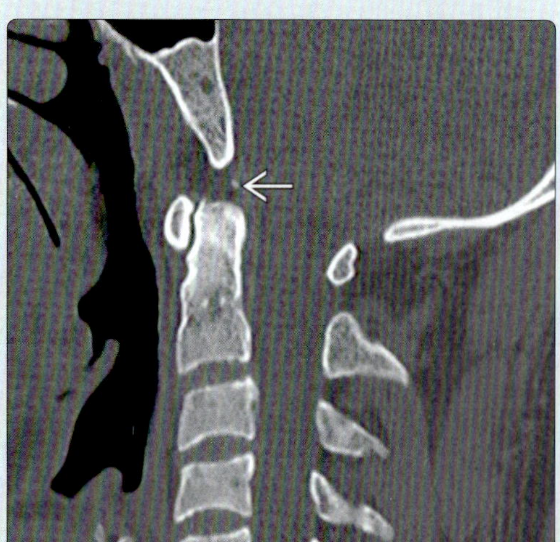

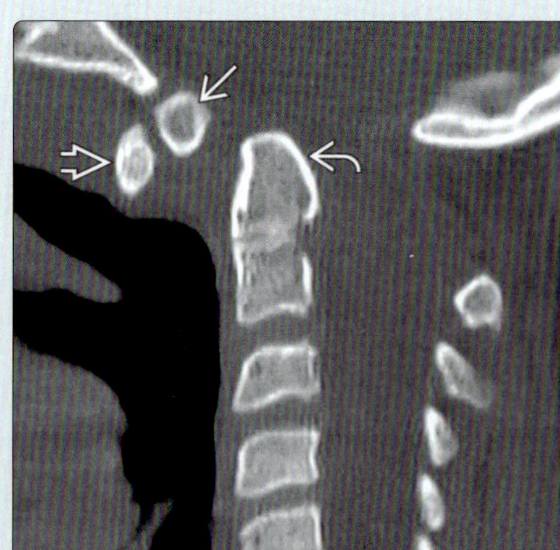

(Left) *Sagittal bone CT reveals a small dystopic ossiculum terminale ➡ positioned between the odontoid tip and clivus. The odontoid tip has remodeled.* **(Right)** *Sagittal bone CT shows subluxation of the anterior C1 ring ➡ relative to the nearly normal-sized odontoid process ➡. There is a large dystopic ossiculum terminale ➡. Although debatable, the nearly normal size of the odontoid process favors classification as an ossiculum terminale rather than os odontoideum.*

TERMINOLOGY

Synonyms

- Ossiculum terminale persistens

Definitions

- Persistence of unfused odontoid tip ossification center into adulthood

IMAGING

General Features

- Best diagnostic clue
  - Separate ossicle with intact cortical margin positioned above normal-sized odontoid process in adolescent or adult
- Size
  - Variable (several mm to > 10 mm)
- Morphology
  - Rounded ossicle at odontoid tip

Radiographic Findings

- Radiography
  - Separate ossicle with intact cortical margin positioned above remainder of odontoid process
  - Flexion/extension radiographs may show ossicle movement relative to odontoid process if unstable

CT Findings

- Bone CT
  - Separate rounded ossicle at odontoid tip
    - Circumferential sclerotic cortical margins
    - May be dystopic or orthotopic

MR Findings

- Remnant of synchondrosis may persist at junction between ossiculum and odontoid proper
  - Cartilage may be visible between ossicle, odontoid
- Soft tissue pannus suggests atlantoaxial instability
- Myelomalacia, brainstem compression in rare cases

Imaging Recommendations

- Best imaging tool
  - Multiplanar bone CT

DIFFERENTIAL DIAGNOSIS

Os Odontoideum

- Rounded, corticated os margins
- Dystopic or orthotopic os position
- Odontoid process dysplastic, hypoplastic
- Atlantoaxial instability more common than with persistent ossiculum terminale

Type I or II Odontoid Fracture

- Inferior margin of odontoid fragment not corticated
- Soft tissue swelling, trauma clinical history helpful

Normal Unfused Odontoid Tip Synchondrosis

- Small terminal ossicle lying within "V" of odontoid tip
- Young patient (< 12 years)

Degenerative Remodeling of Odontoid Process

- Osteophytes, degenerative pannus
- Much more common, especially in adults, than persistent ossiculum terminale

PATHOLOGY

General Features

- Etiology
  - Atlas ossifies from 5 primary ossification centers
    - Odontoid process begins to ossify between 1st and 5th gestational months
  - Odontoid tip arises from separate secondary ossification center
    - Derived from 4th occipital sclerotome
    - Terminal ossicle normally appears by age 3 years, fuses with odontoid body at around age 12 years

Gross Pathologic & Surgical Features

- Terminal ossicle is located above transverse ligament
  - Ossiculum may be mobile if craniovertebral junction (CVJ) instability
  - Atlantoaxial instability less common than with os odontoideum

CLINICAL ISSUES

Presentation

- Most common signs/symptoms
  - Usually asymptomatic
- Other signs/symptoms
  - Neck pain or myelopathy related to CVJ instability

Natural History & Prognosis

- Most patients asymptomatic
- True atlantoaxial instability requiring surgical intervention very rare
  - Unstable ossiculum terminale usually dystopic
  - Present later in life or in association with trisomy 21

Treatment

- Usually none required
- CVJ instability may require surgical fusion

DIAGNOSTIC CHECKLIST

Consider

- Consider ossiculum terminale in patients older than 12 years with persistent terminal ossicle
- Evaluate for atlantoaxial instability if dystopic ossicle, excessive soft tissue pannus, or trisomy 21 patient

SELECTED REFERENCES

1. O'Brien WT Sr et al: The dens: normal development, developmental variants and anomalies, and traumatic injuries. J Clin Imaging Sci. 5:38, 2015
2. Pang D et al: Embryology and bony malformations of the craniovertebral junction. Childs Nerv Syst. 27(4):523-64, 2011
3. Viswanathan A et al: "Orthotopic" ossiculum terminale persistens and atlantoaxial instability in a child less than 12 years of age: a case report and review of the literature. Cases J. 2:8530, 2009
4. Wada E et al: Os odontoideum as a consequence of a posttraumatic displaced ossiculum terminale. A case report. J Bone Joint Surg Am. 91(7):1750-4, 2009
5. Smoker WR et al: Imaging the craniocervical junction. Childs Nerv Syst. 24(10):1123-45, 2008
6. Klimo P Jr et al: Congenital anomalies of the cervical spine. Neurosurg Clin N Am. 18(3):463-78, 2007

Split Atlas

KEY FACTS

TERMINOLOGY

- Synonym: Split C1

IMAGING

- Anterior, posterior C1 arch defects → 2 C1 hemirings
  - Defects usually midline but may be paramedian
  - Wider gaps suggest independent lateral migration of C1 hemirings, instability
- ± hypoplastic ring → spinal canal stenosis, cord compression, myelomalacia, syrinx

TOP DIFFERENTIAL DIAGNOSES

- Jefferson C1 fracture
- Isolated anterior C1 arch defect
- Isolated posterior C1 arch defect

PATHOLOGY

- Simultaneous hypoplasia of C1 hypochordal bow, lateral C1 sclerotomes → combined anterior, posterior C1 arch defects
  - Ring defects usually contain fibrous connective tissue, not cartilage
  - Connective tissue more fragile than cartilage → hemirings may split

CLINICAL ISSUES

- Prognosis largely depends on severity of ring defects, craniovertebral junction (CVJ) stability, C1 ring hypoplasia
- Treatment
  - Asymptomatic patients → observation
  - Unstable, symptomatic patients → surgical stabilization

DIAGNOSTIC CHECKLIST

- Split atlas is rare congenital anomaly
  - Stability depends on anomaly severity, transverse atlantal ligament integrity
- Search for associated skull base, CVJ anomalies

(Left) *Axial bone CT demonstrates short AP dimension of the hypoplastic C1 ring as well as a split ring configuration characterized by midline defects ➡ in both anterior and posterior rings. The dens ➡ is thickened and dysplastic.* **(Right)** *Sagittal bone CT in patient with a split C1 ring shows mildly dysplastic dens ➡ formation and abnormal hypoplastic C1 ring ➡, resulting in severe spinal canal stenosis. Note associated C2/3 segmentation failure ➡.*

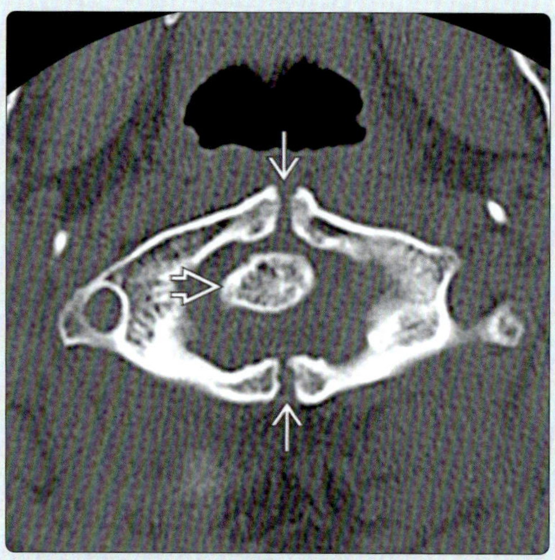

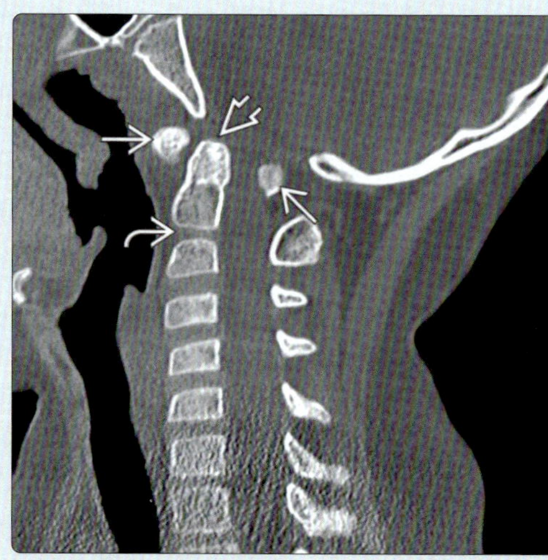

(Left) *Axial bone CT reveals large midline osseous defects ➡ in both the anterior and posterior C1 rings. The wide gaps suggest instability.* **(Right)** *Coronal bone CT shows congenital scoliosis and extensive cervicothoracic vertebral segmentation failure. The C1 lateral masses ➡ are independently displaced laterally in opposite directions, permitted by the split atlas configuration. This is a very unstable configuration necessitating surgical fusion.*

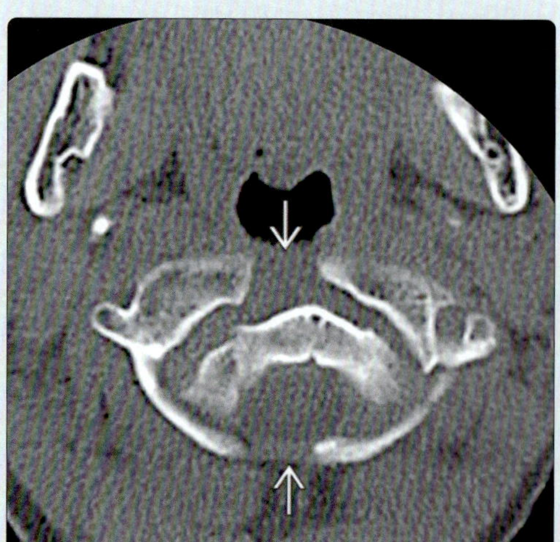

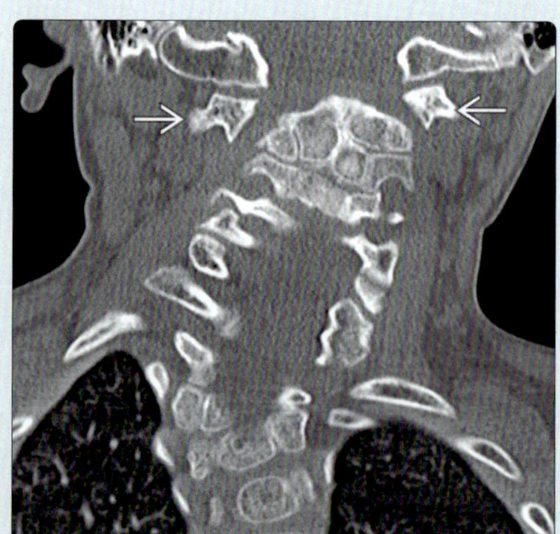

TERMINOLOGY

Synonyms

- Split C1; Congenital clefts of C1

Definitions

- Anterior, posterior C1 arch defects → 2 C1 hemirings

IMAGING

General Features

- Best diagnostic clue
  - Midline gaps in anterior, posterior C1 arches
- Location
  - Craniovertebral junction (CVJ)
- Size
  - Cleft gap ranges from narrow to wide
- Morphology
  - Anterior and posterior C1 arch defects
    - Defects usually midline but can be paramedian

CT Findings

- Bone CT
  - Left and right C1 hemirings
    - ± hypoplastic ring → spinal canal stenosis, cord compression
    - Wider gaps suggest independent lateral migration of C1 hemirings, instability

MR Findings

- T1WI
  - Soft tissue in gaps usually connective tissue, not cartilage
- T2WI
  - Transverse atlantal ligament (TAL) best seen on thin axial T2WI
  - ± cord compression, myelomalacia, syrinx

DIFFERENTIAL DIAGNOSIS

Jefferson C1 Fracture

- Noncorticated osseous fracture margins
- Trauma history, detection of soft tissue injury helpful

Isolated Anterior C1 Arch Defect

- Variable size of C1 ring cleft
- May be associated with clivus anomalies

Isolated Posterior C1 Arch Defect

- Posterior C1 arch rachischisis
- 10x more common than anterior arch defects

PATHOLOGY

General Features

- Etiology
  - Atlas normally forms from 3 primary ossification centers
    - Anterior ossification center → anterior tubercle
    - 2 lateral centers → lateral masses, posterior arch, posterior tubercle (~ 4th year)
    - 4th ossification center (variant, 2% of population) forms posterior tubercle between 2 neural arches
  - Simultaneous hypoplasia of C1 hypochordal bow, lateral C1 sclerotomes → combined anterior, posterior C1 arch defects
- Associated abnormalities
  - Skull base anomalies
  - Klippel-Feil spectrum

Gross Pathologic & Surgical Features

- Anterior and posterior ring defects usually contain fibrous connective tissue, not cartilage
  - Connective tissue more fragile than cartilage → hemirings may split
- Bifid anterior and posterior C1 rings without hypoplasia or significant gap usually stable
  - Anterior arch defect small, insertion tubercles and TAL usually intact
  - Arch gaps usually remain open into adulthood
- If anterior arch defect large or unilateral C1 lateral mass aplastic, insertion tubercle/TAL disrupted → unstable
- Simultaneous C1 ring hypoplasia → spinal cord compression, myelomalacia secondary to canal stenosis

CLINICAL ISSUES

Presentation

- Most common signs/symptoms
  - Simple bifid atlas (minimal gaps) usually asymptomatic, discovered incidentally
  - Split atlas with larger arch defects more likely to be unstable → neck pain, torticollis, myelopathy
- Other signs/symptoms
  - Cervicomedullary ischemia, posttraumatic quadriplegia

Demographics

- Epidemiology
  - 0.1% of autopsy cases show split atlas

Natural History & Prognosis

- Largely depends on severity of ring defects, CVJ stability, C1 ring hypoplasia

Treatment

- Asymptomatic patients → observation
- Unstable, symptomatic patients → surgical stabilization

DIAGNOSTIC CHECKLIST

Consider

- Split atlas is rare congenital anomaly
  - Stability depends on anomaly severity, TAL integrity
- Search for associated skull base, CVJ anomalies

SELECTED REFERENCES

1. Guenkel S et al: Incidence and variants of posterior arch defects of the atlas vertebra. Radiol Res Pract. 2013:957280, 2013
2. Choi JW et al: Congenital cleft of anterior arch and partial aplasia of the posterior arch of the c1. J Korean Neurosurg Soc. 49(3):178-81, 2011
3. Menezes AH: Craniocervical developmental anatomy and its implications. Childs Nerv Syst. 24(10):1109-22, 2008
4. Chambers AA et al: Midline anterior atlas clefts: CT findings. J Comput Assist Tomogr. 16(6):868-70, 1992

Os Odontoideum

KEY FACTS

TERMINOLOGY

- Synonym: Os
- Corticated oval or round ossicle (os) at odontoid process tip

IMAGING

- Well-defined round or oval ossicle at dens tip with smooth, uniform cortex
- ± hypertrophy of anterior C1 (atlas) arch
- ± spinal cord contusion, myelomalacia (if craniocervical instability)

TOP DIFFERENTIAL DIAGNOSES

- Ossiculum terminale
- Odontoid C2 fracture (type II)

PATHOLOGY

- 2 types based on os position
  - Orthotopic: Os in anatomic position
  - Dystopic: Os in any position other than orthotopic (considered less stable)
- Incompetence of transverse atlantal ligament (TAL) → C1/2 instability

CLINICAL ISSUES

- Commonly asymptomatic
  - Os incidentally detected on imaging obtained for other reasons (e.g., trauma)
- Symptomatic patients
  - Local mechanical neck pain, torticollis, headache, or other neurological symptoms
- Prognosis variable; depends in large part on CVJ ligamentous stability

DIAGNOSTIC CHECKLIST

- Evaluate dynamic CVJ stability when os odontoideum is identified

(Left) *Sagittal graphic of the cervical spine demonstrates an orthotopic os odontoideum ➔. There is mild separation of the os away from the odontoid process ➔ toward the clivus ➔. Note the maintenance of normal os distance to the mildly enlarged anterior C1 ring ➔.* **(Right)** *Sagittal T2WI MR of the craniovertebral junction depicts an orthotopic os odontoideum ➔, with close os approximation to the anterior C1 arch ➔. The cervical spinal cord is normal.*

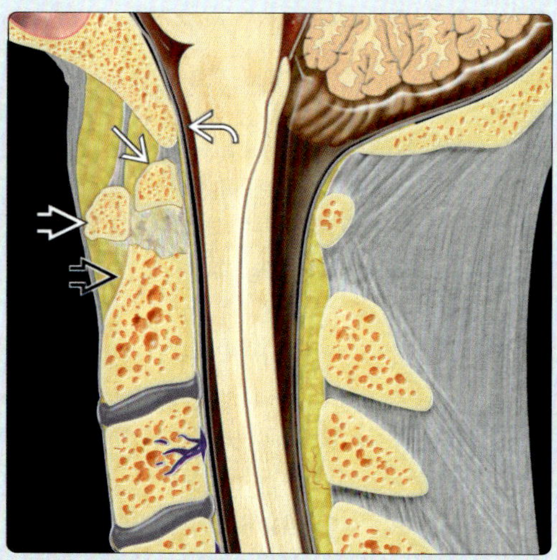

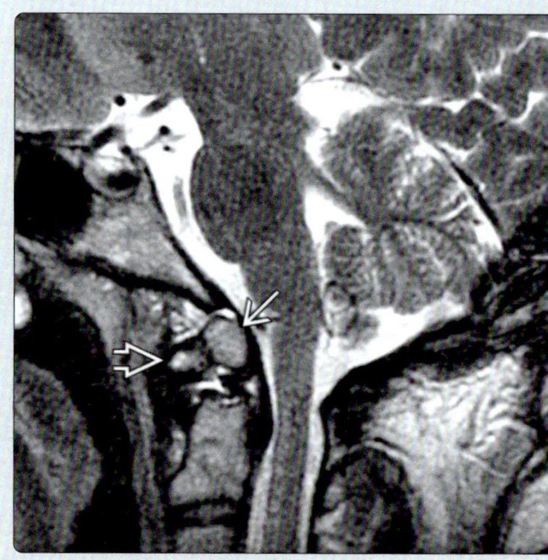

(Left) *Sagittal bone CT reveals enlargement of the C1 anterior ring ➔ in conjunction with mildly dystopic os odontoideum ➔ that is discontiguous with the dysplastic, rounded odontoid process ➔. Note maintenance of os alignment with C1 and the clivus.* **(Right)** *Coronal bone CT confirms discontinuity of the rounded os odontoideum ➔ with the C2 vertebral body. The os is mildly displaced to the left. Alignment of the occipital condyles and C1 lateral masses is normal.*

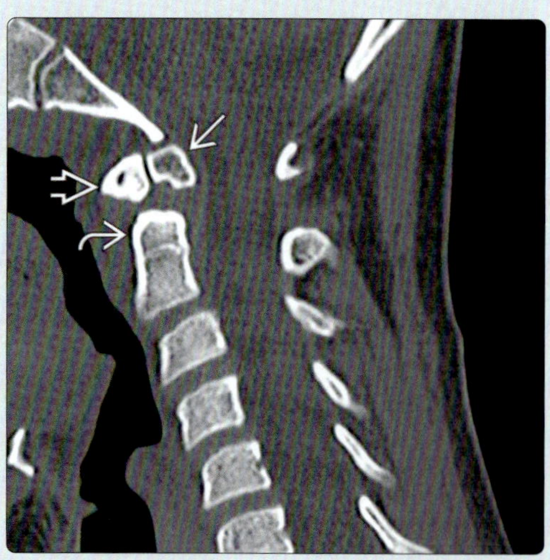

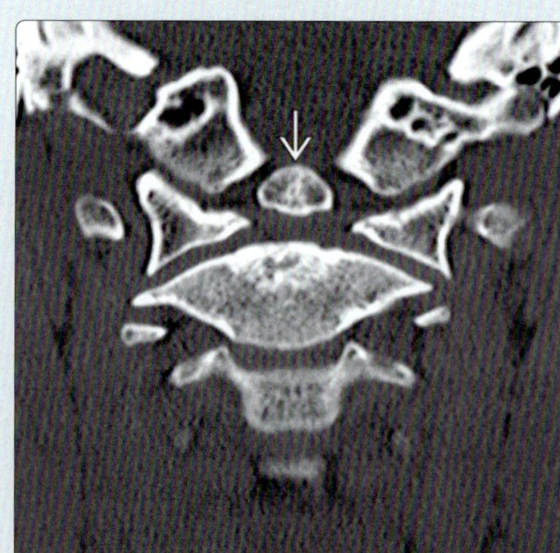

TERMINOLOGY

Synonyms

- Os

Definitions

- Corticated oval or round ossicle (os) at odontoid process tip
- 2 types described based on position of os
  - Orthotopic: Os in normal position of odontoid tip
  - Dystopic: Os in any other location
    - Most commonly os located near foramen magnum, may fuse with clivus (os avis) or anterior C1 ring

IMAGING

General Features

- Best diagnostic clue
  - Ossicle at dysplastic odontoid tip + anterior C1 arch enlargement
- Location
  - CVJ, near dens tip
- Size
  - Variable; typically smaller than normal dens
- Morphology
  - Round or oval ossicle with smooth, uniform cortex
    - Separate from C2 base and odontoid process
    - Ossicle border does not directly match with axis body
  - ± hypertrophy of anterior atlas arch

Radiographic Findings

- Radiography
  - Well-defined ossicle at dens tip + anterior C1 arch enlargement
  - ± atlantoaxial instability on flexion/extension

CT Findings

- Bone CT
  - Well-defined ossicle at dens tip + anterior C1 arch enlargement
  - Os may be fused to clivus or C1 anterior arch

MR Findings

- T1WI
  - Well-defined ossicle at dens tip + anterior C1 arch enlargement
  - Normal marrow signal in os, anterior C1 ring
- T2WI
  - Same as T1WI
  - ± spinal cord contusion, myelomalacia if craniocervical instability

Imaging Recommendations

- Best imaging tool
  - Multiplanar bone CT for osseous anatomy
  - Multiplanar MR for spinal cord, soft tissue evaluation
- Protocol advice
  - Axial bone CT with sagittal, coronal reformats
  - Sagittal, axial, coronal T2WI most helpful
    - May be performed in flexion and extension to assess stability, effect on spinal cord

DIFFERENTIAL DIAGNOSIS

Ossiculum Terminale

- Variant ossification failure of terminal ossicle → incidental "notch" in dens tip, adjacent round ossicle
- Ossicle of ossiculum terminale usually much smaller than os odontoideum; lies at level of C1 ring above transverse atlantal ligament
- Rarely associated with clinical instability

Odontoid C2 Fracture (Type II)

- Dens fracture nonunion
- Normal dens size and shape
- Typically narrow gap between axis base, dens
- Anterior C1 arch normal size

PATHOLOGY

General Features

- Etiology
  - Controversial and actively debated; several theories proposed
    - "Congenital" theory
      - Aberrant embryogenesis of occipital sclerotome, proatlas, and C1 resegmented sclerotome
      - Excessive cartilaginous dens movement at time of ossification → congenital failure of dens fusion to axis body
      - Explains detection of os odontoideum in very young
    - "Traumatic" theory
      - Sequela of prior fracture of odontoid synchondrosis before closure (age 5-6 years) → gradual os odontoideum development
      - With growth, alar ligaments carry dens fragment away from axis base
      - Cranial portion of dens fragment continues to receive blood supply from apical vessels
      - Avascular caudad portion resorbs → typical rounded ossicle
      - Explains os odontoideum detection in patients with previously normal cervical radiographs
- Associated abnormalities
  - ↑ frequency reported in Morquio syndrome, multiple epiphyseal dysplasia, Klippel-Feil syndrome, Down syndrome
- Pertinent embryology of cervicocranium (occiput-C3 sclerotomes) for os odontoideum
  - 4th occipital sclerotome (proatlas) divides into ventral rostral and dorsal caudal portions during normal embryogenesis
    - Ventral proatlas component → anterior foramen magnum, occipital condyles
      - Part of ventral proatlas also detaches to incorporate with pleuricentrum of atlas vertebra → dens
      - Core of proatlas centrum → apical dens ligament
    - Atlas, transverse atlantal ligament (TAL) derived from proatlas
      - Odontoid process represents atlas centrum following separation from C1 ring during 6th-7th gestational weeks, fusion to axis body

- Osseous elements develop through enchondral ossification
  - Dens base ossifies just prior to birth
  - Axis body fuses with odontoid process ~ age 4 years
  - Dens tip fuses to odontoid process ~ age 12 years

Staging, Grading, & Classification

- Orthotopic: Os in anatomic position
- Dystopic: Os in any position other than orthotopic
  - Most commonly os located near foramen magnum, may fuse with clivus or anterior C1 ring
  - Potentially less stable than orthotopic os
- Plain radiograph metrics
  - Anterior atlantodens interval (AADI)
    - Used clinically to measure C1/2 instability
    - Caveat: Os fragment often moves with atlas, even with gross C1/2 instability
  - Posterior atlantodens interval (PADI)
    - Distance between posterior border of dens and anterior border of posterior C1 ring
    - Indirectly reflects space available for cord (SAC)
      - Soft tissue proliferation (synovial cyst, pannus) ↓ SAC but occult on plain radiographs
    - Surrogate for MR or CT, where actual space for spinal cord can be measured
      - MR measurement of cord compression may be more predictive of symptomatology
    - PADI < 13 mm associated with progressive neurologic decline
  - PADI instability index
    - Change in SAC between flexion and extension
  - Direct measurement of C1 motion of C1 on C2 body
    - Space between line superiorly from anterior C2 body and line inferiorly from posterior border of anterior C1 arch
    - > 3 mm separation pathologic

Gross Pathologic & Surgical Features

- Os odontoideum is potentially unstable
  - TAL normally straps around basal dens segment
  - May not normally attach in os odontoideum
    - Incompetence of TAL → C1/2 instability

CLINICAL ISSUES

Presentation

- Most common signs/symptoms
  - Commonly asymptomatic
    - Os incidentally detected on imaging obtained for other reasons (e.g., trauma)
  - Symptomatic patients report local mechanical neck pain, torticollis, headache
    - Because asymptomatic os is common, may be difficult to determine relation of os odontoideum to presenting symptoms
- Other signs/symptoms
  - Transitory or persistent quadriparesis following trauma
  - Progressive myelopathy
  - Weakness
  - Ataxia
  - Lower cranial neuropathies
  - Vertebral artery compression → cervical cord, brainstem ischemia
  - Sudden death (rare)

Demographics

- Age
  - Variable
- Epidemiology
  - Exact prevalence, incidence unknown

Natural History & Prognosis

- Variable; depends in large part on CVJ ligamentous stability
- AADI and PADI prognostic indices for stability

Treatment

- Nonoperative management recommended for most patients incidentally diagnosed with os odontoideum
  - Asymptomatic patients without radiographic evidence for significant instability → observation
  - Symptomatic patients with mechanical symptoms → medical management
    - Cervical traction, physical therapy, firm collar, activity limitation, antiinflammatory medications
- Surgical stabilization for spinal instability, neurologic decline, or intractable pain

DIAGNOSTIC CHECKLIST

Consider

- Evaluate dynamic CVJ stability with flexion/extension radiographs when os odontoideum identified
- Dystopic os considered more likely to be unstable than orthotopic os

SELECTED REFERENCES

1. White D et al: The role of conservative management in incidental os odontoideum. World Neurosurg. 88:695.e15-7, 2016
2. Akpolat YT et al: Treatment of os odontoideum in a patient with spastic quadriplegic cerebral palsy. J Clin Neurosci. 22(8):1239-43, 2015
3. Nguyen JC et al: Os odontoideum. Pediatr Emerg Care. 31(3):225-7, 2015
4. O'Brien WT Sr et al: The dens: normal development, developmental variants and anomalies, and traumatic injuries. J Clin Imaging Sci. 5:38, 2015
5. Rahimizadeh A et al: Atlantoaxial subluxation due to an os odontoideum in an achondroplastic adult: report of a case and review of the literature. Case Rep Orthop. 2015:142586, 2015
6. Pang D et al: Embryology and bony malformations of the craniovertebral junction. Childs Nerv Syst. 27(4):523-64, 2011
7. Arvin B et al: Os odontoideum: etiology and surgical management. Neurosurgery. 66(3 Suppl):22-31, 2010
8. Wada E et al: Os odontoideum as a consequence of a posttraumatic displaced ossiculum terminale. A case report. J Bone Joint Surg Am. 91(7):1750-4, 2009
9. Klimo P Jr et al: Os odontoideum: presentation, diagnosis, and treatment in a series of 78 patients. J Neurosurg Spine. 9(4):332-42, 2008
10. Menezes AH et al: Anatomy and biomechanics of normal craniovertebral junction (a) and biomechanics of stabilization (b). Childs Nerv Syst. 24(10):1091-100, 2008
11. Menezes AH: Craniocervical developmental anatomy and its implications. Childs Nerv Syst. 24(10):1109-22, 2008
12. Smoker WR et al: Imaging the craniocervical junction. Childs Nerv Syst. 24(10):1123-45, 2008
13. Klimo P Jr et al: Congenital anomalies of the cervical spine. Neurosurg Clin N Am. 18(3):463-78, 2007
14. Choit RL et al: Os odontoideum: a significant radiographic finding. Pediatr Radiol. 35(8):803-7, 2005
15. Vargas TM et al: Atlantoaxial instability associated with an orthotopic os odontoideum: a multimodality imaging assessment. Emerg Radiol. 11(4):223-5, 2005

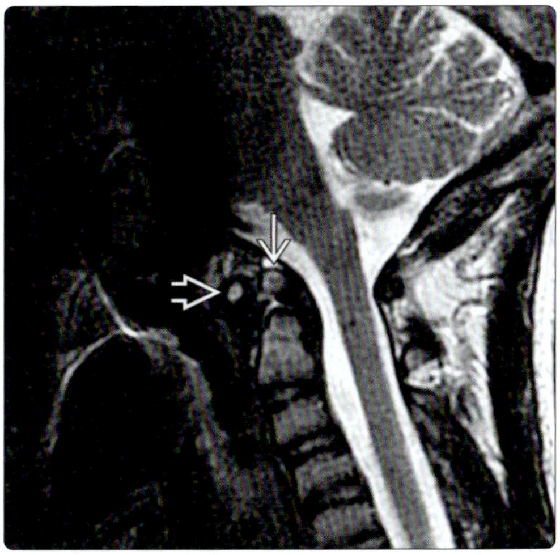

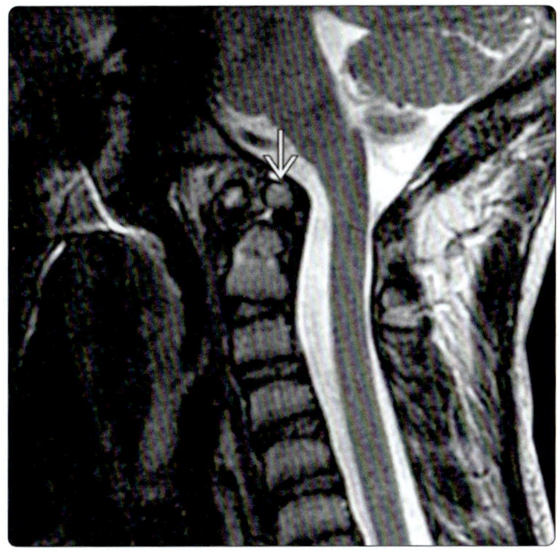

(Left) *Sagittal T2WI MR obtained in flexion shows anterior positioning of the dystopic os ➡ relative to C2. The normal distance between the anterior C1 ring ➡ and the os is preserved, but there was a change in os position relative to C2 (atlantoaxial instability) compared to neutral and extension sagittal images.* **(Right)** *Sagittal T2WI MR (same patient) obtained in extension shows normal os ➡ position. Flexion sagittal T2WI MR showed anterior os translation, indicating atlantoaxial instability.*

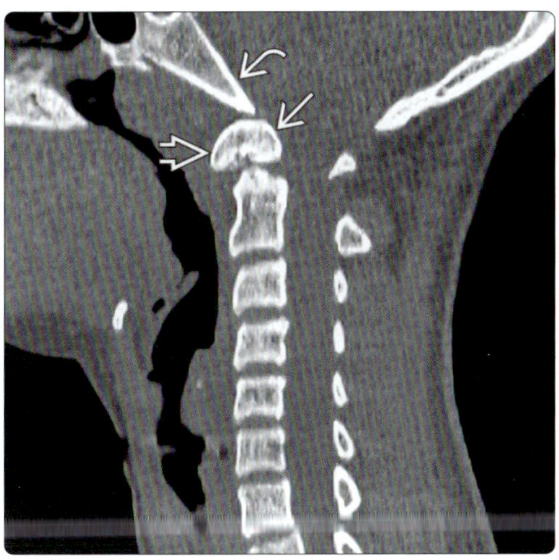

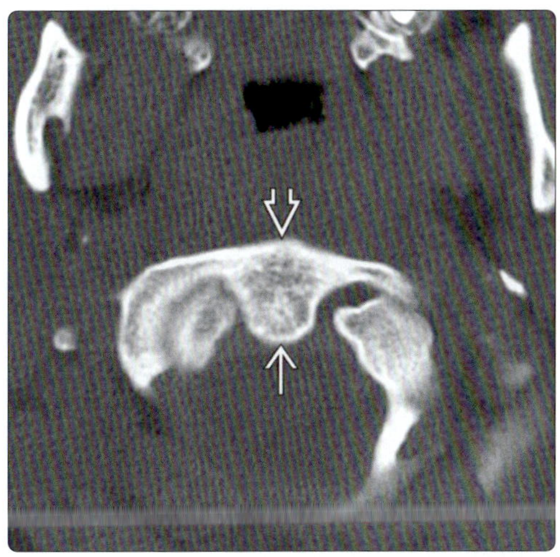

(Left) *Sagittal bone CT of the cervical spine shows congenital fusion of the anterior C1 ring ➡ and a large os odontoideum ➡. Normal clivus ➡ relationship to the os is maintained. The subaxial cervical spine was otherwise normal, and no additional vertebral segmentation anomalies were detected.* **(Right)** *Axial bone CT confirms solid congenital fusion of an orthotopic os ➡ to the midline anterior C1 ring ➡. The posterior C1 ring was complete (not shown).*

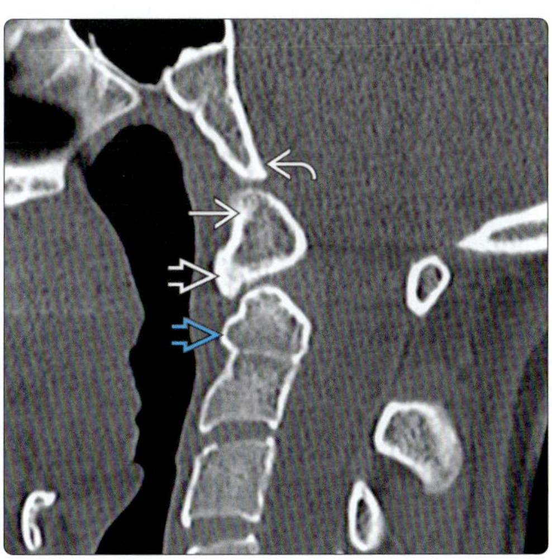

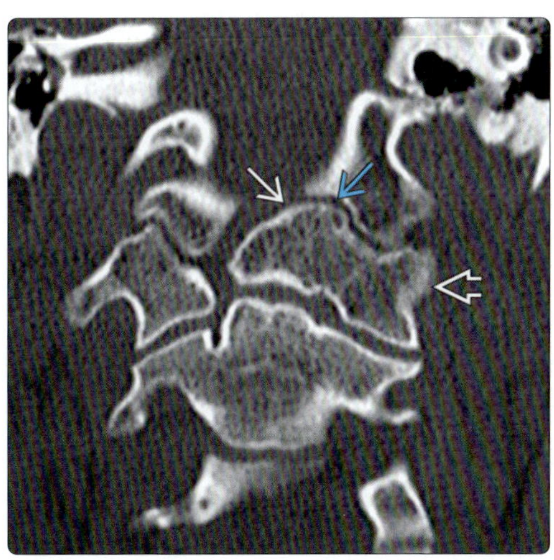

(Left) *Sagittal bone CT demonstrates fusion of a large dystopic os odontoideum ➡ to the anterior C1 arch ➡. The clivus tip ➡ is minimally remodeled (flattened). The short, rounded odontoid process ➡ is dysplastic.* **(Right)** *Coronal bone CT depicts eccentric fusion of a dystopic os odontoideum ➡ to the left C1 ➡ anterior arch and lateral mass. Note also the abnormal pseudoarticulation between the os and the left occipital condyle ➡.*

Os Avis (Fused to Clivus)

KEY FACTS

TERMINOLOGY

- Variant of os odontoideum

IMAGING

- Well-defined ossicle fused to clivus
  - Clivus often dysplastic; may be subtle
- ± spinal cord contusion, myelomalacia (if craniocervical instability)
- Best imaging tool: Bone algorithm CT with multiplanar reformats

TOP DIFFERENTIAL DIAGNOSES

- Os odontoideum
- Odontoid fracture (type II)
- Clival fracture

PATHOLOGY

- Controversial, not well understood

CLINICAL ISSUES

- Often asymptomatic
  - Os avis incidentally detected on imaging obtained for other reasons (e.g., trauma)
- Symptomatic patients report local mechanical neck pain, torticollis, headache, or neurological deterioration
- Exact prevalence, incidence unknown
- Natural history variable
  - Os avis considered at increased risk for neurological deterioration
  - Prognosis depends in large part on craniovertebral junction (CVJ) ligamentous stability

DIAGNOSTIC CHECKLIST

- Evaluate dynamic CVJ stability when os avis is identified

(Left) *Lateral radiography of the cervical spine (neutral position) reveals a dystopic os odontoideum ➡ fused to the clivus. Also demonstrated is a hypoplastic odontoid process ➡.* **(Right)** *Sagittal bone CT confirms that the os odontoideum ➡ is solidly fused to the clivus ➡. Osseous remodeling changes are present in the anterior C1 ring ➡ as well as the os. The hypoplastic posterior C1 ring ⇨ resides within the spinal canal, just below the foramen magnum.*

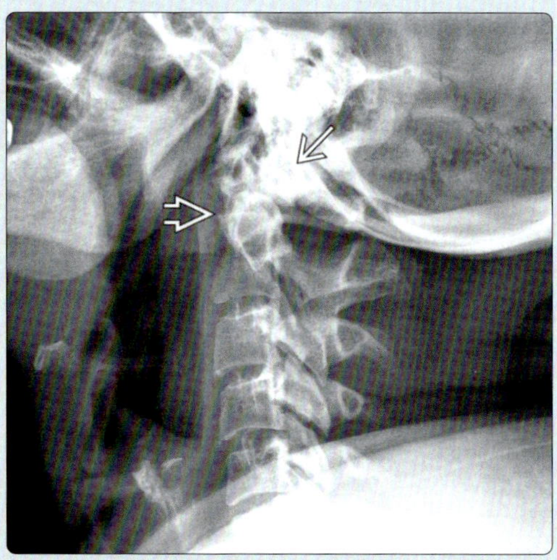

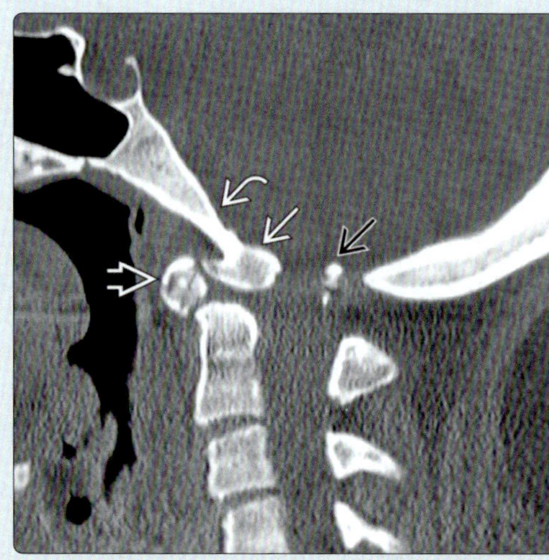

(Left) *Coronal bone CT image depicts fusion of the dystopic os odontoideum ➡ to the clivus ➡ (located eccentric to the right).* **(Right)** *Axial T2 MR image shows abnormal T2 hyperintensity in the cervical spinal cord at the C1 level, reflecting spinal cord injury related to superimposed atlantoaxial instability and mild hypoplasia of the C1 ring in conjunction with an eccentric os avis ➡.*

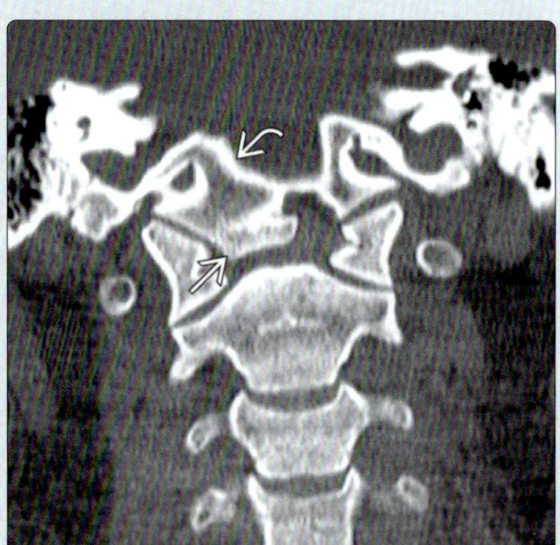

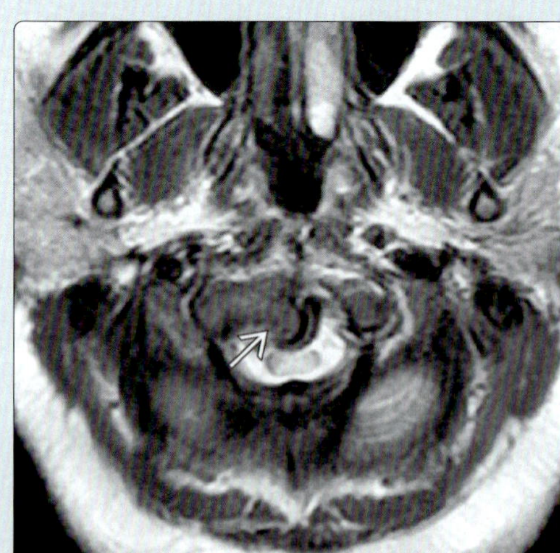

Os Avis (Fused to Clivus)

TERMINOLOGY

Definitions

- Variant of os odontoideum
  - Dystopic os fuses to clivus

IMAGING

General Features

- Best diagnostic clue
  - Os odontoideum with dystopic os fused to clivus
- Location
  - Craniovertebral junction (CVJ), at clivus tip
- Size
  - Variable os size
  - Usually smaller than normal dens
- Morphology
  - Round or oval ossicle with smooth, uniform cortex
    - Os fused to clivus
    - Clivus often dysplastic; may be subtle
  - ± hypertrophy or remodeling of anterior atlas arch

Radiographic Findings

- Radiography
  - Well-defined ossicle fused to clivus
    - Dens usually shorter than normal
    - ± anterior C1 arch enlargement

CT Findings

- Bone CT
  - Same as radiography
  - Clivus often dysplastic

MR Findings

- T1WI
  - Well-defined ossicle fused to clivus
  - Normal marrow signal in os, clivus
- T2WI
  - Same as T1WI
  - ± spinal cord contusion, myelomalacia if craniocervical instability present

Imaging Recommendations

- Best imaging tool
  - Bone algorithm CT with multiplanar reformats
- Protocol advice
  - Thin-section (3.0 mm) axial slices with sagittal and coronal reformats
  - Include clivus and upper cervical spine

DIFFERENTIAL DIAGNOSIS

Os Odontoideum

- Os usually not fused to clivus or anterior C1 ring
  - Os avis is uncommon variant of os odontoideum

Odontoid Fracture (Type II)

- Sharp fracture line through odontoid base without corticated margin
- Dens tip not fused to clivus
- Trauma history helpful

Clival Fracture

- Acute clivus fracture with noncorticated margin
- Edema, hematoma at fracture site
- Clinical history usually helpful

PATHOLOGY

General Features

- Etiology
  - Controversial, not well understood
    - Passionate proponents of both traumatic, congenital etiologies

CLINICAL ISSUES

Presentation

- Most common signs/symptoms
  - Often asymptomatic
    - Os avis incidentally detected on imaging obtained for other reasons (e.g., trauma)
  - Symptomatic patients report local mechanical neck pain, torticollis, headache, or neurological deterioration
- Other signs/symptoms
  - Transitory or persistent paresis following trauma
  - Progressive myelopathy
  - Vertebral artery compression → cervical cord, brainstem ischemia
  - Sudden death (rare)

Demographics

- Age
  - Variable
- Epidemiology
  - Exact prevalence, incidence unknown

Natural History & Prognosis

- Variable; depends in large part on CVJ ligamentous stability
  - Os avis considered at increased risk for neurological deterioration
  - AADI and PADI prognostic indices for stability

Treatment

- Asymptomatic patients without radiographic evidence for significant instability → observation
- Symptomatic patients with mechanical symptoms, stable CVJ → medical management 1st
- Spinal instability, neurologic decline, or intractable pain → surgical stabilization

DIAGNOSTIC CHECKLIST

Consider

- Evaluate dynamic CVJ stability when os avis is identified

SELECTED REFERENCES

1. Pang D et al: Embryology and bony malformations of the craniovertebral junction. Childs Nerv Syst. 27(4):523-64, 2011
2. Arvin B et al: Os odontoideum: etiology and surgical management. Neurosurgery. 66(3 Suppl):22-31, 2010
3. Smoker WR et al: Imaging the craniocervical junction. Childs Nerv Syst. 24(10):1123-45, 2008
4. Klimo P Jr et al: Congenital anomalies of the cervical spine. Neurosurg Clin N Am. 18(3):463-78, 2007

Odontoid Hypoplasia/Aplasia

KEY FACTS

TERMINOLOGY

- Congenital small or absent odontoid process

IMAGING

- Reduced size of odontoid process
  - Odontoid process is small, blunted
  - Hypoplasia > > aplasia
- ± enlargement of anterior C1 ring
- ± spinal cord myelomalacia, syringomyelia

TOP DIFFERENTIAL DIAGNOSES

- Os odontoideum
- Odontoid C2 fracture
- Surgical odontoid resection

PATHOLOGY

- Developmental abnormality
  - More common in patients with skeletal dysplasias, trisomy 21
- Generally nonfamilial, although some reports of autosomal dominant inheritance
- Associated anomalies: Segmentation failure, craniovertebral junction (CVJ) dynamic instability
- Status of transverse atlantal ligament (TAL), other stabilizing ligaments variable

CLINICAL ISSUES

- Most commonly asymptomatic
- Symptomatic patients report neck pain, myelopathy
  - Variable depending on severity, presence of dynamic instability, other associated anomalies

DIAGNOSTIC CHECKLIST

- More common in skeletal dysplasias, trisomy 21, mucopolysaccharidosis
- Severity, status of TAL, & associated anomalies determine CVJ stability

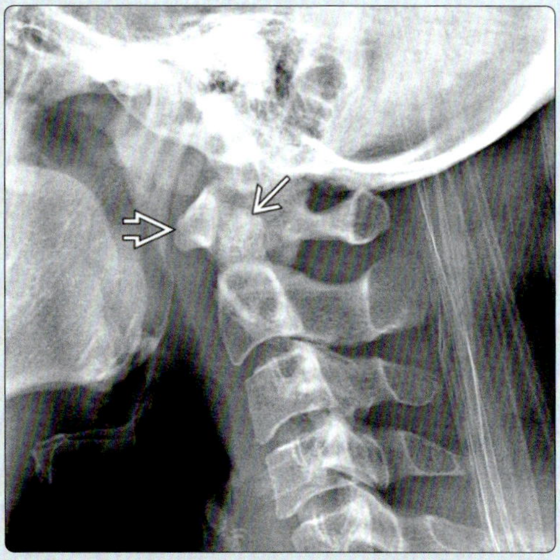

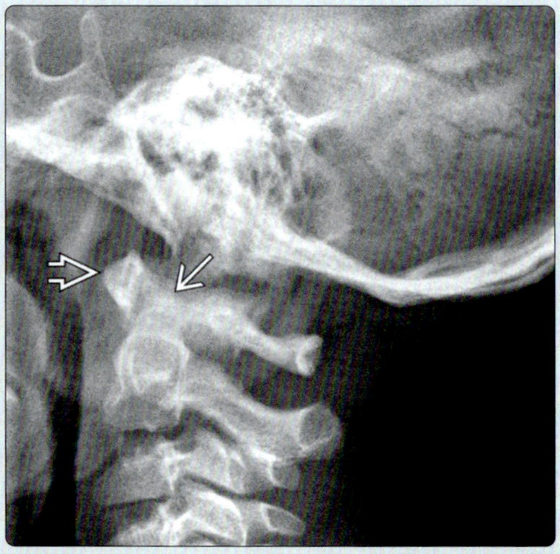

(Left) *Lateral cervical radiograph demonstrates a congenital hypoplastic odontoid process ➡ with normal C1/2 alignment. The anterior C1 ring ➡ is mildly enlarged, likely compensatory hypertrophy. No other cervical spine abnormalities were present.* **(Right)** *Lateral cervical radiograph reveals mild congenital hypoplasia of the dens process ➡. There is compensatory enlargement of the anterior C1 ring ➡. Craniovertebral junction alignment is normal and no additional anomalies are present.*

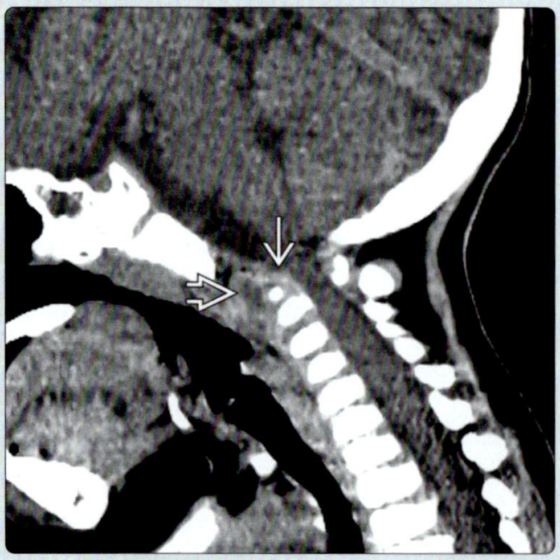

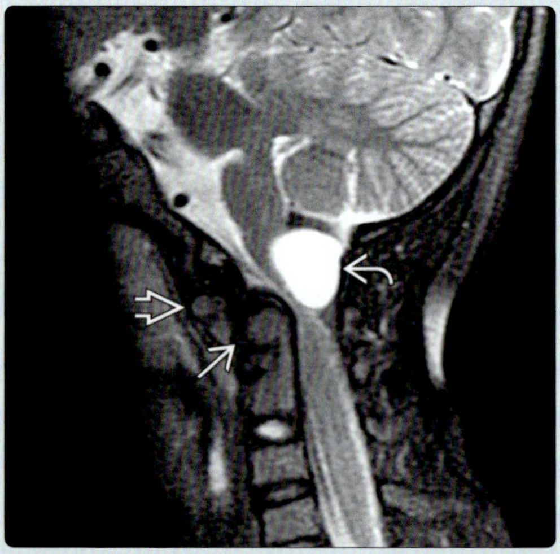

(Left) *Sagittal CECT (spondylometaphyseal dysplasia) confirms odontoid process hypoplasia ➡ and hypoplastic C1 ring, resulting in cervical canal stenosis. The anterior atlas arch ➡ is cartilaginous, representing abnormal delayed ossification.* **(Right)** *Sagittal T2WI MR (neurenteric cyst, ➡) demonstrates congenital craniovertebral junction osseous anomalies, including a short, dysplastic odontoid process ➡. The anterior C1 ring ➡ is anteriorly displaced, reflecting atlantoaxial instability.*

TERMINOLOGY

Definitions

- Congenital small or absent odontoid process

IMAGING

General Features

- Best diagnostic clue
  - Odontoid process is small and blunted ± enlargement of C1 anterior ring
- Location
  - Craniovertebral junction (CVJ)
- Size
  - Variable; absent to nearly normal size
- Morphology
  - Odontoid process shorter, often stubbier than normal dens
  - Hypoplasia > > aplasia

Radiographic Findings

- Radiography
  - Small odontoid process
  - Best appreciated on lateral or odontoid views

CT Findings

- Bone CT
  - Same as radiography
  - Better than radiography to evaluate for C1 ring, other CVJ anomalies

MR Findings

- T1WI
  - Reduced size of odontoid process
  - Normal marrow signal
- T2WI
  - Same as T1WI
  - ± spinal cord myelomalacia, syringomyelia
  - Best to evaluate status of supporting ligaments

Imaging Recommendations

- Best imaging tool
  - Multiplanar bone CT or MR imaging

DIFFERENTIAL DIAGNOSIS

Os Odontoideum

- Rounded ossicle rostral to residual dens
- Anterior C1 ring often enlarged

Odontoid C2 Fracture

- Sharp, noncorticated inferior margination of ossicle rostral to odontoid peg remnant
- Trauma history helpful

Surgical Odontoid Resection

- Usually performed to alleviate ventral cervicomedullary compression
- Surgical history, straight margin of rostral dens, imaging stigmata of prior surgery or instrumentation

PATHOLOGY

General Features

- Genetics
  - Generally nonfamilial, although some reports of autosomal dominant inheritance
  - More common in patients with skeletal dysplasias, trisomy 21
- Associated abnormalities
  - Segmentation anomalies, CVJ dynamic instability
- Developmental abnormality

Gross Pathologic & Surgical Features

- Status of transverse atlantal ligament (TAL), other stabilizing ligaments variable
  - Depends on size of dens remnant, presence of other osseous anomalies

Microscopic Features

- Histologically normal bone

CLINICAL ISSUES

Presentation

- Most common signs/symptoms
  - Asymptomatic
- Other signs/symptoms
  - Neck pain
  - Myelopathy

Natural History & Prognosis

- Variable depending on severity, presence of dynamic instability, other associated anomalies

Treatment

- Asymptomatic patients may be amenable to expectant observation
- Symptomatic, unstable patients may require surgical fusion

DIAGNOSTIC CHECKLIST

Consider

- More common in skeletal dysplasias, trisomy 21, mucopolysaccharidosis
- Severity, status of TAL, associated anomalies determine CVJ stability

SELECTED REFERENCES

1. Jain N et al: CT and MR imaging of odontoid abnormalities: a pictorial review. Indian J Radiol Imaging. 26(1):108-19, 2016
2. Myśliwiec A et al: Atlanto-axial instability in people with Down's syndrome and its Impact on the ability to perform sports activities - a review. J Hum Kinet. 48:17-24, 2015
3. Souza PV et al: Basilar invagination in headache associated with physical exertion and recurrent torticollis. Arq Neuropsiquiatr. 72(11):902-3, 2014
4. Zygourakis CC et al: Delayed development of os odontoideum after traumatic cervical injury: support for a vascular etiology. J Neurosurg Pediatr. 7(2):201-4, 2011
5. Stevens CA et al: Familial odontoid hypoplasia. Am J Med Genet A. 149A(6):1290-2, 2009
6. Menezes AH: Craniocervical developmental anatomy and its implications. Childs Nerv Syst. 24(10):1109-22, 2008
7. Ali FE et al: Cervical spine abnormalities associated with Down syndrome. Int Orthop. 30(4):284-9, 2006
8. Westermeyer RR: Odontoid hypoplasia presenting as torticollis: a discussion of its significance. J Emerg Med. 24(1):15-8, 2003

KEY FACTS

TERMINOLOGY

- Vertebral dysplasia, segmentation, and fusion anomaly (SFA), disorganized spine
- Partial or complete failure of vertebral formation

IMAGING

- Sharply angulated, single curve or focal (kypho)scoliosis
- Hemivertebra, butterfly vertebra generally smaller than normal vertebra

TOP DIFFERENTIAL DIAGNOSES

- Vertebral fracture: History critical
- Inherited spinal dysplasias

PATHOLOGY

- Deranged *PAX1* gene expression in developing vertebral column
- Many syndromes manifest vertebral dysplasia
- Associated anomalies include dysraphism, split notochord syndromes, visceral anomalies (61% of congenital scoliosis patients)

CLINICAL ISSUES

- Many asymptomatic or detected during scoliosis evaluation
- Syndromal patients usually detected in infancy
  - Abnormal spine curvature ± neural deficits, limb or visceral abnormalities
  - Respiratory failure (impeded chest movement 2° to fused ribs, kyphoscoliosis)

DIAGNOSTIC CHECKLIST

- Important to look for and characterize associated visceral anomalies
- Type of deformity determines propensity for scoliosis progression

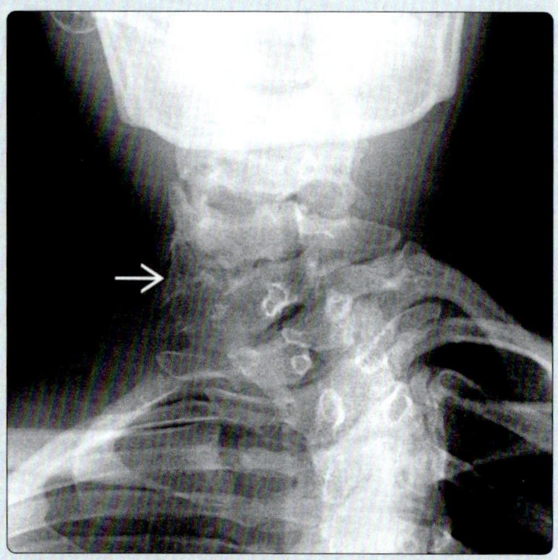

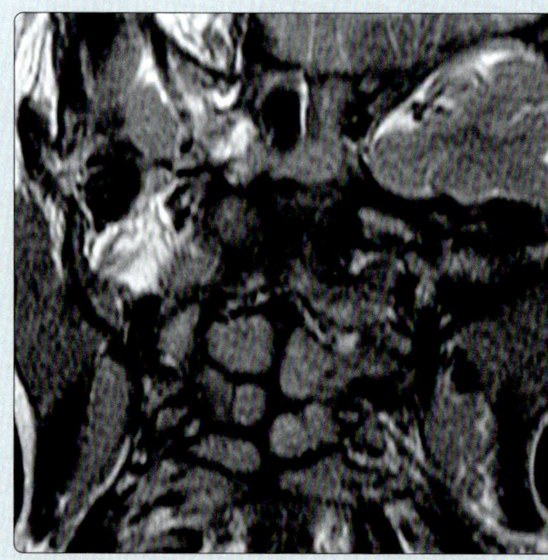

(Left) *Anteroposterior radiograph of the cervical spine demonstrates a right midcervical hemivertebra ➡, which has failed to correctly segment from both the vertebra above and below, resulting in an asymmetric block vertebra and congenital cervical dextroscoliosis.* **(Right)** *Coronal T2WI MR shows extensive cervical hemivertebra and butterfly vertebra in the cervical spine. Marrow signal is normal, but intervertebral disc spaces are absent.*

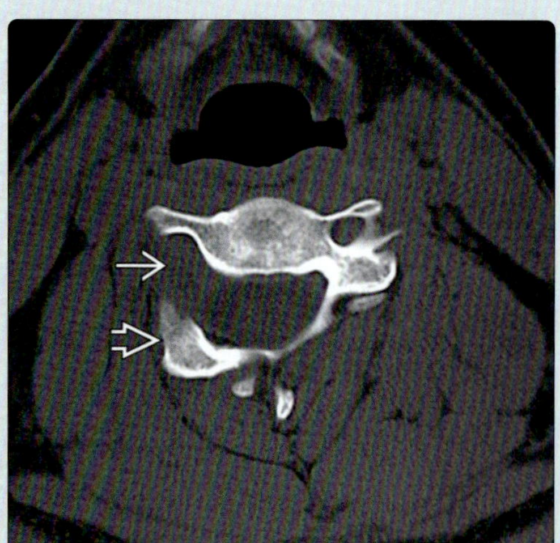

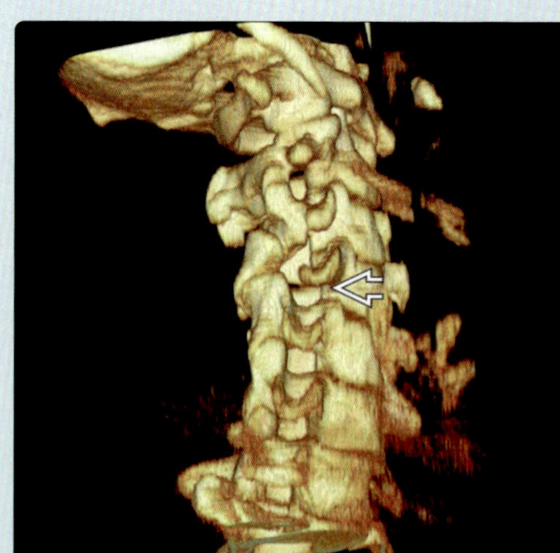

(Left) *Axial bone CT shows expected location ➡ of absent right C4 pedicle. The ipsilateral neural foramen is abnormally large on the side of pedicular formation failure, and the right vertebral posterior elements ⇨ are dysplastic.* **(Right)** *Oblique bone CT 3D reformat shows an enlarged right C4 foramen ⇨ related to an absent right C4 pedicle and dysplastic right posterior elements.*

TERMINOLOGY

Synonyms

- Vertebral dysplasia, segmentation, and fusion anomaly (SFA), disorganized spine

Definitions

- Partial or complete failure of vertebral formation
  - Partial formation failure → wedge vertebra
  - Complete formation failure → vertebral aplasia, hemivertebra, butterfly vertebra

IMAGING

General Features

- Best diagnostic clue
  - Sharply angulated, single curve or focal scoliosis with deformed vertebral bodies
- Location
  - Thoracolumbar most common
- Size
  - Hemivertebra, butterfly vertebra generally smaller than normal vertebra
- Morphology
  - Incompletely formed vertebra; may be missing front, back, side, or middle of vertebral body

Radiographic Findings

- Radiography
  - Vertebral formation failure anomalies
  - ± scoliosis
    - Paired bilateral hemivertebra → "balanced," scoliotic curves cancel out
    - ≥ 1 unilateral hemivertebra → "unbalanced," uncompensated scoliotic curve
  - Best modality for counting vertebral levels, determining presence and severity of scoliosis

CT Findings

- Bone CT
  - Sagittal or coronal vertebral clefts, hemivertebra, butterfly vertebra
    - Abnormal vertebra difficult to evaluate in axial plane; sagittal, coronal reformats helpful
  - ± posterior element dysraphism, fusion anomalies
    - Most readily evaluated in axial plane
  - 3D CT reformatted images best demonstrate vertebral anomalies for surgical planning

MR Findings

- T1WI
  - Vertebral formation failure anomalies
  - Normal marrow, disc signal intensity
- T2WI
  - Similar findings to T1WI
  - ± lipoma, tethered cord, diastematomyelia, spinal cord compression

Imaging Recommendations

- Best imaging tool
  - Multiplanar MR
- Protocol advice
  - Long-cassette weight-bearing radiographs → quantitate scoliosis, counting to definitively localize abnormal vertebral level
  - Multiplanar T1WI, T2WI MR → identify vertebral anomalies, evaluate spinal cord and soft tissues
    - Most vertebral and spinal cord anomalies seen best in coronal, sagittal planes
  - 3D bone CT useful to characterize scoliosis and vertebral anomalies for preoperative planning

DIFFERENTIAL DIAGNOSIS

Vertebral Body Fracture

- Pathologic or traumatic
- 2 pedicles per level
- Noncorticated irregular fracture margins ± soft tissue edema, cord injury
- History helpful

Inherited Spinal Dysplasias

- Mucopolysaccharidosis
- Achondroplasia
- Distinguish by characteristic imaging and clinical and laboratory findings

PATHOLOGY

General Features

- Etiology
  - Total aplasia: Both chondral centers fail to develop early in development
  - Lateral hemivertebra: 1 chondral center does not develop; ossification center subsequently fails to develop on that side
  - Sagittal cleft (butterfly) vertebra: Separate ossification centers form (but fail to unite) in each paired paramedian chondrification center
  - Coronal cleft vertebra: Formation and persistence of separate ventral and dorsal ossification centers
  - Posterior hemivertebra: Later failure during ossification stage
- Genetics
  - Deranged *PAX1* gene expression in developing vertebral column
  - Many syndromes manifest vertebral dysplasia
- Associated abnormalities
  - Dysraphism, split notochord syndromes
    - Diastematomyelia, syrinx, tethered cord/fatty filum, congenital tumor, visceral organ anomalies
  - Other developmental vertebral abnormalities
    - Partial duplication (supernumerary hemivertebra)
    - Segmentation failure (block vertebra, posterior element dysraphism, pediculate bar, neural arch fusion)
  - Visceral abnormalities; 61% of congenital scoliosis patients
- Normal vertebral formation occurs over 3 sequential periods
  - Membrane development: Segmental formation of medial sclerotome (vertebral bodies) and lateral myotome (paraspinal muscles)

- Chondrification: Sclerotomes separate transversely and join with adjacent sclerotomal halves → paired chondrification sites develop in vertebral bodies and neural arches
- Ossification: Chondral skeleton ossifies from single ossification center
- Segmentation and fusion anomalies result from aberrant vertebral column formation
  - Abnormal vertebrae may be supranumerary or replace normal vertebral body
  - More severe SFA → higher likelihood of associated visceral anomalies
- Imaging appearance of vertebral formation failure determined by deficient vertebral body portion
  - Anterior formation failure (common) → sharply angulated kyphosis
  - Posterior formation failure (rare) → hyperlordotic curve
  - Lateral formation failure (common) → classic hemivertebrae of congenital scoliosis
- Hemivertebra variants subclassified as incarcerated, nonincarcerated, segmented, nonsegmented, or semisegmented
  - Incarcerated: Vertebral bodies above and below shaped to accommodate hemivertebrae → do not generally produce scoliosis
  - Nonincarcerated: Found at scoliosis apex, curve magnitude depends on size of wedged segment
  - Segmented ("free"): Normal discs above and below hemivertebra → progressive scoliosis due to unbalanced growth
  - Nonsegmented: Lack disc spaces between wedged, normal adjacent vertebral bodies
  - Semisegmented: Normal disc space on one side, nonsegmented on other side
- Segmental spinal dysgenesis (SSD): Rare congenital abnormality in which 1 segment of vertebral column/spinal cord fails to develop properly
  - Spinal cord thinned or indiscernible at abnormality level; bulky, low-lying cord segment caudad to focal abnormality in most cases
  - Severity of morphologic derangement correlates with residual spinal cord function, severity of clinical deficit

Gross Pathologic & Surgical Features

- Normal bone density unless concurrent metabolic abnormality
- Surgical observations of vertebral configuration matches imaging findings

Microscopic Features

- Normal bone histology unless concurrent metabolic abnormality

CLINICAL ISSUES

Presentation

- Most common signs/symptoms
  - Asymptomatic
  - Abnormal spine curvature ± neural deficits, limb or visceral abnormalities
- Other signs/symptoms
  - Respiratory failure (impeded chest movement 2° to fused ribs, kyphoscoliosis) → rare
- Clinical profile
  - Most are asymptomatic or detected during scoliosis evaluation
  - Syndromal patients usually detected in infancy

Demographics

- Age
  - Usually diagnosed in infancy → early childhood
  - Mild cases may present in adulthood
- Gender
  - M ~ F
- Epidemiology
  - Isolated or syndromal, singular or multiple
  - Incidence increased with parental consanguinity, concurrent multisystem anomalies

Natural History & Prognosis

- Scoliosis is frequently progressive
  - Expectant watching, early intervention if warranted to prevent development of severe deformities

Treatment

- Conservative in mild cases (orthotics, observation)
- Surgical resection &/or fusion to arrest/reverse kyphoscoliosis in moderate to severe cases

DIAGNOSTIC CHECKLIST

Consider

- Syndromal origin or association → important to look for and characterize visceral anomalies

Image Interpretation Pearls

- Look for concurrent segmentation failure, other neural and visceral anomalies
- Type of deformity determines propensity for scoliosis progression

SELECTED REFERENCES

1. Gupta N et al: Vertebral and intraspinal anomalies in Indian population with congenital scoliosis: a study of 119 consecutive patients. Asian Spine J. 10(2):276-81, 2016
2. Pegler JR et al: Clinical description of 41 Brazilian patients with oculo-auriculo-vertebral dysplasia. Rev Assoc Med Bras. 62(3):202-6, 2016
3. Vitković B et al: Airway management with direct laryngoscopy in a child with goldenhar syndrome. Acta Clin Croat. 55 Suppl 1:90-3, 2016
4. Fargen KM et al: Occipitocervicothoracic stabilization in pediatric patients. J Neurosurg Pediatr. 8(1):57-62, 2011
5. Martirosyan NL et al: Aplasia of the anterior arch of atlas associated with multiple congenital disorders: case report. Neurosurgery. 69(6):E1317-20, 2011
6. Winter RB et al: Scoliosis secondary to a hemivertebra: seven patients with gradual improvement without treatment. Spine (Phila Pa 1976). 35(2):E49-52, 2010
7. Noordeen MH et al: The surgical treatment of congenital kyphosis. Spine (Phila Pa 1976). 34(17):1808-14, 2009
8. Patinharayil G et al: Butterfly vertebra: an uncommon congenital spinal anomaly. Spine (Phila Pa 1976). 33(24):E926-8, 2008
9. Wax JR et al: Prenatal sonographic diagnosis of hemivertebrae: associations and outcomes. J Ultrasound Med. 27(7):1023-7, 2008
10. Fernandes T et al: Klippel-Feil syndrome with other associated anomalies in a medieval Portuguese skeleton (13th-15th century). J Anat. 211(5):681-5, 2007
11. Satpathy A et al: Compression fracture or butterfly vertebra: diagnostic importance in a trauma setting. Ann R Coll Surg Engl. 86(6):W41-3, 2004

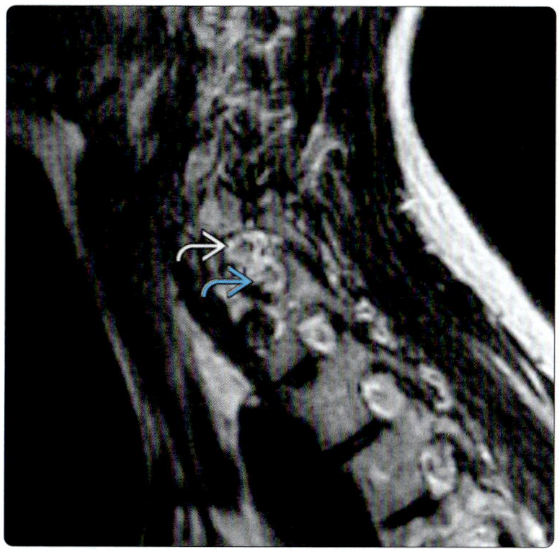
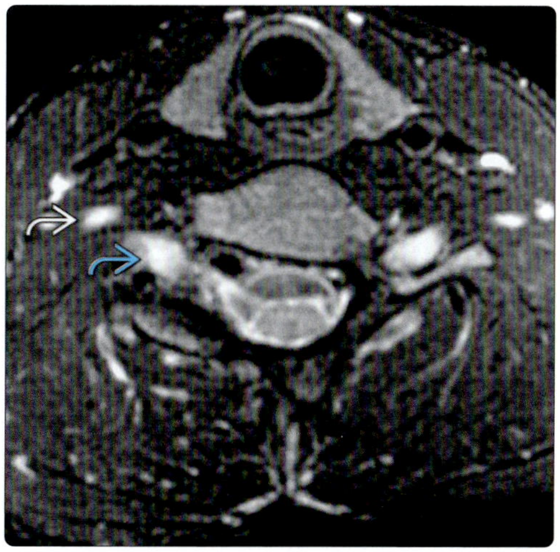

(Left) *Sagittal T2WI MR shows absence of the right C7 pedicle, resulting in an aberrant wide neural foramen containing both the C7 and C8 roots within the same abnormally large foramen that results from absence of the intervening pedicle.* **(Right)** *Axial T2WI FS MR demonstrates absence of the right C7 pedicle with an aberrant wide neural foramen. Both the C7 and C8 roots exit within the same aberrantly large foramen produced by the missing pedicle.*

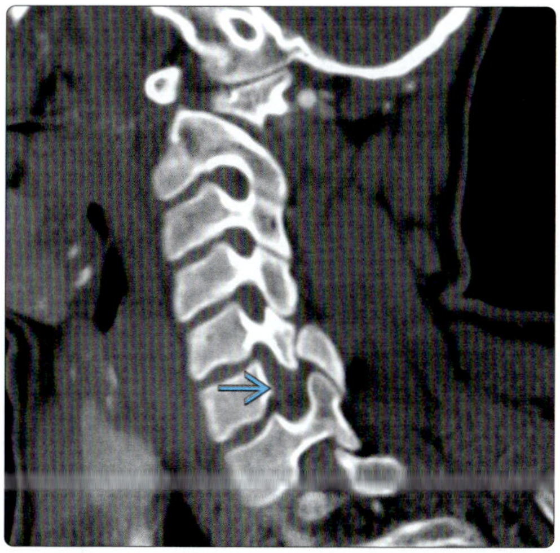
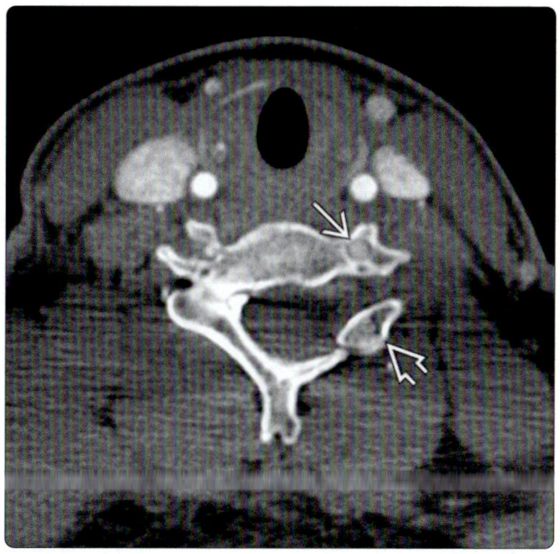

(Left) *Coronal oblique bone CT demonstrates congenital formation failure of the left C6 pedicle with abnormal left posterior arch and a hypoplastic facet. This constellation of anomalies results in formation of an abnormally large neural foramen.* **(Right)** *Axial bone CT reveals congenital failure of formation of the left C6 pedicle with abnormal formation of the left posterior arch and a hypoplastic facet. Note the normal course of the left vertebral artery.*

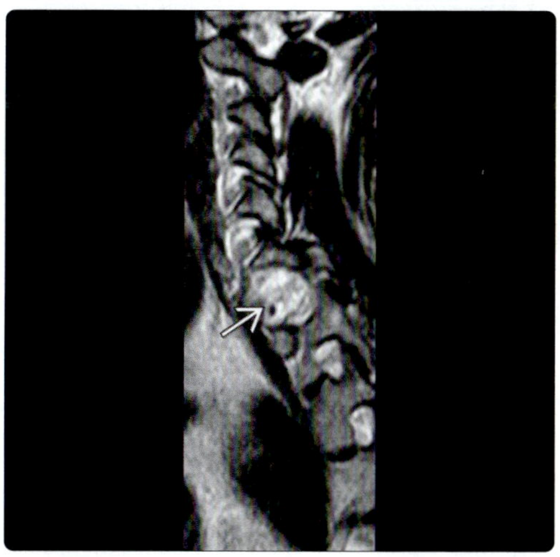
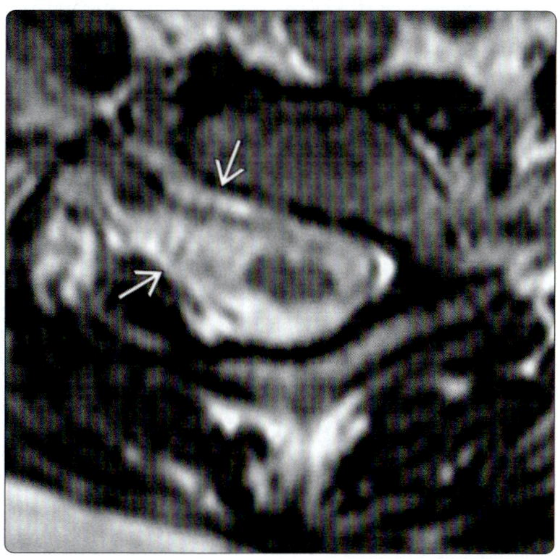

(Left) *Sagittal T2WI MR shows an enlarged right C6-7 neural foramen compared to the normal-sized foramina above and below this level. The right C6-7 foramen is more than 2x the size of the normal left foramen (not shown) at this level. Note that 2 nerves are exiting through the enlarged foramen.* **(Right)** *Axial T2WI MR shows an enlarged right C6-7 neural foramen containing, not just 1, but 2 nerves exiting through the enlarged foramen.*

Failure of Segmentation

KEY FACTS

TERMINOLOGY

- Segmentation anomaly, segmentation and fusion anomaly (SFA), block vertebra, disorganized spine

IMAGING

- Ranges from single level to extensive multilevel involvement
- Search for related fused pedicles, ribs, posterior elements
- ± scoliosis, kyphosis, cord compression

TOP DIFFERENTIAL DIAGNOSES

- Juvenile chronic arthritis
- Surgical vertebral fusion
- Chronic sequelae of discitis
- Ankylosing spondylitis

PATHOLOGY

- Deranged *PAX1* gene expression → abnormal notochord signaling in developing vertebral column
- Many syndromes associated with SFA
- Associations include other neuraxis anomalies, renal, gastrointestinal, congenital cardiac defects

CLINICAL ISSUES

- Usually asymptomatic or present with kyphoscoliosis
- Severe cases detected during infancy/childhood; mild cases may present as adults
- Less commonly neural deficit, limb or visceral anomalies, respiratory failure
- Scoliosis frequently progressive
- Abnormal segments may continue to fuse

DIAGNOSTIC CHECKLIST

- Clinical manifestations variable, determined by type of SFA and syndromal association
- Coronal MR, AP radiography best for detecting and characterizing SFAs, "counting" abnormal vertebral levels

(Left) *Sagittal bone CT depicts odontoid dysplasia and C2-C3 segmentation failure. Note also posterior position of the clivus tip relative to the odontoid tip, suggesting atlantooccipital instability (confirmed on flexion/extension radiographs, not shown).* **(Right)** *Coronal bone CT in a patient with Klippel-Feil syndrome (KFS) demonstrates asymmetric segmentation failure at C2-C3, more severe on the left than the right, resulting in mild congenital scoliosis.*

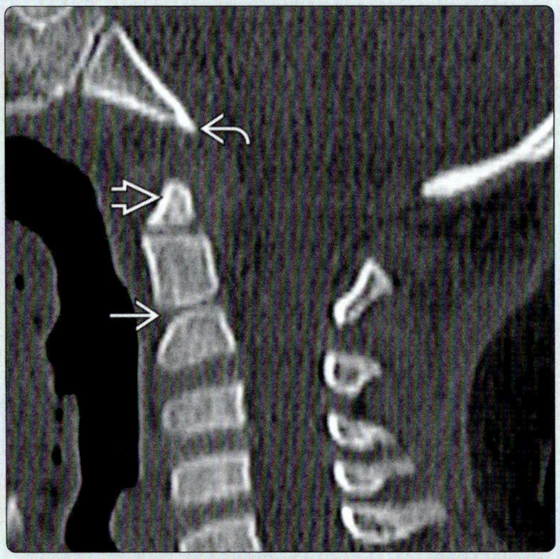

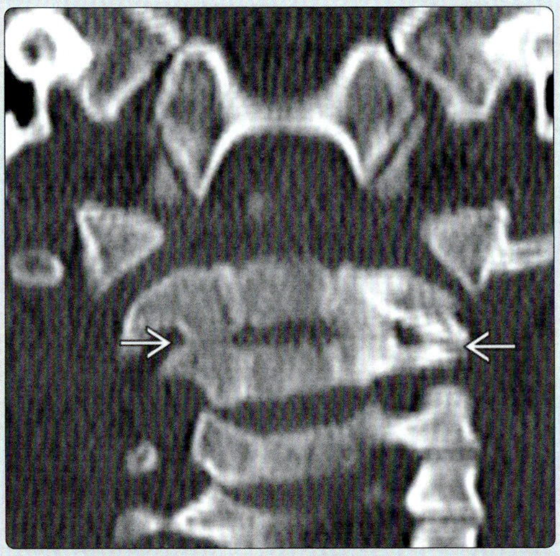

(Left) *Sagittal bone CT in a patient with severe KFS reveals extensive fusion at all cervical levels, as well as assimilation of C1 into the skull base. The narrow vertebra are typical of congenital segmentation failure.* **(Right)** *Coronal bone CT in a patient with severe KFS shows odontoid hypoplasia and fusion of the right occipital condyle, C1 lateral mass, and C2 lateral mass. The left C1 lateral mass is not incorporated into either the occipital condyle or C2 lateral mass.*

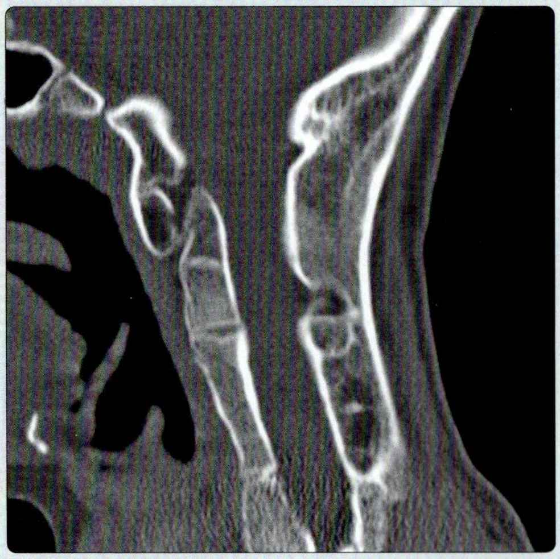

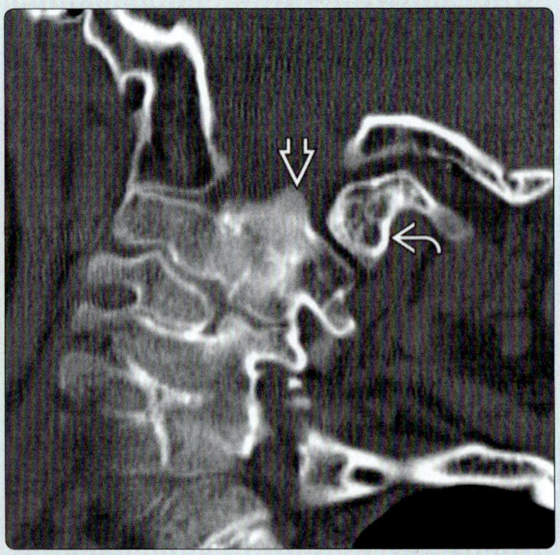

TERMINOLOGY

Synonyms

- Segmentation anomaly, segmentation and fusion anomaly (SFA), block vertebra, disorganized spine

Definitions

- Vertebral column malformations (block vertebra, neural arch fusion, pediculate bar) resulting from deranged embryological development → failure of normal segmentation

IMAGING

General Features

- Best diagnostic clue
  - Sharply angulated focal scoliotic curvature with abnormal fused vertebra
- Location
  - Lumbar > cervical > thoracic
- Size
  - Ranges from single level to extensive multilevel involvement
  - Block vertebra usually larger than 1 single normal vertebral body
- Morphology
  - Incomplete vertebral body segmentation, fused posterior elements, and large misshapen vertebral bodies incorporating 1 or more levels

Radiographic Findings

- Radiography
  - Deformed, fused vertebra ± scoliosis, kyphosis
  - Upright images with lateral and AP bending assess weightbearing effect on scoliosis

CT Findings

- Bone CT
  - Incomplete vertebral body segmentation
    - Large, misshapen vertebral bodies incorporating 1 or more levels
    - ± fused pedicles, ribs, posterior elements

MR Findings

- T1WI
  - Deformed, fused vertebral bodies and posterior elements
  - ± scoliosis
  - Normal marrow signal intensity
- T2WI
  - Findings similar to T1WI
  - ± scoliosis, cord compression

Imaging Recommendations

- Best imaging tool
  - Weightbearing plain radiographs to evaluate scoliosis, "count" abnormal vertebral levels
  - MR imaging
    - Multiplanar T1WI to evaluate vertebral anatomy
      - Vertebral anomalies seen best in coronal, sagittal planes
    - T2WI to evaluate spinal cord pathology, compression
  - 3D CT reformats to characterize osseous structures, preoperative planning

DIFFERENTIAL DIAGNOSIS

Juvenile Chronic Arthritis

- Difficult to distinguish from cervical block vertebra
- Search for other affected joints, appropriate clinical history

Surgical Fusion

- No "waist" at disc space level; facets infrequently ankylosed
- Surgical history key to making diagnosis

Chronic Sequelae of Discitis

- Cortical endplate margins irregular, "waist" absent
- Search for history of prior spinal infection

Ankylosing Spondylitis

- Delicate contiguous syndesmophytes ("bamboo spine") + symmetric SI joint disease
- HLA-B27 positive (95%)

PATHOLOGY

General Features

- Etiology
  - Segmentation and fusion anomalies result from aberrant vertebral column formation
  - Mildest (and most common) form is indeterminate (transitional) vertebrae at thoracolumbar, lumbosacral transition
- Genetics
  - Deranged *PAX1* gene expression → abnormal notochord signaling in developing vertebral column
  - Many syndromes associated with SFA
    - Klippel-Feil (cervical SFA): Common, gene locus 8q22.2
    - Spondylothoracic dysplasia (Jarcho-Levin): Uncommon, thoracic spine fusions in crab like array with multiple rib fusions
- Associated abnormalities
  - Other neuraxis anomalies (40%)
    - Dysraphism, split notochord syndrome
    - Partial or complete failure of formation (vertebral aplasia, hemivertebra, butterfly vertebra)
    - Partial duplication (supernumerary hemivertebra)
  - Scoliosis
  - Renal, gastrointestinal, congenital cardiac defects
- Normal embryology: Vertebral formation occurs over 3 sequential periods
  - Membrane development: Segmental formation of medial sclerotome (vertebral bodies) and lateral myotome (paraspinal muscles)
  - Chondrification: Sclerotomes separate transversely and join with adjacent sclerotomal halves → paired chondrification sites develop in vertebral bodies, neural arches
  - Ossification: Chondral skeleton ossifies from single ossification center

Staging, Grading, & Classification

- Block vertebra: Failure of ≥ 2 vertebral somites to segment
  - Combined vertebrae may be normal height, short, or tall
  - Disc space frequently rudimentary or absent

- Frequent association with hemivertebra/absent vertebra above or below block level, posterior element fusion
- Posterior neural arch anomalies
  - Failure to unite in midline → dysraphism (± unilateral pedicle aplasia/hypoplasia)
  - Unfused spinous processes; L5, S1 > C1 > C7 > T1 > lower thoracic spine
  - Multiple level posterior fusion → congenital vertebral bar

Gross Pathologic & Surgical Features

- Normal bone density unless concurrent metabolic abnormality
- Surgical observations of vertebral configuration matches imaging findings

Microscopic Features

- Normal bone histology unless concurrent metabolic abnormality

CLINICAL ISSUES

Presentation

- Most common signs/symptoms
  - Asymptomatic
  - Kyphoscoliosis
- Other signs/symptoms
  - Neural deficits (usually myelopathic), limb or visceral anomalies
  - Respiratory failure (rare, secondary to impeded chest movement due to severe scoliosis, rib cage fusion)
- Clinical profile
  - Asymptomatic incidental detection or presents for evaluation of abnormal spine curvature

Demographics

- Age
  - Severe cases detected during infancy/childhood; mild cases may present as adults
- Gender
  - M ~ F; dependent on syndromal association
- Epidemiology
  - Isolated or syndromal, singular or multiple
  - SFAs account for 18% of scoliosis; incidence higher with multisystem abnormalities, parental consanguinity

Natural History & Prognosis

- Scoliosis frequently progressive
  - Unilateral unsegmented bar with contralateral hemivertebrae → rapidly progressive, severely deforming congenital scoliosis
  - Isolated block vertebrae rarely produce scoliosis
- Abnormal segments may continue to fuse

Treatment

- Conservative in mild cases (orthotics, observation)
- Surgical fusion to arrest/reverse kyphoscoliosis in moderate to severe cases

DIAGNOSTIC CHECKLIST

Consider

- Clinical manifestations variable, determined by type of SFA and syndromal association

Image Interpretation Pearls

- Coronal MR, AP radiography best for detecting and characterizing SFAs, "counting" abnormal vertebral levels

SELECTED REFERENCES

1. Chang DG et al: Congenital kyphoscoliosis in monozygotic twins: ten-year follow-up treated by posterior vertebral column resection (PVCR): a case report. Medicine (Baltimore). 95(17):e3499, 2016
2. Gupta N et al: Vertebral and intraspinal anomalies in Indian population with congenital scoliosis: a study of 119 consecutive patients. Asian Spine J. 10(2):276-81, 2016
3. Ghiţă RA et al: Burnei-Gavriliu classification of congenital scoliosis. J Med Life. 8(2):239-44, 2015
4. Al Kaissi A et al: Distinctive spine abnormalities in patients with Goldenhar syndrome: tomographic assessment. Eur Spine J. Epub, 2014
5. McMaster MJ et al: Prognosis for congenital scoliosis due to a unilateral failure of vertebral segmentation. J Bone Joint Surg Am. 95(11):972-9, 2013
6. Salunke P et al: Complete segmentation failure causing non-dysjunction of os odontoideum and hypertrophic C1 arch: a case report. Clin Neurol Neurosurg. 115(7):1128-30, 2013
7. Menezes AH: Craniocervical fusions in children. J Neurosurg Pediatr. 9(6):573-85, 2012
8. Giussani C et al: Severely symptomatic craniovertebral junction abnormalities in children: long-term reliability of aggressive management. Pediatr Neurosurg. 45(1):29-36, 2009
9. Kawakami N et al: Classification of congenital scoliosis and kyphosis: a new approach to the three-dimensional classification for progressive vertebral anomalies requiring operative treatment. Spine (Phila Pa 1976). 34(17):1756-65, 2009
10. Menezes AH et al: Remnants of occipital vertebrae: proatlas segmentation abnormalities. Neurosurgery. 64(5):945-53; discussion 954, 2009
11. Menezes AH: Craniocervical developmental anatomy and its implications. Childs Nerv Syst. 24(10):1109-22, 2008
12. Tsirikos AI et al: Congenital anomalies of the ribs and chest wall associated with congenital deformities of the spine. J Bone Joint Surg Am. 87(11):2523-36, 2005
13. Arlet V et al: Congenital scoliosis. Eur Spine J. 12(5):456-63, 2003
14. Cornier AS et al: Controversies surrounding Jarcho-Levin syndrome. Curr Opin Pediatr. 15(6):614-20, 2003
15. Isono M et al: Limited dorsal myeloschisis associated with multiple vertebral segmentation disorder. Pediatr Neurosurg. 36(1):44-7, 2002
16. Kim YJ et al: Surgical treatment of congenital kyphosis. Spine. 26(20):2251-7, 2001
17. Nagashima H et al: No neurological involvement for more than 40 years in Klippel-Feil syndrome with severe hypermobility of the upper cervical spine. Arch Orthop Trauma Surg. 121(1-2):99-101, 2001
18. Suh SW et al: Evaluating congenital spine deformities for intraspinal anomalies with magnetic resonance imaging. J Pediatr Orthop. 21(4):525-31, 2001
19. Jaskwhich D et al: Congenital scoliosis. Curr Opin Pediatr. 12(1):61-6, 2000
20. Yildiran A et al: Semantic and nosological confusions on multiple vertebral segmentation defects. Pediatr Neurosurg. 33(3):168, 2000
21. McMaster MJ et al: Natural history of congenital kyphosis and kyphoscoliosis. A study of one hundred and twelve patients. J Bone Joint Surg Am. 81(10):1367-83, 1999
22. McMaster MJ: Congenital scoliosis caused by a unilateral failure of vertebral segmentation with contralateral hemivertebrae. Spine. 23(9):998-1005, 1998
23. Aslan Y et al: Multiple vertebral segmentation defects. Brief report of three patients and nosological considerations. Genet Couns. 8(3):241-8, 1997
24. Lopez BC et al: Inadequate PAX-1 gene expression as a cause of agenesis of the thoracolumbar spine with failure of segmentation. Case report. J Neurosurg. 86(6):1018-21, 1997
25. Mortier GR et al: Multiple vertebral segmentation defects: analysis of 26 new patients and review of the literature. Am J Med Genet. 61(4):310-9, 1996

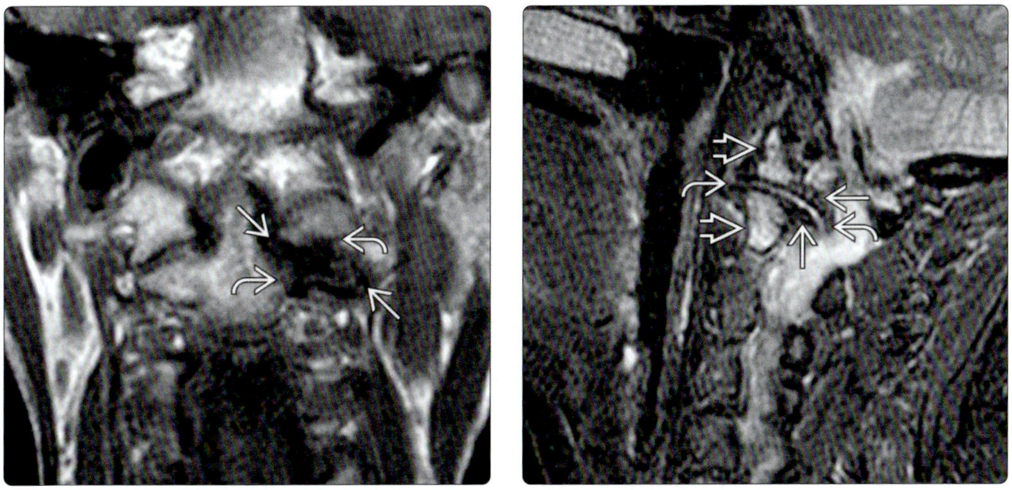

(Left) *Lateral atlantoaxial OA is easily appreciated on this coronal T1WI MR. The joint is narrowing and appears elongated secondary to osteophytes. Extensive subchondral low signal is present along both sides of the joint.* **(Right)** *Sagittal T2WI MR demonstrates advanced OA of the lateral atlantoaxial joint. The joint space is narrowed. Osteophytes are present at the joint margins, and extensive edematous-like signal is present mixed with subchondral foci of low signal.*

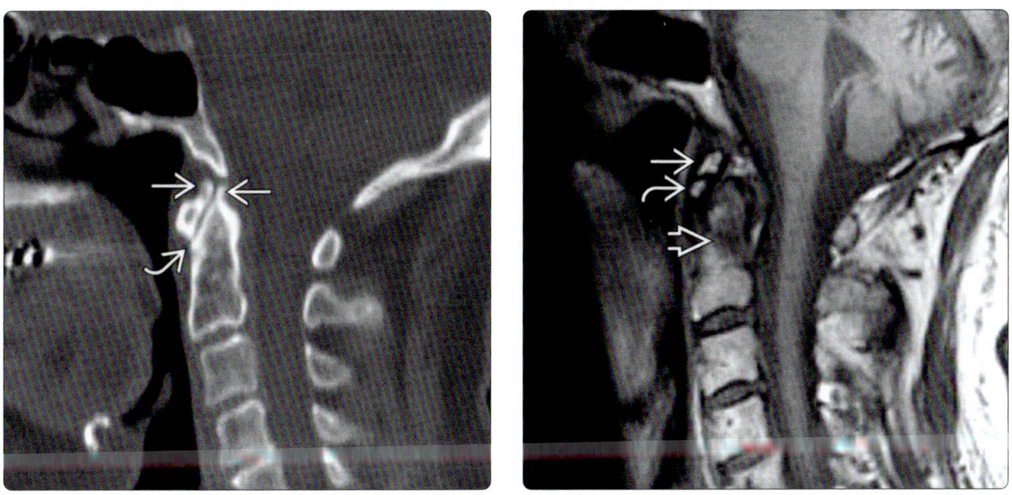

(Left) *On this sagittal reformat bone CT, narrowing of the atlantodental interval is present, accompanied by osteophyte formation superiorly. The lack of mineralization and the presence of osteophytes help exclude CPPD as the etiology.* **(Right)** *Sagittal T1WI MR in the midline shows a large osseous structure superior the the body of C1. The structure is a large osteophyte at the margin of the midline articulation. The extensive low signal within the dens is atypical.*

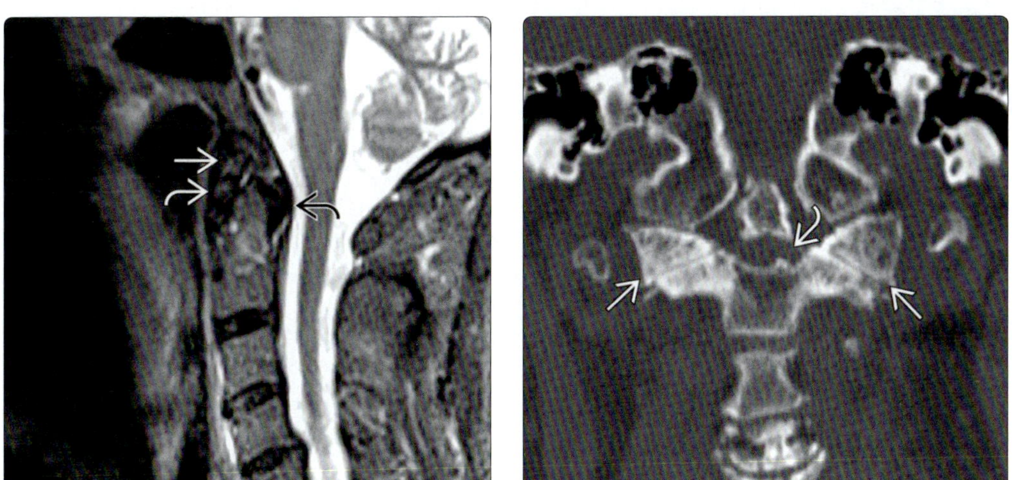

(Left) *On this sagittal T2WI MR, the body of C1 and the osteophyte are difficult to appreciate. What can be appreciated is the thickening of the transverse ligament & synovial hypertrophy, creating slight mass effect.* **(Right)** *Coronal reformat bone CT shows bilateral, symmetric OA of the lateral joints, which is uncommon. In this case, it is likely due to excessive motion from the nonunited dens fracture. The occipitocervical articulations also have mild osteoarthritic changes.*

Ossification of Posterior Longitudinal Ligament

KEY FACTS

IMAGING

- Ossification along posterior surface of vertebra, which may be contiguous over several levels
- At craniovertebral junction: Stalagmite-type extension posterior to C2 from ossification at C3
- Characteristic upside-down T or bowtie posterior longitudinal ligament (PLL) configuration on axial images
- Shows ossification to be midline or laterally deviated
- MR: T1WI and T2WI
  - Mainly low signal ± central fat signal if marrow present

TOP DIFFERENTIAL DIAGNOSES

- Spondylosis
- Calcified herniated disc
- Meningioma
- Cervical peridural calcification of hemodialysis

PATHOLOGY

- Ranges from lamellar bone with no marrow elements to woven bone with marrow elements
- Associated conditions: Ossification in transverse ligament, diffuse idiopathic skeletal hyperostosis, ankylosing spondylitis, ossification of ligamentum flavum

CLINICAL ISSUES

- Radiculopathy (40%), myelopathy (34%), stiffness and axial neck pain (18.5%), asymptomatic (7%)
- M:F = 2:1
- Age: Usually > 50 years; rarely < 30 years
- Patients with mild ossification of PLL at diagnosis rarely present with severe canal stenosis on follow-up
- Asymptomatic patients: Nonoperative management
- Symptomatic or high-grade stenosis patients: Decompression

(Left) *Sagittal graphic shows flowing multilevel ossification within the posterior longitudinal ligament (PLL) producing canal narrowing, cord compression.* **(Right)** *On this lateral radiograph, a thick band of increased density is easily seen posterior to C2. It is more difficult to detect below C2, where it is more often present.*

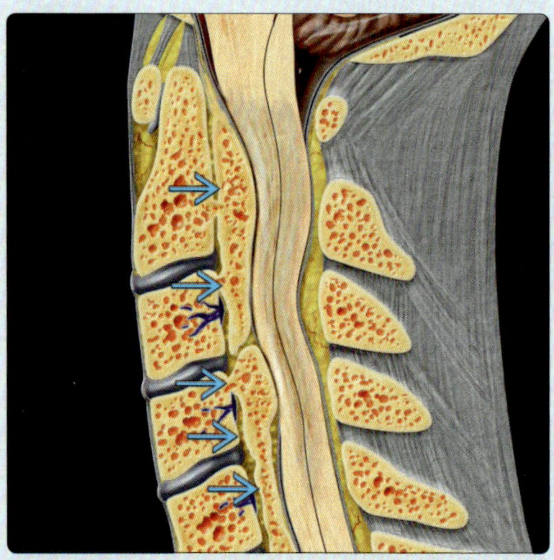

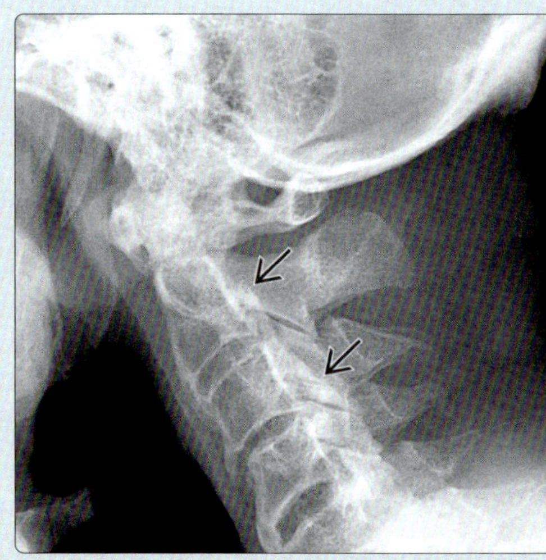

(Left) *On this sagittal bone CT, stalagmite appearance of OPLL posterior to C2 is seen. The ossification extends cephalad from the midcervical spine. Note the separation between the ossification and the posterior cortex of C2. The ossification is closer to the vertebral cortex more inferiorly.* **(Right)** *Sagittal T2WI MR demonstrates bulky PLL ossification with diffuse low-signal intensity. The ossification has created severe central canal stenosis and cord compression. Foci of high signal within the cord indicate cord injury.*

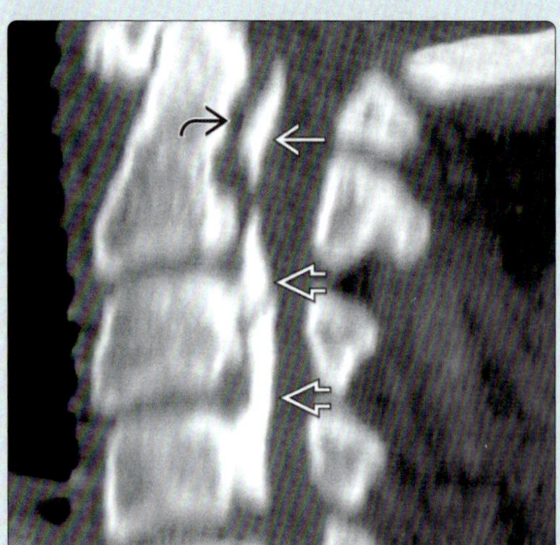

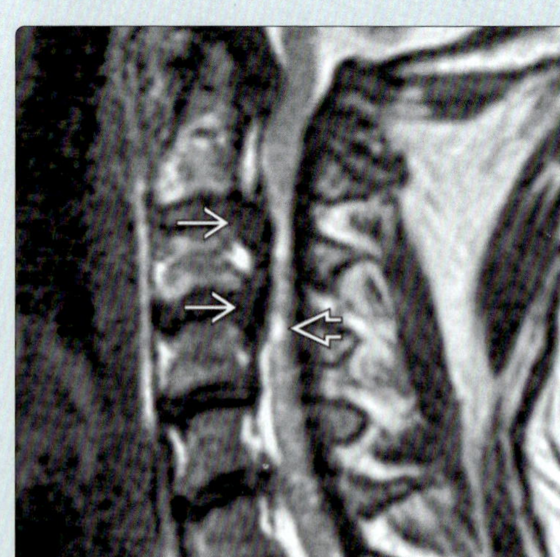

TERMINOLOGY

Abbreviations

- Ossification of posterior longitudinal ligament (OPLL)

IMAGING

General Features

- Best diagnostic clue
  - Ossification along posterior surface of vertebra, which may be contiguous over several levels
- Location
  - Upper cervical spine posterior to C2 vertebra
    - Typically, midcervical > midthoracic
- Size
  - ~ 2- to 5-mm thick
- Morphology
  - Stalagmite-type extension posterior to C2 from ossification at C3 and lower

Radiographic Findings

- Radiography
  - Thick band of increased density posterior to C2
    - Unlike lower levels, not always intimately related to posterior vertebral cortex
    - PLL transitions to tectorial membrane without contacting posterior C2

Fluoroscopic Findings

- Flexion/extension imaging determines dynamic range

CT Findings

- NECT
  - More sensitive than radiography
  - Characteristic upside-down T or bowtie PLL configuration on axial images
  - Shows ossification to be midline or laterally deviated
- Bone CT
  - Similar to NECT findings: Better defines architecture
    - Cortical bone ± central marrow space
    - May appear contiguous with adjacent vertebral cortex or distinct from posterior vertebral body
    - PLL and vertebral marrow spaces are not contiguous

MR Findings

- T1WI
  - Same morphology as on CT
  - Typically low signal; may have central high signal intensity if marrow is present
- T2WI
  - Mainly low signal ± central fat signal if marrow is present
  - ± cord hyperintensity due to myelomalacia or edema
- T2* GRE
  - Hypointense signal intensity within PLL ossification
  - Caveat: Exaggerates severity of stenosis due to magnetic susceptibility effects

Nonvascular Interventions

- Myelography
  - Ossification visible; may compress spinal cord

Imaging Recommendations

- Best imaging tool
  - Multiplanar MR to evaluate status of spinal cord
  - CT is best to assess degree of canal stenosis
- Protocol advice
  - Sagittal T1WI and T2WI to evaluate spinal cord compression and extent of ligamentous ossification
  - Axial T2WI to determine stenosis severity, confirm cord signal abnormality

DIFFERENTIAL DIAGNOSIS

Spondylosis

- Usually centered at disc interspace
  - Rarely contiguous across 4 or more vertebral levels
- More substantial facet, disc degenerative changes

Calcified Herniated Disc

- Focal calcified "mass" posterior to single disc space

Meningioma

- Avidly enhancing dural-based mass + dural "tail"
- Low T2WI signal is secondary to calcification
  - Lacks marrow elements

Cervical Peridural Calcification of Hemodialysis

- Curvilinear dural calcification; may be circumferential

PATHOLOGY

General Features

- Etiology
  - Not conclusively determined
  - Postulated etiologies include genetic conditions, infectious agents, autoimmune disorders, trauma
- Genetics
  - Polymorphisms of chromosome 6 gene (*COL11A2*) → abnormal α chain of type XI collagen → OPLL susceptibility
  - Polymorphisms of collagen 6A1 gene (*COL6A1*) → abnormal α chain of type VI collagen → OPLL susceptibility
- Associated abnormalities
  - 12% of patients with OPLL have ossification in transverse ligament
  - Diffuse idiopathic skeletal hyperostosis is seen in 25% of patients with OPLL
  - OPLL is present in 16% of ankylosing spondylitis cases in Mexico and 23% in Canada
  - OPLL is present in 16-20% of cases of ossification of ligamentum flavum
  - Recently described early-stage "OPLL in evolution" is noted in both Asian and Caucasian populations
    - Hypertrophied PLL with punctate calcifications rather than smooth ossific mass
    - Difficult to distinguish from more common spondylosis at this early stage
  - OPLL patients have higher bone mineral density than age-matched controls
    - Possible predisposition for ↑ bone deposition

Staging, Grading, & Classification

- Established by Investigation Committee on OPLL from Japanese Ministry of Public Health and Welfare
  - Continuous (27%)

- Ossified mass over several vertebral segments
  - Segmental (39%)
    - Noncontiguous (fragmented) ossified lesions behind multiple vertebral bodies
  - Mixed (26%)
    - Combination of continuous and segmental
  - Local or other (8%)
    - Ossification confined to disc level

Gross Pathologic & Surgical Features

- Bulky ossification in ventral epidural space
- OPLL may transgress dura

Microscopic Features

- Ranges from lamellar bone with no marrow elements to woven bone with marrow elements
- Forms primarily via enchondral ossification with some membranous ossification

CLINICAL ISSUES

Presentation

- Most common signs/symptoms
  - Radiculopathy (40%), myelopathy (34%), stiffness and axial neck pain (18.5%), asymptomatic (7%)
  - Symptomatic myelopathy almost universal if canal diameter < 6 mm; rare if > 14 mm
  - Canal diameter: 6- to 14-mm variable presentation
  - Increased myelopathy with lateral deviated pattern
  - Upper extremity symptoms precede lower extremity
- Other signs/symptoms
  - Incidental observation in asymptomatic patient
    - Low rate of subsequent development of symptoms
    - Absent symptoms with significant ossification attributed to slow growth of ossification
    - May have up to 60% canal compromise without neurologic symptoms
- Clinical profile
  - Classic presentation is Japanese patient with progressive quadriparesis or paraparesis

Demographics

- Age
  - Usually > 50 years; rarely < 30 years
- Gender
  - M:F = 2:1
- Ethnicity
  - ↑ prevalence in Asian population
- Epidemiology
  - 2-4% prevalence in Japan; rarer elsewhere

Natural History & Prognosis

- 5% of patients have rapid progression of symptoms
- 11% of patients have chronic symptoms
- Factors associated with progression
  - Younger age at presentation, continuous type, myelopathy
- Continuous type has least associated myelopathy
- Increased mobility stimulates growth
  - More growth at disc level than behind vertebral body
- Mild trauma may exacerbate myelopathy
- Patients with mild OPLL at diagnosis rarely present with severe canal stenosis on follow-up
- May see radiographic progression without development of symptoms
- Growth: 1.5 mm/year

Treatment

- Asymptomatic patients: Careful observation, nonoperative management
- Symptomatic or high-grade stenosis patients: Decompression
- Prophylactic surgery in asymptomatic patients proposed but controversial

DIAGNOSTIC CHECKLIST

Image Interpretation Pearls

- T shape is highly suggestive of this diagnosis
- Overly "thick," hypointense PLL on MR is strongly suggestive of OPLL

SELECTED REFERENCES

1. Chen LF et al: Risk of spinal cord injury in patients with cervical spondylotic myelopathy and ossification of posterior longitudinal ligament: a national cohort study. Neurosurg Focus. 40(6):E4, 2016
2. Chen Y et al: Roles of the Endoplasmic Reticulum Stress Transducer OASIS in Ossification of the Posterior Longitudinal Ligament. Clin Spine Surg. ePub, 2016
3. Fujimori T et al: Prevalence, Concomitance, and Distribution of Ossification of the Spinal Ligaments: Results of Whole Spine CT Scans in 1500 Japanese Patients. Spine (Phila Pa 1976). ePub, 2016
4. Ito K et al: MRI Signal Intensity Classification in Cervical Ossification of the Posterior Longitudinal Ligament -Predictor Of Surgical Outcomes. Spine (Phila Pa 1976). ePub, 2016
5. Kawaguchi Y et al: Characteristics of ossification of the spinal ligament; incidence of ossification of the ligamentum flavum in patients with cervical ossification of the posterior longitudinal ligament - Analysis of the whole spine using multidetector CT. J Orthop Sci. ePub, 2016
6. Tauchi R et al: Cervical Myeloradiculopathy due to Ossification of the Posterior Longitudinal Ligament with versus without Diffuse Idiopathic Spinal Hyperostosis. Global Spine J. 6(4):350-6, 2016
7. Fujimori T et al: Three-dimensional measurement of intervertebral range of motion in ossification of the posterior longitudinal ligament: are there mobile segments in the continuous type? J Neurosurg Spine. 17(1):74-81, 2012
8. Jeon TS et al: Analysis of demographics, clinical, and radiographical findings of ossification of posterior longitudinal ligament of the cervical spine in 146 Korean patients. Spine (Phila Pa 1976). 37(24):E1498-503, 2012
9. Matsunaga S et al: Ossification of the posterior longitudinal ligament of the cervical spine: etiology and natural history. Spine (Phila Pa 1976). 37(5):E309-14, 2012
10. Wu JC et al: Conservatively treated ossification of the posterior longitudinal ligament increases the risk of spinal cord injury: a nationwide cohort study. J Neurotrauma. 29(3):462-8, 2012
11. Matsunaga S et al: Radiographic predictors for the development of myelopathy in patients with ossification of the posterior longitudinal ligament: a multicenter cohort study. Spine (Phila Pa 1976). 33(24):2648-50, 2008
12. Inamasu J et al: Ossification of the posterior longitudinal ligament: an update on its biology, epidemiology, and natural history. Neurosurgery. 58(6):1027-39; discussion 1027-39, 2006
13. Matsunaga S et al: Clinical course of patients with ossification of the posterior longitudinal ligament: a minimum 10-year cohort study. J Neurosurg. 100(3 Suppl):245-8, 2004
14. Shiraishi T et al: Cervical peridural calcification in patients undergoing long-term hemodialysis. Report of two cases. 100(3 Suppl): 284-6, 2004
15. Epstein N: Diagnosis and surgical management of cervical ossification of the posterior longitudinal ligament. Spine J. 2(6):436-49, 2002
16. Epstein NE: Identification of ossification of the posterior longitudinal ligament extending through the dura on preoperative computed tomographic examinations of the cervical spine. Spine. 26(2):182-6, 2001

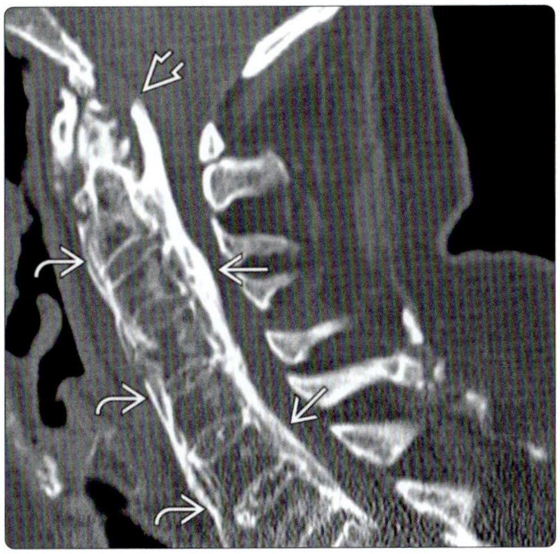

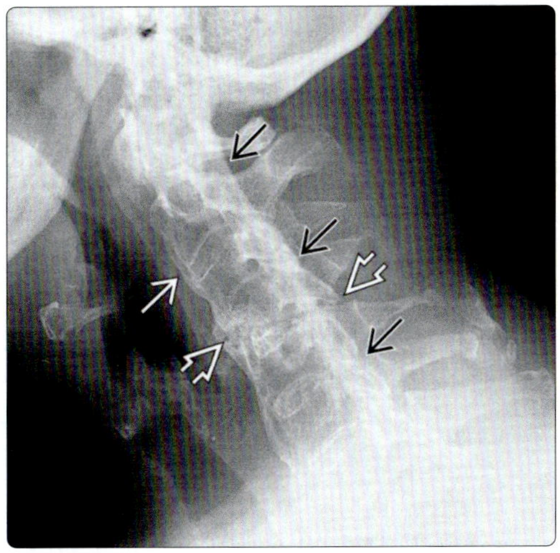

(Left) *Sagittal bone CT shows extensive continuous OPLL. Superiorly, the ossification follows the course of the tectorial membrane. Also noted is concurrent anterior ossification from severe ankylosing spondylitis. The spine is at high risk for pseudoarthrosis following trauma.* **(Right)** *Lateral radiograph shows a patient with both OPLL and anterior ossification due to diffuse idiopathic skeletal hyperostosis. Pseudoarthrosis is present, resulting from previous trauma.*

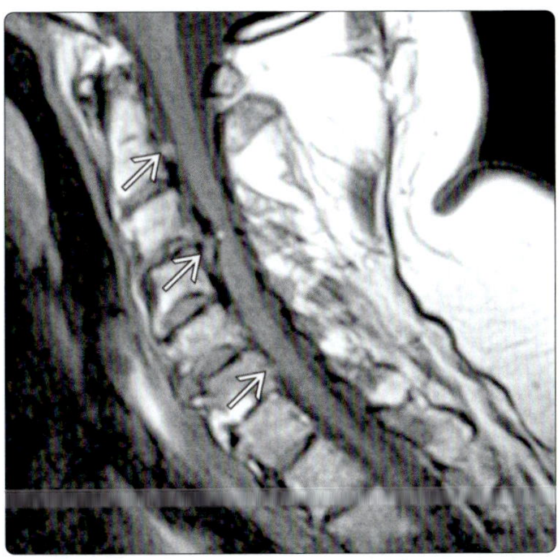

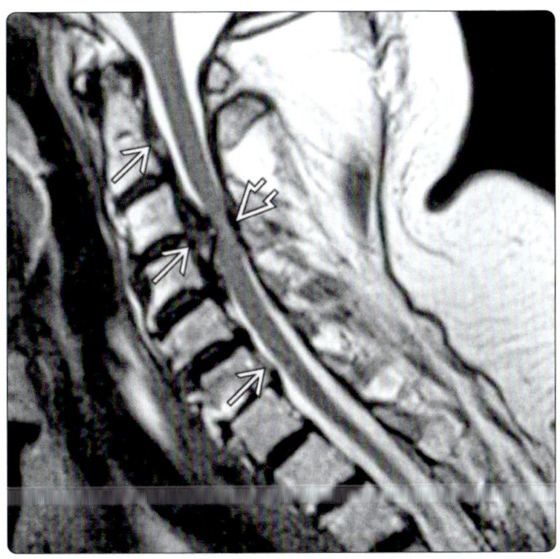

(Left) *Findings of segmental OPLL are evident on this sagittal T1WI MR. Foci of thickened OPLL with marrow signal are seen posterior to the upper and lower levels and behind the disc space at the middle level.* **(Right)** *On this sagittal T2WI MR in the same patient, segmental OPLL is of varying sizes and produces significant cord compression at the middle level. As seen here, the ossification is not always uniform in size. This state may represent an earlier stage of the process.*

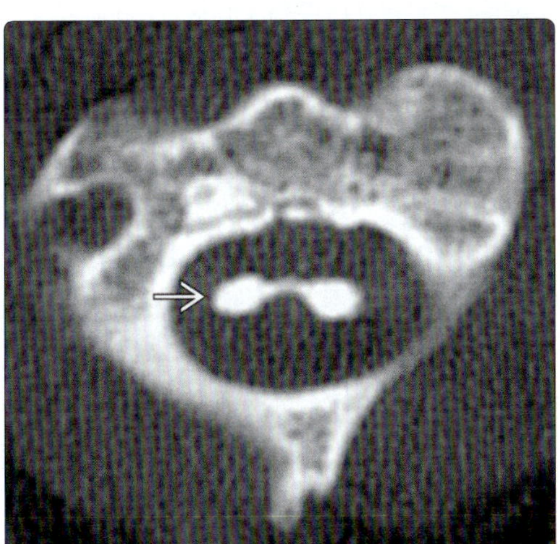

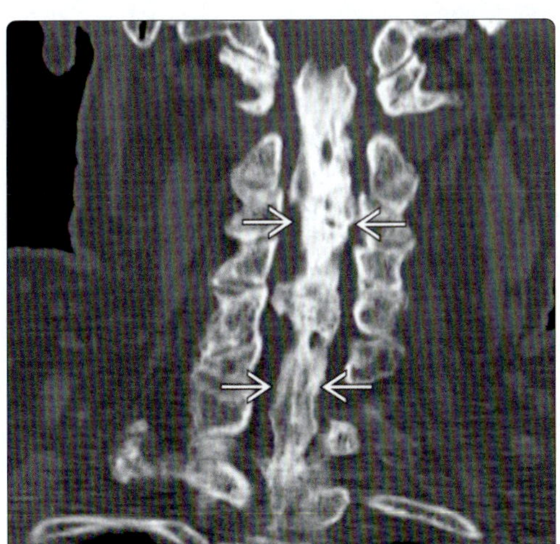

(Left) *Axial bone CT shows classic appearance of OPLL at the craniovertebral junction. Findings include the bowtie shape and the separation from the posterior cortex of C2. Significant canal narrowing is present. At this level, there is a solid appearance of the ossification without evidence of medullary bone (marrow).* **(Right)** *Coronal bone CT presents a unique perspective of OPLL. A large ossified "bar" is present posterior to the vertebral bodies. It has irregular margins and is of varying width.*

Diffuse Idiopathic Skeletal Hyperostosis

KEY FACTS

IMAGING

- Ossification: Thoracic > cervical, lumbar spine
- Primary changes: Flowing anterior vertebral ossification with relatively normal intervertebral discs and facet joints
- Secondary changes: Atlantoaxial subluxation, odontoid fracture
- Other: Ossification of posterior longitudinal ligament (OPLL) may extend up to cervical vertebral joint (CVJ)
- Spinal cord compression if pseudotumor, ligamentous hypertrophy, or OPLL
  - Pseudotumor posterior to odontoid process
  - Hypertrophy of transverse ligament and ligamentum flava

TOP DIFFERENTIAL DIAGNOSES

- Spondylosis
- Ankylosing spondylitis
- Psoriatic or reactive (Reiter) arthritis

PATHOLOGY

- Upper cervical changes result of excessive stress due to immobility of lower cervical spine
- ↓ spine mobility secondary to ALL ossification
  - Relative protection from degenerative disc disease and facet arthropathy
  - Increased fracture risk subsequent pseudoarthrosis
- Dysphagia secondary to diffuse idiopathic skeletal hyperostosis probably multifactorial

CLINICAL ISSUES

- Usually incidental observation
- Most common symptom: Painful stiffness related to disease beyond CVJ
- CVJ disease: Myelopathy
- Cervical spine: Dysphagia and airway obstruction
- Middle-aged and older adults
- M:F = 2:1
- Symptomatic CVJ changes require intervention

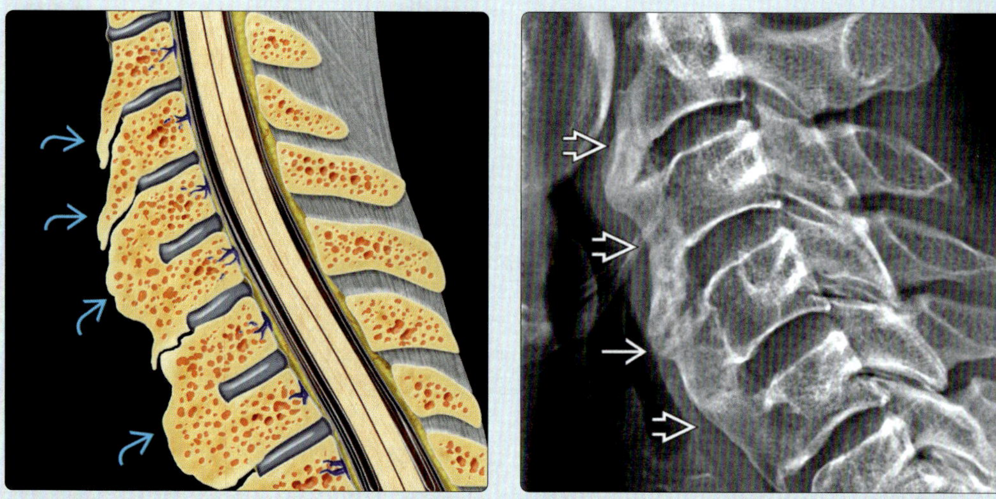

(Left) *Sagittal graphic shows bulky flowing ossification of the anterior longitudinal ligament ⇨ extending over more than 4 contiguous vertebra. Disc spaces are relatively preserved.* **(Right)** *Lateral radiograph shows bulky anterior longitudinal ligament ossification bridging C2 through C5 vertebra ⇨. This ossification severely limits motion. A cleft in the ossification at C3-C4 ⇨ allows limited extension but no flexion at this level.*

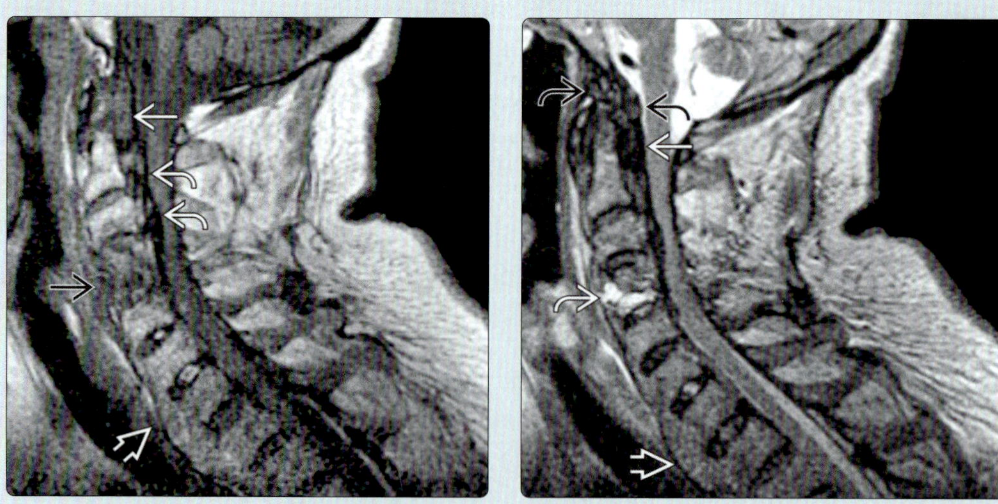

(Left) *Sagittal T1WI MR shows multiple findings of diffuse idiopathic skeletal hyperostosis (DISH), including pseudotumor ⇨, OPLL ⇨, pseudoarthrosis ⇨, and multilevel bridging ALL ossification ⇨. Note normal marrow signal within that ossification.* **(Right)** *Sagittal T2WI MR in the same patient shows multiple ossicles ⇨ from associated osteoarthrosis of C1-C2. Pseudotumor ⇨ has typical ↓ signal, and pseudoarthrosis has ↑ signal ⇨. ALL ossification marrow ⇨ appears contiguous with vertebral marrow, but it is not.*

Diffuse Idiopathic Skeletal Hyperostosis

TERMINOLOGY

Abbreviations

- Diffuse idiopathic skeletal hyperostosis (DISH)

Synonyms

- Forestier disease, senile ankylosing hyperostosis, asymmetrical skeletal hyperostosis

IMAGING

General Features

- Best diagnostic clue
  - Flowing anterior vertebral ossification with relatively normal intervertebral discs and facet joints
- Location
  - Ossification: Thoracic spine (100%) > cervical (65-80%), lumbar spine (68-90%)
    - Cervical spine, typically C4-C7
    - Favors right side: Attributed to aortic pulsations limiting ossification on left
- Size
  - Ossification ranges from small and focal to large and extensive
- Morphology
  - Ossification's greatest point of vertebral body contact
    - Midanterior cortex at attachment site of anterior longitudinal ligament (ALL)
    - Early disease spares anterosuperior and anteroinferior corners
      - Differentiates from syndesmophytes

Radiographic Findings

- Radiography
  - Primary changes
    - Flowing anterior vertebral body ossification
    - Relative preservation of disc spaces, facet joints
    - Earliest sign: New bone formation in midvertebral body
  - Secondary changes
    - Atlantoaxial subluxation
    - Odontoid fracture
  - Other: Ossification of posterior longitudinal ligament (OPLL) may extend up to craniovertebral junction (CVJ)

Fluoroscopic Findings

- Lateral flexion/extension imaging assesses dynamic spinal mobility

CT Findings

- Bone CT
  - ALL ossification, preservation of disc spaces, facet joints
  - OPLL may extend to CVJ, may compress spinal cord
  - Odontoid fracture

MR Findings

- T1WI
  - Flowing ALL ossification along anterior vertebral cortex
    - Hypointense if calcification and not ossification
    - Isointense to hyperintense if marrow is present
    - Marrow not contiguous with vertebral marrow
  - Pseudotumor posterior to odontoid process
  - Hypertrophy of transverse ligament and ligamentum flava
- T2WI
  - Similar findings to T1WI; ALL ossification may be hypointense unless substantial fatty marrow content
- T1WI C+
  - ± minimal enhancement (similar to vertebral marrow)

Nonvascular Interventions

- Myelography
  - Similar osseous findings to plain radiography
  - Spinal cord compression if pseudotumor, ligamentous hypertrophy, or OPLL

Imaging Recommendations

- Best imaging tool
  - Lateral radiography is inexpensive and reliable for detecting primary findings of DISH
  - CT and MR are better in detecting secondary changes at CVJ
- Protocol advice
  - Flexion/extension radiographs detect atlantoaxial instability
  - MR indicated if myelopathic changes are present
  - Bone CT helps confirm OPLL
  - Sagittal and axial planes are most advantageous

DIFFERENTIAL DIAGNOSIS

Spondylosis

- Rarely contiguous across ≥ 4 vertebral levels; usually confined to disc interspace vicinity
- More substantial facet, disc degenerative changes
- No predisposition to right or left side

Ankylosing Spondylitis

- Thin, intervertebral syndesmophytes
  - Arise from anterior vertebral corners
- Symmetric sacroiliac joint facet erosion/ankylosis
- Appropriate clinical history; HLA-B27 ≥ 90%

Psoriatic or Reactive (Reiter) Arthritis

- Large, bulky osteophytes; often lateral with skip areas
- Asymmetric sacroiliitis, erosive arthritis of hands and feet

PATHOLOGY

General Features

- Etiology
  - Ligamentous ossification is unknown
    - Associations postulated, not definitively proven
      - Diabetes mellitus, dyslipidemia, hyperuricemia alcohol intake, poor dietary habits
  - Upper cervical changes result of excessive stress due to immobility of lower cervical spine
- Associated abnormalities
  - OPLL
  - Exuberant entheseal reaction at tendon, ligament, and joint capsule insertions
    - Iliac crest (66%), ischial tuberosities (53%); appears as "pelvic whiskering"
    - Lesser (42%) and greater (36%) femoral trochanters, patellar quadriceps insertion (29%)

- Osseous bridging of fibula → tibia (10%)
- Distal metacarpal, phalangeal periarticular capsular hyperostosis (13%)
- ↓ spine mobility secondary to ALL ossification
  - Relative protection from degenerative disc disease and facet arthropathy
  - Increases fracture risk subsequent pseudoarthrosis
- Dysphagia secondary to DISH is probably multifactorial
  - Combination of direct mechanical compression and inflammation/fibrosis of esophageal wall, esophageal denervation

Staging, Grading, & Classification

- Strict diagnostic criteria: Flowing anterior ossification extending over at least 4 contiguous vertebral bodies
  - Minimal degenerative disc changes, no facet ankylosis

Gross Pathologic & Surgical Features

- Bulky anterior vertebral ossification with normal cortical bone, marrow appearance

Microscopic Features

- Normal-appearing haversian bone and marrow within ossified ligament

CLINICAL ISSUES

Presentation

- Most common signs/symptoms
  - Painful stiffness related to disease beyond CVJ
    - Often worse in morning, after prolonged sitting, or during cold winter weather
    - May be relieved by mild activity
  - Pain related to associated enthesitis, tendinitis
- Other signs/symptoms
  - CVJ disease: Myelopathy
  - Cervical spine: Dysphagia and airway obstruction
    - May have relatively acute onset
    - Stridor (extremely rare) requiring tracheostomy
- Clinical profile
  - Usually incidental observation in asymptomatic white patient imaged for unrelated reasons

Demographics

- Age
  - Middle-aged and older adults
  - Uncommon in patients < 50 years old; common in elderly
- Gender
  - M:F = 2:1
- Ethnicity
  - Whites > > blacks, Native American, or Asian populations
  - ↓ incidence in osteoporotic white populations
- Epidemiology
  - Reported incidence varies widely
    - Conservative estimate: 6-12% of adults > 40 years of age manifest some findings of DISH; actual incidence may be substantially higher

Natural History & Prognosis

- Nearly always incidental finding without additive morbidity or mortality
  - Severe cases may rarely produce dysphagia
  - Suspected ↑ predisposition to fracture due to decreased flexibility
  - ↑ risk of heterotopic ossification after total hip arthroplasty
- Compression of oropharynx, anterior displacement, and mucosal inflammation secondary mechanical irritation

Treatment

- Vast majority of cases are incidental and merit conservative (observational) management
- Consider osteophyte resection if severe symptoms directly referable to DISH
- Symptomatic CVJ changes require intervention
  - Pseudotumor resection
  - Immobilization for atlantoaxial instability or odontoid fracture
- Other: Diet modifications, speech therapy, antacids

DIAGNOSTIC CHECKLIST

Consider

- DISH is largely asymptomatic and incidentally detected
  - Look carefully for signs of associated OPLL that may lead to myelopathy secondary to central canal stenosis

Image Interpretation Pearls

- Flowing ossification is classically more common on right
- Discs/facet joints are relatively preserved
  - No sacroiliac joint erosion or ankylosis
- May coexist with degenerative spondylosis

SELECTED REFERENCES

1. Graves LL et al: Appearance of diffuse idiopathic skeletal hyperostosis on panoramic images. J Oral Maxillofac Surg. 74(9):1712-3, 2016
2. Holgate RL et al: Diffuse idiopathic skeletal hyperostosis: Diagnostic, clinical, and paleopathological considerations. Clin Anat. 29(7):870-7, 2016
3. Macía-Villa CC et al: Simultaneous occurrence of ankylosing spondylitis and diffuse idiopathic skeletal hyperostosis (Forestier-Rotès-Quérol disease). Reumatol Clin. ePub, 2016
4. Yunoki M et al: The importance of recognizing diffuse idiopathic skeletal hyperostosis for neurosurgeons: a review. Neurol Med Chir (Tokyo). 56(8):510-5, 2016
5. Carlson ML et al: Surgical management of dysphagia and airway obstruction in patients with prominent ventral cervical osteophytes. Dysphagia. 26(1):34-40, 2011
6. Verlaan JJ et al: Diffuse idiopathic skeletal hyperostosis of the cervical spine: an underestimated cause of dysphagia and airway obstruction. Spine J. 11(11):1058-67, 2011
7. Storch MJ et al: Cervical myelopathy caused by soft-tissue mass in diffuse idiopathic skeletal hyperostosis. Eur Spine J. 17 Suppl 2:S243-7, 2008
8. Pascal-Moussellard H et al: Myelopathy by lesions of the craniocervical junction in a patient with forestier disease. Spine (Phila Pa 1976). 31(16):E557-60, 2006
9. Jun BY et al: Retro-odontoid pseudotumor in diffuse idiopathic skeletal hyperostosis. Spine (Phila Pa 1976). 27(10):E266-70, 2002
10. Patel NP et al: Forestier disease associated with a retroodontoid mass causing cervicomedullary compression. J Neurosurg. 96(2 Suppl):190-6, 2002
11. Chiba H et al: Atlantoaxial subluxation complicated by diffuse idiopathic skeletal hyperostosis. A case report. Spine (Phila Pa 1976). 17(11):1414-7, 1992
12. Crockard HA et al: Damaged ligaments at the craniocervical junction presenting as an extradural tumour: a differential diagnosis in the elderly. J Neurol Neurosurg Psychiatry. 54(9):817-21, 1991
13. Resnick D et al: Association of diffuse idiopathic skeletal hyperostosis (DISH) and calcification and ossification of the posterior longitudinal ligament. AJR Am J Roentgenol. 131(6):1049-53, 1978

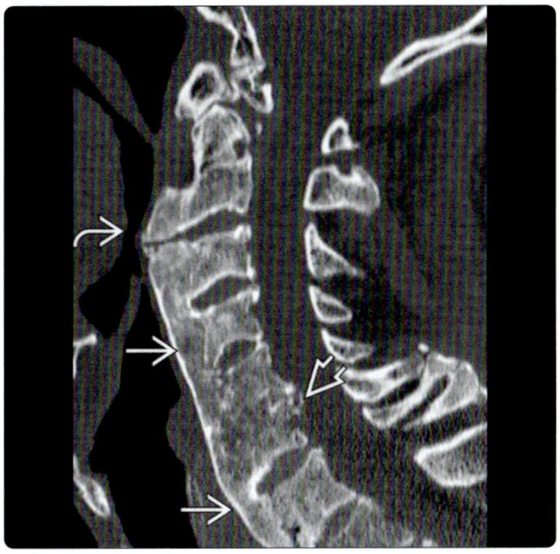

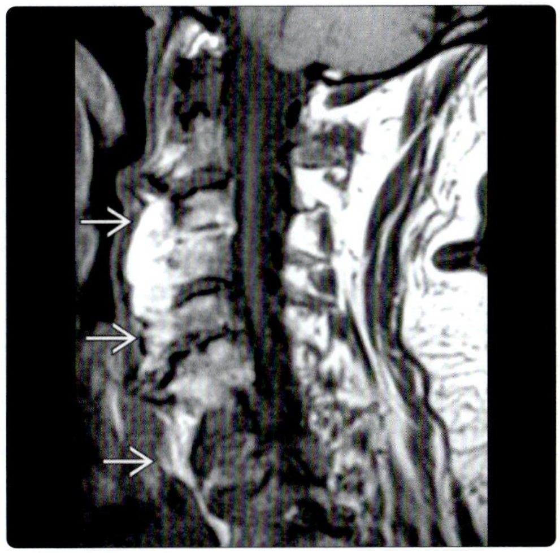

(Left) *Sagittal CT shows large, bulky ALL ossification → that distorts the hypopharynx ⇨. While the ossification of DISH is typically subaxial, it can extend as high as C2. Longstanding immobilization led to ankylosis at the C5-C6 disc space ⇨. Unrelated secondary osteoarthrosis is present at C1-C2.* **(Right)** *Sagittal T1WI MR shows bulky anterior flowing ossification →, consistent with DISH. Fatty marrow is responsible for high T1 signal intensity within the anterior ossification.*

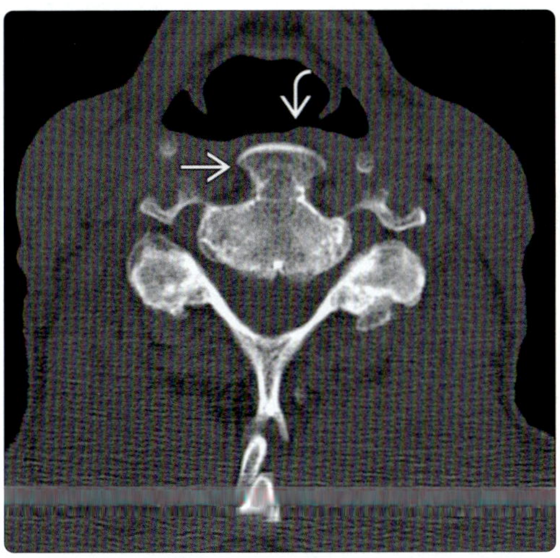

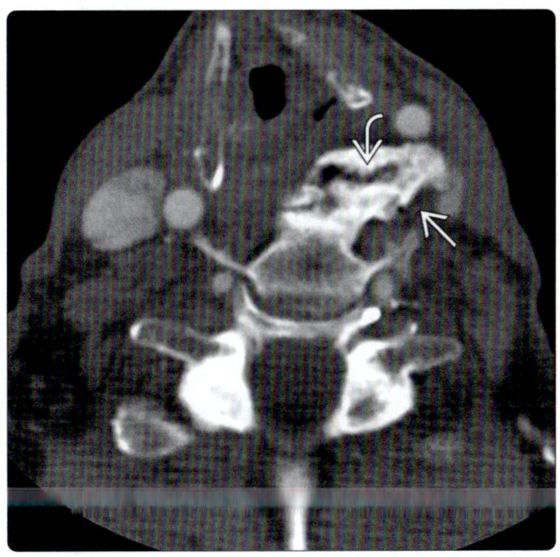

(Left) *Axial NECT shows large, corticated ventral osteophyte → of DISH effacing the hypopharynx ↷. When severe, this effacement can be symptomatic.* **(Right)** *Axial CT shows large, bulky ossification → displacing the left carotid artery and effacing the left hypopharynx. A cleft ↷ within the ossification often occurs at the disc space level. There may be associated dysphagia caused not only by mechanical obstruction of the esophagus but also by resulting inflammation and fibrosis.*

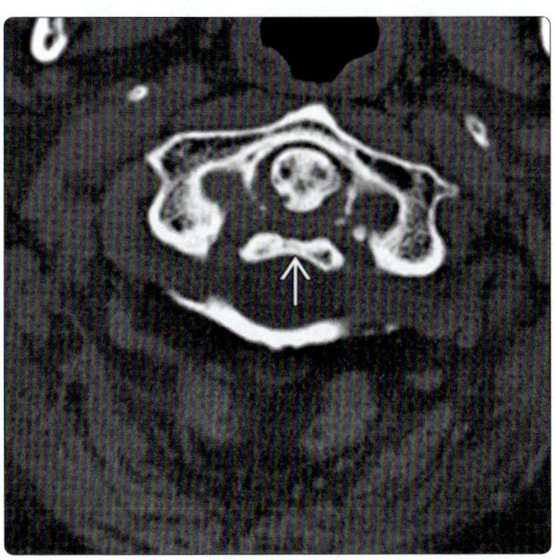

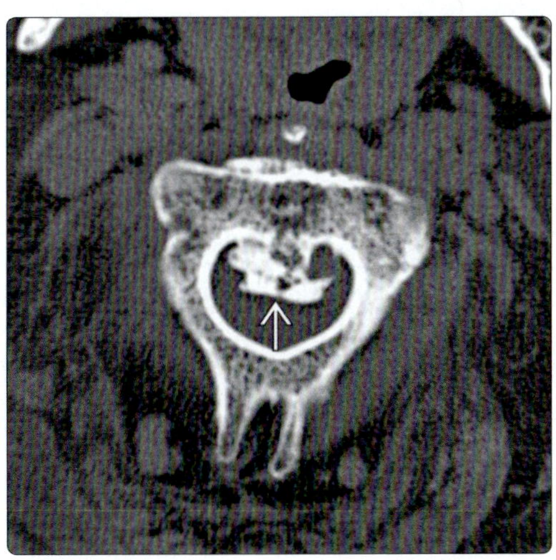

(Left) *Axial bone CT shows the most cephalad extent of OPLL associated with DISH →. At this superior-most level, OPLL is a finger-like projection that usually does not contact the vertebra.* **(Right)** *On this axial bone CT at the base of C2, OPLL → is quite bulky and contiguous with the posterior vertebral cortex. The resulting canal compromise leads to severe spinal cord compression and myelopathic symptoms. These symptoms are some of the few indications for surgical intervention.*

Cervical Facet Arthropathy

KEY FACTS

TERMINOLOGY

- Facet arthrosis, degenerative facet disease, degenerative joint disease

IMAGING

- Osseous facet overgrowth impinging on neural foramina in conjunction with articular joint space narrowing
- Facet joint osteophytes producing foraminal narrowing
- Mushroom cap facet appearance
- Joint space narrowing with sclerosis and bone eburnation
- Intraarticular gas (vacuum phenomenon)
- Enhancing inflammatory soft tissue changes surrounding facet joint are common
- Joint space narrowing, thinning of articular cartilage
- Facet effusions as linear hyperintensity

TOP DIFFERENTIAL DIAGNOSES

- Septic facet
- Healing facet fracture
- Inflammatory arthritides
- Paget disease
- Myositis ossificans
- Metastasis

CLINICAL ISSUES

- Clinical pain aggravated by rest and alleviated by movement
- Poor correlation between duration/severity of pain and extent of facet degeneration
- C2 and C3 nerve impingement may present as TMJ pain

DIAGNOSTIC CHECKLIST

- Best detail with thin-section CT
- T2* images overemphasize degree of foraminal or central narrowing

(Left) *Lateral radiograph shows severe facet hypertrophic degenerative arthropathy at C2-C3 ➔ with marked hypertrophy of the facets.* **(Right)** *Axial NECT shows severe, exuberant right facet degenerative arthropathy ➔. This should not be mistaken for neoplasia.*

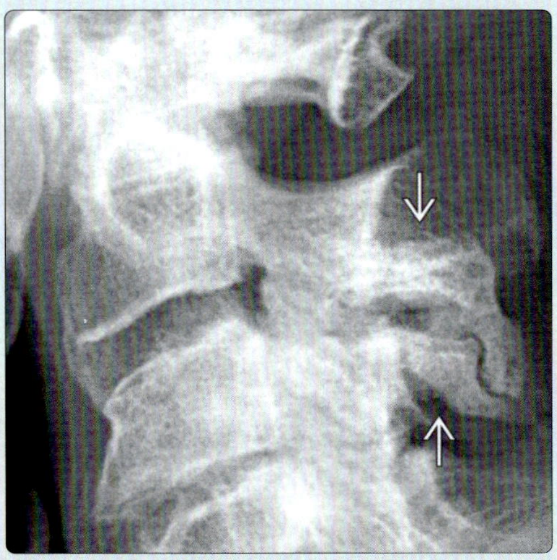

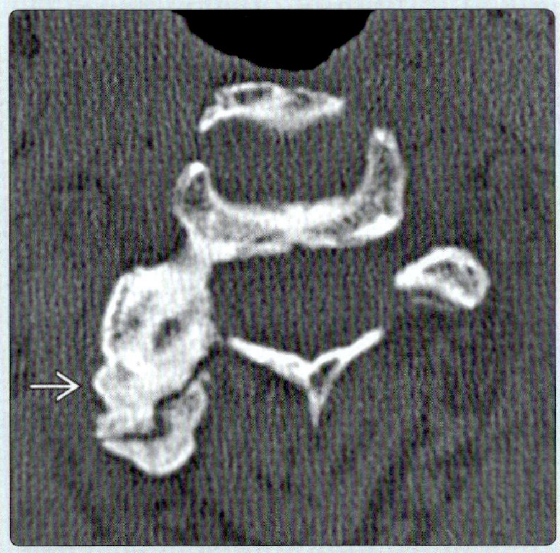

(Left) *Sagittal NECT shows multilevel hypertrophic facet degenerative arthropathy with vacuum phenomenon ➔, bony eburnation, and osteophyte formation ⇨. The C5 neural foramen is narrowed ➔.* **(Right)** *Axial T2* GRE MR shows severe right uncovertebral hypertrophic degenerative arthropathy with severe foraminal stenosis ➔ with facet degenerative change.*

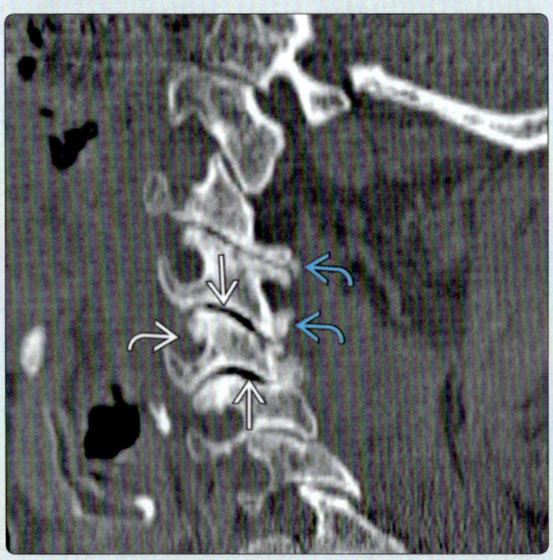

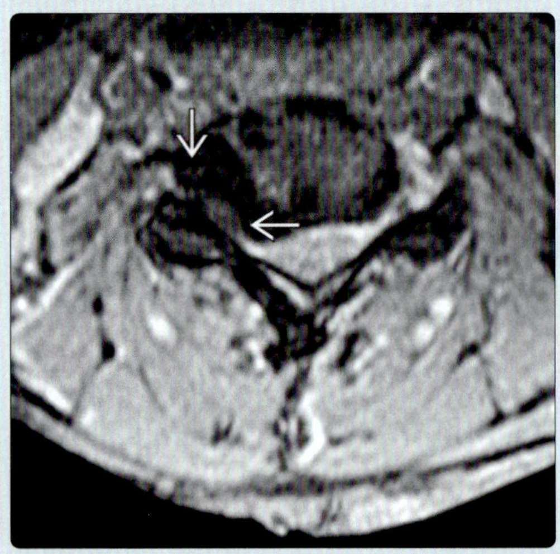

TERMINOLOGY

Synonyms

- Facet arthrosis, degenerative facet disease, degenerative joint disease

Definitions

- Osteoarthritis of synovially lined apophyseal joints

IMAGING

General Features

- Best diagnostic clue
  - Osseous facet overgrowth impinging on neural foramina in conjunction with articular joint space narrowing
- Location
  - Normal anatomy
    - C2 → C7 levels have 2 sets of paired joints
    - Facet or zygapophyseal joints posteriorly, with oblique orientation
    - Uncovertebral joints (joints of Luschka, neurocentral joints) formed by curved edges of vertebral bodies at lateral margins
  - Arthropathy most common in mid/lower cervical spine
- Size
  - Facets may show minimal abnormality or large osteophytes approximating size of facet themselves
- Morphology
  - Osseous facet overgrowth and cartilage erosion with joint space narrowing

Radiographic Findings

- Radiography
  - Poor for demonstrating early facet degeneration
  - Later changes well demonstrated
  - 2D imaging demonstrates facet arthrosis well, not soft tissues
  - Oblique views demonstrate facet joints best
    - Facet joint osteophytes producing foraminal narrowing
    - Joint space narrowing with sclerosis and bone eburnation
    - Intraarticular gas (vacuum phenomenon)

Fluoroscopic Findings

- Same as 2D imaging; can observe motion abnormalities on flexion-extension

CT Findings

- NECT
  - CT more sensitive than 2D imaging for detecting presence and degree of arthrosis
  - Facet joint osteophytes producing foraminal narrowing
  - Mushroom cap facet appearance
  - Joint space narrowing with sclerosis and bone eburnation
  - Intraarticular gas (vacuum phenomenon)
  - CT myelography shows facet relationship to adjacent contrast-opacified thecal sac and nerve root sleeves
- CECT
  - Inflammatory soft tissue changes surrounding facet joint are common
    - May appear aggressive even in absence of infection

MR Findings

- T1WI
  - Enhancing inflammatory soft tissue changes surrounding facet joint are common
    - May appear aggressive even in absence of infection
- T2WI
  - Osteophyte proliferation limiting neural foramina
  - Joint space narrowing, thinning of articular cartilage
  - Facet effusions as linear hyperintensity
- T2* GRE
  - Shows osseous changes well
  - Tends to overemphasize degree of foraminal or central canal narrowing
- T1WI C+
  - Enhancement of synovium, epidural, and foraminal venous plexus

Nonvascular Interventions

- Myelography
  - CT myelography portrays facet relationship to adjacent contrast-opacified thecal sac and nerve root sleeves

Nuclear Medicine Findings

- Bone scan
  - Increased uptake with degenerative disc disease, facet arthropathy

Imaging Recommendations

- 2D imaging useful to demonstrate presence and severity of facet degenerative changes
- Sagittal and axial T1WI and T2WI best demonstrate degenerative facet compression of adjacent thecal sac
  - 3D gradient-echo T2* for foraminal detail

DIFFERENTIAL DIAGNOSIS

Septic Facet

- T2 hyperintensity extending into adjacent soft tissues

Healing Facet Fracture

- Trauma history, search for fracture line

Inflammatory Arthritides

- Look for ankylosis or erosions, cranial settling, atlantoaxial subluxation (rheumatoid arthritis)

Paget Disease

- Thickened cortex, trabeculae, bony expansion

Myositis Ossificans

- Trauma history, circumscribed calcification

Tumor

- Metastasis
- Lymphoma
- Sarcoma

PATHOLOGY

General Features

- Etiology
  - Frequently seen in elderly population

  - Probably related to minor repetitive trauma coupled with abnormal biomechanics
- May see earlier presentation after trauma, with kyphosis/scoliosis, or following surgical fusion at adjacent level
- Genetics
  - Genetic predisposition pondered but not proven
- Associated abnormalities
  - Frequently seen in conjunction with spondylosis
- Degenerative (hypertrophic) inflammatory changes in synovial joints
  - Progression similar to that in other joints except for early focal full-thickness cartilage necrosis
- Normal bone mineralization (in contrast to rheumatoid arthritis)
- Joint traction during subluxation may produce gas in joint (vacuum phenomenon)
- Associated with synovial cysts, degenerative disc disease

Staging, Grading, & Classification

- Grading scale (Pathria scale): Based on imaging studies
  - Grade 0: Normal
  - Grade I: Mild narrowing and joint irregularity
  - Grade II: Moderate narrowing and joint irregularity, sclerosis, and osteophyte formation
  - Grade III: Severe narrowing and almost total loss of joint space, sclerosis, and osteophyte formation

Gross Pathologic & Surgical Features

- Most common locations for facet arthropathy
  - Mid/lower cervical spine, lower lumbar spine
  - Thoracic spine uncommon due to rigidity from ribs/sternum
- Joint space narrowing, capsular laxity may permit subluxation of superior facet on inferior facet (degenerative spondylolisthesis)

Microscopic Features

- Findings are similar to those seen in synovial joints at other locations
  - Osseous proliferation
  - Fibrillation and erosion of articular joint cartilage
  - Preservation of bone density

CLINICAL ISSUES

Presentation

- Most common signs/symptoms
  - Mechanical neck pain (facet arthrosis syndrome)
    - Related to irritation of innervation of joint from medial branch(es) of dorsal primary ramus
    - Capsular distension, inflammatory synovitis, entrapment of synovial villi between 2 articular processes or nerve impingement by osteophytes
    - Aggravated by rest, worse in morning, and relieved by repeated gentle motion
  - Radiculopathy
  - Other signs/symptoms
    - Facet disease may be asymptomatic incidental finding on imaging
    - Myelopathy (rarely)
- Clinical profile
  - Clinical pain syndrome produces symptoms that frequently are aggravated by rest and alleviated by movement
  - Poor correlation between duration and severity of pain, as well as extent of facet degeneration
  - C2 and C3 nerve impingement may present as TMJ pain
    - C2 and C3 dermatomes involve TMJ, angle of mandible, and neck areas

Demographics

- Age
  - Universal after age 60
- Gender
  - No gender preference
- Epidemiology
  - Facet joint degeneration begins in first 2 decades of life

Natural History & Prognosis

- Can show progressive symptoms/signs
- Variable (depending on severity)

Treatment

- Mechanical pain → conservative medical therapy
- Foraminal narrowing with radiculopathy → foraminotomy
- Subluxation
  - Cervical → transarticular fusion with lateral mass screws or anterior cervical discectomy and fusion

DIAGNOSTIC CHECKLIST

Consider

- Best detail of foraminal bony narrowing with thin-section CT with oblique reformats

Image Interpretation Pearls

- 3D gradient-echo T2* images overemphasize degree of foraminal or central canal narrowing

SELECTED REFERENCES

1. Manchikanti L et al: Cervical zygapophysial (facet) joint pain: effectiveness of interventional management strategies. Postgrad Med. 128(1):54-68, 2016
2. Ng A et al: Cervical facet injections in the management of cervicogenic headaches. Curr Pain Headache Rep. 19(5):484, 2015
3. Park MS et al: Facet joint degeneration of the cervical spine: a computed tomographic analysis of 320 patients. Spine (Phila Pa 1976). 39(12):E713-8, 2014
4. Varlotta GP et al: The lumbar facet joint: a review of current knowledge: part 1: anatomy, biomechanics, and grading. Skeletal Radiol. 40(1):13-23, 2011
5. Lehman RA Jr et al: Comparison of magnetic resonance imaging and computed tomography in predicting facet arthrosis in the cervical spine. Spine (Phila Pa 1976). 34(1):65-8, 2009
6. Shedid D et al: Cervical spondylosis anatomy: pathophysiology and biomechanics. Neurosurgery. 60(1 Supp1 1):S7-13, 2007
7. Kettler A et al: Review of existing grading systems for cervical or lumbar disc and facet joint degeneration. Eur Spine J. 15(6):705-18, 2006. Erratum in: Eur Spine J. 15(6):719, 2006
8. Birchall D et al: Evaluation of magnetic resonance myelography in the investigation of cervical spondylotic radiculopathy. Br J Radiol. 76(908):525-31, 2003
9. Roberts CC et al: Oblique reformation in cervical spine computed tomography: a new look at an old friend. Spine. 28(2):167-70, 2003
10. Ross JS: Magnetic resonance imaging of the postoperative spine. Semin Musculoskelet Radiol. 4(3):281-91, 2000
11. Truumees E et al: Cervical spondylotic myelopathy and radiculopathy. Instr Course Lect. 49:339-60, 2000
12. Kaiser JA et al: Imaging of the cervical spine. Spine. 23(24):2701-12, 1998

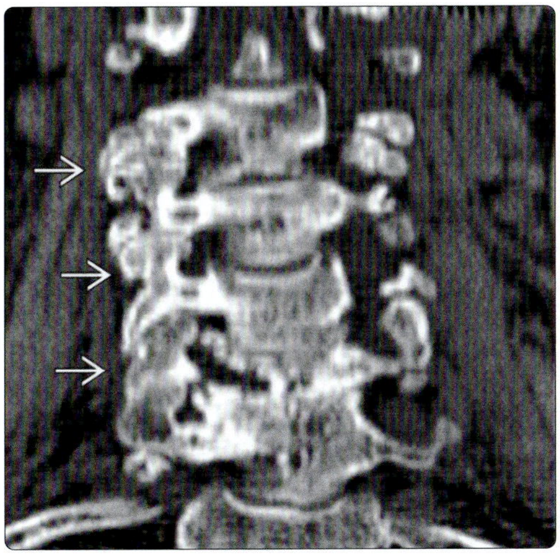

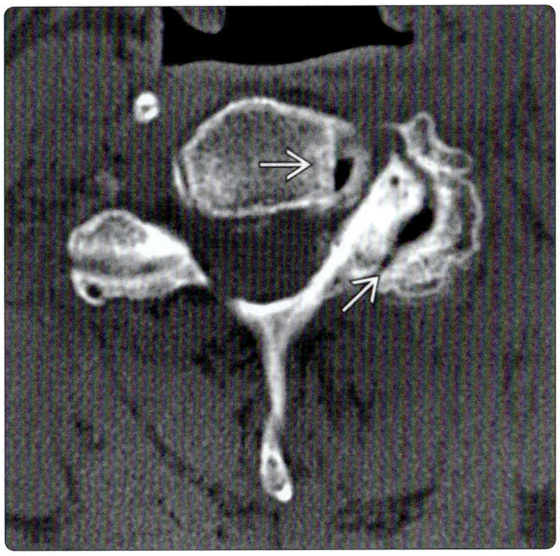

(Left) *Coronal NECT shows multilevel severe facet hypertrophic degenerative arthropathy with foraminal stenosis* ➡. **(Right)** *Axial NECT shows severe left facet degenerative arthropathy and foraminal stenosis. Vacuum phenomenon is present in facet joint and uncovertebral joint* ➡.

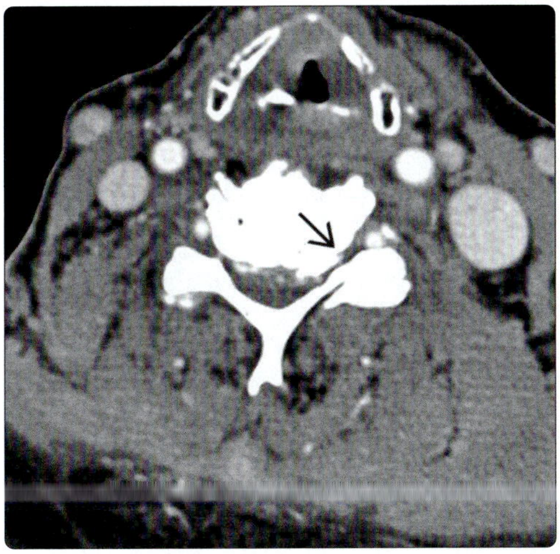

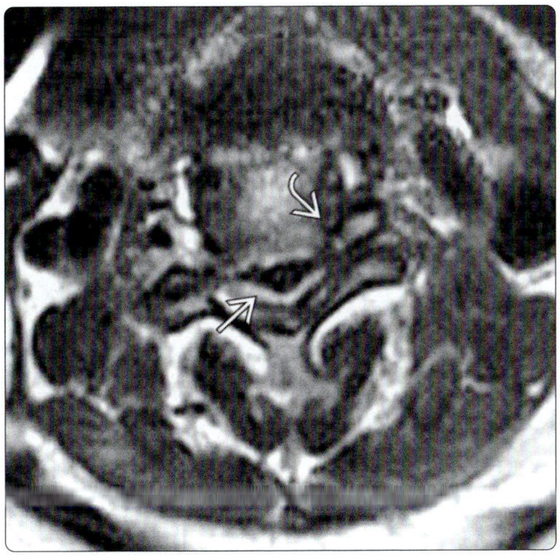

(Left) *Axial CECT shows severe canal stenosis due to diffuse disc bulge and diffuse broad-based herniations anteriorly with associated disc calcification. There is severe bilateral foraminal stenosis with uncovertebral joint hypertrophy* ⇨ *and facet degeneration.* **(Right)** *Axial T2WI MR shows markedly thinned cord as relatively high signal* ➡ *outlined ventrally by disc osteophyte complex and posteriorly by thickened low-signal ligamentum flavum. There is severe bilateral foraminal stenosis* ➡.

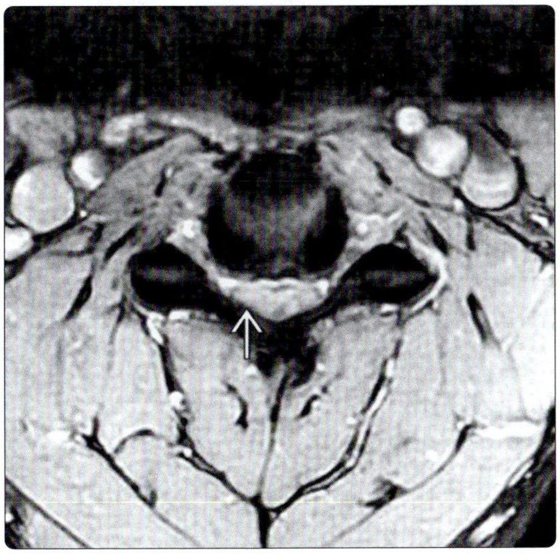

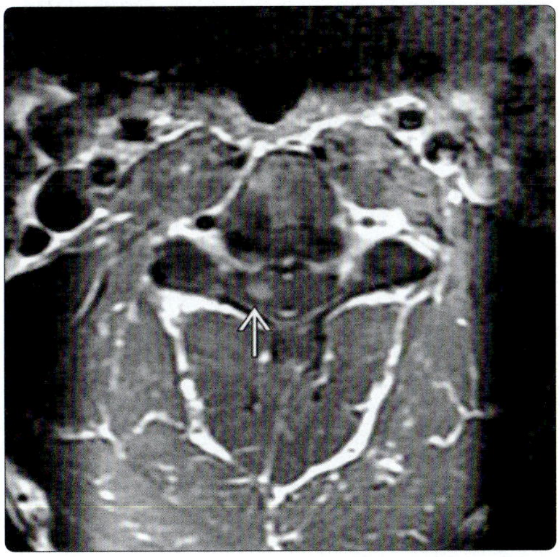

(Left) *Axial T2* GRE MR shows moderate foraminal stenosis from mild facet degenerative change and uncovertebral joint hypertrophy. High signal is present within the cord from chronic compression and myelomalacia* ➡. **(Right)** *Axial T1WI C+ MR shows foraminal stenosis from uncovertebral hypertrophy and facet degeneration with enhancing cord myelomalacia* ➡.

KEY FACTS

TERMINOLOGY

- Common benign venous malformation within vertebrae

IMAGING

- Thoracic location: Lumbar > cervical
- Vertebral body
  - Infrequently extends into posterior elements
  - Usually intraosseous, may have epidural component
- CT: Well-circumscribed lesion of fat density
- Thickened, vertically aligned trabecula
  - Corduroy appearance on sagittal/coronal images
  - Polka-dot appearance on axial images
- T1WI MR: Typical (fatty stroma): Hyperintense
- T2WI MR: Usually hyperintense due to vascular elements
  - May be isointense to fat
- Variable enhancement

TOP DIFFERENTIAL DIAGNOSES

- Focal fatty marrow
- Vertebral metastasis
- Paget disease
- Degenerative endplates, type 2
- Spinal radiation treatment

PATHOLOGY

- Complications in < 1%
  - Pathologic compression fracture
  - Epidural hemangioma component with cord compression

CLINICAL ISSUES

- Peak incidence in 4th-6th decades
- 11% of adult population
- 25-30% multiple, particularly in thoracic spine
- No follow-up typically necessary with pathognomonic imaging

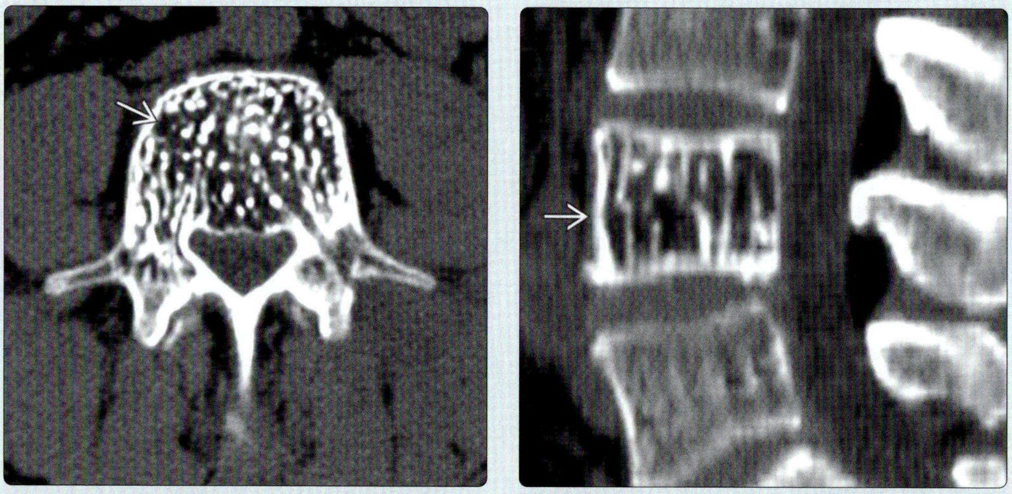

(Left) *Axial NECT shows the classic polka-dot or honeycomb appearance of a hemangioma with fat density ➡ interspersed among the trabecula. The appearance is pathognomonic and can be seen anywhere in the spine.* **(Right)** *Sagittal NECT shows a vertebral hemangioma with the characteristic corduroy appearance resulting from the vertically oriented trabecula. Note the difference in density between the involved vertebral body ➡ and the adjacent vertebra due to the fat stroma.*

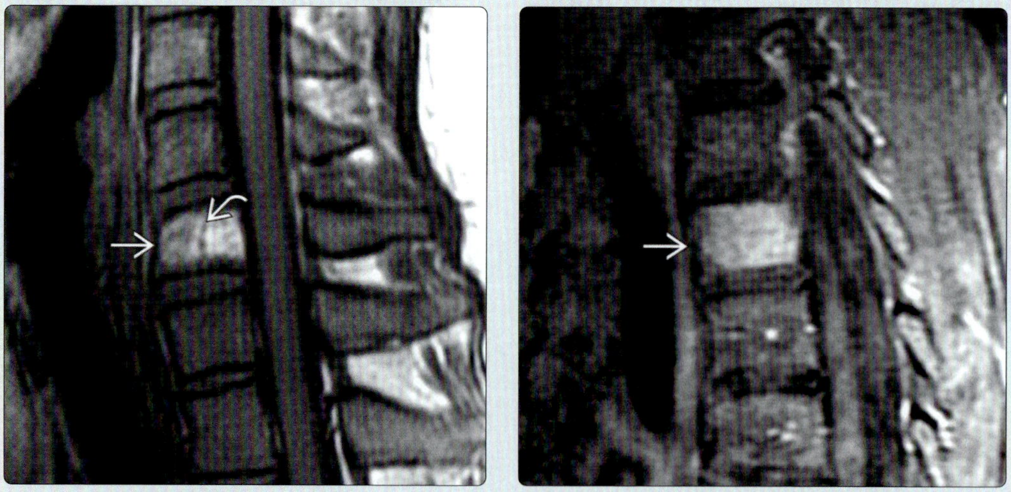

(Left) *A typical hemangioma is evident ➡ on this sagittal T1WI MR. The fat content creates a lesion that is diffusely hyperintense relative to the adjacent marrow. A prominent trabecula is noted in the center of the lesion ↷.* **(Right)** *On this sagittal T1WI C+ FS MR, one can appreciate the intense enhancement of a highly vascular lesion ➡. Contrast enhancement is not necessary to define typical hemangiomas. It may be useful to evaluate atypical hemangiomas.*

TERMINOLOGY

Definitions

- Common benign venous malformation within vertebrae

IMAGING

General Features

- Best diagnostic clue
  - CT: Well-circumscribed, fat-density lesion with coarse vertical trabeculae
    - Polka-dot appearance on axial images
    - Corduroy appearance on sagittal/coronal images
  - MR: Well-defined lesion, follows fat signal on both T1WI and T2WI, with hypointense vertical striations
- Location
  - Thoracic: Lumbar > cervical
  - Often multiple (20-30%)
  - Vertebral body
    - Infrequently extends into posterior elements
    - Usually intraosseous, may have epidural component
    - Rarely, purely epidural spinal hemangioma
- Size
  - Variable, may encompass whole vertebral body
- Morphology
  - Geographic nonsclerotic margins, thick internal trabeculae
  - Infrequently, associated epidural soft tissue

Radiographic Findings

- Radiography
  - Vertebral body of lower density than adjacent vertebra with coarse vertical trabeculae resembling corduroy or honeycomb

CT Findings

- NECT
  - Well-circumscribed lesion of fat density
  - Thickened, vertically aligned trabecula
    - Polka-dot appearance on axial images
    - Corduroy appearance on sagittal/coronal images
  - Aggressive hemangiomas may have no characteristic features; difficult to differentiate from malignant process
    - Density similar to soft tissue rather than fat
    - Ill-defined bone destruction
    - Extensive, enhancing soft tissue component

MR Findings

- T1WI
  - Typical (fatty stroma): Hyperintense
  - Atypical (mostly vascular soft tissue): Isointense or hypointense
    - May simulate malignancy
- T2WI
  - Usually hyperintense due to vascular elements
  - May be isointense to fat
- T1WI C+
  - Variable enhancement
    - Milder enhancement typically seen in lesions with larger fatty component
- Features of aggressive hemangioma
  - T1 isointense to hypointense, with avid contrast enhancement
  - Extraosseous soft tissue extension
  - Pathologic fracture
  - Presence of any fat within lesion is clue to etiology

Angiographic Findings

- Variable enhancement
  - Angiography is unnecessary unless embolization is considered

Nuclear Medicine Findings

- Bone scan
  - Studies are usually normal, lesions are not visualized

Imaging Recommendations

- Best imaging tool
  - Pathognomonic findings usually present on both CT and MR
- Protocol advice
  - Bone CT may supplement MR evaluation of hemangioma with atypical imaging features concerning for neoplasm

DIFFERENTIAL DIAGNOSIS

Focal Fatty Marrow

- Incidental rounded focus of marrow fat conspicuous on MR imaging
- Fat-suppressed sequences (e.g., STIR) will show marked lesion hypointensity; hemangiomas typically retain some high signal due to vascular components

Vertebral Metastasis

- Hypointense on T1WI, hypointense to hyperintense (to marrow) on T2WI
- May be difficult to distinguish from aggressive hemangioma; consider CT
- Typically multiple

Paget Disease

- Expanded body with thickened low-signal cortex, heterogeneous signal containing fat
- No regular pattern of vertically oriented trabeculae
- No epidural soft tissue extension (unless degenerated into sarcoma)

Degenerative Endplates, Type 2

- Abut intervertebral disc
- Adjacent degenerate disc with endplate spondylosis

Spinal Radiation Treatment

- Fatty marrow replacement throughout vertebral body
- Conforms to radiation port
- No coarse, vertical trabeculations as in hemangioma

PATHOLOGY

General Features

- Etiology
  - Developmental, hamartomatous lesions
- Genetics

- Rarely, Krev interaction trapped 1 (*KRIT1*) gene in families with cerebral cavernous malformations, autosomal dominant
- Associated abnormalities
  - Complications in < 1%
    - Pathologic compression fracture
    - Epidural hemangioma component with cord compression

Gross Pathologic & Surgical Features

- Majority confined to vertebral body proper
  - May be small or occupy entire vertebral body
  - Uncommonly involve posterior elements/pedicles (10-15%)
- Thoracic lesions are aggressive more often than those at other locations

Microscopic Features

- Thin-walled sinusoidal channels lined by vascular endothelium
- Interspersed bony trabeculae
- Fatty tissue
  - Atypical lesions have less fat and more vascular stroma
- Slow venous flow
- Similar to venous malformations

CLINICAL ISSUES

Presentation

- Most common signs/symptoms
  - Most commonly incidental finding
  - Aggressive lesions can present with pathologic compression fracture or spinal cord compression
    - Rarely, enlargement of hemangioma during pregnancy resulting in cord compression
- Clinical profile
  - Incidental finding on spine imaging ordered for unrelated reason

Demographics

- Age
  - Peak incidence: 4th-6th decades
- Gender
  - Similar incidence, or up to 2x as frequent in females
- Epidemiology
  - Most common spinal tumor
  - Vertebra most common site of skeletal hemangiomas
  - 11% of adult population
  - 25-30% multiple, particularly in thoracic spine

Natural History & Prognosis

- Benign (fatty) hemangiomas: Incidental lesions, no clinical sequela
- Aggressive vascular hemangiomas: Variable depending on size of lesion, degree of epidural extension, and presence/absence of cord compression

Treatment

- No follow-up necessary with pathognomonic imaging
- Annual neurological and radiological examinations for patients with hemangiomas associated with pain may be appropriate
- Aggressive hemangiomas
  - Direct intralesional injection of ethanol (body collapse post ethanol treatment is reported complication)
  - Embolization with Onyx recently reported
  - Vertebroplasty in conjunction with embolization may be considered if concern for pathologic fracture
  - Surgical resection (corpectomy) or radiation therapy has also been utilized

DIAGNOSTIC CHECKLIST

Consider

- Atypical (fat-poor) hemangioma in low-risk patient with solitary, indeterminate vertebral lesion on MR

Image Interpretation Pearls

- Focused CT of suspected atypical (fat-poor) hemangioma to identify characteristic osseous findings

SELECTED REFERENCES

1. Bouali S et al: Intradural extramedullary capillary hemangioma in the upper cervical spine: first report. World Neurosurg. 92:587.e1-7, 2016
2. Ayhan S et al: Concomitant intramedullary arteriovenous malformation and a vertebral hemangioma of cervical spine discovered by a pathologic fracture during bicycle accident. Eur Spine J. 24(1):187-92, 2015
3. Sade R et al: Cervical hemangioma with neurologic deficit. Spine J. 15(8):1888-9, 2015
4. Miller D et al: Osteolytic mass bridging two cervical vertebrae: Unusual presentation of a vertebral body hemangioma. Radiol Case Rep. 9(4):927, 2014
5. Hurley MC et al: Preoperative Onyx embolization of aggressive vertebral hemangiomas. AJNR Am J Neuroradiol. 29(6):1095-7, 2008
6. Bandiera S et al: Symptomatic vertebral hemangioma: the treatment of 23 cases and a review of the literature. Chir Organi Mov. 87(1):1-15, 2002
7. Gabal AM: Percutaneous technique for sclerotherapy of vertebral hemangioma compressing spinal cord. Cardiovasc Intervent Radiol. 25(6):494-500, 2002
8. Murugan L et al: Management of symptomatic vertebral hemangiomas: review of 13 patients. Neurol India. 50(3): 300-5, 2002
9. Bas T et al: Efficacy and safety of ethanol injections in 18 cases of vertebral hemangioma: a mean follow-up of 2 years. Spine. 26(14): 1577-82, 2001
10. Baudrez V et al: Benign vertebral hemangioma: MR-histological correlation. Skeletal Radiol. 30(8): 442-6, 2001
11. Miszczyk L et al: The efficacy of radiotherapy for vertebral hemangiomas. Neoplasma. 48(1):82-4, 2001
12. Cross JJ et al: Imaging of compressive vertebral haemangiomas. Eur Radiol. 10(6):997-1002, 2000
13. Doppman JL et al: Symptomatic vertebral hemangiomas: treatment by means of direct intralesional injection of ethanol. Radiology. 214(2): 341-8, 2000
14. Lee S et al: Extraosseous extension of vertebral hemangioma, a rare cause of spinal cord compression. Spine. 24(20): 2111-4, 1999
15. Pastushyn AI et al: Vertebral hemangiomas: diagnosis, management, natural history and clinicopathological correlates in 86 patients. Surg Neurol. 50(6): 535-47, 1998
16. Griffith JF et al: Clinics in diagnostic imaging (25). Aggressive vertebral haemangioma. Singapore Med J. 38(5): 226-30, 1997
17. Jayakumar PN et al: Symptomatic vertebral haemangioma: endovascular treatment of 12 patients. Spinal Cord. 35(9): 624-8, 1997
18. Ide C et al: Vertebral haemangiomas with spinal cord compression: the place of preoperative percutaneous vertebroplasty with methyl methacrylate. Neuroradiology. 38(6): 585-9, 1996
19. Fox MW et al: The natural history and management of symptomatic and asymptomatic vertebral hemangiomas. J Neurosurg. 78(1): 36-45, 1993
20. Laredo JD et al: Vertebral hemangiomas: fat content as a sign of aggressiveness. Radiology. 177(2):467-72, 1990
21. Nguyen JP et al: Vertebral hemangiomas presenting with neurologic symptoms. Surg Neurol. 27(4):391-7, 1987
22. Ross JS et al: Vertebral hemangiomas: MR imaging. Radiology. 165(1):165-9, 1987
23. Laredo JD et al: Vertebral hemangiomas: radiologic evaluation. Radiology. 161(1):183-9, 1986

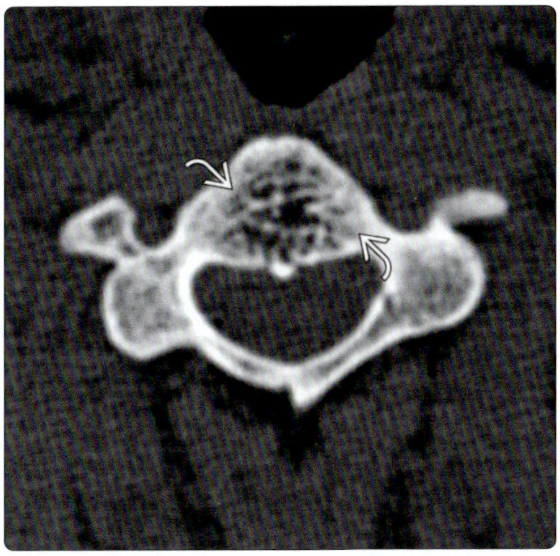

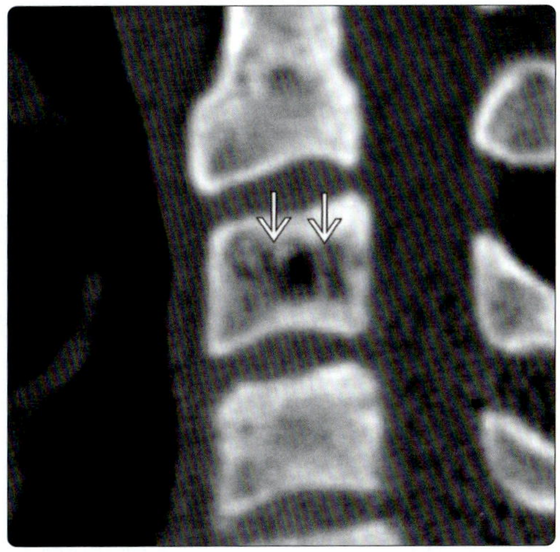

(Left) *Axial NECT shows a lesion that is relatively well defined with nonsclerotic borders. Clues to the diagnosis are the fat density within and the honeycomb appearance.* **(Right)** *Sagittal reformatted CT shows lucency in the C3 vertebral body with a few thickened, vertically oriented trabecula, characteristic CT findings of vertebral hemangioma. The vertical trabecula are not always continuous from one endplate to the other.*

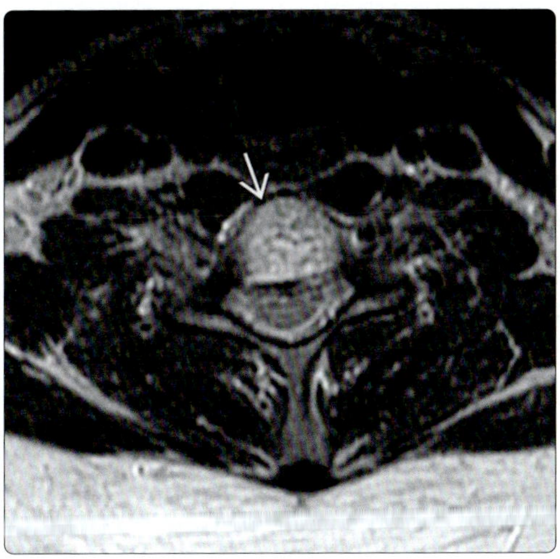

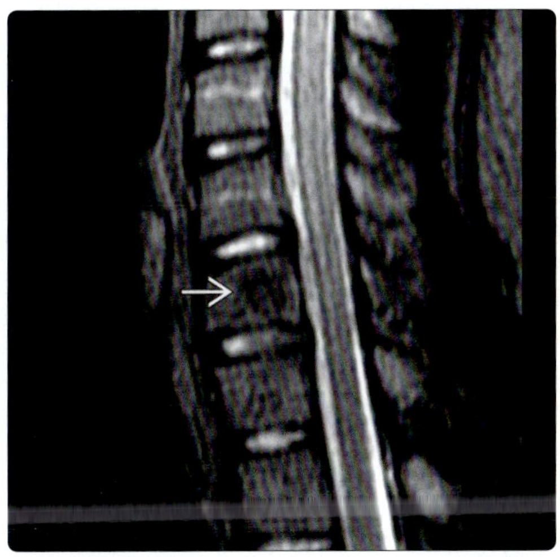

(Left) *Axial T2WI MR nicely shows the expected findings of a vertebral hemangioma. The lesion is confined to the vertebral body, it is isointense with fat, and trabeculae are visible.* **(Right)** *The signal from this typical hemangioma, which is entirely fat, completely suppresses on this sagittal STIR MR. The T2WI appearance of hemangiomas is variable, depending on the mix of fat and vascular elements.*

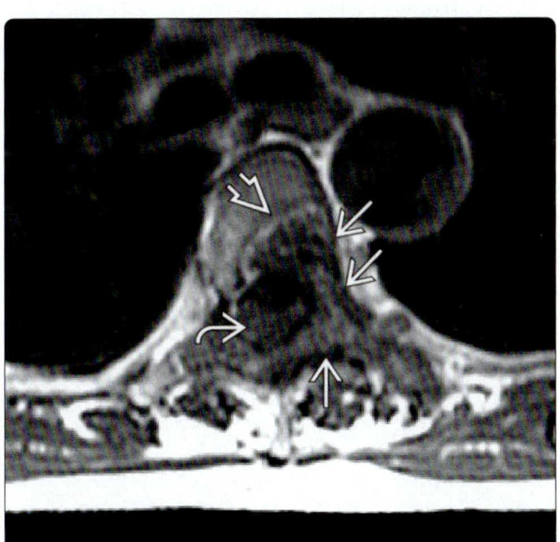

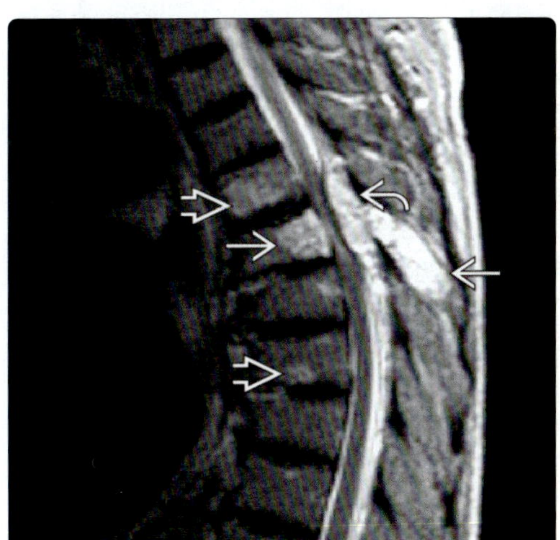

(Left) *Features of an aggressive hemangioma are apparent on this axial T1WI MR. The lesion is in the thoracic spine and extends into the posterior elements and epidural space. Fat is seen in only 1 region. The speckled appearance suggests trabecula of a hemangioma.* **(Right)** *On this sagittal T2WI MR, an aggressive hemangioma is hyperintense. A large epidural component is easily seen. Other hemangiomas are visible.*

Lytic and Blastic Metastases

KEY FACTS

TERMINOLOGY

- Spread of malignancy to spine from primary site

IMAGING

- Multiple lytic or blastic lesions in skeleton
- Radiographs and CT: Lytic lesions have nonsclerotic margins that range from geographic to permeative
    - No tumor matrix
- T1WI: Hypointense metastatic lesion replaces normal T1-hyperintense marrow
- T2WI and STIR: Range from hypointense to hyperintense relative to normal marrow
- Paravertebral and epidural soft tissue extension
- Bone scan and PET: Multiple skeletal foci of radioisotope uptake

TOP DIFFERENTIAL DIAGNOSES

- Hematopoietic malignancy
- Benign (osteoporotic) compression fracture
- Normal heterogeneous marrow
- Spondylodiscitis

PATHOLOGY

- Primary tumor sites in adults include kidney, lung, breast, thyroid, gastrointestinal and genitourinary tracts, ovaries, pancreas; tumor types include melanoma, chordoma, and paraganglioma
- Primary tumor in children: Ewing sarcoma, other sarcoma, neuroblastoma, hematologic malignancies

CLINICAL ISSUES

- Neck pain, stiff neck, &/or headache
- Prognosis varies with histology of primary lesion
- Progressive course leading to pathologic fracture &/or spinal cord compression
- Regardless of tumor histology, radiation therapy and hard collar immobilization are initial forms of treatment

(Left) *On this axial NECT, the classic appearance of a metastatic lesion* ➡ *is evident with destruction of cortical and cancellous bone. The margins of destruction are variable (geographic on the left and permeative on the right).* **(Right)** *Axial NECT shows an expansile, soap bubble lytic lesion of the left side of the neural arch and vertebral body* ➡*. This expansile feature is typical of the underlying primary in this case of thyroid cancer.*

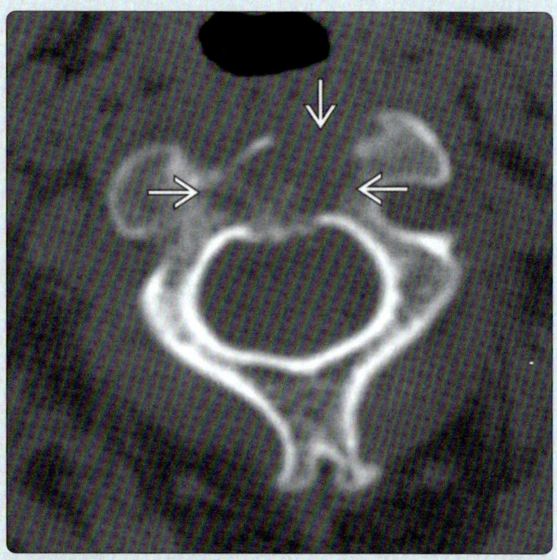

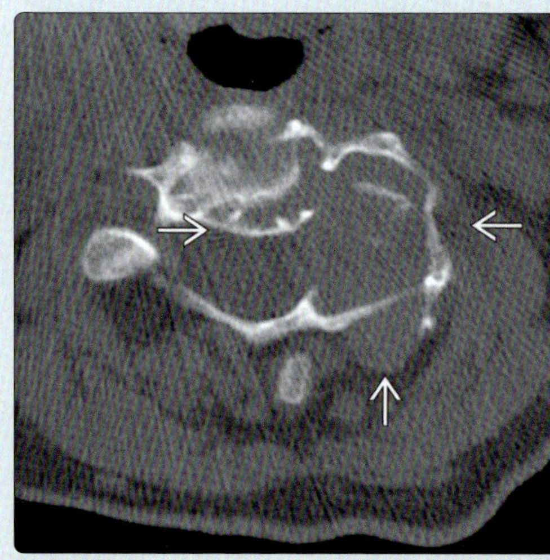

(Left) *On this sagittal T1WI MR, multiple hypointense foci are visible in the vertebral bodies* ➡ *and posterior elements* ➡*. There is an associated collapse of the C6 vertebra. The odontoid process is a typical site of involvement at the craniovertebral junction.* **(Right)** *On this sagittal STIR MR, multiple metastatic lesions are hyperintense relative to suppressed normal fat marrow* ➡*. Absence of an epidural soft tissue mass is a pertinent negative finding.*

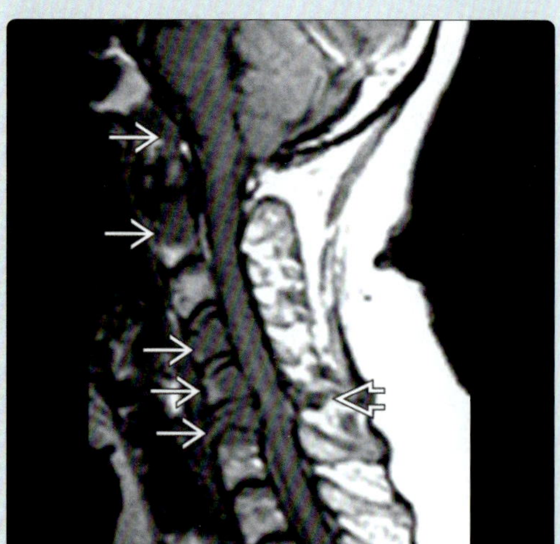

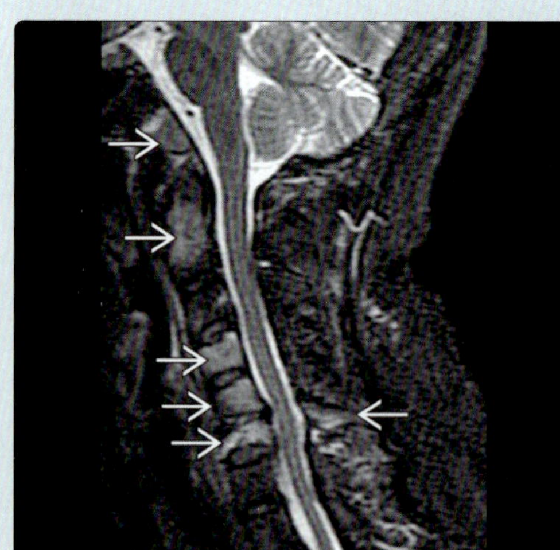

TERMINOLOGY

Synonyms

- Sclerotic metastases = blastic metastases

Definitions

- Spread of malignancy to spine from primary site

IMAGING

General Features

- Best diagnostic clue
  - Multiple lytic or blastic lesions in skeleton
- Location
  - Lesion distribution is proportional to red marrow distribution (lumbar > thoracic > cervical)
    - Involvement of craniovertebral junction (CVJ) is rare
  - Vertebral body and posterior elements
    - Favor anterior vertebra at CVJ
- Size
  - Any size
- Morphology
  - Typically round (due to centrifugal growth) destruction of bone

Radiographic Findings

- Radiography
  - Detection of lytic lesions requires 50-70% bone destruction and tumor size > 1 cm for detection
    - AP: Absent ("missing") pedicle
    - Lateral: Destroyed cortex &/or endplate
  - Sclerotic lesions are more conspicuous and detected earlier

CT Findings

- NECT
  - Destruction of cortical and cancellous bone
    - Lytic lesions have nonsclerotic margins that range from geographic to permeative; no tumor matrix
  - Paravertebral &/or epidural soft tissue mass
  - ± pathologic fracture
    - Soft tissue rim of hematoma/edema can be seen with benign compression fracture, typically < 5 mm
  - Sclerotic metastases are rarely associated with fracture or soft tissue mass
- CECT
  - Variable enhancement

MR Findings

- T1WI
  - Hypointense metastatic lesion replaces normal T1-hyperintense marrow
    - Diffuse osseous involvement causes generalized low marrow signal (discs brighter than bone)
  - Paravertebral and epidural soft tissue extension
    - Curtain sign
  - Intervertebral discs are generally spared
- T2WI
  - Ranges from hypointense to hyperintense relative to normal marrow
- STIR
  - Greater conspicuity of vertebral metastasis than on fast spin-echo T2WI due to fat suppression
- DWI
  - Hyperintense
  - Controversial; technically difficult in spine
    - May help differentiate metastatic disease from osteoporotic compression fracture
    - Many reports of elevated DWI signal seem to be actually due to T2 shine-through
- T1WI C+
  - Diffuse enhancement is typical
  - Without fat saturation, contrast may limit conspicuity relative to normal fatty marrow
- Blastic metastases have low signal on all imaging sequences
  - Rarely have associated epidural/paraspinal soft tissue mass

Nonvascular Interventions

- Myelography
  - Osseous findings as per NECT
  - Extrinsic compression of thecal sac by epidural tumor
    - Better assessment of cord compression than with NECT or CECT
    - Reserve for patients who are unable to undergo MR

Nuclear Medicine Findings

- Bone scan
  - Multiple skeletal foci of radioisotope uptake
  - False-negatives with aggressively lytic tumor and very small lesions
- PET
  - FDG PET has better specificity and lower sensitivity for detecting bone metastases compared to bone scan
  - FDG PET/CT has better specificity for detecting spine metastases compared to FDG PET alone

Imaging Recommendations

- Protocol advice
  - MR imaging of entire spinal axis to evaluate for osseous metastasis, epidural tumor, cord compression
    - Include STIR or fat-suppressed T2WI and contrast-enhanced (± fat-saturated) T1WI
  - Bone scan is useful for screening of entire skeleton

DIFFERENTIAL DIAGNOSIS

Hematopoietic Malignancy

- Diffuse marrow involvement is more common
- Plasmacytoma
  - Solitary expansile lytic lesion
- Multiple myeloma (MM)
  - Bone scan negative/equivocal in 25% of MM cases
- Lymphoma
  - Permeative destruction

Benign (Osteoporotic) Compression Fracture

- Acute osteoporotic compression fracture may mimic metastatic disease (DWI may be helpful)
  - 1/3 of fractures in patients with known primary tumor are benign
  - 1/4 of fractures in apparently osteopenic patients are from malignant disease

- Marrow signal with late subacute/chronic benign fractures similar to normal marrow (suppresses on STIR)
- Follow-up in 6-8 weeks will show resolution of marrow edema aiding differentiation from metastatic disease

Normal Heterogeneous Marrow

- Patchy fatty marrow signal in older patients
- Intact pedicle & vertebral cortex; no soft tissue mass

Spondylodiscitis

- Destruction of disc space with fluid signal, enhancement, and abnormal signal in marrow on either side of disc space

PATHOLOGY

General Features

- Etiology
  - Hematogenous dissemination (arterial or venous via Batson plexus) > perineural, lymphatic, CSF spread
  - Marrow infiltration and tumor growth stimulate osteoclastic response
    - Posterior vertebral body usually 1st, then pedicle
  - Primary tumor sites in adults include kidney, lung, breast, thyroid, GI tract, GU tract, ovaries, pancreas, and tumor types such as melanoma, chordoma, paraganglioma
    - Most common: Breast, lung, prostate, renal
    - Unknown primary in 15-25%
    - Osteoblastic metastases: Prostate, breast, transitional cell, carcinoid
    - Expansile: Renal, thyroid, melanoma
    - Mixed osteolytic and osteoblastic: Breast, lung
  - Primary tumor in children: Ewing sarcoma, other sarcoma, neuroblastoma, hematologic malignancies

Staging, Grading, & Classification

- Surgical stratification
  - 6 parameters scored
    - General condition, number of extraspinal bone metastases, number of metastases in vertebral body, metastases to major internal organs, primary site of cancer, severity of spinal cord palsy
  - Excisional operation > 9 points
  - Palliative operation < 5 points
- Surgical stratification
  - Grade of malignancy (slow growth = 1 point; rapid growth = 4 points)
  - Visceral metastases (no metastasis = 0 points; untreatable = 4 points)
  - Bone metastases (solitary = 1 point; multiple = 2 points)
    - Total of 2-3 points suggests wide excision for long-term local control
    - Total of 8-10 points indicates nonoperative supportive care

Gross Pathologic & Surgical Features

- Softened, eroded bone ± adjacent soft tissue mass

Microscopic Features

- Varies with histology of primary tumor and osseous response

CLINICAL ISSUES

Presentation

- Most common signs/symptoms
  - Neck pain, stiff neck, &/or headache
  - Neurologic symptoms are uncommon
    - When present, more likely from instability than due to epidural tumor
- Clinical profile
  - Neck pain in patient with known primary tumor

Demographics

- Age
  - Most commonly, middle aged to elderly
- Epidemiology
  - Spine is most frequent site of skeletal metastases
    - 10-40% of patients with systemic cancer
    - Account for 40% of all bone metastases

Natural History & Prognosis

- Prognosis varies with histology of primary lesion
- Spine metastases usually indicate advanced disease
- Progressive course leading to pathologic fracture &/or spinal cord compression
- Metastases to odontoid process have prognostic significance
  - When fracture is present, patient has 50% risk of mortality

Treatment

- Local treatment
  - Regardless of tumor histology, radiation therapy and hard collar immobilization are initial forms of treatment
  - If fractured, then likely to require internal stabilization
- Vertebroplasty &/or embolization for adjuvant therapy

DIAGNOSTIC CHECKLIST

Consider

- Metastatic disease is top consideration when destructive lesion is present in spine (even if solitary lesion)

Image Interpretation Pearls

- Persistence of low T1 signal in marrow after therapy may be either residual active tumor or fibrosis

SELECTED REFERENCES

1. De la Garza-Ramos R et al: Vertebroplasty and kyphoplasty for cervical spine metastases: a systematic review and meta-analysis. Int J Spine Surg. 10:7, 2016
2. Rosenberg E et al: Cervical Spine pain as a presenting complaint in metastatic pancreatic cancer: a case report. Postgrad Med. 128(3):331-3, 2016
3. Xu R et al: Metastasis to the occipitocervical junction: A case report and review of the literature. Surg Neurol Int. 1:16, 2010
4. Guillevin R et al: Spine metastasis imaging: review of the literature. J Neuroradiol. 34(5):311-21, 2007
5. Tokuhashi Y et al: A revised scoring system for preoperative evaluation of metastatic spine tumor prognosis. Spine (Phila Pa 1976). 30(19):2186-91, 2005
6. Aebi M: Spinal metastasis in the elderly. Eur Spine J. 12 Suppl 2:S202-13, 2003
7. Lipton A: Bone metastases in breast cancer. Curr Treat Options Oncol. 4(2):151-8, 2003
8. Bilsky MH et al: Diagnosis and management of a metastatic tumor in the atlantoaxial spine. Spine (Phila Pa 1976). 27(10):1062-9, 2002

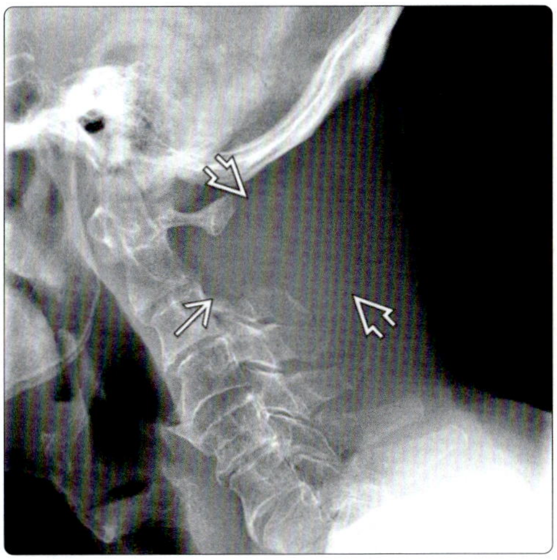

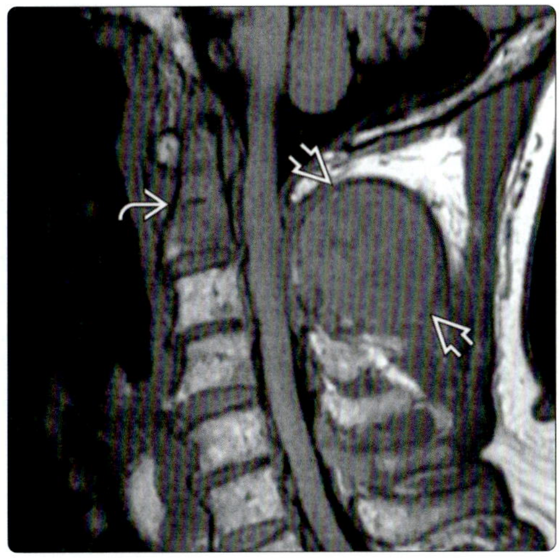

(Left) *Lateral radiograph shows a large soft tissue mass → replacing the C2 neural arch. Destruction of the superior margin of the C3 lateral masses → is also seen. Extension of destruction from one bone to another is not common in metastatic disease.* **(Right)** *Sagittal T1WI MR in the same patient shows a large lesion of the C2 neural arch →. Marrow replacement of the odontoid process is also evident ↷. Radiographs did not reveal the odontoid process involvement. MR is more sensitive for lesion detection.*

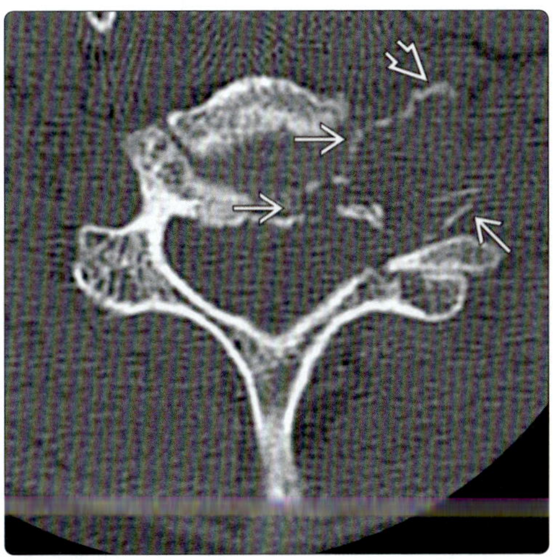

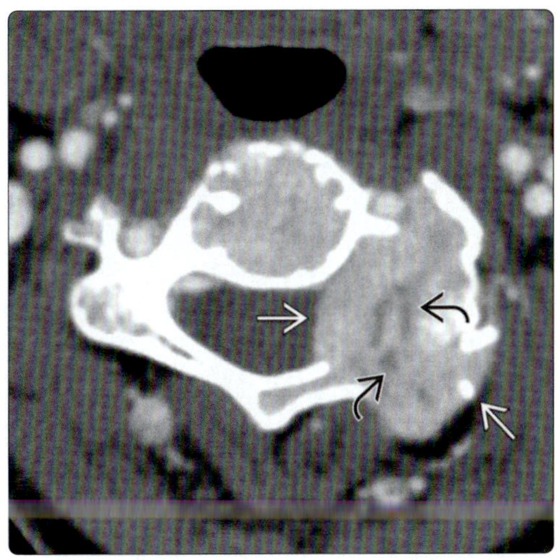

(Left) *Axial NECT shows a typical metastatic lesion with bone destruction →. The eggshell-like fragments → of bone are not tumor mineralization.* **(Right)** *On this axial CTA, the soft tissue mass of this thyroid metastasis shows intense enhancement → indicative of its hypervascular nature. Small, central, nonenhancing foci represent areas of necrosis ↷. Thyroid and renal cell carcinomas and melanomas tend to be hypervascular as well as expansile.*

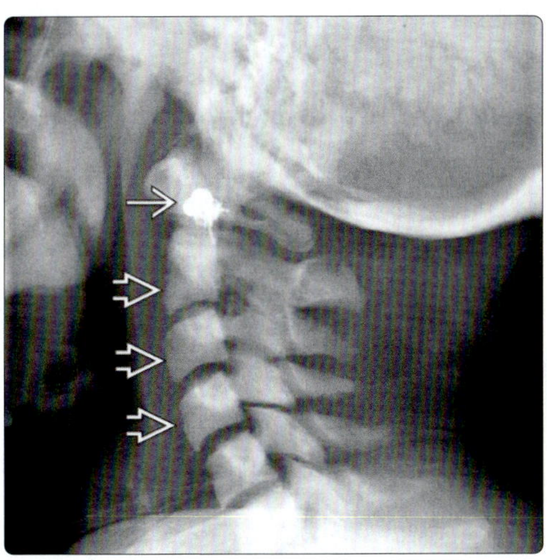

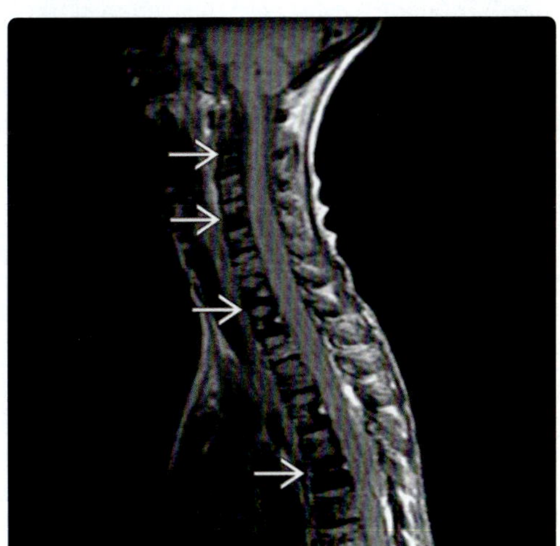

(Left) *Lateral radiograph of a patient with widespread blastic metastases from breast cancer shows that the cervical vertebra and skull base are diffusely sclerotic →. The patient's earrings → create artifact on the study.* **(Right)** *Sagittal T1WI MR shows multiple osteoblastic metastases →. The lesions are all extremely hypointense, indicative of their blastic nature. The same signal intensity should be evident on all sequences.*

Fibrous Dysplasia, Cervical Spine

KEY FACTS

TERMINOLOGY

- Benign fibroosseous lesion with immature woven bone and fibrous stroma

IMAGING

- Neural arch > vertebral body
- Monostotic (70%) more common than polyostotic
  - Cervical spine fibrous dysplasia (FD) more common in polyostotic FD
- Radiography and CT: Fusiform expansion, intact cortex ± cortical thinning
  - Ground-glass matrix ± cystic-appearing foci
  - Matrix ranges from purely lytic to purely sclerotic
  - May contain islands of cartilage
  - Narrow zone of transition ± sclerotic margin
- T1WI: Low to intermediate signal intensity
- T2WI: Heterogeneous intermediate to high signal intensity
  - Low-signal rim reflecting rim of cortical bone
- Variable enhancement

TOP DIFFERENTIAL DIAGNOSES

- Aneurysmal bone cyst
- Paget disease
- Osteoid osteoma
- Osteoblastoma
- Tuberous sclerosis
- Osteosarcoma

PATHOLOGY

- Stroma of bland fibrous tissue
- Small spicules of immature woven bone
- Alphabet soup or Chinese character appearance
- Occasionally has foci of cartilage

CLINICAL ISSUES

- Typically incidental finding; pain if symptomatic
- Growth disturbance, pathologic fracture, and scoliosis (40%) are common in polyostotic form

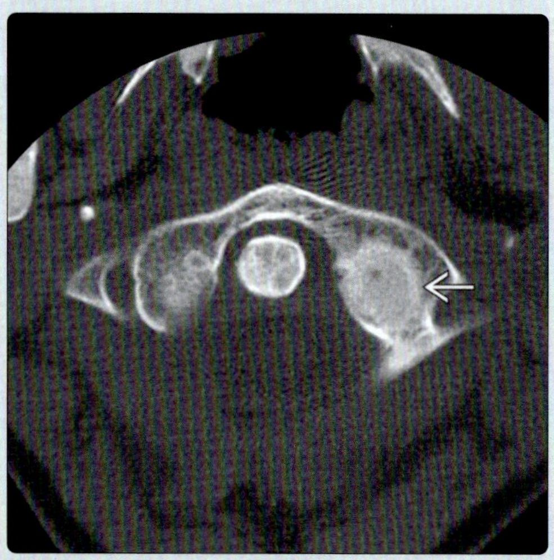

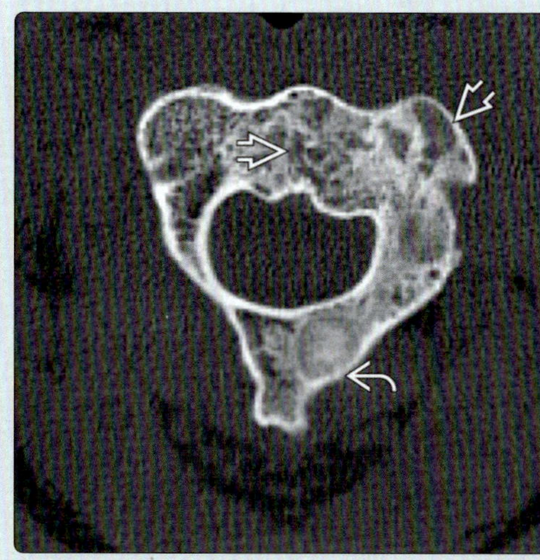

(Left) *Axial bone CT in a patient with polyostotic fibrous dysplasia shows a purely sclerotic lesion in the lateral mass of C1 ➔. This was an incidental discovery.* **(Right)** *Axial NECT shows a lesion of C2 that has several different patterns of internal architecture. The central body and left neural arch have expanded. Ground-glass opacity is seen throughout most of the lesion. A focal area of sclerosis ➔ and small cystic areas ➔ are also present.*

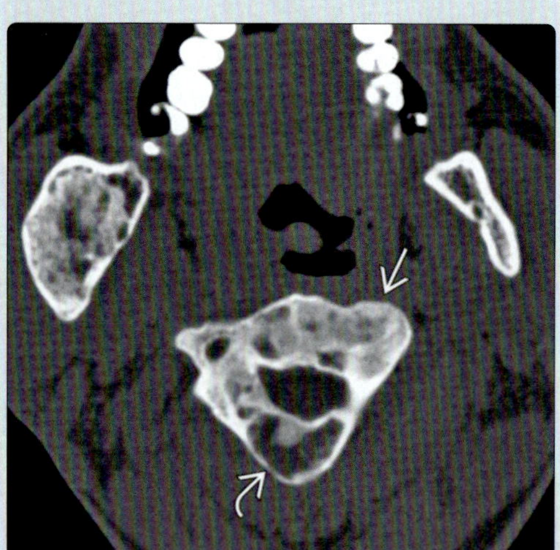

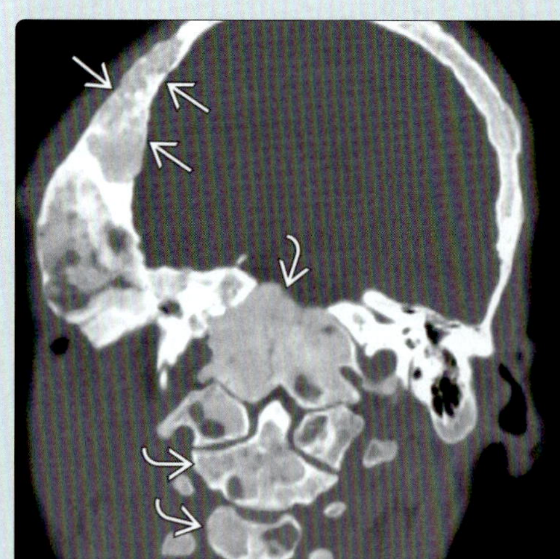

(Left) *Axial bone CT of polyostotic disease shows involvement of C2 and the mandible. Involvement of craniofacial structures is common in polyostotic disease. The involved bones show typical expansion ➔ and ground-glass opacity mixed with lucent foci ➔.* **(Right)** *Coronal bone CT shows loss of normal trabeculae in the majority of the included bones in this polyostotic presentation of fibrous dysplasia, replaced by ground-glass matrix ➔. Thinning of tables of skull ➔ is a characteristic finding.*

TERMINOLOGY

Abbreviations

- Fibrous dysplasia (FD)

Definitions

- Benign fibroosseous lesion with immature woven bone and fibrous stroma

IMAGING

General Features

- Location
  - Neural arch > vertebral body
  - Monostotic (70%) more common than polyostotic
  - Monostotic: Rare in spine, only 1.4% of all FD
    - 36% of monostotic **spine** FD occur in cervical spine
  - Polyostotic: Cervical spine involved in 7%
    - Cervical spine FD more common in polyostotic FD
    - Associated growth disturbances
  - McCune-Albright syndrome: Polyostotic FD, precocious puberty, café au lait skin lesions
  - Mazabraud syndrome: Associated soft tissue myxomas

Radiographic Findings

- Radiography
  - Fusiform expansion, intact cortex ± cortical thinning
  - Ground-glass matrix ± cystic-appearing foci
    - Matrix ranges from purely lytic to purely sclerotic
    - May contain islands of cartilage
  - Narrow zone of transition ± sclerotic margin

CT Findings

- Better visualization of matrix and transition zone than on radiographs

MR Findings

- T1WI
  - Low to intermediate signal intensity
- T2WI FS
  - Heterogeneous intermediate to high signal intensity
  - Low-signal rim reflecting rim of cortical bone
- T1WI C+
  - Variable enhancement

Nuclear Medicine Findings

- Bone scan
  - Mild to marked radionuclide uptake, ↓ with age

Imaging Recommendations

- Best imaging tool
  - CT scan: 1- to 3-mm sections

DIFFERENTIAL DIAGNOSIS

Aneurysmal Bone Cyst

- Balloon-like expansion of neural arch
- Fluid-fluid levels on CT or MR
- Can be associated with fibrous dysplasia

Paget Disease

- Lytic phase may appear similar
- Paget disease thickens cortex and trabeculae
- FD thins cortex and replaces trabeculae

Osteoblastoma

- Usually shows more discrete bone matrix
- May mimic ground-glass matrix

Tuberous Sclerosis

- Sclerotic bone lesions
- Characteristic brain abnormalities

Osteosarcoma

- ± amorphous, immature bone matrix
- Wide zone of transition, periosteal reaction, cortical destruction, soft tissue mass

PATHOLOGY

General Features

- Genetics
  - Sporadic mutation in *GNAS1* gene
- Associated abnormalities
  - Endocrine abnormalities: Hyperparathyroidism, acromegaly, premature puberty, phosphaturia
  - May have associated aneurysmal bone cyst

Gross Pathologic & Surgical Features

- White or tan lesion with gritty consistency

Microscopic Features

- Stroma of bland fibrous tissue
- Small spicules of immature woven bone
  - Alphabet soup or Chinese character appearance
- Occasionally has foci of cartilage

CLINICAL ISSUES

Presentation

- Most common signs/symptoms
  - Typically incidental finding; pain if symptomatic

Demographics

- Age
  - Polyostotic disease: 1st-2nd decades
  - Monostotic spine disease: 3rd-5th decades
- Gender
  - M = F
- Epidemiology
  - 7% of all benign skeletal tumors

Natural History & Prognosis

- Usually no significant sequelae in spine disease
- Growth disturbance, pathologic fracture, and scoliosis (40%) are common in polyostotic form
- Rarely undergoes sarcomatous transformation

SELECTED REFERENCES

1. Zhong H et al: Monostotic fibrous dysplasia of cervical spine. Joint Bone Spine. ePub, 2014
2. Lee SH et al: Cervical fibrous dysplasia presenting as a pathologic fracture in an older patient. J Korean Neurosurg Soc. 50(2):139-42, 2011
3. Meredith DS et al: Twenty-year follow-up of monostotic fibrous dysplasia of the second cervical vertebra: a case report and review of the literature. J Bone Joint Surg Am. 93(13):e74, 2011
4. Mancini F et al: Scoliosis and spine involvement in fibrous dysplasia of bone. Eur Spine J. 18(2):196-202, 2009

Tumoral Calcinosis

KEY FACTS

TERMINOLOGY

- Benign periarticular soft tissue hyperplasia, calcification

IMAGING

- Nonaggressive-appearing calcific mass centered about large synovial joints
- Predilection for large joints
  - Spinal involvement uncommon
- Radiographs/CT
  - Calcific mass with clustered calcific aggregates surrounding joint
- T1/T2/STIR
  - Lobulated low-signal masses centered on facet joint
  - Minimal enhancement

TOP DIFFERENTIAL DIAGNOSES

- Calcium pyrophosphate deposition disease
- Primary bone tumor
- Synovial osteochondromatosis
- Synovial cyst
- Calcific tendinitis, longus coli

PATHOLOGY

- 3 clinical settings
  - Complication of renal dialysis
  - Familial: Painless lesions develop in affected members
  - Sporadic: Patients with degenerated or inflamed tissue

CLINICAL ISSUES

- Symptomatic treatment, rare surgical excision
- Evaluate for underlying metabolic abnormality

DIAGNOSTIC CHECKLIST

- Tumoral calcinosis is diagnosis of exclusion
- Recognition of this entity important
  - Benign nature, potentially confused with malignant bone tumor

(Left) *CT study shows lobulated margins of a mass at the anterior C1 articulation* ➡*, which shows slightly increased attenuation, similar to milk of calcium appearance. There is no bone destruction and no new bone formation.* **(Right)** *MR study shows a low T2 signal intensity mass with well-defined margins ventral to the anterior atlantodental joint* ➡*. The bone marrow signal of C1, C2, and clivus is normal.*

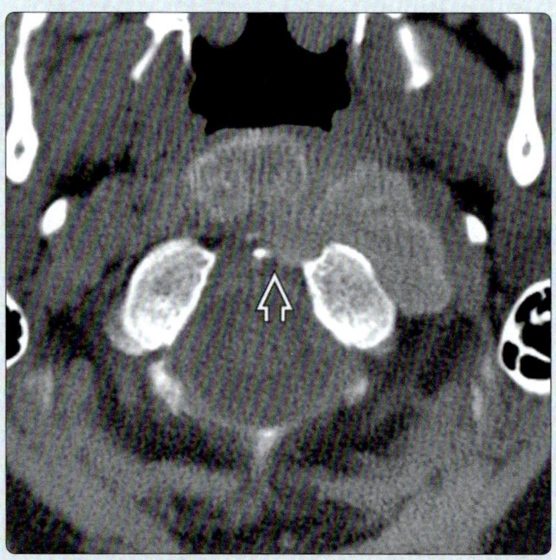

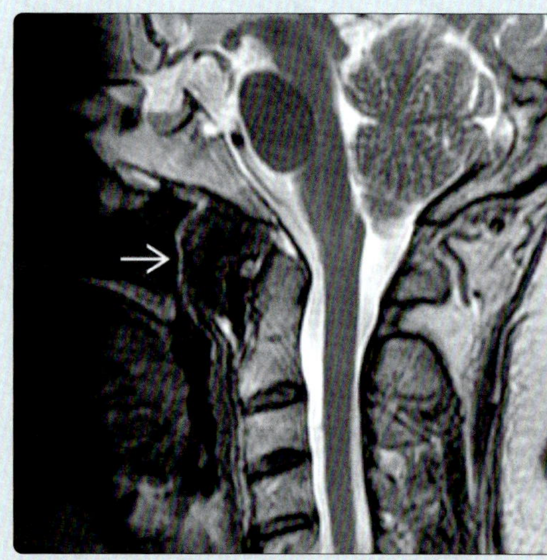

(Left) *Axial T2WI MR study shows a low T2 signal intensity, mildly lobulated mass with well-defined margins ventral to the anterior atlantodental joint* ➡*.* **(Right)** *Axial NECT through the cervical spine shows lobulated density* ➡ *surrounding the facet joint with well-defined margins and no soft tissue component. (Courtesy N. Stence, MD.)*

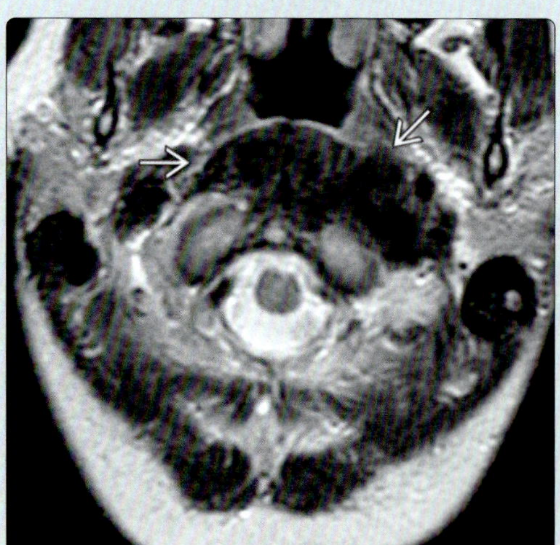

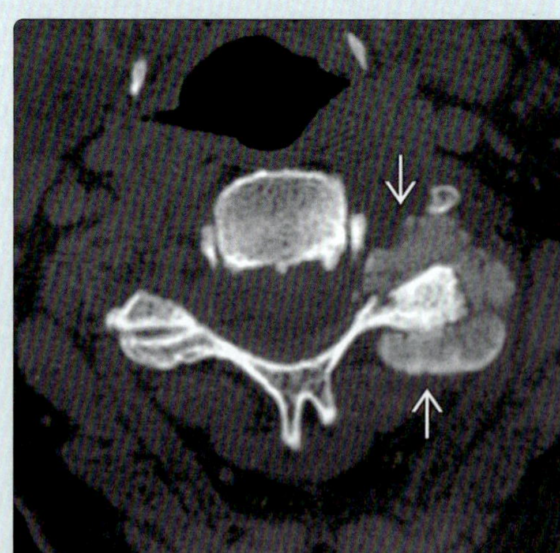

TERMINOLOGY

Definitions

- Benign periarticular soft tissue hyperplasia with calcification

IMAGING

General Features

- Best diagnostic clue
  - Rare nonaggressive-appearing calcific mass centered about large synovial joints
- Location
  - Predilection for large joints: Hip, shoulder, elbow
    - Spinal involvement uncommon
- Size
  - Variable
- Morphology
  - Well-defined calcific mass

Radiographic Findings

- Radiography
  - Calcific mass with clustered calcific aggregates surrounding joint
  - May show bone remodeling, without bone destruction

CT Findings

- NECT
  - Calcific mass with clustered calcific aggregates surrounding joint
  - No evidence of bone destruction
  - No significant soft tissue mass that is **not** calcified

MR Findings

- T1WI
  - Lobulated low-signal masses centered on facet joint
  - May extend into adjacent paraspinal soft tissue
  - Diagnosis difficult on MR; may need CT confirmation
- T2WI
  - Lobulated, low-signal masses
- T1WI C+
  - Minimal enhancement

Imaging Recommendations

- Best imaging tool
  - CT shows calcific lesions, extent, and presence or absence of bone destruction

DIFFERENTIAL DIAGNOSIS

Calcium Pyrophosphate Deposition Disease

- Calcification involving ligamentum flavum and transverse ligament

Primary Bone Tumor

- Ill-defined margins, infiltrative, bone destruction
- Large enhancing soft tissue component

Synovial Osteochondromatosis

- Usually affects larger joints as does tumoral calcinosis
- Multiple intraarticular densities on CT, 2D imaging

Infection/Septic Facet

- Joint effusion, with bone destruction
- Peripheral enhancement of epidural abscess

Synovial Cyst

- Well-defined mass arising from ventral margin of facet joint/ligamentum flavum
- T2 central high signal, peripheral low signal

Calcific Tendinitis, Longus Coli

- More focal, well-defined calcification
- Not centered on joint

PATHOLOGY

General Features

- Etiology
  - 3 clinical settings
    - Complication of renal dialysis
    - Familial: Painless lesions develop in affected members, usually before age of 20 years
      - Heritable abnormality of vitamin D metabolism
    - Sporadic: Patients with degenerated or inflamed tissue
      - No abnormalities in calcium, phosphate, or vitamin D metabolism
      - Traumatic theory: Microtrauma of connective tissues around joints, bleeding, and formation of rudimentary bursae initial event
- Genetics
  - Most cases spontaneous and sporadic
- Associated abnormalities
  - Chronic renal failure
    - Estimated incidence 0.5-7% of hemodialysis patients
  - Systemic sclerosis

Gross Pathologic & Surgical Features

- Calcific mass, with solid and "milk of calcium" components

CLINICAL ISSUES

Presentation

- Most common signs/symptoms
  - Painless enlargement of joint
  - Other signs/symptoms
    - May cause neural compression → radiculopathy, paraparesis, or sensory deficits

Natural History & Prognosis

- Progressive; multiple locations may be involved

Treatment

- Options, risks, complications
  - Symptomatic treatment, rare surgical excision
  - Evaluate for underlying metabolic abnormality

SELECTED REFERENCES

1. Ashraf A et al: Infantile tumoral calcinosis of the cervical spine presenting as torticollis. Clin Imaging. 40(1):161-3, 2016
2. Sambataro D et al: Tumoral calcinosis of the spine in the course of systemic sclerosis: report of a new case and review of the literature. Clin Exp Rheumatol. 33(4 Suppl 91):S175-8, 2015
3. Sasaki O et al: Tumoral calcinosis involving the cervical spine. Surg Neurol Int. 6:109, 2015

PART III
SECTION 1

Teeth

Alterations in Tooth Number

Extra Teeth 844
Missing Teeth 846

Alterations in Tooth Morphology/Shape

Crown Changes 848
Root Changes 850

DIFFERENTIAL DIAGNOSIS

Common

- Hyperdontia: Isolated Teeth

Less Common

- Hyperdontia: Associated With Cleft Palate

Rare but Important

- Cleidocranial Dysplasia
- Gardner Syndrome (Familial Adenomatous Polyposis)

ESSENTIAL INFORMATION

Key Differential Diagnosis Issues

- Isolated supernumerary teeth very common
- Multiple supernumerary teeth may indicate accompanying systemic or inherited disorder

Helpful Clues for Common Diagnoses

- **Hyperdontia: Isolated Teeth**
    - Key facts
        - Mesiodens > distodens > premolars, canines, lateral incisors
        - **Mesiodens** seen in anterior maxilla, most often palatal to incisor teeth
            - Often presents in pairs
        - Will occasionally erupt between central incisors
        - **Distodens** (distomolar, paramolar) seen distal to, lingual to, or buccal to maxillary or mandibular 3rd molar
        - Extra premolars, canines, lateral incisors seen in either jaw
        - May be erupted or unerupted (potential for development of dentigerous cysts)
        - May cause crowding, malocclusion
    - Imaging
        - Often smaller than surrounding teeth (microdonts)
        - Crowns often conical
        - Surrounding follicular space present if unerupted
        - 3D imaging useful for localization

Helpful Clues for Less Common Diagnoses

- **Hyperdontia: Associated With Cleft Palate**
    - Key facts
        - AD-inherited disorder
        - Teeth usually missing in area of cleft
        - Supernumerary teeth sometimes seen in other areas of jaws
    - Imaging
        - May be fully formed or malformed, erupted or unerupted

Helpful Clues for Rare Diagnoses

- **Cleidocranial Dysplasia**
    - Key facts
        - Absent or hypoplastic clavicles along with other skeletal anomalies
        - Multiple supernumerary teeth, often unerupted
        - Retained primary teeth
        - Delayed eruption of permanent teeth
    - Imaging
        - Open skull sutures
        - Wormian bones
        - Dense, coarse trabecular pattern
        - Multiple unerupted teeth, both permanent and supernumerary
- **Gardner Syndrome (Familial Adenomatous Polyposis)**
    - Key facts
        - Familial colorectal polyposis and epidermoid cysts of skin
        - Multiple osteomas
    - Imaging
        - Multiple supernumerary teeth

SELECTED REFERENCES

1. Lubinsky M et al: Syndromes with supernumerary teeth. Am J Med Genet A. 170(10):2611-6, 2016
2. Oliveira MR et al: Gardner syndrome with unusual maxillofacial manifestation. J Craniofac Surg. 27(5):1253-5, 2016
3. Jamilian A et al: Hypodontia and supernumerary and impacted teeth in children with various types of clefts. Am J Orthod Dentofacial Orthop. 147(2):221-5, 2015

Hyperdontia: Isolated Teeth

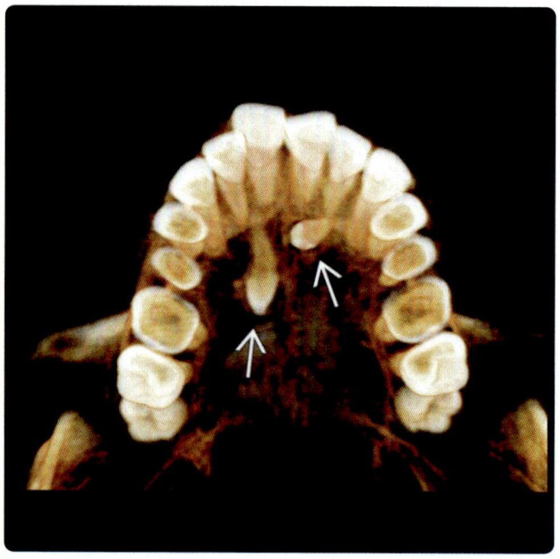

Hyperdontia: Isolated Teeth

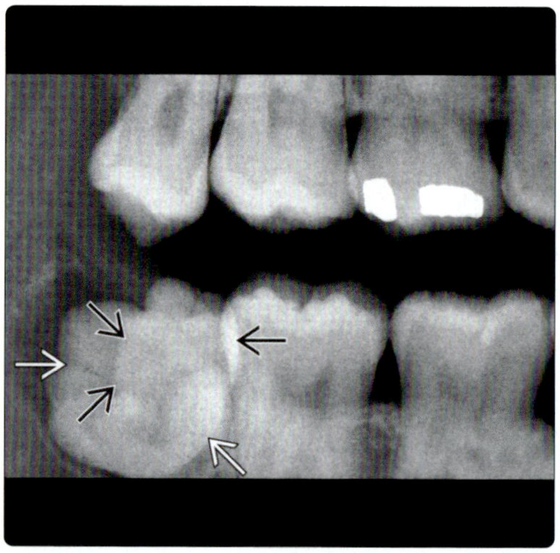

(Left) *Axial format 3D CBCT exhibits 2 mesiodens, both oriented to the posterior* ➡*. It is common that when 1 mesiodens is noted, a 2nd one is present as well.* **(Right)** *Bitewing radiograph shows a horizontally impacted 3rd molar with the occlusal table oriented lingually* ➡ *and a superimposed 4th molar (distodens)* ⇨ *that was located toward the buccal cortical plate.*

Hyperdontia: Isolated Teeth

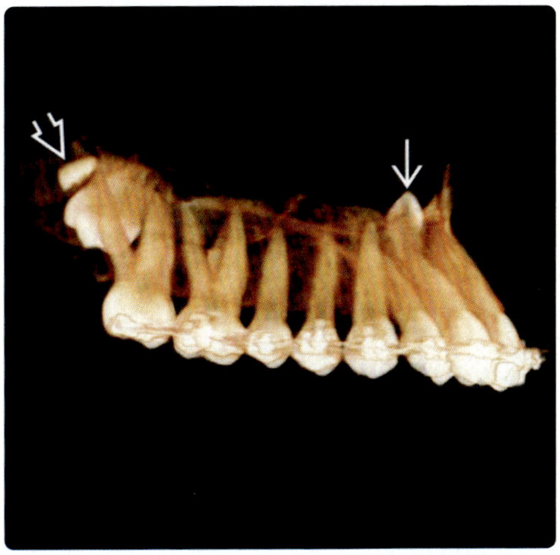

Hyperdontia: Isolated Teeth

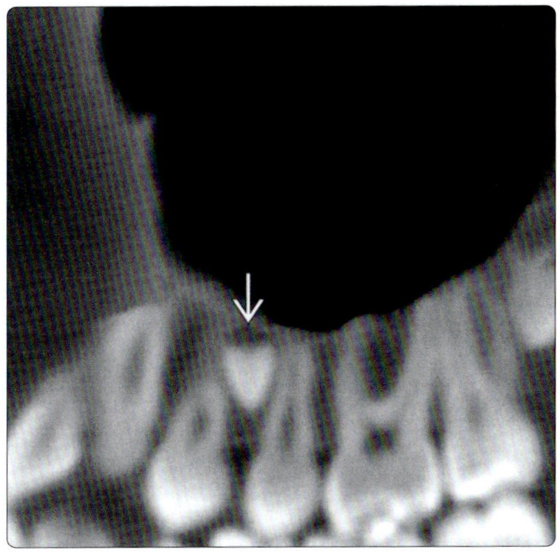

(Left) *Sagittal reformat 3D CBCT of a 14-year-old girl shows an inverted mesiodens* ⇨ *with the crown protruding into the nasal fossa. The patient was imaged to plan for surgical extraction of the mesiodens. Note the developing 4th molar (distodens)* ➡*, which was not visible on panoramic view and was found incidentally.* **(Right)** *Corrected sagittal plane CBCT depicts a small, conical supernumerary tooth in the premolar area* ➡*. There was a similar finding on the contralateral side.*

Hyperdontia: Associated With Cleft Palate

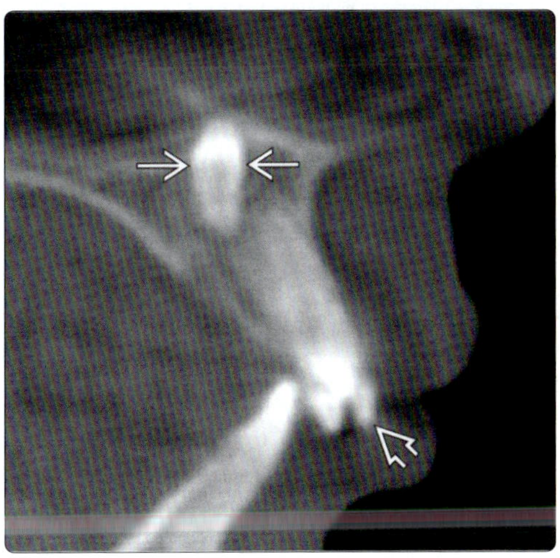

Cleidocranial Dysplasia

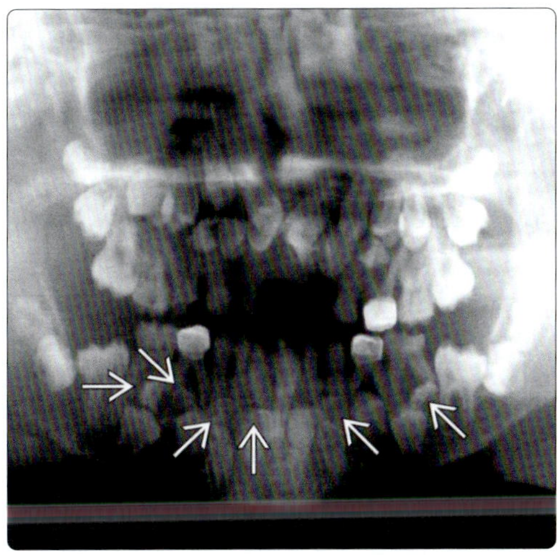

(Left) *Sagittal plane CBCT shows a small supernumerary tooth apical to this cleft palate patient's lateral incisor on the unaffected side* ➡*. There was also an additional erupted lateral incisor* ⇨*.* **(Right)** *Cropped panoramic radiograph demonstrates multiple unerupted teeth in a mixed dentition patient with cleidocranial dysplasia. It is often difficult in these patients to differentiate supernumerary teeth from the normal developing dentition. Supernumerary teeth in the mandible have been identified* ➡*.*

Cleidocranial Dysplasia

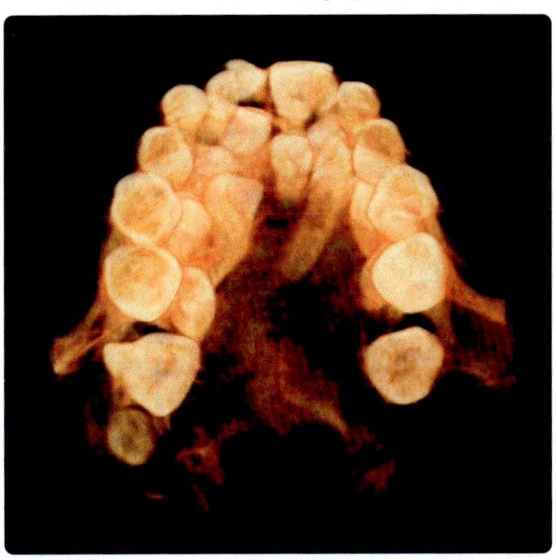

Gardner Syndrome (Familial Adenomatous Polyposis)

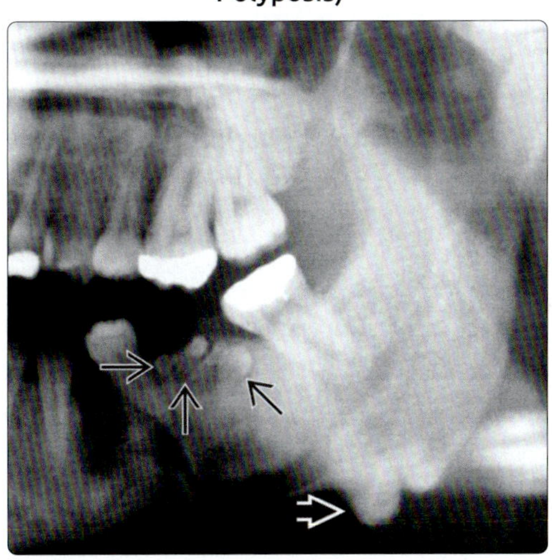

(Left) *3D CBCT reconstruction shows multiple supernumerary teeth in the maxilla of this 14-year-old girl with cleidocranial dysplasia. CBCT is helpful in determining morphology and developmental stage of the unerupted teeth for orthodontic treatment planning.* **(Right)** *Cropped panoramic radiograph shows multiple small, unerupted supernumerary teeth* ➡ *in a patient with Gardner syndrome. Note the presence of an osteoma* ⇨ *at the angle of the mandible. (Courtesy B. Pass, DDS.)*

DIFFERENTIAL DIAGNOSIS

Common

- Hypodontia: Isolated Missing Teeth

Less Common

- Hypodontia: Associated With Cleft Palate

Rare but Important

- Ectodermal Dysplasia
- Basal Cell Nevus Syndrome (Gorlin-Goltz Syndrome)
- Rieger Syndrome
- Focal Dermal Hypoplasia

ESSENTIAL INFORMATION

Key Differential Diagnosis Issues

- Isolated missing teeth very common
    - Familial or sporadic
- Evaluation for syndromes warranted if multiple teeth are missing (especially canines &/or 1st molars)

Helpful Clues for Common Diagnoses

- **Hypodontia: Isolated Missing Teeth**
    - Key facts
        - Most often involves last or most distal of tooth type
        - **Missing 3rd molars > 2nd premolars > lateral incisors**
        - Strong familial tendencies
    - Imaging
        - Intraoral, panoramic images show condition
        - CBCT useful when multiple teeth are affected or when cleft is present

Helpful Clues for Less Common Diagnoses

- **Hypodontia: Associated With Cleft Palate**
    - Key facts
        - Missing teeth in area of cleft; anterior teeth most often affected, especially lateral incisor
    - Imaging
        - CBCT & 3D reconstruction aids in planning treatment

Helpful Clues for Rare Diagnoses

- **Ectodermal Dysplasia**
    - Key facts
        - Decreased number of sweat glands
        - Sparse hair, eyelashes, eyebrows, cleft palate, photophobia
    - Imaging
        - Multiple missing teeth & abnormal (conical) crowns
- **Basal Cell Nevus Syndrome (Gorlin-Goltz Syndrome)**
    - Key facts
        - Multiple basal cell carcinomas
        - Rib (bifid) or vertebral anomalies
        - Missing teeth may or may not occur
    - Imaging
        - Calcification of falx cerebri
        - Odontogenic keratocysts (keratocystic odontogenic tumors) seen bilaterally as uni- or multilocular radiolucencies in jaws
- **Rieger Syndrome**
    - Key facts
        - Ocular abnormalities (cornea, iris, glaucoma)
        - Mild craniofacial abnormalities
    - Imaging
        - Multiple missing teeth frequently seen
- **Focal Dermal Hypoplasia**
    - Key facts
        - Abnormalities of skin, hair, eyes
        - Skeletal abnormalities
    - Imaging
        - Hypodontia, abnormalities of palate

SELECTED REFERENCES

1. Al-Abdallah M et al: Prevalence and distribution of dental anomalies: a comparison between maxillary and mandibular tooth agenesis. Am J Orthod Dentofacial Orthop. 148(5):793-8, 2015
2. Rakhshan V: Congenitally missing teeth (hypodontia): a review of the literature concerning the etiology, prevalence, risk factors, patterns and treatment. Dent Res J (Isfahan). 12(1):1-13, 2015
3. Lasocki AL et al: A case of mosaic Goltz syndrome (focal dermal hypoplasia) in a male patient. Australas J Dermatol. 52(1):48-51, 2011

Hypodontia: Isolated Missing Teeth

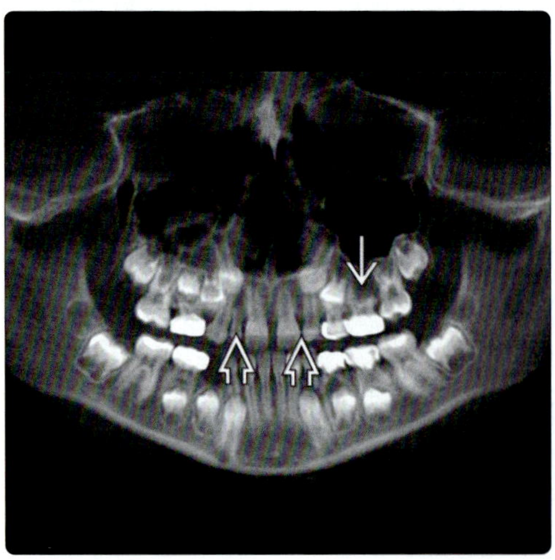

Hypodontia: Isolated Missing Teeth

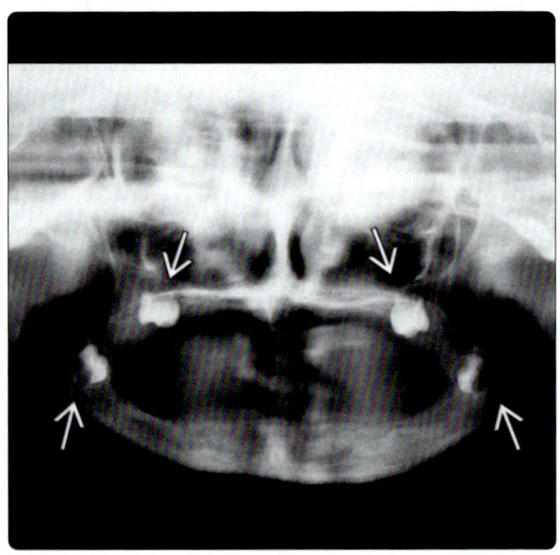

(Left) *Panoramic reformat CBCT shows missing maxillary left 2nd premolar ➔ (primary molar is retained) and permanent lateral incisors ➔ (primary teeth retained). These are both commonly missing permanent teeth.* **(Right)** *Cropped panoramic radiograph of a 13-year-old girl is shown. The patient was congenitally missing all teeth except the developing 3rd molars ➔. There was no known syndrome or medical treatment in childhood associated with this patient.*

Hypodontia: Isolated Missing Teeth

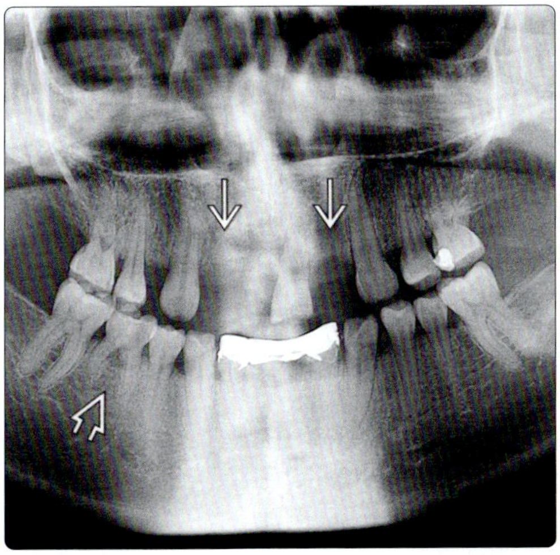

Hypodontia: Isolated Missing Teeth

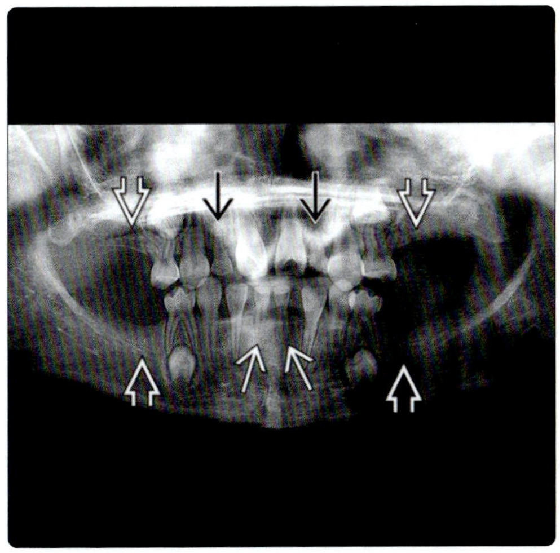

(Left) *Cropped panoramic radiograph shows multiple congenitally missing teeth in this teenager, including permanent molars, maxillary and mandibular premolars, and maxillary lateral incisors.* **(Right)** *Cropped panoramic radiograph in this 11-year-old sibling of the previous patient shows multiple missing teeth, including all permanent molars, 2nd premolars, and permanent maxillary lateral and mandibular central incisors. This similar pattern of missing teeth between siblings suggests an inherited trait.*

Hypodontia: Associated With Cleft Palate

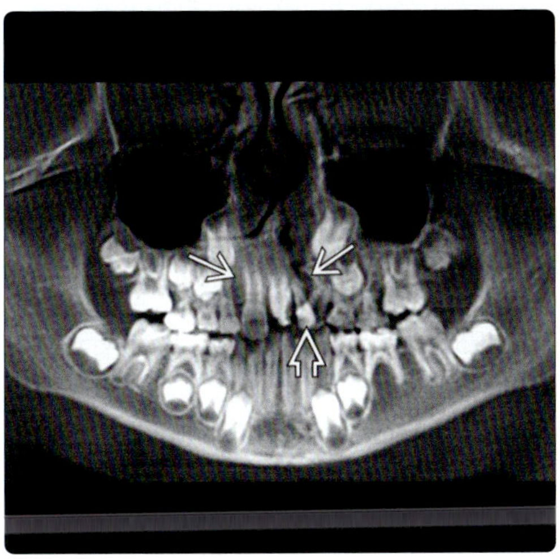

Ectodermal Dysplasia

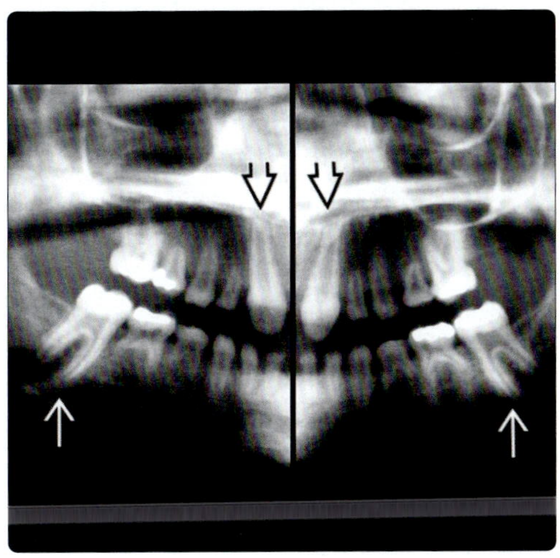

(Left) *Panoramic reformat CBCT shows missing permanent maxillary lateral incisors in a cleft palate patient. It is common for the lateral incisor to be missing on the affected side, but, in this case, it is also missing on the unaffected side. The primary incisor is retained on the affected side.* **(Right)** *Split-image panoramic radiograph in a 9-year-old patient with ectodermal dysplasia depicts the absence of all permanent teeth except the maxillary central incisors and mandibular 1st molars.*

Ectodermal Dysplasia

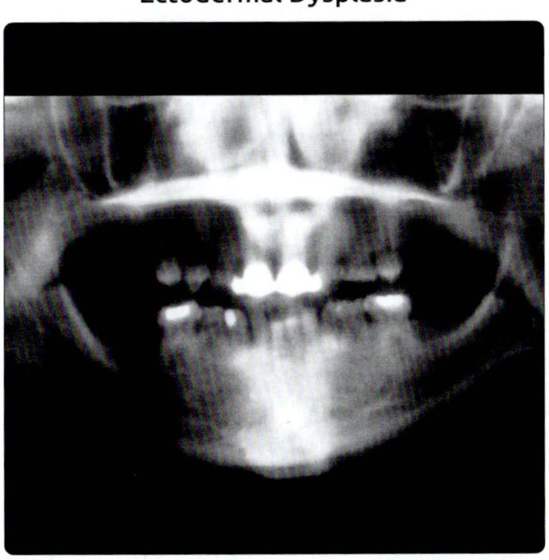

Rieger Syndrome

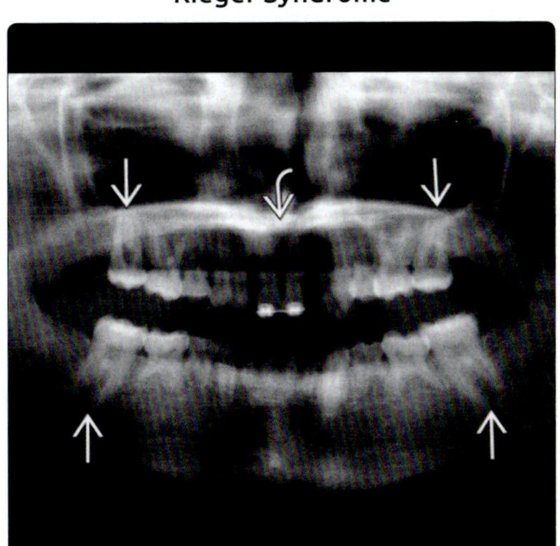

(Left) *Panoramic radiograph shows multiple missing permanent maxillary and mandibular teeth, including molars and premolars in this patient with a rare autosomal-dominant form of ectodermal dysplasia called trichodental dysplasia. Features include fine, dry hair as well as the hypodontia.* **(Right)** *Cropped panoramic radiograph of a 12-year-old girl diagnosed with Axenfeld Rieger syndrome is shown. The only permanent teeth to form were the 1st molars and the maxillary central incisors.*

DIFFERENTIAL DIAGNOSIS

Common

- Dental Caries
- Dental Restorations

Less Common

- Macrodontia
- Microdontia

Rare but Important

- Amelogenesis Imperfecta
- Dentinogenesis Imperfecta
- Dentin Dysplasia
- Regional Odontodysplasia

ESSENTIAL INFORMATION

Helpful Clues for Common Diagnoses

- **Dental Caries**
  - Key facts: More extensive clinically than seen on radiograph
  - Imaging: Intraoral imaging best for detection
- **Dental Restorations**
  - Key facts: Wide variety of materials and types of restorations
  - Imaging
    - May appear radiolucent, mixed, or radiopaque, depending on material used
    - Dense materials create streaking, beam-hardening artifacts on CBCT/CT

Helpful Clues for Less Common Diagnoses

- **Macrodontia**
  - Key facts: Often result of fusion or gemination
  - Imaging: Single large crown or bifid crown with 1 large or 2 separate roots
- **Microdontia**
  - Key facts: Maxillary lateral incisors, 3rd molars, supernumerary teeth most commonly affected
  - Imaging: Unusually small crown, often conical in shape

Helpful Clues for Rare Diagnoses

- **Amelogenesis Imperfecta**
  - Key facts
    - Group of inherited disorders of enamel
    - Appearance ranges from generalized pitting to thin and smooth enamel
  - Imaging
    - Enamel thin or has reduced radiodensity ± visible pitting
- **Dentinogenesis Imperfecta**
  - Key facts
    - Inherited disorder of dentin development
    - Translucent bluish or brownish teeth ("opalescent")
  - Imaging
    - Bulbous crowns, cervical constrictions, thin roots
    - Obliterated pulp chambers and canals
- **Dentin Dysplasia**
  - Key facts
    - Inherited disorders of dentin and pulp
    - Permanent teeth appear normal clinically
  - Imaging
    - Type I: Short roots, crescent-shaped pulps, no root canals; 20% have periapical radiolucencies
    - Type II: Enlarged pulp chambers, pulp stones, thin root canals
- **Regional Odontodysplasia**
  - Key facts
    - **Localized**, noninherited abnormality of teeth (ghost teeth)
  - Imaging
    - Thin enamel and dentin, enlarged pulp, lack of radiographic contrast

SELECTED REFERENCES

1. Al-Abdallah M et al: Prevalence and distribution of dental anomalies: a comparison between maxillary and mandibular tooth agenesis. Am J Orthod Dentofacial Orthop. 148(5):793-8, 2015
2. Lappano R et al: A calixpyrrole derivative acts as an antagonist to GPER, a G-protein coupled receptor: mechanisms and models. Dis Model Mech. 8(10):1237-46, 2015

Dental Caries

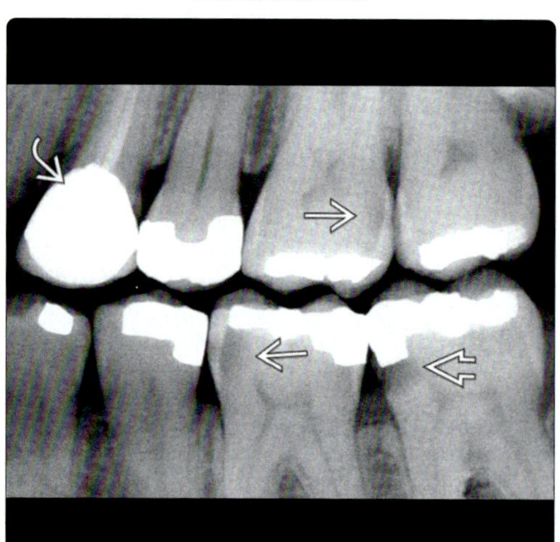

Dental Restorations

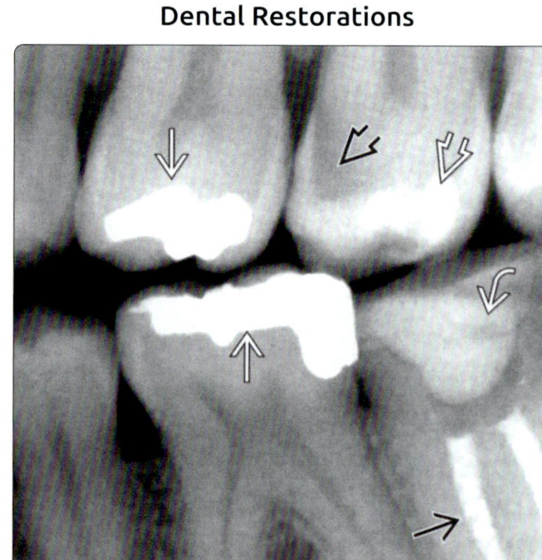

(Left) *Bitewing radiograph shows radiolucent carious lesions in the maxillary and mandibular left 1st molars ➡. There is a recurrent lesion in the mandibular 2nd molar ⇨. Note the porcelain/metal crown on the maxillary 1st premolar ➡.* **(Right)** *Bitewing radiograph depicts a variety of dental materials including amalgam ➡, posterior resin ➡, temporary cement ➡, and gutta percha ⇨ root-filling material. Note caries ⇨ in the maxillary 2nd molar.*

Root Changes

Root Fractures

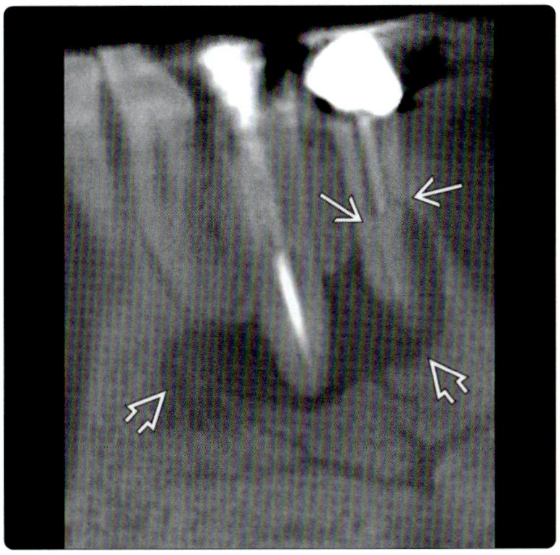

Fused Roots

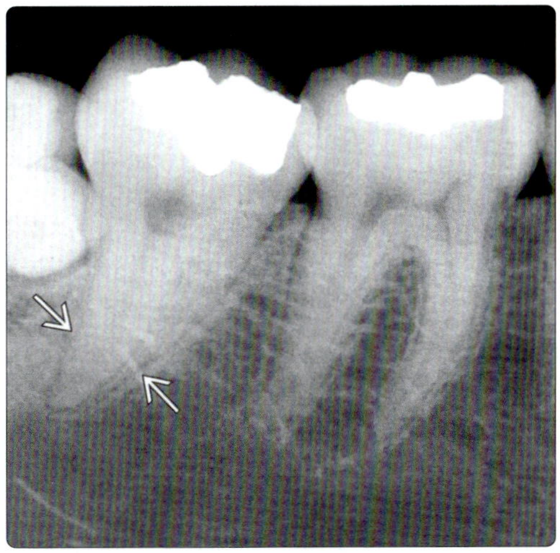

(Left) *Sagittal oblique CBCT exhibits a root fracture on the left mandibular 1st premolar . The fracture lines coincide with the junction of the post and root filling. This is a common site of fracture in endodontically treated teeth. The resulting apical pathosis is extensive and involves multiple teeth .* **(Right)** *Periapical radiograph depicts fused roots on the mandibular right 2nd molar. Most mandibular molars have 2 distinct roots.*

Supernumerary Roots

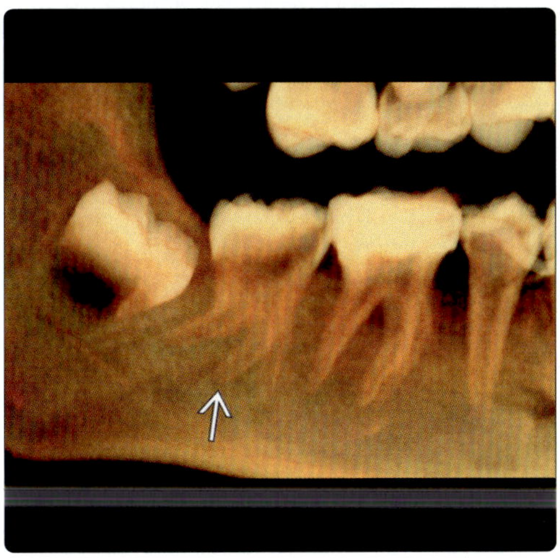

Enamel Pearls

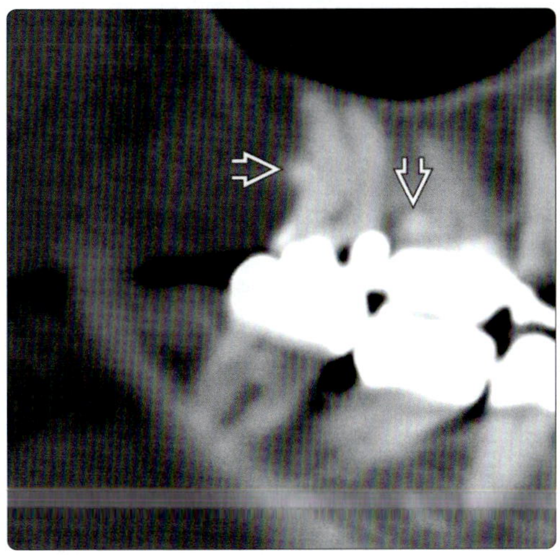

(Left) *3D CBCT viewed from the lingual exhibits a 3-rooted mandibular 2nd molar (radix entomolaris) .* **(Right)** *Corrected sagittal reformat CBCT depicts 2 maxillary molars with enamel pearls at the furcation areas. This is the most common location for enamel pearls. Note the increased density of the pearls compared to the adjacent dentin. Enamel is significantly more mineralized than dentin.*

Dentinogenesis Imperfecta

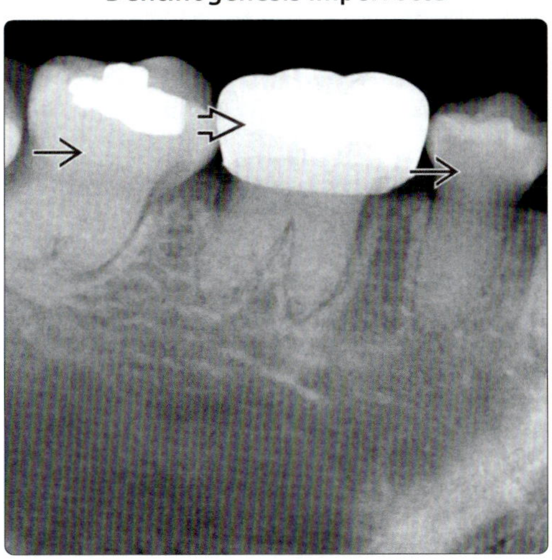

Dentin Dysplasia

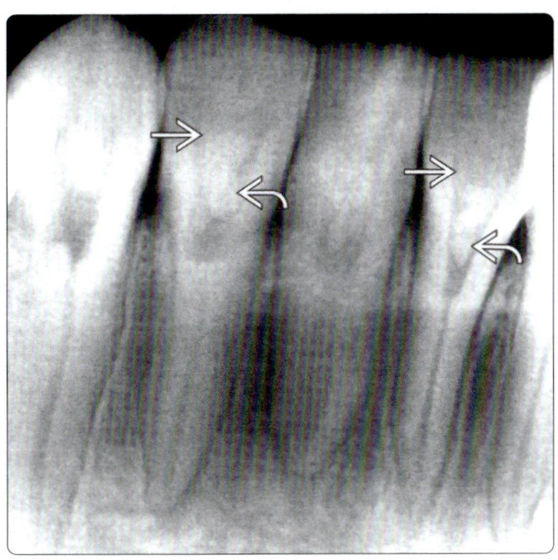

(Left) *Periapical radiograph shows generalized short roots in the right mandible of this patient with dentinogenesis imperfecta. The 1st molar has been restored with a stainless steel crown , most likely as a protective measure. Note the absence of pulp chambers and canals.* **(Right)** *Periapical radiograph shows the thin root canals and enlarged pulp chambers containing calcifications in the mandibular incisors of a patient with dentin dysplasia type II.*

PART III
SECTION 2
Mandible and Maxilla

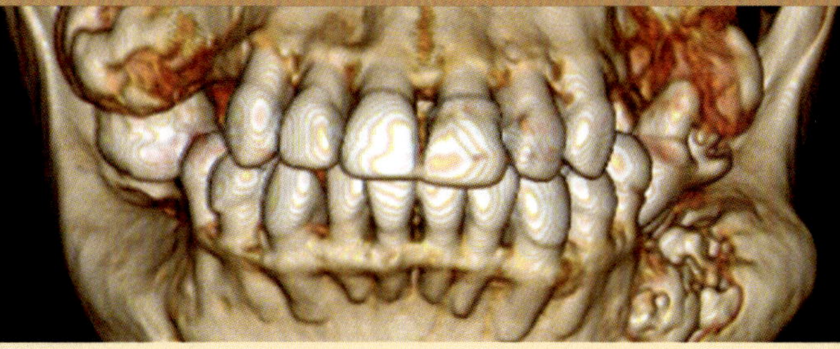

Alterations in Supporting Structures of Teeth

Periapical Radiolucencies 856
Periapical Radiopacities and Mixed Lesions 860
Floating Teeth 862
Widened Periodontal Ligament Space 864
Lamina Dura Changes 866

Radiolucencies

Well-Defined Unilocular Radiolucencies 870
Pericoronal Radiolucencies Without Radiopacities 874
Pericoronal Radiolucencies With Radiopacities 876
Multilocular Radiolucencies 878
Ill-Defined Radiolucencies 882
Generalized Rarefaction 888

Radiopacities

Well-Defined Radiopacities 892
Ground-Glass and Granular Radiopacities [illegible]
Generalized Radiopacities 902

Periosteal Reactions

Periosteal Reactions 906

DIFFERENTIAL DIAGNOSIS

Common

- Periapical Rarefying Osteitis
- Incompletely Formed Root Apex
- Mental Foramen
- Periapical Osseous Dysplasia
- Periapical Scar

Less Common

- Benign Odontogenic Keratocyst
- Osteomyelitis

Rare but Important

- Leukemia
- Metastasis
- Renal osteodystrophy

ESSENTIAL INFORMATION

Key Differential Diagnosis Issues

- **Vitality testing of teeth is key** to differentiating periapical rarefying osteitis from all other lesions

Helpful Clues for Common Diagnoses

- **Periapical Rarefying Osteitis**
  - Key facts
    - Can be abscess, granuloma, or cyst histologically
    - Vitality testing shows nonresponsive tooth
    - Root canal therapy or extraction is treatment
  - Imaging
    - Loss of bone density at apex of tooth
    - Reactive bone (sclerosing osteitis) may surround it
    - **Periapical lamina dura will be eroded** and periodontal ligament space (PDL) space widened
- **Incompletely Formed Root Apex**
  - Key facts
    - Teeth at final stages of development show periapical radiolucencies signifying last of dental papilla
    - Pulp death may occur while apex is still open, superimposing inflammation on dental follicle
    - Correlate to history of trauma and clinical condition of crown
  - Imaging
    - Completely formed root has rounded apex; incompletely formed root has **open, wide apical foramen and pointed dentin**
    - Blunderbuss-shaped apex
- **Mental Foramen**
  - Key facts
    - Normal anatomic landmark in area of mandibular premolar apices
  - Imaging
    - Oval-shaped on periapical radiography
    - Faintly or poorly corticated
    - On 2D imaging, **may superimpose on apices of premolars**
    - 2nd intraoral radiographic image at different horizontal angle will show foramen moving away from apex
    - If apex of tooth is in contact with mandibular canal, may appear similar to draining sinus radiographically
    - Following course of mandibular canal may aid in differentiation
- Periapical Osseous Dysplasia
  - Key facts
    - Teeth are **vital**
    - Common in lower anterior teeth
      - However, can affect any tooth or even multiple teeth
    - Most common in **middle-aged women of African or Asian decent**
    - No biopsy or treatment indicated
    - May be mistaken for periapical rarefying osteitis and erroneously treated with root canal filling
  - Imaging
    - **Early** stage is completely **radiolucent**
    - Small radiopaque flecks may be noted in matrix
    - Calcification becomes more dense with time
    - PDL space and lamina dura may be lost
- **Periapical Scar**
  - Key facts
    - Periapical lesion heals with fibrous connective tissue rather than bone
    - Associated with endodontically treated tooth
    - May also be seen after root amputation (apicoectomy)
  - Imaging
    - Periapical scar looks like periapical rarefying osteitis
    - May be slightly more corticated than inflammatory lesion
    - Amputated root has **blunted apex slanted facially** (seen on CBCT cross sections) and retrograde filling material
    - Facial bone defect (surgical access) may still be present
    - Metallic fragments may be seen in defect

Helpful Clues for Less Common Diagnoses

- **Benign Odontogenic Keratocyst**
  - Key facts
    - Any odontogenic pathology may superimpose on apices of teeth
    - Most commonly odontogenic keratocyst
      - However, may be any odontogenic or nonodontogenic keratocyst
    - Vitality testing of teeth is crucial in diagnosis; **teeth are vital** unless coronal caries or large fillings extending to pulp are present
  - Imaging
    - Corticated expansile lesion
    - May or may not be centered around apex of tooth
    - **Lamina dura** of tooth should be **intact**
    - Odontogenic keratocyst may become infected if root canal treatment to related teeth is done, showing radiographic signs of infection, such as loss of cortication and sclerosis of surrounding bone
- **Osteomyelitis**
  - Key facts
    - Inflammation of bone and bone marrow
    - Patient is febrile, in pain, and may have lymphadenopathy
    - In jawbones, most likely related to infected tooth or tooth socket

- Imaging
  - Early acute osteomyelitis may show **slight decrease in trabeculation**
  - May be progression of periapical rarefying osteitis
  - Other signs of osteomyelitis may be present, such as lamellated periosteal reactions; **sequestra** are hallmark

Helpful Clues for Rare Diagnoses

- **Leukemia**
  - Key facts
    - Malignant tumor of hematopoietic stem cells
    - Acute or chronic myelogenous, acute or chronic lymphoblastic types
    - Chronic leukemia may have no signs and symptoms
    - Acute leukemia patients exhibit malaise, weakness, and bone pain
    - **Teeth may be loose**; gingiva may be swollen, boggy, and ulcerated, and may exhibit petechiae
  - Imaging
    - Most radiographic signs are seen with **acute leukemia**, rarely seen in chronic leukemia
    - Multifocal areas of bone destruction
    - Multiple bilateral ill-defined patchy areas that may coalesce with time
    - May be **centered around apex of tooth**
    - Laminae dura of teeth and cortical boundaries of dental follicles may be effaced
    - May **present apical to developing teeth** and push developing crypts to premature eruption
    - No expansion is noted except in case of chloromas
    - Single lamella of periosteal reaction can be seen, as well as spiculated periosteal reaction
    - **Chloroma**: Foci of destruction may appear as mass and behave like localized malignant tumor; may exhibit spiculated periosteal reaction
- **Metastasis**
  - Key facts
    - May grow within PDL space or at apex of tooth
    - May be mistaken for periapical rarefying osteitis, and tooth may be treated erroneously with root canal filling
    - Vitality testing is recommended; tooth is vital
  - Imaging
    - Ill-defined lytic lesion
    - May or may not be centered over apex of tooth
    - Widening of PDL space may be asymmetric
    - There may be multiple lytic foci
    - Evaluate entire scan or image for other lytic foci signifying seeding of tumor
- **Renal Osteodystrophy**
  - Key facts
    - Secondary to hyperparathyroidism
    - Review of patient's medical history is recommended
  - Imaging
    - Can present as multiple periapical radiolucent lesions
    - Other manifestations: Loss of lamina dura, widened periodontal ligament space, demineralization of bone

SELECTED REFERENCES

1. Bains R et al: Nasopalatine duct cyst mimicking an endodontic periapical lesion: a case report. Gen Dent. 64(1):63-6, 2016
2. Jalali P et al: Multiple periradicular radiolucencies mimicking endodontic lesions in renal osteodystrophy of the mandible: a case report. Int Endod J. 49(7):706-714, 2016
3. Segura-Egea JJ et al: Association between diabetes and the prevalence of radiolucent periapical lesions in root-filled teeth: systematic review and meta-analysis. Clin Oral Investig. 20(6):1133-41, 2016
4. Buraczewski T et al: CLINICOPATHOLOGIC REVIEW: Periapical Radiolucencies & Routine Diagnostic Considerations. Normal anatomy. Pa Dent J (Harrisb). 82(5):36-8, 2015
5. Tatlidil R et al: Mucinous adenocarcinoma of lung presenting as oral metastases: a case report and literature review. J Endod. 37(1):110-3, 2011
6. White SC et al: Oral Radiology: Principles and Interpretation. 6th ed. St. Louis: Mosby Elsevier, 2009
7. Lee JJ et al: Gingival squamous cell carcinoma mimicking a dentoalveolar abscess: report of a case. J Endod. 33(2):177-80, 2007
8. Marmary Y et al: A radiographic survey of periapical jawbone lesions. Oral Surg Oral Med Oral Pathol. 61(4):405-8, 1986

Periapical Rarefying Osteitis

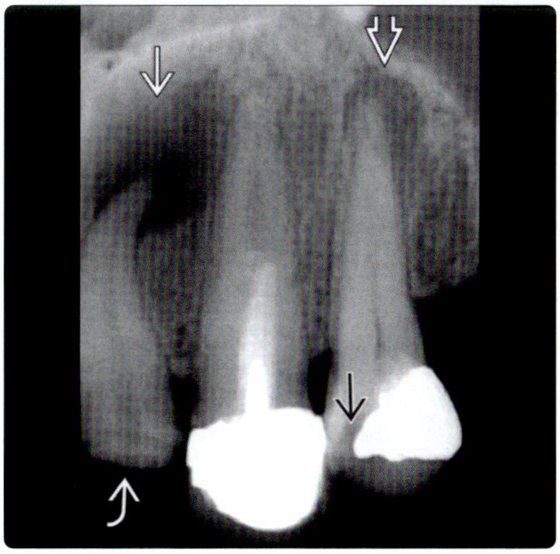

Periapical Rarefying Osteitis

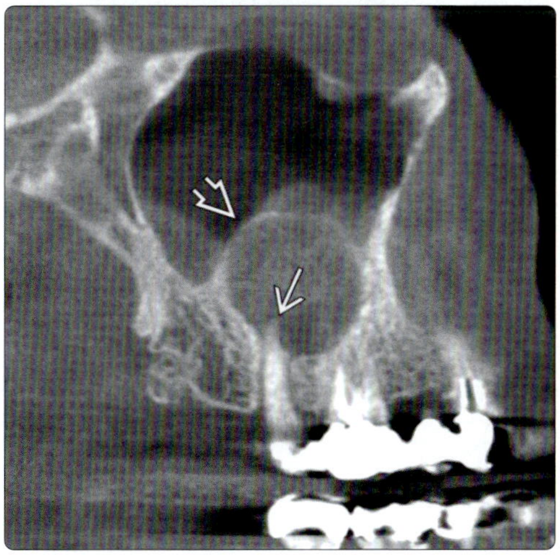

(Left) *Periapical radiograph shows periapical rarefying osteitis on the maxillary left lateral incisor and 1st premolar. These lesions are radiolucent and may or may not be corticated. Note lost crown and coronal caries.* **(Right)** *Sagittal CBCT shows a large unilocular lesion with corticated margins lifting the floor of the maxillary sinus. This is most likely a radicular cyst due to size. Lamina dura of related root apex is lost.*

(Left) *Periapical radiograph shows a maxillary right 2nd premolar that has experienced pulp death prior to closure of the apex due to extensive caries. Compare to 1st premolar with normally developing root and dental papilla. (Courtesy S. Darwish, BDS.)* **(Right)** *Panoramic radiograph shows rarefying osteitis of the mandibular left 1st molar. Compare to the incompletely formed root (open or blunderbuss-shaped) apices of adjacent teeth. Note that dentin comes to a point at the apex.*

Periapical Rarefying Osteitis

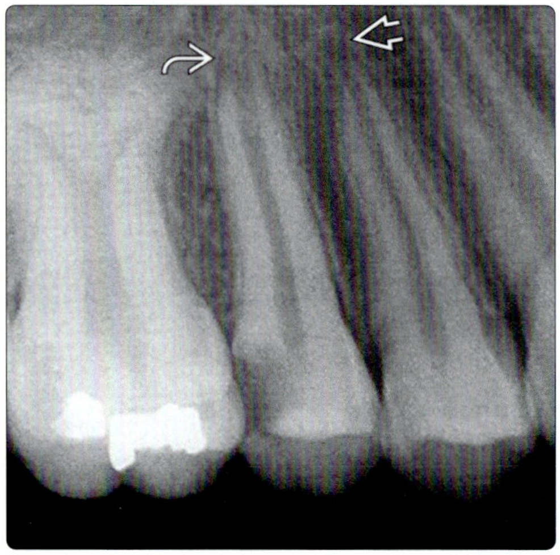

Incompletely Formed Root Apex

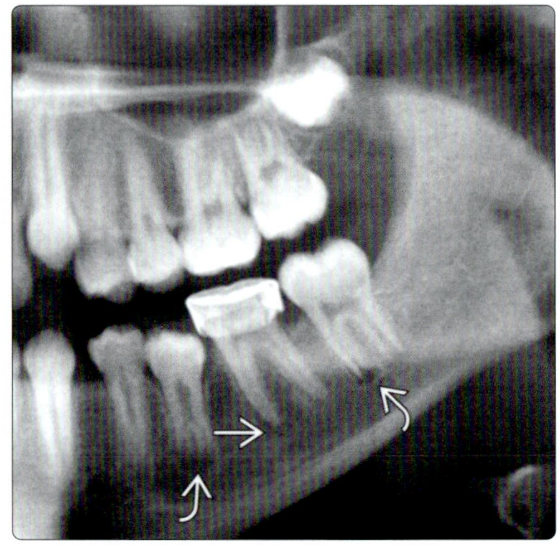

(Left) *Periapical radiograph shows the right mental foramen superimposed on the apex of the mandibular right 2nd premolar. The lamina dura at the apex of the tooth is intact. The tooth does not show any coronal caries or restoration.* **(Right)** *Coronal CBCT shows the apex of the right 2nd premolar in contact with the right mental foramen. Following the course of the mandibular canal along the length of the body of the mandible to the mental foramen aids in excluding periapical pathology.*

Mental Foramen

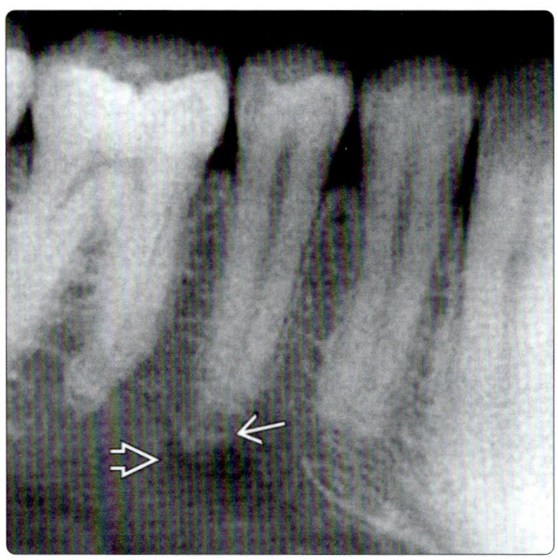

Mental Foramen

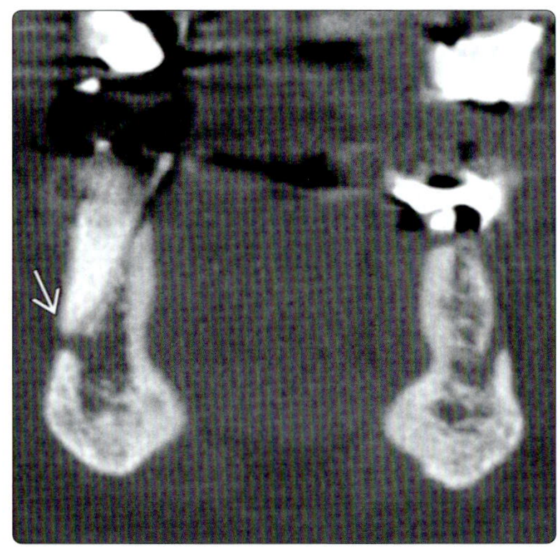

(Left) *Periapical radiograph shows early periapical osseous dysplasia (POD) at the apices of the lower anterior teeth. This is the most common location for PCD. These lesions develop cemental foci gradually over time. Vitality testing differentiates from pulpal pathology.* **(Right)** *Periapical radiograph shows a virgin maxillary right lateral incisor with a well-defined periapical lucent lesion of POD. Vitality testing was normal.*

Periapical Osseous Dysplasia

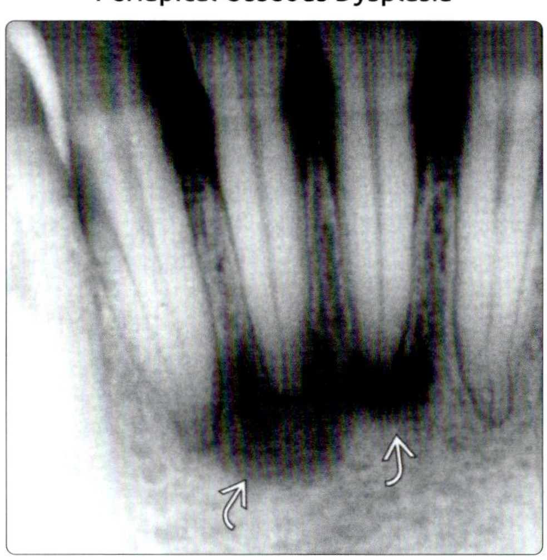

Periapical Osseous Dysplasia

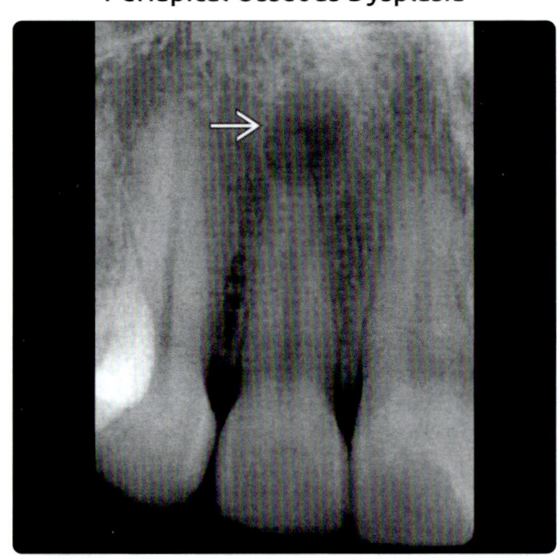

Benign Odontogenic Keratocyst

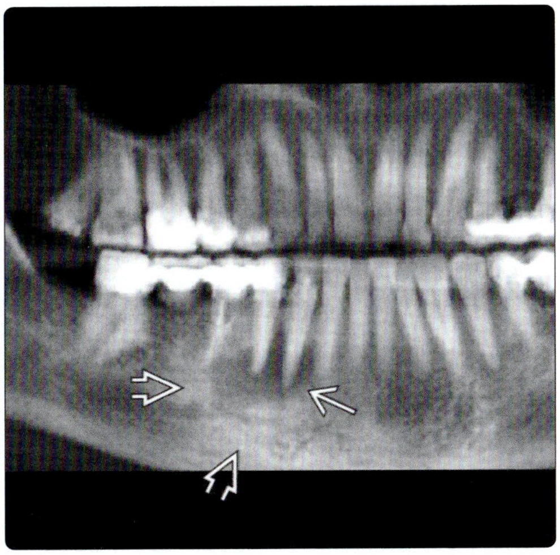

Benign Odontogenic Keratocyst

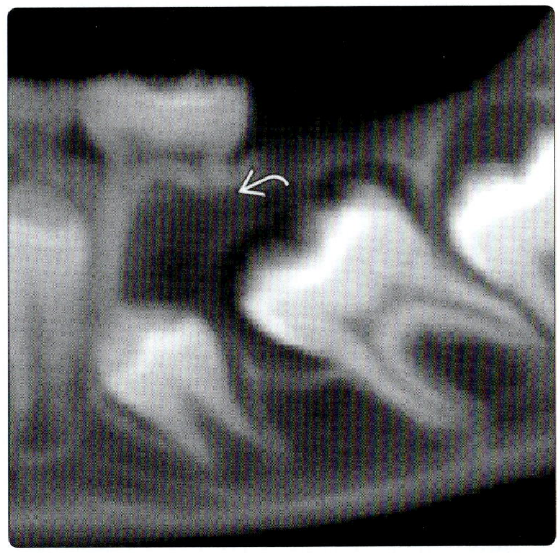

(Left) *CBCT panoramic reformat shows a lesion ➔ that did not heal despite root canal treatment of related teeth over the course of 24 months. The lesion, an odontogenic keratocyst, became infected (note sclerosis of surrounding bone ➔) and showed effacement of the facial cortex of the bone.* **(Right)** *Cropped CBCT panoramic reformat shows an ameloblastic fibroodontoma resorbing the distal apex of the primary left 2nd molar ➔. A hallmark of benign keratocysts is resorption of related teeth.*

Osteomyelitis

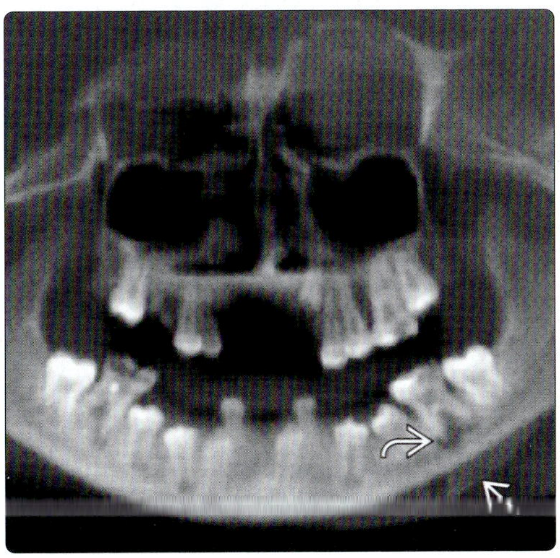

Leukemia

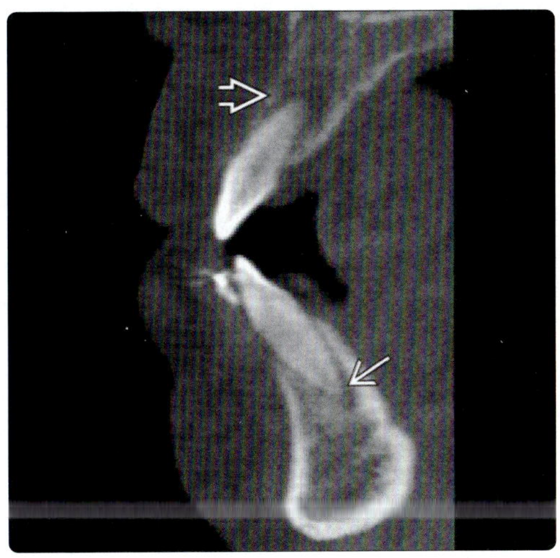

(Left) *Panoramic reformat of CBCT data from a child with periapical rarefying osteitis ➔ that had progressed to osteomyelitis shows periosteal reaction of the inferior border of the mandible ➔. (Courtesy M. Hedesiu, PhD.)* **(Right)** *CBCT cross section of an 11-year-old orthodontic patient with leukemia shows rarefaction at apices of both maxillary and mandibular canines. The maxillary lesion is ill defined ➔. The mandibular lesion appears to be growing along the periodontal ligament space ➔.*

Metastasis

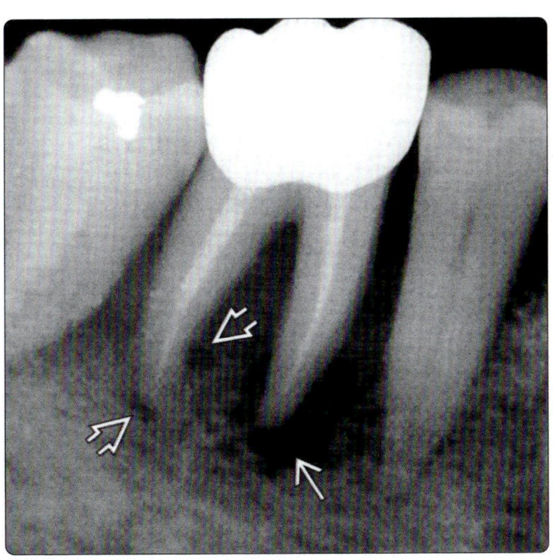

Metastasis

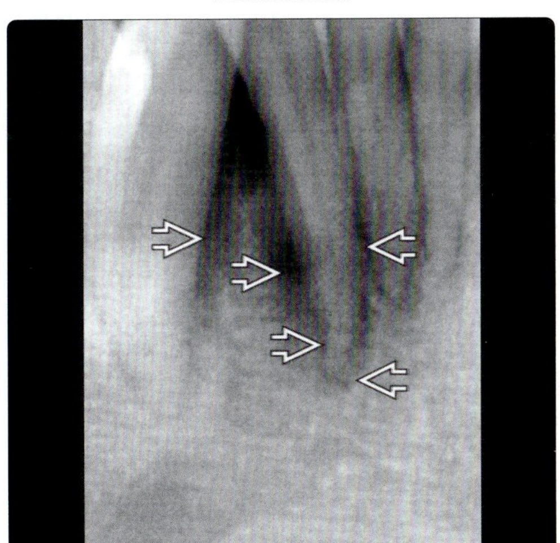

(Left) *Periapical radiograph shows prostate metastasis appearing as widening of the periapical periodontal ligament space ➔ of the mandibular 1st molar. This may have been mistaken for inflammatory disease and inappropriately endodontically treated. Other lytic foci are present ➔.* **(Right)** *Periapical radiograph of the right mandibular cuspid area shows breast cancer metastases. The periodontal ligament spaces of the teeth are widened ➔, and the lamina dura is missing. The trabecular bone pattern is otherwise unremarkable.*

DIFFERENTIAL DIAGNOSIS

Common

- Periapical Sclerosing Osteitis
- Idiopathic Osteosclerosis
- Periapical Osseous Dysplasia
- Hypercementosis
- Odontoma

Less Common

- Florid Osseous Dysplasia
- Cementoblastoma
- Cementoossifying Fibroma

Rare but Important

- Osteoid Osteoma

ESSENTIAL INFORMATION

Key Differential Diagnosis Issues

- **Tooth vitality testing** differentiates periapical sclerosing osteitis from other radiopaque entities

Helpful Clues for Common Diagnoses

- **Periapical Sclerosing Osteitis**
    - Key facts: Inflammatory process producing dense reactive bone at apex of dead or dying tooth
    - Imaging: Periodontal ligament (PDL) space is widened between tooth root and sclerosis
- **Idiopathic Osteosclerosis**
    - Key facts: Localized area of increased radiopacity of unknown cause
    - Imaging: **Well-defined**, nonexpansile, homogeneous radiopacity without radiolucent periphery
- **Periapical Osseous Dysplasia**
    - Key facts: Nonneoplastic replacement of normal bone at tooth apex by dysplastic cementum &/or abnormal bone
    - Imaging: Starts out completely radiolucent and becomes more radiopaque with time; radiopacity is **surrounded by radiolucency**
- **Hypercementosis**
    - Key facts: Excessive production of cementum, primarily around apical area of tooth root
    - Imaging: Normal PDL space surrounds cementum giving **thin, radiolucent periphery**; root looks bulbous or club-like
- **Odontoma**
    - Key facts: Tumor that produces mature tooth structures (**enamel, dentin, cementum, and pulp)**
    - Imaging: Compound odontoma looks like many small **tooth-like structures** surrounded by radiolucent rim
        - Complex odontoma shows **amorphous mass** of tooth-density material

Helpful Clues for Less Common Diagnoses

- **Florid Osseous Dysplasia**
    - Key facts: Similar to periapical osseous dysplasia (POD) but lesions are larger and may involve all quadrants; **teeth vital**
    - Imaging: Radiolucent lesions initially at apical area of roots; gradually becomes more radiopaque
- **Cementoblastoma**
    - Key facts: Attached to root surface; may resorb root; usually associated with mandibular 1st molar
    - Imaging: Radiopacity at apex of tooth surrounded by peripheral zone of radiolucency; tooth apex is resorbed or not visible
- **Cementoossifying Fibroma**
    - Key facts: Slow expansion and tooth displacement
    - Imaging: Well defined with corticated rim; internal radiopaque component fine and evenly distributed

Helpful Clues for Rare Diagnoses

- **Osteoid Osteoma**
    - Key facts: Severe pain
    - Imaging: Reactive sclerotic bone with central nidus of radiolucency; not attached to tooth root

SELECTED REFERENCES

1. Krishnan U et al: Cone beam CT as an aid to diagnosing mixed radiopaque radiolucent lesions in the mandibular incisor region. BMJ Case Rep. 2015, 2015

Periapical Sclerosing Osteitis

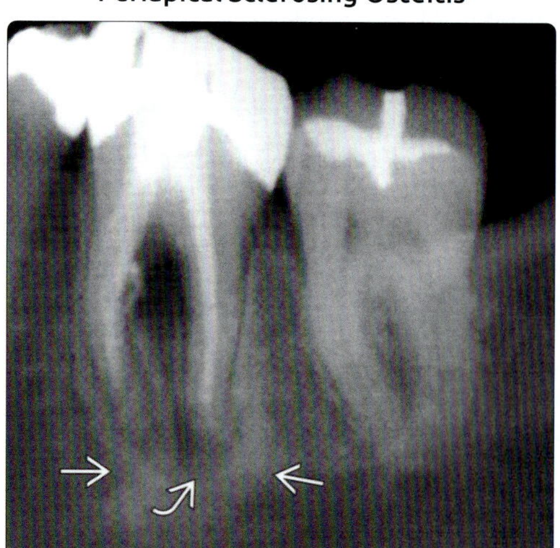

Idiopathic Osteosclerosis

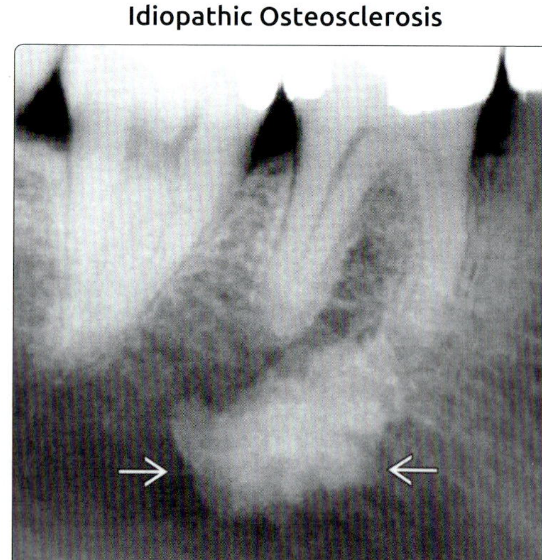

(Left) *Periapical radiograph shows sclerosing osteitis ➡ at the roots of the mandibular left 1st molar. Rarefying osteitis is noted at the apices of the tooth ➚. Note that the sclerotic bone blends into the surrounding normal bone.* **(Right)** *Periapical radiograph shows a well-defined, homogeneous radiopacity with jagged borders ➡ at the apex of the mandibular right 1st molar. Periodontal ligament spaces and laminae dura of roots are normal.*

Periapical Osseous Dysplasia

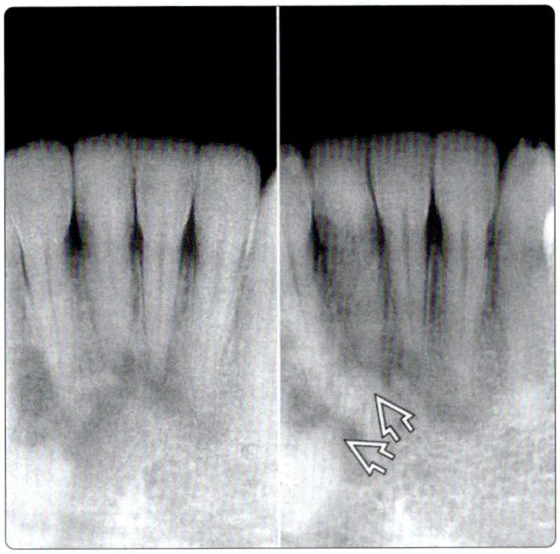

Hypercementosis

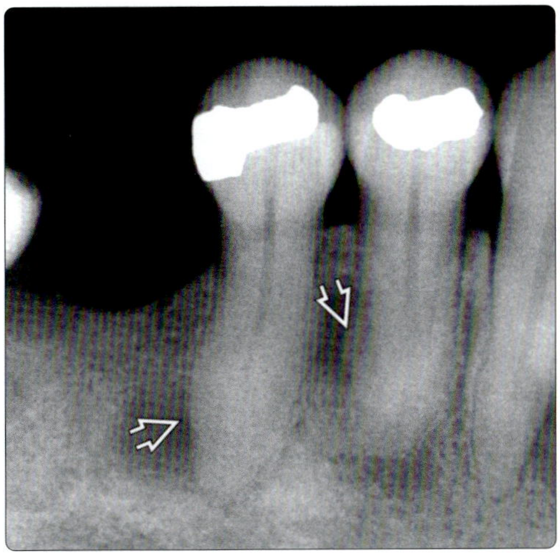

(Left) *Periapical radiographs of the lower anterior region show progression of periapical osseous dysplasia. The image on the right was taken 7 years after the image on the left and shows the gradual mineralization* ➔ *of the lesions.* **(Right)** *Periapical radiograph shows bulbous enlargement of root outline* ➔ *with preservation of the lamina dura and PDL spaces, consistent with hypercementosis.*

Odontoma

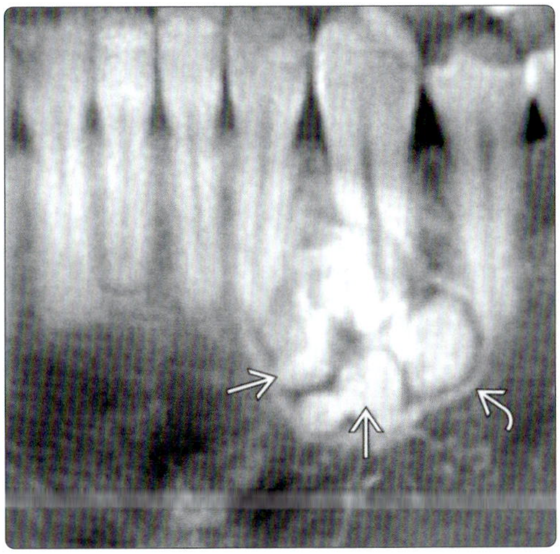

Cementoblastoma

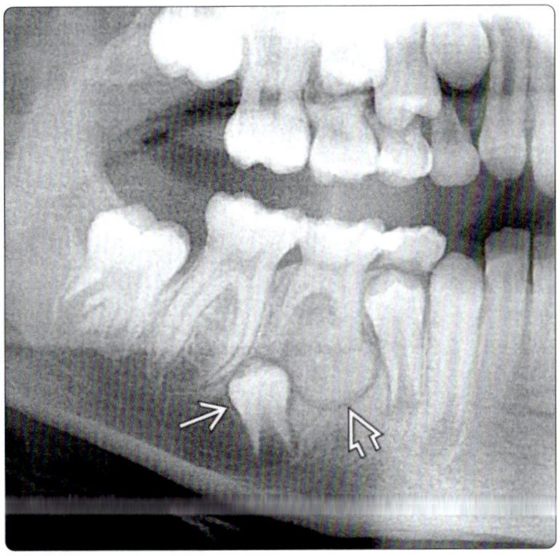

(Left) *CBCT panoramic reformat shows a mixed-density lesion consisting of several small, tooth-like structures* ➔ *surrounded by a radiolucent rim and corticated border* ➔*. This is a compound odontoma and is the most common odontogenic tumor.* **(Right)** *Cropped panoramic radiograph shows a homogeneous radiopacity, surrounded by a radiolucent rim* ➔*, attached to and resorbing the mesial root of the primary mandibular right 2nd molar. Displacement of the 2nd premolar* ➔ *by this cementoblastoma is evident.*

Cementoossifying Fibroma

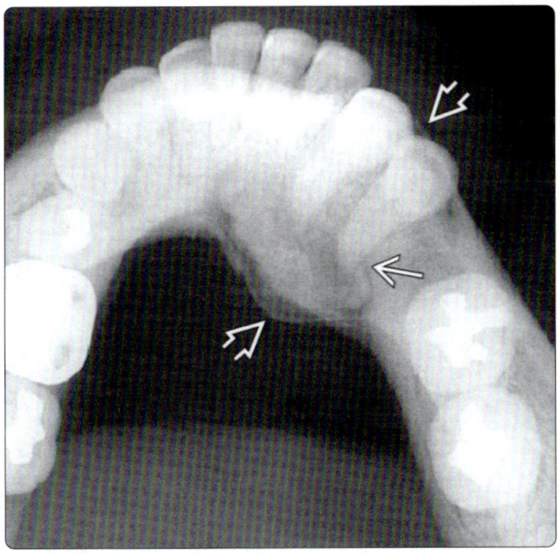

Osteoid Osteoma

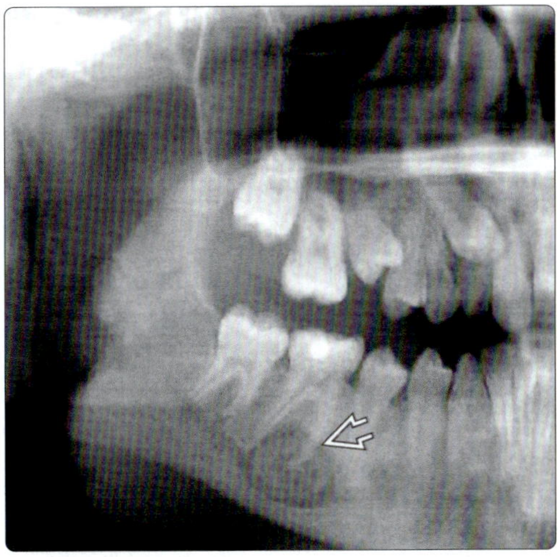

(Left) *Occlusal radiograph shows an expansile* ➔*, homogeneous radiopacity with a radiolucent rim. The roots of the mandibular left canine and 1st premolar are tipped lingually* ➔ *by this cementoossifying fibroma.* **(Right)** *Cropped panoramic radiograph shows a well-defined, mixed-density lesion that was mistakenly diagnosed as cementoblastoma despite the patient's symptom of severe pain and the lesion not being attached to the tooth root* ➔*.*

DIFFERENTIAL DIAGNOSIS

Common

- Advanced Periodontal Disease

Less Common

- Aggressive Periodontitis
- Malignancies
  - Osteosarcoma
  - Chondrosarcoma
  - Lymphoma
  - Primary Intraosseous Carcinoma
  - Metastasis

Rare but Important

- Langerhans Cell Histiocytosis
- Papillon-Lefèvre Syndrome

ESSENTIAL INFORMATION

Key Differential Diagnosis Issues

- Most common is advanced periodontal disease
  - Usually generalized, affecting **most or all teeth**
- Aggressive periodontitis affects specific sites initially
- Malignancies will be solitary
  - May be impossible to differentiate between various malignancies radiographically
- Langerhans cell histiocytosis & Papillon-Lefèvre syndrome in very young patients (1st decade)

Helpful Clues for Common Diagnoses

- **Advanced Periodontal Disease**
  - Key facts
    - Associated with poor oral hygiene ± systemic risk factors (e.g., diabetes)
  - Imaging
    - Generalized bone loss throughout dentition

Helpful Clues for Less Common Diagnoses

- **Aggressive Periodontitis**
  - Key facts
    - Young patients (2nd decade)
  - Imaging
    - Initially specific sites affected: **1st molars & central incisors**; may become generalized as patient ages
    - **Arc defects** may be visible
- **Malignancies**
  - Key facts
    - May be misdiagnosed as periapical pathology
    - Proliferation of soft tissue in socket may occur after extraction of involved tooth
    - Rare for metastatic lesions in jaws to be 1st sign of disease; usually known primary
  - Imaging
    - Ill-defined radiolucency around tooth roots
    - May start as widened periodontal ligament space
    - Chondrosarcoma, osteosarcoma, prostate & breast metastases, may or may not exhibit calcifications

Helpful Clues for Rare Diagnoses

- **Langerhans Cell Histiocytosis**
  - Key facts
    - Group of lesions characterized by proliferation of Langerhans cells
    - Localized form: Eosinophilic granuloma; young males
  - Imaging
    - Bone appears **scooped out**; helps differentiate from periodontal disease
- **Papillon-Lefèvre Syndrome**
  - Key facts
    - a.k.a. hyperkeratosis palmoplantaris
    - Autosomal recessive disorder caused by deficiency in cathepsin C
    - Characterized by destruction of periodontium, loss of teeth, hyperkeratosis of palms & soles of feet
  - Imaging
    - Severe bone loss around multiple or all teeth

SELECTED REFERENCES

1. Golai S et al: Langerhans histiocytosis in a child - diagnosed by oral manifestations. J Clin Diagn Res. 9(4):ZD09-11, 2015

(Left) *Sagittal CBCT shows severe vertical periodontal bone loss on both the mesial & distal root surfaces of the maxillary molar. Clear cortication of remaining bone ➡ helps differentiate from malignancy.* **(Right)** *CBCT panoramic reformat shows severe periodontal bone loss ➡ around the anterior abutment of a 3-unit bridge in the left mandible. The surrounding bone is sclerotic. Torquing forces were likely the etiology.*

Advanced Periodontal Disease

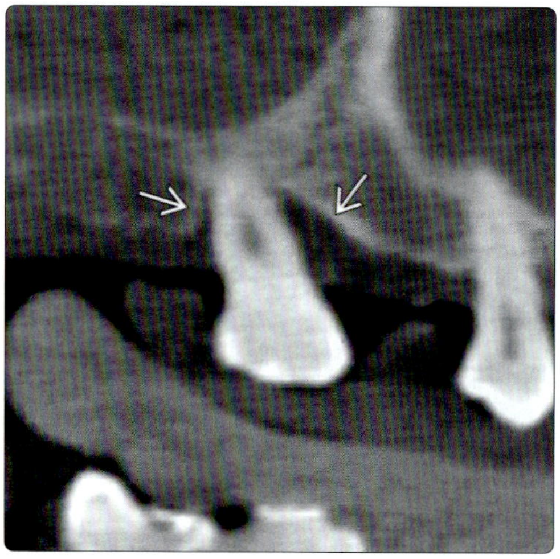

Advanced Periodontal Disease

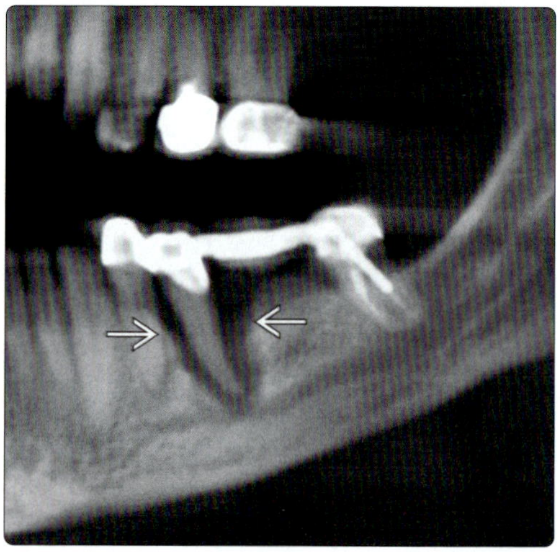

Aggressive Periodontitis

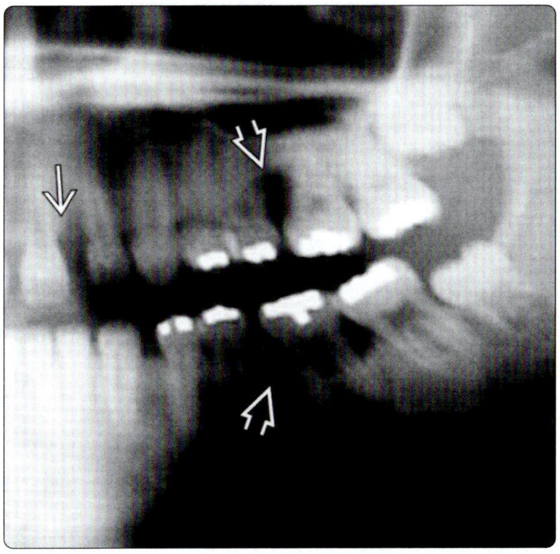

Osteosarcoma

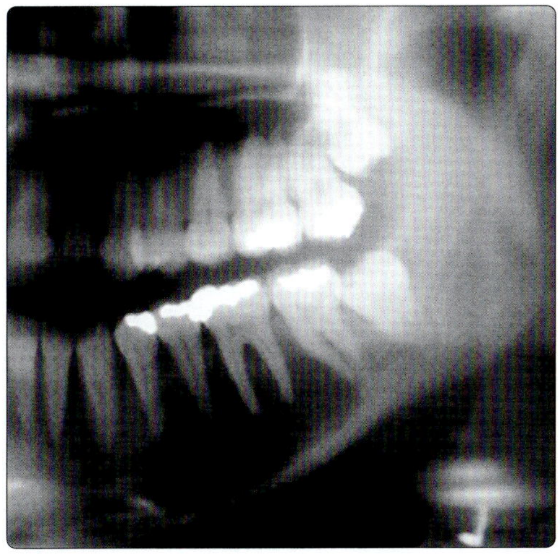

(Left) *Cropped panoramic radiograph of a 19 year old shows periodontal bone loss localized to 1st molars & maxillary anterior teeth. Note arc-shaped defects typical of localized aggressive periodontitis. The localized form is seen in the 2nd decade but may become progressively more generalized as patient ages.* **(Right)** *Panoramic radiograph shows the lytic type of osteosarcoma in the left mandible. The roots of the 2nd premolar & 1st molar appear to be floating. Widened periodontal ligament spaces suggest malignancy.*

Lymphoma

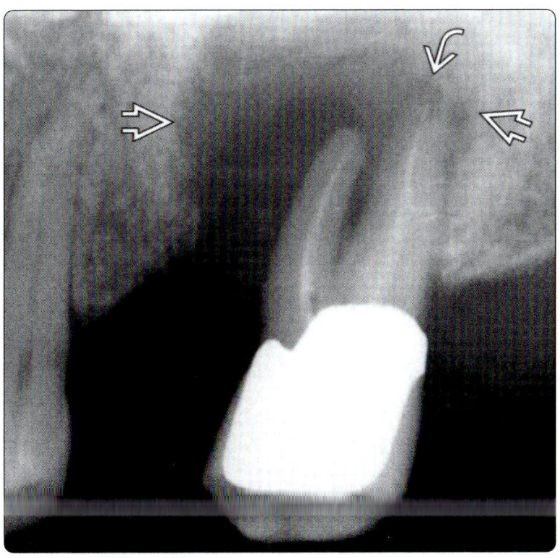

Primary Intraosseous Carcinoma

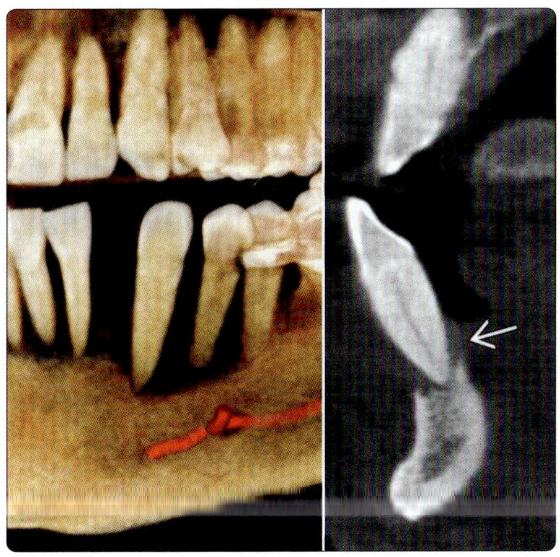

(Left) *Periapical radiograph shows lymphoma masquerading as a periapical inflammatory lesion. Misdiagnosis resulted in the endodontic treatment of a molar tooth. Note ill-defined margins & root resorption at the apex of palatal root.* **(Right)** *3D (left) & sagittal (right) CBCT show a squamous cell carcinoma in the left anterior mandible. The bone loss is localized, helping to differentiate from periodontal disease. The canine is '"floating" in tumor with a thin [illegible]*

Langerhans Cell Histiocytosis

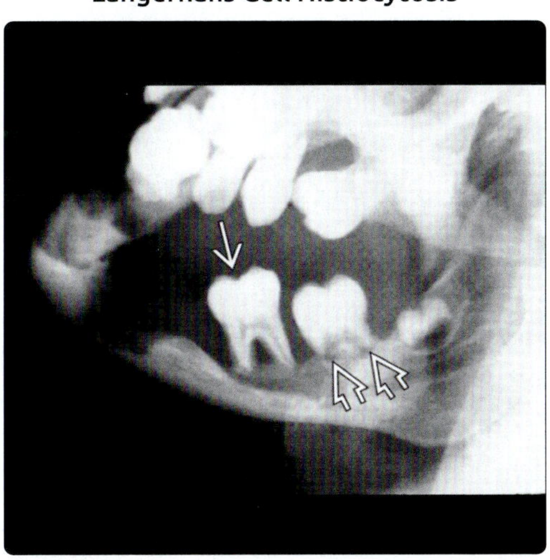

Papillon-Lefèvre Syndrome

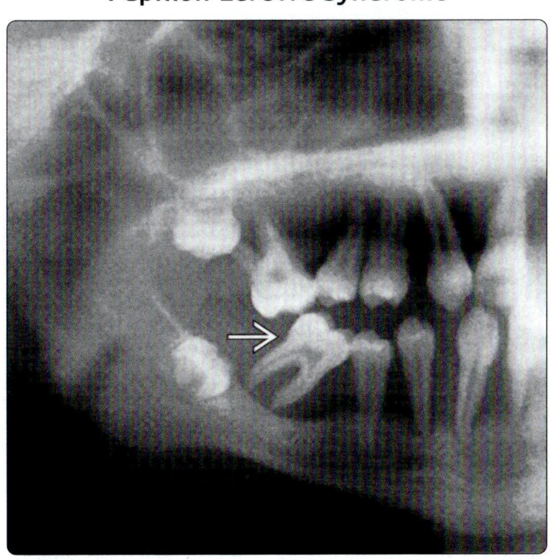

(Left) *Lateral oblique radiograph shows extensive bone loss in posterior mandible in a patient with eosinophilic granuloma. Note that the 1st molar appears to be floating. Radiolucencies at the apices of the 2nd molar are the follicles of the developing tooth roots.* **(Right)** *Cropped panoramic radiograph shows a young patient with Papillon-Lefèvre syndrome. All erupted teeth show severe periodontal bone loss, & the mandibular molar appears to be floating.*

Widened Periodontal Ligament Space

DIFFERENTIAL DIAGNOSIS

Common

- Occlusal Trauma
- Orthodontic Movement

Less Common

- Osteomyelitis
- Osteonecrosis
- Malignancies
  - Osteosarcoma
  - Chondrosarcoma
  - Metastasis

Rare but Important

- Leukemia
- Progressive Systemic Sclerosis (Scleroderma)

ESSENTIAL INFORMATION

Key Differential Diagnosis Issues

- Localized widened periodontal ligament (PDL) spaces: Occlusal trauma, malignancies
- Multiple teeth → whole jaw: Orthodontic movement, osteomyelitis/osteonecrosis, leukemia, scleroderma
- Symmetric widening: Occlusal trauma, osteomyelitis/osteonecrosis, leukemia, **scleroderma**
- Asymmetric widening: Trauma from torquing forces, orthodontic movement, malignancies

Helpful Clues for Common Diagnoses

- **Occlusal Trauma**
  - Key facts: Due to occlusal forces from opposing teeth or torquing forces from fixed or removable prosthesis
  - Imaging: Usually localized symmetric widening; severe bruxism may produce generalized widening
    - Torquing forces may → asymmetric widening
- **Orthodontic Movement**
  - Key facts: Orthodontic forces often result in PDL space widening; asymmetric widening occurs on side away from tooth movement
  - Imaging: Brackets & wires present on teeth

Helpful Clues for Less Common Diagnoses

- **Osteomyelitis/Osteonecrosis**
  - Key facts: Patient may have lymphadenopathy, ↑ temperature, pain & swelling, ± bisphosphonate use
    - Mandible (Md) > maxilla
  - Imaging: Mixed areas of lytic & sclerotic bone: Moth-eaten appearance
    - **Sequestra** & laminated periosteal reactions
- **Malignancies**
  - Key facts: PDL space provides opportunistic growth area for malignancies
    - Age: Osteosarcoma (OS) < chondrosarcoma (CS) & metastasis
    - Metastasis: Usually known primary; posterior Md
  - Imaging: May be impossible to differentiate between various malignancies radiographically
    - OS & CS may not have calcifications
    - Widening may be **symmetric or asymmetric**

Helpful Clues for Rare Diagnoses

- **Leukemia**
  - Key facts: Malignancy of hematopoietic stem cells with acute & chronic subtypes; affects all bones
  - Imaging: Generalized small areas of ill-defined radiolucencies
    - Tooth follicles may be displaced or indistinct
- **Progressive Systemic Sclerosis (Scleroderma)**
  - Key facts: Chronic inflammatory autoimmune disease; deposition of collagen & glycosaminoglycans into skin & internal organs
    - Females > males (4:1); 3rd to 5th decades
  - Imaging: May see mandibular erosions corresponding to insertion of muscles: Lateral pterygoid, temporalis, & masseter
    - **Generalized** PDL space widening; doubled in size

SELECTED REFERENCES

1. Mortazavi H et al: Review of common conditions associated with periodontal ligament widening. Imaging Sci Dent. 46(4):229-237, 2016

Occlusal Trauma

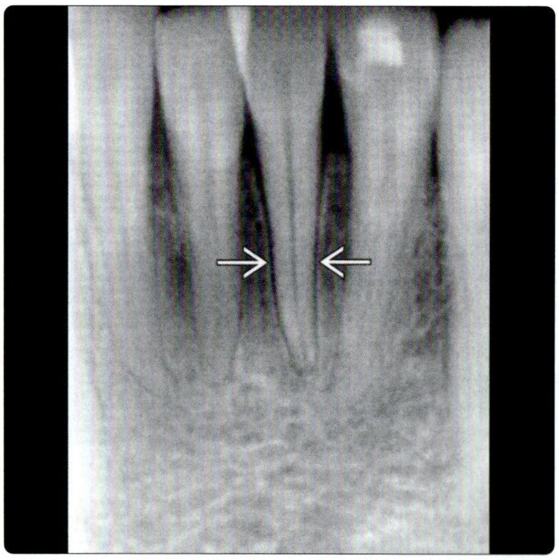

Orthodontic Movement

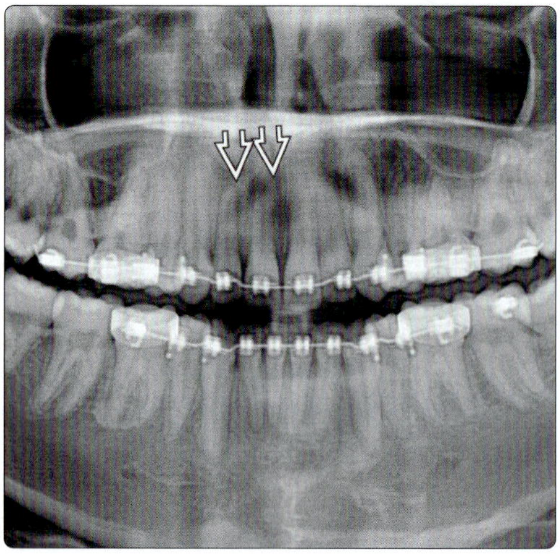

(Left) *Periapical radiograph shows localized symmetrical widening of the periodontal ligament space ➡ around the root of the mandibular left central incisor caused by occlusal trauma from the opposing maxillary central incisor.* **(Right)** *Cropped panoramic radiograph shows asymmetric widening of the periodontal ligament spaces on the mesial aspect of the maxillary right central and lateral incisors ➡. These teeth were being orthodontically moved distally. (Courtesy D. Liu, DDS.)*

Widened Periodontal Ligament Space

Osteonecrosis

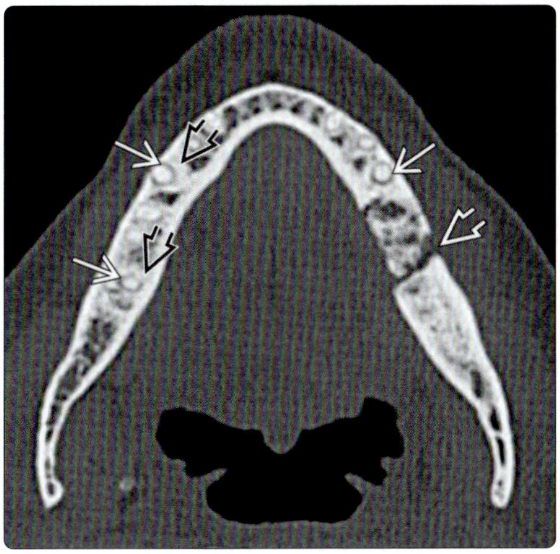

Osteosarcoma

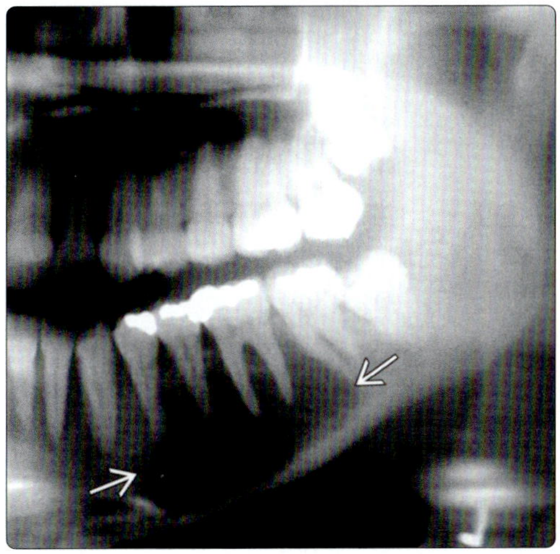

(Left) *Axial bone CT in a patient with medication-related osteonecrosis shows widened periodontal ligament spaces and thickened laminae dura. There are mixed areas of lysis and sclerosis and a pathologic fracture on the left.* **(Right)** *Panoramic radiograph shows the lytic type of osteosarcoma in the left mandible. The lesion is well defined, and the internal aspect is radiolucent, resembling a large cyst. However, there is widening of the periodontal ligament spaces around the teeth, which suggests malignancy.*

Chondrosarcoma

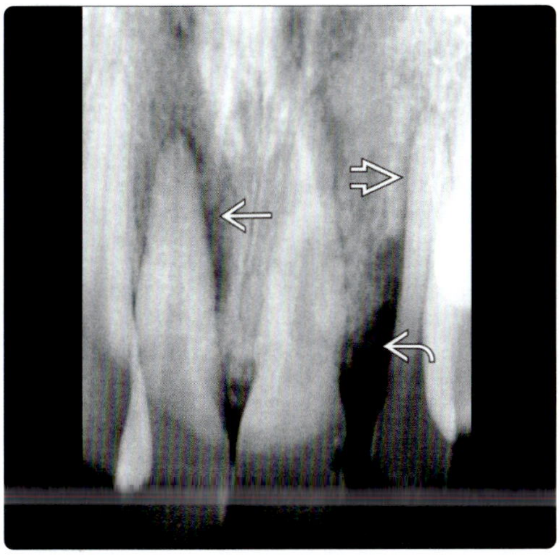

Metastasis

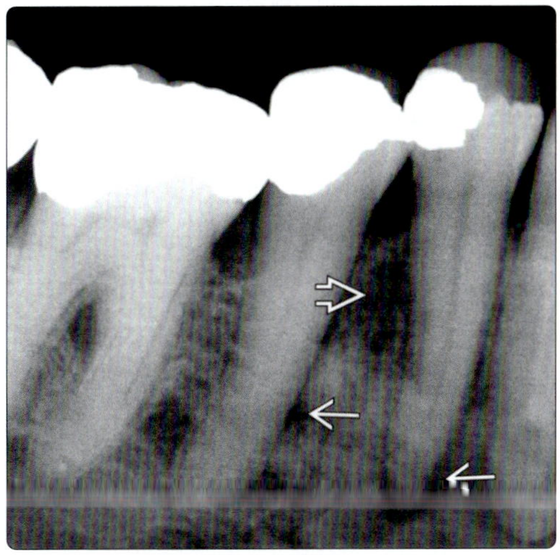

(Left) *Periapical radiograph of anterior maxilla shows a chondrosarcoma causing widening of the periodontal ligament space on the right central and left lateral incisor roots. Note destruction of the interdental bone between the left central and lateral incisor.* **(Right)** *Periapical radiograph shows breast metastases in the right mandible. There is permeative destruction between the premolars near the alveolar crest, sclerotic bone more apically, and asymmetric widening of the periodontal ligament spaces.*

Leukemia

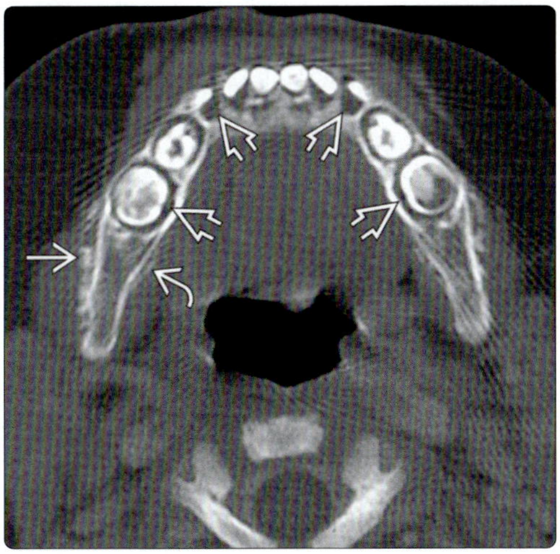

Progressive Systemic Sclerosis (Scleroderma)

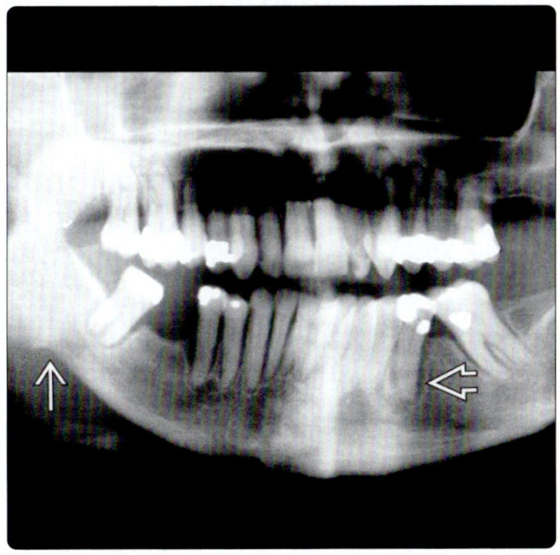

(Left) *Axial bone CT shows a loss of definition of the laminae dura and widening of the periodontal ligament spaces in this young patient with leukemia. Note spiculated pattern of new bone formation on buccal and laminated reaction on lingual.* **(Right)** *Panoramic radiograph of a woman with scleroderma shows generalized symmetric widening of periodontal ligament spaces, some of which are more than doubled in width. Note antegonial notching at insertion of masseter.*

Lamina Dura Changes

DIFFERENTIAL DIAGNOSIS

Common

- Osteoporosis
- Osteomyelitis
- Osteonecrosis
- Fibrous Dysplasia

Less Common

- Hyperparathyroidism
- Paget Disease
- Gardner Syndrome
- Malignancies
    - Osteosarcoma
    - Chondrosarcoma
    - Metastasis

Rare but Important

- Osteopetrosis
- Rickets/Osteomalacia
- Leukemia
- Hypophosphatasia
- Renal Osteodystrophy
- Hypophosphatemia

ESSENTIAL INFORMATION

Key Differential Diagnosis Issues

- Most often, lamina dura is lost or blends into altered bone pattern
- Lamina dura may be thickened in bisphosphonate-related osteonecrosis and osteopetrosis
- Loss of lamina dura associated with periodontal disease and pulpal pathology not discussed here

Helpful Clues for Common Diagnoses

- **Osteoporosis**
    - Key facts
        - Generalized decrease in bone mass
        - Most common in postmenopausal women
    - Imaging
        - Generalized reduced bone density
        - Cortical boundaries and laminae dura may be thinned or absent
- **Osteomyelitis**
    - Key facts
        - **Mandible** > > maxilla
        - Localized to involvement of whole jaw
        - Source of infection is often **odontogenic**
    - Imaging
        - Ill-defined mixed lytic and sclerotic changes
        - **Sequestra and laminated periosteal reactions**
        - Cortical boundaries and laminae dura may be thinned or absent
- **Osteonecrosis**
    - Key facts
        - Necrosis of jaws associated with bisphosphonate use
        - Exposed bone > 8 weeks
        - Mandible > maxilla
    - Imaging
        - Mixed sclerotic and lytic changes
        - When highly sclerotic, **lamina dura may become thickened**
        - Most often at nonhealing extraction site
        - Sequestra; pathologic fracture in severe cases
- **Fibrous Dysplasia**
    - Key facts
        - Nonneoplastic replacement of normal bone with cellular fibrous tissue
        - Monostotic most common in jaws
        - Maxilla > mandible; posterior more common
        - Usually unilateral
    - Imaging
        - Expansion is typical, but bone maintains its overall shape
        - Bone pattern described as granular, ground glass or orange peel
        - Periodontal ligament spaces may be narrowed
        - Laminae dura altered to abnormal bone pattern

Helpful Clues for Less Common Diagnoses

- **Hyperparathyroidism**
    - Key facts
        - Increased production of parathormone
        - Primary is due to adenoma in parathyroid gland
        - Secondary is compensatory to decreased serum calcium, most often caused by renal disease or vitamin D deficiency or malabsorption
        - F > M; 4th to 6th decade
    - Imaging
        - Overall rarefaction of bone initially; teeth may appear prominent
        - Lamina dura loss may be generalized or localized
        - Loss of cortical boundaries: Inferior cortex and mandibular canal
        - Bone may become granular or take on **ground-glass** appearance
        - Brown tumors seen in later stage: Radiolucent, well defined, unilocular, or occasionally multilocular
- **Paget Disease**
    - Key facts
        - Disease of osteoclasts causing bone remodeling in waves of osteoclastic and osteoblastic activity
        - Most common sites: Pelvis, skull, lumbosacral spine, femur, and vertebrae
        - Maxilla > mandible; affects entire jaw
        - M > F; > 40 years
    - Imaging
        - Radiographic appearance depends on disease phase
        - Begins as radiolucency and becomes progressively more sclerotic (**cotton wool** appearance)
        - Laminae dura not distinct and **altered to lesion bone pattern**
        - May see hypercementosis
- **Gardner Syndrome**
    - Key facts
        - Autosomal dominant inherited condition (familial adenomatous polyposis)
        - Multiple osteomas precede intestinal polyposis, which have **100% potential for malignant change**
    - Imaging
        - Central osteomas may obscure laminae dura

- Peripheral osteomas most often posterior mandible at angle or ramus
- Unerupted supernumerary teeth

- **Malignancies**
  - Key facts
    - Age: Osteosarcoma (OS) < chondrosarcoma (CS) and metastasis
    - Metastasis: Usually known primary; predilection for posterior mandible
  - Imaging
    - May be impossible to differentiate between various malignancies radiographically
    - OS and CS may not have calcifications
    - Loss of laminae dura may be in conjunction with widened periodontal ligament spaces

Helpful Clues for Rare Diagnoses

- **Osteopetrosis**
  - Key facts
    - Osteoclasts are dysfunctional, resulting in increased bone density and mass
    - Fragility of bones with increased susceptibility to infection and fracture
    - Osteopetrosis congenita (autosomal recessive): Seen in infants and invariably fatal
    - Osteopetrosis tarda (autosomal dominant): Appears later in life and is milder
  - Imaging
    - Bone may be so dense that teeth, periodontal ligament, and lamina dura not evident
    - Lamina dura and cortical boundaries may be thickened
- **Rickets/Osteomalacia**
  - Key facts
    - Abnormal activity of vitamin D metabolites causes failure of gastric absorption of calcium; leads to decreased calcium and phosphate levels
    - Rickets in young patients; osteomalacia in adult patients (usually no radiographic signs)
    - Bowing of legs; greenstick fractures in rickets
  - Imaging
    - Thinning of cortical boundaries and thinned or absent laminae dura
    - Delayed development and eruption of teeth
- **Leukemia**
  - Key facts
    - > 60% of acute leukemia patients have jaw lesions
  - Imaging
    - Laminae dura and developing tooth follicles may become indistinct due to generalized osteopenia
- **Hypophosphatasia**
  - Key facts
    - Rare inherited disorder, often fatal within 1st year
    - Abnormal production or function of alkaline phosphatase
    - Premature loss of deciduous teeth
  - Imaging
    - Generalized rarefaction of bone with loss of cortical boundaries and thinning or loss of lamina dura
- **Renal Osteodystrophy**
  - Key facts
    - Results from chronic renal failure
    - Secondary hyperparathyroidism ensues
  - Imaging
    - Radiographic appearance similar to secondary hyperparathyroidism or rickets
    - Laminae dura and cortical boundaries absent or thinned
- **Hypophosphatemia**
  - Key facts
    - Inherited condition resulting in excessive excretion of phosphorus in kidney
    - Ricket-like symptoms, including bowing of legs
  - Imaging
    - May be indistinguishable from rickets
    - Laminae dura and cortical boundaries absent or thinned

SELECTED REFERENCES

1. White SC et al: Oral Radiology: Principles and Interpretation. 7th ed. St. Louis: Mosby Elsevier, 2014

Osteoporosis

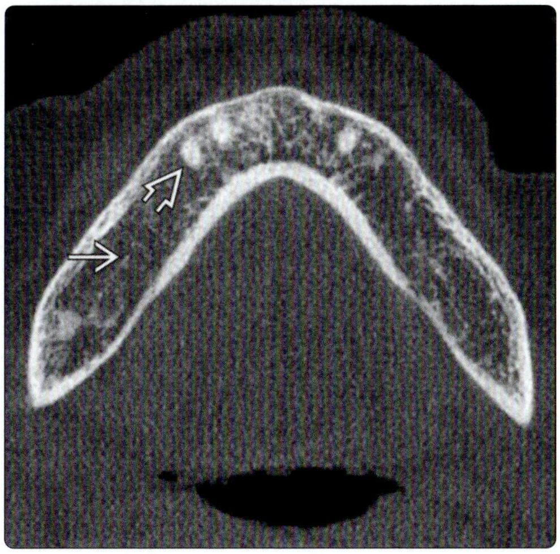

Osteomyelitis

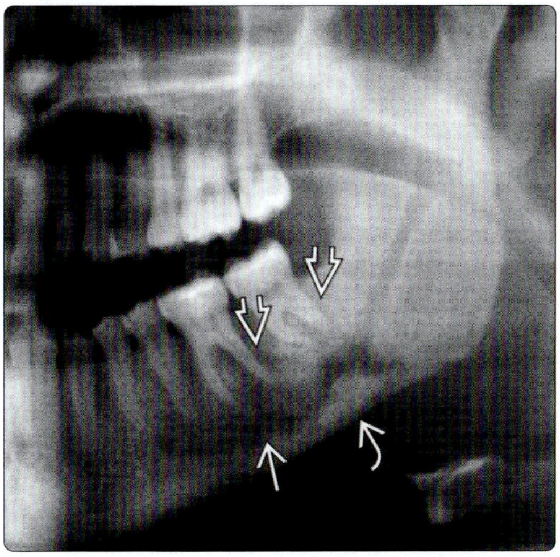

(Left) *Axial CBCT of a 90-year-old woman with a diagnosis of osteoporosis shows osteopenic changes in the mandible, including sparse trabeculation ➡ and thinned or absent ➡ lamina dura around the remaining teeth.* **(Right)** *Panoramic radiograph shows mixed lytic and sclerotic appearance in left mandible. Note loss of laminae dura of involved teeth ➡ and cortical boundary of mandibular canal ➡. Sequestration is seen at the inferior border ➡.*

(Left) *Cropped panoramic radiograph of left mandible shows appearance of bone prior to extraction of the 1st molar. Note sclerosis and thickening of laminae dura of premolar and molar, suggestive of bisphosphonate-related changes. BRONJ developed in extraction site.* **(Right)** *Cropped panoramic radiograph shows mandibular canal superiorly displaced, a pathognomic feature of fibrous dysplasia. Bone has appearance of ground glass. Expanded inferior cortex and laminae dura are altered to lesion bone pattern.*

Osteonecrosis

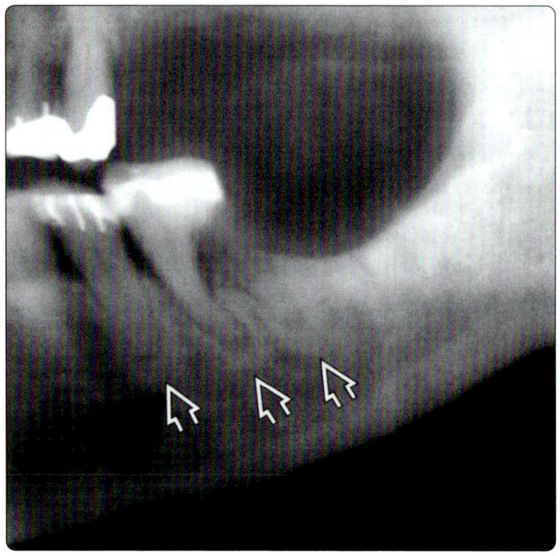

Fibrous Dysplasia

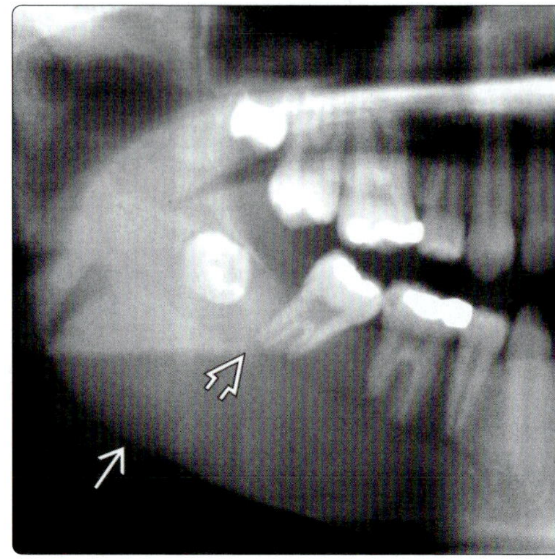

(Left) *Panoramic radiograph shows the ground-glass appearance and loss or thinning of the lamina dura around all the teeth in a 27-year-old woman with 2° hyperparathyroidism related to renal disease. (Courtesy S. Friedlander-Barenboim, DMD.)* **(Right)** *Periapical radiograph of the right mandible in the same patient shows loss of laminae dura and a small radiolucency in the 1st premolar area. This is a "brown tumor," which appears in the later stage of disease. (Courtesy S. Friedlander-Barenboim, DMD.)*

Hyperparathyroidism

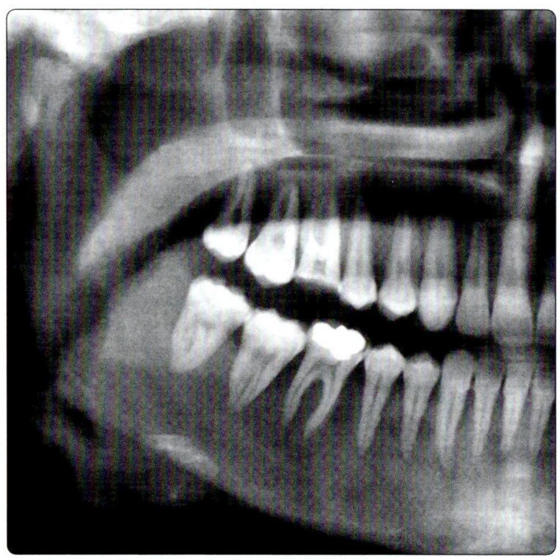

Hyperparathyroidism

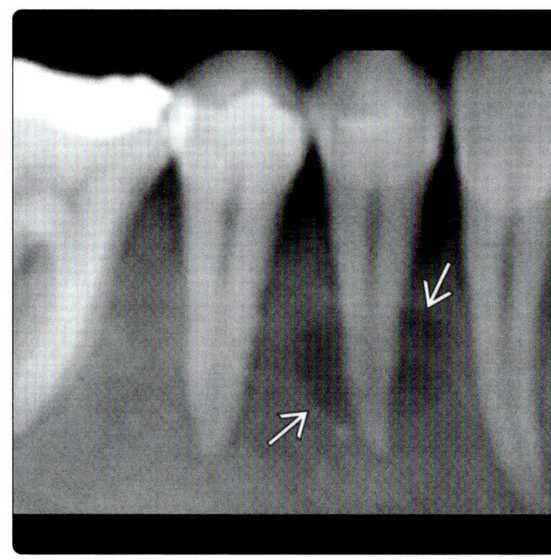

(Left) *Panoramic radiograph shows late phase of Paget disease in the right mandible. The trabecular pattern is coarse and sclerotic, and inferior cortex and lamina dura cannot be distinguished. The mandibular canal is visible, but corticated margins are absent.* **(Right)** *Panoramic radiograph shows an osteoma at inferior border of the left mandible in a patient with Gardner syndrome. Increased density of mandible caused by central osteomas has obscured the laminae dura. Note small supernumerary teeth. (Courtesy B. Pass, DDS.)*

Paget Disease

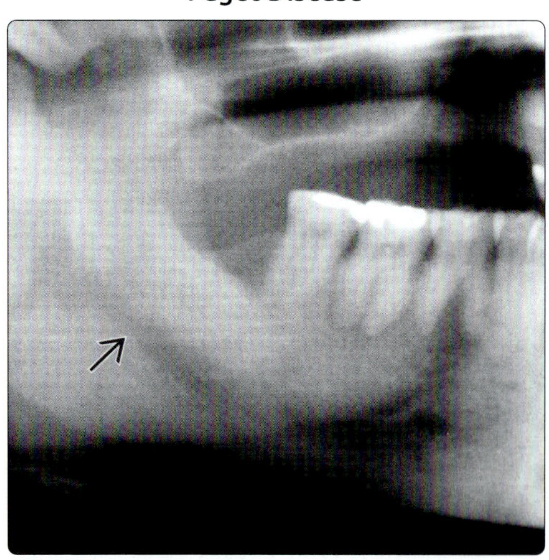

Gardner Syndrome

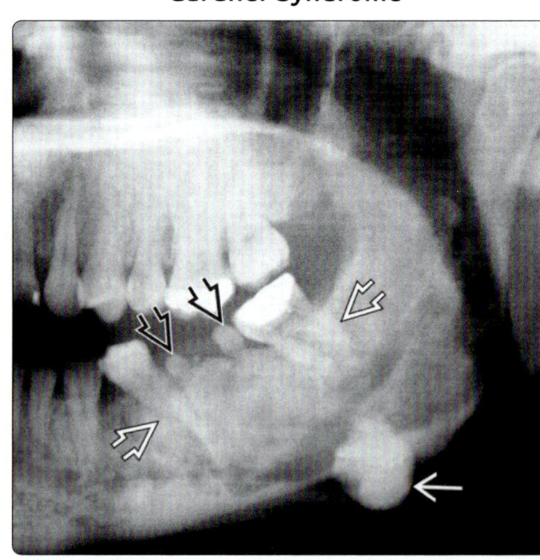

Osteosarcoma

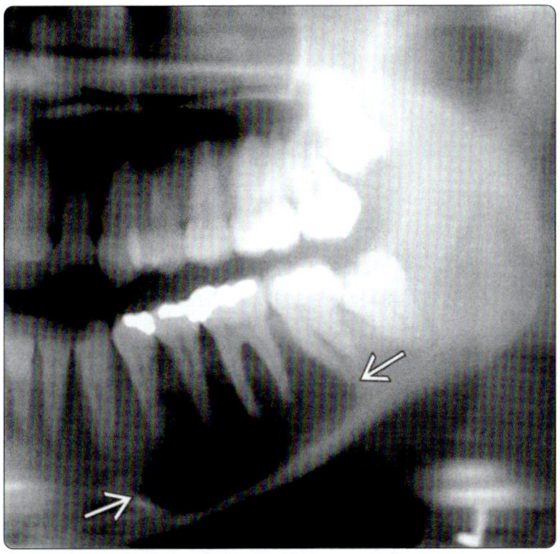

Chondrosarcoma

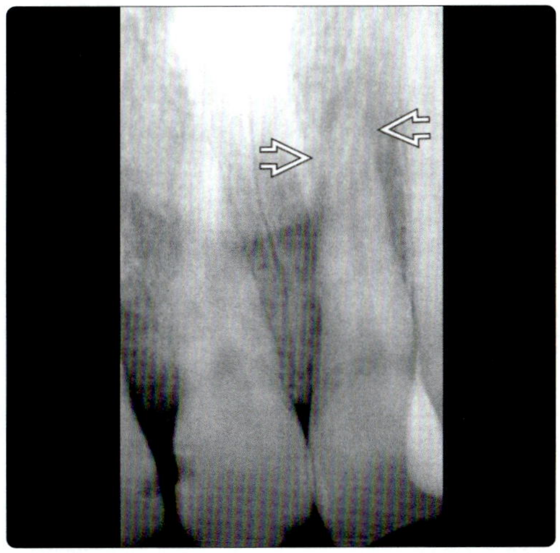

(Left) *Panoramic radiograph shows the lytic type of osteogenic sarcoma in the left mandible. The lesion is mostly well defined, but there is widening of the periodontal ligament spaces and loss of lamina dura around the teeth, which suggests malignancy.* **(Right)** *Periapical radiograph shows a chondrosarcoma in the anterior maxilla. There is increased radiolucency with shortening of the trabeculae. The periodontal ligament space around the root of the left maxillary incisor is symmetrically widened, and the lamina dura is missing.*

Metastasis

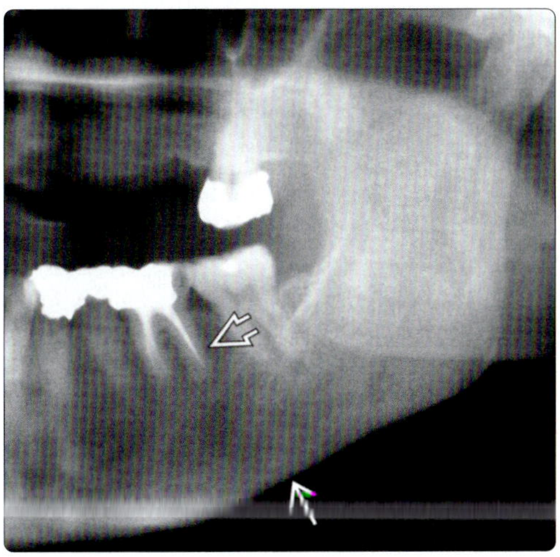

Osteopetrosis

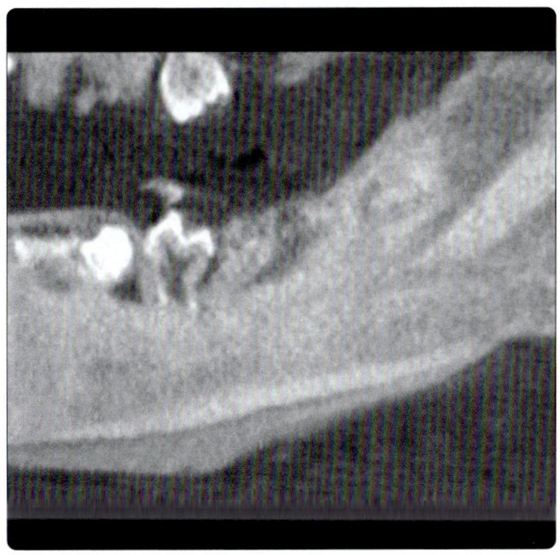

(Left) *Panoramic radiograph shows breast metastases affecting left mandible and ramus. There is loss of the inferior cortical border, laminae dura, and normal trabecular architecture. It is rare for jaw metastasis to be the 1st sign of disease.* **(Right)** *Panoramic CBCT reformat of a 4 year old with malignant infantile osteopetrosis shows dense trabecular bone. The teeth are malformed, eruption is impeded, and the outline of the inferior alveolar canal and laminae dura has been effaced. (Courtesy D. Hung, DDS.)*

Rickets/Osteomalacia

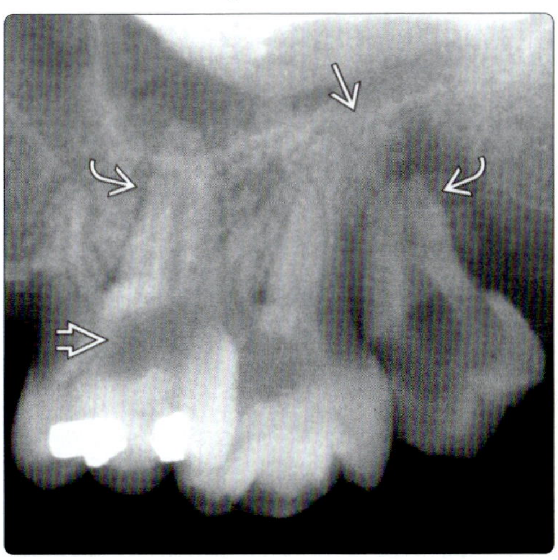

Leukemia

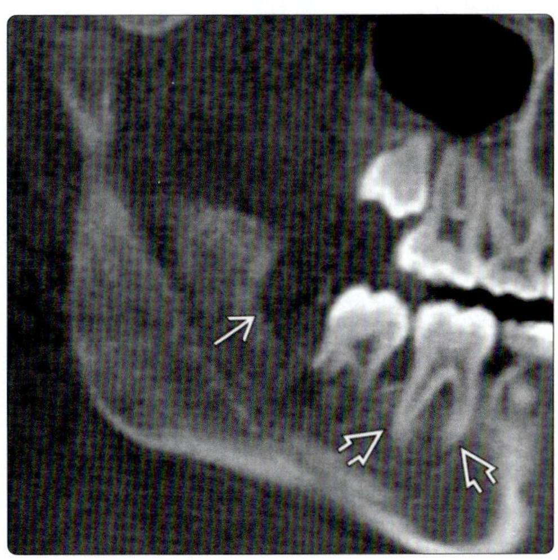

(Left) *Periapical radiograph of a 30-year-old woman with rickets shows characteristic enlarged pulp chambers, a decrease in density of the floor of the maxillary sinus, and loss of laminae dura around all teeth. Patient had severe leg bowing. (Courtesy A. Potluri, DMD.)* **(Right)** *Panoramic reformat CBCT shows minimally corticated mandibular right 3rd molar tooth follicle in an 11-year-old boy with leukemia. There is loss of the lamina dura around the 1st molar tooth. (Courtesy M. Noujeim, DDS.)*

DIFFERENTIAL DIAGNOSIS

Common

- Periapical (Radicular) Cyst
- Residual Cyst
- Mandibular Salivary Gland Defect (Stafne)

Less Common

- Dentigerous Cyst
- Nasopalatine Duct Cyst
- Simple (Traumatic) Bone Cyst
- Odontogenic Keratocyst (Keratocystic Odontogenic Tumor)
- Lateral Periodontal Cyst
- Unicystic Ameloblastoma

Rare but Important

- Multiple Myeloma
- Eosinophilic Granuloma

ESSENTIAL INFORMATION

Key Differential Diagnosis Issues

- **Foramina** of jaws appear as well-defined unilocular radiolucencies; **location and size** help differentiate from pathology
- **Enlarged marrow spaces** may also present as corticated unilocular radiolucencies; presence of any internal trabeculae helps to differentiate from pathology
  - If in doubt, radiographic follow-up is recommended to monitor for change
- Most benign unilocular radiolucencies are cystic lesions and **corticated**
  - Cystic lesions: Usually round due to hydraulic expansion
- Benign unilocular radiolucencies are usually **solitary**; however, bilateral nasopalatine duct cysts reported
- Dentigerous cyst and odontogenic keratocyst (OKC) can be bilateral/multiple and nonsyndromic
  - Multiple OKCs associated with basal cell nevus syndrome
  - Multiple dentigerous cysts found in Maroteaux-Lamy syndrome (mucopolysaccharidosis type VI)
- Multiple myeloma (MM) and eosinophilic granuloma (EG) may appear well-defined but **not corticated**
  - Often described as **punched out**
- MM and EG most often present with **multiple lesions** in jaws; EG more likely to be solitary than MM
  - MM in much older age group

Helpful Clues for Common Diagnoses

- **Periapical (Radicular) Cyst**
  - Key facts
    - Associated with pulpal pathology and **nonvital tooth**
    - Most common odontogenic cyst
  - Imaging
    - Located at apex of tooth: Apical lamina dura is missing
    - If associated with lateral canal, epicenter may be on lateral surface of root close to apex
- **Residual Cyst**
  - Key facts
    - Remains after tooth extraction and incomplete removal of periapical cyst
    - Maxilla > mandible; anterior > posterior
    - Male > female
  - Imaging
    - **Tooth** or teeth will be **missing**
    - Well-corticated radiolucency
    - Symptomatic lesions may be less corticated
    - Can become very large
- **Mandibular Salivary Gland Defect (Stafne)**
  - Key facts
    - Defects contain salivary gland or fatty soft tissue
    - Defect on posterior lingual aspect of mandible most common; submandibular fossa area
    - Anterior defects associated with lingual salivary glands may be confused with odontogenic cysts
    - Parotid defects may be lingual or buccal; rare
    - Male > female (6:1); 5th and 6th decades most common
  - Imaging
    - All variants appear as corticated radiolucency **without expansion**
    - Posterior variant most common: At angle of mandible
    - **Below mandibular canal**
    - Anterior variant will be **above mylohyoid muscle**

Helpful Clues for Less Common Diagnoses

- **Dentigerous Cyst**
  - Key facts
    - Unilocular pericoronal radiolucency
    - **Mandibular 3rd molars** > maxillary 3rd molars > maxillary canines; 5% associated with supernumerary teeth
  - Imaging
    - Well-defined corticated unilocular radiolucency around crown of impacted/unerupted tooth
    - Radiolucency attaches at or close to cementoenamel junction
    - Significant displacement of associated tooth characteristic
- **Nasopalatine Duct Cyst**
  - Key facts
    - Most common nonodontogenic cyst
    - Anterior maxilla, palatal to maxillary central incisors
    - Teeth are **vital**
  - Imaging
    - Corticated radiolucency between maxillary central incisors in intraoral images
    - May appear **heart-shaped** in intraoral images due to superimposition of anterior nasal spine
    - Rounded enlargement of nasopalatine canal and foramen on CBCT/CT: Size > 1 cm differentiates normal foramen/canal from pathology
    - Homogeneous hyperintense T2 signal
- **Simple (Traumatic) Bone Cyst**
  - Key facts
    - Solitary and empty or partially empty bone cavity; not true cyst because no epithelial lining
    - History of trauma < 1/2 cases
    - Male > female; 2nd decade; if associated with florid osseous dysplasia, older women
  - Imaging
    - Usually posterior mandible
    - Lesion may **scallop between teeth**

- May see **endosteal scalloping**
- Usually only mild expansion if present

- **Odontogenic Keratocyst (Keratocystic Odontogenic Tumor)**
  - Key facts
    - Mandible > maxilla (2:1); posterior > anterior
    - Can also be pericoronal and multilocular; loculations large and few if present
    - High recurrence rate: **Recurrent lesions** most likely to be **unilocular**
    - Multiple lesions associated with basal cell nevus syndrome
  - Imaging
    - Epicenter above inferior alveolar canal
    - **Minimal expansion in mandible** relative to size; tends to creep along mandible and up ramus
    - May have scalloping periphery or scallop between teeth
    - OKC and simple bone cyst have similar radiographic findings in mandible
- **Lateral Periodontal Cyst**
  - Key facts
    - Odontogenic developmental cyst lateral to erupted **vital tooth**
    - May be confused with lateral radicular cyst; testing vitality of adjacent teeth is key
    - Mandible > maxilla; premolar area most common
    - Wide age range; peak in 6th decade
  - Imaging
    - Well-defined, corticated, **interradicular radiolucency** with rounded or **teardrop shape**
    - Usually < 1 cm in size
    - Occasionally buccal expansion and rarely cortical perforation
- **Unicystic Ameloblastoma**
  - Key facts
    - Arises from epithelium in cyst wall or de novo
    - Typically younger patients than ameloblastoma
    - Majority pericoronal and resemble dentigerous cyst
    - Less aggressive course and less recurrence
  - Imaging
    - Unilocular, but scalloping margins may give multilocular appearance on 2D imaging
    - T1WI C+ MR: Enhancement of mural nodules

Helpful Clues for Rare Diagnoses

- **Multiple Myeloma**
  - Key facts
    - Monoclonal malignant proliferation of plasma cells
    - Most common malignancy of bone in adults: Skull lesions in 45% of cases; jaw lesions, 20-30%
    - Mandible > maxilla; posterior > anterior
    - Male > female; mean age: **60 years**
  - Imaging
    - **Multiple** small, unilocular, round, or oval radiolucencies
    - **Punched out without corticated border**
    - Lesions usually < 1 cm at diagnosis but may coalesce to form larger lesions
    - Lesions that coalesce may appear multilocular
    - Examine skull and spine for additional lesions
- **Eosinophilic Granuloma**
  - Key facts
    - Localized form of Langerhans histiocytosis
    - Jaws involved in 10-20% of cases
    - Mandible > maxilla; posterior > anterior
    - **Older children** to young adults
  - Imaging
    - Round or oval radiolucencies at onset
    - **Punched out without corticated border**
    - Larger lesions become irregular and may coalesce; teeth may appear to be **floating**
    - Alveolar bone may appear **scooped out**
    - Examine skull for additional lesions

SELECTED REFERENCES

1. Agani Z et al: Maxillary unicystic ameloblastoma: a case report. BMC Res Notes. 9(1):469, 2016
2. Langlais RP et al: Diagnostic Imaging of the Jaws. Malvern, PA: Williams & Wilkins, 1995

Periapical (Radicular) Cyst

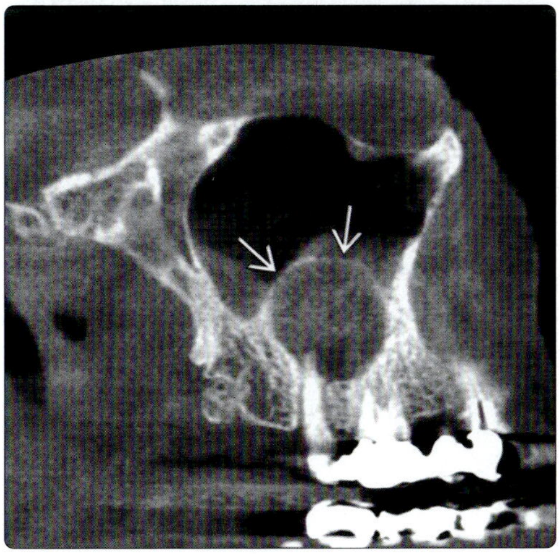

Residual Cyst

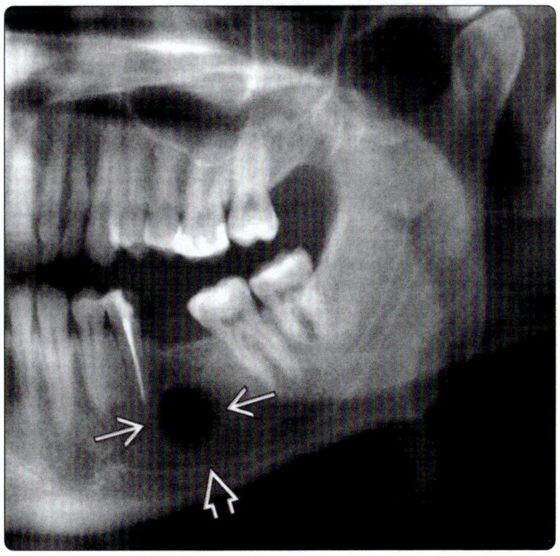

(Left) *Sagittal CBCT shows a large radicular cyst associated with the palatal root of a maxillary molar. Lesion elevates floor of sinus ➡. Corticated border indicates growth from outside sinus rather than from within the sinus.* **(Right)** *Cropped panoramic radiograph of the left mandible shows a well-defined round radiolucency ➡ in the apical area of the missing 1st molar. The lesion is unilocular and thinly corticated consistent with residual cyst. Note location above the mandibular canal ➡.*

(Left) *Panoramic radiograph shows mandibular salivary gland defect* ➡ *appearing as a well-defined, corticated, round radiolucency in the angle of the mandible. The defect is located inferior to the mandibular canal* ➡. **(Right)** *Cross section CBCT shows mandibular salivary gland defect* ➡ *invaginating into the medullary bone. Note that the defect is well corticated. The mandibular canal* ➡ *is in close proximity and was visible through the defect in sagittal views. (Courtesy M. Noujeim, DDS.)*

Mandibular Salivary Gland Defect (Stafne)

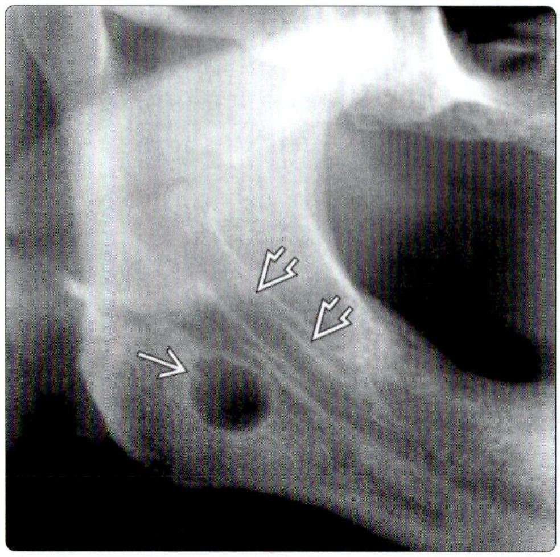

Mandibular Salivary Gland Defect (Stafne)

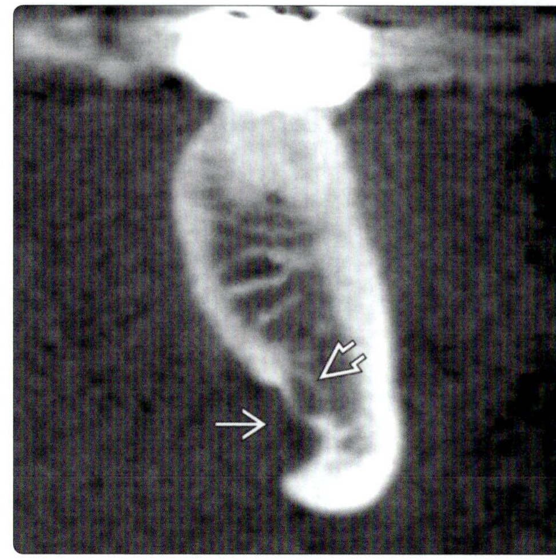

(Left) *Ray-sum CT rendering shows classic appearance of a dentigerous cyst as a well-defined unilocular radiolucency pericoronal to the impacted mandibular 3rd molar* ➡ *in a 38-year-old woman. The mandibular canal* ➡ *is displaced inferiorly. (Courtesy J. Curé, MD.)* **(Right)** *Axial bone CT shows a corticated uniform and concentric expansion of the nasopalatine canal in the midline maxillary alveolus* ➡ *typical of a nasopalatine duct cyst. Size greater than 1 cm presumes development of pathology.*

Dentigerous Cyst

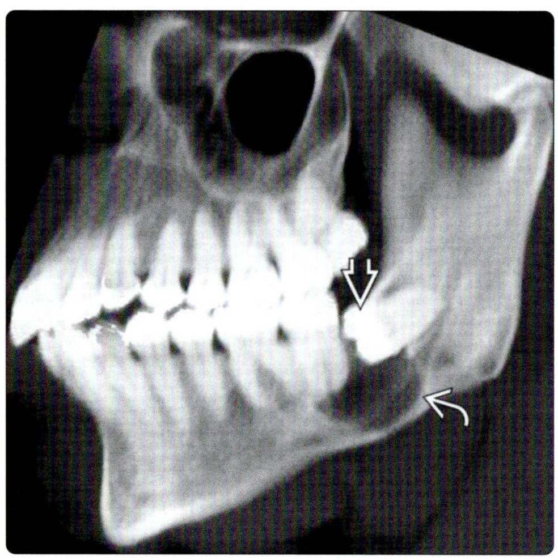

Nasopalatine Duct Cyst

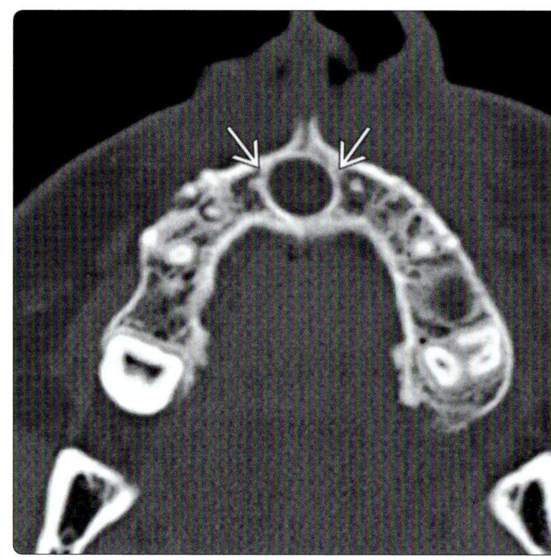

(Left) *Cropped panoramic radiograph of the anterior mandible shows a large well-defined unilocular radiolucency* ➡ *representing a simple bone cyst in a 17-year-old boy.* **(Right)** *Axial CBCT in the same patient shows endosteal scalloping* ➡ *along the buccal cortex typical of simple bone cyst. This scalloping may cause the lesion to appear to have septa on plain radiographs resulting in an inaccurate multilocular differential diagnosis.*

Simple (Traumatic) Bone Cyst

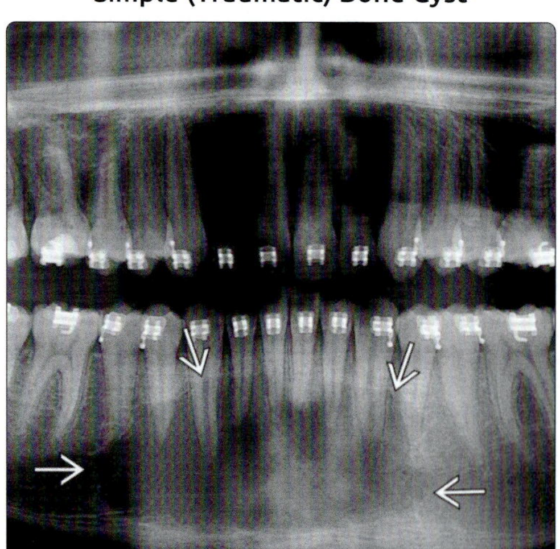

Simple (Traumatic) Bone Cyst

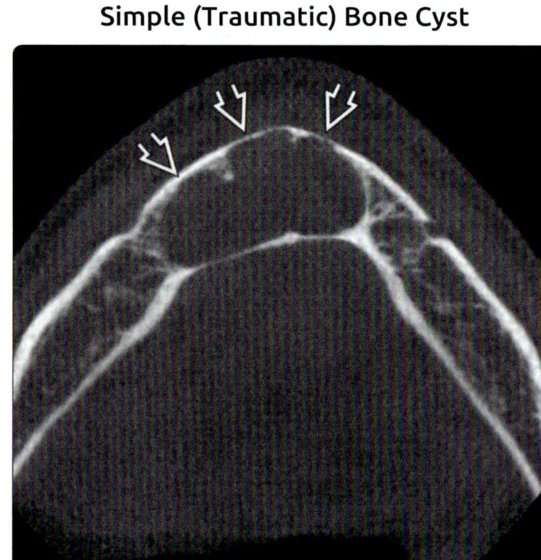

Odontogenic Keratocyst (Keratocystic Odontogenic Tumor)

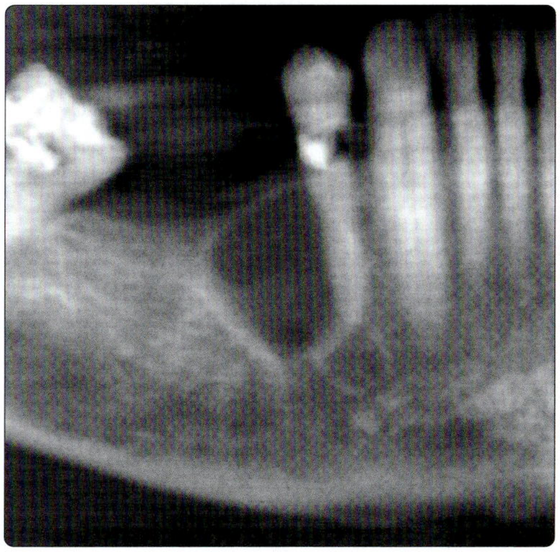

Odontogenic Keratocyst (Keratocystic Odontogenic Tumor)

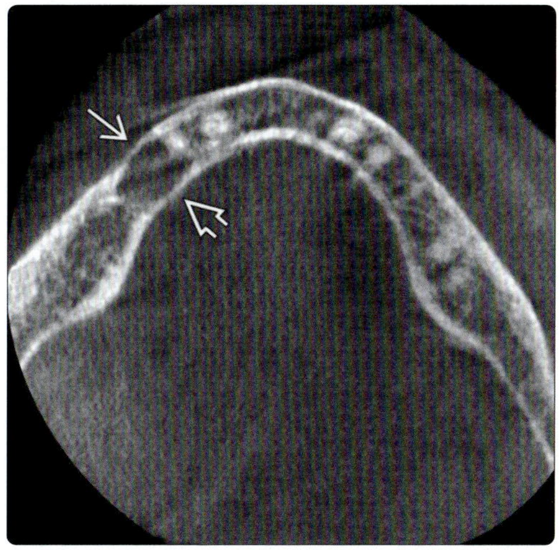

(Left) *Panoramic reformat CBCT shows a unilocular, well-defined, corticated odontogenic keratocyst (OKC) in the mandibular right premolar area. The lesion is in the alveolar bone above the mandibular canal.* **(Right)** *Axial CBCT in same patient shows the unilocular nature of the lesion and thinning of the buccal and lingual cortices. No expansion is noted, which is typical of OKC in the mandible. OKC and simple bone cyst may appear very similar radiographically.*

Lateral Periodontal Cyst

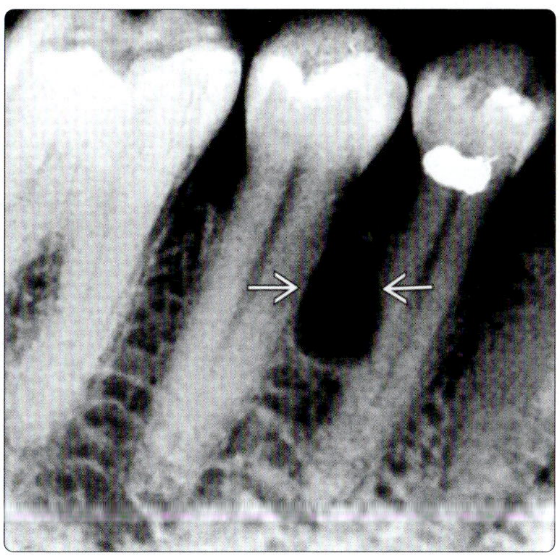

Unicystic Ameloblastoma

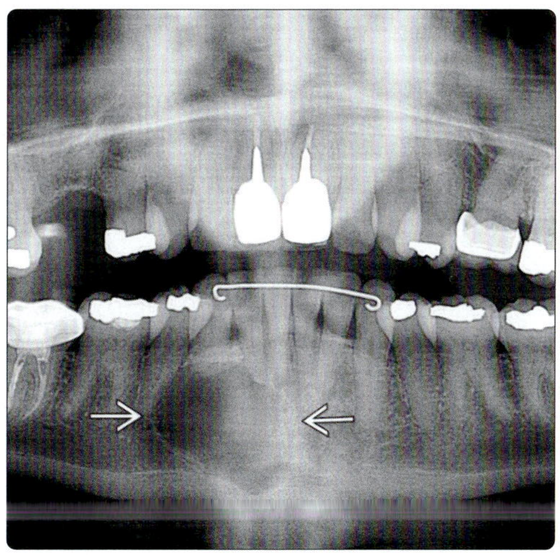

(Left) *Periapical radiograph shows a lateral periodontal cyst (LPC) between the 1st and 2nd mandibular premolars. This is the most common location for an LPC. Note the teardrop appearance of the lesion. (Courtesy M. Ahmad, DDS.)* **(Right)** *Panoramic image shows large unicystic ameloblastoma in the anterior mandible of a 50-year-old woman. Note absence of loculations and well-defined corticated margins. This lesion is less aggressive and has less recurrence than ameloblastoma. (Courtesy J. Zimmet, DDS.)*

Multiple Myeloma

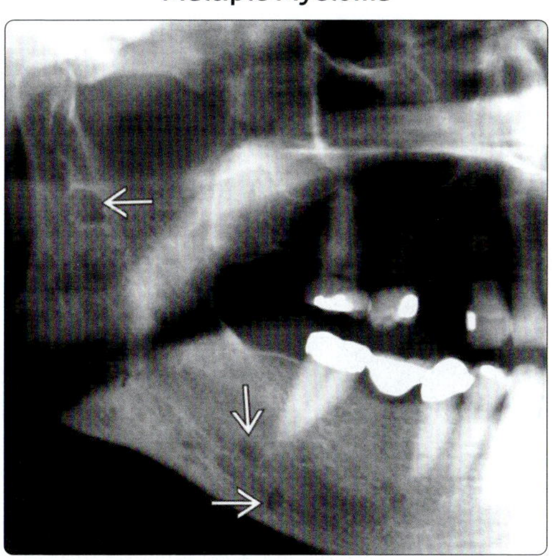

Eosinophilic Granuloma

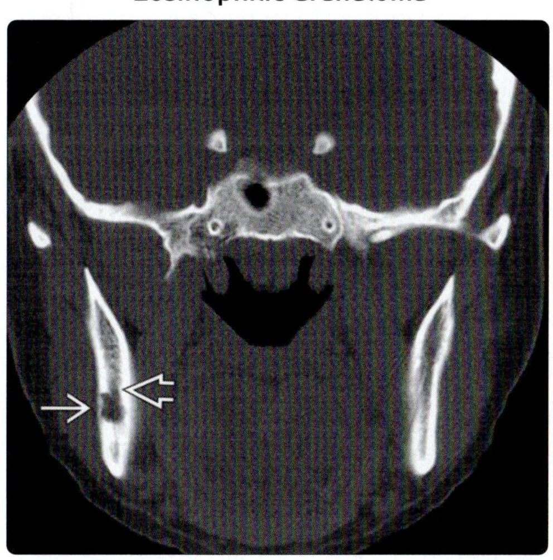

(Left) *Panoramic radiograph shows multiple well-defined, punched-out radiolucencies in right mandibular body and ramus of an 80-year-old man with undiagnosed multiple myeloma (MM). 20-30% of patients with MM develop jaw lesions, but it is rare that these are 1st presentation of disease.* **(Right)** *Coronal bone CT shows a small well-defined lesion of eosinophilic granuloma in the right mandibular ramus. The buccal cortex is thinned but not perforated. The lesion extends buccally to the mandibular canal.*

Pericoronal Radiolucencies Without Radiopacities

DIFFERENTIAL DIAGNOSIS

Common

- Dentigerous Cyst

Less Common

- Unicystic Ameloblastoma
- Odontogenic Keratocyst
- Ameloblastic Fibroma
- Buccal Bifurcation Cyst

Rare but Important

- Melanotic Neuroectodermal Tumor of Infancy

ESSENTIAL INFORMATION

Key Differential Diagnosis Issues

- Difficult to differentiate between lesions when small
- As lesion enlarges, will see typical hydraulic cystic expansion with dentigerous cyst: Lesion forms obtuse and equal angles with normal cortex at both sides of cyst
- Neoplastic expansion tends to meet normal cortex at acute &/or unequal angles
- Pericoronal lesions with calcifications (radiopacities) may initially appear completely radiolucent

Helpful Clues for Common Diagnoses

- **Dentigerous Cyst**
  - Key facts
    - 2nd and 3rd decades; M:F = 3:2
    - **Mandibular 3rd molars** most common
  - Imaging
    - Well-defined, **unilocular**, corticated radiolucency around entire crown, attaching at CEJ
    - Uniform round expansion and thinning of cortex
    - Associated tooth is often significantly displaced

Helpful Clues for Less Common Diagnoses

- **Unicystic Ameloblastoma**
  - Key facts
    - Begins as mural nodule in lining of existing cyst
    - Once in bone, behaves like typical ameloblastoma
    - 3rd decade: Primarily mandibular 3rd molars
  - Imaging
    - **Unilocular** (faint septa) **or multilocular** radiolucency with significant expansion
    - Smaller tumors: **Enhancing mural nodule** on T1WI C+
- **Odontogenic Keratocyst**
  - Key facts
    - Pericoronal odontogenic keratocyst is orthokeratinized variant
    - 2nd and 3rd decades; M > F
  - Imaging
    - Little expansion in mandible: May exhibit **scalloping**
    - Radiolucency attaches apical to CEJ
    - **Lumen may be milky** due to presence of keratin
- **Ameloblastic Fibroma**
  - Key facts
    - Childhood/adolescence: Mean age: ~ 15 years
    - Slow growing but can reach large size
  - Imaging
    - Unilocular or multilocular radiolucency
    - Typical neoplastic expansion
- **Buccal Bifurcation Cyst**
  - Key facts
    - Usually < 11 years
    - Mandibular molars: 1st > 2nd > 3rd; maxilla rare
  - Imaging: Radiolucency **lateral to crown of tipped molar tooth**: Does not surround entire crown

Helpful Clues for Rare Diagnoses

- **Melanotic Neuroectodermal Tumor of Infancy**
  - Key facts
    - Infants: Usually < 6 months up to 1 year
    - Maxilla > mandible: Anterior > posterior
  - Imaging
    - Pericoronal to developing **primary tooth**

SELECTED REFERENCES

1. Langlais RP et al: Diagnostic Imaging of the Jaws. Malvern, PA: Williams & Wilkins, 2005

Dentigerous Cyst

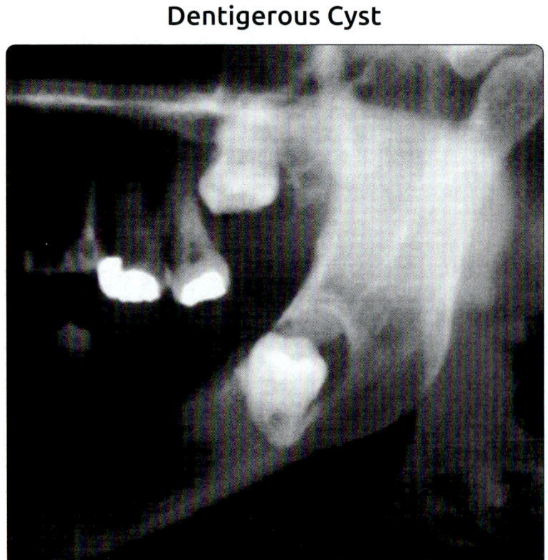

Dentigerous Cyst

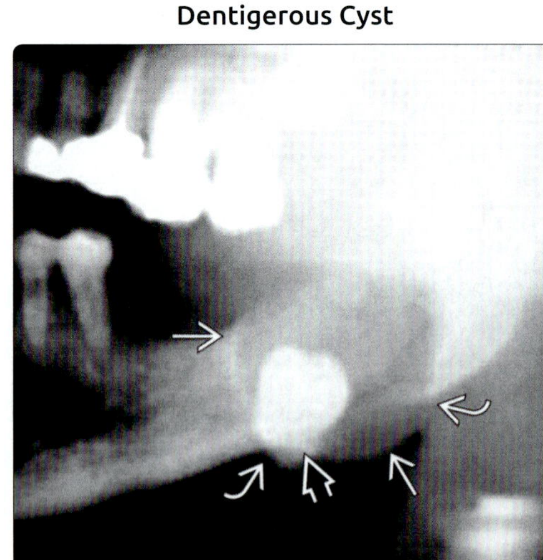

(Left) *Panoramic radiograph shows a dentigerous cyst associated with the impacted mandibular left 3rd molar. When small, all lesions in the differential diagnosis may look similar. Also consider immature pericoronal lesions containing radiopacities.* **(Right)** *Panoramic radiograph in the same patient 4 years later shows round, unilocular, hydraulic expansion* ➡ *typical of a dentigerous cyst. Note the obtuse angle with normal cortex* ➡ *and displacement of the affected tooth* ➡.

Dentigerous Cyst

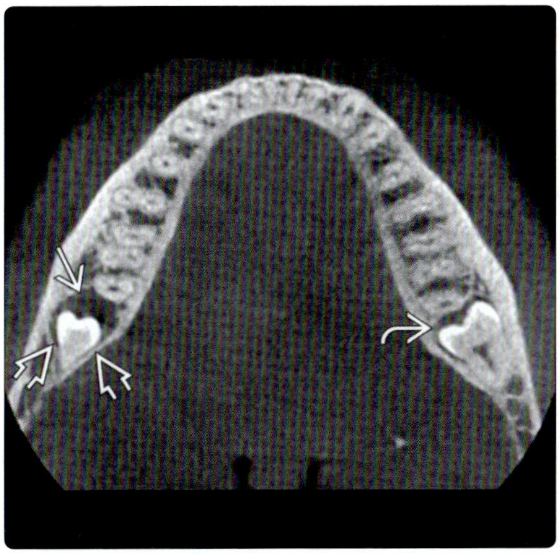

Unicystic Ameloblastoma

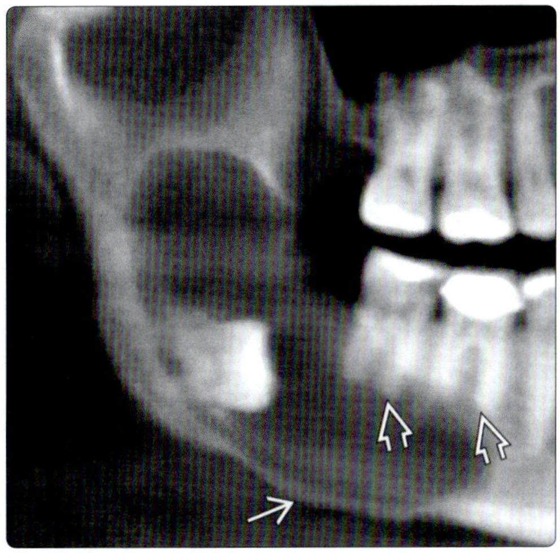

(Left) *Axial CBCT shows an impacted right mandibular 3rd molar with a pericoronal radiolucency ➡ measuring > 3 mm. This is the most common location for dentigerous cyst. Note attachment at the CEJ ➡. Compare to normal follicular space on the left ➡.* **(Right)** *Panoramic reformat CBCT shows unicystic ameloblastoma associated with the impacted mandibular right 3rd molar. The lesion has expanded the inferior cortex ➡ and caused knife-edge root resorption ➡ typical of ameloblastoma. (Courtesy M. Noujeim, DDS.)*

Odontogenic Keratocyst

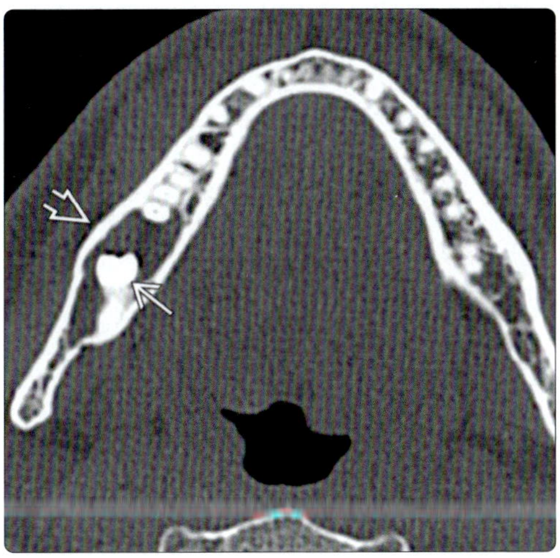

Odontogenic Keratocyst

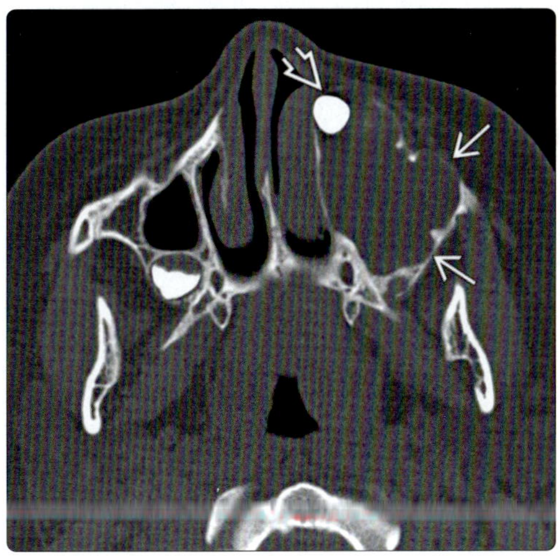

(Left) *Axial bone CT shows an odontogenic keratocyst (OKC) as a pericoronal radiolucency associated with the impacted mandibular right 3rd molar ➡. Note minimal expansion ➡ for a lesion this size, characteristic of OKCs, which favor anteroposterior growth in the mandible.* **(Right)** *Axial bone CT shows OKC associated with the maxillary left canine, which is displaced superiorly, medially, and anteriorly ➡. Note the lesion is expansile, filling the left maxillary sinus and smoothly scalloping and thinning the walls ➡.*

Ameloblastic Fibroma

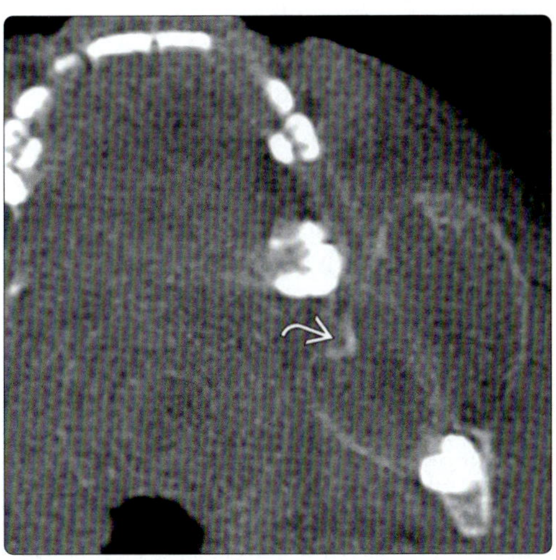

Buccal Bifurcation Cyst

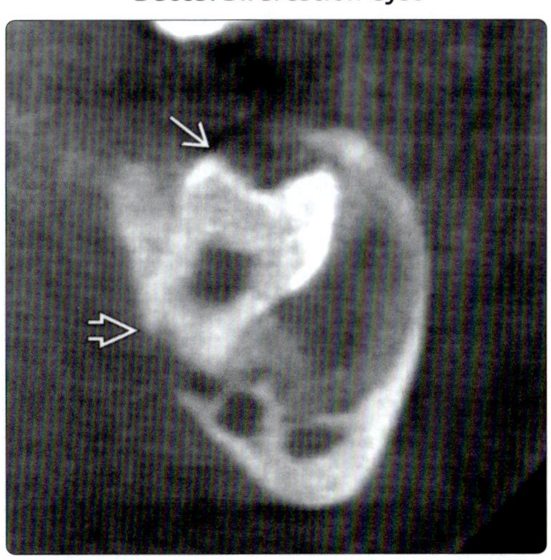

(Left) *Axial CBCT shows ameloblastic fibroma associated with the mandibular left 2nd molar. The lesion makes an acute angle ➡ with a normal cortex, typical of neoplastic expansion. (Courtesy M. Noujeim, DDS.)* **(Right)** *Cross-section CBCT shows buccal bifurcation cyst associated with the mandibular left 2nd molar. The lesion encompasses the occlusal surface of the tooth but terminates at the lingual cusp ➡. Note the characteristic tipping of the tooth with roots at the lingual cortex ➡.*

DIFFERENTIAL DIAGNOSIS

Common

- Odontoma

Less Common

- Adenomatoid Odontogenic Tumor (AOT)
- Calcifying Odontogenic Cyst (COC)
- Calcifying Epithelial Odontogenic Tumor (CEOT)

Rare but Important

- Ameloblastic Fibroodontoma (AFO)
- Ameloblastic Odontoma (AO)

ESSENTIAL INFORMATION

Key Differential Diagnosis Issues

- Lesions may be totally radiolucent initially & confused with pericoronal radiolucencies without radiopacities
- Density, quantity, & location of calcifications helpful
  - Odontoma, AFO, & AO calcifications more dense
  - CCOT, CEOT, & AFO calcifications often sparse
  - CEOT, CCOT, AOT, & AO calcifications tend to cluster around incisal or occlusal aspect of crown
  - AOT may have peripheral zone/band of radiolucency

Helpful Clues for Common Diagnoses

- **Odontoma**
  - Key facts
    - Young patients: 2nd decade
  - Imaging
    - Narrow radiolucent rim surrounded by thin cortex
    - **Compound odontoma:** Calcifications **resemble small teeth**; predilection for anterior jaws
    - **Complex odontoma:** Calcifications are dense but do not resemble teeth; posterior jaws

Helpful Clues for Less Common Diagnoses

- **Adenomatoid Odontogenic Tumor (AOT)**
  - Key facts
    - 2nd decade; anterior > posterior
  - Imaging
    - Calcifications: **Snowflakes** or small pebbles
    - May have peripheral zone of radiolucency
    - Attachment apical to cementoenamel junction
- **Calcifying Odontogenic Cyst (COC)**
  - Key facts
    - 10-30 years
    - Anterior > posterior
  - Imaging
    - Calcifications appear as flecks & may be clustered around occlusal/incisal surface of tooth or oriented along periphery
- **Calcifying Epithelial Odontogenic Tumor (CEOT)**
  - Key facts
    - Older age group: Mean 5th decade; M > F
    - Location: Posterior mandible
  - Imaging
    - Calcifications may be clustered at occlusal surface of associated tooth & often described as **driven snow**

Helpful Clues for Rare Diagnoses

- **Ameloblastic Fibroodontoma (AFO)**
  - Key facts
    - Young patient: 1st & 2nd decades
    - Very benign; does not behave as ameloblastoma
  - Imaging
    - Tooth density calcifications that are sparse & do not resemble teeth; lesion mostly radiolucent
    - Calcifications may be **donut** shaped
- **Ameloblastic Odontoma (AO)**
  - Key facts
    - 2nd decade or younger; anterior > posterior
    - Rare & more aggressive because ameloblastic component identical to ameloblastoma histologically
  - Imaging
    - May see **washer-like** structures

SELECTED REFERENCES

1. Langlais RP et al: Diagnostic Imaging of the Jaws. Malvern, Pennsylvania: Williams & Wilkins, 2005

Odontoma

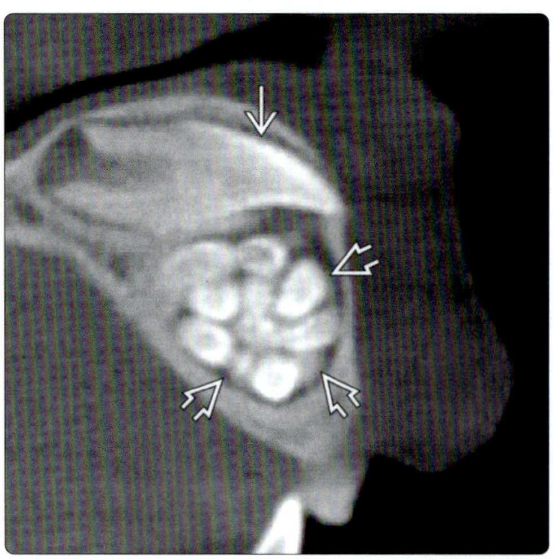

Odontoma

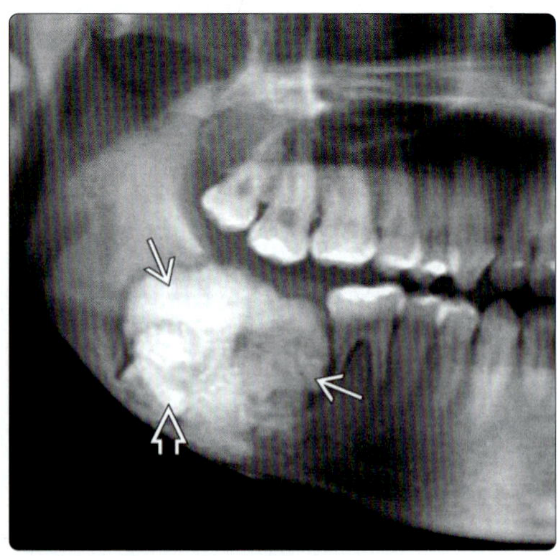

(Left) *Sagittal CBCT shows a compound odontoma pericoronal to the permanent maxillary left central incisor* ➡*. Note contents look like teeth & odontoma has thin peripheral radiolucency* ➡ *with corticated margin.* **(Right)** *Panoramic radiograph shows a complex odontoma* ➡ *associated with the crown of the mandibular 2nd molar* ➡*. Note no resemblance to teeth, but the lesion exhibits density of enamel. Complex odontomas favor the posterior jaws. (Courtesy M. Noujeim, DDS.)*

Adenomatoid Odontogenic Tumor (AOT)

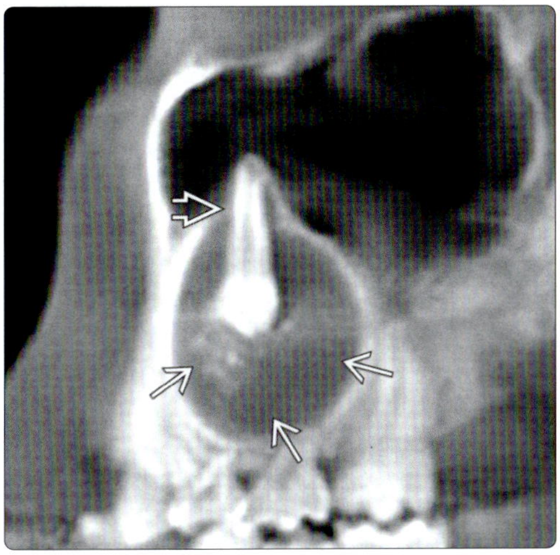

Adenomatoid Odontogenic Tumor (AOT)

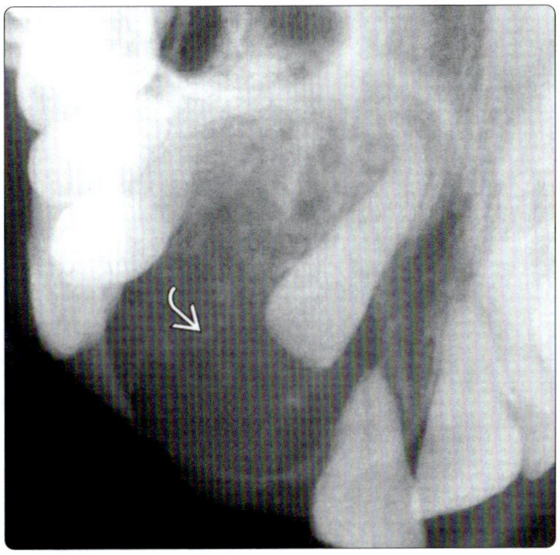

(Left) *Sagittal CBCT shows an adenomatoid odontogenic tumor (AOT) pericoronal to a maxillary premolar. The cortex of the lesion is attached to the midroot of the tooth ➡. Note calcifications are in the center of the lesion, & there is a peripheral zone of radiolucency often seen in AOT ➡. (Courtesy M. Noujeim, DDS.)* **(Right)** *Occlusal radiograph shows a large, expansile AOT associated with the maxillary right lateral incisor. Note the faint calcifications ➡. This is a common location for AOT. (Courtesy M. Noujeim, DDS.)*

Calcifying Odontogenic Cyst (COC)

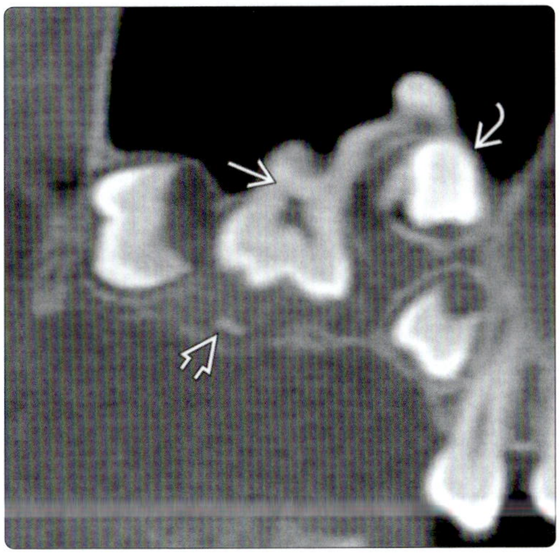

Calcifying Epithelial Odontogenic Tumor (CEOT)

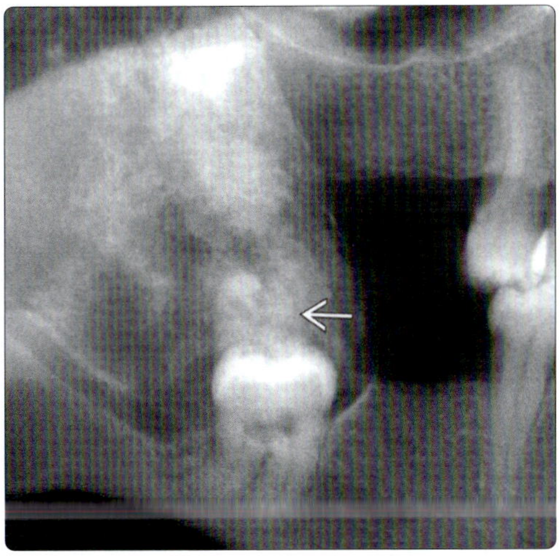

(Left) *Sagittal CBCT shows COC around crown of the maxillary 1st molar ➡. Note small calcification ➡. Calcifications may be sparse & should be looked for carefully. Lesion has impeded eruption of the 1st molar, & the 2nd premolar follicle ➡ is displaced. (Courtesy M. Ahmad, DDS.)* **(Right)** *Cropped panoramic radiograph shows large CEOT around crown of mandibular 2nd molar. Diffuse radiopacities give a driven-snow appearance & calcifications are clustered at occlusal surface ➡. (Courtesy K. Ambramovitch, DDS.)*

Ameloblastic Fibroodontoma (AFO)

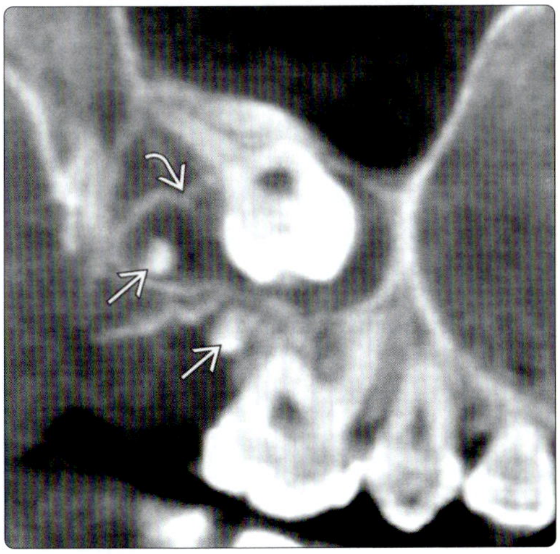

Ameloblastic Fibroodontoma (AFO)

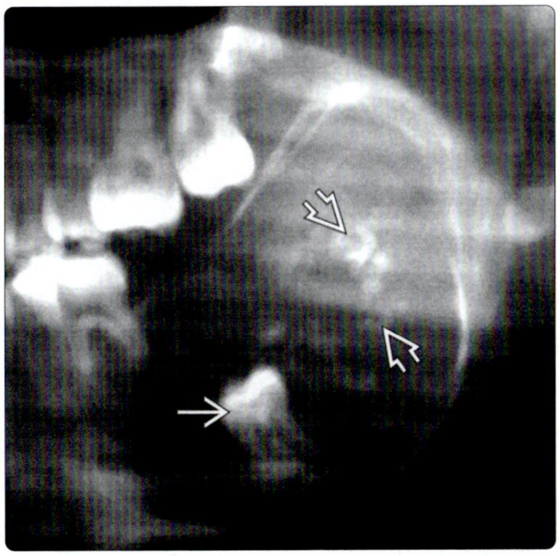

(Left) *Sagittal CBCT shows an ameloblastic fibroodontoma (AFO) presenting as a well-defined, corticated, pericoronal radiolucency containing 2 small, high-density areas that are comparable to tooth structure ➡. Note the hint of loculation ➡.* **(Right)** *Panoramic radiograph shows a large expansile AFO associated with the mandibular left 2nd molar ➡. Note donut-shaped calcifications ➡ signifying enamel & dentin deposition.*

DIFFERENTIAL DIAGNOSIS

Common

- Odontogenic Keratocyst (Keratocystic Odontogenic Tumor)
- Ameloblastoma
- Central Giant Cell Granuloma

Less Common

- Aneurysmal Bone Cyst
- Hemangioma, Facial Bones
- Odontogenic Myxoma (Myxofibroma)

Rare but Important

- Cherubism
- Central Mucoepidermoid Carcinoma
- Glandular Odontogenic Cyst

ESSENTIAL INFORMATION

Key Differential Diagnosis Issues

- Characteristics of internal septa help differentiate similar-appearing lesions
  - Coarse, curved septa: Ameloblastoma, glandular odontogenic cyst, central mucoepidermoid carcinoma
  - Thin, curved septa: Odontogenic keratocyst, cherubism
  - Straight, geometric septa: Odontogenic myxoma; may also contain coarse, curved septa
  - Septa at right angles to periphery: Central giant cell granuloma (CGCG), hemangioma, aneurysmal bone cyst
- Bilateral appearance: Cherubism
- Lesions with radiating septa or pseudoperiosteal reaction must be differentiated from more aggressive condition such as osteogenic sarcoma
- Central mucoepidermoid carcinoma can mimic benign multilocular conditions
- All multilocular lesions should be **aspirated prior to biopsy** to avoid excessive bleeding if lesion vascular

Helpful Clues for Common Diagnoses

- **Odontogenic Keratocyst (Keratocystic Odontogenic Tumor)**
  - Key facts
    - May displace, extrude, or resorb teeth
    - Rapid growth and **high recurrence** rate
    - Consider **basal cell nevus syndrome** if multiple and bilateral
  - Imaging
    - Sclerotic, scalloped border; often **pericoronal**
    - Roughly half are unilocular
    - Few and large loculations; septa often thin, curved
    - Little expansion in mandible; grows along bone
    - T1WI MR: Intermediate to high signal intensity
    - T2WI MR: Heterogeneous, low to high signal intensity
- **Ameloblastoma**
  - Key facts
    - Most often posterior mandible
    - **Expansile**; displaces teeth
    - **Angled root resorption** common
    - High recurrence unless unicystic
  - Imaging
    - Well-defined, corticated border
    - Septa thick, curved; **soap-bubble** appearance
    - Cortical expansion, impingement, perforation
    - Displacement of adjacent anatomic structures
    - T1WI MR: Low to intermediate signal intensity
    - T2WI MR: High signal intensity
    - Enhanced MR to define extraosseous components &/or association with neurovascular structures
- **Central Giant Cell Granuloma**
  - Key facts
    - **Expansile**; may displace teeth
    - **Anterior to molars** in adolescents & young adults
      - May cross midline, which is uncharacteristic for other multilocular radiolucencies
    - Similar lesion seen in hyperparathyroidism (Brown tumor)
  - Imaging
    - Wispy septa, often at **right angles to edge of lesion**
    - Scalloped margins, may not be corticated
    - Occasional cortical perforation, especially in maxilla
    - Indistinguishable from Brown tumor (osteitis fibrosa cystica) of hyperparathyroidism, radiographically and histologically

Helpful Clues for Less Common Diagnoses

- **Aneurysmal Bone Cyst**
  - Key facts
    - Posterior mandible favored; young patients
    - Pseudocyst; lacks epithelial lining
    - Frequently painful
  - Imaging
    - Expansion and thinning of cortex ("ballooning")
    - Thin septa at right angles to edge of lesion
    - Often mimics CGCG
    - Low-density areas (vascular spaces) on CT soft tissue window
    - T1WI MR: Hyperintense signal
    - T2WI MR: Fluid-fluid levels
- **Hemangioma, Facial Bones**
  - Key facts
    - Uncommon vascular neoplasm
      - Most should be considered as venous or arteriovenous malformation and not tumor
    - Depressible or displaced teeth
    - Spontaneous gingival bleeding
  - Imaging
    - Ill-defined, irregular margins
    - Thin septa, often **radiating** like spokes of wheel
    - T2WI MR: High signal intensity
    - Phleboliths may be seen
- **Odontogenic Myxoma (Myxofibroma)**
  - Key facts
    - Expansile; may displace teeth
      - Rapid growth pattern
    - More common in posterior mandible
    - Rarely in ramus, condyle, zygoma
    - Does not metastasize but **high recurrence rate**
  - Imaging
    - Lobular, scalloped edges
    - Thin septa, may form **right angles or geometric shapes** with each other

- Coarse and curved septa also common
- Straight septa may produce **pseudoperiosteal reaction** at periphery
- Borders may be well or ill defined, corticated or not

Helpful Clues for Rare Diagnoses

- **Cherubism**
  - Key facts
    - Rare, hereditary, bilateral jaw expansion in children
    - Most often in mandible
    - May involve coronoid process; condyles often spared
    - Painless
    - Self-limiting; regresses after puberty
      - Surgical correction for cosmetic reasons possible
  - Imaging
    - **Expansile, bilateral**
    - Septa thick, curved
    - Displaced teeth or tooth buds, unerupted teeth
    - Missing or malformed teeth, especially 1st and 2nd molars
    - Mandibular canal displaced inferiorly
    - Root resorption
    - Cortical thinning but no perforation
    - Lesions replaced by sclerotic or granular-appearing bone following regression
    - T1WI MR: Hypointense or intermediate signal
    - T2WI MR: Hypo-, hyper-, or intermediate signal intensity
- **Central Mucoepidermoid Carcinoma**
  - Key facts
    - Uncommon tumor of mucus-producing epithelium
    - Painless swelling
    - Posterior mandible most common
    - **Mimics benign cyst or tumor**
  - Imaging
    - Expansile, but cortical plates usually intact and thin
    - Thick, corticated periphery, often undulating or scalloped
    - Internal septa often thick, curved, similar to ameloblastoma
    - Rarely contains thin, wispy septa
    - Displacement of adjacent structures possible
- **Glandular Odontogenic Cyst**
  - Key facts
    - **Rare** cyst of odontogenic epithelium with mucus-producing cells
    - Aggressive behavior
    - Tendency to recur
    - Most common in anterior mandible and anterior maxilla
  - Imaging
    - Scalloped corticated borders
    - May be multilocular
    - Expansion of outer cortex with possible perforation
    - Displacement of teeth

SELECTED REFERENCES

1. Robinson RA: Diagnosing the most common odontogenic cystic and osseous lesions of the jaws for the practicing pathologist. Mod Pathol. 30(s1):S96-S103, 2017
2. von Stempel C et al: Imaging of palatal lumps. Clin Radiol. 72(2):97-107, 2017
3. Ali IK et al: Non-familial cherubism with bilateral maxilla and mandible Involvement - clinicoradiographic findings. Cureus. 8(7):e709, 2016
4. Chrcanovic BR et al: Recurrence probability for keratocystic odontogenic tumors: An analysis of 6427 cases. J Craniomaxillofac Surg. ePub, 2016
5. da Silva LP et al: Central mucoepidermoid carcinoma radiographically mimicking an odontogenic tumor: A case report and literature review. J Oral Maxillofac Pathol. 20(3):518-522, 2016
6. Davanian H et al: Ameloblastoma RNA profiling uncovers a distinct non-coding RNA signature. Oncotarget. ePub, 2016
7. Dolanmaz D et al: Management of central giant cell granuloma of the jaws with intralesional steroid injection and review of the literature. Oral Maxillofac Surg. 20(2):203-9, 2016
8. Kalaiselvan S et al: "Evaluation of safety margin" in ameloblastoma of the mandible by surgical, radiological, and histopathological methods: An evidence-based study. J Pharm Bioallied Sci. 8(Suppl 1):S122-S125, 2016
9. MacDonald D: Lesions of the jaws presenting as radiolucencies on cone-beam CT. Clin Radiol. 71(10):972-85, 2016
10. Dhiman NK et al: Central cavernous hemangioma of mandible: Case report and review of literature. Natl J Maxillofac Surg. 6(2):209-13, 2015
11. Faisal M et al: Glandular odontogenic cyst - Literature review and report of a paediatric case. J Oral Biol Craniofac Res. 5(3):219-25, 2015
12. Urs AB et al: Aneurysmal Bone Cyst of the Jaws: Clinicopathological Study. J Maxillofac Oral Surg. 13(4):458-63, 2014

Odontogenic Keratocyst (Keratocystic Odontogenic Tumor)

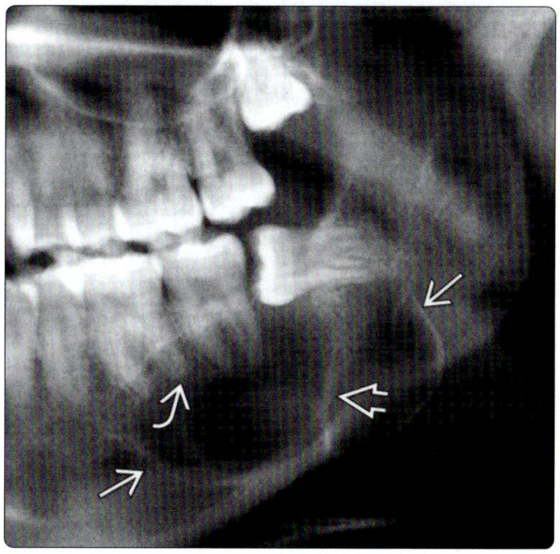

Odontogenic Keratocyst (Keratocystic Odontogenic Tumor)

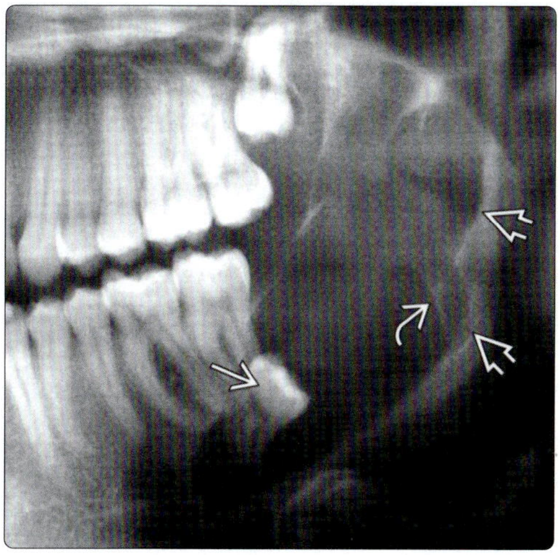

(Left) *Cropped panoramic radiograph shows a well-defined, radiolucent, corticated odontogenic keratocyst (OKC) in the posterior left mandible ➡. Single septum partially divides the lesion into 2 large loculations ➡. Note mild root resorption ➡.* **(Right)** *Cropped panoramic radiograph shows a large OKC pericoronal to the displaced impacted mandibular 3rd molar ➡ and occupying the entire ramus with minimal expansion. Note scalloping ➡ and small septa ➡.*

Ameloblastoma | **Ameloblastoma**

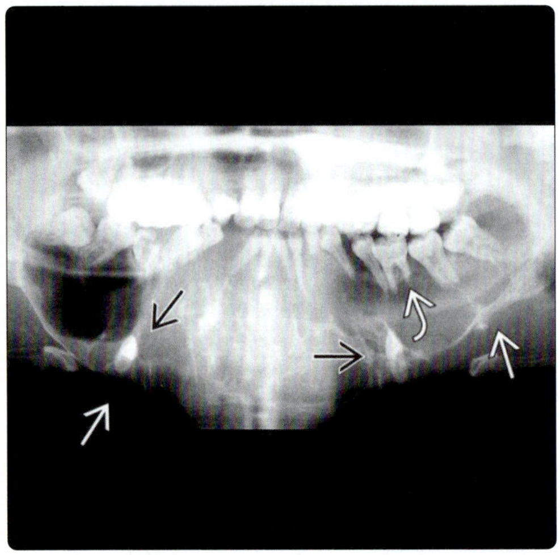

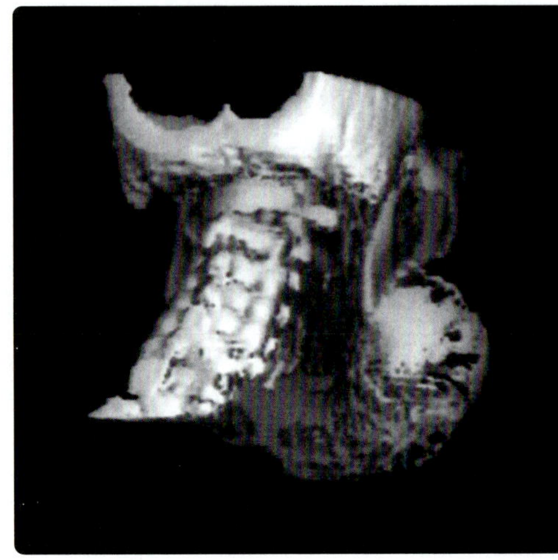

(Left) *Cropped panoramic radiograph of a 19-year-old woman exhibits an extensive multilocular radiolucency involving the entire mandible. There is significant expansion ➡, tooth displacement ⇨, and root resorption ➦. Postoperative evaluation of the right radiolucency demonstrated a cavity filled with a serous exudate.* **(Right)** *3D CT reconstruction of the same patient shows significant mandibular expansion. The expanded cortex exhibits effacement and perforation.*

Central Giant Cell Granuloma | **Central Giant Cell Granuloma**

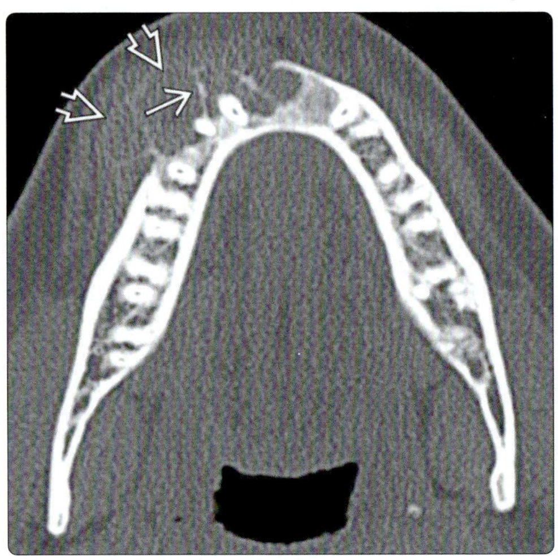

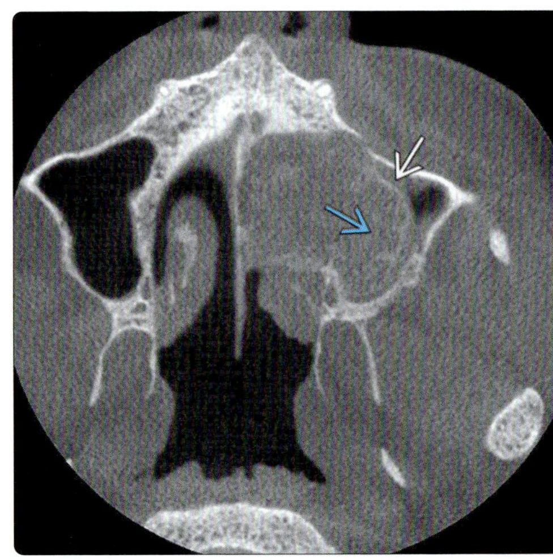

(Left) *Axial bone CT shows granular, wispy septa, some of which are oriented at right angles to the periphery ➡. This is the most common site for central giant cell granuloma, and buccal expansion is typical. Notice that the peripheral cortex is very faint and grainy ➡.* **(Right)** *Axial CBCT shows a multilocular lesion with extension from alveolar ridge into maxillary sinus and nasal fossa. Note fine corticated border ➡ and wispy septa ⇨. Patient tested positive for hyperparathyroidism; this is Brown tumor.*

Aneurysmal Bone Cyst | **Aneurysmal Bone Cyst**

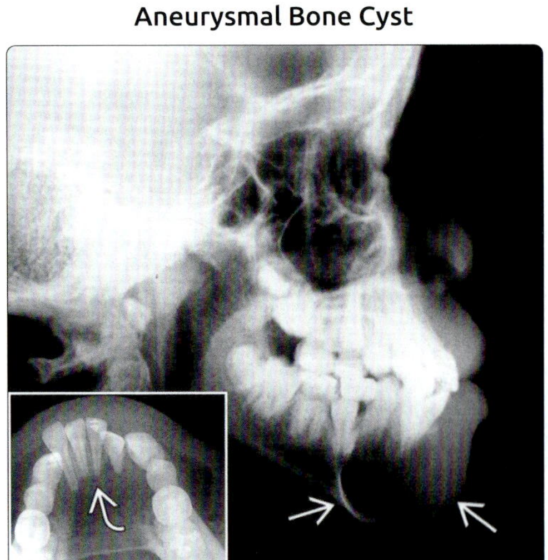

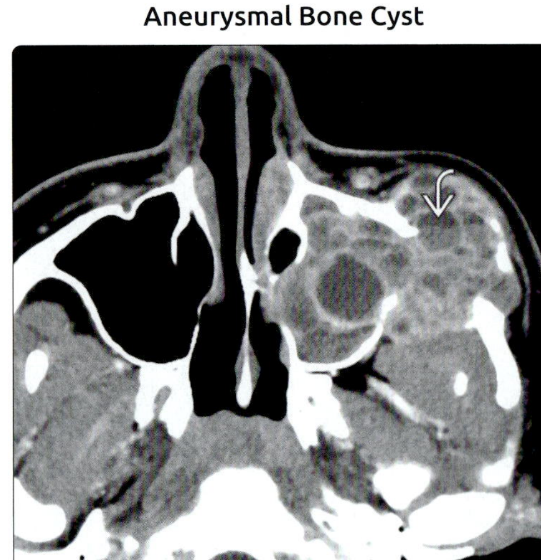

(Left) *Lateral cephalometric & occlusal images of an 11-year-old boy show rounded expansion of the anterior mandible ➡, tooth displacement, and external root resorption ➦. Moderate pain was noted.* **(Right)** *Axial CECT shows marked expansion protruding beyond the margins of the zygomatic arch into the subcutaneous tissues, obliterating the maxillary sinus. Fluid-fluid levels ➦ are evident. A rapidly expanding multilocular lesion in a young person is highly suggestive of aneurysmal bone cyst. (Courtesy S. Blaser, MD.)*

Non-Hodgkin Lymphoma

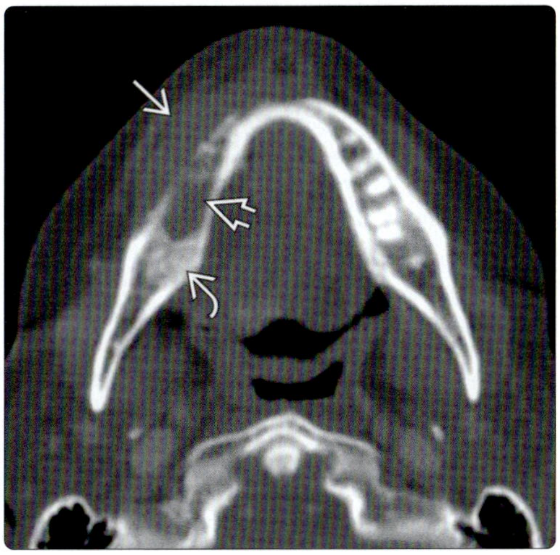

Non-Hodgkin Lymphoma

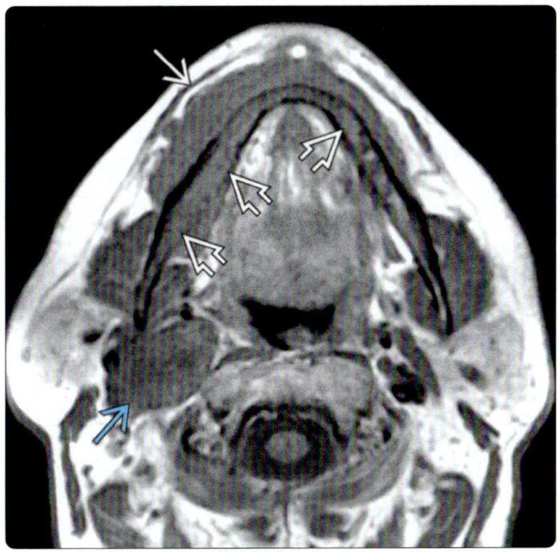

(Left) *Axial CECT with bone window demonstrates a poorly marginated lytic right hemimandibular lesion with destruction of the buccal cortex and sclerosis at the posterior margin. An associated soft tissue mass is evident.* **(Right)** *Axial T1WI MR in the same patient better illustrates the soft tissue component but also reveals more extensive marrow involvement. A markedly enlarged right level II node is also evident.*

Non-Hodgkin Lymphoma

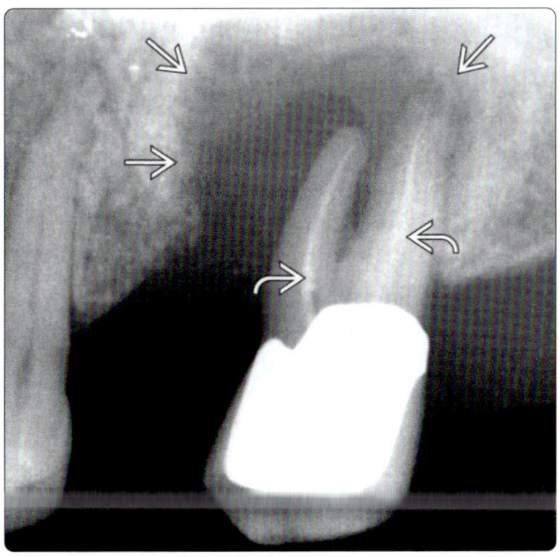

Multiple Myeloma

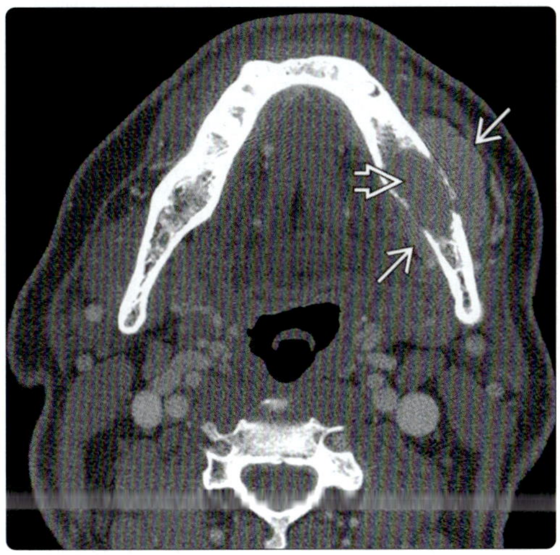

(Left) *Periapical radiograph shows lymphoma masquerading as a periapical inflammatory lesion. The lesion was misdiagnosed, and the molar was treated endodontically. Vitality testing of teeth is key in differentiating pulpal pathosis from more serious conditions.* **(Right)** *Axial bone CT shows a poorly marginated lytic lesion in the left mandible with patchy destruction of the lingual and buccal cortices. Note the associated soft tissue mass. Lesions of flat bones, such as the cranium, are typically more prominent.*

Osteonecrosis (Medication Related)

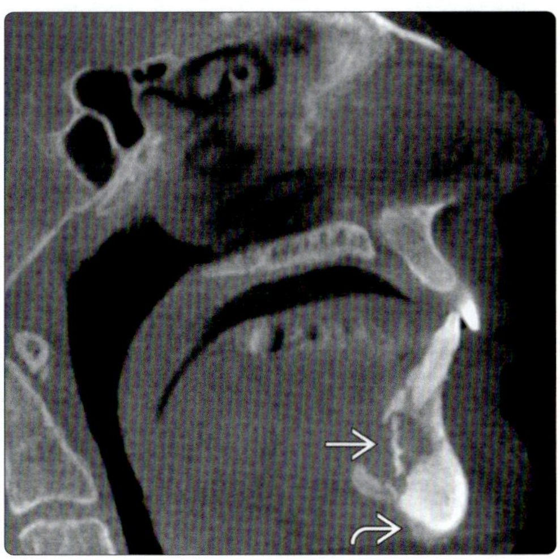

Osteonecrosis (Medication Related)

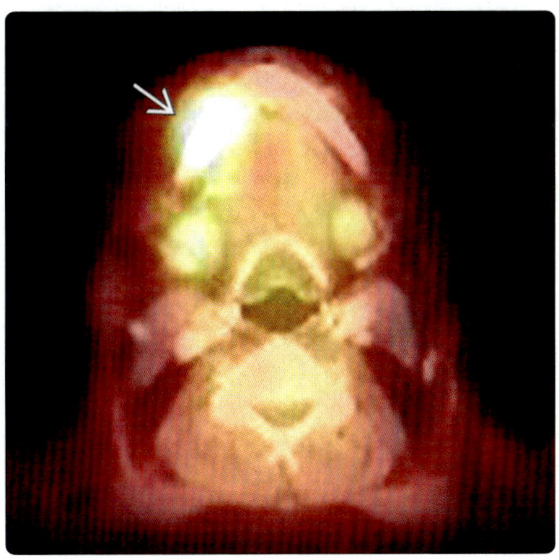

(Left) *Sagittal CBCT shows sequestration and periosteal reaction in the area of the genial tubercles and inferior border of the mandible. Exposed bone is usually the 1st clinical sign and precedes radiographic changes.* **(Right)** *Fused FDG PET/CT shows marked new uptake in the right body of the mandible adjacent to failing dental implants (not shown). The patient was using IV bisphosphonates to manage bone carcinoma.*

(Left) *Cropped panoramic radiograph reveals an expansile, multilocular lesion with moderately ill-defined margins ➡. The lesion has a granular bone pattern with wispy septa. Mild apical external root resorption ➡ is present on the distal root of the 1st mandibular molar. The diagnosis was proven with biopsy. These lesions are more common anterior to the 1st molars.* **(Right)** *Axial CBCT shows destruction of the lingual cortex ➡ and alveolar bone adjacent to the mandibular anterior teeth ➡.*

Central Giant Cell Tumor/Granuloma

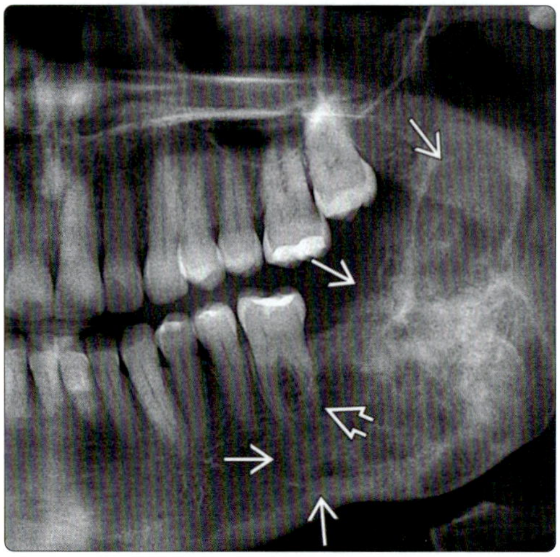

Central Giant Cell Tumor/Granuloma

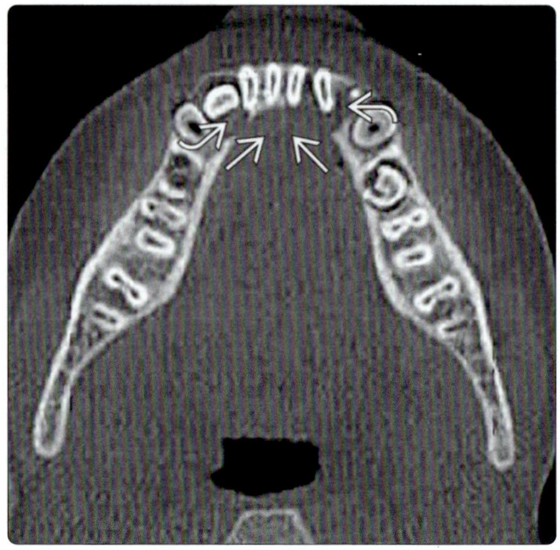

(Left) *Axial bone CT shows a solitary bone metastasis. The mass is painful and palpable. The osteolytic destructive process is centered in the posterior body of the left mandible with clear cortical perforation ➡ and subtle fullness of the left cheek, suggesting involvement of the masseter muscle ➡.* **(Right)** *Coronal fusion PET/CT of the same patient shows abnormal bone signal in the left mandible where intense FDG avidity was demonstrated ➡. Work-up revealed a primary bronchogenic tumor.*

Metastasis

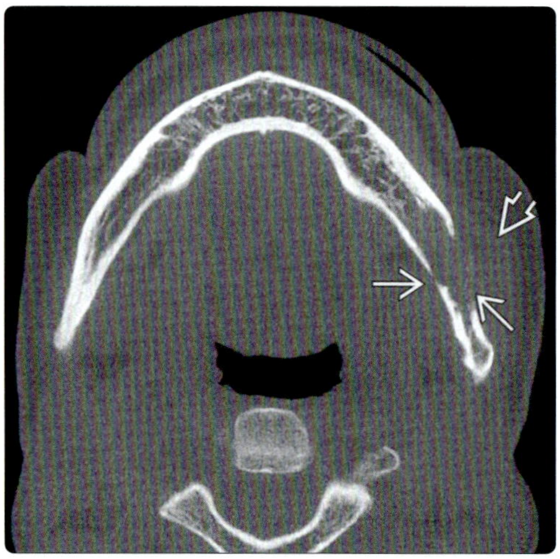

Metastasis

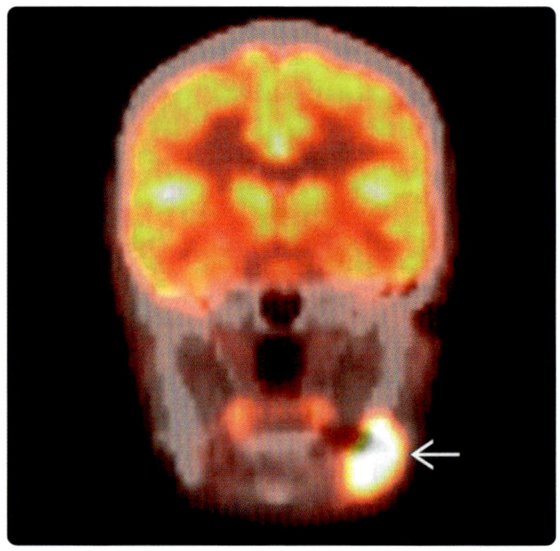

(Left) *Coronal T2WI MR of mucoepidermoid carcinoma of the hard palate shows a well-circumscribed mass ➡. Note that the signal intensity is higher than muscle intensity on T2. The tumor is immediately adjacent to a maxillary molar ➡.* **(Right)** *Coronal T1WI C+ FS MR in the same patient shows a well-circumscribed mass ➡ involving the adjacent molar ➡. It also shows extension into the alveolar recess of the left maxillary sinus ➡. The margins of the mass would typically appear less defined on bone CT.*

Minor Salivary Gland Malignancy

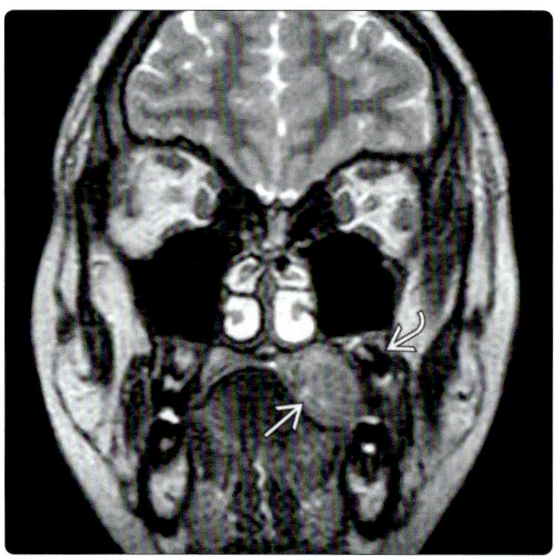

Minor Salivary Gland Malignancy

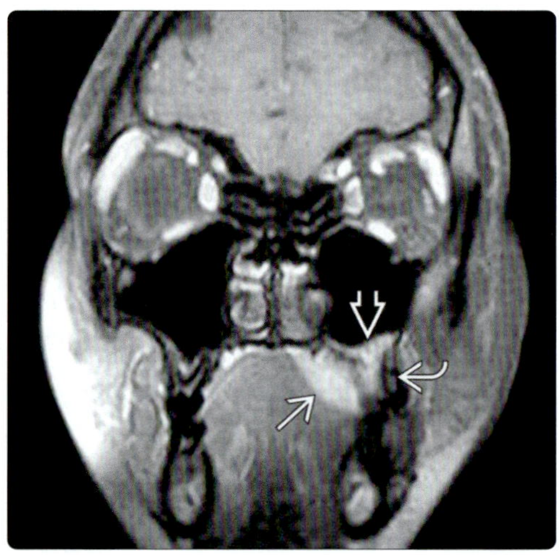

Ewing Sarcoma

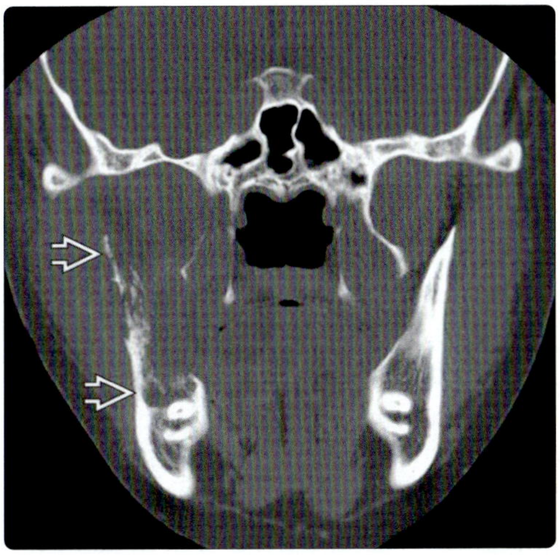

Ewing Sarcoma

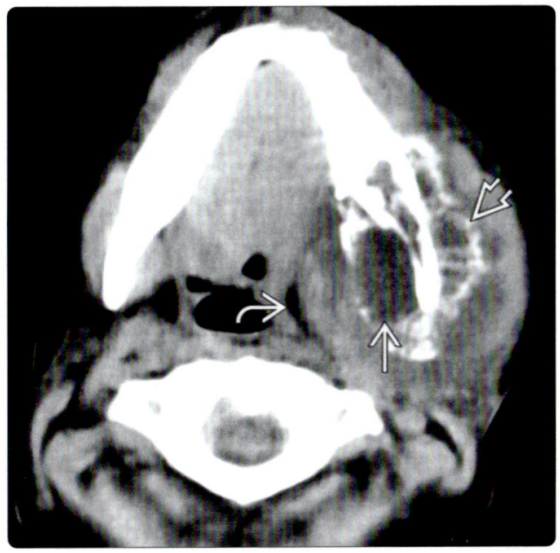

(Left) *Coronal bone CT reveals an ill-defined lytic lesion destroying the right mandibular ramus and coronoid process* ➡. *A periosteal reaction is not evident.* **(Right)** *Axial NECT shows a distended left cheek and a lytic mandibular lesion* ➡. *Sunburst periosteal new bone formation is evident, extending from the buccal cortex* ➡. *A medial soft tissue mass displaces parapharyngeal fat* ➡.

Osteosarcoma

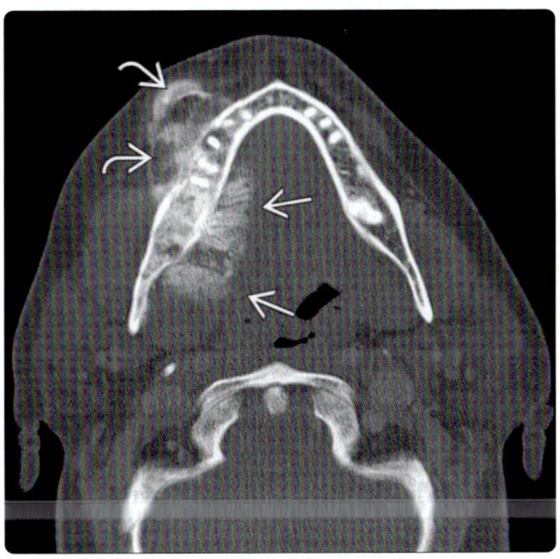

Osteosarcoma

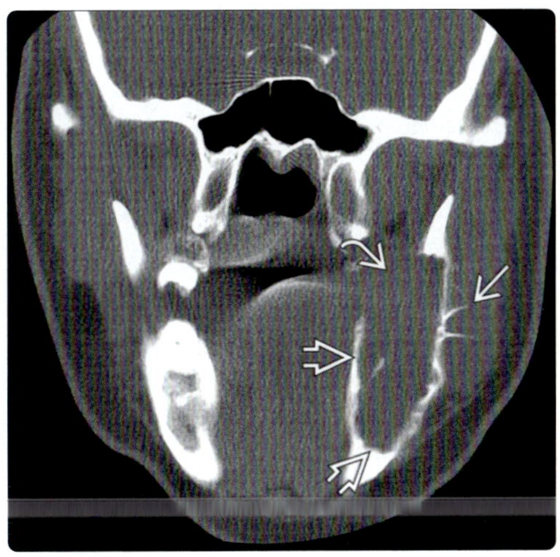

(Left) *Axial CECT shows a large, heterogeneous mass centered about the right mandibular body. The classic "sunburst" periosteal reaction is noted medially* ➡ *with an exophytic component along the buccal surface of the mandible* ➡. **(Right)** *Coronal bone CT shows an expansile mass involving the left mandibular body and ramus with irregular margins* ➡ *and cortical destruction* ➡. *Spiculated new bone formation* ➡ *(sunburst pattern) is seen on the lateral margin.*

Leukemia

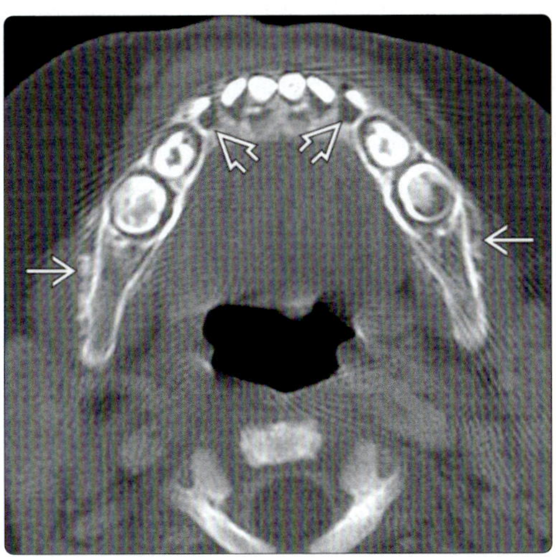

Langerhans Cell Histiocytosis

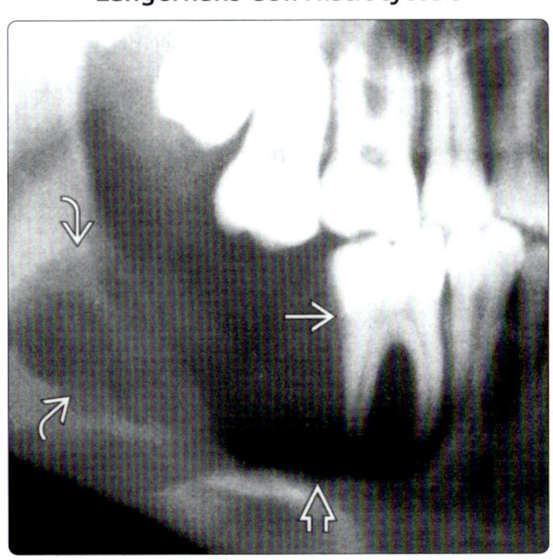

(Left) *Axial bone CT shows loss of definition of the dental laminae dura and widening of the periodontal ligament spaces around the teeth* ➡. *Diffuse osseous radiolucency is also evident with hair on end pattern of new bone formation* ➡. **(Right)** *Panoramic radiograph shows floating tooth appearance of the mandibular right 1st molar* ➡. *This high-contrast postprocessed image helps delineate the ill-defined lesion typical of Langerhans cell histiocytosis, which extends into the ramus* ➡ *and mandibular body* ➡.

DIFFERENTIAL DIAGNOSIS

Common

- Osteoporosis
- Osteomyelitis

Less Common

- Hyperparathyroidism
- Leukemia
- Vitamin D Deficiency
- Sickle Cell Anemia
- Thalassemia
- Cushing Syndrome

Rare but Important

- Hypophosphatasia
- Hypophosphatemia
- Massive Osteolysis (Vanishing Bone Disease)
- Gaucher Disease

ESSENTIAL INFORMATION

Key Differential Diagnosis Issues

- When generalized rarefaction of bone is noted, systemic disease can be suspected; the exception is osteomyelitis, which may span entire jaw without affecting any others

Helpful Clues for Common Diagnoses

- **Osteoporosis**
  - Key facts
    - Generalized **decrease** in bone **mass** with **histologically normal bone** that occurs gradually with age and more commonly in postmenopausal women
    - Secondary osteoporosis may occur with nutritional deficiencies, lack of osteoblast stimulation through weight-bearing exercise such as in cases of paralysis, corticosteroid or heparin therapy, or hormonal imbalance
  - Imaging
    - Diagnosis of "osteoporosis" is not confirmed through dental imaging but by dual energy x-ray absorption (DEXA) scan
    - Reduced density of bone (osteopenia) and thinning of inferior border of mandible ± lacunae formation in cortex
- **Osteomyelitis**
  - Key facts
    - Inflammation of bone and bone marrow due to bacterial infection; source of infection is usually identifiable (odontogenic, surgical, trauma)
    - May superimpose on osteoradionecrosis or bisphosphonate-related osteonecrosis of jaw
    - Although localized to one area of jaw bone, may cross midline and become extensive, involving entire jaw
  - Imaging
    - Acute osteomyelitis presents as ill-defined lucency of bone
    - **Sequestrae** (bone within bone appearance) and **periosteal bone reaction** become noticeable with time, giving more mixed density appearance

Helpful Clues for Less Common Diagnoses

- **Hyperparathyroidism**
  - Key facts
    - Endocrine disorder with excess circulating parathyroid hormone (PTH) causing ↑ osteoclastic activity
    - Primary hyperparathyroidism usually caused by tumor (most commonly adenoma) of parathyroid glands resulting in excess production of PTH
    - Secondary hyperparathyroidism occurs in response to hypocalcemia, usually due to poor intake or absorption of vitamin D, or due to deficient vitamin D metabolism in liver or kidney
    - Tertiary hyperparathyroidism occurs with longstanding secondary hyperparathyroidism that no longer responds to medication
  - Imaging
    - Demineralization and thinning of cortical boundaries
    - **Teeth appear to "stand out"** in contrast to demineralized bone; loss of lamina dura of teeth may occur
    - Trabecular pattern may be fine and random or granular appearing
- **Leukemia**
  - Key facts
    - Malignant tumor of hematopoietic stem cells that displaces normal bone marrow
  - Imaging
    - Can present as patchy areas of radiolucency or generalized decrease in density of bone
- **Vitamin D Deficiency**
  - Key facts
    - Defect in activity of vitamin D metabolites, leading to vitamin D deficiency; vitamin D is required for absorption of calcium in intestine; no vitamin D = ↓ calcium and phosphate in serum
  - Imaging
    - **Rickets**: In growing skeleton in children
      - Jaw cortices are thin and trabeculation in medullary spaces is reduced
      - Development and eruption of dentition is delayed; enamel hypoplasia is common if occurs before 3 years of age
      - Lamina dura and follicle cortex thinned or missing
    - **Osteomalacia**: In mature skeleton of adults
      - Generally no radiographic signs; may rarely cause generalized rarefaction and thin laminae dura
- **Sickle Cell Anemia**
  - Key facts
    - Autosomal recessive chronic hemolytic blood disorder that damages red blood cells (RBCs) and reduces their capability to carry oxygen
    - Hemapoietic system responds by increasing production of RBCs, which causes hyperplasia of marrow spaces
  - Imaging
    - Radiographic features include generalized osteoporosis
    - In skull: Widening of diploic space and thinning of inner and outer tables; hair on end appearance may occur in extreme cases
- **Thalassemia**
  - Key facts

- Hereditary disorder causing defect in hemoglobin synthesis; RBCs have shortened life span, causing hemopoietic system to produce more RBCs → hyperplasia of marrow spaces
- Prominent cheekbone and protrusive premaxilla develops: **Rodent facies**
- Imaging
  - Marked marrow hyperplasia preventing pneumatization of paranasal sinuses; obliteration of maxillary sinus
  - Expansion of maxilla → malocclusion
  - Generalized rarefaction with thinning of cortical boundaries and laminae dura; large marrow spaces; coarse and large trabeculae
- **Cushing Syndrome**
  - Key facts
    - Excess secretion of glucocorticoids by adrenal glands, causing reduced osteoblastic function & direct or indirect ↑ in osteoclastic function
  - Imaging
    - Generalized osteoporosis with granular bone pattern; skull may be mottled and thinned
    - Pathologic fractures may occur
    - Tooth eruption accelerated (if occurs in younger patient); partial loss of laminae dura seen

Helpful Clues for Rare Diagnoses

- **Hypophosphatasia**
  - Key facts
    - Rare inherited disorder resulting in reduced production or defective function of alkaline phosphatase (required to make osteoid)
  - Imaging
    - Generalized radiolucency of jaw bones; cortical bone and laminae dura are thin
    - Teeth have thin enamel layer and large pulp
- **Hypophosphatemia**
  - Key facts
    - Inherited condition causing renal tubular disorders → excessive loss of phosphorus
    - Also called vitamin D resistant rickets
  - Imaging
    - **In children**: Similar appearance as rickets
    - **Teeth**: Enamel is thin and pulp chambers are large
    - Periapical and periodontal abscesses occur frequently without visible cause
    - Laminae dura and cortices of follicles of developing teeth may be thin or absent
- **Massive Osteolysis (Vanishing Bone Disease)**
  - Key facts
    - Rare disorder characterized by proliferation of vascular channels that result in destruction and resorption of osseous matrix
    - Progressive in most patients; in some cases disease process is self-limiting
  - Imaging
    - During initial stage of lesion, radiolucent foci appear in intramedullary or subcortical regions, resembling findings seen in patchy osteoporosis
    - Slow, progressive atrophy, dissolution, fracture, fragmentation, and disappearance of portion of bone occurs with tapering or "pointing" of remaining osseous tissue and atrophy of soft tissues
    - Disease process can extend to contiguous bones; intervening joints afford no protection to extension of disease
- **Gaucher disease**
  - Key Facts
    - Genetic disorder in which glucocerebroside (a sphingolipid, also known as glucosylceramide) accumulates in cells and certain organs
  - Imaging
    - Osteoporosis is 75% of patients with disease due to accumulation of glucocerebroside in bone

SELECTED REFERENCES

1. Hekmatin E et al: Prediction of lumbar spine bone mineral density from the mandibular cortical width in postmenopausal women. J Res Med Sci. 18(11):951-5, 2013

Osteoporosis

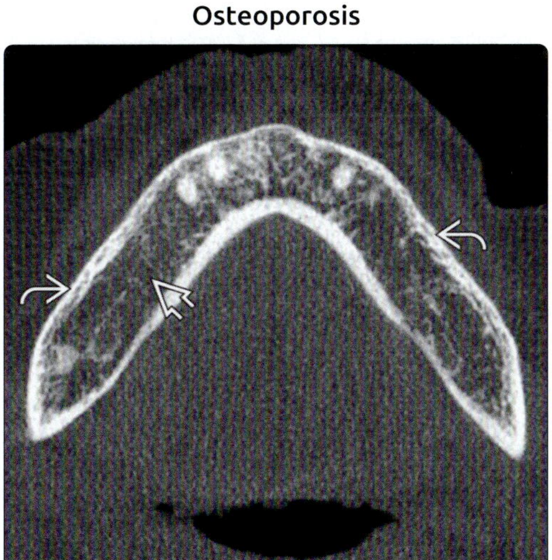

Osteoporosis

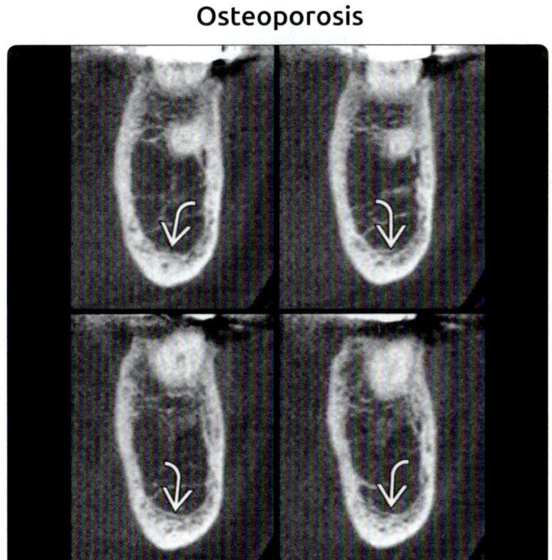

(Left) *Axial CBCT of a 90-year-old woman with osteoporosis shows osteopenic changes in the mandible. Note sparse trabeculation ➔ and semilunar defects (lacunar resorption) ➔ in the internal surface of the buccal cortex.* **(Right)** *Cross sections of CBCT data in the same patient show the semilunar resorption ➔ of the internal surface and thinning of the inferior cortex of the mandible, typical of osteoporosis.*

(Left) *Sagittal oblique thick ray-sum image shows osteomyelitis of the mandible complicating a preexisting advanced osteoradionecrosis of the mandible, represented as diffuse heterogeneous multifocal lucency and fragmentation of the coronoid process and mandibular neck .* **(Right)** *This 3D CT of mandibular osteomyelitis superimposing on osteoradionecrosis shows diffuse rarefaction and a pathologic fracture of the mandibular body just posterior to the level of the mental foramen.*

Osteomyelitis

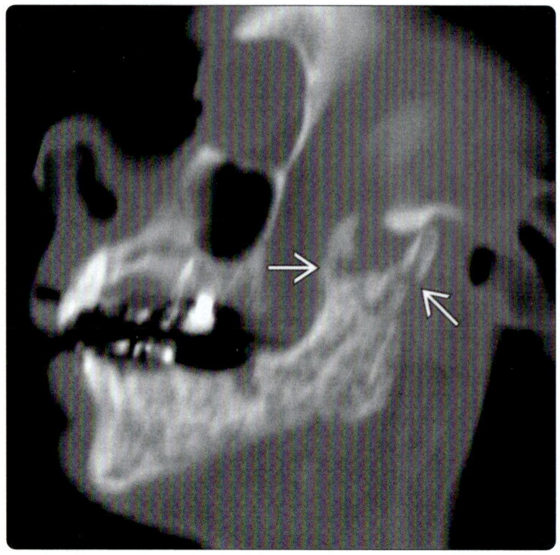

Osteomyelitis

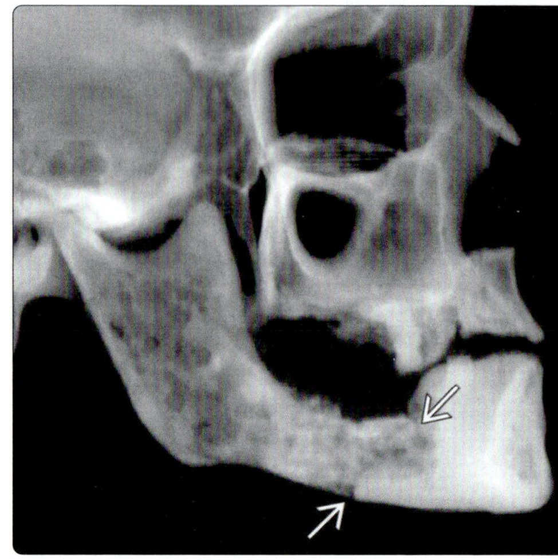

(Left) *NECT of the same patient demonstrates scattered intraosseous gas bubbles and an evolving bone within a bone appearance where radiolucencies within the bone appear to be carving out intraosseous bone sequestra. There are multiple foci of cortical bone interruption .* **(Right)** *Generalized granular rarefaction of bone with loss of laminae dura and mandibular cortices is seen with 2° hyperparathyroidism due to renal disease. (Courtesy S. Friedlander-Barenboim, DMD.)*

Osteomyelitis

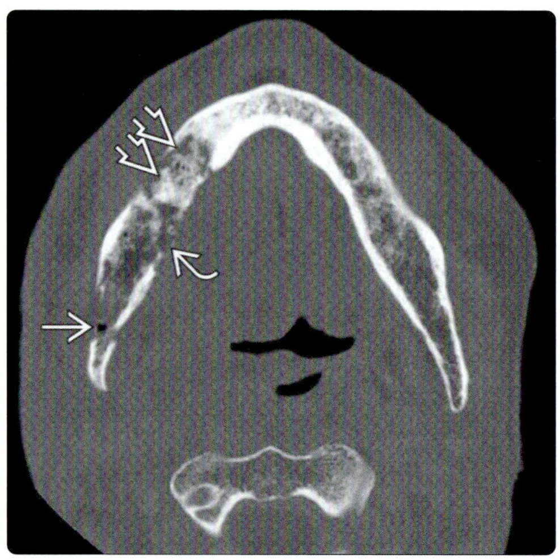

Hyperparathyroidism

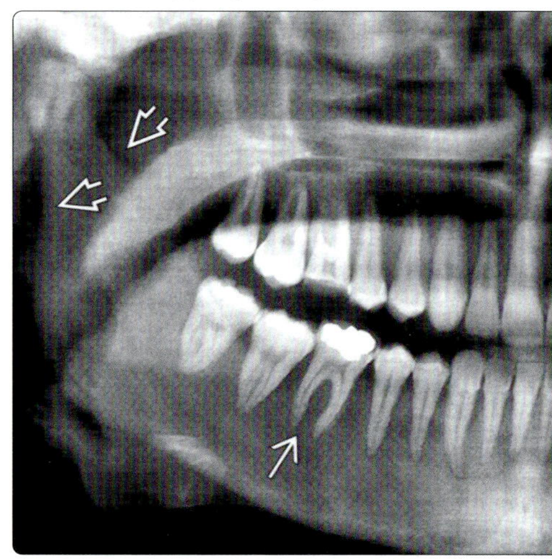

(Left) *Photograph shows a 30-year-old woman with pronounced physical and dental abnormalities. The patient presents with short stature and marked bowing of the legs. (Courtesy A. Potluri, DMD.)* **(Right)** *Cropped panoramic radiograph of the same patient shows generalized demineralization of bone with thinning of the cortices of the mandibular canal and rampant decay and periapical lesions . (Courtesy A. Potluri, DMD.)*

Vitamin D Deficiency

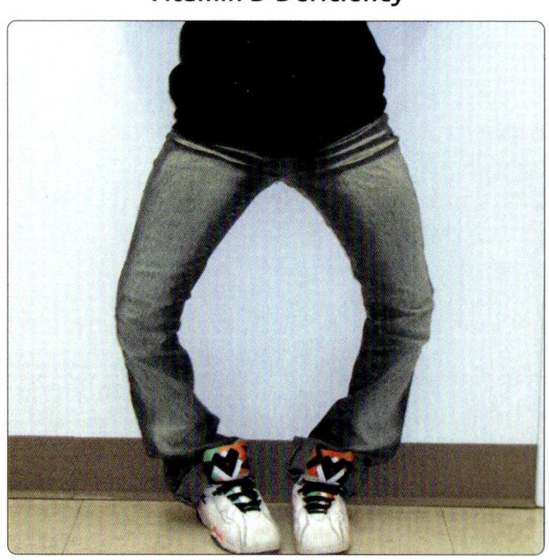

Vitamin D Deficiency

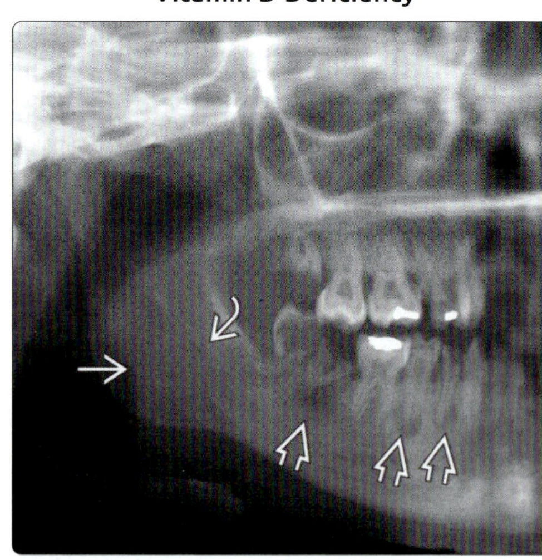

Vitamin D Deficiency

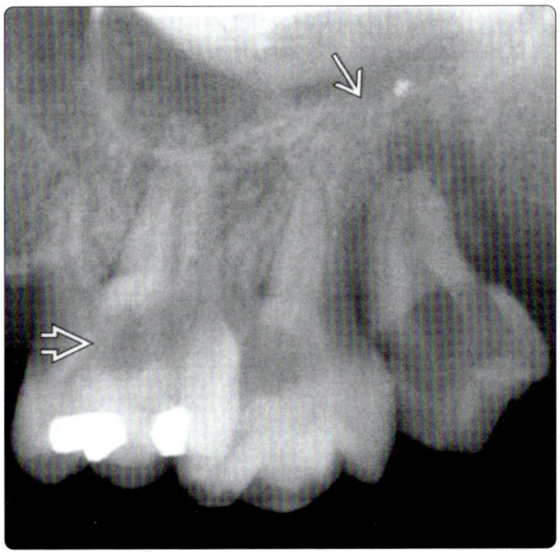

Sickle Cell Anemia

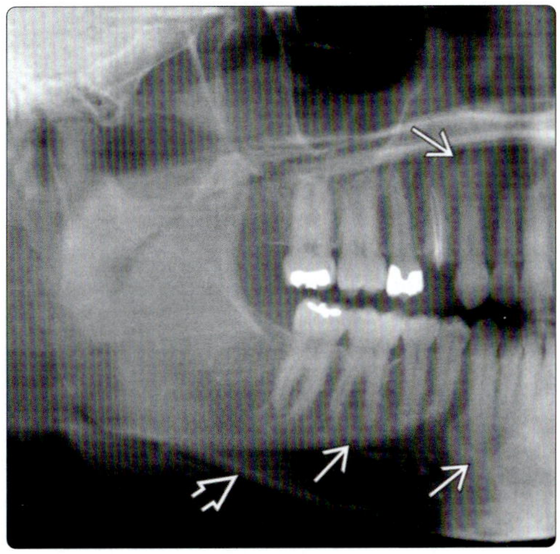

(Left) *Periapical radiograph of the same patient shows the characteristic enlarged pulp chambers ➔, lowered density of the maxillary sinus floor ➔, and thin or absent laminae dura. (Courtesy A. Potluri, DMD.)* **(Right)** *Panoramic radiograph shows thinning of the mandibular cortices ➔ and generalized rarefaction of the mandible. Florid osseous dysplasia (FOD) is noted ➔. Both sickle cell anemia and FOD are seen in people of African descent, but neither condition is associated with the other. (Courtesy A. Potluri, DMD.)*

Thalassemia

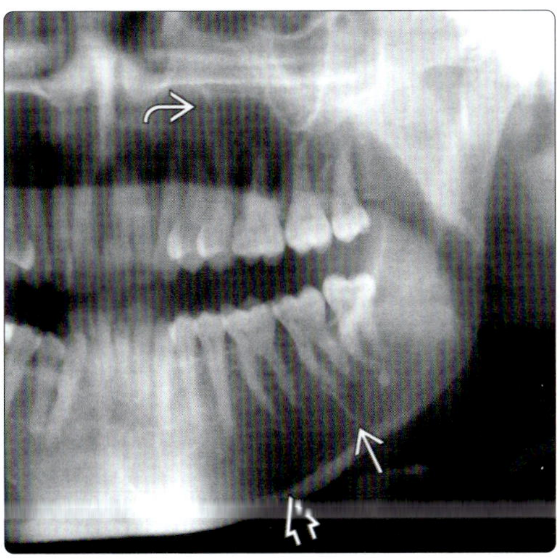

Thalassemia

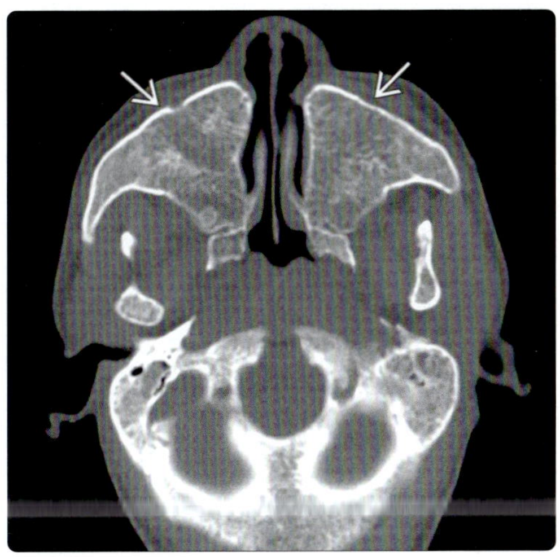

(Left) *Cropped panoramic radiograph shows a patient with thalassemia. The mandibular body is thickened with increased vertical dimension ➔ and thick trabeculae ➔ within the enlarged marrow spaces. The maxillary sinus is opacified ➔.* **(Right)** *Axial NECT demonstrates obliteration of the maxillary sinuses ➔. This obliteration is a result of marrow hyperplasia. Generalized expansion of the maxilla is present.*

Thalassemia

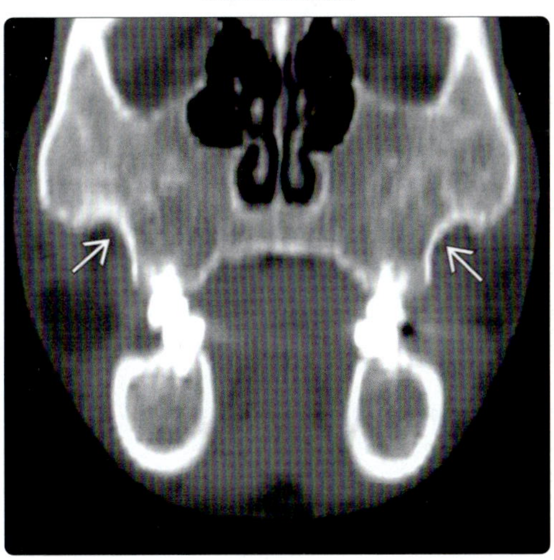

Thalassemia

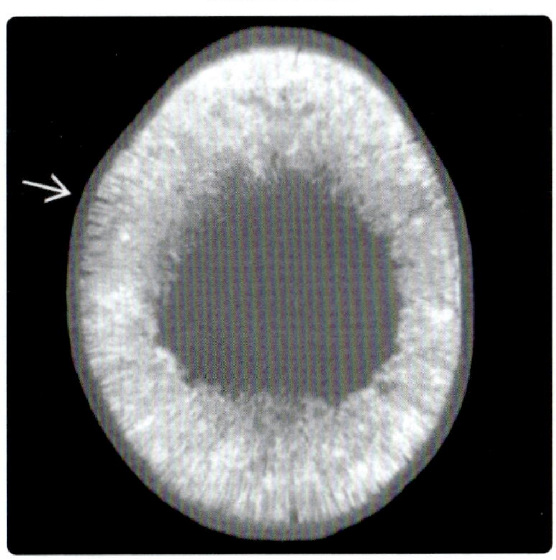

(Left) *Coronal NECT reconstruction demonstrates obliteration of the maxillary sinuses ➔ and expansion of the maxilla (result of marrow hyperplasia). This expansion leads to a distortion of the facial features, which is typical of thalassemia and is known as rodent facies.* **(Right)** *Axial NECT shows typical CT appearance of the head in an adult with thalassemia. The hair on end appearance ➔ of the skull secondary to marked thickening of the diploic marrow space is appreciated. The occipital bone is typically spared.*

DIFFERENTIAL DIAGNOSIS

Common

- Condensing Osteitis
- Idiopathic Osteosclerosis
- Retained Root Tip
- Mandibular Torus
- Palatal Torus
- Exostosis
- Foreign Object

Less Common

- Osteoma, Mandible-Maxilla
- Proliferative Periostitis

Rare but Important

- Osteoid Osteoma, Mandible-Maxilla
- Osteoblastoma

ESSENTIAL INFORMATION

Key Differential Diagnosis Issues

- Tori, exostoses, and osteomas often radiographically similar
  - Location is helpful
    - Mandibular torus: Lingual to mandibular premolars
    - Palatal torus: Midline of palate
    - Exostoses: Buccal and lingual alveolar process
      - Subpontic hyperostosis variant
    - Osteoma: Commonly seen in angle and ramus of mandible
- Multiple osteomas suggest familial colorectal polyposis **(Gardner syndrome)**
  - Skeletal abnormalities
  - Cutaneous abnormalities (cysts)
  - Adenomatous colorectal polyps with high malignant potential
- Proliferative periostitis radiographically similar to some malignant conditions (Ewing sarcoma, osteosarcoma)
  - Has inflammatory etiology

Helpful Clues for Common Diagnoses

- **Condensing Osteitis**
  - Synonyms: Chronic focal sclerosing osteomyelitis; focal periapical osteopetrosis; periapical sclerosing osteitis; **sclerosing osteitis**
  - Key facts
    - Associated with tooth with extensive caries &/or pulpal necrosis
    - Innocuous proliferative bony response to **chronic inflammation**
    - Frequently seen in 2nd and 3rd decades
  - Imaging
    - More common in posterior mandible
    - Uniform radiopacity with no separation from surrounding bone
    - Marrow spaces absent or very small in affected area
    - Irregular shape or follows outline of root adjacent to periodontal ligament
- **Idiopathic Osteosclerosis**
  - Synonyms: Hyperostosis, enostosis, dense bone island
  - Key facts
    - Innocuous incidental finding of unknown etiology
    - Common in mandibular canine-premolar areas
  - Imaging
    - Not necessarily associated with tooth
    - Uniform radiopacity, often with irregular borders
    - No separation from surrounding bone; no radiolucent phase
- **Retained Root Tip**
  - Key facts
    - Root fragment remaining after extraction or gross carious destruction of tooth crown
  - Imaging
    - Uniform radiopaque density of dentin surrounded by periodontal ligament space
    - Remnants of mandibular primary molars may persist in mandibular premolar area of adults
- **Mandibular Torus**
  - Key facts
    - Common exostosis on lingual aspect of mandible
    - Prevalence: ~ 10-15% in USA
    - Often bilateral but may be larger on one side than other
    - May gradually increase in size over time
  - Imaging
    - Uniformly dense, rounded radiopacity seen superimposed over midroot area of premolars and panoramic images; **no radiolucent rim**
    - Most commonly seen on periapical images
    - CBCT images will demonstrate exophytic nature
- **Palatal Torus**
  - Key facts
    - Common exostosis in midline of palate
    - Prevalence: ~ 20-35% in USA
    - F:M = 2:1
  - Imaging
    - Uniformly dense radiopacity with smooth borders and **no radiolucent periphery**
    - Seen on 2D imaging and maxillary periapicals when image receptor placed behind torus
- **Exostosis**
  - Key facts
    - Bony protuberance from cortical plate of alveolar process
      - Subpontic hyperostosis is variant under fixed prosthetic appliances (bridges)
    - Frequently seen in jaws; size varies
    - Prevalence: ~ 1:1,000 adults, but may be higher
    - Multiple buccal exostoses thought to be related to parafunctional habits (bruxism)
    - Differentiated from torus by location
  - Imaging
    - Rounded radiopacity seen superimposed on alveolar bone of maxilla or mandible on 2D imaging; **no radiolucent rim**
    - Mandibular buccal exostosis may resemble lingual mandibular torus on intraoral images
- **Foreign Object**
  - Key facts
    - Metal, some plastics, and glass appear radiopaque
    - Dental amalgam most common implanted metal

- Remnants of dental cements &/or plastic filling materials also seen
- Glass fragments embedded in soft tissue may superimpose over bone
  - Seen in motor vehicle accident patients
- Imaging
  - May be seen in any area of bone or superimposed on bone

Helpful Clues for Less Common Diagnoses

- **Osteoma, Mandible-Maxilla**
  - Key facts
    - Benign neoplasm of cancellous or compact bone
    - Most common on angle/ramus of mandible or condyle
    - May be associated with **Gardner syndrome** (skeletal abnormalities, epidermoid cysts, familial adenomatous polyposis)
  - Imaging
    - Well-defined, radiopaque mass
    - May be uniform in radiodensity or have sclerotic periphery with central trabeculation
    - Small osteomas resemble idiopathic osteosclerosis or tori
- **Proliferative Periostitis**
  - Synonyms: Garré osteomyelitis, periostitis ossificans of Garré, nonsuppurative ossifying periostitis, osteomyelitis with proliferative periostitis
  - Key facts
    - Bone formation within periosteum in **response to inflammation**
    - Seen mostly in **children and young adults**; mean age of 13
    - Often related to periapical or periodontal inflammation especially in mandible
    - Also seen with nonodontogenic infection: Fracture
    - Usually resolves in 6-12 months after elimination of source of inflammation
  - Imaging
    - **Laminations of bone** parallel to each other
    - Creates **onion skin** appearance
    - May also be seen as fine spicules radiating perpendicularly from periosteum (hair-on-end)
    - Must be differentiated from malignancies such as Ewing sarcoma or osteosarcoma

Helpful Clues for Rare Diagnoses

- **Osteoid Osteoma, Mandible-Maxilla**
  - Key facts
    - M > F (3:1 up to 2:1)
    - Most common in 2nd decade
    - < 2 cm in size
    - **Painful** condition alleviated with **aspirin**
    - Histologically identical to osteoblastoma
  - Imaging
    - Well defined with varying amount of mineralization
    - Frequently has reactive sclerosis surrounding central **radiolucent nidus**
- **Osteoblastoma**
  - Key facts
    - Rare (< 1% of all bone tumors
    - In jaws, most common in posterior mandible, usually 2-4 cm in size
    - M > F, usually prior to age 30
    - **Painful** condition but **not** alleviated well with aspirin
    - Histologically identical to osteoid osteoma
  - Imaging
    - Well defined with varying amounts of mineralized tissue (patchy to very dense)
    - Border may be corticated or uncorticated
    - May resemble cementoblastoma or osteoid osteoma

SELECTED REFERENCES

1. Emanuelsson J et al: Osteoblastoma of the temporal articular tubercle misdiagnosed as a temporomandibular joint disorder. Int J Oral Maxillofac Surg. ePub, 2016
2. Infante-Cossio P et al: Mandibular osteoid osteoma. J Emerg Med. ePub, [illegible]
3. Cortes AR et al: Mandibular tori are associated with mechanical stress and mandibular shape. J Oral Maxillofac Surg. 72(11):2115-25, 2014

Condensing Osteitis

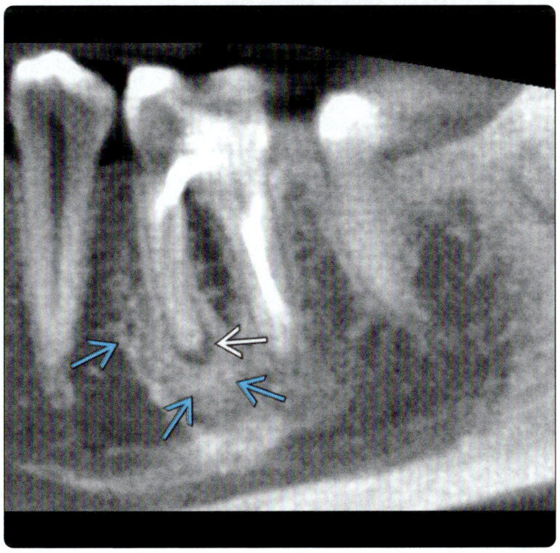

Idiopathic Osteosclerosis

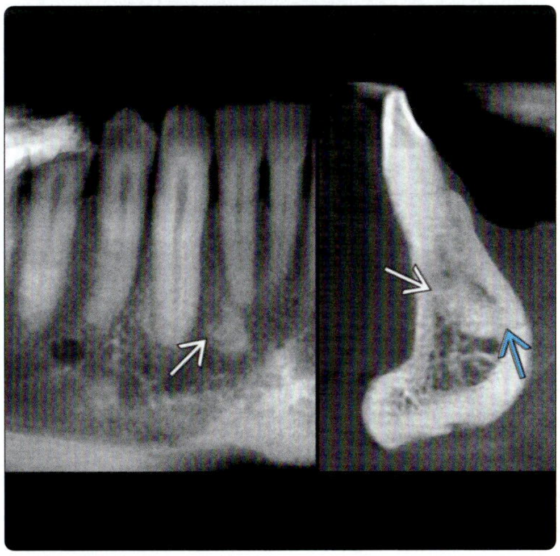

(Left) *Limited FOV slice CBCT of the left mandibular 1st molar exhibits rarefying osteitis ➡ with hyperdensity of the adjacent lamina dura and trabecular bone. The hyperdense bone is condensing osteitis (sclerosing osteitis) ➡.* **(Right)** *Sagittal and cross-sectional CBCT images of the right mandibular canine area exhibit a well-defined hyperdensity ➡. The hyperdensity blends into the surrounding bone and is continuous with the lingual endosteal cortex ➡, and there is no expansion.*

Idiopathic Osteosclerosis

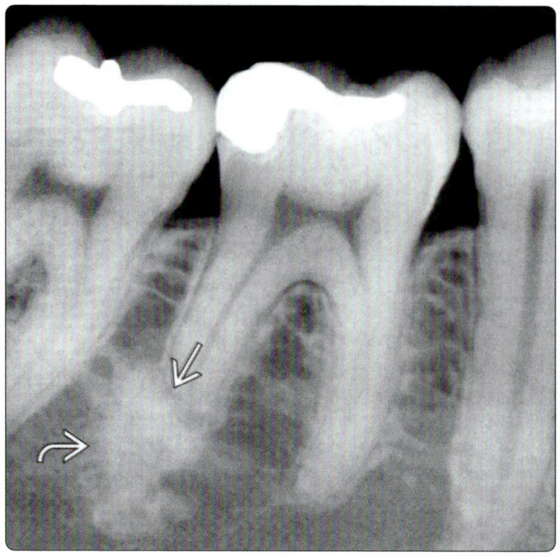

Retained Root Tip

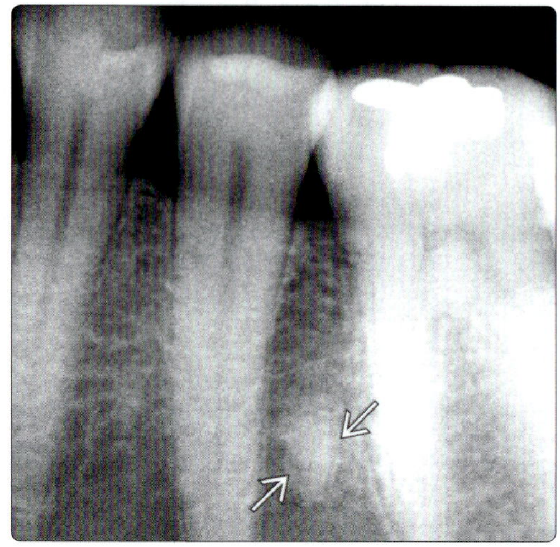

(Left) *Periapical radiograph shows irregular area of increased density ➔ at the apex of the resorbed distal root of the mandibular 1st molar. Root resorption is sometimes seen with osteosclerosis. Visible apical periodontal ligament space ➔ is normal.* **(Right)** *Periapical radiograph shows a remnant of the distal root of the 2nd primary molar ➔. Note the periodontal ligament space around it. Primary root remnants are relatively common in the mandible compared to the maxilla.*

Mandibular Torus

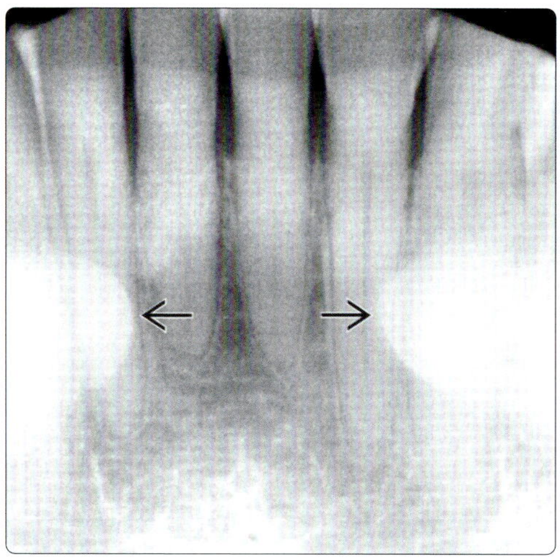

Mandibular Torus

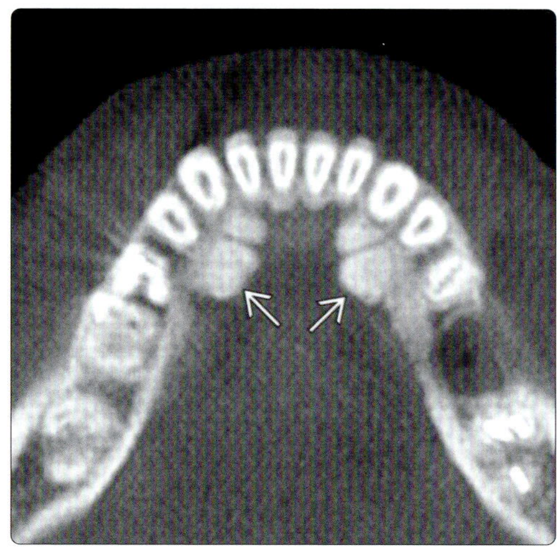

(Left) *Periapical radiograph shows bilateral rounded, dense radiopacities superimposed over the midroot area of the canines ➔. This is the typical appearance for mandibular torus on anterior periapical views.* **(Right)** *Axial CBCT shows the lobulated, dense cortical bone of mandibular tori ➔. Mandibular tori are usually bilateral and located anterior to the 1st molar. The overlying mucosa is often thin and easily injured. These tori may need to be removed prior to the placement of dentures.*

Palatal Torus

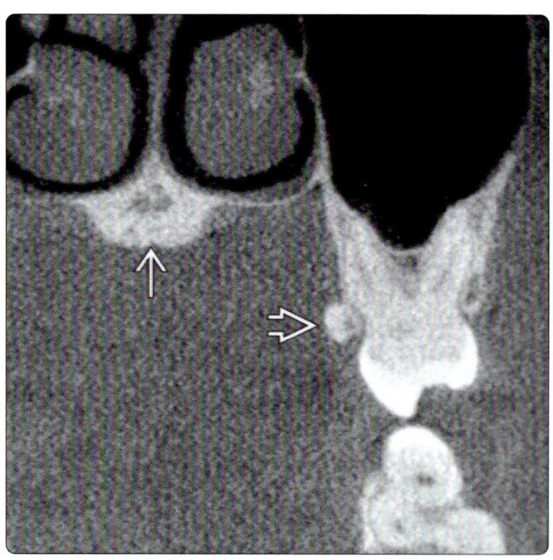

Exostosis

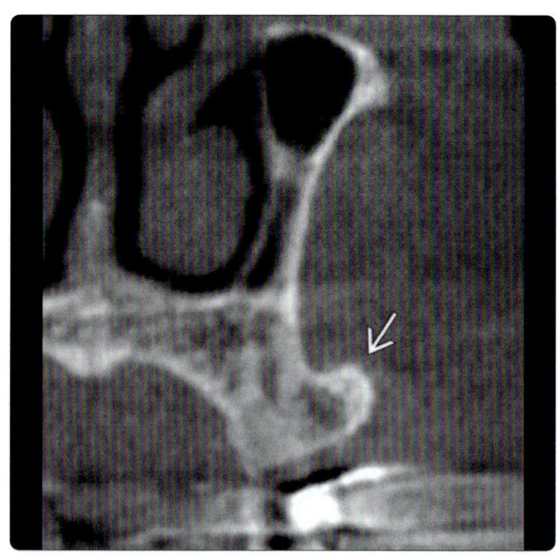

(Left) *Coronal reformat CBCT shows the dense compact bone of a palatal torus ➔. In addition, there is a palatal exostosis adjacent to the molar ➔. Exostoses may occur on either the buccal or palatal aspect of the alveolus.* **(Right)** *Coronal reformatted CBCT of the maxillary left canine-premolar area exhibits pronounced facial exostosis ➔. There is a thickened layer of cortical bone covering the outgrowth. There is a correlation between excessive occlusal forces and alveolar exostoses.*

Foreign Object

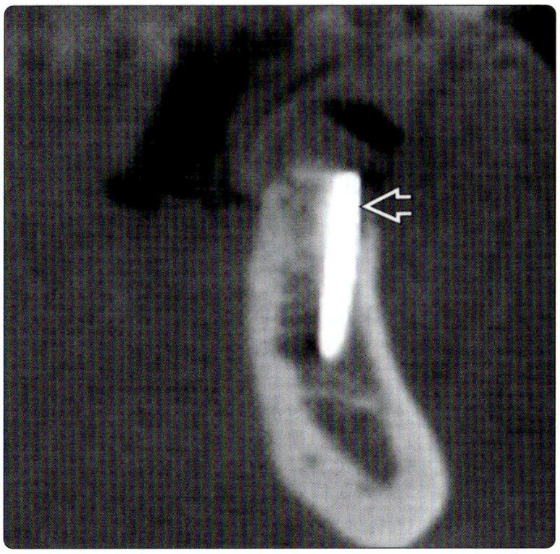

Foreign Object

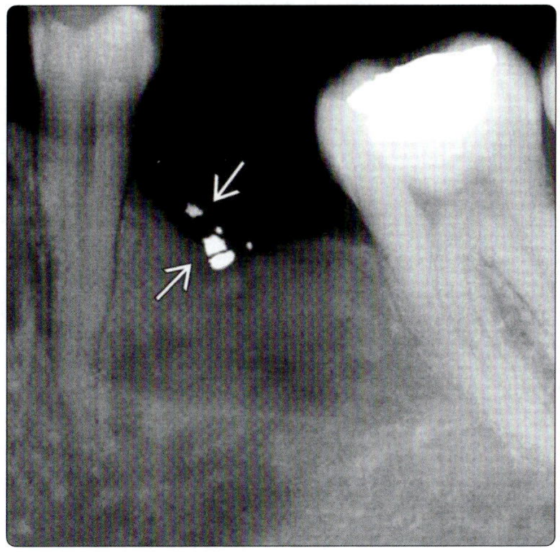

(Left) *Cross-sectional CBCT of the anterior mandible reveals metallic hyperdensity with similar morphology to an endosseous implant ⇨. Upon removal, this was a fractured-off surgical instrument.* **(Right)** *Periapical radiograph shows very dense, irregular radiopacities →. These are fragments of dental amalgam, likely fractured off during extraction of the molar. These fragments may stain the overlying mucosa, creating a bluish "tattoo."*

Osteoma, Mandible-Maxilla

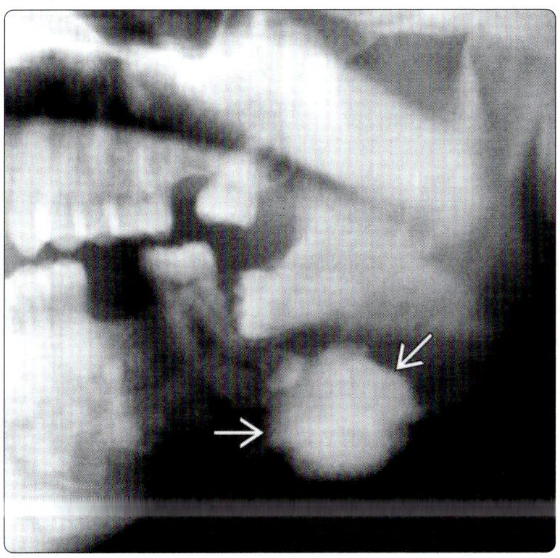

Proliferative Periostitis

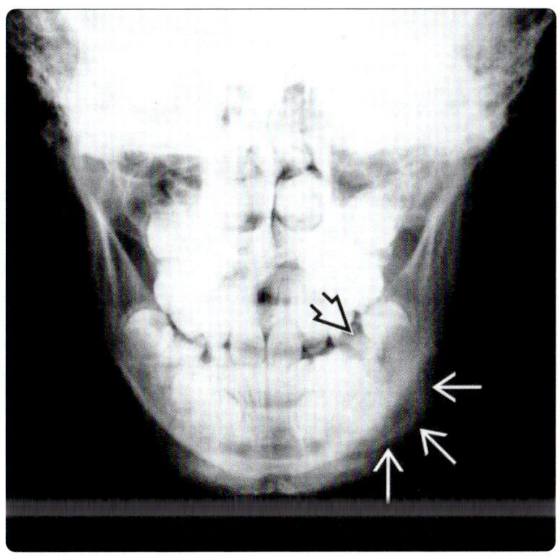

(Left) *Cropped panoramic radiograph shows a large osteoma → in a patient with Gardner syndrome. Osteomas are commonly seen at the angle and on the ramus of the mandible.* **(Right)** *Anteroposterior radiograph shows lamellar expansion of the left mandible in a child with a carious tooth ⇨. The radiograph was deliberately underexposed in order to show the proliferative periostitis →.*

Osteoid Osteoma, Mandible-Maxilla

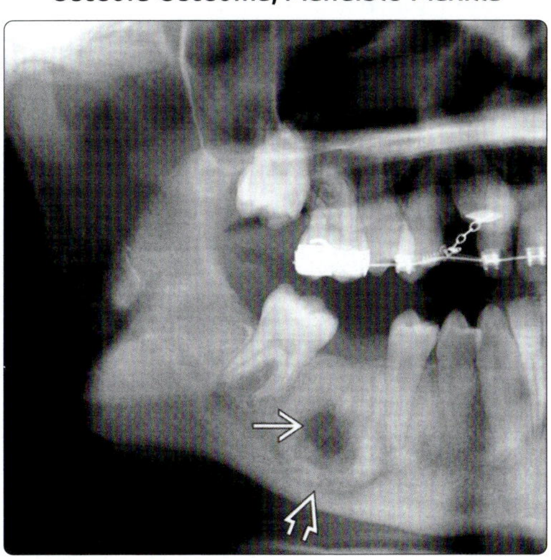

Osteoblastoma

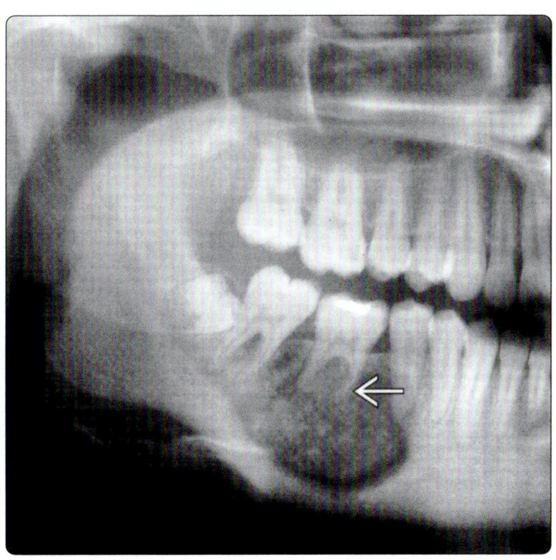

(Left) *Panoramic radiograph shows an osteoid osteoma with radiolucent nidus → and surrounding zone of sclerosis. Note displacement of the inferior alveolar canal ⇨.* **(Right)** *Panoramic radiograph shows that a mixed-density lesion consistent with an osteoblastoma appears similar to cementoblastoma. The periodontal ligament space → around the roots differentiates. The radiographic appearance of osteoblastoma ranges from radiolucent to densely radiopaque. (Courtesy K. Martonffy, MD.)*

DIFFERENTIAL DIAGNOSIS

Common

- Fibrous Dysplasia
- Graft Material for Ridge Augmentation Procedure

Less Common

- Florid Osseous Dysplasia
- Periapical Osseous Dysplasia
- Cementoossifying Fibroma

Rare but Important

- Hyperparathyroidism
- Paget Disease
- Leukemia
- Cushing Disease

ESSENTIAL INFORMATION

Key Differential Diagnosis Issues

- Ground-glass lesions: Mass-like, calcified, matrix-producing bone lesions
  - May be homogeneous or heterogeneous intermediate CT attenuation
  - Fibroosseous lesions account for majority
  - Aggressive bone destruction, periosteal reactive new bone formation, & extraosseous soft tissue components are absent
- **Particulate graft material** used for augmenting atrophied alveolar processes prior to implant placement may be **similar to fibroosseous lesions in radiographic appearance**
  - Clinical history of implant treatment planning
    - Sinus lift surgeries show granular opacities in floor of maxillary sinus

Helpful Clues for Common Diagnoses

- **Fibrous Dysplasia**
  - Key facts
    - Monostotic (80-85%), polyostotic (15-20%)
    - "Monostotic" term difficult to apply in craniofacial fibrous dysplasia (FD) where otherwise isolated FD may cross sutures to involve adjacent bones
    - Most cases become quiescent at bone maturity (early adulthood)
    - Infrequently presents or reactivates in adulthood
    - Craniofacial region is most common site for sarcomatous degeneration of FD
  - Imaging
    - Often less well defined, more radiopaque in craniofacial region than long bones
    - Ground-glass matrix expands involved bone (especially mandible) in fusiform fashion
    - Maintains native shape of affected bone unless complicated by cystic degeneration (aneurysmal bone cyst)
    - May encroach on neural & vascular foramina & canals; **displaced mandibular canal superiorly**
    - FD and teeth: Periodontal ligament space narrowed; lamina dura involved
    - Teeth surrounded but often not displaced or resorbed, though entire alveolar ridge may be displaced by massive lesion
    - FD and sarcomatous degeneration: Permeative lytic pattern, destroyed cortex, widening of periodontal ligament space, spiculated periosteal new bone formation
- **Graft Material for Ridge Augmentation Procedure**
  - Key facts
    - There are 3 types of graft materials used for pre-implant ridge augmentation
    - **Autografts**: Graft is harvested from patient and may be used as block fixed with screws or may be ground up to create bone particles
    - **Allografts**: Freeze-dried or demineralized, freeze-dried cadaver bone provided as particles
    - **Xenografts**: Calcium phosphate minerals, calcium carbonates, bioactive glass ceramics, calcium sulfate, and polymers
  - Imaging
    - All particulate graft materials appear as granular radiopacities, similar to ground-glass appearance; placed in sinus, within dental socket or on facial surface of alveolar process
    - Graft material does not expand or remodel walls of maxillary sinus as fibroosseous lesions do
    - Dental socket grafts look like granular tooth roots

Helpful Clues for Less Common Diagnoses

- **Florid Osseous Dysplasia**
  - Key facts
    - Diffuse (3 or more quadrants) form of periapical cementoosseous dysplasia
  - Imaging
    - "Fluffy" sclerotic lesions in periapical alveolar bone or in edentulous areas
    - Often symmetric, expansile, lobulated, larger than periapical form
    - May be accompanied by simple bone cysts or complicated by osteomyelitis
- **Periapical Osseous Dysplasia**
  - Key facts
    - Middle-aged women; blacks, Asians more prevalent than whites
  - Imaging
    - Most common site = mandibular incisors; often multifocal, between adjacent teeth, usually < 1 cm
    - Initially lucent, progressing to sclerosis with lucent margin; intermediate stage may be granular
    - May be accompanied by simple bone cysts that may heal spontaneously, giving granular appearance
- **Cementoossifying Fibroma**
  - Key facts
    - Clinical: Occurs predominantly in women; more common in blacks
    - Presents in 3rd-4th decade; later than FD
    - Histologically characterized by lamellar bone and osteoblastic rimming, cementum-like tissue
    - Rarely, OF lesions are multiple; may be confused with polyostotic FD
  - Imaging

- Circumscribed, spherical, & focally more expansile than FD (due to centrifugal expansion) with thin intact cortex
- Teeth often displaced and resorbed

Helpful Clues for Rare Diagnoses

- **Hyperparathyroidism**
  - Increased production of parathyroid hormone → ↑ osteoclast activity & population
  - Primary due to parathyroid adenoma, parathyroid hyperplasia, hereditary hyperparathyroidism, parathyroid carcinoma
  - Secondary is compensatory to ↓ in serum calcium and may be due to inadequate intake or poor intestinal absorption of vitamin D or from deficient metabolism of vitamin D in liver or kidney
  - Osteitis fibrosa cystica (OFC): Progression of hyperparathyroidism in bone without treatment; occurs in 50% of end-stage renal disease (ESRD) patients
    - Over-activity of osteoclastic resorption results in loss of bone mass, weakening of bones due to calcified supporting structures replaced with fibrous tissue (peritrabecular fibrosis), and formation of cyst-like **brown tumors**
    - Noncystic form mimics diffuse FD
  - Brown tumors: Histologically and radiographically similar to central giant cell granuloma
  - Renal osteodystrophy
    - Thought to be result of hyperparathyroidism secondary to hyperphosphatemia combined with hypocalcemia, both of which are due to ↓ excretion of phosphate by damaged kidney
  - **OFC common presentation** of renal osteodystrophy
  - Imaging
    - Diffuse demineralization, lace-like subperiosteal resorption, with **ground-glass** or **"salt and pepper" granular** enlargement of bones
    - Multifocal cortical thinning, loss of definition of lamina dura
    - Teeth may appear prominent due to loss of surrounding bone density
    - Focal enlargement with brown tumor in osteitis fibrosa cystica
- **Paget Disease**
  - Key facts
    - 17% of cases involve mandible or maxilla
    - Older males
    - Usually seen with skull involvement
  - Imaging
    - Often bilateral and symmetric, maxilla involved 2x as commonly as mandible
    - Cortical and trabecular thickening, ground-glass density interspersed with sclerotic islands of dense bone
    - Hypercementosis around tooth roots mimicking cementoosseous dysplasia; may obliterate periodontal ligament space
- **Leukemia**
  - Key facts
    - Malignant tumor of hematopoietic stem cells
  - Imaging
    - Very rarely, granular bone may be seen within rarefaction associated with displacement of normal bone marrow with malignant cells
- **Cushing Disease**
  - Key facts
    - Excess secretion of glucocorticoids by adrenal glands
  - Imaging
    - Generalized osteoporosis, which may have granular bone pattern

SELECTED REFERENCES

1. Dagistan S et al: Changes in jawbones of male patients with chronic renal failure on digital panoramic radiographs. Eur J Dent. 10(1):64-8, 2016
2. Demirtas N et al: Recurrent cherubism in an adult patient. J Craniofac Surg. 26(3):e225-7, 2015
3. Fusconi M et al: Fibrous dysplasia of the maxilla: diagnostic reliability of the study image. Literature review. J Neurol Surg B Skull Base. 74(6):364-8, 2013
4. Garlini G et al: Maxillary sinus elevation with an alloplastic material and implants: 11 years of clinical and radiologic follow-up. J Oral Maxillofac Surg. 68(5):1152-7, 2010

Fibrous Dysplasia

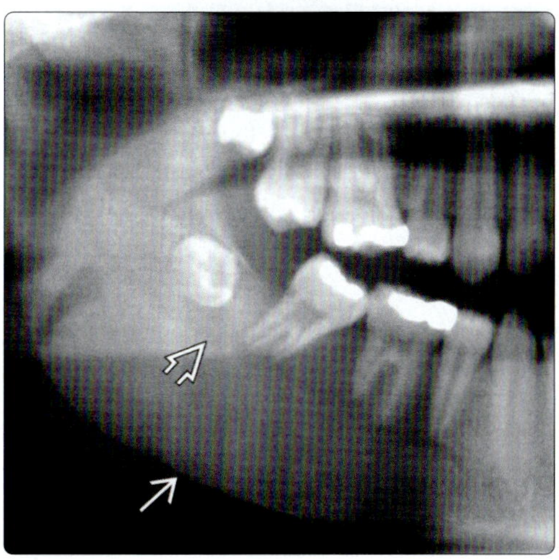

Fibrous Dysplasia

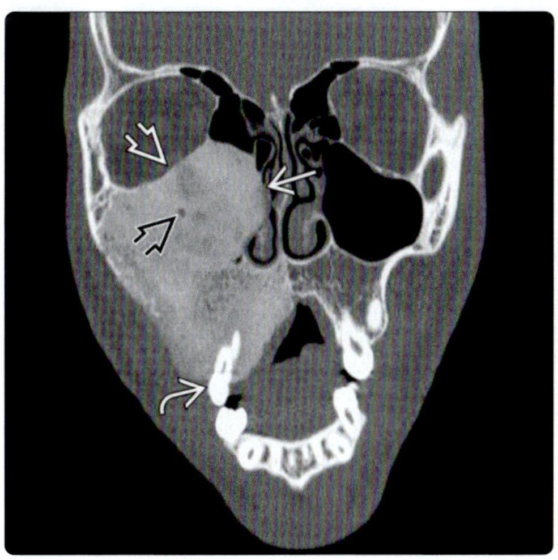

(Left) *Cropped panoramic radiograph shows the mandibular canal superiorly displaced ➡, pathognomonic of fibrous dysplasia. Bone has the appearance of ground glass. Inferior cortex ➡ and laminae dura are not evident.* **(Right)** *Coronal bone CT shows expansile maxillary bone lesion. Note orbital ➡ & nasal cavity ➡ encroachment, maxillary antrum obliteration, inferior displacement of maxillary teeth ➡, & engulfed infraorbital canal ➡.*

(Left) *Right anterior oblique 3D CT shows diffuse pagetoid heterogeneous ground-glass density in this patient with polyostotic fibrous dysplasia.* **(Right)** *CBCT cross section shows the granular appearance of a tooth socket graft ➔. The contours of the bone are preserved as resorption and remodeling of the bone is prevented.*

Fibrous Dysplasia

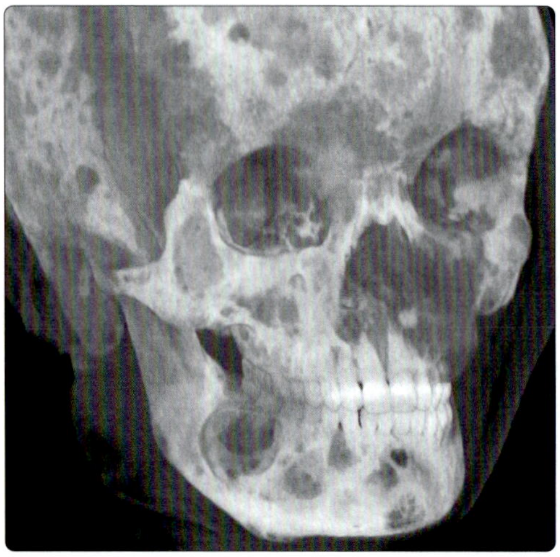

Graft Material for Ridge Augmentation Procedure

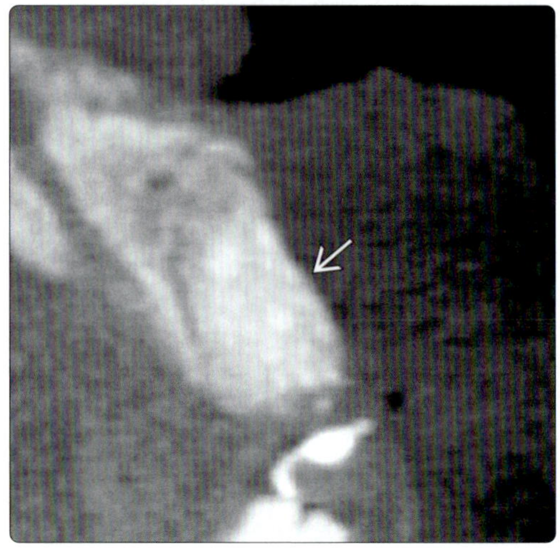

(Left) *CBCT panoramic format of an implant planning case shows graft material ➔ has been introduced into the floor of the maxillary sinus ("sinus lift") to augment the severely atrophied posterior alveolar process. The radiographic markers ➔ can be seen indicating the location of the proposed implants.* **(Right)** *Axial CBCT in the same patient shows the granular nature of the graft material in the floor of the maxillary sinus. Mucosal thickening is noted surrounding the graft. The cortices and outline of the sinus are intact ➔.*

Graft Material for Ridge Augmentation Procedure

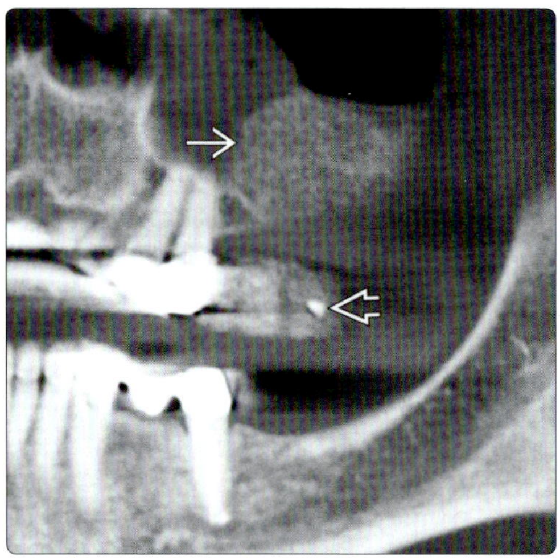

Graft Material for Ridge Augmentation Procedure

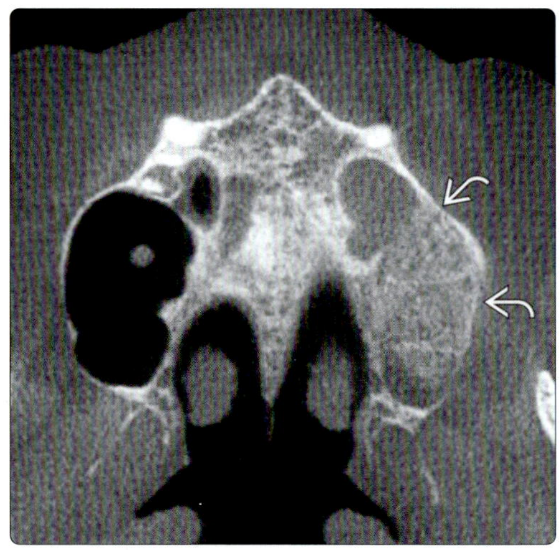

(Left) *Axial bone CT shows florid osseous dysplasia (FOD) affecting the left posterior mandible. The cemental masses are indistinct and inhomogeneous ➔, giving the lesion a granular appearance. Note radiolucent component at the posterior aspect of the lesion ➔. (Courtesy S. Mardini, DDS.)* **(Right)** *Periapical radiograph shows FOD. The granular appearance ➔ of the lesion in the edentulous area can be appreciated. An additional radiolucent lesion ➔ and hypercementosis ➔ are also seen.*

Florid Osseous Dysplasia

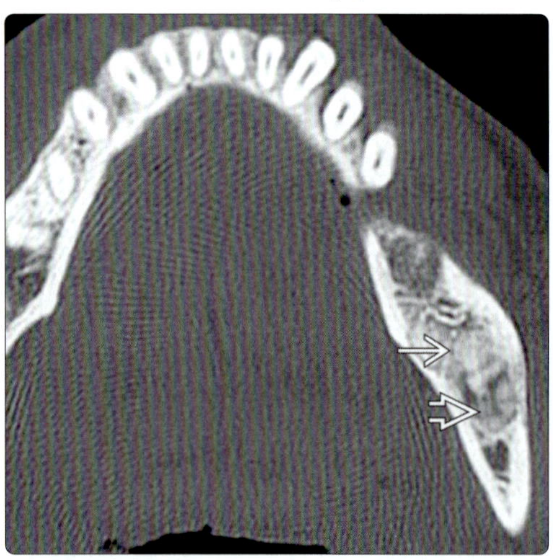

Florid Osseous Dysplasia

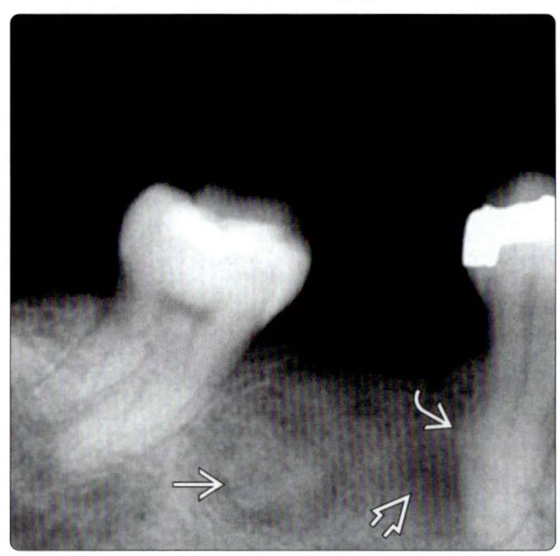

Florid Osseous Dysplasia

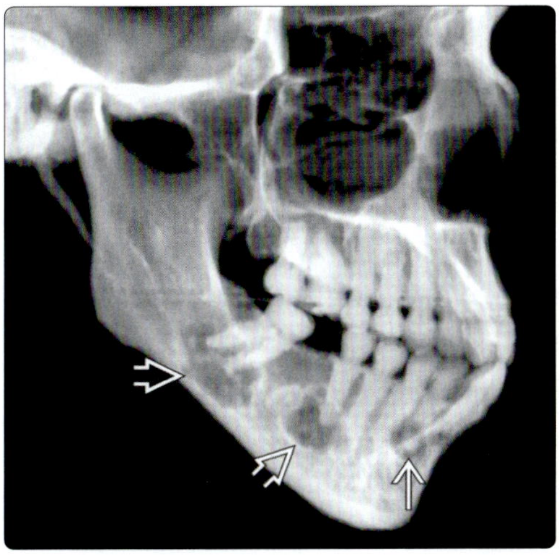

Florid Osseous Dysplasia

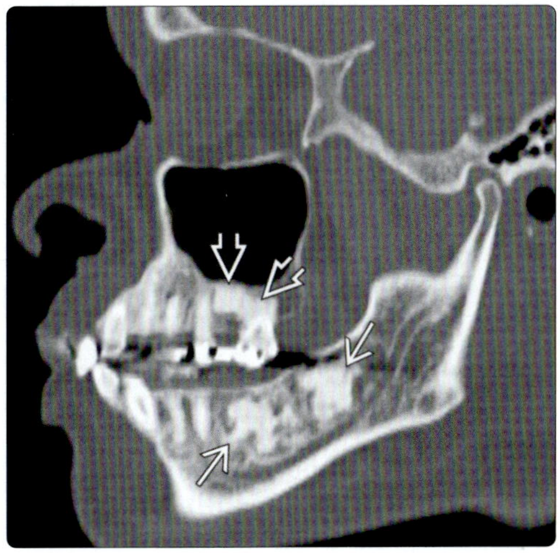

(Left) *Right anterior oblique maximum-intensity projection CT shows early pattern of periapical lucencies associated with vital teeth . Subtle periapical calcification of 1 lesion is visible.* **(Right)** *Sagittal oblique bone CT demonstrates patchy areas of increased density in the left mandible and left maxilla . This example demonstrates the late-stage appearance of these lesions.*

Florid Osseous Dysplasia

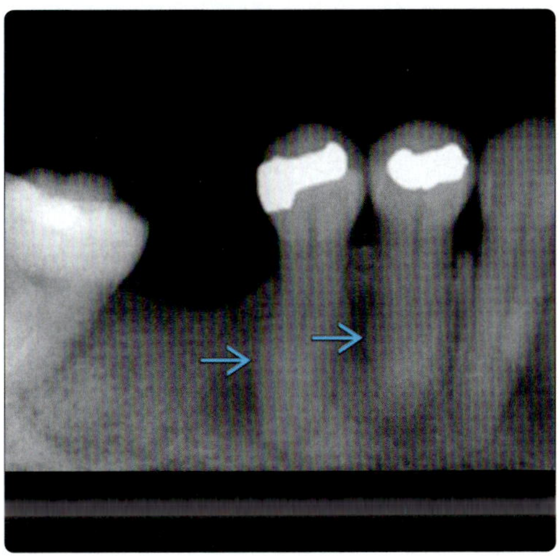

Periapical Osseous Dysplasia

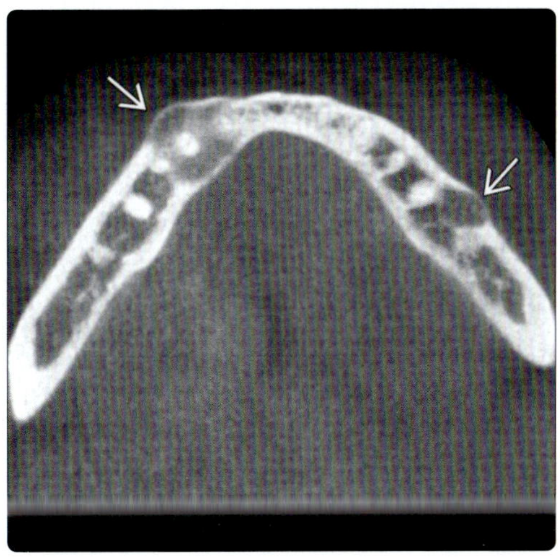

(Left) *Periapical radiograph shows the granular appearance of the alveolar process in mid to late stage FOD. It is common for the roots of the teeth to exhibit hypercementosis in this condition.* **(Right)** *Axial CBCT shows 2 separate PCD lesions in a 30-year-old white woman . Expansion and thinning of the cortices of the mandible are noted, as well as faint granular internal structure.*

Periapical Osseous Dysplasia

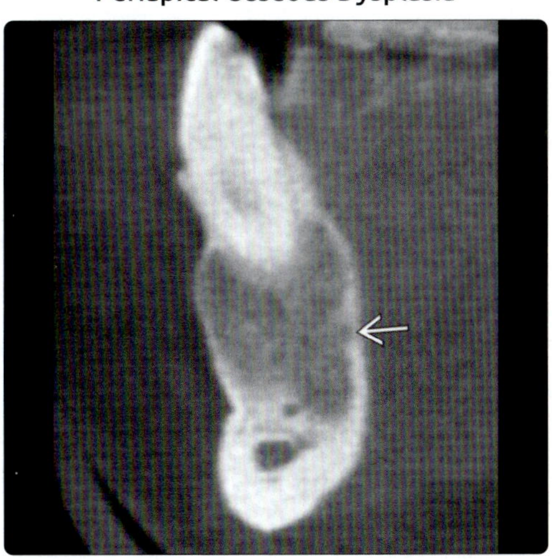

Periapical Osseous Dysplasia

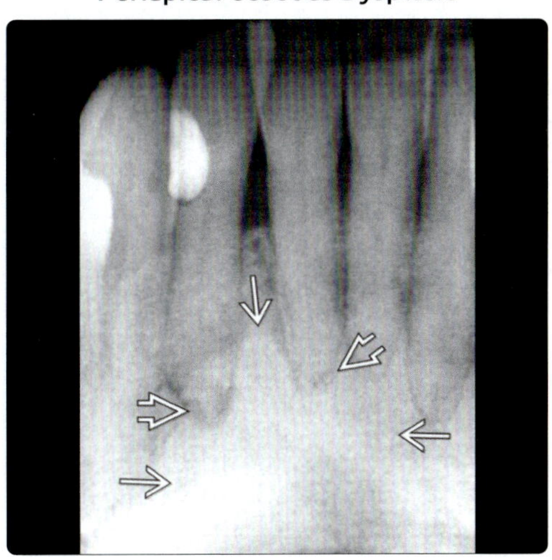

(Left) *CBCT cross section of the lesion on the right canine in the same patient shows expansion and thinning of the cortices, as well as granular internal structure. Endosteal scalloping of the lingual cortex is noted , an appearance typical of simple bone cysts, which can occur with these lesions.* **(Right)** *Periapical radiograph shows late-stage periapical osseous dysplasia. Dense, granular, calcified material at the apices of the mandibular anterior teeth can be appreciated . Note the periodontal ligament spaces of the teeth are preserved .*

Cementoossifying Fibroma

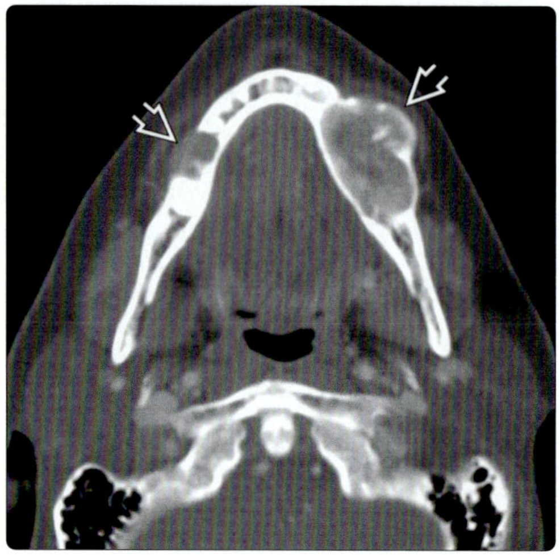

Cementoossifying Fibroma

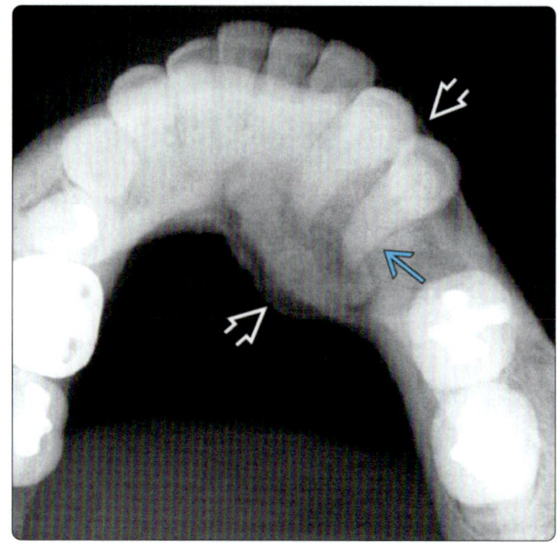

(Left) *Axial CECT shows bilateral expansile ground-glass cementoossifying fibroma lesions ; patient has hyperparathyroidism due to a parathyroid carcinoma. While brown tumors are possible, there is also an association between cementoossifying fibromas and hyperparathyroidism.* **(Right)** *Occlusal radiograph shows a localized, expansile ground-glass cementoossifying fibroma lesion surrounded by a radiolucent rim . Lingual displacement of the roots of the associated teeth can be appreciated.*

Cementoossifying Fibroma

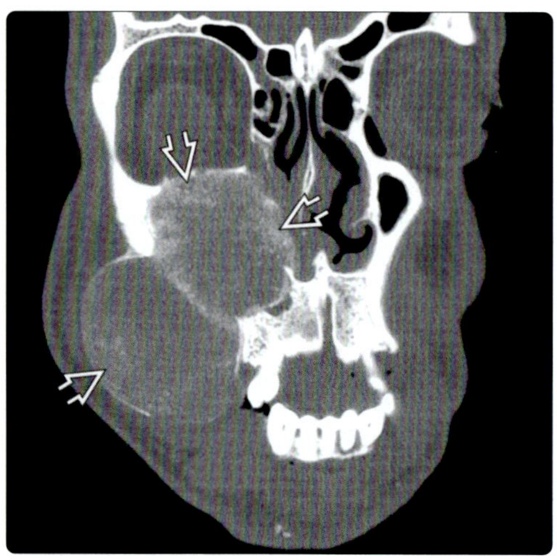

Cementoossifying Fibroma

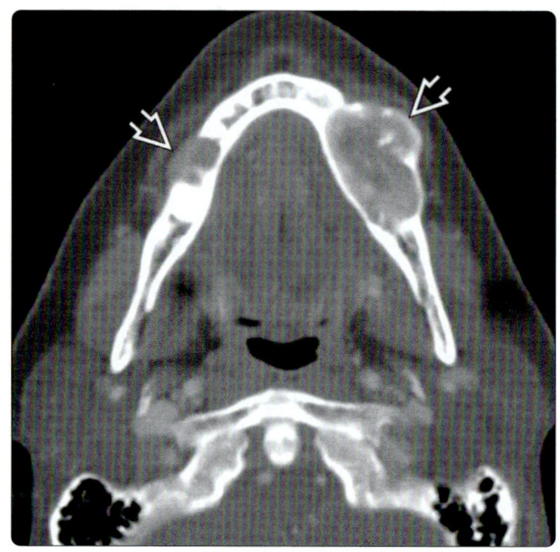

(Left) *Coronal bone CT reveals a bilobed cementoossifying fibroma with innumerable foci of psammomatoid calcifications , most prominent along the lesion's periphery.* **(Right)** *Axial CECT shows bilateral expansile ground-glass cementoossifying fibroma lesions in this patient with hyperparathyroidism due to a parathyroid carcinoma. While brown tumors are possible, there is also an association between cementoossifying fibromas and hyperparathyroidism.*

Cementoossifying Fibroma

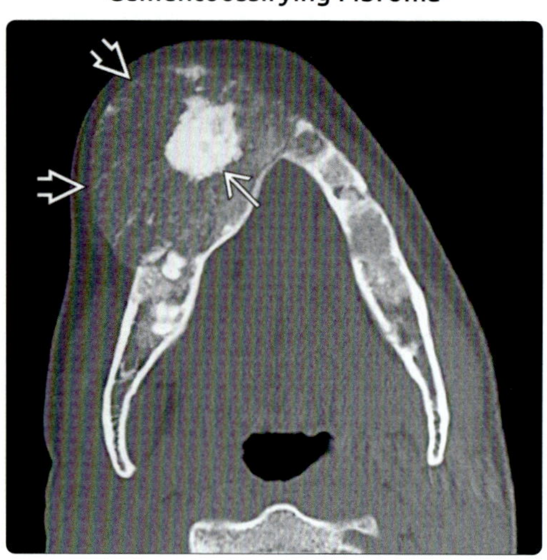

Cementoossifying Fibroma

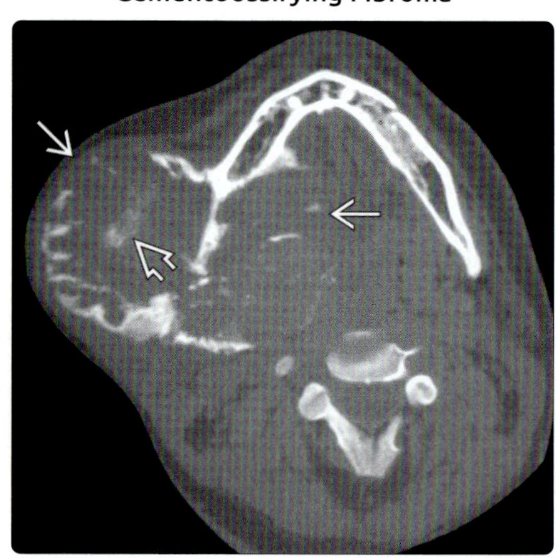

(Left) *Axial bone CT reveals a focally expansile ground-glass density lesion with a thick intact cortex and a central focus of coarse calcification .* **(Right)** *Axial bone CT reveals an aggressive-appearing mandibular mass with central increased density but multiple areas of apparent cortical breakthrough . An osteosarcoma was suspected but juvenile aggressive ossifying fibroma was the final pathological diagnosis.*

Hyperparathyroidism

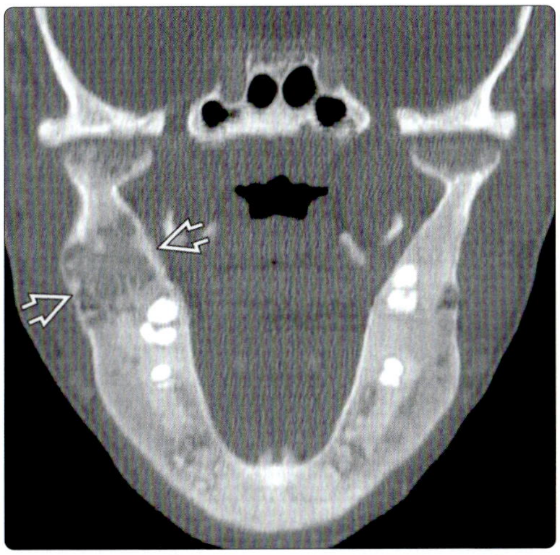

Hyperparathyroidism

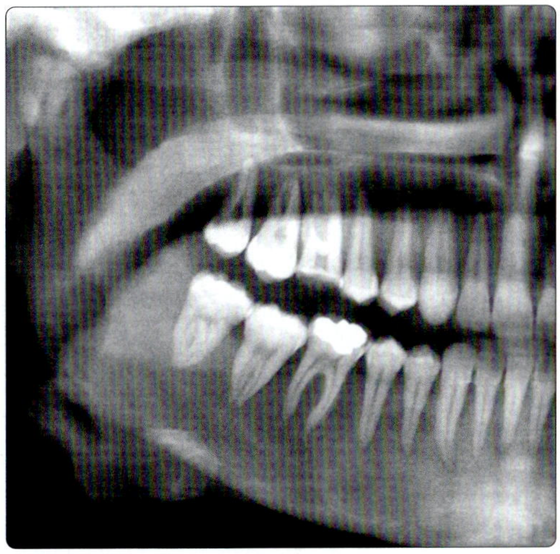

(Left) *Coronal oblique bone CT shows diffuse expansion and uniform increased density of the mandible in renal osteodystrophy. More focal expansion is seen on the right due to a coexisting brown tumor.* **(Right)** *Panoramic radiograph shows ground-glass appearance and loss or thinning of lamina dura around all the teeth in a 27-year-old woman with secondary hyperparathyroidism related to renal disease. (Courtesy S. Friedlander-Barenboim, DMD.)*

Hyperparathyroidism

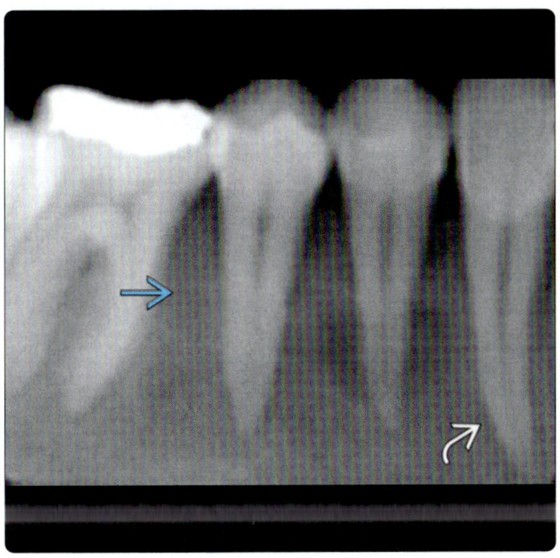

Paget Disease

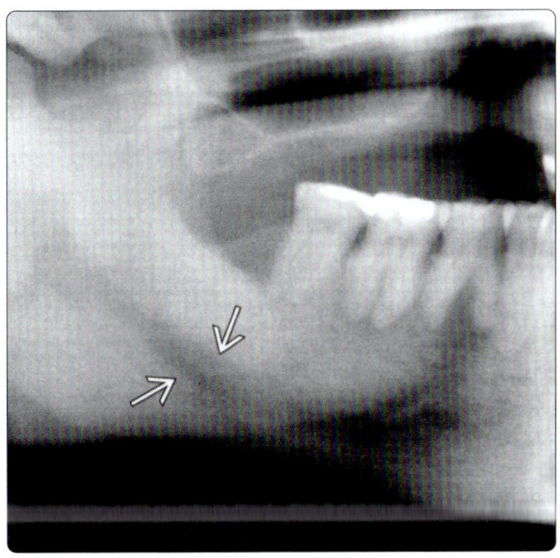

(Left) *Periapical radiograph in the same patient shows the loss of the lamina dura and the ground-glass appearance of the alveolar process.* **(Right)** *Panoramic radiograph shows the late sclerotic phase of Paget disease in the right mandible. The bone is homogeneously radiopaque and the inferior cortex cannot be distinguished. The mandibular canal is easily seen, but corticated borders and laminae dura are missing.*

Paget Disease

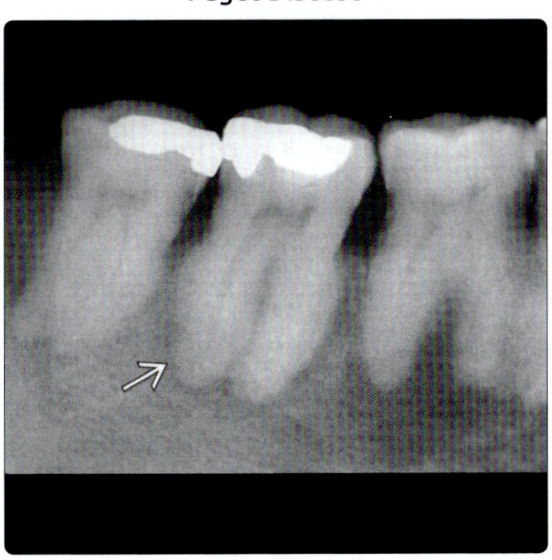

Paget Disease

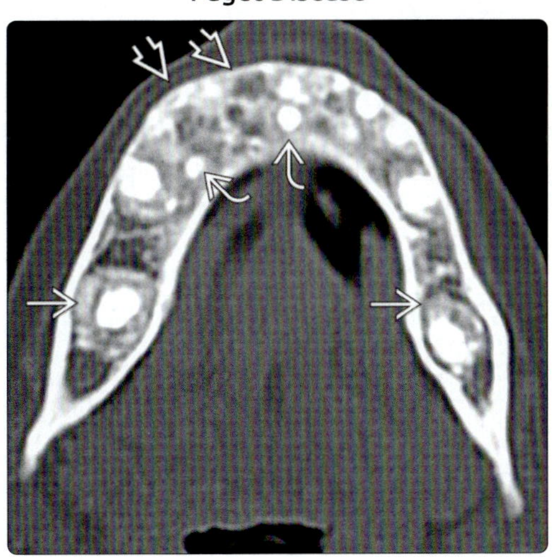

(Left) *Periapical radiograph in the same patient shows hypercementosis of the right 2nd mandibular molar tooth roots and alteration of lamina duras to the pagetoid bone pattern. The periodontal ligament spaces are narrowed or absent.* **(Right)** *Axial bone CT shows diffuse expansion & heterogeneous increased density/cotton wool appearance of the mandible. Note thinned and expanded anterior cortex, clumps of calcification resembling cotton wool, & sclerotic foci.*

DIFFERENTIAL DIAGNOSIS

Common

- Florid Osseous Dysplasia
- Osteomyelitis
- Chronic Recurrent Multifocal Osteomyelitis
- Fibrous Dysplasia

Less Common

- Paget Disease
- Gardner Syndrome
- Secondary Hyperparathyroidism

Rare but Important

- Osteopetrosis
- Sclerosing Bone Dysplasias
- Infantile Cortical Hyperostosis
- Fluorosis

ESSENTIAL INFORMATION

Helpful Clues for Common Diagnoses

- **Florid Osseous Dysplasia**
  - Key facts
    - Extensive form of periapical osseous dysplasia affecting 3 or more quadrants or widespread involvement in 1 jaw
    - Tooth-bearing areas only
    - **Above inferior alveolar nerve canal** in mandible
  - Imaging
    - Normal trabecular bone replaced with dense acellular cemental and osseous tissue in fibrous tissue stroma
- **Osteomyelitis**
  - Key facts
    - Inflammation of bone marrow
    - Patient is often symptomatic: Febrile, lymphadenopathy, sinus tracts
  - Imaging
    - **Sequestra** are hallmark; diffuse or lamellated periosteal reactions
- **Chronic Recurrent Multifocal Osteomyelitis**
  - Key facts
    - Recurrent episodes of multifocal sterile autoinflammatory disorder that affects bones and soft tissues
    - Synonym: **Chronic nonbacterial osteomyelitis**
    - Skeletal inflammation occurring primarily in childhood and adolescence
    - Etiology is unknown
      - Suspect both autoinflammatory and genetic susceptibility (chronic recurrent multifocal osteomyelitis locus on chromosome 18q21.3-18q22)
  - Imaging
    - 3 appearance types
      - Focal lytic lesion
      - Mixed lytic and sclerotic lesions
      - Sclerotic lesions
- **Fibrous Dysplasia**
  - Key facts
    - Nonneoplastic condition of bone with formation of dysplastic bone in fibrous connective tissue
    - Young females most affected
    - Can be monostotic or polyostotic
  - Imaging
    - Borders blend with surrounding bone
    - Internal structure is granular and often described radiographically as **ground glass**

Helpful Clues for Less Common Diagnoses

- **Paget Disease**
  - Key facts
    - Affects all bones, especially skull
    - Maxilla > mandible; affects entire jaw
    - Caucasian men
    - 50-60 years
    - Increased serum alkaline phosphatase
  - Imaging
    - Depends on disease phase
      - Becomes more sclerotic as matures, described as **cotton wool**
- **Gardner Syndrome**
  - Key facts
    - Autosomal dominant genetic disease
    - Multiple osteoma formation precedes presentation of intestinal polyps (100% potential for malignant change); epidermoid cysts
  - Imaging
    - ↑ in alveolar bone density and loss of periodontal ligament spaces
    - Supernumerary teeth
    - Hypercementosis and odontoma also associated
- **Secondary Hyperparathyroidism**
  - Key facts
    - Response to decrease in serum calcium caused by vitamin D deficiency, malabsorption, or inadequate metabolism by liver or kidney
    - Females > males
    - 30-60 years
    - Clinical history may aid in diagnosis
  - Imaging
    - Usually rarefaction of bone with prominence of teeth; however, some severe cases produce generalized granular or sclerotic appearance

Helpful Clues for Rare Diagnoses

- **Osteopetrosis**
  - Key facts
    - Inherited as autosomal recessive type (osteopetrosis congenita) and autosomal dominant type (osteopetrosis tarda)
    - Dysfunctional osteoclasts result in abnormal formation of 1° skeleton and ↑ in bone mass
    - Dense, fragile bones → fracture and infection
    - Hematopoiesis is retarded and cranial nerves may be compressed
  - Imaging
    - ↑ density of bone is bilaterally symmetric
    - **Bone** may be **so dense** that teeth **roots** and other structures within bone **may not be apparent**

  - Lamina dura and cortical boundaries thickened or blended into surrounding dense bone
  - Delayed eruption of teeth, missing teeth, and hypocalcification of teeth may occur
- **Sclerosing Bone Dysplasias**
  - Key facts
    - Pycnodysostosis
      - Short stature, hypoplastic lateral ends of clavicles, hypoplastic terminal phalanges, bulging cranium, and delayed closure of anterior fontanelle
    - Craniotubular dysplasias
      - Abnormal skeletal modeling ± increased bone density
      - Examples: Metaphyseal dysplasia, craniometaphyseal dysplasia, craniodiaphyseal dysplasia, frontometaphyseal dysplasia, osteodysplasty (Melnick-Needles)
    - Craniotubular hyperostoses
      - Overgrowth of bone with alteration of contours and increased bone density
      - Examples: Endosteal hyperostosis (van Buchem type and Worth type), sclerosteosis, and diaphyseal dysplasia (Camurati-Engelmann)
    - Osteopetrosis is considered bone dysplasia
  - Imaging
    - Generalized increased bone density in mainly children
- **Infantile Cortical Hyperostosis**
  - Key facts
    - Infants up to 6 months of age
    - Most frequently mandible, ribs, and clavicles
  - Imaging
    - Increased density of bones due to massive periosteal new bone
- **Fluorosis**
  - Key facts
    - Fluoride poisoning in adults
    - Usually not in head and neck
  - Imaging
    - Generalized increased density of bone with periosteal reaction
    - Prominent muscle attachments
    - Calcification of ligaments and interosseous membranes

SELECTED REFERENCES

1. Kuperstein AS et al: Systemic diseases and conditions affecting jaws. Dent Clin North Am. 60(1):235-64, 2016
2. Aygun D et al: Chronic recurrent multifocal osteomyelitis: a rare skeletal disorder. BMJ Case Rep. 2015, 2015
3. Patel R et al: Parotid swelling and chronic recurrent multifocal osteomyelitis of mandible in children. Int J Pediatr Otorhinolaryngol. 79(1):47-52, 2015
4. Acikgoz G et al: Chronic recurrent multifocal osteomyelitis: typical patterns of bone involvement in whole-body bone scintigraphy. Nucl Med Commun. 35(8):797-807, 2014
5. Chiellini G et al: The importance of stereochemistry on the actions of vitamin d. Curr Top Med Chem. 11(7):840-59, 2011
6. Cortis K et al: Imaging Paget's disease of bone-from head to toe. Clin Radiol. 66(7):662-72, 2011
7. Dlouhy BJ et al: Osteopetrosis with Chiari I malformation: presentation and surgical management. J Neurosurg Pediatr. 7(4):369-74, 2011
8. Russell RG: Bisphosphonates: The first 40years. Bone. 49(1):2-19, 2011
9. Waller S: Parathyroid hormone and growth in chronic kidney disease. Pediatr Nephrol. 26(2):195-204, 2011
10. Zati A et al: Pain in Paget's disease: a retrospective study of treatment efficacy. Neuro Endocrinol Lett. 32(2), 2011
11. Fusaro M et al: Vertebral fractures in dialysis: Endocrinological disruption of the bone-kidney axis. J Endocrinol Invest. 33(5):347-52, 2010
12. Mazzaferro S et al: The bone and the kidney. Arch Biochem Biophys. 503(1):95-102, 2010
13. Monsour PA et al: Chronic recurrent multifocal osteomyelitis involving the mandible: case reports and review of the literature. Dentomaxillofac Radiol. 39(3):184-90, 2010
14. Rajathi M et al: Autosomal-dominant osteopetrosis: an incidental finding. Indian J Dent Res. 21(4):611-4, 2010
15. Gómez García EB et al: Gardner's syndrome (familial adenomatous polyposis): a cilia-related disorder. Lancet Oncol. 10(7):727-35, 2009
16. Half E et al: Familial adenomatous polyposis. Orphanet J Rare Dis. 4:22, 2009
17. Scaramuzzo L et al: Clinical and histological modifications in osteopetrotic bone: a review. J Biol Regul Homeost Agents. 23(2):59-63, 2009
18. Curran AE et al: Autosomal dominant osteosclerosis: report of a kindred. Oral Surg Oral Med Oral Pathol Oral Radiol Endod. 87(5):600-4, 1999
19. Abramovitch K: Generalized radiopacities. Dent Clin North Am. 38(1):137-53, 1994

Florid Osseous Dysplasia

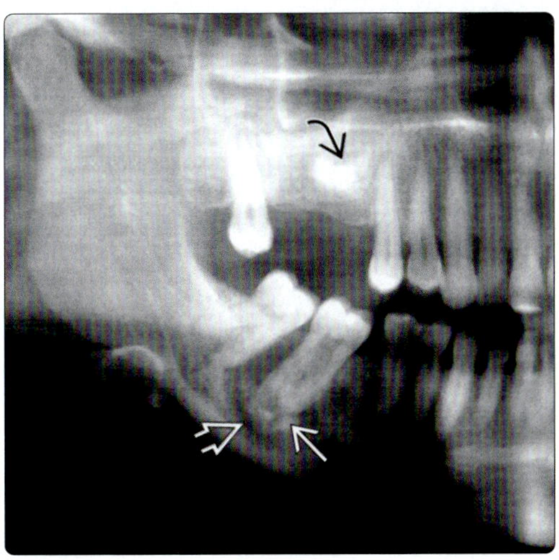

Osteomyelitis

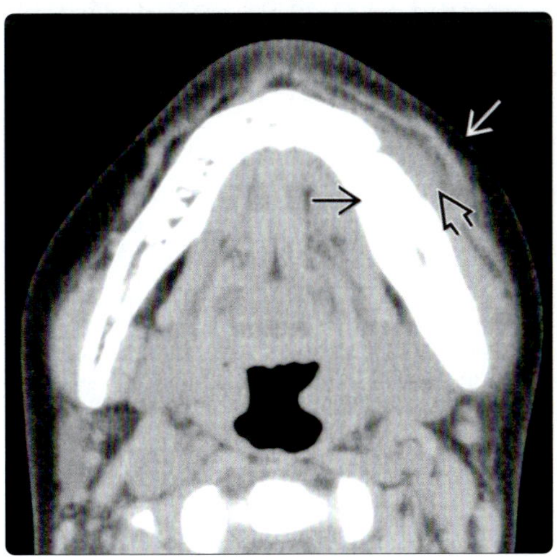

(Left) *Panoramic radiograph shows lesions of florid osseous dysplasia in the right mandible and maxilla. Mandibular cemental masses are globular and surrounded by a zone of radiolucency.* **(Right)** *Axial NECT demonstrates associated facial swelling and thickening of the soft tissues surrounding the mandible and fat stranding secondary to osteomyelitis. The bone marrow spaces are sclerotic.*

(Left) *CBCT coronal reformat at the level of the mandibular rami in a patient with osteomyelitis shows sclerosis of the medullary spaces* → *on the left with marked periosteal reaction* ↗*. Compare to the normal right cortical and medullary bone.* **(Right)** *Coronal CBCT through the anterior ramus in a child with chronic recurrent multifocal osteomyelitis shows the periosteal new bone* ↗ *has increased the overall dimensions of the left side. Generalized sclerosis of the left mandible is noted. (From SI: TMJ.)*

Osteomyelitis

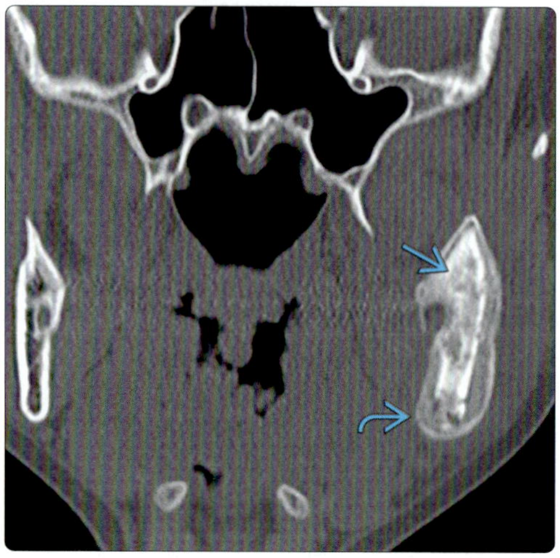

Chronic Recurrent Multifocal Osteomyelitis

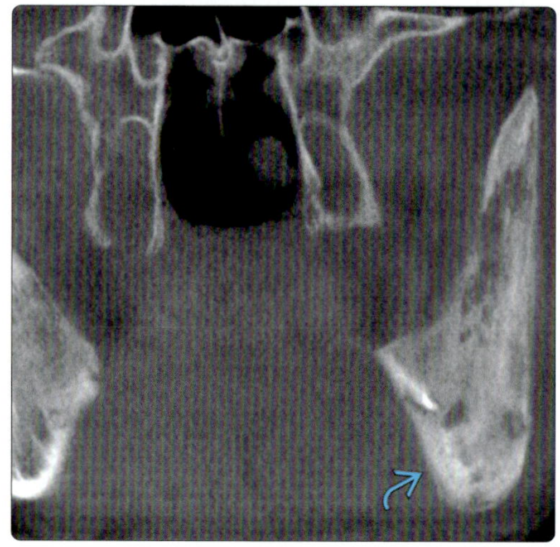

(Left) *CBCT panoramic reconstruction of the right mandible in the same patient demonstrates 2 separate lytic areas* → *without surrounding sclerosis. (From SI: TMJ.)* **(Right)** *CBCT sagittal oblique view of the left mandible in the same patient shows generalized sclerotic bone* → *with multiple lytic islands* → *and periosteal new bone* →*. (From SI: TMJ.)*

Chronic Recurrent Multifocal Osteomyelitis

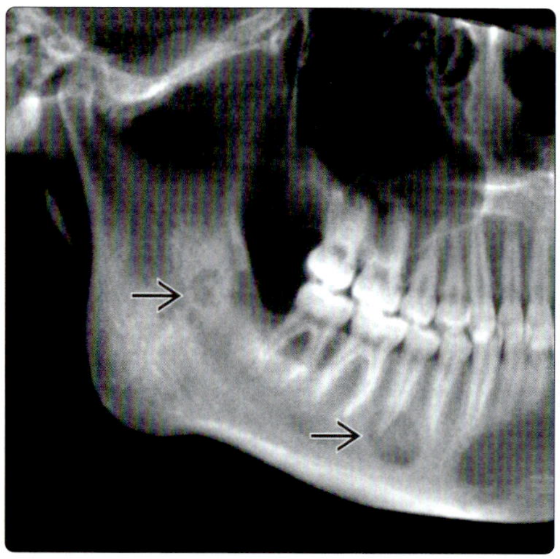

Chronic Recurrent Multifocal Osteomyelitis

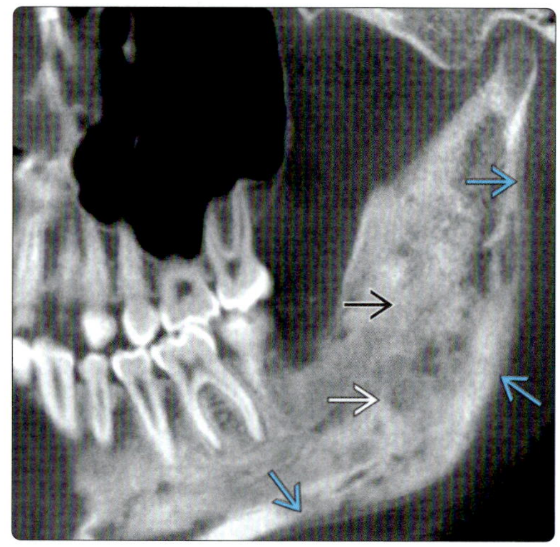

(Left) *McCune-Albright syndrome in a teenaged boy shows ground-glass opacification and expansion affecting all of the visible bones. Scattered lucencies are present* → *as can sometimes be seen in fibrous dysplasia. The mandibular condyles* → *and coronoid processes* → *are affected. (From SI: TMJ.)* **(Right)** *Axial CT in the same patient shows expansion of the medullary cavity of the mandible* ↗*. This appearance is very similar to the ground-glass appearance of fibrous dysplasia. (From: SI TMJ.)*

Fibrous Dysplasia

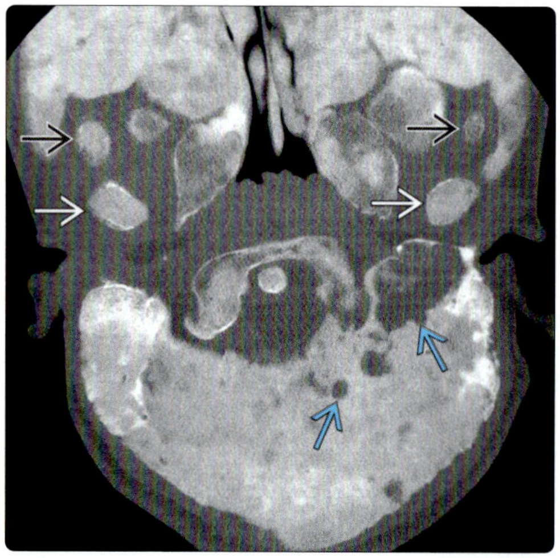

Fibrous Dysplasia

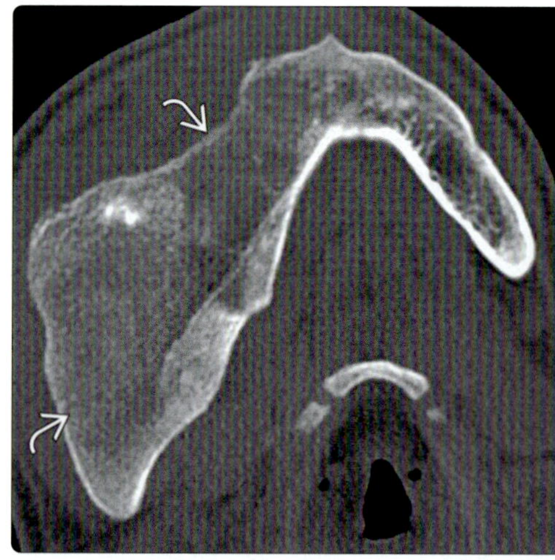

Paget Disease

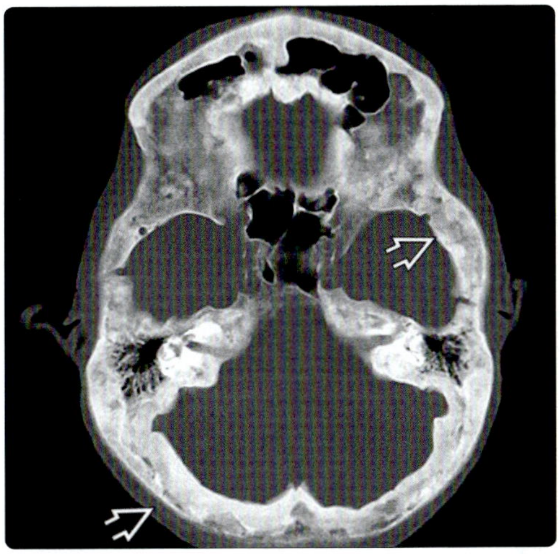

Paget Disease

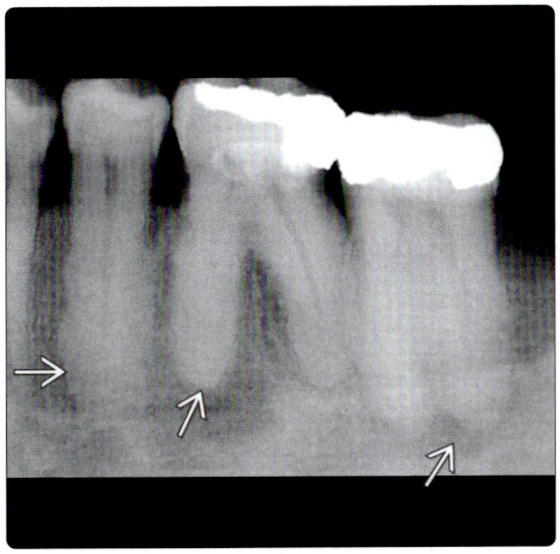

(Left) *Axial NECT demonstrates diffuse skull base Paget disease involvement with diploic widening, coarsened trabeculae, and thick cortices ➡. Cotton wool appearance is typical of late stage.* **(Right)** *Periapical radiograph of a patient with Paget disease shows hypercementosis ➡ of the roots of the teeth and generalized increased density of bone and loss of lamina dura.*

Gardner Syndrome

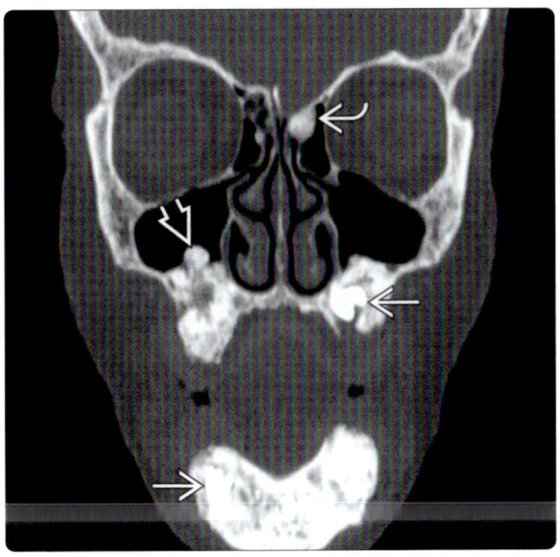

Gardner Syndrome

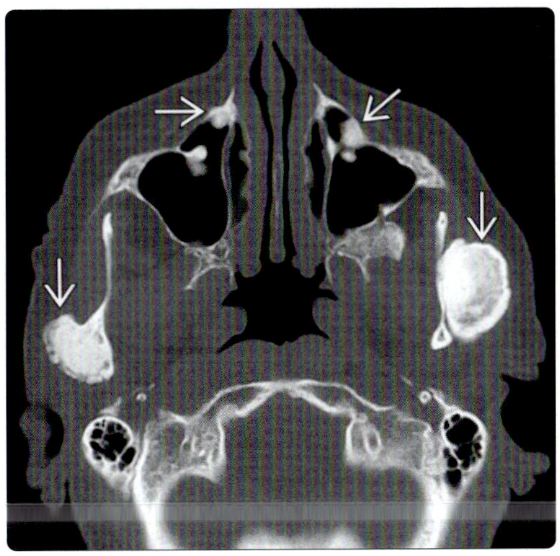

(Left) *Coronal bone CT shows dense alveolar bone with impacted teeth ➡ and peripheral osteomas present in the maxillary ➡ and ethmoid sinuses ➡ in a patient with Gardner syndrome. Jaw osteomas precede development of intestinal polyps that are premalignant.* **(Right)** *Axial CBCT of a patient with Gardner syndrome shows multiple osteomas ➡ in the maxilla and mandible.*

Secondary Hyperparathyroidism

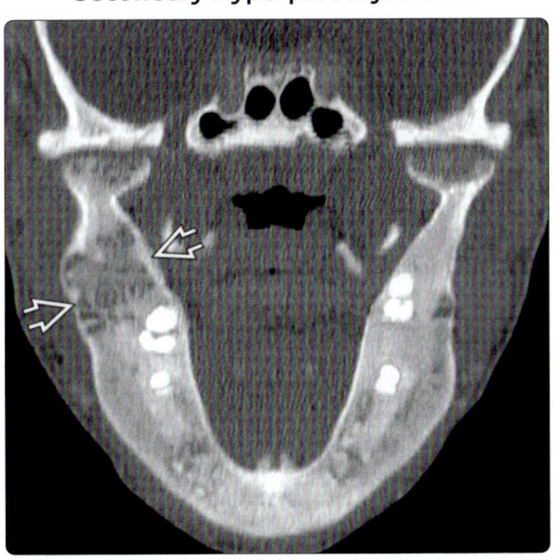

Osteopetrosis

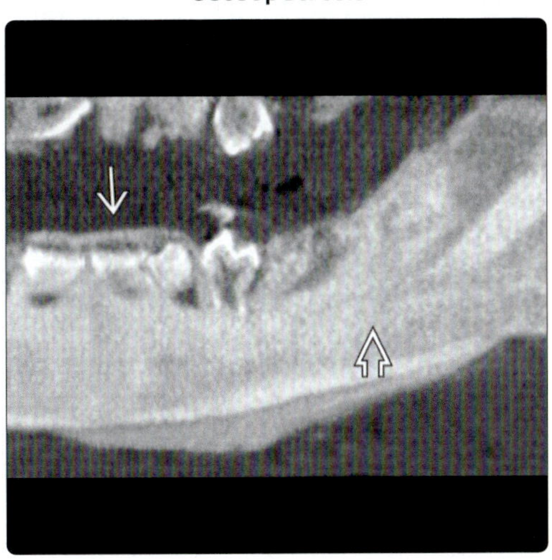

(Left) *Coronal oblique bone CT shows diffuse expansion and uniform increased density of the mandible. Note more focal expansion on the right due to a coexisting brown tumor ➡.* **(Right)** *Cropped CBCT panoramic reformat in a 4-year-old child with malignant infantile osteopetrosis shows replacement of trabecular bone with dense bone. The teeth are malformed and eruption is impeded ➡. The outline of the inferior alveolar canal has been effaced ➡. (Courtesy P. Hung, DDS.)*

DIFFERENTIAL DIAGNOSIS

Common

- Osteomyelitis
  - Chronic Osteomyelitis
  - Garré Osteomyelitis
- Trauma
- Osteonecrosis (Bisphosphonate Related)

Less Common

- Reaction to Longstanding Esthetic Implants
- Bone Remodeling
- Chronic Recurrent Multifocal Osteomyelitis
- Odontogenic Myxoma (Myxofibroma)
- Hemangioma
- Osteosarcoma
- Chondrosarcoma
- Metastases

Rare but Important

- Ewing Sarcoma
- Leukemia

ESSENTIAL INFORMATION

Key Differential Diagnosis Issues

- **Periosteum**: Membrane several cell layers thick that covers every surface of bone that is not covered by cartilage
- **Periosteal reactions by location**
  - **Asymmetric/unilateral**
    - Infections
    - Arthritic inflammation (psoriatic, Reiter, juvenile rheumatoid arthritis): Not usually seen in head and neck
    - Trauma (healing process of fractures): Examine populations prone to fractures, such as patients with osteoporosis and osteomalacia
    - Tumors (benign and malignant): Expansion of cortices as result of benign tumors is considered periosteal reaction
    - Vascular (subperiosteal hemorrhage)
  - **Symmetric/bilateral** (usually in long bones)
    - Vascular insufficiency (venous > arterial), hypertrophic pulmonary osteoarthropathy, pachydermoperiostitis, fluorosis, thyroid acropathy
- **Periosteal reaction by appearance**
  - There are different appearances for periosteal reactions that are generally nonspecific and could have multiple etiologies; there are some exceptions
  - **Continuous expansion with original bone cortex outline and thickness effaced**
    - Benign tumor
  - **Lamellated onion skin**
    - Garré osteomyelitis
  - **Codman triangle** (low-density triangle between original cortex and periosteal reaction); can be single lamina or lamellated
    - Aggressive malignant tumor extending into soft tissues such as osteosarcoma and Ewing sarcoma, infection (occasionally)
  - **Parallel spiculated "hair on end"**
    - Ewing sarcoma, congenital syphilis (in long bones), infantile cortical hyperostosis (Caffey disease)
  - **Divergent spiculated "sunray"**
    - Osteosarcoma, chondrosarcoma, metastases (especially from sigmoid colon, rectum, and prostate), Ewing sarcoma, hemangioma, odontogenic myxoma, meningioma, tuberculosis, tropical ulcer
  - **Solid smooth**
    - Healing fracture (callus formation), chronic osteomyelitis, bone remodeling
- **Bone sclerosis with periosteal reaction**
  - **Traumatic**
    - Healing fracture with callus
  - **Neoplastic**
    - Metastasis, lymphoma, osteoid osteoma/osteoblastoma, osteosarcoma, Ewing sarcoma, chondrosarcoma
  - **Infective**
    - Osteomyelitis, syphilis
  - **Idiopathic**
    - Infantile cortical hyperostosis, melorheostosis (long bones)

Helpful Clues for Common Diagnoses

- **Osteomyelitis**
  - Key facts
    - Usually caused by dental infection
    - **Chronic osteomyelitis**: Longstanding infection of bone marrow
    - **Garré osteomyelitis**: Occurs in young patients
  - Imaging
    - **Chronic osteomyelitis**: Will show sequestra formation within rarefied bone; **periosteal reaction morphology is nonspecific**
    - **Garré osteomyelitis**: Lamellated reaction giving **onion skin** appearance
- **Trauma**
  - Key facts
    - Healing fracture can produce callus formation (**solid smooth** periosteal reaction)
  - Imaging
    - Fracture line is usually evident; for small pathologic fractures due to osteoporosis and osteomalacia, callus formation may aid in diagnosis
- **Osteonecrosis (Bisphosphonate Related)**
  - Key facts
    - History of taking bisphosphonates
  - Imaging
    - Radiographically similar to chronic osteomyelitis

Helpful Clues for Less Common Diagnoses

- **Reaction to Longstanding Esthetic Implants**
  - Key facts
    - Implants used to enhance facial esthetics may develop calcification on external surface with time
    - **Pseudoperiosteal reaction**
  - Imaging
    - Chin implants are horseshoe-shaped, moderate-density entity on facial surface of mandible from molar-to-molar regions

- External surface develops thin layer of calcification that appears to be parallel to cortex of mandible and **mimics** periosteal reaction

- **Bone Remodeling**
  - Key facts
    - Changes in bone loading will lead to redistribution of forces through remodeling of bone
    - Osteoblast and osteoclast action to change shape of bone in response to new biomechanical situation
  - Imaging
    - Can appear similar to periosteal reaction
- **Chronic Recurrent Multifocal Osteomyelitis**
  - Key facts
    - Recurrent episodes of multifocal sterile autoinflammatory disorder that affects bones and soft tissues
    - Skeletal inflammation occurring primarily in childhood and adolescence
  - Imaging
    - **3 appearance types**: Focal lytic, mixed lytic and sclerotic lesions, and sclerotic lesions
    - Periosteal reaction common; **often mistaken for infection/osteomyelitis**
- **Odontogenic Myxoma (Myxofibroma)**
  - Key facts
    - Rare odontogenic tumor; tooth-bearing areas
  - Imaging
    - **Multilocular** radiolucency
    - Orientation of **straight septa** at periphery of lesion may give **pseudoperiosteal sunray** appearance
- **Hemangioma**
  - Key facts
    - Cortical or periosteal reaction is not unusual in areas adjacent to soft tissue (peripheral) hemangioma
  - Imaging
    - Divergent, spiculated **sunray** appearance may be seen on surface of adjacent bone
- **Osteosarcoma**
  - Key facts
    - Destructive, malignant lesion with osteoid formation
  - Imaging
    - Bone destruction with aggressive **"sunray"** periosteal reaction ± tumor bone formation
- **Chondrosarcoma**
  - Key facts
    - Malignant tumor arising from cartilage cells
    - May occur centrally in bone, on periphery of bone (parosteal chondrosarcoma), or in soft tissue
  - Imaging
    - Irregular shape that may be well defined and corticated or permeative
    - If periosteal involvement, spicules perpendicular to bone surface: **"Sunray"**
- **Metastases**
  - Key facts
    - Spread of malignant disease from distant primary
  - Imaging
    - Ill-defined destruction with invasive margins
    - Generally **spiculated** or **sunray** appearance
    - May show **solid, smooth periosteal reaction**

Helpful Clues for Rare Diagnoses

- **Ewing Sarcoma**
  - Key facts
    - Very rare; preferred location not established
  - Imaging
    - **Sunray** appearance may or may not be seen
- **Leukemia**
  - Key facts
    - Acute leukemia in young children
  - Imaging
    - May cause **diffuse spiculated** appearance on surface of bone, widening of periodontal ligament spaces of teeth, and low density of bone

SELECTED REFERENCES

1. Padwa BL et al: Pediatric chronic nonbacterial osteomyelitis of the jaw: clinical, radiographic, and histopathologic features. J Oral Maxillofac Surg. ePub, 2016

Chronic Osteomyelitis

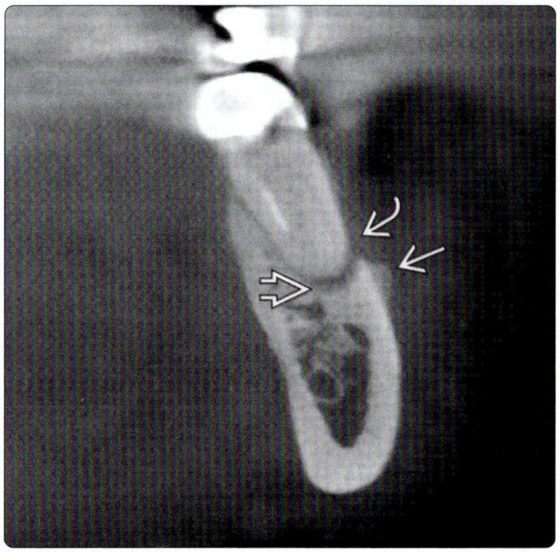

Chronic Osteomyelitis

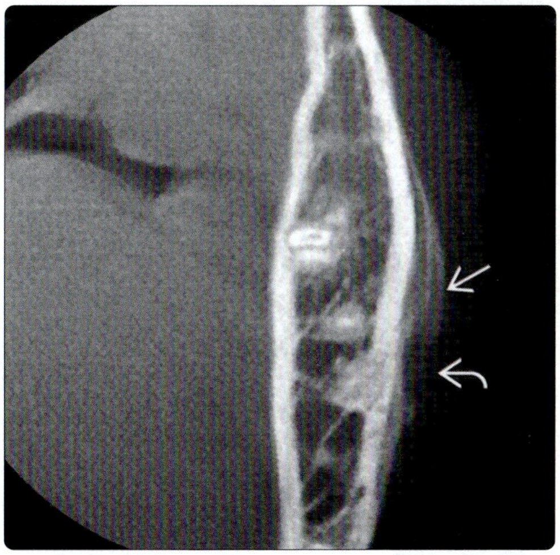

(Left) *Cross section CBCT shows an endodontically treated tooth with periapical rarefying osteitis ➡ that is eroding the buccal cortex ➡. A periosteal reaction is noted ➡. (Courtesy A. Briner, DDS.)* **(Right)** *Axial CBCT of the left posterior mandible shows lamellated onion skin periosteal reaction ➡ with disruption ➡ developing in a patient after 3rd molar extraction. (Courtesy A. Briner, DDS.)*

Chronic Osteomyelitis

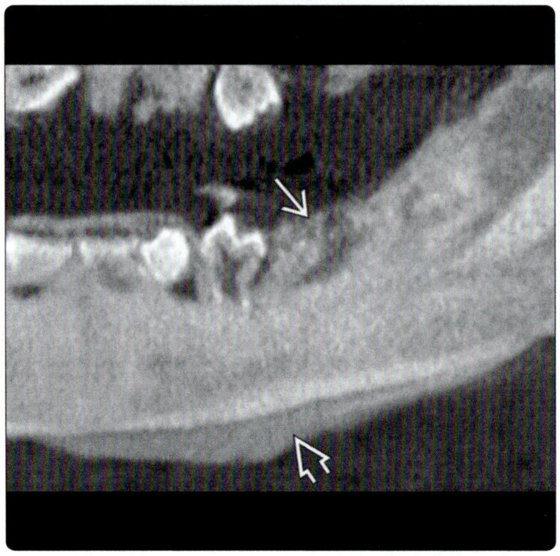

Garré Osteomyelitis

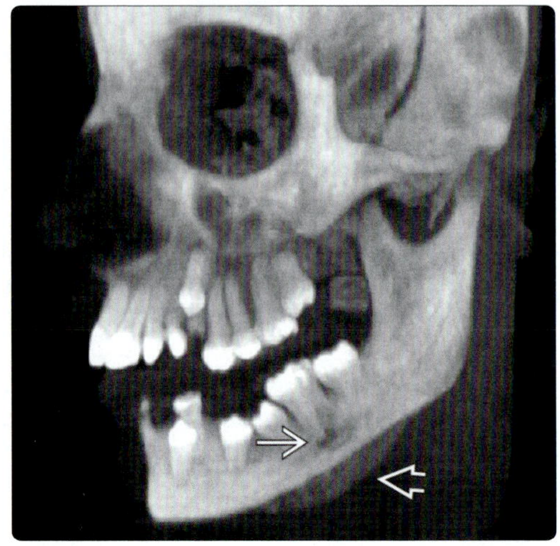

(Left) *Panoramic reformat CBCT shows osteomyelitis of the posterior left mandible → in a child with osteopetrosis. A solid, smooth periosteal reaction ⇨ is noted at the inferior border of the mandible. (Courtesy P. Hung, DDS.)* **(Right)** *Sagittal maximum-intensity projection shows that dental infection from the left mandibular molar → has progressed to osteomyelitis in this young patient. A periosteal reaction is noted at the inferior border of the mandible ⇨. (Courtesy M. Hedesiu, PhD.)*

Garré Osteomyelitis

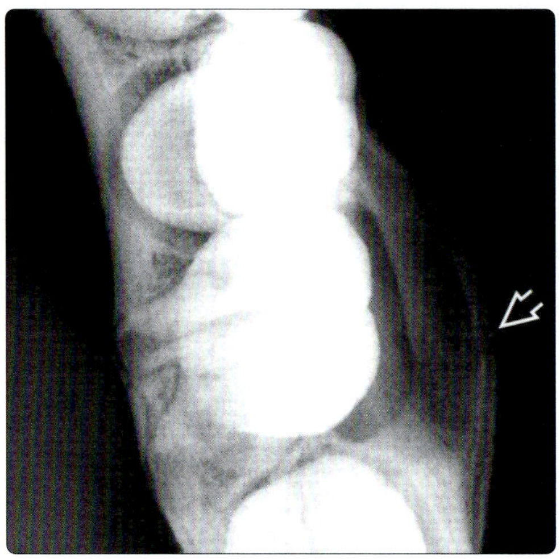

Garré Osteomyelitis

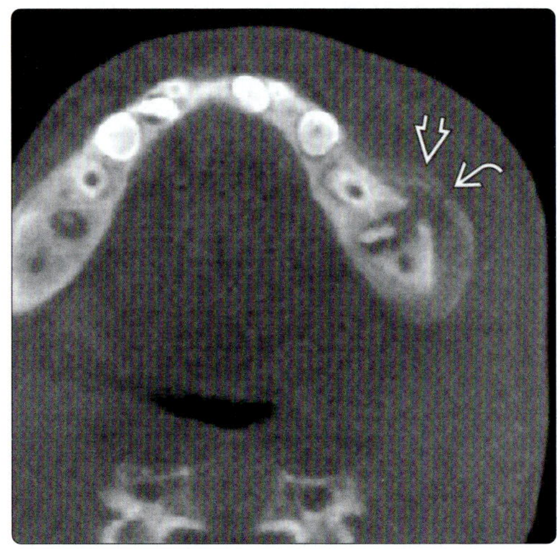

(Left) *Occlusal radiograph of the left posterior mandible of a young child shows the onion skin lamellated bone appearance ⇨ seen in Garré osteomyelitis. Osteomyelitis can occur secondary to infected odontogenic cysts. (Courtesy A. Wenzel, DDS.)* **(Right)** *Axial CBCT shows lamellated periosteal reaction ↶. Interruption of cortex is noted in both the periosteal reaction ⇨ and buccal cortex of the mandible adjacent to the dental infection. (Courtesy M. Hedesiu, PhD.)*

Trauma

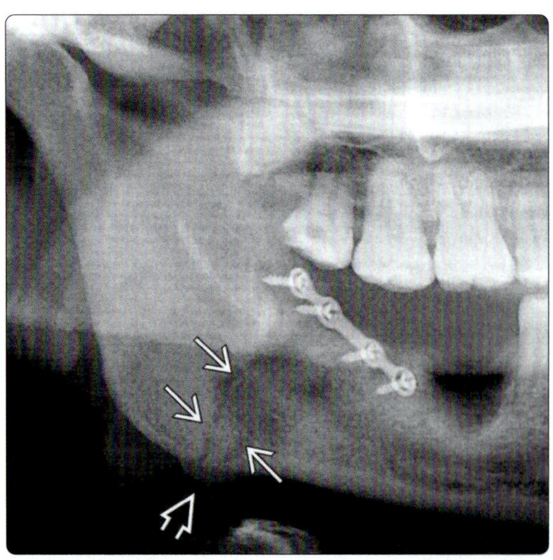

Osteonecrosis (Bisphosphonate Related)

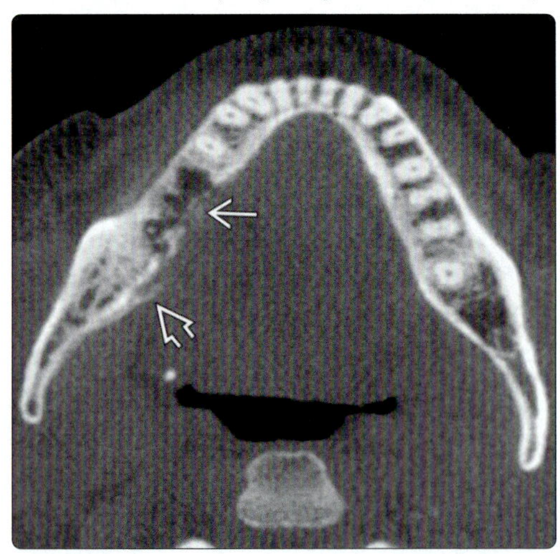

(Left) *Panoramic radiograph shows a fracture → through both the buccal and lingual cortices of the right mandibular angle. A bony callus ⇨ is seen on the inferior aspect of the mandible, indicating healing.* **(Right)** *Axial CBCT shows bisphosphonate-related osteonecrosis of the jaw. Interruption of the lingual cortex of the mandible → as well as a periosteal reaction ⇨ are appreciated. (Courtesy M. Ahmad, DDS.)*

Osteonecrosis (Bisphosphonate Related)

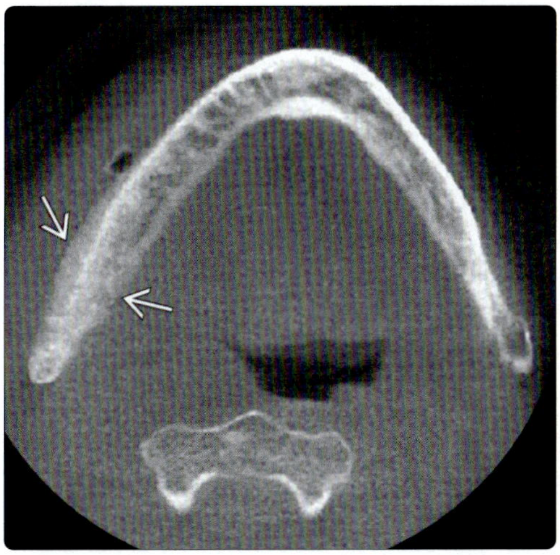

Osteonecrosis (Bisphosphonate Related)

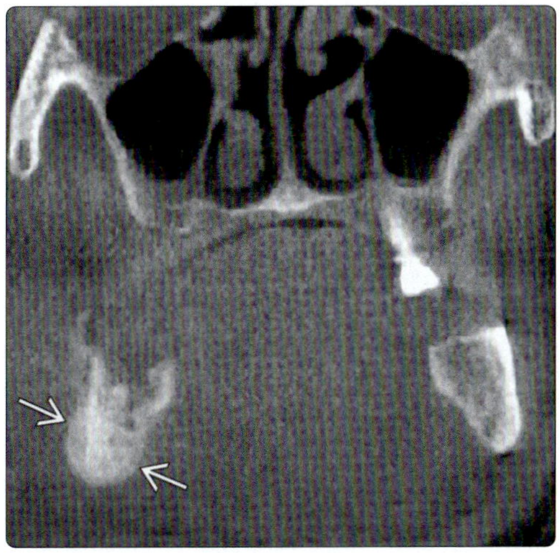

(Left) *Axial CBCT shows diffuse periosteal reaction on the buccal and lingual aspects* ➔ *of the right mandibular body after extraction of the 3rd molar. This patient has a history of taking bisphosphonates. (Courtesy M. Hedesiu, PhD.)* **(Right)** *Coronal CBCT in the same patient shows diffuse periosteal reactions seen along the lingual, inferior, and buccal aspects* ➔ *of the right posterior mandibular body. This radiographic appearance is similar to osteomyelitis. (Courtesy M. Hedesiu, PhD.)*

Reaction to Longstanding Esthetic Implants

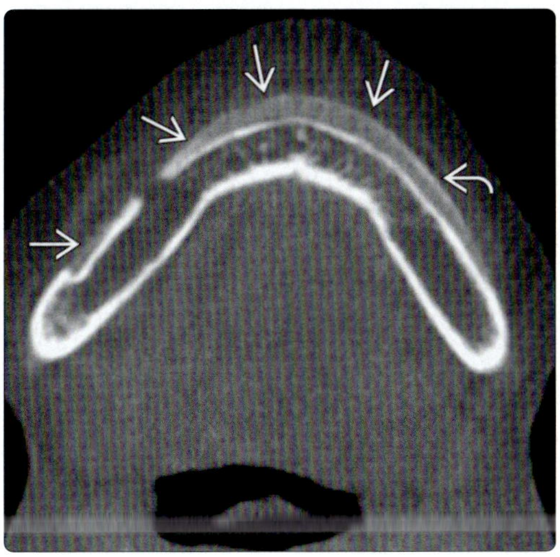

Reaction to Longstanding Esthetic Implants

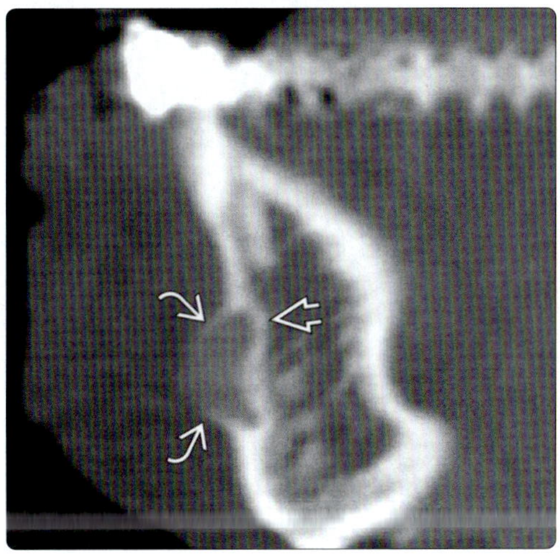

(Left) *Axial CBCT shows a longstanding genial implant* ➔ *on the buccal surface of the mandible. The surface of esthetic implants tends to calcify with time, giving the appearance of a periosteal reaction* ↷. **(Right)** *CBCT cross section shows a chin implant with a calcified surface* ↷. *With time, these implants tend to remodel the underlying bone* ⇨. *The evaluation of such implants should include the integrity of the adjacent structures, such as teeth, neurovascular canals, and foramina*

Bone Remodeling

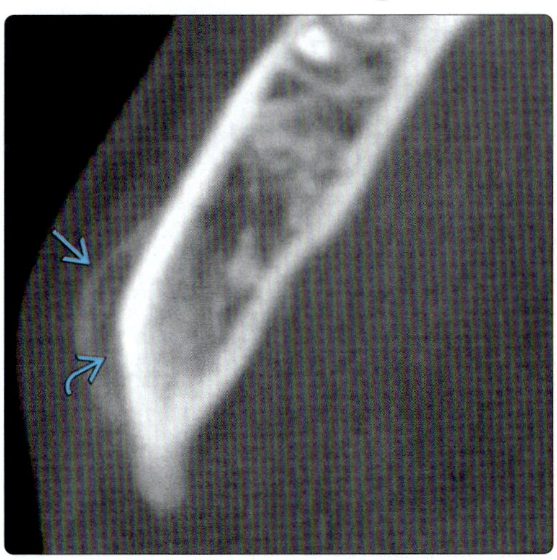

Chronic Recurrent Multifocal Osteomyelitis

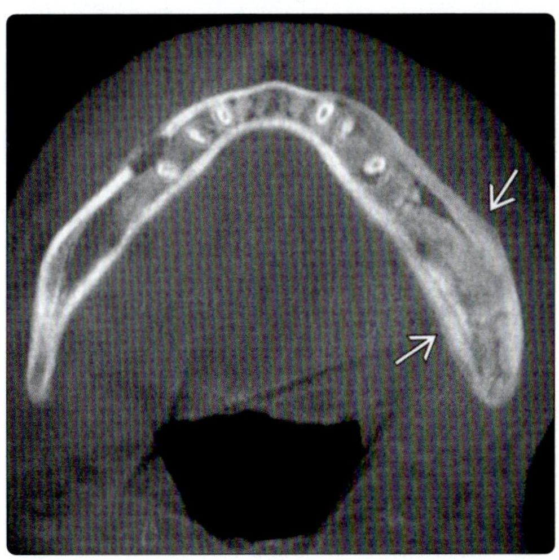

(Left) *Axial CBCT of the posterior mandible shows periosteal new bone* ➔. *Note the trabecular bone* ↷ *between the native cortex and outer surface of periosteal new bone. This is a modeling response to high stresses at the periosteal surface following an ipsilateral condylectomy (change in bone loading). (From SI: TMJ.)* **(Right)** *Axial CBCT of a mandible with CRMO shows sclerotic medullary bone in the left 1/2. Periosteal new bone is evident on the left side of the mandible* ➔. *(From SI: TMJ.)*

(Left) *Axial NECT in the same patient shows the spiculated sunray appearance of a pseudoperiosteal reaction* ➡. *Careful examination reveals an intact thin margin* ➡. *(Courtesy S. Kalathingal, BDS, MS.)* **(Right)** *Axial bone CT shows intraosseous hemangioma of the left maxilla. Notice the spiculated, honeycomb appearance of the expanded bone, typical of this lesion. Faint spiculation* ➡ *of the posterior surface is noted. This reaction is more common in soft tissue hemangiomas abutting bone.*

Odontogenic Myxoma (Myxofibroma)

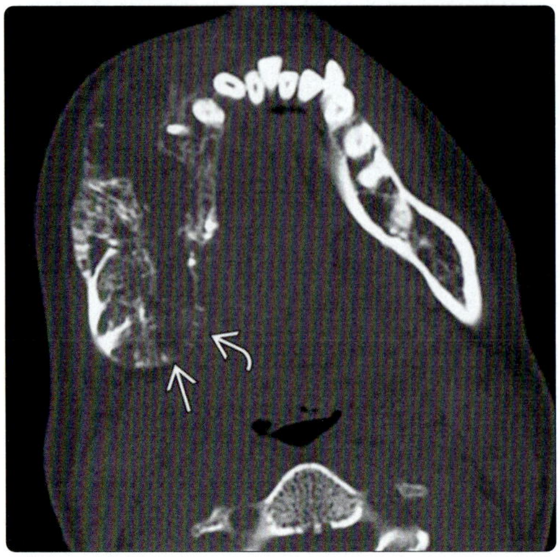

Hemangioma

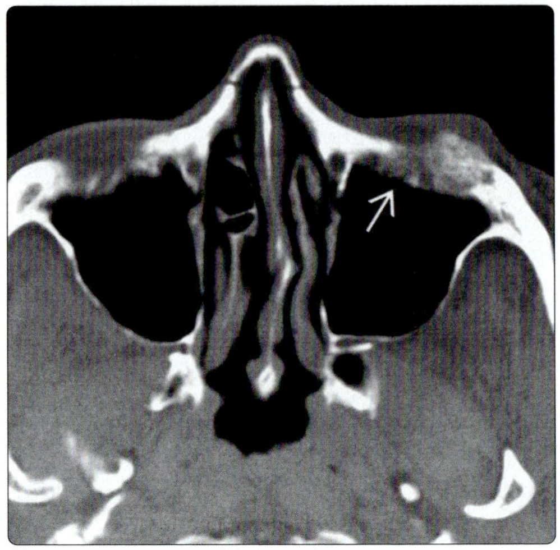

(Left) *Axial bone CT shows osteosarcoma involving the right mandibular ramus and condyle. The cortical margins are thickened, and there is a spiculated periosteal reaction* ➡. **(Right)** *Axial NECT of 11-year-old boy with osteosarcoma of the left posterior mandible shows nonuniform and patchy periosteal reaction* ➡. *The internal structure of the mandible is heterogeneous* ➡. *Note asymmetric swelling of the overlying soft tissues. (Courtesy M. Ayadi, MD.)*

Osteosarcoma

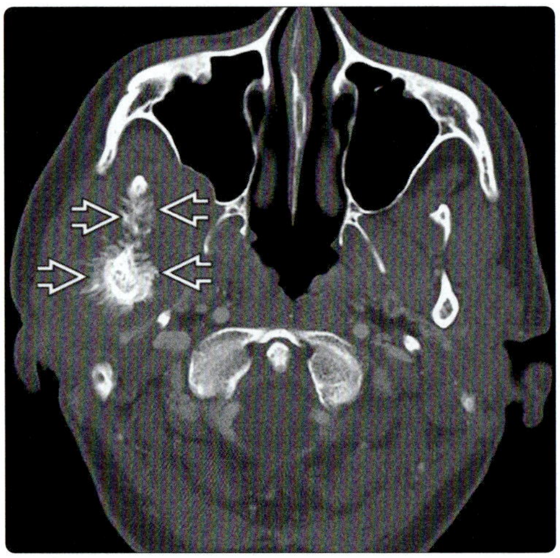

Osteosarcoma

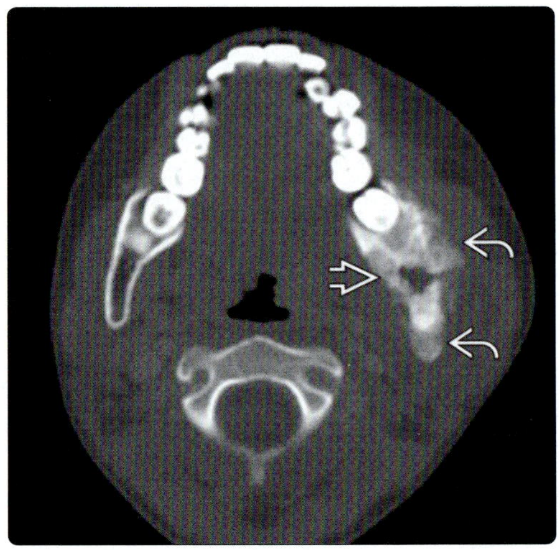

(Left) *Axial CBCT scan illustrates periosteal sunray appearance in chondrosarcoma of the mandible. The bony spicules are aligned perpendicular to the buccal* ➡ *and lingual* ➡ *cortices, more exuberant on the lingual aspect.* **(Right)** *Coronal CECT shows diffuse periosteal new bone formation* ➡ *seen with malignant metastasis to the right mandibular ramus and neck of the condyle.*

Chondrosarcoma

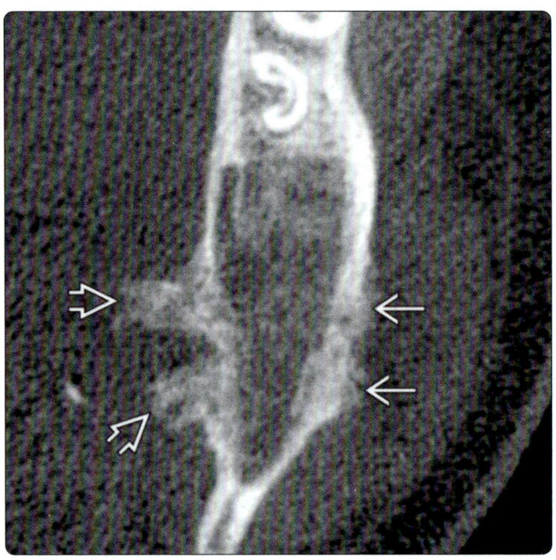

Metastases

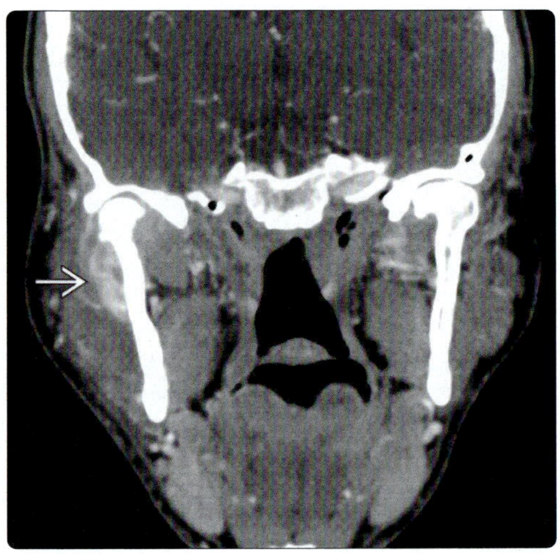

Metastases

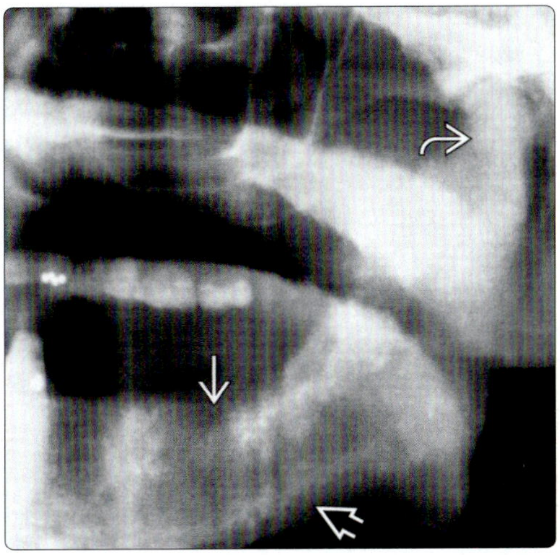

Metastases

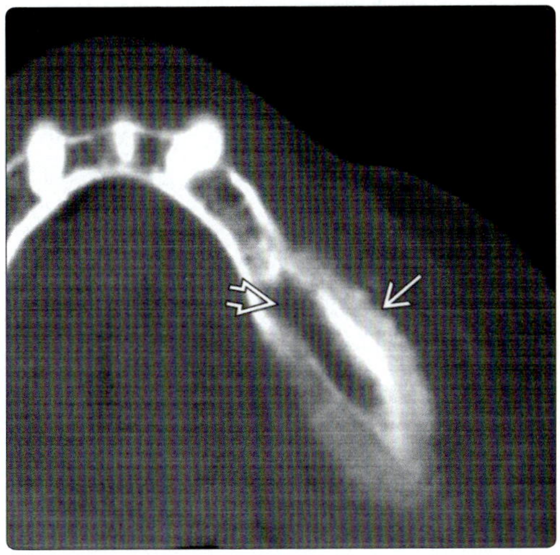

(Left) *Cropped panoramic radiograph shows moth-eaten bone pattern in the left mandibular body →, with sclerotic metastases in the upper ramus and condyle →. The mandibular cortex is irregular due to a spiculated periosteal response →. (Courtesy E. Lam, DMD.)* **(Right)** *Axial bone CT in the same patient shows the spiculated (beard-like) periosteal reaction → and a very radiolucent body of the mandible → due to bone destruction from the prostate metastases. (Courtesy E. Lam, DMD.)*

Metastases

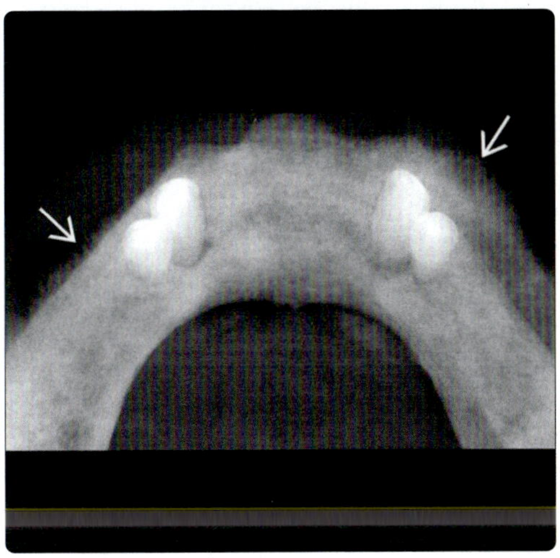

Ewing Sarcoma

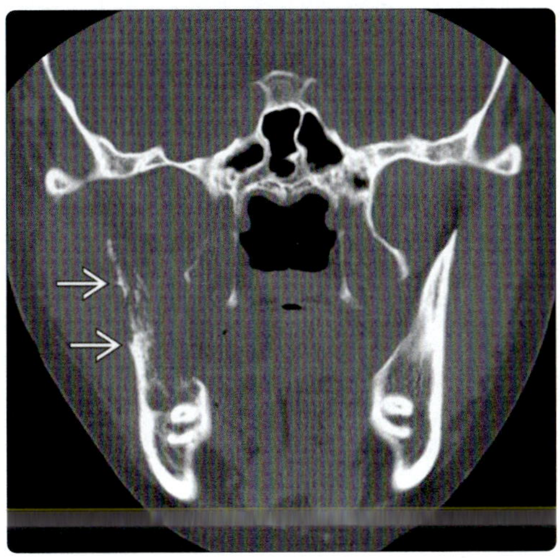

(Left) *Occlusal radiograph shows prostate metastases in the mandible. Note the bilateral, finely spiculated periosteal reaction → frequently seen with prostate metastases. Prostate periosteal reactions tend to grow along the mandible rather than from an epicenter.* **(Right)** *Coronal NECT shows destruction of the ramus of the mandible by a lytic lesion with faint periosteal spiculation noted on the lateral surface →. The lesion was proven histologically to be a Ewing sarcoma.*

Ewing Sarcoma

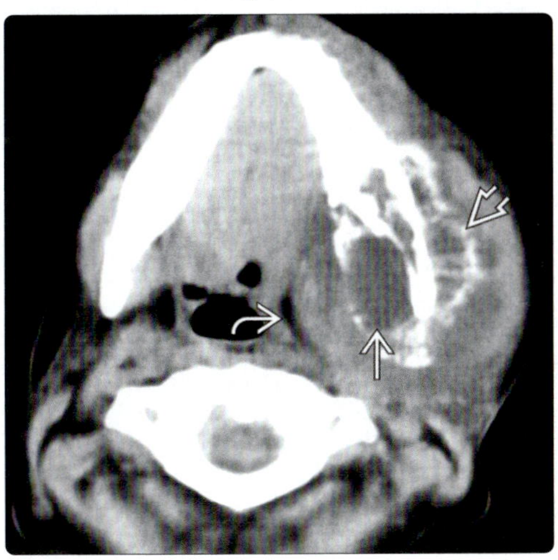

Leukemia

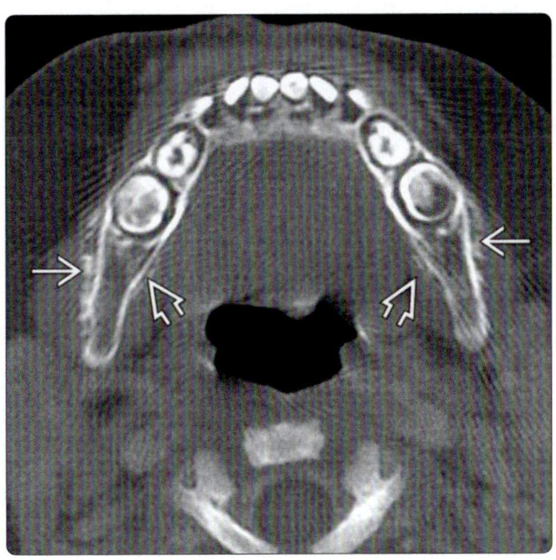

(Left) *Axial NECT shows a distended left cheek with underlying lytic mandibular mass →. "Sunburst" periosteal new bone formation is evident within the lateral extraosseous component →. Medial component displaces parapharyngeal fat →.* **(Right)** *Axial bone CT of the mandible of a young child shows diffuse osseous radiolucency. Periosteal reaction is also evident with spiculated → and lamellar → pattern of new bone formation as can be seen in acute leukemia.*

Ranula, Diving

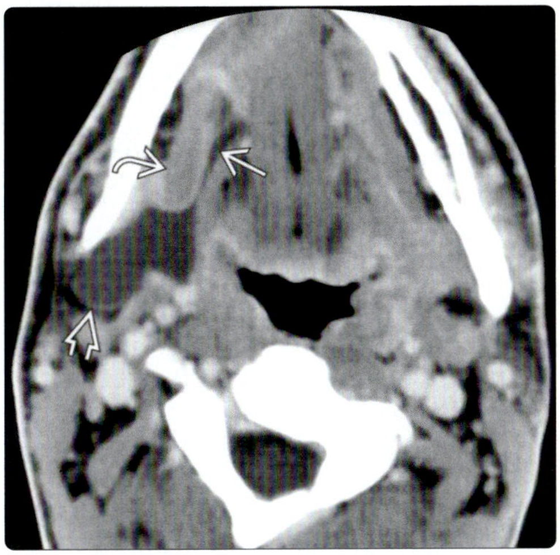

Benign Mixed Tumor, Submandibular Gland

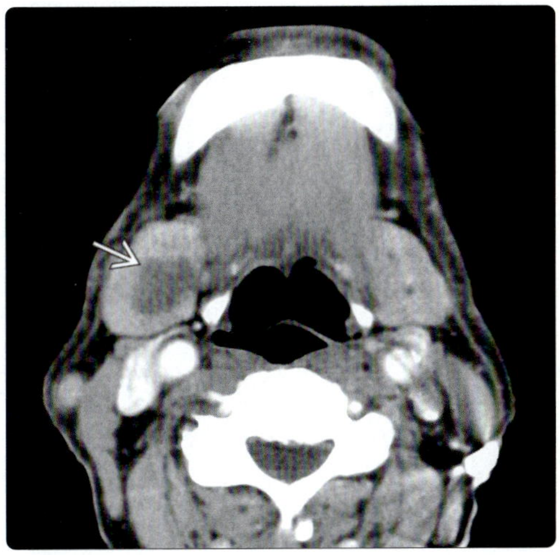

(Left) *Axial CECT shows a smoothly marginated cystic lesion with a narrow tail component extending into the SLS. The tail represents the collapsed portion of the ranula. The mylohyoid muscle is lateral to the tail. More posteriorly, there is a larger extravasation pseudocyst component extending into the SMS.* **(Right)** *Axial CECT shows a mass within the right SMG. This tumor is well defined and low density in comparison to the SMG.*

Carcinoma, Submandibular Gland

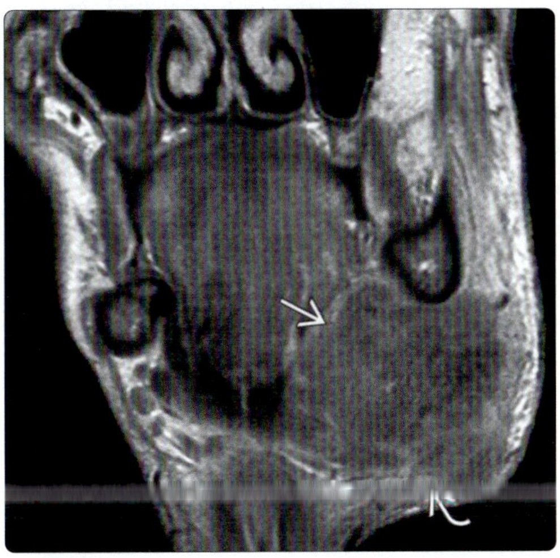

Suppurative Lymph Nodes

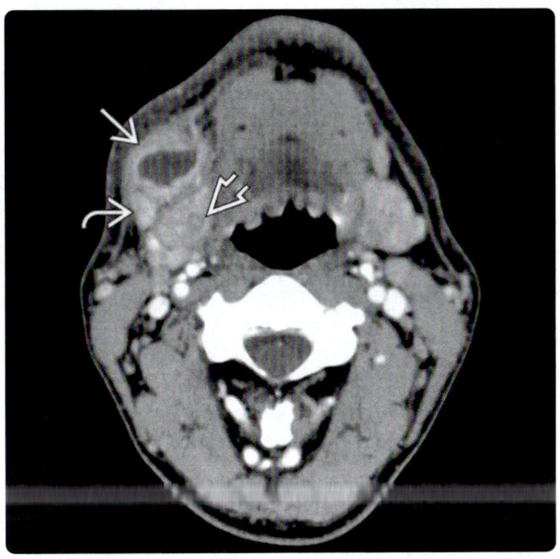

(Left) *Axial postgadolinium T1WI MR shows left SMG carcinoma invasion of the left mandible and the left floor of the mouth. The large, heterogeneously enhancing mass replaces the left SMG.* **(Right)** *Axial CECT shows an irregular, rim-enhancing, thick-walled suppurative lymph node. Suppurative nodal change has resulted in abscess, displacing the SMG posteroinferiorly, and is associated with reactive, nonsuppurative nodes.*

Non-Hodgkin Lymphoma, Nodal

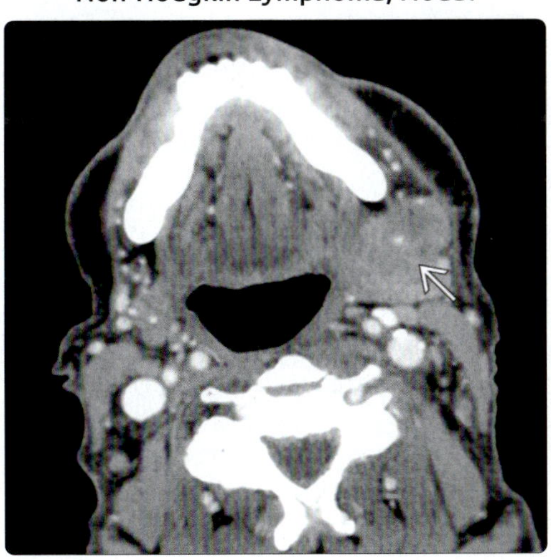

Tuberculosis, Lymph Nodes

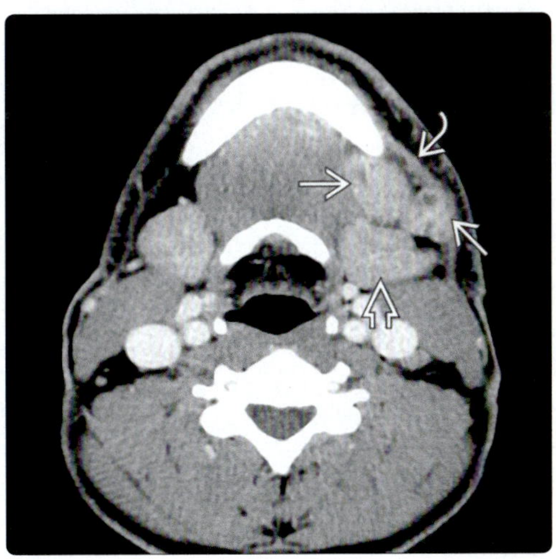

(Left) *Axial CECT shows a large, heterogeneously enhancing mass with irregular margins within the SMS. Subtle surrounding hyperdensity in adjacent fat raises the possibility of local invasion or adjacent inflammation. The SMG is not visualized separately.* **(Right)** *Axial CECT shows a small, heterogeneous level 2 node and multiple larger, heterogeneous submandibular nodes displacing the SMG.*

DIFFERENTIAL DIAGNOSIS

Common

- Benign Mixed Tumor
- Warthin Tumor
- Metastatic Disease, Nodal

Less Common

- Salivary Gland Malignancies
  - Mucoepidermoid Carcinoma
  - Adenoid Cystic Carcinoma
  - Malignant Mixed Tumor
  - Acinic Cell Carcinoma
  - Adenocarcinoma
  - Ductal Carcinoma
  - Squamous Cell Carcinoma
- Non-Hodgkin Lymphoma
- Schwannoma
- Infantile Hemangioma
- Lipoma

Rare but Important

- Oncocytoma, Parotid
- Venous Malformation
- Lymphatic Malformation
- 1st Branchial Cleft Cyst
- Neurofibromatosis Type 1
- Rhabdomyosarcoma

ESSENTIAL INFORMATION

Key Differential Diagnosis Issues

- **Boundaries of parotid space (PS)**
  - Superior: External auditory canal & mastoid tip
  - Inferior: Angle of mandible
  - Confined within superficial layers of deep cervical fascia
- **PS contents**
  - Parotid gland, intraparotid & extraparotid lymph nodes, retromandibular vein, external carotid, and extracranial branches of facial nerve
- **General interpretation issues**
  - Overlapping features of PS masses can make imaging diagnosis difficult
    - Different malignancies are radiologically indistinguishable
  - Many lesions require FNA/resection for diagnosis, but imaging can localize & guide surgeon to likely diagnosis
    - Caveat: Beware of FNA pitfalls in parotid
  - Small, well-defined lesion of PS
    - Almost impossible to distinguish node from benign or low-grade neoplasm
  - Large lesions of PS
    - Any loss of margin definition suggests malignancy
- **Imaging recommendations**
  - CT can localize, enumerate, determine cystic vs. solid, assess for neck nodes
  - MR best characterizes lesions
    - T1: Evaluate lesion margins & extent
    - T1 C+ FS: Clarify solid or cystic, evaluate CNVII for perineural tumor
    - MR T2 FS: Solid lesion signal intensity can suggest benign or malignant
      - ↑ T2 signal in solid lesion suggests benign [benign mixed tumor (BMT)] or low-grade malignancy
      - ↓ T2 signal seen with higher grade solid tumors
  - US guides FNA of superficial lobe lesion
  - FDG PET of little use in characterization of parotid masses

Helpful Clues for Common Diagnoses

- **Benign Mixed Tumor**
  - Key facts: a.k.a. **pleomorphic adenoma**
    - 80% of parotid tumors
    - Arises from ductal epithelium with epithelial and mesenchymal components
    - Slow-growing, unilateral, encapsulated, painless mass
    - 50% recurrence after excision
    - Malignant transformation in up to 15% if untreated
  - Imaging: Sharply marginated, essentially round mass
    - MR: Heterogeneous if large; hypointense on T1 C+
      - Solid, mostly hyperdense on T2
    - CT: Internal calcifications commonly seen and are strongly suggestive of BMT over other parotid masses
    - Nuclear medicine: Does not usually concentrate Tc-99m pertechnetate
- **Warthin Tumor**
  - Key facts: a.k.a. papillary cystadenoma lymphomatosum
    - Tobacco-linked benign tumor
    - 2-6% of parotid tumors
    - Slow-growing, painless, round to ovoid mass
    - Can be **bilateral**
  - Imaging: Typically at tail of parotid
    - May be multiple, solid, or cystic
    - T2 MR: Bright if cystic or solid
    - Nuclear medicine: Typically intense high signal with Tc-99m pertechnetate
- **Metastatic Disease, Nodal**
  - Key facts: Scalp, external auditory canal (EAC), or cheek skin squamous cell carcinoma or melanoma
    - Systemic metastases rarely occur in PS
  - Imaging: ≤ 1.5 cm superficial mass(es)
    - Other periparotid, occipital, or level II or VA nodes often found

Helpful Clues for Less Common Diagnoses

- **Salivary Gland Malignancies**
  - Multiple less common lesions included
  - Typically, no imaging features distinguish these carcinomas
  - When small or low grade, these may appear well defined and mimic node or BMT
    - Look for ill-defined margin as clue to malignancy
    - ↓ T2 signal in solid mass as clue to malignancy
    - Always look for **perineural tumor spread along CNVII** in temporal bone!
  - **Mucoepidermoid carcinoma**
    - Key facts: Most common salivary gland tumor (35%); more common in parotid than submandibular gland
      - Movable, slow-growing, painless nodule

- Imaging: Low grade is indistinguishable from other benign salivary tumors; cystic areas and calcifications sometimes seen
  - High grade shows ill-defined irregular margins
- **Malignant mixed tumor**
  - Key facts: a.k.a. carcinoma ex BMT and malignant pleomorphic adenoma
    - Most often arises in longstanding BMT
    - Early metastasis with unfavorable prognosis
  - Imaging: Indistinguishable from other high-grade malignancies on CT and MR
- **Squamous cell carcinoma**
  - Key facts: De novo or extranodal spread of metastatic parotid nodal disease
  - Imaging: If de novo, mimics other high-grade parotid neoplasms; if in parotid nodes, typically multiple coalescent nodules

- **Non-Hodgkin Lymphoma**
  - Key facts: With parotid nodes or gland
  - Imaging: If in parotid nodes, mimics other metastatic nodal disease
    - Primary parotid lymphoma mimics other salivary malignancies
- **Schwannoma**
  - Key facts: Often arises from small nerves, not from facial nerve itself
  - Imaging: Well-defined oval mass in superficial lobe
    - MR: Target appearance with peripheral lower T2 signal, T1 C+ enhancement
- **Infantile Hemangioma**
  - Key facts: Clinical history is key
    - Rapidly enlarging mass in 1st year of life
  - Imaging: Diffusely enlarged gland with marked C+
- **Lipoma**
  - Imaging: Clearly defined margins
    - MR: T1 and T2 hyperintense on MR, but hypointense with FS
    - CT: Markedly low density

Helpful Clues for Rare Diagnoses

- **Oncocytoma, Parotid**
  - Key facts: Benign lesion
    - Associated with prior radiation
  - Imaging: Small, well defined, possibly lobular; mimics node
    - Enhancing tumor with non-C+ curvilinear cleft on CT
    - Hypointense on T1 and T2 MR
- **Venous Malformation**
  - Key facts: Often transspatial
    - Multilobulated, loculations ± fluid levels
  - Imaging: Diffusely enhancing; phleboliths on CT and MR; MR: T2 hyperintense with diffuse C+
- **Lymphatic Malformation**
  - Key facts: Often transspatial
    - Multilobulated, cystic, ± fluid levels
  - Imaging: Cystic, lobulated without C+ on CT and MR; Bright T2 on MR, ± blood-fluid levels
- **1st Branchial Cleft Cyst**
  - Key facts: 2 cyst types
    - Type 1: Preauricular or intraparotid; ± sinus tract to middle ear or medial EAC
    - Type 2: Posterior or inferior to angle of mandible; ± sinus tract to lateral EAC
- **Neurofibromatosis Type 1**
  - Key facts: Plexiform neurofibroma characteristic
  - Imaging: Lobulated, infiltrating lesion
- **Rhabdomyosarcoma**
  - Key facts: Enlarging PS mass in child
  - Imaging: Infiltrating, patchy C+ mass

SELECTED REFERENCES

1. Prasad RS: Parotid gland imaging. Otolaryngol Clin North Am. 49(2):285-312, 2016
2. Kanekar SG et al: Parotid space: anatomic imaging. Otolaryngol Clin North Am. 45(6):1253-72, 2012
3. Wong KT et al: Vascular lesions of parotid gland in adult patients: diagnosis with high-resolution ultrasound and MRI. Br J Radiol. 77(919):600-6, 2004
4. Yousem DM et al: Major salivary gland imaging. Radiology. 216(1):19-29, 2000

Benign Mixed Tumor

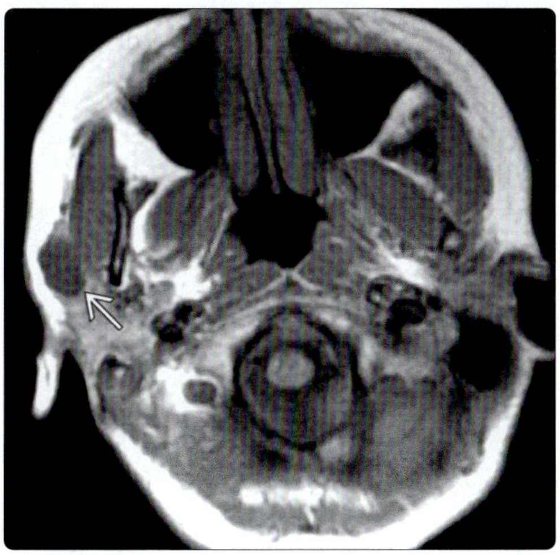

Benign Mixed Tumor

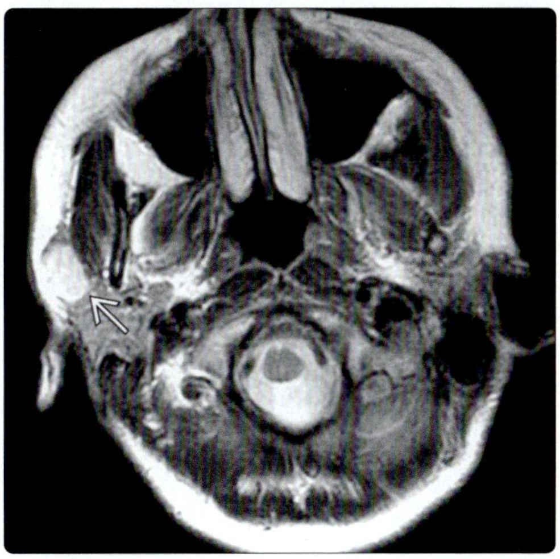

(Left) *Axial T1WI MR reveals a hypointense, well-defined mass ➡ within the anterior aspect of the superficial lobe of the right parotid gland.* **(Right)** *Axial T1WI MR in the same patient shows a uniformly hyperintense mass with well-defined margins ➡. The high signal intensity is suggestive of a benign parotid tumor or a lymph node within the parotid.*

Differential Diagnoses: Oral Cavity

(Left) *Axial T2WI FS MR shows a solitary, diffusely intense mass in superficial lobe of the left parotid. The ill-defined margin raises concern for a malignant neoplasm, although the high T2 signal of this solid lesion favors a benign process.* **(Right)** *Axial CECT shows heterogeneous, well-defined mass within right parotid, which is posterior to the retromandibular vein. The contralateral retromandibular vein is evident with an adjacent small, well-defined intraparotid nodule. Note: 20% of Warthin tumors are multicentric or bilateral.*

Warthin Tumor

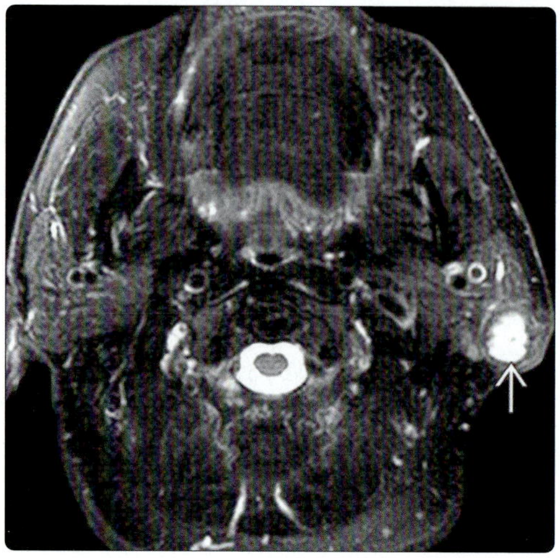

Warthin Tumor

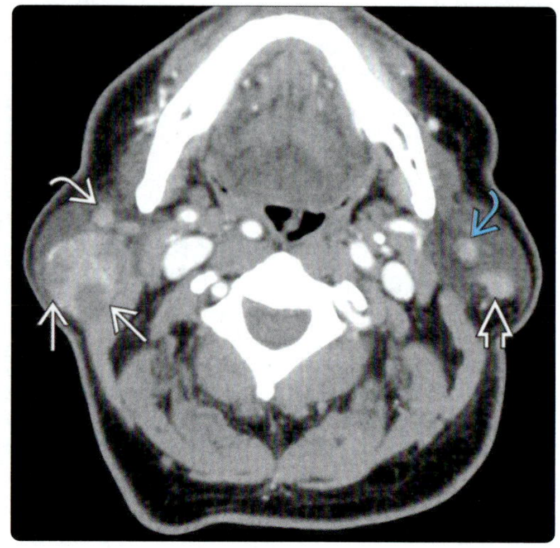

(Left) *Axial T1WI C+ FS MR shows bilateral, well-defined, round parotid masses. Necrosis within one of the masses was only evident on this contrast-enhanced fat-suppressed image.* **(Right)** *CECT shows heterogeneously enhancing masses in the left and right parotid glands. The left mass has an irregular contour and marked central necrosis which, in association with the history of squamous cell carcinoma, is most suggestive of metastatic disease.*

Metastatic Disease, Nodal

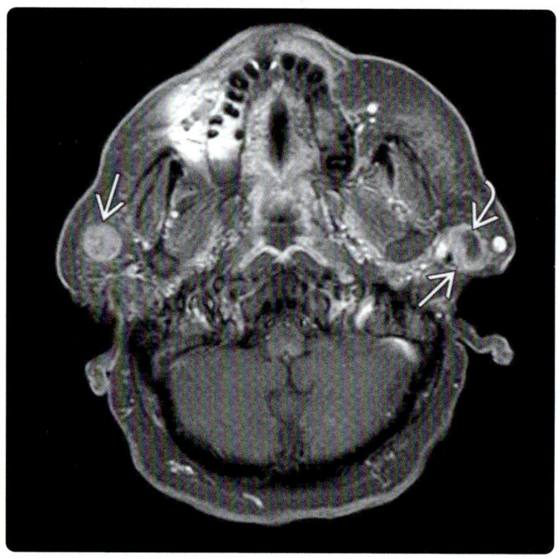

Metastatic Disease, Nodal

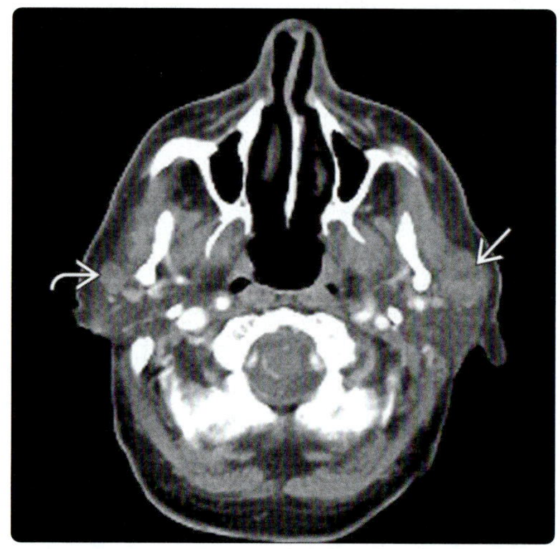

(Left) *Axial T1WI MR shows a small, well-defined solid mass in superficial lobe of left parotid. Low-grade mucoepidermoid carcinoma is often indistinguishable from more common benign neoplasms like benign mixed tumor.* **(Right)** *Axial CECT shows a large, hyperdense mass infiltrating the left parotid gland. High-grade mucoepidermoid carcinoma has an aggressive infiltrative appearance. Always look for perineural tumor spread along the facial nerve and auriculotemporal branch of CNV in these cases.*

Mucoepidermoid Carcinoma

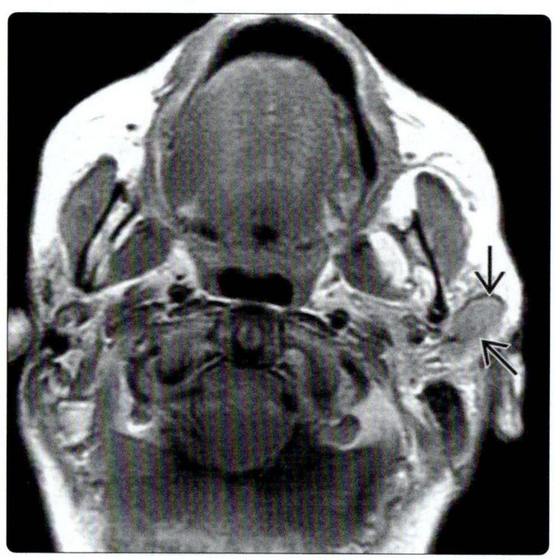

Mucoepidermoid Carcinoma

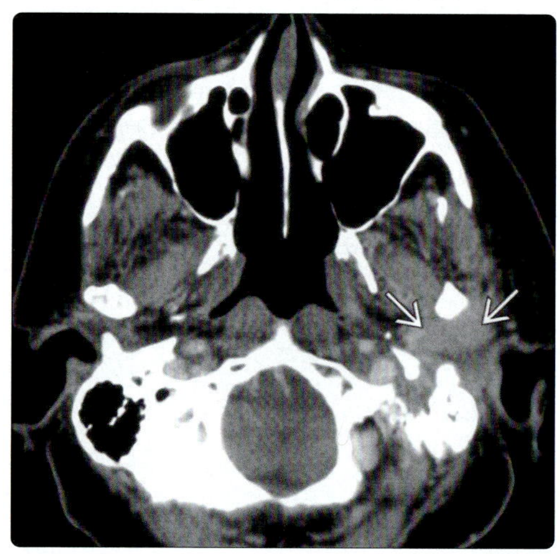

Acinic Cell Carcinoma

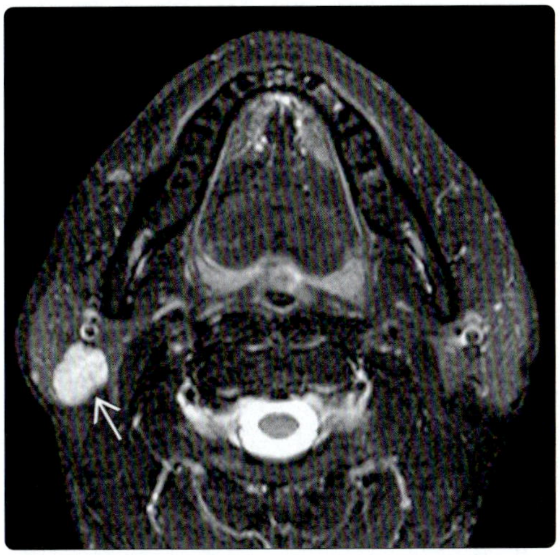

Acinic Cell Carcinoma

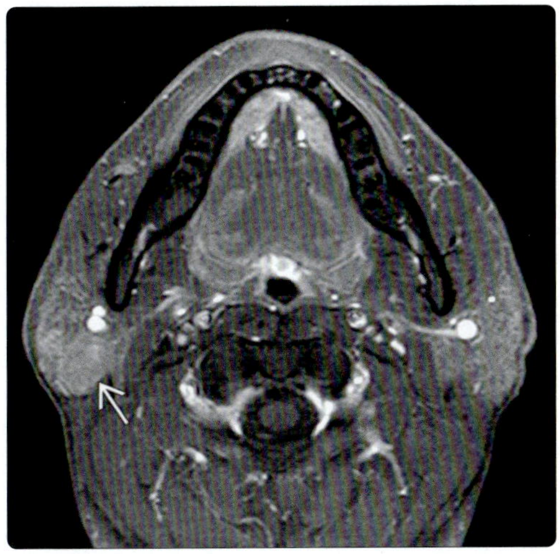

(Left) *Axial T2WI FS MR depicts a well-circumscribed mass at the posterior margin of the superficial lobe of the right parotid gland* ➡*, suggesting a benign mixed tumor.* **(Right)** *Axial T1WI C+ FS MR in the same patient shows minimal enhancement* ➡*, making benign mixed tumor less likely. It is usually not possible to differentiate the multiple types of malignancies of the parotid gland with imaging alone.*

Non-Hodgkin Lymphoma

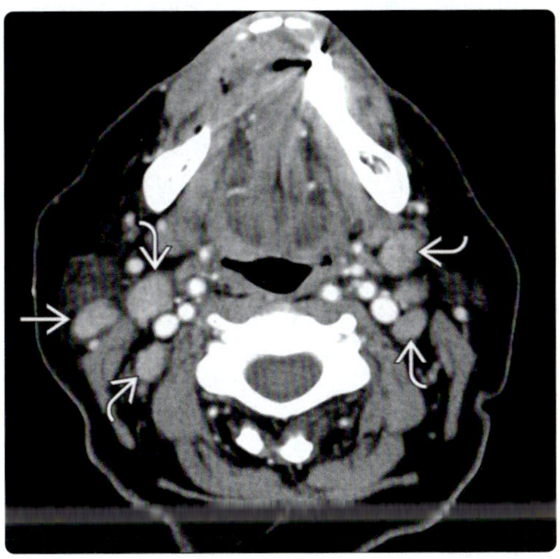

Non-Hodgkin Lymphoma

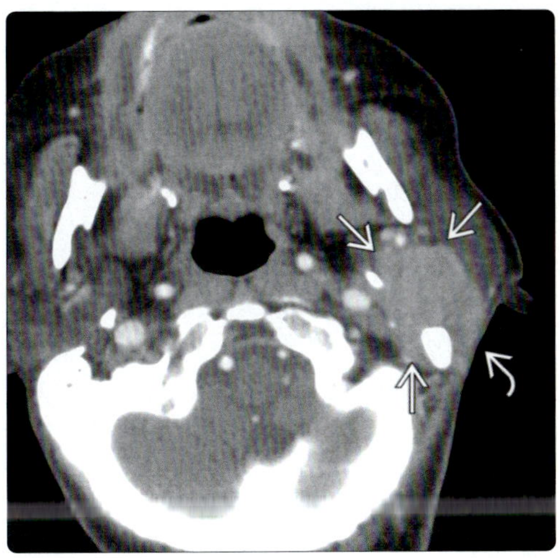

(Left) *CECT shows multiple uniformly enhancing nodules* ➡ *within the right parotid gland of a patient with non-Hodgkin lymphoma. Bilateral neck adenopathy* ↪ *is also seen.* **(Right)** *Axial NECT shows an asymmetrically dense left parotid gland with a well-defined mass* ➡*. The mass extends to the skin* ↪*. MR is necessary to evaluate the intratemporal and intracranial facial nerve for perineural tumor spread.*

Schwannoma

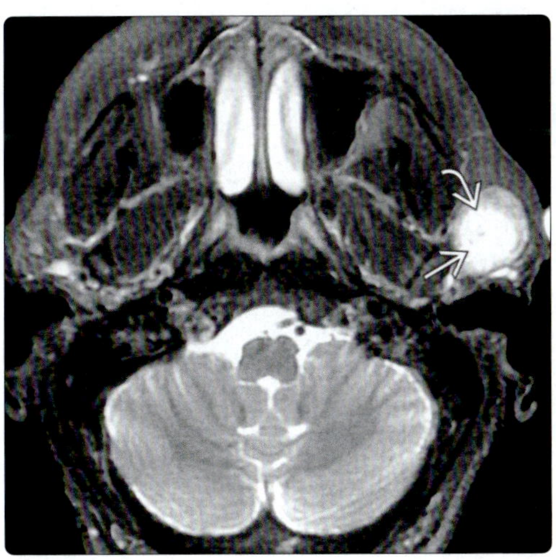

Lipoma

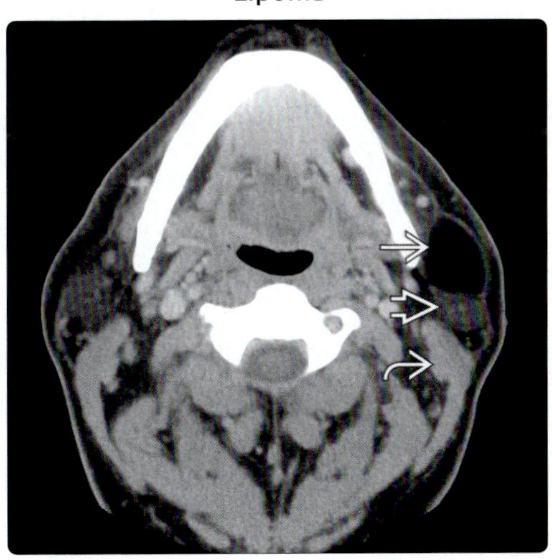

(Left) *Axial T2WI FS MR shows a solitary, well-defined mass in the left parotid. Note central hyperintensity* ➡ *with a peripheral intermediate signal rim* ↪*, giving a target-like appearance considered by some as typical for schwannoma of the parotid.* **(Right)** *Axial CECT shows a benign-appearing mass within the inferior aspect of the left parotid space* ➡ *separate from the normal parotid parenchyma* ➡ *and anterior to the sternocleidomastoid muscle* ↪*. The density is homogeneous and follows fat density.*

DIFFERENTIAL DIAGNOSIS

Common

- Simple Ranula
- Abscess, Sublingual Space
- Dilated Wharton Duct
- Squamous Cell Carcinoma, Floor of Mouth
- Squamous Cell Carcinoma, Oral Tongue, Invasive
- Sialadenitis, Sublingual Gland
- Acute Radiation Changes, Sublingual Gland

Less Common

- Sublingual Space Sialocele
- Hypoglossal Nerve Atrophy
- Dermoid and Epidermoid Cysts, Sublingual Space
- Venous Malformation, Sublingual Space
- Lymphatic Malformation, Sublingual Space

Rare but Important

- Carcinoma, Sublingual Gland
- Benign Mixed Tumor, Sublingual Gland

ESSENTIAL INFORMATION

Key Differential Diagnosis Issues

- **Boundaries of sublingual space (SLS)**
  - Superior: Floor of mouth and mucosa
  - Inferior: Mylohyoid muscle
  - Anterolateral: Medial surface of mandible
  - Posterior: Geniohyoid and genioglossus muscles
  - Medial: Instrinsic tongue and genioglossus muscles separate left and right SLS, which communicate at anterior isthmus
  - No fascial encapsulation: **Communicates with posterosuperior submandibular and inferior parapharyngeal spaces**
- **SLS contents**
  - Anterosuperior hyoglossus muscle
  - Lingual nerve (distal CNV3 and chordae tympani branch CNVII), distal CNIX, CNXII
  - Lingual artery and vein
  - Sublingual gland (SLG) and minor salivary glands
  - Deep submandibular gland (SMG) and Wharton duct
- **Imaging recommendations**
  - CECT with coronal reformations best initial choice
  - NECT, CBCT, cross-sectional mandibular occlusal radiograph adequate for sialoliths with at least moderate calcification
  - MR for staging malignancies and complex disease involving multiple anatomic spaces
  - US with high-resolution liner array to delineate muscles and possible herniation as well as sialoliths
  - Angiography for vascular anomalies in floor of mouth lesions involving lingual artery/vein

Helpful Clues for Common Diagnoses

- **Simple Ranula**
  - Key facts: Postinflammatory, unilateral SLG mucous retention cyst usually
    - Closely mimics lymphatic malformation, epidermoid, and sialocele
    - Superior to mylohyoid muscle near SLG; may also be associated with minor salivary glands in floor of mouth
  - Imaging: Cystic lesion in SLS usually < 3 cm
- **Abscess, Sublingual Space**
  - Key facts: Secondary to dental abscess, Wharton duct sialolith, or mandibular osteomyelitis
    - Superomedial to mylohyoid muscle
  - Imaging: CECT is study of choice
    - Rim-enhancing fluid collection ± Wharton duct sialolith ± dental abscess
    - If bilateral, **horseshoe-shaped fluid collection** with anterior isthmus
    - If caused by osteomyelitis, look for focal osseous destruction or periosteal reaction
    - Panoramic or CBCT to evaluate mandible for dental source (periapical dental inflammatory lesion or focal cortical dehiscence)
- **Dilated Wharton Duct**
  - Key facts: Wharton duct enlargement secondary to sialolith or stenosis
  - Imaging
    - CT/MR: High-density/low-intensity sialolith causes proximal Wharton duct enlargement with swollen, enhancing SMG (sialadenitis)
    - CBCT or underpenetrated mandibular occlusal radiograph are appropriate to define sialolith
    - Conventional sialography presents ductal morphology with best resolution
- **Squamous Cell Carcinoma, Floor of Mouth**
  - Key facts: Invasive squamous cell carcinoma (SCCa) under anterior tongue invades SLS
  - Imaging
    - CT/MR: Enhancing anterior SLG; SCCa directly invades SLS
- **Squamous Cell Carcinoma, Oral Tongue, Invasive**
  - Key facts: SCCa on epithelial surface of oral tongue invades SLS
    - Assess mandibular cortex, hyoglossus and mylohyoid invasion as well as contralateral spread
    - Typically 70% malignant nodes at presentation
  - Imaging
    - CT/MR: Enhancing tongue **SCCa follows hyoglossus into SLS**
- **Sialadenitis, Sublingual Gland**
  - Key facts: Focal inflammation of SLG in SLS
  - Imaging: Enlarged, enhancing SLG
- **Acute Radiation Changes, Sublingual Gland**
  - Key facts: Suprahyoid radiation causes sialadenitis in all salivary glands
    - Acute inflammation → xerostomia
  - Imaging
    - CT/MR: Enhancing, enlarged SLG
    - Skin thickened with adjacent edema

Helpful Clues for Less Common Diagnoses

- **Sublingual Space Sialocele**
  - Key facts: SLS cystic lesion secondary to trauma, surgery, obstructing sialolith, or stenosis of Wharton duct
    - True sialocele: Distended proximal Wharton duct

- False sialocele: Ruptured duct, extravasated saliva develops pseudocyst (fluid collection adjacent to duct in SLS without enhancing wall)
- Imaging
  - CT/MR: Fluid density/intensity in dilated Wharton duct (true) or adjacent to duct (false)
  - May peripherally enhance after 2 weeks

- **Hypoglossal Nerve Atrophy**
  - Key facts: Unilateral atrophy of tongue, secondary to CNXII dysfunction
    - Evaluate course of CNXII from medulla to SLS
    - Contralateral muscular hypertrophy may be hypermetabolic on PET
  - Imaging
    - CT/MR: Fatty replacement of genioglossus-geniohyoid
- **Dermoid and Epidermoid Cysts, Sublingual Space**
  - Key facts: Tissue rests in SLS
    - Epidermoid (ectoderm only) vs. dermoid (ectoderm and mesoderm) contents
  - Imaging (CT/MR)
    - Epidermoid: Fluid density/intensity; DWI restriction, high signal
    - Dermoid: Mixed density/intensity; fatty or calcified elements possible
- **Venous Malformation, Sublingual Space**
  - Key facts: Poorly circumscribed dilated venous channels, transspatial
    - Slow flow; invisible on angiography
    - No enlarged feeding arteries
  - Imaging: Transspatial variably enhancing lesion and phleboliths
- **Lymphatic Malformation, Sublingual Space**
  - Key facts: Varied spectrum of dilated lymphatic spaces
    - Presentation: Pediatric to early adult
  - Imaging (CT/MR)
    - Cystic nonenhancing lesion with imperceptible walls
    - Multilocular; often transspatial
    - Fluid-fluid levels possible
    - No mass effect when small

Helpful Clues for Rare Diagnoses

- **Carcinoma, Sublingual Gland**
  - Key facts: SLG masses 90% malignant
    - Most commonly adenoid cystic, mucoepidermoid, or acinic cell carcinoma
  - Imaging (CT/MR)
    - Invasive SLS mass with heterogeneous density/intensity
    - Variable enhancement
    - 5- to 10-year follow-up; late recurrence
- **Benign Mixed Tumor, Sublingual Gland**
  - Key facts
    - Synonym: Pleomorphic adenoma
    - Arises from ductal components of SLG or minor salivary gland within SLS
  - Imaging (CT/MR)
    - Well-circumscribed SLS lesion with homogeneous enhancement
    - MR: T2/STIR high signal

Alternative Differential Approaches

- Imaging appearance
  - Transspatial lesions: Lymphatic and venous malformations
  - Cystic lesions: Ranula, sialocele, lymphatic malformation, epidermoid, dermoid
  - Solid lesions: Sialadenitis, SCCa, benign mixed tumor, tongue atrophy

SELECTED REFERENCES

1. Agarwal AK et al: Submandibular and sublingual spaces: diagnostic imaging and evaluation. Otolaryngol Clin North Am. 45(6):1311-23, 2012
2. Gadodia A et al: MR sialography of iatrogenic sialocele: comparison with conventional sialography. Dentomaxillofac Radiol. 40(3):147-53, 2011
3. La'porte SJ et al: Imaging the floor of the mouth and the sublingual space. Radiographics. 31(5):1215-30, 2011
4. Jain P: High resolution sonography of sublingual space. J Med Imaging Radiat Oncol. 52(2):101-8, 2008
5. Yu T et al: Malignant sublingual gland tumors: a retrospective clinicopathologic study of 28 cases. Oncology. 72(1-2):39-44, 2007
6. De Ponte FS et al: Sublingual epidermoid cyst. J Craniofac Surg. 13(2):308-10, 2002

Simple Ranula

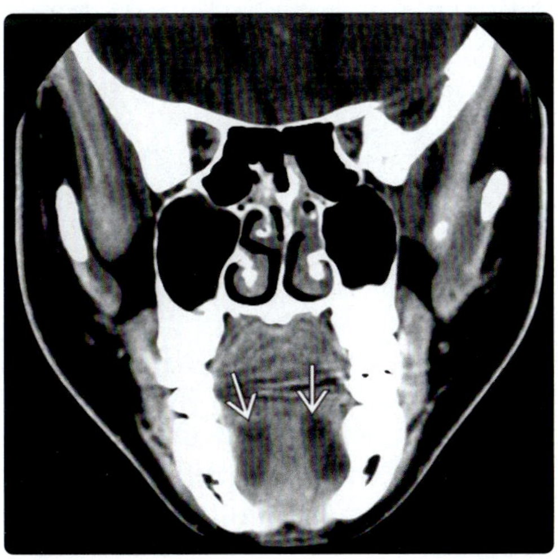

Abscess, Sublingual Space

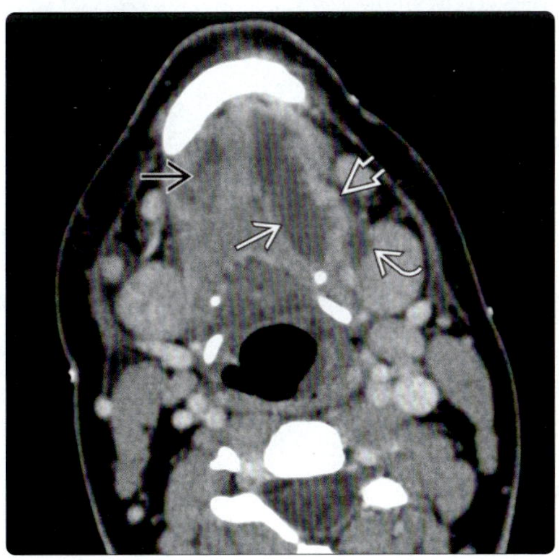

(Left) *Coronal CECT shows a simple ranula involving SLS on both sides ➡. A simple ranula is an epithelial-lined retention cyst of the SLG. This simple ranula extends into the SMS. In this case, the cyst must be clinically differentiated from a floor of mouth abscess.* **(Right)** *Axial CECT shows a predominantly SLS abscess ➡ secondary to an infected molar. A smaller, deep SMS abscess ➡ is seen as pus escapes the SLS posterior to the mylohyoid muscle ➡. A small contralateral anterior SLS abscess ➡ is also present.*

Dilated Wharton Duct

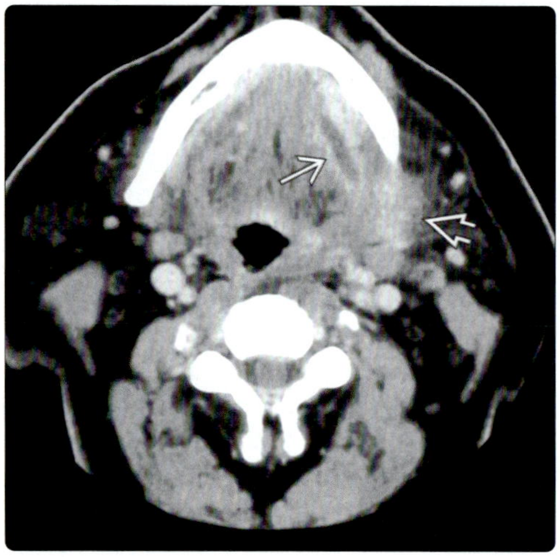

Squamous Cell Carcinoma, Floor of Mouth

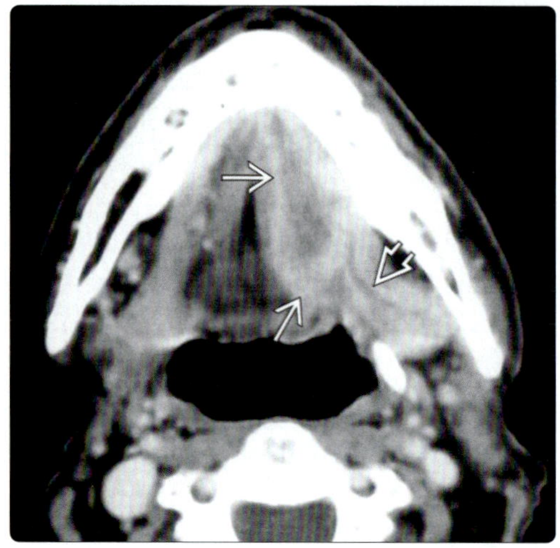

(Left) *Axial CECT reveals an enlarged SMG duct ➡ secondary to a calculus (not shown) with associated SMG postobstructive sialadenitis ➡.* **(Right)** *Axial CECT reveals extensive invasion of the left SLS by squamous cell carcinoma ➡ in the left floor of the mouth. The submandibular duct ➡ is obstructed by the tumor with enlargement and secondary submandibular sialadenitis visible.*

Squamous Cell Carcinoma, Oral Tongue, Invasive

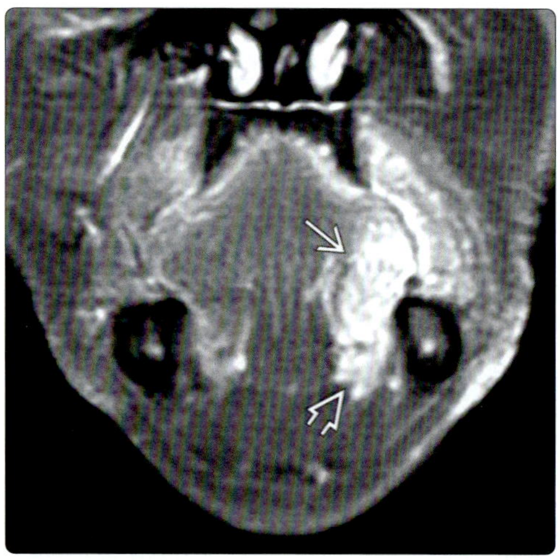

Sialadenitis, Sublingual Gland

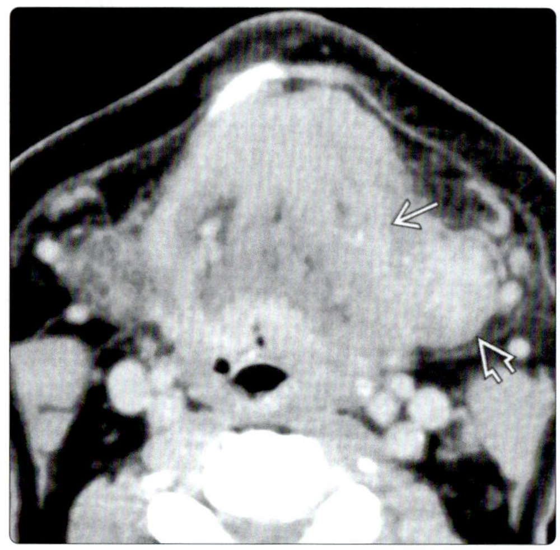

(Left) *Coronal T1 C+ FS MR demonstrates an enhancing squamous cell carcinoma primary tumor extending inferiorly from the lateral oral tongue ➡ into the SLS ➡.* **(Right)** *Axial CECT shows enlarged, enhancing left submandibular ➡ and sublingual ➡ glands secondary to the SMG duct obstruction (not seen). Note loss of distinction of normal SLS fat separating the genioglossus-geniohyoid from SLG secondary to inflammatory stranding.*

Acute Radiation Changes, Sublingual Gland

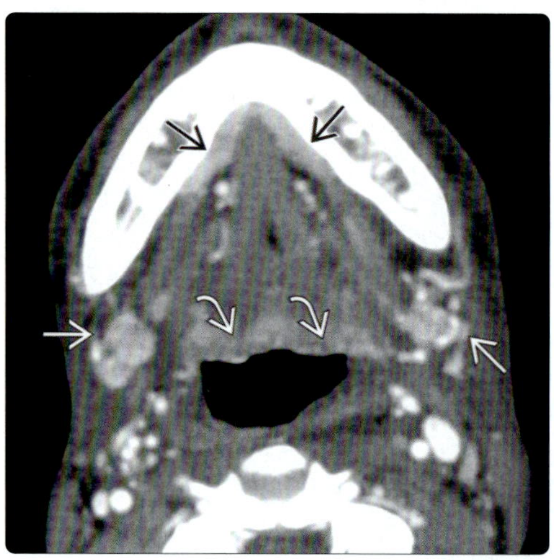

Sublingual Space Sialocele

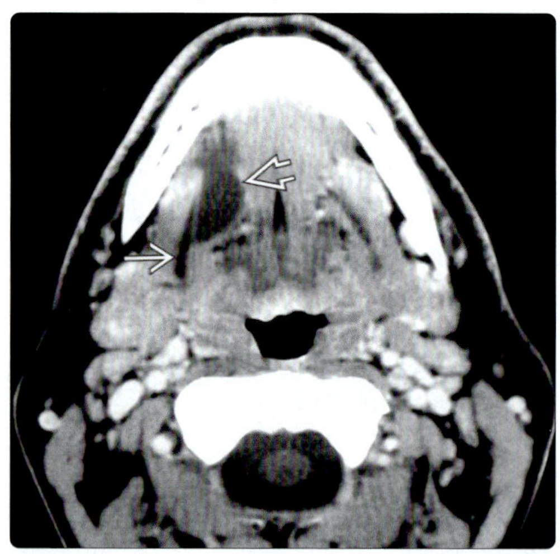

(Left) *Axial CECT reveals enhancing SLGs ➡, SMGs ➡, and lingual tonsils ➡. Note the diffuse stranding of the subcutaneous fat.* **(Right)** *Axial CECT reveals a dilated Wharton duct ➡ secondary to a distal ductal stenosis. Larger fluid density within the right SLS ➡ represents a resultant "false sialocele" from a Wharton duct rupture and extravasated saliva contained within a fibrous pseudocapsule.*

Hypoglossal Nerve Atrophy

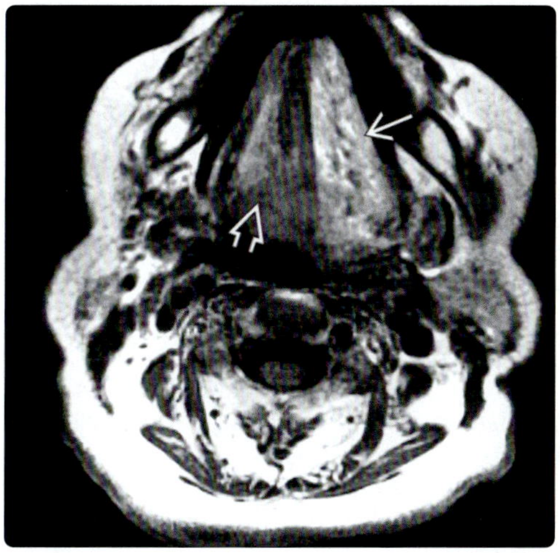

Dermoid and Epidermoid Cysts, Sublingual Space

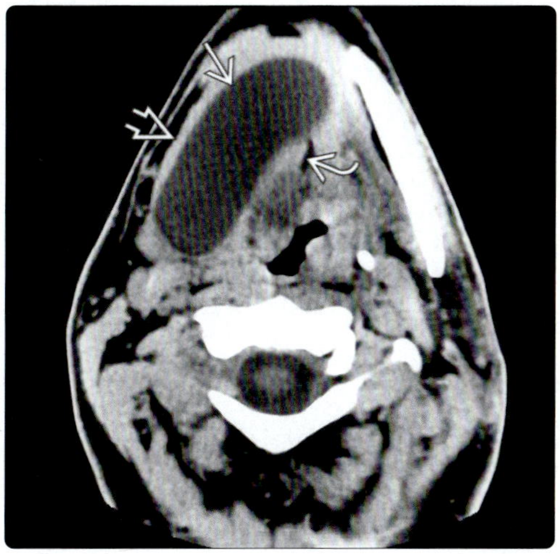

(Left) *Axial T1WI MR shows atrophy and fatty replacement of the left hyoglossus and genioglossus/geniohyoid musculature →. Note mild hypertrophy of the contralateral root of the tongue musculature →.* **(Right)** *Axial NECT shows a well-defined, homogeneous, low-density mass within the right SLS →. The mass bows the mylohyoid muscle laterally → and genioglossus muscle medially →. This is a classic presentation of an epidermoid cyst. Note the lack of internal calcification or fat consistent with this epidermoid.*

Venous Malformation, Sublingual Space

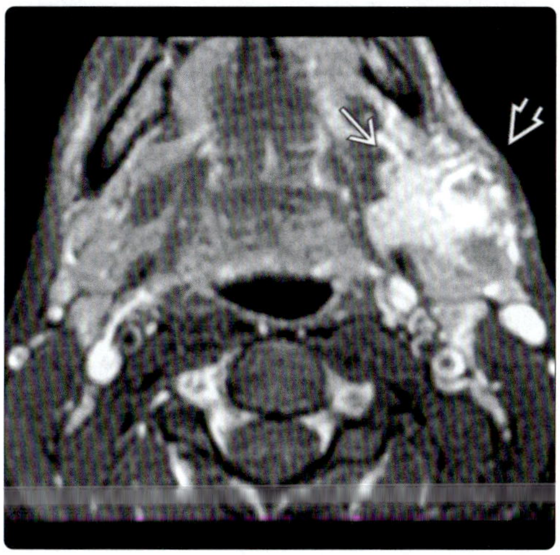

Lymphatic Malformation, Sublingual Space

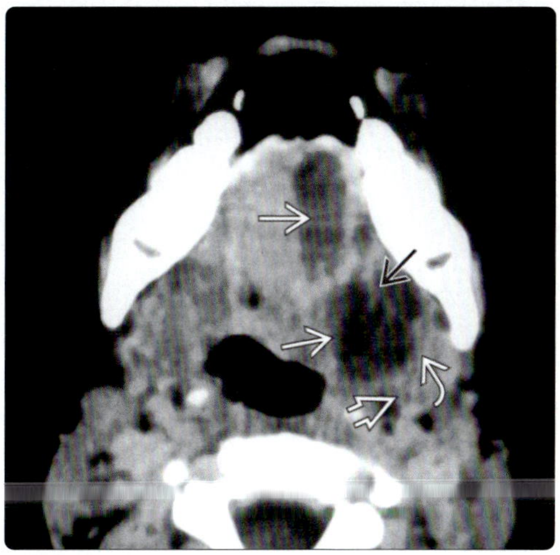

(Left) *Axial T1 C+ FS MR shows an enhancing transspatial venous malformation that involves both the sublingual → and submandibular → spaces.* **(Right)** *Axial CECT in a child shows typical lymphatic malformation appearing as a well-defined, lobulated, low-density mass within the left SLS → extending posteriorly into the SMS →. The mass displaces the left SMG posteriorly →. Fine septations are also identified within the lesion →.*

Carcinoma, Sublingual Gland

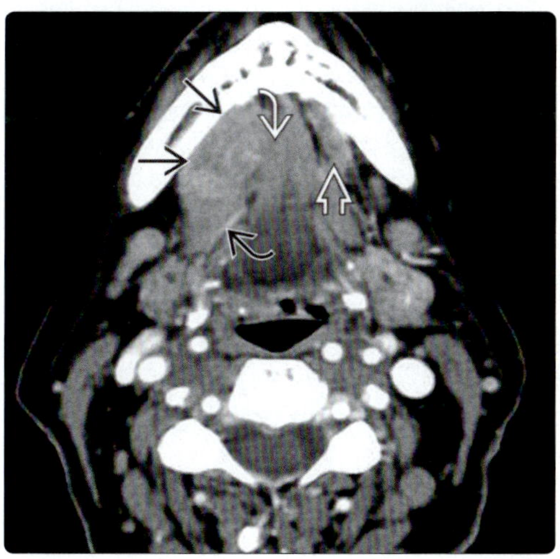

Benign Mixed Tumor, Sublingual Gland

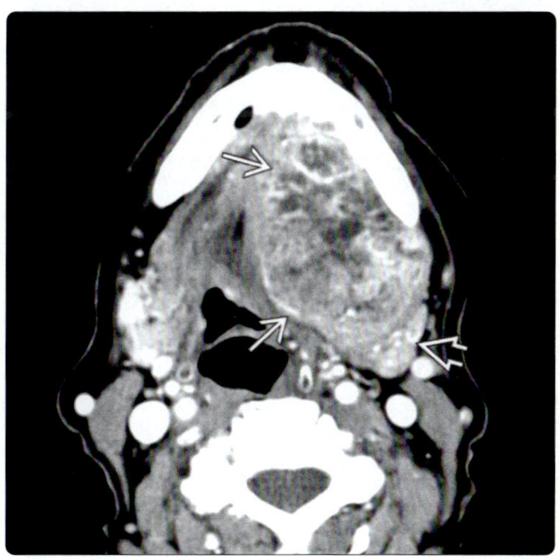

(Left) *Axial CECT shows a heterogeneous mass on the right side →. This infiltrative mass replaces the SLG but also spreads to the adjacent genioglossus muscle → and neurovascular bundle →. The normal left SLG → is clearly defined. At resection, this was adenoid cystic carcinoma.* **(Right)** *Axial CECT demonstrates a large heterogeneous mass in the left SLS → that displaces the SMG posterolaterally →. The mylohyoid muscle is hard to see laterally as it has been thinned over many years.*

DIFFERENTIAL DIAGNOSIS

Common

- Oral Tongue SCCa
- Floor of Mouth SCCa
- Retromolar Trigone SCCa
- Gingival SCCa
- Buccal Mucosa SCCa
- Denture Adhesive

Less Common

- Palatal Torus
- Mandibular Torus
- Buccal and Palatal Exostoses
- Minor Salivary Gland Malignancy, Oral
- Benign Mixed Tumor, Oral

Rare but Important

- Hard Palate SCCa
- Radiation Mucositis

ESSENTIAL INFORMATION

Key Differential Diagnosis Issues

- **Boundaries of oral mucosal space (OMS)**
  - Mucosal lining of entire oral cavity, including buccal, gingival, palatal, and lingual surfaces
  - Anterior: Skin/vermilion junction of lips
  - Posterosuperior: Junction of hard and soft palate
  - Posteroinferior: Junction of anterior 2/3 of tongue and posterior 1/3 of tongue at circumvallate papillae
  - Lateral: Cheeks
- **Patient signs & symptoms**
  - "Sore," ulceration, &/or swelling in mouth
  - Boring pain (bone involvement)
  - Dysesthesias (perineural tumor)
- **Imaging recommendations**
  - OMS lesions are usually clinically known and imaging is objectively ordered to assess mass size, deep tissue extent, and nodal involvement
  - Best work-up: MR for primary tumor; CECT for nodal disease
    - Imaging primarily used for deep tongue & bone invasion + nodal metastases
    - CECT: Dental metallic artifact may obscure primary tumor; better than MR for detecting metastatic lymph nodes
    - MR: Best for interface between tumor & normal tissue
  - Oral cavity SCCa subsites (nearby locations with different treatment and prognosis)
    - SCCa of oral tongue, floor of mouth (FOM), buccal mucosa surgically treated with wide resection
    - SCCa of retromolar trigone, alveolar ridge, hard palate treated with composite resection (bone resection in addition to soft tissues & mucosal surface)
  - Imaging must stage primary and nodes
    - Usually in levels IA, IB, and IIA/B

Helpful Clues for Common Diagnoses

- **Oral Tongue SCCa**
  - Key facts: Most common oral cavity SCCa
    - Lateral tongue subsite most common
    - Management of small lesion is resection
    - Management of lesions > 2 mm deep to mucosal surface is neck dissection
  - Imaging: Enhancing mass on oral tongue
    - Depth of extension to other subsites important
    - Small/superficial lesions difficult to detect on imaging
    - Staging MR is best study for larger lesions (> 3 cm) that require more extensive surgery
- **Floor of Mouth SCCa**
  - Key facts: Mucosa-covered space over mylohyoid & hyoglossus muscles
    - Undersurface of tongue, extending to anterior tonsillar pillar
    - Hyoglossus muscle in sublingual portion of FOM important landmark marking neurovascular bundle (CNXII)
  - Imaging: Note size & extent of tumor
    - Assess lingual mandible cortex erosion & determine if tumor crosses lingual septum
    - Involvement of neurovascular bundle affects surgical approach; check for tumor adjacent to hyoglossus muscle
- **Retromolar Trigone SCCa**
  - Key facts: Small, triangular area distal to mandibular 3rd molars
    - Rapid spread with multiple potential sites/routes
    - Pterygomandibular raphe spread reaches hamulus of medial pterygoid plate
  - Imaging: Note size & extent of tumor
    - Assess spread anteriorly along mandibular alveolar ridge, laterally to buccal sulcus, medially to lingual sulcus, & to FOM
    - Look for posterior extension to anterior tonsillar pillar, superior extension to pterygoid plates or buccal space
    - Bone windows may show buccal or lingual mandibular invasion, erosion of pterygoid plates, maxillary tuberosity, or posterior maxillary sinus wall
- **Gingival SCCa**
  - Key facts: Invasive malignant neoplasm of squamous epithelium arising in gingiva
    - Nonhealing, painless gingival ulcer
    - No image findings if confined to gingiva
  - Imaging: Best to assess mandible or maxilla bone invasion
    - Widened periodontal ligament space; discontinuous lamina dura
    - May progress to floating tooth appearance with DDx of malignancy/inflammatory lesion/Langerhans cell histiocytosis
    - Simultaneous nodal metastasis assessment done at time of imaging; nodal metastasis ↓ survival by 50%
- **Buccal Mucosa SCCa**
  - Key facts: Tobacco/alcohol use are risk factors for all oral cavity SCCa
    - Betel nut chewing (popular in South Africa & Asia) predisposes to buccal SCCa
  - Imaging: May be hard to visualize on CECT because of dental metallic artifact
    - Assess extension to buccinator muscle, subcutaneous fat, skin
    - Check for posterior spread into buccal space

- **Denture Adhesive**
  - Key facts: Patient should always remove dentures prior to CECT to avoid this artifact
  - Imaging: Denture adhesive is seen as high-density, thin symmetric line along alveolar ridge mucosa
    - Assure all denture adhesive is removed from mucosa, as residual material may be visualized

Helpful Clues for Less Common Diagnoses

- **Palatal Torus**
  - Key facts: Incidental hard midline submucosal mass on hard palate
  - Imaging: Midline lobulated cortical & subcortical bone thickening on oral surface of hard palate
- **Mandibular Torus**
  - Key facts: Incidental hard submucosal mass on lingual surface of mandible
    - Typical location is in canine/premolar area
    - If located more posteriorly or on buccal surface, more commonly referred to as exostosis
    - Typically bilateral, can occur unilaterally
  - Imaging: Lobulated cortical bone thickening, uni- or bilateral, on lingual mandibular cortex
- **Buccal and Palatal Exostoses**
  - Key facts: Incidental hard submucosal mass on buccal or palatal/lingual surface of maxillary alveolar processes
    - Maxilla > mandible; posterior > anterior
  - Imaging: Lobulated cortical bone on buccal or palatal/lingual cortex of maxilla or mandible; may be multiple
- **Minor Salivary Gland Malignancy, Oral**
  - Key facts: 2nd most common primary oral cavity malignancy
    - Adenoid cystic carcinoma or mucoepidermoid carcinoma
    - Most common oral location is junction of hard and soft palates
  - Imaging: Submucosal, so imaging needed to stage tumor
    - Determine local extension, presence of perineural spread
    - Palate most common location; look for CNV-V2 branch tumor spread
    - CECT: Homogeneous enhancement
    - Bone CT/CBCT: Erosion of hard palate, enlargement of greater palatine foramen
    - T1WI MR: Similar signal intensity relative to muscle
    - T2WI MR: High signal intensity relative to muscle
    - T1WI C+ MR: Homogeneous enhancement; best to assess perineural spread (V2)
- **Benign Mixed Tumor, Oral**
  - Key facts: Most common location is submucosal at junction of hard and soft palates
  - Imaging: Smooth, well-defined, enhancing submucosal mass of hard palate
    - May also occur in sublingual space; rare in other oral cavity subsites
    - May pedunculate into airway if large

Helpful Clues for Rare Diagnoses

- **Hard Palate SCCa**
  - Key facts: Most rare oral cavity SCCa subsite
  - Imaging: Invasive hard palate mass with ill-defined margins
- **Radiation Mucositis**
  - Key facts: Acute-subacute radiation phase
  - Imaging: Diffuse mucosal enhancement

SELECTED REFERENCES

1. Law CP et al: Imaging the oral cavity: key concepts for the radiologist. Br J Radiol. 84(1006):944-57, 2011
2. Mosel D et al: Oral complications in the treatment of cancer patients. Oral Dis. Epub ahead of print, 2011
3. Park JO et al: Diagnostic accuracy of magnetic resonance imaging (MRI) in the assessment of tumor invasion depth in oral/oropharyngeal cancer. Oral Oncol. 47(5):381-6, 2011
4. Trotta BM et al: Oral cavity and oropharyngeal squamous cell cancer: key imaging findings for staging and treatment planning. Radiographics. 31(2):339-51, 2011
5. García-García AS et al: Current status of the torus palatinus and torus mandibularis. Med Oral Patol Oral Cir Bucal. 15(2):e353-60, 2010
6. Lalla RV et al: Management of oral mucositis in patients who have cancer. Dent Clin North Am. 52(1):61-77, viii, 2008
7. Pons Vicente O et al: Minor salivary gland tumors: A clinicopathological study of 18 cases. Med Oral Patol Oral Cir Bucal. 13(9):E582-8, 2008

Oral Tongue SCCa

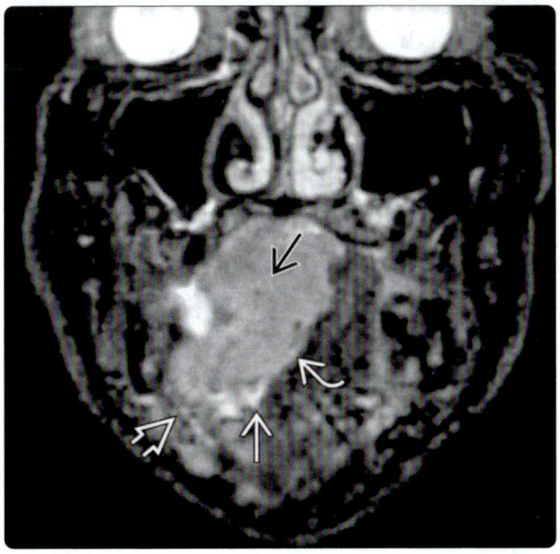

Oral Tongue SCCa

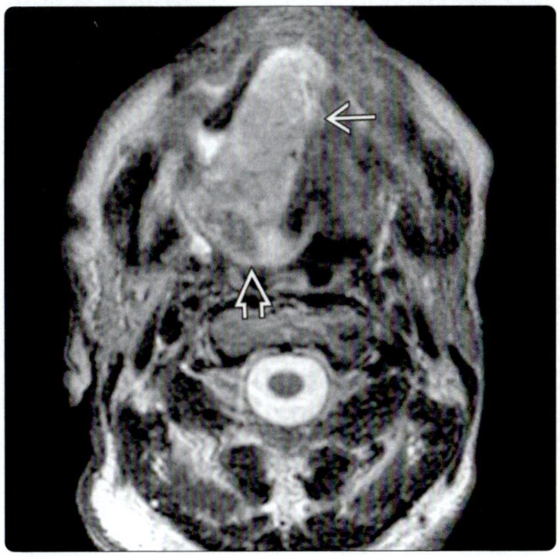

(Left) *Coronal T1WI MR of advanced T4 oral tongue squamous cell carcinoma (SCCa) shows the typical appearance of a large lesion of the right lateral portion of the tongue with extension into the adjacent sublingual space (SLS), genioglossus muscle, and mylohyoid muscle.* **(Right)** *Axial T2WI MR demonstrates a large right oral tongue SCCa, which crosses the midline and extends posterior to the base of the tongue/lingual tonsil area.*

(Left) *Axial CECT shows a poorly defined soft tissue mass involving the base of tongue and floor of mouth. Fatty infiltration of the right hemitongue is related to denervation atrophy; the denervated portion with decreased muscle tone bulges posteriorly into the oropharyngeal airway.* **(Right)** *Typical axial PET/CT fusion shows invasive retromolar trigone SCCa that spreads superiorly along the pterygomandibular raphe.*

Floor of Mouth SCCa

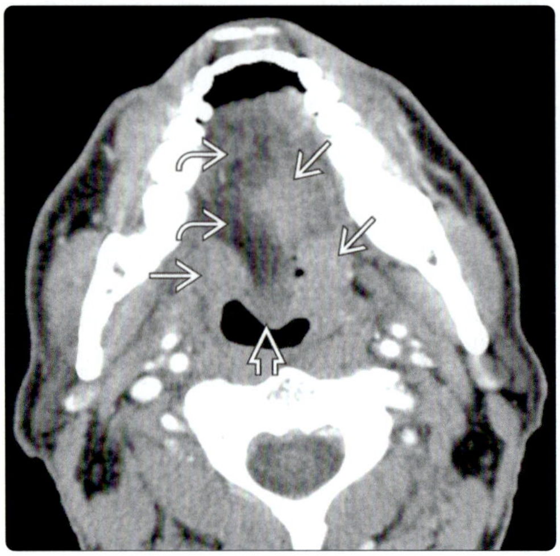

Retromolar Trigone SCCa

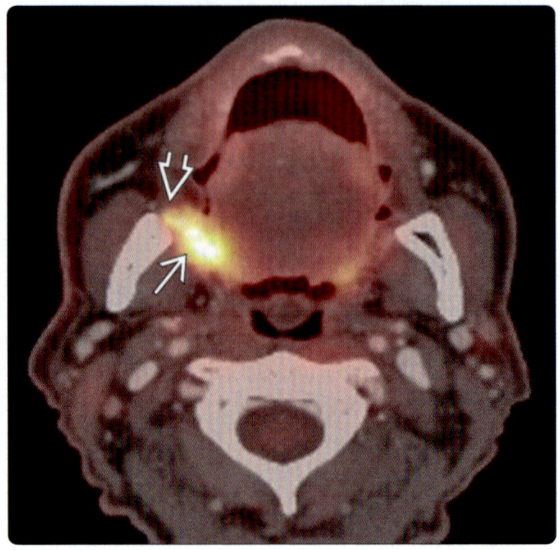

(Left) *Axial CBCT shows gingival SCCa invading the mandibular right alveolar ridge.* **(Right)** *Axial T1WI MR shows a small left buccal mucosa SCCa. Note the loss of fat beneath the buccinator muscle and erosion of the maxilla. The lesion is so subtle that it probably would have been missed if clinical examination results were not available.*

Gingival SCCa

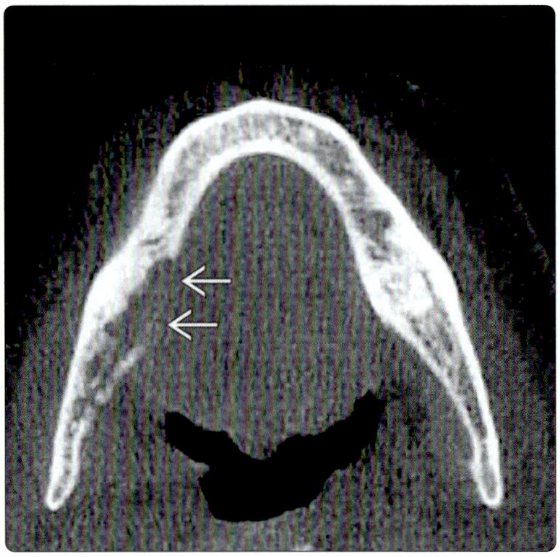

Buccal Mucosa SCCa

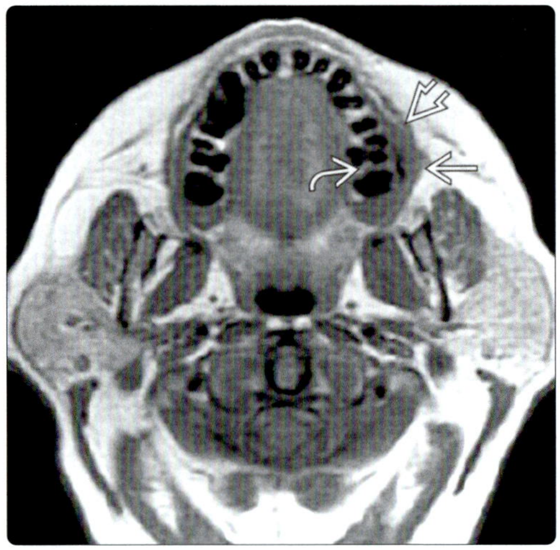

(Left) *Axial CECT shows a thin, straight line of high density on the buccal side of the sulcus in a patient who removed dentures prior to image acquisition; however, the denture adhesive was not adequately cleaned off.* **(Right)** *Panoramic radiograph shows palatal torus. Note periapical inflammatory lesion on endodontically treated right maxillary lateral incisor. Sclerotic bone of inflammatory origin is seen in the mandible.*

Denture Adhesive

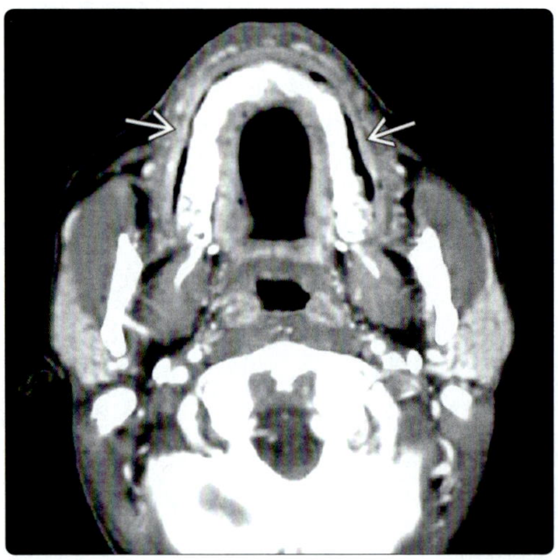

Palatal Torus

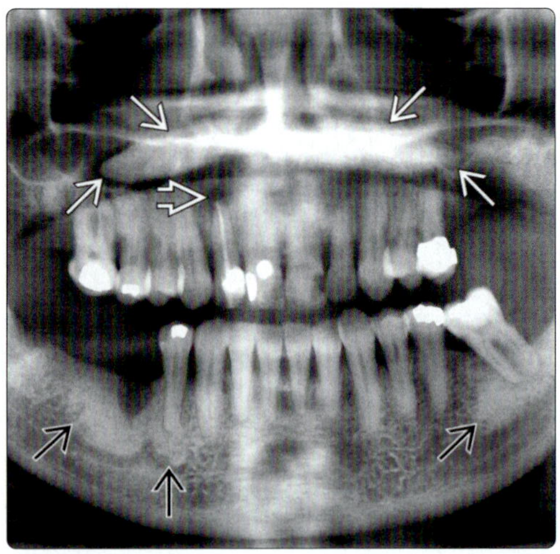

Thyroglossal Duct Cyst

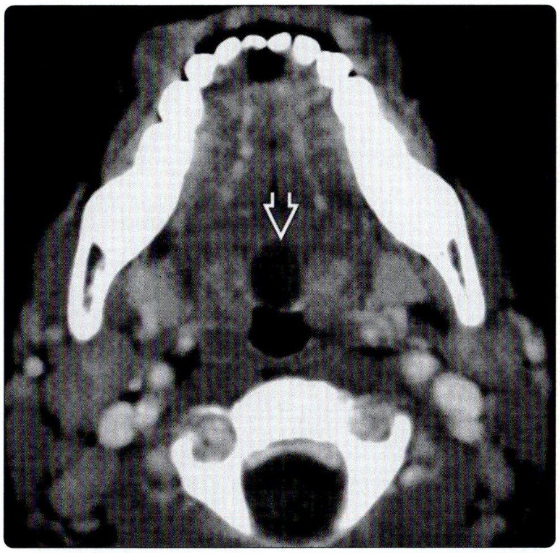

Thyroglossal Duct Cyst

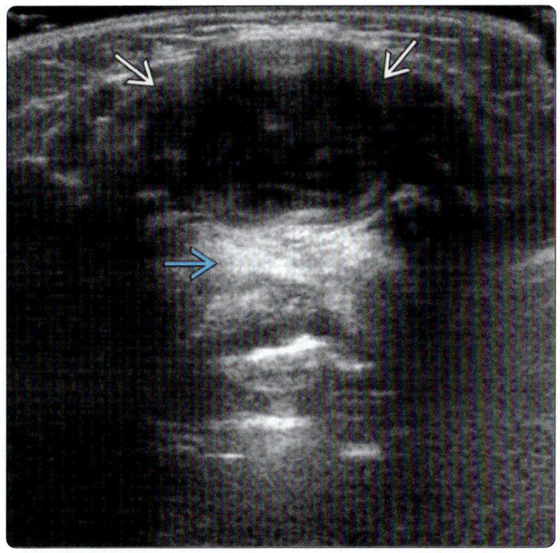

(Left) *Axial CECT shows a well-defined round, low attenuation, nonenhancing midline tongue base mass in the region of the foramen cecum →. This is typical CT appearance of thyroglossal duct cyst at the ROT.* **(Right)** *Sonographic image through the midline neck shows an ovoid, thick-walled, hypoechoic mass → with heterogeneous internal echotexture and posterior acoustic enhancement →. This presentation is compatible with thyroglossal duct cyst.*

Ectopic Thyroid

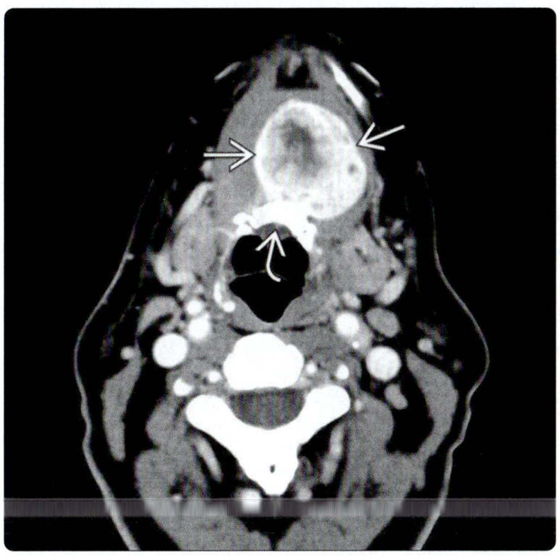

Lymphatic Malformation, Oral Cavity

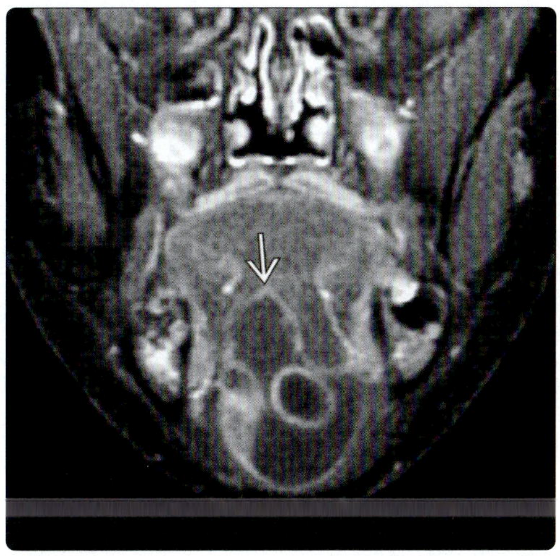

(Left) *Axial CECT demonstrates a heterogeneously enhancing mass centered near the ROT →, which extends inferiorly to the hyoid → into the infrahyoid neck.* **(Right)** *Coronal T1WI C+ FS MR reveals a complex root of tongue cystic mass → with enhancing septations. No significant enhancement of the rest of the lesion was present after the administration of contrast.*

Venous Malformation

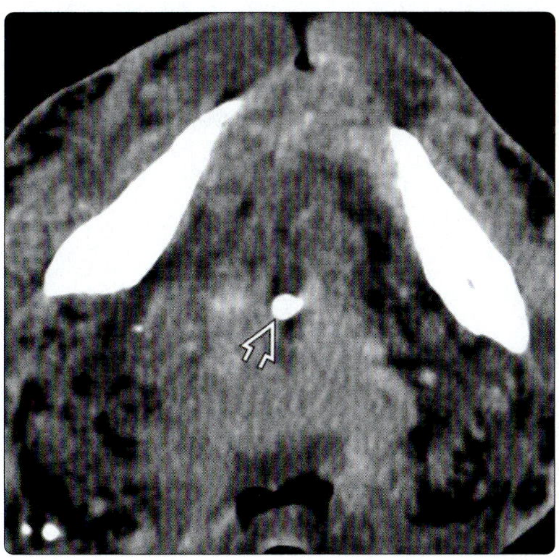

Foregut Duplication Cyst, Tongue

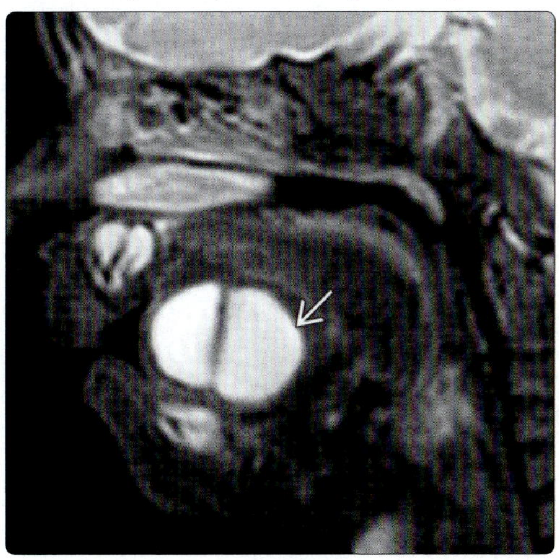

(Left) *Axial NECT shows a trans-spatial venous malformation involving the sublingual & submandibular spaces bilaterally. A lingual septum phlebolith → indicates involvement of the root of tongue.* **(Right)** *Sagittal T2WI FS MR shows a septated foregut duplication cyst → located in the root of tongue. The homogeneously thick wall may suggest the differentiation from other ROT cystic lesions, such as an epidermoid cyst or a thyroglossal duct cyst.*

DIFFERENTIAL DIAGNOSIS

Common

- Calcified Stylohyoid Ligament
- Calcified Triticeous Cartilage
- Calcified Thyroid Cartilage

Less Common

- Calcified Lymph Node
- Sialolith
- Antrolith
- Tonsillolith
- Rhinolith
- Atherosclerosis, Carotid Artery, Neck
- Ossified Spinal Ligaments

Rare but Important

- Arteriosclerosis
- Phlebolith
- Myositis Ossificans
- Calcinosis Cutis

ESSENTIAL INFORMATION

Key Differential Diagnosis Issues

- Calcified atherosclerosis must be differentiated from other calcifications due to serious nature of condition
- Calcified lymph nodes, sialoliths, and phleboliths often resemble each other radiographically

Helpful Clues for Common Diagnoses

- **Calcified Stylohyoid Ligament**
    - Key facts
        - Common incidental finding, innocuous unless symptomatic
        - Incidence ranges from 3-90% depending on population
        - When symptomatic, known as **Eagle syndrome**: Facial pain, otalgia, dysphagia, headache, vertigo
    - Imaging
        - Extension of styloid process (> 30 mm), may appear pseudoarticulated
        - Long, tapered, often with borders more radiopaque than interior
        - On axial CBCT view, seen as round radiopacities flanking oropharynx at level of C2-C4
        - On panoramic image, arises from region of mastoid and crosses posterior-inferior aspect of ramus
- **Calcified Triticeous Cartilage**
    - Key facts
        - Triticeous cartilage located centrally in lateral thyrohyoid ligament
        - At level of C3-C4; superior to superior cornua of thyroid cartilage
    - Imaging
        - Well-defined border with smooth outline
        - **Oval or round** appearance: Morphology helps differentiate from calcified carotid atheroma that most commonly appears on panoramic radiograph as **irregular linear** radiopacity
- **Calcified Thyroid Cartilage**
    - Key facts
        - Superior cornua of thyroid cartilage mineralize with age
        - Innocuous incidental finding
    - Imaging
        - Seen adjacent to pharyngeal airway, inferior to hyoid, and adjacent to C4
        - Smooth periphery, uniform radiopacity or may see outer shell only
        - Must be differentiated from calcified carotid atheroma

Helpful Clues for Less Common Diagnoses

- **Calcified Lymph Node**
    - Key facts
        - Result of chronic inflammation in node
        - Frequently seen in patients with tuberculosis, sarcoidosis, fungal infections, lymphoma treated with radiation therapy
        - Most common in submandibular and cervical nodes
    - Imaging
        - Irregular, **cauliflower-shaped** radiopacity
        - May be superimposed over mandibular body or ramus
- **Sialolith**
    - Key facts
        - Aggregation of mineralized material within salivary gland ducts or glandular tissue
        - Usually occurs singly but may be multiple, especially in parotid gland
        - Peak incidence between 4th and 6th decades
        - Submandibular gland (80%) > parotid gland (19%) > sublingual gland (1%)
        - May be asymptomatic or associated with swelling and pain
    - Imaging
        - Round, ovoid, or cylindrical radiopacity
        - Submandibular: Differentiate from calcified lymph node
        - Parotid: Differentiate from tonsilloliths
        - Localization enhanced with CBCT, occlusal images
- **Antrolith**
    - Key facts
        - Dystrophic calcification of chronically inflamed mucosa
        - Nidus may be endogenous foreign object (root tip, bone fragment)
    - Imaging
        - Small homogeneous radiopacity, some have radiopaque rim or shell
        - Seen on panoramic, periapical, or CBCT images
- **Tonsillolith**
    - Key facts
        - Mineralization of material in tonsillar crypts
        - Most frequent in palatine tonsils
        - Small calcifications usually asymptomatic
        - Larger calcification may cause pain, swelling, fever, fetid breath, dysphagia
    - Imaging
        - Small round radiopacities flanking oropharynx in axial CBCT
        - Superimposed over posterior midramus area in panoramic images

- **Rhinolith**
  - Key facts
    - Nidus for calcification often exogenous foreign object
  - Imaging
    - Variety of shapes
    - Homogeneous or heterogeneous radiopacity, depending on nidus
- **Atherosclerosis, Carotid Artery, Neck**
  - Key facts
    - Usually begins in bifurcation of carotid artery
    - Often affects > 1 vessel
    - **Patients should be referred to physician for cardiovascular/cerebrovascular evaluation**
  - Imaging
    - Panoramic image: Irregular, vertical, linear radiopacity near hyoid or epiglottis
    - Axial CBCT: Circular or semicircular ring of radiopacity in soft tissue at level of C3 or C4
- **Ossified Spinal Ligaments**
  - Key Facts
    - Distinct linear hyperdensities anterior or posterior to vertebrae
    - Associated with idiopathic skeletal hyperostosis (DISH), ankylosing spondylitis
  - Imaging
    - CT, CBCT of cervical spine
    - T2 MR for cord compression

Helpful Clues for Rare Diagnoses

- **Arteriosclerosis**
  - Key facts
    - Degeneration of elastic fibers in vessel wall
    - Intracranial lesions in patients with Sturge-Weber syndrome
    - Also seen in patients with hyperparathyroidism
  - Imaging
    - Parallel radiopaque outlines (pipe stem or railroad-track appearance)
    - Outlines may follow tortuous path, depending on course of vessel
- **Phlebolith**
  - Key facts
    - Calcified thrombi in veins, venules, sinusoidal vessels of hemangiomas (common)
  - Imaging
    - Round or oval radiopacity most often with smooth periphery, often mobile
    - May have lamellar or target-like appearance
- **Myositis Ossificans**
  - Key facts
    - Heterotopic bone within interstitial muscle, tendons, ligaments
    - Muscle atrophies secondary to formation, often related to trauma
    - Common in masseter, sternocleidomastoid, and lateral pterygoid muscles
  - Imaging
    - Radiopaque periphery with less radiopaque internal structure
    - Irregular, ovoid, linear streaks running in same direction as muscle fibers
- **Calcinosis Cutis**
  - Key facts
    - Soft tissue calcification in skin of scar or chronic inflammation
    - Secondary to chronic acne, also seen on tongue
  - Imaging
    - Smooth radiopacities from 0.1-0.5 cm in diameter
    - Common in cheeks, lips, chin

SELECTED REFERENCES

1. Hooker JD et al: Carotid stent fracture from stylocarotid syndrome. J Radiol Case Rep. 10(6):1-8, 2016
2. Mori K et al: Prevalence and distribution of ossification of the supra/interspinous ligaments in symptomatic patients with cervical ossification of the posterior longitudinal ligament of the spine: a CT-based multicenter cross-sectional study. BMC Musculoskelet Disord. 17(1):492, 2016
3. Nonin S et al: Plaque surface irregularity and calcification length within carotid plaque predict secondary events in patients with coronary artery disease. Atherosclerosis. 256:29-34, 2016

Calcified Stylohyoid Ligament

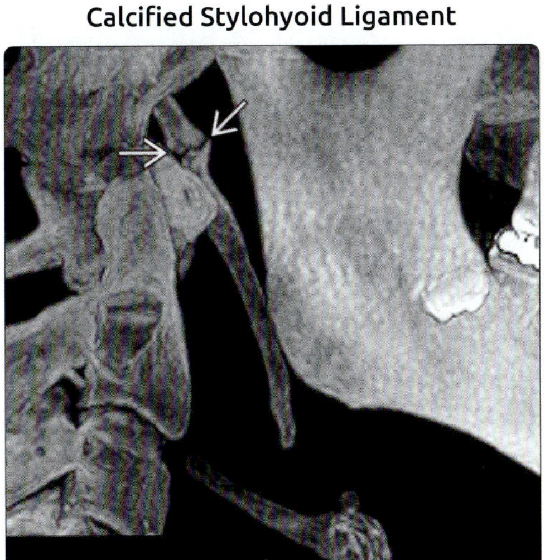

Calcified Stylohyoid Ligament

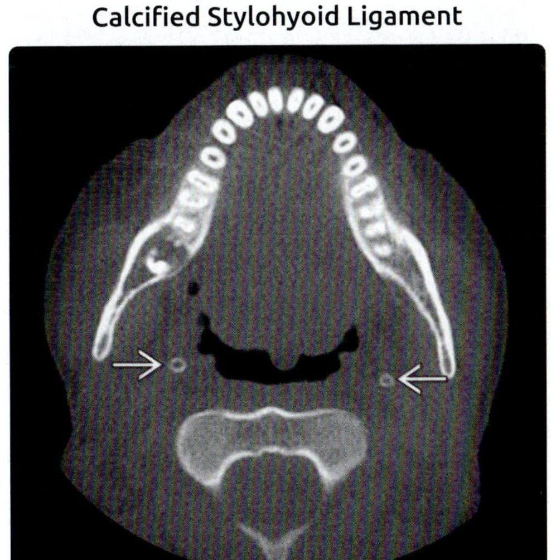

(Left) *Sagittal CBCT view shows an elongated styloid process with an area of pseudoarticulation →. The patient was asymptomatic and the finding was incidental. When symptomatic, e.g., pain or dysphagia, the condition is known as Eagle syndrome.* **(Right)** *Axial CBCT shows bilateral, round, ring-like radiopacities → that represent calcification in the stylohyoid ligament or an elongated process. Note the periphery is more calcified than the interior.*

Calcified Triticeous Cartilage

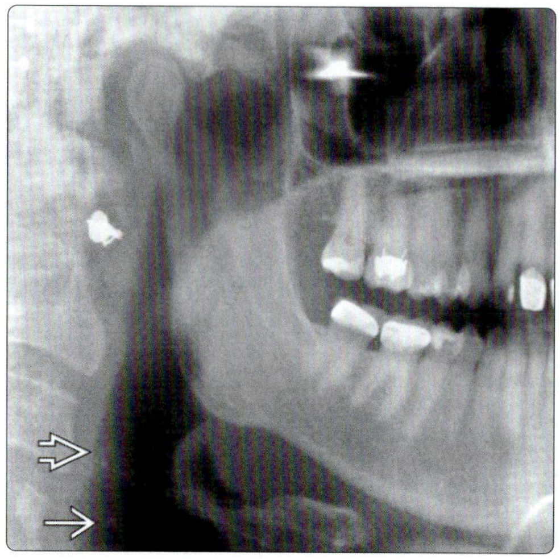

Calcified Thyroid Cartilage

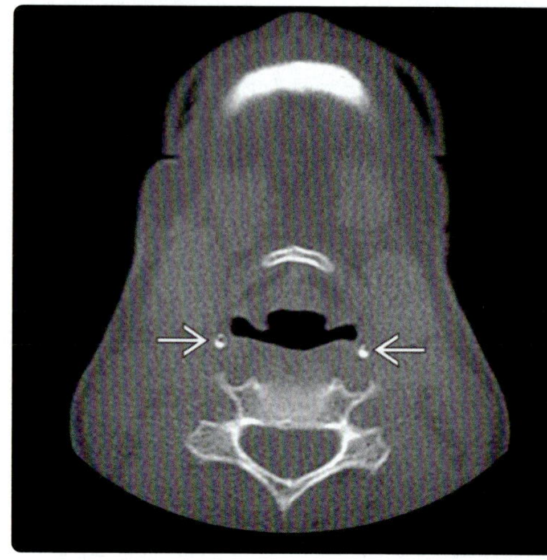

(Left) *Panoramic radiograph shows a calcified triticeous cartilage* ➔ *inferior to the greater cornu* ➔ *of the hyoid bone. Triticeous means grain of wheat. When calcified, the cartilage appears as a small, round or oval radiopacity differentiating it from carotid atheroma, which appears irregularly linear.* **(Right)** *Axial CBCT shows 2 round radiopacities* ➔ *flanking the oropharynx representing calcification of the superior cornua of the thyroid cartilage. These must be differentiated from calcified atheromas.*

Calcified Lymph Node

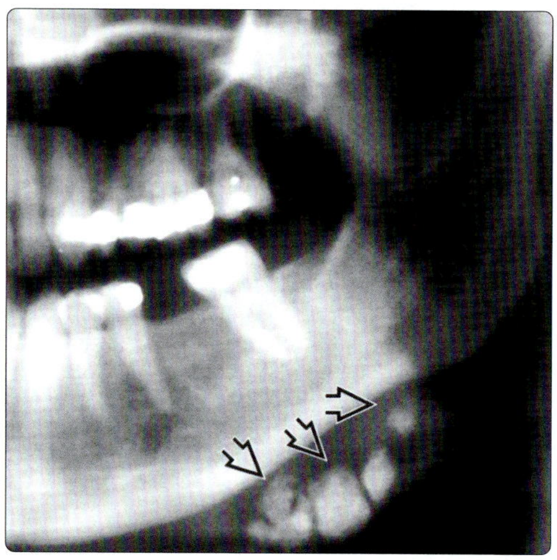

Sialolith

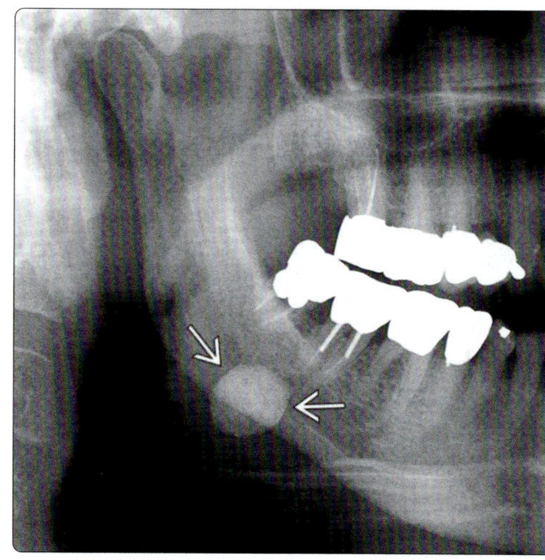

(Left) *Cropped panoramic radiograph shows multiple irregular, cauliflower-like radiopacities* ⇨ *inferior to the left mandible. Note the irregular outline compared to a submandibular sialolith. These calcified submandibular nodes were clinically palpable.* **(Right)** *Panoramic radiograph shows large radiopacity* ➔ *located over the inferior border of the mandible just anterior to the angle. Differential includes a calcified lymph node; however, smooth border favors submandibular sialolith.*

Sialolith

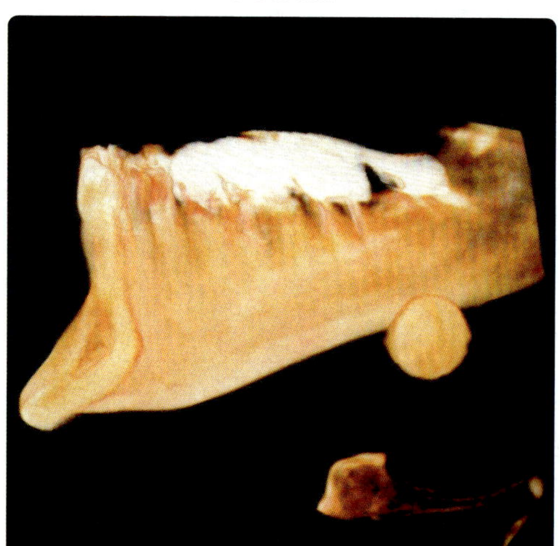

Antrolith

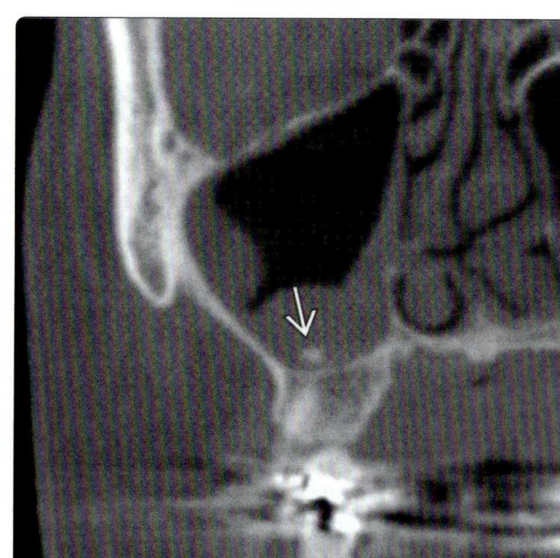

(Left) *Sagittal reformat CBCT of the right mandible, viewed from the medial aspect in the same patient, shows the radiopacity is located lingual to the mandibular ramus in the submandibular gland area.* **(Right)** *Coronal CBCT exhibits oval opacification in the mucoperiosteum of the right maxillary sinus* ➔*. It is important to differentiate opacities associated with inflammatory sinusitis from fungal sinusitis. Fungal sinusitis typically exhibits finer, punctate calcifications.*

Tonsillolith

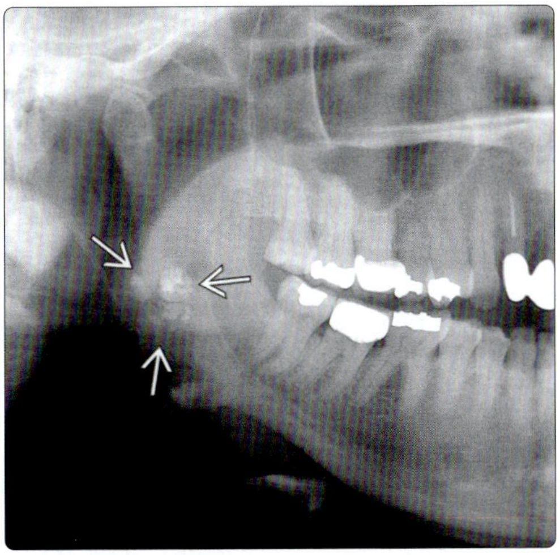

Atherosclerosis, Carotid Artery, Neck

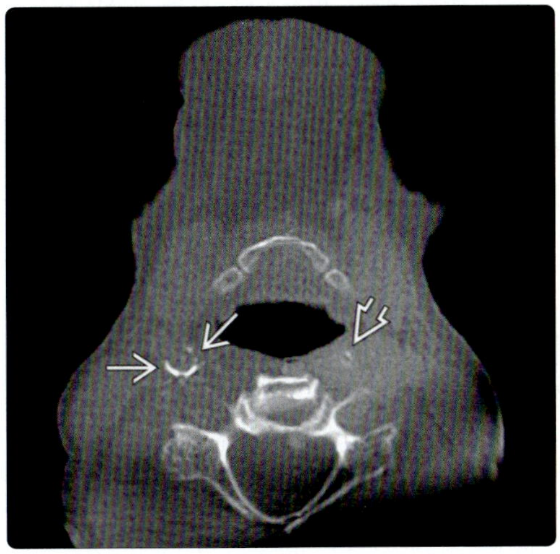

(Left) *Panoramic radiograph shows multiple radiopacities* ➡ *superimposed over the right ramus. Parotid calcifications are in the differential but more likely to ghost in panoramic imaging. Axial CBCT images proved these radiopacities to be palatine tonsilloliths.* **(Right)** *Axial CBCT view shows a circular radiopacity indicating calcification in a vessel wall* ➡ *(right carotid artery). Note smaller, more medial circular calcification on the left* ⇨*, which represents calcified superior cornu of thyroid cartilage.*

Ossified Spinal Ligaments

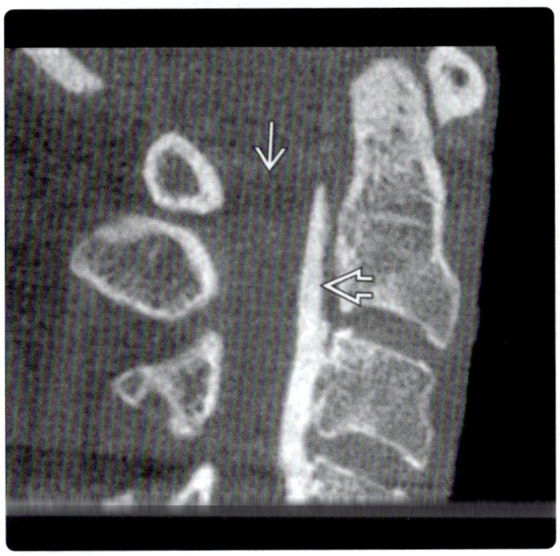

Arteriosclerosis

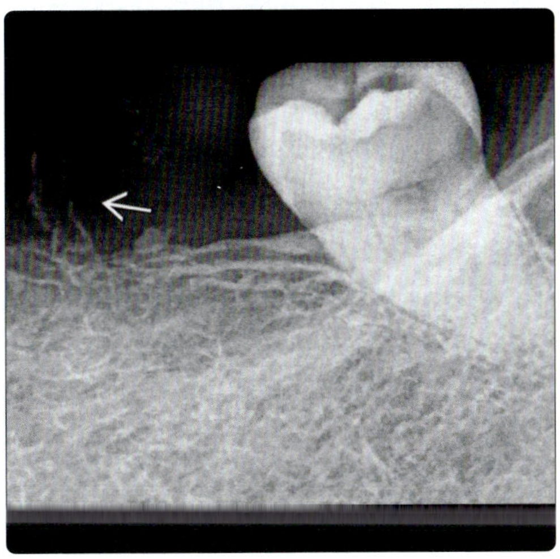

(Left) *Sagittal CBCT of a patient complaining of mild numbness in her arms shows a linear hyperdensity on the dorsal side of the bodies of C2, C3, and C4* ⇨ *with narrowing of the spinal canal* ➡*. This is an ossified posterior longitudinal ligament.* **(Right)** *Intraoral periapical image of an 85-year-old woman shows indistinct parallel linear opacities extending superior to the alveolar ridge and then curving* ➡*. This is a calcified facial artery.*

Phlebolith

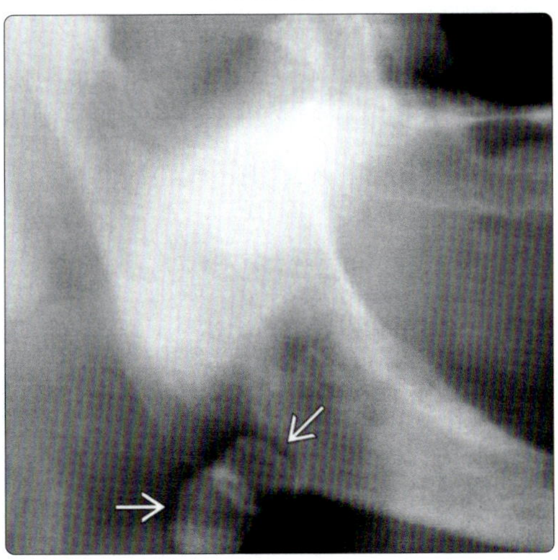

Calcinosis Cutis

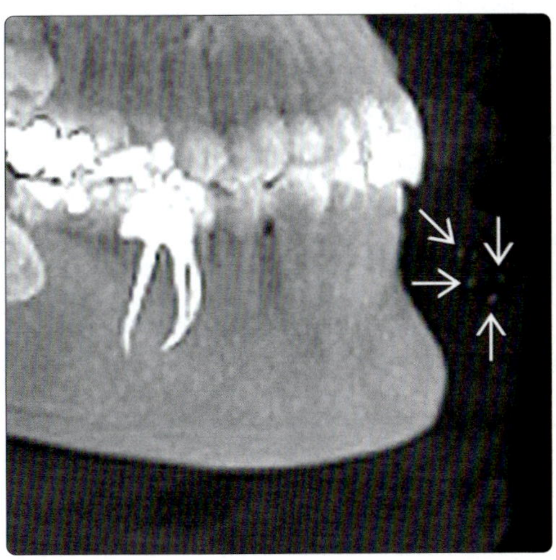

(Left) *Cropped panoramic radiograph shows 2 round radiopacities* ➡ *with target-like lamellae, which is a typical presentation for phleboliths. This patient had a soft tissue hemangioma, which is often associated with phleboliths.* **(Right)** *Sagittal reformat (lateral cephalometric) CBCT shows several small, punctate radiopacities* ➡ *in the soft tissue of the patient's chin. These represent calcifications in acne scars.*

PART III
SECTION 4

Temporomandibular Joint

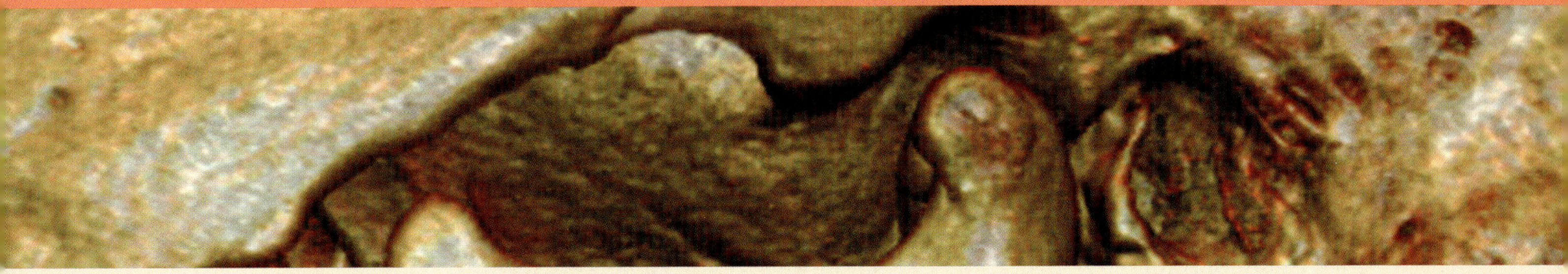

Changes in Condylar Size and Function

Small Condyle 940
Large Condyle 946
Limited Condylar Translation 950

Mass Lesions

TMJ Radiolucencies 954
TMJ Radiopacities 956

Miscellaneous

TMJ Articular Loose Bodies 960

DIFFERENTIAL DIAGNOSIS

Common

- Degenerative Joint Disease (Adult)
- Progressive Condylar Resorption
- Regressive Remodeling
- Condylar Hypoplasia
- Condylar Fracture

Less Common

- Rheumatoid Arthritis
- Juvenile Idiopathic Arthritis
- Hemifacial Microsomia

Rare but Important

- Chondrosarcoma
- Metastatic Disease

ESSENTIAL INFORMATION

Key Differential Diagnosis Issues

- Determine whether condylar morphology is normal or whether there are other osseous abnormalities in condyle or temporal component of joint
  - Check ipsilateral mandible, midface, and skull for signs of **impaired growth**
  - Abnormal condylar morphology may be associated with arthritic condition or indicate fracture
    - Check entire mediolateral dimension of joint since "abnormal condyle" seen in one CT slice may represent ramus stump, and condyle may be medially &/or anteriorly displaced
- Erosions and osteophyte formation suggest **arthritis** but may be **secondary** to other predisposing abnormality
- Must differentiate erosions and loss of condylar volume in arthritis from **malignant** process destroying condylar bone
  - Malignancy has **permeative** appearance and is often associated with **periosteal reaction**
- Joint space usually **normal** unless primary or secondary degenerative joint disease or other arthritis

Helpful Clues for Common Diagnoses

- **Degenerative Joint Disease (Adult)**
  - Key facts
    - Localized, noninflammatory degenerative disorder of synovial joints characterized by destruction and repair of articular fibrocartilage and underlying subchondral bone
  - Imaging
    - Reduction in condylar size from **superior surface** ± evidence of sclerosis, flattening, erosions, osteophytes, and subchondral bone cyst, joint space narrowing, disc displacement
    - Starts as focal defect in articular soft tissues and subjacent bone; may enlarge to involve entire condyle
    - Progressive vertical loss of condylar height resulting in decreased condylar size
    - **Narrowed** joint space due to disc displacement or perforation
- **Progressive Condylar Resorption**
  - Key facts
    - Localized, noninflammatory degenerative disorder of TMJs characterized by lysis and repair of articular fibrocartilage and underlying subchondral bone following onset of **puberty** in **females**
    - Limited jaw development on ipsilateral side
    - Closely follows onset of puberty; rare after age 20 compared with degenerative joint disease, which develops later
  - Imaging
    - Unilateral but often bilateral resorption of superior aspects of condyles, resulting in decreased condylar size
    - Occasionally affects articular eminence: Initiates as focal defect with loss of articular soft tissue and subjacent bone
- **Regressive Remodeling**
  - Key facts
    - Remodeling of condyle that may precede degenerative changes
  - Imaging
    - Thinning of anteroposterior dimension of condyle **without** reduction of condylar height
    - Condyle is usually posteriorly positioned in fossa
- **Condylar Hypoplasia**
  - Key facts
    - Developmental abnormality resulting in abnormally small condyle with underdevelopment of ipsilateral ramus and mandibular body
    - Degree of asymmetry worse if affected at young age
    - Unilateral more common than bilateral
    - Degenerative joint disease often long-term sequela
  - Imaging
    - Small condyle with **normal shape and structure**
    - Mandibular fossa small
    - Condyle and neck are proportionately small, therefore neck will not be elongated or relatively slender
    - Normal joint space
- **Condylar Fracture**
  - Key facts
    - Usually occurs at condylar neck; often accompanied by dislocation of condyle
    - Unilateral or bilateral
    - Fracture at young age results in mandibular hypoplasia on affected side with deviation of mandible due to damage to condylar growth center
  - Imaging
    - Condylar angle altered or condyle displaced from normal position
    - Fractured condyle often anteromedially displaced and remaining **ramus stump** may simulate abnormally small condyle
    - Degenerative joint disease may be long-term sequela

Helpful Clues for Less Common Diagnoses

- **Rheumatoid Arthritis**
  - Key facts
    - Chronic inflammatory disease manifesting as synovial membrane inflammation in several joints; characterized by progressive bony erosions and cartilage destruction
    - Preauricular swelling, pain, tenderness

- Bilateral and symmetrical involvement
  - Imaging
    - Condyle appears small due to erosion and flattening of anterior and posterior surfaces, giving **sharpened pencil** appearance
    - Erosions can destroy entire condyle and articular eminence
    - Generalized osteopenia of condyle and temporal component
    - Often secondary degenerative joint disease with narrowed joint space
- **Juvenile Idiopathic Arthritis**
  - Key facts
    - Autoimmune musculoskeletal inflammatory disease of childhood, which can also affect TMJs
    - Affected TMJs may be asymptomatic
    - Retrognathia, micrognathia, malocclusion, limited opening
  - Imaging
    - Condyles appear small, flat, and deformed with wide glenoid fossae
    - Condylar concavity or bifid appearance
    - Bilateral more common
    - May have secondary degenerative joint disease with joint space narrowing and osteophyte formation
- **Hemifacial Microsomia**
  - Key facts
    - Underdevelopment of mandibular condyle ranging from small condyle to condylar aplasia with reduced development of ipsilateral half of mandible
    - Facial asymmetry with chin deviation to affected side
    - May have associated ear abnormalities such as atresia, microtia, preauricular tags or pits
  - Imaging
    - Fossa development proportional to condylar development and function
    - Occlusal plane elevated on involved side ± cleft palate
    - Small malar bone and zygomatic arch; hypoplasia of mastoid process; orbit displaced laterally and inferiorly

Helpful Clues for Rare Diagnoses

- **Chondrosarcoma**
  - Key facts
    - Malignant tumor arising from cartilage cells
    - Preauricular swelling, mandibular deviation, pain, limited opening
  - Imaging
    - Condyle may appear small due to destruction by tumor
    - **Ringlet** pattern of calcification in and around condyle ± spiculated periosteal reaction
    - Nonenhancing soft tissue **mass** in widened joint space with erosion of surrounding anatomical structures
- **Metastatic Disease**
  - Key facts
    - Most common primary malignancies metastasizing to TMJ are breast, lung, and prostate
    - Symptoms mimic TMJ dysfunction and may have preauricular swelling, mandibular paresthesia, and pathological fracture
    - Most cases > 40 years old
  - Imaging
    - Condyle appears small due to radiolucent destruction by metastases
    - Some metastases cause bone formation and mixed or sclerotic radiographic appearance
    - Usually **poorly defined, invasive** margins; may also see destruction of neighboring anatomic structures
    - May have associated soft tissue **mass**
    - Usually unilateral in TMJ
    - Solitary metastasis to TMJ rare: TMJ involvement usually associated with mandibular or generalized skeletal metastases

SELECTED REFERENCES

1. Sansare K et al: Management-related outcomes and radiographic findings of idiopathic condylar resorption: a systematic review. Int J Oral Maxillofac Surg. 44(2):209-16, 2015
2. Garzino-Demo P et al: Chondrosarcoma of the temporomandibular joint: a case report and review of the literature. J Oral Maxillofac Surg. 68(8):2005-11, 2010

Degenerative Joint Disease (Adult)

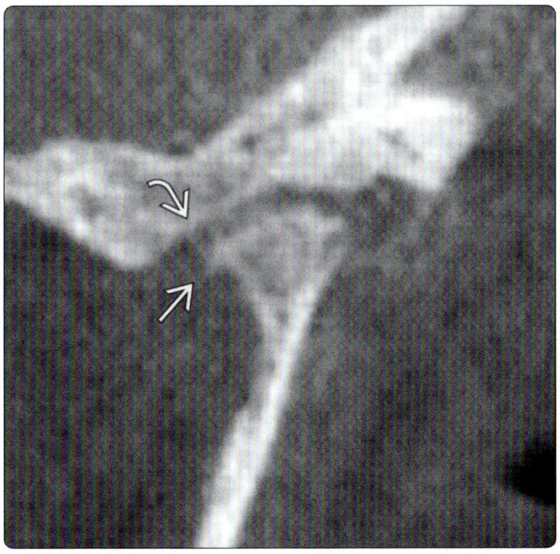

Degenerative Joint Disease (Adult)

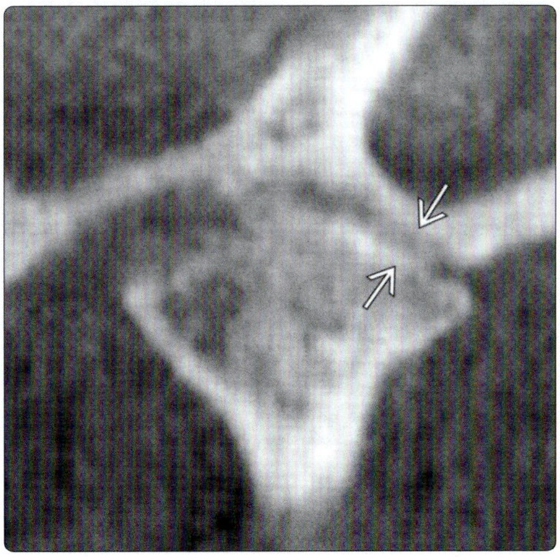

(Left) *Sagittal oblique CBCT of the left TMJ affected with adult degenerative joint disease shows a condyle that is reduced in height and volume, with flattening of the superior aspect and anterior osteophyte formation ➡. Congruent articulation with the flattened posterior slope of the eminence ➡ is seen.* **(Right)** *Coronal oblique CBCT in the same patient shows reduction of the condylar mass above the lateral and medial poles of the condyle with congruency in the lateral superior articulation ➡.*

Differential Diagnoses: Temporomandibular Joint

(Left) *Panoramic reformatted CBCT of a patient with progressive condylar resorption shows growth disturbance on the right side. The right ramus is shorter than the left, the right coronoid process is elongated, and the right condylar neck is short.* **(Right)** *Panoramic reformatted CBCT of the same patient shows normal development of the left side. The vertical height of the left mandibular body is greater than the right and the antegonial notch is shallower.*

Progressive Condylar Resorption

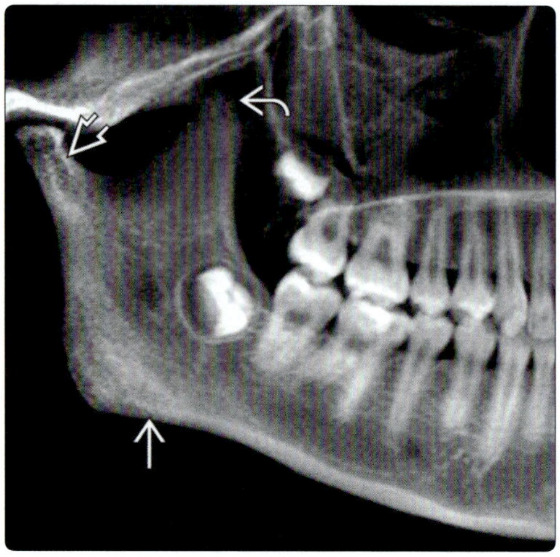

Progressive Condylar Resorption

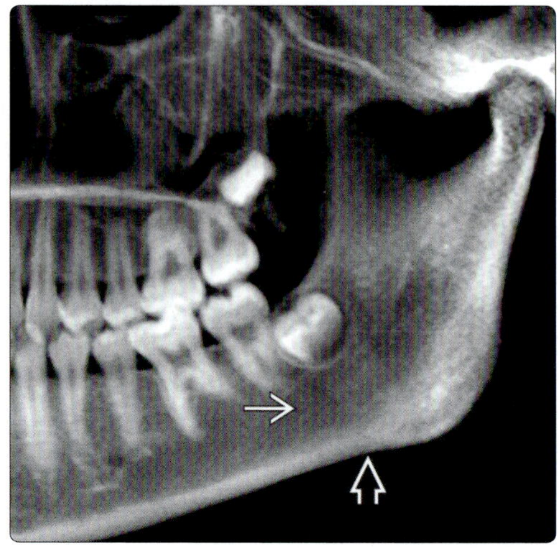

(Left) *Coronal oblique and sagittal oblique cross sections of a TMJ affected by progressive condylar resorption shows flattening of the superior aspect with loss of condylar height.* **(Right)** *Sagittal oblique T1WI MR of a TMJ with progressive condylar resorption shows a small condyle, and anterior disc displacement. Disc displacement almost always precedes the degenerative changes that occur in the bone.*

Progressive Condylar Resorption

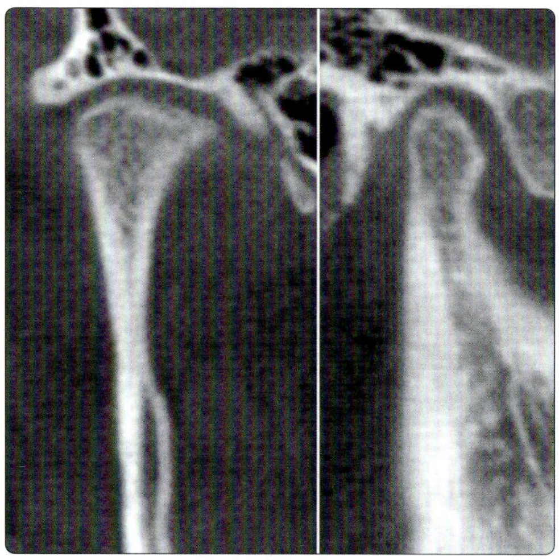

Progressive Condylar Resorption

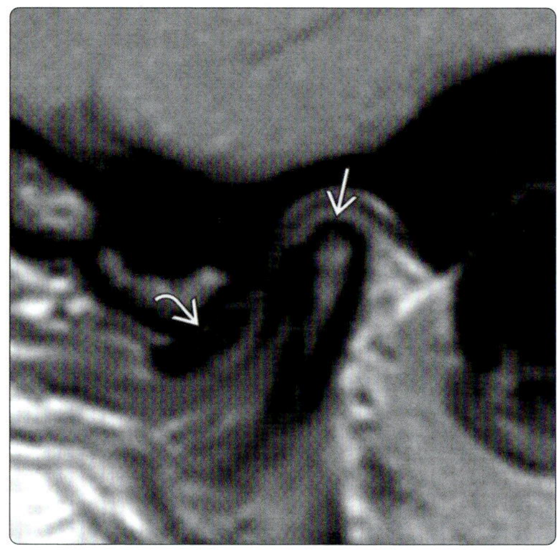

(Left) *Panoramic reformatted CBCT shows bilateral small condyles with thinned anteroposterior dimensions due to regressive remodeling. The heights of the condylar processes and the rami are unchanged.* **(Right)** *Sagittal oblique CBCT cross sections in the same patient show reduction of the anteroposterior dimension of the condyles without loss of condylar height. These changes occur with increased biomechanical forces that approximate the degenerative threshold of the bone.*

Regressive Remodeling

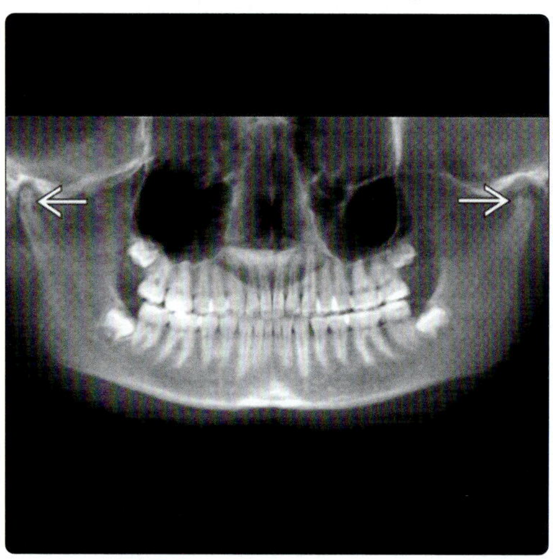

Regressive Remodeling

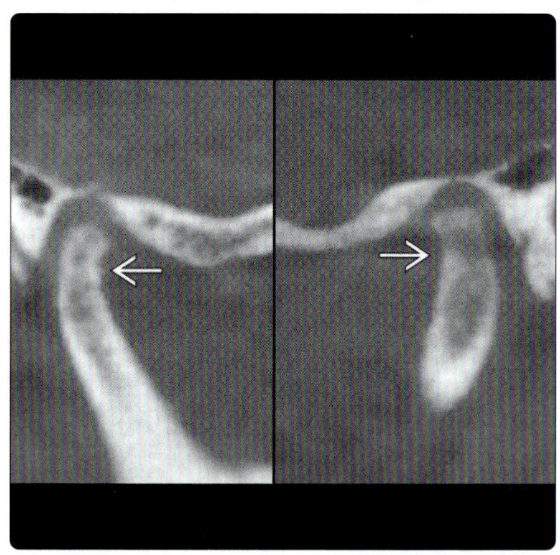

Condylar Hypoplasia

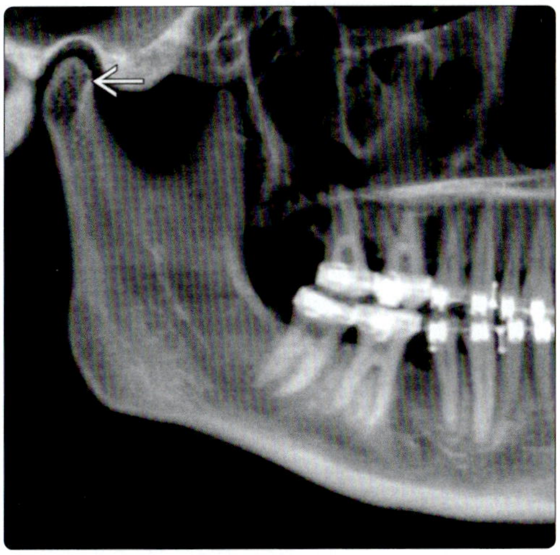

Condylar Hypoplasia

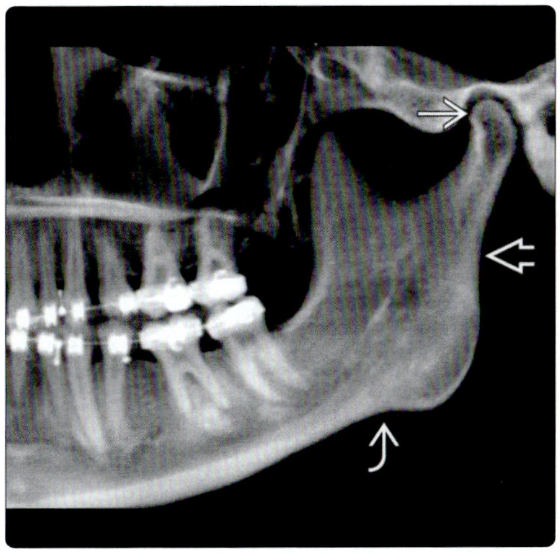

(Left) *Panoramic reformatted CBCT of the right side of a patient with left condylar hypoplasia shows a small, but normal condyle ➔ and a normal right mandible.* **(Right)** *Panoramic reformatted CBCT of the left side in the same patient shows a small condyle ➔ with otherwise normal morphology. Note the signs of a small mandible, including short ramus, a pronounced dorsal bend ➔ of the ramus, and a deepened antegonial notch ➔.*

Condylar Fracture

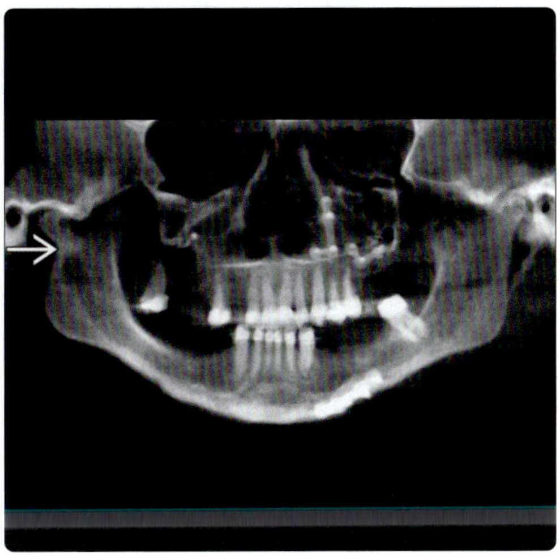

Condylar Fracture

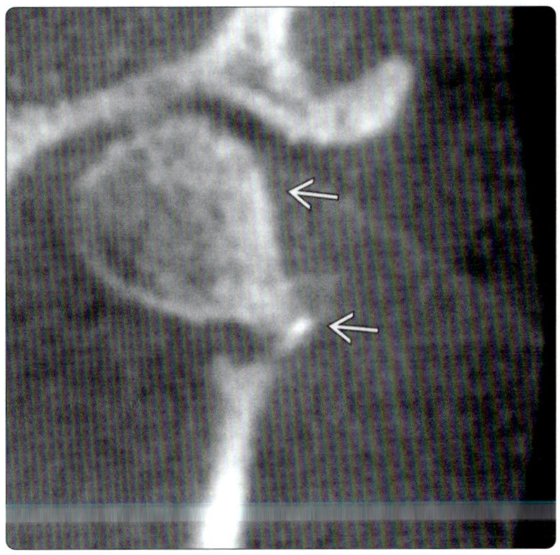

(Left) *Panoramic reformatted CBCT shows a patient with multiple fractures, including subcondylar fracture of the right condyle, which appears shortened. The excessive dorsal angulation of the condyle and the increased attenuation in this area ➔ are indicative of fracture.* **(Right)** *Coronal oblique CBCT cross section of a subcondylar fracture of the left TMJ shows that although the condylar size is unchanged, the fracture and reorientation of the condylar process ➔ can give the appearance of a small condyle.*

Condylar Fracture

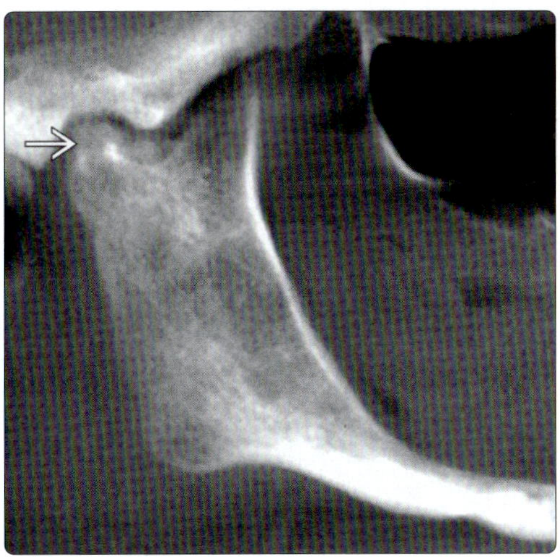

Condylar Fracture

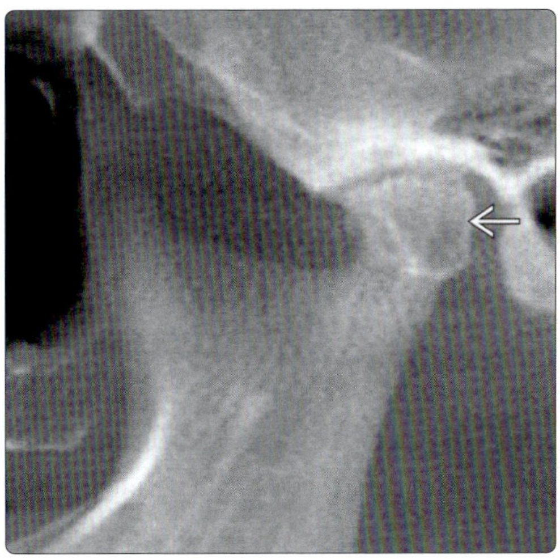

(Left) *Panoramic reformatted CBCT of a right condylar fracture shows the condyle ➔ appears small with an absent condylar neck. This appearance is misleading, and the "small condyle" likely represents the ramus stump. The actual condyle is medially displaced, out of the plane of this section.* **(Right)** *Panoramic reformatted CBCT of the left TMJ shows a condylar crush fracture ➔. The condyle appears small and the condylar neck is short. Degenerative changes may ensue after this type of fracture.*

(Left) *Panoramic reformatted CBCT shows a small condyle due to rheumatoid arthritis. The condyle has characteristic flattening* ➔ *("sharpened pencil") that is often seen in this condition.* **(Right)** *Cropped panoramic reformatted CBCT in the same patient shows rheumatoid arthritis also affecting the left TMJ. Bilateral involvement is characteristic. The inflammatory process affects both the condyle and the fossa* ➔.

Rheumatoid Arthritis

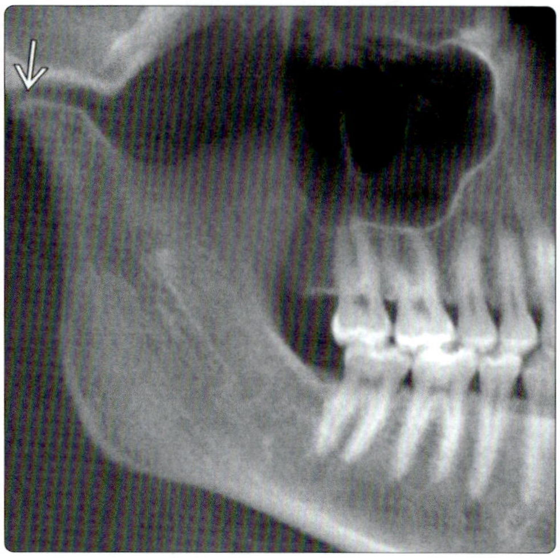

Rheumatoid Arthritis

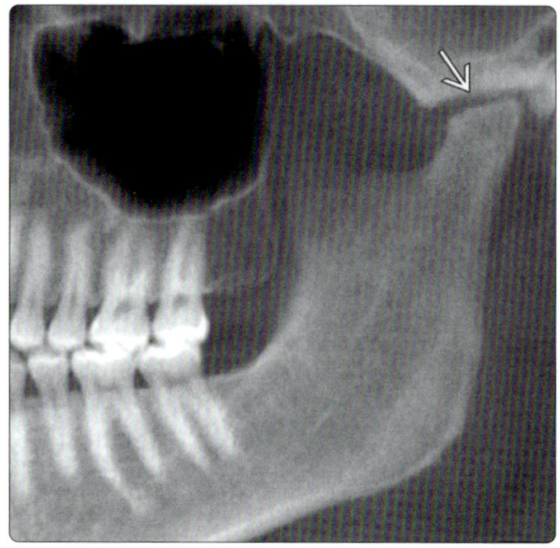

(Left) *Sagittal oblique CBCT cross sections in the same patient show flattening and irregularity of the anterior-superior aspect of the condyle, resulting in a characteristic pointed shape of the posterior aspect of the condyle* ➔. **(Right)** *Sagittal oblique T1WI MR in the same patient shows the pannus formation* ➔ *in the joint space destroying the articular surfaces of the fossa and condyle* ➔.

Rheumatoid Arthritis

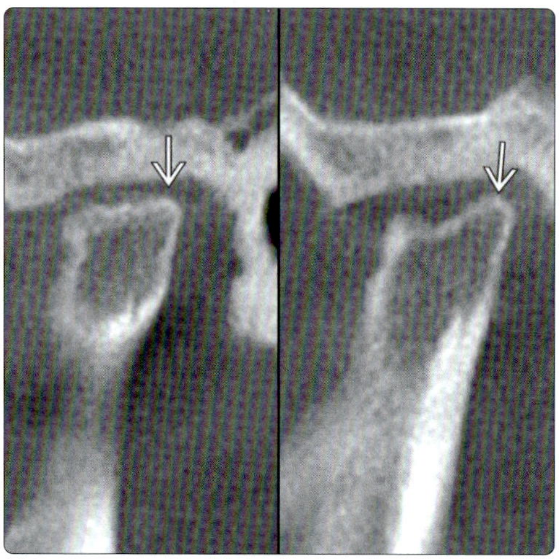

Rheumatoid Arthritis

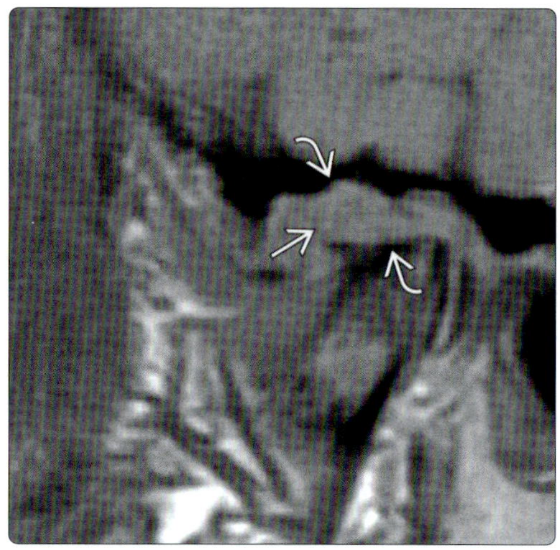

(Left) *Sagittal oblique CBCT of the right condyle shows irregular articular surfaces of the fossa and the condyle* ➔ *often seen with rheumatoid arthritis. Reduction of condylar height and volume occurs due to this inflammatory process.* **(Right)** *Coronal oblique CBCT in the same patient shows irregular articular surfaces* ➔*, condylar size reduction, and narrowing of the joint space. This appearance may be indistinguishable from degenerative joint disease.*

Rheumatoid Arthritis

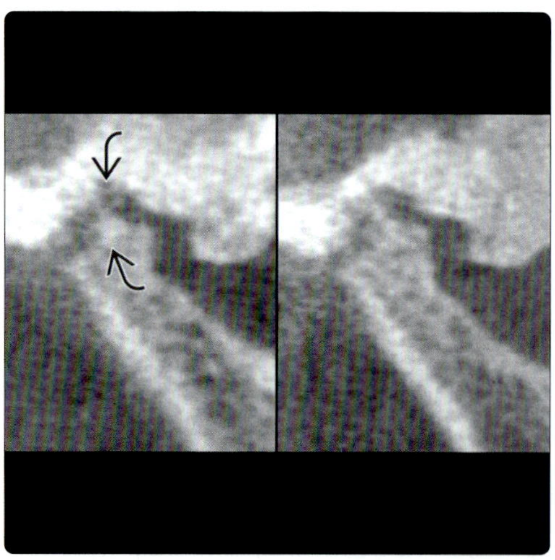

Rheumatoid Arthritis

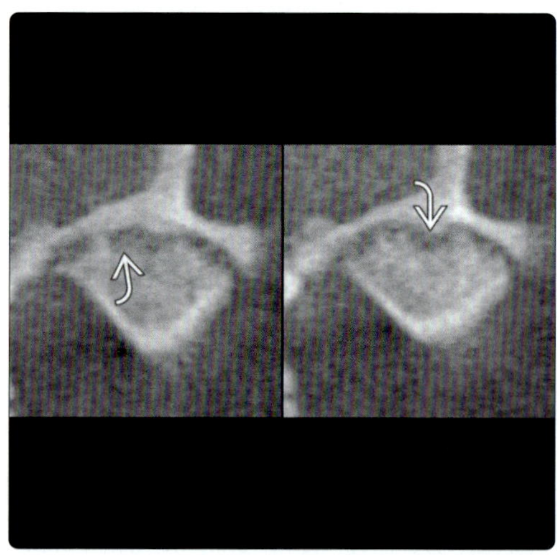

Juvenile Idiopathic Arthritis

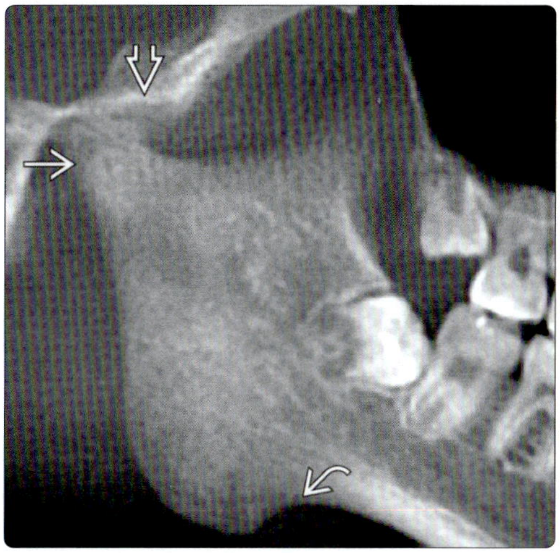

Juvenile Idiopathic Arthritis

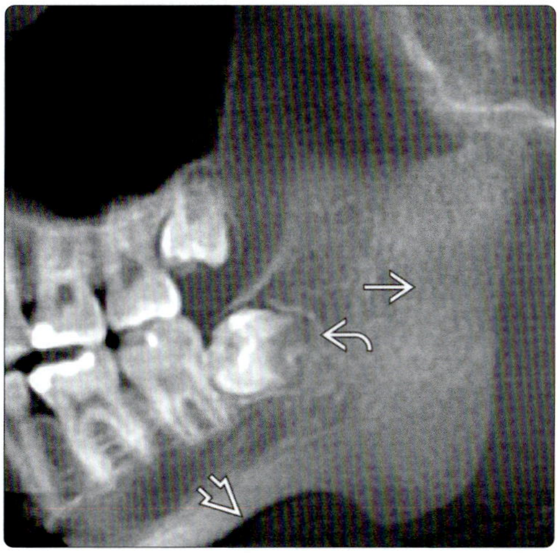

(Left) *Panoramic reformatted CBCT of the right mandible in a case of bilateral TMJ juvenile idiopathic arthritis shows the condyle appears small and the condylar neck ➡ is short. The posterior slope of the articular eminence is flat and horizontal ➡ and the antegonial notch is deep ➡.* **(Right)** *Panoramic reformatted CBCT in the same patient shows a short left ramus ➡. The 3rd molar is developing in the ramus ➡, and the mandibular plane is steep ➡.*

Hemifacial Microsomia

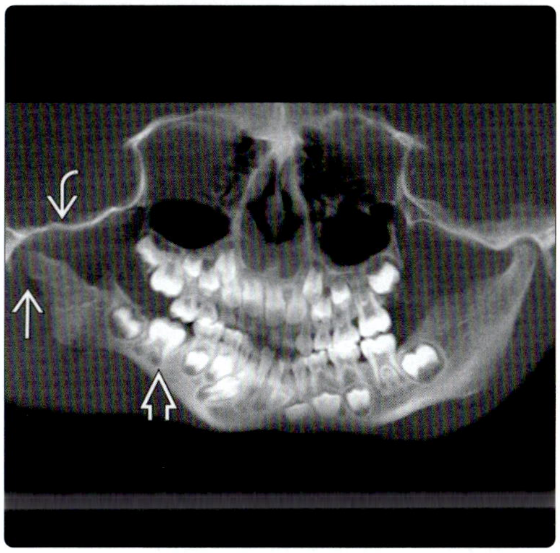

Chondrosarcoma

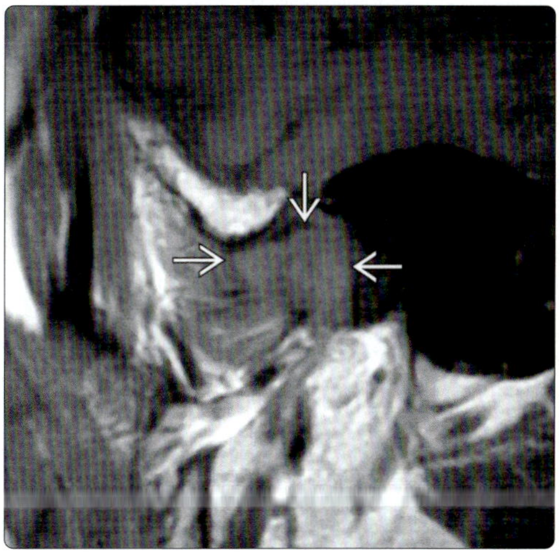

(Left) *Panoramic reformatted CBCT of hemifacial microsomia shows a small, deformed right condyle with posterior inclination ➡. Note the decreased vertical right mandibular body height ➡, short ramus, and no articular eminence development ➡.* **(Right)** *Sagittal oblique T1WI MR of chondrosarcoma in the left TMJ shows a soft tissue mass ➡ destroying the condyle and filling the condylar fossa. Typical ring-like calcifications are not seen in this case.*

Metastatic Disease

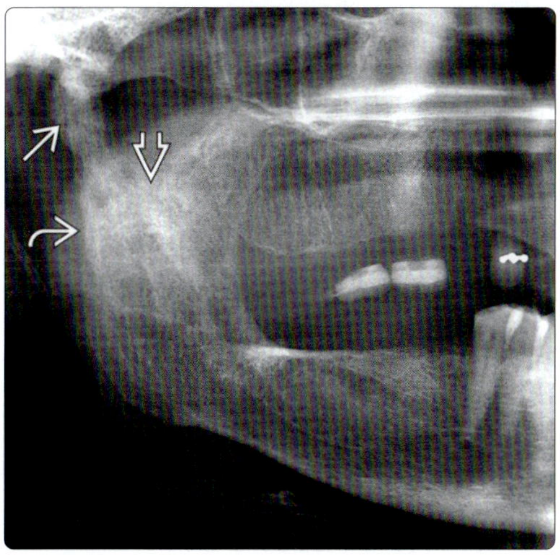

Metastatic Disease

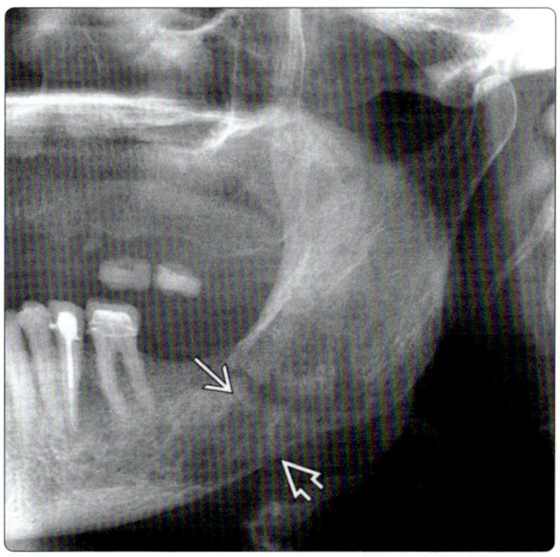

(Left) *Panoramic radiograph of breast metastases to the mandible shows the right condyle ➡ appears small and sclerotic with patchy areas of destruction. The upper ramus is sclerotic ➡ with loss of cortical boundaries and irregularity of the posterior border ➡.* **(Right)** *Panoramic radiograph in the same patient shows ill-defined bone destruction in the left molar area ➡ with irregular destruction of the inferior cortex ➡. Metastatic disease to the TMJ is rarely solitary.*

DIFFERENTIAL DIAGNOSIS

Common

- Proliferative Degenerative Joint Disease
- Condylar Hyperplasia
- Condylar Fracture

Less Common

- Osteochondroma
- Osteoma
- Bifid Condyle
- Bony Ankylosis

Rare but Important

- Fibrous Dysplasia
- Chondrosarcoma
- Osteosarcoma

ESSENTIAL INFORMATION

Key Differential Diagnosis Issues

- Large condyle with normal condylar morphology suggests hyperplasia, especially if accompanied by enlargement of ipsilateral mandible
- Osteochondroma can simulate condylar hyperplasia but is not accompanied by mandibular enlargement
  - Osteochondroma often results in condylar displacement out of normal-sized fossa
  - Glenoid fossa may remodel (enlarge) to accommodate enlarged condyle with condylar hyperplasia
- History helpful if suspect old condylar fracture
  - Fracture may result in bifid condyle or bony ankylosis
- Permeative changes in bone pattern suggest malignancy
  - Malignancy may be accompanied by spiculated periosteal reaction

Helpful Clues for Common Diagnoses

- **Proliferative Degenerative Joint Disease**
  - Key facts
    - Degenerative changes that result in increased proliferation of bone
    - Increase in condylar mass but without mass effect
  - Imaging
    - Overgrowth of bone on condyle and sometimes fossa without mass effect
    - Congruent articulation with fossa occurs
    - Loose articular bodies can occur (secondary synovial chondromatosis)
- **Condylar Hyperplasia**
  - Key facts
    - Slowly developing unilateral **overgrowth** of mandibular condyle
    - May have elongation of condylar neck
    - Enlargement of **ipsilateral** 1/2 of **mandible** proportional to condylar overgrowth
    - Most common between 10-25 years of age
    - M > F
    - Clinical signs: Facial **asymmetry**, depression of occlusal plane on involved side ± open bite
    - Self-limiting but growth may continue to 3rd decade
  - Imaging
    - Unilateral enlargement of mandibular condyle and ipsilateral ascending ramus and mandibular body
    - Cortical borders and subchondral bone **normal**
    - Condylar enlargement greatest in anteroposterior and vertical dimensions
    - Condylar shape: Conical, spherical, elongated, lobulated, or irregular
    - Fossa may enlarge to accommodate enlarged condyle
- **Condylar Fracture**
  - Key facts
    - Usually occurs at condylar neck and often accompanied by **dislocation** of condyle
    - May be **asymptomatic**, especially in young patients
    - Clinical findings: Swelling over TMJ, limited range of motion, malocclusion, often chin contusion
  - Imaging
    - Fractured fragment may **ankylose** to stump of condylar neck on medial aspect, simulating enlarged condyle with abnormal morphology
    - Mandibular fossa flattens
    - Degenerative changes may occur over time in TMJ on affected side
    - If fracture at young age: **Mandibular hypoplasia** on affected side with deviation of mandible

Helpful Clues for Less Common Diagnoses

- **Osteochondroma**
  - Key facts
    - Slow-growing, cartilage-capped **exophytic** lesion arising from bone
    - Mean age at diagnosis: 40 years; F > M
    - May present with swelling over TMJ, facial asymmetry, ± pain
    - Posterior open bite on affected side, deviation of mandible to unaffected side
    - Hypomobility
  - Imaging
    - Often mistaken for condylar hyperplasia or degenerative joint disease osteophytes
    - Irregular, distorted, enlarged condyle but ipsilateral 1/2 of mandible **not** enlarged
    - Appears as pedunculated mass of mixed density attached to condyle or coronoid process
    - May appear at bony projection following direction of lateral pterygoid muscle fibers (medially and anteriorly)
    - Often extends from anterior or anteromedial surface of condyle
    - Border between lesion and underlying normal bone usually **indistinct**
- **Osteoma**
  - Key facts
    - Benign tumor of bone
    - May deviate mandible to unaffected side
  - Imaging
    - Usually occurs on surfaces covered by periosteum (condylar neck and posterior condyle)
    - Can be cortical or cancellous
    - Can be pedunculated or sessile
    - May cause displacement of condyle in direction away from mass

- **Bifid Condyle**
  - Key facts
    - Uncommon entity characterized by partial division of condyle
    - Unilateral:bilateral = 4:1
    - Usually asymptomatic, may have pain or joint noises
  - Imaging
    - Condyle appears **lobulated** &/or **enlarged**
    - Depression or notch on superior condylar surface or duplication of condyle
    - Mandibular fossa may remodel to accommodate altered condylar morphology
    - May be accompanied by bony **ankylosis** if etiology is trauma
- **Bony Ankylosis**
  - Key facts
    - Joint immobility characterized by formation of osseous, fibrous, or fibroosseous mass fused to skull
    - Unilateral or bilateral
    - History of progressively restricted jaw opening or longstanding history of limited opening
    - If ankylosis occurs in young patient, mandibular **growth** affected
    - Etiology may be trauma (fracture), infection, systemic disease, rheumatoid arthritis
  - Imaging
    - Markedly reduced or absent joint space
    - Irregular, enlarged joint margins with fibrous or bony bridging
    - Enlarged **condyle**, may see elongation of **coronoids**, deepened antegonial notch on affected side

Helpful Clues for Rare Diagnoses

- **Fibrous Dysplasia**
  - Key facts
    - Rare in TMJ
  - Imaging
    - Uniform expansion of condyle with ground-glass appearance
    - Usually additional sites affected
- **Chondrosarcoma**
  - Key facts
    - Rare malignant tumor arising from cartilage cells
    - Mean age: 50 years
    - F:M = 2:1 in TMJ
    - Clinical findings: Preauricular swelling, mandibular deviation, pain, limitation of motion
  - Imaging
    - Condyle may appear enlarged and lengthened but **flocculent calcifications** around condyle and joint space ± osseous destruction
    - Articular fossa may also enlarge
    - Soft tissue mass
    - Internal calcifications may be cloud-like with calcified whorls and arcs
    - May have spiculated **periosteal reaction**
- **Osteosarcoma**
  - Key facts
    - Malignant tumor of bone in which osteoid is produced by malignant stroma
    - Mean age: 35 years
    - M:F = 2:1
    - Clinical findings: Swelling, limitation of motion, malocclusion, pain, headaches
  - Imaging
    - Bone destruction with aggressive spiculated **periosteal reaction** ± tumor formation
    - Condyle may appear enlarged and composed of **mottled** bone pattern

SELECTED REFERENCES

1. Sekhar MM et al: Giant osteochondroma of the mandibular condyle. J Oral Maxillofac Pathol. 19(3):407, 2015
2. Villanueva-Alcojol L et al: Hyperplasia of the mandibular condyle: clinical, histopathologic, and treatment considerations in a series of 36 patients. J Oral Maxillofac Surg. 69(2):447-55, 2011
3. Garzino-Demo P et al: Chondrosarcoma of the temporomandibular joint: a case report and review of the literature. J Oral Maxillofac Surg. 68(8):2005-11, 2010
4. Shintaku WH et al: Imaging modalities to access bony tumors and hyperplasic reactions of the temporomandibular joint. J Oral Maxillofac Surg. 68(8):1911-21, 2010

Proliferative Degenerative Joint Disease

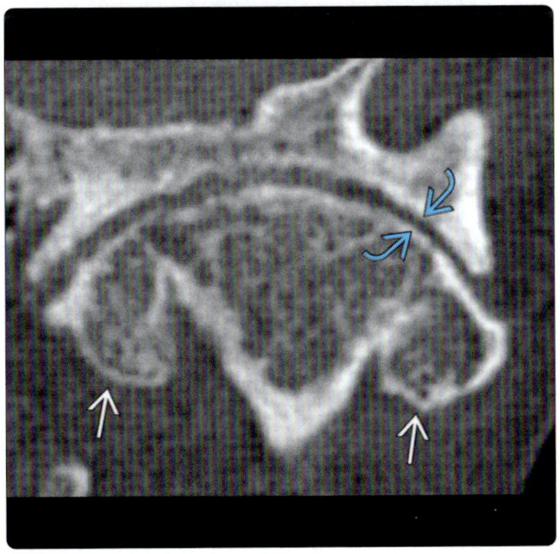

Condylar Hyperplasia

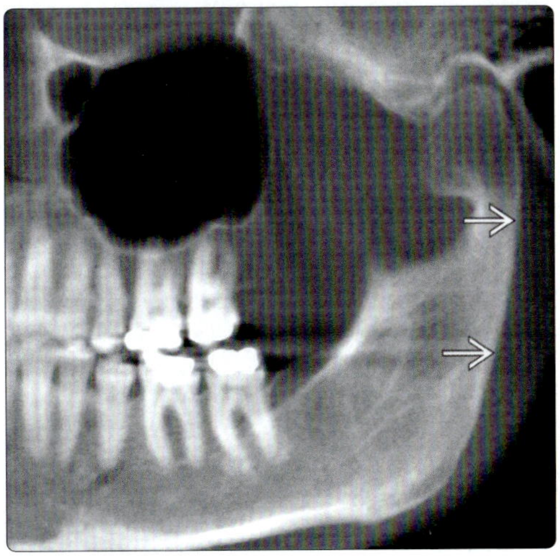

(Left) *Coronal oblique CBCT of the TMJ shows proliferative degenerative changes* ➡*. This proliferation can become large and mimic tumor. The presence of a congruent articulation* ⮫ *and other DJD signs, as well as absence of mass effect, may aid in the diagnosis.* **(Right)** *Panoramic reformatted CBCT shows left condylar hyperplasia. The condyle exhibits normal cortical outline and subchondral trabeculation. Note the convex shape (bowing)* ➡ *of the neck of the condyle and posterior border of the ramus.*

(Left) *Panoramic radiograph of left condylar fracture shows enlargement of the condyle due to overlap of the fractured fragment on the condylar neck stump.* **(Right)** *Sagittal CBCT of a left condylar fracture shows unusual condylar morphology and enlargement. The fractured fragment has reattached to the ramus, resulting in a "step" defect. The glenoid fossa has remodeled to accommodate the enlarged condyle and is flattened and sclerotic.*

Condylar Fracture

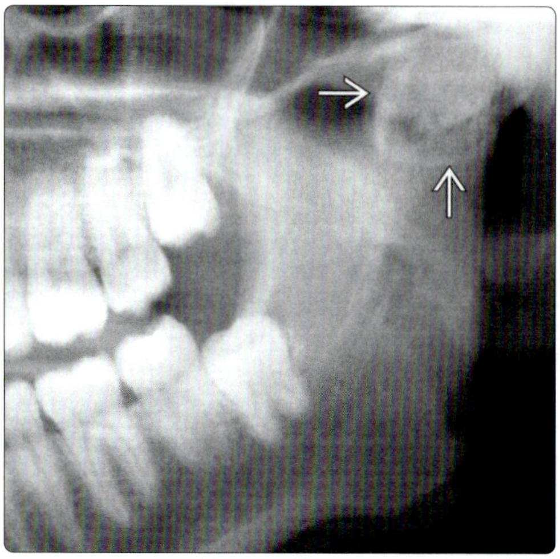

Condylar Fracture

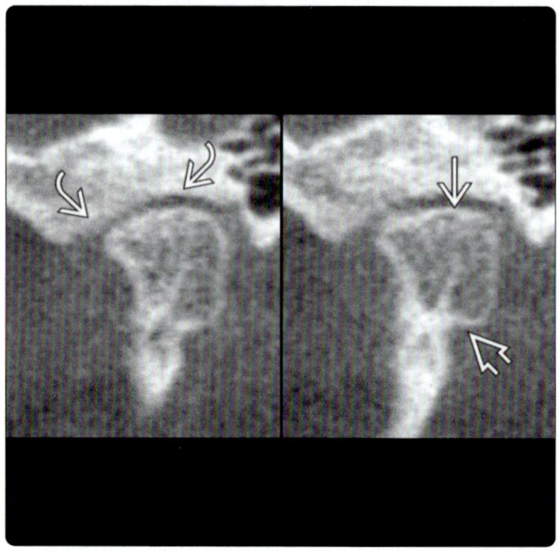

(Left) *Panoramic radiograph shows an osteochondroma of the right condyle. The condyle is enlarged, but the ipsilateral ramus is normal, which rules out condylar hyperplasia.* **(Right)** *Panoramic radiograph shows osteochondroma of the left condyle. The lesion extends from the anterior condylar surface and articulates with the articular eminence, preventing seating of the condyle in the fossa. The trabecular bone of the lesion is continuous with the trabecular bone of the condyle.*

Osteochondroma

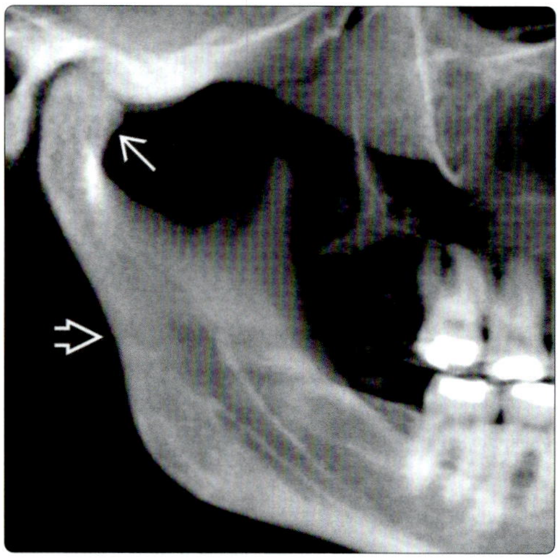

Osteochondroma

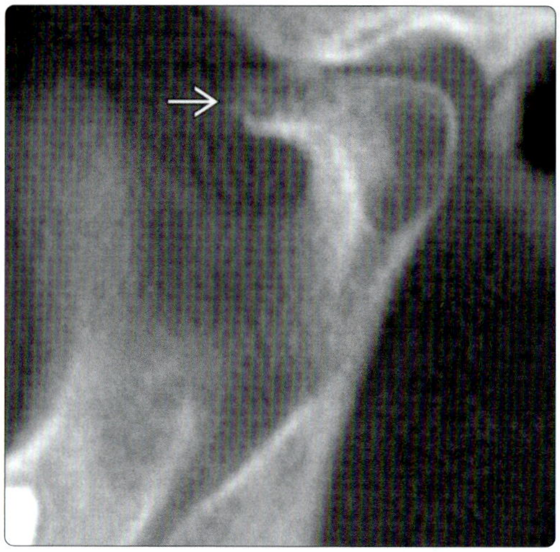

(Left) *Axial CBCT shows a TMJ osteoma extending from the posterior and medial aspects of the condyle. This mass has both cortical and cancellous components and originates from the periosteal surface of the condyle.* **(Right)** *Lateral 3D surface rendering in the same patient shows the portion of the lesion originating from the posterior aspect of the condyle and displacing the condyle anteriorly.*

Osteoma

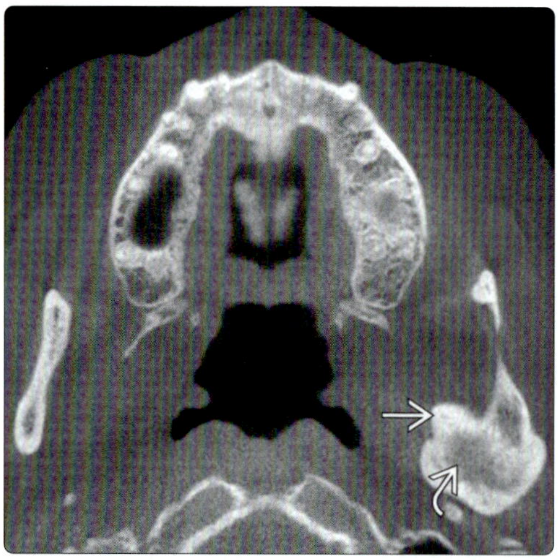

Osteoma

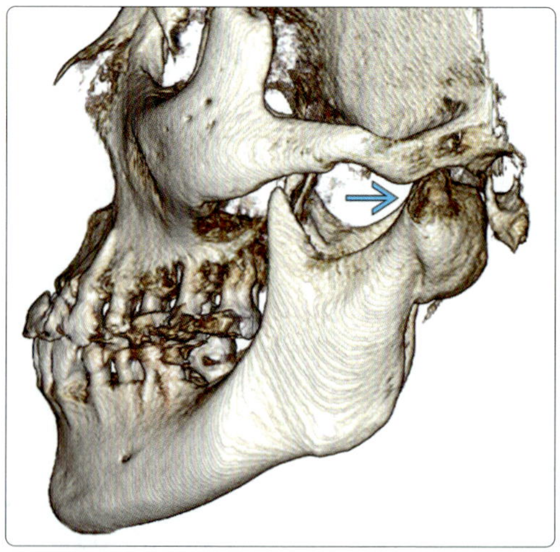

Large Condyle

Bifid Condyle

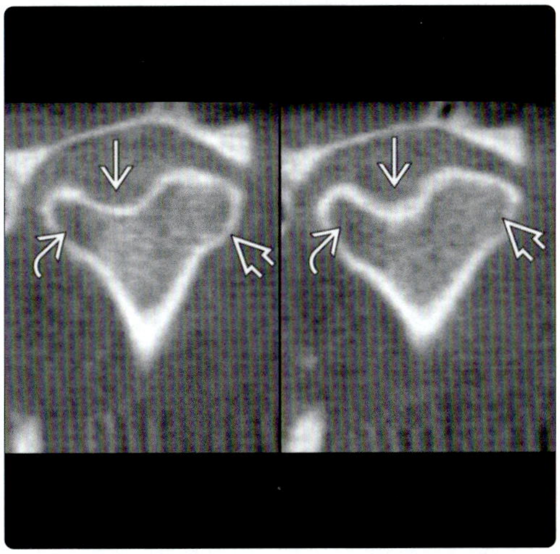

Bony Ankylosis

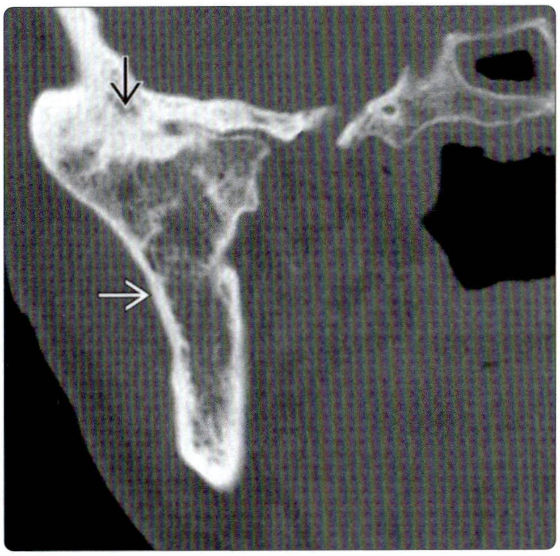

(Left) *Coronal CBCT shows a bifid condyle with a moderately deep and wide central depression* ➔ *dividing the condyle into a larger lateral lobe* ➔ *and smaller medial lobe* ➔*. The condyle appears enlarged and heart-shaped.* **(Right)** *Coronal CBCT shows enlargement of the right condyle, which is fused to the temporal bone by an osseous bridge* ⇨ *on the lateral aspect. The joint space is obliterated. The condylar neck and ramus* ➔ *are thick.*

Chondrosarcoma

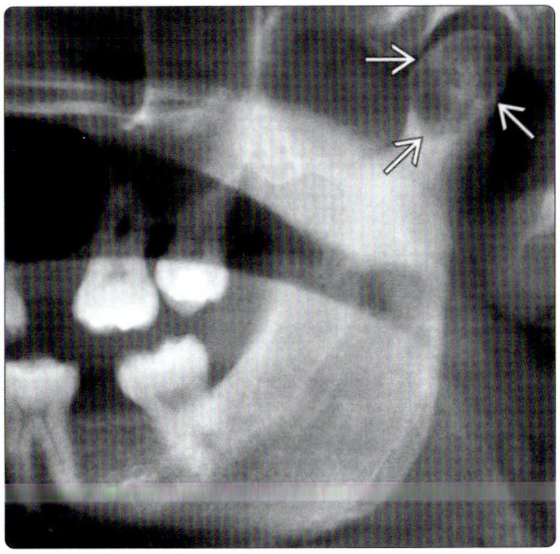

Chondrosarcoma

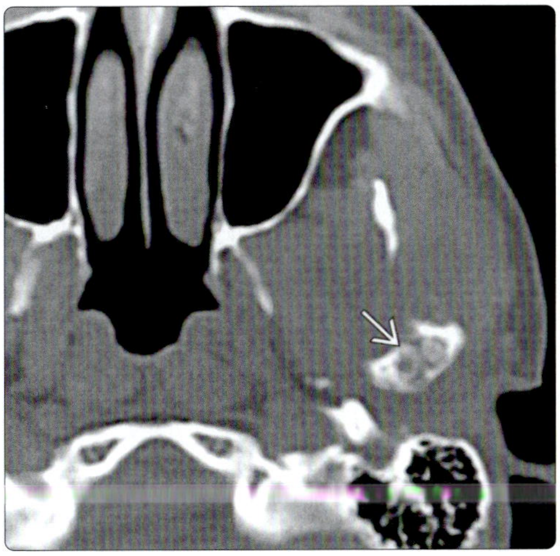

(Left) *Cropped panoramic radiograph shows a chondrosarcoma of the left condyle. The condyle is enlarged, but the lesion is radiolucent with well-defined borders* ➔ *and a lobulated appearance.* **(Right)** *Axial bone CT of the same patient shows condylar enlargement, but the internal aspect has a radiolucent bubbly appearance* ➔ *instead of a normal trabecular pattern, which helps to distinguish this from condylar hyperplasia.*

Osteosarcoma

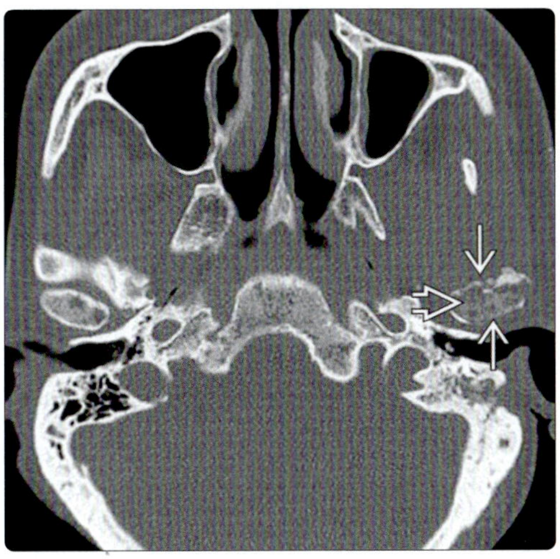

Osteosarcoma

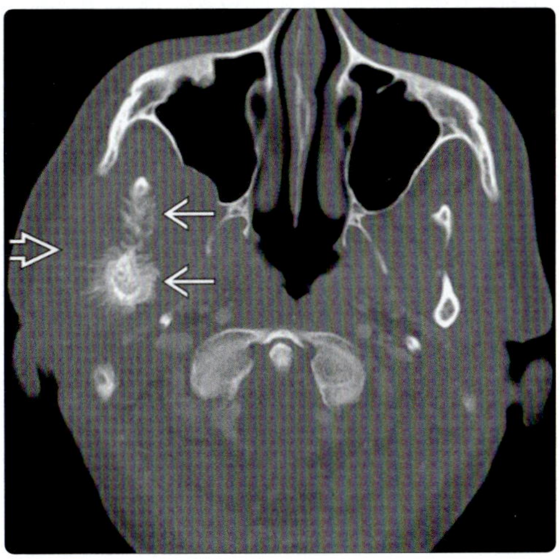

(Left) *Axial bone CT shows osteosarcoma of the left condyle appearing as an overall enlargement but with destruction of trabecular bone* ➔ *in the condyle. The condylar cortex* ➔ *is thinned and irregular.* **(Right)** *Axial bone CT shows osteosarcoma involving the right mandibular ramus and condyle* ➔*. A spiculated periosteal reaction, which is typical of osteosarcoma, has caused enlargement of the condyle and thickening of the ramus. There is an associated soft tissue mass* ➔ *lateral to the mandible.*

DIFFERENTIAL DIAGNOSIS

Common

- Disc Derangement Without Reduction
- Degenerative Joint Disease
- Condylar Fracture

Less Common

- Adhesions
- Fibrous Ankylosis
- Bony Ankylosis
- Coronoid Hyperplasia
- Osteochondroma

Rare but Important

- Myositis Ossificans

ESSENTIAL INFORMATION

Key Differential Diagnosis Issues

- Determine whether limited translation due to muscular, osseous, or soft tissue abnormality
  - Consider that other causes of limited translation may be unrelated to TMJ itself, such as scleroderma, torticollis, scar tissue of face or mouth, submucous fibrosis, tissue damage secondary to high-dose radiation treatment
- Abnormality on one side may also limit translation of contralateral condyle
- Consider MR in conjunction with CBCT or CT to image soft tissues in and around TMJ
- Check coronoid processes because coronoid hyperplasia or osteochondroma can cause limited translation due to mechanical interference

Helpful Clues for Common Diagnoses

- **Disc Derangement Without Reduction**
  - Key facts
    - Disc displaced or misaligned with condyle in mandibular closed ± open position
    - Displaced disc may interfere with condylar motion resulting in limited translation
    - With time, mandibular opening may improve due to stretching of posterior disc ligaments, allowing disc to translate further anteriorly
  - Imaging
    - T1-weighted MR open mandibular position: Condyle translates to point posterior to summit of articular eminence, but disc remains anterior to condyle
    - Disc may be deformed or folded and is mechanical barrier to further condylar translation
- **Degenerative Joint Disease**
  - Key facts
    - Limited translation may be due to associated muscle spasm or displaced disc
    - Osseous signs of degenerative joint disease (DJD) usually preceded by nonreducing anteriorly displaced disc
    - End-stage DJD often accompanied by normal motion and pain-free function
  - Imaging
    - Reduction in condylar size from superior surface ± sclerosis, flattening, erosions, osteophytes, subchondral bone cyst, joint space narrowing
    - Often associated disc displacement
- **Condylar Fracture**
  - Key facts
    - Most common at condylar neck and accompanied by dislocation of condylar head
    - Dislocated condylar head may impede condylar motion
    - Consider that condylar fracture often accompanied by fracture of mandible and facial skeleton
  - Imaging
    - Condylar angle altered or condyle displaced from normal position
    - Fractured fragment often anterior-medially dislocated due to pull of lateral pterygoid muscle
    - Occasionally disc disruption, capsular tear, retrodiscal tissue tear, hemarthrosis, all of which may cause limited condylar translation

Helpful Clues for Less Common Diagnoses

- **Adhesions**
  - Key facts
    - Connection of disc to fossa or eminence by fibrous connective tissue in superior joint compartment
    - May restrict condylar translation
    - May have pain on maximum opening
    - May have joint sounds
  - Imaging
    - No disc translation and no or reduced condylar translation
    - Joint space visible in superior joint compartment
    - Posterior band of disc may remain adhered to temporal bone in open position
- **Fibrous Ankylosis**
  - Key facts
    - Restriction of condylar movement due to intraarticular fibrous tissue
    - Condyle adhered to temporal bone
    - Painless
    - No joint sounds
  - Imaging
    - Limited or no condylar translation
    - Joint space maintained
    - No joint effusion
    - May have cortical irregularities
- **Bony Ankylosis**
  - Key facts
    - Limited condylar translation due to formation of osseous or fibroosseous mass fused to skull
    - Often some degree of opening possible, but range of motion markedly decreased
  - Imaging
    - Markedly reduced or absent joint space with irregular, enlarged joint margins with fibrous or bony bridging
    - Bridge may fuse condyle to cranial base and obliterate joint space
    - Associated changes: Elongation of coronoids, deepened antegonial notch on affected side due to muscle function during attempted opening

- **Coronoid Hyperplasia**
  - Key facts
    - Unilateral or bilateral
    - Slowly developing elongation of coronoid, so may have progressive reduction in opening
  - Imaging
    - Coronoid tip may be enlarged but normal or curved anteriorly and extends ≥ 1 cm above inferior rim of zygomatic arch
    - Coronoid process impinges on medial surface of zygomatic arch during opening, restricting condylar translation
- **Osteochondroma**
  - Key facts
    - Can occur in condyle or coronoid process; either location can result in limited mandibular opening
    - Slow-growing so may have gradual reduction in opening over long period of time
  - Imaging
    - Condyle: Irregular, distorted, enlarged; lesion may be pedunculated
    - Coronoid: May have mushroom-shaped enlargement
    - Lesion cortex and internal aspect continuous with those of originating bone
    - Border between lesion and underlying normal bone indistinct

Helpful Clues for Rare Diagnoses

- **Myositis Ossificans**
  - Key facts
    - Most common subsequent to trauma (localized) but is rarely genetic (generalized)
    - Injury to muscle → hemorrhage into muscle or associated tendons and fascia with metaplasia to cartilage and bone during healing
    - If affects one of muscles of mastication, results in limited mandibular opening
  - Imaging
    - Single: Radiopaque oval mass may lie along long axis of muscle
    - Multiple: Linear streaks parallel to direction of normal muscle fibers

SELECTED REFERENCES

1. Braimah RO et al: A multidisciplinary approach to the management of temporomandibular joint ankylosis in a sickle-cell anemia patient in a resource-limited setting. Ann Maxillofac Surg. 6(1):130-4, 2016
2. Pasetti M et al: Temporomandibular joint ankylosis as part of the clinical spectrum of Carey-Fineman-Ziter syndrome? Am J Med Genet A. 170(8):2191-5, 2016
3. Rozeboom AV et al: Closed treatment of unilateral mandibular condyle fractures in adults: a systematic review. Int J Oral Maxillofac Surg. ePub, 2016
4. Çorumlu U et al: Bilateral elongated mandibular coronoid process in an Anatolian skull. Anat Cell Biol. 49(3):217-220, 2016
5. Alajbeg IZ et al: Mandibular range of movement and pain intensity in patients with anterior disc displacement without reduction. Acta Stomatol Croat. 49(2):119-27, 2015
6. Malik AH et al: Efficacy of temporomandibular joint arthrocentesis on mouth opening and pain in the treatment of internal derangement of TMJ-a clinical study. J Maxillofac Oral Surg. 13(3):244-8, 2014
7. Sporniak-Tutak K et al: Management of temporomandibular ankylosis - compromise or individualization - a literature review. Med Sci Monit. 17(5):RA111-116, 2011
8. Zhang S et al: Arthroscopic treatment for intra-articular adhesions of the temporomandibular joint. J Oral Maxillofac Surg. 69(8):2120-7, 2011
9. Arayasantiparb R et al: Quantification of disc displacement in internal derangement of the temporomandibular joint using magnetic resonance imaging. Odontology. 98(1):73-81, 2010
10. Etöz OA et al: Osteochondroma of the mandibular coronoid process: a rare cause of limited mouth opening. Br J Oral Maxillofac Surg. 47(5):409-11, 2009
11. Kaban LB et al: A protocol for management of temporomandibular joint ankylosis in children. J Oral Maxillofac Surg. 67(9):1966-78, 2009
12. Wang P et al: MR imaging assessment of temporomandibular joint soft tissue injuries in dislocated and nondislocated mandibular condylar fractures. AJNR Am J Neuroradiol. 30(1):59-63, 2009
13. Zhang S et al: Magnetic resonance imaging in the diagnosis of intra-articular adhesions of the temporomandibular joint. Br J Oral Maxillofac Surg. 47(5):389-92, 2009
14. Avinash KR et al: Computed tomographic features of mandibular osteochondroma. Dentomaxillofac Radiol. 36(7):434-6, 2007
15. Izumi M et al: Computed tomographic features of bilateral coronoid process hyperplasia with special emphasis on patients without interference between the process and the zygomatic bone. Oral Surg Oral Med Oral Pathol Oral Radiol Endod. 99(1):93-100, 2005
16. Pregarz M et al: Computed tomography and magnetic resonance imaging in the management of coronoid process hyperplasia: review of five cases. Dentomaxillofac Radiol. 27(4):215-20, 1998
17. Spinazze RP et al: Chronic, progressive limitation of mouth opening. J Oral Maxillofac Surg. 56(10):1178-86, 1998

Disc Derangement Without Reduction

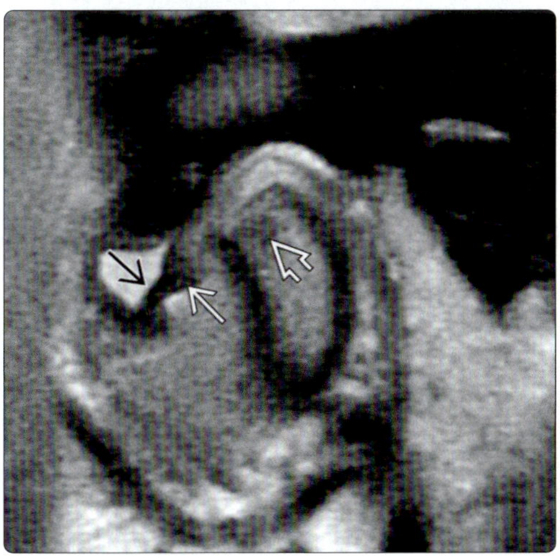

Disc Derangement Without Reduction

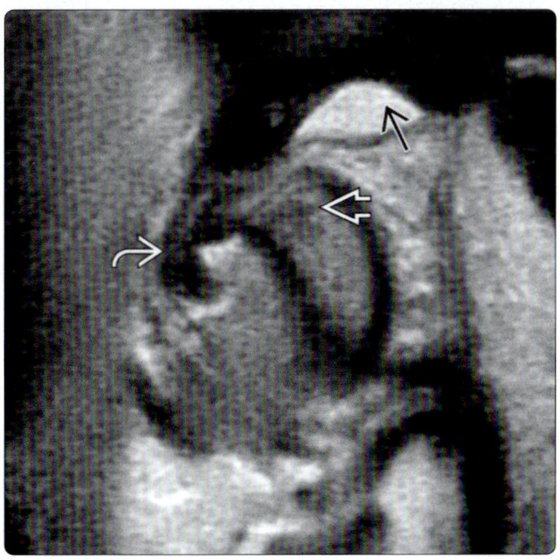

(Left) *Parasagittal T2WI MR of the TMJ in closed position shows the disc ➔ located anteriorly to the condyle with a shortened AP dimension and relatively small intermediate zone ⇨. There are erosions and subchondral signal changes ➔ in the condyle.* **(Right)** *Parasagittal T2WI MR of the same patient, in open position, shows that the disc ➔ remains anterior to the condyle ➔. Note limited condylar translation and fluid signal in the superior joint compartment ⇨.*

Degenerative Joint Disease

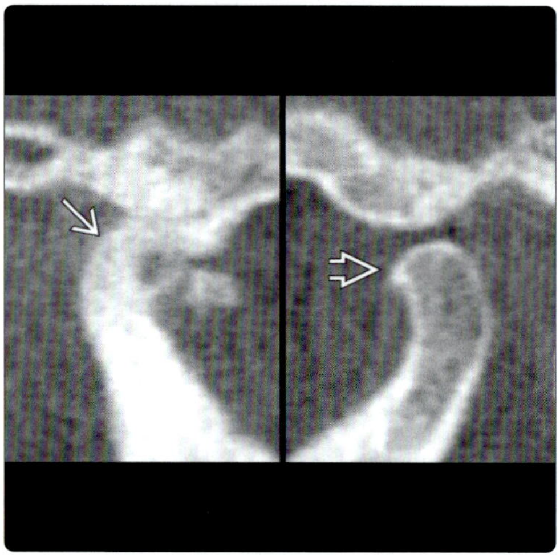

Degenerative Joint Disease

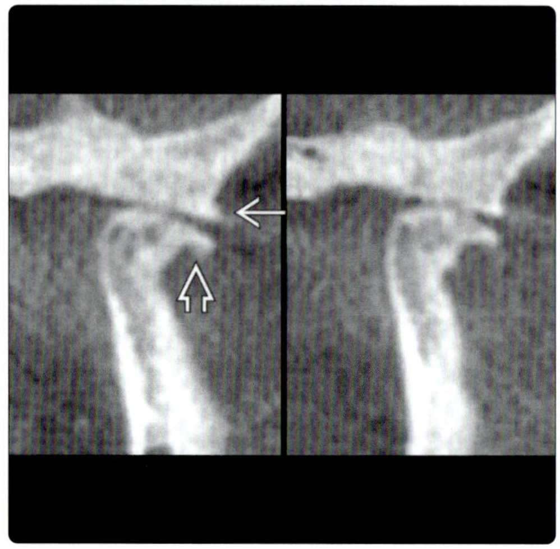

(Left) *Sagittal CBCT of degenerative joint disease (DJD) in the right TMJ shows limited right condylar translation posteriorly and superiorly to the articular eminence. The left condyle translates further than the right. There is likely an associated disc displacement on one or both sides.* **(Right)** *Sagittal CBCT of DJD shows limited condylar translation. The articular eminence is absent, and the joint components are flattened. A large osteophyte extends from the anterior aspect of the condyle.*

Condylar Fracture

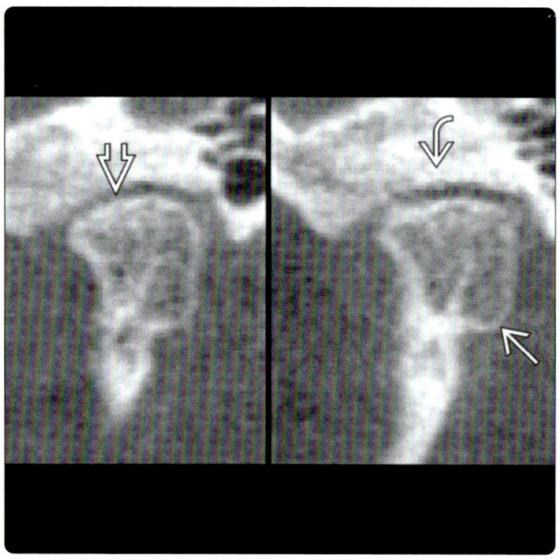

Condylar Fracture

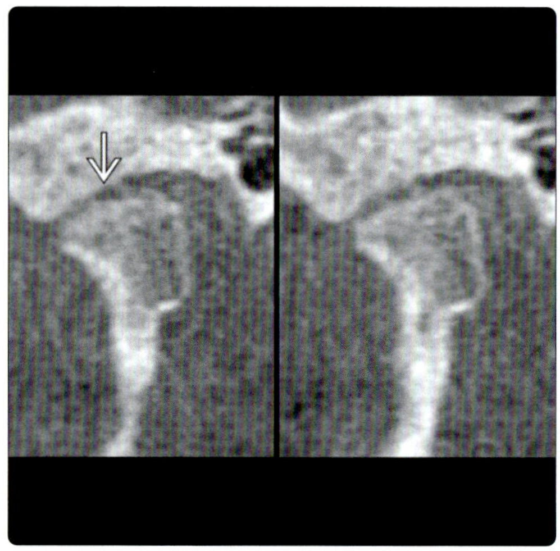

(Left) *Sagittal CBCT images of a longstanding condylar fracture, with the teeth in occlusion, show the condylar morphology is abnormal due to the fracture. The condyle is centered in the glenoid fossa, but the joint space is narrowed. The temporal component of the joint is sclerotic and flattened due to secondary DJD.* **(Right)** *Sagittal CBCT of the same patient, in the open position, shows the condyle is hypomobile and translates only to a point posterior and superior to the articular eminence.*

Adhesions

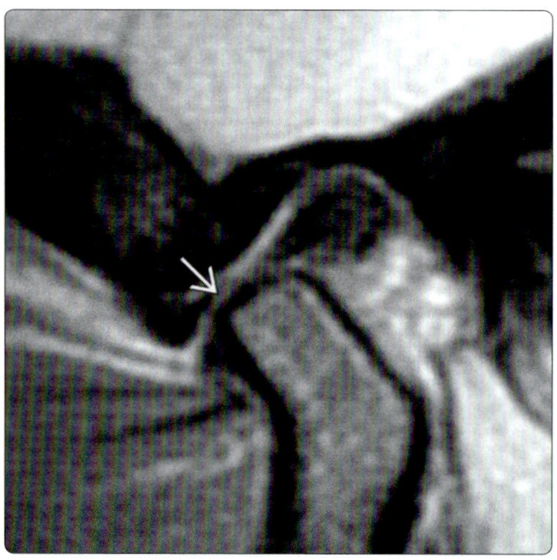

Fibrous Ankylosis

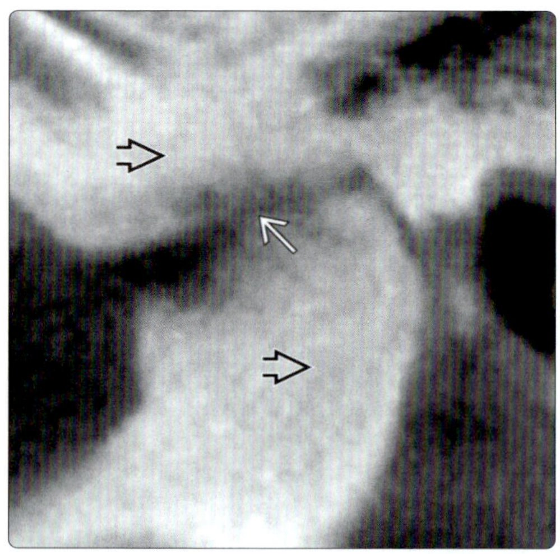

(Left) *Parasagittal T2WI MR, in open mouth position, shows limited condylar translation due to adhesions. There is no disc translation. The junction between the intermediate zone and anterior band is interposed between the condyle and articular eminence.* **(Right)** *Parasagittal CBCT, in open mouth position, shows fibrous ankylosis of the TMJ. There is no translation, but joint space is maintained. Subchondral bone has an attenuation value similar to cortical bone.*

Bony Ankylosis

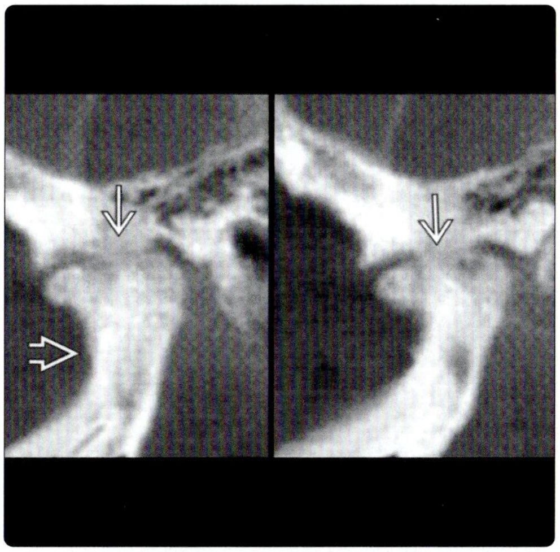

Coronoid Hyperplasia

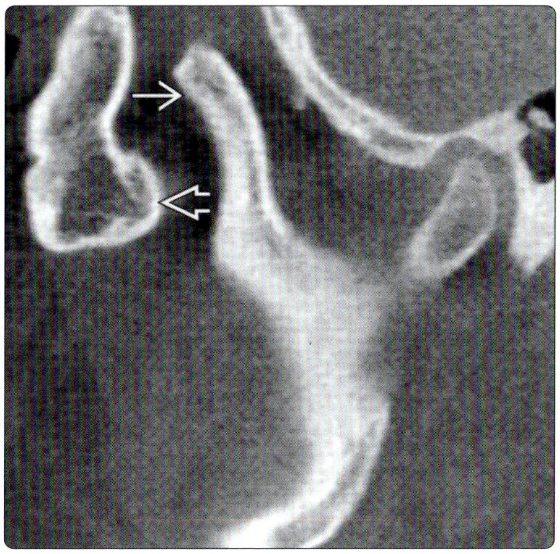

(Left) *Parasagittal CBCT of bony ankylosis shows an osseous bridge connecting the condyle with the glenoid fossa roof, preventing condylar translation. The condylar neck is thickened.* **(Right)** *Sagittal CBCT of coronoid hyperplasia shows an elongated and thickened coronoid process, which curves anteriorly and extends above the level of the zygomatic arch. The coronoid impinges on the medial surface of the zygomatic arch on opening, limiting condylar translation.*

Osteochondroma

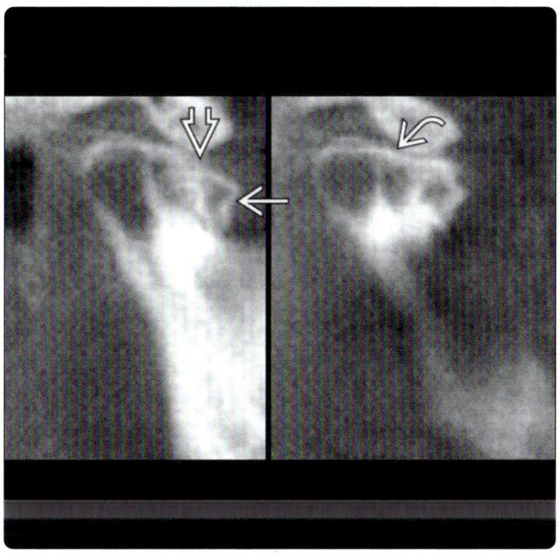

Osteochondroma

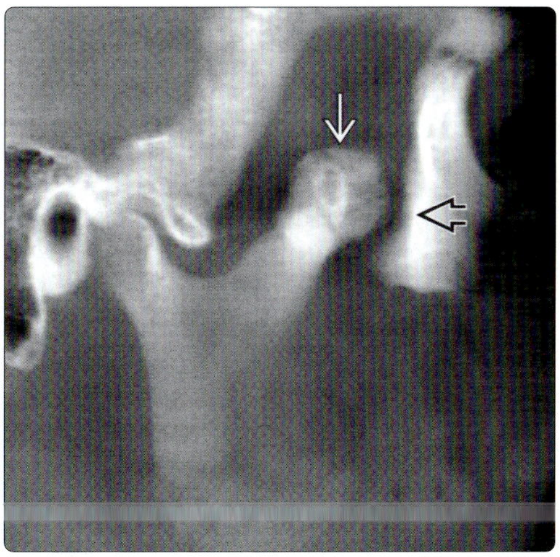

(Left) *Sagittal CBCT shows a condylar osteochondroma causing limited condylar translation due to impingement of the lesion with the articular eminence. The lesion is attached to the condyle by a narrow stalk.* **(Right)** *Sagittal CBCT shows a large coronoid osteochondroma. The lesion has a bulbous mushroom-shaped morphology and interferes with the mandibular opening as it articulates with the zygomatic process of the maxilla*

Myositis Ossificans

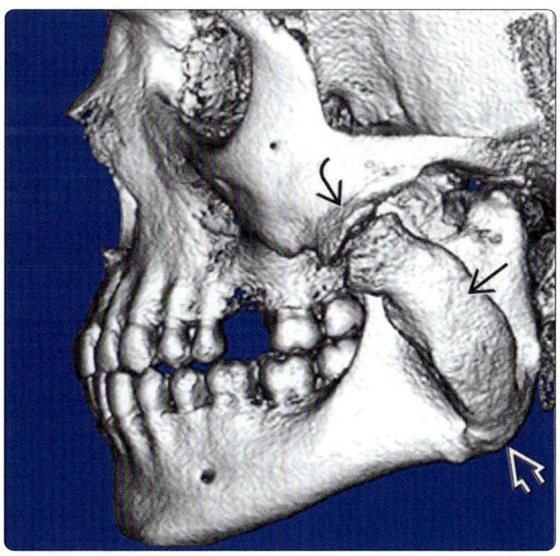

Myositis Ossificans

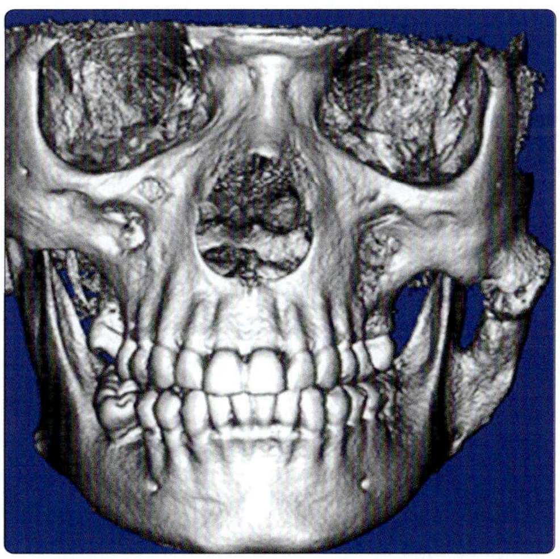

(Left) *Lateral 3D reformation of myositis ossificans of the superficial masseter muscle shows a large portion of the muscle is ossified, resulting in a bony bridge between the mandibular angle and zygomatic process, which prevents mandibular opening. The ossification lies along the axis of the muscle.* **(Right)** *Anteroposterior 3D reformation of the same patient shows the degree and position of the ossification. A facial asymmetry is clinically visible.*

DIFFERENTIAL DIAGNOSIS

Common

- Degenerative Joint Disease

Less Common

- Simple Bone Cyst
- Multiple Myeloma
- Langerhans Histiocytosis

Rare but Important

- Metastatic Disease
- Chondrosarcoma
- Osteosarcoma

ESSENTIAL INFORMATION

Key Differential Diagnosis Issues

- Degenerative joint disease very common; destructive and permeative changes suggest malignancy
- Check mandible since radiolucent lesion from posterior mandible/ramus (e.g., odontogenic keratocyst, central giant cell granuloma, osteomyelitis) may extend to condyle

Helpful Clues for Common Diagnoses

- **Degenerative Joint Disease**
  - Key facts
    - Large subchondral erosions (Ely cysts) simulate other condylar radiolucencies
  - Imaging
    - Erosions, often with osteophyte formation, flattening, subchondral sclerosis, joint space narrowing

Helpful Clues for Less Common Diagnoses

- **Simple Bone Cyst**
  - Key facts
    - Usually incidental finding, most common in posterior mandible and ramus; uncommon in condyle
  - Imaging
    - Single, corticated, usually nonexpansile radiolucency in condyle
- **Multiple Myeloma**
  - Key facts
    - Calvaria and mandible common sites
  - Imaging
    - Multiple punched-out, noncorticated, round, radiolucent lesions that may coalesce
- **Langerhans Histiocytosis**
  - Key facts
    - Condylar involvement rare
  - Imaging
    - Usually sharply defined, punched-out area but occasionally poorly defined

Helpful Clues for Rare Diagnoses

- **Metastatic Disease**
  - Key facts
    - Radiolucent destruction of condyle; history of distant primary malignancy
  - Imaging
    - Poorly defined invasive radiolucency and bony destruction ± soft tissue mass
- **Chondrosarcoma**
  - Key facts
    - Appearance varies depending on degree of tumor calcification
  - Imaging
    - Nonenhancing soft tissue mass with ringlet pattern of calcification ± spiculated periosteal reaction
- **Osteosarcoma**
  - Key facts
    - Can be radiolucent, mixed, or sclerotic
  - Imaging
    - Poorly defined destructive lesion of condyle with cortical erosion and occasional spiculated periosteal reaction

SELECTED REFERENCES

1. Petrikowski CG: Diagnostic Imaging of the Temporomandibular Joint. In White SC et al: Oral Radiology Principles and Interpretation, 6th ed. St. Louis: Mosby Elsevier. 473, 2009

Degenerative Joint Disease

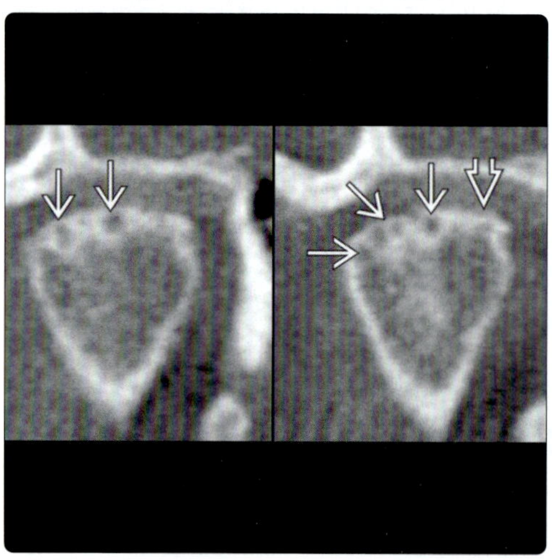

Degenerative Joint Disease

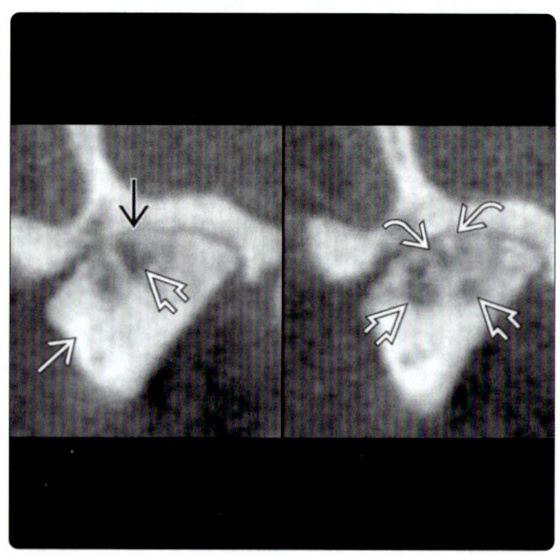

(Left) *Coronal CBCT shows degenerative joint disease of the right condyle. Several subchondral cysts ➡ are surrounded by a thick zone of sclerosis, differentiating from malignancy. The medial condylar surface is flattened ➡.* **(Right)** *Coronal CBCT of degenerative joint disease shows condylar sclerosis ➡, large radiolucencies representing subchondral (Ely) cysts ➡, and surface erosions ➡ with markedly narrowed joint space ➡.*

Simple Bone Cyst

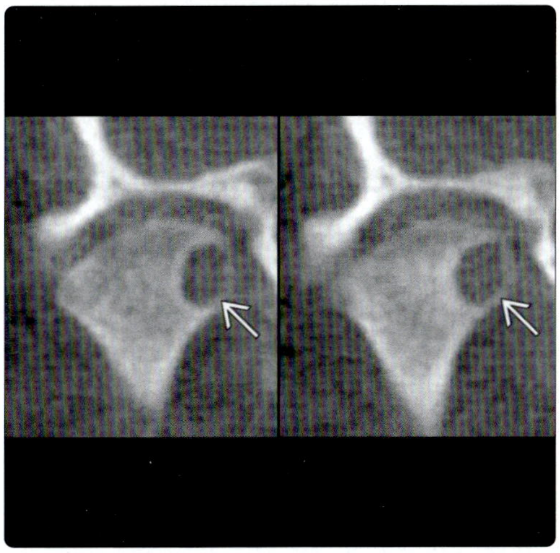

Simple Bone Cyst

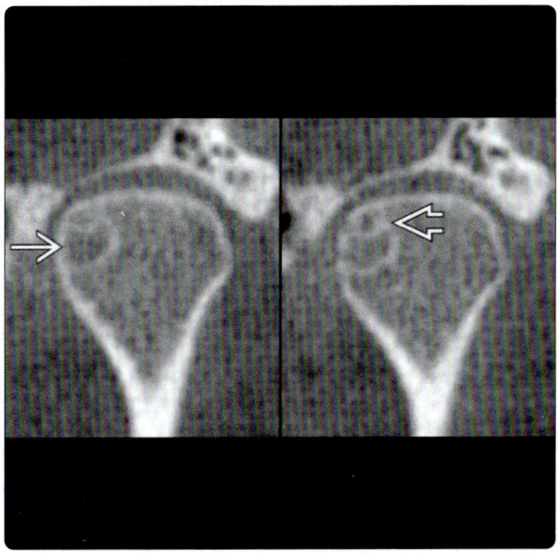

(Left) *Coronal CBCT of a simple bone cyst shows a large, corticated, nonexpansile radiolucency on the medial pole* ➡ *of the right condyle in a 15-year-old girl. The cyst spontaneously healed within 2 years.* **(Right)** *Coronal CBCT of a simple bone cyst shows a corticated, nonexpansile radiolucency* ➡ *at the medial pole of the left condyle. This cyst has a multilocular "cyst within a cyst" appearance* ⇨ *due to scalloping of the lesion. Note absence of degenerative changes, which differentiates from a subchondral cyst.*

Multiple Myeloma

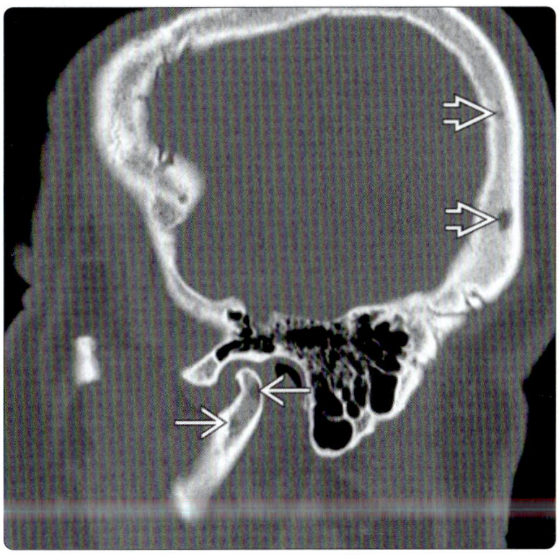

Chondrosarcoma

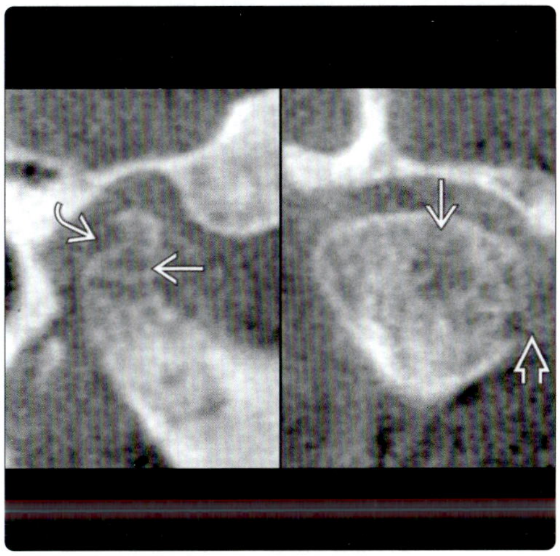

(Left) *Sagittal bone CT of multiple myeloma shows well-defined lesions in the condyle and condylar neck* ➡ *with additional skull lesions* ⇨. *The calvaria and mandible are common sites for multiple myeloma in the head and neck.* **(Right)** *Sagittal and coronal CBCT of prostate metastases to the right condyle shows permeative bone destruction* ➡ *and loss of cortical boundaries at the medial* ➡ *and posterior aspects* ⇨. *Metastases were also seen in the right ramus. Note the lack of a periosteal reaction in this case.*

Chondrosarcoma

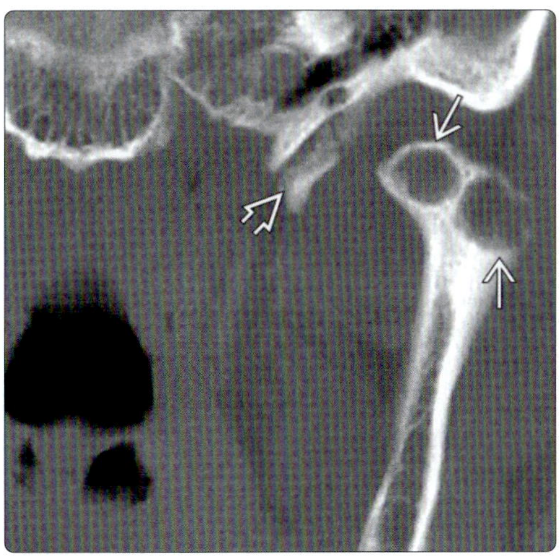

Osteosarcoma

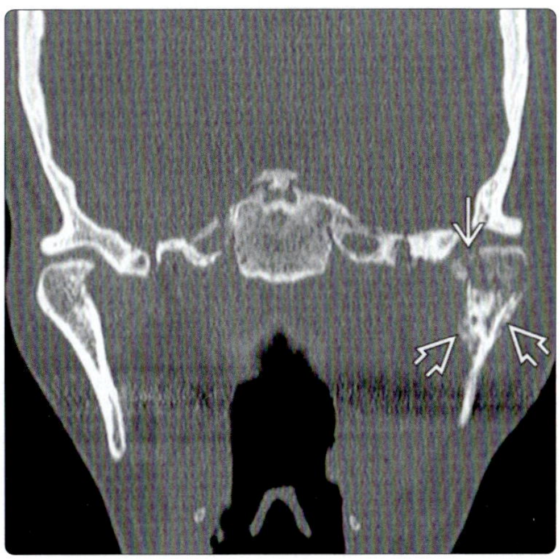

(Left) *Coronal bone CT of chondrosarcoma of the left condyle shows 2 well-defined corticated radiolucencies* ➡ *in the condyle that simulate simple bone cysts. Note calcifications* ⇨ *medial to the condyle and increased joint space, suggestive of soft tissue tumor extension.* **(Right)** *Coronal bone CT of osteosarcoma shows a permeative lytic appearance of the left condyle* ➡ *with associated pathological fracture. Note thickening and periosteal reactions* ⇨ *of the condylar neck.*

DIFFERENTIAL DIAGNOSIS

Common

- Subchondral Sclerosis
- Degenerative Joint Disease

Less Common

- Osteochondroma
- Osteoma
- Idiopathic Osteosclerosis
- Bony Ankylosis

Rare but Important

- Chondrosarcoma
- Osteosarcoma
- Metastatic Disease

ESSENTIAL INFORMATION

Key Differential Diagnosis Issues

- Determine if radiopacity is located within condyle, is exophytic, or effaces condylar outlines
  - DDx for opacity within condyle outlines
    - Subchondral sclerosis
    - Degenerative joint disease (DJD)
  - DDx for exophytic lesions
    - Osteoma
    - Osteochondroma
    - Bony ankylosis
    - DJD (proliferative variation)
  - Does opacity efface normal outlines of TMJ osseous components?
    - If yes, consider malignancy

Helpful Clues for Common Diagnoses

- **Subchondral Sclerosis**
  - **Key facts**
    - Adaptive change of TMJ components to forces acting upon them
    - Bone responds to excessive biomechanical forces by increasing trabeculation
    - May or may not be associated with degenerative changes
    - May be 1st indication that biomechanical forces have exceeded functional threshold
      - May indicate that fibrocartilaginous cap has broken down
      - Fibrocartilage acts as shock absorbent
      - Degenerative changes may subsequently ensue
  - **Imaging**
    - Increased bone density in normal or flattened (remodeled) TMJ osseous components
    - May appear as minimal thickening of articular surface cortex
      - Normal subchondral cortex under healthy fibrocartilage is eggshell thin
    - May appear as diffuse, irregular sclerosis of medullary portion of bone
    - Entire condylar process may increase in density with increased trabeculation in condyle and neck
    - Should differentiate from idiopathic osteosclerosis, which can occur independent of articular surfaces (such as condylar neck)
- **Degenerative Joint Disease**
  - **Key facts**
    - Localized, noninflammatory, degenerative disorder of synovial joints
    - Loss of articular fibrocartilage integrity after chronic disc displacement may result in subchondral sclerosis superimposed on other degenerative changes, such as erosions, subchondral bone cysts, and osteophytes
    - Proliferative DJD
      - Shows features of DJD with exophytic masses ± loose articular bodies
      - Differentiate from osteochondroma and osteoma
  - **Imaging**
    - Overgrowth of bone on condyle ± fossa without mass effect
    - Possible evidence of sclerosis, flattening, erosions, osteophytes, and subchondral (Ely) bone cyst and joint space narrowing
    - Condyle may appear radiopaque due to sclerosis or superimposition of osteophyte

Helpful Clues for Less Common Diagnoses

- **Osteochondroma**
  - **Key facts**
    - Cartilage-capped exophytic lesion arising from bone
    - Painless, hard swelling over TMJ with facial asymmetry
  - **Imaging**
    - Condyle appears radiopaque because lesion resembles enlarged sclerotic mass
    - Lesion cortex and internal aspect continuous with trabecular portion and cortex of originating bone
    - Osteochondromas usually originate from fibrocartilage-lined articular surfaces on condyle and eminence
      - Evaluate location in relation to normal osseous anatomy and histology to differentiate from osteomas
    - Osteochondromas tend to follow orientation of lateral pterygoid fibers
      - Differentiate from osteophytes in degenerative changes
- **Osteoma**
  - **Key facts**
    - Benign, slow-growing, bone-forming tumor characterized by proliferation of either compact or cancellous bone
    - Ipsilateral open bite if condyle involved
    - Must differentiate from osteochondroma
    - Multiple osteomas associated with Gardner syndrome
  - **Imaging**
    - Well-defined, bone-density lesion extending from condyle, condylar neck, or upper ramus
    - Osteomas originate from periosteum-lined surfaces
      - Evaluate location in relation to normal osseous anatomy and histology to differentiate from osteochondroma
    - May be corticated

- May simulate condylar radiopacity if lesion superimposed over condyle in 2D imaging
- Globular: Grow from wide base or attached to cortex by pedicle

- **Idiopathic Osteosclerosis**
  - **Key facts**
    - Localized area of increased bone density
    - Unknown cause
    - Not associated with inflammatory, neoplastic, or dysplastic processes
  - **Imaging**
    - Well-defined, nonexpansile, homogeneous high-density area within bone
    - Isodense to cortical bone
    - Blends with cortical bone; no low-density rim
- **Bony Ankylosis**
  - **Key facts**
    - Joint immobility characterized by formation of osseous mass fused to skull
    - Often secondary to trauma
      - Hematoma formation results in fibrosis and excessive bone formation
    - Fractured condyle may ankylose to temporal component of TMJ
    - Ankylosis can occur secondary to chronic inflammatory arthritides
  - **Imaging**
    - Markedly reduced or absent joint space
    - Irregular, enlarged joint margins with bony bridging
    - Condyle may appear radiopaque and enlarged with bony bridge to temporal bone
    - Associated changes
      - Elongation of coronoids
      - Deepened antegonial notch on affected side due to muscle function during attempted opening

Helpful Clues for Rare Diagnoses

- **Chondrosarcoma**
  - **Key facts**
    - Malignant tumor arising from cartilage cells
    - Preauricular swelling; may have pain, mandibular deviation, limitation of motion
  - **Imaging**
    - Appearance depends on degree of tumor calcification
    - Ringlet or flocculent pattern of calcification in and around condyle ± spiculated periosteal reaction
    - May be well defined and corticated or permeative
    - Often, erosion of articular fossa with involvement of infratemporal fossa, temporal bone, and middle cranial fossa
    - Soft tissue **mass**
- **Osteosarcoma**
  - **Key facts**
    - Malignant tumor of bone
    - Symptoms of TMJ dysfunction, preauricular swelling
  - **Imaging**
    - Can be radiolucent, mixed, or sclerotic
    - Poorly defined destructive lesion of condyle with cortical erosion
    - Condyle may be enlarged and composed of mottled bone pattern and spiculated periosteal reaction
- **Metastatic Disease**
  - **Key facts**
    - Breast, prostate, and lung mets may be radiopaque
    - Metastases to TMJ rare and usually unilateral
    - TMJ involvement usually associated with mandibular or generalized skeletal metastases
  - **Imaging**
    - May have sclerosis with poorly defined, invasive margins
    - Destruction of condyle
    - May have associated soft tissue mass
    - May see destruction of neighboring anatomic structures

SELECTED REFERENCES

1. Cömert Kiliç S et al: Temporomandibular joint osteoarthritis: cone beam computed tomography findings, clinical features, and correlations. Int J Oral Maxillofac Surg. 44(10):1268-74, 2015
2. Uchiyama Y et al: MRI in a case of osteosarcoma in the temporomandibular joint. Dentomaxillofac Radiol. 43(2):20130280, 2014

Subchondral Sclerosis

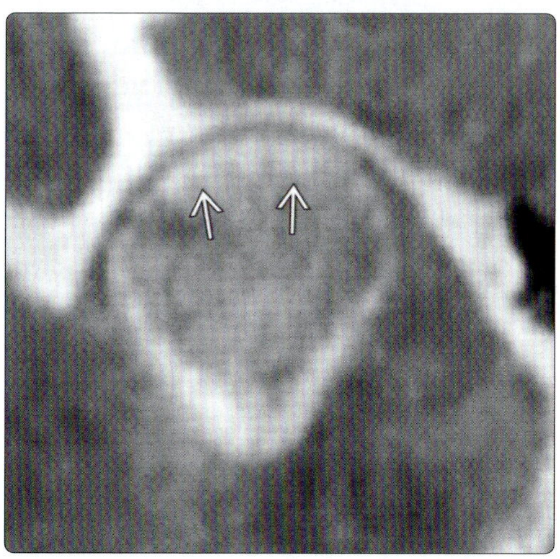

Subchondral Sclerosis

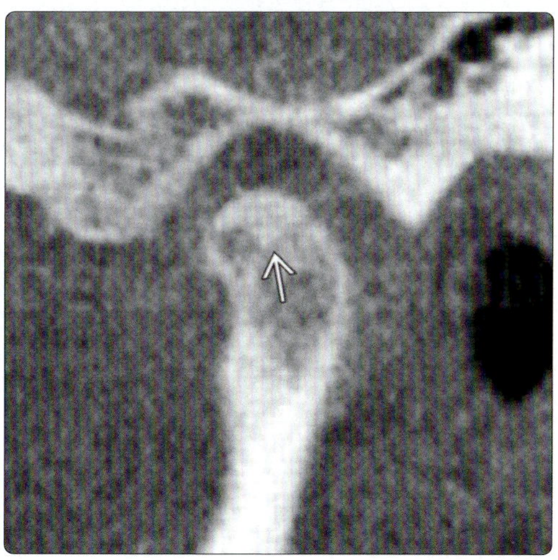

(Left) *Coronal oblique CBCT shows normal osseous contours of the condyle and the fossa with narrowing of the superior joint space, which may indicate disc displacement or thinning. There is thickening of the superior cortex ➡ of the articular surface of the condyle.* **(Right)** *Sagittal oblique CBCT shows normal osseous contours and spatial relationships of the TMJ osseous components with increased bone density ➡ noted beneath the subchondral surface of the condyle.*

(Left) *Coronal CBCT shows flattening ➡ and sclerosis ➡ of the condyle due to remodeling, which increases the surface area and bone density of the articulating surface.* (Right) *Coronal and sagittal CBCT of degenerative joint disease show an osteophyte ➡ extending from the anterior condylar surface. Coronal view shows diffuse sclerosis in center of condyle ➡ corresponding to the osteophyte and sclerosis.*

Degenerative Joint Disease

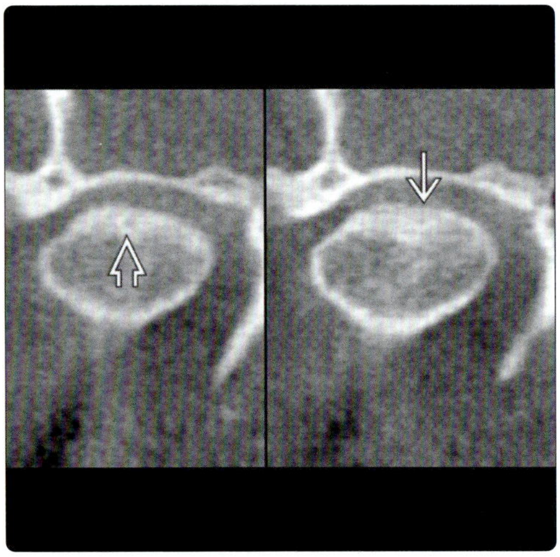

Degenerative Joint Disease

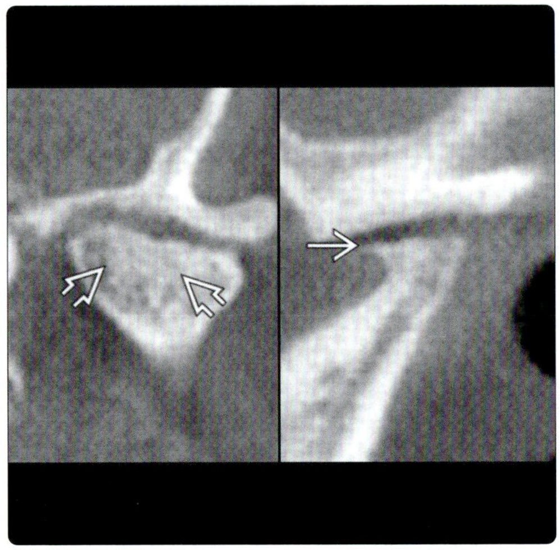

(Left) *Coronal oblique CBCT shows a condyle with proliferative degenerative changes. The articular surfaces are congruent, and the joint space is uniformly narrowed ➡. Exophytic bone ➡ is noted extending from the medial and lateral poles of the condyle without condylar displacement.* (Right) *Bone CT shows a sclerotic condyle and glenoid fossa. The sclerosis involves the temporal bone ➡ and ramus ➡ of the mandible. Extensive sclerosis can be seen with chronic degenerative joint disease.*

Degenerative Joint Disease

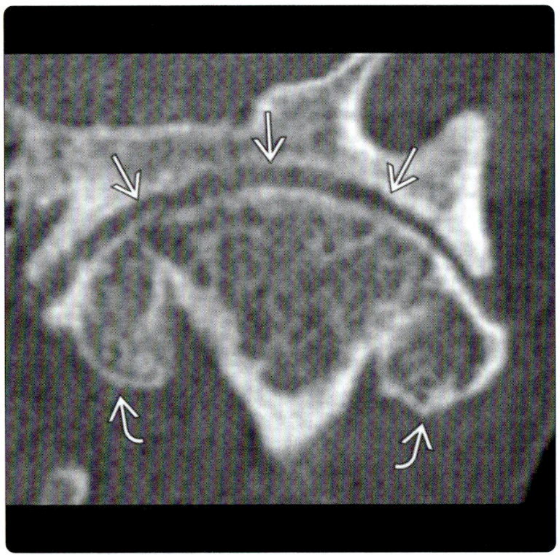

Degenerative Joint Disease

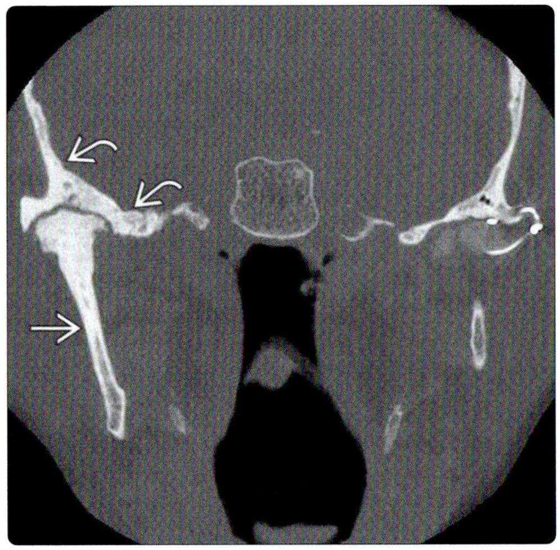

(Left) *Axial CBCT of the TMJ shows an osteochondroma ➡ extending medially from the anterior surface of the condyle. The lesion is continuous with the cortex of the condyle and could be confused with sclerosis if viewed in the coronal plane.* (Right) *Axial CBCT shows an osteoma ➡ extending from the posterior-lateral condylar surface. It arises from the cortex and is symmetric in shape. The condylar morphology is normal. (Courtesy M. Noujeim, DDS.)*

Osteochondroma

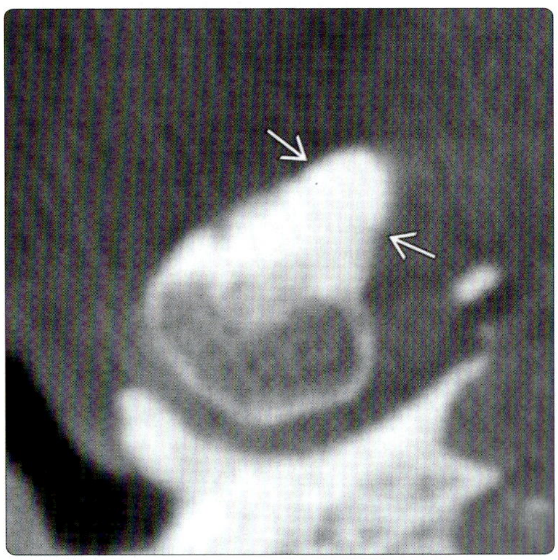

Osteoma

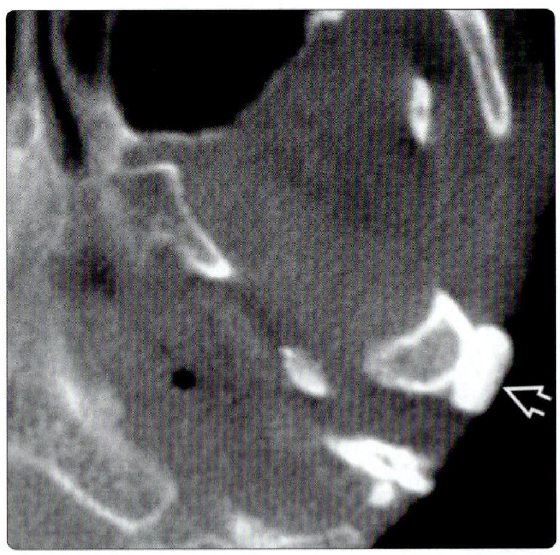

Idiopathic Osteosclerosis

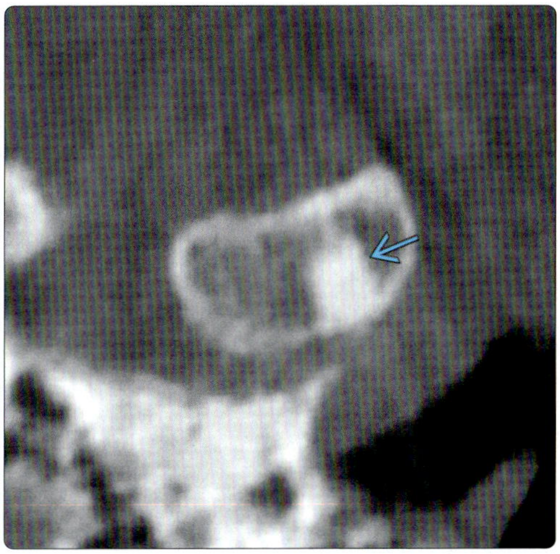

Idiopathic Osteosclerosis

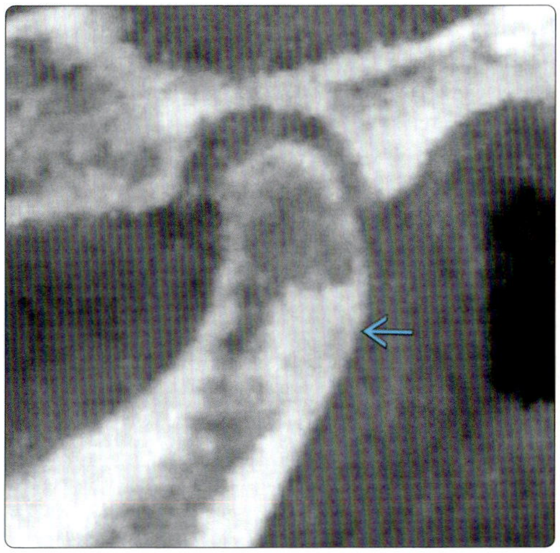

(Left) *Axial CBCT shows a homogeneous high-density area in the medullary bone of the left condyle. It is isodense to cortical bone and blends into the posterior cortex of the condyle. No osseous expansion is noted.* **(Right)** *Sagittal oblique CBCT in the same TMJ shows the high-density area blending into the posterior cortex of the condylar neck. This lesion should not be confused with subchondral sclerosis since this condylar neck lesion does not involve the articular surface of the condyle.*

Bony Ankylosis

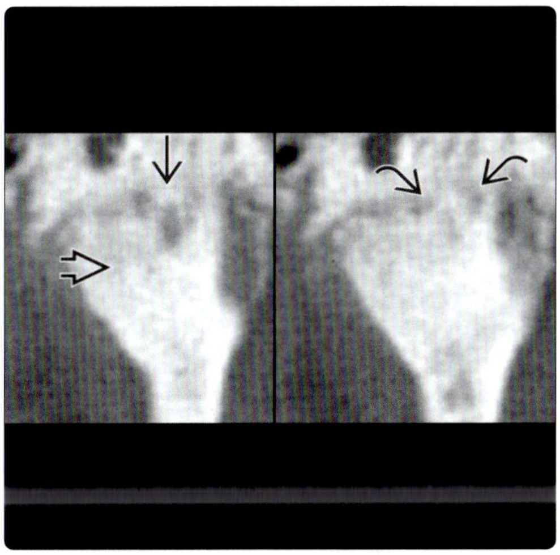

Chondrosarcoma

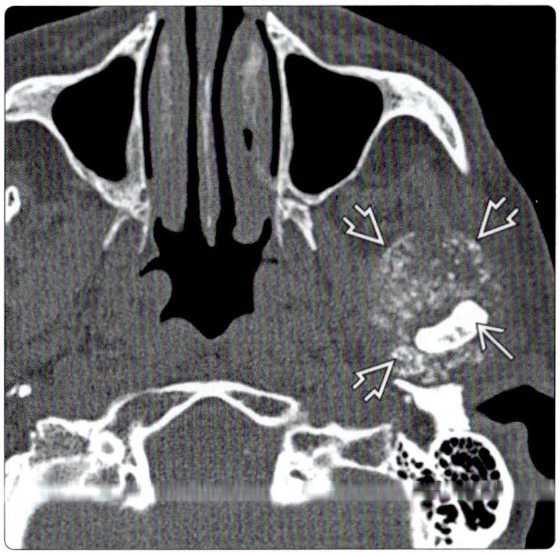

(Left) *Coronal CBCT images show bony ankylosis of the right condyle. There is a bony bridge between the condyle and glenoid fossa roof with severe condylar sclerosis and erosions.* **(Right)** *Axial bone CT of chondrosarcoma (CS) shows irregular sclerosis of the condyle surrounded by multiple flocculent calcifications. No periosteal reaction is noted. CS is often associated with erosion of the articular fossa with involvement of the infratemporal fossa, temporal bone, and middle cranial fossa.*

Osteosarcoma

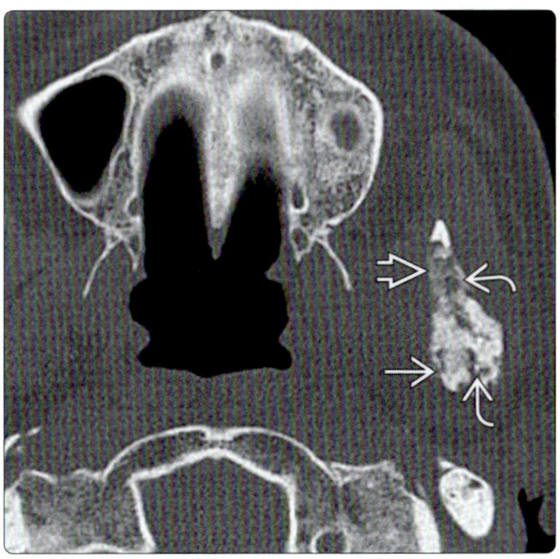

Metastatic Disease

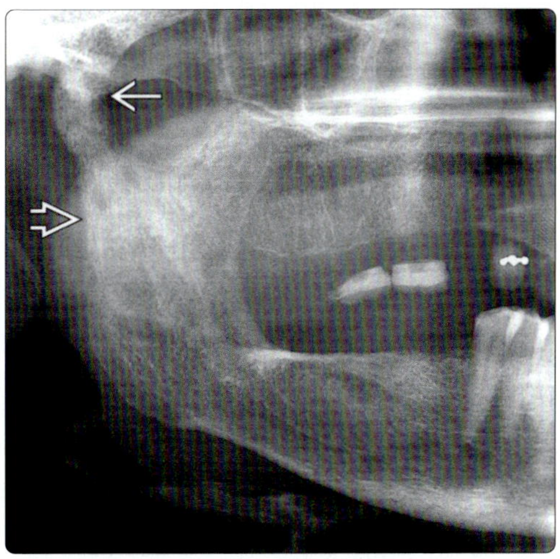

(Left) *Axial bone CT shows an osteosarcoma presenting as sclerosis and enlargement of the left condyle and condylar neck with areas of bone destruction.* **(Right)** *Panoramic radiograph shows breast metastases to the right mandible and TMJ. The condyle is sclerotic with patchy areas of destruction, and there is sclerosis of the ramus with loss of cortical boundaries. TMJ involvement is rare and usually associated with mandibular or generalized skeletal metastases.*

TMJ Articular Loose Bodies

DIFFERENTIAL DIAGNOSIS

Common

- Degenerative Joint Disease
- Calcified Cartilaginous External Auditory Canal

Less Common

- Calcium Pyrophosphate Deposition Disease
- Synovial Chondromatosis

Rare but Important

- Chondrosarcoma

ESSENTIAL INFORMATION

Key Differential Diagnosis Issues

- Condylar erosion and symptoms of temporomandibular dysfunction may be seen in all of these conditions
- Determine whether loose body is single or multiple

Helpful Clues for Common Diagnoses

- **Degenerative Joint Disease**
  - Key facts
    - Osteophyte may detach from condyle and lie free in joint space **("joint mouse")**
    - Joint mouse is usually single in contrast to other conditions in which multiple calcifications are seen
    - Secondary synovial chondromatosis may occur in degenerative joint disease, resulting in joint space radiopacity, and appear identical to joint mouse
  - Imaging
    - Joint mouse may be large or small
    - Joint mouse usually moves with condylar translation since it lies within joint space
    - Will see other degenerative changes, such as flattening, sclerosis, erosions, narrowed joint space
- **Calcified Cartilaginous External Auditory Canal**
  - Key facts
    - Cartilaginous external auditory canal (EAC) may calcify to various degrees
    - In close proximity to posterior aspect of condyle
      - Calcification should not be mistaken for loose articular bodies
  - Imaging
    - On CBCT sagittal oblique cross sections: Calcified linear or oval calcifications in anterior wall of EAC

Helpful Clues for Less Common Diagnoses

- **Calcium Pyrophosphate Deposition Disease**
  - Key facts
    - Calcium pyrophosphate crystals deposited in synovial fluid resulting in calcification of articular cartilage
  - Imaging
    - Fine cloud-like synovial calcifications with even distribution in joint space, often encircling condyle
    - Associated remodeling, erosion, or mass effect on condyle and adjacent structures
- **Synovial Chondromatosis**
  - Key facts
    - Synovial metaplasia with formation of hyaline cartilage foci
    - Can be primary or secondary (in response to degenerative changes, osteochondroma, or trauma)
  - Imaging
    - Soft tissue mass consisting of multiple calcified loose bodies in superior joint space
    - Degenerative changes of condylar articular surface (irregularity and sclerosis) may be seen in secondary synovial chondromatosis

Helpful Clues for Rare Diagnoses

- **Chondrosarcoma**
  - Key facts
    - Mass around condyle, often with erosion of articular fossa and condyle ± spiculated periosteal reaction
  - Imaging
    - Mass consists of ringlet pattern of calcification and radiolucent center in each radiopacity
    - Appearance varies depending on degree of tumor calcification
    - Destructive behavior and invasion

Degenerative Joint Disease

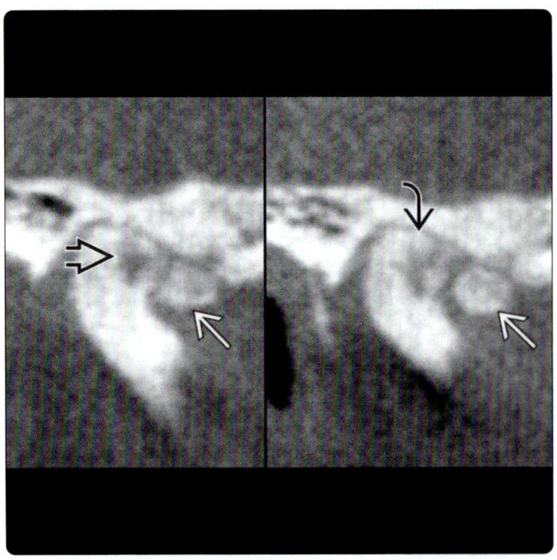

Calcified Cartilaginous External Auditory Canal

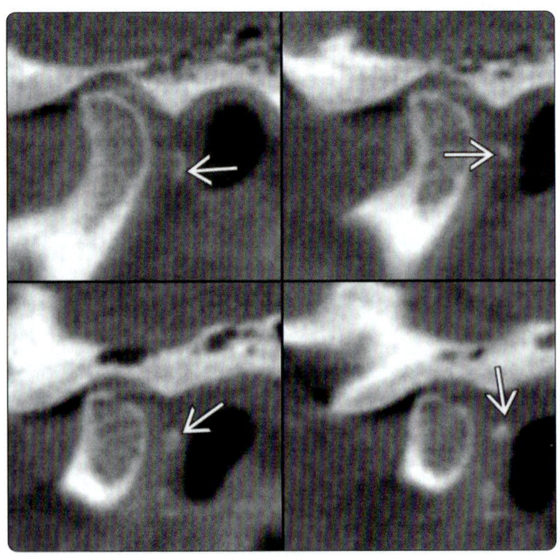

(Left) *Sagittal CBCT of degenerative joint disease shows a large "joint mouse" ➡ located anteriorly to the condyle. The condyle is sclerotic with a large subchondral erosion ⇨. The superior joint space ↷ is narrowed.* **(Right)** *Sagittal oblique cross sections of the left TMJ show calcification of the cartilaginous EAC that may appear radiographically as calcified, loose articular bodies ➡. The location of the calcifications, which are an anatomic variant, is in the anterior wall of the EAC and not in the joint spaces.*

Calcium Pyrophosphate Deposition Disease

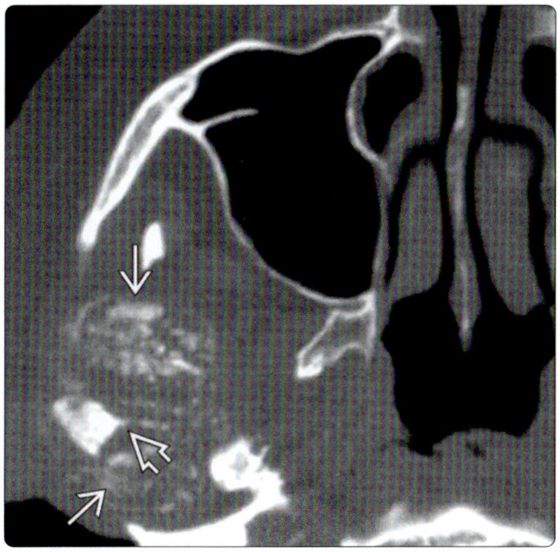

Calcium Pyrophosphate Deposition Disease

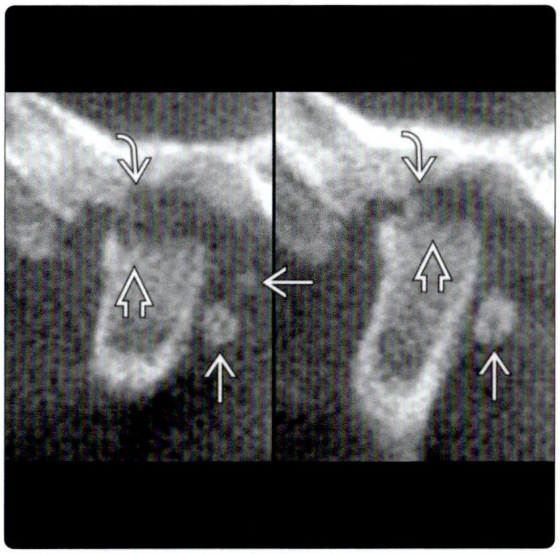

(Left) *Axial bone CT of calcium pyrophosphate deposition disease (CPPD) shows a well-defined mass ➡ anterior and posterior to the right condyle. Calcifications within the mass are fine and evenly distributed. A large radiolucent erosive defect ➡ is visible at the medial aspect of the condyle.* **(Right)** *Sagittal CBCT reformats of CPPD disease of the left TMJ show large radiopaque masses ➡ in the joint space and erosions of the condyle ➡ and fossa ➡ with sclerosis. The masses should not be confused with calcified EAC cartilage.*

Synovial Chondromatosis

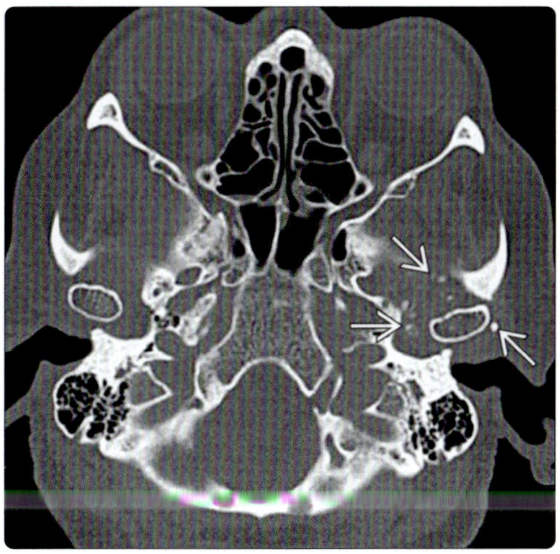

Synovial Chondromatosis

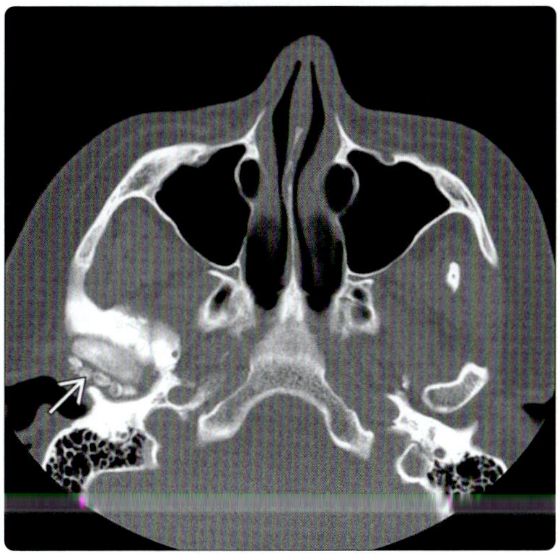

(Left) *Axial bone CT of synovial chondromatosis in the left TMJ shows a mass with multiple punctate calcifications ➡ anterior and posterior to the condyle. The uneven distribution helps to distinguish this from CPPD disease.* **(Right)** *Axial bone CT of synovial chondromatosis shows multiple calcified nodules posterior to the right condyle ➡. The nodules are discrete and relatively large with an irregular shape and may be difficult to distinguish from those seen in CPPD disease.*

Chondrosarcoma

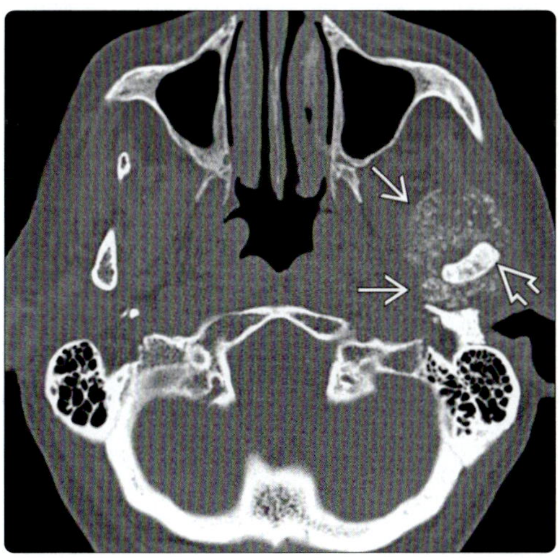

Chondrosarcoma

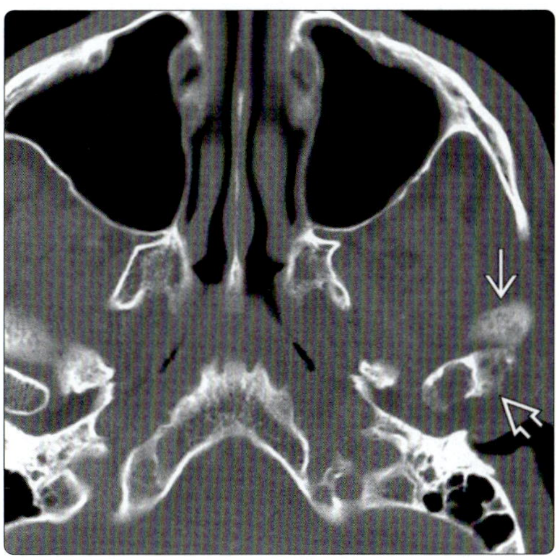

(Left) *Axial bone CT of chondrosarcoma in the left TMJ shows multiple flocculent calcifications ➡ around the condyle and irregular sclerosis ➡ of the condyle.* **(Right)** *Axial bone CT of chondrosarcoma in the left TMJ shows fine calcifications ➡ anterior and lateral to the condyle. These have the appearance of a solid mass. There is bone destruction of the condyle, and the lateral aspect is expanded ➡.*

PART III
SECTION 5

Maxillary Sinus and Nasal Cavity

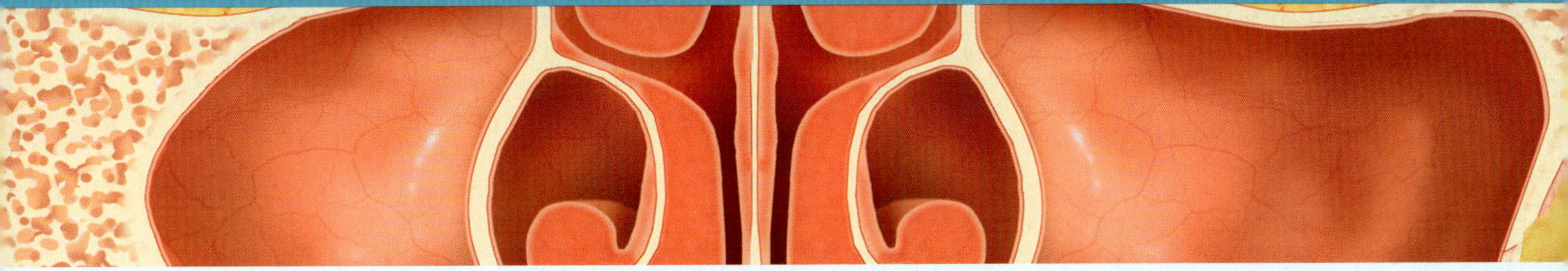

Nasal Lesions

Perforated Nasal Septum 964
Nasal Lesion Without Bony Destruction 966
Nasal Lesion With Bony Destruction 970
Sinonasal Fibroosseous and Cartilaginous Lesions 974

Sinus Lesions

Paranasal Sinus Lesions Without Bony Destruction 976
Paranasal Sinus Lesions With Bony Destruction 980

Miscellaneous

Displaced Dental Structures Into Antrum 984

Perforated Nasal Septum

DIFFERENTIAL DIAGNOSIS

Common

- Trauma
- Rhinitis Medicamentosa (Topical Nasal Spray Overuse)
- Cocaine Necrosis, Nose
- Granulomatosis With Polyangiitis, Sinonasal

Less Common

- Fungal Sinusitis, Invasive
- Sarcoidosis, Sinonasal
- Squamous Cell Carcinoma, Sinonasal
- Non-Hodgkin Lymphoma, Sinonasal
- Hexavalent (Cr VI) or Trivalent Arsenic (As III) Exposure

Rare but Important

- Melanoma, Sinonasal
- Syphilis
- Nasal Septal Abscess
- Ruthenium and Platinum Salts, Mercury Fulminate, Cement Exposure

ESSENTIAL INFORMATION

Key Differential Diagnosis Issues

- Insult to mucoperichondrium compromises blood supply to septal quadrangular cartilage leading to ischemic necrosis
- Trauma and inhaled substances more common than infectious/neoplastic etiologies
- Patient history important to determine potential cause

Helpful Clues for Common Diagnoses

- **Trauma**
  - Septal fracture → hematoma → ischemic necrosis **or** mucosal laceration with cartilage exposure
  - Iatrogenic: Postseptoplasty, intubation, packing, transsphenoid and modified Lothrop surgeries
  - Habitual (nose picking)
  - Jewelry magnet compression and cosmetic piercing
- **Rhinitis Medicamentosa (Topical Nasal Spray Overuse)**
  - Vasoconstrictive and steroid nasal sprays cause ischemic necrosis
- **Cocaine Necrosis, Nose**
  - Vasoconstriction leads to ischemic necrosis; chemical irritants damage mucosa
- **Granulomatosis With Polyangiitis, Sinonasal**
  - Vasculitis and necrotizing granulomatous disorder; nodular soft tissue erodes septum and turbinates

Helpful Clues for Less Common Diagnoses

- **Fungal Sinusitis, Invasive**
  - Angioinvasion compromises blood supply or fungi directly invade septum
- **Sarcoidosis, Sinonasal**
  - Granulomatous disease similar to Wegener on imaging
- **Squamous Cell Carcinoma, Sinonasal**
  - 30-35% arise in nasal cavity and invade septum
- **Non-Hodgkin Lymphoma, Sinonasal**
  - Prefers nasal cavity over sinuses
  - Dense on CT, ↓ T2 signal on MR
- **Hexavalent (Cr VI) or Trivalent Arsenic (As III) Exposure**
  - History of occupational exposure
  - Chrome holes (ulcers on hands and arms) for chromium

Helpful Clues for Rare Diagnoses

- **Melanoma, Sinonasal**
  - Nasal cavity preferred site of origin; may remodel or destroy septum
    - MR: ↑ T1, ↓ T2 signal
- **Syphilis**
  - Affects bony septum rather than cartilaginous portion
- **Nasal Septal Abscess**
  - Etiologies: Superinfected hematoma, sinusitis, or dental
- **Ruthenium and Platinum Salts, Mercury Fulminate, Cement Exposure**
  - History of occupational exposure

SELECTED REFERENCES

1. Boynuegri S et al: The effect of nasal septal perforation and its treatment on objective sleep and breathing parameters. Med Sci Monit. 22:501-7, 2016

Trauma

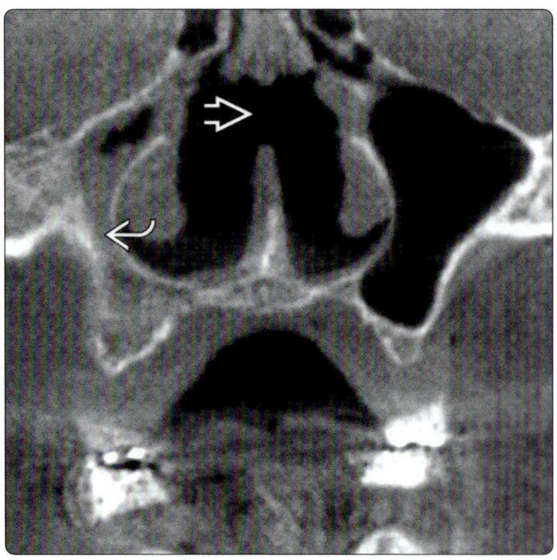

Trauma

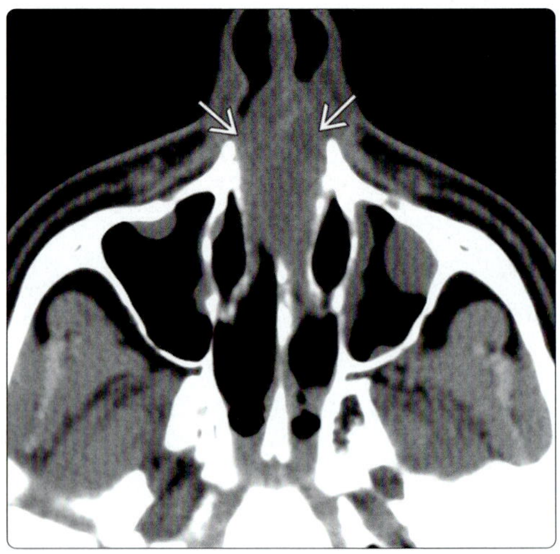

(Left) *Coronal CBCT shows post chronic sinusitis surgical perforation of the septum ➡. There is sinusitis in the right maxillary sinus ↩.* **(Right)** *Axial NECT shows an expansile lesion ➡ involving the cartilaginous and bony nasal septum, clinically consistent with a hematoma, although not hyperdense on CT. The hematoma is a result of trauma to the area. (Courtesy W. Smoker, MD.)*

Cocaine Necrosis, Nose

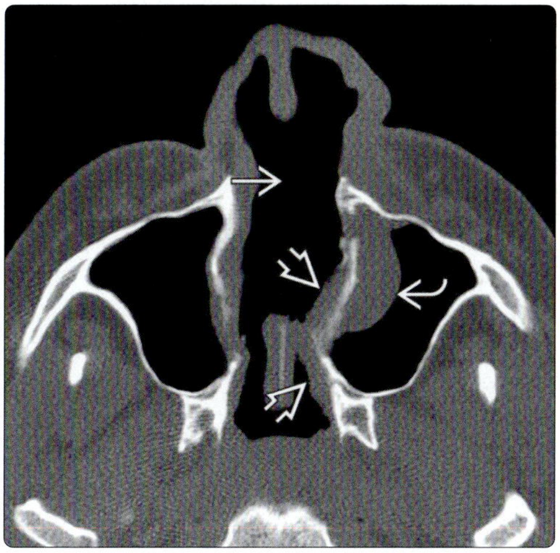

Granulomatosis With Polyangiitis, Sinonasal

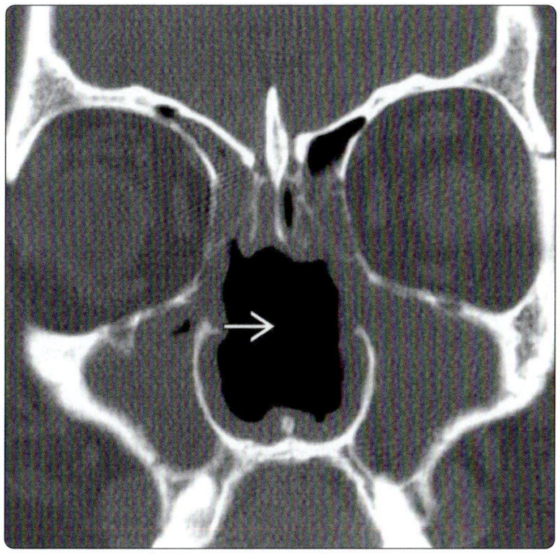

(Left) *Axial bone CT shows a very large perforation of the cartilaginous and bony nasal septum* ➡ *related to cocaine abuse. Mucosal thickening is noted in the nasal cavity* ➡ *and maxillary antrum* ➡*.* **(Right)** *Coronal bone CT shows a large septal perforation* ➡ *in a patient with Wegener granulomatosis. There is middle and inferior turbinate erosion. Soft tissue thickening is present in the adjacent maxillary sinuses.*

Fungal Sinusitis, Invasive

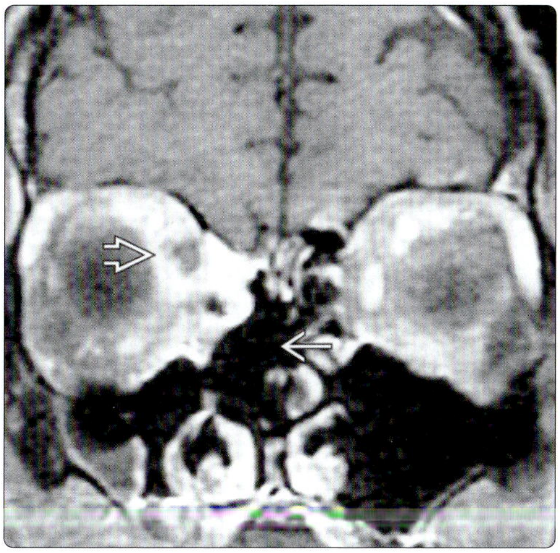

Sarcoidosis, Sinonasal

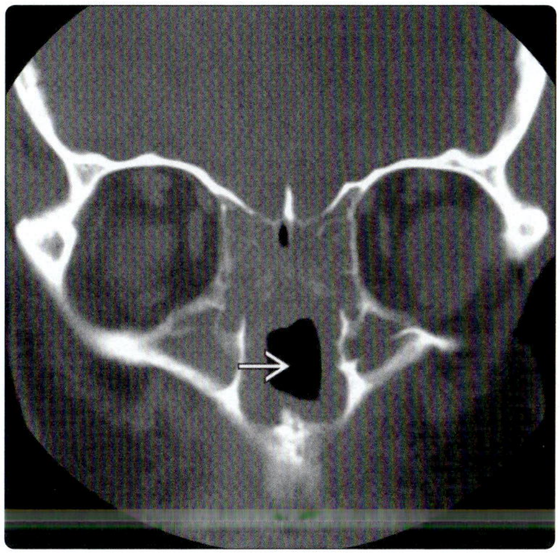

(Left) *Coronal T1 C+ FS MR shows a septal perforation* ➡ *related to invasive fungal sinusitis. Disease persists in the right ethmoid sinuses, and there is extension into the orbit* ➡*.* **(Right)** *Coronal bone CT shows extensive sinus opacification and nasal cavity soft tissue thickening in a sarcoidosis patient. A large septal perforation is present anteriorly* ➡*.*

Squamous Cell Carcinoma, Sinonasal

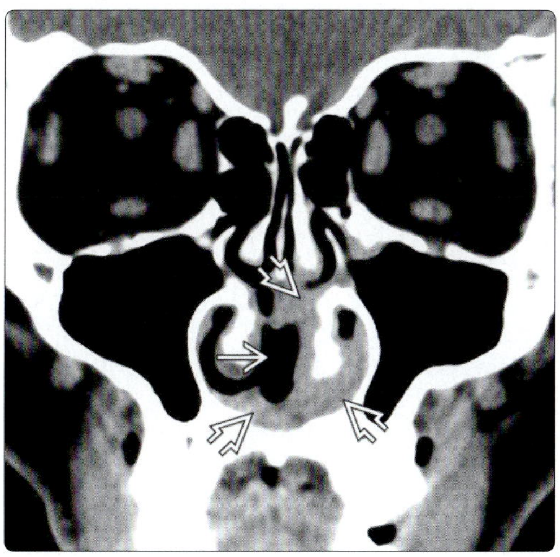

Nasal Septal Abscess

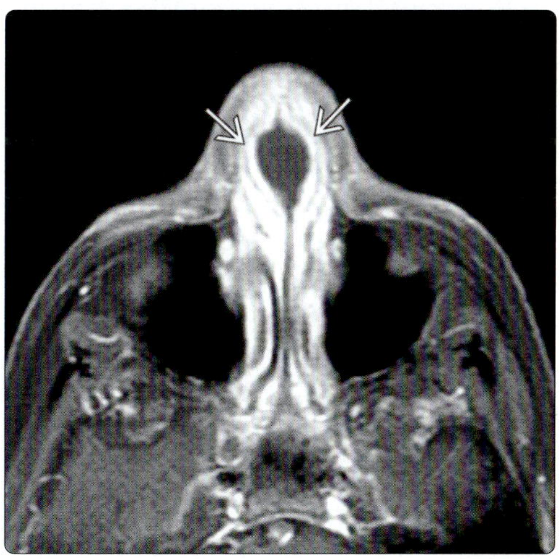

(Left) *Coronal NECT shows inferior nasal septal perforation* ➡ *related to erosion caused by a squamous carcinoma* ➡ *of the floor of the nasal cavity and inferior turbinate.* **(Right)** *Axial T1 C+ FS MR shows a nasal septal abscess. There is peripheral enhancement of the septal abscess wall* ➡ *with central hypointense signal consistent with pus.*

DIFFERENTIAL DIAGNOSIS

Common

- Polyposis, Sinonasal
- Fungal Sinusitis, Allergic
- Polyps, Solitary, Sinonasal
- Juvenile Angiofibroma
- Inverted Papilloma, Sinonasal
- Fibrous Dysplasia, Craniofacial Type

Less Common

- Osteoma, Sinonasal
- Nasolacrimal Duct Cyst/Dacryocystocele
- Arteriovenous Vascular Malformation, Sinonasal
- Benign Mixed Tumor, Sinonasal
- Rhinolith
- Non-Hodgkin Lymphoma, Sinonasal

Rare but Important

- Nerve Sheath Tumor, Sinonasal
- Melanoma, Sinonasal
- Giant Cell Granuloma, Mandible-Maxilla

ESSENTIAL INFORMATION

Key Differential Diagnosis Issues

- Patient demographics and findings at nasal endoscopy very helpful for narrowing differential diagnosis
- Imaging suggestions
  - CT most useful for visualizing bone remodeling produced by these lesions
  - MR helpful for further characterizing lesions (signal characteristics, vascularity, architecture, presence of mucoid material or melanin)
    - For lesions in superior nasal cleft with possible cribriform plate erosion, MR indicated to evaluate for intracranial extension & to exclude cephalocele
- In pediatric population, congenital lesions may also present as nasal mass without bone destruction
  - Nasal dermal sinus, nasal glioma, & nasoethmoid cephaloceles included here

Helpful Clues for Common Diagnoses

- **Polyposis, Sinonasal**
  - Key facts: Patient > 20 years, often with history of allergies; when lesion large & expansile, can produce significant cosmetic deformity
  - Imaging: Usually involves nasal cavity and paranasal sinuses; multiple and bilateral; anterior > posterior
    - Predominantly along lateral nasal wall & roof of nasal cavity
- **Fungal Sinusitis, Allergic**
  - Key facts: Severe form of chronic rhinosinusitis most often seen in young adults
  - Imaging: Unilateral or bilateral sinonasal opacification; multiple sinuses involved
    - CT: Central hyperdensity with low attenuation peripherally
    - MR: Signal variable on T1 related to protein/water content; hypointense/signal void on T2
- **Polyps, Solitary, Sinonasal**
  - Key facts: Teenager or young adult with unilateral nasal obstruction
  - Imaging: Well-defined, dumbbell-shaped lesion arising from antrum; widens middle meatus and extends into nasal cavity
    - CT: Mucoid density, rarely osseous metaplasia occurs
    - MR: Low T1 and high T2 signal with peripheral enhancement
- **Juvenile Angiofibroma**
  - Key facts: Adolescent male patient presenting with unilateral nasal obstruction and epistaxis; vascular lesion in nasal cavity on endoscopy
  - Imaging: On CT, appears as enhancing mass centered at sphenopalatine foramen with nasal cavity, nasopharyngeal, and pterygopalatine fossa extension; bone remodeling or erosion may be present
    - MR: Hyperintense on T2; salt & pepper appearance due to flow voids on T2 or postcontrast T1 sequences
- **Inverted Papilloma, Sinonasal**
  - Key facts: Male patient, 40-70 years of age; polypoid mass centered on lateral nasal wall near middle meatus
  - Imaging: On CT involves both nasal cavity and maxillary antrum; may contain Ca++ and erode and remodel bone
    - Typically along lateral nasal wall centered at middle meatus ± extension into maxillary sinus
    - MR: Convoluted cerebriform architecture
- **Fibrous Dysplasia, Craniofacial Type**
  - Key facts: Usually < 20 years old, more common in females
    - Enlargement of associated bones may compromise nasal airway
  - Imaging: Altered bone pattern toward ground-glass appearance on plain radiographs, granular on CT

Helpful Clues for Less Common Diagnoses

- **Osteoma, Sinonasal**
  - Key facts: Located more commonly in paranasal sinuses than nasal cavity
  - Imaging: On CT, attaches to or arises within bones surrounding sinonasal cavities
    - Cortical (dense) type is classic, but density variable due to mixture of fibrous and osseous components
    - Cancellous type has mixture of more and less dense areas like cancellous bone
    - MR: T2 hypointense
- **Nasolacrimal Duct Cyst/Dacryocystocele**
  - Key facts: Located anywhere along nasolacrimal apparatus from lacrimal sac to inferior meatus (valve of Hasner)
    - Usually in inferior part of duct or meatus as congenital lesion in newborns but have been found in adults
    - May cause nasal obstruction; serious in neonates who are obligate nasal breathers
  - Imaging: On CT/MR, mucoid or fluid density/signal; expands nasolacrimal duct; cystic mass at sac or inferior meatus
- **Arteriovenous Vascular Malformation, Sinonasal**
  - Key facts: Soft, red-blue mass usually in anterior nasal cavity arising from septum near Kiesselbach venous plexus; more common in pediatric population
  - Imaging: On CT, remodels adjacent bone; intraosseous form has more permeative, lytic appearance

- MR: T2 hyperintense; diffuse enhancement
- May require histopathology to differentiate arteriovenous vascular malformation (AVM) from hemangioma
  - Nerve bundles consistently found in AVM and absent in hemangiomas
- AVMs may present with continuous loud roaring murmur and palpable thrill

- **Benign Mixed Tumor, Sinonasal**
  - Key facts: Arises from minor rests of salivary tissue in nasal cavity or palate mucosa
  - Imaging: Well-defined mass; may contain Ca++ on CT; T2 hyperintensity characteristic on MR with variable enhancement
- **Rhinolith**
  - Key facts: Usually found in children, but are seen in adults
    - Often found incidentally on panoramic, occlusal, and lateral skull radiographs made for other dental treatment
    - May present with chronic purulent rhinitis; imaging often not necessary
  - Imaging: Standard occlusal and lateral skull radiographs are best imaging study
    - As calcium is deposited on foreign body or inspissated mucus, rhinoliths are radiopaque
    - Less radiation than more advanced imaging techniques
    - CBCT preferred over CT because of ↓ radiation
- **Non-Hodgkin Lymphoma, Sinonasal**
  - Key facts: Most common in older patients; prefers nasal cavity origin over paranasal sinuses
  - Imaging: On CT, although malignant, this tumor may show bone remodeling &/or bone destruction
    - MR: Homogeneous; decreased T2 signal; homogeneous enhancement

Helpful Clues for Rare Diagnoses

- **Nerve Sheath Tumor, Sinonasal**
  - MR: Well-circumscribed mass with variable signal & enhancement; schwannoma most common
- **Melanoma, Sinonasal**
  - Key facts: Nasal cavity site of origin more common than paranasal sinus
  - Imaging: On CT, although malignant, this tumor may show bone remodeling &/or bone destruction
    - MR: T1 shortening in highly melanotic form (blood products, melanin); T2 hypointense (blood products, melanin, free radicals)
- **Giant Cell Granuloma, Mandible-Maxilla**
  - Key facts: Nonodontogenic tumor occurring only in maxilla and mandible; benign, expansile lesion, most commonly anterior mandible
  - Imaging: On CBCT or CT, well-defined soft tissue mass arising from maxilla with expansion into nasal cavity; loculations, if present, orient at right angles to outer cortex

SELECTED REFERENCES

1. Breik O et al: Survival outcomes of mucosal melanoma in the head and neck: case series and review of current treatment guidelines. J Oral Maxillofac Surg. ePub, 2016
2. Cahill KN et al: Impaired E prostanoid2 expression and resistance to prostaglandin E2 in nasal polyp fibroblasts from subjects with aspirin-exacerbated respiratory eisease. Am J Respir Cell Mol Biol. 54(1):34-40, 2016
3. Houette A et al: Prognostic value of two tumour staging classifications in patients with sinonasal mucosal melanoma. Eur Ann Otorhinolaryngol Head Neck Dis. ePub, 2016
4. Jalilvand S et al: The prevalence of human papillomavirus infection in Iranian patients with sinonasal inverted papilloma. J Chin Med Assoc. 79(3):137-40, 2016
5. Lisan Q et al: Sinonasal inverted papilloma: From diagnosis to treatment. Eur Ann Otorhinolaryngol Head Neck Dis. ePub, 2016
6. Lombardi D et al: Sinonasal mucosal melanoma: A 12-year experience of 58 cases. Head Neck. 38 Suppl 1:E1737-45, 2016
7. Nicolae V et al: Clinical and histological aspects of malignant inverted sinonasal papilloma. Two case reports. Rom J Morphol Embryol. 57(1):289-94, 2016
8. Roh HJ et al: Smoking, not human papilloma virus infection, is a risk factor for recurrence of sinonasal inverted papilloma. Am J Rhinol Allergy. 30(2):79-82, 2016
9. Samstein RM et al: Localized sinonasal mucosal melanoma: Outcomes and associations with stage, radiotherapy, and positron emission tomography response. Head Neck. ePub, 2016
10. Adegboyega PA et al: Hemangioma versus vascular malformation: presence of nerve bundle is a diagnostic clue for vascular malformation. Arch Pathol Lab Med. 129(6):772-5, 2005

Polyposis, Sinonasal

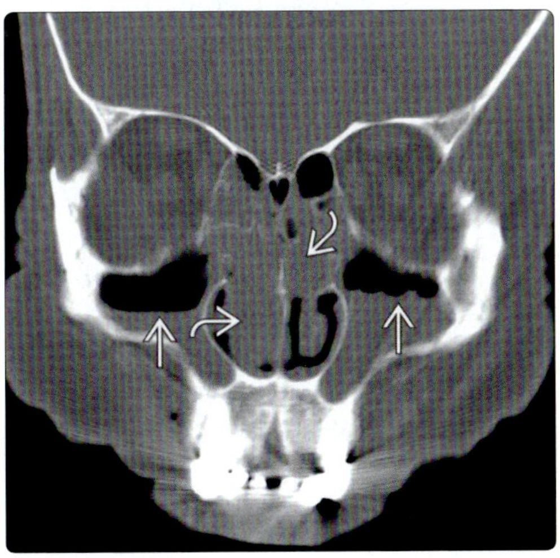

Fungal Sinusitis, Allergic

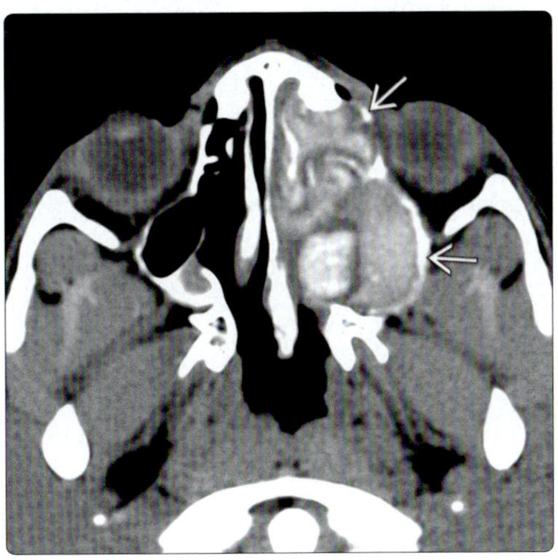

(Left) *Coronal bone CT shows diffuse sinonasal polyposis with bilateral nasal polyps* ➡ *and sinus mucosal thickening. There are maxillary fluid levels* ➡ *consistent with acute inflammation.* **(Right)** *Axial NECT shows the typical appearance of allergic fungal sinusitis. Note unilateral expansion of the sinonasal cavities* ➡ *with central increased density and peripheral low-density material.*

(Left) *Axial T1 C+ MR shows a solitary sinonasal (antrochoanal) polyp extending from the maxillary antrum through the middle meatus into the nasal cavity and nasopharynx.* **(Right)** *Axial CECT shows a small juvenile angiofibroma of the left nasal cavity projecting into the nasopharynx. Taken early in the injection, this image shows that the tumor enhances before the muscles enhance.*

Polyps, Solitary, Sinonasal

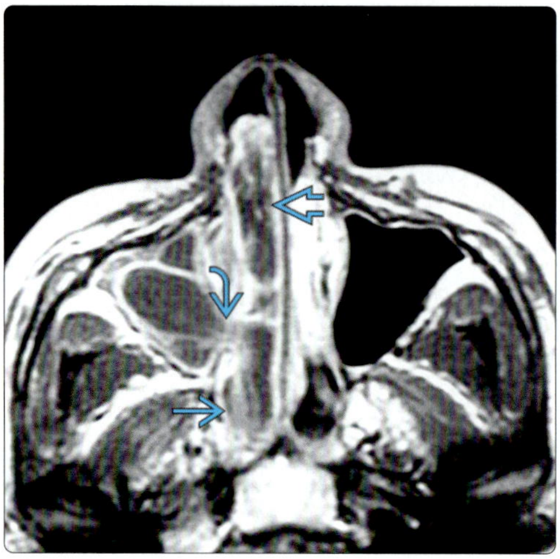

Juvenile Angiofibroma

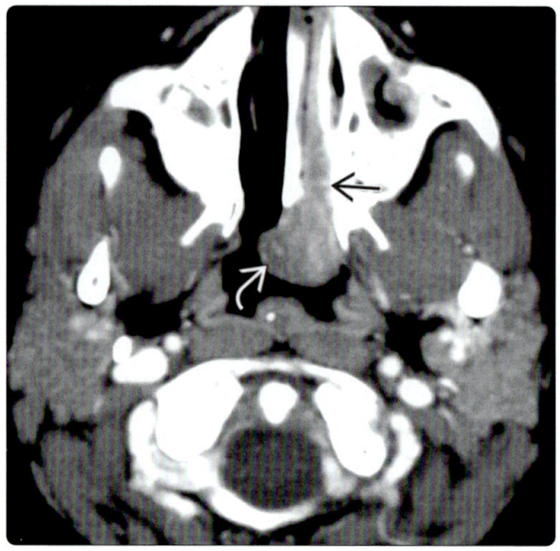

(Left) *Coronal bone CT shows an inverted papilloma arising near the middle meatus and extending into the maxillary antrum. The septum is slightly deviated toward the left.* **(Right)** *Coronal bone CT shows an osteoma of the left nasal cavity. This osteoma originated from the middle concha and is of mixed bone and soft tissue density.*

Inverted Papilloma, Sinonasal

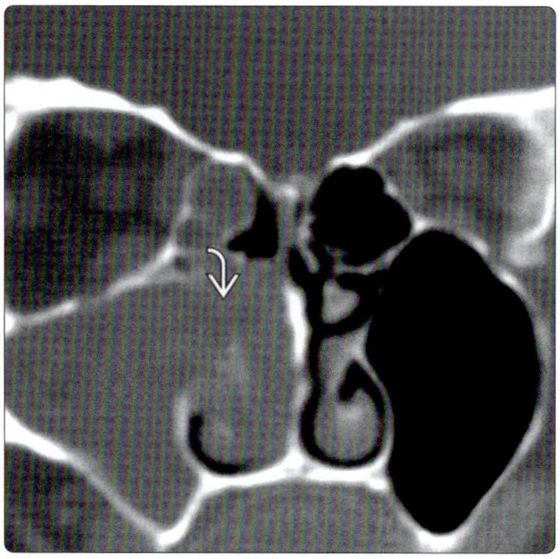

Osteoma, Sinonasal

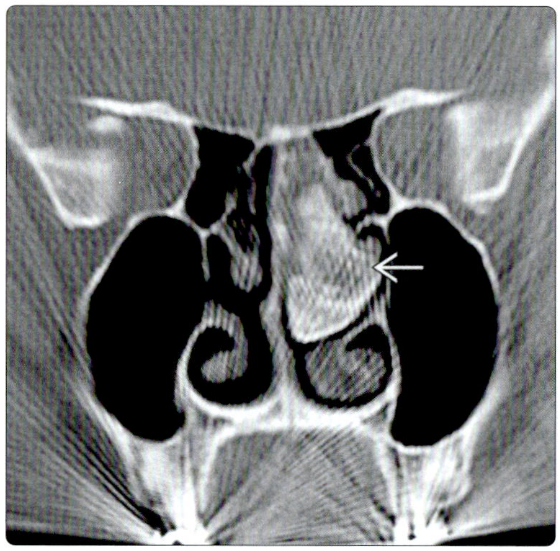

(Left) *Coronal bone CT shows a nasolacrimal cyst with expansion of the right nasolacrimal duct and extension to the level of the inferior meatus just beneath the inferior turbinate.* **(Right)** *Coronal CECT shows the features of a posterior nasal cavity arteriovenous vascular malformation in an adult patient. Note the well-circumscribed, lobular, enhancing mass in the left nasal cavity at the choana.*

Nasolacrimal Duct Cyst/Dacryocystocele

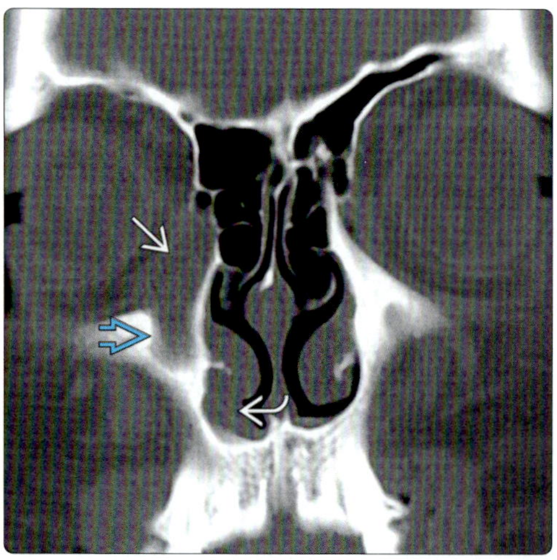

Arteriovenous Vascular Malformation, Sinonasal

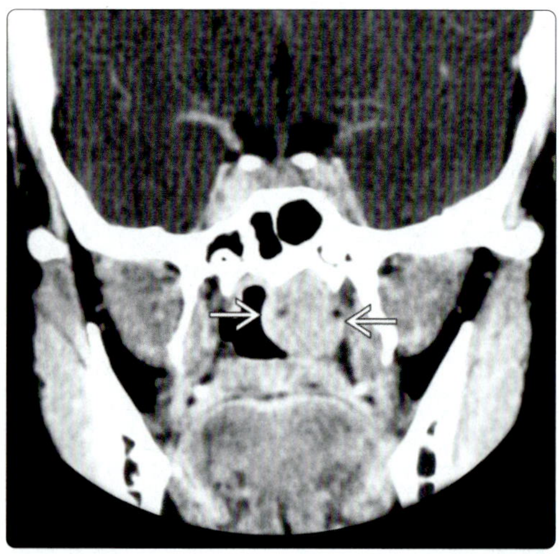

Benign Mixed Tumor, Sinonasal

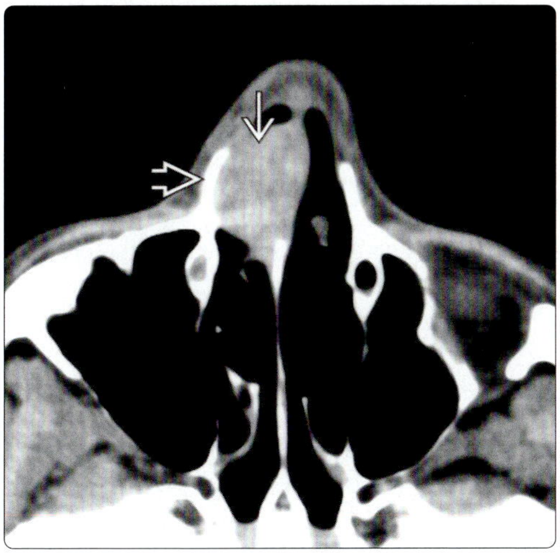

Rhinolith

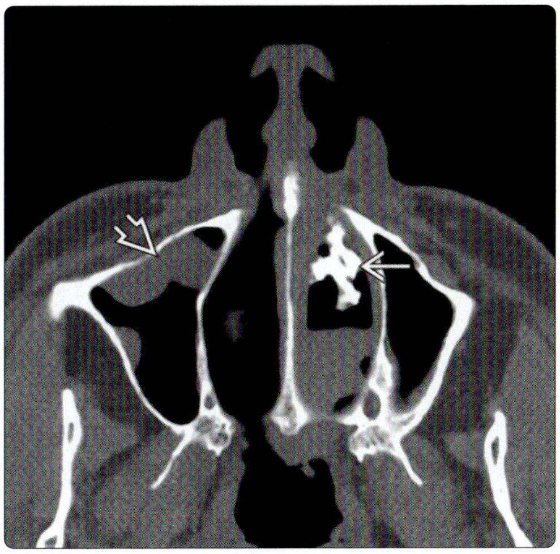

(Left) *Axial NECT shows a benign mixed tumor (pleomorphic adenoma) in the right nasal vestibule ➡ arising from the septum. There is slight remodeling of the nasal process of the maxilla ➡.* **(Right)** *Axial bone CT shows an irregular, dense rhinolith in the left nasal cavity ➡. Mucosal thickening is noted in the alveolar recess of the right maxillary sinus ➡.*

Non-Hodgkin Lymphoma, Sinonasal

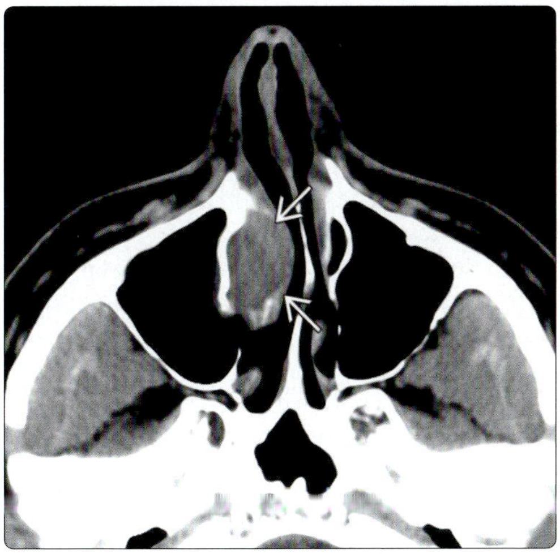

Nerve Sheath Tumor, Sinonasal

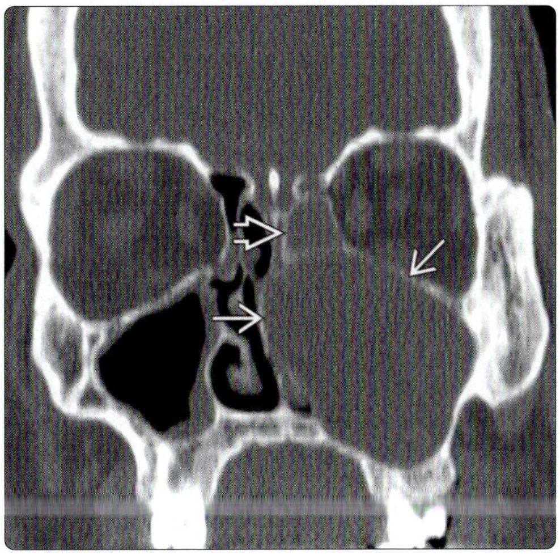

(Left) *Axial NECT shows a homogeneous soft tissue mass ➡ in the right nasal cavity at the level of the inferior meatus. This lymphoma of the nasolacrimal duct expands the surrounding bone.* **(Right)** *Coronal bone CT shows a neurofibroma within the left maxillary sinus. There is remodeling of the sinus walls ➡. Obstructed secretions are noted in the left ethmoid sinuses ➡.*

Melanoma, Sinonasal

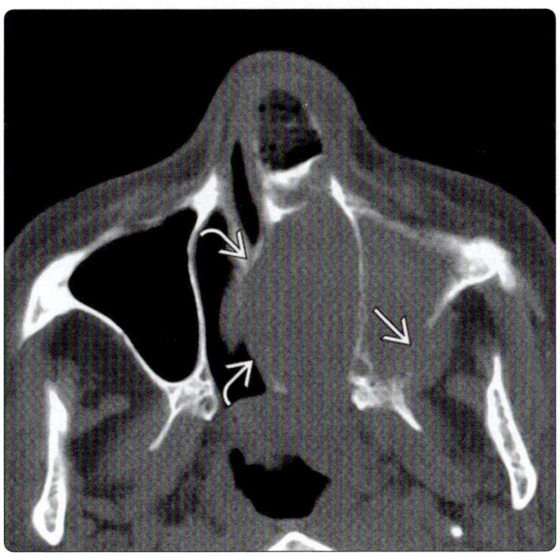

Giant Cell Granuloma, Mandible-Maxilla

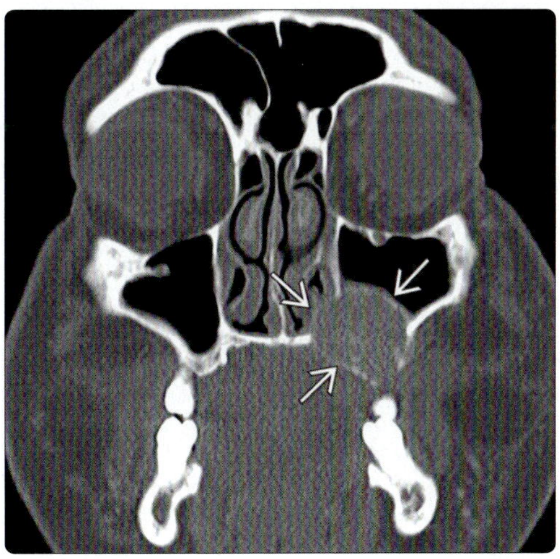

(Left) *Axial bone CT shows a sinonasal melanoma with both bone remodeling ➡ and destruction ➡. Although highly malignant, melanoma may show benign changes within surrounding bone.* **(Right)** *Coronal bone CT shows a maxillary alveolar giant cell granuloma bulging into the left nasal cavity. A thin rim of intact bone is seen at the periphery of the lesion ➡.*

Nasal Lesion With Bony Destruction

DIFFERENTIAL DIAGNOSIS

Common

- Squamous Cell Carcinoma, Sinonasal
- Non-Hodgkin Lymphoma, Sinonasal
- Inverted Papilloma, Sinonasal
- Fungal Sinusitis, Invasive
- Esthesioneuroblastoma

Less Common

- Granulomatosis With Polyangiitis, Sinonasal
- Adenocarcinoma, Sinonasal
- Undifferentiated Carcinoma, Sinonasal
- Sarcoidosis, Sinonasal
- Juvenile Angiofibroma
- Melanoma, Sinonasal

Rare but Important

- Chondrosarcoma, Sinonasal
- Osteosarcoma, Sinonasal
- Rhabdomyosarcoma, Sinonasal
- Langerhans Histiocytosis, Skull Base
- Plasmacytoma, Skull Base
- Metastasis, Mandible-Maxilla

ESSENTIAL INFORMATION

Key Differential Diagnosis Issues

- Knowledge of patient demographics and clinical history is critical for narrowing differential diagnosis
- Presenting symptoms may be nonspecific and mimic chronic rhinosinusitis
- Best imaging tools
    - Sinonasal CT without contrast to identify Ca++ and early cortical bone destruction
    - Enhanced MR to determine vascularity, transspatial spread

Helpful Clues for Common Diagnoses

- **Squamous Cell Carcinoma, Sinonasal**
    - Key facts: Adult patient (95% > 40 years); M > F
        - Maxillary antrum origin more common than nasal cavity, but most antral lesions involve nasal cavity
    - Imaging: Poorly defined with aggressive bone destruction; heterogeneous enhancement
        - Moderate tendency to invade nerves (22%)
        - IR FSE MR: Hyperintense to muscle, isointense with cortex
- **Non-Hodgkin Lymphoma, Sinonasal**
    - Key facts: B-cell phenotype more common in North America and Europe; presents in 6th decade; M:F = 3:1
    - Imaging: Centered in nasal cavity with nasal septal destruction
        - CT: Homogeneous and may be hyperdense relative to other soft tissue
        - MR: Homogeneous signal and enhancement; decreased T2 signal due to high nuclear:cytoplasmic ratio of cells
- **Inverted Papilloma, Sinonasal**
    - Key facts: Adult man (40-70 years)
        - Rhinoscopy: Firm, vascular polypoid lesion on lateral nasal wall
    - Imaging: On CT, polypoid mass near middle meatus with extension into maxillary antrum; intratumoral Ca++
        - MR: "Convoluted, cerebriform" architecture on T1 and T2 C+ sequences
- **Fungal Sinusitis, Invasive**
    - Key facts: Immunocompromised patient; rapidly progressive infection
    - Imaging: Maxillary or ethmoid sinus origin with spread into nasal cavity
        - Infiltration of retroantral or premaxillary fat; decreased T2 signal due to fungal hyphae, metal chelates
        - Most common organisms: Aspergillosis and mucormycosis
- **Esthesioneuroblastoma**
    - Key facts: Adolescent or middle-aged patient with unilateral nasal obstruction and mild epistaxis; may bleed profusely on biopsy
        - No sex predilection
    - Imaging: Morphology is dumbbell-shaped mass centered at cribriform plate
        - CT: Intralesional Ca++
        - MR: Avid enhancement; foci of hemorrhage; intracranial cyst formation

Helpful Clues for Less Common Diagnoses

- **Granulomatosis With Polyangiitis, Sinonasal**
    - Key facts: Wide age range (6th decade most common); M > F
    - Imaging: On CT, lobular soft tissue lesions on nasal septum and turbinates; septal perforation is common complication
- **Adenocarcinoma, Sinonasal**
    - Key facts: Adult (40-60 year old) man patient; indolent disease; may have occupational exposure history
    - Imaging: Nonspecific imaging features, but may be more well defined than squamous cell carcinoma and esthesioneuroblastoma
- **Undifferentiated Carcinoma, Sinonasal**
    - Key facts: Wide age range (6th decade most common); M:F = 2:1
        - Aggressive rapid growth pattern
    - Imaging: Nasal cavity and paranasal sinus involvement with spread into adjacent compartments
- **Sarcoidosis, Sinonasal**
    - Key facts: Incidence considered to be underreported
        - Usually systemic disease with lung and kidney involvement; sinonasal involvement less often than in Wegener granulomatosis
        - Anosmia in 70% of cases
    - Imaging: Nasal septum and turbinate involvement common; less "mass-like" with superficial, nodular soft tissue involvement
- **Juvenile Angiofibroma**
    - Key facts: Adolescent boy patient with nasal obstruction and epistaxis
    - Imaging: Centered at sphenopalatine foramen with spread into pterygopalatine fossa, nasal cavity, and nasopharynx
        - Vascular mass with flow voids and avid enhancement
- **Melanoma, Sinonasal**

- Key facts: Adult patient with epistaxis; pigmented lesion in nasal cavity at rhinoscopy
  - Age range 20-80 years; mean 65
- Imaging: Attached to septum, lateral nasal wall, or inferior turbinate
  - CT: Bone may be remodeled or destroyed
  - MR: ↑ T1, ↓ T2 signal

Helpful Clues for Rare Diagnoses

- **Chondrosarcoma, Sinonasal**
  - Key facts: Younger age group than conventional chondrosarcoma: 80% < 40 years
  - Imaging: Site of origin most often in skull base with secondary nasal cavity involvement
    - Chondroid matrix of Ca++ on CT; T1WI hypointense, T2WI hyperintense, T1WI C+ isointense
- **Osteosarcoma, Sinonasal**
  - Key facts: Rare lesion; originates in maxilla or palate
  - Imaging: On CT, osseous mass with periosteal reaction
- **Rhabdomyosarcoma, Sinonasal**
  - Key facts: 70% < 12 years; ~ 4% of H&N rhabdomyosarcoma
  - Imaging: Arise near skull base with extension into nasopharynx and nasal cavity
- **Langerhans Histiocytosis, Skull Base**
  - Key facts: Presents in 1st decade; M > F
  - Imaging: Originates in skull base or maxilla with extension into nasal cavity
- **Plasmacytoma, Skull Base**
  - Key facts: 5th to 9th decades; M > F; more common in blacks
  - Imaging: Originates in skull base with extension into nasal cavity
- **Metastasis, Mandible-Maxilla**
  - Key facts: Breast and lung carcinoma most common primaries; widespread skeletal metastases present

Other Essential Information

- Although nodal spread from sinonasal malignancies is uncommon (< 20%), be sure to look at retropharyngeal and L2 and L3 lymph nodes
- Imaging features of these lesions (particularly in adults) may be nonspecific, and histologic confirmation is essential for diagnosis

SELECTED REFERENCES

1. Breik O et al: Survival Outcomes of Mucosal Melanoma in the Head and Neck: Case Series and Review of Current Treatment Guidelines. J Oral Maxillofac Surg. ePub, 2016
2. Houette A et al: Prognostic value of two tumour staging classifications in patients with sinonasal mucosal melanoma. Eur Ann Otorhinolaryngol Head Neck Dis. ePub, 2016
3. Jalilvand S et al: The prevalence of human papillomavirus infection in Iranian patients with sinonasal inverted papilloma. J Chin Med Assoc. 79(3):137-40, 2016
4. Lewis JS Jr: Sinonasal Squamous Cell Carcinoma: A Review with Emphasis on Emerging Histologic Subtypes and the Role of Human Papillomavirus. Head Neck Pathol. 10(1):60-7, 2016
5. Lisan Q et al: Sinonasal inverted papilloma: From diagnosis to treatment. Eur Ann Otorhinolaryngol Head Neck Dis. ePub, 2016
6. Lombardi D et al: Sinonasal mucosal melanoma: A 12-year experience of 58 cases. Head Neck. 38 Suppl 1:E1737-45, 2016
7. Nicolae V et al: Clinical and histological aspects of malignant inverted sinonasal papilloma. Two case reports. Rom J Morphol Embryol. 57(1):289-94, 2016
8. Park SH et al: Outcome of definitive and postoperative radiotherapy in patients with sinonasal squamous cell carcinomas. Tumori. 102(4):426-32, 2016
9. Prasad H et al: Inverted Sinonasal Papilloma Masquerading as a Malignancy - Report of an Unusual Case. Cureus. 8(3):e526, 2016
10. Roh HJ et al: Smoking, not human papilloma virus infection, is a risk factor for recurrence of sinonasal inverted papilloma. Am J Rhinol Allergy. 30(2):79-82, 2016
11. Samstein RM et al: Localized sinonasal mucosal melanoma: Outcomes and associations with stage, radiotherapy, and positron emission tomography response. Head Neck. ePub, 2016
12. Suzuki H et al: The Charlson comorbidity index is a prognostic factor in sinonasal tract squamous cell carcinoma. Jpn J Clin Oncol. 46(7):646-51, 2016
13. Unsal AA et al: Squamous cell carcinoma of the nasal cavity: A population-based analysis. Laryngoscope. 126(3):560-5, 2016
14. Zhao RW et al: Human papillomavirus infection and the malignant transformation of sinonasal inverted papilloma: A meta-analysis. J Clin Virol. 79:36-43, 2016
15. Zhu W et al: Clinicopathological Features and Prognosis of Sinonasal Mucosal Malignant Melanoma: A Retrospective Study of 83 Cases in a Chinese Population. ORL J Otorhinolaryngol Relat Spec. 78(2):94-104, 2016
16. Aleksić A et al: Melanoma of the sinonasal mucosa: A report on the two cases and a review of the literature. Vojnosanit Pregl. 72(10):937-41, 2015

Squamous Cell Carcinoma, Sinonasal

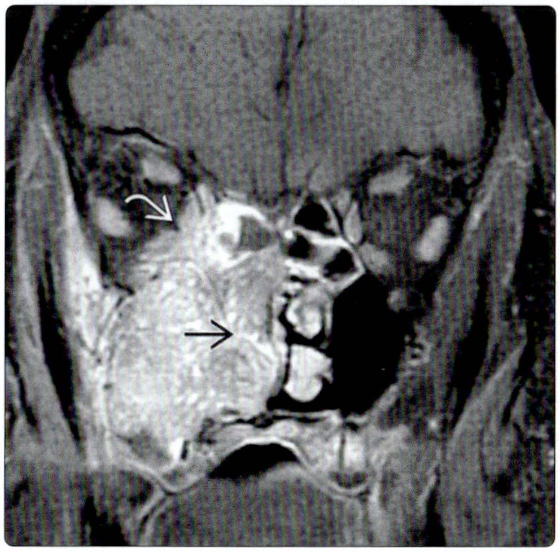

Non-Hodgkin Lymphoma, Sinonasal

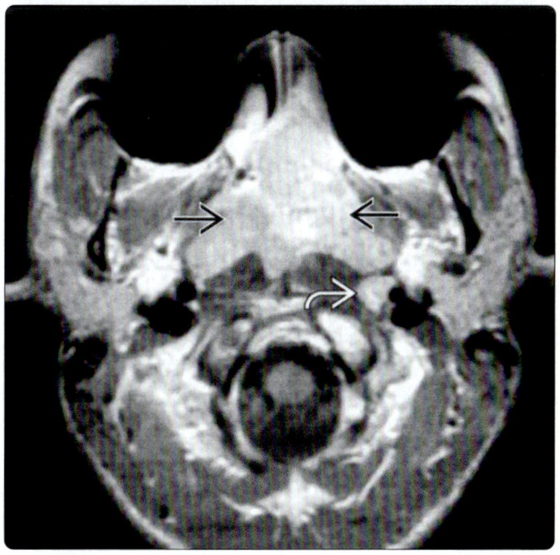

(Left) *Coronal T1WI C+ FS MR shows large antral squamous cell carcinoma with extension into the right nasal cavity ⇒ and orbit ➡. The middle and inferior turbinates are invaded by a tumor.* **(Right)** *Axial T1WI C+ MR shows the typical location and homogeneous enhancement pattern of sinonasal lymphoma with extension into the nasopharynx ⇒. Note the small retropharyngeal node on the left ➡.*

Nasal Lesion With Bony Destruction

(Left) *Axial T1WI C+ FS MR shows typical inverted papilloma centered near the middle meatus ⇨ extending into the antrum ➡ and nasal cavity ➡. A "convoluted" architecture is appreciated.* **(Right)** *Axial T2WI FS MR shows fungal sinusitis with spread from the antrum into the nasal cavity ⇨ and masticator space ➡. Decreased T2 signal and the mass-like appearance are typical.*

Inverted Papilloma, Sinonasal

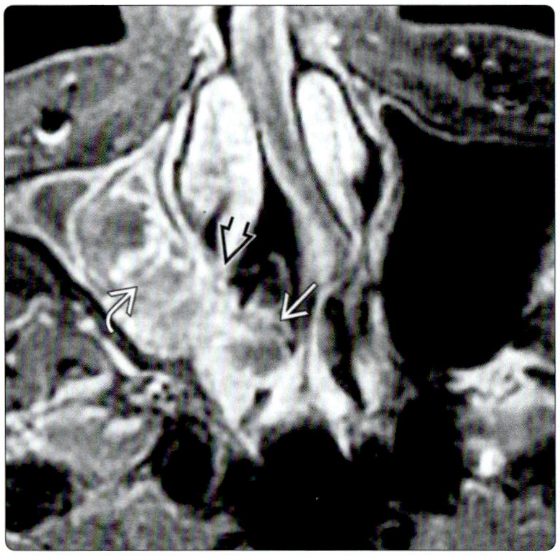

Fungal Sinusitis, Invasive

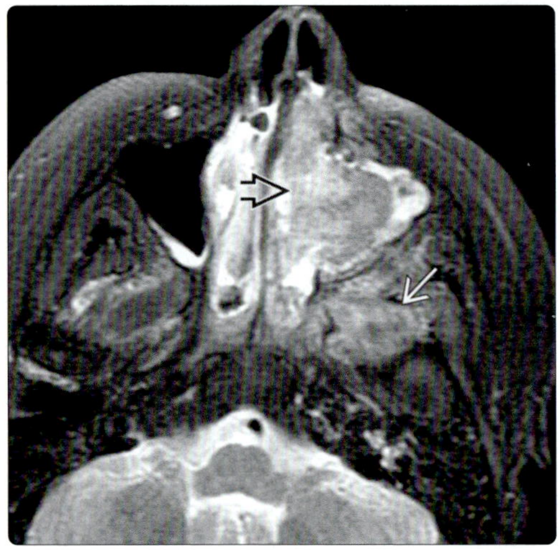

(Left) *Coronal T1 C+ FS MR shows an invasive tumor with extension into the anterior cranial fossa ➡. Diffuse enhancement is noted in this vascular neoplasm. Extension into the right orbit ➡ is also present.* **(Right)** *Coronal bone CT shows lobular soft tissue thickenings centered on the septum and turbinates, characteristic of granulomatous diseases with septal perforation ➡. Lobular tissue ➡ is noted in the maxillary antrum.*

Esthesioneuroblastoma

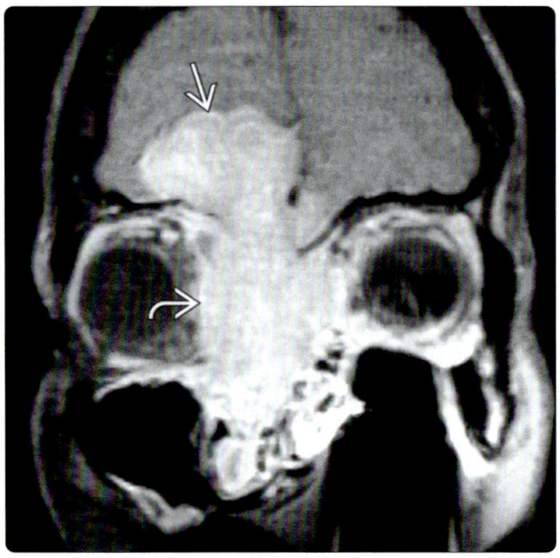

Granulomatosis With Polyangiitis, Sinonasal

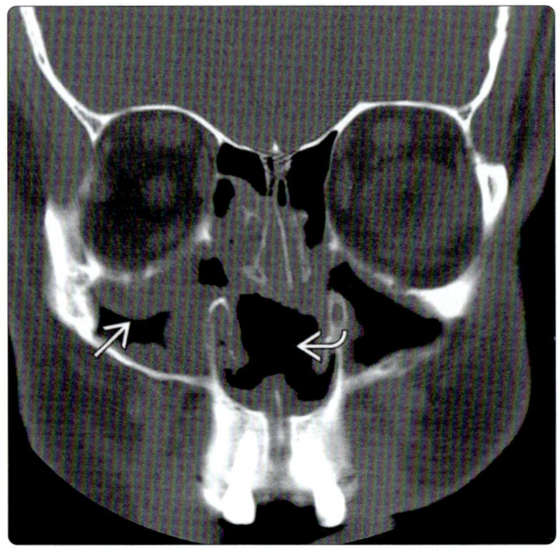

(Left) *Coronal T1 C+ MR shows a large sinonasal adenocarcinoma with heterogeneous enhancement and marked intracranial extension ➡. The site of origin was likely the superior nasal cavity.* **(Right)** *Coronal bone CT shows a sinonasal undifferentiated carcinoma involving the nasal cavity and ethmoid sinuses with anterior skull base ➡ and orbital ➡ invasion.*

Adenocarcinoma, Sinonasal

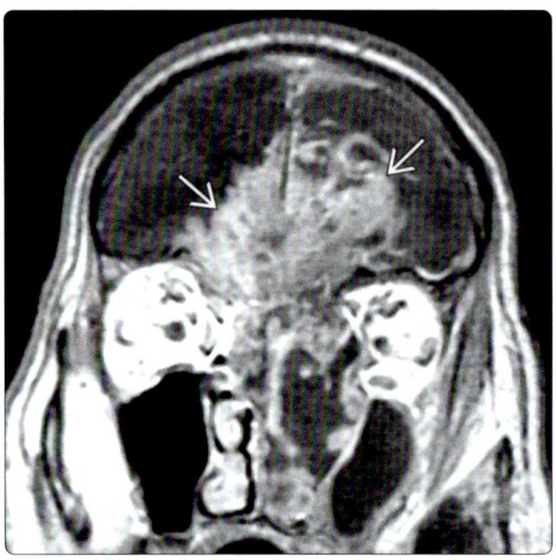

Undifferentiated Carcinoma, Sinonasal

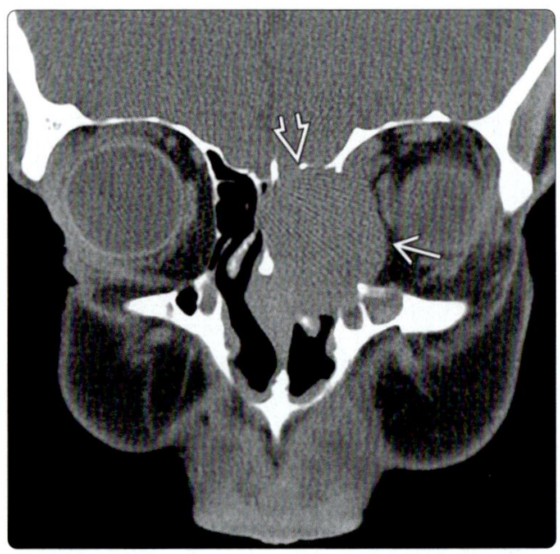

Sarcoidosis, Sinonasal

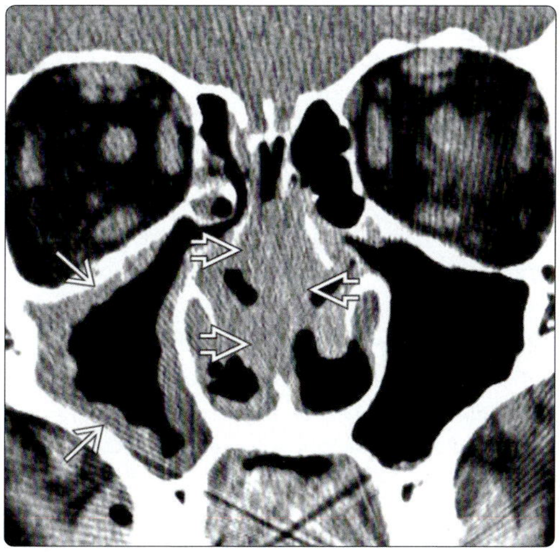

Juvenile Angiofibroma

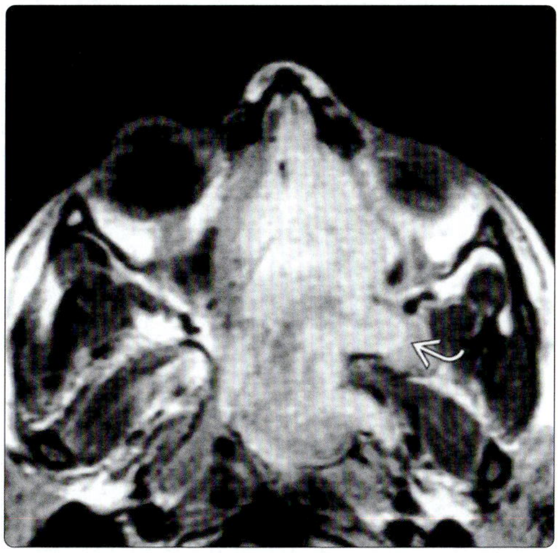

(Left) *Coronal NECT shows typical appearance of sinonasal sarcoid involvement with lobular soft tissue along the nasal septum ➡ and involving the right maxillary sinus ➡.* **(Right)** *Axial T1WI C+ MR shows large juvenile angiofibroma involving the nasal cavity, nasopharynx, and pterygopalatine fossa ➡. Diffuse enhancement is seen throughout this vascular lesion.*

Melanoma, Sinonasal

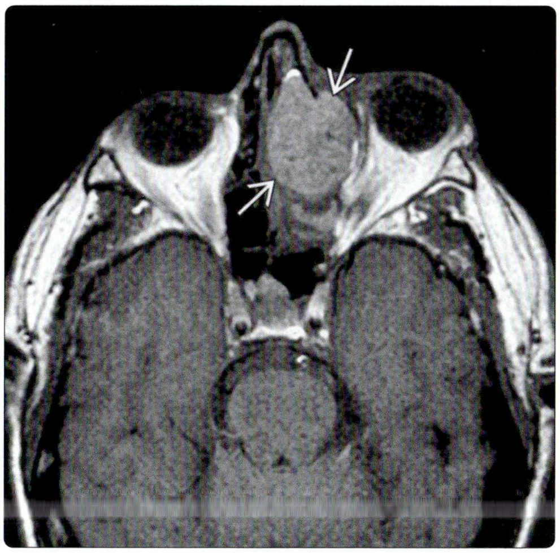

Chondrosarcoma, Sinonasal

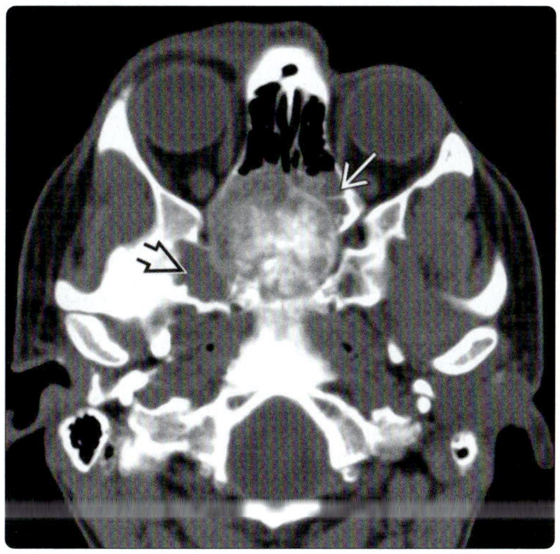

(Left) *Axial T1WI MR shows fairly well-defined sinonasal melanoma ➡ involving the left ethmoids and upper nasal cavity. Note increased T1 signal in the mass relative to other soft tissue (muscle, brain).* **(Right)** *Axial bone CT shows a typical chondrosarcoma arising from the vomer area of the nasal septum with chondroid matrix. Note obstructed secretions in the sphenoid ➡ and ethmoid ➡ sinuses.*

Osteosarcoma, Sinonasal

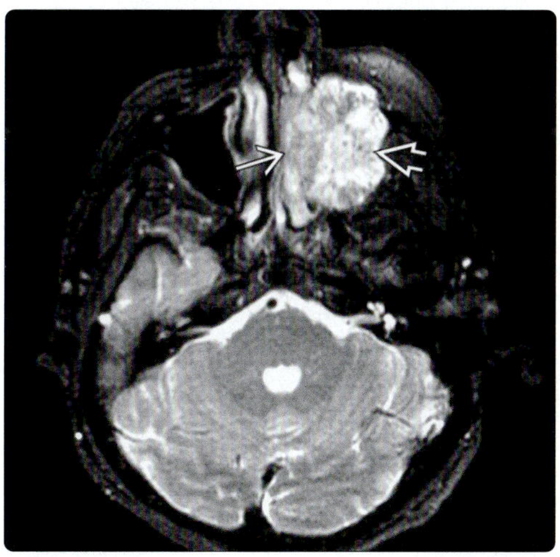

Rhabdomyosarcoma, Sinonasal

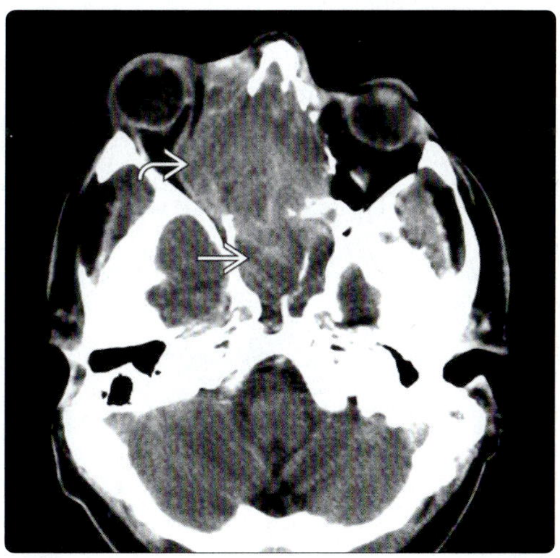

(Left) *Axial T2WI FS MR reveals an osteosarcoma arising from the maxilla, involving the nasal cavity ➡ and maxillary antrum ➡. The ossific matrix creates low signal areas in the tumor matrix.* **(Right)** *Axial CECT shows aggressive midface alveolar rhabdomyosarcoma with bilateral nasal cavity involvement. There is extension into the sphenoid sinus ➡ and orbit ➡.*

DIFFERENTIAL DIAGNOSIS

Common

- Osteoma, Sinonasal
- Fibrous Dysplasia, Sinonasal
- Ossifying Fibroma, Sinus

Less Common

- Osteomyelitis, Maxilla
- Chondrosarcoma, Sinonasal
- Osteosarcoma, Sinonasal

Rare but Important

- Chordoma, Clivus
- Central Giant Cell Granuloma, Maxilla
- Cherubism, Mandible-Maxilla

ESSENTIAL INFORMATION

Key Differential Diagnosis Issues

- Fibroosseous lesions may have similar imaging and histologic features

Helpful Clues for Common Diagnoses

- **Osteoma, Sinonasal**
  - Key facts: Frontal > ethmoid > maxillary > sphenoid
  - Imaging: On CT, density varies from dense (compact type) to less ossified (fibrous type)
- **Fibrous Dysplasia, Sinonasal**
  - Key facts: Medullary bone replaced by woven bone
    - Facial bone involvement ↑ in polyostotic form
  - Imaging: On CT/MR appearance varies with amount of fibrous tissue (classic = ground-glass appearance)
    - Intraoral radiographs: Appearance also varies (classic = orange peel appearance)
- **Ossifying Fibroma, Sinus**
  - Key facts: Benign expansile tumor
  - Imaging: Lesion ossifies from periphery
    - Better demarcated fibrous and osseous zones than fibrous dysplasia

Helpful Clues for Less Common Diagnoses

- **Osteomyelitis, Maxilla**
  - Key facts: Most often related to dental disease
  - Imaging: Osteolytic or sclerotic
    - ± sequestra or periosteal reaction
- **Chondrosarcoma, Sinonasal**
  - Key facts: Most in anterior maxillary alveolar process
  - Imaging: Expansile with bony remodeling
    - ± Ca++ tumor matrix; ↑ water content → ↑ T2 signal
- **Osteosarcoma, Sinonasal**
  - Key facts: ≤ 1% of sinonasal tumors
  - Imaging: Appearance varies with degree of osteo/chondroid/fibroblastic components
    - "Sunburst" periosteal reaction possible
    - May have widened periodontal ligament spaces if involving teeth

Helpful Clues for Rare Diagnoses

- **Chordoma, Clivus**
  - Key facts: Malignant notochordal tumor
  - Imaging: If from clivus, can extend into sphenoid sinus
    - Rarely, 1% arises in nasal cavity or nasopharynx without clivus involvement
    - Destructive midline mass with ↑ T2 signal
- **Central Giant Cell Granuloma, Maxilla**
  - Key facts: < 30 years; M:F = 1:2; anterior > posterior
  - Imaging: Expansile and remodels bone; septa, if present, form "T" with outer cortex
  - MR: Low to intermediate T1/T2 signal
- **Cherubism, Mandible-Maxilla**
  - Key facts: Autosomal dominant; M > F; mutation in *SH3BP2* gene found in 80%; giant cell lesion
  - Imaging: Bilateral, multilocular, expansion of mandible, then maxilla; multiple displaced, unerupted teeth
    - Can displace intact border of maxillary sinus

SELECTED REFERENCES

1. Ali IK et al: Non-familial cherubism with bilateral maxilla and mandible involvement - clinicoradiographic Findings. Cureus. 8(7):e709, 2016

Osteoma, Sinonasal

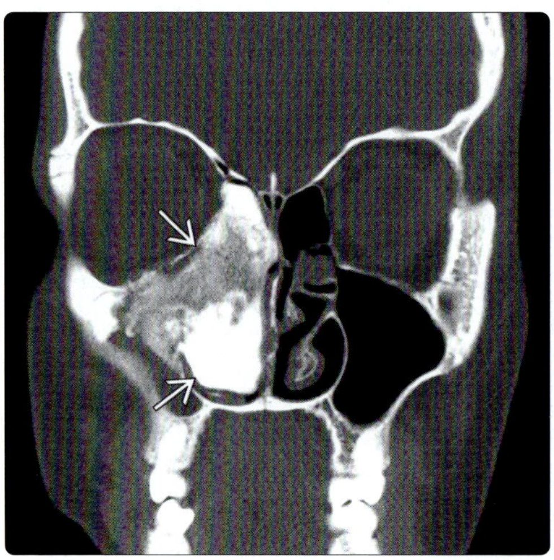

Fibrous Dysplasia, Sinonasal

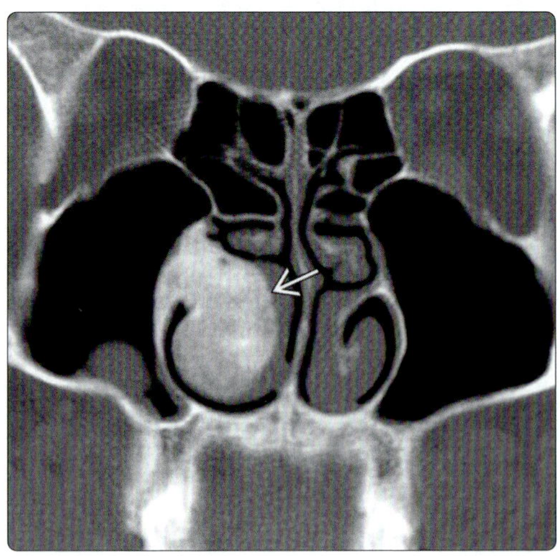

(Left) *Coronal bone CT shows a large, mixed osseous and soft tissue density mass within the nasal cavity and adjacent sinuses ➡. This osteoma could be confused with other fibroosseous lesions.* **(Right)** *Coronal bone CT shows monostotic fibrous dysplasia involving the inferior turbinate ➡. The concha of the turbinate is expanded and has a ground-glass appearance.*

Ossifying Fibroma, Sinus

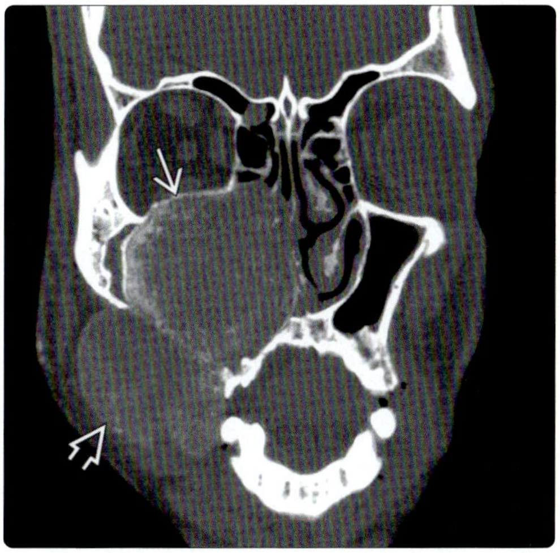

Osteomyelitis, Maxilla

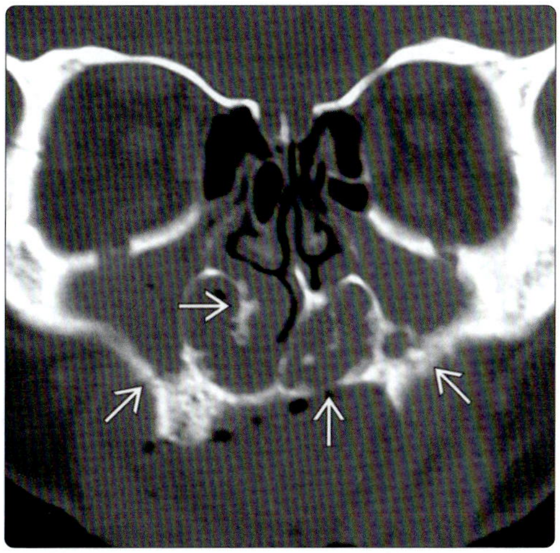

(Left) *Coronal bone CT shows a bilobed ossifying fibroma in the superficial soft tissues ➡ of the buccal space and maxillary sinus ➡. Note increased ossification along the superficial aspect of the maxillary sinus portion.* **(Right)** *Coronal bone CT shows a permeative bone erosion ➡ involving the palate, maxillary alveolar process, sinus and lateral nasal walls, and inferior conchae in this elderly patient with osteomyelitis.*

Chondrosarcoma, Sinonasal

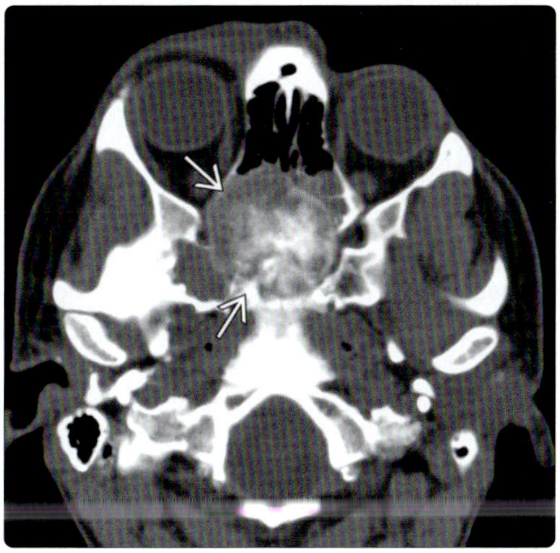

Osteosarcoma, Sinonasal

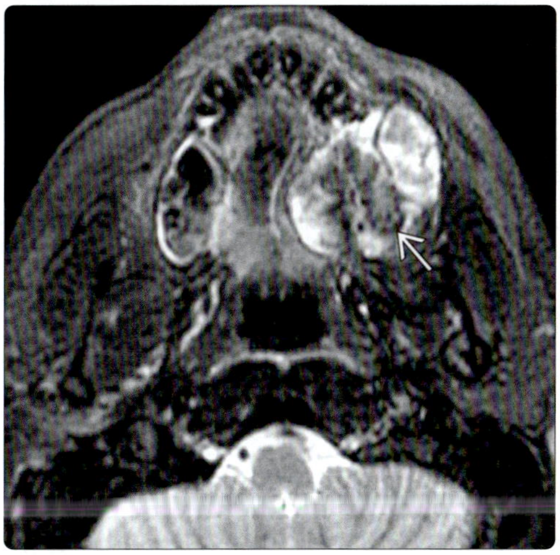

(Left) *Axial bone CT shows a large vomer nasal septal chondrosarcoma ➡. The mass shows calcifications that are not characteristic of chondroid calcifications.* **(Right)** *Axial T2WI FS MR demonstrates an osteosarcoma arising within the left maxillary alveolar process with extension into the antrum. The ossific matrix ➡ creates areas of hypointense signal on MR images.*

Chordoma, Clivus

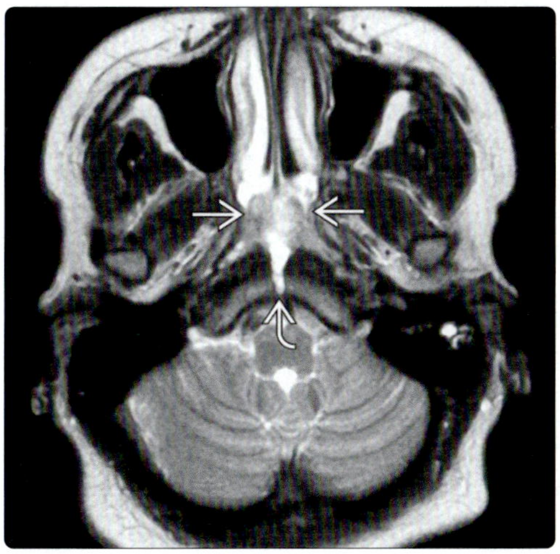

Central Giant Cell Granuloma, Maxilla

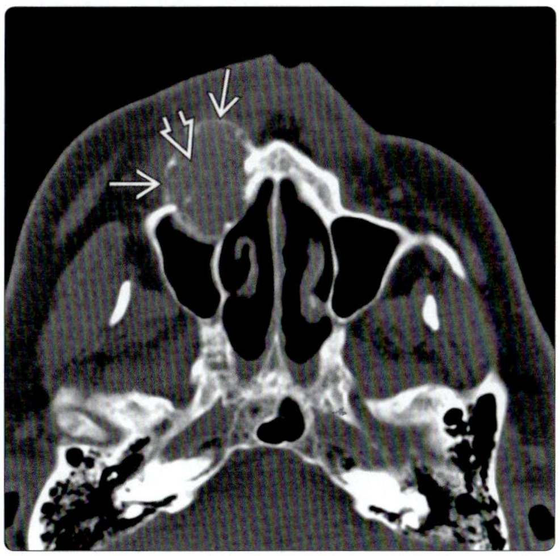

(Left) *Axial T2WI MR shows an atypical chordoma ➡ presenting as a posterior nasal cavity/nasopharyngeal mass. The midline clival defect ➡ correlates with the path of the primitive notochord.* **(Right)** *Axial bone CT shows a maxillary giant cell granuloma ➡. An "eggshell" wall indicates its probable benign nature. Note the hint of loculation with septa ➡ oriented at right angles to the outer cortex.*

Paranasal Sinus Lesions Without Bony Destruction

DIFFERENTIAL DIAGNOSIS

Common

- Mucus Retention Pseudocyst
- Rhinosinusitis, Chronic
- Rhinosinusitis, Acute
- Odontogenic Cyst
- Mucocele, Sinonasal
- Polyposis, Sinonasal
- Fungal Sinusitis, Mycetoma
- Osteoma, Sinonasal

Less Common

- Fungal Sinusitis, Allergic
- Inverted Papilloma, Sinonasal
- Fibrous Dysplasia, Sinonasal
- Ossifying Fibroma, Sinus
- Polyps, Solitary, Sinonasal
- Juvenile Angiofibroma
- Antrolith/Sinolith

Rare but Important

- Benign Mixed Tumor, Sinonasal
- Nerve Sheath Tumor, Sinonasal
- Silent Sinus Syndrome

ESSENTIAL INFORMATION

Key Differential Diagnosis Issues

- Infectious/inflammatory disorders & benign neoplasms are majority of lesions in this differential
- Malignant neoplasms such as lymphoma & melanoma can cause bone remodeling rather than destruction

Helpful Clues for Common Diagnoses

- **Mucus Retention Pseudocyst**
  - Key facts: Incidental finding
    - Most common sinus: Maxillary > sphenoid > ethmoid & frontal
    - Most common in spring & fall
  - Imaging: Usually solitary but may be multiple & bilateral
    - Usually no other soft tissue thickening
    - **No cortical border** around lesion
- **Rhinosinusitis, Chronic**
  - Key facts: Involves multiple sinuses
    - Sinusitis > 3 months
  - Imaging: Mucosal thickening, bone sclerosis, & thickening of sinus walls (osteitis)
    - Look for anatomic variants or obstructing lesions of drainage pathways
- **Rhinosinusitis, Acute**
  - Key facts: Viral or bacterial infection
    - Sinusitis < 1 month
  - Imaging: Normal-sized sinus lumen with mucosal thickening ± air-fluid levels
    - Look for odontogenic source if isolated to 1 maxillary sinus
- **Odontogenic Cyst**
  - Key facts: Radicular cyst associated with root of carious tooth
    - Dentigerous cyst associated with crown of impacted tooth
    - Both may encroach upon, but are not within, sinus
  - Imaging: Radiolucent lesion with **corticated border** encroaching upon, but not within, maxillary sinus
- **Mucocele, Sinonasal**
  - Key facts: Most common expansile sinus lesion arising from chronic obstruction
    - Adult > children
    - Frontal > ethmoid > maxillary > sphenoid
    - If secondarily infected → **mucopyocele**
  - Imaging
    - CT: Opacified, expanded sinus with intact bony rim
    - MR: ↓ T1, ↑ T2 with peripheral enhancement; if ↑ T1, high protein content secretions
- **Polyposis, Sinonasal**
  - Key facts: Commonly allergic patients
    - Involves nasal cavity & sinuses
    - Chronic inflammatory condition
  - Imaging: Lobular soft tissue lesions that can opacify & expand sinonasal cavities
- **Fungal Sinusitis, Mycetoma**
  - Key facts: Often asymptomatic
    - Colonization of obstructed secretions by noninvasive fungi in immunocompetent patient
  - Imaging: Opacified, nonexpanded sinus with increased density material ± calcifications
    - Maxillary > sphenoid
    - T1WI & T2WI ↓ intensity → fungus ball invisible
- **Osteoma, Sinonasal**
  - Key facts: Most common benign sinus tumor; frontal > ethmoid sinuses
  - Imaging: Well-defined, densely ossified mass attached to sinus wall
    - May be mixed fibrous & osseous

Helpful Clues for Less Common Diagnoses

- **Fungal Sinusitis, Allergic**
  - Key facts: Form of chronic sinusitis with eosinophilic mucin & noninvasive fungi
    - Often seen in allergic patients & those with polyposis
  - Imaging
    - CT: Opacified, expanded sinuses (unilateral or bilateral) with central ↑ density & peripheral ↓ density
    - MR signal variable; ↓ T2 signal mimics air
- **Inverted Papilloma, Sinonasal**
  - Key facts: Benign epithelial neoplasm with endophytic growth pattern
    - M:F = 4:1; nasal cavity > sinuses
    - May contain squamous cell carcinoma
  - Imaging: Lobular mass in nasal cavity near middle meatus with extension into antrum
    - "Convoluted" or "cerebriform" architecture on T2 or C+ MR
- **Fibrous Dysplasia, Sinonasal**
  - Key facts: Mesenchymal developmental anomaly forming weak woven bone
    - Mono- or polyostotic; focal or diffuse
    - Encroaches on sinuses & decreases their volume
  - Imaging

- CT or CBCT: Commonly expansile, ill-defined, bony lesion with ground-glass matrix
- MR: Variable signal; ↓ T2 common
- Intraoral radiographs: May be radiolucent or have orange-peel or ground-glass matrix

- **Ossifying Fibroma, Sinus**
  - Key facts: Benign fibroosseous tumor of mature bone & fibrous tissue
    - Maxilla < mandible
  - Imaging
    - CT: Well-demarcated, expansile mass with mixed soft tissue (central fibrous) & osseous (peripheral) density
    - MR: Fibrous component ↑ T2 & osseous ↓ T2 signal; heterogeneous enhancement
- **Polyps, Solitary, Sinonasal**
  - Key facts: Antrochoanal polyp common
  - Imaging
    - CT: Well-defined, low-density lesion arising in antrum, widening ostium, & protruding into nasal cavity/nasopharynx
    - MR: ↓ T1 & ↑ T2 signal with peripheral mucosal enhancement
- **Juvenile Angiofibroma**
  - Key facts: Benign but locally invasive vascular neoplasm
    - Occurs in adolescent boys with nasal obstruction & epistaxis
  - Imaging: Lesion centered in sphenopalatine foramen with extension into nasal cavity, nasopharynx, & pterygopalatine fossa
    - CT: Bone remodeling; pterygopalatine fossa expansion common
    - MR: Heterogeneous ↓ T1 & ↑ T2 MR signal with avid enhancement
- **Antrolith/Sinolith**
  - Key facts: Benign, slow growing, & not invasive
  - Imaging: Lesion usually on floor of sinus but separated from osseous border
    - Usually associated sort tissue thickening
    - Laminated appearance: Less dense layers = proteinaceous; more dense layers = calcium salts

Helpful Clues for Rare Diagnoses

- **Benign Mixed Tumor, Sinonasal**
  - Key facts: 8% of benign mixed tumors (pleomorphic adenoma) occur outside of major salivary glands
    - Most arise on nasal septum
    - 30-60 years at presentation
  - Imaging
    - CT: Well-defined mass with adjacent bone remodeling
    - MR: Intermediate T1 & ↑ T2 signal; variable enhancement
- **Nerve Sheath Tumor, Sinonasal**
  - Key facts: Benign tumors (schwannoma > neurofibroma)
    - ~ 10% of H&N schwannomas
    - Nasoethmoid > maxillary > nasal cavity > sphenoid
    - Neurofibroma more common in NF1
  - Imaging
    - CT: Well-defined mass with bone expansion/remodeling
    - MR: ↓ T1, ↑ T2 MR signal; variable enhancement; ± intramural cysts
- **Silent Sinus Syndrome**
  - Key facts: Chronic maxillary obstruction results in painless wall retraction from negative intrasinus pressure
  - Imaging: Opacified maxillary sinus with decreased volume & inward bowing of all walls + enophthalmos

SELECTED REFERENCES

1. Cahill KN et al: Impaired E prostanoid2 expression and resistance to prostaglandin E2 in nasal polyp fibroblasts from subjects with aspirin-exacerbated respiratory disease. Am J Respir Cell Mol Biol. 54(1):34-40, 2016
2. Dass K et al: Diagnosis and management of rhinosinusitis: Highlights from the 2015 Practice Parameter. Curr Allergy Asthma Rep. 16(4):29, 2016
3. Jalilvand S et al: The prevalence of human papillomavirus infection in Iranian patients with sinonasal inverted papilloma. J Chin Med Assoc. 79(3):137-40, 2016
4. Lisan Q et al: Sinonasal inverted papilloma: From diagnosis to treatment. Eur Ann Otorhinolaryngol Head Neck Dis. ePub, 2016
5. Loftus PA et al: Anatomic variants of the paranasal sinuses in patients with recurrent acute rhinosinusitis. Int Forum Allergy Rhinol. 6(3):328-33, 2016
6. Nicolae V et al: Clinical and histological aspects of malignant inverted sinonasal papilloma. Two case reports. Rom J Morphol Embryol. 57(1):289-94, 2016

Mucus Retention Pseudocyst

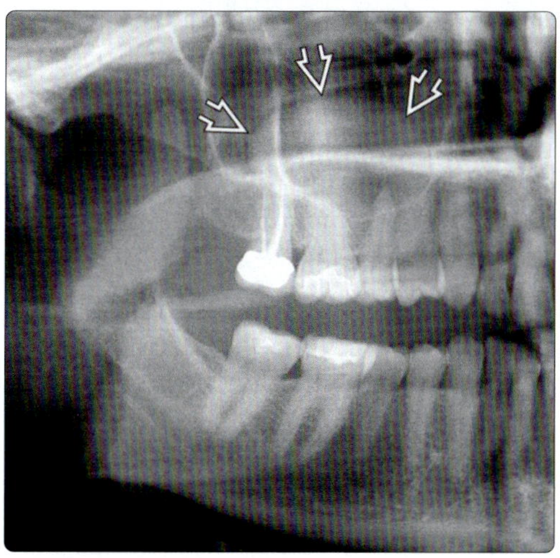

Rhinosinusitis, Chronic

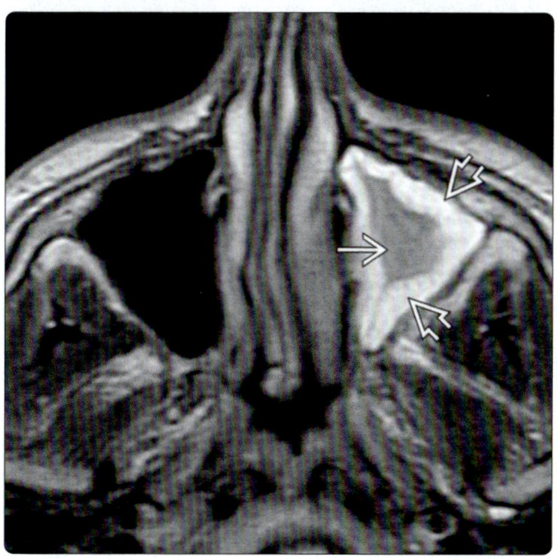

(Left) *Cropped panoramic radiograph shows a rounded "hydraulic" mucus retention pseudocyst ➡ on the floor of the right maxillary sinus. Note lack of a corticated border, indicating lesion is within the sinus, not encroaching upon it.* **(Right)** *Axial T2WI MR shows filling of the left maxillary sinus air space. The sinus volume is decreased, the walls are thickened, & central proteinaceous secretions ➡ with peripheral edematous mucosa ➡ are visible.*

(Left) *Coronal bone CT shows mucosal thickening & air-fluid level in the left maxillary sinus of a patient with clinical symptoms of acute sinusitis. There is occlusion of the ostiomeatal unit at the infundibulum.* **(Right)** *Axial CBCT shows a dentigerous cyst (arising from around the crown of the 3rd molar) encroaching on the left maxillary sinus. Note the corticated border of the cyst, indicating it is extending from outside the sinus, unlike the noncorticated border of the retention pseudocyst in the right sinus.*

Rhinosinusitis, Acute

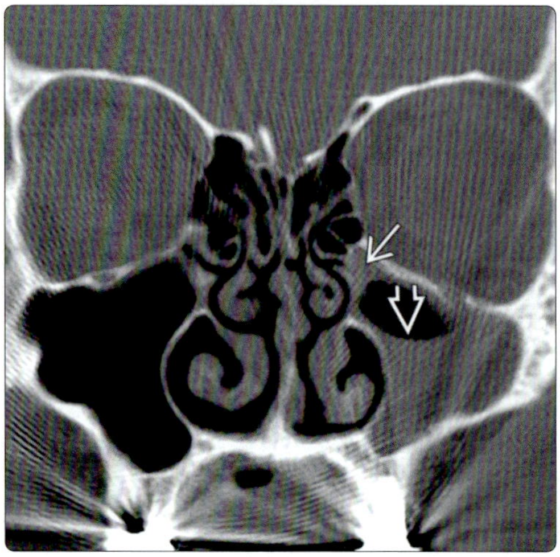

Odontogenic Cyst

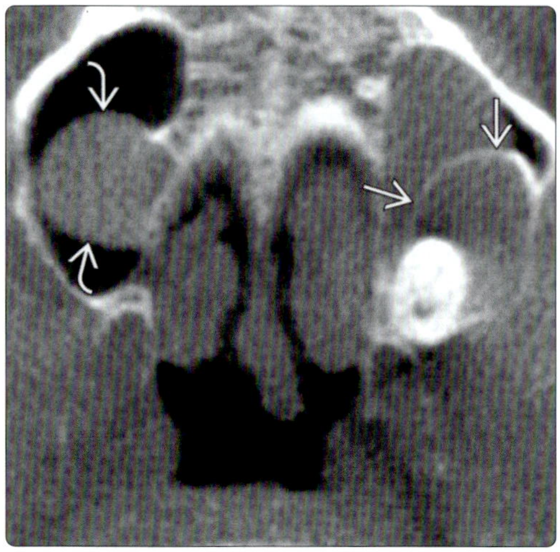

(Left) *Coronal bone CT shows an expanded, opacified right maxillary sinus in a patient with granulomatosis with polyangiitis. There is circumferential bony remodeling consistent with a mucocele.* **(Right)** *Coronal bone CT shows opacification & expansion of the right ethmoid cells and a polyp in the nasal cavity. Bubbly secretions in the right maxillary sinus suggest acute inflammation.*

Mucocele, Sinonasal

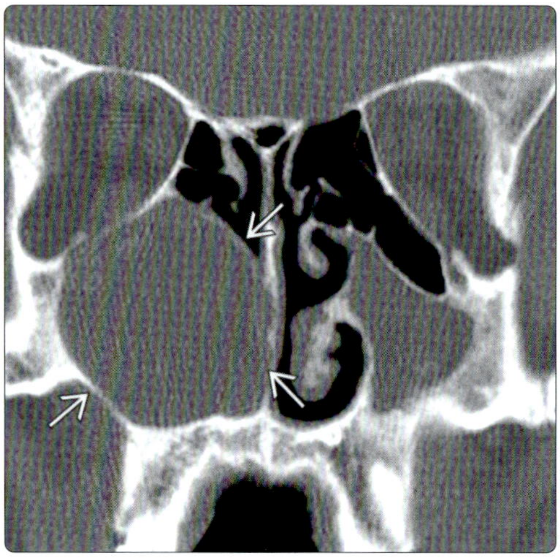

Polyposis, Sinonasal

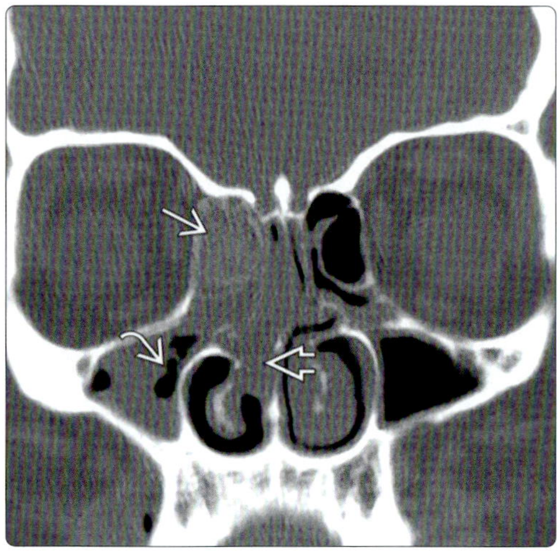

(Left) *Axial NECT shows a high-attenuation mycetoma (fungus ball) in the right maxillary sinus with multiple calcifications centrally. Mucosal thickening is seen peripherally.* **(Right)** *Coronal bone CT shows a well-defined, dense, osseous lesion in the right frontal sinus, consistent with an osteoma. The lesion did not obstruct sinus drainage. The frontal sinus is the most common location for osteoma.*

Fungal Sinusitis, Mycetoma

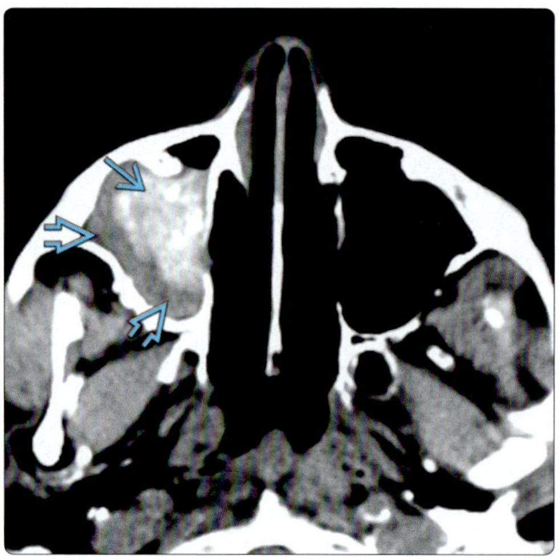

Osteoma, Sinonasal

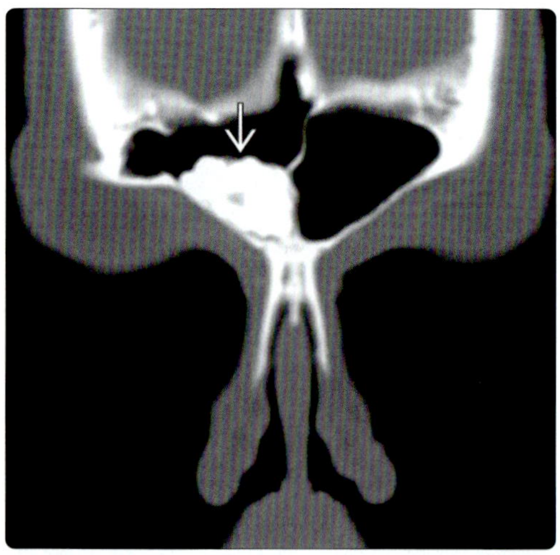

Fungal Sinusitis, Allergic

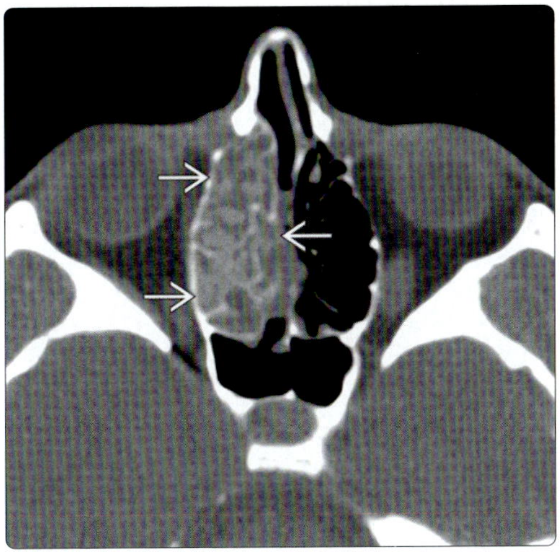

Inverted Papilloma, Sinonasal

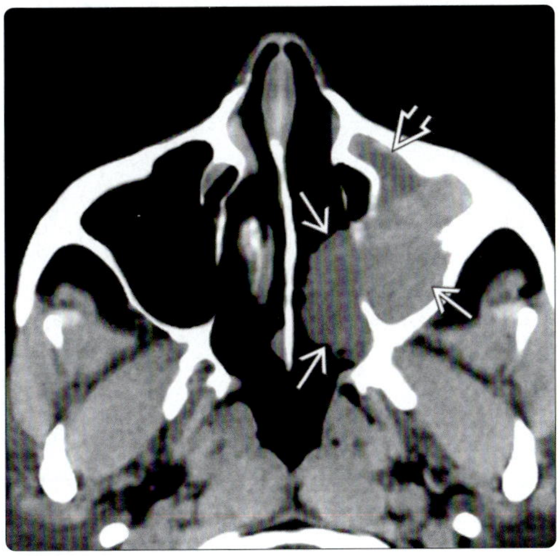

(Left) *Axial bone CT shows opacified, expanded right ethmoid sinuses ➡ with centrally dense material characteristic of allergic fungal sinusitis. The surrounding bone is remodeled, not destroyed.* **(Right)** *Axial NECT shows a nasal cavity inverted papilloma ➡ that has widened the maxillary ostium & extended into the left antrum. Secretions trapped anterior to the lesion ➡ are less dense.*

Fibrous Dysplasia, Sinonasal

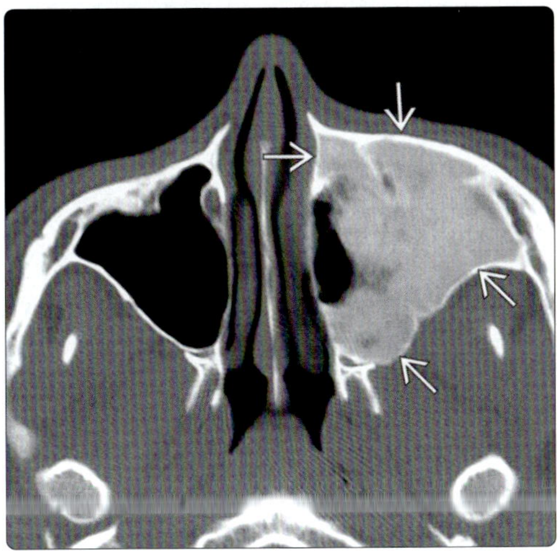

Ossifying Fibroma, Sinus

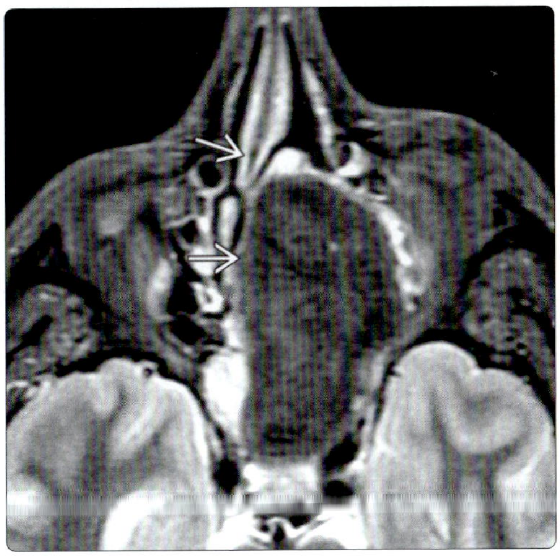

(Left) *Axial bone CT shows a typical ground-glass appearance of fibrous dysplasia involving the left maxillary sinus. There is marked bone expansion, but the cortex ➡ remains intact.* **(Right)** *Axial T2WI MR shows a large, hypointense, left ethmoid ossifying fibroma. The nasal septum ➡ is deviated to the right. The low T2 signal is characteristic of an ossified lesion.*

Polyps, Solitary, Sinonasal

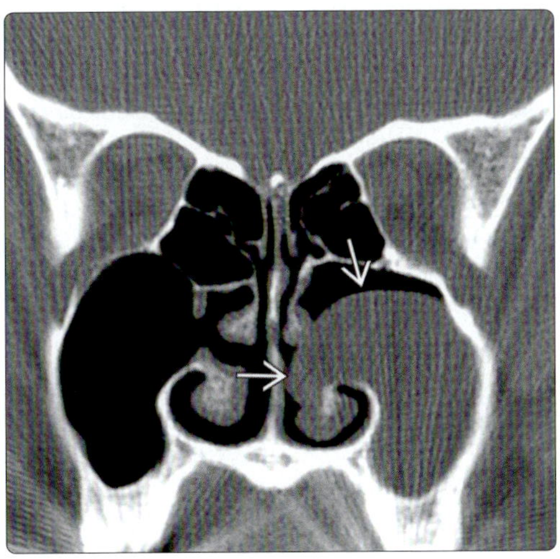

Juvenile Angiofibroma

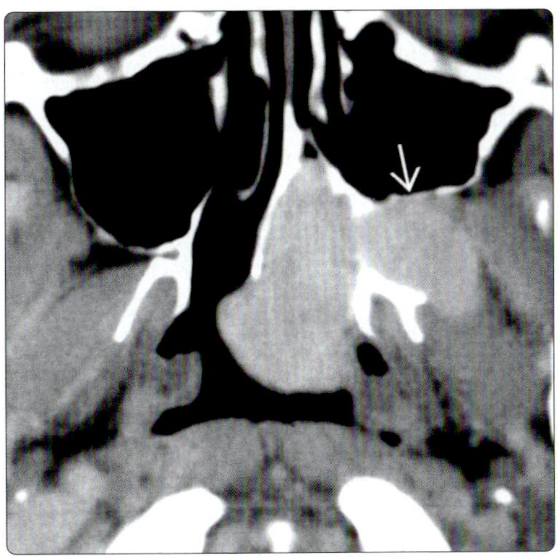

(Left) *Coronal bone CT reveals a sharply marginated polyp ➡ arising from the left antrum & extending through a widened maxillary ostium into the left nasal cavity.* **(Right)** *Axial CECT reveals a dumbbell-shaped, homogeneously enhancing juvenile angiofibroma in the left nasal cavity, nasopharynx, & pterygopalatine fossa & displacing the posterior maxillary sinus wall ➡.*

DIFFERENTIAL DIAGNOSIS

Common

- Squamous Cell Carcinoma, Sinonasal
- Fungal Sinusitis, Invasive (Fulminant Sinusitis)
- Esthesioneuroblastoma (Olfactory Neuroblastoma)
- Non-Hodgkin Lymphoma, Sinonasal

Less Common

- Granulomatosis With Polyangiitis, Sinonasal
- Undifferentiated Carcinoma, Sinonasal
- Adenocarcinoma, Sinonasal
- Sarcoidosis, Sinonasal
- Rhabdomyosarcoma
- Adenoid Cystic Carcinoma, Sinonasal

Rare but Important

- Osteosarcoma, Sinonasal
- Chondrosarcoma, Sinonasal
- Langerhans Cell Histiocytosis, Skull Base
- Metastasis

ESSENTIAL INFORMATION

Key Differential Diagnosis Issues

- Differential includes primarily neoplasms & aggressive infectious/granulomatous disorders

Helpful Clues for Common Diagnoses

- **Squamous Cell Carcinoma, Sinonasal**
  - Key facts: Most common sinonasal (SN) malignancy
    - 80% involve maxillary sinus
    - May coexist in inverted papilloma
    - Predominantly in males
  - Imaging: Ill-defined mass
    - Aggressive bone destruction (rarely remodeling) & heterogeneous, mild enhancement
    - Large lesions with necrosis & hemorrhage
- **Fungal Sinusitis, Invasive (Fulminant Sinusitis)**
  - Key facts: Aggressive infection in immunocompromised or debilitated patient
    - Most common clinical findings: Cranial nerve deficits, facial swelling, proptosis, palatal ulceration
    - Most commonly in adults
    - Aspergillus & mucormycosis most common
  - Imaging: Infiltrating mucosal or mass lesion ± bone destruction
    - MR for early signs of arterial & cavernous sinus thrombosis
    - ↓ T2 signal with spread into adjacent compartments
- **Esthesioneuroblastoma (Olfactory Neuroblastoma)**
  - Key facts: Neural crest tumor of olfactory origin with good prognosis
    - No sex predilection
    - 2 age peaks: 11-20 years & 50-60 years
    - 2-3% of all intranasal neoplasms
    - Originates in superior nasal cavity
    - Presents with epistaxis or bleeding upon biopsy
    - Kadish classification stage B involves sinuses
  - Imaging: Avidly enhancing nasoethmoid mass
    - Intratumoral matrix calcification
    - Intracranial extension with cysts at tumor-brain interface
- **Non-Hodgkin Lymphoma, Sinonasal**
  - Key facts: < 50% of extranodal H&N non-Hodgkin lymphoma arise in SN cavities
    - Curable with radiotherapy; prefers nasal cavity site of origin
    - All ages but peaks in 6th decade; most common pediatric H&N neoplasm
    - M > F
  - Imaging: High nucleus:cytoplasm ratio results in ↑ CT density & ↓ T2 MR signal
    - Homogeneously enhancing; causes bone remodeling or destruction

Helpful Clues for Less Common Diagnoses

- **Granulomatosis With Polyangiitis, Sinonasal**
  - Key facts: Necrotizing granulomatous disease with frequent nasal involvement
    - Prefers septum & turbinates
    - Most common in middle age
  - Imaging: Nodular soft tissue lesions in nasal cavity
    - Septal perforation & erosion of ethmoid septations
- **Undifferentiated Carcinoma, Sinonasal**
  - Key facts: Extremely malignant neoplasm with rapid growth, distant metastases, & poor prognosis
    - Presents at advanced stage
  - Imaging: Aggressive expansile mass with ill-defined margins, bone destruction, & spread into adjacent compartments
- **Adenocarcinoma, Sinonasal**
  - Key facts: 10-20% of SN malignancies
    - Salivary & intestinal types; M > F
    - Average age: 64 years
    - Higher incidence with inhalational exposures
    - Predilection for nasoethmoid region
  - Imaging: Nonspecific; well- to poorly defined soft tissue mass with bone destruction
    - Variable MR signal with heterogeneous enhancement
- **Sarcoidosis, Sinonasal**
  - Key facts: Granulomatous disorder with less frequent SN involvement than granulomatosis with polyangiitis but similar features
    - SN sarcoidosis in 1-4% of patients with sarcoidosis
  - Imaging: Nodular soft tissue lesions in nasal cavity > paranasal sinuses
- **Rhabdomyosarcoma**
  - Key facts: Malignancy of striated muscle
    - Most common childhood sarcoma
    - 40% in H&N (orbit, SN, temporal bone)
  - Imaging: Soft tissue mass ± bone destruction with variable enhancement
    - MR best for evaluating perineural & intracranial spread
- **Adenoid Cystic Carcinoma, Sinonasal**
  - Key facts: Accounts for < 10% of SN malignancies
    - Median age of incidence is 50 years
    - No sex predilection
    - Palate primaries may extend into maxillary antrum & nasal cavity

- Perineural spread, late recurrences, & distant metastases more common than other SN malignancies
- Maxillary sinus & nasal cavity most common sites

o Imaging: Nonspecific; well- to poorly defined soft tissue mass ± bone destruction
- Variable MR signal with heterogeneous enhancement
- Look for perineural spread (may be extensive despite small primary site)

Helpful Clues for Rare Diagnoses

- **Osteosarcoma, Sinonasal**
  - o Key facts: ≤ 1% of SN tumors
    - ↑ risk if prior radiation therapy & ThO_2 (Thorotrast) exposure
    - Can arise in Paget disease of bone, fibrous dysplasia, or osteoblastoma
    - Males in 3rd & 4th decades
  - o Imaging
    - CT: Aggressive mass with bone destruction, irregular calcification ± osteoid matrix, "sunburst" periosteal reaction
    - MR: Low to intermediate T1 & T2 signals (ossified areas ↓ signal)
- **Chondrosarcoma, Sinonasal**
  - o Key facts: Most arise in anterior maxilla with antral extension; M:F = 3:2
    - 2nd-8th decade; most in 5th-7th decade
    - Most subtypes no strong sex predilection; mesenchymal subtype F > M (2:1)
  - o Imaging: Ca++ matrix (< 50%)
    - Expansile with variable bone destruction/remodeling
    - MR: ↑ T2 signal common
- **Langerhans Cell Histiocytosis, Skull Base**
  - o Key facts: Skull & T-bone most common
    - Skull base; mandible/maxilla less common
    - Presents in 1st decade (more severe cases present earlier)
  - o Imaging
    - CT: Focal or diffuse mass + bone destruction; punched-out or irregular margins
    - MR: ↓ T1, ↑ T2 signal; heterogeneous enhancement ± blood products
- **Metastasis**
  - o Key facts: Very rare; renal > lung > breast; systemic metastases usually present
  - o Imaging: Aggressive bone-destroying soft tissue masses with variable enhancement

SELECTED REFERENCES

1. Lewis JS Jr: Sinonasal squamous cell carcinoma: a review with emphasis on emerging histologic subtypes and the role of human papillomavirus. Head Neck Pathol. 10(1):60-7, 2016
2. Park SH et al: Outcome of definitive and postoperative radiotherapy in patients with sinonasal squamous cell carcinomas. Tumori. 102(4):426-32, 2016
3. Suzuki H et al: The Charlson comorbidity index is a prognostic factor in sinonasal tract squamous cell carcinoma. Jpn J Clin Oncol. 46(7):646-51, 2016
4. Tabrizi R et al: Association between clinical features, treatment, and recurrence rate of adenoid cystic carcinoma of the palate: a 10-year retrospective study. Br J Oral Maxillofac Surg. ;54(6):648-51, 2016
5. Unsal AA et al: Squamous cell carcinoma of the nasal cavity: a population-based analysis. Laryngoscope. 126(3):560-5, 2016
6. Banuchi V et al: Cancers of the nose, sinus, and skull base. Surg Oncol Clin N Am. 24(3):563-77, 2015
7. Doescher J et al: Epstein-Barr virus infection is strictly associated with the metastatic spread of sinonasal squamous-cell carcinomas. Oral Oncol. 51(10):929-34, 2015
8. Janisiewicz AM et al: Higher antineutrophil cytoplasmic antibody (C-ANCA) titers are associated with increased overall healthcare use in patients with sinonasal manifestations of granulomatosis with polyangiitis (GPA). Am J Rhinol Allergy. 29(3):202-6, 2015
9. Knopf A et al: Clinical aspects of granulomatosis with polyangiitis affecting the head and neck. Eur Arch Otorhinolaryngol. 272(1):185-93, 2015
10. Pakalniskis MG et al: The many faces of granulomatosis with polyangiitis: a review of the head and neck imaging manifestations. AJR Am J Roentgenol. 205(6):W619-29, 2015
11. Zhang SC et al: Inability of PET/CT to identify a primary sinonasal inverted papilloma with squamous cell carcinoma in a patient with a submandibular lymph node metastasis: A case report. Oncol Lett. 10(2):749-753, 2015
12. Garg D et al: Clinico-pathological study of space occupying lesions of nasal cavity, paranasal sinuses and nasopharynx. J Clin Diagn Res. 8(11):FC04-7, 2014
13. Kuo CY et al: Changes in sinonasal mucosa in Wegener granulomatosis. CMAJ. 186(11):854, 2014

Squamous Cell Carcinoma, Sinonasal

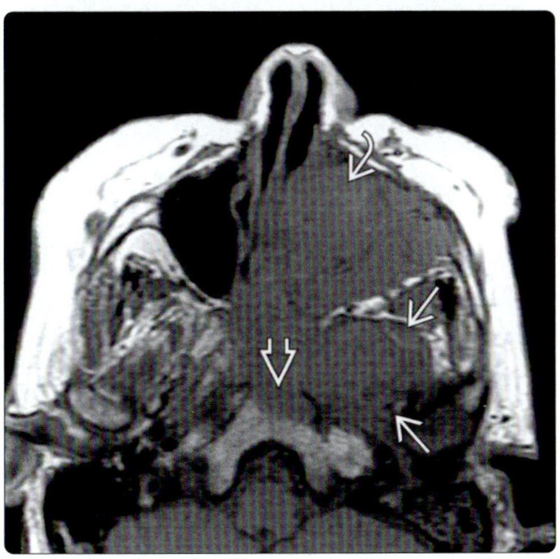

Fungal Sinusitis, Invasive (Fulminant Sinusitis)

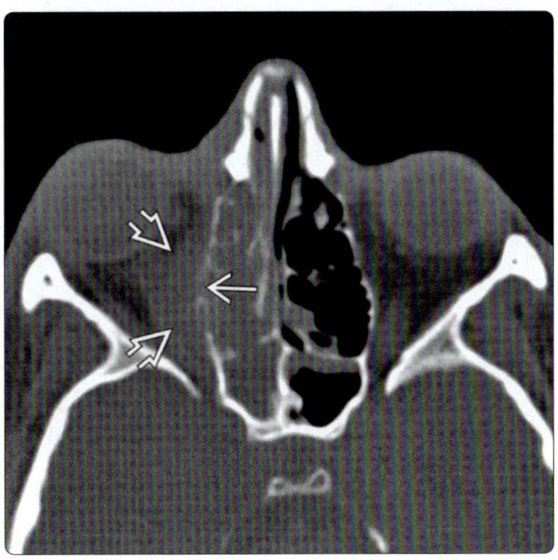

(Left) *Axial T1WI MR shows a large maxillary squamous cell carcinoma ➡. The lesion destroys the maxillary sinus walls and invades the masticator space ➡ and clivus ➡. Squamous cell carcinoma is the most common sinonasal malignancy.* **(Right)** *Axial bone CT shows extension of fungal sinusitis of the ethmoid sinuses into the orbit ➡. A small area of bone erosion by the fungus is noted in the lamina papyracea ➡. Aspergillus and mucormycosis are most common.*

Paranasal Sinus Lesions With Bony Destruction

(Left) *Axial CECT demonstrates a large esthesioneuroblastoma involving the ethmoid sinuses bilaterally and extending into the orbits* ➡ *and anterior skull base* ⇨. **(Right)** *Coronal bone CT reveals a lymphoma originating in the nasal cavity and causing obstruction of multiple ethmoid air cells* ➡. *Destruction of the bony nasal septum* ⇨ *is present. Less than 50% of extranodal H&N non-Hodgkin lymphomas arise in the sinonasal cavities.*

Esthesioneuroblastoma (Olfactory Neuroblastoma)

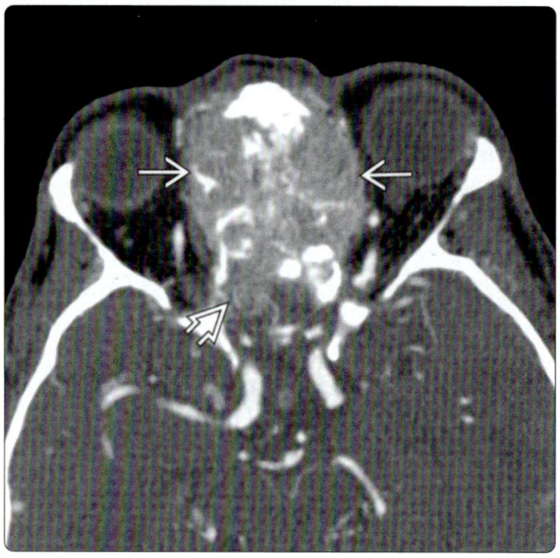

Non-Hodgkin Lymphoma, Sinonasal

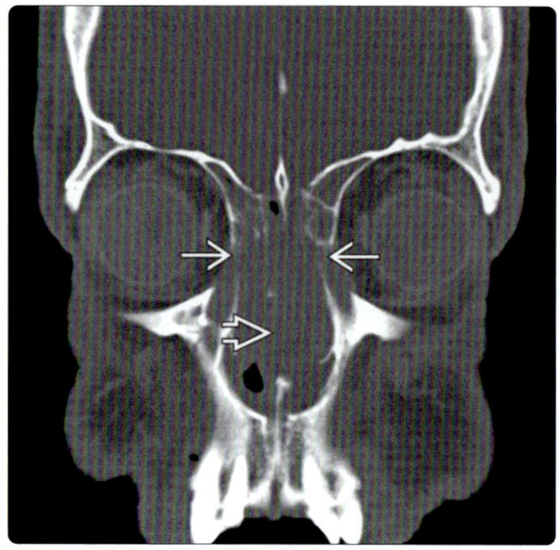

(Left) *Axial CECT shows extensive nodular soft tissue in the sinonasal cavities and bone destruction of the septum* ➡ *and medial maxillary sinus walls* ⇨ *related to granulomatosis with polyangiitis.* **(Right)** *Coronal NECT demonstrates a large sinonasal undifferentiated carcinoma (SNUC) that originated in the maxillary sinus and spread into the nasal cavity* ➡, *orbit* ↪, *and soft tissues of the cheek. SNUCs are extremely malignant with rapid growth, distant metastases, and poor prognosis.*

Granulomatosis With Polyangiitis, Sinonasal

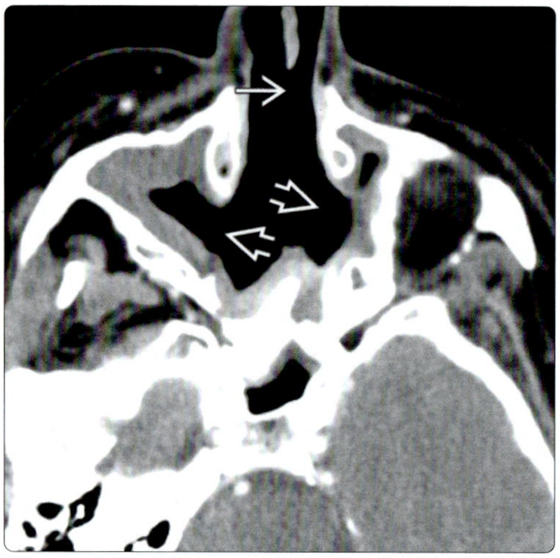

Undifferentiated Carcinoma, Sinonasal

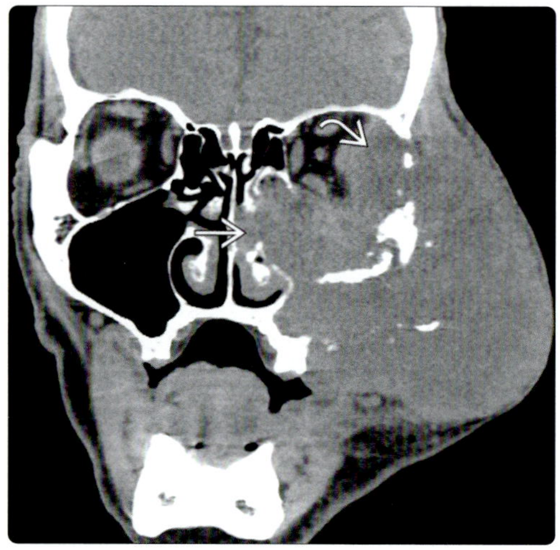

(Left) *Axial CECT shows a heterogeneous ethmoid sinus adenocarcinoma with cystic foci that invade the orbits* ➡. *Invasion of the subcutaneous soft tissues is noted anteriorly* ⇨. *Adenocarcinoma accounts for ~ 10-20% of all sinonasal malignancies.* **(Right)** *Coronal bone CT shows extensive sarcoidosis with nodular sinonasal soft tissue thickening. Large nasal septal perforation* ➡ *is present as well as erosion of turbinates and ethmoid trabecula* ⇨.

Adenocarcinoma, Sinonasal

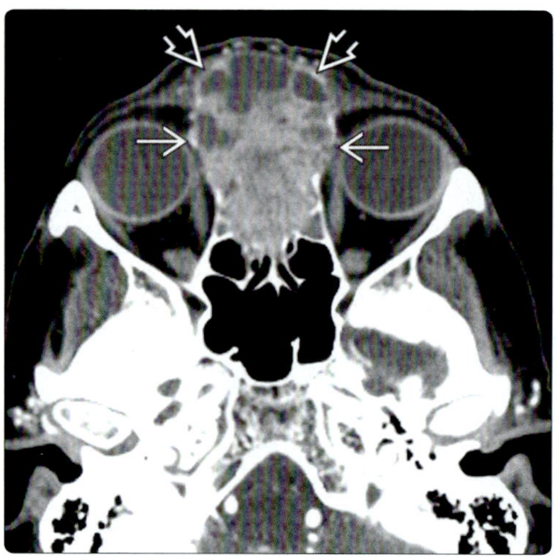

Sarcoidosis, Sinonasal

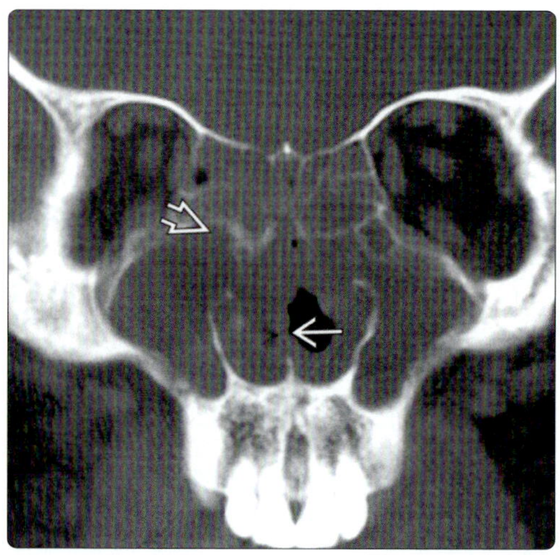

Rhabdomyosarcoma

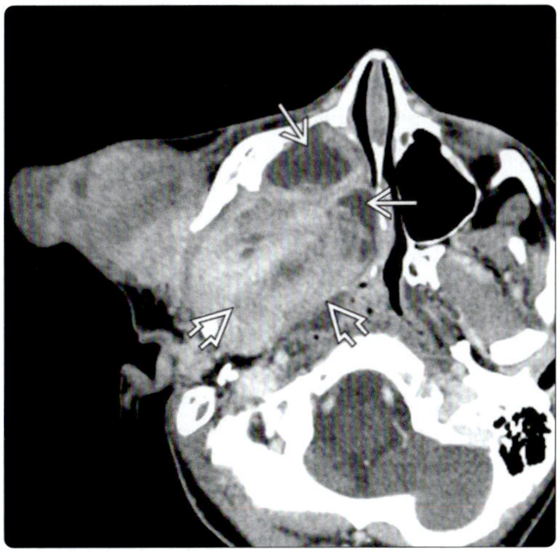

Adenoid Cystic Carcinoma, Sinonasal

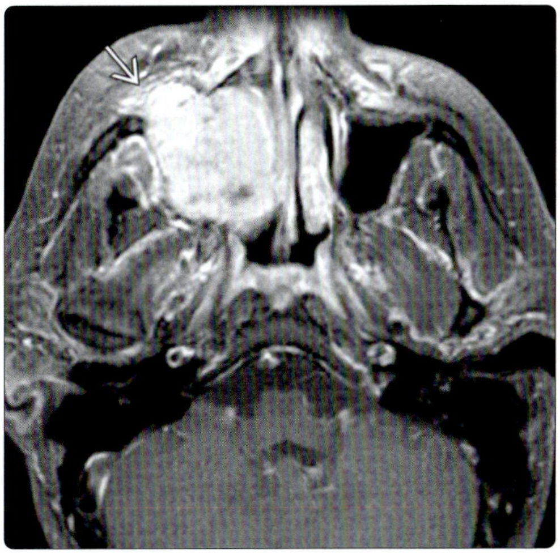

(Left) *Axial CECT of a child reveals a large rhabdomyosarcoma involving the right maxillary sinus, infratemporal fossa, and soft tissues of the cheek. Rhabdomyosarcoma is the most common childhood sarcoma. (Courtesy L. Ginsberg, MD.)* **(Right)** *Axial T1WI C+ FS MR reveals a heterogeneously enhancing adenoid cystic carcinoma of the right maxillary antrum. There is extension through the anterior wall into soft tissues of the cheek.*

Osteosarcoma, Sinonasal

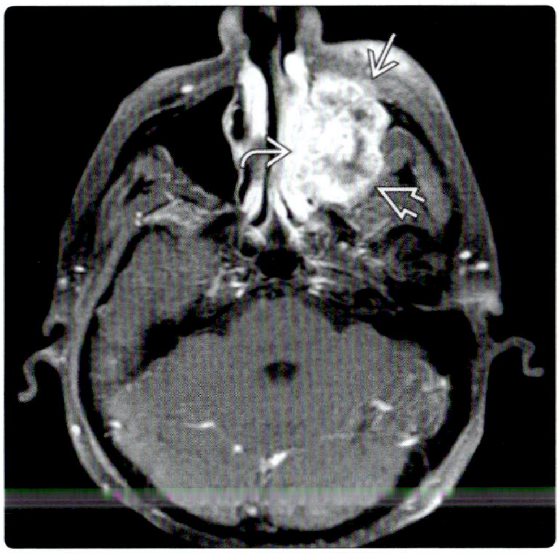

Chondrosarcoma, Sinonasal

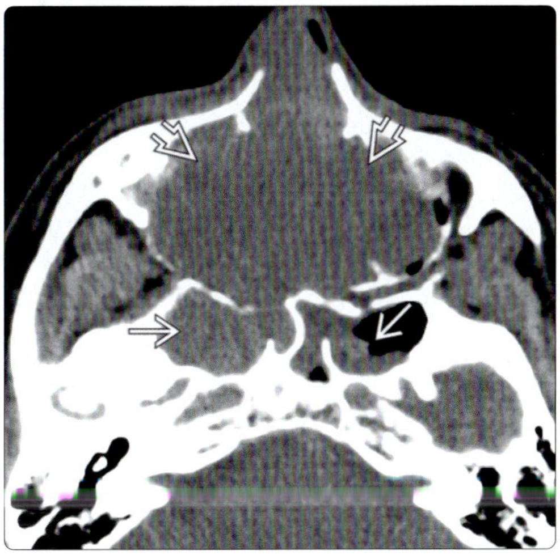

(Left) *Axial T1WI C+ FS MR shows a heterogeneously enhancing osteosarcoma involving the maxillary ridge, hard palate, and antrum. Note the spread through anterior, posterior, and medial walls.* **(Right)** *Axial NECT shows a large myxoid chondrosarcoma with bone destruction involving the nasal cavity and maxillary sinuses bilaterally. The nasal septum is eroded, and trapped secretions are present in the sphenoid sinuses. Most sinonasal chondrosarcomas arise in the anterior maxilla.*

Langerhans Cell Histiocytosis, Skull Base

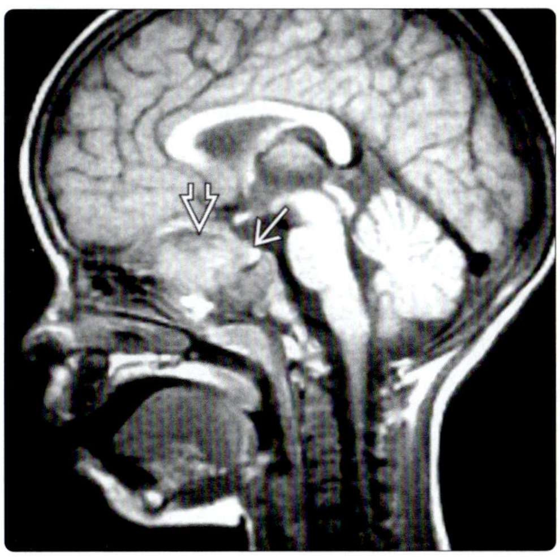

Metastasis

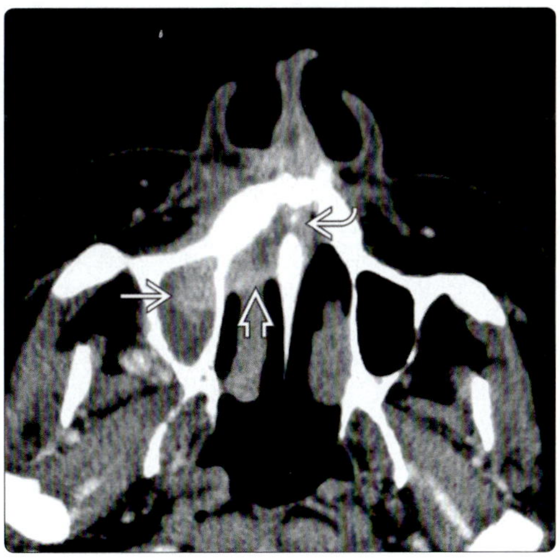

(Left) *Sagittal T1WI MR in a child reveals Langerhans cell histiocytosis of the central skull base that invades the sella turcica, anterior cranial fossa, and posterior ethmoid sinuses.* **(Right)** *Axial CECT shows an enhancing lesion involving the right antrum and nasal cavity. This prostate carcinoma metastasis erodes the septum and extends into the contralateral nasal cavity. Metastasis to the sinonasal area is very rare, and systemic metastases are usually present.*

Displaced Dental Structures Into Antrum

DIFFERENTIAL DIAGNOSIS

Common

- Root or Root Fragment
- Whole Tooth

Less Common

- Implant
- Dental Amalgam
- Endodontic Filling Material: Gutta Percha, Cement
- Bone Grafting Material
- Denture Lining Material

Rare but Important

- Surgical Bur
- Surgical Screws and Hardware
- Syringe Needle
- Dental Impression Material

ESSENTIAL INFORMATION

Key Differential Diagnosis Issues

- Antral projections (exostoses) may mimic root fragments
- Displaced structure between oral soft tissue and bone, outside sinus
- Displaced structure between antral soft tissue and bone, outside sinus lumen
- Antrolith (maxillary sinolith) less homogeneously radiopaque

Helpful Clues for Common Diagnoses

- **Root or Root Fragment**
  - Key facts
    - Missing tooth in arch unless supernumerary or deciduous tooth was extracted
    - History of extraction
  - Imaging
    - Object with radiopacity of root, size variable
    - Coronal or axial CT or CBCT shows it in sinus
- **Whole Tooth**
  - Key facts
    - Missing tooth in arch unless supernumerary or deciduous tooth was displaced
    - History of attempted extraction
  - Imaging
    - Object should have morphology and density of tooth, most often molar or premolar

Helpful Clues for Less Common Diagnoses

- **Implant**
  - Key facts
    - History of implant placement in maxilla
  - Imaging
    - Cylindrical object with radiopacity of metal
- **Dental Amalgam**
  - Key facts
    - History of extraction of carious but restored tooth
    - History of retrograde amalgam
  - Imaging
    - Dental amalgam has radiopacity of metal
    - Usually irregular small mass
- **Endodontic Filling Material: Gutta Percha, Cement**
  - Key facts
    - History of endodontic treatment
    - Gutta percha (GP) and cement less radiopaque than metal; silver points radiopacity of metal
    - GP or silver point extends from apex into sinus
    - Cement usually discrete entity; may be multiple
- **Bone Grafting Material**
  - Key facts
    - History of bone augmentation
  - Imaging
    - Heterogeneous radiopacity similar to bone
    - If properly placed, located just below mucoperiosteum
    - If displaced, within lumen of sinus
    - Stippled heterogeneous radiopacity if hydroxyapatite
- **Denture Lining Material**
  - History of maxillary posterior dental extraction with possible oroantral fistula
  - Recent relining of maxillary denture

Helpful Clues for Rare Diagnoses

- **Surgical Bur**
  - Key facts
    - History of osseous surgery and missing bur
  - Imaging
    - Long cylindrical homogeneous metal rod
    - Bur head may be spherical, cylindrical, or tapered
- **Surgical Screws and Hardware**
  - Key facts
    - History of osseous surgery and missing hardware
  - Imaging
    - Surgical screws: Recognizable screw shape with head and thread
    - Surgical plates: Recognizable metallic surgical hardware shape
      - Multiple possible shapes
      - Usually smooth edges and perforations
    - Metallic sutures: Thin, linear, metallic entity
      - May be straight or loop with twisted tail
- **Syringe Needle**
  - Key facts
    - History of needle breaking during injection or aspiration
  - Imaging
    - Thin, linear, metallic entity with beveled (pointed) end
    - Less radiopaque lumen
- **Dental Impression Material**
  - Key facts
    - History of impression that was hard to remove; presence of oroantral fistula
  - Imaging
    - Irregular smooth mass of variable density

SELECTED REFERENCES

1. Deniz Y et al: An unusual foreign body in the maxillary sinus: Dental impression material. Niger J Clin Pract. 19(2):298-300, 2016
2. Lari SS et al: Comparative sensitivity assessment of cone beam computed tomography and digital radiography for detecting foreign bodies. J Contemp Dent Pract. 17(3):224-9, 2016
3. Nogami S et al: Removal of dental implant displaced into maxillary sinus by combination of endoscopically assisted and bone repositioning techniques: a case report. J Med Case Rep. 10(1):1, 2016

4. Sugiura T et al: Chronic maxillary sinusitis caused by denture lining material. Open Dent J. 10:261-7, 2016
5. Yousefi J et al: Penetrating nose and maxillary sinus injury with a metal part of a military gun. J R Army Med Corps. 162(2):137-8, 2016
6. Ding X et al: Displacement of a dental implant into the maxillary sinus after internal sinus floor elevation: report of a case and review of literature. Int J Clin Exp Med. 8(4):4826-36, 2015
7. Yamashita Y et al: Removal of migrated dental implants from maxillary sinus 4 years 10 months after implant placement. Oral Maxillofac Surg. 19(3):315-9, 2015
8. Alons-ter Hoeven J et al: Silent sinus syndrome secondary to a radix relicta in the antrum. J Craniofac Surg. 21(2):607-9, 2010
9. Borgonovo A et al: Displacement of a dental implant into the maxillary sinus: case series. Minerva Stomatol. 59(1-2):45-54, 2010
10. Chandrasena F et al: Removal of a root from the maxillary sinus using functional endoscopic sinus surgery. Br J Oral Maxillofac Surg. 48(7):558-9, 2010
11. Chrcanovic BR et al: Traumatic displacement of maxillary permanent incisor into the nasal cavity. Oral Maxillofac Surg. 14(3):175-82, 2010
12. Griffa A et al: Endoscopic-assisted removal of an intraorbital dislocated dental implant. Clin Oral Implants Res. 21(7):778-80, 2010
13. Kitamura A et al: Migrated maxillary implant removed via semilunar hiatus by transnasal endoscope. Implant Dent. 19(1):16-20, 2010
14. Mostafa YA et al: Four curious cases of cone-beam computed tomography. Am J Orthod Dentofacial Orthop. 137(4 Suppl):S136-40, 2010
15. Ramsey RA et al: Re: root fragment in the ostium of the maxillary sinus [Br. J. Oral Maxillfac. Surg. 47 (2009) 572-573]. Br J Oral Maxillofac Surg. 48(2):154-5, 2010
16. Saleem T et al: Supernumerary, ectopic tooth in the maxillary antrum presenting with recurrent haemoptysis. Head Face Med. 6:26, 2010
17. Chappuis V et al: Displacement of a dental implant into the maxillary sinus: report of an unusual complication when performing staged sinus floor elevation procedures. Int J Periodontics Restorative Dent. 29(1):81-7, 2009
18. Chiapasco M et al: The management of complications following displacement of oral implants in the paranasal sinuses: a multicenter clinical report and proposed treatment protocols. Int J Oral Maxillofac Surg. 38(12):1273-8, 2009
19. Dennis MJ: Exodontia for the general dentist: complications. Todays FDA. 21(10):14-9, 2009
20. Flanagan D: A method to retrieve a displaced dental implant from the maxillary sinus. J Oral Implantol. 35(2):70-4, 2009
21. Ridaura-Ruiz L et al: Accidental displacement of dental implants into the maxillary sinus: a report of nine cases. Clin Implant Dent Relat Res. 11 Suppl 1:e38-45, 2009
22. Rodrigues MT et al: Chronic maxillary sinusitis associated with dental impression material. Med Oral Patol Oral Cir Bucal. 14(4):E163-6, 2009
23. Segal N et al: Paranasal sinus complications caused by dental implants and complementary procedures. B-ENT. 5(3):153-7, 2009
24. Sethi A et al: Root fragment in the ostium of the maxillary sinus. Br J Oral Maxillofac Surg. 47(7):572-3, 2009

Whole Tooth

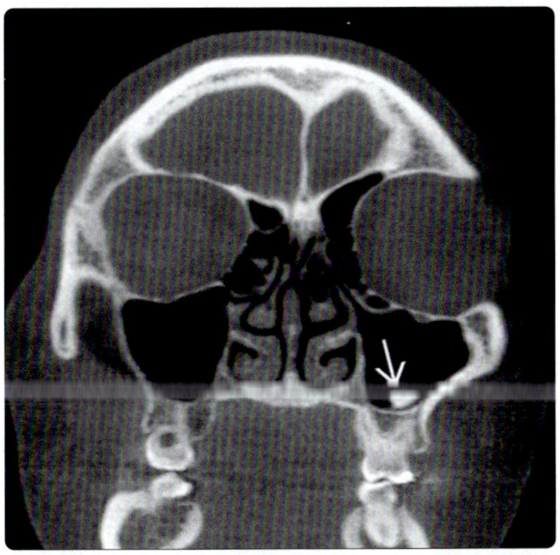

Whole Tooth

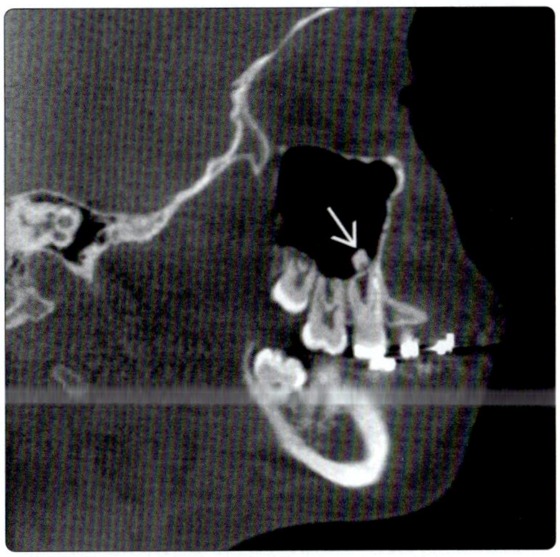

(Left) *Reconstructed coronal CBCT shows a supernumerary tooth ➡ in the left maxillary sinus. (Courtesy S. Vijayan, BDS.)* **(Right)** *Reconstructed sagittal CBCT in the same patient shows a supernumerary tooth ➡ in the left maxillary sinus. (Courtesy S. Vijayan, BDS.)*

Whole Tooth

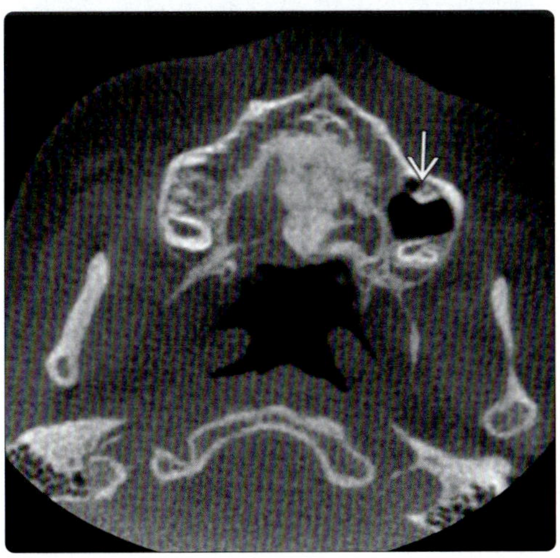

Implant

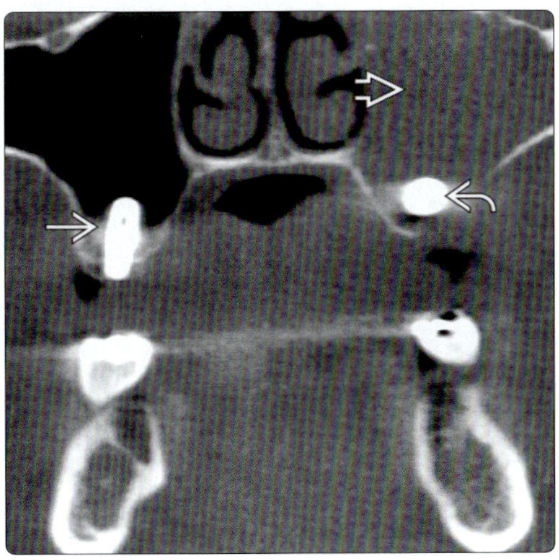

(Left) *Reconstructed axial CBCT in the same patient shows a supernumerary tooth ➡ in the left maxillary sinus. (Courtesy S. Vijayan, BDS.)* **(Right)** *Coronal CBCT shows an implant ➡ entirely within the left maxillary sinus with sinusitis ➡ and an implant ➡ protruding into the right maxillary sinus. If an implant protrudes > 4 mm into the sinus, it will likely breach the mucosa and cause inflammation.*

(Left) *Sagittal reformat CBCT in the same patient shows left implant entirely within maxillary sinus. Note that the implant is not homogeneously radiopaque. There is an associated sinusitis, resulting in almost complete opacification of sinus air space.* **(Right)** *Coronal reconstructed CBCT shows a metallic foreign body, consistent with a displaced dental implant in the left maxillary sinus. There is soft tissue thickening, consistent with inflammation. (Courtesy D. Alhazmi, BDS.)*

Implant

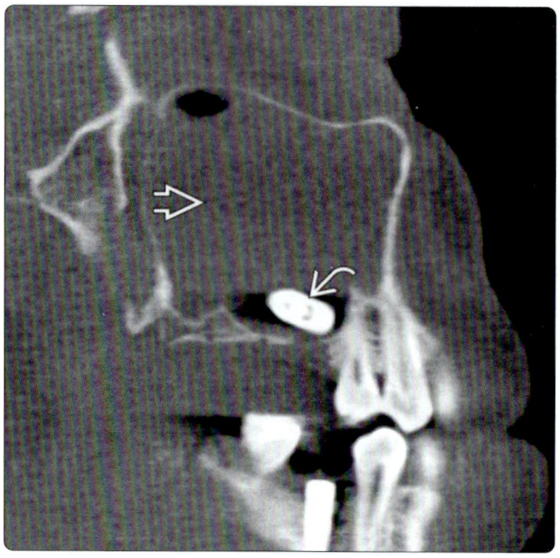

Implant

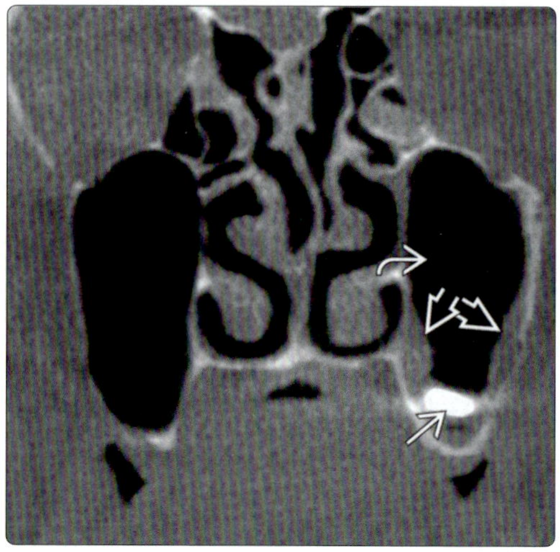

(Left) *Axial reconstructed CBCT in the same patient shows the metallic foreign body, consistent with a displaced dental implant in the left maxillary sinus. There is soft tissue thickening, consistent with inflammation. (Courtesy D. Alhazmi, BDS.)* **(Right)** *Axial reconstructed CBCT in the same patient shows the displaced implant in the left maxillary sinus. There is soft tissue thickening, consistent with inflammation. (Courtesy D. Alhazmi, BDS.)*

Implant

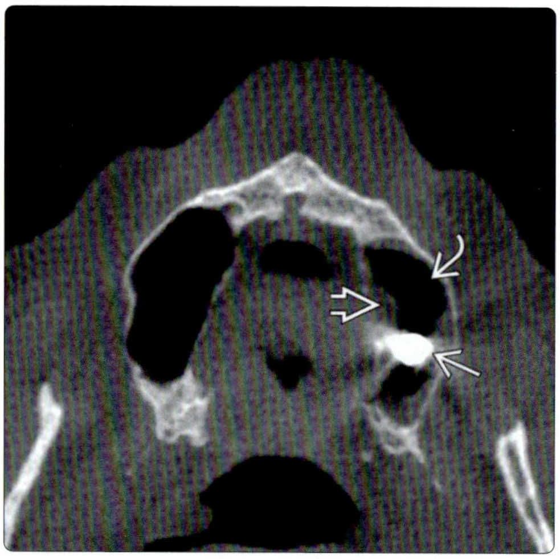

Implant

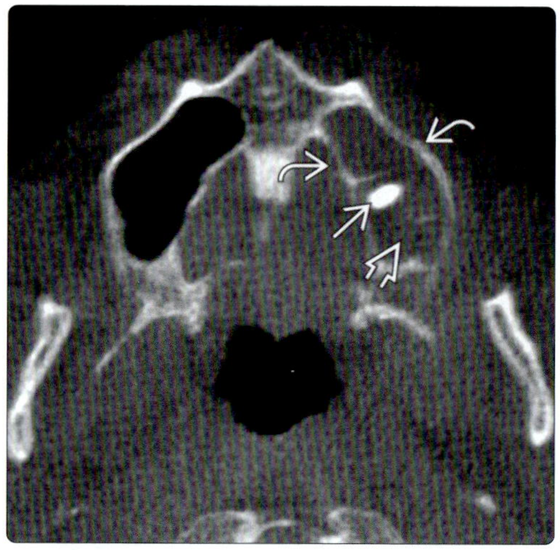

(Left) *Periapical radiograph of the right maxillary posterior dentition shows an endodontically treated 1st permanent molar. The apex is near the sinus border. There is extruded endodontic cement at the floor of the sinus.* **(Right)** *CBCT composite shows a surgical bur in the right maxillary sinus in the coronal and sagittal views. The patient had a history of sinus-lift surgery prior to implants with subsequent poor healing and discomfort.*

Endodontic Filling Material: Gutta Percha, Cement

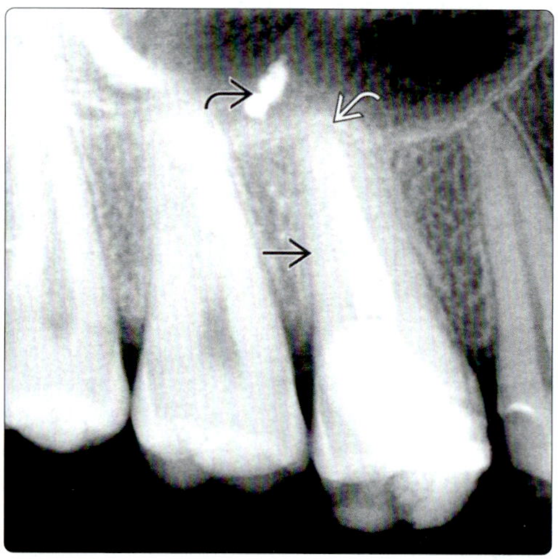

Surgical Bur

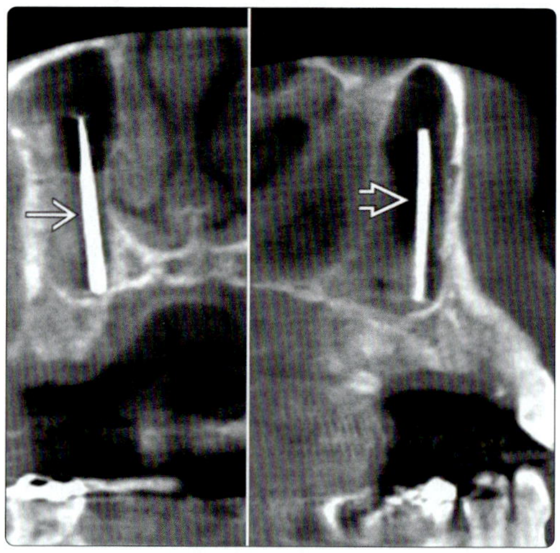

Surgical Bur

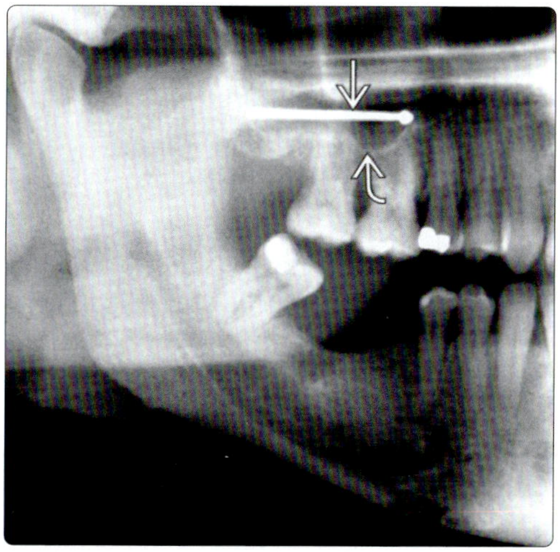

Syringe Needle

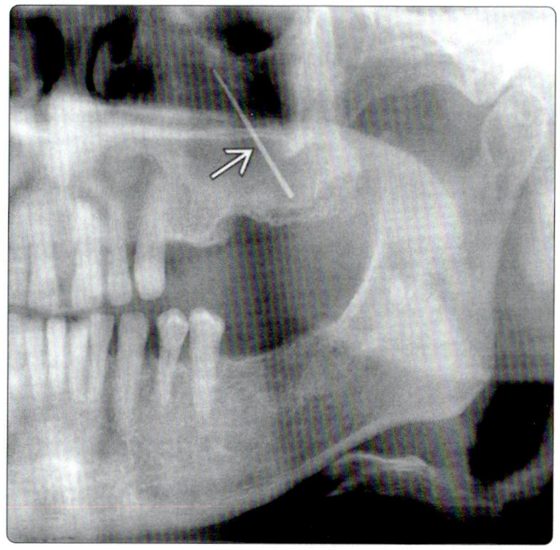

(Left) *Cropped panoramic radiograph shows a surgical bur ➡ in the right maxillary sinus ➡. (Courtesy R. Santilli, DDS.)* **(Right)** *A cropped panoramic radiograph of the left maxillary sinus shows a long tapered metallic radiopacity ➡, consistent with a broken needle. (Courtesy M. Hansen, DDS.)*

Syringe Needle

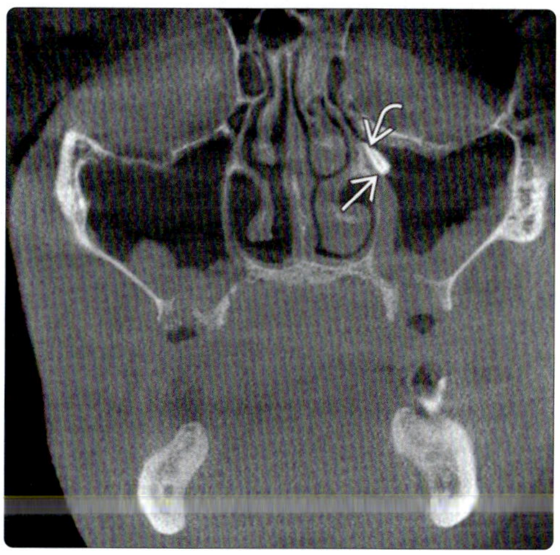

Syringe Needle

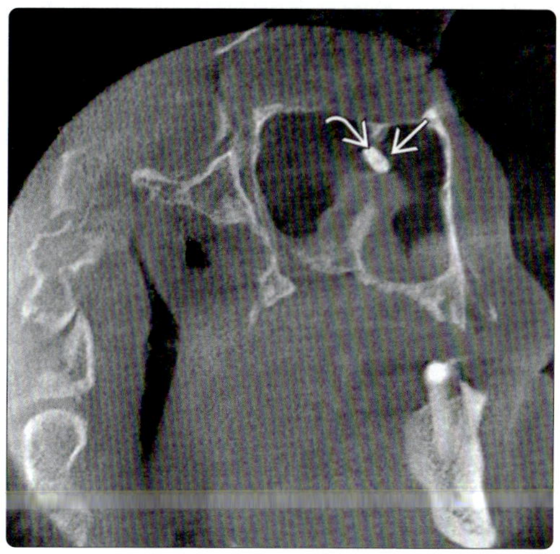

(Left) *Coronal CBCT reconstruction shows a metallic radiopaque mass ➡ with a radiolucent lumen ➡, suggestive of a possible broken needle or other metallic object. (Courtesy M. Hansen, DDS.)* **(Right)** *Sagittal CBCT reconstruction in the same patient shows a metallic radiopaque mass ➡ with a radiolucent lumen ➡, suggestive of a broken needle or other metallic object. (Courtesy M. Hansen, DDS.)*

Syringe Needle

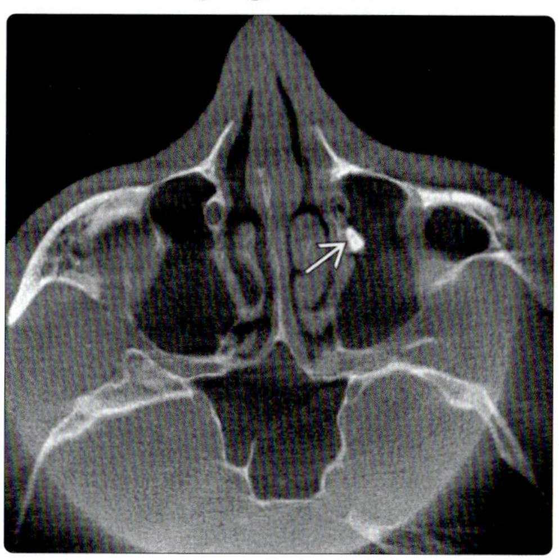

Dental Impression Material

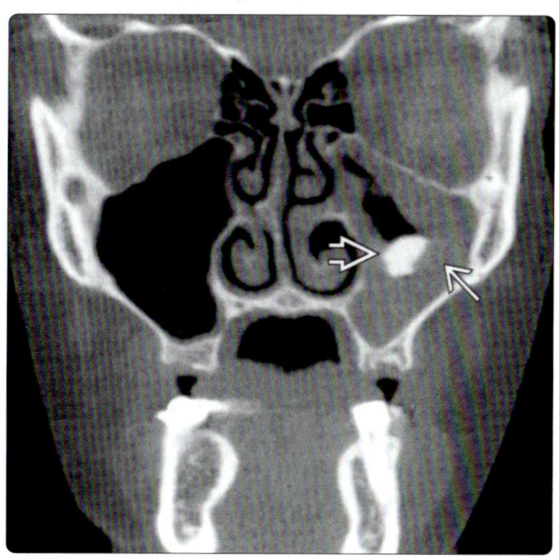

(Left) *Axial CBCT reconstruction in same patient shows a metallic radiopaque mass ➡. Visualizing structures displaced into the antrum in multiple planes is necessary to determine proximity to important anatomy. (Courtesy M. Hansen, DDS.)* **(Right)** *Coronal CBCT shows dental impression material ➡ in the lumen of the left maxillary sinus. The dentist was unaware of the presence of an oroantral fistula from prior extraction, and impression material was expressed into the sinus. Note the marked mucosal thickening ➡.*

INDEX

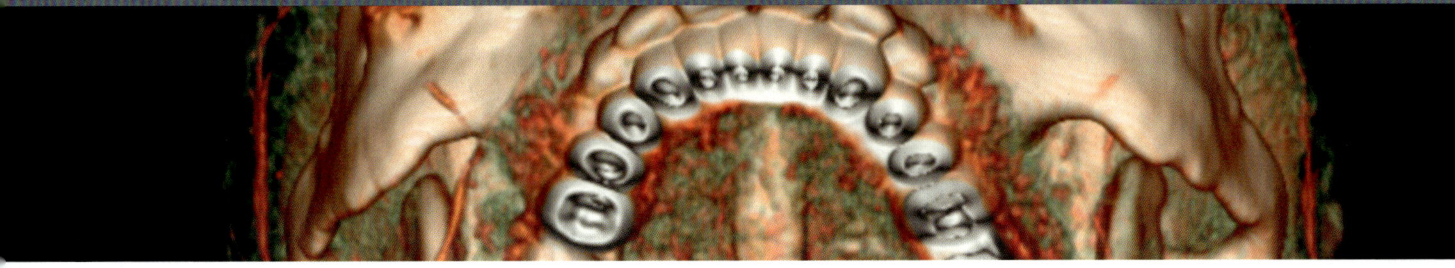

A

AA. *See* Aortic arch.
AADI. *See* Anterior atlantodens interval.
ABC. *See* Aneurysmal bone cyst, mandible-maxilla.
Abducens nerve, **132**
- CNVI, **127, 132**

Abducens nucleus (CNVI), **140**
Abfraction, **240**
- diagnostic checklist, **240**
- differential diagnosis, **240**

Abrasion, **238**
- abfraction vs., **240**
- attrition vs., **237**
- erosion vs., **239**
- internal and external resorption vs., **243–244**

Abscess
- dermoid and epidermoid cysts vs., **285**
- floor of mouth, sublingual gland benign mixed tumor vs., **307**
- masticator space, **724–727**
  - benign masticator muscle hypertrophy vs., **747**
  - diagnostic checklist, **726**
  - differential diagnosis, **725–726**
  - masticator muscle atrophy vs., **729**
  - masticator space sarcoma vs., **739**
  - prognosis, **726**
  - retromolar trigone squamous cell carcinoma vs., **329**
- oral cavity
  - floor of mouth squamous cell carcinoma vs., **325**
  - ranula vs., **297**
  - root of tongue lesions vs., **930, 931**
  - sublingual gland carcinoma vs., **315**
  - submandibular space lesions vs., **914, 916**
- palatal, palate benign mixed tumor vs., **311**
- periapical. *See* Periapical rarefying osteitis.
- periodontal, **271**
- radicular. *See* Periapical rarefying osteitis.
- sublingual space, sublingual space lesions vs., **922, 923**
- submandibular space, submandibular space accessory salivary tissue vs., **281**

Abutment tooth, **16**
ACCa. *See* Adenoid cystic carcinoma.
Accessory atlantoaxial ligament, **151**
Accessory inferior alveolar canal (IAC). *See* Accessory mandibular canal.
Accessory mandibular canal, **348–349**
- associated abnormalities, **349**
- diagnostic checklist, **349**
- differential diagnosis, **349**
- gubernaculum dentis vs., **277**
- prognosis, **349**

Accessory maxillary ostia. *See* Accessory ostia.
Accessory meningeal artery, **206**
Accessory nerve (CNXI), **111, 189, 190**
Accessory openings. *See* Accessory ostia.
Accessory ostia, **656–657**
- associated abnormalities, **657**
- differential diagnosis, **657**
- staging, grading, and classification, **657**

Accessory parotid gland, **183**
Accessory salivary tissue, in mylohyoid boutonnière. *See* Submandibular space accessory salivary tissue.
Accessory sinus ostia. *See* Accessory ostia.
Acinic cell carcinoma, parotid space lesions vs., **921**
Acrocephalosyndactyly, hypoplasia/aplasia associated, **660**
Acute apical periodontitis. *See* Periapical rarefying osteitis.
Acute bacterial rhinosinusitis (ABRS). *See* Rhinosinusitis, acute.
Acute invasive fungal rhinosinusitis (AIFRS). *See* Fungal sinusitis, invasive.
Acute lymphoblastic leukemia (ALL). *See* Leukemia.
Acute necrotizing FRS. *See* Fungal sinusitis, invasive.
Acute necrotizing ulcerative periodontitis, **271, 272**
Acute nonlymphoblastic leukemia (ANL). *See* Leukemia.
Acute osteomyelitis, periapical rarefying osteitis vs., **266**
Acute radiation changes, sublingual gland, sublingual space lesions vs., **922, 924**
Acute sialadenitis, **301**
Acute suppurative osteomyelitis. *See* Osteomyelitis, mandible-maxilla.
Adamantinoma. *See* Ameloblastoma.
Adamantoblastoma. *See* Ameloblastoma.
Adenoameloblastoma. *See* Adenomatoid odontogenic tumor.
Adenocarcinoma, sinonasal
- intestinal type, sinonasal adenoid cystic carcinoma vs., **707**
- nasal lesion with bony destruction vs., **970, 972**
- paranasal sinus lesions with bony destruction vs., **980, 982**

Adenoid cystic carcinoma (ACCa), **313, 315**
- parotid, **772–773**
  - diagnostic checklist, **773**
  - differential diagnosis, **773**
  - parotid malignant mixed tumor vs., **767**
  - parotid mucoepidermoid carcinoma vs., **769**
  - prognosis, **773**
  - staging, grading, & classification, **773**
  - Warthin tumor vs., **761**
- sinonasal, **706–707**
  - differential diagnosis, **707**

INDEX

paranasal sinus lesions with bony destruction vs., **980–981, 983**
prognosis, **707**
staging, grading, & classification, **707**
- sublingual gland benign mixed tumor vs., **307**

Adenoidal benign lymphoid hyperplasia, nasopharyngeal carcinoma vs., **709**
Adenoids, **109, 175, 176, 177, 178**
Adenolymphoma. *See* Warthin tumor.
Adenoma
- palate pleomorphic. *See* Palate benign mixed tumor.
- pleomorphic. *See* Submandibular gland benign mixed tumor.
  of sublingual gland. *See* Sublingual gland benign mixed tumor.

Adenomatoid odontogenic tumor (AOT), **454–455**
- ameloblastic fibroodontoma vs., **465**
- calcifying epithelial odontogenic tumor vs., **467**
- calcifying odontogenic cyst vs., **413**
- differential diagnosis, **455**
- gubernaculum dentis, **277**
- pericoronal radiolucencies with radiopacities vs., **876, 877**
- prognosis, **455**
- staging, grading, & classification, **455**

Adhesions, **616–617**
- diagnostic checklist, **617**
- differential diagnosis, **617**
- disc displacement without reduction vs., **612**
- fibrous ankylosis vs., **561**
- limited condylar translation vs., **950, 952**
- prognosis, **617**
- staging, grading, & classification, **617**

Aditus ad antrum, **90, 92**
Advanced periodontal disease, floating teeth vs., **862**
Aerated tip uncinate process, **74**
AF. *See* Ameloblastic fibroma.
AFO. *See* Ameloblastic fibroodontoma.
African jaw lymphoma. *See* Burkitt lymphoma.
Agger nasi cells, **66, 68, 72, 75**
- sinonasal overview, **56**

Aggressive fibromatosis. *See* Desmoplastic fibroma.
Aggressive periodontitis, **271, 272**
- floating teeth vs., **862, 863**

Air in nasolacrimal sac, **66**
Alae nasi, **26**
Alar fascia, **163, 193, 194**
Alar ligament, **151**
Albers Schönberg disease, hypoplasia/aplasia associated, **660**
Alisphenoid, **106**
Allergy
- chronic rhinosinusitis associated, **682**
- sinonasal polyposis associated, **674**

Alveolar bone, **10**
Alveolar canal, inferior, anatomy, **35**
Alveolar foramen, middle superior, **26**
Alveolar interdental bone, **11**
Alveolar nerve
- of mandible, inferior, anatomy, **31**
- of maxilla, anatomy
  anterior superior, **22**
  middle superior, **22**
  posterior superior, **22**
- posterior, middle, and anterior superior, **128**

Alveolar process
- anatomy, **31, 34**
  mandible, **30**
  maxilla, **22**
- around molar tooth, pneumatization of, **63**
- fractures of, dentoalveolar fractures vs., **255**
- implant centered in, **20**
- of maxilla, **58**

Alveolar ridge (gingiva), **53**
Alveolar/mandibular canal, inferior, anatomy, **30**
Amalgam restoration
- class I, **15**
- class II, **15**

Ameloblastic adenomatoid tumor. *See* Adenomatoid odontogenic tumor.
Ameloblastic carcinoma, malignant ameloblastoma and, **492–493**
- differential diagnosis, **493**
- prognosis, **493**

Ameloblastic carcinosarcoma, ameloblastic fibroma transformation, **462**
Ameloblastic fibroma, **460–463**
- ameloblastic fibroodontoma vs., **465**
- associated abnormalities, **462**
- dentigerous cyst vs., **397**
- diagnostic checklist, **462**
- differential diagnosis, **461**
- genetics, **462**
- malignant transformation, **462**
- pericoronal radiolucencies without radiopacities vs., **874, 875**
- prognosis, **462**

Ameloblastic fibroodontoma, **464–465**
- adenomatoid odontogenic tumor vs., **455**
- calcifying epithelial odontogenic tumor vs., **467**
- calcifying odontogenic cyst vs., **413**
- diagnostic checklist, **465**
- differential diagnosis, **465**
- immature, ameloblastic fibroma vs., **461**
- odontoma vs., **452**
- pericoronal radiolucencies with radiopacities vs., **876, 877**

Ameloblastic fibrosarcoma, ameloblastic fibroma transformation, **462**
Ameloblastic odontoma
- immature, ameloblastic fibroma vs., **461**
- pericoronal radiolucencies with radiopacities vs., **876**

Ameloblastoma, **456–459**
- ameloblastic carcinoma and, malignant, **492–493**
  differential diagnosis, **493**
  prognosis, **493**
- ameloblastic fibroma vs., **461**
- central giant cell granuloma vs., **531**
- central hemangioma vs., **475**
- central mucoepidermoid carcinoma vs., **511**
- desmoplastic fibroma vs., **491**

INDEX

- diagnostic checklist, **458**
- differential diagnosis, **457–458**
- lateral periodontal cyst vs., **405**
- malignant ameloblastoma and ameloblastic carcinoma vs., **493**
- mandible-maxilla aneurysmal bone cyst vs., **415**
- multilocular radiolucencies vs., **878, 880**
- odontogenic keratocyst vs., **401**
- odontogenic myxoma vs., **471**
- prognosis, **458**
- unicystic (mural)
    ameloblastic fibroma vs., **461**
    dentigerous cyst vs., **397**

Ameloblasts, **6**
- secreting enamel matrix, **6**

Amelogenesis imperfecta, **226–229**
- crown changes vs., **848, 849**
- differential diagnosis, **227**
- genetics, **227**
- staging, grading, & classification, **227–228**
- Turner dysplasia vs., **241**

American Burkitt lymphoma. *See* Burkitt lymphoma.
American Joint Committee on Cancer (AJCC)
- staging forms (2010), oral tongue squamous cell carcinoma, **321–322**
- submandibular gland carcinoma, **317**

Aneurysmal bone cyst, **644–647**
- ameloblastoma vs, **458**
- central giant cell granuloma vs., **531**
- central hemangioma vs., **475**
- desmoplastic fibroma vs., **491**
- diagnostic checklist, **645**
- differential diagnosis, **645**
- fibrous dysplasia, cervical spine vs., **839**
- mandible-maxilla, **414–417**
    differential diagnosis, **415**
    prognosis, **415**
    staging, grading, & classification, **415**
- mandible-maxilla simple (traumatic) bone cyst vs., **425**
- multilocular radiolucencies vs., **878, 880**
- odontogenic myxoma vs., **471**
- prognosis, **645**
- sinonasal fibrous dysplasia associated, **716**
- of TMJ, TMJ osteosarcoma vs., **635**
- TMJ simple (traumatic) bone cyst vs., **643**

Angiofibroma, juvenile, sinonasal inverted papilloma vs., **697**
Angle of mandible, **31, 33, 84, 121, 209**
Ankylosed tooth, **7**
Ankylosing spondylitis
- diffuse idiopathic skeletal hyperostosis vs., **823**
- failure of segmentation vs., **811**

Ankylosis, false, adhesions vs., **617**
Anodontia. *See* Hypodontia.
Antegonial notch, **31, 33**
Anterior arch, **152**
- C1, **117, 151, 152, 156, 159, 166**

Anterior atlantodens interval, os odontoideum, **800**
Anterior atlantodental joint, **156**
Anterior atlantooccipital membrane, **151**
Anterior band of disc, **86**
Anterior belly digastric muscle, **53, 129, 182, 202**
Anterior border of mandibular ramus, **142**
Anterior C1 arch defect, isolated, split atlas vs., **797**
Anterior choroidal artery, **206**
Anterior composite restorations, **15**
- radiolucent, **16**

Anterior cranial fossa, **69**
Anterior epitympanic recess, **90, 92**
Anterior ethmoid air cells, **57, 65, 66, 67, 68, 70**
Anterior ethmoid artery, **70**
- canal, **65**

Anterior ethmoid complex, **69, 73, 74**
Anterior ethmoid foramen, **99**
Anterior ethmoid nerve (CNV1), lateral internal nasal branch of, **128**
Anterior ethmoid ostia, **73**
Anterior ethmoids, **75**
Anterior genu
- cavernous (C4) ICA, **206**
    segments, **208**
- CNVII, **140**

Anterior height of contour, **87**
Anterior loculus of maxillary sinus, **60**
Anterior longitudinal ligament, **151**
Anterior mallear ligament, **92**
Anterior mandibular salivary gland defect (Stafne), residual cyst vs., **407**
Anterior median atlantoaxial joint, **151**
Anterior middle cyst. *See* Nasopalatine duct cyst.
Anterior middle palatine cyst. *See* Nasopalatine duct cyst.
Anterior nasal spine, **11, 137**
Anterior neuropore, **100, 103**
Anterior open bite, **179**
Anterior parotid space, **169**
Anterior recess inferior meatus, **67**
Anterior ridge, **88**
Anterior skull base (ASB), **98–103, 105**
Anterior slope of eminence, **88**
Anterior stapes crura, **91**
Anterior tonsillar pillar, **37, 174**
Anterior tympanic segment of CNVII, **93, 94, 143, 146**
Anterior vertical (C4) ICA, **206**
Antibiotics, intravenous, oral cavity soft tissue infections, **294**
Antrochoanal polyps, mucus retention pseudocyst vs., **663**
Antrolith
- paranasal sinus lesions without bony destruction vs., **977**
- sinonasal osteoma vs., **701**
- soft tissue calcifications vs., **934, 936**

Aortic arch (AA), **204**
AOT. *See* Adenomatoid odontogenic tumor.
Apert syndrome, hypoplasia/aplasia associated, **660**
Apex of maxillary canine, **28**
Apical foramen, **10**
Apical ligament, **151, 159**
Apical periodontal cyst. *See* Periapical rarefying osteitis.
Apical periodontitis
- acute. *See* Periapical rarefying osteitis.
- chronic. *See* Periapical rarefying osteitis.
- nasopalatine duct cyst vs., **420**

INDEX

Apical rarefying osteitis, periapical osseous dysplasia vs., **429**
Apical/periradicular radiolucency, **221**
Apicoectomy, periapical scar, **265–266**
Arcuate eminence, **145, 146**
Arcuate foramen. *See* Ponticulus posticus.
Arnott grading system, cherubism, **359–360**
Arteriosclerosis, soft tissue calcifications vs., **935, 937**
Arteriovenous fistula, central hemangioma vs., **475**
Arteriovenous vascular malformation, sinonasal, nasal lesion without bony destruction vs., **966–967, 968**
Arthritides, inflammatory, cervical facet arthropathy vs., **827**
Arthritis, juvenile, condylar hypoplasia vs., **557**
Arthrosis deformans (AD). *See* Degenerative joint disease; Progressive condylar resorption.
Articular disc, **82, 89**
- anterior band of, **89**
- posterior band of, **89**
Articular eminence, **82, 84, 88, 89**
Articular facet for dens, **152**
Articulating surfaces, deviations of form and shape of, disc replacement with reduction vs., **605**
ASB. *See* Anterior skull base.
Ascending pharyngeal artery, **204, 205**
Aspergilloma. *See* Mycetoma.
Aspirin sensitivity, sinonasal polyposis associated, **674**
Asthma
- chronic rhinosinusitis associated, **682**
- sinonasal polyposis associated, **674**
Asymmetrical skeletal hyperostosis. *See* Diffuse idiopathic skeletal hyperostosis.
Atherosclerosis, carotid artery, neck, soft tissue calcifications vs., **935, 937**
Atlantal assimilation. *See* C1 assimilation.
Atlantal posterior foramen. *See* Ponticulus posticus.
Atlantoaxial joints, **157, 158**
- anterior articular facet for, **153**
- lateral, anatomy, **150**
- median, anatomy, **150**
- posterior median, articular facet for, **153**
Atlantodental joint, anterior, **159**
Atlantooccipital assimilation. *See* C1 assimilation.
Atlantooccipital joint, **116, 150, 151, 156, 158**
- angle, **154**
Atlantooccipital membrane
- anterior, anatomy, **150, 159**
- posterior, anatomy, **150**
Atlas (C1), anatomy, **150**
Attrition, **236–237**
- abrasion vs., **238**
- diagnostic checklist, **237**
- differential diagnosis, **237**
- prognosis, **237**
Auricularis muscles, anterior, superior, and posterior, **142**
Auriculocondylar syndrome, condylar hypoplasia, **557**
Auriculotemporal nerve, **85, 128, 129, 131**
Autoimmune sialadenitis, **301**
Autosomal dominant neurofibromatosis. *See* Neurofibromatosis type 1.
Axis (C2), anatomy, **150**

B

BA. *See* Basilar artery.
Bacterial rhinitis, nasopalatine duct cyst associated, **420**
Basal cell carcinoma syndrome, nevoid, cherubism vs., **359**
Basal cell nevus syndrome, **362–363**
- associated abnormalities, **363**
- coronoid hyperplasia associated, **553**
- diagnostic checklist, **363**
- differential diagnosis, **363**
- genetics, **363**
- hypodontia vs., **213**
- missing teeth vs., **846**
- odontogenic keratocyst associated, **402**
- prognosis, **363**
Basal lamella of middle turbinate, **68, 75**
Basal turn of cochlea, **144, 145, 146**
Basilar artery (BA), **127, 132, 204**
Basilar occipital bone (clivus), **115**
Basiocciput, **106, 114, 117**
- part of clivus, **108**
Basion, **151, 158, 159**
Basisphenoid, **64, 169, 177, 178**
BBC. *See* Buccal bifurcation cyst.
BCNS. *See* Basal cell nevus syndrome.
BCT. *See* Brachiocephalic trunk.
Benign cementoblastoma. *See* Cementoblastoma.
Benign central giant cell tumor. *See* Aneurysmal bone cyst.
Benign compression fracture, lytic and blastic metastases vs., **835–836**
Benign lymphoepithelial cysts, HIV, parotid sialadenitis vs., **755**
Benign lymphoepithelial lesions
- HIV, **750–753**
  - associated abnormalities, **752**
  - diagnostic checklist, **752**
  - differential diagnosis, **751**
  - metastatic disease of parotid nodes vs., **779**
  - parotid non-Hodgkin lymphoma vs., **775**
  - prognosis, **752**
  - Warthin tumor vs., **761**
- Sjögren syndrome vs., **783**
Benign masseteric hypertrophy. *See* Benign masticator muscle hypertrophy.
Benign masticator muscle hypertrophy, **746–747**
- diagnostic checklist, **747**
- differential diagnosis, **747**
- prognosis, **747**
Benign mixed tumor (BMT)
- malignant degeneration of, **315**
- oral, oral mucosal space/surface lesions vs., **927, 929**
- palate, **310–311**
  - differential diagnosis, **311**
  - hard palate squamous cell carcinoma vs., **335**
  - oral cavity minor salivary gland malignancy vs., **313**
  - prognosis, **311**

INDEX

- parotid, **756–759**
  diagnostic checklist, **758**
  differential diagnosis, **757–758**
  parotid malignant mixed tumor vs., **767**
  parotid mucoepidermoid carcinoma vs., **769**
  parotid schwannoma vs., **765**
  prognosis, **758**
  space, parotid adenoid cystic carcinoma vs., **773**
  Warthin tumor vs., **761**
- parotid space lesions vs., **918, 919**
- parotid tail, submandibular space lesions vs., **914, 916**
- recurrent parotid, metastatic disease of parotid nodes vs., **779**
- sinonasal
  nasal lesion without bony destruction vs., **967, 969**
  paranasal sinus lesions without bony destruction vs., **977**
- sublingual gland, **306–307**
  diagnostic checklist, **307**
  differential diagnosis, **307**
  sublingual space lesions vs., **923, 925**
- submandibular gland, **308–309**
  diagnostic checklist, **309**
  differential diagnosis, **309**
  prognosis, **309**
  submandibular gland carcinoma vs., **317**
  submandibular gland sialadenitis vs., **301**
  submandibular space lesions vs., **914–915, 917**

Benign odontogenic keratocyst, periapical radiolucencies vs., **856, 859**
Bicuspid. *See* Teeth.
Bifid condyle, **572–575**
- diagnostic checklist, **573**
- differential diagnosis, **573**
- large condyle vs., **947, 949**
- prognosis, **573**
- TMJ fractures vs., **565**

Bifid mandibular canal. *See* Accessory mandibular canal.
Bifid mandibular condyle (BMC). *See* Bifid condyle.
Bifid rib syndrome. *See* Basal cell nevus syndrome.
Bifid spinous process, C2, **157**
Bilateral acoustic schwannomas, **483**
Bilateral facial microsomia, Treacher Collins syndrome vs., **369**
Bimaxillary protrusion, **23**
Binder syndrome, hypoplasia/aplasia associated, **660**
Bisphosphonate-related osteonecrosis of jaws. *See* Osteonecrosis, mandible-maxilla.
Blastic metastases, **834–837**
- diagnostic checklist, **836**
- differential diagnosis, **835–836**
- prognosis, **836**
- staging, grading, & classification, **836**

Block vertebra. *See* Failure of segmentation.
Blowout fracture
- inferior orbital, zygomaticomaxillary complex fracture vs., **379**
- medial orbital, nasoethmoid complex fracture vs., **375**

Blue sclera, dentinogenesis imperfecta vs., **231**
BMMH. *See* Benign masticator muscle hypertrophy.
Body of incus, **92**
Body of mandible, **32, 84, 135**
Body of tongue, **119**
Bone, **7**
- developing, **6**
- facial aspect of implant not covered with, **20**

Bone eburnation. *See* Mandible-maxilla idiopathic osteosclerosis.
Bone grafting material, displaced dental structures into antrum vs., **984**
Bone level, **21**
Bone marrow defect, osteoporotic
- lateral periodontal cyst vs., **405**
- mandible-maxilla simple (traumatic) bone cyst vs., **425**

Bone remodeling, periosteal reactions vs., **907, 909**
Bone restoration stage, cherubism, **360**
Bone scar. *See* Mandible-maxilla idiopathic osteosclerosis.
Bone tumor, primary, tumor calcinosis vs., **841**
Bone whorl. *See* Mandible-maxilla idiopathic osteosclerosis.
Bony ankylosis, **562–563**
- differential diagnosis, **563**
- fibrous ankylosis vs., **561**
- large condyle vs., **947, 949**
- limited condylar translation vs., **950, 953**
- prognosis, **563**
- staging, grading, & classification, **563**
- TMJ radiopacities vs., **957, 959**

Botryoid odontogenic cyst (BOC). *See* Lateral periodontal cyst.
Brachial plexus, in perivertebral space, **196**
Brachiocephalic trunk (BCT), **204**
Brachium pontis, **132**
Branch to distobuccal root, **29**
Branches to teeth, **131**
Branchial arch anomalies, 1st and 2nd, submandibular gland aplasia-hypoplasia associated, **289**
Branchial arch syndrome. *See also* Hemifacial microsomia.
- condylar aplasia associated, **541**

Branchial cleft anomaly
- 2nd, ranula vs., **297**
- submandibular gland mucocele vs., **305**

Branchial cleft cyst, 1st, benign lymphoepithelial lesions: HIV vs., **751**
Branchiootorenal syndrome, Treacher Collins syndrome vs., **369**
Breathing, difficulty, deviated nasal septum associated, **651**
Bridges (prosthetic), **14**
Broad C1 posterior arch, ponticulus posticus vs., **793**
Brown tumor of hyperparathyroidism
- central giant cell granuloma vs., **531**
- cherubism vs., **359**

Buccal and lingual exostoses, mandible-maxilla osteoma vs., **481**
Buccal and palatal exostoses, **342–343**
- associated abnormalities, **343**
- differential diagnosis, **343**
- genetics, **343**
- oral mucosal space/surface lesions vs., **927, 929**
- prognosis, **343**

INDEX

Buccal bifurcation cyst, **408–411**
- diagnostic checklist, **410**
- differential diagnosis, **409–410**
- pericoronal radiolucencies without radiopacities vs., **874, 875**
- prognosis, **410**

Buccal branch, of CNVII, **141, 142, 186**
Buccal exostosis, mandibular torus vs., **345**
Buccal lipping. *See* Buccal and palatal exostoses.
Buccal mucosa, **52, 53**
Buccal mucosa squamous cell carcinoma, **332–333**
- diagnostic checklist, **333**
- differential diagnosis, **333**
- oral mucosal space/surface lesions vs., **926, 928**
- prognosis, **333**
- retromolar trigone squamous cell carcinoma vs., **329**
- staging, grading, & classification, **333**

Buccal nerve, **131**
Buccal plate, **10**
Buccal shelf, **32, 33**
Buccal space, **181, 183**
Buccinator, **26, 38, 39, 41, 42, 43, 53, 130, 131, 139, 142, 166, 183, 187**
Buccinator node, **201**
"Bull tooth," **223**
Burkitt lymphoma, **512–515**
- associated abnormalities, **514**
- diagnostic checklist, **514**
- differential diagnosis, **513**
- prognosis, **514**
- staging, grading, & classification, **514**
- variants, **513**

Burkitt tumor. *See* Burkitt lymphoma.
Burnout, cervical, dental caries vs., **261**

C

C1 assimilation, **790–791**
- associated abnormalities, **791**
- diagnostic checklist, **791**
- differential diagnosis, **791**
- prognosis, **791**
- staging, grading, & classification, **791**

C1 fracture, Jefferson, split atlas vs., **797**
C1 posterior arch, broad, ponticulus posticus vs., **793**
C2 fracture, odontoid
- odontoid hypoplasia/aplasia vs., **805**
- os odontoideum vs., **799**

C2 vertebra, **121**
C2-C3 fusion, **788–789**
- diagnostic checklist, **789**
- differential diagnosis, **789**
- genetics, **789**
- prognosis, **789**

C2-C3 neural foramen, **157**
Calcific tendinitis, longus coli, tumor calcinosis vs., **841**
Calcified cartilaginous external auditory canal, TMJ articular loose bodies vs., **960**
Calcified herniated disc, ossification of posterior longitudinal ligament vs., **819**
Calcified lymph node, soft tissue calcifications vs., **934, 936**
Calcified mixed odontoma. *See* Odontoma.
Calcified stylohyoid ligament, soft tissue calcifications vs., **934, 935**
Calcified thyroid cartilage, soft tissue calcifications vs., **934, 936**
Calcified triticeous cartilage, soft tissue calcifications vs., **934, 936**
Calcifying cystic odontogenic tumor. *See* Calcifying odontogenic cyst.
Calcifying epithelial odontogenic cyst. *See* Calcifying odontogenic cyst.
Calcifying epithelial odontogenic tumor, **466–467**
- adenomatoid odontogenic tumor vs., **455**
- ameloblastic fibroodontoma vs., **465**
- associated abnormalities, **467**
- calcifying odontogenic cyst vs., **413**
- diagnostic checklist, **467**
- differential diagnosis, **467**
- pericoronal radiolucencies with radiopacities vs., **876, 877**
- prognosis, **467**

Calcifying odontogenic cyst, **412–413**
- adenomatoid odontogenic tumor vs., **455**
- ameloblastic fibroma associated, **462**
- ameloblastic fibroodontoma vs., **465**
- associated abnormalities, **413**
- calcifying epithelial odontogenic tumor vs., **467**
- diagnostic checklist, **413**
- differential diagnosis, **413**
- genetics, **413**
- pericoronal radiolucencies with radiopacities vs., **876, 877**
- prognosis, **413**
- staging, grading, & classification, **413**

Calcinosis cutis, soft tissue calcifications vs., **935, 937**
Calcium pyrophosphate deposition disease
- degenerative joint disorders of craniovertebral junction vs., **815**
- TMJ articular loose bodies vs., **960, 961**
- tumor calcinosis vs., **841**

Calcium pyrophosphate dihydrate deposition disease
- temporomandibular joint, **626–629**
  - associated abnormalities, **628**
  - diagnostic checklist, **628**
  - differential diagnosis, **627**
  - prognosis, **628**
  - staging, grading, & classification, **628**
- TMJ chondrosarcoma vs., **637**
- TMJ juvenile idiopathic arthritis vs., **585**
- TMJ primary synovial chondromatosis vs., **631**

Calculus
- enamel pearls vs, **222**
- periodontal disease, **272**

Camurati-Engelmann disease, hypoplasia/aplasia associated, **660**
Canaliculus innominatus, **104**

INDEX

Canalis vertebralis. *See* Ponticulus posticus.
Canine (C), **4**
Canine eminence, **24, 27**
Canine fossa, **26**
Capsulitis, TMJ juvenile idiopathic arthritis vs., **585**
Carcinoma
- sublingual gland, sublingual space lesions vs., **923, 925**
- submandibular gland, **316–317**
  submandibular gland benign mixed tumor vs., **309**
  submandibular gland sialadenitis vs., **301**
  submandibular space lesions vs., **915, 917**

Carcinoma ex dentigerous cyst, malignant ameloblastoma and ameloblastic carcinoma vs., **493**
Carcinoma ex pleomorphic adenoma. *See* Parotid malignant mixed tumor.
Carcinosarcoma, ameloblastic, ameloblastic fibroma transformation, **462**
Caries, **19**
Carotid arteries, external and internal, **167, 204–209**
- arterial calcifications on panoramic and CBCT, **209**
- axial NECT, **207–208**
- in carotid space, **184, 189**
- cervical, **204**
- graphics, **205–206**
- intracranial, **204**
- normal variants, anomalies, **204**

Carotid bifurcation
- calcifications, **209**
- carotid body location in, **190**

Carotid body location, **191**
Carotid bulb, internal carotid artery, **205**
Carotid calcification, **209**
Carotid canal, **119, 170, 207**
- of central skull base, **104**
- entrance, **114**
- internal carotid artery, **164, 190**

Carotid sheath, **189**
Carotid space (CS), **169, 170, 171, 173, 174, 181, 182, 185, 186, 188–191, 193, 194, 195, 199**. *See also* Parapharyngeal space (PPS)
- anatomy, **163, 164, 165, 166**
  imaging, **162**
  relationships, **188**
- fascia of, **188**
- internal contents, **188**
- skull base, angiography, CT venography, **190**
- superior margin, **117**
- suprahyoid carotid space on CECT, **191**
- suprahyoid neck, carotid space graphics, **189**

Carotid space mass, **189**
Carotid sulcus, **208**
Caudal loop of CNXII, submandibular space, **48**
Cavernous (C4) segment, **204**
Cavernous carotid artery, **70**
Cavernous internal carotid artery, **101, 107, 127, 133**
Cavernous sinus, **112, 126, 127, 204**
Cavities. *See* Dental caries.
Cavity preparation
- abfraction vs., **240**
- abrasion vs., **238**
- unfilled, dental caries vs., **261**

Cellulitis, oral cavity soft tissue infections, **293**
Cellulitis-phlegmon of masticator space, masticator space abscess vs., **725**
Cement, **17**
- exposure, perforated nasal septum vs., **964**

Cemental dysplasia. *See* Periapical osseous dysplasia.
Cemental fracture, dentoalveolar fractures, **255**
Cementifying fibroma. *See* Ossifying fibroma; Sinonasal ossifying fibroma.
Cementoblastoma, **468–469**
- differential diagnosis, **469**
- hypercementosis vs., **248**
- ossifying fibroma vs., **437**
- osteoblastoma vs., **479**
- osteoid osteoma vs., **477**
- periapical osseous dysplasia vs., **429**
- periapical radiopacities and mixed lesions vs., **860, 861**
- periapical sclerosing osteitis vs., **269**
- sinonasal ossifying fibroma vs., **719**

Cementoenamel junction, **10, 11, 18**
- future, **6**

Cementoma. *See* Periapical osseous dysplasia.
Cementoosseous dysplasia. *See also* Periapical osseous dysplasia.
- mandible-maxilla osteomyelitis associated, **386**
- sinonasal ossifying fibroma vs., **719**

Cementoossifying fibroma. *See also* Sinonasal ossifying fibroma.
- ground-glass and granular radiopacities vs., **896–897, 900**
- periapical radiopacities and mixed lesions vs., **860, 861**

Cemento-ossifying fibroma. *See also* Ossifying fibroma.
- osteoblastoma vs., **479**
- osteoid osteoma vs., **477**

Cementum, **6, 10**
  anatomy, **5**

Central desmoplastic fibroma, central odontogenic fibroma vs., **473**
Central giant cell granuloma
- ameloblastic carcinoma vs., **493**
- ameloblastic fibroma vs., **461**
- ameloblastoma vs, **458**
- central hemangioma vs., **475**
- central odontogenic fibroma vs., **473**
- cherubism vs., **359**
- malignant ameloblastoma vs., **493**
- mandible-maxilla aneurysmal bone cyst vs., **415**
- mandible-maxilla simple (traumatic) bone cyst vs., **425**
- maxilla, sinonasal fibroosseous and cartilaginous lesions vs., **974, 975**
- multilocular radiolucencies vs., **878, 880**
- nasopalatine duct cyst vs., **419**
- odontogenic myxoma vs., **471**

Central giant cell lesion. *See* Aneurysmal bone cyst.
Central giant cell tumor, ill-defined radiolucencies vs., **882–883, 886**
Central hemangioma, **474–475**
- desmoplastic fibroma vs., **491**
- diagnostic checklist, **475**
- differential diagnosis, **475**

INDEX

- odontogenic myxoma vs., **471**
- prognosis, **475**

Central incisor teeth, maxillary and mandibular, **137**
Central mucoepidermoid. *See* Mucoepidermoid carcinoma, central.
Central mucoepidermoid carcinoma, multilocular radiolucencies vs., **879, 881**
Central mucoepidermoid tumor, malignant ameloblastoma and ameloblastic carcinoma vs., **493**
Central odontogenic fibroma, **472–473**
- desmoplastic fibroma vs., **491**
- differential diagnosis, **473**
- types, **473**

Central ossifying fibroma, periapical osseous dysplasia vs., **429**
Central skull base (CSB), **99, 104–109**
Central squamous cell carcinoma. *See* Intraosseous squamous cell carcinoma, primary.
CEOT. *See* Calcifying epithelial odontogenic tumor.
Cephalad clivus, **134**
Cephalocele, frontoethmoidal, dermoid and epidermoid vs., **286**
Ceramic on PFM bridge, **16**
Cerebellopontine angle cistern (CNVII), **140**
Cervical branch of CNVII, **141, 142, 186**
Cervical burnout, dental caries vs., **261**
Cervical caries (class V)
- abfraction vs., **240**
- erosion vs., **239**

Cervical facet arthropathy, **826–829**
- associated abnormalities, **828**
- diagnostic checklist, **828**
- differential diagnosis, **827**
- genetics, **828**
- prognosis, **828**
- staging, grading, & classification, **828**

Cervical line, posterior, **150**
Cervical loop, **6**
Cervical peridural calcification of hemodialysis, ossification of posterior longitudinal ligament vs., **819**
Cervical resorption, idiopathic
- dental caries vs., **261**
- internal and external resorption vs., **243–244**

Cervical space, posterior, **191**
- anatomy, **162**

Cervical spine, **120, 121**
- anatomy. *See* Craniocervical junction.

Cervical VAs, **204**
Cervical vertebra, **176**
- 2nd, **176**

Cervical vertebral body, 3rd, **179**
CFFx. *See* Complex midfacial fracture.
Chamberlain line, **150, 154, 155**
Chédiak-Higashi syndrome, periodontal disease associated, **272**
Chemical tooth wear. *See* Erosion.
Cherubism, **358–361**
- associated abnormalities, **359**
- basal cell nevus syndrome vs., **363**
- Burkitt lymphoma vs., **513**
- central giant cell granuloma vs., **531**
- diagnostic checklist, **360**
- differential diagnosis, **359**
- genetics, **359**
- mandible-maxilla, sinonasal fibroosseous and cartilaginous lesions vs., **974**
- multilocular radiolucencies vs., **879, 881**
- prognosis, **360**
- sinonasal fibrous dysplasia vs., **715**
- staging, grading, & classification, **359–360**

Chiasmatic sulcus, of central skull base, **104**
Chondrification, failure of formation, **808**
Chondroblastoma, calcium pyrophosphate dihydrate deposition disease vs., **627**
Chondrocalcinosis. *See also* Calcium pyrophosphate dihydrate deposition disease, temporomandibular joint.
- TMJ pigmented villonodular synovitis vs., **591**

Chondrogenic sarcoma. *See* Chondrosarcoma, mandible-maxilla; Chondrosarcoma, temporomandibular joint.
Chondrosarcoma
- calcium pyrophosphate dihydrate deposition disease vs., **627**
- floating teeth vs., **862**
- lamina dura changes vs., **867, 869**
- large condyle vs., **947, 949**
- mandible-maxilla, **504–507**
  - diagnostic checklist, **506**
  - differential diagnosis, **505–506**
  - prognosis, **506**
  - staging, grading, & classification, **506**
- mandible-maxilla osteosarcoma vs., **501**
- masticator space, **734–737**
  - diagnostic checklist, **736**
  - differential diagnosis, **735**
  - masticator muscle atrophy vs., **729**
  - prognosis, **736**
  - staging, grading, & classification, **735–736**
- mesenchymal, Ewing sarcoma vs., **525**
- periosteal reactions vs., **907, 910**
- sinonasal
  - nasal lesion with bony destruction vs., **971, 973**
  - paranasal sinus lesions with bony destruction vs., **981, 983**
  - sinonasal fibroosseous and cartilaginous lesions vs., **974, 975**
- small condyle vs., **941, 945**
- temporomandibular joint, **636–639**
  - diagnostic checklist, **638**
  - differential diagnosis, **637**
  - prognosis, **638**
  - staging, grading, & classification, **638**
- TMJ
  - TMJ osteochondroma vs., **621**
  - TMJ osteosarcoma vs., **635**
- TMJ articular loose bodies vs., **960, 961**
- TMJ metastasis vs., **641**
- TMJ pigmented villonodular synovitis vs., **591**
- TMJ primary synovial chondromatosis vs., **631**
- TMJ radiolucencies vs., **954, 955**
- TMJ radiopacities vs., **957, 959**

- widened periodontal ligament space vs., **864, 865**
Chorda tympani nerve, **129, 131, 140, 141, 182, 186**
- as branch of CN7, **138–139**
- CNVII, **128**
Chordoma, clivus, sinonasal fibroosseous and cartilaginous lesions vs., **974, 975**
Choristomatic cyst. *See* Foregut duplication cyst in tongue.
Chromosome anomalies, clefts, **357**
Chronic apical periodontitis. *See* Periapical rarefying osteitis.
Chronic arthritis, juvenile, failure of segmentation vs., **811**
Chronic lymphocytic leukemia (CLL). *See* Leukemia.
Chronic myelocytic leukemia (CML). *See* Leukemia.
Chronic osteomyelitis, periosteal reactions vs., **907, 908**
Chronic recurrent multifocal osteomyelitis
- generalized radiopacities vs., **902, 904**
- periosteal reactions vs., **907, 909**
Chronic sclerosing osteomyelitis. *See* Osteomyelitis, mandible-maxilla.
Chronic sclerosing sialadenitis, **301**
Chronic sequelae of discitis
- C2-C3 fusion vs., **789**
- failure of segmentation vs., **811**
Chronic sialadenitis, **301**
Ciliary ganglion, **128**
Circumferential dentigerous cyst. *See* Buccal bifurcation cyst.
Circumvallate papilla, **37, 53**
Cisternal abducens nerve (CNVI), **140**
Classic syndrome, **118**
Cleft lip (CL), **357**
Cleft palate, **357**
- deviated nasal septum associated, **651**
- hypoplasia/aplasia associated, **660**
Clefts, **356–357**
- associated abnormalities, **357**
- differential diagnosis, **357**
- genetics, **357**
Cleidocranial dysostosis. *See* Cleidocranial dysplasia.
Cleidocranial dysplasia, **364–365**
- differential diagnosis, **365**
- extra teeth vs., **844, 845**
- genetics, **365**
- hyperdontia vs., **215**
Clicking jaw. *See* Disc replacement, with reduction.
Clinoid (C5) segment, **204**
- ICA, **206**
Clinoid process
- anterior, **99, 102, 107, 109, 209**
  of anterior skull base, **98**
  of central skull base, **104**
- posterior, **107**
  of central skull base, **104**
Clival fracture, os avis vs., **803**
Clival occipital bone, **114**
Clival venous plexus, **112**
Clivus, **113, 127, 133, 134, 151, 178, 208**
- basiocciput, **115**
- canal angle, **150**
Closed lock. *See* Disc displacement, without reduction.
CNIII, **105**
CNIV, **105**
CNV. *See* Cranial nerve V (CNV).
CNV3, **189**
- motor innervation, **729**
- neurofibroma, masticator space CNV3 perineural tumor vs., **743**
- normal fat pad, masticator space CNV3 perineural tumor vs., **744**
- schwannoma in MS, masticator space CNV3 perineural tumor vs., **743**
CNVI, **105**
- sulcus, **134**
CNVII. *See* Cranial nerve VII (CNVII).
COC. *See* Calcifying odontogenic cyst.
Cocaine necrosis, nose, perforated nasal septum vs., **964, 965**
Cochlea, **143, 146**
Cochlear aqueduct, **116, 144**
Cochlear nerve, **147**
Cochleariform process, **92, 94, 146**
COF. *See* Central odontogenic fibroma.
Common carotid artery, **204, 205**
- at aortic arch, **190**
Communicating (C7) segment, **204**
- ICA, **206**
Complex composite odontoma. *See* Odontoma.
Complex facial fracture, transfacial fracture (Le Fort) vs., **381**
Complex midfacial fracture, **376–377**
- associated abnormalities, **377**
- differential diagnosis, **377**
- nasoethmoid complex fracture vs., **375**
- prognosis, **377**
- staging, grading, & classification, **377**
- zygomaticomaxillary complex fracture vs., **379**
Complex odontoma, **451, 452**
- mandible-maxilla idiopathic osteosclerosis vs., **355**
Compound composite odontoma. *See* Odontoma.
Compound odontoma, **451, 452**
- hyperdontia vs., **215**
Compressor naris muscle, **26**
Concha bullosa, **63, 72, 74, 75, 652–655**
- diagnostic checklist, **653**
- prognosis, **653**
Concha pneumatization. *See* Concha bullosa.
Conchal crest, **25**
Concrescence, **219**
Concussion, **249**
- diagnostic checklist, **249**
- differential diagnosis, **249**
- luxation vs., **251**
- prognosis, **249**
Condensing osteitis. *See also* Periapical sclerosing osteitis.
- mandible-maxilla idiopathic osteosclerosis vs., **355**
- supernumerary roots vs., **225**
- well-defined radiopacities vs., **892, 893**
Condylar aplasia, **540–541**
- associated abnormalities, **541**
- diagnostic checklist, **541**
- differential diagnosis, **541**
- prognosis, **541**

Condylar fibrocartilage, **86**
Condylar fossa, **117**
- temporomandibular joint, **182**
Condylar fracture
- bifid condyle vs., **573**
- large condyle vs., **946, 948**
- limited condylar translation vs., **950, 952**
- small condyle vs., **940, 943**
Condylar hyperplasia, **546–551**
- diagnostic checklist, **548**
- differential diagnosis, **547–548**
- large condyle vs., **946, 947**
- prognosis, **548**
- TMJ osteochondroma vs., **621**
- TMJ osteoma vs., **619**
Condylar hypoplasia, **556–559**
- diagnostic checklist, **557**
- differential diagnosis, **557**
- hemifacial microsomia vs., **543**
- prognosis, **557**
- small condyle vs., **940, 943**
- TMJ, condylar hyperplasia vs., **547**
- TMJ fractures vs., **565**
- TMJ juvenile idiopathic arthritis vs., **585**
Condylar (lateral) occipital bone, **116**
Condylar neck, **31, 32, 84, 86, 88**
Condylar osteoarthritis, calcium pyrophosphate dihydrate deposition disease vs., **627**
Condylar process, **33**
- mandibular, anatomy, **30**
Condylar subluxation, disc replacement with reduction vs., **605**
Condyle, **31, 32, 84**
- bifid, TMJ fractures vs., **565**
Condylysis. *See* Progressive condylar resorption
Congenital clefts of C1. *See* Split atlas.
Congenital external ear dysplasia, Treacher Collins syndrome vs., **369**
Connective tissue, **7**
Continuous apical lamina dura, **35**
Core, **14, 17**
Coronoid hyperplasia, **552–555**
- associated abnormalities, **553**
- diagnostic checklist, **553**
- differential diagnosis, **553**
- limited condylar translation vs., **950, 953**
- prognosis, **553**
- TMJ osteochondroma vs., **621**
Coronoid notch, **31, 33**
Coronoid process, **31, 32, 84**
- of mandible, **183**
  - anatomy, **30**
- tip of, **87**
Corrugator supercilii, **139**
Cotton roll, **15**
Cranial nerve V (CNV), **124–137**
- axial & coronal T2 MR, **133**
- axial bone CT, **134**
- axial T2 MR, **132**
- CBCT reformats, **135**
- cisternal (preganglionic) segment, **124**
- coronal CBCT, **136**
- divisions (post ganglionic) of CNV, **124**
  - mandibular nerve, **124–125**
  - maxillary nerve (CNV2), **124**
- graphics, **126–131**
- interdural segment, **124**
- sagittal CBCT, **137**
Cranial nerve VII (CNVII), **138–147**
- axial bone CT, **143–144**
- branches of CN7, **138**
- cisternal segment, **138**
- coronal bone CT, **145–146**
- extracranial segment, **138**
- graphics, **140–142**
- intraaxial segment, **138**
- intratemporal segment, **138**
- T2 & T1 MR, **147**
Craniocervical junction (CCJ), **150–159**
- axial bone CT, **156–157**
- bone CT & T1 MR craniometry, **155**
- C1 graphics, **152**
- C2 graphics, **153**
- components of, **150**
- coronal bone CT, **158**
- craniometry graphics, **154**
- frontal assessment of, **150**
- graphics, **151**
- lateral assessment of, **150**
- sagittal CT & MR, **159**
Craniodiaphyseal dysplasia, hypoplasia/aplasia associated, **660**
Craniofacial complex, cleidocranial dysplasia, **365**
Craniofacial dysostosis, hypoplasia/aplasia associated, **660**
Craniofacial microsomia. *See* Hemifacial microsomia
Craniometaphyseal dysplasia, hypoplasia/aplasia associated, **660**
Craniopharyngeal canal, **106**
- persistent, **104**
Craniovertebral junction
- degenerative joint disorders of, **814–817**
  - diagnostic checklist, **816**
  - differential diagnosis, **815–816**
  - prognosis, **816**
- surgical fusion, C1 assimilation vs., **791**
Crest of alveolar bone (crestal lamina dura), **10, 11**
Cretinism, hypoplasia/aplasia associated, **660**
Cribriform plate, **65, 66, 99, 101, 102, 208**
Cricoid cartilage, **201**
- plane, **201**
Crista galli, **25, 65, 66, 99, 101, 103**
- of anterior skull base, **98**
- area, **103**
- ethmoid bone, **102**
- normal fatty marrow in, dermoid and epidermoid vs., **286**
- site of future, **100**
Crouzon syndrome, condylar hypoplasia, **557**
Crowe sign, **487**
Crown, **10, 14**
- on abutment tooth, **16**
- anatomy, **5**

- changes, **848–849**
 differential diagnosis, **848**
- in contact with opposing crown, **20**
- prosthetic, preparation, Turner dysplasia vs., **241**
- on tilted abutment, **20**
Crown dilaceration, **224**
Crown-root fracture. *See* Dentoalveolar fractures.
Cruciate ligament, anatomy, **150, 151, 159**
- superior extension of, **159**
CS. *See* Cavernous sinus; Chondrosarcoma, mandible-maxilla.
CSB. *See* Central skull base (CSB).
CS-MS. *See* Masticator space chondrosarcoma.
Cushing disease, ground-glass and granular radiopacities vs., **897**
Cushing syndrome, generalized rarefaction vs., **889**
Cuspid. *See* Teeth.
Cylindrical epithelioma. *See* Sinonasal inverted papilloma.
Cylindroma. *See* Adenoid cystic carcinoma.
Cystadenoma lymphomatosum, papillary. *See* Warthin tumor.
Cystic fibrosis, sinonasal polyposis associated, **674**
Cystic hygroma
- foregut duplication cyst in tongue vs., **291**
- submandibular gland mucocele vs., **305**
Cystic lesion mimicking maxillary sinus, **61**
Cystic lymphangioma, foregut duplication cyst in tongue vs., **291**
Cystic odontoma. *See* Odontoma.
Cystic submandibular lymph node, submandibular gland mucocele vs., **305**

D

Dacryocystocele, nasal lesion without bony destruction vs., **966**
Danger space, **174, 194, 197**
- anatomy, **162, 163, 165**
Deep cervical fascia, **165**
- deep layer, **165, 189, 193, 194, 197, 198**
- middle layer, **164, 165, 169, 173, 174, 175, 193, 194, 197**
- superficial layer, **165, 169, 175, 181, 182, 186, 189, 197**
Deep lobe parotid, **187**
- mass, **185**
Deep temporal artery, **85**
Degenerative disease
- calcium pyrophosphate dihydrate deposition disease vs., **627**
- hemifacial microsomia vs., **543**
- temporomandibular joint, masticator space abscess vs., **725**
- TMJ
 TMJ primary synovial chondromatosis vs., **631**
 TMJ rheumatoid arthritis vs., **579**
 TMJ simple (traumatic) bone cyst vs., **643**
- TMJ juvenile idiopathic arthritis vs., **585**
Degenerative endplates, type 2, hemangioma, cervical spine vs., **831**
Degenerative facet disease. *See* Cervical facet arthropathy.
Degenerative joint disease, **592–595**. *See also* Cervical facet arthropathy.
- condylar hypoplasia vs., **557**
- diagnostic checklist, **593**
- differential diagnosis, **593**
- limited condylar translation vs., **950, 952**
- prognosis, **593**
- progressive condylar resorption vs., **599**
- small condyle vs., **940, 941**
- TMJ articular loose bodies vs., **960**
- TMJ osteochondritis dissecans vs., **577**
- TMJ osteochondroma vs., **621**
- TMJ radiolucencies vs., **954**
- TMJ radiopacities vs., **956, 958**
Degenerative joint disorders of craniovertebral junction, **814–817**
- diagnostic checklist, **816**
- differential diagnosis, **815–816**
- prognosis, **816**
Degenerative remodeling of odontoid process, ossiculum terminale vs., **795**
Demarcated opacities, amelogenesis imperfecta vs., **227**
Denervation atrophy. *See* Masticator muscle atrophy.
Dens in dente. *See* Dens invaginatus.
Dens invaginatus, **220, 221**
Dense bone island. *See also* Mandible-maxilla idiopathic osteosclerosis.
- periapical osseous dysplasia vs., **430**
Dental amalgam, displaced dental structures into antrum vs., **984**
Dental anomalies, dental caries vs., **261**
Dental caries, **260–263**
- abrasion vs., **238**
- cervical caries (class V)
 abfraction vs., **240**
 erosion vs., **239**
- crown changes vs., **848**
- diagnostic checklist, **261**
- differential diagnosis, **261**
- internal and external resorption vs., **243**
Dental concussion. *See* Concussion.
Dental corrosion. *See* Erosion.
Dental decay. *See* Dental caries.
Dental fluorosis, amelogenesis imperfecta vs., **227**
Dental follicle, **5**
- hyperplastic, buccal bifurcation cyst vs., **409**
Dental impression material, displaced dental structures into antrum vs., **984, 986, 987**
Dental infection, submandibular gland sialadenitis vs., **301**
Dental lamina, **6**
Dental papilla, **5, 6**
Dental problems, cleidocranial dysplasia vs., **365**
Dental restorations, **14–21**
- CBCT axial and periapicals, **15–16**
- CBCT reformats, **17–21**
- crown changes vs., **848**
- endodontics, **14**

- orthodontics, **14**
- pediatrics, **14**
- periapical radiograph, **21**
- prosthetic, **14**
- restorative materials, **14**

Dental sac, **6**
Dentigerous cyst, **396–399**
- adenomatoid odontogenic tumor vs., **455**
- ameloblastic fibroma vs., **461**
- ameloblastoma vs, **458**
- associated abnormalities, **397**
- buccal bifurcation cyst vs., **409**
- calcifying epithelial odontogenic tumor vs., **467**
- calcifying odontogenic cyst vs., **413**
- central mucoepidermoid carcinoma vs., **511**
- circumferential. *See* Buccal bifurcation cyst
- diagnostic checklist, **397**
- differential diagnosis, **397**
- encroaching sinus, mucus retention pseudocyst vs., **663**
- nasopalatine duct cyst vs., **420**
- odontogenic keratocyst vs., **401**
- oral cavity minor salivary gland malignancy vs., **313**
- pericoronal radiolucencies without radiopacities vs., **874, 875**
- prognosis, **397**
- well-defined unilocular radiolucencies vs., **870, 872**

Dentin, **7, 10, 11**
- anatomy, **4–5**

Dentin dysplasia, **232**
- crown changes vs., **848, 849**
- dentinogenesis imperfecta vs., **231**
- differential diagnosis, **232**
- root changes vs., **851, 853**

Dentin matrix, **6**
Dentinoenamel junction (DEJ), **10, 11, 261**
Dentinogenesis imperfecta, **230–231**
- crown changes vs., **848, 849**
- dentin dysplasia vs., **232**
- differential diagnosis, **231**
- genetics, **231**
- root changes vs., **851, 853**
- staging, grading, & classification, **231**

Dentoalveolar fractures, **254–259**
- differential diagnosis, **255**

Denture adhesive, oral mucosal space/surface lesions vs., **927, 928**
Dentures, complete and partial, **14**
Deposition disease, calcium pyrophosphate, degenerative joint disorders of craniovertebral junction vs., **815**
Depressor alae nasi, **26**
Depressor anguli oris, **139, 142**
Depressor labii inferioris, **139, 142**
Depressor septi nasi, **139, 142**
Dermoid and epidermoid cyst, oral cavity, **284–287**
- diagnostic checklist, **286**
- differential diagnosis, **285–286**
- foregut duplication cyst in tongue vs., **291**
- nasolabial cyst vs., **423**
- oral cavity minor salivary gland malignancy vs., **313**
- oral cavity soft tissue infections vs., **293**
- prognosis, **286**
- ranula vs., **297**
- root of tongue lesions vs., **930, 932**
- staging, grading, & classification, **286**
- sublingual space
  - oral cavity sialocele vs., **303**
  - sublingual space lesions vs., **923, 925**
- submandibular gland mucocele vs., **305**
- submandibular space lesions vs., **915**

Dermoid cyst. *See* Dermoid and epidermoid.
Desmoplastic fibroma, **490–491**
- associated abnormalities, **491**
- central, central odontogenic fibroma vs., **473**
- diagnostic checklist, **491**
- differential diagnosis, **491**
- prognosis, **491**

Developing apices, root changes vs., **850, 852**
Developmental cyst. *See* Dermoid and epidermoid cyst, oral cavity.
Deviated nasal septum, **650–651**
- associated abnormalities, **651**
- diagnostic checklist, **651**
- differential diagnosis, **651**
- staging, grading, & classification, **651**

DF. *See* Desmoplastic fibroma.
Diaphragma sella, **127**
Diffuse idiopathic skeletal hyperostosis, **822–825**
- associated abnormalities, **823–824**
- diagnostic checklist, **824**
- differential diagnosis, **823**
- prognosis, **824**
- staging, grading, & classification, **824**

Diffuse opacities, amelogenesis imperfecta vs., **227**
Diffuse rough type, amelogenesis imperfecta and, **228**
Diffuse smooth type, amelogenesis imperfecta and, **228**
Digastric muscle
- anterior belly of, **38, 39**
  - submandibular space, **48, 50, 51**
- posterior belly of, **39, 170, 171, 185, 187**
  - submandibular space, **49**

Dilaceration, **224**
- root changes vs., **850, 852**

Dilated Wharton duct, sublingual space lesions vs., **922, 924**
Disc derangement
- with reduction, disc displacement without reduction vs., **612**
- without reduction, limited condylar translation vs., **950, 951**

Disc displacement
- calcium pyrophosphate dihydrate deposition disease associated, **628**
- with recapture. *See* Disc replacement, with reduction.
- without reduction, **610–615**
  - differential diagnosis, **612**
  - prognosis, **612**
  - staging, grading, & classification, **612**

Disc replacement
- with reduction, **604–609**
  - diagnostic checklist, **606**
  - differential diagnosis, **605**
  - prognosis, **606**

INDEX

staging, grading, & classification, **606**
- without reduction, disc replacement with reduction vs., **605**

DISH. *See* Diffuse idiopathic skeletal hyperostosis.
Disintegration of Hertwig root sheath, **6**
Dislocation, temporomandibular joint, **570–571**
- diagnostic checklist, **571**
- differential diagnosis, **571**
- prognosis, **571**
- staging, grading, & classification, **571**

Disorganized spine. *See* Failure of formation; Failure of segmentation.
Displaced dental structures, into antrum, **984–987**
- differential diagnosis, **984**

Displaced ZMC fracture. *See* Zygomaticomaxillary complex fracture.
Displacement without recapture. *See* Disc displacement, without reduction.
Diving ranula. *See also* Ranula.
- oral cavity soft tissue infections vs., **293–294**
- submandibular space accessory salivary tissue vs., **281**

DL-DCF completely circumscribes PVS, **196**
Dorsum of tongue, **33**
Dorsum sellae, **99, 101, 107, 111, 113, 208**
Double tooth. *See* Macrodontia.
Down syndrome
- hypoplasia/aplasia associated, **660**
- microdontia vs., **218**
- periodontal disease associated, **272**

Ductal carcinoma, parotid, parotid mucoepidermoid carcinoma vs., **769**
Duplication/division of mandibular canal. *See* Accessory mandibular canal.
Dura, **100**
Dysplasia
- dentin, **232**
- ectodermal, microdontia vs., **218**
- fibrous, segmental odontomaxillary dysplasia vs., **235**
- segmental odontomaxillary, **234–235**

Dysraphism, failure of formation vs., **807**
Dystrophic calcification of lymph nodes
- parotid sialoliths vs., **785**
- submandibular sialoliths vs., **339**

E

Ear dysplasia, congenital external, Treacher Collins syndrome vs., **369**
Early destructive phase, Paget disease, **447**
Early stage, periapical osseous dysplasia, **429**
Eburnation, bone. *See* Mandible-maxilla idiopathic osteosclerosis.
Ectoderm, oral epithelium arising from, **6**
Ectodermal dysplasia
- hypodontia vs., **213**
- microdontia vs., **218**
- missing teeth vs., **846, 847**
- submandibular gland aplasia-hypoplasia associated, **289**

Ectodermal inclusion cyst. *See* Dermoid and epidermoid cyst, oral cavity.
Ectomesenchyme, **6**
Ectopic thyroid
- root of tongue lesions vs., **930–931, 933**
- tissue. *See* Lingual thyroid.

Edentulous span exhibiting bone loss, **27**
Ekman-Westborg and Julin trait, macrodontia, gemination, and fusion vs., **217**
Elevated sinus floor, **61**
Elfin face syndrome, hypoplasia/aplasia associated, **660**
Elongated pars interarticularis, **153**
Eminence click, disc replacement with reduction vs., **605**
Eminence fibrocartilage, **86**
Enamel, **7, 10, 11**
- anatomy, **4**
- matrix, **6**
- organ, **6**

Enamel agenesis, amelogenesis imperfecta and, **228**
Enamel hypoplasia, environmental, Turner dysplasia vs., **241**
Enamel pearls, **222, 271**
- diagnostic checklist, **222**
- differential diagnosis, **222**
- root changes vs., **851, 853**

Endodontic filling material, displaced dental structures into antrum vs., **984, 986**
Endophytic papilloma. *See* Sinonasal inverted papilloma.
Enlarged adenoids, **179**
Enostosis. *See also* Mandible-maxilla idiopathic osteosclerosis.
- cementoblastoma vs., **469**
- mandibular torus vs., **345**
- periapical sclerosing osteitis vs., **269**
- submandibular sialoliths vs., **339**

Enteric duplication cyst. *See* Foregut duplication cyst in tongue.
Environmental defects of enamel, amelogenesis imperfecta vs., **227**
Environmental enamel hypoplasia, Turner dysplasia vs., **241**
Eosinophilic angiocentric fibrosis, invasive pseudotumor vs., **695**
Eosinophilic granuloma. *See also* Langerhans histiocytosis.
- desmoplastic fibroma vs., **491**
- mandibular salivary gland defect vs., **351**
- well-defined unilocular radiolucencies vs., **871, 873**

Eosinophilic mucin rhinosinusitis, allergic fungal sinusitis vs., **687**
Epidermoid. *See* Dermoid and epidermoid cyst, oral cavity.
Epidural tumor, **198**
- compressing spinal cord, **198**

Epiglottis, **39, 119, 120, 175, 176, 177**
- free margin, **167**

Epithelial odontogenic cyst, calcifying. *See* Calcifying odontogenic cyst.
Epithelial rests of Malassez, **6**
Epitympanic cog, **92**
Epitympanum, **90, 91, 92, 93**

Erosion, **239**
- abfraction vs., **240**
- abrasion vs., **238**
- attrition vs., **237**
- diagnostic checklist, **239**
- differential diagnosis, **239**
- internal and external resorption vs., **243–244**
Erupting tooth, **6**
- cusp, **7**
ES family of tumors (ESFT). *See* Ewing sarcoma.
Esophagus, **165, 194**
ES/primitive neuroectodermal tumor (ES/PNET). *See* Ewing sarcoma.
Esthesioneuroblastoma
- nasal lesion with bony destruction vs., **970, 972**
- paranasal sinus lesions with bony destruction vs., **980, 982**
- sinonasal adenoid cystic carcinoma vs., **707**
- sinonasal inverted papilloma vs., **697**
- sinonasal malignant melanoma vs., **713**
- sinonasal squamous cell carcinoma vs., **705**
Ethmoid, cribriform plate of, **99**
Ethmoid air cells, **58, 63**
- anterior, **101, 103**
- posterior, **101, 103, 107**
Ethmoid bone, **25, 100, 103**
- perpendicular plate of, **25**
Ethmoid bullae, **57, 58, 62, 65, 66, 67, 68, 70, 72, 73, 74, 75**
Ethmoid foramen
- anterior, **101**
  anatomy, **98**
- posterior, anatomy, **98**
Ethmoid nerves, anterior & posterior, **105, 128**
Ethmoid sinus, **134**
- sinonasal overview, **56**
Ethmoidal crest, of maxilla, **25**
Ethmoidomaxillary suture, **24**
Eustachian tube opening, **173, 175, 178**
Ewing sarcoma, **524–527**. *See also* Sarcoma.
- diagnostic checklist, **526**
- differential diagnosis, **525**
- genetics, **525**
- ill-defined radiolucencies vs., **883, 887**
- mandible-maxilla osteosarcoma vs., **501**
- periosteal reactions vs., **907, 911**
- prognosis, **526**
Exocciput, **106**
Exostoses
- buccal, mandibular torus vs., **345**
- buccal and lingual, mandible-maxilla osteoma vs., **481**
- buccal and palatal, **342–343**
  associated abnormalities, **343**
  differential diagnosis, **343**
  genetics, **343**
  prognosis, **343**
- palatal torus vs., **347**
- well-defined radiopacities vs., **892, 894**
External auditory canal, **84, 87, 88, 89, 144, 182, 186**
- tympanic bone of, **84**
External auditory meatus, **88, 119, 120, 121**
External carotid artery, **85, 166, 185, 187, 190, 191, 202**
External ear, **90–95, 121**
- axial bone CT, **92–93**
- coronal bone CT, **94–95**
- embryology, **90**
- graphics, **91**
External (ECA) carotid arteries, **204**
External oblique ridge, **31, 33**
External resorption, **242–247**
- root changes vs., **850, 852**
Extra teeth, **844–845**
- differential diagnosis, **844**
Extraconal fat, **70**
Extracranial facial nerve (CNVII), **184**
Extracranial motor (CNVII), **140**
Extravasation cyst. *See* Simple (traumatic) bone cyst, mandible-maxilla; Simple (traumatic) bone cyst, temporomandibular joint.
Extrusive luxation. *See* Luxation.

F

Facet arthropathy, cervical, **826–829**
- associated abnormalities, **828**
- diagnostic checklist, **828**
- differential diagnosis, **827**
- genetics, **828**
- prognosis, **828**
- staging, grading, & classification, **828**
Facet arthrosis. *See* Cervical facet arthropathy.
Facet joint, **157**
Facial alveolar bone thickness, **20**
Facial artery, **51, 204, 205**
- calcification of, **209**
Facial bone loss, **271**
Facial colliculus, **140**
Facial expression, muscles of, **139**
Facial fracture, complex, transfacial fracture (Le Fort) vs., **381**
Facial nerve (CNVII), **111, 129, 147, 186**. *See also* Cranial nerve VII (CNVII).
- in stylomastoid foramen, **147**
Facial nerve recess, **92, 143, 144**
Facial neuroma. *See* Parotid schwannoma.
Facial nodal group, **200**
Facial "smash" injury. *See* Complex midfacial fracture.
Facial vein, **50, 51, 167**
Failure of formation, **806–809**
- associated abnormalities, **807**
- diagnostic checklist, **808**
- differential diagnosis, **807**
- genetics, **807**
- prognosis, **808**
Failure of segmentation, **810–813**
- associated abnormalities, **811**
- diagnostic checklist, **812**
- differential diagnosis, **811**
- genetics, **811**

INDEX

- prognosis, **812**
- staging, grading, & classification, **811–812**

Faintly calcified atheroma, **209**
False ankylosis
- adhesions vs., **617**
- fibrous ankylosis vs., **561**

False sialocele, oral cavity soft tissue infections vs., **294**
Familial adenomatous polyposis
- extra teeth vs., **844, 845**
- TMJ osteoma associated, **619**

Familial benign giant cell tumor of jaw. *See* Cherubism.
Familial fibrous dysplasia (FD). *See* Cherubism.
Familial gigantiform cementoma. *See* Florid osseous dysplasia.
Familial multilocular cystic disease of jaw. *See* Cherubism.
Familial multiple cementomas. *See* Florid osseous dysplasia.
Fascial "trap door," **165, 194**
Fat
- in crista galli, **70**
- in nasal bone, **70**

Fat pad, CNV3, masticator space CNV3 perineural tumor vs., **744**
Fatty marrow
- in crista galli, normal, dermoid and epidermoid vs., **286**
- focal, hemangioma, cervical spine vs., **831**

FD. *See* Fibrous dysplasia; Fibrous dysplasia, mandible-maxilla.
Fibroadamantoblastoma. *See* Ameloblastic fibroma.
Fibrocementoma. *See* Periapical osseous dysplasia.
Fibroma, ameloblastic, ameloblastic fibroodontoma vs., **465**
Fibromatosis
- aggressive. *See* Desmoplastic fibroma.
- gingiva, segmental odontomaxillary dysplasia vs., **235**

Fibromyxoma. *See* Odontogenic myxoma.
Fibroodontoma, ameloblastic, **464–465**
- calcifying epithelial odontogenic tumor vs., **467**
- calcifying odontogenic cyst vs., **413**
- diagnostic checklist, **465**
- differential diagnosis, **465**
- odontoma vs., **452**

Fibro-osteoma. *See* Ossifying fibroma.
Fibroosteoma, periapical. *See* Periapical osseous dysplasia.
Fibrosarcoma. *See also* Sarcoma.
- ameloblastic, ameloblastic fibroma transformation, **462**

Fibrous ankylosis, **560–561**
- adhesions vs., **617**
- bony ankylosis vs., **563**
- diagnostic checklist, **561**
- differential diagnosis, **561**
- limited condylar translation vs., **950, 952**
- staging, grading, & classification, **561**

Fibrous bands and adhesions (stuck disc), disc replacement with reduction vs., **605**
Fibrous dysplasia
- cervical spine, **838–839**
    - associated abnormalities, **839**
    - differential diagnosis, **839**
    - genetics, **839**
    - prognosis, **839**
- cherubism vs., **359**
- chronic rhinosinusitis vs., **681**
- condylar hyperplasia vs., **548**
- craniofacial type, nasal lesion without bony destruction vs., **966**
- dentin, dentin dysplasia vs., **232**
- florid osseous dysplasia vs., **433**
- generalized radiopacities vs., **902, 904**
- ground-glass and granular radiopacities vs., **896, 897, 898**
- hypoplasia/aplasia vs., **659**
- lamina dura changes vs., **866, 868**
- large condyle vs., **947**
- mandible-maxilla, **440–445**
    - associated abnormalities, **442**
    - diagnostic checklist, **442**
    - differential diagnosis, **441–442**
    - genetics, **442**
    - prognosis, **442**
    - staging, grading, & classification, **442**
- mandible-maxilla chondrosarcoma vs., **505–506**
- mandible-maxilla osteomyelitis vs., **386**
- mandible-maxilla osteosarcoma vs., **501**
- ossifying fibroma vs., **437**
- Paget disease vs., **448**
- segmental odontomaxillary dysplasia vs., **235**
- sinonasal, **714–717**
    - associated abnormalities, **716**
    - diagnostic checklist, **716**
    - differential diagnosis, **715–716**
    - paranasal sinus lesions without bony destruction vs., **976–977, 979**
    - prognosis, **716**
    - sinonasal fibroosseous and cartilaginous lesions vs., **974**
    - sinonasal ossifying fibroma vs., **719**
    - sinonasal osteoma vs., **701**
    - staging, grading, & classification, **716**

Fibrous osteodysplasia. *See* Fibrous dysplasia, mandible-maxilla.
Fibrous osteoma. *See* Fibrous dysplasia, mandible-maxilla.
5th cranial nerve. *See* Cranial nerve V (CNV).
1st branchial cleft cyst
- benign lymphoepithelial lesions: HIV vs., **751**
- parotid space lesions vs., **919**

1st premolar, **13**
Fixed appliances (orthodontics), **14**
Floating teeth, **862–863**
- differential diagnosis, **862**

Flocculus, **132**
- of cerebellum, **147**

Floor
- of maxillary sinus, **29, 59, 60**
- of nasal cavity, **24**
- of nasal fossa, **59, 60, 61**
- of orbit, **24, 26, 58, 61, 62**
- of sella, **107**

Floor carotid canal, **164**
Floor of mouth, **36, 52, 53**
- abscess, sublingual gland benign mixed tumor vs., **307**

Floor of mouth sialocele. *See* Sialocele, oral cavity.

INDEX

Floor of mouth squamous cell carcinoma, **324–325**
- differential diagnosis, **325**
- oral mucosal space/surface lesions vs., **926, 928**
- prognosis, **325**
- staging, grading, & classification, **325**
- sublingual gland carcinoma vs., **315**

Florid cementoosseous dysplasia. *See* Florid osseous dysplasia.
Florid osseous dysplasia, **432–435**
- diagnostic checklist, **434**
- differential diagnosis, **433**
- generalized radiopacities vs., **902, 903**
- ground-glass and granular radiopacities vs., **896, 898, 899**
- Paget disease vs., **448**
- periapical osseous dysplasia vs., **429**
- periapical radiopacities and mixed lesions vs., **860**
- prognosis, **434**
- staging, grading, & classification, **434**

Florid-ossifying dysplasia. *See* Florid osseous dysplasia.
Fluorosis, generalized radiopacities vs., **903**
Focal cementoosseous dysplasia. *See* Periapical osseous dysplasia.
Focal dermal hypoplasia
- hypodontia vs., **213**
- missing teeth vs., **846**

Focal fatty marrow, hemangioma, cervical spine vs., **831**
Focal osteopetrosis. *See* Mandible-maxilla idiopathic osteosclerosis.
Focal sclerosing osteitis. *See* Periapical sclerosing osteitis.
Focal sclerosing osteomyelitis. *See* Periapical sclerosing osteitis.
FOD. *See* Florid osseous dysplasia.
Follicular cyst. *See* Dentigerous cyst.
Follicular space, hyperplastic, ameloblastic fibroma vs., **461**
Fonticulus frontalis, **100**
Foramen artery, **206**
Foramen cecum, **100**
- anterior skull base, anatomy, **98, 99**
- area, **103**
- nonossified, dermoid and epidermoid vs., **286**
- remnant, **99, 100**
    pit, **101, 103**

Foramen lacerum, **105, 108, 109, 114, 164, 170, 174, 175, 207**
- of central skull base, **104**
- lacerum (C3) ICA segment, **207**

Foramen magnum, **110, 111, 114, 116, 156**
Foramen of Vesalius, **104**
Foramen ovale, **64, 78, 105, 108, 109, 115, 119, 127, 144, 170, 174, 182, 206, 207, 209**
- calcification of, **209**
- of central skull base, **104**
- CNV3, **134, 164, 169, 182**

Foramen rotundum, **28, 64, 77, 78, 79, 105, 107, 108, 109, 137, 206, 207**
- artery of, **205, 206**
- of central skull base, **104**
- CNV2, **102, 134**

Foramen spinosum, **78, 105, 108, 115, 119, 134, 144, 170, 207**
- of central skull base, **104**
- middle meningeal artery, **164, 182**

Foramina of cribriform plate, **98**
Foregut duplication cyst in tongue, **290–291**
- diagnostic checklist, **291**
- differential diagnosis, **291**
- options, risks, complications, **291**
- root of tongue lesions vs., **931, 933**

Foreign object, well-defined radiopacities vs., **892–893, 895**
Forestier disease. *See* Diffuse idiopathic skeletal hyperostosis.
"Forme fruste," nerve sheath tumor, **484**
Forming periodontal ligaments, **6**
Fossa of Rosenmüller, **177**
4th ventricle, **132, 147**
Fovea ethmoidalis, **65, 66, 101, 102**
Fractures
- clefts vs., **357**
- hemifacial microsomia vs., **543**
- mandible, **370–373**
- temporomandibular joint, **564–569**
    associated abnormalities, **565**
    diagnostic checklist, **565**
    differential diagnosis, **565**
    prognosis, **565**

Frontal bone, **68, 99, 100, 102, 103**
Frontal crest, **102**
- of anterior skull base, **98**

Frontal lobe, **100**
Frontal nerve, **105, 128**
Frontal process, **24**
- in maxilla, **26**
- maxillary bone, **22**

Frontal recess, **68, 75**
- of frontal sinus, **68**

Frontal sinus, **57, 66, 67, 69, 75, 99, 101, 102, 103**
- drainage, **57, 66**
- septum, **69**
- sinonasal overview, **56**

Frontoethmoidal cephalocele, dermoid and epidermoid vs., **286**
Frontomaxillary suture, **24**
Full metal crown, **16**
Fulminant sinusitis, paranasal sinus lesions with bony destruction vs., **980, 981**
Functional tooth wear. *See* Attrition.
Fungal sinusitis
- allergic, **686–687**
    chronic rhinosinusitis vs., **681**
    diagnostic checklist, **687**
    differential diagnosis, **687**
    mycetoma vs., **693**
    nasal lesion without bony destruction vs., **966, 967**
    odontogenic sinusitis vs., **685**
    paranasal sinus lesions without bony destruction vs., **976, 979**
    prognosis, **687**
    sinonasal mucocele vs., **665**

sinonasal polyposis vs., **673**
- invasive, **688–691**
  diagnostic checklist, **690**
  differential diagnosis, **689**
  mycetoma vs., **693**
  nasal lesion with bony destruction vs., **970, 972**
  paranasal sinus lesions with bony destruction vs., **980, 981**
  perforated nasal septum vs., **964, 965**
  prognosis, **690**
  sinonasal granulomatosis with polyangiitis vs., **669**
  sinonasal squamous cell carcinoma vs., **705**
  staging, grading, & classification, **690**
- mycetoma, paranasal sinus lesions without bony destruction vs., **976, 978**
- sinonasal, chronic rhinosinusitis vs., **681**

Fungus ball. *See* Mycetoma.
Furcal bone, **11**
Furcation bone loss, periodontal, **271**
Fused roots, root changes vs., **851, 853**
Fusion, concrescence and, **219**

G

Ganglion cyst, TMJ synovial cyst vs., **597**
Gardner syndrome, **343**
- cleidocranial dysplasia vs., **365**
- extra teeth vs., **844, 845**
- florid osseous dysplasia vs., **434**
- generalized radiopacities vs., **902, 905**
- hyperdontia vs., **215**
- lamina dura changes vs., **866–867, 868**
- mandible-maxilla idiopathic osteosclerosis vs., **355**
- sinonasal osteoma associated, **701**
- TMJ osteoma associated, **619**

Garré osteomyelitis, periosteal reactions vs., **908**
Gastrointestinal cyst. *See* Foregut duplication cyst in tongue.
Gaucher disease
- generalized rarefaction vs., **889**
- hypoplasia/aplasia vs., **659**

Gemination, concrescence and, **219**
Generalized cortical hyperostosis, hypoplasia/aplasia associated, **660**
Generalized pitted pattern, amelogenesis imperfecta and, **227**
Generalized radiopacities, **902–905**
- differential diagnosis, **902–903**

Generalized rarefaction, **888–891**
- differential diagnosis, **888–889**

Genetic counseling, clefts, **357**
Genial tubercle, **32, 34**
Geniculate fossa, **143**
Geniculate ganglion, **92, 94, 138, 140, 186**
- of CNVII, **141**
- in geniculate fossa, **146**

Genioglossus, **45, 46, 53, 119**
- anatomy, **36, 37, 38, 39**

Geniohyoid, **32, 38, 39, 46, 53**
Genu of petrous (C2) ICA, **206, 207**
Ghost cell carcinoma, odontogenic, **413**
Ghost teeth. *See* Regional odontodysplasia.
Giant cell granuloma
- central, **530–533**
  aneurysmal bone cyst vs., **645**
  associated abnormalities, **531**
  differential diagnosis, **531**
  prognosis, **531**
- mandible-maxilla, nasal lesion without bony destruction vs., **967, 969**
- TMJ simple (traumatic) bone cyst vs., **643**

Giant cell lesion of hyperparathyroidism, mandible-maxilla aneurysmal bone cyst vs., **415**
Giant cell reparative granuloma. *See* Giant cell granuloma, central.
Giant cell tumor
- Paget disease, **448, 449**
- TMJ pigmented villonodular synovitis vs., **591**

Giant dense bone island, **355**
Giant osteogenic fibroma. *See* Osteoblastoma.
Giant osteoid osteoma. *See* Osteoblastoma.
Gigantiform cementoma. *See* Florid osseous dysplasia.
Gingiva, anatomy, **5**
Gingival embrasure, **11**
Gingival epithelium, basal cell layer of, **5**
Gingival fibromatosis, segmental odontomaxillary dysplasia vs., **235**
Gingival squamous cell carcinoma, **326–327**
- diagnostic checklist, **327**
- differential diagnosis, **327**
- oral mucosal space/surface lesions vs., **926, 928**
- prognosis, **327**
- staging, grading, & classification, **327**

Gingivitis. *See* Periodontal disease.
Glandular odontogenic cyst
- central mucoepidermoid carcinoma vs., **511**
- multilocular radiolucencies vs., **879**
- residual cyst vs., **407**

Glass ionomer, **14**
Glass ionomer cement, **18**
Glenoid fossa, **82, 84, 88, 89**
- lateral ridge of, **87**
- roof of, **87**

Glossoepiglottic fold, **174**
Glossoepiglottic ligament, **37**
Glossopharyngeal nerve (CNIX), **53, 111, 189, 190**
- sublingual space, anatomy, **44**

Goldenhar syndrome. *See also* Hemifacial microsomia.
- condylar aplasia associated, **541**
- hypoplasia/aplasia associated, **660**

Gorlin cyst. *See* Calcifying odontogenic cyst.
Gorlin syndrome. *See* Basal cell nevus syndrome.
Gorlin-Goltz syndrome. *See also* Basal cell nevus syndrome.
- hypodontia vs., **213**
- missing teeth vs., **846**

Graft material, for ridge augmentation procedure, ground-glass and granular radiopacities vs., **896, 898**
Granular cell AF. *See* Ameloblastic fibroma.

INDEX

Granular radiopacities, **896–901**
- differential diagnosis, **896–897**

Granuloma
- ill-defined radiolucencies vs., **882–883, 886**
- periapical. *See* Periapical rarefying osteitis.
- radicular. *See* Periapical rarefying osteitis.

Granulomatosis with polyangiitis
- invasive fungal sinusitis vs., **689**
- sinonasal, **668–671**
  - associated abnormalities, **669–670**
  - diagnostic checklist, **670**
  - differential diagnosis, **669**
  - nasal lesion with bony destruction vs., **970, 972**
  - paranasal sinus lesions with bony destruction vs., **980, 982**
  - perforated nasal septum vs., **964, 965**
  - prognosis, **670**
  - sinonasal polyposis vs., **673**

Granulomatous invasive fungal rhinosinusitis (GIFRS). *See* Fungal sinusitis, invasive.
Greater and lesser palatine nerves, **128**
Greater palatine canal, **25, 28, 79, 136, 137**
- part of, **24**

Greater palatine foramen, **26, 27, 28, 65, 67, 78, 79**
Greater palatine nerve, **27, 77, 105, 128**
Greater petrosal nerve, **129**
Greater superficial petrosal nerve, **140, 141, 186**
- facial hiatus for, **143**

Greater wing, of sphenoid bone, **101, 105, 107, 109**
Gross caries, **60**
Ground-glass radiopacities, **896–901**
- differential diagnosis, **896–897**

Gubernacular canal. *See* Gubernaculum dentis.
Gubernacular cord. *See* Gubernaculum dentis.
Gubernaculum dentis, **276–277**
- accessory mandibular canal vs., **349**
- associated abnormalities, **277**
- differential diagnosis, **277**

Gum disease. *See* Periodontal disease.
Gutta percha, **14, 15, 16**
- cement, displaced dental structures into antrum vs., **984, 986**

Gyrus rectus, **99, 101**

H

Haller air cell (infraorbital extramural ethmoid air cell), **74**
Haller cell, **72**
Hamulus, **64, 109**
Hamulus of medial pterygoid plate, **28, 41, 42, 43, 166**
Hard palate, **136, 137**
Hard palate minor salivary gland carcinoma, hard palate squamous cell carcinoma vs., **335**
Hard palate minor salivary gland malignancy, sinonasal adenoid cystic carcinoma vs., **707**
Hard palate mucosal surface, **52**
Hard palate squamous cell carcinoma, **334–335**
- diagnostic checklist, **335**
- differential diagnosis, **335**
- oral mucosal space/surface lesions vs., **927, 929**
- palate benign mixed tumor vs., **311**
- prognosis, **335**
- staging, grading, & classification, **335**

Hashimoto thyroiditis, non-Hodgkin lymphoma of pharyngeal space associated, **518**
Head of malleus, **92, 143**
Healing facet fracture, cervical facet arthropathy vs., **827**
Hemangioma
- central, **474–475**
  - desmoplastic fibroma vs., **491**
  - diagnostic checklist, **475**
  - differential diagnosis, **475**
  - odontogenic myxoma vs., **471**
  - prognosis, **475**
- cervical spine, **830–833**
  - associated abnormalities, **832**
  - diagnostic checklist, **832**
  - differential diagnosis, **831**
  - genetics, **831–832**
  - prognosis, **832**
- facial bones, multilocular radiolucencies vs., **878, 881**
- masticator space CNV3 schwannoma vs., **733**
- neurofibromatosis type 1 vs., **487**
- periosteal reactions vs., **907, 910**
- upper airway, lingual thyroid vs., **283**

Hematopoietic malignancy, lytic and blastic metastases vs., **835**
Hemifacial hypertrophy. *See* Condylar hyperplasia.
Hemifacial microsomia, **542–545**
- condylar hypoplasia, **557**
- diagnostic checklist, **543**
- differential diagnosis, **543**
- hypoplasia/aplasia associated, **660**
- prognosis, **543**
- small condyle vs., **941, 945**
- staging, grading, & classification, **543**
- TMJ fractures vs., **565**
- TMJ juvenile idiopathic arthritis vs., **585**
- type III, condylar aplasia associated, **541**

Hemignathia. *See* Condylar aplasia.
Hemimandibular elongation, condylar hyperplasia vs., **547**
Hemimandibular hyperplasia. *See* Condylar hyperplasia.
Hemimaxillofacial dysplasia. *See* Segmental odontomaxillary dysplasia (SOD).
Hemimaxillofacial enlargement, asymmetry of face, teeth abnormalities, skin findings (HATS). *See* Segmental odontomaxillary dysplasia (SOD).
Hemivertebra, failure of formation vs., **808**
Hemodialysis, cervical peridural calcification , ossification of posterior longitudinal ligament vs., **819**
Hemorrhagic bone cyst. *See* Simple (traumatic) bone cyst, mandible-maxilla; Simple (traumatic) bone cyst, temporomandibular joint.
Hereditary opalescent dentin. *See* Dentinogenesis imperfect.
Hertwig root sheath, **6**
Heterogeneous marrow, lytic and blastic metastases vs., **836**

INDEX

Heterotopia, nasal glial, dermoid and epidermoid vs., **286**
Hexavalent exposure, perforated nasal septum vs., **964**
Hiatus semilunaris, **57, 67, 68, 72, 73, 74, 75**
High internal jugular lymph nodes, **201**
- level II, **202**
- level IIA, **202, 203**
- level IIB, **202**
High spinal accessory lymph nodes, **201**
High submandibular node, **51**
High-force trauma, nasoethmoid complex fracture, **375**
High-grade B-cell lymphoma. *See* Burkitt lymphoma.
Histiocytosis, Langerhans, periodontal disease vs., **272**
Histiocytosis X. *See* Langerhans histiocytosis.
HIV-related benign lymphoepithelial cysts, parotid sialadenitis vs., **755**
Horizontal bone loss, **271**
Horizontal fracture. *See* Dentoalveolar fractures.
Horizontal petrous internal carotid artery, **113, 114**
- canal, **108, 117**
Horizontal process, **24**
Horizontal segment of carotid canal, **78**
Horizontal segment of cavernous (C4) ICA, **206**
- calcification of, **209**
Horizontal segment of petrous internal carotid artery, **146, 206**
Horizontally impacted 3rd molar, **12**
Horizontally oriented permanent canines, **13**
Hyoglossus, **38, 39, 45, 46, 49, 51, 53, 119**
- anatomy, **36, 37**
Hyoid bone, **32, 39, 119, 120, 121, 165, 176, 177, 191, 194, 197, 199**
- greater cornu of, **209**
- lesser horn of, **121**
Hyoid bone plane, **201**
Hypercementosis, **248**
- cementoblastoma vs., **469**
- differential diagnosis, **210**
- mandible-maxilla idiopathic osteosclerosis vs., **355**
- periapical radiopacities and mixed lesions vs., **860, 861**
- periapical sclerosing osteitis vs., **269**
- root changes vs., **850, 851**
- supernumerary roots vs., **225**
Hyperdontia, **214–215**
- associated abnormalities, **215**
- diagnostic checklist, **215**
- differential diagnosis, **215**
- extra teeth vs., **844, 845**
- genetics, **215**
- odontoma vs., **451**
- prognosis, **215**
Hyperkeratosis palmoplantaris, periodontal disease associated, **272**
Hypermobility, temporomandibular joint, TMJ dislocation vs., **571**
Hyperostoses. *See* Buccal and palatal exostoses.
Hyperparathyroidism
- brown tumor of, cherubism vs., **359**
- generalized rarefaction vs., **888, 890**
- giant cell lesion of, mandible-maxilla aneurysmal bone cyst vs., **415**
- ground-glass and granular radiopacities vs., **897, 901**
- lamina dura changes vs., **866, 868**
- multiple myeloma vs., **521**
Hyperplasia, segmental hemifacial, segmental odontomaxillary dysplasia vs., **235**
Hyperplastic cingulum. *See* Talon cusp.
Hyperplastic dental follicles, buccal bifurcation cyst vs., **409**
Hyperplastic follicular space, ameloblastic fibroma vs., **461**
Hypertrophic polypoid rhinosinusitis. *See* Sinonasal polyposis.
Hypodontia, **212–213**
- diagnostic checklist, **213**
- differential diagnosis, **213**
- genetics, **213**
- missing teeth vs., **846, 847**
- prognosis, **213**
Hypoglossal canal, **110, 111, 116, 144, 145, 158, 164**
- external opening, **117**
- inferior margin, **115**
Hypoglossal nerve (CNXII), **36, 53, 111, 189, 190**
- atrophy, sublingual space lesions vs., **923, 925**
- paralysis. *See* Motor denervation CNXII.
- sublingual space, anatomy, **44**
Hypoglossal nerve (CNXII) palsy. *See* Motor denervation CNXII.
Hypoglossus, **38**
Hypomaturation amelogenesis imperfecta (type II), **227**
Hypomaturation types, amelogenesis imperfecta and, **228**
Hypomaturation/hypoplastic amelogenesis imperfecta (type IV), **27**
Hypomaturation-hypoplastic types, amelogenesis imperfecta and, **228**
Hypomineralized amelogenesis imperfecta (type III), **227**
Hypomineralized types, amelogenesis imperfecta and, **228**
Hypopharynx, **194**
Hypophosphatasia
- generalized rarefaction vs., **889**
- lamina dura changes vs., **867**
Hypophosphatemia
- generalized rarefaction vs., **889**
- lamina dura changes vs., **867**
- periodontal disease associated, **272**
Hypoplasia
- amelogenesis imperfecta vs., **227**
- environmental enamel, Turner dysplasia vs., **241**
- focal dermal, hypodontia vs., **213**
Hypoplasia/aplasia, **658–661**. *See also* Submandibular gland aplasia-hypoplasia.
- associated abnormalities, **660**
- diagnostic checklist, **660**
- differential diagnosis, **659**
- genetics, **659–660**
- staging, grading, & classification, **660**
- submandibular gland, submandibular space lesions vs., **915**
Hypoplastic amelogenesis imperfecta, type I, **227**
Hypoplastic left maxillary sinus, **63**
Hypotympanum, **90, 91, 93**

INDEX

I

Idiopathic bone cavity. *See* Mandibular salivary gland defect (Stafne); Simple (traumatic) bone cyst, mandible-maxilla; Simple (traumatic) bone cyst, temporomandibular joint.
Idiopathic cervical resorption, dental caries vs., **261**
Idiopathic condylar resorption. *See* Progressive condylar resorption.
Idiopathic histiocytosis. *See* Langerhans histiocytosis.
Idiopathic osteosclerosis
- buccal and palatal exostoses vs., **343**
- cementoblastoma vs., **469**
- mandible-maxilla, **354–355**
- mandible-maxilla osteoma vs., **481**
- mandibular torus vs., **345**
- odontoma vs., **452**
- periapical osseous dysplasia vs., **430**
- periapical radiopacities and mixed lesions vs., **860**
- TMJ radiopacities vs., **957, 959**
- well-defined radiopacities vs., **892, 893, 894**
Idiopathic osteosclerosis/enostosis
- periapical sclerosing osteitis vs., **269**
- submandibular sialoliths vs., **339**
Idiopathic skeletal hyperostosis, diffuse, **822–825**
- associated abnormalities, **823–824**
- diagnostic checklist, **824**
- differential diagnosis, **823**
- prognosis, **824**
- staging, grading, & classification, **824**
IgG4-related disease (IgG4-RD). *See* Invasive pseudotumor.
IHN. *See* Infrahyoid neck.
IJC. *See* Internal jugular chain.
Ill-defined radiolucencies, **882–887**
- differential diagnosis, **882–883**
Immature ameloblastic fibroodontoma, ameloblastic fibroma vs., **461**
Immature ameloblastic odontoma, ameloblastic fibroma vs., **461**
Immature odontoma
- ameloblastic fibroma vs., **461**
- dentigerous cyst vs., **397**
Immature ossifying fibroma, mandibular salivary gland defect vs., **351**
Impacted 3rd molar, **27, 61**
Impacted canine, **13, 61**
Impacted teeth, **220**
Impactions, **12–13**
Impaired collagen maturation, inherited disorder of, dentinogenesis imperfecta vs., **231**
Implant
- apex, **21**
- displaced dental structures into antrum vs., **984, 986**
- prosthetic, **14**
Inc. *See* Incisor (Inc).
Incisal edge, **11**
Incisal embrasure, **11**
Incisive canal, **25, 27, 136**
- meeting in midline, **33**
- nasopalatine nerve in, **128, 137**
Incisive canal cyst. *See* Nasopalatine duct cyst.
Incisive foramen, **28, 137**
Incisive (nasopalatine) canal, **25**
Incisive (nasopalatine) foramen (V2), **24**
Incisive nerve, **31, 131, 135**
- of mandible, anatomy, **30**
Incisor duct cyst. *See* Nasopalatine duct cyst.
Incisor (Inc), **4**
Incompletely formed root apex
- periapical radiolucencies vs., **856, 858**
- periapical rarefying osteitis vs., **266**
Incudostapedial articulation, **91, 92**
Incus, **88**
- anatomy, **90**
- body, **91, 92, 93, 94**
Incus lenticular process, **91, 93**
Incus long process, **91, 93**
Incus short process, **91, 92, 93**
Indolent fungal sinusitis. *See* Fungal sinusitis, invasive.
Infantile cortical hyperostosis, generalized radiopacities vs., **903**
Infantile hemangioma
- orbital, dermoid and epidermoid vs., **285–286**
- parotid space lesions vs., **919**
Infection, tumor calcinosis vs., **841**
Inferior alveolar artery, **85, 205**
Inferior alveolar canal, **10, 21, 35**
- accessory. *See* Accessory mandibular canal.
- mandible fracture vs., **371**
Inferior alveolar nerve (IAN), **13, 30, 43, 46, 50, 53, 105, 128, 129, 131, 182**
- canal, **33**
- in mandibular canal, **131**
Inferior articular facet, **152, 153**
- C1, **157**
Inferior articular process, **153**
- C2, **157**
Inferior body C2, **157**
Inferior concha, **58**
Inferior extension cruciate ligament, **151**
Inferior hypophyseal arteries, **205, 206**
Inferior lamina, posterior attachment, **86**
Inferior meatus, **25, 65, 73, 74, 75**
Inferior nasal concha, **25, 177, 179**
Inferior oblique muscle, **26**
Inferior orbital (blowout) fracture, zygomaticomaxillary complex fracture vs., **379**
Inferior orbital fissure, **64, 65, 70, 78, 79, 101, 102, 107, 134, 137, 207**
Inferior orbital rim, **58, 60**
Inferior petrosal sinus, **112**
Inferior posterior lateral nasal branch, **128**
Inferior rectus, **70**
Inferior turbinate, **57, 62, 63, 64, 65, 66, 67, 68, 69, 71, 73, 74, 75**
Inferior vestibular nerve, **147**
Inferolateral trunk, **205, 206**

INDEX

Inflammatory arthritides, cervical facet arthropathy vs., **827**
Inflammatory collateral cyst. *See* Buccal bifurcation cyst.
Inflammatory myofibroblastic tumor. *See* Invasive pseudotumor.
Inflammatory paradental cyst. *See* Buccal bifurcation cyst.
Inflammatory pseudotumor. *See also* Invasive pseudotumor.
- IgG4 disease, non-Hodgkin lymphoma of pharyngeal mucosal space vs., **517**
- orbital idiopathic, dermoid and epidermoid vs., **286**
Inflammatory (rheumatoid) arthritis, degenerative joint disease vs., **593**
Infrahyoid internal jugular vein, **190**
Infrahyoid neck (IHN), **162, 165, 188**
Infraorbital artery, **205**
Infraorbital canal, **24, 58, 62, 136, 137**
Infraorbital ethmoid (Haller) cell, **62**
- sinonasal overview, **56**
Infraorbital foramen, **24, 26, 33, 58, 137**
Infraorbital groove, **26**
Infraorbital nerve, **65, 66, 69, 70, 77, 105, 108, 128**
- of maxilla, anatomy, **22**
Infraorbital node, **201**
Infrazygomatic masticator space, **164, 169**
Infundibulum, **63**
Inherited spinal dysplasias, failure of formation vs., **807**
Initial junctional epithelium, **7**
Injury, dilaceration, **224**
Inner ear, **90–95**
- axial bone CT, **92–93**
- coronal bone CT, **94–95**
- embryology, **90**
- graphics, **91**
Interdental craters, **271**
Intermaxillary suture, **11, 24**
Intermediate phase, Paget disease, **447**
Intermediate stage, periapical osseous dysplasia, **429**
Intermediate zone of disc, **86**
Internal auditory canal, **92, 113, 117, 143, 145, 146**
- anterior margin of, **147**
- CNVII, **140**
- segment, **138**
Internal carotid artery, **166, 167, 171, 189, 190, 191, 195, 202, 204**
- enters carotid canal, **190**
Internal jugular chain (IJC), **200**
- node, **203**
Internal jugular lymph nodes
- low, **201**
- middle, **201**
Internal jugular nodal group, **201**
Internal jugular vein, **112, 166, 167, 171, 189, 190, 191, 202**
Internal maxillary artery, **71, 77, 206**
Internal occipital crest, **111, 113**
Internal occipital protuberance, **114**
Internal resorption, **242–247**
- root changes vs., **850–851, 852**
Interproximal contact, **11**
Intersphenoidal suture, **106**
Intersphenoidal synchondrosis, **106**
Intervertebral disc, C2-3, **157, 158, 159**
Intraalveolar squamous cell carcinoma, ill-defined radiolucencies vs., **882, 884**
Intraarticular adhesions (IA). *See* Adhesions.
Intranasal neoplasm, deviated nasal septum vs., **651**
Intraoral plain film, dentoalveolar fractures, **255**
Intraosseous carcinoma, primary, multiple myeloma vs., **521**
Intraosseous squamous cell carcinoma, primary, **508–509**
- diagnostic checklist, **509**
- differential diagnosis, **509**
- prognosis, **509**
Intraparotid facial nerve, **185**
Intraparotid lymph nodes, **184, 185**
Intraparotid metastatic nodal disease, parotid adenoid cystic carcinoma vs., **773**
Intraparotid neurilemmoma. *See* Parotid schwannoma.
Intravenous antibiotics, oral cavity soft tissue infections, **294**
Intrinsic muscles, **37**
Intrinsic tongue muscles, **36, 39, 45, 46, 53, 170**
Intrusive luxation. *See* Luxation.
Invasive cervical resorption, **243**
Invasive pseudotumor, **694–695**
- diagnostic checklist, **695**
- differential diagnosis, **695**
- prognosis, **695**
Invasive squamous cell carcinoma, masticator space sarcoma vs., **739**
Inverted papilloma
- sinonasal
  - nasal lesion with bony destruction vs., **970, 972**
  - nasal lesion without bony destruction vs., **966, 968**
  - paranasal sinus lesions without bony destruction vs., **976, 979**
- sinonasal squamous cell carcinoma vs., **705**
Isolated anterior C1 arch defect, split atlas vs., **797**
Isolated missing teeth, missing teeth vs., **846, 847**
Isolated occurrence, hypodontia and, **213**
Isolated posterior C1 arch defect, split atlas vs., **797**
Isolated teeth, extra teeth vs., **844, 845**

J

Jacob disease. *See* Coronoid hyperplasia.
Jefferson C1 fracture, split atlas vs., **797**
Joint capsule, **82, 85**
Joint effusion, TMJ synovial cyst vs., **597**
Jugular bulb, **112, 113**
- roof, **113**
Jugular foramen, **110, 111, 114, 116, 117, 119, 134, 145, 158, 170, 186, 190, 207**
- CNIX-XI, **116, 164**
Jugular spine, **111, 113**
Jugular tubercle, **111, 114, 116, 117**
- occipital bone, **114**

INDEX

Jugular vein, internal, anatomy, **189**
Jugulodigastric node, **46, 167, 200, 201, 202**
- level II, **202**

Jugulodigastric reactive node, **51**
Junction base of odontoid with body C2, **157**
Juvenile angiofibroma
- nasal lesion with bony destruction vs., **970, 973**
- nasal lesion without bony destruction vs., **966, 968**
- paranasal sinus lesions without bony destruction vs., **977, 979**
- sinonasal malignant melanoma vs., **713**

Juvenile arthritis, condylar hypoplasia vs., **557**
Juvenile chronic arthritis. *See also* Juvenile idiopathic arthritis, temporomandibular joint.
- failure of segmentation vs., **811**

Juvenile degenerative joint disease. *See* Progressive condylar resorption.
Juvenile idiopathic arthritis
- C1 assimilation vs., **791**
- C2-C3 fusion vs., **789**
- progressive condylar resorption vs., **599**
- small condyle vs., **941, 945**
- temporomandibular joint, **584–589**
  - differential diagnosis, **585**
  - genetics, **585**
  - staging, grading, & classification, **585–586**
- TMJ rheumatoid arthritis vs., **579**

Juvenile ossifying fibroma, sinonasal fibrous dysplasia vs., **715**
Juvenile psammomatoid ossifying fibroma. *See* Sinonasal ossifying fibroma.
Juvenile rheumatoid arthritis (JRA). *See* Juvenile idiopathic arthritis, temporomandibular joint.
Juvenile trabecular ossifying fibroma. *See* Sinonasal ossifying fibroma.
Juvenile-aggressive ossifying fibroma. *See* Sinonasal ossifying fibroma.

K

KBG syndrome, macrodontia, gemination, and fusion vs., **217**
Keratocyst, odontogenic, **400–403**
- adenomatoid odontogenic tumor vs., **455**
- ameloblastic fibroma vs., **461**
- ameloblastoma vs, **458**
- associated abnormalities, **402**
- buccal bifurcation cyst vs., **409**
- diagnostic checklist, **402**
- differential diagnosis, **401**
- genetics, **402**
- lateral periodontal cyst vs., **405**
- mandible-maxilla simple (traumatic) bone cyst vs., **425**
- nasopalatine duct cyst vs., **419**
- periapical rarefying osteitis vs., **266**
- prognosis, **402**
- residual cyst vs., **407**
- staging, grading, & classification, **402**

Keratocystic odontogenic tumor. *See also* Odontogenic keratocyst.
- multilocular radiolucencies vs., **878, 879**
- well-defined unilocular radiolucencies vs., **871, 873**

Klestadt cyst. *See* Nasolabial cyst.
Koerner septum, **92**

L

Labyrinthine segment, **138**
- of CNVII, **92, 140, 143, 146**

Lacerum (C3) segment, **204**
- ICA, **206**

Lacrimal nerve, **105, 128**
Lacrimal puncta, atresia/absence of, submandibular gland aplasia-hypoplasia associated, **289**
Lacrimo-auriculo-dento-digital (LADD) syndrome, submandibular gland aplasia-hypoplasia associated, **289**
Lacrimomaxillary suture, **24**
Lamina, **153, 157**
- C2, **157**

Lamina dura, **11**
- changes, **866–869**
  - differential diagnosis, **866–867**

Lamina papyracea, **65, 66, 69, 70, 101, 102**
Langerhans cell disease. *See* Langerhans histiocytosis.
Langerhans cell granuloma. *See* Langerhans histiocytosis.
Langerhans cell granulomatosis. *See* Langerhans histiocytosis.
Langerhans histiocytosis, **534–537**
- basal cell nevus syndrome vs., **363**
- buccal bifurcation cyst vs., **409**
- Burkitt lymphoma vs., **513**
- diagnostic checklist, **536**
- differential diagnosis, **535**
- floating teeth vs., **862, 863**
- ill-defined radiolucencies vs., **883, 887**
- mandible-maxilla simple (traumatic) bone cyst vs., **425**
- multiple myeloma vs., **521**
- orbital, dermoid and epidermoid vs., **285**
- periodontal disease vs., **272**
- prognosis, **536**
- skull base
  - nasal lesion with bony destruction vs., **971**
  - paranasal sinus lesions with bony destruction vs., **981, 983**
- staging, grading, & classification, **535–536**
- TMJ radiolucencies vs., **954**
- TMJ simple (traumatic) bone cyst vs., **643**

Large condyle, **946–949**
- differential diagnosis, **946–947**

Large nasopalatine foramen, nasopalatine duct cyst vs., **419**
Large pulp chamber in young permanent teeth, internal and external resorption vs., **243**
Late sclerotic phase, Paget disease, **447**
Late stage, periapical osseous dysplasia, **429**

Latent bone cyst. *See* Mandibular salivary gland defect (Stafne).
Lateral atlantoaxial joint, **151**
Lateral canal, **10**
Lateral capsule, **86, 89**
Lateral collateral ligament, **86, 89**
Lateral cortical margins C1 & C2, normal alignment of, **158**
Lateral dural margin of Meckel cave, **132**
Lateral facial cleft, **357**
Lateral facial dysplasia. *See* Hemifacial microsomia.
Lateral lamella, **102**
Lateral luxation. *See* Luxation.
Lateral malleal ligament, **94**
Lateral mass, **153**
- C1, **117, 156, 158**
  vertebral body, **116**
Lateral periapical cyst, lateral periodontal cyst vs., **405**
Lateral periodontal cyst, **404–405**
- buccal bifurcation cyst vs., **409**
- central odontogenic fibroma vs., **473**
- diagnostic checklist, **405**
- differential diagnosis, **405**
- mandible-maxilla simple (traumatic) bone cyst vs., **425**
- prognosis, **405**
- well-defined unilocular radiolucencies vs., **871, 873**
Lateral pharyngeal recess, **173, 177**
Lateral pole, **87**
Lateral process of malleus, **94**
Lateral pterygoid muscle, **86, 129, 133, 166, 171, 181, 182, 183**
- inferior head, **130**
- and nerve, **131**
- superior head, **130**
Lateral pterygoid plate, **27, 29, 64, 71, 78, 79, 109, 171, 177, 182, 183**
Lateral radicular cyst
- buccal bifurcation cyst vs., **409**
- lateral periodontal cyst vs., **405**
Lateral retropharyngeal space, **189**
Lateral semicircular canal, **92, 93, 140, 141, 145, 146, 186**
Lateral temporomandibular ligament, **85**
Le Fort fracture. *See* Transfacial fracture (Le Fort).
Left mandibular condyle, **87**
Left maxillary sinus, **58**
Leiomyosarcoma. *See* Sarcoma.
Lenticular process of incus, **92**
Lesser horn of hyoid bone, **119**
Lesser palatine foramen, **26, 78**
Lesser palatine nerve, **27, 105, 128**
Lesser petrosal nerve, **129**
Lesser wing, sphenoid bone, **99, 105**
Leukemia, **528–529**
- diagnostic checklist, **529**
- differential diagnosis, **529**
- generalized rarefaction vs., **888**
- genetics, **529**
- ground-glass and granular radiopacities vs., **897**
- ill-defined radiolucencies vs., **883, 887**
- lamina dura changes vs., **867, 869**
- Langerhans histiocytosis vs., **535**
- periapical radiolucencies vs., **857, 859**
- periodontal disease vs., **272**
- periosteal reactions vs., **907, 911**
- staging, grading, & classification, **529**
- widened periodontal ligament space vs., **864, 865**
Levator anguli oris, **26, 139**
Levator labii superioris, **26, 139, 142**
Levator labii superioris alaeque nasi, **142**
Levator scapulae muscle, **199**
Levator veli palatini, **171, 173, 178**
Level IA node, **53**
Liesegang rings, **467**
Ligamentum nuchae, **151, 197**
Limited condylar translation, **950–953**
- differential diagnosis, **950–951**
Lingual alveolar bone thickness, **20**
Lingual artery, **45, 46, 204, 205**
- and vein, sublingual space, anatomy, **44**
Lingual bone loss, **271**
Lingual canal, **34**
Lingual foramen, **32, 34, 137**
Lingual nerve, **31, 32, 53, 105, 128, 129, 131, 141, 182**
- sublingual space, anatomy, **44**
Lingual periodontal ligament space, widening of, **19**
Lingual plate, **10**
Lingual salivary gland depression. *See* Mandibular salivary gland defect (Stafne).
Lingual septum, **37, 39, 46**
Lingual thyroid, **282–283**
- associated abnormalities, **283**
- diagnostic checklist, **283**
- differential diagnosis, **283**
- prognosis, **283**
Lingual tonsil, **37, 39, 46, 52, 170, 174, 175, 176, 178, 195, 203**
Lingual tonsil squamous cell carcinoma
- motor denervation CNXII vs., **337**
- non-Hodgkin lymphoma of pharyngeal mucosal space vs., **517**
Lingula, **32, 135**
Lip, cleft, **357**
Lipoma, parotid space lesions vs., **919, 921**
Liposarcoma. *See* Sarcoma.
Localized pitted pattern, amelogenesis imperfecta and, **227–228**
Long bones deformities, dentinogenesis imperfecta vs., **231**
Long ciliary nerve, **128**
Long process incus, **92**
Longitudinal fracture. *See* Dentoalveolar fractures.
Longitudinal ligament
- anterior, **159**
- posterior, **159**
Longstanding esthetic implants, reaction to, periosteal reactions vs., **906–907, 909**
Longus colli/capitis muscle, **42**
Loose bodies, disc replacement with reduction vs., **605**
Low palatine tonsil, **46**
Lower alveolar ridge mucosal surface, **52**
LPC. *See* Lateral periodontal cyst.

Luxation, **250–253**. *See also* Temporomandibular joint, dislocation.
- diagnostic checklist, **251**
- differential diagnosis, **251**
- extrusive, concussion vs., **249**
- prognosis, **251**

Lymph nodes
- anatomy, **200–203**
  - axial CECT, **202**
  - axial T1 & T2 MR, **203**
  - graphics, **201**
  - internal contents, **200**
- dystrophic calcification of, submandibular sialoliths vs., **339**
- reactive, submandibular space nodal non-Hodgkin lymphoma vs., **319**
- sarcoidosis, submandibular space nodal non-Hodgkin lymphoma vs., **319**
- tuberculosis, submandibular space nodal non-Hodgkin lymphoma vs., **319**

Lymphangioma
- foregut duplication cyst in tongue vs., **291**
- submandibular gland mucocele vs., **305**

Lymphatic malformation
- neurofibromatosis type 1 vs., **487**
- oral cavity
  - motor denervation CNXII vs., **337**
  - ranula vs., **297**
  - root of tongue lesions vs., **931, 933**
  - sublingual gland benign mixed tumor vs., **307**
  - sublingual gland carcinoma vs., **315**
  - submandibular space lesions vs., **915**
- orbital, dermoid and epidermoid vs., **285–286**
- parotid space lesions vs., **919**
- sublingual space
  - oral cavity sialocele vs., **303**
  - sublingual space lesions vs., **923, 925**
- submandibular space, submandibular space accessory salivary tissue vs., **281**

Lymphatic tissue, nasopharynx and oropharynx, **172**

Lymphoepithelial cysts, HIV, benign, parotid sialadenitis vs., **755**

Lymphoepithelial lesions, benign
- HIV, **750–753**
  - associated abnormalities, **752**
  - diagnostic checklist, **752**
  - differential diagnosis, **751**
  - metastatic disease of parotid nodes vs., **779**
  - parotid non-Hodgkin lymphoma vs., **775**
  - prognosis, **752**
  - Warthin tumor vs., **761**
- Sjögren syndrome vs., **783**

Lymphoma
- cervical facet arthropathy vs., **827**
- floating teeth vs., **862, 863**
- Langerhans histiocytosis vs., **535**
- leukemia vs., **529**

Lymphomatous adenoma. *See* Warthin tumor.

Lytic metastases, **834–837**
- diagnostic checklist, **836**
- differential diagnosis, **835–836**
- prognosis, **836**
- staging, grading, & classification, **836**

M

Mach band effect, dental caries vs., **261**

Macrodontia
- crown changes vs., **848, 849**
- gemination, and fusion, **216–217**
  - diagnostic checklist, **217**
  - differential diagnosis, **217**

Main motor nucleus CNV, **126**

Main sensory nucleus
- area of, **132**
- CNV, **126**

Malar node, **201**

Malignancies
- enter stylomastoid foramen, **186**
- floating teeth vs., **862**
- lamina dura changes vs., **867**
- periapical rarefying osteitis vs., **266**
- primary, periodontal disease vs., **272**
- widened periodontal ligament space vs., **864**

Malignancy recurrence, mandible-maxilla osteoradionecrosis vs., **389**

Malignant degeneration of benign mixed tumor, **315**

Malignant mixed tumor
- parotid, **766–767**
  - diagnostic checklist, **767**
  - differential diagnosis, **767**
  - prognosis, **767**
- parotid space lesions vs., **919**

Malignant neoplasm, sinus, mucus retention pseudocyst vs., **663**

Malignant parotid tumor, Warthin tumor vs., **761**

Malignant peripheral nerve sheath tumor (MPNST), **487, 488**

Malignant tumor
- parotid sialadenitis vs., **755**
- V2 perineural spread of, **23**

Malleoincudal articulation, **91, 92**

Malleus, **88, 90, 146**
- anterior process, **91**
- head, **91, 92, 94**
- lateral process, **91**
- manubrium of, **91, 92, 94**
- neck, **91, 92, 94**
- umbo, **91, 93**

Malocclusion, luxation vs., **251**

Mandible, **30–35, 119, 179**
- 3D reformation, panoramic, panoramic reformat, **33**
- angle of, **130**
- CBCT, periapical radiograph, **34, 35**
- graphics, **31, 32**
- inferior border of, **31, 34**
- internal contents, **30**

INDEX

Mandible and maxilla
- accessory mandibular canal, **348–349**
- adenomatoid odontogenic tumor, **454–455**
- ameloblastic fibroma, **460–463**
- ameloblastic fibroodontoma, **464–465**
- ameloblastoma, **456–459**
- aneurysmal bone cyst, **414–417**
- basal cell nevus syndrome, **362–363**
- buccal and palatal exostoses, **342–343**
- buccal bifurcation cyst, **408–411**
- Burkitt lymphoma, **512–515**
  - associated abnormalities, **514**
  - diagnostic checklist, **514**
  - differential diagnosis, **513**
  - prognosis, **514**
  - staging, grading, & classification, **514**
  - variants, **513**
- calcifying epithelial odontogenic tumor, **466–467**
- calcifying odontogenic cyst, **412–413**
- cementoblastoma, **468–469**
- central giant cell granuloma, **530–533**
  - associated abnormalities, **531**
  - differential diagnosis, **531**
  - prognosis, **531**
- central hemangioma, **474–475**
- central mucoepidermoid carcinoma, **510–511**
- central odontogenic fibroma, **472–473**
- cherubism, **358–361**
- chondrosarcoma, **504–507**
- clefts, **356–357**
- cleidocranial dysplasia, **364–365**
- complex midfacial fracture, **376–377**
- dentigerous cyst, **396–399**
- desmoplastic fibroma, **490–491**
- Ewing sarcoma, **524–527**
  - diagnostic checklist, **526**
  - differential diagnosis, **525**
  - genetics, **525**
  - prognosis, **526**
- fibrous dysplasia, **440–445**
- florid osseous dysplasia, **432–435**
- idiopathic osteosclerosis, **354–355**
- intraosseous carcinoma, primary, multiple myeloma vs., **521**
- lateral periodontal cyst, **404–405**
- malignant ameloblastoma and ameloblastic carcinoma, **492–493**
- mandible fracture, **370–373**
- mandibular salivary gland defect (Stafne), **350–353**
- mandibular torus, **344–345**
- multiple myeloma, **520–523**
  - diagnostic checklist, **522**
  - differential diagnosis, **521**
  - genetics, **521**
  - prognosis, **522**
  - staging, grading, & classification, **521**
- nasoethmoid complex fracture, **374–375**
- nasolabial cyst, **422–423**
- nasopalatine duct cyst, **418–421**
- nerve sheath tumor, **482–485**
- neurofibromatosis type 1, **486–489**
- non-Hodgkin lymphoma of pharyngeal mucosal space, **516–519**
  - associated abnormalities, **518**
  - diagnostic checklist, **518**
  - differential diagnosis, **517**
  - genetics, **518**
  - prognosis, **518**
  - staging, grading, & classification, **518**
  - subtypes, **517**
- odontogenic keratocyst, **400–403**
- odontogenic myxoma, **470–471**
- odontoma, **450–453**
- ossifying fibroma, **436–439**
- osteoblastoma, **478–479**
- osteoid osteoma, **476–477**
- osteomyelitis, **384–387**
- osteonecrosis, **392–395**
- osteoradionecrosis, **388–391**
- osteosarcoma, **500–503**
- Paget disease, **446–449**
- palatal torus, **346–347**
- periapical osseous dysplasia, **428–431**
- Pierre Robin sequence, **366–367**
- primary intraosseous squamous cell carcinoma, **508–509**
  - diagnostic checklist, **509**
  - differential diagnosis, **509**
  - prognosis, **509**
- residual cyst, **406–407**
- simple (traumatic) bone cyst, **424–427**
- transfacial fracture (Le Fort), **380–383**
- Treacher Collins syndrome, **368–369**
- zygomaticomaxillary complex fracture, **378–379**

Mandible fracture, **370–373**
- associated abnormalities, **371**
- differential diagnosis, **371**

Mandible-maxilla aneurysmal bone cyst, vascular malformation, **415**

Mandible-maxilla chondrosarcoma, **504–507**
- diagnostic checklist, **506**
- differential diagnosis, **505–506**
- prognosis, **506**
- staging, grading, & classification, **506**

Mandible-maxilla idiopathic osteosclerosis, **354–355**
- diagnostic checklist, **355**
- differential diagnosis, **355**
- prognosis, **355**

Mandible-maxilla metastasis, **494–499**
- diagnostic checklist, **495**
- differential diagnosis, **495**
- gingival squamous cell carcinoma vs., **327**
- prognosis, **495**

Mandible-maxilla osteoma, **480–481**
- associated abnormalities, **481**
- diagnostic checklist, **481**
- differential diagnosis, **481**
- prognosis, **481**
- staging, grading, & classification, **481**

Mandible-maxilla osteomyelitis, gingival squamous cell carcinoma vs., **327**

INDEX

Mandible-maxilla osteonecrosis, gingival squamous cell carcinoma vs., **327**
Mandible-maxilla osteoradionecrosis, gingival squamous cell carcinoma vs., **327**
Mandible-maxilla osteosarcoma, **500–503**
- associated abnormalities, **502**
- diagnostic checklist, **502**
- differential diagnosis, **501**
- gingival squamous cell carcinoma vs., **327**
- prognosis, **502**
- staging, grading, & classification, **502**

Mandibular 1st molar, **8**
Mandibular 1st premolar, **8**
Mandibular 2nd molar, **8**
Mandibular 2nd premolar, **8, 135**
Mandibular 3rd molar, **8**
Mandibular alveolar process, **33**
Mandibular alveolar ridge, **43**
Mandibular body, anatomy, **30, 31**
Mandibular branch of CNVII, **141, 142, 186**
Mandibular canal, **135, 136, 137**
- accessory, **348–349**
  - associated abnormalities, **349**
  - diagnostic checklist, **349**
  - differential diagnosis, **349**
  - gubernaculum dentis vs., **277**
  - prognosis, **349**
- containing inferior alveolar nerve, **135**
- duplication/division of. *See* Accessory mandibular canal.

Mandibular canine, **8**
- apices of, **35**
- developing, **7**

Mandibular central incisor, **8**
- apices of, **34**

Mandibular condyle, **82, 84, 86, 88, 89, 115, 119, 120, 121, 130, 133, 144, 183**
Mandibular division (CNV3), **105, 126, 127, 129**
- entering foramen ovale, **128**

Mandibular foramen, **32, 33, 43, 64, 129, 135, 166, 183**
Mandibular fossa, **119**
Mandibular head, **117**
Mandibular infected buccal cyst. *See* Buccal bifurcation cyst.
Mandibular lateral incisor, **8**
Mandibular lingula, mandible fracture vs., **371**
Mandibular metastasis
- masticator space chondrosarcoma vs., **735**
- masticator space sarcoma vs., **739**

Mandibular nerve, **133, 181, 182**
- anatomy, **30**
- CNV3, **31, 105, 124, 133, 173, 180**

Mandibular node, **201**
Mandibular notch, **32, 84**
Mandibular osteomyelitis, **293**
- masticator space sarcoma vs., **739**

Mandibular osteoradionecrosis, masticator space abscess vs., **725**
Mandibular osteosarcoma, masticator space chondrosarcoma vs., **735**
Mandibular ramus, **43, 171, 177**
- anatomy, **30, 31, 183**

Mandibular salivary gland defect (Stafne), **350–353**
- diagnostic checklist, **351**
- differential diagnosis, **351**
- prognosis, **351**
- well-defined unilocular radiolucencies vs., **870, 872**

Mandibular (sigmoid) notch, **31, 33**
Mandibular teeth, **43**
Mandibular torus, **344–345**
- associated abnormalities, **345**
- buccal and palatal exostoses vs., **343**
- diagnostic checklist, **345**
- differential diagnosis, **345**
- genetics, **345**
- mandible-maxilla idiopathic osteosclerosis vs., **355**
- mandible-maxilla osteoma vs., **481**
- oral mucosal space/surface lesions vs., **927, 929**
- prognosis, **345**
- well-defined radiopacities vs., **892, 894**

Mandibulofacial dysostosis. *See also* Treacher Collins syndrome.
- hypoplasia/aplasia associated, **660**
- submandibular gland aplasia-hypoplasia associated, **289**

Manson classification system, nasoethmoid complex fracture, **375**
Marfan syndrome, deviated nasal septum vs., **651**
Masseter, **42, 49, 50, 129, 142, 166, 167, 171, 187, 199**
- anatomy, **181, 183**
- deep head, **130**
- superficial head, **130**

Masseteric hypertrophy, benign. *See* Benign masticator muscle hypertrophy.
Masseteric nerve, **85, 131**
Massive osteolysis, generalized rarefaction vs., **889**
Mast cell granuloma. *See* Invasive pseudotumor.
Masticator muscle atrophy, **728–731**
- associated abnormalities, **729–730**
- diagnostic checklist, **730**
- differential diagnosis, **729**
- masticator space abscess vs., **725**
- prognosis, **730**

Masticator muscle hypertrophy
- benign, **746–747**
  - diagnostic checklist, **747**
  - differential diagnosis, **747**
  - prognosis, **747**
- masticator muscle atrophy vs., **729**
- masticator space abscess vs., **725**

Masticator nerve, **182**
Masticator space, **45, 49, 69, 169, 170, 171, 173, 174, 178, 180–183, 185, 186, 187, 190, 193**
- anatomy, **163, 164, 167**
  - imaging anatomy, **162**
  - relationships, **180**
- chondrosarcoma, masticator muscle atrophy vs., **729**
- internal contents, **180**
- malignancy, **182**
- masticator muscle atrophy, **728–731**
  - associated abnormalities, **729–730**
  - diagnostic checklist, **730**
  - differential diagnosis, **729**
  - prognosis, **730**

INDEX

- masticator muscle hypertrophy, masticator space abscess vs., **725**
- muscles of, **180**
- normal axial CECT of, **183**
- normal masticator space; MS mass, **181**
- perineural tumor, V3, masticator muscle atrophy vs., **729**
- skull base interactions, CNV3, perineural tumor, **182**

Masticator space abscess, **724–727**
- benign masticator muscle hypertrophy vs., **747**
- diagnostic checklist, **726**
- differential diagnosis, **725–726**
- masticator muscle atrophy vs., **729**
- masticator space sarcoma vs., **739**
- prognosis, **725**
- retromolar trigone squamous cell carcinoma vs., **329**

Masticator space chondrosarcoma, **734–737**
- diagnostic checklist, **736**
- differential diagnosis, **735**
- prognosis, **736**
- staging, grading, & classification, **735–736**

Masticator space CNV3 perineural tumor, **742–745**
- diagnostic checklist, **744**
- differential diagnosis, **743–744**
- prognosis, **744**

Masticator space CNV3 schwannoma, **732–733**
- differential diagnosis, **733**
- genetics, **733**
- prognosis, **733**

Masticator space infection, masticator space chondrosarcoma vs., **735**

Masticator space pseudolesion, benign masticator muscle hypertrophy vs., **747**

Masticator space sarcoma, **738–741**
- benign masticator muscle hypertrophy vs., **747**
- diagnostic checklist, **740**
- differential diagnosis, **739**
- genetics, **739**
- masticator space CNV3 schwannoma vs., **733**
- prognosis, **740**
- staging, grading, & classification, **740**

Masticator space squamous cell carcinoma, benign masticator muscle hypertrophy vs., **747**

Masticator space venous malformation, masticator space sarcoma vs., **739**

Mastoid air cells, **88, 113, 116**

Mastoid antrum, **92, 143, 145**

Mastoid node, **201**

Mastoid process, **84, 87, 89, 116, 119, 120**

Mastoid segment, **138**
- of CNVII, **92, 116, 142, 144, 145**

Mastoid sinuses, **147**

Mastoid tip, **115, 144, 145, 166, 185, 186, 187**

Maxilla (Mx), **22–29**
- alveolar process of, **26, 63**
- anatomy relationships, **22**
- axial and coronal CBCT, **28**
- graphics, **24–26**
  - and bone CT, **27**
- horizontal (palatine) process of, **25**
- innervation, **22–23**
- internal contents, **22–23**
- maxillary bone, **22**
- minor salivary glands, **23**
- palatine processes of, **26**
- periapical and panoramic, **29**
- zygomatic process of, **26, 29**

Maxillary 1st molar, **8**

Maxillary 1st premolar, **8**

Maxillary 2nd molar, **8**

Maxillary 2nd premolar, **8**

Maxillary 3rd molar, **8, 23**

Maxillary alveolar process, **33, 42, 43**

Maxillary alveolar ridge, **42**

Maxillary artery, **85, 204, 205**
- internal, **205**

Maxillary bone, **25**

Maxillary canine, **8**
- developing, **7**

Maxillary central incisor, **8**

Maxillary division (CNV2), **105, 126, 127**
- entering foramen rotundum, **128**

Maxillary hard palate, posterior margin of, **25**

Maxillary hiatus, **25**

Maxillary hypoplasia (micrognathia), **23**

Maxillary infundibulum, **65, 67, 72, 73, 74**

Maxillary lateral incisor, **8**

Maxillary midline cyst. *See* Nasopalatine duct cyst.

Maxillary midline suture, **23**

Maxillary nerve
- CNV1, **141**
- CNV2, **70, 77, 105, 128, 129**
  - as division of cranial nerve 5, **124**

Maxillary ostium, **73**

Maxillary ridge, **166**

Maxillary sinus, **27, 61, 62, 63, 65, 66, 67, 69, 70, 71, 73, 74, 77, 78, 134, 136, 137, 177**
- drainage, **57**
- floor, **60**
- infundibulum, **62**
- ostium, **58, 63**
- outline of, **24**
- proximity of apices of, **23**
- sinonasal overview, **56**

Maxillary sinus and nasal cavity
- accessory ostia, **656–657**
  - associated abnormalities, **657**
  - diagnostic checklist, **657**
  - differential diagnosis, **657**
  - prognosis, **657**
  - staging, grading, and classification, **657**
- adenoid cystic carcinoma, sinonasal, **706–707**
  - differential diagnosis, **707**
  - prognosis, **707**
  - staging, grading, & classification, **707**
- allergic fungal sinusitis, **686–687**
  - diagnostic checklist, **687**
  - differential diagnosis, **687**
  - prognosis, **687**
- chronic rhinosinusitis, **680–683**
  - associated abnormalities, **682**
  - diagnostic checklist, **682**

differential diagnosis, **681**
genetics, **682**
prognosis, **682**
staging, grading, & classification, **682**
- concha bullosa, **652–655**
diagnostic checklist, **653**
prognosis, **653**
- deviated nasal septum, **650–651**
associated abnormalities, **651**
diagnostic checklist, **651**
differential diagnosis, **651**
staging, grading, & classification, **651**
- hypoplasia/aplasia, **658–661**
associated abnormalities, **660**
diagnostic checklist, **660**
differential diagnosis, **659**
genetics, **659–660**
staging, grading, & classification, **660**
- invasive fungal sinusitis, **688–691**
diagnostic checklist, **690**
differential diagnosis, **689**
prognosis, **690**
staging, grading, & classification, **690**
- invasive pseudotumor, **694–695**
diagnostic checklist, **695**
differential diagnosis, **695**
prognosis, **695**
- mucus retention pseudocyst, **662–663**
diagnostic checklist, **663**
differential diagnosis, **663**
prognosis, **663**
- mycetoma, **692–693**
differential diagnosis, **693**
prognosis, **693**
- nasopharyngeal carcinoma, **708–711**
diagnostic checklist, **710**
differential diagnosis, **709**
prognosis, **710**
staging, grading, & classification, **709–710**
- odontogenic sinusitis, **684–685**
diagnostic checklist, **685**
differential diagnosis, **685**
prognosis, **685**
staging, grading, & classification, **685**
- rhinosinusitis, acute, **676–679**
associated abnormalities, **677–678**
diagnostic checklist, **678**
differential diagnosis, **677**
genetics, **677**
prognosis, **678**
staging, grading, & classification, **678**
- sinonasal fibrous dysplasia, **714–717**
associated abnormalities, **716**
diagnostic checklist, **716**
differential diagnosis, **715–716**
prognosis, **716**
staging, grading, & classification, **716**
- sinonasal granulomatosis with polyangiitis (Wegener granulomatosis), **668–671**
associated abnormalities, **669–670**
diagnostic checklist, **670**
differential diagnosis, **669**
prognosis, **670**
sinonasal polyposis vs., **673**
- sinonasal inverted papilloma, **696–699**
associated abnormalities, **698**
diagnostic checklist, **698**
differential diagnosis, **697–698**
prognosis, **698**
staging, grading, & classification, **698**
- sinonasal malignant melanoma, **712–713**
diagnostic checklist, **713**
differential diagnosis, **713**
genetics, **713**
prognosis, **713**
staging, grading, & classification, **713**
- sinonasal mucocele, **664–667**
associated abnormalities, **666**
diagnostic checklist, **666**
differential diagnosis, **665**
prognosis, **666**
staging, grading, & classification, **666**
- sinonasal ossifying fibroma, **718–721**
associated abnormalities, **720**
diagnostic checklist, **720**
differential diagnosis, **719**
prognosis, **720**
staging, grading, & classification, **720**
- sinonasal osteoma, **700–703**
associated abnormalities, **701**
associated syndromes, **701**
diagnostic checklist, **701**
differential diagnosis, **701**
genetics, **701**
staging, grading, & classification, **701**
- sinonasal polyposis, **672–675**
associated abnormalities, **674**
diagnostic checklist, **674**
differential diagnosis, **673**
genetics, **674**
prognosis, **674**
- squamous cell carcinoma, sinonasal, **704–705**
diagnostic checklist, **705**
differential diagnosis, **705**
prognosis, **705**
Maxillary sinusitis, accessory ostia associated, **657**
Maxillary teeth, proximity of apices of, **23**
Maxillary tuberosity, **24, 26, 27, 29**
Maxillary wall, destruction by malignant lesion, accessory ostia vs., **657**
Maxillofacial dysostosis, X-linked, Treacher Collins syndrome vs., **369**
Maxillomandibular dysplasia, hypoplasia/aplasia associated, **660**
Maxillovomerine suture, **24**
Mazabraud syndrome, fibrous dysplasia, **442**
McCune-Albright syndrome
- café au lait spots, sinonasal fibrous dysplasia associated, **716**
- cherubism vs., **359**
- endocrinopathies, sinonasal fibrous dysplasia associated, **716**

- fibrous dysplasia, **442**
McGregor line, **150, 154, 155**
McRae foramen magnum line, **154**
McRae line, **150**
Md. *See* Mandible.
ME. *See* Middle ear.
Meati, **56**
MECa. *See* Mucoepidermoid carcinoma.
Meckel cave, **129, 132, 182**
- dural margin to, **133**
- with trigeminal fascicles, **132, 133**
- with trigeminal ganglion, **126**
- trigeminal nerve fascicles in, **132**
- trigeminal nerve rootlets within, **127**
Medial capsule, **86, 89**
Medial collateral ligament, **86, 89**
Medial orbital blowout fracture, nasoethmoid complex fracture vs., **375**
Medial pole, **87**
Medial pterygoid muscle, **42, 43, 49, 86, 129, 166, 167, 171, 182, 183, 187, 199**
- anatomy, **181**
- deep head, **130**
- superficial head, **130**
Medial pterygoid nerve, **129**
Medial pterygoid plate, **27, 64, 71, 78, 79, 109, 137, 171, 182, 183**
Medial pterygoid plate hamulus, **183**
Medial rectus, **70**
Medial wall of maxillary sinus, **60**
Median cleft of upper lip, **357**
Median maxillary anterior alveolar cleft, **357**
Median palatal cyst, nasopalatine duct cyst vs., **420**
Median raphe, **195**
Median sulcus, **37**
Medication-related osteonecrosis, mandible-maxilla osteomyelitis vs., **386**
Medication-related osteonecrosis of jaws (MRONJ). *See* Osteonecrosis, mandible-maxilla.
Medulloblastomas, basal cell nevus syndrome associated, **363**
Megadontia. *See* Macrodontia.
Megalodontia. *See* Macrodontia.
Melanoma, sinonasal
- malignant, **712–713**
  - diagnostic checklist, **713**
  - differential diagnosis, **713**
  - genetics, **713**
  - prognosis, **713**
  - staging, grading, & classification, **713**
- nasal lesion with bony destruction vs., **970–971, 973**
- nasal lesion without bony destruction vs., **967, 969**
- perforated nasal septum vs., **964**
Melanotic neuroectodermal tumor of infancy, pericoronal radiolucencies without radiopacities vs., **874**
Melkersson-Rosenthal syndrome, submandibular gland aplasia-hypoplasia associated, **289**
Melnick-Needles syndrome, hypoplasia/aplasia associated, **660**
Meningeal artery, middle, **205**
Meningeal nerve, **129**
Meningioma
- ossification of posterior longitudinal ligament vs., **819**
- skull base, masticator space CNV3 perineural tumor vs., **744**
Meningohypophyseal arteries, **205**
Meningohypophyseal trunk (MHT), **206**
Mental foramen, **11, 31, 33, 35, 84, 131, 135, 136, 137, 142**
- mandible fracture vs., **371**
- periapical radiolucencies vs., **856, 858**
- periapical rarefying osteitis vs., **266**
Mental foramina, **35**
Mental nerve, **131**
- anatomy, **30, 31**
Mental protuberance, **31, 33**
Mental tubercle, **31, 33, 34**
Mentalis, **142**
Mercury fulminate exposure, perforated nasal septum vs., **964**
Mesencephalic nucleus CNV, **126**
Mesial root, inferior alveolar nerve running through, **12**
Mesioangularly impacted 3rd molar, **12**
Mesiobuccal root of 1st molar, branch to, **29**
Mesiodens, **214**
Mesio-occluso-distal amalgam build-up, **15**
Mesotympanum, **90, 91, 94**
- middle ear, **88**
Metabolic disorders, leukemia vs., **529**
Metastases
- lytic and blastic, **834–837**
  - diagnostic checklist, **836**
  - differential diagnosis, **835–836**
  - prognosis, **836**
  - staging, grading, & classification, **836**
- nodal, from systemic primary, submandibular space nodal non-Hodgkin lymphoma vs., **319**
- osteolytic, Paget disease vs., **448**
- osteosclerotic, Paget disease vs., **448**
- periosteal reactions vs., **907, 910, 911**
Metastasis
- cervical facet arthropathy vs., **827**
- floating teeth vs., **862**
- ill-defined radiolucencies vs., **883, 886**
- lamina dura changes vs., **867, 869**
- Langerhans histiocytosis vs., **535**
- mandible-maxilla, **494–499**
  - diagnostic checklist, **495**
  - differential diagnosis, **495**
  - gingival squamous cell carcinoma vs., **327**
  - nasal lesion with bony destruction vs., **971**
  - prognosis, **495**
- mandible-maxilla osteomyelitis vs., **386**
- mandible-maxilla osteonecrosis vs., **393**
- mandible-maxilla osteosarcoma vs., **501**
- mandibular
  - masticator space chondrosarcoma vs., **735**
  - masticator space sarcoma vs., **739**
- multiple myeloma vs., **521**
- paranasal sinus lesions with bony destruction vs., **981, 983**

INDEX

- periapical radiolucencies vs., **857, 859**
- periodontal disease vs., **272**
- temporomandibular joint, **640–641**
  diagnostic checklist, **641**
  differential diagnosis, **641**
  prognosis, **641**
- vertebral, hemangioma, cervical spine vs., **831**
- widened periodontal ligament space vs., **864, 865**

Metastatic disease
- Burkitt lymphoma vs., **513**
- of parotid nodes, **778–781**
  benign lymphoepithelial lesions: HIV vs., **751**
  diagnostic checklist, **780**
  differential diagnosis, **779**
  parotid benign mixed tumor vs., **758**
  parotid non-Hodgkin lymphoma vs., **775**
  prognosis, **780**
- periapical rarefying osteitis vs., **266**
- small condyle vs., **941, 945**
- to TMJ, TMJ osteosarcoma vs., **635**
- TMJ chondrosarcoma vs., **637**
- TMJ radiolucencies vs., **954**
- TMJ radiopacities vs., **957, 959**

Metastatic lesion, primary intraosseous squamous cell carcinoma vs., **509**

Metastatic nodal disease
- intraparotid, parotid adenoid cystic carcinoma vs., **773**
- parotid
  parotid mucoepidermoid carcinoma vs., **769**
  parotid schwannoma vs., **765**
  Warthin tumor vs., **761**
- parotid space lesions vs., **918, 920**

Metastatic tumor, mandible-maxilla chondrosarcoma vs., **506**

Microdontia, **218**
- crown changes vs., **848, 849**

Micrognathia, condylar hypoplasia, **557**

Microsomia, bilateral facial, Treacher Collins syndrome vs., **369**

Microstomia, hemifacial, submandibular gland aplasia-hypoplasia associated, **289**

Mid internal auditory canal facial nerve, **147**

Middle cerebellar peduncle, **133**

Middle cranial fossa, **69, 78, 89**

Middle ear, **90–95**
- axial bone CT, **92–93**
- coronal bone CT, **94–95**
- embryology, **90**
- graphics, **91**

Middle meatus, **25, 58, 63, 65, 71, 72, 73, 74, 75**

Middle meningeal artery, **85, 205, 206**

Middle superior alveolar canal, **29**

Middle superior alveolar foramen, **24**

Middle turbinate, **63, 64, 65, 66, 68, 71, 73, 74, 75**
- attachment, **57**
- cut margin, **73**

Midfacial fracture, complex, **376–377**
- associated abnormalities, **377**
- differential diagnosis, **377**
- prognosis, **377**
- staging, grading, & classification, **377**

Midpalatal suture, **26**

Minor salivary gland
- maxilla, anatomy, **23**
- pathology, **23**

Minor salivary gland carcinoma, hard palate, hard palate squamous cell carcinoma vs., **335**

Minor salivary gland malignancy
- ill-defined radiolucencies vs., **883, 886**
- nasopharyngeal, nasopharyngeal carcinoma vs., **709**
- oral
  oral mucosal space/surface lesions vs., **927, 929**
  retromolar trigone squamous cell carcinoma vs., **329**
- oral cavity, **312–313**
  buccal mucosa squamous cell carcinoma vs., **333**
  diagnostic checklist, **313**
  differential diagnosis, **313**
  prognosis, **313**
  staging, grading, & classification, **313**

Minor salivary glands, **52**
- nasopharynx and oropharynx, anatomy, **172**

Missing teeth, **846–847**
- differential diagnosis, **846**

Mixed dentition, **4**

Mixed odontogenic tumor. *See* Ameloblastic fibroma.

MMT. *See* Malignant mixed tumor.

Modiolus, **142**

Molar (M), **4**

Monoclonal gammopathy, **521**

Morquio syndrome, amelogenesis imperfecta vs., **227**

Motor denervation CNXII, **336–337**
- diagnostic checklist, **337**
- differential diagnosis, **337**

Motor nucleus
- CNV, **126**
  area of, **132**
- CNVII, **140**
- of facial nerve, **138**

Motor root, **129**

MS. *See* Masticator space.

MSGM. *See* Minor salivary gland malignancy, oral cavity.

Mucin rhinosinusitis, eosinophilic, allergic fungal sinusitis vs., **687**

Mucocele
- mucus retention pseudocyst vs., **663**
- nasolacrimal duct, nasolabial cyst vs., **423**
- sinonasal
  allergic fungal sinusitis vs., **687**
  paranasal sinus lesions without bony destruction vs., **976, 978**
- sublingual gland. *See* Ranula.
- submandibular gland, **304–305**
  associated abnormalities, **305**
  diagnostic checklist, **305**
  differential diagnosis, **305**
  prognosis, **305**
  ranula vs., **297**
  submandibular gland benign mixed tumor vs., **309**
  submandibular gland carcinoma vs., **317**
  submandibular space accessory salivary tissue vs., **281**

Mucoepidermoid carcinoma, **313, 315**
- central, **510–511**
  - diagnostic checklist, **511**
  - differential diagnosis, **511**
  - primary intraosseous squamous cell carcinoma vs., **509**
  - prognosis, **511**
- parotid, **768–771**
  - diagnostic checklist, **770**
  - differential diagnosis, **769**
  - parotid malignant mixed tumor vs., **767**
  - parotid schwannoma vs., **765**
  - prognosis, **770**
  - staging, grading, & classification, **770**
  - Warthin tumor vs., **761**
- parotid benign mixed tumor vs., **758**
- parotid space, parotid adenoid cystic carcinoma vs., **773**
- parotid space lesions vs., **918–919, 920**

Mucoepidermoid tumor, central, malignant ameloblastoma and ameloblastic carcinoma vs., **493**

Mucosa, **178**

Mucosa-associated lymphoid tissue lymphoma. *See* Non-Hodgkin lymphoma.

Mucosal lip, **52**

Mucosal thickening, **60**

Mucositis, localized, mucus retention pseudocyst vs., **663**

Mucus plug. *See* Parotid sialoliths; Submandibular sialoliths.

Mucus retention cyst. *See* Mucus retention pseudocyst.

Mucus retention cyst, sublingual gland. *See* Ranula.

Mucus retention phenomenon. *See* Mucus retention pseudocyst.

Mucus retention pseudocyst, **17, 71, 662–663**
- diagnostic checklist, **663**
- differential diagnosis, **663**
- multiple, odontogenic sinusitis vs., **685**
- paranasal sinus lesions without bony destruction vs., **976, 977**
- prognosis, **663**
- sinonasal polyposis vs., **673**

Multidisciplinary approach, clefts, **357**

Multifocal osteomyelitis, chronic recurrent, generalized radiopacities vs., **902**

Multilocular radiolucencies, **878–881**
- differential diagnosis, **878–879**

Multiple basal cell carcinomas, basal cell nevus syndrome associated, **363**

Multiple dentigerous cysts, basal cell nevus syndrome vs., **363**

Multiple fractures, dentinogenesis imperfecta vs., **231**

Multiple myeloma, **520–523**
- diagnostic checklist, **522**
- differential diagnosis, **521**
- genetics, **521**
- ill-defined radiolucencies vs., **882, 885**
- mandible-maxilla metastasis vs., **495**
- prognosis, **522**
- staging, grading, & classification, **521**
- TMJ metastasis vs., **641**
- TMJ radiolucencies vs., **954, 955**
- well-defined unilocular radiolucencies vs., **871, 873**

Multiple odontogenic keratocysts, nonsyndromic, basal cell nevus syndrome vs., **363**

Multiple periapical osteofibromatosis. *See* Florid osseous dysplasia.

Muscles of mastication, **83**
- anterior division, **129**

Mx. *See* Maxilla (Mx).

Mycetoma, **692–693**
- chronic rhinosinusitis vs., **681**
- differential diagnosis, **693**
- prognosis, **693**
- sinus fungal, allergic fungal sinusitis vs., **687**

Myeloma. *See also* Multiple myeloma.
- multiple, mandible-maxilla metastasis vs., **495**

Mylohyoid, **32, 37, 38, 39, 45, 46, 49, 51, 53, 119, 129, 169, 170, 182**
- cleft with vessel, **51**
- nerve and artery to, **32**
- posterior margin, **46**

Mylohyoid boutonnière, accessory salivary tissue in. *See* Submandibular space accessory salivary tissue.

Mylohyoid cleft, **49**
- with vessel, **46**

Mylohyoid groove, **32**

Mylohyoid (internal oblique) ridge, **32, 35**

Mylohyoid nerve, **129, 131, 182**

Mylohyoid ridge, **46, 50**
- of mandible, **50**

Myoepithelial sialadenitis. *See* Sjögren syndrome.

Myositis, oral cavity soft tissue infections, **293**

Myositis ossificans
- cervical facet arthropathy vs., **827**
- limited condylar translation vs., **950, 953**
- soft tissue calcifications vs., **935**

Myxofibroma. *See also* Central odontogenic fibroma; Odontogenic myxoma.
- ameloblastoma vs, **457**
- multilocular radiolucencies vs., **878–879, 881**
- periosteal reactions vs., **907, 910**

Myxoma. *See* Odontogenic myxoma.

N

Nager syndrome, Treacher Collins syndrome vs., **369**

Nasal bone, **99, 100, 102**
- fracture, nasoethmoid complex fracture vs., **375**

Nasal capsule, cartilage of developing, **100**

Nasal cartilage, **100**

Nasal cavity, **71, 179**
- implant apices in, **21**
- proximity of apices of, **23**
- root apex in, **13**

Nasal choanae, **177**

Nasal cocaine necrosis, sinonasal granulomatosis with polyangiitis vs., **669**

Nasal fossa, **58, 60, 136**
- floor of, **136**

INDEX

Nasal glial heterotopia, dermoid and epidermoid vs., **286**
Nasal glioma, dermoid and epidermoid vs., **286**
Nasal lesion
- with bony destruction, **970–973**
  differential diagnosis, **970–971**
- without bony destruction, **966–969**
  differential diagnosis, **966–967**
Nasal notch, **25**
Nasal septal abscess, perforated nasal septum vs., **964, 965**
Nasal septum, **65, 66, 69, 71, 136, 177**
- deviated, **650–651**
  associated abnormalities, **651**
  diagnostic checklist, **651**
  differential diagnosis, **651**
  staging, grading, & classification, **651**
Nasal spine
- anterior, **25, 26, 27**
- hypoplasia, anterior, **23**
- posterior, **25**
Nasalis, **139, 142**
Nasoalveolar cyst. *See* Nasolabial cyst.
Nasoethmoid complex fracture, **374–375**
- associated abnormalities, **375**
- diagnostic checklist, **375**
- differential diagnosis, **375**
- staging, grading, & classification, **375**
Nasolabial cyst, **422–423**
- diagnostic checklist, **423**
- differential diagnosis, **423**
- prognosis, **423**
Nasolacrimal duct, **57, 66, 67, 69, 70, 71, 75**
- cyst, nasal lesion without bony destruction vs., **966, 968**
- groove for, **25**
- mucocele, nasolabial cyst vs., **423**
- opening, **57, 73**
  into inferior meatus, **71**
Nasolacrimal sac, **66**
Nasomaxillary suture, **24**
Naso-orbital-ethmoid fracture
- complex midfacial fracture vs., **377**
- transfacial fracture (Le Fort) vs., **381**
Nasopalatine canal, **27, 28, 60**
Nasopalatine duct cyst, **418–421**
- associated abnormalities, **420**
- diagnostic checklist, **420**
- differential diagnosis, **419–420**
- nasolabial cyst vs., **423**
- oral cavity minor salivary gland malignancy vs., **313**
- palate benign mixed tumor vs., **311**
- prognosis, **420**
- residual cyst vs., **407**
- well-defined unilocular radiolucencies vs., **870, 872**
Nasopalatine foramen, large, nasopalatine duct cyst vs., **419**
Nasopalatine (incisive) nerve, **27**
Nasopalatine nerve, of maxilla, **22**
Nasopharyngeal airway, **71, 109**
Nasopharyngeal carcinoma, **708–711**
- diagnostic checklist, **710**
- differential diagnosis, **709**
- non-Hodgkin lymphoma of pharyngeal mucosal space vs., **517**
- prognosis, **710**
- staging, grading, & classification, **709–710**
Nasopharyngeal carotid space, **115, 189**
Nasopharyngeal mucosal space, **169, 175**
- adenoids of, **109**
Nasopharynx, **64, 75, 137, 172–179**
- anatomy relationships, **172**
- CBCT airway analysis, **179**
- CBCT of nasopharynx and oropharynx, **177**
- fascia of pharyngeal mucosal space, **172**
- graphics
  of axial oropharynx, skull base interactions, coronal pharynx, **174**
  of coronal, **175**
  of normal axial nasopharynx and PMS mass, **173**
- internal contents, **172**
- lateral cephalometric and panoramic of, **176**
- normal axial & coronal MR, **178**
Neck lesions, pediatric, dermoid and epidermoid vs., **286**
Nerve sheath tumor, **482–485**
- associated abnormalities, **483**
- diagnostic checklist, **484**
- differential diagnosis, **483**
- prognosis, **484**
- sinonasal
  nasal lesion without bony destruction vs., **967, 969**
  paranasal sinus lesions without bony destruction vs., **977**
- staging, grading, & classification, **483–484**
Nerve to stapedius muscle, **140**
Neural arch anomalies, posterior, failure of segmentation vs., **812**
Neural foramen, **158**
- C2-3, **157**
Neurilemmoma. *See* Nerve sheath tumor; Schwannoma.
Neurinoma. *See* Nerve sheath tumor; Schwannoma.
Neuroblastoma
- leukemia vs., **529**
- olfactory, Ewing sarcoma vs., **525**
Neurofibroma. *See also* Nerve sheath tumor.
- CNV3
  masticator space CNV3 perineural tumor vs., **743**
  masticator space CNV3 schwannoma vs., **733**
Neurofibromatosis, autosomal dominant. *See* Neurofibromatosis type 1.
Neurofibromatosis type 1, **486–489**
- associated abnormalities, **488**
- central giant cell granuloma associated, **531**
- diagnostic checklist, **488**
- differential diagnosis, **487**
- genetics, **488**
- nerve sheath tumor associated, **483**
- parotid space lesions vs., **919**
- prognosis, **488**
- staging, grading, & classification, **488**
Neuroma. *See* Schwannoma.
Nevoid basal cell carcinoma syndrome. *See also* Basal cell nevus syndrome.
- cherubism vs., **359**

INDEX

NHL. *See* Non-Hodgkin lymphoma.
Nodal drainage, regional, parotid benign mixed tumor vs., **758**
Nodal metastases
- squamous cell carcinoma, submandibular gland sialadenitis vs., **301**
- systemic, parotid benign mixed tumor vs., **758**
- from systemic primary, submandibular space nodal non-Hodgkin lymphoma vs., **319**

Nodal metastatic disease, parotid, parotid non-Hodgkin lymphoma vs., **775**
Nodal non-Hodgkin lymphoma, submandibular space, **318–319**
- associated abnormalities, **319**
- diagnostic checklist, **319**
- differential diagnosis, **319**
- prognosis, **319**
- submandibular gland carcinoma vs., **317**
- submandibular space nodal non-Hodgkin lymphoma vs., **319**
- submandibular space nodal squamous cell carcinoma vs., **331**

Nodal SSCa in submandibular space, submandibular gland benign mixed tumor vs., **309**
NOE fx. *See* Nasoethmoid complex fracture.
Non-Hodgkin lymphoma
- ill-defined radiolucencies vs., **882, 885**
- lingual tonsil, lingual thyroid vs., **283**
- nasopharyngeal, nasopharyngeal carcinoma vs., **709**
- nodal, submandibular space lesions vs., **915, 917**
- parotid, **774–777**
    benign lymphoepithelial lesions: HIV vs., **751**
    diagnostic checklist, **776**
    differential diagnosis, **775**
    metastatic disease of parotid nodes vs., **779**
    parotid benign mixed tumor vs., **758**
    parotid mucoepidermoid carcinoma vs., **769**
    prognosis, **776**
    Sjögren syndrome vs., **783**
    staging, grading, & classification, **776**
    Warthin tumor vs., **761**
- parotid space lesions vs., **919, 921**
- periodontal disease vs., **272**
- of pharyngeal mucosal space, **516–519**
    associated abnormalities, **518**
    diagnostic checklist, **518**
    differential diagnosis, **517**
    genetics, **518**
    prognosis, **518**
    staging, grading, & classification, **518**
    subtypes, **517**
- sinonasal
    allergic fungal sinusitis vs., **687**
    invasive fungal sinusitis vs., **689**
    nasal lesion with bony destruction vs., **970, 971**
    nasal lesion without bony destruction vs., **967, 969**
    paranasal sinus lesions with bony destruction vs., **980, 982**
    perforated nasal septum vs., **964**
    sinonasal granulomatosis with polyangiitis vs., **669**
    sinonasal malignant melanoma vs., **713**
- sinonasal squamous cell carcinoma vs., **705**

Nonreducing displaced disc (NRDD). *See* Disc displacement, without reduction.
Nontuberculosis mycobacterium, lymph nodes, submandibular space lesions vs., **915**
Noonan syndrome, central giant cell granuloma associated, **531**
Normal sinus floor, **61**
Nose
- shadow of, **21**
- and sinus anatomy
    ostiomeatal complex, **72–75**
    pterygopalatine fossa, **76–79**
    sinonasal overview, **56–71**

NPDC. *See* Nasopalatine duct cyst.
Nutrient canal, **10, 11**
Nutrient/neurovascular canal, mandible fracture vs., **371**

O

OA. *See* Ophthalmic artery.
Oblique coronal plane, **87**
Oblique facial cleft, **357**
Oblique fracture, dentoalveolar fractures, **255**
Oblique sagittal plane, **87**
Occipital artery, **204, 205**
Occipital bone, **110, 114, 174**
- anatomy, **150**
- basilar portion (clivus), **115**
- condylar portion, **114, 115**
- squamous part, **113, 114**

Occipital condyle, **115, 116, 156, 158**
Occipital node, **201**
Occipitalization. *See* C1 assimilation.
Occipitofrontalis, frontal belly of, **139, 142**
Occipitomastoid suture, **111, 113, 114**
Occlusal trauma, widened periodontal ligament space vs., **864**
Oculoauriculovertebral dysplasia. *See also* Hemifacial microsomia.
- condylar aplasia associated, **541**

Oculofaciocardiodental syndrome, macrodontia, gemination, and fusion vs., **217**
Oculomotor nerve (CNIII), **127**
Odontoblasts, **6**
- secreting dentin matrix, **6**

Odontodysplasia, regional, **233**
- differential diagnosis, **233**
- segmental odontomaxillary dysplasia vs., **235**

Odontogenic cyst, **61**
- calcifying
    ameloblastic fibroodontoma vs., **465**
    calcifying epithelial odontogenic tumor vs., **467**
- hypoplasia/aplasia vs., **659**
- paranasal sinus lesions without bony destruction vs., **976, 978**
- primary intraosseous squamous cell carcinoma vs., **509**

Odontogenic fibroma. *See also* Central odontogenic fibroma.
- central, **472–473**
  - differential diagnosis, **473**
  - types, **473**

Odontogenic ghost cell carcinoma, **413**
Odontogenic hamartoma. *See* Odontoma.
Odontogenic infection, oral cavity soft tissue infections, **293**
Odontogenic keratocyst, **400–403**
- adenomatoid odontogenic tumor vs., **455**
- ameloblastic fibroma vs., **461**
- ameloblastoma vs, **458**
- associated abnormalities, **402**
- benign, periapical radiolucencies vs., **856, 859**
- buccal bifurcation cyst vs., **409**
- central odontogenic fibroma vs., **473**
- dentigerous cyst vs., **397**
- diagnostic checklist, **402**
- differential diagnosis, **401**
- genetics, **402**
- lateral periodontal cyst vs., **405**
- malignant ameloblastoma and ameloblastic carcinoma vs., **493**
- mandible-maxilla simple (traumatic) bone cyst vs., **425**
- multilocular radiolucencies vs., **878, 879**
- multiple, nonsyndromic, basal cell nevus syndrome vs., **363**
- nasopalatine duct cyst vs., **419**
- periapical rarefying osteitis vs., **266**
- pericoronal radiolucencies without radiopacities vs., **874, 875**
- prognosis, **402**
- residual cyst vs., **407**
- staging, grading, & classification, **402**
- well-defined unilocular radiolucencies vs., **871, 873**

Odontogenic lesions, extending into condyle, condylar hyperplasia vs., **547**
Odontogenic myxoma, **470–471**
- ameloblastic fibroma vs., **461**
- ameloblastoma vs, **457**
- central giant cell granuloma vs., **531**
- central hemangioma vs., **475**
- central odontogenic fibroma vs., **473**
- desmoplastic fibroma vs., **491**
- diagnostic checklist, **471**
- differential diagnosis, **471**
- malignant ameloblastoma and ameloblastic carcinoma vs., **493**
- multilocular radiolucencies vs., **878–879, 881**
- periosteal reactions vs., **907, 910**
- prognosis, **471**

Odontogenic origin, sinusitis of. *See* Odontogenic sinusitis.
Odontogenic sinusitis, **684–685**
- diagnostic checklist, **685**
- differential diagnosis, **685**
- prognosis, **685**
- staging, grading, & classification, **685**

Odontogenic squamous cell carcinoma. *See* Intraosseous squamous cell carcinoma, primary.
Odontogenic tumor
- adenomatoid, **277, 454–455**
  - differential diagnosis, **455**
  - prognosis, **455**
  - staging, grading, & classification, **455**
- calcifying cystic. *See* Calcifying odontogenic cyst.
- calcifying epithelial, **466–467**
  - associated abnormalities, **467**
  - diagnostic checklist, **467**
  - differential diagnosis, **467**
  - prognosis, **467**

Odontoid, **156**
- anterior to cruciate ligament, **151**

Odontoid aplasia, **804–805**
- associated abnormalities, **805**
- diagnostic checklist, **805**
- differential diagnosis, **805**
- genetics, **805**
- prognosis, **805**

Odontoid C2 fracture
- odontoid hypoplasia/aplasia vs., **805**
- os odontoideum vs., **799**

Odontoid fracture
- os avis vs., **803**
- type I or II, ossiculum terminale vs., **795**

Odontoid hypoplasia, **804–805**
- associated abnormalities, **805**
- diagnostic checklist, **805**
- differential diagnosis, **805**
- genetics, **805**
- prognosis, **805**

Odontoid ligaments, anatomy, **150**
Odontoid process, **116, 151, 153, 158**
- base of, **159**
- degenerative remodeling of, ossiculum terminale vs., **795**

Odontoid resection, surgical, odontoid hypoplasia/aplasia vs., **805**
Odontoid tip, **156, 159**
Odontoid tip synchondrosis, unfused, ossiculum terminale vs., **795**
Odontoma, **220, 450–453**
- ameloblastic fibroodontoma vs., **465**
- associated abnormalities, **452**
- complex, **451, 452**
  - mandible-maxilla idiopathic osteosclerosis vs., **355**
- compound, **451, 452**
- diagnostic checklist, **452**
- differential diagnosis, **451–452**
- immature
  - ameloblastic fibroma vs., **461**
  - dentigerous cyst vs., **397**
- periapical osseous dysplasia vs., **430**
- periapical radiopacities and mixed lesions vs., **860, 861**
- pericoronal radiolucencies with radiopacities vs., **876**
- prognosis, **452**
- soft. *See* Ameloblastic fibroma.
- staging, grading, & classification, **452**

Odontome. *See* Odontoma.
Oehlers classification, **221**
OKC. *See* Odontogenic keratocyst.

Olfactory bulb, **99**
- and nerves, **128**
Olfactory nerve (CN1), **99**
Olfactory neuroblastoma
- Ewing sarcoma vs., **525**
- paranasal sinus lesions with bony destruction vs., **980, 982**
Olfactory recess, **208**
- nasal vault, **65, 66**
Oligodontia. *See* Hypodontia.
Olivary eminence, **106**
OMC. *See* Ostiomeatal complex (OMC).
Oncocytoma, parotid, parotid space lesions vs., **919**
Opalescent teeth, dentinogenesis imperfecta vs., **231**
Ophthalmic artery (OA), **204, 205, 206**
Ophthalmic (C6) segment, **204**
- calcification of, **209**
- ICA, **206**
Ophthalmic division CNV (CNV1), **105, 126, 127, 128**
Ophthalmic nerve (CNV1), **105**
- as division of cranial nerve, **124**
Opisthion, **151, 156, 159**
Optic canal, **28, 64, 79, 101, 102, 105, 107, 208**
- of central skull base, **104**
Optic chiasm, **133**
Optic hamartomas, **487**
Optic nerve (CNII), **70, 99, 105**
Optic tract, **127**
Oral cavity
- anatomy
    dental restorations, **14–21**
    mandible, **30–35**
    maxilla, **22–29**
    oral mucosal space/surface, **52–53**
    retromolar trigone, **40–43**
    sublingual space, **44–47**
    submandibular space, **48–51**
    teeth, **4–13**
    tongue, **36–39**
- buccal mucosa squamous cell carcinoma, **332–333**
- dermoid and epidermoid, **284–287**
- floor of mouth squamous cell carcinoma, **324–325**
- foregut duplication cyst in tongue, **290–291**
- gingival squamous cell carcinoma, **326–327**
- hard palate squamous cell carcinoma, **334–335**
- lingual thyroid, **282–283**
- minor salivary gland malignancy, **312–313**
- motor denervation CNXII, **336–337**
- oral tongue squamous cell carcinoma, **320–323**
- palate benign mixed tumor, **310–311**
- ranula, **296–299**
- retromolar trigone squamous cell carcinoma, **328–329**
- sialocele, **302–303**
    diagnostic checklist, **303**
    differential diagnosis, **303**
- soft tissue infections, **292–295**
    diagnostic checklist, **294**
    differential diagnosis, **293–294**
- sublingual gland benign mixed tumor, **306–307**
- sublingual gland carcinoma, **314–315**
- submandibular gland aplasia-hypoplasia, **288–289**
- submandibular gland benign mixed tumor, **308–309**
- submandibular gland carcinoma, **316–317**
- submandibular gland mucocele, **304–305**
- submandibular gland sialadenitis, **300–301**
- submandibular sialoliths, **338–339**
- submandibular space accessory salivary tissue, **280–281**
- submandibular space nodal non-Hodgkin lymphoma, **318–319**
- submandibular space nodal squamous cell carcinoma, **330–331**
Oral cavity abscess
- floor of mouth squamous cell carcinoma vs., **325**
- sublingual gland carcinoma vs., **315**
Oral cavity infection, buccal mucosa squamous cell carcinoma vs., **333**
Oral cavity lymphatic malformation
- motor denervation CNXII vs., **337**
- sublingual gland benign mixed tumor vs., **307**
- sublingual gland carcinoma vs., **315**
Oral cavity minor salivary gland malignancy, buccal mucosa squamous cell carcinoma vs., **333**
Oral cavity venous malformation, motor denervation CNXII vs., **337**
Oral epithelium, **7**
- fusion of reduced enamel epithelium to, **7**
Oral minor salivary gland malignancy, retromolar trigone squamous cell carcinoma vs., **329**
Oral mucosal space/surface (OMS), **36, 50, 52–53**
- graphics, **53**
- lesions, **926–929**
Oral tongue, **43, 52, 53, 178**
Oral tongue lymph vessels, **36**
Oral tongue squamous cell carcinoma, **320–323**
- diagnostic checklist, **322**
- differential diagnosis, **321**
- floor of mouth squamous cell carcinoma vs., **325**
- genetics, **321**
- motor denervation CNXII vs., **337**
- oral cavity soft tissue infections vs., **294**
- oral mucosal space/surface lesions vs., **926, 927**
- prognosis, **322**
- staging, grading, & classification, **321–322**
Orbicularis oculi, **26, 139, 142**
- palpebral portion of, **26**
Orbicularis oris, **139, 142**
Orbit, **62, 63, 136**
- floor of, **136**
Orbital branch, **128**
Orbital fissure
- inferior, of central skull base, **104**
- superior, of central skull base, **104**
Orbital idiopathic inflammatory pseudotumor, dermoid and epidermoid vs., **286**
Orbital infantile hemangioma, dermoid and epidermoid vs., **285–286**
Orbital Langerhans cell histiocytosis, dermoid and epidermoid vs., **285**
Orbital lesions, pediatric, dermoid and epidermoid vs., **285**
Orbital lymphatic malformation, dermoid and epidermoid vs., **285–286**

INDEX

Orbital roof, frontal bone, **102**
Orbital venous malformation, dermoid and epidermoid vs., **286**
Orbitosphenoid, **106**
ORN. *See* Osteoradionecrosis, mandible-maxilla.
Oropharyngeal airway, **195**
Oropharyngeal mucosal space, **49, 169, 175**
Oropharynx, **46, 137, 172–179, 203**
- anatomy relationships, **172**
- CBCT airway analysis, **179**
- CBCT of nasopharynx and oropharynx, **177**
- fascia of pharyngeal mucosal space, **172**
- graphics
  - of axial oropharynx, skull base interactions, coronal pharynx, **174**
  - of coronal, **175**
  - of normal axial nasopharynx and PMS mass, **173**
- internal contents, **172**
- lateral cephalometric and panoramic of, **176**
- normal axial & coronal MR, **178**

Orthodontic archwire, **19**
Orthodontic band, **19**
Orthodontic bracket, **19**
Orthodontic movement
- periodontal disease vs., **272**
- widened periodontal ligament space vs., **864**

Orthodontic spacers, **18**
Os avis, **802–803**
- diagnostic checklist, **803**
- differential diagnosis, **803**
- prognosis, **803**

Os odontoideum, **798–801**
- associated abnormalities, **799**
- diagnostic checklist, **800**
- differential diagnosis, **799**
- odontoid hypoplasia/aplasia vs., **805**
- os avis vs., **803**
- ossiculum terminale vs., **795**
- prognosis, **800**
- staging, grading, & classification, **800**

Osseous dysplasia
- florid, ground-glass and granular radiopacities vs., **896, 898, 899**
- periapical
  - ground-glass and granular radiopacities vs., **896, 899**
  - mandible-maxilla idiopathic osteosclerosis vs., **355**
  - periapical rarefying osteitis vs., **265**
  - periapical sclerosing osteitis vs., **269**

Ossicles of middle ear, anatomy, **90**
Ossiculum terminale, **794–795**
- diagnostic checklist, **795**
- differential diagnosis, **795**
- os odontoideum vs., **799**
- prognosis, **795**

Ossiculum terminale persistens. *See* Ossiculum terminale.
Ossification
- failure of formation, **808**
- of posterior longitudinal ligament, **818–821**
  - associated abnormalities, **819**
  - diagnostic checklist, **820**
  - differential diagnosis, **819**
  - genetics, **819**
  - prognosis, **820**
  - staging, grading, & classification, **819–820**

Ossified spinal ligaments, soft tissue calcifications vs., **935, 937**
Ossified stylohyoid ligament, **120, 121**
Ossifying fibroma, **436–439**
- associated abnormalities, **438**
- diagnostic checklist, **438**
- differential diagnosis, **437**
- genetics, **438**
- immature, mandibular salivary gland defect vs., **351**
- mandible-maxilla fibrous dysplasia vs., **442**
- odontoma vs., **451**
- prognosis, **438**
- sinonasal fibrous dysplasia vs., **715**
- sinus
  - paranasal sinus lesions without bony destruction vs., **977, 979**
  - sinonasal fibroosseous and cartilaginous lesions vs., **974, 975**
- staging, grading, & classification, **438**

Osteitis
- apical rarefying, periapical osseous dysplasia vs., **429**
- condensing
  - mandible-maxilla idiopathic osteosclerosis vs., **355**
  - supernumerary roots vs., **225**
- periapical rarefying, central odontogenic fibroma vs., **473**
- periapical sclerosing. *See also* Periapical sclerosing osteitis.
  - condensing, cementoblastoma vs., **469**
- sclerosing
  - mandible-maxilla idiopathic osteosclerosis vs., **355**
  - odontoma vs., **452**

Osteitis deformans. *See* Paget disease.
Osteitis fibrosa. *See* Fibrous dysplasia, mandible-maxilla.
Osteoarthritis. *See* Degenerative joint disease; Degenerative joint disorders of craniovertebral junction; Progressive condylar resorption.
Osteoarthrosis (OA). *See* Degenerative joint disease.
Osteoblastoma, **478–479**
- associated abnormalities, **479**
- cementoblastoma vs., **469**
- diagnostic checklist, **479**
- differential diagnosis, **479**
- fibrous dysplasia, cervical spine vs., **839**
- mandible-maxilla, sinonasal osteoma vs., **701**
- osteoid osteoma vs., **477**
- staging, grading, & classification, **479**
- well-defined radiopacities vs., **893, 895**

Osteocartilaginous exostosis. *See* Osteochondroma, temporomandibular joint.
Osteochondral defects. *See* Osteochondritis dissecans, temporomandibular joint.
Osteochondritis. *See* Osteochondritis dissecans, temporomandibular joint.
Osteochondritis dissecans
- temporomandibular joint, **576–577**
  - differential diagnosis, **577**

prognosis, **577**
staging, grading, & classification, **577**
- TMJ primary synovial chondromatosis vs., **631**

Osteochondroma
- coronoid hyperplasia vs., **553**
- large condyle vs., **946, 948**
- limited condylar translation vs., **950, 953**
- temporomandibular joint, **620–625**
  bony ankylosis vs., **563**
  condylar hyperplasia vs., **547**
  diagnostic checklist, **621**
  differential diagnosis, **621**
  prognosis, **621**
  TMJ osteoma vs., **619**
- TMJ radiopacities vs., **956, 958**

Osteochondromatosis. *See* Synovial chondromatosis, temporomandibular joint.
Osteodysplasia, fibrous. *See* Fibrous dysplasia, mandible-maxilla.
Osteodystrophia fibrosa. *See* Fibrous dysplasia, mandible-maxilla.
Osteodystrophy, hypoplasia/aplasia associated, **660**
Osteofibroma. *See* Ossifying fibroma.
Osteofibromatosis, multiple periapical. *See* Florid osseous dysplasia.
Osteogenesis imperfecta, dentinogenesis imperfecta vs., **231**
Osteogenic fibroma, giant. *See* Osteoblastoma.
Osteogenic sarcoma. *See also* Osteosarcoma, mandible-maxilla.
- ossifying fibroma vs., **437**

Osteoid osteoma, **476–477**
- cementoblastoma vs., **469**
- differential diagnosis, **477**
- mandible-maxilla, well-defined radiopacities vs., **893, 895**
- osteoblastoma vs., **479**
- periapical radiopacities and mixed lesions vs., **860, 861**
- staging, grading, & classification, **477**

Osteolytic metastases, Paget disease vs., **448**
Osteolytic stage, cherubism, **360**
Osteoma
- buccal and palatal exostoses vs., **343**
- condylar hyperplasia vs., **547**
- coronoid hyperplasia vs., **553**
- large condyle vs., **946, 948**
- mandible-maxilla, **480–481**
  associated abnormalities, **481**
  diagnostic checklist, **481**
  differential diagnosis, **481**
  prognosis, **481**
  staging, grading, & classification, **481**
  well-defined radiopacities vs., **893, 895**
- mandibular torus vs., **345**
- odontoma vs., **452**
- osteoid, **476–477**
  cementoblastoma vs., **469**
  differential diagnosis, **477**
  osteoblastoma vs., **479**
  staging, grading, & classification, **477**
- palatal torus vs., **347**
- sinonasal, **700–703**
  associated abnormalities, **701**
  associated syndromes, **701**
  diagnostic checklist, **701**
  differential diagnosis, **701**
  genetics, **701**
  nasal lesion without bony destruction vs., **966, 968**
  paranasal sinus lesions without bony destruction vs., **976, 978**
  sinonasal fibroosseous and cartilaginous lesions vs., **974**
  sinonasal ossifying fibroma vs., **719**
  staging, grading, & classification, **701**
- sinonasal fibrous dysplasia vs., **715**
- temporomandibular joint, **618–619**
  associated abnormalities, **619**
  bony ankylosis vs., **563**
  diagnostic checklist, **619**
  differential diagnosis, **619**
  prognosis, **619**
  staging, grading, & classification, **619**
  TMJ osteochondroma vs., **621**
- TMJ radiopacities vs., **956–957, 958**

Osteomalacia, lamina dura changes vs., **867, 869**
Osteomyelitis
- acute, periapical rarefying osteitis vs., **266**
- Burkitt lymphoma vs., **513**
- chronic, periapical osseous dysplasia vs., **430**
- florid osseous dysplasia vs., **433**
- generalized radiopacities vs., **902, 903, 904**
- generalized rarefaction vs., **888, 890**
- ill-defined radiolucencies vs., **882, 884**
- lamina dura changes vs., **866, 867**
- Langerhans histiocytosis vs., **535**
- mandible-maxilla, **293, 384–387**
  associated abnormalities, **386**
  diagnostic checklist, **386**
  differential diagnosis, **385–386**
  gingival squamous cell carcinoma vs., **327**
  masticator space sarcoma vs., **739**
  prognosis, **386**
  sinonasal fibroosseous and cartilaginous lesions vs., **974, 975**
  staging, grading, & classification, **386**
- mandible-maxilla fibrous dysplasia vs., **441**
- mandible-maxilla metastasis vs., **495**
- mandible-maxilla osteonecrosis vs., **393**
- mandible-maxilla osteoradionecrosis vs., **389**
- mandible-maxilla osteosarcoma vs., **501**
- multiple myeloma vs., **521**
- periapical radiolucencies vs., **856–857, 859**
- periosteal reactions vs., **906**
  chronic, **907, 908**
  Garré, **908**
- sinonasal fibrous dysplasia vs., **715**
- TMJ metastasis vs., **641**
- widened periodontal ligament space vs., **864**

Osteonecrosis
- ill-defined radiolucencies vs., **882, 885**
- lamina dura changes vs., **866, 868**

- mandible-maxilla, **392–395**
    - diagnostic checklist, **393**
    - differential diagnosis, **393**
    - gingival squamous cell carcinoma vs., **327**
    - prognosis, **393**
    - staging, grading, & classification, **393**
- medication-related
    - mandible-maxilla osteomyelitis vs., **386**
    - mandible-maxilla osteoradionecrosis vs., **389**
- periosteal reactions vs., **906, 908, 909**
- widened periodontal ligament space vs., **864, 865**

Osteopenia
- leukemia vs., **529**
- TMJ rheumatoid arthritis vs., **579**

Osteopetrosis
- focal. *See* Mandible-maxilla idiopathic osteosclerosis.
- generalized radiopacities vs., **902–903, 905**
- hypoplasia/aplasia associated, **660**
- lamina dura changes vs., **867, 869**

Osteoporosis
- generalized rarefaction vs., **888, 889**
- lamina dura changes vs., **866, 867**
- leukemia vs., **529**

Osteoporotic bone marrow defect
- lateral periodontal cyst vs., **405**
- mandible-maxilla simple (traumatic) bone cyst vs., **425**

Osteoporotic compression fracture, lytic and blastic metastases vs., **835–836**

Osteoradionecrosis
- ill-defined radiolucencies vs., **882, 884**
- mandible-maxilla, **388–391**
    - diagnostic checklist, **389**
    - differential diagnosis, **389**
    - gingival squamous cell carcinoma vs., **327**
    - masticator space abscess vs., **725**
    - prognosis, **389**
- mandible-maxilla osteomyelitis vs., **386**
- mandible-maxilla osteonecrosis vs., **393**

Osteosarcoma
- Burkitt lymphoma vs., **513**
- central hemangioma vs., **475**
- Ewing sarcoma vs., **525**
- fibrous dysplasia, cervical spine vs., **839**
- floating teeth vs., **862, 863**
- ill-defined radiolucencies vs., **883, 887**
- lamina dura changes vs., **867, 869**
- large condyle vs., **947, 949**
- mandible-maxilla, **500–503**
    - associated abnormalities, **502**
    - diagnostic checklist, **502**
    - differential diagnosis, **501**
    - gingival squamous cell carcinoma vs., **327**
    - masticator space chondrosarcoma vs., **735**
    - prognosis, **502**
    - staging, grading, & classification, **502**
- mandible-maxilla chondrosarcoma vs., **505**
- mandible-maxilla fibrous dysplasia vs., **442**
- mandible-maxilla osteomyelitis vs., **385–386**
- odontogenic myxoma vs., **471**
- osteoblastoma vs., **479**
- periodontal disease vs., **272**
- periosteal reactions vs., **907, 910**
- sinonasal
    - nasal lesion with bony destruction vs., **971, 973**
    - paranasal sinus lesions with bony destruction vs., **981, 983**
    - sinonasal fibroosseous and cartilaginous lesions vs., **974, 975**
    - sinonasal ossifying fibroma vs., **719**
    - sinonasal osteoma vs., **701**
- sinonasal fibrous dysplasia vs., **716**
- temporomandibular joint, **634–635**
    - diagnostic checklist, **635**
    - differential diagnosis, **635**
    - prognosis, **635**
    - staging, grading, & classification, **635**
- TMJ chondrosarcoma vs., **637**
- TMJ metastasis vs., **641**
- TMJ radiolucencies vs., **954, 955**
- TMJ radiopacities vs., **957, 959**
- widened periodontal ligament space vs., **864, 865**

Osteosclerosis, idiopathic
- buccal and palatal exostoses vs., **343**
- cementoblastoma vs., **469**
- mandible-maxilla, **354–355**
    - diagnostic checklist, **355**
    - differential diagnosis, **355**
    - prognosis, **355**
- mandible-maxilla osteoma vs., **481**
- mandibular torus vs., **345**
- odontoma vs., **452**
- periapical osseous dysplasia vs., **430**
- periapical sclerosing osteitis vs., **269**
- submandibular sialoliths vs., **339**
- supernumerary roots vs., **225**
- TMJ radiopacities vs., **957, 959**

Osteosclerosis/enostosis/dense bone island, idiopathic, hypercementosis vs., **248**

Osteosclerotic metastases, Paget disease vs., **448**

Ostia maxillare accessoria. *See* Accessory ostia.

Ostiomeatal complex (OMC), **72–75**
- coronal and sagittal graphics, **73**
- normal coronal bone CT, **74**
- normal sagittal bone CT, **75**

Otic ganglion, **129**

Outer enamel epithelium, **6**

Oval window, **91, 92, 93, 145, 146**

Overinstrumentation of pulp canal, internal and external resorption vs., **243**

P

PADI. *See* Posterior atlantodens interval.

Paget disease, **446–449**
- cervical facet arthropathy vs., **827**
- diagnostic checklist, **448**
- differential diagnosis, **448**
- fibrous dysplasia, cervical spine vs., **839**
- florid osseous dysplasia vs., **433**

- generalized radiopacities vs., **902, 905**
- ground-glass and granular radiopacities vs., **897, 901**
- hemangioma, cervical spine vs., **831**
- lamina dura changes vs., **866, 868**
- mandible-maxilla fibrous dysplasia vs., **441**
- prognosis, **448**
- sinonasal fibrous dysplasia vs., **715**

Palatal abscess, palate benign mixed tumor vs., **311**
Palatal cyst, median, nasopalatine duct cyst vs., **420**
Palatal minor salivary gland malignancy, palate benign mixed tumor vs., **311**
Palatal process of maxilla, **58**
Palatal torus, **346–347**
- associated abnormalities, **347**
- buccal and palatal exostoses vs., **343**
- diagnostic checklist, **347**
- differential diagnosis, **347**
- genetics, **347**
- oral mucosal space/surface lesions vs., **927, 928**
- palate benign mixed tumor vs., **311**
- prognosis, **347**
- well-defined radiopacities vs., **892, 894**

Palate, cleft, **357**
Palate benign mixed tumor, **310–311**
- differential diagnosis, **311**
- hard palate squamous cell carcinoma vs., **335**
- oral cavity minor salivary gland malignancy vs., **313**
- prognosis, **311**

Palate pleomorphic adenoma. *See* Palate benign mixed tumor.
Palatine bone, **25**
- articulation with tuberosity portion of, **24**

Palatine nerve of maxilla, greater, anatomy, **22–23**
Palatine nerves, **77**
Palatine process, anatomy, **22**
Palatine tonsil, **37, 41, 43, 167, 171, 195**
Palatine tonsil squamous cell carcinoma, non-Hodgkin lymphoma of pharyngeal mucosal space vs., **517**
Palatine tonsillolith, parotid sialoliths vs., **785**
Palatine tonsils, **174, 175, 177, 178, 179**
Palatoglossal airway, mandible fracture vs., **371**
Palatoglossus muscle, **174**
- anatomy, **36, 37, 38, 39**

Panfacial fracture. *See* Complex midfacial fracture.
Papillary cystadenoma lymphomatosum. *See* Warthin tumor.
Papillon-Lefèvre syndrome
- floating teeth vs., **862, 863**
- periodontal disease associated, **272**

Paradental cyst. *See* Buccal bifurcation cyst.
Parafunctional tooth wear. *See* Attrition.
Paranasal sinus lesions
- with bony destruction, **980–983**
  - differential diagnosis, **980–981**
- without bony destruction, **976–979**
  - differential diagnosis, **976–977**

Parapharyngeal space (PPS), **168–171, 173, 174, 175, 178, 181, 182, 183, 185, 186, 187, 189, 190, 191, 193, 194, 195**
- anatomy, **163, 164, 166, 167**
  - abuts skull base, **164**
  - imaging anatomy, **162**
  - relationships, **168**
- axial CECT & coronal T1 MR images of normal PPS, **171**
- fascial margins of, **168**
- fat, **185**
- internal contents, **168**
- masticator space mass enters, **181**
- normal axial & coronal space, **169**
- skull base interaction; normal axial PPS, **170**

Paraspinal component, perivertebral space, **167, 197**
Paraspinal muscles, **197, 199**
Paraspinal-PVS, in perivertebral space, **196**
Parotid adenoid cystic carcinoma, **772–773**
- diagnostic checklist, **773**
- differential diagnosis, **773**
- parotid benign mixed tumor vs., **758**
- parotid malignant mixed tumor vs., **767**
- parotid mucoepidermoid carcinoma vs., **769**
- prognosis, **773**
- staging, grading, & classification, **773**
- Warthin tumor vs., **761**

Parotid benign mixed tumor, **756–759**
- diagnostic checklist, **758**
- differential diagnosis, **757–758**
- parotid malignant mixed tumor vs., **767**
- parotid mucoepidermoid carcinoma vs., **769**
- parotid schwannoma vs., **765**
- prognosis, **758**
- recurrent, metastatic disease of parotid nodes vs., **779**
- Warthin tumor vs., **761**

Parotid carcinoma, primary, parotid benign mixed tumor vs., **758**
Parotid duct, **142, 166, 184, 187**
Parotid ductal carcinoma, parotid mucoepidermoid carcinoma vs., **769**
Parotid gland, **142, 147**
- accessory, **184**
- deep lobe, **171, 185, 187**
- superficial lobe, **187**

Parotid gland tail, **51**
Parotid hypoplasia, submandibular gland aplasia-hypoplasia associated, **289**
Parotid malignant mixed tumor, **766–767**
- diagnostic checklist, **767**
- differential diagnosis, **767**
- prognosis, **767**

Parotid malignant tumor, **186**
Parotid mass, TMJ synovial cyst vs., **597**
Parotid metastatic nodal disease
- parotid schwannoma vs., **765**
- Warthin tumor vs., **761**

Parotid metastatic nodes, parotid mucoepidermoid carcinoma vs., **769**
Parotid mucoepidermoid carcinoma, **768–771**
- diagnostic checklist, **770**
- differential diagnosis, **769**
- parotid malignant mixed tumor vs., **767**
- parotid schwannoma vs., **765**
- prognosis, **770**
- staging, grading, & classification, **770**
- Warthin tumor vs., **761**

INDEX

Parotid nodal group, **200**
Parotid nodal metastatic disease, parotid non-Hodgkin lymphoma vs., **775**
Parotid nodes, **201**
- metastatic disease of, **778–781**
  diagnostic checklist, **780**
  differential diagnosis, **779**
  prognosis, **780**
- tail area, **202**
Parotid non-Hodgkin lymphoma, **774–777**
- diagnostic checklist, **776**
- differential diagnosis, **775**
- metastatic disease of parotid nodes vs., **779**
- parotid benign mixed tumor vs., **758**
- parotid mucoepidermoid carcinoma vs., **769**
- prognosis, **776**
- staging, grading, & classification, **776**
- Warthin tumor vs., **761**
Parotid sarcoidosis, benign lymphoepithelial lesions: HIV vs., **751**
Parotid schwannoma, **764–765**
- diagnostic checklist, **765**
- differential diagnosis, **765**
- prognosis, **765**
- staging, grading, & classification, **765**
Parotid sialadenitis, **754–755**
- diagnostic checklist, **755**
- differential diagnosis, **755**
Parotid sialoliths, **784–785**
- diagnostic checklist, **785**
- differential diagnosis, **785**
- prognosis, **785**
Parotid Sjögren syndrome
- benign lymphoepithelial lesions: HIV vs., **751**
- parotid non-Hodgkin lymphoma vs., **775**
Parotid space, **169, 170, 171, 181, 182, 183, 190**
- anatomy, **163, 164, 166, 167**
  imaging anatomy, **162**
Parotid space benign mixed tumor, parotid adenoid cystic carcinoma vs., **773**
Parotid space lesions, **918–921**
- differential diagnosis, **918–919**
Parotid space mucoepidermoid carcinoma, parotid adenoid cystic carcinoma vs., **773**
Parotid space (PS), **184–187**
- anatomy relationships, **184**
- embryology, **184**
- fascia of, **184**
- internal contents, **184**
- normal axial PS CECT, **187**
- normal parotid space, deep lobe mass, **185**
- skull base interaction, facial nerve, perineural tumor, **186**
Parotid tail, **186**
Parotid tumor, malignant, Warthin tumor vs., **761**
Parotitis. *See* Parotid sialadenitis.
Pars nervosa, **110, 114**
- jugular foramen, **111, 112, 113**
Pars vascularis, **110, 114**
- jugular foramen, **111, 113**
Partial agnathia. *See* Condylar aplasia.
PD. *See* Paget disease.
Pediatric orbital lesions, dermoid and epidermoid vs., **285–286**
Pedicle, **157**
Peg-shaped lateral incisors, **220**
Perforated nasal septum, **964–965**
- differential diagnosis, **964**
Periapical cemental dysplasia
- florid osseous dysplasia vs., **433**
- osteoid osteoma vs., **477**
Periapical cyst. *See also* Periapical rarefying osteitis.
- lateral, lateral periodontal cyst vs., **405**
Periapical dysplasia. *See* Periapical osseous dysplasia.
Periapical fibroosteoma. *See* Periapical osseous dysplasia.
Periapical fibrous dysplasia. *See* Periapical osseous dysplasia.
Periapical granuloma. *See* Periapical rarefying osteitis.
Periapical inflammation, mandible-maxilla metastasis vs., **495**
Periapical inflammatory lesion, ill-defined radiolucencies vs., **882, 883**
Periapical osseous dysplasia, **428–431**
- associated abnormalities, **430**
- cemental, cementoblastoma vs., **469**
- diagnostic checklist, **430**
- differential diagnosis, **429–430**
- ground-glass and granular radiopacities vs., **896, 899**
- mandible-maxilla idiopathic osteosclerosis vs., **355**
- mature, hypercementosis vs., **248**
- odontoma vs., **451**
- ossifying fibroma vs., **437**
- periapical radiolucencies vs., **856, 858**
- periapical radiopacities and mixed lesions vs., **860, 861**
- periapical rarefying osteitis vs., **265**
- periapical sclerosing osteitis vs., **269**
- prognosis, **430**
- staging, grading, & classification, **430**
Periapical osteofibrosis. *See* Periapical osseous dysplasia.
Periapical periodontal ligament space, **11**
Periapical (radicular) cyst
- mandible-maxilla simple (traumatic) bone cyst vs., **425**
- nasolabial cyst vs., **423**
- nasopalatine duct cyst vs., **419**
- well-defined unilocular radiolucencies vs., **870, 871**
Periapical radiography, **265**
Periapical radiolucencies, **856–859**
- differential diagnosis, **856–857**
Periapical radiopacities and mixed lesions, **860–861**
- differential diagnosis, **860**
Periapical rarefying osteitis, **17, 264–267**
- central odontogenic fibroma vs., **473**
- diagnostic checklist, **265–266**
- differential diagnosis, **265–266**
- nerve sheath tumor vs., **483**
- periapical radiolucencies vs., **856, 857, 858**
Periapical scar
- periapical radiolucencies vs., **856**
- periapical rarefying osteitis vs., **265–266**
Periapical sclerosing osteitis, **268–269**
- condensing, cementoblastoma vs., **469**
- diagnostic checklist, **269**

- differential diagnosis, **269**
- osteoid osteoma vs., **477**
- periapical radiopacities and mixed lesions vs., **860**
- prognosis, **269**

Pericoronal radiolucencies
- with radiopacities, **876–877**
  differential diagnosis, **876**
- without radiopacities, **874–875**
  differential diagnosis, **874**

Perineural malignancy on mastoid CNVII, **186**
Perineural tumor
- CNV3, masticator space, **742–745**
  diagnostic checklist, **744**
  differential diagnosis, **743–744**
  masticator muscle atrophy vs., **729**
  masticator space CNV3 schwannoma vs., **733**
  masticator space sarcoma vs., **739**
  nerve sheath tumor vs., **483**
  prognosis, **744**
- on mandibular nerve, **182**
- spread along CN5, **125**

Periodontal abscess, **271**
Periodontal bone, anatomy, **5**
Periodontal cyst, lateral, **404–405**
- buccal bifurcation cyst vs., **409**
- central odontogenic fibroma vs., **473**
- diagnostic checklist, **405**
- differential diagnosis, **405**
- mandible-maxilla simple (traumatic) bone cyst vs., **425**
- prognosis, **405**

Periodontal disease, **270–275**
- associated abnormalities, **272**
- diagnostic checklist, **272**
- differential diagnosis, **272**

Periodontal furcation bone loss, **271**
Periodontal ligament, anatomy, **5**
Periodontal ligament space, **10, 11**
- widened, **864–865**
  differential diagnosis, **864**

Periodontal therapy, periodontal disease, **272**
Periodontitis. *See also* Periodontal disease.
- apical, nasopalatine duct cyst vs., **420**
- localized aggressive, Langerhans histiocytosis vs., **535**

Periodontium, anatomy, **5**
Perioendo lesions, **271**
Periosteal new bone, **385**
Periosteal reactions, **906–911**
- differential diagnosis, **906–907**

Peripheral fibroblastoma. *See* Nerve sheath tumor.
Perivertebral space (PVS), **165, 167, 169, 189, 196–199**
- anatomy, imaging anatomy, **162**
- axial and sagittal graphics, **197**
- fascia of, **196**
- generic mass, axial T1 MR tumor graphics, **198**
- normal axial CECT prevertebral space, **199**
- paraspinal component, **163, 165**
- prevertebral component, **163, 165, 193**

Permanent 1st molar, **9**
Permanent central incisor, **9**
Permanent incisors, **9**
Permanent tooth bud, **6**
Perpendicular plate, **102**
Petrooccipital fissure, **108, 111, 114, 117**
Petrosal nerve, greater, as branch of CN7, **138**
Petrotympanic fissure, **88**
Petrous apex, **113, 114, 208**
Petrous apex marrow, **133**
Petrous internal carotid artery, **204**
- horizontal segment, **206**
- vertical segment, **144**

Petrous ridge, **105, 106, 107, 111**
Phakomatosis, **487**
Pharyngeal constrictor muscle, **39**
Pharyngeal mucosal space, **163, 164, 166, 167, 169, 170, 171, 173, 174, 178, 182, 193, 195**
- abuts basisphenoid, **175**
- anatomy, **162**
- benign mixed tumor, non-Hodgkin lymphoma of pharyngeal mucosal space vs., **517**
- mass, **173**
- minor salivary gland malignancy, non-Hodgkin lymphoma of pharyngeal mucosal space vs., **517**
- muscles, anatomy, **172**
- nasopharynx level, **164**
- oropharynx level, **164**

Pharyngeal mucosal space sarcoma, nasopharyngeal carcinoma vs., **709**
Pharyngeal recess/fossa of Rosenmüller, anatomy, **172**
Pharyngobasilar fascia, anatomy, **172**
Pharyngoepiglottic fold, **175**
Phlebolith
- parotid sialoliths vs., **785**
- soft tissue calcifications vs., **935, 937**
- submandibular sialoliths vs., **339**

Phlegmon, oral cavity soft tissue infections, **293**
Phrenic nerve location, **199**
Physiologic tooth wear. *See* Attrition.
Pierre Robin sequence, **366–367**
- clefts associated, **357**
- condylar hypoplasia, **557**
- diagnostic checklist, **367**
- differential diagnosis, **367**
- genetics, **367**
- prognosis, **367**

Pierre Robin syndrome, TMJ juvenile idiopathic arthritis vs., **585**
Pigmented villonodular synovitis, temporomandibular joint, **590–591**
- diagnostic checklist, **591**
- differential diagnosis, **591**
- prognosis, **591**

Pindborg tumor. *See* Calcifying epithelial odontogenic tumor.
Pituitary dwarfism, microdontia vs., **218**
Pituitary gland, **127**
Pituitary macroadenoma, nasopharyngeal carcinoma vs., **709**
Planum sphenoidale, **99, 102**
- of anterior skull base, **98**

Plasma cell granuloma. *See* Invasive pseudotumor.
Plasma cell myeloma. *See* Multiple myeloma.

Plasmacytoma. *See also* Multiple myeloma.
- skull base, nasal lesion with bony destruction vs., **971**
Platysma, **37, 38, 39, 49, 50, 51, 142, 167, 171**
Pleomorphic adenoma. *See* Parotid benign mixed tumor; Submandibular gland benign mixed tumor.
- palate. *See* Palate benign mixed tumor.
- of sublingual gland. *See* Sublingual gland benign mixed tumor.
PM. *See* Premolar.
Pneumatized anterior clinoid, **64**
Pneumatized pterygoid wing, **71**
POD. *See* Periapical osseous dysplasia.
Polypoid sinusitis. *See* Sinonasal polyposis.
Polyposis, sinonasal
- nasal lesion without bony destruction vs., **966, 967**
- paranasal sinus lesions without bony destruction vs., **976, 978**
Polyposis nasi. *See* Sinonasal polyposis.
Polyps, solitary, sinonasal
- nasal lesion without bony destruction vs., **966, 968**
- paranasal sinus lesions without bony destruction vs., **977, 979**
Pons, **132**
Pontic, **16**
Ponticulus posticus, **792–793**
- associated abnormalities, **793**
- diagnostic checklist, **793**
- differential diagnosis, **793**
- staging, grading, & classification, **793**
Pontomedullary junction, **147**
Porcelain crown, **17**
Porcelain fused to metal crown, **17**
Porus acusticus, **111, 113, 117**
- posterior margin, **116**
Porus trigeminus, **126, 132, 133**
Post angled lingual to pulp canal, **17**
Post (dental), **14, 17**
Posterior arch, **152**
- C1, **156, 157, 159**
Posterior atlantodens interval, os odontoideum, **800**
Posterior atlantooccipital membrane, **151**
Posterior auricular artery, **204, 205**
Posterior auricular branch of CNVII, **141, 186**
Posterior auricular nerve, **142**
Posterior band of disc, **86**
Posterior belly of digastric muscle, **119, 163, 167, 191, 195**
- nerve to stylohyoid and, **142**
Posterior body cortical margin, **153**
Posterior C1 arch defect, isolated, split atlas vs., **797**
Posterior cerebral artery, **127**
Posterior cervical space, **163, 167, 197, 199**
Posterior communicating artery, **206**
Posterior composite restoration
- radiolucent, **15**
- radiopaque, **15**
Posterior elements, vertebrae, **197**
Posterior ethmoid air cells, **67, 68, 70, 107**
Posterior ethmoid complex, **69**
Posterior ethmoid drainage, **57**
Posterior ethmoid foramen, **99**
Posterior ethmoids, **75**
Posterior genu, **138**
- cavernous (C4) ICA, **206**
  segment, **207**
- of CNVII, **92, 140, 145**
- of facial nerve canal, **143**
Posterior height of contour, **87**
Posterior longitudinal ligament, **151**
- ossification of, **818–821**
  associated abnormalities, **819**
  diagnostic checklist, **820**
  differential diagnosis, **819**
  genetics, **819**
  prognosis, **820**
  staging, grading, & classification, **819–820**
Posterior median atlantoaxial joint, **151**
Posterior middle meatus, **65**
Posterior nasal cavity, **71, 175**
Posterior neural arch anomalies, failure of segmentation vs., **812**
Posterior semicircular canal, **145**
Posterior skull base (PSB), **105, 110–117**
Posterior slope of eminence, **88**
Posterior stapes crura, **91**
Posterior superior alveolar canal, **59**
Posterior temporal nerve, **85**
Posterior tonsillar pillar, **174**
Posterior tympanic artery, **85**
Posterior wall of maxillary sinus, **60**
Postfunctional dental lamina, **5**
Postobstructive secretions, acute rhinosinusitis vs., **677**
Postsphenoid, **106**
- basisphenoid, **106**
"Poststyloid parapharyngeal space." *See* Parapharyngeal space (PPS).
Posttraumatic blood level, acute rhinosinusitis, **677**
PPF. *See* Pterygopalatine fossa (PPF).
PPS. *See* Parapharyngeal space.
Preaxial acrofacial dysostosis, Treacher Collins syndrome vs., **369**
Prefunctional dental lamina, **5**
Preganglionic segment, **105, 128**
- CNV, **126, 132, 133**
Premolar, **4, 9**
- 2nd, **61**
  branch to, **29**
Prenasal space, **100**
Prepontine cistern, **132**
Presphenoid, **106**
"Prestyloid parapharyngeal space." *See* Parapharyngeal space (PPS).
Prevertebral component, perivertebral space, **167, 178, 193, 194, 195, 197, 198, 199**
Prevertebral muscles, **171, 178, 195, 197, 198, 199**
- anteriorly displaced, **198**
Prevertebral space. *See* Perivertebral space (PVS).
Prevertebral-perivertebral space
- anatomy, **196**
- tumor, **198**
Previous cyst removal, **61**
Primary 1st molar, **9**
Primary bone tumor, tumor calcinosis vs., **841**

INDEX

Primary canine crown, **13**
Primary central incisor, **9**
Primary ciliary dyskinesia, sinonasal polyposis associated, **674**
Primary dentition, **4**
Primary intraalveolar carcinoma. *See* Intraosseous squamous cell carcinoma, primary.
Primary intraosseous carcinoma. *See also* Intraosseous squamous cell carcinoma, primary.
- floating teeth vs., **862, 863**

Primary lateral incisor crown, **13**
Primary malignancy, periodontal disease vs., **272**
Primary odontogenic carcinoma. *See* Intraosseous squamous cell carcinoma, primary.
Primary paranasal granuloma. *See* Fungal sinusitis, invasive.
Primary parotid carcinoma, parotid benign mixed tumor vs., **758**
Procerus, **139**
Progressive condylar resorption, **598–603**
- diagnostic checklist, **599**
- differential diagnosis, **599**
- prognosis, **599**
- small condyle vs., **940, 942**
- TMJ juvenile idiopathic arthritis vs., **585**

Progressive diaphyseal dysplasia, hypoplasia/aplasia associated, **660**
Progressive systemic sclerosis, widened periodontal ligament space vs., **864, 865**
Projected CNVII course, **187**
Proliferative degenerative joint disease, large condyle vs., **946, 947**
Proliferative periostitis. *See also* Osteomyelitis, mandible-maxilla.
- well-defined radiopacities vs., **893, 895**

Prominent zygomatic sutures, zygomaticomaxillary complex fracture vs., **379**
PRS. *See* Pierre Robin sequence.
Prussak space, **90, 91, 92, 93**
PS. *See* Parotid space.
Psammomatoid ossifying fibroma. *See* Sinonasal ossifying fibroma.
PSB. *See* Posterior skull base (PSB).
Pseudocyst, mandible-maxilla aneurysmal bone cyst, **415**
Pseudo-fluid level, acute rhinosinusitis, **677**
Pseudogout. *See* Calcium pyrophosphate dihydrate deposition disease, temporomandibular joint.
Pseudolesion, masticator space, benign masticator muscle hypertrophy vs., **747**
Pseudosarcomatous myofibroblastic proliferation. *See* Invasive pseudotumor.
Pseudosubluxation, **150**
Pseudotumor
- degenerative joint disorders of craniovertebral junction vs., **815–816**
- invasive, **694–695**
  - diagnostic checklist, **695**
  - differential diagnosis, **695**
  - prognosis, **695**

Psoriatic arthritis
- diffuse idiopathic skeletal hyperostosis vs., **823**
- TMJ, rheumatoid arthritis vs., **579**

PT. *See* Palatal torus.
Pterygoid canal, nerve of, **128**
Pterygoid fovea, **32, 82, 88**
Pterygoid plate, **58**
- avulsion, transfacial fracture (Le Fort) vs., **381**
- medial and lateral, **135**

Pterygoid process marrow, **133**
Pterygoid venous plexus
- anatomy, **180**
- asymmetry, masticator space CNV3 perineural tumor vs., **743**

Pterygomandibular raphe, **41, 42, 43, 53, 130, 183**
- anatomy, **40**
  - axial & sagittal graphics, **41**
  - cephalad attachment, **42**
  - inferior attachment, **41**
  - normal axial T2 MR, **42**
  - superior attachment, **41**
- cephalad attachment, **43**

Pterygomaxillary fissure, **29, 64, 65, 69, 78, 79, 102, 107, 108**
Pterygopalatine fossa (PPF), **28, 64, 65, 67, 69, 71, 76–79, 102, 107, 108, 133, 134, 137, 183, 205, 207**
- descending palatine artery in, **205**
- normal axial bone CT of, **78**
- normal coronal bone CT of, **79**
- sagittal graphics, **77**

Pterygopalatine ganglion, **77, 105, 128, 129, 141**
Puffed cheek method, buccal mucosa squamous cell carcinoma, **333**
Pulp, anatomy, **5**
Pulp canal, **10, 11**
- overinstrumentation, internal and external resorption vs., **243**

Pulp chamber, **10, 11**
- elongation of, **223**
- large, in young permanent teeth, internal and external resorption vs., **243**

Pulp horn, **10, 11**
Pulp (root) canal, **11**
Pulp stones, enamel pearls vs., **222**
Pulpal dysplasia, dentin dysplasia vs., **232**
Pulpal sclerosis, root changes vs., **850, 852**
PVS. *See* Perivertebral space.
Pycnodysostosis
- cleidocranial dysplasia vs., **365**
- hypoplasia/aplasia associated, **660**

Pyramidal eminence, **92, 143, 144, 145**

Q

Quadramalar fracture. *See* Zygomaticomaxillary complex fracture.
Quadripod fracture. *See* Zygomaticomaxillary complex fracture.

INDEX

R

Radiation mucositis, oral mucosal space/surface lesions vs., **927, 929**
Radiation necrosis. *See* Osteoradionecrosis, mandible-maxilla.
Radiation osteitis. *See* Osteoradionecrosis, mandible-maxilla.
Radicular abscess. *See* Periapical rarefying osteitis.
Radicular cyst. *See also* Periapical rarefying osteitis.
- encroaching sinus, mucus retention pseudocyst vs., **663**
- lateral
  buccal bifurcation cyst vs., **409**
  lateral periodontal cyst vs., **405**
- odontogenic keratocyst vs., **401**
- well-defined unilocular radiolucencies vs., **870, 871**
Radicular granuloma. *See* Periapical rarefying osteitis.
Radiography, periapical, **265**
Radiolucencies
- ill-defined, **882–887**
  differential diagnosis, **882–883**
- multilocular, **878–881**
  differential diagnosis, **878–879**
Radiolucent fillings, dental caries vs., **261**
Radiopacities, ground-glass and granular, **896–901**
- differential diagnosis, **896–897**
Ramus, **32**
- of mandible, **42, 43, 84, 135, 209**
Ranula, **296–299**
- diagnostic checklist, **298**
- differential diagnosis, **297**
- diving
  submandibular space accessory salivary tissue vs., **281**
  submandibular space lesions vs., **914, 917**
- floor of mouth squamous cell carcinoma vs., **325**
- foregut duplication cyst in tongue vs., **291**
- oral cavity sialocele vs., **303**
- prognosis, **298**
- simple or diving, oral cavity soft tissue infections vs., **293–294**
- staging, grading, & classification, **298**
- sublingual gland benign mixed tumor vs., **307**
- sublingual gland carcinoma vs., **315**
- submandibular gland mucocele vs., **305**
Rapid palatal expander, **18**
Raposo-Amaral system, cherubism, **360**
Rarefying osteitis
- concussion vs., **249**
- periapical. *See* Periapical rarefying osteitis.
Reactive arthritis, diffuse idiopathic skeletal hyperostosis vs., **823**
Reactive lymph nodes
- submandibular gland benign mixed tumor vs., **309**
- submandibular gland carcinoma vs., **317**
- submandibular space lesions vs., **914, 915**
- submandibular space nodal non-Hodgkin lymphoma vs., **319**
Reactive nodal disease, submandibular space, submandibular space accessory salivary tissue vs., **281**
Reciprocal clicking. *See* Disc replacement, with reduction.
Recurrent multifocal osteomyelitis, chronic, generalized radiopacities vs., **902, 904**
Recurrent parotid benign mixed tumor, metastatic disease of parotid nodes vs., **779**
Redlund-Johnell line, **150, 154**
Reduced enamel epithelium, **7**
Reducing displaced disc. *See* Disc replacement, with reduction.
Region of constriction, **179**
Regional nodal drainage, parotid benign mixed tumor vs., **758**
Regional odontodysplasia, **233**
- crown changes vs., **848, 849**
- differential diagnosis, **233**
- segmental odontomaxillary dysplasia vs., **235**
Regressive remodeling, small condyle vs., **940, 942**
Reiter arthritis, diffuse idiopathic skeletal hyperostosis vs., **823**
Relatively even joint space, **87**
Renal osteodystrophy
- lamina dura changes vs., **867**
- periapical radiolucencies vs., **857**
Residual cyst, **406–407**
- diagnostic checklist, **407**
- differential diagnosis, **407**
- mandibular salivary gland defect vs., **351**
- nasopalatine duct cyst vs., **419**
- prognosis, **407**
- well-defined unilocular radiolucencies vs., **870, 871**
Resorption
- external
  abfraction vs., **240**
  erosion vs., **239**
- idiopathic cervical, internal and external resorption vs., **244**
- internal and external, **242–247**
  diagnostic checklist, **244**
  differential diagnosis, **243–244**
  prognosis, **244**
- normal, of primary teeth, internal and external resorption vs., **244**
Retained root tip, well-defined radiopacities vs., **892, 894**
Retention cyst, submandibular gland. *See* Submandibular gland mucocele.
Retroarticular canal. *See* Ponticulus posticus.
Retroarticular vertebral artery ring. *See* Ponticulus posticus.
Retrocondylar vein, **156**
Retrocondylar vertebral artery ring. *See* Ponticulus posticus.
Retrodiscal tissues, **86, 89**
Retromandibular vein, **166, 191**
- anatomy, **184, 185, 187**
Retromaxillary fat pad, **69, 71, 181**
- buccal space, **163, 166, 171**
Retromolar trigone (RMT), **40–43, 52, 53**
- axial & sagittal graphics, RMT & PMR, **41**

- axial T1 MR, **43**
- muscle of, **41**
- normal axial T2 MR pterygomandibular raphe, **42**

Retromolar trigone squamous cell carcinoma, **328–329**
- diagnostic checklist, **329**
- differential diagnosis, **329**
- oral mucosal space/surface lesions vs., **926, 928**
- prognosis, **329**
- staging, grading, & classification, **329**

Retropharyngeal node, **201**
- lateral, **193, 195**
- middle, **193**

Retropharyngeal (RPS) nodal group, **200**

Retropharyngeal space (RPS), **163, 165, 167, 169, 170, 173, 174, 178, 192–195, 197, 198, 199**
- anatomy relationships, **192**
- fascia of, **192**
- fat, **167**
- imaging anatomy, **162**
- internal contents, **192**
- lateral, **191**
- mass, lateral, **193, 194, 195**
  air in, **195**
- normal axial T2 MR, T1 MR, & bone CT, **195**
- normal graphic, RPS mass graphic, **193**
- skull base graphic; sagittal RPS graphic, **194**

Retrozygomatic node, **201**

Rhabdomyosarcoma. *See also* Sarcoma.
- dermoid and epidermoid vs., **285**
- Ewing sarcoma vs., **525**
- neurofibromatosis type 1 vs., **487**
- paranasal sinus lesions with bony destruction vs., **980, 983**
- parotid space lesions vs., **919**
- sinonasal, nasal lesion with bony destruction vs., **971, 973**

Rheumatoid arthritis
- adult, degenerative joint disorders of craniovertebral junction vs., **815**
- small condyle vs., **940–941, 944**
- temporomandibular joint, **578–583**
  associated abnormalities, **579**
  diagnostic checklist, **580**
  differential diagnosis, **579**
  prognosis, **580**
  staging, grading, & classification, **579–580**

Rhinitis, bacterial, nasopalatine duct cyst associated, **420**

Rhinitis medicamentosa, perforated nasal septum vs., **964**

Rhinolith
- nasal lesion without bony destruction vs., **967, 969**
- soft tissue calcifications vs., **935**

Rhinosinusitis
- acute, **676–679**
  associated abnormalities, **677–678**
  chronic rhinosinusitis vs., **681**
  diagnostic checklist, **678**
  differential diagnosis, **677**
  genetics, **677**
  paranasal sinus lesions without bony destruction vs., **976, 978**
  prognosis, **678**
  staging, grading, & classification, **678**
- chronic, **680–683**
  associated abnormalities, **682**
  diagnostic checklist, **682**
  differential diagnosis, **681**
  genetics, **682**
  hypoplasia/aplasia vs., **659**
  invasive pseudotumor vs., **695**
  mycetoma vs., **693**
  paranasal sinus lesions without bony destruction vs., **976, 977**
  prognosis, **682**
  sinonasal granulomatosis with polyangiitis vs., **669**
  sinonasal polyposis associated, **674**
  staging, grading, & classification, **682**
- complicated, invasive fungal sinusitis vs., **689**
- deviated nasal septum associated, **651**

Rib abnormalities, basal cell nevus syndrome associated, **363**

Rickets, lamina dura changes vs., **867, 869**

Ridge augmentation procedure, graft material for, ground-glass and granular radiopacities vs., **896, 898**

Rieger syndrome
- hypodontia vs., **213**
- missing teeth vs., **846, 847**

Right mandibular condyle, **87**

Right maxillary sinus, **58, 63**

Risorius, **139**

RMT. *See* Retromolar trigone.

Robin sequence. *See* Pierre Robin sequence.

Roof of glenoid fossa, **86**

Root, **10**
- anatomy, **5**
- supernumerary, **225**
  differential diagnosis, **225**

Root apex, **17**
- incompletely formed
  periapical radiolucencies vs., **856, 858**
  periapical rarefying osteitis vs., **266**

Root canal filling, **16**
- short of apex, **16**

Root canal overfill, **17**

Root (cemental) caries, root changes vs., **850, 852**

Root changes, **850–853**
- differential diagnosis, **850–851**

Root dilaceration, **224**

Root entry zone, **105, 126, 128, 132**
- CNV, **132**
- lateral pons, **133**

Root fractures, root changes vs., **851, 853**

Root fragment, displaced dental structures into antrum vs., **984**

Root of tongue, **36, 46, 50, 53**
- abscess, **293**
- lesions, **930–933**
  differential diagnosis, **930–931**

Root-filling materials, root changes vs., **850, 851**

Rotundum notch, **79**

Round window membrane, **92**

Round window niche, **145**

RPS. *See* Retropharyngeal space (RPS).

Ruthenium and platinum salts exposure, perforated nasal septum vs., **964**

S

SAC. *See* Spinal accessory chain (SAC).
Sagittal foramen. *See* Ponticulus posticus.
Salivary calculus of parotid. *See* Parotid sialoliths.
Salivary gland malignancy
- minor. *See also* Minor salivary gland malignancy, oral cavity.
  ill-defined radiolucencies vs., **883, 886**
- palatal minor, palate benign mixed tumor vs., **311**
- parotid space lesions vs., **918–919**
Salivary stone. *See* Parotid sialoliths.
Salivary stone/calculus. *See* Submandibular sialoliths.
Sa-MS. *See* Sarcoma, masticator space.
Sarcoidosis
- lymph nodes, submandibular space nodal non-Hodgkin lymphoma vs., **319**
- parotid, benign lymphoepithelial lesions: HIV vs., **751**
- sinonasal
  chronic rhinosinusitis vs., **681**
  invasive pseudotumor vs., **695**
  nasal lesion with bony destruction vs., **970, 973**
  paranasal sinus lesions with bony destruction vs., **980, 982**
  perforated nasal septum vs., **964, 965**
  sinonasal granulomatosis with polyangiitis vs., **669**
  sinonasal polyposis vs., **673**
- Sjögren syndrome vs., **783**
Sarcoma
- cervical facet arthropathy vs., **827**
- chondrogenic. *See* Chondrosarcoma, mandible-maxilla.
- masticator space, **738–741**
  benign masticator muscle hypertrophy vs., **747**
  diagnostic checklist, **740**
  differential diagnosis, **739**
  genetics, **739**
  masticator space abscess vs., **725**
  masticator space CNV3 schwannoma vs., **733**
  prognosis, **740**
  staging, grading, & classification, **740**
- osteogenic. *See also* Osteosarcoma, mandible-maxilla.
  ossifying fibroma vs., **437**
- synovial, Ewing sarcoma vs., **525**
Scalene muscle
- anterior, **199**
- middle, **199**
SCCa. *See* Squamous cell carcinoma.
Scheuthauer-Marie-Sainton syndrome. *See* Cleidocranial dysplasia.
Schizodontia. *See* Macrodontia.
Schneiderian papilloma. *See* Sinonasal inverted papilloma.
Schwannoma. *See also* Nerve sheath tumor.
- CNV3
  masticator space, **732–733**
  in MS, masticator space CNV3 perineural tumor vs., **743**
- neurofibromatosis type 1 vs., **487**
- parotid, **764–765**
  diagnostic checklist, **765**
  differential diagnosis, **765**
  prognosis, **765**
  staging, grading, & classification, **765**
- parotid space lesions vs., **919, 921**
Scleroderma, widened periodontal ligament space vs., **864, 865**
Sclerosing bone dysplasias, generalized radiopacities vs., **903**
Sclerosing cementoma. *See* Periapical osseous dysplasia.
Sclerosing osteitis, **265**. *See also* Periapical sclerosing osteitis.
- hypercementosis vs., **248**
- mandible-maxilla idiopathic osteosclerosis vs., **355**
- mandible-maxilla osteoma vs., **481**
- odontoma vs., **452**
- periapical, osteoid osteoma vs., **477**
Sclerosing osteomyelitis, chronic. *See* Osteomyelitis, mandible-maxilla.
Sclerotic cemental masses. *See* Florid osseous dysplasia.
Sclerotic metastases. *See* Blastic metastases.
Scutum, **91, 92, 146**
Sealer cement, **14**
2nd branchial cleft cyst, submandibular space lesions vs., **915**
2nd molar, developing root of, **13**
2nd premolar, **13**
Secondary hyperparathyroidism, generalized radiopacities vs., **902, 905**
Secondary malignancy. *See* Metastasis, mandible-maxilla; Metastasis, temporomandibular joint.
Secondary SMG sialadenitis, **301**
Segmental hemifacial hyperplasia, segmental odontomaxillary dysplasia vs., **235**
Segmental odontomaxillary dysplasia (SOD), **234–235**
- diagnostic checklist, **235**
- differential diagnosis, **235**
- prognosis, **235**
- staging, grading, & classification, **235**
Segmental spinal dysgenesis, failure of formation vs., **808**
Segmentation and fusion anomaly. *See* Failure of formation; Failure of segmentation.
Segmentation anomaly. *See* Failure of segmentation.
Sella, **101**
Sella turcica, **208**
- of central skull base, **104**
Senile ankylosing hyperostosis. *See* Diffuse idiopathic skeletal hyperostosis.
Septal spine, anterior, **24**
Septal tubercle, deviated nasal septum vs., **651**
Septic facet
- cervical facet arthropathy vs., **827**
- tumor calcinosis vs., **841**
Septum, **62**
- fracture, deviated nasal septum vs., **651**
- nasopalatine nerve heading to, **128**

Sequelae of discitis, chronic
- C2-C3 fusion vs., **789**
- failure of segmentation vs., **811**

SFA (segmentation and fusion anomaly). *See* Failure of formation; Failure of segmentation.
Shadow of nose, **11**
Shadow of soft palate, **33**
SHN. *See* Suprahyoid neck.
Short ciliary nerve, **128**
Short process of incus, **143**
- in fossa incudius, **92**

Short roots, root changes vs., **851**
Sialadenitis
- parotid, **754–755**
    - diagnostic checklist, **755**
    - differential diagnosis, **755**
- sublingual gland, sublingual space lesions vs., **922, 924**
- submandibular gland, **300–301**
    - diagnostic checklist, **301**
    - differential diagnosis, **301**
    - submandibular gland benign mixed tumor vs., **309**
    - submandibular gland carcinoma vs., **317**
    - submandibular space lesions vs., **914, 916**

Sialadenosis, **301**
Sialocele. *See also* Submandibular gland mucocele.
- oral cavity, **302–303**
    - diagnostic checklist, **303**
    - differential diagnosis, **303**
    - prognosis, **303**
    - ranula vs., **297**
- oral cavity soft tissue infections vs., **294**

Sialolithiasis, **301**. *See also* Parotid sialoliths; Submandibular sialoliths.
- submandibular gland aplasia-hypoplasia associated, **289**

Sialoliths
- parotid, **784–785**
    - diagnostic checklist, **785**
    - differential diagnosis, **785**
    - prognosis, **785**
- soft tissue calcifications vs., **934, 936**
- submandibular, **338–339**
    - diagnostic checklist, **339**
    - differential diagnosis, **339**
- submandibular gland mucocele associated, **305**
- in Wharton duct, mandibular torus vs., **345**

Sicca syndrome. *See* Sjögren syndrome.
Sickle cell anemia
- generalized rarefaction vs., **888, 891**
- hypoplasia/aplasia associated, **660**

Sigmoid plate, **113**
Sigmoid sinus, **112, 113, 114, 190**
- groove for, **110**

"Signal" (Virchow) node, **200**
Silent sinus syndrome
- hypoplasia/aplasia vs., **659**
- paranasal sinus lesions without bony destruction vs., **977**

Simple bone cyst
- nerve sheath tumor vs., **483**
- odontogenic keratocyst vs., **401**
- periapical osseous dysplasia associated, **430**
- sinonasal fibrous dysplasia associated, **716**
- sinonasal ossifying fibroma associated, **720**
- TMJ radiolucencies vs., **954, 955**

Simple odontogenic fibroma. *See* Central odontogenic fibroma.
Simple ranula. *See also* Ranula.
- oral cavity soft tissue infections vs., **293–294**
- sublingual space lesions vs., **922, 923**

Simple (traumatic) bone cyst
- desmoplastic fibroma vs., **491**
- lateral periodontal cyst vs., **405**
- mandible-maxilla, **424–427**
    - associated abnormalities, **425**
    - differential diagnosis, **425**
    - prognosis, **425**
- multiple myeloma vs., **521**
- temporomandibular joint, **642–643**
    - differential diagnosis, **643**
    - prognosis, **643**
- well-defined unilocular radiolucencies vs., **870–871, 872**

Simulated crown, **20**
Simulated implant, **20**
Single gene defects, clefts, **357**
Sinolith, paranasal sinus lesions without bony destruction vs., **977**
Sinonasal anatomy, overview, **56–71**
- anatomy relationships, **56**
- axial bone CT, **69**
- axial T1 MR, **70–71**
- coronal bone CT, **64–66**
- graphics, **57–58**
- maxillary sinus variations, **59–61**
- sagittal bone CT, **67–68**
- sinonasal variations, **62–63**

Sinonasal fibroosseous and cartilaginous lesions, **974–975**
- differential diagnosis, **974**

Sinonasal inverted papilloma, **696–699**
- associated abnormalities, **698**
- diagnostic checklist, **698**
- differential diagnosis, **697–698**
- mycetoma vs., **693**
- prognosis, **698**
- staging, grading, & classification, **698**

Sinonasal mucocele, **664–667**
- allergic fungal sinusitis vs., **687**
- associated abnormalities, **666**
- diagnostic checklist, **666**
- differential diagnosis, **665**
- mycetoma vs., **693**
- prognosis, **666**
- staging, grading, & classification, **666**

Sinonasal ossifying fibroma, **718–721**
- associated abnormalities, **720**
- diagnostic checklist, **720**
- differential diagnosis, **719**
- prognosis, **720**
- sinonasal osteoma vs., **701**
- staging, grading, & classification, **720**

Sinonasal polyposis, **672–675**
- allergic fungal sinusitis vs., **687**
- associated abnormalities, **674**

- chronic rhinosinusitis vs., **681**
- diagnostic checklist, **674**
- differential diagnosis, **673**
- genetics, **674**
- prognosis, **674**
- sinonasal inverted papilloma vs., **697**
- sinonasal mucocele vs., **665**

Sinonasal solitary polyps
- allergic fungal sinusitis vs., **687**
- sinonasal inverted papilloma vs., **697**
- sinonasal mucocele vs., **665**
- sinonasal polyposis vs., **673**

Sinonasal squamous cell carcinoma, hard palate squamous cell carcinoma vs., **335**
Sinuous canal, **28, 136**
- containing anterior superior alveolar nerve, **136**

Sinus
- dentigerous cyst encroaching, mucus retention pseudocyst vs., **663**
- malignant neoplasm, mucus retention pseudocyst vs., **663**
- radicular cyst encroaching, mucus retention pseudocyst vs., **663**

Sinus confluence (torcular Herophili), **112**
Sinus fungal mycetoma, allergic fungal sinusitis vs., **687**
Sinus loculation, **61**
Sinus opacification, transfacial fracture (Le Fort), **381**
Sinus septum, **59**
Sinus tract
- accessory mandibular canal vs., **349**
- gubernaculum dentis vs., **277**

Sinus tympani, **92, 143, 144, 145**
Sinusitis
- mucus retention pseudocyst vs., **663**
- nonodontogenic origin, odontogenic sinusitis vs., **685**

Sjögren syndrome, **782–783**
- differential diagnosis, **783**
- non-Hodgkin lymphoma of pharyngeal space associated, **518**
- parotid
  - benign lymphoepithelial lesions: HIV vs., **751**
  - metastatic disease of parotid nodes vs., **779**
  - parotid non-Hodgkin lymphoma vs., **775**
- parotid sialadenitis vs., **755**
- prognosis, **783**
- staging, grading, & classification, **783**

Skeletal hyperostosis, diffuse idiopathic, **822–825**
- associated abnormalities, **823–824**
- diagnostic checklist, **824**
- differential diagnosis, **823**
- prognosis, **824**
- staging, grading, & classification, **824**

Skull base, anatomy
- anterior, **98–103**
  - axial bone CT, **101**
  - bony landmarks of, **98**
  - coronal bone CT, **102**
  - development of, **98**
  - foramina and fissures of, **98**
  - graphics, **99–100**
- central, **104–109**
  - axial bone CT, **107–108**
  - bony landmarks of, **104**
  - coronal bone CT, **109**
  - development of, **104**
  - graphics, **105–106**
  - variant anatomy, **104**
- posterior, **110–117**
  - axial bone CT, **113–115**
  - bony landmarks of, **110**
  - coronal bone CT, **116–117**
  - development of, **110**
  - foramina and fissures of, **110**
  - graphic and MR of dural sinuses, **112**
  - graphics, **111**
  - variant anatomy of, **110**

Skull base marrow around foramen ovale, masticator space CNV3 perineural tumor vs., **744**
Skull base meningioma, masticator space CNV3 perineural tumor vs., **744**
SLS. *See* Sublingual space.
Small condyle, **940–945**
- differential diagnosis, **940–941**

Small noncleaved cell lymphoma. *See* Burkitt lymphoma.
SMS. *See* Submandibular space.
Snow-capped patterns, amelogenesis imperfecta and, **228**
SOD. *See* Segmental odontomaxillary dysplasia.
Soft odontoma. *See* Ameloblastic fibroma.
Soft palate, **137, 175, 176, 177, 179**
- of tongue, **39**

Soft tissue calcifications, **934–937**
- differential diagnosis, **934–935**

Soft tissue infections, oral cavity, **292–295**
- diagnostic checklist, **294**
- differential diagnosis, **293–294**

Soft tissue structures, superimposition of, dentoalveolar fractures vs., **255**
Solitary bone cyst. *See* Simple (traumatic) bone cyst, mandible-maxilla; Simple (traumatic) bone cyst, temporomandibular joint.
Solitary tract nucleus, **138, 140**
- taste, **140**

Space maintainer, **14**
Sphenoethmoidal cells (Onodi), sinonasal overview, **56**
Sphenoethmoidal recess, **57, 65, 68, 75**
Sphenoid body, **107, 109**
Sphenoid bone, **100, 115, 174**
- lesser wing, of anterior skull base, **98**

Sphenoid ostium, **57**
Sphenoid sinus, **57, 64, 65, 67, 68, 69, 70, 75, 78, 79, 99, 101, 102, 103, 107, 127, 134, 177, 179, 208, 209**
- drainage, **57**
- extensive pneumatization, **104**
- sinonasal overview, **56**

Sphenomandibular ligament, **85**
Sphenooccipital fissure, **134**
Sphenooccipital synchondrosis, **106, 107, 108, 113, 114**
Sphenopalatine artery, **205**
Sphenopalatine foramen, **57, 64, 71, 78, 79, 102, 108**
Sphenopalatine fossa. *See* Pterygopalatine fossa (PPF).
Spinal accessory chain (SAC), **200**

INDEX

Spinal accessory lymph nodes, low, **201**
Spinal accessory nodal group, **201**
Spinal accessory nodes, **201**
- level VA, **202**
Spinal canal, **157**
Spinal dysplasias, inherited, failure of formation vs., **807**
Spinal nucleus CNV, **126**
Spinal radiation treatment, hemangioma, cervical spine vs., **831**
Spindle cell pseudotumor. *See* Invasive pseudotumor.
Spinous process, **153, 157**
- C2, **159**
Split atlas, **796–797**
- associated abnormalities, **797**
- diagnostic checklist, **797**
- differential diagnosis, **797**
- prognosis, **797**
Split C1. *See* Split atlas.
Split notochord syndromes, failure of formation vs., **807**
Split palatal suture, **18**
Spondylodiscitis, lytic and blastic metastases vs., **836**
Spondylosis
- diffuse idiopathic skeletal hyperostosis vs., **823**
- ossification of posterior longitudinal ligament vs., **819**
Squamotympanic fissure, **88**
Squamous cell carcinoma
- buccal mucosa, **332–333**
  diagnostic checklist, **333**
  differential diagnosis, **333**
  prognosis, **333**
  retromolar trigone squamous cell carcinoma vs., **329**
  staging, grading, & classification, **333**
- floor of mouth, **324–325**
  differential diagnosis, **325**
  prognosis, **325**
  root of tongue lesions vs., **930, 932**
  staging, grading, & classification, **325**
  sublingual gland carcinoma vs., **315**
  sublingual space lesions vs., **922, 924**
- gingival, **326–327**
  diagnostic checklist, **327**
  differential diagnosis, **327**
  prognosis, **327**
  staging, grading, & classification, **327**
- hard palate, **334–335**
  diagnostic checklist, **335**
  differential diagnosis, **335**
  palate benign mixed tumor vs., **311**
  prognosis, **335**
  staging, grading, & classification, **335**
- intraalveolar, ill-defined radiolucencies vs., **882, 884**
- invasive, masticator space sarcoma vs., **739**
- Langerhans histiocytosis vs., **535**
- lingual tonsil, motor denervation CNXII vs., **337**
- mandible-maxilla osteomyelitis vs., **385**
- masticator space, benign masticator muscle hypertrophy vs., **747**
- nodal, submandibular space lesions vs., **914, 915, 916**
- nodal metastases, submandibular gland sialadenitis vs., **301**
- oral cavity minor salivary gland malignancy vs., **313**
- oral tongue, **320–323**
  diagnostic checklist, **322**
  differential diagnosis, **321**
  floor of mouth squamous cell carcinoma vs., **325**
  genetics, **321**
  invasive, sublingual space lesions vs., **922, 924**
  invasive into submandibular space, submandibular space lesions vs., **915**
  motor denervation CNXII vs., **337**
  oral cavity soft tissue infections vs., **294**
  prognosis, **322**
  root of tongue lesions vs., **930, 932**
  staging, grading, & classification, **321–322**
- parotid space lesions vs., **919**
- pterygomandibular raphe, **40**
- retromolar trigone, **328–329**
  diagnostic checklist, **329**
  differential diagnosis, **329**
  prognosis, **329**
  staging, grading, & classification, **329**
- sinonasal, **704–705**
  diagnostic checklist, **705**
  differential diagnosis, **705**
  hard palate squamous cell carcinoma vs., **335**
  invasive fungal sinusitis vs., **689**
  invasive pseudotumor vs., **695**
  nasal lesion with bony destruction vs., **970, 971**
  paranasal sinus lesions with bony destruction vs., **980, 981**
  perforated nasal septum vs., **964, 965**
  prognosis, **705**
  sinonasal adenoid cystic carcinoma vs., **707**
  sinonasal inverted papilloma vs., **697**
  sinonasal malignant melanoma vs., **713**
- submandibular space nodal, **330–331**
  diagnostic checklist, **331**
  differential diagnosis, **331**
  prognosis, **331**
  submandibular gland carcinoma vs., **317**
Squamous cell papilloma. *See* Sinonasal inverted papilloma.
Squamous odontogenic tumor, buccal bifurcation cyst vs., **410**
Squamous portion of temporal bone, **86**
SS. *See* Sjögren syndrome.
SSD. *See* Segmental spinal dysgenesis.
Stafne bone cyst/cavity. *See* Mandibular salivary gland defect (Stafne).
Stapedius head, **92**
Stapedius muscle, **144**
- anatomy, **90, 92**
Stapedius nerve, **141, 186**
- greater, as branch of CN7, **138**
Stapes, anatomy, **90**
Stapes anterior crura, **93**
Stapes footplate, **91, 92**
Stapes head, **91, 93**
Stapes posterior crus, **92**
Static bone cavity. *See* Mandibular salivary gland defect (Stafne).
Stellate reticulum, **6**

INDEX

Sternocleidomastoid, **51, 142, 167, 170, 187, 199, 202, 209**
Stickler and related syndromes, Pierre Robin sequence vs., **367**
Straight sinus, **112**
Stratum intermedium, **6**
Stylocarotid artery syndrome, **118**
Styloglossus, **119, 171**
- anatomy, **36, 38, 39**
Stylohyoid, **38, 119**
- ligament, anatomy, **118–121**
Styloid process, **84, 88, 115, 119, 120, 156, 166, 171, 185, 186, 187, 189, 190, 191, 209**
- anatomy, **118–121**
  3D CT, panoramic, **120**
  graphics, **119**
  panoramic, CBCT, **121**
- elongated, and Eagle syndrome, **118**
- inferior tip, **191**
Stylomandibular gap, **185**
Stylomandibular ligament, **85, 119**
Stylomastoid foramen, **88, 110, 115, 116, 140, 144, 145, 170, 186, 187**
- CNVII, **142, 164**
- fat, **141, 186**
Stylopharyngeus muscle, **38, 39, 119, 171**
Subchondral sclerosis
- TMJ radiopacities vs., **956, 957**
- TMJ rheumatoid arthritis vs., **579**
Sublingual gland, **45, 53, 129, 141**
- and ducts, anatomy, **44**
- mucocele. *See* Ranula.
- mucus retention cyst. *See* Ranula.
- pleomorphic adenoma of. *See* Sublingual gland benign mixed tumor.
- transoral excision, **298**
Sublingual gland benign mixed tumor, **306–307**
- diagnostic checklist, **307**
- differential diagnosis, **307**
Sublingual gland carcinoma, **314–315**
- diagnostic checklist, **315**
- differential diagnosis, **315**
- floor of mouth squamous cell carcinoma vs., **325**
- prognosis, **315**
- staging, grading, & classification, **315**
Sublingual sialocele. *See* Sialocele, oral cavity.
Sublingual space epidermoid, oral cavity sialocele vs., **303**
Sublingual space sialocele, sublingual space lesions vs., **922–923, 924**
Sublingual space (SLS), **39, 44–47, 46, 49, 53**
- abscess, **293, 294**
- anatomy relationship, **44**
- axial graphic, normal axial CECT of, **45**
- coronal graphic, normal coronal T1 MR of, **46**
- internal contents, **44**
- lesions, **922–925**
  differential diagnosis, **922–923**
- normal axial CECT of, **46**
- oral cavity abscess in, oral cavity sialocele vs., **303**
- pediatric lesions, dermoid and epidermoid vs., **285**
Subluxation. *See also* Temporomandibular joint, dislocation.
- luxation vs., **251**
Submandibular duct, **32, 53, 129**
- dilation of, oral cavity soft tissue infections vs., **294**
Submandibular duct injury, **303**
Submandibular duct (SMD) sialocele. *See* Sialocele, oral cavity.
Submandibular ganglion, **129, 141**
Submandibular gland, **46, 51, 129, 141, 167, 171, 191, 199, 202, 203**
- anatomy, submandibular space, **48**
- deep portion, **45, 46, 49, 51**
  anatomy, sublingual space, **44**
- superficial portion, **45, 46, 49, 50**
Submandibular gland aplasia-hypoplasia, **288–289**
- associated abnormalities, **289**
- diagnostic checklist, **289**
- genetics, **289**
- prognosis, **289**
Submandibular gland benign mixed tumor, **308–309**
- diagnostic checklist, **309**
- differential diagnosis, **309**
- prognosis, **309**
- submandibular gland carcinoma vs., **317**
- submandibular gland sialadenitis vs., **301**
Submandibular gland carcinoma, **316–317**
- diagnostic checklist, **317**
- differential diagnosis, **317**
- staging, grading, & classification, **317**
- submandibular gland benign mixed tumor vs., **309**
- submandibular gland sialadenitis vs., **301**
Submandibular gland duct, sublingual space, anatomy, **44**
Submandibular gland fossa, **35**
Submandibular gland mucocele, **304–305**
- associated abnormalities, **305**
- diagnostic checklist, **305**
- differential diagnosis, **305**
- prognosis, **305**
- ranula vs., **297**
- submandibular gland benign mixed tumor vs., **309**
- submandibular gland carcinoma vs., **317**
- submandibular space accessory salivary tissue vs., **281**
Submandibular gland sialadenitis, **300–301**
- diagnostic checklist, **301**
- differential diagnosis, **301**
- submandibular gland benign mixed tumor vs., **309**
- submandibular gland carcinoma vs., **317**
Submandibular gland (SMG) retention cyst. *See* Submandibular gland mucocele.
Submandibular lymph nodes, **201**
Submandibular nodal groups, submandibular space, **48**
Submandibular node, **49, 50, 51**
- level IB, **201, 202, 203**
Submandibular sialoliths, **338–339**
- diagnostic checklist, **339**
- differential diagnosis, **339**
Submandibular space, **44, 45, 46, 48–51, 53, 163, 164, 165, 169, 170**
- abscess, **293, 294**
  submandibular space accessory salivary tissue vs., **281**

INDEX

- anatomy relationships, **48**
- axial graphic, normal axial T2 MR, **49**
- coronal graphic, normal coronal T1 MR, **50**
- internal contents, **48**
- lymphatic malformation, submandibular space accessory salivary tissue vs., **281**
- nodal non-Hodgkin lymphoma of, submandibular space nodal squamous cell carcinoma vs., **331**
- nodal squamous cell carcinoma, **330–331**
  diagnostic checklist, **331**
  differential diagnosis, **331**
  prognosis, **331**
  submandibular gland benign mixed tumor vs., **309**
  submandibular gland carcinoma vs., **317**
  submandibular space nodal non-Hodgkin lymphoma vs., **319**
- normal axial CECT suprahyoid SMS, **51**
- pediatric lesions, dermoid and epidermoid vs., **285**
- reactive nodal disease, submandibular space accessory salivary tissue vs., **281**

Submandibular space accessory salivary tissue, **280–281**
- diagnostic checklist, **281**
- differential diagnosis, **281**
- submandibular space lesions vs., **914, 916**

Submandibular space lesions, **914–917**
- differential diagnosis, **914–915**

Submandibular space nodal non-Hodgkin lymphoma, **318–319**
- associated abnormalities, **319**
- diagnostic checklist, **319**
- differential diagnosis, **319**
- prognosis, **319**

Submaxillary space. *See* Submandibular space.
Submental lymph nodes, **201**
Submental nodal groups, submandibular space, **48**
Submental nodes, level IA, **201, 202**
Suboccipital venous plexus, **112**
Summit of eminence, **88**
Superficial layer, deep cervical fascia, **164, 165, 185**
Superficial temporal artery, **85, 204, 205**
Superimposition, of soft tissue structures, dentoalveolar fractures vs., **255**
Superior alveolar artery, **205**
Superior alveolar canal
- anterior, **28**
- posterior, **29**

Superior alveolar foramen, posterior, **26**
- V2, **24**

Superior articular facet, **152, 153**
- C1, **156**
- C2, **157**

Superior articular process, C3, **157**
Superior cerebellar artery, **127**
Superior constrictor muscle, **43, 53, 171, 173**
Superior cortex of anterior arch C1, **156**
Superior extension cruciate ligament, **151**
Superior hypophyseal arteries, **206**
Superior lamina, posterior attachment, **86**
Superior malleal ligament, **94**
Superior mediastinal nodes, **201**
Superior orbital fissure, **64, 79, 101, 105, 107, 134, 208**
- CNV1, CNIII, CNIV, & CNVI, **134**

Superior petrosal sinus, **112**
Superior pharyngeal constrictor muscle, **41, 42, 119, 130, 173, 174**
Superior posterior lateral nasal branches, **128**
Superior sagittal sinus, **112**
Superior salivatory nucleus, **138, 140**
- parasympathetic, **140**

Superior semicircular canal, **146**
Superior thyroid artery, **204, 205**
Superior turbinate, **75**
- attachment, **57**
- cut margin, **73**

Superior vestibular nerve, **147**
Supernumerary cusp, **220**
Supernumerary impacted tooth, **12**
Supernumerary microdont, enamel pearls vs., **222**
Supernumerary roots, **225**
- differential diagnosis, **225**
- root changes vs., **851, 853**

Supernumerary teeth, **220**. *See also* Hyperdontia.
- cleidocranial dysplasia, **365**
- odontoma vs., **451**

Supplementary ostia. *See* Accessory ostia.
Suppurative lymph nodes
- ranula vs., **297**
- submandibular space lesions vs., **915, 917**
- submandibular space nodal squamous cell carcinoma vs., **331**

Suppurative osteomyelitis, acute. *See* Osteomyelitis, mandible-maxilla.
Suprahyoid internal jugular vein, **190**
Suprahyoid neck, **162, 165, 188**
- anatomy
  external and internal carotid arteries, **204–209**
  lymph nodes, **200–203**
  masticator space, **180–183**
  nasopharynx and oropharynx, **172–179**
  parotid space, **184–187**
  perivertebral space, **196–199**
  retropharyngeal space, **192–195**
- carotid space, **188–191**
- overview, **162–167**
  axial & coronal skull base-space interactions graphics, **164**
  axial CECT images of normal suprahyoid neck, **166–167**
  axial nasopharynx & oropharynx space graphics, **163**
  key spatial relationships, **162**
  sagittal & 3D longitudinal spatial relationships graphics, **165**
  spaces of suprahyoid and infrahyoid neck, **162**

Suprahyoid thyroglossal duct cyst, foregut duplication cyst in tongue vs., **291**
Supraorbital nerve, **105, 128**
Suprazygomatic masticator space, **164**
Surgical bur, displaced dental structures into antrum vs., **984, 986**
Surgical ciliated cyst, residual cyst vs., **407**

Surgical defect
- accessory ostia vs., **657**
- periodontal disease vs., **272**
Surgical fusion
- C2-C3 fusion vs., **789**
- failure of segmentation vs., **811**
Surgical odontoid resection, odontoid hypoplasia/aplasia vs., **805**
Surgical screws and hardware, displaced dental structures into antrum vs., **984**
Sympathetic chain, **197**
Sympathetic plexus, **189**
Sympathetic trunk, **189**
Synovial chondromatosis
- calcium pyrophosphate dihydrate deposition disease vs., **627**
- disc replacement with reduction vs., **605**
- primary, temporomandibular joint, **630–633**
  diagnostic checklist, **632**
  differential diagnosis, **631**
  prognosis, **632**
  staging, grading, & classification, **631**
- temporomandibular joint, masticator space chondrosarcoma vs., **735**
- TMJ articular loose bodies vs., **960, 961**
- TMJ chondrosarcoma vs., **637**
- TMJ juvenile idiopathic arthritis vs., **585**
- TMJ osteochondritis dissecans vs., **577**
- TMJ pigmented villonodular synovitis vs., **591**
- TMJ synovial cyst vs., **597**
Synovial chondrometaplasia. *See* Synovial chondromatosis, temporomandibular joint.
Synovial chondrosis. *See* Synovial chondromatosis, temporomandibular joint.
Synovial cyst
- temporomandibular joint, **596–597**
  differential diagnosis, **597**
- tumor calcinosis vs., **841**
Synovial osteochondromatosis, tumor calcinosis vs., **841**
Synovial sarcoma. *See also* Sarcoma.
- Ewing sarcoma vs., **525**
Synovitis, TMJ juvenile idiopathic arthritis vs., **585**
Syphilis, perforated nasal septum vs., **964**
Syringe needle, displaced dental structures into antrum vs., **984**
Systemic nodal metastases, parotid benign mixed tumor vs., **758**

T

T3 vertebral body, **165**
Talon cusp, **220**
Tapering cortex, **87**
Taurodont, **223**
Taurodontism, **223**
T-bone. *See* Temporal bone.
TCS. *See* Treacher Collins syndrome.
Tectorial membrane, anatomy, **150, 151, 159**
Teeth, **4–13**
- abfraction, abrasion vs., **238**
- anatomy
  mandible, **30–35**
  maxilla, **22–29**
  oral mucosal space/surface, **52–53**
  relationships, **4**
  retromolar trigone, **40–43**
  sublingual space, **44–47**
  submandibular space, **48–51**
  tongue, **36–39**
- attrition, **236–237**
  abrasion vs., **238**
  differential diagnosis, **237**
- cementum, **5**
- concrescence, **219**
- concussion, **249**
  luxation vs., **251**
- crown, **5**
- dens invaginatus, **221**
- dental anatomy graphic, **10**
- dental caries, **260–263**
- dentin, **4–5**
- dentoalveolar fractures, **254–259**
- devitalization of, **266**
- dilacerated, hypercementosis vs., **248**
- dilaceration, **224**
- double. *See* Macrodontia
- enamel, **4**
- enamel pearls, **222**
- eruption graphic, **7**
- eruption patterns, **4**
- human dentitions scan, **9**
- impactions graphic, **12–13**
- luxation, **250–253**
  diagnostic checklist, **251**
  differential diagnosis, **251**
  extrusive, concussion vs., **249**
  prognosis, **251**
- microdontia, **218**
- nomenclature and eruption ages, **8**
- numbering, **4**
- periapical rarefying osteitis, **264–267**
- periodontal disease, **270–275**
- periodontium, **5**
- pulp, **5**
- radiographic anatomy, **11**
- regional odontodysplasia, **233**
- root, **5**
- supernumerary roots, **225**
- talon cusp, **220**
- taurodontism, **223**
- tooth development and tumorigenesis, **5**
- tooth development graphic, **6**
- Turner dysplasia, **241**
Tegmen tympani, **90, 117, 145, 146**
Temporal bone, **90**
- anatomy, external, middle, and inner ear, **90–95**
- zygomatic process of, **119**
Temporal branch of CNVII, **141, 142, 186**
Temporal lobe of brain, **89**

INDEX

Temporal nerves, anterior and posterior, **131**
Temporalis, **42, 129, 130, 131, 133, 166**
- anatomy, **181, 182, 183**
- fascia, **142**
- tendon, **43, 183**

Temporary filling, **15**
Temporomandibular component, congenital malformations of, submandibular gland aplasia-hypoplasia associated, **289**
Temporomandibular joint (TMJ), **82–89, 114**
- 3D-VRT bone CT, **84**
- adhesions, **616–617**
  - diagnostic checklist, **617**
  - differential diagnosis, **617**
  - prognosis, **617**
  - staging, grading, & classification, **617**
- aneurysmal bone cyst, **644–647**
  - diagnostic checklist, **645**
  - differential diagnosis, **645**
  - prognosis, **645**
  - TMJ osteosarcoma vs., **635**
- bifid condyle, **572–575**
  - diagnostic checklist, **573**
  - differential diagnosis, **573**
  - prognosis, **573**
- bony ankylosis, **562–563**
  - differential diagnosis, **563**
  - prognosis, **563**
  - staging, grading, & classification, **563**
- calcium pyrophosphate dihydrate deposition disease, **626–629**
  - associated abnormalities, **628**
  - diagnostic checklist, **628**
  - differential diagnosis, **627**
  - prognosis, **628**
  - staging, grading, & classification, **628**
- CBCT of normal, **87–88**
- chondrosarcoma, **636–639**
  - calcium pyrophosphate dihydrate deposition disease vs., **627**
  - diagnostic checklist, **638**
  - differential diagnosis, **637**
  - prognosis, **638**
  - staging, grading, & classification, **638**
  - TMJ osteochondroma vs., **621**
  - TMJ osteosarcoma vs., **635**
- compartments, **82**
- condylar aplasia, **540–541**
  - associated abnormalities, **541**
  - diagnostic checklist, **541**
  - differential diagnosis, **541**
  - prognosis, **541**
- condylar hyperplasia, **546–551**
  - diagnostic checklist, **548**
  - differential diagnosis, **547–548**
  - prognosis, **548**
- condylar hypoplasia, **556–559**
  - condylar hyperplasia vs., **547**
  - diagnostic checklist, **557**
  - differential diagnosis, **557**
  - prognosis, **557**
  - TMJ fractures vs., **565**
- coronoid, TMJ osteochondroma vs., **621**
- coronoid hyperplasia, **552–555**
  - associated abnormalities, **553**
  - diagnostic checklist, **553**
  - differential diagnosis, **553**
  - prognosis, **553**
- degenerative disease, TMJ primary synovial chondromatosis vs., **631**
- degenerative joint disease, **592–595**
  - diagnostic checklist, **593**
  - differential diagnosis, **593**
  - prognosis, **593**
- disc derangement with reduction, disc displacement without reduction vs., **612**
- disc displacement without reduction, **610–615**
  - differential diagnosis, **612**
  - prognosis, **612**
  - staging, grading, & classification, **612**
- disc replacement with reduction, **604–609**
  - diagnostic checklist, **606**
  - differential diagnosis, **605**
  - prognosis, **606**
  - staging, grading, & classification, **606**
- dislocation, **570–571**
  - diagnostic checklist, **571**
  - differential diagnosis, **571**
  - prognosis, **571**
  - staging, grading, & classification, **571**
- fibrous ankylosis, **560–561**
  - diagnostic checklist, **561**
  - differential diagnosis, **561**
  - staging, grading, & classification, **561**
- fractures, **564–569**
  - associated abnormalities, **565**
  - diagnostic checklist, **565**
  - differential diagnosis, **565**
  - prognosis, **565**
- graphics, **85–86**
- hemifacial microsomia, **542–545**
  - diagnostic checklist, **543**
  - differential diagnosis, **543**
  - prognosis, **543**
  - staging, grading, & classification, **543**
  - TMJ fractures vs., **565**
- hypermobility, dislocation vs., **570–571**
- internal content, **82**
- juvenile idiopathic arthritis, **584–589**
  - differential diagnosis, **585**
  - genetics, **585**
  - staging, grading, & classification, **585–586**
- ligaments, **82–83**
- metastasis, **640–641**
  - diagnostic checklist, **641**
  - differential diagnosis, **641**
  - prognosis, **641**
- metastatic disease, TMJ osteosarcoma vs., **635**
- MR of normal, **89**
- osteochondritis dissecans, **576–577**
  - differential diagnosis, **577**
  - prognosis, **577**

staging, grading, & classification, **577**
TMJ primary synovial chondromatosis vs., **631**
- osteochondroma, **620–625**
condylar hyperplasia vs., **547**
diagnostic checklist, **621**
differential diagnosis, **621**
prognosis, **621**
TMJ osteoma vs., **619**
- osteoma, **618–619**
associated abnormalities, **619**
diagnostic checklist, **619**
differential diagnosis, **619**
prognosis, **619**
staging, grading, & classification, **619**
TMJ osteochondroma vs., **621**
- osteosarcoma, **634–635**
diagnostic checklist, **635**
differential diagnosis, **635**
prognosis, **635**
staging, grading, & classification, **635**
- peripheral components, **82–83**
- pigmented villonodular synovitis, **590–591**
diagnostic checklist, **591**
differential diagnosis, **591**
prognosis, **591**
- primary synovial chondromatosis, **630–633**
diagnostic checklist, **632**
differential diagnosis, **631**
prognosis, **632**
staging, grading, & classification, **631**
- progressive condylar resorption, **598–603**
diagnostic checklist, **599**
differential diagnosis, **599**
prognosis, **599**
- rheumatoid arthritis, **578–583**
associated abnormalities, **579**
diagnostic checklist, **580**
differential diagnosis, **579**
prognosis, **580**
staging, grading, & classification, **579–580**
- simple (traumatic) bone cyst, **642–643**
differential diagnosis, **643**
prognosis, **643**
- synovial chondromatosis, masticator space chondrosarcoma vs., **735**
- synovial cyst, **596–597**
differential diagnosis, **597**
Temporosphenoidal suture, **86**
Tendo occuli, **26**
Tensor tympani, **92, 144, 146**
- anatomy, **90**
- belly, **144**
- nerve, **129**
- tendon, **92, 94, 146**
Tensor veli palatini, **173, 178**
- nerve, **129**
Tentorial branch, MHT, **206**
Teratoid cyst, **286**
Tetracycline staining, dentinogenesis imperfecta and, **231**
Thalassemia
- generalized rarefaction vs., **888–889, 891**
- hypoplasia/aplasia associated, **660**
3rd mandibular molar, **41, 42**
- tooth, **43**
3rd molar follicles, **9**
Thyroglossal duct cyst
- dermoid and epidermoid vs., **285**
- root of tongue lesions vs., **930, 933**
- submandibular gland mucocele vs., **305**
Thyroid cartilage, **119**
Thyroid gland, **199**
Tic douloureux (trigeminal neuralgia), **125**
Tissue disintegration, **7**
TMJ articular loose bodies, **960–961**
- differential diagnosis, **960**
TMJ radiolucencies, **954–955**
- differential diagnosis, **954**
TMJ radiopacities, **956–959**
- differential diagnosis, **956–957**
Tongue, **36–39, 179**
- anatomy relationships, **36**
- anterior 2/3 of, **52**
- base of, **176, 177, 179**
- foregut duplication cyst in, **290–291**
diagnostic checklist, **291**
differential diagnosis, **291**
options, risks, complications, **291**
- internal contents, **36**
- intrinsic muscles of, **38**
- sagittal,coronal, & axial T1 MR, **39**
- squamous cell carcinoma, **320–323**
diagnostic checklist, **322**
differential diagnosis, **321**
genetics, **321**
oral cavity soft tissue infections vs., **294**
prognosis, **322**
staging, grading, & classification, **321–322**
- vasculature of, **36**
Tongue denervation. *See* Motor denervation CNXII.
Tonsillar lymphoid hyperplasia, non-Hodgkin lymphoma of pharyngeal mucosal space vs., **517**
Tonsillar tissue, prominent/asymmetric, lingual thyroid vs., **283**
Tonsilloliths, **177**
- soft tissue calcifications vs., **934, 937**
Tooth fracture, attrition vs., **237**
Tooth furcation, **10, 11**
Tooth impactions, **12–13**
Tooth wear, dental caries vs., **261**
Tophaceous pseudogout. *See* Calcium pyrophosphate dihydrate deposition disease, temporomandibular joint.
Tophaceous (tumoral) CPPD deposition disease, **627**
Topical nasal spray overuse, perforated nasal septum vs., **964**
Torus, palatal, palate benign mixed tumor vs., **311**
Torus mandibularis. *See* Mandibular torus.
Torus palatinus. *See* Palatal torus.
Torus tubarius, **109, 173, 175, 177, 178**
- of nasopharynx and oropharynx, **172**
Trachea, **165**
Transfacial fracture (Le Fort), **380–383**
- complex midfacial fracture vs., **377**

- diagnostic checklist, **381**
- differential diagnosis, **381**
- prognosis, **381**
- zygomaticomaxillary complex fracture vs., **379**

Transitional cell papilloma. *See* Sinonasal inverted papilloma.
Transverse cervical nodes, **201**
Transverse facial artery, **85**
Transverse foramen, **152, 156, 157**
Transverse fracture. *See* Dentoalveolar fractures.
Transverse ligament, **151, 156**
Transverse process, **152, 153, 156, 157, 197**
- anterior tubercle of, **152**
- C1, **158**
- posterior tubercle of, **152**

Transverse sinus, **112**
Trapezius, **167, 199**
Trauma
- dilaceration, **224**
- perforated nasal septum vs., **964**
- periosteal reactions vs., **906, 908**

Traumatic bone cyst. *See also* Simple (traumatic) bone cyst, temporomandibular joint.
- well-defined unilocular radiolucencies vs., **870–871, 872**

Treacher Collins syndrome, **368–369**
- condylar aplasia associated, **541**
- condylar hypoplasia, **557**
- diagnostic checklist, **369**
- differential diagnosis, **369**
- genetics, **369**
- hypoplasia/aplasia associated, **660**
- Pierre Robin sequence vs., **367**
- submandibular gland aplasia-hypoplasia associated, **289**
- TMJ juvenile idiopathic arthritis vs., **585**

Treacher Collins-Franceschetti syndrome. *See* Treacher Collins syndrome.
Tricho-dento-osseous dysplasia, hypoplasia/aplasia associated, **660**
Trichodentoosseous syndrome, amelogenesis imperfecta vs., **227**
Tricolor carotid sheath, **169**
Trigeminal fascicles, **133**
Trigeminal ganglion, **77, 105, 126, 128, 129, 133, 182**
- within Meckel cave, **127**

Trigeminal nerve. *See also* Cranial nerve V (CNV).
- division, mandibular, **180**

Trigeminal neuralgia (tic douloureux), **125**
Trimalar fracture. *See* Zygomaticomaxillary complex fracture.
Tripod fracture. *See* Zygomaticomaxillary complex fracture.
Trismus-pseudocamptodactyly syndrome, coronoid hyperplasia associated, **553**
Trisomy 21, hypoplasia/aplasia associated, **660**
Trivalent arsenic exposure, perforated nasal septum vs., **964**
Trochlear nerve (CNIV), **127**
True cementoblastoma. *See* Cementoblastoma.
True sialocele, oral cavity soft tissue infections vs., **294**
Tuberculosis, lymph nodes
- submandibular space lesions vs., **915, 917**
- submandibular space nodal non-Hodgkin lymphoma vs., **319**

Tuberculum sellae, **99, 101, 105, 107**
- of central skull base, **104**

Tuberous sclerosis, fibrous dysplasia, cervical spine vs., **839**
Tumor, cervical facet arthropathy vs., **827**
Tumor calcinosis, **840–841**
- associated abnormalities, **841**
- differential diagnosis, **841**
- genetics, **841**
- prognosis, **841**

Turbinate pneumatization. *See* Concha bullosa.
Turbinates, **56**
Turner dysplasia, **241**
- diagnostic checklist, **241**
- differential diagnosis, **241**

Turner hypoplasia. *See* Turner dysplasia.
Turner tooth. *See* Turner dysplasia.
Twinning. *See* Macrodontia.
2 holes syndrome. *See* Accessory ostia.
Tympanic annulus, **91, 93, 94, 145, 146**
Tympanic membrane, **146**
Tympanic plate, **87, 88**
Tympanic segment, **138**
- CNVII, **93, 145, 146, 186**
- facial nerve canal, **143**

U

Umbo of malleus, **92**
Uncinate process, **58, 62, 63, 65, 67, 72, 73, 74, 158**
- C3, **157**

Undifferentiated carcinoma, sinonasal
- nasal lesion with bony destruction vs., **970, 972**
- paranasal sinus lesions with bony destruction vs., **980, 982**
- sinonasal adenoid cystic carcinoma vs., **707**

Unerupted 3rd molar, **29**
Unfilled cavity preparations, dental caries vs., **261**
Unfused odontoid tip synchondrosis, ossiculum terminale vs., **795**
Unicameral bone cyst. *See* Simple (traumatic) bone cyst, mandible-maxilla; Simple (traumatic) bone cyst, temporomandibular joint.
Unicystic (mural) ameloblastoma
- ameloblastic fibroma vs., **461**
- dentigerous cyst vs., **397**
- pericoronal radiolucencies without radiopacities vs., **874, 875**
- well-defined unilocular radiolucencies vs., **871, 873**

Unilocular radiolucencies, well-defined, **870–873**
- differential diagnosis, **870–871**

Unique tumor spread patterns, retromolar trigone squamous cell carcinoma, **329**
Unossified chondrocranium, **100**
Upper alveolar ridge mucosal surface, **52**

Upper lip, median cleft of, **357**
Upper retroarticular foramen. *See* Ponticulus posticus.
Uvula, **39, 175, 178, 179**

V

VA. *See* Vertebral artery.
Vagus nerve (CNX), **111, 190**
- in carotid space, **188**
- location, **191**
Vallecula, **167, 174**
van Buchem disease, hypoplasia/aplasia associated, **660**
Vanishing bone disease, generalized rarefaction vs., **889**
Vasa nervosa CNV3, masticator space CNV3 perineural tumor vs., **744**
Vascular malformation
- mandible-maxilla aneurysmal bone cyst, **415**
- nerve sheath tumor vs., **483**
- parotid sialoliths vs., **785**
Vein of Labbé, **112**
Velocardiofacial syndrome, Pierre Robin sequence vs., **367**
Venolymphatic malformation, floor of mouth squamous cell carcinoma vs., **325**
Venous malformation
- lingual thyroid vs., **283**
- masticator space, masticator space sarcoma vs., **739**
- neurofibromatosis type 1 vs., **487**
- oral cavity, motor denervation CNXII vs., **337**
- orbital, dermoid and epidermoid vs., **286**
- parotid space lesions vs., **919**
- root of tongue lesions vs., **931, 933**
- sublingual space, sublingual space lesions vs., **923, 925**
- submandibular space lesions vs., **915**
Vertebral abnormalities, failure of formation vs., **807**
Vertebral artery, **111, 190, 197, 198, 199, 204**
- loop, **191**
Vertebral body, **197**
- destruction, **198**
- fracture, failure of formation vs., **807**
- T3, **194**
Vertebral canal, **152**
Vertebral dysplasia. *See* Failure of formation.
Vertebral metastasis, hemangioma, cervical spine vs., **831**
Vertebral vein, **198**
Vertical (angular) bone loss, **271**
Vertical fracture. *See* Dentoalveolar fractures.
Vertical petrous internal carotid artery canal, **108, 114**
Vertical plate, ethmoid bone, **103**
Vertical segment petrous internal carotid artery, **133, 134, 146, 206**
Vestibule, **92, 143**
Vestibulocochlear nerve (CNVIII), **111, 147**
Vidian artery, **205, 206**
Vidian canal, **64, 78, 79, 108, 109, 115**
- of central skull base, **104**
- pterygoid nerve and artery, **134**
- vidian artery, **207**
Vidian nerve, **77**
- in vidian canal, **105, 128**
Visceral abnormalities, failure of formation vs., **807**
Visceral space, **199**
- anatomy, **162, 165**
Visceral space nodes, **201**
Vitality testing, periapical rarefying osteitis, **266**
Vitamin D deficiency, generalized rarefaction vs., **888, 890, 891**
Volume averaging artifact, internal and external resorption vs., **243**
von Recklinghausen disease, **483**. *See also* Neurofibromatosis type 1.

W

Wackenheim line, **150, 154, 155**
Warthin tumor, **760–763**
- associated abnormalities, **762**
- benign lymphoepithelial lesions: HIV vs., **751**
- diagnostic checklist, **762**
- differential diagnosis, **761**
- metastatic disease of parotid nodes vs., **779**
- parotid adenoid cystic carcinoma vs., **773**
- parotid benign mixed tumor vs., **757**
- parotid malignant mixed tumor vs., **767**
- parotid mucoepidermoid carcinoma vs., **769**
- parotid non-Hodgkin lymphoma vs., **775**
- parotid schwannoma vs., **765**
- parotid space lesions vs., **918, 920**
- prognosis, **762**
- Sjögren syndrome vs., **783**
Wegener granulomatosis, **668–671**
- associated abnormalities, **669–670**
- chronic rhinosinusitis vs., **681**
- diagnostic checklist, **670**
- differential diagnosis, **669**
- invasive pseudotumor vs., **695**
- prognosis, **670**
- sinonasal polyposis vs., **673**
Welcher basal angle, **150, 154**
Well-defined radiopacities, **892–895**
- differential diagnosis, **892–893**
Well-defined unilocular radiolucencies, **870–873**
- differential diagnosis, **870–871**
Wharton duct, sialolith in, mandibular torus vs., **345**
Whole tooth, displaced dental structures into antrum vs., **984**
Widened periodontal ligament space, **864–865**
- differential diagnosis, **864**
Williams-Beuren syndrome, hypoplasia/aplasia associated, **660**

X

Xanthogranuloma. *See* Invasive pseudotumor.
Xerostomia, submandibular gland aplasia-hypoplasia, **289**
X-linked dominant diffuse smooth type, amelogenesis imperfecta and, **228**
X-linked maxillofacial dysostosis, Treacher Collins syndrome vs., **369**
X-linked pattern, amelogenesis imperfecta and, **228**

Z

ZMC. *See* Zygomaticomaxillary complex fracture.
Zygomatic arch, **58, 84, 87, 130, 164, 182**
- fracture, zygomaticomaxillary complex fracture vs., **379**
Zygomatic bone, inferior border of, **29**
Zygomatic branch of CNVII, **141, 142, 186**
Zygomatic process, **24, 26**
- anatomy, **22**
- of maxilla, **24, 58, 59, 60, 61, 142**
Zygomatic sutures, prominent, zygomaticomaxillary complex fracture vs., **379**
Zygomaticomaxillary complex fracture, **378–379**
- complex midfacial fracture vs., **377**
- differential diagnosis, **379**
- prognosis, **379**
- staging, grading, & classification, **379**
- transfacial fracture (Le Fort) vs., **381**
Zygomaticomaxillary suture, **24**
Zygomaticus major, **139, 142**
Zygomaticus minor, **142**